WILLARD & SPACKMAN'S

Occupational Therapy

TWELFTH EDITION

WILLARD & SPACKMAN'S

Occupational Therapy

Barbara A. Boyt Schell, PhD, OT/L, FAOTA

Associate Dean, College of Health and Science
Director, School of Occupational Therapy
Professor
Brenau University
Gainesville, Georgia

Glen Gillen, EdD, OTR/L, FAOTA

Associate Director, Programs in Occupational Therapy
Associate Professor
Department of Rehabilitation and Regenerative Medicine
Columbia University
New York, New York

Marjorie E. Scaffa, PhD, OTR/L, FAOTA

Chair, Department of Occupational Therapy
Professor
University of South Alabama
Mobile, Alabama

Ellen S. Cohn, ScD, OTR/L, FAOTA (consulting editor)

Clinical Professor and MSOT Program Director
Department of Occupational Therapy
Boston University College of Health & Rehabilitation Sciences: Sargent College
Boston University
Boston, Massachusetts

Wolters Kluwer | Lippincott Williams & Wilkins
Health

Philadelphia • Baltimore • New York • London
Buenos Aires • Hong Kong • Sydney • Tokyo

Acquisitions Editor: Michael Nobel
Product Manager: Linda G. Francis
Marketing Manager: Shauna Kelley
Project Manager: Laura Horowitz
Design Coordinator: Stephen Druding
Compositor: Absolute Service, Inc.
Composition Project Manager: Harold Medina

12th Edition

351 West Camden Street
Baltimore, MD 21201

Two Commerce Square
2001 Market Street
Philadelphia, PA 19103

Printed in China

9 8 7 6 5 4

Library of Congress Cataloging-in-Publication Data

Willard & Spackman's occupational therapy. — 12th ed. / [edited by] Barbara A. Boyt Schell ... [et al.].
p. ; cm.
Willard and Spackman's occupational therapy
Occupational therapy
Includes bibliographical references and index.
ISBN 978-1-4511-1080-7
I. Willard, Helen S. II. Schell, Barbara A. Boyt. III. Title: Willard and Spackman's occupational therapy. IV. Title: Occupational therapy.
[DNLM: 1. Occupational Therapy. 2. Rehabilitation, Vocational. WB 555]

615.8'515—dc23

2012042507

To purchase additional copies of this book, call our customer service department at **(800) 638-3030** or fax orders to **(301) 223-2320**. International customers should call **(301) 223-2300**.

Visit Lippincott Williams & Wilkins on the Internet: http://www.lww.com. Lippincott Williams & Wilkins customer service representatives are available from 8:30 am to 6:00 pm, EST.

When citing chapters from this book, please use the appropriate form. The APA format is as follows:

[Chapter author last name, I.] (2014). Chapter title. In B. A. B. Schell, G. Gillen, & M. E. Scaffa (Eds). *Willard and Spackman's occupational therapy* (12th ed., pp. x–x). Philadelphia: Lippincott Williams & Wilkins.

Dickie, V. (2014). What is occupation? In B. A. B. Schell, G. Gillen, & M. E. Scaffa (Eds). *Willard and Spackman's occupational therapy* (12th ed., pp. 2–8). Philadelphia: Lippincott Williams & Wilkins.

Dedication

Elizabeth Blesedell Crepeau, PhD, OT, FAOTA
Professor Emerita, Occupational Therapy Department, University of New Hampshire
Co-Editor, *Willard and Spackman's Occupational Therapy* 9th Edition
Lead Editor, *Willard and Spackman's Occupational Therapy* 10th & 11th Editions

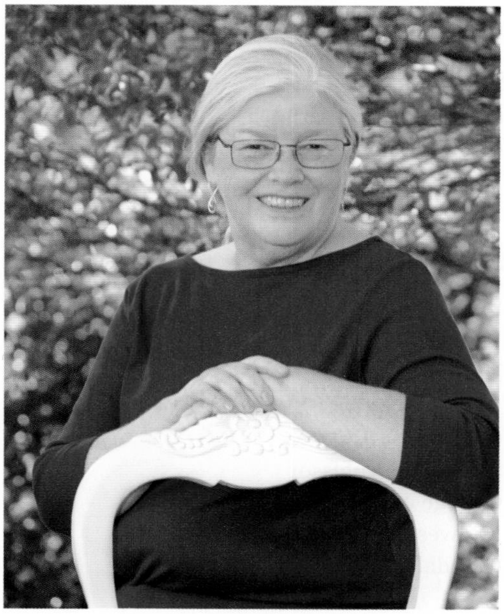

Dr. Crepeau leaning on a chair that originally belonged to Claire Spackman. Two of these chairs were refurbished and given to Betty as a gift upon her retirement from UNH. (Photo by Rod Crepeau.)

We are pleased to dedicate this edition to Dr. Elizabeth "Betty" Crepeau. Dr. Crepeau, a careful and thoughtful scholar, has made a significant contribution to the occupational therapy profession. Through her scholarship, teaching, and mentoring, she has enhanced our understanding of the ways in which people construct meaning in their lives. Drawing from the fields of sociology and anthropology, she has enriched our appreciation of the impact of socially constructed experience and reminds us to attend to the broader social worlds in which others live. In all of her work, she has consistently advocated for practitioners to strive to understand the privately composed subjective experience of others and honor that experience in interactions and interventions. Her challenge to analyze our own perspectives in order to better understand others has enriched the practice of many.

Dr. Crepeau's contributions to *Willard and Spackman's Occupational Therapy* are numerous and long lasting. She and Dr. Maureen Neistadt became editors during an explosion of knowledge about occupational science and occupational therapy. They responded by reconceptualizing and reorganizing the knowledge presented in this textbook to provide both emerging and current practitioners with a strong foundation in the centrality of occupation to practice. With characteristic grace and wit, Dr. Crepeau assumed the lead editor role for the 10th and subsequent 11th editions, where she effectively championed revisions of the text to reflect the continuing scholarship about the many facets of occupation and occupational therapy. We are grateful for her decades of service to the profession and for the many years she dedicated to this text.

Contributors

DIANE E. ADAMO, PhD
Assistant Professor
Department of Health Care Sciences
Wayne State University
Detroit, MI

NANCY BAKER, ScD, MPH, OTR/L
Associate Professor
Department of Occupational Therapy
University of Pittsburgh
Pittsburgh, PA

KATE BARRETT
Associate Professor
Department of Occupational Science and Occupational Therapy
St. Catherine University
St. Paul, MN

SUE BERGER, PhD, OTR/L, BCG, FAOTA
Assistant Clinical Professor
Department of Occupational Therapy
Boston University College of Health & Rehabilitation Sciences: Sargent College
Boston, MA

CHRISTY BILLOCK, PhD, OTR/L
Associate Professor
Department of Occupational Therapy
Loma Linda University
Loma Linda, CA

ROXIE M. BLACK, PhD, OTR/L, FAOTA
Professor and Program Chair
Master of Occupational Therapy Program
University of Southern Maine
Lewiston, ME

BETTE R. BONDER, PhD
Special Assistant to the Dean for the NEOMED-CSU Partnership
Professor, School of Health Sciences and Department of Psychology
Cleveland State University
Cleveland, OH

ALISSA BONJUKLIAN
MSOT Student, Department of Occupational Therapy
Boston University College of Health & Rehabilitation Sciences: Sargent College
Boston, MA

CHERYL LYNNE TRAUTMANN BOOP, MS, OTR/L
Occupational Therapist
Cooperative School Services
Rensselaer, IN

BRENT BRAVEMAN, PhD, OTR/L, FAOTA
Director of Rehabilitation Services
University of Texas MD Anderson Cancer Center
Houston, TX

CATANA E. BROWN, PhD, OTR/L
Associate Professor
College of Health Sciences
Midwestern University Glendale
Glendale, AZ

CHRISTINE M. CARIFIO
MSOT Student, Department of Occupational Therapy
Boston University College of Health & Rehabilitation Sciences: Sargent College
Boston, MA

TINA CHAMPAGNE, OTD, OTR/L
Program Director
Center for Human Development
Institute for Dynamic Living
Springfield, MA

JIM CHARLTON
Research Assistant Professor
University of Chicago
Founder, Access Living
Chicago, IL

DENISE CHISHOLM, PhD, OTR/L, FAOTA
Associate Professor and Vice Chair
Department of Occupational Therapy
School of Health and Rehabilitation Sciences
University of Pittsburgh
Pittsburgh, PA

CHARLES H. CHRISTIANSEN, EdD, OTR, OT(C), FAOTA
Executive Director
American Occupational Therapy Foundation
Bethesda, MD

SHERRILENE CLASSEN, PhD, MPH, OTR/L, FAOTA
Director
Institute for Mobility, Activity, and Participation
Associate Professor
Department of Occupational Therapy
College of Public Health and Health Professions
University of Florida
Gainesville, FL

ELLEN S. COHN, ScD, OTR/L, FAOTA
Clinical Professor and MSOT Program Director
Department of Occupational Therapy
Boston University College of Health & Rehabilitation Sciences: Sargent College
Boston, MA

WENDY J. COSTER, PhD, OTR/L, FAOTA
Professor and Chair
Department of Occupational Therapy
Boston University College of Health & Rehabilitation Sciences: Sargent College
Boston, MA

ELIZABETH BLESEDELL CREPEAU, PhD, OT, FAOTA
Professor Emerita
Occupational Therapy Department
University of New Hampshire
Durham, NH

PATRICIA A. HICKERSON CRIST, PhD, PC, OTR/L, FAOTA
Professor
Department of Occupational Therapy
Duquesne University
Pittsburgh, PA

GLORIA F. DICKERSON, BS
Recovery Specialist
Center for Social Innovation
Newton Centre, MA

VIRGINIA DICKIE, PhD, OTR/L, FAOTA
Associate Professor Emerita
Division of Occupational Science
University of North Carolina at Chapel Hill
Chapel Hill, NC

REGINA F. DOHERTY, OTD, MS, OTR/L
Associate Professor and Director
Occupational Therapy Department
School of Health and Rehabilitation Sciences
MGH Institute of Health Professions
Boston, MA

MARY E. EVENSON, OTD, MPH, OTR/L
Clinical Associate Professor and Director of Clinical Education
Department of Occupational Therapy
MGH Institute of Health Professions
Boston, MA

JANET FALK-KESSLER, EdD, OTR, FAOTA
Director
Programs in Occupational Therapy
Associate Professor
Department of Rehabilitation and Regenerative Medicine
Columbia University
New York, NY

MARY FELDHAUS-WEBER
Boston, MA

ANNE G. FISHER, ScD, OT, FAOTA
Professor
Division of Occupational Therapy
Department of Community Medicine and Rehabilitation
Umeå University
Umeå, Sweden

KIRSTY FORSYTH, PhD, OTR, FCOT
Professor
Department of Occupational Therapy
School of Health Sciences
Queen Margaret University
Edinburgh, Scotland, United Kingdom

KAREN ROE GARREN, MS, OTR/L, CHT
Senior Staff Occupational Therapist
Select Physical Therapy
New Milford, CT

GLEN GILLEN, EdD, OTR/L, FAOTA
Associate Director
Programs in Occupational Therapy
Associate Professor
Department of Rehabilitation and Regenerative Medicine
Columbia University
New York, NY

KATHLEEN M. GOLISZ, OTD, OTR
Professor and Associate Director
Occupational Therapy Program
Mercy College
Dobbs Ferry, NY

YAEL GOVEROVER, PhD, OT
Associate Professor
Department of Occupational Therapy
Steinhardt School of Culture, Education, and Human Development
New York University
New York, NY

THERESA GRIFFIN
MSOT Student, Department of Occupational Therapy
Boston University College of Health & Rehabilitation Sciences: Sargent College
Boston, MA

LOU ANN GRISWOLD, PhD, OTR, FAOTA
Associate Professor
Department of Occupational Therapy
University of New Hampshire
Durham, NH

KRISTINE HAERTL, PhD, OTR/L, FAOTA
Professor
Department of Occupational Science and Occupational Therapy
St. Catherine University
St. Paul, MN

JOY HAMMEL, PhD, OTR/L, FAOTA
Professor
University of Illinois at Chicago
Chicago, IL

CHRISTINE A. HELFRICH, PhD, OTR/L, FAOTA
Assistant Professor
Department of Occupational Therapy
Boston University
Boston, MA

CLARE HOCKING, DipOT, AdvDipOT, MHSc(OT), PhD
Department of Occupational Science and Therapy
Auckland University of Technology
Auckland, New Zealand

WENDY M. HOLMES, PhD, OTR/L
Associate Professor
School of Occupational Therapy
Brenau University
Gainesville, GA

BARBARA HOOPER, PhD, OTR, FAOTA
Assistant Professor
Department of Occupational Therapy
Colorado State University
Fort Collins, CO

RUTH HUMPHRY, PhD, OTR/L, FAOTA
Professor and Division Director
Division of Occupational Science and Occupational Therapy
Department of Allied Health, School of Medicine
University of North Carolina at Chapel Hill
Chapel Hill, NC

ANNE BIRGE JAMES, PhD, OTR/L
Professor
Occupational Therapy Department
University of Puget Sound
Tacoma, WA

ROBIN A. JONES, MPA, COTA/L, ROH
Project Director and Instructor
DBTAC-Great Lakes ADA Center
Department of Disability and Human Development
University of Illinois at Chicago
Chicago, IL

MARY ALUNKAL KHETANI, ScD, OTR
Assistant Professor
Department of Occupational Therapy
Colorado State University
Fort Collins, CO

PHYLLIS M. KING, PhD, OT, FAOTA
Professor
Department of Occupational Science and Technology
College of Health Sciences
University of Wisconsin-Milwaukee
Milwaukee, WI

JESSICA M. KRAMER, PhD, OTR/L
Assistant Professor
Department of Occupational Therapy
Boston University
Boston, MA

ALAINA KRUMBACH
MSOT Student, Department of Occupational Therapy
Boston University College of Health & Rehabilitation Sciences: Sargent College
Boston, MA

TERRY KRUPA, PhD, OT Reg (Ont), FCAOT
Professor
School of Rehabilitation Therapy
Queen's University
Kingston, Ontario, Canada

SHELLY J. LANE, PhD, OTR/L, FAOTA
Professor
Department of Occupational Therapy
School of Allied Health Professions
Virginia Commonwealth University
Richmond, VA

MARY C. LAWLOR, ScD, OTR/L, FAOTA
Division of Occupational Science and Occupational Therapy
Herman Ostrow School of Dentistry
University of Southern California
Los Angeles, CA

ANNE LEBORGNE
MSOT Student, Department of Occupational Therapy
Boston University College of Health & Rehabilitation Sciences: Sargent College
Boston, MA

CLAUDIA LEONARD, OTD, MBA, OT/L
Associate Professor
School of Allied Health
Western New Mexico University
Silver City, NM

LORI LETTS, PhD, OT Reg (Ont)
Assistant Dean
Occupational Therapy Program
Associate Professor
School of Rehabilitation Science
McMaster University
Hamilton, Ontario, Canada

HELENE LOHMAN, OTD, OTR/L
Professor
Department of Occupational Therapy
Creighton University
Omaha, NE

CATHERINE L. LYSACK, PhD
Professor and Deputy Director
Institute of Gerontology
Wayne State University
Detroit, MI

CHERYL MATTINGLY, PhD
Department of Anthropology
Division of Occupational Science and Occupational Therapy
University of Southern California
Los Angeles, CA

KATHLEEN MATUSKA, PhD, OTR/L, FAOTA
Professor and Chair
Department of Occupational Science and Occupational Therapy
St. Catherine University
St. Paul, MN

ALEXANDER MCINTOSH
Dover, NH

LAURIE S. MCINTOSH, MS, OTR/L
Occupational Therapist
Supervisory Union 16
Exeter, NH

LOU MCINTOSH
Portsmouth Naval Shipyard
Portsmouth, ME

EMILY MEIBEYER
MSOT Student, Department of Occupational Therapy
Boston University College of Health & Rehabilitation Sciences: Sargent College
Boston, MA

JANE MELTON, PhD, FCOT
Clinical Director
Social Inclusion
Together NHS Foundation Trust
Gloucestershire and Herefordshire Trust Headquarters, Rikenel
Montpellier, Gloucester, United Kingdom

DONALD M. MURRAY (DECEASED)
Professor Emeritus
English Department
University of New Hampshire
Durham, NH

DARCIE L. OLSON, MHS, OTR
Instructor
Occupational Therapy Assistant Program
Madison Area Technical College
Madison, WI

CHRISTINE OWEN, Msc
Head Occupational Therapist
Children's Occupational Therapy Service
St Johns Hospital
Livingston, Scotland, United Kingdom

SHAWN PHIPPS, PhD, MS, OTR/L, FAOTA
Chief Strategic Development Officer
Rancho Los Amigos National Rehabilitation Center
Los Angeles, CA

LOREE A. PRIMEAU, PhD, OTR, FAOTA
Executive Director
Autism Community Network
San Antonio, TX

SUSAN PRIOR, BSc PgCert
Lead Research Practitioner
Department of Occupational Therapy
School of Health Sciences
Queen Margaret University
Edinburgh, Scotland, United Kingdom

RUTH RAMSEY, EdD, OTR/L
Chair and Associate Professor
Department of Occupational Therapy
Dominican University of California
San Rafael, CA

S. MAGGIE REITZ, PhD, OTR/L, FAOTA
Chairperson and Professor
Department of Occupational Therapy and Occupational Science
Towson University
Towson, MD

LYNN RICHIE, BSc
Lead Occupational Therapist
The WORKS, NHS Lothian
Edinburgh, Scotland, United Kingdom

PATRICIA RIGBY, PhD, OT(C)
Associate Professor
Department of Occupational Science and Occupational Therapy
Faculty of Medicine, University of Toronto
Toronto, Ontario, Canada

PAMELA S. ROBERTS, PhD, OTR/L, SCFES, FAOTA, CPHQ
Manager-Rehabilitation and Neuropsychology
Department of Rehabilitation
Cedars-Sinai Medical Center
Los Angeles, CA

SUSANNE SMITH ROLEY, OTD, OTR/L, FAOTA
Project Director
Sensory Integration Certification Program
Division of Occupational Science and Occupational Therapy
University of Southern California
Los Angeles, CA

LARISSA SACHS
MSOT Student, Department of Occupational Therapy
Boston University College of Health & Rehabilitation Sciences: Sargent College
Boston, MA

KAREN M. SAMES, MBA, OTR/L, FAOTA
Associate Professor
Occupational Science and Occupational Therapy
St. Catherine University
St. Paul, MN

MARJORIE E. SCAFFA, PhD, OTR, FAOTA
Professor and Chair
Department of Occupational Therapy
University of South Alabama
Mobile, AL

BARBARA A. BOYT SCHELL, PhD, OT/L, FAOTA
Associate Dean
College of Health and Science
Professor & Director
School of Occupational Therapy
Brenau University
Gainesville, GA

SALLY A. SCHREIBER-COHN, MTS
Editor and friend
Marblehead, MA

SALLY W. SCHULTZ, PhD, OTR, LPC-S
Professor
School of Occupational Therapy
Texas Woman's University
Dallas, TX

DAVID SEAMON, PhD
Professor
Department of Architecture
Kansas State University
Manhattan, KS

MARY P. SHOTWELL, PhD, OT/L
Associate Professor and Chair
Department of Occupational Therapy—North Atlanta Norcross
Brenau University
Gainesville, GA

C. DOUGLAS SIMMONS, PhD, OTR/L
Assistant Professor
Department of Occupational Therapy
University of New Hampshire
Nottingham, NH

SAMANTHA SLOCUM
MSOT Student, Department of Occupational Therapy
Boston University College of Health and Rehabilitation Sciences: Sargent College
Boston, MA

THERESA M. SMITH, PhD
Assistant Professor
Department of Occupational Therapy and Occupational Science
Towson University
Towson, MD

JO M. SOLET, MS, EdM, PhD, OTR/L
Harvard Medical School
Division of Sleep Medicine
Cambridge Health Alliance
Department of Medicine
Cambridge, MA

DANIELLE SOTELO
MSOT Student, Department of Occupational Therapy
Boston University College of Health & Rehabilitation Sciences: Sargent College
Boston, MA

SARAH STULTZ
MSOT Student, Department of Occupational Therapy
Boston University College of Health & Rehabilitation Sciences: Sargent College
Boston, MA

PEGGY SWARBRICK, PhD, OT, CPRP
Assistant Professor
Psychiatric Rehabilitation and Counseling Professions
School of Health Related Professions
University of Medicine and Dentistry of New Jersey
Scotch Plains, NJ

YVONNE L. SWINTH, PhD, OTR/L, FAOTA
Professor and Chair
School of Occupational Therapy
University of Puget Sound
Tacoma, WA

RENÉE R. TAYLOR, PhD
Professor
Department of Occupational Therapy
University of Illinois at Chicago
Chicago, IL

LINDA TICKLE-DEGNEN, PhD, OTR/L, FAOTA
Professor and Chair
Department of Occupational Therapy
Tufts University
Medford, MA

JOAN PASCALE TOGLIA, PhD, OTR/L
Professor and Program Director
Graduate Occupational Therapy Program
Mercy College
Dobbs Ferry, NY

SCOTT D. TOMCHEK, PhD, OTR/L, FAOTA
Associate Professor of Pediatrics
Assistant Director
Chief Occupational Therapist
Weisskopf Child Evaluation Center
University of Louisville Pediatrics
Louisville, KY

ELIZABETH A. TOWNSEND, PhD, OT(C), Reg. PEI, FCAOT
Professor Emerita
School of Occupational Therapy
Dalhousie University
Halifax, Nova Scotia, Canada

BARRY TRENTHAM, PhD, OT Reg (Ont)
Department of Occupational Science and Occupational Therapy
Toronto, Ontario, Canada

DEBRA TUPE, PhD, MPH, OTR, FAOTA
Assistant Professor in Clinical Occupational Therapy
Columbia University
New York, NY

PAMELA VAUGHN
MSOT Student, Department of Occupational Therapy
Boston University College of Health & Rehabilitation Sciences: Sargent College
Boston, MA

CRAIG A. VELOZO, PhD, OTR/L
Professor and Associate Chair
Department of Occupational Therapy
University of Florida
Gainesville, FL

STEVEN D. WHEELER, PhD, OTR/L
Associate Professor
Occupational Therapy Division
West Virginia University School of Medicine
Morgantown, WV

JAQUELINE WHITEHEAD, BA(Hons) PgDip OT
Research Practitioner
Department of Occupational Therapy
School of Health Sciences
Queen Margaret University
Edinburgh, Scotland, United Kingdom

ANN A. WILCOCK, PhD, FCOT, GradDipPubHealth, BAppScOT
Retired Inaugural Professor
Occupational Science and Therapy
Deakin University, Geelong
Victoria, Australia

TOM WILSON, MA
Personal Assistant and Health Care Team Leader
Access Living
Chicago, IL

JENNIFER WOMACK, MS, OTR/L
Associate Professor
Division of Occupational Science and Occupational Therapy
Department of Allied Health, School of Medicine
University of North Carolina at Chapel Hill
Chapel Hill, NC

WENDY WOOD, PhD, OTR/L, FAOTA
Professor and Department Head
Department of Occupational Therapy
Colorado State University
Fort Collins, CO

VALERIE A. WRIGHT-ST CLAIR, PhD, DipProfEthics, MPH, DipBusStud (HEALTH MANAGEMENT), DipOT
Department of Occupational Sciences and Therapy
School of Rehabilitation and Occupation Studies
Faculty of Health and Environmental Sciences
Auckland University of Technology
Auckland, New Zealand

MARY JANE YOUNGSTROM, MS, OTR/L, FAOTA
Assistant Professor of Occupational Therapy
Rockhurst University
Kansas City, MO

Editorial Review Board

Preface

This 12th edition of *Willard & Spackman's Occupational Therapy* continues a long tradition in the field that started in the 1940s when Helen Willard and Clare Spackman edited a textbook designed to educate occupational therapy students about the core knowledge of the field. That first edition of *Willard and Spackman's Occupational Therapy* was published in 1947. In the more than half century since that first edition, this textbook has become an icon in the field. It is the text that welcomes students into the complexities of their newly chosen profession while also serving as a resource to the field by documenting the central knowledge and practices of occupational therapy. It has gained this iconic status in no small part due to the work of previous editors (see Figure) and the many contributors.

Chapters in this text summarize important and complex material in a way that is accessible and which challenges budding practitioners to think deeply about the many facets of occupation that emerge in the daily rounds of life. Furthermore, the process of occupational therapy is described across a wide array of practice arenas. This 12th edition continues these traditions, as Barbara A. Boyt Schell assumes the role of lead editor, Glen Gillen and Marjorie E. Scaffa join as new co-editors, and Ellen S. Cohn shifts into the role of consulting editor.

This revision of *Willard and Spackman's Occupational Therapy* builds on the successful revisions done in the last edition. To identify needed changes, students and faculty who use the book were surveyed. Additionally, both students and faculty from a range of programs participated in focus groups at the 2010 American Occupational Therapy Association (AOTA) Annual Conference and Exposition in Orlando, Florida. Several leaders and scholars in the field also graciously provided advice through individual consultations. Although users generally expressed strong satisfaction with the text, several concerns did arise—some related to content and some

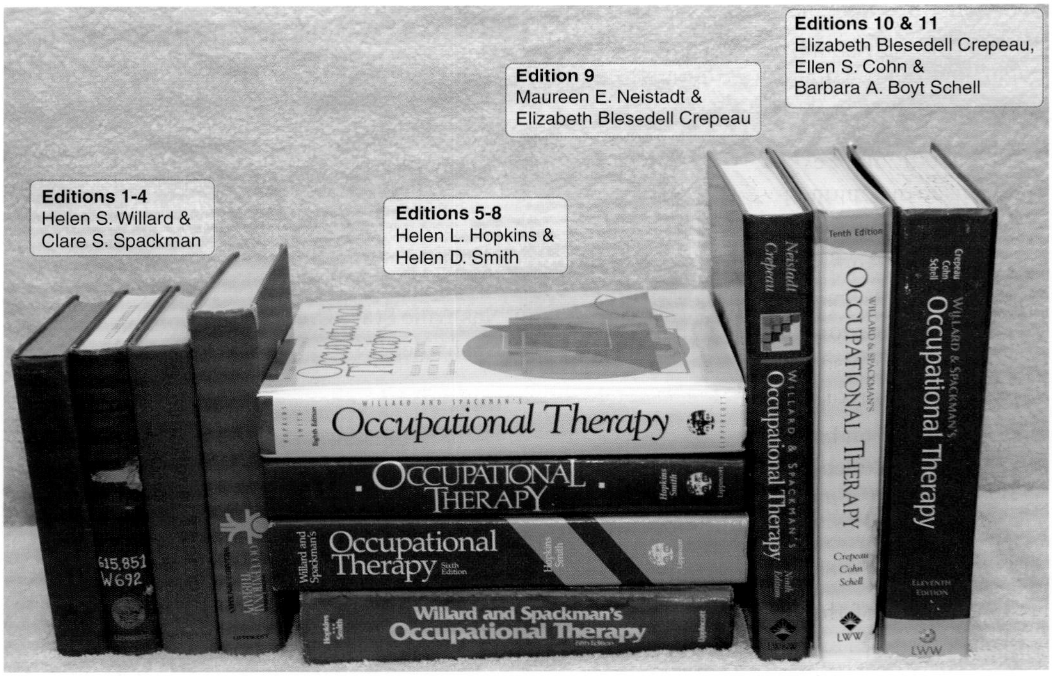

Editions 10 & 11
Elizabeth Blesedell Crepeau,
Ellen S. Cohn &
Barbara A. Boyt Schell
Edition 9
Maureen E. Neistadt &
Elizabeth Blesedell Crepeau
Editions 1-4
Helen S. Willard &
Clare S. Spackman
Editions 5-8
Helen L. Hopkins &
Helen D. Smith

Willard & Spackman's Occupational Therapy, editions 1 to 11, with editors noted.

related to the need for expanded Web-based resources. This information, in addition to the perspectives of the editors, informed the reorganization of this edition as well as the addition of new materials. An overall summary of these changes is provided next, followed by an overview of each unit, highlighting the materials included in each.

Overall Changes in the Text and Web-Based Materials

Because feedback on many aspects of the 11th edition was quite positive, *Willard and Spackman's* 12th edition retained materials focused on the centrality of occupation as the basis for practice, both as a means and an end of therapy. In this edition, we continue to acknowledge that evaluation and intervention processes are integrated with the theoretical perspectives of practitioners and the influences of the broader social and political environment on the day-to-day lives of both the practitioner and the clients they serve. Attempts were made to provide a diverse range of examples across cultures, life course, and occupational performance concerns.

As in previous editions, we maintain that effective occupational therapy requires a collaborative process between or among occupational therapy practitioners and the clients they serve. For therapy to be optimally effective, a blending of current best evidence with therapist experience and client preferences must guide the process. Because of these complexities, contributors were asked to provide many illustrations of the professional reasoning and underlying assumptions that guide practice. Furthermore, contributors were asked to acknowledge the challenges in implementing best practice and suggest approaches for overcoming these challenges.

As authors and editors, we acknowledge the power of language. Throughout this book, we have attempted to use language that is inclusive. That extends to appreciating the many different ways that humans are configured and the ways in which they engage in occupations. We also attempted to be inclusive of international perspectives by acknowledging when content is particularly reflective of U.S perspectives versus content that appears to be fairly applicable across occupational therapy as it is practiced throughout the world. Because this is the first full color edition of *Willard and Spackman's*, a special effort was made to update photos and to be inclusive from a visual perspective.

In addition to the overall guiding principles just described, there were some noticeable changes in the book which include

1. The addition of expanded Web-based materials, including video cases of clients which can be used in conjunction with the book to provide students with opportunities to observe and analyze applications of concepts and techniques;
2. The restructuring of units to improve clarity of organization and make the relationship of materials to the AOTA Occupational Therapy Practice Framework: Domain and Process, 2nd Edition more apparent while retaining an appreciation for broader international perspectives by also relating materials to the World Health Organization (WHO) International Classification of Functioning, Disability and Health (ICF);
3. A new unit on broad theories which come from outside the field that inform occupational therapy practices;
4. A new unit on the occupational therapy process which adds specific chapters detailing the evaluation process as well as separate chapters for individual versus group and population-level intervention;
5. Expansion of the focused intervention theory unit to include more materials related to mental health aspects of practice; and
6. A new unit entitled *Practice Context: Therapists in Action*, which showcases how practitioners design occupational therapy interventions for actual clients in specific settings. Each chapter addresses the continuum of care for people with particular health conditions commonly seen by occupational therapists.

Unit-by-Unit Summary

As noted earlier, the units in this edition were reorganized and, in some cases, renamed to clarify the contents and to improve cohesion of the materials in the unit. In the description that follows, new chapters added to the text will be highlighted. Except where noted, all chapters returning from the 11th edition were either updated or completely rewritten; and with few exceptions, all chapters were externally reviewed by a member of our faculty reviewer panel and a member of our student reviewer panel.

- *Unit I* profiles the profession by opening with a chapter on occupation followed by a newly written history of the profession, which places occupational therapy history in the context of larger world events. Next, a new chapter on the philosophical assumptions guiding the profession is added to this unit to help students appreciate the core beliefs which are embedded in the profession. The final chapter in this unit profiles contemporary practice in the United States and worldwide. By placing this material together in the opening unit, students are provided with important foundational material for the rest of the book.
- *Unit II* describes the occupational nature of humans. The opening chapter explores how participation in occupation changes over the course of life, thus expanding on the previous version of this chapter which primarily focused on child development and occupation. The next chapter explaining the relationships among occupation and health has been updated. And finally, a new author for the occupational science chapter provides insight into the ongoing research about occupation.
- *Unit III* continues to have first-person narratives of people with various occupational challenges after an opening chapter explaining the importance of client narratives to effective practice. Narratives provided range from Mary Feldhaus-Weber's experience of a head injury to Alex and his parents' views of their child growing up with cerebral palsy and Donald Murray's poignant description of caring for his wife during her days with dementia. Most of these powerful accounts remain as they were in the 11th edition, although Gloria F. Dickerson has updated her narrative of surviving the challenges of mental illness. The chapter on programs in different countries that closed the unit in the last edition has been moved to the Web for continued availability but has been replaced in the text by a new series of first-person narratives collected from individuals in Ecuador.
- *Unit IV* on occupations in context represents a reorganization of existing chapters to make a clearer connection with the broad array of contextual factors discussed in the Occupational Therapy Practice Framework: Domain and Process, 2nd Edition and the WHO's ICF. An updated chapter on family perspectives opens the unit, followed by a new chapter on the temporal aspects of occupation entitled "Patterns of Occupation." A new author provides a fresh look at the impact of culture, race, and ethnicity on occupation, followed by an updated chapter on socioeconomic factors. Finally, a newly synthesized chapter on "Physical and Virtual Environments" broadens the content from the previous edition.
- *Unit V* focuses on personal factors affecting occupation and represents a reorganization of chapters into a unit that closely parallels the Occupational Therapy Practice Framework: Domain and Process, 2nd Edition. The opening chapter on individual factors has been significantly expanded to provide more examples to students about how body functions and structures impact performance. The updated chapter on spirituality and beliefs explains how these individual differences impact the meaning of occupation.
- *Unit VI* focuses on analyzing occupation, with an updated and expanded chapter on occupational analysis, followed by a new chapter on performance skills that provides additional information on ways to consider occupational performance.

- *Unit VII* expands the discussion of the occupational therapy process in the previous edition and is compatible with the AOTA Occupational Therapy Practice Framework: Domain and Process, 2nd Edition. The introductory chapter to this unit is expanded to include outcomes of care. A new chapter on determining client needs provides detailed examples of client evaluation across a variety of contexts. This is followed by a new chapter on critiquing assessments that not only speaks to assessing traditional measures but also introduces considerations relevant to new psychometric approaches as they relate to current occupational therapy assessments. The process of intervention for individuals and for organizations, communities, and populations is more fully explored in two new chapters. Finally, a new chapter on modifying performance contexts consolidates several chapters which were in the 11th edition.
- *Unit VIII* clusters together several updated chapters that address core concepts and skills such as professional reasoning, group process and intervention, evidence-based practice, and ethical practice. Two new chapters consolidate related material in one place, one on therapeutic relationships and client collaboration, and the other on professional communications and documentation.
- *Unit IX* discusses theories of occupational performance, including ecological models, the Model of Human Occupation, and Occupational Adaptation. In addition to updates, improvements include a new version of the theory and practice chapter which sets up the range of theories discussed in this unit and subsequent units. Occupational justice is included in this unit as a theoretical perspective. The final chapter is a new one devoted to emerging theories within occupational therapy.
- *Unit X* is a new unit providing descriptions of broad theories that inform practice but which are not occupational therapy theories per se. These include the recovery model, health promotion theories, and theories on learning and behavior change.
- *Unit XI* starts with a new introductory chapter that provides an overview of evaluation, intervention, and outcomes for the major areas of occupation. Basic and instrumental activities of daily living are combined into one new chapter, followed by updated chapters on education, work, play, and leisure. A new chapter on sleep and rest along with a new chapter on social participation round out this unit.
- *Unit XII* provides a survey of focused theories that are commonly used in conjunction with occupational performance theories to guide intervention. Included is a newly reworked chapter on motor function/control by a new author, an updated chapter on cognition and perception, and a newly reworked chapter on sensory processing. The unit ends with two new chapters, one on emotional regulation and the other addressing communication and social interaction.
- *Unit XIII*, entitled *Practice Context: Therapists in Action*, is a new unit which displays therapist decision making as it is implemented in different therapy settings across various continuums of care. The first chapter explains how clients may receive therapy across a wide range of settings, although clusters of settings may be more associated with some health or participation challenges than others. Subsequent chapters each provide a therapist narrative explaining the thinking behind the evaluation and intervention strategies implemented for a particular client. Additionally, each chapter addressed how services commonly occur across different settings. Separate chapters address services for individuals with autism spectrum disorders, traumatic brain injury, and schizophrenia, followed by additional chapters focused on injured workers, older adults with changing needs, and disaster survivors. The intent of this unit is to "bring alive" the various theories and intervention approaches by displaying real-world situations.
- *Unit XIV* addresses professional development in the transition from student to practitioner as well as the role of professional organizations in supporting professional development and advocacy. The chapter on fieldwork has been expanded to address the process of professional entry. The chapter on professional development and continuing

competency has been expanded by a new author to include a discussion of the variety of advanced education options. The final chapter, again by a new author, includes information about professional organizations in the United States and worldwide.

- *Unit XV* addresses occupational therapy management, supervision, and related topics such as payment for service and advocacy. The content in all of these chapters has been updated. The social and health policy chapter was moved into this unit. The chapter on payment includes the current information on changes in health policy in the United States. The chapter on consultation, written by a new author, provides a discussion of opportunities and issues to consider in becoming an occupational therapy consultant.
- There are two appendices in the book. The first includes either new or completely updated summaries of resources and evidence related to common conditions for which occupational therapy services are provided. The second appendix is an updated table of assessments.
- The glossary contains definitions of key words from chapters and important terminology from official documents such as the WHO ICF and the AOTA Occupational Therapy Practice Framework: Domain and Process, 2nd Edition.

Special Features

Special features are found both in the text and in the Web materials associated with this text. Special features include the following:

- **Practice Dilemma:** A practice situation related to chapter content with one to three questions designed to challenge students. Answers are not provided to the student.
- **Ethical Dilemma:** A scenario relevant to chapter content which poses an ethical challenge for practitioners.
- **Case Study:** An example of occupational therapy evaluation and intervention modeling expert practice. Note that these are available both in text and in the form of video vignettes online.
- **Commentary on the Evidence:** A succinct discussion about available evidence to support practice, including identification of where evidence is lacking or inconclusive and where further research required.

With this edition, we are pleased to offer specially selected video clips from International Clinical Educators, Inc. These may be found on our Website, http://thePoint.lww.com/Willard-Spackman12e. Also on the Web are PowerPoint slides for each chapter, quiz and test banks, additional learning materials, and several professionally developed video clips.

Final Notes

As a new team of editors, we are grateful for the guidance provided by many experienced colleagues as we have created this edition and the support of Ellen S. Cohn as consulting editor as well as Elizabeth "Betty" Crepeau, the former senior editor. It is our hope that we have created a work that honors the heritage of this book and that serves the profession well by lighting the way for the next generation of occupational therapy practitioners.

Barbara A. Boyt Schell
Glen Gillen
Marjorie E. Scaffa

Acknowledgments

This edition of *Willard & Spackman* was accomplished through the collective efforts of the contributors, focus group members, editorial review board, photographers, students, colleagues, friends, and family. Well over 150 people have directly contributed to the development of this book. We are grateful for their many contributions to this effort and know that their commitment, scholarship and generosity in sharing these traits have improved the quality of the work presented here.

Editing a book such as this becomes an occupation in and of itself. Like all occupations, it is interwoven within the larger tapestry of activities that comprise our lives. Indeed, there is the "text" and the "subtext" of each edition. The text you see before you. The subtext is hidden behind the scenes. This edition started in the midst of changing editorial responsibilities which resulted in our new team of editors. We inaugurated our partnership as a group through an initial shared weekend with our consulting editor Ellen who dubbed herself our "transition object." We cemented our team over the years with conference calls, emails, shared meals, and celebrations at AOTA conferences, along with occasional visits for a mix of work and pleasure. As the book progressed, each of our own life stories evolved as well. Health challenges involving ourselves, family members, and colleagues served to personalize many of the concepts in this book as we took turns both supporting and covering for each other. We said goodbye to beloved pets (Eve and Smoky for Barb, Ginger for Glen), while welcoming new ones (Max for Glen). At this writing, Barbara is anxiously awaiting the holidays when Santa has promised to bring her a new puppy. Each of us is fortunate to have a life partner who supports us and who knows when to let us work and when to suggest that it is time to play.

- Barbara thanks her husband John W. Schell, PhD, who is both playmate and professional partner in education and scholarship; photographer extraordinaire; and father/grandfather to our wonderful family, Brad, Trina, Sophie & Izzy Schell, and Alyxius, Marcus, Adrian, Rooke, Akhasa and Samarra Young, all of whom give meaning to our lives. Finally, thanks to Helen Clayton for her service in our household.
- Glen thanks Michael P. Lawrence, partner, best friend, father to Max, and amazing uncle to Avery, Harry, Julianna, Marley, Lizzy, Matthew, Todd, and Zachary.
- Marjorie thanks S. Blaise Chromiak, MD, husband and professional colleague for his overall love and support, his expertise in reviewing, proofing, and organizing chapters I was writing or editing, and his willingness to cook, do laundry and whatever else I needed done to enable me to dedicate large amounts of time to this project.

Thanks to each of you for your commitment to each of us.

Finally, each of us are very proud of our universities and occupational therapy programs which sustain us in our work and encourage us to greater accomplishments. Our students, faculty, and practitioners in our professional communities provide a background of inspiration for taking on a task such as this. We thank all those listed below for their generous assistance in helping us to think through needed changes and for imagining how to best extend Willard and Spackman into new technologies and Web-based resources.

Professional Colleagues and Students

We thank our colleagues for their assistance, support, and insightful feedback. We are grateful for the large group of faculty and students who responded to surveys in Spring, 2010, and those are participated in focus groups at the AOTA Annual Conference in 2010. They validated what was working, identified content gaps, and helped us to organize the flow of the book for a better fit with important documents and ideas currently guiding the profession. Additionally, their encouragement provided increase impetus for the high quality Web-based companion materials that are newly available with this text. Beyond our larger community of professional colleagues and students, we are particularly grateful for those closer to home and who are listed below. They have lived with this project for several years, participated in endless conversations about *Willard & Spackman* and steadily backed our efforts. To you we are most grateful:

Brenau University

- Mary Shotwell & Robin Underwood for taking up much of the school's administrative work when I needed to focus on editing, and for being sounding boards for ideas large and small.
- Kay Graham, Wendy Holmes, Rosalie Miller for critical feedback and support "on demand."
- Carol Eggerding and Adam Bruce for keeping it all going at work.
- Gale Starich for being the most supportive dean ever.
- The rest of the occupational therapy faculty, who with the folks above, make me proud to be an occupational therapist and educator: Irma Alvarado, Jennifer Allison, Jenene Craig, Marsey Waller Devoto, Nancy Fowler, Tamara Mills, Kris Probert, Lisa Schubert, Susan Stallings-Sahler, Debbie Weissman-Miller.
- Occupational Therapy students in our Brenau day and weekend programs for providing ongoing inspiration and reality checks.

Columbia University

- Janet Falk-Kessler, my director, for ongoing support, encouragement, and letting me know when my work load was exceeding "just the right challenge."
- My occupational therapy faculty colleagues for creating a stimulating (and fun!) work environment.
- Emily Raphael-Greenfield, Pamela A. Miller, Dawn M. Nilsen, and Debra Tupe for sage advice on chapter content.
- Marilyn Harper and Brenda Spivey-Nieves for keeping it all going.
- My students, who teach me on a daily basis.

University of South Alabama

- Cherie McGee, my administrative assistant, for protecting my writing and editing time from interruptions.
- Courtney Sasse, MS, OTR/L for collegial, emotional, and instrumental support throughout the process of text development.
- Occupational therapy students for providing feedback on the chapters I was writing and assisting in the development of context-rich case studies.

And

- Jan Davis of International Clinical Educators, Inc. for her willingness to work with us to make Web-based video cases a reality.
- Betty Crepeau for moral support and encouragement that we were doing fine, and indeed would arrive "in the barn, warm and dry."

Editorial Review Board

We thank our invited editorial review board who gave generously of their time and knowledge to review chapters in this book to assure that each chapter met our standards for both scholarship and accessibility. They are listed by name earlier in this front matter, but we wish to once again thank them for their service.

Lippincott Williams & Wilkins
Current and former Lippincott Williams & Wilkins personnel contributed to the development of this book and we appreciate their ongoing support.

- Linda Francis, Mike Nobel, Kelley Squazzo, Renee Thomas, Rachel Stark, Tish Oglesby, Courtney Shell, Shauna Kelley, Tim Serpico.
- Harold Medina of Absolute Service, Inc., our newly met colleague in the Philippines for his thoroughness in copy editing and page formatting, willingness to remind us (again!) what he is missing from us, and overall generosity of spirit.

Hearthside Publishing Services
Our thanks to LWW for allowing us once again to have the special attentions of this group. This is the second time that Laura and her staff have served to support us in this text and their contributions are invaluable.

- Laura Horowitz provided overall guidance of the development of the manuscript through the production of the book. Her steady guidance, expertise, patience, and good humor provided significant support to our efforts.
- Gretchen Miller who helped us with her careful tracking of manuscripts, photos, and all other editorial details needed to bring the book to fruition.
- Christine Mercer Vernon who had the daunting task of either drawing or converting all the artwork in the book to their 4-color versions. Thanks for adding color to our work!

Brief Contents

Contents

Features

PRACTICE DILEMMA

ETHICAL DILEMMA

COMMENTARY ON THE EVIDENCE

CASE STUDIES

Online Video Clips

In addition to the features listed above, this edition of *Willard and Spackman's Occupational Therapy* will feature a video library on thePoint (visit http://thePoint.lww.com/Willard-Spackman12e). The videos are from the library of International Clinical Educators, Inc. (http://www.icelearningcenter.com/) and were chosen to supplement various chapters. Although chapter suggestions are listed in the descriptions below, these suggestions are not exhaustive. The videos take place in various contexts (acute care hospitals, home-based services, outpatient services, school-based services, etc.) but are not meant to represent all of the contexts and population that are served by occupational therapy practitioners. Video clips are listed by their titles.

Acute Care: How to Awaken a Lethargic Patient
The therapist demonstrates methods of how to arouse a lethargic patient in the acute care setting. *Recommended as a supplement to Chapter 55.*

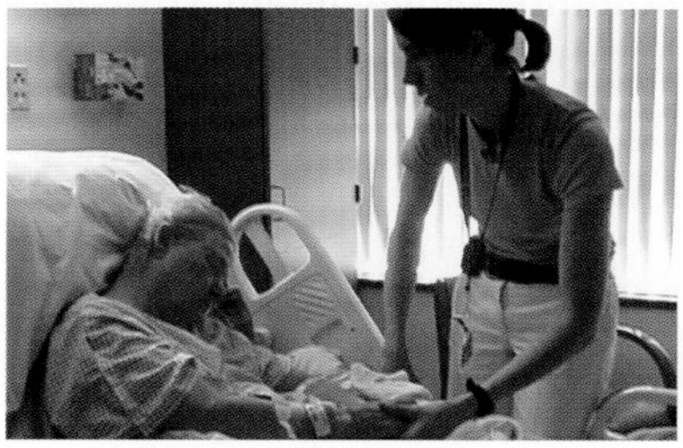

IADL: Sweeping the Sidewalk
Functioning at a high level, this stroke survivor attempts to use his involved hand during an IADL task: sweeping the sidewalk. *Recommended as a supplement to Chapter 47.*

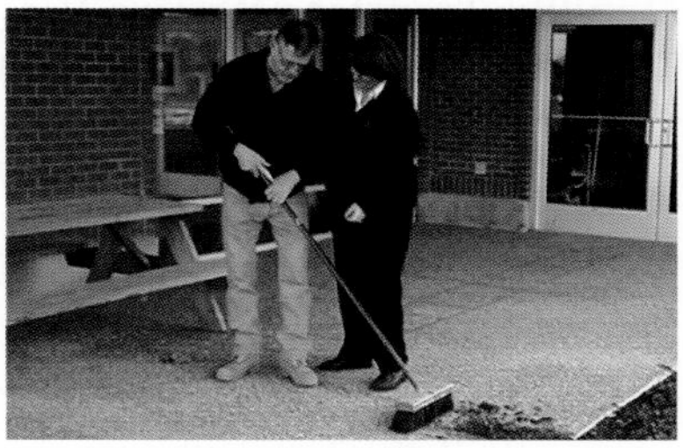

ICU: Co-treatment
The PT and OT work together, demonstrating bed mobility techniques (rolling, sidelying to sitting) with a stroke survivor in the ICU. *Recommended as a supplement to Chapters 35, 47, 54, and 59.*

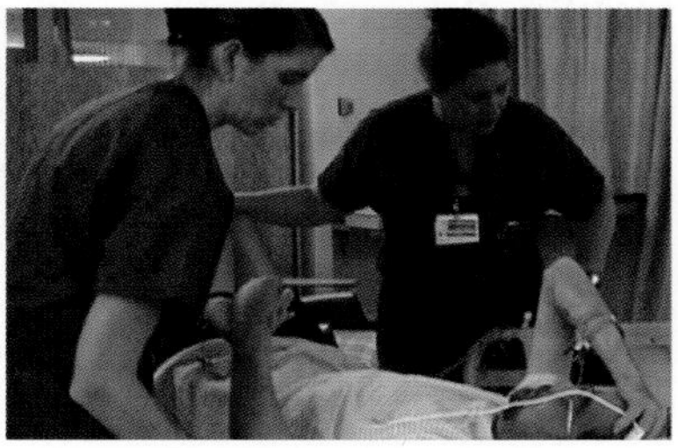

ICU: Initial Contact
As the therapist begins her treatment session in the ICU, she quickly assesses the stroke survivor's visual and sensory status. *Recommended as a supplement to Chapters 19 and 24.*

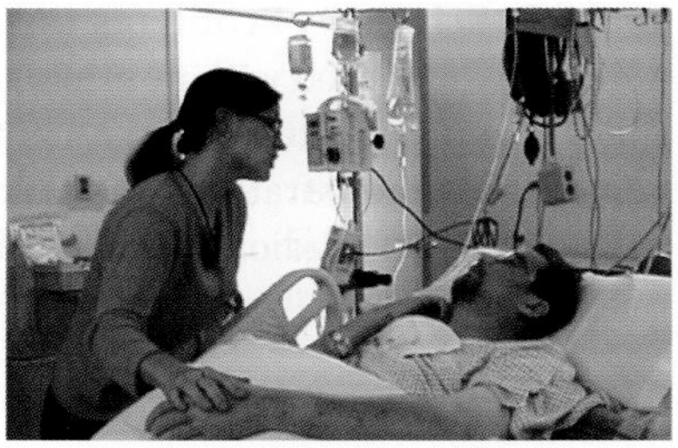

Initial Interview: Outpatient
The therapist begins her initial assessment and gathers information while she observes this stroke survivor maneuver his wheelchair into the clinic, try to move his hand, and describe his medical condition. *Recommended as a supplement to Chapters 23, 33, and 24.*

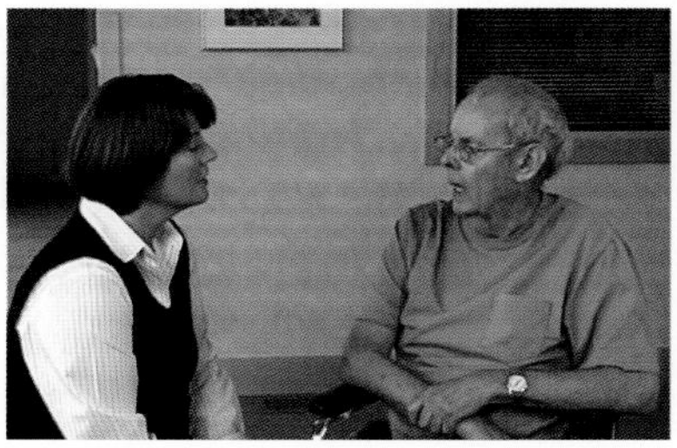

Initiating Treatment Bedside: Self-Care
The therapist introduces self-care tasks with a stroke survivor while working on sitting balance, weight shifts, and visual field deficits in the acute care hospital. *Recommended as a supplement to Chapters 47 and 59.*

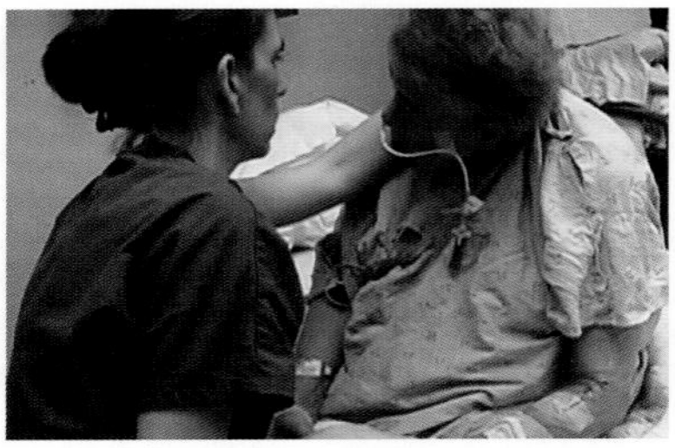

Mobility: Independent Transfer from Bed to Wheelchair
A stroke survivor transfers safely and independently from his bed to his wheelchair. *Recommended as a supplement to Chapter 47.*

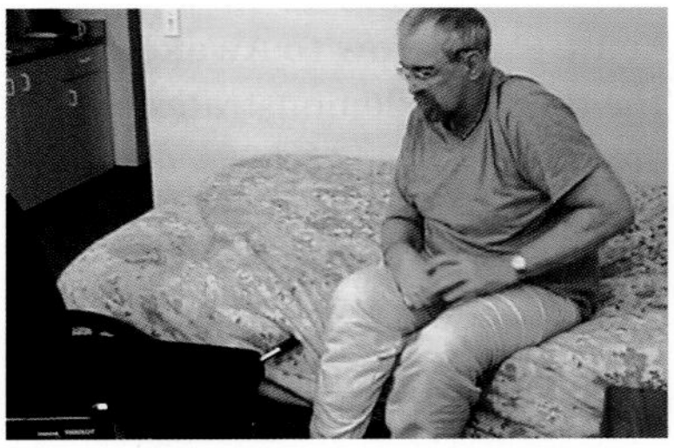

Mobility: Transfer with Two-Person Assist
The therapist teaches a family member how to safely transfer a stroke survivor from her wheelchair to the sofa with the assistance of two persons. *Recommended as a supplement to Chapters 28, 33, and 47.*

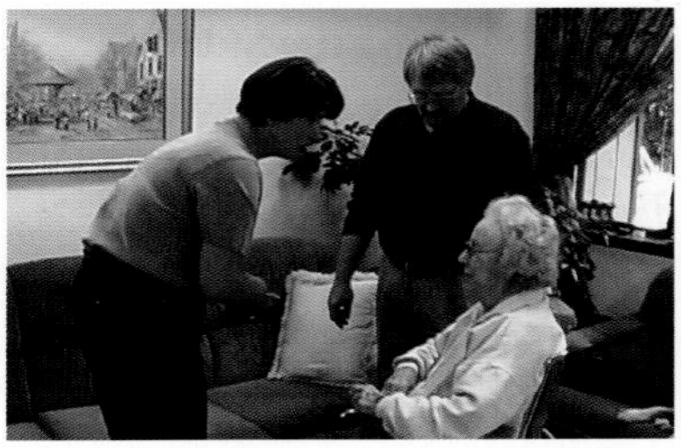

Multiple Sclerosis, Problems Observed in the Home
An artist, diagnosed with multiple sclerosis, has difficulty standing because of fatigue. She shares her concerns about safety and the need to modify her work environment. She asked for help in determining the best solutions. *Recommended as a supplement to Chapters 18, 24, and 29.*

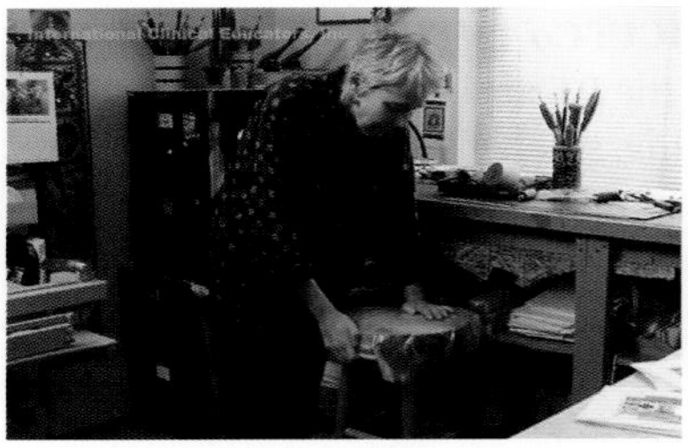

Multiple Sclerosis, Problems Observed in the Home: Part 1
A woman diagnosed with multiple sclerosis describes how weakness, fatigue, and the symptoms of her disease impact her work as an artist and her life at home. She demonstrates how she has adapted her tools to make them easier to use in her art studio. *Recommended as a supplement to Chapters 33 and 49.*

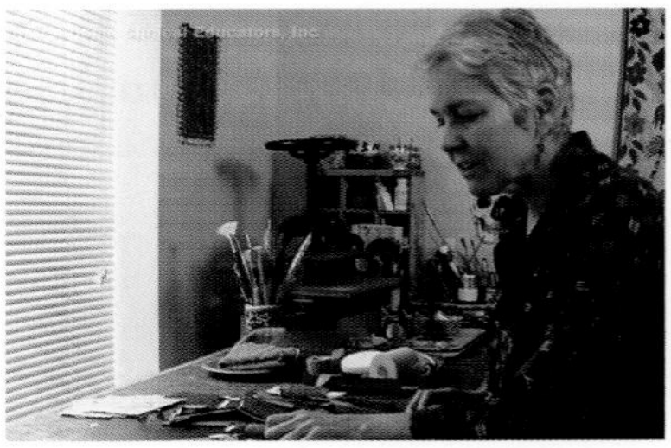

Multiple Sclerosis, Problems Observed in the Home: Part 5
The need to do physically demanding activities at home, such as cleaning the bathtub, may require the help of a therapist to problem solve and determine the best solution. This client, a woman with multiple sclerosis, asks for assistance in finding an optimal solution to this problem. *Recommended as a supplement to Chapters 18, 29, 47, and 59.*

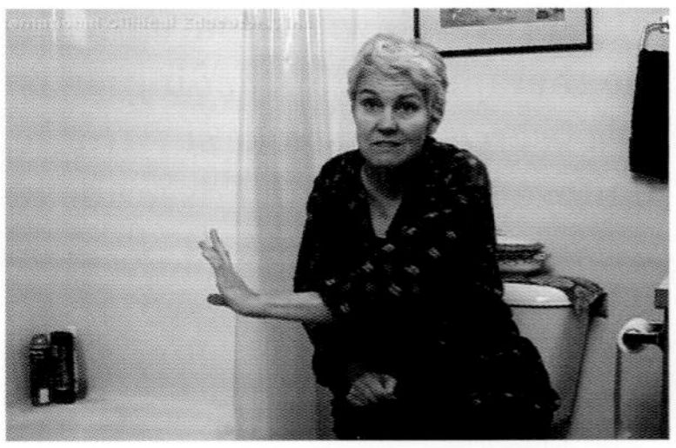

Patient Education: Answering Patient Questions
As the initial treatment session ends, the patient asks a common question: "How long will this take?" The therapist explains how end range of motion feels and the importance of continuing active range of motion (AROM) to minimize loss of hand function following her surgical repair for a distal radial fracture. *Recommended as a supplement to Chapters 23, 28, and 33.*

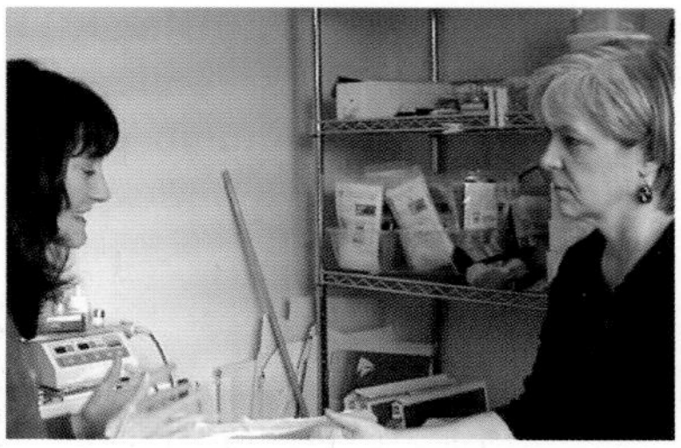

Pediatric Assessment: Administration of the Test of Visual Motor Skills
The therapist administers the Test of Visual Motor Skills to a 6-year-old with fine motor, attention and developmental vision challenges. *Recommended as a supplement to Chapters 24 and 48.*

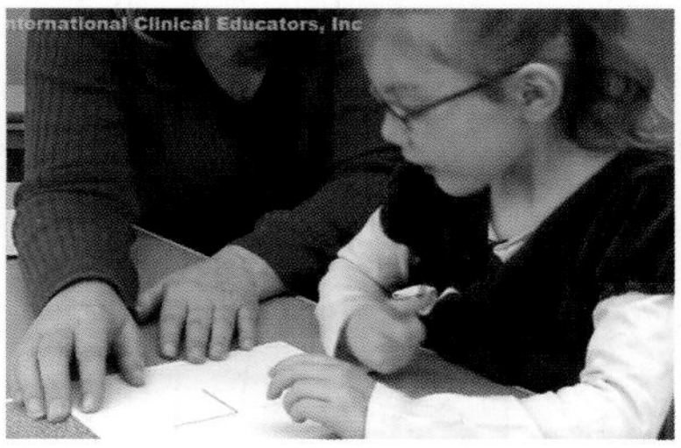

Pediatric Fine Motor: Ocular Motor and Visual Perception
The therapist uses an iPad to help a 6-year-old child develop visual motor, eye–hand coordination, and developmental vision skills by practicing her letter formation. This intervention strategy, developed in collaboration with a developmental optometrist, uses a colored filter so all letters in red can only be seen by the weaker (left) eye, thus requiring that eye to work harder. *Recommended as a supplement to Chapter 48.*

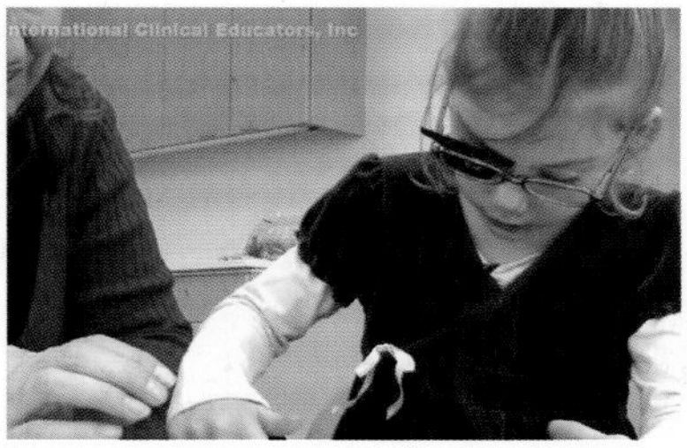

Pediatric Mat Activity: Hand Function
A series of short clips illustrate hand function, grasp, and reaching in a 4-year-old diagnosed with a chromosomal abnormality. *Recommended as a supplement to Chapter 54.*

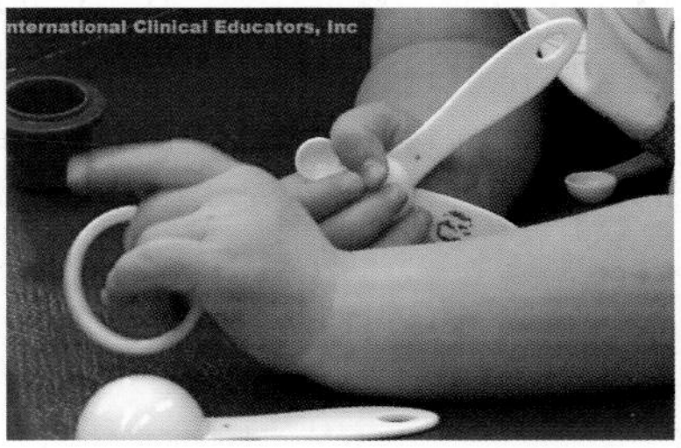

Pediatric Sensory Integration/Sensory Processing: Scooter-board and Letter Recognition Activity
The therapist uses a play activity with a scooter board and ramp as part of an intervention plan to support the development of letter recognition, auditory memory, and attention in a 6-year-old with fine motor, visual motor, and attention difficulties. *Recommended as a supplement to Chapter 56.*

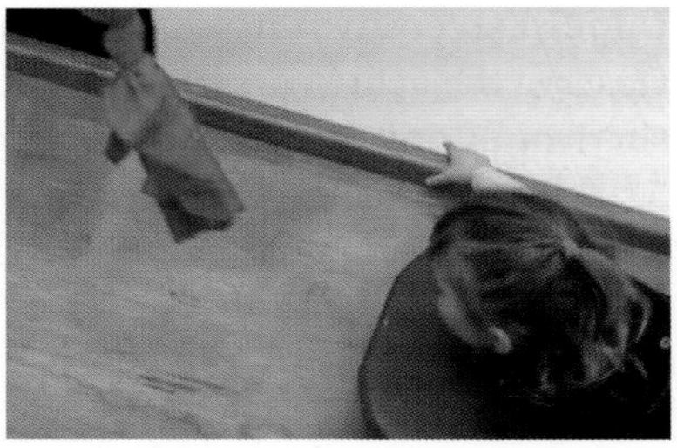

Pediatrics: Behavior Management: Developing a Therapy Plan
A 6-year-old with fine and visual motor challenges and her therapist develop a therapy plan to help with behavior management. Writing vertically on the board helps with wrist position, and phonetic spelling is used because it reinforces what is done in the classroom. *Recommended as a supplement to Chapters 56 and 57.*

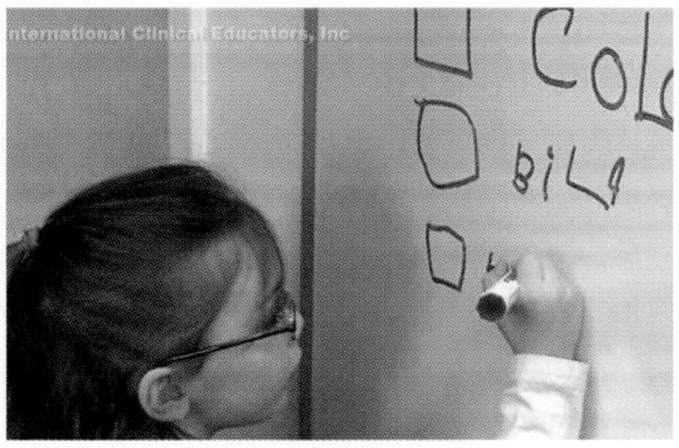

Radial Fracture: Measuring ROM

During the initial assessment, the therapist measures range of motion (ROM) of the wrist, thumb, and forearm to determine a baseline for treatment. The patient is 8 weeks postsurgery. *Recommended as a supplement to Chapters 19 and 24.*

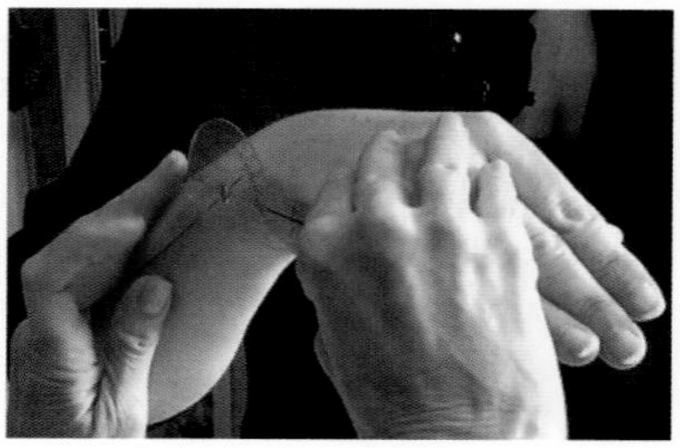

Self-Care: Dressing in Acute Care

A young stroke survivor becomes frustrated as he attempts to dress himself. The therapist demonstrates ADL training and upper extremity dressing techniques with a patient exhibiting expressive aphasia, cognitive/perceptual deficits, and right hemiplegia in the acute care hospital. *Recommended as a supplement to Chapters 47, 54, 55, and 57.*

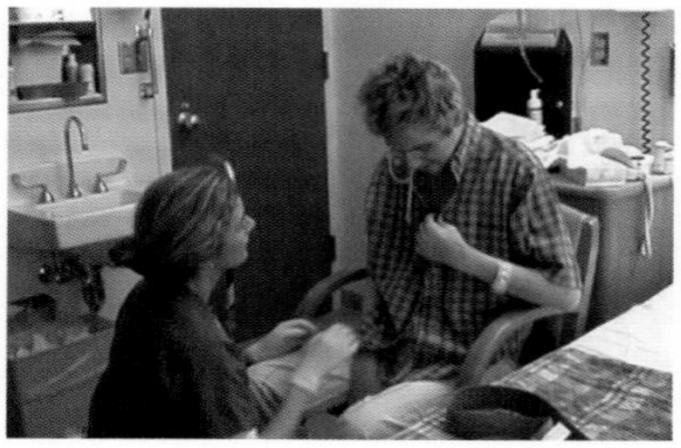

Self-Care: One-Handed Shoe Tying

Many stroke survivors are unable to tie their own shoes. A very simple method of how to tie shoes with the use of one hand is demonstrated to a stroke survivor in the outpatient clinic. *Recommended as a supplement to Chapter 47.*

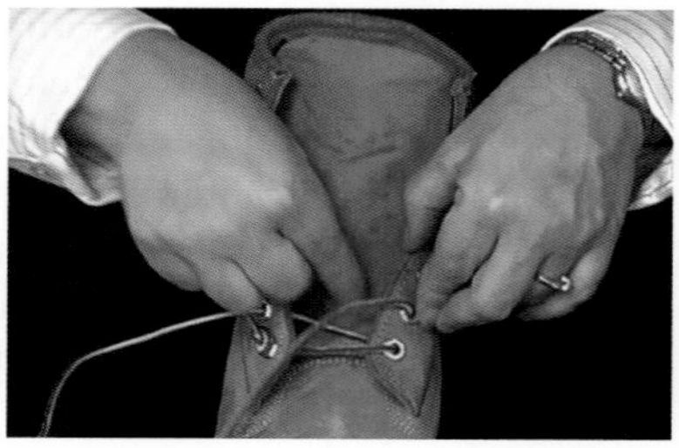

Standing at the Kitchen Counter

As a stroke survivor comes from sit to stand at the kitchen counter, the therapist teaches the importance of safety to a family member. *Recommended as a supplement to Chapters 18, 23, and 28.*

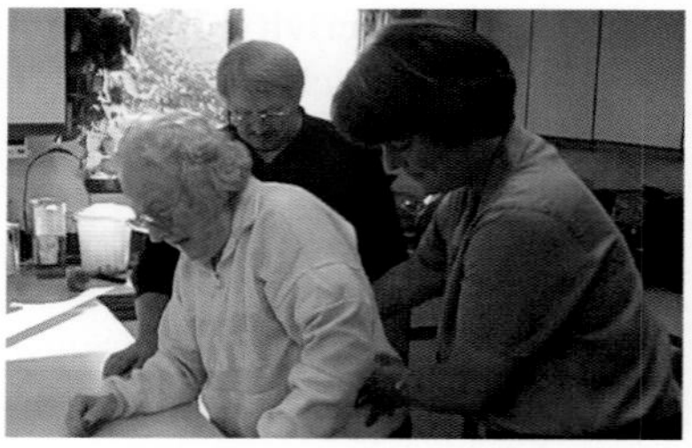

Upper Extremity: Initial Assessment in Acute Care

Observe the acute care therapist continue a bedside assessment of a stroke survivor during mealtime. *Recommended as a supplement to Chapters 24 and 54.*

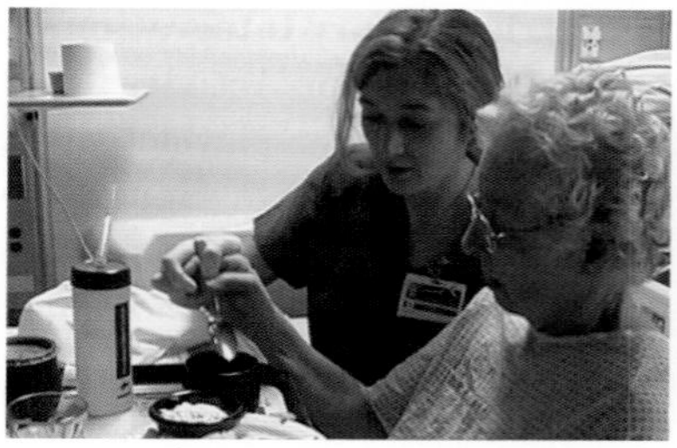

Visual Field Deficits: Examples in Acute Care

Just 48-hours poststroke, a patient in the acute care hospital exhibits disregard of her left side. *Recommended as a supplement to Chapters 24 and 55.*

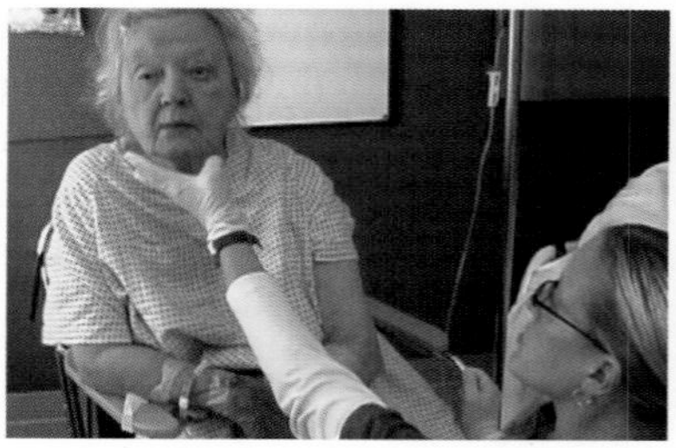

Occupation Therapy: Profile of the Profession

UNIT I

"The object of the society shall be the advancement of occupation as a therapeutic measure; the study of the effects of occupation upon the human being; and the dissemination of scientific knowledge of this subject." (Article I, Section 3, Constitution; National Society for the Promotion of Occupational Therapy, 1917)

CHAPTER 1

What Is Occupation?

Virginia Dickie

OUTLINE

*"**Mr. Jourdain**. You mean to say that when I say, 'Nicole, fetch me my slippers' or 'Give me my nightcap' that's prose?*

***Philosopher**. Certainly, sir.*

***Mr. Jourdain**. Well, my goodness! Here I've been talking prose for forty years and never known it. . . . "*

—MOLIERE (1670)

LEARNING OBJECTIVES

After reading this chapter, you will be able to:

1. Identify and evaluate ways of knowing occupation
2. Articulate different ways of defining and classifying occupation
3. Describe the relationship between occupation and context

Knowing and Learning about Occupation

Reading the paper, washing hands, throwing a Frisbee, walking through a colorful market in a foreign country, telling a story (in poetry or prose)—all are occupations people do without ever thinking about them as being occupations. Many occupations are ordinary and become part of the context of daily living. Such occupations are generally taken for granted and most often are habitual (Aarts & Dijksterhuis, 2000; Bargh & Chartrand, 1999; Wood, Quinn, & Kashy, 2002). In the myriad of activities people do every day, they do *occupation* all their lives, perhaps without ever knowing it.

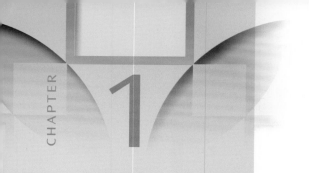

Occupations are ordinary, but they can also be special when they represent a new achievement such as driving a car or when they are part of celebrations and rites of passage. Preparing and hosting a holiday dinner for the first time and baking the pies for the annual family holiday for the twentieth time are examples of special occupations. Occupations tend to be special when they happen infrequently and carry symbolic meanings such as representing achievement of adulthood or one's love for family. Occupations are also special when they form part of a treasured routine such as reading a bedtime story to one's child, singing "Twinkle, Twinkle, Little Star," and tucking the covers around the small, sleepy body. But even special occupations, although heavy with tradition, may change over time. Hocking, Wright-St. Clair, and Bunrayong (2002) illustrated the complexity of traditional occupations in their study of holiday food preparation by older women in Thailand and New Zealand. The study identified many similarities between the groups (such as the activities the authors named "recipe work"), but the Thai women valued maintenance of an invariant tradition in what they prepared and how they did it, whereas the New Zealand women changed the foods they prepared over time and expected such changes to continue. Nevertheless, the doing of food-centered occupations around holidays was a tradition for both groups.

To be human is to be occupational. Occupation is a biological imperative, evident in the evolutionary history of humankind, the current behaviors of our primate relatives, and the survival needs that must be met through occupation (Clark, 1997; Krishnagiri, 2000; Wilcock, 2006; Wood, 1998). Fromm (as cited by Reilly, 1962) asserted that people have a "physiologically conditioned need" to work as an act of self-preservation (p. 4). Humans also have occupational needs beyond survival. Addressing one type of occupation, Dissanayake (1992, 1995) argued that making art, or as she describes it, "making special," is a biological necessity of human existence. According to Molineux (2004), occupational therapists now understand humans, their function, and their therapeutic needs in an occupational manner in which *occupation is life itself* [emphasis added]. Townsend (1997) described occupation as the "active process of living: from the beginning to the end of life, our occupations are all the active processes of looking after ourselves and others, enjoying life, and being socially and economically productive over the lifespan and in various contexts" (p. 19).

The Need to Understand Occupation

Occupational therapy practitioners need to base their work on a thorough understanding of occupation and its role in health. Understanding occupation is more than having an easy definition (which is a daunting challenge in its own right). To know what occupation is, it is necessary to examine what humans do with their time, how such activities are organized, what purposes they serve, and what they mean for individuals and society.

Personal experience of doing occupation, whether consciously attended to or not, provides a fundamental understanding of occupation—what it is, how it happens, what it means, what is good about it, and what is not. This way of knowing is both basic and extraordinarily rich. It is the way we learn to participate in the social worlds we inhabit.

Looking Inward to Know Occupation

If you had asked me about gardening when I was young, I would have described the hard work of weeding the family garden on hot summer days, emphasizing that gardening was a *chore*. In my parents' garden I learned a great deal about how to garden, such as varieties of flowers and vegetables, sunshine and rain requirements, weed identification, and how to grasp a weed to pull it out with all its roots. This is *knowledge* of rules and techniques, of how to *do* gardening. Now, many years later, I know gardening in a very different way. Weeding is one of my great pleasures. I understand the challenges of learning to garden in new places, the patience required to discover what will grow where, and the right time of year to plant. Between my youth and the present, gardening has taken on a different *form* (no longer a chore assigned by my parents but now creating and maintaining a low-tillage series of small gardens with herbs, shrubs, flowers, and selected vegetables on my own initiative or with my husband), *function* (then I gardened to avoid displeasing my parents, and now I garden to meet my own needs for aesthetic pleasures and satisfying "doing"), and *meaning* (from being a neutral to disagreeable series of chores to being a source of relaxation, reflection, shared time, and gratifying hard work). These elements—the form, function, and meaning of occupation—are the basic areas of focus for the science of occupation (Larson, Wood, & Clark, 2003).

To be useful to occupational therapy practitioners, knowledge of occupation based on personal experience demands examination and reflection. What do we do, how do we do it, when and where does it take place, and what does it mean? Who else is involved directly and indirectly? What capacities does it require in us? What does it cost? Is it challenging or easy? How has this occupation changed over time? What would it be like if we no longer had this occupation? My gardening example illustrates how occupation is a *transaction* with the *environment* or *context* of other people, plants, earth, and weather. It includes the *temporal* nature of occupation—seasonal variations but also change over time and perhaps some notion of occupation filling time. That I call myself a gardener exemplifies how occupation has become part of my *identity* and suggests that it might be difficult for me to give up gardening.

Basic as it is, however, understanding derived from personal experience is insufficient as the basis for practice. Reliance solely on this source of knowledge has the risk of expecting everyone to experience occupation in the same manner as the therapist. So while occupational therapy practitioners will profit in being attuned to their own occupations, they must also turn their view to the occupation around them and to understanding occupation through study and research.

Looking Outward to Know Occupation

Observation of the world through an occupational lens is another rich source of occupational knowledge. Connoisseurs of occupation can train themselves to new ways of seeing a world rich with occupations: the way a restaurant hostess manages a crowd when the wait for seating is long, the economy of movement of a construction worker doing a repetitive task, the activities of musicians in the orchestra pit when they are not playing, the almost aimless tossing of a ball as students take a break from class. Furthermore, people like to talk about what they do, and the student of occupation can learn a great deal by asking for information about people's work and play. By being observant and asking questions, people increase their repertoire of occupational knowledge far beyond the boundaries of personal interests, practices, and capabilities.

Observation of others' occupations enriches the occupational therapy practitioner's knowledge of the range of occupational possibilities and of human responses to occupational opportunities. But although this sort of knowledge goes far beyond the limits of personal experience, it is still bounded by the world any one person is able to access; and it lacks the depth of knowledge that is developed through research and scholarship.

Turning to Research and Scholarship to Understand Occupation

Knowledge of occupation that comes from personal experience and observation must be augmented with the understanding of occupation drawn from research in occupational therapy and occupational science as well as other disciplines. Hocking (2000) developed a framework of needed knowledge for research in occupation, organized into the categories of the "essential elements of occupation . . . occupational processes . . . [and the] relationship of occupation to other phenomena" (p. 59). This research is being done within occupational therapy and occupational science, but there is also a wealth of information to be found in the work of other disciplines. For example, in anthropology, Orr (1996) studied the work of copy machine repairmen, and Downey (1998) studied computer engineers and what they did. Consumer researchers have studied Christmas shopping (Sherry & McGrath, 1989), motorcycle riding (Schouten & McAlexander, 1995), and many other occupations of consumption. Psychologists have studied habits (Aarts & Dijksterhuis, 2000; Bargh & Chartrand, 1999; Wood et al., 2002) and a wealth of other topics that relate to how people engage in occupation. Understanding of occupation will benefit from more research within occupational therapy and occupational science and from accessing relevant works of scholars in other fields. Hocking (2009) recently called for more occupational science research focused on occupations themselves rather than people's experiences of occupations.

Defining Occupation

For many years, the word *occupation* was not part of the daily language of occupational therapists; nor was it prominent in the profession's literature (Hinojosa, Kramer, Royeen, & Luebben, 2003). According to Kielhofner and Burke (1977), the founding paradigm of occupational therapy was occupation, and the occupational perspective focused on people and their health "in the context of the culture of daily living and its activities" (p. 688). But beginning in the 1930s, occupational therapy strove to become more like the medical profession, entering into a paradigm of **reductionism** that lasted into the 1970s. During that time, occupation, both as a concept and as a means and/or outcome of intervention, was essentially absent from professional discourse. With time, a few professional leaders began to call for occupational therapy to return to its roots in occupation (Schwartz, 2003); and since the 1970s, acceptance of occupation as the foundation of occupational therapy has grown (Kielhofner, 2009). With that growth, professional debates about the definition and nature of occupation emerged and continue to this day.

Defining occupation in occupational therapy is challenging because the word is part of common language with meanings that the profession cannot control. The term *occupation* and related concepts such as *activity*, *task*, *employment*, and *work* are used in many ways within occupational therapy. It seems quite logical to think of a job, or cleaning house, or bike riding as an occupation; but the concept is fuzzier when we think about the smaller components of these larger categories. Is dusting an occupation, or is it part of the occupation of house cleaning? Is riding a bike a skill that is part of some larger occupation such as physical conditioning or getting from home to school, or is it an occupation in its own right? Does this change over time?

The founders of occupational therapy used the word *occupation* to describe a way of "properly" using time that included work and worklike activities and recreational activities (Meyer, 1922/1977). Breines (1995) pointed out that the founders chose a term that was both ambiguous and comprehensive to name the profession; a choice, she argued, that was not accidental. The term was open to holistic interpretations that supported the diverse areas of practice of the time, encompassing the elements of occupation defined by Breines (1995) as "mind, body, time, space, and others" (p. 459). The term *occupation* spawned ongoing examination, controversy, and redefinition as the profession has matured.

Nelson (1988, 1997) introduced the terms *occupational form*, "the preexisting structure that elicits, guides, or structures subsequent human performance," and *occupational performance*, "the human actions taken in response to an occupational form" (Nelson, 1988, p. 633). This distinction separates individuals and their actual doing of occupations from the general notion of an occupation and what it requires of anyone who does it.

Yerxa et al. (1989) defined occupation as "specific 'chunks' of activity within the ongoing stream of human behavior which are named in the lexicon of the culture. . . . These daily pursuits are self-initiated, goal-directed (purposeful), and socially sanctioned" (p. 5). Yerxa (1993) further elaborated this definition to incorporate an environmental perspective and a greater breadth of characteristics. "Occupations are units of activity which are classified and named by the culture according to the purposes they serve in enabling people to meet environmental challenges successfully. . . . Some essential characteristics of occupation are that it is self-initiated, goal-directed (even if the goal is fun or pleasure), experiential as well as behavioral, socially valued or recognized, constituted of adaptive skills or repertoires, organized, essential to the quality of life experienced, and possesses the capacity to influence health" (p. 5).

According to the Canadian Association of Occupational Therapists (as cited in Law, Steinwender, & Leclair, 1998), occupation is "groups of activities and tasks of everyday life, named, organized and given value and meaning by individuals and a culture." In a somewhat circular definition, they went on to state "occupation is everything people do to occupy themselves, including looking after themselves (self-care), enjoying life (leisure), and contributing to the social and economic fabric of their communities (productivity)" (p. 83). More recently, occupational scientists Larson et al., (2003) provided a simple definition of occupation as "the activities that comprise our life experience and can be named in the culture" (p. 16).

The previous definitions of occupation from occupational therapy literature help in explaining why occupation is the profession's focus (particularly in the context of therapy), yet they are open enough to allow continuing research on the nature of occupation. Despite, and perhaps because of, the ubiquity of occupation in human life, there is still much to learn about the nature of occupation through systematic research using an array of methodologies (Dickie, 2010; Hocking, 2000, 2009; Molke, Laliberte-Rudman, & Polatajko, 2004). Such research should include examination of the premises that are built into the accepted definitions of occupation.

At a more theoretical level, such an examination has begun. Several authors have recently challenged the unexamined assumptions and beliefs about occupation of Western occupational therapists (cf., Hammell, 2009a, 2009b; Iwama, 2006; Kantartzis & Molineux, 2011). This critiques center on the Western cultural bias in the definition and use of occupation and the inadequacy of the conceptualization of occupation as it is used in occupational therapy in Western countries to describe the daily activities of most of the world's population. Attention to these arguments will strengthen our knowledge of occupation.

Context and Occupation

The photograph of the two young boys playing in the garden sprinkler evokes a sense of a hot summer day and the experience of icy cold water coming out of the sprinkler, striking and stinging the boys' faces and tongues (Figure 1.1). Playing in the sprinkler has a context with temporal elements (summer, the play of children, and the viewer's memories of doing it in the past), a physical environment (grass, hot weather, hose, sprinkler, cold water), and a social environment (a pair of children and the likelihood of an indulgent parent). Playing in the sprinkler cannot be described or understood—or even happen—without its context. It is difficult to imagine that either boy would enjoy the activity as much doing it alone; the social context is part of the experience. A sprinkler might be set up for play on an asphalt driveway but not in a living room. Parents would be unlikely to allow their children to get soaking wet in cold weather. The contexts of the people viewing the picture are important, too; many will relate the picture to their own past experiences, but someone who lives in a place where lawn sprinklers are never used might find the picture meaningless and/or confusing. In this example, occupation and context are enmeshed with one another.

It is generally accepted that the specific *meaning* of an occupation is fully known only to the individual engaged in the occupation (Larson et al., 2003; Pierce, 2001; Weinblatt, Ziv, & Avrech-Bar, 2000). But it is also well accepted that occupations take place in *context* (sometimes referred to as the environment) (e.g., Baum & Christiansen, 2005; Kielhofner, 2002; Law et al., 1996; Schkade & Schultz, 2003; Yerxa et al., 1989) and thus

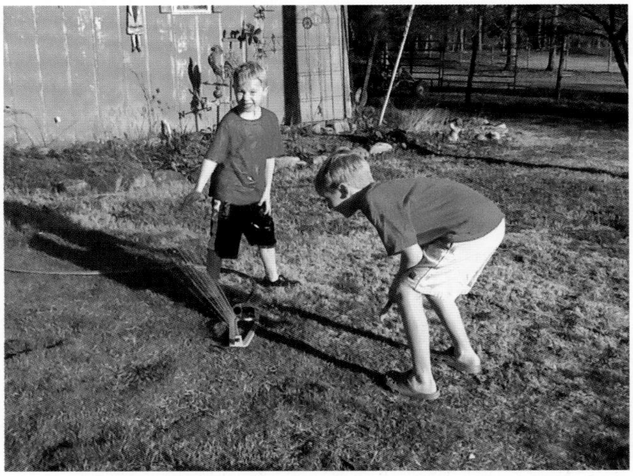

FIGURE 1.1 Two boys on a hot summer day.

have dimensions that consider other humans (in both social and cultural ways), temporality, the physical environment, and even virtual environments (American Occupational Therapy Association, 2008).

Description of occupation as taking place *in* or *with* the environment or context implies a separation of person and context that is problematic. In reality, person, occupation, and context are inseparable. Context is changeable but always present. Cutchin (2004) offered a critique of occupational therapy theories of adaptation-to-environment that separate person from environment and proposed that John Dewey's view of human experience as "always situated and contextualized" (p. 305) was a more useful perspective. According to Cutchin (2004), "situations are always inclusive of us, and us of them" (p. 305). Occupation occurs at the level of the situation and thus is inclusive of the individual and context (Dickie, Cutchin, & Humphry, 2006). Occupational therapy interventions cannot be context-free. Even when an occupational therapy practitioner is working with an individual, contextual elements of other people, the culture of therapist and client, the physical space, and past experiences are present.

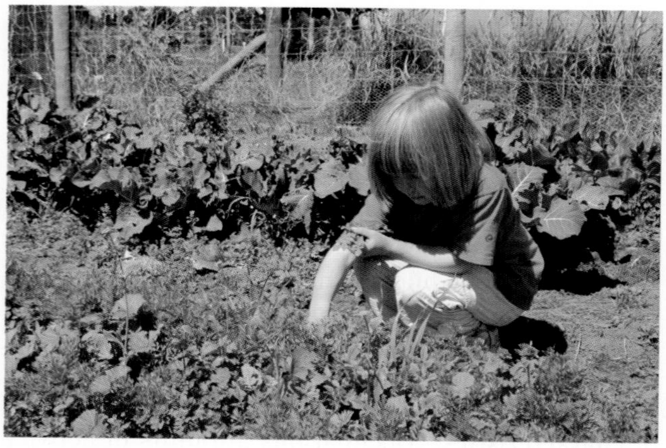

FIGURE 1.2 Child in the family garden.

Is Occupation Always Good?

In occupational therapy, occupation is associated with health and well-being, both as a means and as an end. But occupation can also be unhealthy, dangerous, maladaptive, or destructive to self or others and can contribute to societal problems and environmental degradation (Hammell, 2009a, 2009b). For example, the seemingly benign act of using a car to get to work, run errands, and pursue other occupations can limit one's physical activity and risk injury to self and others. Furthermore, Americans' reliance on the automobile contributes to urban sprawl, the decline of neighborhoods, air pollution, and overuse of nonrenewable natural resources. Industry and the work that provides monetary support to individuals and families cause serious air pollution in expanding economies such as that of China (Facts and Details, 2012).

Personal and societal occupational choices have consequences, good and bad. In coming to understand occupation, we need to acknowledge the breadth of occupational choices and their effects on individuals and the world.

Organizing Occupation

Categorization of occupations (e.g., into areas of activities of daily living, work, and leisure) is often problematic. Attempts to define work and leisure demonstrate that distinctions between the two are not always clear (Csikszentmihalyi & LeFevre, 1989; Primeau, 1996). Work may be defined as something people *have* to do, an unpleasant necessity of life, but many people enjoy their work and describe it as "fun." Indeed, Hochschild (1997) discovered that employees in the work setting she studied often preferred the homelike qualities of work to being in their actual homes and consequently spent more time at work than was necessary. The concept of leisure is problematic as well. Leisure might involve activities that are experienced as hard work, such as helping a friend to build a deck on a weekend.

Similar problems can be described with any categorization scheme. The photographs of the young girl, her father, and her mother (Figures 1.2, 1.3, & 1.4) each show activity in the same family garden. Categorizing the activity presents a challenge. The girl is intent on pulling weeds, which might mean she is engaging in work or productive activity. But she might also be

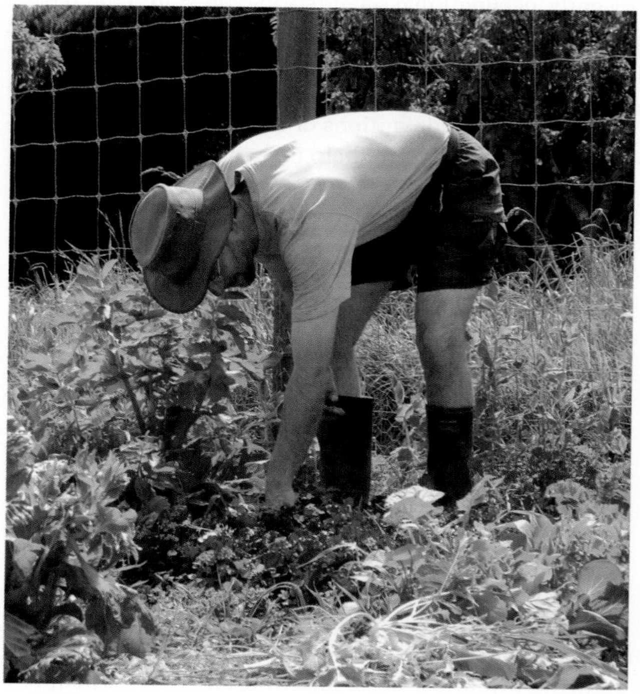

FIGURE 1.3 Father in the family garden.

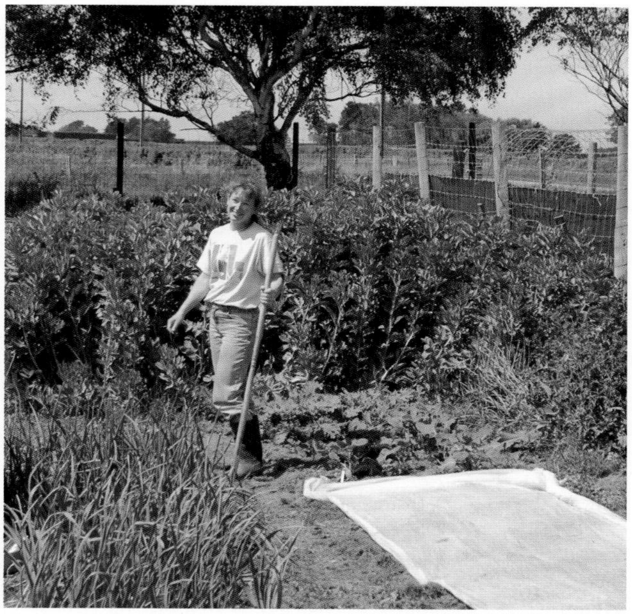

FIGURE 1.4 Mother in the family garden.

pretending to be like her mother—in that case playing. Her father is also weeding, clearly doing work. What sort of work is it though—paid work, caregiving work, the sort of leisure weed-pulling I enjoy? Both of the parents are dressed for dirty gardening activity, and the mother has gardening tools. But she is also posing for the picture. The gardening of all three is being captured to send to grandparents on the other side of the world. Categorizing the totality of this occupational situation is complicated, in contrast to the children gardening in Figure 1.5 who are clearly playing. No simple designation of what is happening in the pictures will suffice.

Another problem with categories is that an individual may experience an occupation as something entirely different from what it appears to be to others. Weinblatt et al. (2000) described how an elderly woman used the supermarket for purposes quite different from provisioning (that would likely be called an instrumental activities of daily living). Instead, this woman used her time in the store as a source of new knowledge and interesting information about modern life. What should we call her occupation in this instance?

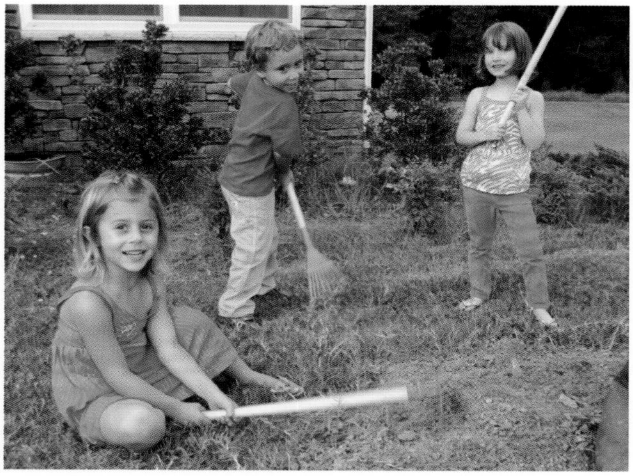

FIGURE 1.5 Children playing in a garden.

The construct of occupation might very well defy efforts to reduce it to a single definition or a set of categories. Many examples of occupations can be found that challenge other theoretical approaches and definitions. Nevertheless, the richness and complexity of occupation will continue to challenge occupational therapists to know and value it through personal experience, observations, and scholarly work. The practice of occupational therapy depends on this knowledge.

References

Aarts, J., & Dijksterhuis, A. (2000). Habits as knowledge structures: Automaticity in goal-directed behavior. *Journal of Personality and Social Psychology, 78*, 53–63.

American Occupational Therapy Association. (2008). Occupational therapy practice framework: Domain and process, 2nd edition. *American Journal of Occupational Therapy, 62*, 625–683.

Bargh, J. A., & Chartrand, T. L. (1999). The unbearable automaticity of being. *American Psychologist, 54*, 462–479.

Baum, C. M., & Christiansen, C. H. (2005). Person-environment-occupation-performance: An occupation-based framework for practice. In C. H. Christiansen, C. M. Baum, & J. Bass-Haugen (Eds.), *Occupational therapy: Performance, participation, and well-being* (3rd ed., pp. 243–266). Thorofare, NJ: SLACK.

Breines, E. B. (1995). Understanding "occupation" as the founders did. *British Journal of Occupational Therapy, 5*, 458–460.

Clark, F. A. (1997). Reflections on the human as an occupational being: Biological need, tempo and temporality. *Journal of Occupational Science: Australia, 4*, 86–92.

Csikszentmihalyi, M., & LeFevre, J. (1989). Optimal experience in work and leisure. *Journal of Personality and Social Psychology, 56*, 815–822.

Cutchin, M. P. (2004). Using Deweyan philosophy to rename and reframe adaptation-to-environment. *American Journal of Occupational Therapy, 58*, 303–312.

Dickie, V. A. (2010). Are occupations 'processes too complicated to explain'? What we can learn by trying. *Journal of Occupational Science, 17*, 195–203.

Dickie, V., Cutchin, M., & Humphry, R. (2006). Occupation as transactional experience: A critique of individualism in occupational science. *Journal of Occupational Science, 13*, 83–93.

Dissanayake, E. (1992). *Homo aestheticus: Where does art comes from and why*. Seattle, WA: University of Washington Press.

Dissanayake, E. (1995). The pleasure and meaning of making. *American Craft, 55*(2), 40–45.

Downey, G. (1998). *The machine in me*. New York, NY: Routledge.

Facts and Details. (2012). *Air pollution in China*. Retrieved from http://factsanddetails.com/china.php?itemid=392&catid=10&subcatid=66

Hammell, K. (2009a). Sacred texts: A sceptical exploration of the assumptions underpinning theories of occupation. *Canadian Journal of Occupational Therapy, 76*, 6–22.

Hammell, K. (2009b). Self-care, productivity, and leisure, or dimensions of occupational experience? Rethinking occupational "categories." *Canadian Journal of Occupational Therapy, 76*, 107–114.

Hinojosa, J., Kramer, P., Royeen, C. B., & Luebben, A. J. (2003). Core concept of occupation. In P. Kramer, J. Hinojosa, & C. B. Royeen (Eds.), *Perspectives in human occupation: Participation in life* (pp. 1–17). Philadelphia, PA: Lippincott Williams & Wilkins.

Hochschild, A. R. (1997). *The time bind: When work becomes home and home becomes work.* New York, NY: Metropolitan Books.

Hocking, C. (2000). Occupational science: A stock take of accumulated insights. *Journal of Occupational Science, 7,* 58–67.

Hocking, C. (2009). The challenge of occupation: Describing the things people do. *Journal of Occupational Science, 16,* 140–150.

Hocking, C., Wright-St. Clair, V., & Bunrayong, W. (2002). The meaning of cooking and recipe work for older Thai and New Zealand women. *Journal of Occupational Science, 9,* 117–127.

Iwama, M. (2006). *The Kawa model: Culturally relevant occupational therapy.* Philadelphia, PA: Churchill Livingston, Elsevier.

Kantartzis, S., & Molineux, M. (2011). The influence of Western society's construction of a healthy daily life on the conceptualization of occupation. *Journal of Occupational Science, 18,* 62–80.

Kielhofner, G. (2002). *Model of human occupation: Theory and application* (3rd ed.). Philadelphia, PA: Lippincott Williams & Wilkins.

Kielhofner, G. (2009). *Conceptual foundations of occupational therapy practice* (4th ed.). Philadelphia, PA: F. A. Davis.

Kielhofner, G., & Burke, J. P. (1977). Occupational therapy after 60 years: An account of changing identity and knowledge. *American Journal of Occupational Therapy, 31,* 675–689.

Krishnagiri, S. (2000). Occupations and their dimensions. In J. Hinojosa & M. L. Blount (Eds.), *The texture of life: Purposeful activities in occupational therapy* (pp. 35–50). Bethesda, MD: American Occupational Therapy Association.

Larson, E., Wood, W., & Clark, F. (2003). Occupational science: Building the science and practice of occupation through an academic discipline. In E. B. Crepeau, E. Cohn, & B. Schell (Eds.), *Willard & Spackman's occupational therapy* (10th ed., pp. 15–26). Philadelphia, PA: Lippincott Williams & Wilkins.

Law, M., Cooper, B., Strong, S., Stewart, D., Rigby, P., & Letts, L. (1996). The person-environment-occupation model: A transactive approach to occupational performance. *Canadian Journal of Occupational Therapy, 63,* 9–23.

Law, M., Steinwender, S., & Leclair, L. (1998). Occupation, health and well-being. *Canadian Journal of Occupational Therapy, 65,* 81–91.

Meyer, A. (1977). The philosophy of occupational therapy. *American Journal of Occupational Therapy, 31,* 639–642. (Original work published 1922)

Molineux, M. (2004). Occupation in occupational therapy: A labour in vain? In M. Molineux (Ed.), *Occupation for occupational therapists* (pp. 1–14). Oxford, UK: Blackwell.

Molke, D., Laliberte-Rudman, D., & Polatajko, H. J. (2004). The promise of occupational science: A developmental assessment of an emerging academic discipline. *Canadian Journal of Occupational Therapy, 71,* 269–281.

Nelson, D. L. (1988). Occupation: Form and performance. *American Journal of Occupational Therapy, 42,* 633–641.

Nelson, D. L. (1997). Why the profession of occupational therapy will flourish in the 21st century. The 1996 Eleanor Clarke Slagle Lecture. *American Journal of Occupational Therapy, 51,* 11–24.

Orr, J. E. (1996). *Talking about machines: An ethnography of a modern job.* Ithaca, NY: Cornell University Press.

Pierce, D. (2001). Untangling occupation and activity. *American Journal of Occupational Therapy, 55,* 138–146.

Primeau, L. A. (1996). Work and leisure: Transcending the dichotomy. *American Journal of Occupational Therapy, 50,* 569–577.

Reilly, M. (1962). Occupational therapy can be one of the great ideas of 20th century medicine. *American Journal of Occupational Therapy, 16,* 1–9.

Schkade, J. K., & Schultz, S. (2003). Occupational adaptation. In P. Kramer, J. Hinojosa, & C. B. Royeen (Eds.), *Perspectives in human occupation: Participation in life* (pp. 181–221). Philadelphia, PA: Lippincott Williams & Wilkins.

Schouten, J. W., & McAlexander, J. H. (1995). Subcultures of consumption: An ethnography of the new bikers. *Journal of Consumer Research, 22,* 43–61.

Schwartz, K. B. (2003). History of occupation. In P. Kramer, J. Hinojosa, & C. B. Royeen (Eds.), *Perspectives in human occupation: Participation in life* (pp. 18–31). Philadelphia, PA: Lippincott Williams & Wilkins.

Sherry, J. F., Jr., & McGrath, M. A. (1989). Unpacking the holiday presence: A comparative ethnography of two gift stores. In E. C. Hirschmann (Ed.), *Interpretative consumer research* (pp. 148–167). Provo, UT: Association for Consumer Research.

Townsend, E. (1997). Occupation: Potential for personal and social transformation. *Journal of Occupational Science: Australia, 4,* 18–26.

Weinblatt, N., Ziv, N., & Avrech-Bar, M. (2000). The old lady from the supermarket—Categorization of occupation according to performance areas: Is it relevant for the elderly? *Journal of Occupational Science, 7,* 73–79.

Wilcock, A. A. (2006). *An occupational perspective of health* (2nd ed.). Thorofare, NJ: SLACK.

Wood, W. (1998). Biological requirements for occupation in primates: An exploratory study and theoretical synthesis. *Journal of Occupational Science, 5,* 68–81.

Wood, W., Quinn, J. M., & Kashy, D. A. (2002). Habits in everyday life: Thought, emotion, and action. *Journal of Personality and Social Psychology, 83,* 1281–1297.

Yerxa, E. J. (1993). Occupational science: A new source of power for participants in occupational therapy. *Journal of Occupational Science: Australia, 1,* 3–9.

Yerxa, E. J., Clark, F., Frank, G., Jackson, J., Parham, D., Pierce, D., . . . Zemke, R. (1989). An introduction to occupational science, a foundation for occupational therapy in the 21st century. In J. A. Johnson & E. J. Yerxa (Eds.), *Occupational science: The foundation for new models of practice* (pp. 1–17). New York, NY: Haworth Press.

For additional resources on the subjects discussed in this chapter, visit http://thePoint.lww.com/Willard-Spackman12e.

CHAPTER 2

A Contextual History of Occupational Therapy

Charles H. Christiansen, Kristine Haertl

OUTLINE

LEARNING OBJECTIVES

After reading this chapter, you will be able to:

1. Appreciate that historical accounts are retrospective attempts to reconstruct and understand the events of the past with the purpose of gaining improved insight into the present
2. Identify key personalities and events that influenced the founding and development of occupational therapy
3. Recognize that wars, social movements, and legislation were associated with significant developments in occupational therapy
4. Discern how mind/body dualism and the competition between social and biomedical approaches to health care have been persistent points of tension since occupational therapy's founding

Introduction

Occupational therapy has a rich but complicated history. It has been influenced, as all professions have, by world events, personalities, and social movements. In this chapter, we have attempted to identify some of these factors as a way of explaining how occupational therapy came into being and evolved as a profession. Important examples that have influenced the evolution of occupational therapy include industrialization, women's rights, wars, economic downturns, health care legislation, and the digital age. Occupational therapy's history demonstrates that just as the development of knowledge does not always steadily progress with logical continuity (Kuhn, 1996), neither do events in history progress in logical, uninterrupted, or predictable ways. History is replete with examples of ideas that fail to take root when first introduced, only to become truly influential at a much later time, as though the several conditions necessary for their success needed to occur simultaneously in order for them to fully germinate.

What Is a Contextual History?

It sounds obvious, but it is often overlooked that historical events happen in larger contexts. The conditions that have influenced occupational therapy during its history often have very little to do with health care or therapy, yet they set the stage for ways of thinking that make people and societies more or less amenable to ideas, innovations, and actions. Aside from events influenced by nature, such as tornadoes, floods, droughts, or epidemics, no one can know with certainty why people acted the way they did in earlier years. By providing a description of the contexts for events, historians offer *possible* explanations for why events occurred when they did and why they unfolded the way they did. These questions are of vital importance if people are to derive lessons from the past. To present a history without context would be to oversimplify an important story that deserves to be told and appreciated.

The Periods Covered by This Chapter

The periods we have demarcated for this chapter include 1700–1899 (which we label a prehistory), 1900–1919, 1920–1939, 1940–1959, 1960–1979, 1980–1999, and 2000–present. No two eras can claim equivalent impact on the field because the people, ideas, contexts, and events influencing occupational therapy during each time period vary greatly in their impact and significance.

To begin, we have chosen to follow the late occupational therapy historian Robert K. Bing. He identified the Age of Enlightenment as a particularly fruitful time in the generation of ideas that influenced the field (Bing, 1981). We describe these ideas in the opening section referred to as occupational therapy's "prehistory."

Occupational Therapy Prehistory: 1700–1899

Historical Context

Considerable advancements were made in civilization between 1700 and 1899. During the first hundred years of this period (roughly 1700–1799), significant social movements sprang up in Western civilization that challenged authority and conventional thinking. This was the Age of Enlightenment (sometimes known as the Age of Reason), given this name because the idea that logical thinking was the most trustworthy way of knowing was gaining dominance (Paine, 1794).

During this era, leaders in several European countries embraced the idealism and egalitarian views that were prevalent and instituted reforms to strengthen their nations. Support of the arts and sciences was also a predominant theme. Little wonder, then, that some of the great artists, composers, and thinkers that ever lived flourished during this period.

Although the enlightenment cannot easily be summarized, common themes of the period included goals of progress, increased tolerance, and dedication to removal of the historical abuses of church and state, such as persecution and corruption. Because this was the beginning of the Industrial Revolution, methods of mass production led to the printing and wide distribution of books, helping to spread ideas broadly (Hackett, 1992).

Industrialization brought new opportunities, yet there is evidence that its influence on human migration overwhelmed social infrastructures and created conflict as workers rebelled against being subjected to exploitation and poor working conditions. Great social change also challenged the ability of people to adapt; many relocated from rural to urban areas, encountered new cultures, and became factory workers.

In the United States, the middle decades of the 19th century were marred by conflict, which can be linked to the egalitarian and humanitarian ideas brought forward from the enlightenment. A collision of moral values and economic traditions resulted in the great Civil War. Tensions between moral values and economics have recurred at several points in American history, and these tensions are important to occupational therapy because the philosophy of the field has such a strong moral core (Bing, 1981).

Nowhere is this moral influence more apparent than in treatment for persons with mental illness. During the late 18th century, dramatic changes in how people with mental illness were viewed resulted in more humane treatment, first in Europe and later in the United States (Whiteley, 2004). An emerging belief influencing this change was that the "insane" were creatures of reason and therefore must be treated with compassion (Gordon, 2009).

Although often associated with mental illness, **moral treatment** was also applied to physical illness because health and illness were viewed as related to patient character and spiritual development (Luchins, 2001). This emergence of humanitarian treatment influenced the development of therapeutic communities and the emphasis on engagement of groups in productive activities (Whiteley, 2004).

The ideas of moral treatment were also influential outside health care, especially in social services as exemplified by the settlement house movement. A notable and influential example was the Hull House, a settlement house in Chicago started by Jane Addams and Ellen Gates

Starr. Funded through philanthropy, the Hull House was formed to create opportunity, participation, and dignity for poor people living in urban areas of Chicago. Volunteers often lived in the communities and taught practical skills of living. Eventually, settlement houses led to community development efforts that continue to this day (Husock, 1992). Hull House and the Henry Street Settlement in New York were funded by wealthy donors to help people escape poverty and become productive, self-reliant members of society (Kreutziger, Ager, Lewis, & England, 2001). These concepts would later become the basis for a movement to use curative occupations in mental illness and ultimately influence the creation and development of occupational therapy.

People and Ideas Influencing Occupational Therapy

In his Eleanor Clarke Slagle Lecture, Bing (1981) recounted many of the historical figures and ideas of the 18th and 19th centuries that he believed influenced the founding of occupational therapy. The figures he identified from the 18th century were John Locke, Philippe Pinel, and William Tuke.

John Locke, a physician and philosopher who lived in the late 17th century and died in 1704, is credited with advancing many ideas that later influenced the philosophy and practices of occupational therapy, including sensory learning and pragmatism (Faiella, 2006).

Philippe Pinel, superintendent of the Bicetre and Salpetriere asylums in Paris, reportedly ordered the removal of chains from some of the inmates held in these places and is widely regarded as a pioneer of a more humanitarian treatment of the insane. His actions are repeatedly described as emblematic of the societal movement known as moral treatment (Weissmann, 2008).

William Tuke, an English businessman and philanthropist who founded the York retreat, is credited with being the father of the moral treatment movement. Tuke was appalled by the inhumane conditions he observed at the York lunatic asylum and sought a radical, more compassionate approach to mental health treatment. He eliminated restraints and physical punishment and encouraged conditions where patients could learn self-control and improve self-esteem through participation in leisure and work activities (Digby, 1985).

Adolf Meyer was a Swiss-educated physician who emigrated to the United States in 1892 seeking an academic appointment at the University of Chicago. Unable to get a faculty appointment, Meyer landed at the Eastern Illinois Asylum at Kankakee, a large mental institution typical of those during the era. As the head *alienist* (a term used for psychiatrists of the day), Meyer introduced an individualized approach to treatment and in so doing began a decades-long career of innovation and leadership in American psychiatry (Figure 2.1). While on a trip to the Chicago World's Fair in 1893, Meyer injured his leg and, during a brief convalescence in the city, visited Hull House and was impressed with the practical programs of activity and teaching that were used there. It is likely that this experience influenced Meyer's thinking about the connections between occupation and mental illness, concepts to appear in an important paper (the philosophy of occupation therapy) he would deliver three decades later an early meeting of the newly created American Occupational Therapy Association (AOTA; Lief, 1948; Meyer, 1922).

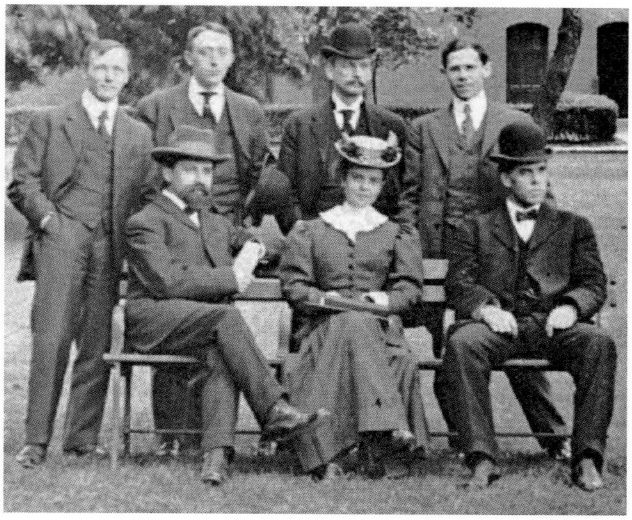

FIGURE 2.1 Dr. Adolf Meyer, a Swiss immigrant known as the father of American Psychiatry, is shown with his staff at the Eastern Illinois Asylum at Kankakee, Illinois around 1895. Dr. Meyer later became the head of psychiatry at Johns Hopkins University and was a strong advocate for occupational therapy after its founding. His philosophy paper on occupational therapy, delivered at the Fifth Annual Meeting of the American Occupational Therapy Association, continues to be widely cited even today. (Photo credit: Meyer Collection, Allen Chesney Memorial Library, Johns Hopkins University. Used with permission.)

Influences on the Evolution of Occupational Therapy

During occupational therapy's prehistory, the seeds had clearly been planted for the ideas that would lead to the founding of the profession (see Box 2.1). However, by 1899, its time had not yet come. In fact, the rise of large public asylums teeming with inmates, the shortage of well-trained physicians, and cost concerns led to a standard of care that fell far short of the individualized treatment and conditions idealized by the moral treatment movement. In fact, the ideas that were later to come together in the formal beginning of the Society for the Promotion of Occupational Therapy would have to be nurtured and applied by several different people in different settings before the profession of occupational therapy would take root in the United States.

BOX 2.1 Key Occupational Therapy Implications of the Periods

Occupational Therapy's Prehistory (1700–1899)

- The Age of Reason emphasized logical ways of knowing, ultimately leading to scientific health care and today's evidence-based practice.
- Early roots of social justice led to moral treatment and more humane care for persons with mental illness, ultimately leading to curative treatment involving work.
- Industrialization and technological advances led to global migration and the settlement house movement, a birthplace of many ideas influencing occupational therapy.
- Key persons during this period included John Locke, Philippe Pinel, William Tuke, and Adolf Meyer

1900–1919

Historical Context

The first two decades of the 20th century provided the context and circumstances needed to enable the founding of occupational therapy. This was a period of bold optimism in the ability of the United States to innovate and produce ideas and products that would make it a world leader. The century began with the assassination of President McKinley by an anarchist protesting corruption and social inequities tied to industrialization. McKinley was succeeded by Theodore Roosevelt, a bold reformer who championed consumer protection and antitrust legislation, supported worker rights, started the Panama Canal project, created a powerful navy, and established a national park system to preserve federal lands (DiNunzio, 1994).

The **progressive era** was rounded out by Presidents William Taft and Woodrow Wilson, each of whom was a highly educated and task-oriented leader. Taft continued Theodore Roosevelt's agenda, whereas Wilson focused on the regulation of commerce, the financing of World War I, and promoting international diplomacy (Cooper, 1990). Yet, significant social progress, including reforms in education and mental health, occurred during this period; thanks to the influence of John Dewey's pragmatism (Schutz, 2011) and Clifford Beers's accounts of inhumane treatment in large mental institutions. The 19th Amendment of the U.S. Constitution ratified in 1920 afforded women the right to vote, providing a springboard for the advancement of women throughout the culture, particularly in the workplace (Greenwald, 2005).

In 1917, after a period of neutrality and unsuccessful efforts to broker peace, the United States was drawn into the "The Great War," a horrendous world conflict centered in Europe that had begun in 1914 and ended on November 11, 1918. Overall, the war resulted in more than 15 million deaths, with 7 million soldiers sustaining wounds resulting in permanent disability (Votaw, 2005). As the American Expeditionary Forces prepared for battle, the War Department, at the request of General John J. Pershing, mobilized plans for the care of wounded soldiers whose disabilities would require rehabilitation and vocational reeducation (collectively called *reconstruction* at the time) to return them to civilian employment (Quiroga, 1995). Given the horrors of the battle, with its protracted trench warfare, inadequate tactics, and unthinkable casualties from artillery and poisonous gas (Votaw, 2005), the idea of sending untested **reconstruction aides** to Europe was both novel and somewhat incongruous, reflecting the sense of bold optimism permeating American culture. Yet, because the war ended in November 1918, casualties for the American Expeditionary Force were relatively modest in comparison to the losses of other countries, and swept up in the wave of pride following the allied victory, the reconstruction aide experiment was deemed a success. This propelled reconstruction aides (and later a field called *rehabilitation*) into a permanent place within American medicine.

People and Ideas Influencing Occupational Therapy (1900–1919)

The death of President William McKinley by preventable infection illustrated the variable quality of American medicine in 1900 (Fisher, 2001). The event was a precursor to reform efforts affecting general medicine as well as psychiatry. Reform in mental health was spurred by ***Clifford Beers***, a businessman who wrote *A Mind That Found Itself*, a critical and widely read account of his treatment in an asylum and eventual recovery (Beers, 1908). This led to the creation of the mental hygiene movement (Dain, 1980).

Shortly thereafter (in 1910), Abraham Flexner completed a report for the Carnegie Foundation that led to significant reforms in medical education. His critical indictment of substandard medical schools effectively closed scores of "storefront" schools and situated medical schools in large universities (Beck, 2004). Increased public awareness about the connection between science and its application in health care set medicine on a firm course connecting it to research and fostering a reductionistic approach that emphasized observable science to the exclusion of other factors such as social, psychological, and spiritual influences on health (Kielhofner & Burke, 1977). It also increased the public standing and political power of organized medicine, to an extent insulating it from legitimate criticism (Starr, 1983). But scientific medicine was not universally welcomed by the public, many of whom believed that illness needed to be understood in spiritual and psychological terms. These sentiments produced conditions where movements that involved patients in the healing process and also considered spiritual and psychological factors were likely to gain supporters and did.

One such movement was **Emmanuelism**, started by an Episcopal minister named Elwood Worcester in Boston as part of an effort to provide community-based treatment for indigent persons with tuberculosis (Quiroga, 1995). The Emmanuel movement was patient centered, holistic, community based, and comprehensive, involving social services and lay practitioners. In 1909, public awareness of the movement increased with a series of articles in the popular magazine, *Ladies Home Journal* (Quiroga, 1995). This increased visibility brought criticism from conservative physicians, who questioned its church-based delivery and its use of lay practitioners (Williams, 1909).

Simultaneously, during this period, Massachusetts-based physician ***Herbert J. Hall*** adopted a work-based approach to treating **neurasthenia**, a functional nervous disorder resulting in fatigue and listlessness thought to be caused by the stress of societal change and the cultural emphasis on productivity and efficiency (Beard, 1880). Hall agreed that the rest cure was the wrong treatment for neurasthenia (Figure 2.2). Instead, Hall's work cure at the Marblehead sanatorium in Massachusetts sought to actively engage patients in arts and crafts such as weaving, basketry, and pottery taught by skilled artisans, such as Jessie Luther, who had worked at Hull House in Chicago (Anthony, 2005). The new "work cure" approach became a suitable response to calls for improved mental health care. The use of occupations to treat neurasthenia had also been embraced at the Adams Nervine Asylum in Jamaica Plain, Massachusetts, where nurse ***Susan E. Tracy*** was hired to train nurses and to develop an active approach to treating patients (Quiroga, 1995).

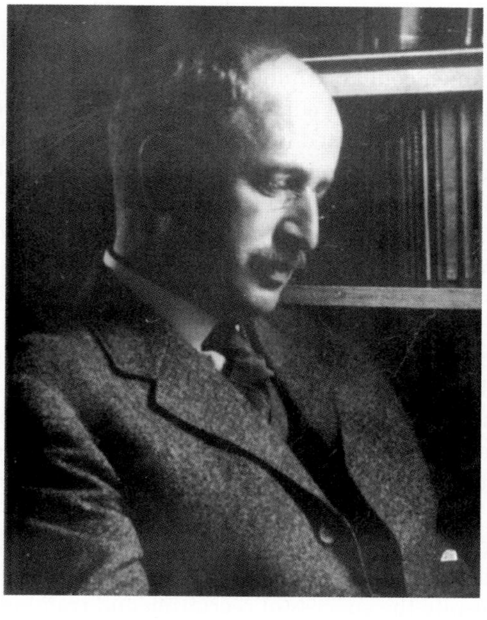

FIGURE 2.2 Dr Herbert J. Hall, Massachusetts psychiatrist and proponent of curative occupations, played a prominent role in the evolution of occupational therapy. (Photo credit: Archives of the American Occupational Therapy Association [AOTA], Wilma L. West Library, American Occupational Therapy Foundation [AOTF], Bethesda, MD. Used with permission.)

In 1910, based on her work at the asylum, Tracy wrote the first book on the "work cure approach" called *Studies in Invalid Occupations* (Tracy, 1910). Although primarily a craft book, Tracy's work applied the ideas of William James's pragmatism and led to her involvement in the first course on occupations for patients in a general hospital setting at the Massachusetts General Hospital (Quiroga, 1995).

Tracy's book influenced ***William Rush Dunton Jr.***, a psychiatrist practicing at the Sheppard and Enoch Pratt Asylum in Baltimore, to teach his own course on occupations and recreations for nurses working there. In 1912, Dunton was placed in charge of programs in occupation and later wrote his own book on occupational therapy (Bing, 1961). Dunton's enthusiasm was such that he later became a significant advocate and leader in developing the occupational therapy profession.

As the first decade of the 20th century ended, many state mental hospitals were using occupations as a regular part of their treatment. Under the auspices of the Hull House in Chicago and influenced by the mental hygiene movement, coursework in occupations and amusements for attendants at public hospitals and asylums began under the newly formed Chicago School of Civics and Philanthropy (Quiroga, 1995).

One of the social work students in a course called *curative occupations and recreations*, **Eleanor Clarke Slagle**, believed that the principles taught there could be applied usefully to idle patients in the state mental hospital at Kankakee (Quiroga, 1995). Slagle's interest in curative occupations gave her impetus to do more study and later develop the curative occupations therapy program with Adolf Meyer at the Phipps Clinic in Baltimore, where she collaborated with Dr. William Rush Dunton Jr. at the nearby Sheppard and Enoch Pratt Asylum (Bing, 1961).

Meanwhile, in 1912, Elwood Worcester of Boston, one of the founders of the Emmanuelism movement, was invited to the Clifton Springs Sanitarium in upstate New York to teach courses to the patients there. One of the patients was an architect, ***George Edward Barton***, who was recovering from tuberculosis and hysterical paralysis and suffered during work assignments in the Western United States. Barton was so influenced by his personal experiences with the work cure that he became a zealot for using occupations in the recovery of physical illness. On his discharge, he studied nursing at the sanitarium's school and opened "Consolation House," a convalescence center in which he hoped to apply the ideas of the emerging curative occupation philosophy (Figure 2.3) (Quiroga, 1995).

Barton began corresponding with prominent advocates for curative occupations, including Susan Tracy, Susan Cox

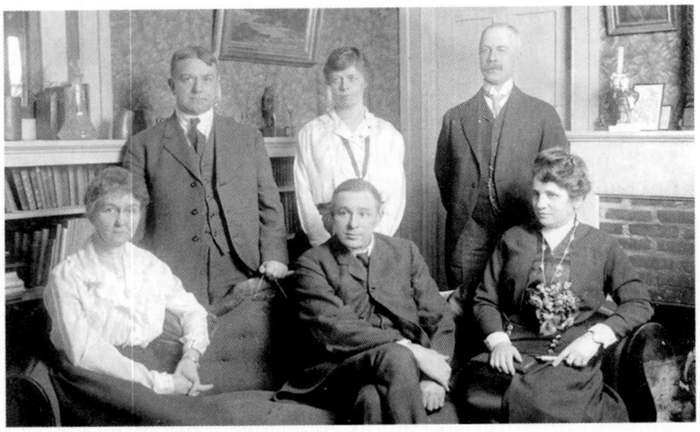

FIGURE 2.3 Society for the Promotion of Occupational Therapy Founders at Consolation House, Clifton Springs, New York, March 1917. Front row (left to right): Susan Cox Johnson, George Edward Barton, and Eleanor Clarke Slagle. Back row (left to right): William Rush Dunton Jr., Isabelle Newton, and Thomas Bessell Kidner. (Photo credit: Archives of American Occupational Therapy Association [AOTA], Wilma L. West Library, American Occupational Therapy Foundation [AOTF], Bethesda, MD. Used with permission.)

Johnson, and William Rush Dunton Jr. From 1914 to 1917, Barton wrote articles and developed plans for establishing a profession of caregivers dedicated to the use of occupations in therapy. Dr. Dunton assisted him, but Barton was initially hesitant to use the physician's help, fearing that his own lack of medical credentials might diminish his leadership role. Finally, in March 1917, the first organizing meeting of the Society for the Promotion of Occupational Therapy was hosted by George Barton at Consolation House in Clifton Springs, New York (Bing, 1961).

In attendance at that meeting were Barton, his secretary Isabel Newton, William Rush Dunton Jr., Eleanor Clarke Slagle, Thomas Kidner, and Susan Cox Johnson, who had organized many curative occupation programs in New York City. Susan Tracy of Massachusetts had been invited but was not able to attend. The meeting at Consolation House drew up a charter of incorporation, drafted a constitution for the new society, named committees, planned for an annual conference, and elected officers, with Barton becoming the inaugural president and Slagle as the vice-president (Bing, 1961).

In the following month, America entered World War I. Because of its massive scale and immense number of casualties, World War I raised government interest in reconstruction efforts (a term used to refer to physical rehabilitation and vocational reeducation) (Quiroga, 1995).

Efforts in North America were given a head start through work by the Canadians, who had been involved in the war since its inception. The vocational secretary for the Canadian Military Hospitals Commission, ***Mr. Thomas B. Kidner***, an architect who had trained in vocational rehabilitation in England, was loaned to the U.S. government to assist with vocational rehabilitation efforts (Friedland & Silva, 2008). Emerging medical specialties, such as orthopedics, also sought to improve their standing during the war, creating some political resistance to the inclusion of an untested group of occupation workers (Quiroga, 1995, p. 152).

Developments in Occupational Therapy (1900–1919)

In the period before World War I, several activities pursued independently by different individuals in different locations would come together in 1917 in Clifton Springs, New York at Consolation House, the convalescent center and home of George Edward Barton. Although Barton was instrumental in organizing occupational therapy as a profession through establishment of the Society for the Promotion of Occupational Therapy, he resigned his presidency of the organization within a year and for unknown reasons never resumed an active role in the continued evolution of the profession.

By the time the United States entered the war, several programs for training occupation workers had been established in the United States, some of which were organized for nurses and others that were freestanding or organized under the auspices of settlement houses. The need for occupation workers in asylums had received significant impetus from the mental hygiene movement, reform efforts in mental health, and for patients recovering from physical injuries and chronic illnesses such as tuberculosis.

Because of the casualties already experienced by other countries during the war, the United States anticipated the need for a significant number of facilities and rehabilitation workers. Although there were efforts to recruit men to these roles, the military soon realized that women could be trained to support the effort. Some existing programs for curative occupations added courses to meet the anticipated standards of the surgeon general, whereas others were established in large East Coast cities explicitly for the war effort (Figure 2.4) (Quiroga, 1995).

Success in quickly establishing these important war-training courses for reconstruction aides was made possible through the efforts of committed and prominent individuals who were able to organize the financial and political resources necessary to establish high-quality schools (Quiroga, 1995). Separate supervisors, reflecting a separation of roles, headed the reconstruction aide service in the military. Physical therapists did orthopedic work, corrective exercise, and massage, whereas occupational therapists provided handicrafts and assisted with orthopedic patients but also worked with those having psychiatric problems.

Despite the success in recruiting and training qualified reconstruction aides for the war effort, the initial placement of these trained aides proved to be difficult because some physicians viewed occupational therapy as a fad, failing to appreciate that it may have a worthwhile role in the reconstruction and rehabilitation efforts. However, after occupational therapy reconstruction aides

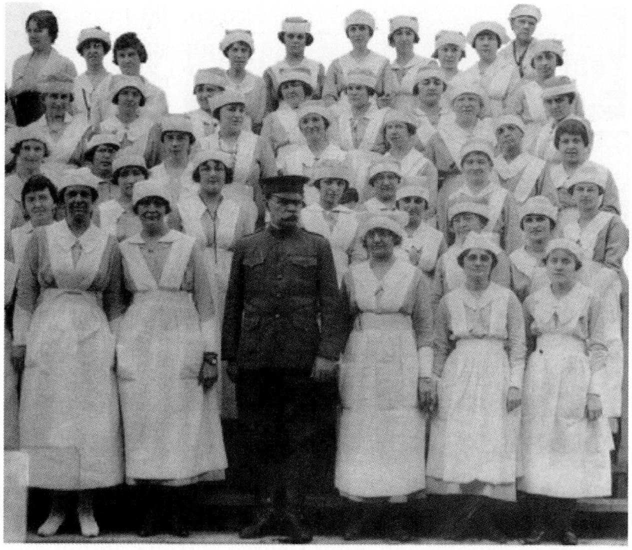

FIGURE 2.4 General W. C. Gorgas (surgeon general, U.S. Army) and reconstruction aides pictured in 1918. (Photo credit: Archives of American Occupational Therapy Association [AOTA], Wilma L. West Library, American Occupational Therapy Foundation [AOTF], Bethesda, MD. Used with permission.)

were assigned to a base hospital in Bordeaux, France, attitudes began to change when the benefits of their services became fully apparent (Figure 2.5) (Quiroga, 1995).

By November 1918, when Germany and its allies surrendered, at least 200 reconstruction aides were serving in 20 base hospitals in France (Quiroga, 1995). The war ended on November 11, 1919. Between 1917 and January 1, 1920, nearly 148,000 sick and wounded men were treated upon their return to the United States at 53 reconstruction hospitals (Office of the Surgeon General, 1918). The military specifications governing occupational therapy declared that it should have a purely medical function and be prescribed for the early stages of convalescence to occupy the soldier's minds. Even at this early date, there was a lack of clarity and considerable ambiguity in the roles and functions of the reconstruction aides providing occupational therapy. However, leadership in the newly formed professional association for occupational therapy, which was now known as the AOTA, provided wise advocacy for the recruitment of high-quality trainees. Dr. William Dunton Jr. succeeded Barton as president in 1917, and his friend, Eleanor Clarke Slagle, succeeded him in the role. Success in the deployment of the reconstruction aides in Europe provided momentum and legitimacy for the fledgling profession as it began the third decade of the 20th century (Quiroga, 1995). See Box 2.2 for a summary of important influences and social movements from this period that impacted occupational therapy's development.

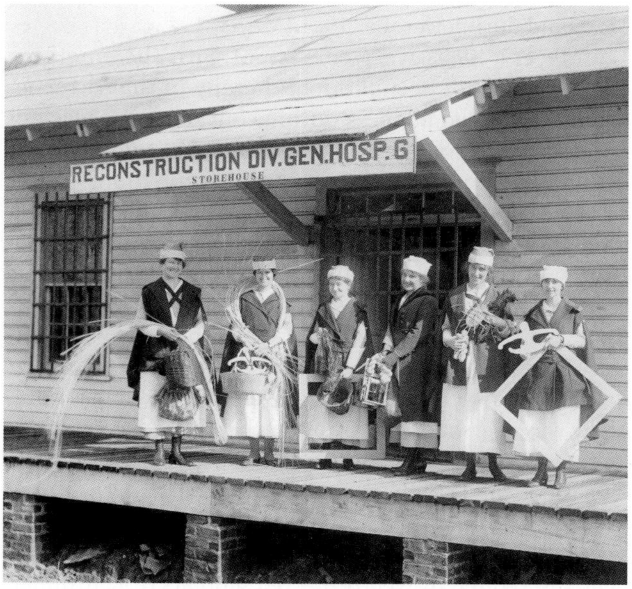

FIGURE 2.5 Reconstruction aides preparing projects at a field hospital in France during World War I. (Photo credit: Image Archive, History of Medicine Collection, National Library of Medicine.)

1920–1939

Historical Context

As the Treaty of Versailles following World War I was negotiated by the allies, President Woodrow Wilson proposed a League of Nations to prevent such wars from recurring. Wilson was successful in getting these terms into the treaty, but he suffered a severe stroke and the U.S. Congress never ratified them. Ultimately, the harsh conditions and reparations imposed on Germany in the treaty created resentment and hardship that may have indirectly led to a second world conflict less than 20 years later when in September 1939, Germany invaded Poland (Stokesbury, 1980).

Within the United States, the period from 1920 to 1939 witnessed the continuation of significant societal transformations as women asserted their right to vote. The 18th amendment, which prohibited the manufacture, transportation, and sale of alcohol, created a period from 1919 to 1933 during which organized crime flourished to capitalize on a black market in liquor. The first decade of this period is sometimes called the "roaring twenties" because the advancements of the era in manufacturing, transportation, and communication encouraged a sense of optimism and excess (Cooper, 1990). Profits in industry allowed increased earnings for workers, and the introduction of installment buying led to a very high level of consumerism that fueled a robust economy. Yet, new wealth encouraged widespread and irrational speculation in the stock market, which contributed to the crash of 1929 and a long period of hardship that followed, known as the *Great Depression*. In rural areas, the economic situation was made more difficult by a persistent drought that was worsened in some areas by poor conservation (Egan, 2006). With unemployment at

BOX 2.2 Occupational Therapy's Early Years and World War I (1900–1919)

- A period of progressive movements in the United States brought political and social reform to improve working conditions, advance women's rights, and improve medicine and psychiatry.
- The arts and crafts and curative occupation movements, which were reactions to industrialization and modernization, led to the formation of a formal occupational therapy professional society in 1917.
- The U.S. entry into World War I created the need for services to reconstruct wounded soldiers, giving occupational therapy an early opportunity to advance its cause.
- Key people during the era included Herbert Hall, George Barton, Eleanor Clarke Slagle, William Rush Dunton Jr., Susan Tracy, Adolf Meyer, and General J. J. Pershing.

25% and family incomes sliced in half, many people were desperate (McElvaine, 1993). President Herbert Hoover, an engineer, humanitarian, and respected administrator, was unable to contend with a crisis made worse by a financial disaster in Europe. In 1932, Franklin D. Roosevelt was elected to the first of four terms, and he quickly moved ahead with economic and social reform programs, collectively called the "New Deal" (Figure 2.6). These included Social Security, higher taxes on the wealthy, new controls over banks and public utilities, and enormous work relief programs for the unemployed, including the Civilian Conservation Corps for rural conservation and environment projects and the Works Progress Administration focusing on constructing or repairing bridges, libraries, and public buildings (Kennedy, 1999).

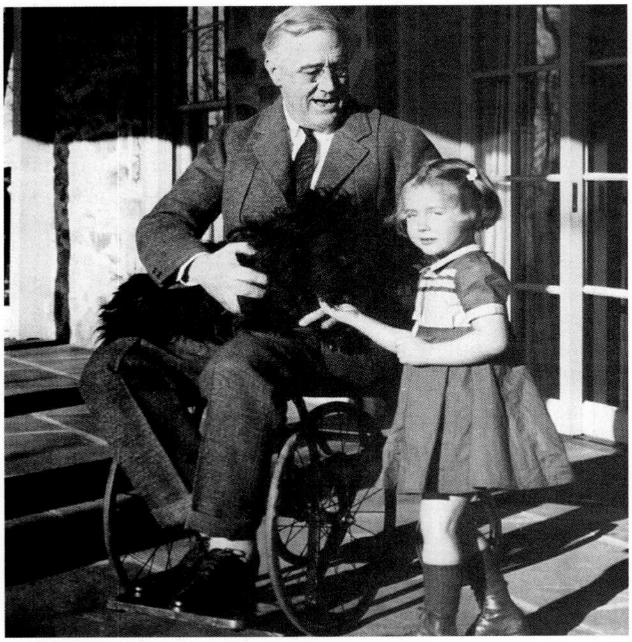

FIGURE 2.6 Franklin D. Roosevelt, president of the United States from 1933 to 1945, pictured with Ruthie Bie (a friend's granddaughter) and his dog Fala at the Roosevelt Cottage in Hyde Park, New York in 1941. Roosevelt's legs became paralyzed at age 39 after an acute illness. Elected for four terms, he is known for many accomplishments, including the Social Security Act of 1935. (Photo credit: Franklin Delano Roosevelt Library, Library ID 73113:61.)

People and Ideas Influencing Occupational Therapy (1920–1939)

The founders of the National Occupational Therapy Society had set events in motion for the rapid evolution of their new profession. After George Barton's abrupt resignation in 1917, his successor, Dr. William Rush Dunton Jr., helped to advance the new society, which was then focusing on standardizing educational programs. Dunton embraced Adolf Meyer's theory of psychobiology, which provided a common sense approach to treating mental illness (Lief, 1948). Psychobiology was holistic and practical, emphasizing that mental disease was reflective of habit disorganization in the lives of those affected. Meyer believed that humans organized time through doing things and that a balance of activities involving work and rest was essential for well-being (Figure 2.7). More importantly, Meyer and Dunton shared the belief that occupational therapists had an important role in helping patients reorganize their daily habits and regain a sense of optimism. Meyer expressed these ideas in a paper given at the Fifth Annual Meeting of the AOTA held in Baltimore, Maryland during October 1921 (Meyer, 1922).

Meyer's ideas were consistent with the emerging central tenets of occupational therapy in that it recognized that forced idleness during convalescence was not only morally wrong but also disorienting and physically debilitating. Through engagement in occupations, Meyer asserted that patients could ward off depression and gain a sense of self-confidence that would help motivate them further (Christiansen, 2007). There were also economic motivations to normalize lives by enabling individuals to develop skills that would help them become economically independent of assistance by the state.

Within psychiatry, Adolf Meyer's theory of psychobiology was overshadowed by other theoretical perspectives including the work of Sigmund Freud, whose psychoanalytic theory and emphasis on unconscious drives captured the interest of many psychiatrists as well as the general public (Burnham, 2006). Some of Freud's theory has now been discredited by well-respected scholars (e.g., Brunner, 2001) and remains a contentious topic; however, many view the distraction it created as a scientific setback (Eysenck, 1985). The progress made in general medicine in treating common diseases during that era encouraged

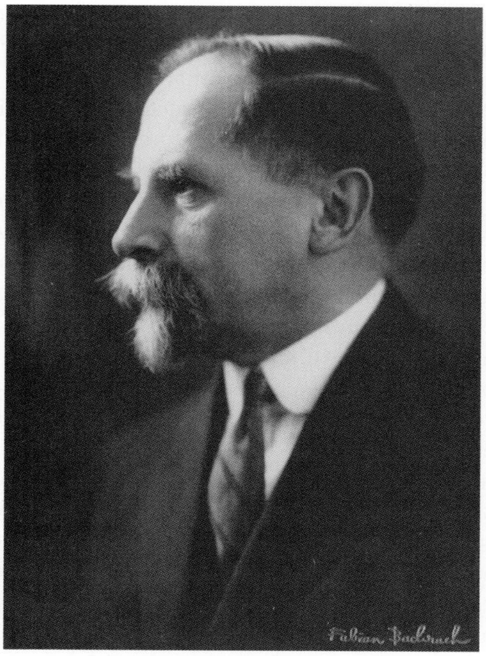

FIGURE 2.7 Dr. Adolf Meyer, a renowned psychiatrist and advocate for occupational therapy, shown at the Henry Phipps Clinic at Johns Hopkins University around 1915. (Photo credit: Meyer Collection, Alan Chesney Memorial Library, Johns Hopkins University.)

pursuit of biological explanations in the treatment of mental illness. One theory held that mental conditions were caused by focal infections in the body and led to unnecessary and sometimes harmful surgeries to some institutionalized mental patients because patient consent was not yet required for experimental procedures (Scull, 2005). Electroconvulsive treatments and lobotomies began to be used with both positive and negative consequences and these treatments remain controversial even today (Fink &Taylor 2007; Pressman, 1998).

The trend toward medicalization in occupational therapy that occurred in the 1920s and 1930s was influenced by strategic decisions of the profession's leaders. In its quest for professional legitimacy, occupational therapists perceived that there would be benefit in allying more closely with organized medicine. The rise of physical medicine and rehabilitation as a specialty of medicine and the leadership of ***Frank H. Krusen, MD*** had a clear influence on the practice of occupational therapists in rehabilitation. Krusen believed that occupational therapy was simply a special application of physical therapy (Krusen, 1934) and that the two disciplines should merge. This point of view had adherents in Canada, where training programs combined the theory and practices of both professions and produced graduates who could be dually credentialed (Friedland, 2011).

During the 1920s and 1930s, the principles of occupational therapy were also viewed as beneficial in the care of persons with tuberculosis, a disease stigmatized through its association with immigrants and poverty. Thomas B. Kidner, the Canadian architect turned vocational education expert who had been a member of the American Occupational Therapy founder's group at Clifton Springs, decided to remain in the United States after his temporary assignment to advise the surgeon general. Kidner, who served two separate terms as president of the AOTA, used his consulting practice to design hospitals and sanitoria, which included work spaces for occupational therapy and vocational training (Friedland & Silva, 2008). Kidner had a keen interest in the relationship between occupational therapy and vocational training, yet a firm conclusion about the appropriate relationship of these two important areas of social benefit remained undecided well beyond his death in 1932. The issue would reemerge in an area of applied theoretical emphasis 30 years later known as "occupational behavior" (Kielhofner & Burke, 1977; Reilly, 1962).

Occupational Therapy (1920–1939)

In occupational therapy, the early part of this era was dominated by the continued "reconstruction" of wounded soldiers from World War I, which occurred at more than 50 hospitals established with reconstruction in mind (Quiroga, 1995). These facilities provided employment for occupational therapists in the early 1920s as did the curative occupation programs in place at mental hospitals (Hall, 1922).

The AOTA became an effective organization for promoting the profession through its network of members, annual meetings, and the publication of a journal under three different names between 1917 and 1925, at which time the association had nearly 900 members (Dunton, 1925) (Figure 2.8).

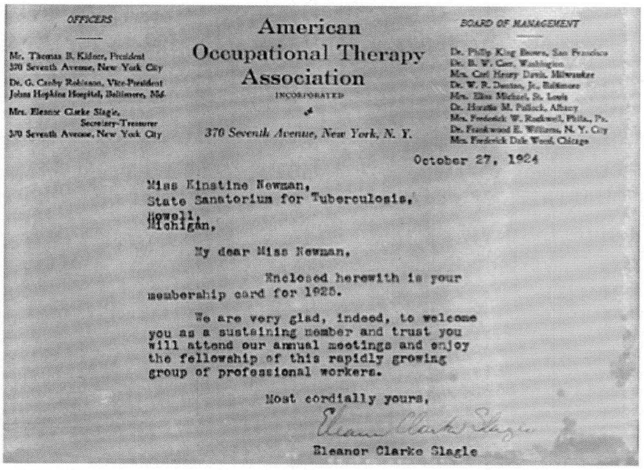

OFFICERS

Mr. Thomas B. Kidner, President
370 Seventh Avenue, New York City

Dr. G. Canby Robinson, Vice-President
Johns Hopkins Hospital, Baltimore, Md.

Mrs. Eleanor Clarke Slagle, Secretary-Treasurer
370 Seventh Avenue, New York City

American Occupational Therapy Association
INCORPORATED

370 Seventh Avenue, New York, N. Y.

BOARD OF MANAGEMENT

Dr. Philip King Brown, San Francisco
Dr. B. W. Carr, Washington
Mrs. Carl Henry Davis, Milwaukee
Dr. W. R. Dunton, Jr., Baltimore
Mrs. Elias Michael, St. Louis
Dr. Horatio M. Pollock, Albany
Mrs. Frederick W. Rockwell, Phila., Pa.
Dr. Frankwood E. Williams, N. Y. City
Mrs. Frederick Dale Wood, Chicago

October 27, 1924

Miss Kinstine Newman,
State Sanatorium for Tuberculosis,
Howell,
Michigan,

My dear Miss Newman,

Enclosed herewith is your membership card for 1925.

We are very glad, indeed, to welcome you as a sustaining member and trust you will attend our annual meetings and enjoy the fellowship of this rapidly growing group of professional workers.

Most cordially yours,

Eleanor Clarke Slagle

Eleanor Clarke Slagle

FIGURE 2.8 Letter from Eleanor Clarke Slagle, secretary-treasurer of American Occupational Therapy Association (AOTA), acknowledging dues receipt to a new sustaining member from Michigan (October 27, 1924). (Photo credit: Archives of the AOTA, Wilma L. West Library, American Occupational Therapy Foundation [AOTF], Bethesda, MD. Used with permission.)

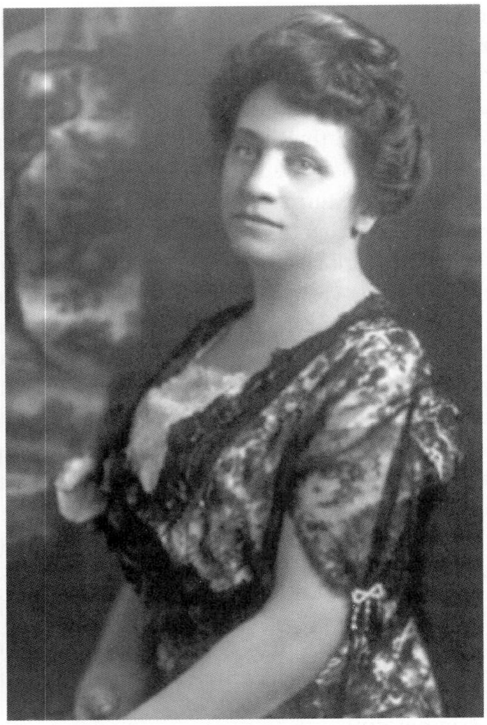

FIGURE 2.9 Eleanor Clarke Slagle. Her work as founder and tireless leader is recognized through a prestigious lectureship named in her honor. (Photo credit: Archives of the American Occupational Therapy Association [AOTA], Wilma West Library, American Occupational Therapy Foundation [AOTF], Bethesda, MD. Used with permission.)

In order to continue the development and growth of the new profession during the 1920s, Eleanor Clarke Slagle, who served as president and later secretary-treasurer of the new society for 15 years, found creative ways to continue promoting the field through networking through women's clubs and the establishment of a national office in New York (Metaxas, 2000; Quiroga, 1995) (**Figure 2.9**). Attendance in the association and in the society grew steadily during this time so that by 1929, there were 18 state and local occupational therapy associations and approximately 1,000 members of the AOTA (Slagle, 1934) (Figure 2.9). The association leadership continued to foster stability and quality in the profession by establishing standards for professionals and for educational programs. In many respects, the profession wished to gain legitimacy through aligning itself with other health professionals (Quiroga, 1995).

In 1935, after several years of negotiation, the accreditation of occupational therapy programs was initiated in concert with the American Medical Association (Quiroga, 1995). During this period, male physicians dominated association leadership in occupational therapy; still, many more positions for occupational therapists were being created in specialized facilities for physical rehabilitation, mental health, and tuberculosis.

The emergence of physical medicine and rehabilitation in the mid-1930s, which had been influenced by physicians who used physical agents and practiced physical therapy, was reflected in many of the publications during this era (Slagle, 1934). Because occupational therapists assumed roles in rehabilitation units, they adopted goniometry and began adapting tools and equipment to enable patients to gain strength, endurance, and range of motion while doing crafts.

During this period, polio epidemics and President Franklin Roosevelt's presumed polio-related paralysis brought visibility and public awareness to the disease, leading to treatment facilities and research as well as specialized centers that employed occupational therapists and others for the care of patients. Epidemics peaked in 1952 and diminished after development of a vaccine by Jonas Salk (Oshinsky, 2005).

Aided by the advocacy of Thomas B. Kidner, tuberculosis hospitals had also become settings where many occupational therapists assumed roles providing recuperative, diversional, and vocational therapy for long periods of convalescence (Friedland & Silva, 2008). The principle of activity graded to provide appropriate challenge and physical demand for patients was by this time a well-established part of the occupational therapy regimen in physical rehabilitation. See Box 2.3 for a summary of social challenges and the profession's responses during this period.

BOX 2.3 Postwar Growth and Advancement during Challenging Times (1920–1939)

- In the aftermath of the treaty ending World War I, advances in manufacturing and great optimism led to consumerism and speculation, leading to a stock market crash and the Great Depression.
- The American Occupational Therapy Association, led by wise leaders, focused on allying itself with physicians and hospitals and developing and standardizing its educational programs while distinguishing itself from vocational and medical rehabilitation.
- Occupational therapy practice expanded into specialized hospitals treating tuberculosis and polio.
- Key people during the era included Eleanor Clarke Slagle, William Rush Dunton Jr., Thomas Kidner, and Adolf Meyer.

1940–1959

Historical Context

With the onset of World War II, the economic and social toll of the war was felt around the world. Germany invaded nearby countries, and Hitler's reign led to the Nazi Holocaust and the concentration camps. Despite the Neutrality Acts of the 1930s designed to prevent the United States from entering another major war, the United States openly opposed Hitler; and when the Japanese attacked Pearl Harbor in 1941, the United States entered World War II. With the numbers of men drafted to armed service, the workforce surpluses of the late 1930s gave way to a shortage of "manpower," leading to an influx of women in the workforce. Shortages plagued all areas of industry leaving many hospitals understaffed and ill equipped to meet health care needs of those at home as well as soldiers returning from combat. Health challenges of returning veterans included not only diseases of the time such as tuberculosis, hepatitis, and rheumatic fever but also injuries from warfare, amputations, and new to this war, exposure to toxic chemicals (Richards, 2011).

According to the U.S. Department of Veterans Affairs (2011), World War II killed more people, destroyed more property, and was among the most devastating in history, with more than 16 million serving in the armed forces and more than 291,000 American deaths (Veterans Affairs); total estimates of global fatalities vary by source, but it is generally accepted that they exceed 60 million. The economic and social effects of World War II brought changes in health care and the passage of a number of U.S. legislative acts to fund research and services to returning veterans. The Public Health Service Act gave the National Institutes of Health (NIH) permission to grant awards for nonfederal research, the GI Bill of 1944 funded efforts to aid veterans to transition back to civilian life, and in 1946, Harry Truman signed the Mental Health Act designed to provide funding for mental health services and research (Harlow, 2007). Rehabilitation also expanded to assist veterans to return to work. The amendments in 1943 and 1954 of the Vocational Rehabilitation Act emphasized physical and mental restoration leading to a rise in the development of curative workshops (Gainer, 2008). Additional mental health challenges and posttraumatic stress required medical services to address the psychological effects of war, yet they were given less priority than care for physical injuries from war (Jarvis, 2009).

The post–World War II era marked the start of the Cold War, during which tensions between the United States and Russia were high. These were caused by the conflicting ideals of the democratic philosophies of the United States and the communist beliefs of Russia. Cold War tensions included the space race; global disagreements brought forth by the United States led efforts to encourage free trade, and the competition between the United States and Russia for power. Globally, as Japan started to rebuild post–World War II, the Korean War again brought armed forces from the United Nations (including the United States) to support the Republic of Korea (now South Korea).

Domestically, post–World War II brought tremendous economic growth, and although the United States had only 6% of the world's population, it was producing half of the world's goods (American Machinist, 2000). Yet, despite the economic affluence, more than 36 million Americans remained impoverished and the social concerns identified by social workers, statisticians, and economists were given new political emphasis (Huret, 2010).

As new economic growth and postwar social concerns marked the 1950s, major health care advances took place, including triumph over polio, the discovery of the DNA double helix, the development of the pacemaker, and the formation of the Joint Commission of Accreditation of Health Care Organizations (Gerber, 2007). Yet, despite these advances, there were still areas of health care in dire need of change. Mental health institutions were overcrowded and the rate of alcoholism and juvenile delinquency skyrocketed (Dworkin, 2010). As the stigmatizing effects of mental illness plagued the decade, patients and their families began organizing, and efforts were made to address concerns not only of the clients but also of their families (Brown, Shepherd, Wituk, & Meissen, 2008). This, paired with the discovery of the antipsychotic effects of chlorpromazine (Thorazine), ushered in a new era of psychiatric treatments for those with mental illness. Although, perhaps helpful, the reliance on pharmaceutical interventions and **deinstitutionalization** brought a new set of social and health care challenges.

Occupational Therapy (1940–1959)

World War II created increased demand for most health professions, including occupational therapists, in order to treat veterans returning from war. This was a time of immense growth and change in occupational therapy (Gordon, 2009) because the focus shifted from the use of arts and crafts toward rehabilitation techniques based on scientific methods. Occupational therapists imported techniques from other professionals such as physical therapy (Bissel & Mailloux, 1981). Additional emphasis was placed on reintegrating veterans into society, and therefore the use of activities of daily living, ergonomics, and vocational rehabilitation gained favor in therapeutic communities (Gainer, 2008). With battlefield medicine focused on saving severely wounded soldiers, the development of prosthetics and orthotics gained momentum during this period (Ott, Serlin, & Mihm, 2002). Occupational therapists became involved in prosthetic training, which often entailed the use of adapted tools and involved strengthening and conditioning (**Figure 2.10**).

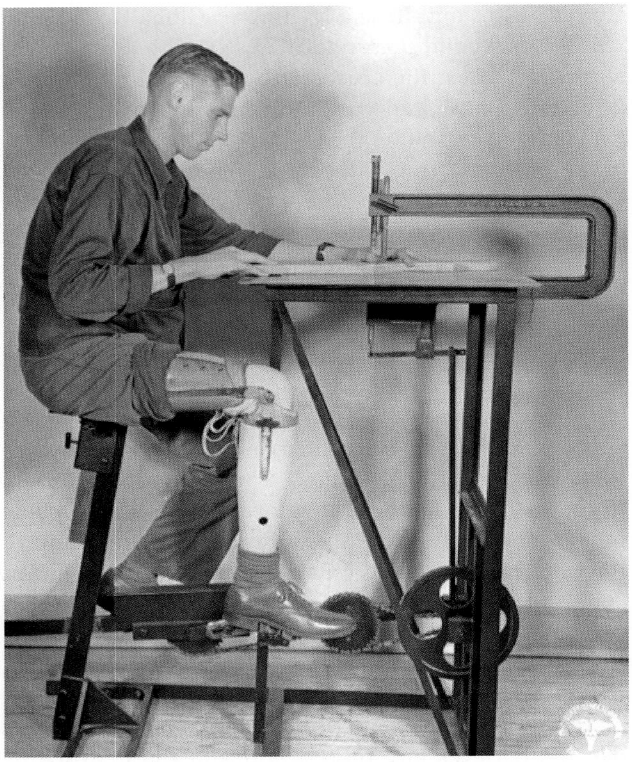

FIGURE 2.10 Bicycle jigsaw, common in physical rehabilitation occupational therapy clinics from the 1940s through the 1960s. (Photo credit: Archives of the American Occupational Therapy Association [AOTA], Wilma L. West Library, American Occupational Therapy Foundation [AOTF], Bethesda, MD. Used with permission.)

With the shift toward hospital-based therapy and the growth of rehabilitation, occupational therapy educational programs reorganized their curricula (Gordon, 2009) supported by the publication of the first occupational therapy textbook written in the United States, edited by Helen Willard and Clare Spackman (Spackman, 1968).

In 1956, the occupational therapy assistant was created to help meet workforce needs, and in 1958, the AOTA took responsibility for accrediting assistant level occupational therapy programs (AOTA, 2009). Although the term *certified occupational therapy assistant* did not take hold internationally, countries such as Canada, Australia, and the United Kingdom developed positions similar to the occupational therapy assistant in order to augment the workforce demands of the profession (Nancarrow & Mackey, 2005; Salvatori, 2001).

Globally, the number of occupational therapists continued to increase as educational programs expanded, and by 1950, there were seven occupational therapy educational courses in England and one in Scotland (Oxford Brookes University, 2011). In 1952, preliminary discussions took place for the eventual formation of the World Federation of Occupational Therapists (WFOT; 2011) recognized in 1959 by the World Health Organization, which was at that time just over a decade old. See Box 2.4 summarizing important challenges and the profession's responses.

People and Ideas Influencing Occupational Therapy (1940–1959)

Influences on the profession during this period came from occupational therapy leaders in the Army as well as from therapists working with individuals having motor paralysis. Here, we include the Bobaths (physiotherapists practicing in England), Ruth Robinson, and Margaret Rood.

Karl and Berta Bobath: The Bobaths were physiotherapists who developed the popular neurodevelopmental treatment (NDT), originally designed for persons with cerebral palsy but later applied to others with various neurological deficits and developmental conditions. Although the technique originally used manual techniques to control tone and movement patterns, once they noticed a lack of generalization, the Bobaths expanded their intervention to use normal play environments and natural contexts to encourage neurological development (Patel, 2005). Although studies question the effectiveness of NDT for various populations, the Bobath techniques are still used widely by occupational and physical therapists throughout the world.

Ruth A. Robinson, an army colonel, helped create occupational therapy educational programs for those preparing to serve in the military. Robinson proposed an accelerated training program to meet the needs for expansion during the Korean War (U.S. Army Medical Department, 2012). She continued in leadership positions, serving as the president of AOTA from 1955 to 1958 (Peters, 2011b) (Figure 2.11).

Margaret Rood was an occupational and physical therapist credited as one of the earliest theorists on

BOX 2.4 World War II and Continued Development (1940–1959)

- World War II, fought in European and Pacific theatres, causes the mobilization of men and material as the United States enters the war in 1941 following the attack on Pearl Harbor.
- Occupational therapy, still influenced greatly by its ties to medical rehabilitation, once again plays a key role in the care of wounded soldiers.
- Developments in prosthetics, assistive technology, neurodevelopmental care, and compensatory techniques for therapy accelerate as part of the war effort.
- Key personalities of the period include Ruth Robinson, Margaret Rood, and Karl and Berta Bobath.

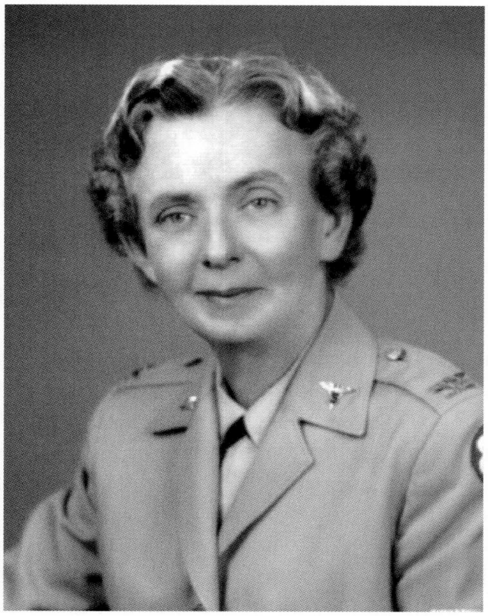

FIGURE 2.11 Colonel Ruth A. Robinson. Robinson established accelerated programs in the U.S. Army to train therapists for the Korean War and served several leadership roles in the American Occupational Therapy Association (AOTA), including that of president from 1955 to 1958. (Photo credit: Archives of the AOTA, Wilma L. West Library, American Occupational Therapy Foundation [AOTF], Bethesda, MD. Used with permission.)

motor control. Rood stressed the importance of reflexes in early development and emphasized the use of facilitation and inhibition techniques, which were soon after used and expanded on by the Bobaths. In addition to clinical work, Margaret Rood took on leadership and educational positions including the development of the Occupational Therapy Department of the University of Southern California (USC), where she served as the first chair (USC, n.d.).

1960–1979

Historical Context

During this period, Martin Luther King's famous "dream speech" (King, 1963) symbolized decades of the civil rights movement seeking equality and justice for black Americans. This was also an era of unrest and change marked by the construction of the Berlin wall, the advancement in space science, the Cuban Missile Crisis, and the Vietnam War. In 1964, President Johnson signed the ***Civil Rights Act*** into law, protecting individual rights and freedom from discrimination in areas such as voting, education, and employment (Pedriana & Stryker, 2004). Concerns were raised regarding poverty, access to health care, and quality education for all, leading President Johnson to institute a number of other domestic programs commonly known as the "Great Society," aimed at reducing poverty and providing increased funding in areas such as education and health care (Warner, 2012). Perhaps foremost among these was legislation in 1965, establishing Medicare and Medicaid (Figure 2.12), which provided health care access to millions of seniors and disabled and impoverished American citizens, many of whom previously did not have access to such care (Bakken, 2009).

By the 1960s, American health care had been modernized greatly with updated equipment, electric beds, advanced communication systems, and innovative laboratories; it was a system readily compared with industrial corporations (Stevens, 1996). The demographics of hospitalization shifted because new medicines were discovered and medical advances escalated. With the mass production of antibiotics and other pharmaceutical treatments for physical and mental health conditions, there was a move away from the treatment of acute epidemic illness (e.g., polio and smallpox) toward increased need for care of chronic conditions such as rheumatism, arthritis, and heart conditions (U.S. Department of Health, Education, and Welfare, 1965). During this period, private health insurance provided by employers as a benefit to attract workers was well established; typically, these insurance plans had low deductibles and negligible requirements for co-payments by the insured (Thomasson, 2002). This, alongside the legislation providing government payments under Medicare and Medicaid, contributed to an overuse of services and further stimulated the growth and cost of health care. Yet, there were confusing laws regarding coverage for services, difficulty with health care access for all, and demographic shifts with more people older than the age of 65, causing a shortage of housing options and lack of acceptable nursing home beds (Stevens, 1996).

A move to close state institutions for the infirmed, particularly those with mental illness, caused additional challenges. The emergence of psychotropic medications paired with the overcrowding and deplorable

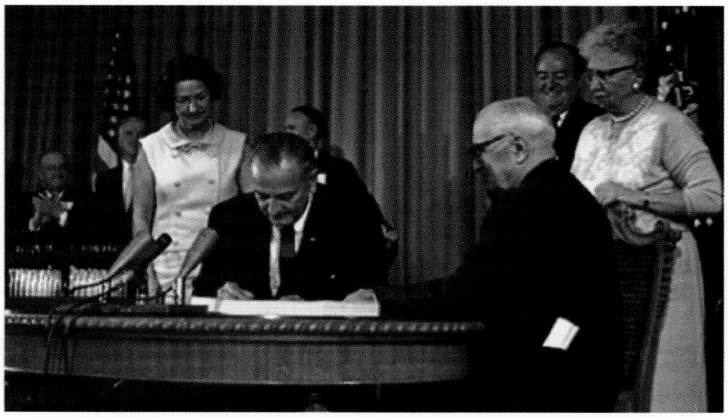

FIGURE 2.12. Lyndon B. Johnson signing the 1965 Medicare and Medicaid Legislation with former President Harry S. Truman, Mrs. Truman, Mrs. Lady Bird Johnson, and members of Congress. (Photo credit: National Archives, photograph collection.)

conditions of many state hospital systems led to the deinstitutionalization movement and subsequent closure of state and psychiatric hospitals both in Canada and the United States (Koyangi, 2007; Sealy & Whitehead, 2004). Although the aim was to contain costs and provide improved care in the community, the development of community mental health services was inadequate to address the demands (Koyangi, 2007). Many of those affected by deinstitutionalization wound up homeless or in the criminal justice systems (McGrew, Wright, Pescosolido, & McDonel, 1999). Efforts to shift the care for those with mental illness to the community have continued to present day. Along with changes in service delivery, health care workers and rehabilitation providers such as occupational therapists saw shifts in areas of practice and increased emphasis toward science-driven therapy. Practices were heavily influenced by the medical model because professions fought to gain recognition and access to payment from third-party systems such as Medicare and Medicaid.

Occupational Therapy (1960–1979)

The decades from 1960 to 1979 brought significant change to occupational therapy practice (see Box 2.5). During the reorganization of the AOTA in 1964 under the presidency of Wilma West, renewed emphasis was placed on supporting scientific endeavors in occupational therapy (Yerxa, 1967b). The board supported the idea of reorganization and expansion; and in 1965, the American Occupational Therapy Foundation (AOTF) was established to advance the science of the field and improve its public recognition (AOTA, 1969). Efforts to emphasize science and theory development led to increased graduate education in the field and later led to a proliferation of models, theories, and frames of references for practice. Continued emphasis on the legitimacy of the profession increased efforts to regulate practice through state licensure legislation as the government, concerned about costs for outpatient therapy services, initiated the first caps on payments for services in 1972.

The practice of occupational therapy during this period was heavily influenced by medical rehabilitation, which continued the post–World War II mechanistic paradigm emphasizing neuromotor and musculoskeletal systems and their impact on function (Kielhofner, 2009). Advances in neuroscience motivated A. Jean Ayres to expand on the work of the Bobaths and Rood . Ayres used neuroscience to study perceptual motor issues in children and develop and apply a theory of sensory integration (Ayres, 1966, 1972). Influences on practice shifted from the holistic mind–body occupation-based philosophies to those with bottom-up approaches focusing on the underlying source of the problem, often with emphasis on reflex integration and motor function (Figure 2.13).

Various Great Society programs and the ***Education for All Handicapped Children Act* (*P.L. 94-142, 1975*)** expanded the scope and areas of practice for occupational therapists. Medicare and Medicaid laid the foundation for expanded services to the elderly, those with disabilities, and the poor; and P.L. 94-142 mandated access to education for all children, including those with disabilities. These laws, governing provision for health care and educational services to expanded populations, led to expansion of work areas for occupational therapists as the need for therapists in educational systems continued to grow (Coutinho & Hunter, 1988).

Internationally, occupational therapy was guided by the conceptualizations of theorists but, similar to the United States, was also driven by the medical profession and the social and health care institutions because these were the main employers of occupational therapists (Clouston & Whitcombe, 2008). ADL tools and adaptations were developed to accommodate for dysfunctions (Hocking, 2008), and the profession continued to emphasize scientific endeavors. There was also an increase in educational programs throughout the world, fostered in part by international efforts of representatives to the WFOT (Cockburn, 2001).

People and Ideas Influencing Occupational Therapy (1960–1979)

Mary Reilly became a distinguished clinician in the U.S. Army Medical Corps during the war (see Figure 2.14) (Brown, 1996) and went on to earn her doctorate in education, serving as the chief of the Rehabilitation Department at the Neuropsychiatric Institute at

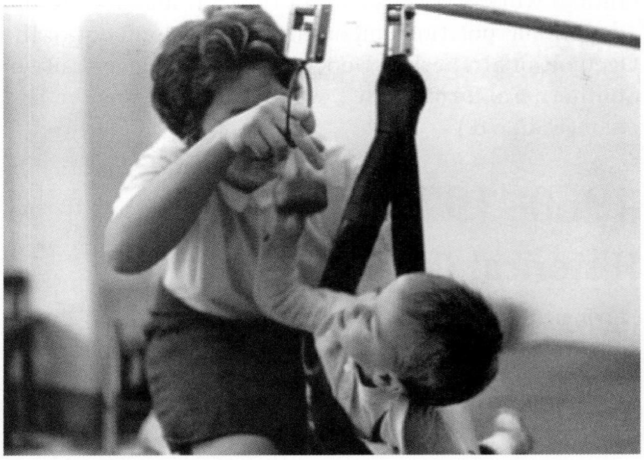

FIGURE 2.13 Therapy for developmental disabilities grew rapidly in the 1980s because therapists applied theories of reflex integration from the neurosciences. In this undated photo from the period, an unidentified therapist works with a young child. (Photo credit: Archives of the American Occupational Therapy Association [AOTA], Wilma L. West Library, American Occupational Therapy Foundation [AOTF], Bethesda, MD. Used with permission.)

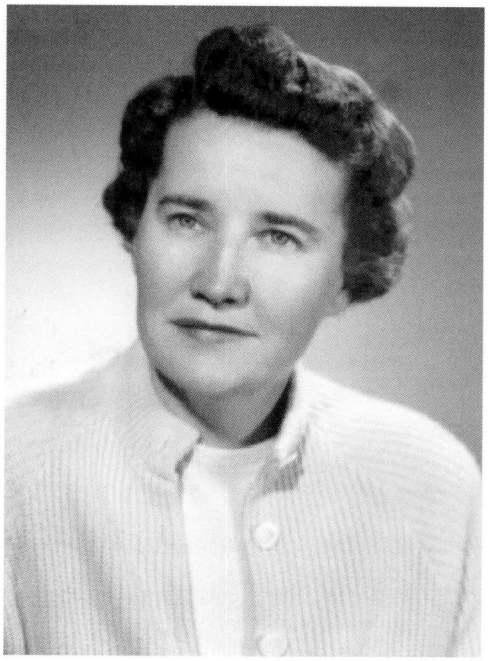

FIGURE 2.14 Dr. Mary Reilly created a frame of reference known as occupational behavior. She was the Eleanor Clarke Slagle lecturer in 1961 and a charter member of the Academy of Research of the American Occupational Therapy Foundation (AOTF). (Photo credit: Archives of American Occupational Therapy Association [AOTA], Wilma L. West Library, AOTF, Bethesda, MD. Used with permission.)

University of California, Los Angeles. She later served as a professor at the USC, where she developed her philosophy that occupational behavior should serve as the foundation for occupational therapy (Kielhofner, 2009). Reilly became a prominent clinician and academician, gaining international attention with her development of the occupational behavior frame of reference, which took a holistic view of humans and their daily occupations. In her 1961 Eleanor Clark Slagle Lecture, Reilly challenged the profession to reclaim its roots in occupation and famously proclaimed, "Man, through the use of his hands as they are energized by mind and will, can influence the state of his own health" (Reilly, 1962, p. 2). Reilly's advocacy for an occupational behavior frame of reference emphasized that promoting the field's contribution to human productivity through occupation was of paramount importance. She emphasized that important occupational skills began in children as forms of play (Reilly, 1974).

A. Jean Ayres, an occupational therapist and licensed educational psychologist, applied neuroscience to practice (Figure 2.15). Dr. Ayres was educated at the USC, where she served as a student, scientist, practitioner, and educator. Within her research, Ayres developed tools for practice, including assessments of integrated sensory processing, later forming a battery known as the Sensory Integration and Praxis Tests (Bowman, 1989). In 1976, Ayres founded the Ayres Clinic, in which she combined teaching, research, and practice to develop her practice model of sensory integration (Kielhofner, 2009). Her theories and influence continue to present day.

Another influential therapist, ***Gail Fidler*** (Figure 2.16), emphasized the use of occupation as a means for emotional expression. Fidler, a teacher and occupational therapist with a background in psychology, was influenced by her studies of interpersonal theory, self-esteem, and ego development (Miller & Walker, 1993). Gail Fidler became a leader in mental health occupational therapy, studied with her mentor Helen Willard, and worked in a settlement house while a student at the Philadelphia School of Occupational Therapy (Peters, 2011a). She and her husband wrote *Introduction to Psychiatric Occupational Therapy* (Fidler & Fidler, 1954), a groundbreaking book that promoted the application of ego theory and therapeutic use of self in practice.

Ann Mosey advanced Fidler's ideas by developing the object relations/psychodynamic frame of reference that offered concepts integral to understanding the use of activities and groups in therapy (Mosey, 1973) (Figure 2.17). Other prominent theorists emerged at the time, increasing the theory base of occupational therapy. ***Lorna Jean King*** (1974) applied sensory integrative

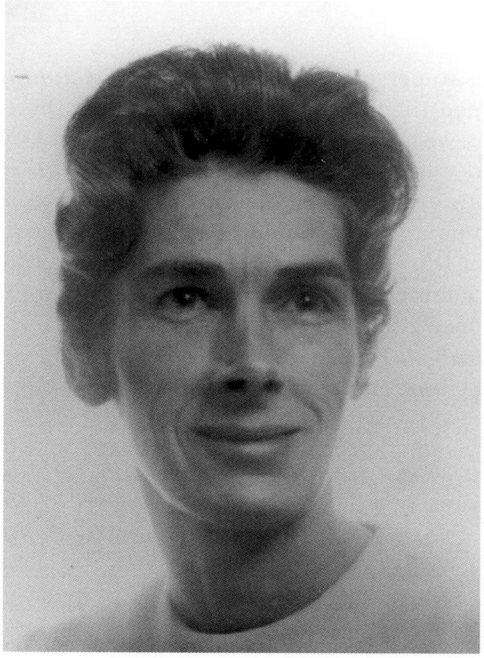

FIGURE 2.15 A. Jean Ayres, PhD, was one of the first occupational therapists to use basic science to develop applied theory in occupational therapy. Her area of interest was sensory processing in children with developmental disorders. (Photo credit: Archives of American Occupational Therapy Association [AOTA], Wilma L. West Library, American Occupational Therapy Foundation [AOTF], Bethesda, MD. Used with permission.)

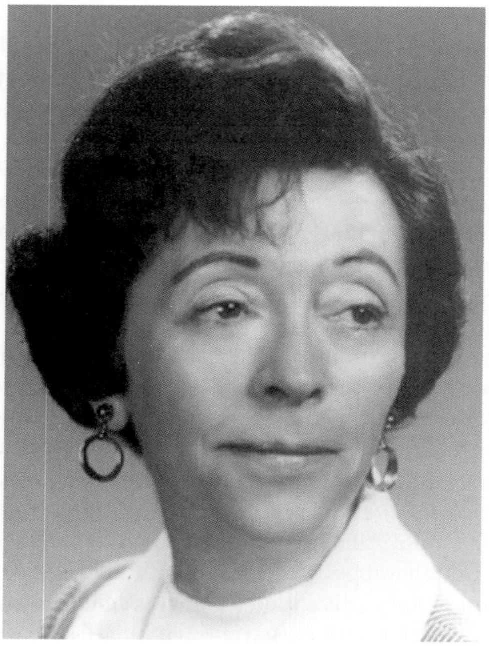

FIGURE 2.16 Gail Fidler was a leading spokesperson for the application of psychodynamic theory in occupational therapy, publishing (with her husband, a psychiatrist) one of the first textbooks in the field dedicated to practice in mental health. (Photo credit: Archives of the American Occupational Therapy Association [AOTA], Wilma L. West Library, American Occupational Therapy Foundation [AOTF], Bethesda, MD. Used with permission.)

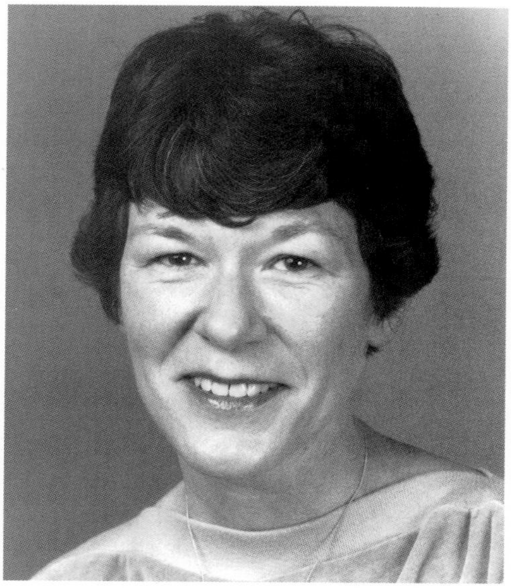

FIGURE 2.17 Ann Mosey, PhD, a widely respected scholar and professor of occupational therapy at New York University, published frequently on topics related to the evolution of theory in the field of occupational therapy as well as on topics in mental health. (Photo credit: Archives of the American Occupational Therapy Association [AOTA], Wilma L. West Library, American Occupational Therapy Foundation [AOTF], Bethesda, MD. Used with permission.)

theories to persons with schizophrenia, ***Claudia Allen*** developed theories of cognition to guide therapy for persons with chronic mental illness (Allen Cognitive Network, 2011), and Kielhofner and Burke (1977) advocated an occupational therapy paradigm to refocus on human adaptation and occupation. The core concepts of this work later became the foundation of a widely adopted Model of Human Occupation (MOHO) (Kielhofner & Burke, 1980).

Elizabeth Yerxa, a successor to Mary Reilly, emphasized the importance of advancing theory to the benefit of practice (Figure 2.18). In her 1966 Eleanor Clark Slagle Lecture, she asserted the need for occupational therapists to take steps toward professionalism, produce research, and focus on the unique assets of the profession, including purposeful activity and the practice of authentic occupational therapy (Yerxa, 1967a). Yerxa later became involved in active promotion of research efforts and in promoting the development of occupational science as an academic discipline and foundation for practice. Yerxa retired in 1988 and was recognized as a distinguished professor emerita at the USC. See Box 2.5 for a summary of the key events and professional developments of this period.

BOX 2.5 Medicare, Vietnam, and Further Evolution of the Profession (1960–1979)

- The civil rights movement and the ***Great Society*** lead to historic legislation that infuences health care and social justice.
- In occupational therapy, educational programs continue to mature and school-based practice gains great momentum with passage of the Education for Handicapped Children Act; large mental institutions begin to close, affecting the number of therapists employed in longer term mental health settings; and the American Occupational Therapy foundation is founded to foster scientific development.
- Increased emphasis is placed on sensorimotor therapies, particularly driven by neurodevelopmental theorists, and occupational behavior emerges as a counterbalance to the medicalization of therapy.
- Key personalities of the period are A. Jean Ayres, Mary Reilly, and Gail Fidler; and Wilma West.

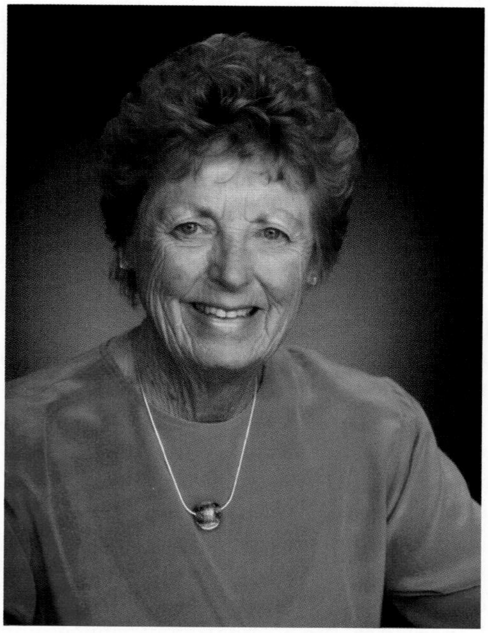

FIGURE 2.18 Dr. Elizabeth J. Yerxa led the initial development of the academic discipline of occupational science. Dr. Yerxa received many awards for her work, including the American Occupational Therapy Association (AOTA) Award of Merit for her leadership of the profession. (Photo credit: Archives of AOTA, Wilma L. West Library, American Occupational Therapy Foundation [AOTF], Bethesda, MD. Used with permission.)

1980–1999

Historical Context

The onset of the 1980s brought international change with the end of the Cold War, the collapse of the Soviet Union, and the removal of the Berlin wall. Internationally, the Treaty of Maastricht was signed in formation of the European Union, later paving the way for the development of the European Free Trade Association. Within the United States, Ronald Reagan took office and the era of the space shuttle began along with the initiation of "star wars," a highly technological strategic defense system. With the advancement of the scientific age, perhaps one of the most pronounced shifts was the onset of a new technological era.

In 1981, IBM released the first personal computer (PC) launching the modern age of digital technology. It was an era of proliferation of computer languages and technology (Bergin, 2007). Because computer use extended to the World Wide Web, the Internet provided opportunities for cross-cultural communication and knowledge sharing like never before as digital networks connected people from all over the world instantaneously (Palfrey, 2010). By the 1990s, the computers were integral to all areas of society, including business, education, and health care.

Along with scientific and technological advances, the health care industry grew and expanded. Trends in health concerns shifted during the era as the World Health Organization declared small pox eradicated and the first case of HIV was identified (Hospitals and Health Networks, 2012). Advanced digital imaging technology (such as computed tomography [CT] and magnetic resonance imaging [MRI]) brought increased diagnostic capabilities and costs. Between 1980 and 2000, annual age-adjusted costs per person for health care in the United States nearly tripled (Centers for Medicare and Medicaid Services, 2012). Hospital stays grew shorter, telemedicine emerged, and increased emphasis was placed on patient choice and participation in health care decisions. Not only did telemedicine provide health professionals the opportunity to extend medical care, maintain records, and efficiently transfer information from one provider to another but patients also began increasingly using the Internet to gather their own information on health care and medical conditions (Hernandez, 2005).

Outside of physical medicine, advances in psychiatric rehabilitation were influenced by a paradigm shift away from an expert model toward inclusion of the consumer in treatment decisions. Within mental health, the recovery model emerged (Anthony, 1993), highlighting the importance of skill training, consumer empowerment, and the development of cooperative alliances in psychiatric rehabilitation. Within this model, concepts of self-determination are emphasized along with empowerment, consumer rights, and community involvement (Tilsen & Nylund, 2008). Goals of mental health recovery included reduced symptoms, enhanced quality of life, and emphasis on personal meaning, purpose, and values (Gagne, White, & Anthony, 2007).

The changing nature of the health care system, along with the renaming and reformulation of the Education for All Handicapped Children Act to the **Individuals with Disabilities Education Act** (IDEA) and President H. W. Bush's signing the **Americans with Disabilities Act** (ADA) in 1990, influenced access for persons with disabilities to educational systems and employment. The shifts in health care and education further influenced areas of practice as increasing numbers of occupational therapists served in the school systems (AOTA, 2006).

Occupational Therapy (1980–1999)

During this period, significant public attention was given to health care, especially following the election of William Jefferson Clinton as president. Clinton's health care reform agenda created much discussion but did not result in significant action, primarily due to heavy lobbying by the private health insurance industry, the complexity of the administration's plan, and lack of consensus among members of the majority party in Congress (Birn, Brown, Fee, & Lear, 2003). In occupational therapy, state professional associations continued their lobbying for legislative acts and licensure to regulate the practice of occupational therapy and increase the public safety, visibility, and legitimacy of the profession. During this period, emphasis was placed on research, efficacy, and defining the scope of practice for occupational therapists. For example, one significant controversy related to the appropriate use of physical agent modalities by occupational therapists, with some leaders arguing that use of these procedures blurred the distinction between physical and occupational therapy (West, 1991).

Also during this time, the AOTF (under the leadership of President Wilma West) hired a full time executive director and began a series of programs to advance research and education. The most significant initiatives included the starting of a professional journal *Occupational Therapy Journal of Research* in 1980 (AOTF, 2012b) and the creation of the Academy of Research in 1983, an honorary body to recognize outstanding scientists in occupational therapy (AOTF, 2012a).

Within the professional association (AOTA), discussions took place regarding the governance of certification activities. In 1986, the AOTA board of directors determined that certification activities and membership functions were not sufficiently independent to avoid potential liability under antitrust legislation. Accordingly, the board voted to create the American Occupational Therapy Certification Board, which later became known as the National Board for Certification in Occupational Therapy (Low, 1997). This action eventually led to a decline in the membership of the AOTA because membership was no longer required for certification purposes.

In addition to activities of the professional association, legislation of the period affecting practicing therapists in the United States included the IDEA (1997), the ADA (1990), and the Balanced Budget Act P.L. 95-33, enacted August 5, 1997).

In 1997, the Individuals with Disabilities Education Act Amendments were signed into law providing strength and accountability for the education of children and adolescents with disabilities. Occupational therapy was one of the specialized services provided for under this Act. The provisions for rehabilitation services in the law gave rise to an increase in therapists practicing in the school system such that by the mid-2000s, education and early intervention was the area with the highest number of practicing therapists (AOTA, 2006).

The ADA of 1990 became the most comprehensive piece of legislation in U.S. history to provide protection against discrimination for persons with disabilities (Karger & Rose, 2010). The law defined disability and addressed issues of employment accommodation and ensured that persons with disabilities could access public services, transportation, and telecommunications (Hein & VanZante, 1993). Many occupational therapists were well qualified to advocate for clients and consult with organizations seeking to comply with ADA mandates (AOTA, 2000). Yet, despite legislation providing opportunities during this era (such as IDEA and ADA), occupational therapy employment growth slowed because of legislation to contain health care costs. The ***Balanced Budget Act of 1997*** was enacted largely to control Medicare's subacute care costs (Qaseem, Weech-Maldonado, & Mkanta, 2007). However, it reduced positions and led to a decrease in applicants to occupational therapy programs, a few of which were eventually closed as a result of low enrollment.

During this era, occupational science was proposed as an academic discipline to provide an underlying foundation for occupational therapy (Yerxa, 1990). Although occupation had long been the core of the profession, it had never formed the basis of a discipline worthy of study in its own right. This changed in 1989, when Elizabeth Yerxa and colleagues developed the first occupational science PhD program at the USC (Gordon, 2009). Occupational science was developed to closely study occupation as a human behavioral science and to gain perspectives that would lead to new insights to inform practice (Clark, Wood, & Larson, 1998; Gordon, 2009). Shortly thereafter, the occupational science movement expanded steadily and globally. In Australia, Ann Wilcock and colleagues launched the *Journal of Occupational Science* in 1993 to be followed over the next decade by the creation of societies in several countries dedicated to the study of occupation. These groups were organized to bring together scientists from multiple disciplines (e.g., social geography, anthropology, social psychology, occupational science, and occupational therapy), but widespread participation by outside professions has been slow to develop. (Refer to Box 2.6 for a summary of important trends during this era.

Individuals during this period who were influential in advancing the study of occupation included Ann Wilcock and Gary Kielhofner. In 1980, Kielhofner and his colleagues published a series of articles on the MOHO (Kielhofner, 1980a, 1980b; Kielhofner & Burke, 1980). Influenced by Mary Reilly's work in occupational behavior and general systems theory, the Kielhofner model emphasized motivation, performance, and patterns or routines. Wilcock's (1998) book, *An Occupational Perspective of Health*, emphasized the need for promoting health globally through a focus on the occupational nature of humans. Her work led to an improved recognition that if engagement in meaningful occupation is necessary for health, a truly just world must ensure human opportunities for such engagement (Stadnyk, Townsend, & Wilcock, 2010). Additional occupation-based models such as the Person-Environment-Occupational Performance Model (PEOP) (Christiansen & Baum, 1997), the Ecology of Human Performance Model (Dunn, Brown, & McGuigan, 1994), the Occupational Performance Process Model (Fearing, Law, & Clark, 1997), and the Canadian Model of Occupational Performance (Canadian Association of Occupational Therapists [CAOT], 1997; Townsend, 2002) laid foundation for the growth of occupation-based practice.

In Canada, the government funded programs to increase independence of older adults; in the early 1990s, a 30-month project began to emphasize health prevention and promotion in occupational therapy (CAOT, 1993). Soon after, a collaborative group from CAOT, the Client-Centered Practice committee, met to develop guidelines on consulting, research, education, and practice. Initial representatives included Helene Polatajko, Tracey Thompson-Franson, Cary Brown, Christine Kramer, Liz Townsend, Mary Law, Sue Stanton, and Sue Baptiste. The eventual work resulted in publication of the monograph, *Enabling Occupation: An Occupational Therapy Perspective* (CAOT, 1997), that was foundational to the Canadian Model of Occupational Performance and helped guide organized occupational therapy efforts in Canada.

People and Ideas Influencing Occupational Therapy (1980–1999)

Florence Clark completed her PhD in Education at USC and went on to serve as a faculty member, chair, and administrator (Figure 2.19). Clark is a respected scientist in occupational therapy and was among a group of faculty who argued that occupational science, the study of humans as occupational beings, is an appropriate academic discipline to serve as a foundation for occupational therapy practice. Clark and colleagues have gained recognition for studying the effect of lifestyle-oriented activity programs for maintaining health and preventing cognitive decline in elders with an aim of helping them remain in their homes and communities (Clark et al., 1997, 2011).

Gary Kielhofner, a student of Mary Reilly at USC, developed the MOHO (Figure 2.20). His work emphasized humans as occupational beings guided by performance subsystems including volition, habituation, and performance. Kielhofner was a prolific writer, publishing more than 19 books and 140 articles (Suarez-Balcazar, 2010). He spent most of his academic career as head of the Department of Occupational Therapy at the University of Illinois at Chicago. Kielhofner also spoke and consulted widely and assisted therapists in Sweden, England, and other countries to implement the MOHO in practice. Kielhofner died in 2010 after a brief illness. In a published memorial, his colleagues (Braveman, Fisher, & Suarez-Balcazar, 2010) described him as one of the most "influential and multifaceted occupational therapy scholars of the past 30 years" (p. 828). (For a summary of key events and people during the period 1980–1999, see Box 2.6).

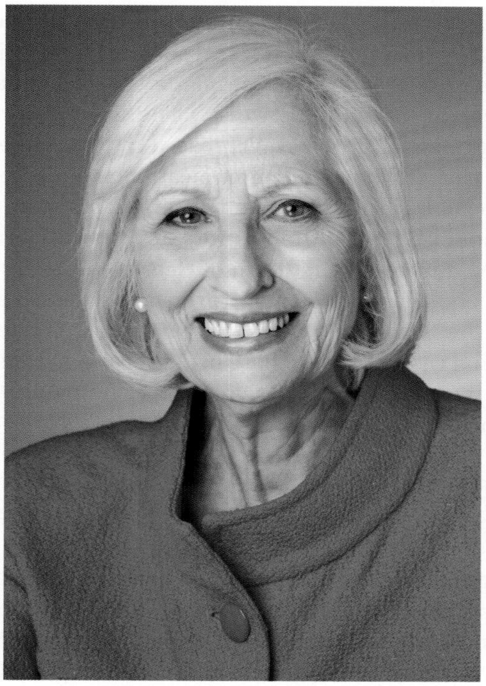

FIGURE 2.19 Florence Clark, scientist, scholar, and association leader, is a strong proponent of science-driven, evidence-based practice. Clark, from the University of Southern California, is a member of The Academy of Research of the American Occupational Therapy Foundation (AOTF). (Photo courtesy of Archives of American Occupational Therapy Association [AOTA], Wilma L. West Library, AOTF, Bethesda, MD. Used with permission.)

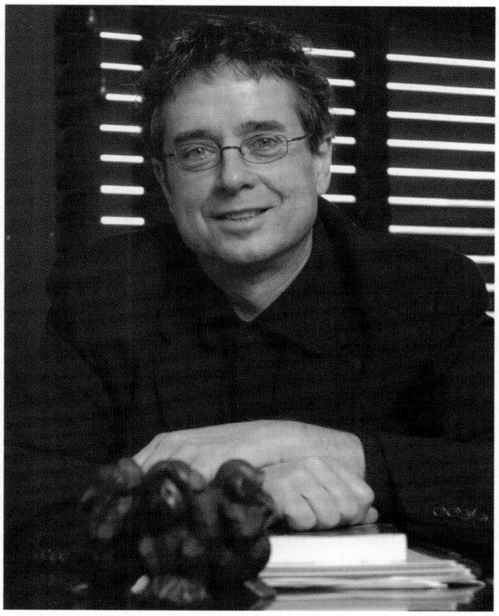

FIGURE 2.20 Gary Kielhofner (1949–2010) worked with colleagues in graduate school to develop a model of human occupation, which amalgamated knowledge from the social and behavioral sciences to provide an occupation-based approach to occupational therapy practice. During his career, Kielhofner's lectures and publications became internationally known and had a significant influence on practice in Europe, Asia, and South America. (Photo credit: Renee R. Taylor, PhD. Used with permission.)

BOX 2.6 The Conceptual Renaissance, Americans with Disabilities Act, and Occupational Science (1980–1999)

- The aftermath of the Vietnam War leads to a period of dramatic growth for occupational therapy, and the Americans with Disabilities Act extends civil rights to persons with disabilities.
- The demand for therapists increases dramatically, only to be interrupted by the Balanced Budget Act; key changes regarding the regulation of practice through licensure and certification characterize the era.
- Graduate education in the field develops and theory-driven practice further evolves, with several new conceptual models emerging to influence practice. The idea of a core discipline to provide a foundation for applied science begins with the development of occupational science. Client-centered practice gains emphasis.
- Key people during the era include Gary Kielhofner, Elizabeth Yerxa, and Florence Clark.

2000–Present

Historical Context

A new century is commonly approached with anticipation for the changes it will bring, and this anticipation is even greater as a new millennium begins. In the United States, the 21st century began with remarkable events. In 2000, the outcome of a historically close presidential election was decided by the Supreme Court, and George W. Bush became the 43rd president under contentious circumstances.

During the first year of his presidency, the United States experienced a dramatic terrorist attack on the World Trade Center in New York City on September 11, 2001. This unprecedented foreign attack on U.S. soil reverberated profoundly in nationwide efforts to increase security. These included passage of the Patriot Act, which suspended some individual liberties in the service of national defense, and led to the beginning of controversial wars in Afghanistan and Iraq aimed at tracking down terrorist leader Osama Bin Laden and eliminating the ability of terrorist groups to train personnel and plan attacks. The creation of a Department of Homeland Security was an additional part of this initiative.

The economy was recovering from a stock market decline in 2000 resulting from speculative investment in digital communications, which was followed by prodigious defense spending that stimulated speculative investments in real estate and the equity markets leading to a profound collapse of the market in 2008. This resulted in a serious and continuing global recession having profound economic consequences for the nation and world. Meanwhile, economic developments abroad, particularly in China, India, South America, and Europe, made it increasingly apparent that the U.S. economy could no longer be viewed outside a global context (Friedman, 2006). As global oil production struggled to keep pace with demand, the interest in the development of alternative sources of energy was spurred both by increasing prices and concerns about climate changes affected by a scientific phenomenon known colloquially as "global warming."

Barack Obama, the country's first African-American president, was elected in 2008, inheriting a difficult economic and political situation brought about by a global economic crisis, spending on the wars in Iraq and Afghanistan, and the need for urgent efforts by the government to spur economic development (American Recovery and Reinvestment Act of 2009). Mr. Obama's presidential challenges were made more difficult during the second half of his first term through a divided Congress and an inability to achieve political compromises across a range of key issues, especially regarding economic growth and health care.

The growth of digital communication accelerated through sales of digital devices such as smart phones, tablets and e-readers, which made use of cellular and wireless broadband networks. The growth of social networking Websites and Web-based commerce began to create changes in mass communication and marketing.

Social legislation during the period included a prescription drug benefit for seniors on Medicare (Part D), enacted during the first term of George W. Bush's presidency, and a historic but controversial bill passed in 2010 called the "Affordable Care Act" to reform health care by requiring citizens to purchase health insurance and instituting regulations for health insurance companies to protect consumers.

Occupational Therapy (2000–Present)

During the first decade of the 21st century, occupational therapy practice continued to be influenced by federal and state legislation and policy changes aimed at achieving cost containment and increasing quality, as determined by measurable outcomes and demonstrated effectiveness. In 2004, the NIH introduced a strategic plan to guide biomedical research called the NIH Roadmap (Zerhouni, 2003). Its purpose was to focus and coordinate biomedical research efforts toward areas deemed important to the health of the nation.

Increasingly, the federal Centers for Medicare and Medicaid Services (CMS) and the Agency for Healthcare

Research and Quality (AHRQ) began to exert influence on health care practices and research by linking clinical studies of effectiveness to reimbursement through its Effective Health Care Program (Slutsky, Atkins, Chang, & Sharp, 2010). Also, health care experts recommended that the country needed to pay more attention to population-based approaches to deliver health care that would emphasize prevention and promotion. Because of shifts in demographics in the United States and Canada showing more cultural diversity and an aging population (Lasser, Himmelstein, & Woolhandler, 2006), it became necessary to increase attention to health disparities, and the delivery of care to enable consumers to manage chronic conditions at home. Internationally, focus increased on global health, disparities, and public health conditions that transcend national boundaries (Macfarlane, Jacobs, & Kaaya, 2008).

Within the United States, the increased emphasis of the federal government and private health insurers on cost containment and evidence-based practice led to greater emphasis on research within organized occupational therapy. Because hospitals experienced pressures to reduce patient lengths of stay in order to contain costs, the types of procedures offered to inpatients began to focus more on those needed for discharge. More therapy was offered on an outpatient basis or in the home as part of home health services.

Because occupational therapy developed globally, it was natural that existing conceptual models would be examined and challenged by the growing numbers of professionals internationally, particularly in the Asia Pacific region, South America, and the European Union. A key development in this regard was the Kawa Model (Iwama, 2006, 2009), which offered a different but culturally relevant view of occupational therapy through the lens of Asian Pacific and other collectivist cultures. The influence of international perspectives was also fostered through the emergence of international societies for occupational science. The inaugural organizing meeting of the first Society for the Study of Occupation in the United States (SSO:USA) was held in Galveston, Texas in 2002; this was followed by developments in the Asia Pacific region as well as in Canada and the European Communities.

In 2007, the AOTA and the AOTF published the Research Agenda for Occupational Therapy, recommended by a joint panel of occupational therapy scientists serving the two organizations (AOTA/AOTF Research Advisory Panel, 2011). This agenda emphasized the importance of providing a strong infrastructure for supporting research in occupational therapy that will demonstrate the efficacy of services. Key areas of practice in the United States during 2010 as reflected in association membership data include school-based services and early intervention (27%), hospitals (28%), long-term care facilities (16%), and home health and community (7%), whereas the number of therapists practicing in the United States that reported their primary area of practice as mental health decreased to 3% (AOTA, 2010).

During this period, the wars abroad resulted in significant and challenging injuries for many survivors of combat. These returning wounded warriors impelled innovations in military occupational therapy and called attention to the need for services to reintegrate soldiers sustaining blast injuries that resulted in polytrauma, including brain injuries, severe burns, and amputations (Howard & Doukas, 2006).

In occupational therapy education, the growth of clinical doctorate programs escalated during the period. Online and hybrid educational programs also increased, offering a significant portion of curricular content to be delivered over the Internet. This trend accelerated with the growth of online social networking and the development of new digital learning technologies and the advent of mobile wireless smartphones and tablet computing devices.

People and Ideas Influencing Occupational Therapy (2000–Present)

In 2004, ***M. Carolyn Baum***, (Figure 2.21), president of the AOTA, worked with her board members to initiate strategic planning in order to develop a Centennial Vision. The aim was to identify suitable goals necessary to position the profession for success in the year 2017 (the 100th anniversary of occupational therapy) and beyond. The Centennial Vision has served as an ongoing goal-setting device for the AOTA since that time, emphasizing research, evidence-based practice, diversity, and leadership as key areas of

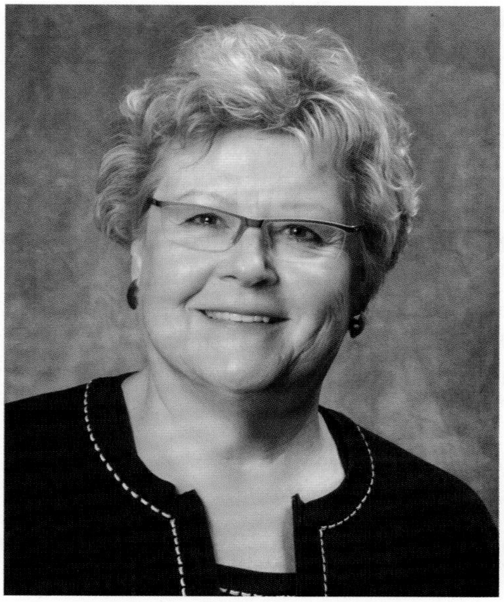

FIGURE 2.21 M. Carolyn Baum, PhD, is professor and Elias Michael Director of the Program in Occupational Therapy at Washington University School of Medicine in St. Louis. As a widely recognized leader and scientist, Baum has advocated strongly for the important links between practice, education, and research. (Photo credit: Washington University in St. Louis. Used with permission.)

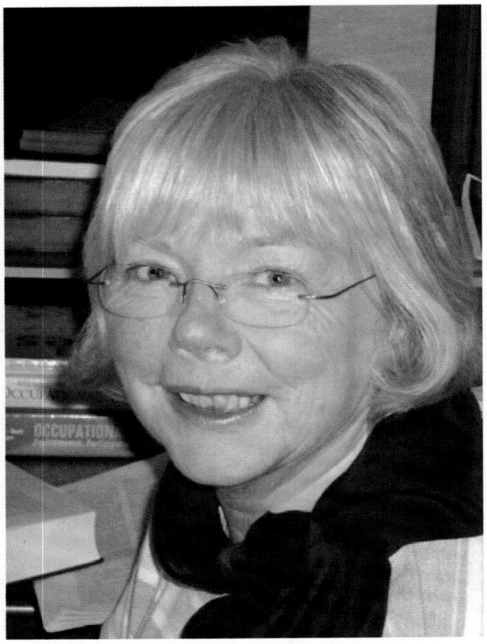

FIGURE 2.22 Ann Wilcock, PhD, DipCOT, BAppSCiOT, GradDipPH of Australia. Dr. Wilcock is the author of *An Occupational Perspective of Health* and other works, and is a developer of the concept of occupational justice. (Photo courtesy of Ann Wilcock.)

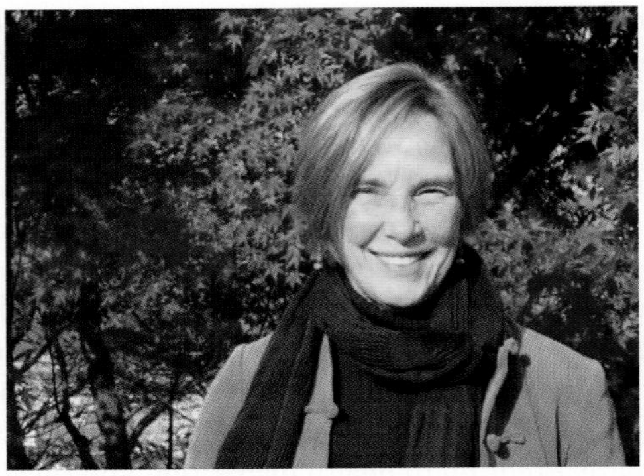

FIGURE 2.23 Elizabeth Townsend, PhD, OT(C), FCAOT, professor emerita of Dalhousie University, Halifax, Nova Scotia, Canada. Dr. Townsend is a coauthor of the Canadian guide to practice known as *Enabling Occupation* and a developer, with Ann Wilcock of Australia, of the concept of occupational justice. (Photo courtesy of Elizabeth Townsend.)

focus in the years ahead (AOTA, 2006). Baum was succeeded in her presidency by other leaders (Penelope Moyers Cleveland and Florence Clark) who continued to emphasize the importance of leadership development and research capacity building in occupational therapy.

Ann Wilcock, of Australia, one of the first scholars to emphasize the idea of occupational therapy as a key contribution to population health (Figure 2.22), and ***Elizabeth Townsend*** (Figure 2.23), a Canadian who partnered with Wilcock to develop and advance the concept of occupational justice (Townsend & Wilcock, 2004), jointly had a significant global influence on occupational therapy. The concept was grounded in the belief that opportunities to engage in meaningful occupation are a prerequisite to health and well-being. Their concept was given additional impetus when the revised version of the World Health Organization's International Classification of Impairment, Disability, and Handicap was dramatically revised to become the International Classification of Functioning, Disability, and Health (ICF) (World Health Organization, 2001). Townsend, of Dalhousie University in Halifax, Nova Scotia, was also a leading figure in the development of an influential Canadian document called *Enabling Occupation* (Townsend, 2002). (For a summary of significant events and people during this era, see Box 2.7)

Summary

In this chapter, more than a century of occupational therapy history has been reviewed, beginning with a description of important ideas and personalities prior to the 20th century that influenced the birth of the profession. For each of five eras, a contextual backdrop was provided to describe the historical circumstances under which different events occurred, with the aim of emphasizing that professions, like individuals, are best understood in situational contexts.

Occupational therapy began during a progressive era that was auspicious for bold ideas and new approaches.

BOX 2.7 The New Millennium, Digital Transformation, and Globalization (2000–Present)

- Terrorism, globalization, digital technologies, and economic turbulence characterize the early part of the era, leading to dramatic societal changes and political upheaval.
- Occupational therapy expands dramatically in emerging regions, augmented by digital technologies; this leads to models based on different cultural perspectives, the development of online education, and the emergence of clinical doctorates.
- In the United States, practice is increasingly driven by federal reimbursement regulations influenced by cost containment and evidence-based practice, a Centennial Vision is created to guide organized national efforts, research begins to mature.
- Key people during the era included Carolyn Baum, Elizabeth Townsend, and Ann Wilcock.

Although its fundamental principles were already being applied by professionals and nonprofessionals in different settings, it was not until an enthusiastic and ambitious consumer (George Barton) took the initiative to bring an interdisciplinary group of like-minded advocates together that the profession of occupational therapy was officially launched. Within weeks, a nation's preparations for caring for its wounded soldiers as it entered a great war provided a rare opportunity for the profession to organize around a patriotic cause and demonstrate its value. Because women were just emerging as a political force in the country and so few women held professional roles at the time, the recruits to occupational therapy were uncertain about how to manifest their opportunities. Occupational therapy had to compete with medical specialties, vocational educators, nurses, and others who believed that they were equally entitled to the use of curative occupations as part of their treatment regimens.

For the entirety of their history, occupational therapists have been doers, often little interested in explaining or proving the theoretical ideas and practical benefits of their actions. This has placed the profession at a disadvantage to medicine and other disciplines, where science-based practice has become increasingly the norm. Yet, the inherent flexibility of occupations as a therapeutic medium has continued to offer creative opportunities for benefiting a wide range of patients and clients. Although once daunting health problems served by occupational therapists (e.g., tuberculosis [TB], HIV, and polio) have faded into the history books of biomedical success, occupational therapists have been able to mobilize in the service of emerging health problems and concerns deemed important by the public (such as dementia and autism spectrum disorders). Moreover, the cooperative nature of the therapeutic relationship has afforded a bridge to connect the body and mind—providing occupational therapists with a rare, important, and enduring place in the lives of their patients—serving as healers as well as technologists, a role not easily appreciated by the casual observer.

As occupational therapy moves ahead into the 21st century, one must ask if these themes will continue to shape the story of the profession. Will there continue to be role ambiguity and underappreciation for the importance of science and theory? Will therapists continue to reinvent new approaches for serving the emerging diseases of the 21st century, and will they capitalize on the unique position they have, but perhaps underuse, as technologists and custodians of meaning (Engelhardt, 1983)? Only the histories yet to be written will tell.

References

Allen Cognitive Network. (2011). *Brief history.* Retrieved from the Allen Cognitive Network website: http://www.allen-cognitive-network.org/

American Machinist. (2000). 1950s. *American Machinist, 144,* 130.

American Occupational Therapy Association. (1969). American occupational therapy organizations. *American Journal of Occupational Therapy, 23,* 519.

American Occupational Therapy Association. (2000). Occupational therapy and the Americans with Disabilities Act (ADA). *American Journal of Occupational Therapy, 54,* 622–625. doi:10.5014/AJOT.54.6.622

American Occupational Therapy Association. (2006). 2006 AOTA workforce and compensation survey: Occupational therapy salaries and job opportunities continue to improve. *OT Practice Online,* 9-11-06. Retrieved from the American Occupational Therapy Association website: http://www.aota.org/Pubs/OTP/1997–2007/Features/2006/f-091106.aspx

American Occupational Therapy Association. (2009). *History of AOTA accreditation.* Retrieved from the American Occupational Therapy Association website: http://www.aota.org/Educate/Accredit/Overview/38124.aspx

American Occupational Therapy Association. (2010). Practice survey. *OT Practice, 15,* 8–11.

American Occupational Therapy Association/American Occupational Therapy Foundation Research Advisory Panel. (2011). Occupational therapy research agenda. *OTJR: Occupation, Participation and Health, 31,* 52–54.

American Occupational Therapy Foundation. (2012a). *Academy of Research in Occupational Therapy.* Retrieved from the AOTF website: http://www.aotf.org/awardshonors/forresearch/academyofresearchinoccupationaltherapy.aspx

American Occupational Therapy Foundation. (2012b). *OTJR: Occupation, participation, and health.* Retrieved from the AOTF website: http://www.aotf.org/awardshonors/forresearch/academyofresearchinoccupationaltherapy.aspx

American Recovery and Reinvestment Act of 2009, Pub. L. No. 111-5, 123 Stat. 115, H.R. 1 (2009).

Americans with Disabilities Act of 1990, 42 U.S.C.A. § 12101 *et seq.*

Anthony, S. H. (2005). Dr. Herbert J. Hall: Originator of honest work for occupational therapy 1904–1923 [Part I]. *Occupational Therapy in Health Care, 19,* 3–19.

Anthony, W. A. (1993). Recovery from mental illness: Setting some system level standards. *Psychiatric Rehabilitation Journal, 24,* 159–168.

Ayres, A. J. (1966). Interrelationships among perceptual-motor functions in children. *American Journal of Occupational Therapy, 20,* 68–71.

Ayres, A. J. (1972). *Sensory integration and learning disorders.* Los Angeles, CA: Western Psychological Services.

Bakken, K. (2009). Health care coverage: The mark of a great society? *Journal of Illinois Nursing,* 7–8.

Balanced Budget Act of 1997, Pub. L. No. 105–33, 111 Stat. 269 (1997).

Beard, G. M. (1880). *A practical treatise on nervous exhaustion (neurasthenia).* New York, NY: William Wood.

Beck, A. H. (2004). The Flexner report and the standardization of American medical education. *Journal of the American Medical Association, 291,* 2139–2140.

Beers, C. (1908). *A mind that found itself: An autobiography.* New York, NY: Longmans, Green and Company.

Bergin, T. J. (2007). A history of the history of programming languages. *Communications of the ACM, 50,* 69–74.

Bing, R. K. (1961). *William Rush Dunton, Jr.: American psychiatrist—A Study in self* (Unpublished doctoral dissertation). College Park, MD: University of Maryland.

Bing, R. K. (1981). Occupational therapy revisited: A paraphrastic journey. *American Journal of Occupational Therapy, 35,* 499–518.

Birn, A., Brown, T. M., Fee, E., & Lear, W. J. (2003). Struggles for National Health Reform in the United States. *American Journal of Public Health, 93,* 86–91.

Bissel, J. C., & Mailloux, Z. (1981). The use of crafts in occupational therapy for the physically disabled. *American Journal of Occupational Therapy, 35,* 369–374.

Bowman, O. J. (1989). In memoriam: A. Jean Ayres: 1920–1988: Therapist, scholar, scientist, and teacher. *American Journal of Occupational Therapy, 43,* 479–480.

Braveman, B., Fisher, G., & Suarez-Balcazar, Y. (2010). In memoriam: "Achieving the ordinary things: A tribute to Gary Kielhofner." *American Journal of Occupational Therapy, 64,* 828–831.

Brown, E. J. (1996). Mary Reilly: A true bonafide character. *Advance,* April 1, 1996 edition.

Brown, L. D., Shepherd, M. D., Wituk, S. A., & Meissen, G. (2008). Introduction to the special issue on mental health self-help. *American Journal of Community Psychology, 42*, 105–109. doi:10.1007/s10464-008-9187-7

Brunner, J. (2001). *Freud and the politics of psychoanalysis.* New Brunswick, NY: Transaction.

Burnham, J. C. (2006). The "New Freud Studies": A historiographical shift. *Journal of the Historical Society, 6*, 213–233. doi:10.1111/j.1540-5923-2006.00176.x

Canadian Association of Occupational Therapists. (1993). *Seniors' health promotion project: Responding to the challenge of an aging population's final report.* Ottawa, Canada: Author.

Canadian Association of Occupational Therapists. (1997). *Enabling occupation: An occupational therapy perspective.* Ottawa, Canada: Author.

Centers for Medicare and Medicaid Services. (2012). *Office of the Actuary, National Health Statistics Group, National Health Care Expenditures Data.* Retrieved from https://www.cms.gov/Research-Statistics-Data-and-Systems/Statistics-Trends-and-Reports/NationalHealthExpendData/downloads/tables.pdf

Christiansen, C. (2007). Adolf Meyer revisited: Connections between lifestyles, resilience and illness. *Journal of Occupational Science, 14*(2), 63–76.

Christiansen, C., & Baum, C. (Eds.). (1997). Person-environment occupational performance: A conceptual model for practice. In *OT: Enabling function and well being* (2nd ed., pp. 47–70). Thorofare, NJ: Slack.

Clark, F., Azen, S.P., Zemke, R., Jackson, J., Carlson, M., Mandel, D., . . . Lipson, L. (1997). Occupational therapy for independent-living older adults. A randomized controlled trial. *The Journal of the American Medical Association, 278*, 1321–1326.

Clark, F., Jackson, J., Carlson, M., Chou, C.P., Cherry, B.J., Jordan-Marsh, M., . . . Azen, S.P. (2011). Effectiveness of a lifestyle intervention in promoting the well-being of independently living older people: Results of the Well Elderly 2 Randomised Controlled Trial. *Journal of Epidemiology and Community Health.* Advance online publication. doi:10.1136/jech.2009.099754

Clark, F., Wood, W., & Larson, E. A. (1998). Occupational science: Occupational therapy's legacy for the 21st century. In M. Neistadt & E. Crepeau (Eds.), *Willard and Spackman's occupational therapy* (9th ed., pp. 13–21). Philadelphia, PA: Lippincott Williams & Wilkins.

Clouston, T. J., & Whitcombe, S. W. (2008). The professionalization of occupational therapy: A continuing challenge. *British Journal of Occupational Therapy, 71*, 314–320.

Cockburn, L. (2001, May–June). The professional era: CAOT in the 1950's and 1960's. *Occupational Therapy Now*, 5–9.

Cooper, J. M. (1990). *Pivotal decades: The United States, 1900–1920.* New York, NY: Norton.

Coutinho, M. J., & Hunter, D. L. (1988). Special education and occupational therapy: Making the relationship work. *American Journal of Occupational Therapy, 42*, 706–712.

Dain, N. (1980). *Clifford W. Beers, advocate for the insane.* Pittsburgh, PA: University of Pittsburgh Press.

Digby, A. (1985). *Madness, morality, and medicine: A study of the York retreat, 1796–1914.* Cambridge, NY: Cambridge University Press.

DiNunzio, M. (1994). *Theodore Roosevelt: An American mind.* New York, NY: Penguin Books.

Dunn, W., Brown, C., & McGuigan, A. (1994). The ecology of human performance: A framework for considering the effect of context. *American Journal of Occupational Therapy, 48*, 595–607.

Dunton, W. R., Jr. (1925). Editorial. *Occupational Therapy and Rehabilitation, 4*, 73–75.

Dworkin, R. W. (2010). The rise of the caring industry. *Policy Review, 161*, 45–59.

Education for All Handicapped Children Act of 1975, Pub. L. No. 94-142, 20 U.S.C. § 1401 (1975).

Egan, T. (2006). *The worst hard time: The untold story of those who survived the great American dust bowl.* New York, NY: Houghton Mifflin.

Engelhardt, H. T. (1983). Occupational therapists as technologists and custodians of meaning. In G. Kielhofner (Ed.), *Health through occupation* (pp. 130–144). Philadelphia, PA: F. A. Davis.

Eysenck, H. (1985). *Decline and fall of the Freudian empire.* Harmondsworth, United Kingdom: Pelican.

Faiella, G. (2006). *John Locke: Champion of modern democracy.* New York, NY: Rosen.

Fearing,V. G., Law, M., & Clark, J. (1997). An occupational performance process model: Fostering client and therapist alliances. *Canadian Journal of Occupational Therapy, 64*, 7–15.

Fidler, G., & Fidler, J. (1954). *Introduction to psychiatric occupational therapy.* New York, NY: McMillan.

Fink, M., & Taylor, M. A. (2007). Electroconvulsive therapy: Evidence and challenges. *The Journal of the American Medical Association, 298*, 330–332.

Fisher, J. (2001). *Stolen glory: The McKinley assassination.* La Jolla, CA: Alamar Books.

Friedland, J. (2011). *Restoring the spirit: The beginnings of occupational therapy in Canada, 1890–1930.* Montreal, Canada: McGill-Queens University Press.

Friedland, J., & Silva, J. (2008). Evolving identities: Thomas Bessell Kidner and occupational therapy in the United States. *American Journal of Occupational Therapy, 62*, 349–360.

Friedman, T. L. (2006). *The world is flat. A brief history of the 21st century.* New York, NY: Farar, Strauss, and Giroux.

Gagne, C., White, W., & Anthony, W. A. (2007). Recovery: A common vision for the fields of mental health and addictions. *Psychiatric Rehabilitation, 31*, 32–37.

Gainer, R. D. (2008). History of ergonomics and occupational therapy. *Work, 31*, 5–9.

Gerber, K. M. (2007). Eight decades of health care: The 1950's. *Hospitals & Health Networks, 81*, 10–13.

Gordon, D. M. (2009). The history of occupational therapy. In E. B. Crepeau, E. S. Cohn, & B. A. Boyt Schell (Eds.), *Willard and Spackman's occupational therapy* (11th ed., pp. 202–215). Philadelphia, PA: Lippincott Williams & Wilkins.

Greenwald, R. A. (2005). *The triangle fire, the protocols of peace, and industrial democracy in progressive era New York.* Philadelphia, PA: Temple University Press.

Hackett, L. (1992). *The age of enlightenment: The European dream of progress and enlightenment.* Chicago, IL: Chicago Press.

Hall, H. J. (1922). *What is occupation therapy?* Paper written for the general federation of women's clubs. Chataqua, NY: Official Archives, American Occupational Therapy Foundation, Bethesda, MD.

Harlow, J. (2007). Eight decades of health care: The 1940's. *Hospitals and Health Networks, 81*, 10–13.

Hein, C. D., & VanZante, N. R. (1993). A manager's guide: Americans with Disabilities Act of 1990. *SAM: Advanced Management Journal, 58*, 40–45.

Hernandez, N. (2005). Telemedicine and the future of telemedicine. *AMT Events, 22*, 74–75; 116–117.

Hocking, C. (2008). The way we were. *British Journal of Occupational Therapy, 71*, 185–195.

Hospital and Health Networks. (2012). Eight decades of health care. Retrieved from http://www.hhnmag.com/hhnmag_app/jsp/articledisplay.jsp?dcrpath=HHNMAG/Article/data/07JUL2007/0707HHN_FEA_timeline&domain=HHNMAG

Howard, W. J., III, & Doukas, W. C. (2006). Process of care for battle casualties at Walter Reed Army Medical Center: Part IV. Occupational therapy service. *Military Medicine, 171*, 209–210.

Huret, R. (2010). Poverty in Cold War America: A problem that has no name? The invisible network of poverty experts in the 1950s and 1960s. *History of Political Economy, 2*(Suppl. 1), 53–76. doi:10.1215/00182702-2009-072

Husock, H. (1992). Bringing back the settlement house. *National Affairs, 109.* Retrieved from: http://www.nationalaffairs.com/public_interest/detail/bringing-back-the-settlement-house

Individuals with Disabilities Education Act of 1997, Pub. L. No. 105-117, 20 U.S.C., §614, 672, 20 U.S.C. (1997). Retrieved from http://www2.ed.gov/offices/OSERS/Policy/IDEA/index.html

Iwama, M. (2006). *The Kawa model: Culturally relevant occupational therapy.* Edinburgh, United Kingdom: Churchill Livingstone Elsevier Press.

Iwama, M. (2009). The Kawa model: The power of culturally responsive occupational therapy. *Disability and Rehabilitation, 31*, 1125–1135.

Jarvis, C. (2009). "If he comes home nervous": U.S. World War II neuropsychiatric casualties and postwar masculinities. *The Journal of Men's Studies, 17,* 97–115.

Karger, H., & Rose, S. R. (2010). Revisiting the Americans with Disabilities Act after two decades. *Journal of Social Work in Disability and Rehabilitation, 9,* 73–86. doi:10.1080/1536710X.2010.493468

Kennedy, D. M. (1999). *1929–1945. Freedom from fear: The American people in depression and war.* Oxford, NY: Oxford University Press.

Kielhofner, G. (1980a). A model of human occupation, part two. Ontogenesis from the perspective of temporal adaptation. *American Journal of Occupational Therapy, 34,* 657–663.

Kielhofner, G. (1980b). A model of human occupation, part three. Benign and vicious cycles. *American Journal of Occupational Therapy, 34,* 731–737.

Kielhofner, G. (2009). *Conceptual foundations of occupational therapy* (4th ed.). Philadelphia, PA: F. A. Davis.

Kielhofner, G., & Burke, J. P. (1977). Occupational therapy after 60 years: An account of changing identity and knowledge. *American Journal of Occupational Therapy, 31,* 675–689.

Kielhofner, G., & Burke, J. P. (1980). A model of human occupation part 1: Conceptual framework and content. *American Journal of Occupational Therapy, 34,* 572–581.

King, L. J. (1974). A sensory integrative approach to schizophrenia. *American Journal of Occupational Therapy, 28,* 529–536.

King, M. L. (1963). *I had a dream.* Text of speech delivered August 28, 1963. Washington DC.

Koyangi, C. (2007). *Learning from history: Deinstitutionalization of people with mental illness as precursor to long-term care reform.* Washington, DC: Kaiser Foundation on Medicaid and Uninsured.

Kreutziger, S. S., Ager, R., Lewis, J. S., & England, S. (2001). A critical look at a contemporary welfare-to-work program in light of the historical settlement ideal. *Journal of Community Practice, 9,* 49–69.

Krusen, F. H. (1934). The relationship of physical therapy and occupational therapy. *Occupational Therapy and Rehabilitation, 13,* 69–77.

Kuhn, T. S. (1996). *The structure of scientific revolutions* (3rd ed.). Chicago, IL: University of Chicago Press.

Lasser, K. E., Himmelstein, D. U., & Woolhandler, S. (2006). Access to care, health status, and health disparities in the United States and Canada: Results of a cross national population-based survey. *American Journal of Public Health, 96,* 1300–1307.

Lief, A. (1948). *The commonsense psychiatry of Adolf Meyer.* New York, NY: McGraw-Hill.

Low, J. F. (1997). The issue is: NBCOT and state regulatory agencies: Allies or adversaries? *American Journal of Occupational Therapy, 51,* 74–75.

Luchins, A. S. (2001). Moral treatment in asylums and general hospitals in 19th-century America. *The Journal of Psychology, 123,* 585–607.

Macfarlane, S. B., Jacobs, M., & Kaaya, E. E. (2008). In the name of global health trends in academic institutions. *Journal of Public Health Policy, 29,* 383–401.

McElvaine, R. S. (1993). *The Great Depression: America 1929–1941.* New York, NY: Random House.

McGrew, J. H., Wright, E. R., Pescosolido, B. A., & McDonel, E. C. (1999). The closing of Central State Hospital: Long-term outcomes for persons with severe mental illness. *The Journal of Behavioral Health Services and Research, 26,* 246–261.

Metaxas, V. A. (2000). Eleanor Clarke Slagle and Susan E. Tracy: Personal and professional identity and the development of occupational therapy in progressive era America. *Nursing History Review, 8,* 39–70.

Meyer, A. (1922). The philosophy of occupation therapy. *Archives of Occupational Therapy, 1,* 1–10.

Miller, R. J., & Walker, K. F. (1993). *Perspectives on theory for practice in occupational therapy.* Gaithersburg, MD: Aspen.

Mosey, A. (1973). *Activities therapy.* Nashville, TN: Raven Press.

Nancarrow, S., & Mackey, H. (2005). The introduction and evaluation of an occupational therapy assistant practitioner. *Australian Journal of Occupational Therapy, 52,* 293–301.

Office of the Surgeon General. (1918). *Carry on. A Magazine on the reconstruction of disabled soldiers and sailors.* Washington, DC: American Red Cross.

Oshinsky, D. M. (2005). *Polio: An American story.* New York, NY: Oxford University Press.

Ott, K., Serlin, D., & Mihm, S. (2002). *Artificial parts, practical lives.* New York, NY: New York University Press.

Oxford Brookes University. (2011). *The Churchill Hospital years.* Retrieved from http://www.brookes.ac.uk/library/speccoll/dorset/dorsethist3.html

Paine, T. (1794). *The age of reason: Being an investigation of true and fabulous theology.* Paris, France: Barras.

Palfrey, J. (2010). Four phases of Internet regulation. *Social Research, 77,* 981–996.

Patel, D. R. (2005). Therapeutic interventions in cerebral palsy. *Indian Journal of Pediatrics, 72,* 979–983.

Pedriana, N., & Stryker, R. (2004). The strength of a weak agency: Enforcement of Title VII of the 1964 Civil Rights Act and the expansion of state capacity, 1965–1971. *American Journal of Sociology, 110,* 709–760.

Peters, C. (2011a). History of mental health: Perspectives of consumers and practitioners. In C. Brown & V. C. Stoffel (Eds.), *Occupational therapy in mental health: A vision for participation* (pp. 17–30). Philadelphia, PA: F. A. Davis.

Peters, C. (2011b). Powerful occupational therapists: A community of professionals. 1950–1980. *Occupational Therapy in Mental Health, 27,* 199–410. doi:10.1080/0164212X.2011.597328

Pressman, J. D. (1998). *Last resort: Psychosurgery and the limits of medicine.* Cambridge, NY: Cambridge University Press.

Qaseem, A., Weech-Maldonado, R., & Mkanta, W. (2007). The Balanced Budget Act (1997) and the supply of nursing home subacute care. *Journal of Health Care Finance, 34,* 38–47.

Quiroga, V. A. (1995). *Occupational therapy: The first 30 years 1900–1930.* Bethesda, MD: American Occupational Therapy Association.

Reilly, M. (1962). Occupational therapy can be one of the great ideas of 20th century medicine. *American Journal of Occupational Therapy, 20,* 61–67.

Reilly, M. (Ed.). (1974). *Play as exploratory learning.* Beverly Hills, CA: Sage.

Richards, E. E. (2011). Responses to occupational and environmental exposures in the U.S. military—World War II to the present. *Military Medicine, 176,* 22–28.

Salvatori, P. (2001). The history of occupational therapy assistants in Canada: A comparison with the United States. *Canadian Journal of Occupational Therapy, 68,* 217–227.

Schutz, A. (2011). Power and trust in the public realm: John Dewey, Saul Alinsky, and the limits of progressive democratic education. *Educational Theory, 61,* 491–512.

Scull, A. (2005). *Madhouse: A tragic tale of megalomania and modern medicine.* New Haven, CT: Yale University Press.

Sealy, P., & Whitehead, P. C. (2004). Forty years of deinstitutionalization of psychiatric services in Canada: An Empirical Assessment. *Canadian Journal of Psychiatry, 49,* 249–257.

Slagle, E. C. (1934). Occupational therapy: Recent methods and advances in the United States. *Occupational Therapy and Rehabilitation, 13,* 289–298.

Slutsky, J., Atkins, D., Chang, S., & Sharp B. A., (2010). Comparing medical interventions: AHRQ and the Effective Healthcare Program. *Journal of Clinical Epidemiology, 63*(5), 471–473.

Spackman, C. S. (1968). A history of the practice of occupational therapy for restoration of physical function: 1917–1967. *American Journal of Occupational Therapy, 22,* 67–71.

Stadnyk, R., Townsend, E. A., & Wilcock, A. (2010). Occupational justice. In C. H. Christiansen & E. A. Townsend (Eds.), *Introduction to occupation: The art and science of living* (2nd ed., pp. 329–358). Upper Saddle River, NJ: Prentice Hall.

Starr, P. (1983). *The social transformation of American medicine.* New York, NY: Basic Books.

Stevens, R. A. (1996). Healthcare in the early 1960s. *Healthcare Financing Review, 18,* 11–22.

Stokesbury, J. L. (1980). *A short history of World War II*. New York, NY: Harper Collins.

Suarez-Balcazar, Y. (2010). *OT community mourns the loss of Dr. Gary Kielhofner*. Retrieved from the AOTA website: http://www.aota.org/News/AOTANews/Gary-Kielhofner.aspx

Thomasson, M. A. (2002). From sickness to health: The twentieth-century development of U.S. health insurance. *Explorations in Economic History, 39*, 233–253.

Tilsen, J., & Nylund, D. (2008). Psychotherapy research, the recovery movement and practiced based evidence in psychiatric rehabilitation. *Journal of Social Work in Disability and Rehabilitation, 7*, 340–354.

Townsend, E. (Ed.). (2002). *Enabling occupation: An occupational therapy perspective*. Ottawa, Canada: Canadian Association of Occupational Therapists.

Townsend, E., & Wilcock, A. A. (2004). Occupational justice and client-centered practice. A dialogue in progress. *Canadian Journal of Occupational Therapy, 71*, 75–87.

Tracy, S. (1910). *Studies in invalid occupation*. Boston, MA: Whitcomb and Barrows.

University of Southern California. (n.d.). USC occupational therapy: The 20th century. Retrieved from the USC website: http://ot.usc.edu/images/uploads/ot_timeline.pdf

U.S. Army Medical Department. (2012). *Occupational therapy educational programs April 1947–January 1961*. Retrieved from the U.S. Army Medical Department Office of Medical History: http://history.amedd.army.mil/corps/medical_spec/chapterxv.html

U.S. Department of Health, Education, and Welfare. (1965). *Part I: National trends in health education and welfare trends*. Washington, DC: Author.

U.S. Department of Veterans Affairs. (2011). *Military health history pocket card for clinicians*. Retrieved from http://www.va.gov/oaa/pocket-card/worldwar.asp

Votaw, J. F. (2005). *Battle orders: The American expeditionary forces in World War I*. New York, NY: Osprey.

Warner, D. C. (2012). Access to health services for immigrants in the USA: From the Great Society to the 2010 health care reform and after. *Ethnic and Racial Studies, 35*, 40–55. doi:10.1080/01419870.2011.594171

Weissmann, G. (2008). Citizen Pinel and the madman at Bellevue. *Federation of American Societies for Experimental Biology Journal, 22*(5), 1289–1293.

West, W. L. (1991). The issue is: Should the Representative Assembly have voted as it did, when it did, on occupational therapists' use of physical agent modalities? *American Journal of Occupational Therapy, 45*, 1143–1147.

Whiteley, S. (2004). The evolution of the therapeutic community. *Psychiatric Quarterly, 75*, 233–248. doi:0033-2720/040900/0233/0

Wilcock, A. A. (1998). *An occupational perspective on health*. Thorofare, NJ: Slack.

Williams, T. A. (1909). Requisite for the treatment of psycho-neuroses. *The Kansas City Medical Index-Lancet, 32*, 353–354.

World Federation of Occupational Therapists. (2011). *History*. Retrieved from the WFOT website: http://www.wfot.org/AboutUs/History.aspx

World Health Organization. (2001). *International classification of functioning disability and health (ICF)*. Geneva, Switzerland: Author.

Yerxa, E. J. (1967a). The 1966 Eleanor Clark Slagle Lecture: Authentic occupational therapy. *American Journal of Occupational Therapy, 21*, 155–173.

Yerxa, E. J. (1967b). The American Occupational Therapy Foundation is born. *American Journal of Occupational Therapy, 21*, 299–300.

Yerxa, E. J. (1990). An introduction to occupational science: A foundation for occupational therapy in the 21st century. *Occupational Therapy in Health Care, 6*, 1–17.

Zerhouni, E. (2003). Medicine. The NIH roadmap. *Science, 302*, 63–72.

For additional resources on the subjects discussed in this chapter, visit http://thePoint.lww.com/Willard-Spackman12e.

CHAPTER 3

The Philosophy of Occupational Therapy

A Framework for Practice

Barbara Hooper, Wendy Wood

LEARNING OBJECTIVES

After reading this chapter, you will be able to:

1. Describe elements of a philosophical framework and their transactions with each other
2. Explain how a philosophical framework is a guide for practice
3. Using a comprehensive philosophical framework, articulate occupational therapy's basic philosophical assumptions and their transactions
4. Given a practice scenario or your own experiences, evaluate the fit of occupational therapy's philosophy with practice
5. Given a practice scenario or your own experiences, create one or two strategies that could strengthen the congruence between occupational therapy's philosophy and practice

OUTLINE

Introduction

Occupational therapy has a philosophy, and it may be the most basic element of practice. The profession's philosophy is the foundation upholding all that practitioners and researchers do; indeed, it provides the necessary footing on which to make decisions and select actions when theory, evidence, and experience are insufficient to fully guide practice (Ruona & Lynham, 2004). Philosophy further helps practitioners (1) develop a clear and coherent professional identity as an *occupational* therapist; (2) hone a practice that is and looks unique among health care providers; and (3) explain the hidden and often underestimated complexity of the profession, both to themselves and others. Emphasizing how basic philosophy is, Wilcock (1999) stated that "the first essential for each individual in any profession is the acceptance of a philosophy that is the profession's keystone" (p. 192).

Proponents of occupational therapy have long been dedicated to articulating and promoting the profession's philosophy, often drawing from established formal philosophies. For example, Adolph Meyer, a psychiatrist, first published "The Philosophy of Occupation Therapy" in 1922.

TABLE 3.1 Select Resources on the Influences of Formal Philosophies on Occupational Therapy

Formal Philosophy	Select Resources
Pragmatism	Breines, 1986, 1987; Cutchin, 2004; Hooper & Wood, 2002; Ikiugu & Schultz, 2006
Arts & crafts movement	Friedland, 2003; Hocking, 2008; Levine, 1987; Reed, 1986, 2005
European enlightenment	Ikiugu & Schultz, 2006; Wilcock, 2006
Structuralism	Hooper & Wood, 2002
Existentialism	Yerxa, 1967
Humanism	Bruce & Borg, 2002; Devereaux, 1984; Nelson, 1997
Holism	Finlay, 2001
See also	Nelson, 1997; Peloquin, 2005; Punwar & Peloquin, 2000; Reed & Sanderson, 1999; West, 1984

In this classic work, Meyer described the young profession as "a very important manifestation of a very general gain in human philosophy" (p. 4). It is likely that Meyer was addressing how occupational therapy was influenced by **pragmatism**, a formal philosophy of his day that has shaped occupational therapy's philosophical foundations to the present day (Breines, 1986; Cutchin, 2004; Hooper & Wood, 2002; Ikiugu & Schultz, 2006). Specific influences of many formal philosophies on the field have been carefully detailed elsewhere (Table 3.1) and are beyond the scope of this chapter. Yet many beliefs, **values**, principles, and perspectives originally imported from these formal philosophies have melded into a compelling profession-specific philosophy, which is the focus here.

Influential writers have elaborated single elements within this profession-specific philosophy, such as beliefs about humans, knowledge, values, and principles for best practice. To our knowledge, however, these elements, often addressed apart from one another, have yet to be assembled into a philosophical framework. Thus, our purpose in this chapter is to describe the profession's philosophy using a comprehensive philosophical framework. To do so, we introduce the meaning of philosophy and three elements of a philosophical framework: ontology, epistemology, and axiology. We next explore the profession-specific philosophy of occupational therapy related to these elements, each of which suggests a question as captured in the headings:

- Ontology: What Is Most Real for Occupational Therapy?
- Epistemology: What Is Knowledge in Occupational Therapy?
- Axiology: What Is Right Action in Occupational Therapy?

We conclude the chapter with a comparison of philosophical and nonphilosophical thinking and practice scenarios as opportunities to use the philosophical framework.

The Meaning of Philosophy

At its root, the word *philosophy* refers to "love (philo) of knowledge or wisdom (sophia)" (Philosophy, n.d.). Philosophy is both a framework for thinking and a mode of thinking. As a ***framework for thinking***, philosophy means thinking within and acting from a "network" of assumptions and beliefs (Paul, 1995). **Assumptions** are ideas or principles that are "taken for granted as the basis for argument and action" (Hooper, 2008, p. 15). Assumptions are sometimes referred to as "first principles" that form a bedrock for beliefs (Ikiugu & Schultz, 2006). **Beliefs** are convictions about what is true (Rogers, 1982b; Yerxa, 1979). When assumptions and beliefs are consciously examined and organized into a coherent framework for thought and action, they begin to take shape as supporting a philosophical mode of thinking. A philosophical mode of thinking refers to "thinking with a clear sense of the ultimate foundations of one's thinking" (Paul, 1995, p. 436). We thus define **philosophy** as (1) a conscious framework of assumptions and beliefs that guides actions and (2) as a mode of thinking that actively relies on the framework for processing ideas and decisions.

A Philosophical Framework: Ontology, Epistemology, and Axiology

A philosophical framework is often presented as having at least three elements: ontology, epistemology, and axiology (Lincoln, Lynham, & Guba, 2011; Ruona & Lynham, 2004; J. Schell, 2008; Yerxa, 1979). In this section, we define each element, identify the big questions each addresses, and then describe how they function as part of a dynamic system.

Ontology is concerned with the question, *what is most real*? Ontology is defined as the "science or study of being; that branch of metaphysics concerned with the nature or essence of being or existence" (http://www.oed.com).

Occupational therapy's ontology can be discerned by examining how the field's scholars and practitioners have addressed the following questions:

- What is occupational therapy's view of the human?
- What are the *most* real dimensions of life from an occupational therapy perspective?

Yerxa (1979) phrased the question, "what is 'really' real in the world" (p. 26). Yerxa thus referred to reality as having multiple dimensions; those dimensions in the foreground for occupational therapists constitute what is "most" real. Other philosophers (e.g., Sire, 2009) have phrased the question, "What is prime reality—the really real?" (p. 18), again referring to the aspects of reality that are illuminated and foregrounded by one's perspective.

Epistemology asks the question, *what is knowledge*? Epistemology is defined as the theory of knowledge (http://www.oed.com). Occupational therapy's epistemology can be discerned by examining how the field's scholars and practitioners have addressed the following questions:

- What knowledge is most important to know and demonstrate in occupational therapy?
- How is knowledge in occupational therapy organized?
- How is knowledge acquired and used?
- What is an occupational therapy view of the essence or nature of knowledge?

Axiology asks the question, *what are right actions*? Axiology is defined as "the study of values including what is good, beautiful, and morally desirable" (Yerxa, 1979, p. 26). Values in turn help "make explicit how we ought to act" (Ruona & Lynham, 2004, p. 154). Thus, axiology also entails directly observable manifestations of values; that is, actions referred to as methodologies and methods. A **methodology** is a general approach to practice. **Methods** are the actual processes and procedures used when working within a given methodology. Occupational therapy's axiology can be discerned by examining how the field's scholars and practitioners have addressed the following questions:

- What are occupational therapy's enduring values?
- What are the core methodologies and methods that practitioners use in practice that manifest its enduring values?

The elements of a philosophical framework are dynamic and each helps cocreate the other. We borrow an illustration from Parker Palmer (2009). Figure 3.1 uses a Mobius strip to depict the dynamic nature and ongoing transactions among occupational therapy's ontological, epistemological, and axiological premises. Beliefs about reality and knowledge are commonly more internal to the profession and individual practitioners and may be held without full conscious awareness; they are, therefore, depicted on what seems to be the "inside" of the

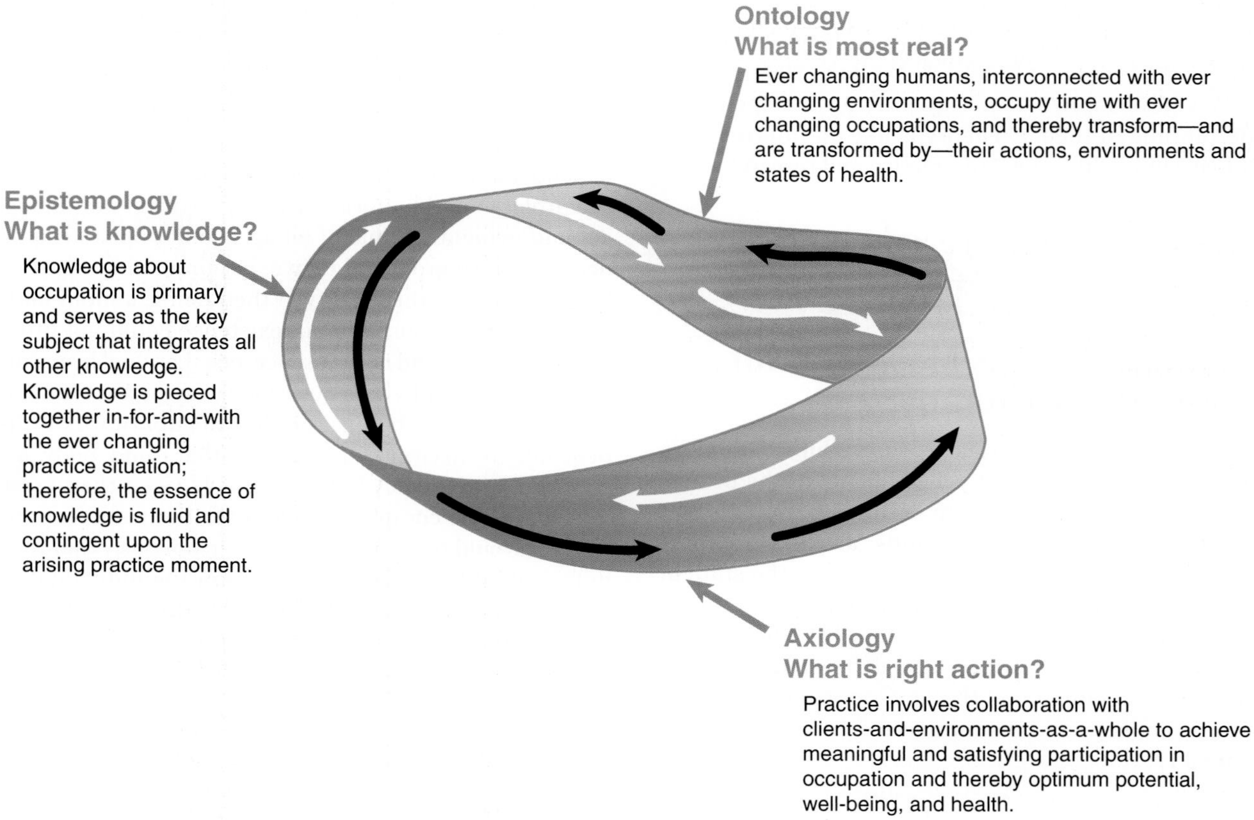
Ontology
What is most real?
Ever changing humans, interconnected with ever changing environments, occupy time with ever changing occupations, and thereby transform—and are transformed by—their actions, environments and states of health.
Epistemology
What is knowledge?
Knowledge about occupation is primary and serves as the key subject that integrates all other knowledge. Knowledge is pieced together in-for-and-with the ever changing practice situation; therefore, the essence of knowledge is fluid and contingent upon the arising practice moment.
Axiology
What is right action?
Practice involves collaboration with clients-and-environments-as-a-whole to achieve meaningful and satisfying participation in occupation and thereby optimum potential, well-being, and health.

FIGURE 3.1 An occupational therapy philosophical framework for practice.

Mobius strip. Beliefs about what actions to take, which are expressed in observable methodologies and methods, are depicted on what seems to be the "outside" of the strip. On closer examination, however, there is no dichotomy between an inside and outside on a Mobius strip. Rather, according to Palmer, the two sides keep cocreating each other. All three elements are fluid, mutually influential, and continually interacting. Ruona and Lynham (2004) accordingly argued that through their dynamic interactions, these elements form "a guiding framework for a congruent and coherent system of thought and action" (p. 154).

If Figure 3.1 were made into a three-dimensional object (we encourage readers to do so using instructions found in the web content), one's finger could continuously move from ontology to epistemology to axiology and so on, indicating that these three elements can be considered one whole. That is, professional beliefs about reality flow into and shape beliefs about knowledge, which flow into and shape actions manifest in practice. In reverse, professional actions and values flow into, reflect, and shape one's beliefs about reality, and continue around the Mobius strip reflecting and influencing beliefs about knowledge.

The Relationship of Philosophy to Theory

As argued in Chapter 37, it is not possible to construct theories in the absence of assumptions about the nature of reality and what it means to be human. This is because theory helps people understand their worlds; this understanding is inextricably linked to particular ways of seeing (ontology), thinking about (epistemology), and acting in the world (axiology) (Ruona & Lynham, 2004). A profession's philosophy is consequently an indispensable underpinning of theory. Theory is like an intermediary that helps bind philosophy to practice and research.

The Philosophy of Occupational Therapy

Ontology: What Is Most Real for Occupational Therapy?

In her 1961 Eleanor Clarke Slagle lectureship, Mary Reilly (1962) posed that the most central belief of the profession could be stated in the form of this hypothesis: "That man, through the use of his hands, as they are energized through mind and will, can influence the state of his own health" (p. 6). Influenced by Reilly's hypothesis, and also having considered ideas that have been more recently refined or introduced (as elaborated later), we propose that occupational therapy's most central ontological premises can be summarized today as follows (Figure 3.1):

> Ever changing humans, interconnected with ever changing environments, occupy time with ever changing occupations, and thereby transform—and are transformed by—their actions, environments and states of health.

We next elaborate on each element in the earlier statement, beginning with the ever changing occupational human.

The Nature of Humans, Ever Changing Occupational Beings

A profound view of human beings has served as a cornerstone of occupational therapy since its inception: Human beings are infused with an innate, biological need for occupation; as humans engage in daily occupations, they seek to meet needs for survival, growth, development, health, and well-being (Wilcock, 2006; Wood, 1993; 1998a; Yerxa, 1998). Dunton (1919) described humans' biological need for occupation quite simply, "Occupation is as necessary to life as food and drink" (p. 17). Reilly (1962) described humans' biological requirement for occupation in neurological terms. If the human organism is to grow and become productive, then there is a vital need for occupation; indeed, in her view, the central nervous system "demands the rich and varied stimuli that solving life problems provides" (p. 5). Wilcock (2006) likewise argued that occupation activates the integrative functions of the central nervous system, making it possible not only for individuals to develop and experience health and well-being but also for the species to survive.

Embedded in these descriptions of humans' need for occupation is another long-standing belief: Humans are an indivisible whole who possess an "inextricable union of the mind and body" (Bing, 1981, p. 306; Damasio, 1994). Mind, body, and spirit can be united in humans' pursuit of and engagement with occupation (Bing, 1981; Reed & Sanderson, 1999). A core philosophical assumption of the profession, therefore, is that by virtue of our biological endowment, people of all ages and abilities require occupation to grow and thrive; in pursuing occupation, humans express the totality of their being, a mind-body-spirit union. Because human existence could not otherwise be, humankind is, in essence, occupational by nature.

Yet as noted by Wilcock (2000), saying that humans are occupational beings, or that occupation is indispensable to survival and health, or that mind, body, and spirit are inextricably linked, is much easier than grasping what these complex articles of faith mean. Stopping there, it would be easy to conclude erroneously that these human qualities solely reside within the individual. As next discussed, one must also, therefore, consider how the environment calls forth, develops, and sustains the occupational essence of humans.

The Nature of Humans as Interconnected with Ever Changing Environments

Being interconnected with the environment does not denote either being in harmony with the environment or being fully determined by the environment. Occupational therapy's view of reality includes simply the belief that human beings, as indivisible wholes, are part and parcel of their daily living environments (Reed & Sanderson, 1999). Kielhofner (1983) posited, for example, that "unity of the human system with the social environment is not a platitude but is an essential part of the human condition" (p. 76). In Yerxa's (1998) words, people are "complex, multileveled (biological, psychological, social, spiritual) open systems who interact with their environments" (p. 411). She maintained that just like "water cannot be reduced to hydrogen and oxygen and still be wet and drinkable" neither can human beings be viewed as separate from their environments nor "be reduced to a single level, say that of the motor system, and retain their richness or identity" (p. 413).

Although an enduring belief of occupational therapy is that human beings are best understood in the context of their environments, beliefs about the person-environment relationship have evolved. Earlier conceptions of this relationship have been critiqued for separating the person and environment too much. According to Cutchin (2004), occupational therapy historically embraced a view of the environment "as a container" in which an individual carries out occupation. The individual was the focus; the environment the background. This view allowed understandings of people to be too easily separated from understandings of environments as eliciting people's actions and influencing how they perform and experience occupation. As an alternative, scholars advocate for a closer adherence to Dewey's transactionalism, in which the human is viewed as an "organism-in-environment-as-a-whole" (Dickie, Cutchin, & Humphry, 2006, p. 83). Or, as expressed in this chapter, human beings are interconnected with their environments.

The Nature of Transformation and Health

As humans, interconnected with their environments, enact their biological need for occupation, they continuously change. Thus, through occupation, people transform and are transformed by their actions and their environments. Transformation refers to change on both small and grand scales, change for both better and worse, and subtle change such as new manifestations of an unchanging essence. On a small scale, for example, recall a time when participating in a favorite occupation transformed your outlook, emotional state, and body sense. For me (Barb), I can be in the throes of anxiety, feeling out of shape and out of time. Yet, if I can convince myself to go for a bike ride, I am, almost immediately, transformed. My anxiety falls away, joy emerges, strength returns, and time opens. In such fashion, consider how often clients express that they feel much better after working in an occupational therapy to wash their face and brush their teeth for the first time after surgery. As Hasselkus (2011) persuasively illustrated, these taken-for-granted experiences and interactions reflect small scale, yet still very important, transformations through occupation; they can even be epiphanous.

Especially prominent in occupational therapy is the more grand-scale belief that people's health changes as a function of their occupations over time (e.g., Blanche & Henny-Kohler, 2000; Friedland, 2011; Hasselkus, 2011; Kielhofner, 2004; Meyer, 1922; Peloquin, 2005; Quiroga, 1995; Reed & Sanderson, 1999; Reilly, 1962; West, 1984). In occupational therapy, health is not viewed as the absence of disease or pathology but rather as being able to engage in valued occupations. Consequently, health encompasses a dynamic state of thriving and well-being, considerations of human dignity, realization of potential, functional competence, a good quality of life, and finding meaning and satisfaction in life (Hasselkus, 2011; Peloquin, 2005; Rogers, 1982a; Yerxa, 1983, 1998). People are viewed as being able to favorably influence these states of their health through occupation. Thus, occupational therapy's ontological view of human beings is an optimistic view.

This is not to say that the occupations in which people engage are seen as inevitably positive in either their subjective experiences or consequences. Because engagement in occupation is a biological necessity, when people fail to use—for whatever reasons—their powers to act, when they are unable to develop their potentials, when they are thwarted in being able to express their capacities for doing, then the change is toward states of dysfunction, dissatisfaction, poor health, and ill-being. What people do each day can lead to boredom, anxiety, depression, alienation, dysfunction, and ill-health. So, too, can what they do lead to excitement, happiness, satisfaction, competence, and good health.

Ultimately, changes on a grand scale over time, whether for better or worse, can be understood to result from transformations that occur on a small scale each day. Furthermore, people's persistent "doings" can change not only themselves for both better and worse, but their doings can also change communities, societies, and the health of the planet for both better and worse (Wilcock, 2006). Although occupational therapy's optimistic view of humans does not deny these realities, it does foreground attention to the inherent potential of all people to experience and cultivate, through occupation, a better life for themselves and others. As well summarized by Peloquin (2005), a core belief of occupational therapy is that there is, in occupation, a "capacity to help individuals become hale and whole" (p. 614).

Epistemology: What Is Knowledge in Occupational Therapy?

Occupational therapy's dominant perspective of reality and the nature of humans "sets priorities for knowledge"

(Kielhofner & Burke, 1983, p. 43). As shown in Figure 3.1, we propose that the profession's most central epistemological premises today can be summarized as follows:

> Knowledge about occupation is primary and serves as the key subject that integrates all other knowledge and clarifies the desired consequences of action. Toward that end, knowledge is pieced together in-for-and-with the present practice situation that is continuously changing; therefore, the essence of knowledge is both bound and fluid, contingent upon the arising practice moment.

We elaborate on this epistemological premise by discussing each of its elements.

Knowledge of Occupation Is Primary for Occupational Therapists

Given occupational therapy's ontological premises, what is most important to know? Overwhelmingly, the answer is knowledge about occupation. As proclaimed by Weimer (1979), "Ours is, and must be, the basic knowledge of occupation" (p. 43). Reilly (1962) advised that knowledge about anatomy, neurophysiology, personality theory, social processes, and medical conditions that affect these functions, while relevant, are not our unique content. Rather, in Reilly's (1962, 1974) view, the unique knowledge of occupational therapy is a deep understanding of the nature of work and productive activity, including the play–work continuum, a belief that she believed aligned with what the founders of occupational therapy saw as most central to the new field. That occupation continues to be held today as the foremost subject matter of occupational therapy has been corroborated extensively (e.g., Hasselkus, 2011; Hooper, 2006; Molineux, 2004; Townsend, 1999; Wilcock, 2006; Wood et al., 2000).

As the Primary Subject, Knowledge about Occupation Organizes and Integrates All Other Knowledge

In addition to what's most important to know, epistemology entails questions such as does knowledge have a structure? If so, then how is the structure to be conceptualized? Such questions are of particular interest because knowledge of occupation entails so many, and sometimes seemingly disparate, topics ranging from kinesiology to ethics and culture. Students can feel lost in the field's wide array of topics and, not seeing an organization among them, may mistakenly think that they can pick and choose based on personal interests. It is reassuring, therefore, that scholars have promoted the view that knowledge in occupational therapy has a structure.

For example, Kielhofner (1983) conceptualized occupational therapy knowledge as a matrix consisting of three integrated and hierarchical domains: biological, psychological, and social knowledge. Neuromusculoskeletal and kinematic knowledge was placed at the bottom of the biologic hierarchy, not because it was considered basic knowledge for the field but because it was viewed as being influenced by knowledge at higher levels of the hierarchy, namely, the psychological, social, and symbolic dimensions of occupation. Given this structure, biologic knowledge *works* for occupational therapists when it is understood to be regulated by the psychological, social, and symbolic dimensions of occupation. For example, although two people may have an identical injury, "A hand injury to an accountant is not the same as a hand injury to a clock maker" (p. 79). In the same way, a hip fracture for a retired married man is not the same as a hip fracture for a woman who is the caregiver for an ailing spouse. Each situation is unique because of the roles, values, goals, interests, and culture (i.e., psychological, social, and symbolic levels of Kielhofner's structure) into which the injury is introduced and for which it has consequences. Conversely, although two people may have disparate diagnoses, say, schizophrenia or spinal cord injury, they may both share the identical *occupational* diagnosis of limited occupational choice, again due to what is occurring at higher psychologic, symbolic, and social levels of each person.

Kielhofner (2004) later modified the relationship between knowledge domains from hierarchical to heterarchical, yet the transactional structure among biologic, psychological, social, and symbolic domains remained central to understanding human performance and participation. That is, the arrangements of musculoskeletal components during performance occur in spontaneous dynamic transaction with internal and external components such as intention and contours of an object.

As the Primary Subject, Knowledge about Occupation Clarifies Desired Consequences of Action

What is most important to know and how that knowledge is organized is often linked to a group's vision for society or a set of desired consequences that a group would like to see realized (MacIntyre, 1990). Pragmatist philosophers described knowledge as continually being developed and evaluated in light of "a coveted future" (Hooper & Wood, 2002, p. 42). Thus, knowledge about occupation and how it is structured reflects a future, a set of desired consequences toward which the profession aims. That future is the optimal participation of individuals and populations in health-promoting occupations (Wilcock, 2006). This desired future serves as the beacon toward which practitioners aim their knowledge. The exact path for arriving at this distant beacon is discovered through active experimentation that involves piecing occupational therapy knowledge together for a given practice situation and evaluating the results in light of how well it contributed to the desired consequence of participation in occupation.

Knowledge is Pieced Together In-for-and-with the Ever Changing Practice Situation

Knowledge in occupational therapy is bound by subject, structure, and consequence. However, working within that boundary, practitioners continuously compose knowledge domains and modes of reasoning for each practice situation. For example, in Chapter 30, Schell illustrates how practitioners assimilate and use knowledge in multiple domains, including knowledge of (1) their own beliefs, values, abilities, and experiences; (2) professional theories, evidence, and skills; (3) clients' beliefs, values, abilities, and experiences; (4) clients' goals, expectations for therapy, and how health conditions impact clients' occupations; and (5) the practice culture and its influence on services. Additionally, practitioners shift rapidly among and integrate multiple modes of reasoning including scientific, narrative, pragmatic, ethical, and interactive reasoning (Mattingly & Fleming, 1994; B. Schell, 2009).

Practitioners not only integrate multiple knowledge domains through multiple reasoning processes but they also do so again and again with each practice situation. Even if on the surface the situation seems routine, it is likely unique in subtle ways such as the emotional state of the therapist or client, a change in schedule, or a change in the social environment, all of which can make the present practice situation one of a kind. Practitioners recognize that each practice situation is unique and changing even within a single therapy session. Thus, practitioners continuously assemble knowledge with and in response to each practice situation as it presents itself in each moment. Another way of saying this is: Practitioners use occupational therapy knowledge by configuring it for and with each practice situation.

The Essence of Knowledge Is Tentative, Fluid, and Contingent with the Arising Practice Moment

The earlier discussion culminates in the central consideration in epistemology: What is the nature of knowledge? In sum, knowledge in occupational therapy is bounded by its subject, occupation, and its desired consequence, health-promoting occupational engagement of individuals and populations. Additionally, there are structures for how knowledge about occupation relates to knowledge about its various elements. The subject, structure, and consequence of knowledge serve as boundaries for knowledge in the field. On the surface, these boundaries seem somewhat stable, yet they are always evolving in how we understand and talk about them. Thus, they are paradoxically enduring and tentative. On these seemingly stable foundations, occupational therapy knowledge is newly pieced together in-for-and-with each practice situation. Such an understanding of knowledge is highly compatible with views of knowledge associated with pragmatism (Hooper & Wood, 2002, p. 42).

> Pragmatists promoted a view of knowledge as flexible, fallible, and contingent. . . . Knowledge was flexible because it was determined in the making and doing of direct experience and, therefore, could not be "found" or become fixed. Knowledge was fallible because it was always being overturned by better ways of explaining or understanding things. . . . Knowledge was likewise contingent because it issued from an iterative process between action and particular contexts.

The essence of knowledge in occupational therapy is, thus, like a musical score. The practice of music is bounded by notes, music theory, and principles. These seemingly stable boundaries (understood and described in new ways over time) are continuously assembled into new pieces of music, and even the same pieces of music are experimented with and played with, given new interpretations in-for-and-with changing audiences and sociocultural situations. This tentative, fluid, and contingent view of knowledge means that practice is bounded within the unique knowledge base and philosophy of occupational therapy and, within that boundary, is fluid, contingent on the practice moment.

That knowledge arises from the practice moment in a fluid and contingent manner is important for occupational therapy students to understand because it has everything to do with how students learn. That is, along with learning discrete content and skills, students need also to learn how to assemble knowledge, evaluate knowledge, and create knowledge in-for-and-with practice situations. To meet this epistemological challenge, some students find they have to dramatically shift how they have viewed themselves for many years from a learner who receives knowledge from experts to a learner who thoughtfully and reflectively acquires and integrates knowledge and uses it flexibly according to what is needed for a practice situation.

Axiology: What Is Right Action in Occupational Therapy?

The profession's axiology answers the questions, *Given occupational therapy's central beliefs about reality and knowledge, how then shall we live day to day in practice? What do we value? What will we do?* As illustrated in Figure 3.1, views of reality and of knowledge "shape and direct how we *act* in the world. . ." (Ruona & Lynham, 2004, p. 154). Coherence between how we act in practice and the other aspects of the field's philosophy is important to work out because as Wilcock (1999) cautioned,

> Skills without a philosophy can be a problem. It allows poaching outside a domain of concern, duplication of skills already available to those being served, the dropping of established skills for different ones when some other discipline

changes its direction, or sticking to familiar skills because of no mandate to inform the direction to be taken. (p. 193)

To illustrate links between skills and philosophy, we discuss three key practice methodologies. We do not believe that these methodologies are comprehensive; for example, they do not encompass important values and actions outlined in the Occupational Therapy Code of Ethics (American Occupational Therapy Association, 2010). We do believe, however, that these methodologies help to illustrate how actions flow from the field's ontological and epistemological premises. In accordance with those premises, we propose that occupational therapy's axiology can be summarized as follows (Figure 3.1):

> Practice involves collaboration with clients-and-environments-as-a-whole to achieve meaningful and satisfying participation in occupation and thereby optimal potential, well-being, and health.

Collaborative Practice

Because ever changing humans, environments and occupations are central to occupational therapy's beliefs about reality, it follows that entering into a personal collaboration with clients is a fundamental methodology for practice. Students will recognize this as client-centered practice but may not have considered how client-centered practice is an outward manifestation of a broader philosophical framework. Considered in light of the philosophical framework in Figure 3.1, collaborative relationships are a natural extension from the profession's ontology. Through collaborative relationships, practitioners explore the occupations and environments that each client has found engaging over time, the occupational hopes of each client, the occupations that will and will not serve as therapeutic experiences for each client, and how clients have changed, are changing now, and view future change. Similarly, if occupational therapy's central belief about knowledge involves piecing knowledge together in-for-and-with each situation, it follows that collaboration is necessary in order for the practitioner to determine which elements of knowledge and experience to assemble for the current situation. Thus, collaborative, relationship-centered practice constitutes a methodology that manifests occupational therapy values and beliefs about reality and knowledge.

By using the term, *methodology*, we do not mean to portray collaborative practice as a technical procedure; it is, rather, a long-standing, normative way of practicing occupational therapy and exhibiting the profession's values. As Peloquin (2005) stated, "occupational therapy *is* [emphasis added] personal engagement." Watson (2006) elaborated, stating that if we are true to the field's philosophy,

> We will make a personal connection with people in a personal way. The people we are, who we have become . . . and our earnest desire to be of service, will lead us to reach out to the "being" of the "other." (p. 156)

This textbook has much to say about occupational therapy's use of collaboration as a methodology in practice. Our purpose here is to highlight how collaborative practice as a methodology stems directly from and manifests the field's views of reality, knowledge, and right action. Collaborative practice can, therefore, serve as a stimulus for reflecting on the congruence between philosophy and practice by asking the following:

- Does this assessment or intervention or my way of being with this client reflect collaborative, relationship-centered care?
- Is collaboration at the center of my actions as an occupational therapist?

Each practitioner will have to work out specific methods for collaborative practice within the parameters of client populations served, cultural contexts for services, and practice setting, among others. But whatever challenges present, collaborative, relationship-centered care is one methodology that naturally expresses the field's core values, ontology, and epistemology.

Occupation-Centered Practice

Because occupation is at the very center of an occupational therapy view of reality and what practitioners most need to know, it follows that a core methodology for practice is to help clients participate in meaningful, satisfying, and health-promoting occupations. Since the field's origin, practitioners have provided opportunities for people to engage in occupation and, in so doing, to develop and transform their skills and potential. Students may recognize this methodology as occupation-centered or occupation-based practice (see e.g., Christiansen, Baum, & Bass-Haugen, 2005; Kielhofner, 2004; West, 1984; Wood, 1998b). This methodology means that practitioners focus on occupational performance issues and experiences. Right from the start of care, practitioners seek to understand the things that clients want and need to do and use those as intervention. Short of that, practitioners make explicit how their therapeutic approaches relate to and support the occupations that clients want and need to do. According to Price and Miner (2007), placing occupational performance issues and occupation itself front and center of one's actions is a complex process that emerges from within each practice situation through collaborative relationships with clients. Therefore, like collaborative practice, occupation-centered practice is grounded in and manifests beliefs about the occupational nature of humans and about knowledge as continuously being put together in-and-with each situation.

This textbook has much to say about the use of occupation-centered practice as a methodology. Our purpose here is to highlight how occupation-centered practice is a natural right action directly stemming from and manifesting the field's views of reality and knowledge.

Occupation-centered practice can, thus, serve as a stimulus for reflecting on the congruence between philosophy and practice by asking the following:

- Does this assessment or intervention or my way of being with this client reflect occupation-centered practice?
- Is occupation at the center of my actions as an occupational therapist?
- Am I making a credible and meaningful connection for clients between occupation and each therapeutic approach that I use?

Once again, although each practitioner will have to work out specific methods for occupation-centered practice within the parameters of client populations served, cultural contexts for services, and practice settings, among others, occupation-centered practice is a methodology that naturally expresses the field's core values, ontology, and epistemology.

Context in Practice: Clients-and-environments-as-a-whole

The emphasis in occupational therapy's central belief about reality as an essential unity existing between people and environments leads to a third important methodology for practice, referred to here as clients-and-environments-as-a-whole. Occupations that are meaningful to clients—where they occur and with whom, the habits with which occupations are carried out, and the routines that help organize them, and even the musculoskeletal patterns used to perform them—occur in an interconnection between the environment and the client. This is equally true for the environments in which clients live and the environments in which they receive occupational therapy services, for example, the hospital, rehabilitation center, outpatient clinic, skilled nursing facility, home, work, school, or community (Cutchin, 2004).

According to Hasselkus (2011), seeing clients as tightly knit together with their environments through memories of places, occupation, meanings, roles, routines, and intentions, can positively influence therapy outcomes related to adoption and follow-through with environmental modifications. Conversely, when practitioners view clients as separate from environments, they may overly focus on clients' performance. For example, practitioners may make recommendations for environmental modifications from a template such as widen doorways, put in stair lifts, remove throw rugs, add medical equipment, rearrange furniture, and move items to within easy reach. But because these recommendations have been considered as separate from the client-environment-as-a-whole, the family may refuse to implement them.

Like the other methodologies presented, this textbook has much to say about occupational therapy's use of the performance context as a methodology in practice. Our purpose here is to illustrate how clients-and-environments-as-a-whole constitute a natural right action stemming directly from and manifesting the field's views of reality and knowledge. Clients-and-environments-as-a-whole can, therefore, serve as a stimulus for reflecting on the congruence between philosophy and practice by asking the following:

- Does this assessment or intervention or my way of being with this client reflect the unity reflected in clients-and-environments-as-a-whole?

Although each practitioner will, again, have to work out specific methods associated with this methodology within the multiple parameters previously mentioned, clients-and-environments-as-a-whole is a methodology that naturally expresses the field's core values, ontology, and epistemology.

Core Values in Occupational Therapy's Axiology

Lastly, though perhaps most importantly, the methodologies briefly presented earlier uphold and manifest core values of the profession that have been prominent throughout its history (see e.g., Bing, 1981; Meyer, 1922; Peloquin, 1995, 2005, 2007; Yerxa, 1983). More specifically, inherent in these methodologies is a distinct valuing of and respect for

- The essential humanity and dignity of all people;
- The perspectives and subjective experiences of clients and their significant others;
- Empathy, caring, and genuine engagement in the therapeutic encounter;
- The use of imagination and integrity in creating occupational opportunities; and
- The inherent potential of people to experience well-being.

Application to Practice: From a Philosophical Framework to a Philosophical Mode of Thinking

Application of the philosophy of occupational therapy to practice requires a philosophical mode of thinking. A philosophical mode of thinking is bidirectional. In other words, this mode of thinking requires that a practitioner reflect on occupational therapy's philosophical assumptions about reality, knowledge, values, and action and walk those assumptions forward into practices that intentionally manifest them; it also involves reflecting on one's practice and identifying the assumptions about reality, knowledge, values, and action that it seems to manifest. Practicing this mode of thinking will help a practitioner develop a philosophical mind, which may be the most indispensable element of practice.

To further illustrate, consider Paul's (1995) contrast between a philosophical and nonphilosophical mind. The nonphilosophical mind is largely unaware that it thinks within a framework of assumptions and beliefs. Without a clear sense of the foundations that direct it, the nonphilosophical mind cannot critique those foundations; it is, therefore, somewhat trapped or run by its own unconscious, inherited system of thinking. The nonphilosophical mind tends to conform to how things are done, preferring straightforward methods and procedures without realizing that those also stem from systems of thinking. There is little awareness of a broader framework in light of which methods and procedures need to be evaluated.

Conversely, the philosophical mind is aware that all thinking occurs within and from a set of assumptions, beliefs, and values. It is keen on probing those, seeking congruence among them, and realizing them in action. The philosophical mind probes the systems of thinking reflected in methods and procedures and seeks to continuously refine those in light of its chosen broader framework of thinking. Because the philosophical mind does not confuse its own thinking with reality, it continuously considers alternative and refined thinking frameworks.

The two scenarios in the Practice Dilemma box (and additional learning activities on the Web) provide opportunities to build a philosophical mode of thinking, hence, to become more philosophically minded. The two scenarios are real, and we have portrayed them as accurately as possible based on direct knowledge of typical practices in each setting. We selected the scenarios because of their contrasts related to application of the philosophy of occupational therapy.

Specifically, the practices in Setting A suggest that practitioners are well grounded in the philosophy of occupational therapy and apply a philosophical mode of thinking to how they conceive and deliver services. The practices in Setting B suggest only weak links to the profession's

Practice Dilemma

Setting A

In Setting A, occupational therapy practitioners meet each morning to determine how the client caseload will be distributed and, as opportunities permit, collaborate across the day on intervention ideas. Priorities for self-care are determined with clients and only prioritized activities of daily living (ADL) tasks are addressed. In response to the many priorities of clients beyond basic and instrumental ADL, new occupational spaces have been created in the rehab "gym"; these include an office area with computers and Internet access and a work area in which various mechanical, leisure, or work-related activities occur. The kitchen is in constant use for clients whose priorities involve aspects of home management. After morning ADL, the day is filled with individual sessions, which range from 30 minutes to 1 hour, in addition to one group session. This scheduling approach meets productivity requirements. The occupational therapists played a leadership role in designing the group in which clients commit to completing one realistic occupational project over 3 to 5 days such as, for instance, outdoor picnics for clients and their families, collecting clothing for a women's shelter, and visiting a local flea market. Steps and tasks within these projects are assigned based on clients' interests and the likelihood that they will be both challenged and successful. Although individual sessions may include exercises as a "warm-up," the focus is on either an individual occupational goals or aspects of the group occupational project. Clients are also often given "occupational homework" for weekends. Significant others are encouraged to take part in both individual and group therapy sessions. When possible, home visits are undertaken to help identify what occupations take place in what spaces and to collaborate with clients and their significant others about acceptable modifications. Discharge planning involves setting up environments and tasks as closely as possible to clients' usual contexts and performance patterns.

Setting B

In Setting B, occupational therapy practitioners meet each morning to determine how the client caseload will be distributed and then go about their day largely independent of each other. All clients receive occupational therapy for basic ADL in the morning; practitioners emphasize ADL independence and typically complete the same ADL tasks with all clients. The rest of the day consists of consecutive 30-minute individual sessions followed by brief documentation breaks; this way of scheduling sessions is sufficient to meet the high productivity demand of the setting. Sessions emphasize physical components of function such as range of motion, strength, and endurance; prominently used modalities include theraband or putty, the range of motion arc, cones, wrist weights, the upper extremity ergometer, pulleys, dowel exercises, various physical agent modalities, and ball or balloon toss. Also addressed are visual-perceptual and cognitive components of function using modalities such as paper and pencil activities, puzzles, peg boards, and computer-based exercises. Intervention seldom varies from client to client, and some clients question why they need to see the occupational therapist because they already had their "therapy," that is, physical therapy that day. There is a kitchen that is used for splinting and staff meetings. Significant others are discouraged from attending therapy so that clients will not be distracted. When a client needs two people to complete a transfer or ambulate, an occupational therapist and a physical therapist may see the client together. Discharge planning may include a kitchen activity such as making a cup of tea to determine safety for returning home. Significant others receive training the last day of service before a client is discharged.

philosophy and little evidence of a philosophical mode of thinking. Despite this divergence, both scenarios are from fast-paced, for-profit hospitals with subacute adult neurorehabilitation programs in which demands for productivity are equally high. Also in both settings, clients have various neurological conditions and many have suffered from strokes or other brain injuries. Occupational therapy is provided two or three times daily in both settings and length of stay typically ranges from 3 to 10 days.

As you read each of these practice dilemmas, consider how philosophy contributes to the different practice approaches in each setting. Specifically,

1. Identify both ontological and epistemological assumptions and beliefs that are manifested in how occupational therapy is understood and practiced in each scenario.
2. Identify core values that underlie the predominant practice methodologies and methods in each scenario.
3. Guided by Figure 3.1, identify areas of congruence and incongruence with the philosophy of occupational therapy in each scenario.
4. For Setting A, identify strategies that practitioners may have used to help them practice in a philosophically minded manner. Do you believe these same strategies might have been possible in Setting B? Why or why not?

Conclusion

We presented a philosophical framework consisting of three elements: ontology, epistemology, and axiology. Each element can be thought of as a "resting place," if you will, on the Mobius strip in Figure 3.1. At each rest, corresponding philosophical assumptions were identified and described. Having identified and described philosophical assumptions about reality at the ontology resting place, we traced them into assumptions about knowledge. Having then identified and described philosophical assumptions about knowledge, we traced those, along with the ontology, into assumptions about right action. Finally, a few sample methodologies and values were identified and described at the axiology resting place. The philosophical framework was applied to two practice scenarios.

As is true of all professions, belonging to and working in occupational therapy requires fidelity to its unique philosophy and practice approaches and, additionally, building congruence between those and one's personal philosophies. Wilcock (1999) urged that if examination suggests strong *in*compatibility between professional and personal philosophies, then engagement with occupational therapy should likely cease for the good of the professional (or student), future clients, and the profession itself. Conversely, Wilcock related congruence between one's personal philosophy and one's professional philosophy with the possibility for meaningful, satisfying, sustaining, and impactful work. Thus are the stakes high for engaging in philosophical modes of thinking.

References

American Occupational Therapy Association. (2010). Occupational therapy code of ethics and ethics standards. *American Journal of Occupational Therapy, 64*(Suppl), S17–S26.

Bing, R. K. (1981). Eleanor Clarke Slagle Lectureship—1981. Occupational therapy revisited: a paraphrastic journey. *American Journal of Occupational Therapy, 35*, 499–518.

Blanche, E. I., & Henny-Kohler, E. (2000). Philosophy, science and ideology: A proposed relationship for occupational science and occupational therapy. *Occupational Therapy International, 7*, 99–110.

Breines, E. (1986). *Origins and adaptations: A philosophy of practice.* Lebanon, NJ: Geri-Rehab.

Breines, E. (1987). Pragmatism as a foundation for occupational therapy curricula. *American Journal of Occupational Therapy, 41*, 522–525.

Bruce, M. A., & Borg, B. (2002). *Psychosocial occupational therapy: Frames of reference for intervention.* Thorofare, NJ: Slack.

Christiansen, C. H., Baum, C. M., & Bass-Haugen, J. (Eds.). (2005). *Occupational therapy: Performance, participation, and well-being.* Thorofare, NJ: Slack.

Cutchin, M. P. (2004). Using Deweyan philosophy to rename and reframe adaptation-to-environment. *American Journal of Occupational Therapy, 58*, 303–312.

Damasio, A. (1994). *Descartes' error: Emotion, reason, and the human brain.* New York, NY: Putnam.

Devereaux, E. B. (1984). Occupational therapy's challenge: The caring relationship. *American Journal of Occupational Therapy, 38*, 791–798.

Dickie, V., Cutchin, M. P., & Humphry, R. (2006). Occupation as transactional experience: A critique of individualism in occupational science. *Journal of Occupational Science, 13*, 83–93.

Dunton, W. R. (1919). *Reconstruction therapy.* Philadelphia, PA: W.B. Saunders.

Finlay, L. (2001). Holism in occupational therapy: Elusive fiction an ambivalent struggle. *American Journal of Occupational Therapy, 55*, 268–276.

Friedland, J. (2003). Muriel Driver Memorial lecture: Why crafts? Influences on the development of occupational therapy in Canada from 1890 to 1930. *Canadian Journal of Occupational Therapy, 70*, 204–212.

Friedland, J. (2011). *Restoring the spirit: The beginnings of occupational therapy in Canada, 1890–1930.* Montreal, Canada: McGill-Queen's University Press.

Hasselkus, B. R. (2011). *The meaning of everyday occupation* (2nd ed.). Thorofare, NJ: Slack.

Hocking, C. (2008). The way we were: Romantic assumptions of pioneering occupational therapists in the United Kingdom. *British Journal of Occupational Therapy, 71*, 146–154.

Hooper, B. (2006). Beyond active learning: A case study of teaching practices in an occupation-centered curriculum. *American Journal of Occupational Therapy, 60*, 551–562.

Hooper, B. (2008). Therapists' assumptions as a dimension of professional reasoning. In B. A. Schell & J. W. Schell (Eds.), *Clinical and professional reasoning in occupational therapy* (pp. 13–35). Baltimore, MD: Lippincott, Williams & Wilkins.

Hooper, B., & Wood, W. (2002). Pragmatism and structuralism in occupational therapy: The long conversation. *American Journal of Occupational Therapy, 56*, 40–50.

Ikiugu, M., & Schultz, S. (2006). An argument for pragmatism as a foundational philosophy of occupational therapy. *Canadian Journal of Occupational Therapy, 73*, 86–96.

Kielhofner, G. (1983). *Health through occupation: Theory and practice in occupational therapy.* Philadelphia, PA: F. A. Davis.

Kielhofner, G. (2004). *Conceptual foundations of occupational therapy* (3rd ed.). Philadelphia, PA: F. A. Davis.

Kielhofner, G., & Burke, J. (1983). The evolution of knowledge and practice in occupational therapy: Past, present, and future. In G. Kielhofner (Ed.), *Health through occupation: Theory and practice in occupational therapy* (pp. 3–54). Philadelphia, PA: F. A. Davis.

Levine, R. E. (1987). The influence of the arts-and-crafts movement on the professional status of occupational therapy. *American Journal of Occupational Therapy, 41*, 248–254.

Lincoln, Y. S., Lynham, S. A., & Guba, E. G. (2011). Paradigmatic controversies, contradictions, and emerging confluences, revisited. In N. K. Denzin & Y. S. Lincoln (Eds.), *Handbook of qualitative research*. Thousand Oaks, CA: Sage.

MacIntyre, A. C. (1990). *First principles, final ends and contemporary philosophical issues*. Milwaukee, WE: Marquette University Press.

Mattingly, C., & Fleming, M. H. (1994). *Clinical reasoning: Forms of inquiry in a therapeutic practice*. Philadelphia, PA: F. A. Davis.

Meyer, A. (1922). The philosophy of occupation therapy. *Archives of Occupational Therapy, 1*, 1–10.

Molineux, M. (2004). *Occupation for occupational therapists*. Oxford, United Kingdom: Blackwell.

Nelson, D. L. (1997). Why the profession of occupational therapy will flourish in the 21st century: The 1996 Eleanor Clarke Slagle Lecture. *American Journal of Occupational Therapy, 51*, 11–24.

Palmer, P. J. (2009). *Hidden wholeness: The journey toward an undivided life*. San Francisco, CA: Wiley & Sons.

Paul, R. (1995). *Critical thinking: How to prepare students for a rapidly changing world*. Santa Rosa, CA: Foundation for Critical Thinking.

Peloquin, S. M. (1995). The fullness of empathy: Reflections and illustrations. *American Journal of Occupational Therapy, 49*, 24–31.

Peloquin, S. M. (2005). The 2005 Eleanor Clark Slagle Lecture—Embracing our ethos, reclaiming our heart. *American Journal of Occupational Therapy, 59*, 611–625.

Peloquin, S. M. (2007). A reconsideration of occupational therapy's core values. *American Journal of Occupational Therapy, 61*, 474–478.

Philosophy. (n.d.). In *Online etymology dictionary*. Retrieved from http://www.etymonline.com/index.php?allowed_in_frame=0&search=philosophy&searchmode=none

Price, P., & Miner, S. (2007). Occupation emerges in the process of therapy. *American Journal of Occupational Therapy, 61*, 441–450.

Punwar, A. J., & Peloquin, S. (2000). *Occupational therapy principles and practice* (3rd ed.). Baltimore, MD: Lippincott Williams & Wilkins.

Quiroga, V. A. M. (1995). *Occupational therapy: The first 30 years 1900 to 1930*. Bethesda, MD: American Occupational Therapy Association.

Reed, K. L. (1986). Tools of practice: Heritage or baggage? 1986 Eleanor Clarke Slagle Lecture. *American Journal of Occupational Therapy, 40*, 597–605.

Reed, K. L. (2005). Dr. Hall and the work cure. *Occupational Therapy in Health Care, 19*, 33–50.

Reed, K. L., & Sanderson, S. N. (1999). *Concepts of occupational therapy* (4th ed.). Philadelphia, PA: Lippincott, Williams & Wilkins.

Reilly, M. (1962). Eleanor Clarke Slagle Lecture—Occupational therapy can be one of the greatest ideas of 20th century medicine. *American Journal of Occupational Therapy, 16*, 1–9.

Reilly, M. (1974). *Play as exploratory learning*. Beverly Hills, CA: Sage.

Rogers, J. C. (1982a). Order and disorder in medicine and occupational therapy. *American Journal of Occupational Therapy, 36*, 29–35.

Rogers, J. C. (1982b). The spirit of independence: The evolution of a philosophy. *American Journal of Occupational Therapy, 36*, 709–715.

Ruona, W. E. A., & Lynham, S. A. (2004). A philosophical framework for thought and practice in human resource development. *Human Resource Development International, 7*, 151–164.

Schell, B. (2009). Professional reasoning in practice. In E. B. Crepeau, E. S. Cohn, & B. Schell (Eds.), *Willard & Spackman's occupational therapy* (11th ed., pp. 314–327). Philadelphia, PA: Lippincott Williams & Wilkins.

Schell, J. W. (2008). Epistemology: Knowing how you know. In B. A. Schell & J. W. Schell (Eds.), *Clinical and professional reasoning in occupational therapy* (pp. 229–257). Philadelphia, PA: Lippincott Williams & Wilkins.

Sire, J. W. (2009). *Universe next door: A basic worldview catalog*. Madison, WI: Inter-Varsity Press.

Townsend, E. (1999). Enabling occupation in the 21st century: Making good intentions a reality. *Australian Occupational Therapy Journal, 46*, 147–159.

Watson, R. M. (2006). Being before doing: The cultural identity (essence) of occupational therapy. *Australian Occupational Therapy Journal, 53*, 151–158.

Weimer, R. (1979). Traditional and nontraditional practice arenas. In *Occupational therapy: 2001 AD*. Rockville, MD: American Occupational Therapy Association.

West, W. L. (1984). A reaffirmed philosophy and practice of occupational therapy for the 1980s. *American Journal of Occupational Therapy, 38*, 15–23.

Wilcock, A. A. (1999). Reflections on doing, being and becoming. Republished with kind permission from the Canadian Journal of Occupational Therapy, *65*, 248–257. *Australian Occupational Therapy Journal, 46*, 1–11.

Wilcock, A. A. (2000). Development of a personal, professional and educational occupational philosophy: An Australian perspective. *Occupational Therapy International, 7*, 79–86.

Wilcock, A. A. (2006). *An occupational perspective on health* (Vol. 2). Thorofare, NJ: Slack.

Wood, W. (1993). Occupation and the relevance of primatology to occupational therapy. *American Journal of Occupational Therapy, 47*, 515–522.

Wood, W. (1998a). Biological requirements for occupation in primates: An exploratory study and theoretical analysis. *Journal of Occupational Science, 5*, 66–81.

Wood, W. (1998b). Special issue—Occupation centered practice. *American Journal of Occupational Therapy, 52*.

Wood, W., Nielson, C., Humphry, R., Coppola, S., Baranek, G., & Rourk, J. (2000). A curricular renaissance: Graduate education centered on occupation. *American Journal of Occupational Therapy, 54*, 586–597.

Yerxa, E. J. (1967). 1966 Eleanor Clarke Slagle lecture. Authentic occupational therapy. *American Journal of Occupational Therapy, 21*, 1–9.

Yerxa, E. J. (1979). The philosophical base of occupational therapy. In *Occupational therapy: 2001 AD* (pp. 26–30). Rockville, MD: American Occupational Therapy Association.

Yerxa, E. J. (1983). Audacious values: The energy source for occupational therapy practice. In G. Kielhofner (Ed.), *Health through occupation: Theory and practice in occupational therapy* (pp. 149–162). Philadelphia, PA: F. A. Davis.

Yerxa, E. J. (1998). Health and the human spirit for occupation. *American Journal of Occupational Therapy, 52*, 412–422.

For additional resources on the subjects discussed in this chapter, visit http://thePoint.lww.com/Willard-Spackman12e.

CHAPTER 4

Contemporary Occupational Therapy Practice

*Barbara A. Boyt Schell, Marjorie E. Scaffa,
Glen Gillen, Ellen S. Cohn*

"People are most true to their humanity when engaged in occupation."

—Yerxa et al. (1989)

OUTLINE

LEARNING OBJECTIVES

After reading this chapter, you will be able to:

1. Define occupational therapy
2. Explain the focus of the profession using professionally relevant terminology
3. Discuss the occupational therapy process including core aspects of practice
4. Describe aspects of the workforce of the profession in the United States and worldwide
5. Consider possible futures for the profession

Occupational Therapy in Action

Contemporary occupational therapists work with a vast array of clients in many settings. A selection of clients and settings are outlined in Case Study 4.1.

These six scenarios represent the diversity of occupational therapy intervention for occupational therapy clients, be they individuals, groups, organizations, or populations. Maxine wants to continue to enjoy her friends and her creative activities while dealing with the challenges of aging. Her daughter wants to know that she is safe in a supportive environment. Lydia wants to show that she is responsible so that she can be a good mother, find fulfilling work, and stay a welcome member of her church while avoiding the temptations to start drinking again. Linda wants to be able to work and be competitive so that she can earn as much as possible in her job. Lauro wants to be more autonomous from his parents, use public transportation, live in his own apartment someday, and learn job skills to prepare him for life after high school. Larry wants to adjust to life after injury while

CASE STUDY 4.1 Examples of Clients and Settings

Maxine

Maxine is a retired librarian who lives in a life care community. She moved into a duplex there shortly after her husband's death because her sons all lived in another state and she didn't feel she could manage all the house and yard work. Shortly after she moved in, the occupational therapist met with her to help her with her transition to her new home. The occupational therapist encouraged her to explore the crafts room because quilting and making furnishings for miniature doll houses were long time hobbies of hers. Over time, Maxine became the leader of a crafts group of several women, sharing her files of patterns and showing others how to do needlework.

After about 3 years, some of the women in her group began to notice that Maxine was becoming very anxious and forgetful and alerted the nursing staff. Eventually, Maxine was diagnosed with multi-infarct dementia. The occupational therapist and the nurse both evaluated Maxine and recommended that she be placed on a program where her medications were managed by the nursing staff. Additionally because Maxine still had her driver's license, the occupational therapist conducted a screening of key factors related to driving, including vision, cognition, coordination, and reaction time. Maxine demonstrated significant deficits in all of these areas. Based on the results of the evaluation, the occupational therapist counseled Maxine and her family that she either cease driving or be retested by an on-road driving evaluation. After exploring community mobility alternatives, Maxine and her family decided that she would stop driving, and she sold her car. The occupational therapists worked with Maxine on using the life care community van so that she could continue to go on regular community outings, and her family assisted her by driving her when she needed to go shopping.

Lauro

Lauro is a 14-year-old junior high school student with developmental disabilities. He has been successfully included in the public school setting, but he, his family, and his educational team must begin planning for his transition from school to life after graduation. At a recent educational planning meeting, Lauro stated that he would like to take the local bus with his peers to his weekly after-school sports program rather than driving with his mother each week. Lauro has never used public transportation and has little understanding of how to manage money. He is not sure what he would like to do when he grows up but knows he wants to live in his own apartment someday. Based on these goals, his occupational therapist worked with Lauro on how to manage money. They then started planning short trips on the bus to his sports program, with the occupational therapist going with him and a friend. Once the occupational therapist observed Lauro' s performance, she met with the family to plan how they could support him as he learns to ride the bus and pay for his fare. For now, Lauro is being accompanied by a friend or family member until he gains more confidence and is able to reliably use the bus.

Lydia

Lydia is a 39-year-old mother with a diagnosis of bipolar disorder. She came from a difficult family situation; her father was abusive and her mother was addicted to prescription medications. Lydia herself has a history of depression since age 13 at which time she became withdrawn, started drinking a lot, and even attempted suicide. When she was 23, she sought treatment for alcoholism and has been consistently sober for the past 9 years. Lydia is recently divorced from her husband, and their three surviving children live with their father. Their oldest son was killed last year in a motorcycle wreck. Although she has visitation rights, Lydia rarely sees her children because she does not drive. She doesn't have a regular job but has worked as a maid at a local hotel. Although she only went through eighth grade in school, she later obtained her high school diploma by passing the General Educational Development (GED) test.

After her latest episode, Lydia attended a community-based partial hospitalization program called Harborplace, where she was evaluated by an occupational therapist.

The therapist noted that Lydia was pleasant, appeared clean and well groomed, and seemed willing to participate in therapy. Lydia did demonstrate some problematic interpersonal skills such as recognizing and responding to feedback and taking responsibility for her actions. Although Lydia indicated she was interested in many things (i.e., gardening, hiking, cross-stitch, singing, and playing the piano), it was apparent that Lydia did not actually do very much on a daily basis and seemed to have trouble following through on tasks. Her only regular routines were to attend Alcoholic Anonymous (AA) meetings and church on a weekly basis. The occupational therapist worked with Lydia to develop better interpersonal and task skills and to expand her participation in all aspects of life. An important part of therapy was to help Lydia shape some goals for herself related to all her daily activities and to help her problem-solve how to actually follow through on these goals. As a result, Lydia was able to find part-time work in the garden center at a local home improvement store. She participates in several social and charitable church activities and has learned to use public transportation for community mobility and is now able to visit her children.

Linda Jo

Linda Jo works at a chicken processing plant. After a serious hand injury on one of the machines, a hand surgeon referred her for occupational therapy at a private outpatient clinic specializing in people with hand injuries. There, John, her occupational therapist, made her a hand splint to protect the areas where she had surgery and showed her the daily wound care routines she would need to do to support healing. He also talked with her about problems she was having managing her activities at home while she recovered and made suggestions on how to manage with one hand. Once her surgeon indicated it was safe for Linda to begin gentle movements, John helped Linda regain use of her hand through focused exercise and light activities. Next, John talked with

CASE STUDY 4.1 Examples of Clients and Settings *(continued)*

the human resources department to find out her exact duties so that he could gradually have her perform those work activities. From the company health nurse, he learned that although injuries such as Linda's were less common, there was a relatively larger number of employees at the processing plant experiencing various work-related repetitive trauma injuries. John arranged to conduct a worksite assessment to fully understand Linda's job and to arrange for her to return to a modified job until she was able to do her old job. Later, he returned to identify how the various workstations could be changed to avoid repetitive trauma injuries. He also has been working with the company health nurse to develop and implement an employee-training program to prevent the onset of these injuries.

Larry

Larry is a 26-year-old man who returned from an overseas war after surviving being hit by the shrapnel of a rocket-propelled grenade. He is missing his right upper limb, has burns across his chest wall, and loss of hearing in his right ear. Prior to deployment, Larry worked in a supermarket and was living with his girlfriend. Larry began receiving outpatient occupational therapy to prepare for and then train with using his new upper limb prosthesis. While waiting on his new artificial arm, Larry's occupational therapist taught Larry how to care for his wounds from the burn and his surgical incisions. Larry also worked on activities to strengthen his remaining arm and residual limb. Larry's occupational therapy assistant taught him one-handed techniques to perform self-care and introduced assistive devices to help him be more independent in everyday tasks. Larry was hesitant to accept these devices saying, "I would rather wait for my new arm."

Larry began missing therapy sessions. When he did attend he looked fatigued and disheveled. He reported being unable to sleep and concentrate due to reliving the war over and over again in the form of unwanted memories and nightmares. He reported that he and his girlfriend were now fighting and that she was resentful of the assistance that he required. The occupational therapy assistant reported these signs of post-traumatic stress disorder (PTSD) to his supervising occupational therapist who, in turn, encouraged Larry to contact the Wounded Warrior Project for a referral to a mental health worker specialized in treating PTSD. Larry's occupational therapist worked with him to identify triggers to these unwanted memories and to structure his day so that he remained active. She suggested that Larry begin swimming daily (because his wounds had healed) as well as begin journaling activities. Larry was encouraged to focus on any positive changes/events that occurred from serving in the war and document these changes in his journal. Larry reported that since his service, he "could face any challenge." This became Larry's new mantra, as he began the difficult task of working with his occupational therapist on learning to use his new prosthesis. See Figure 4.1 for an example of occupational therapy for a wounded warrior.

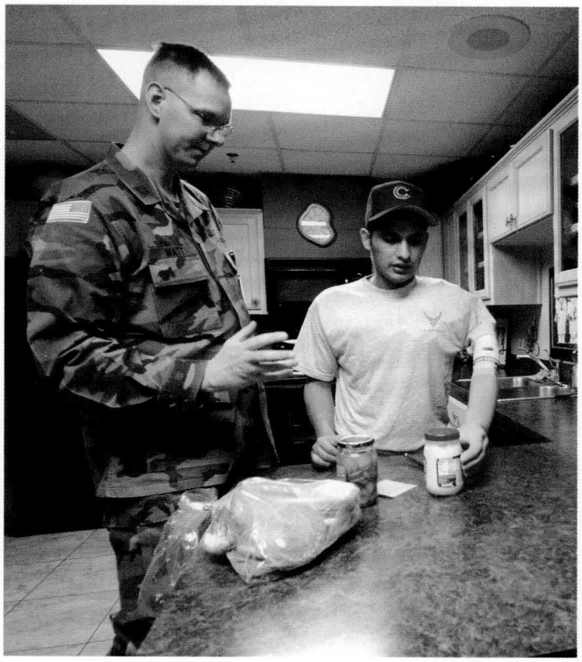

FIGURE 4.1 Army Capt. James Watt, an occupational therapist, helps Senior Airman Dan Acosta make a sandwich in the life skills area of the amputee rehabilitation clinic at Brooke Army Medical Center in San Antonio. A mock apartment in the center helps patients get used to completing common tasks with their prosthetic limbs. (U.S. Air Force photo/Steve White).

Mary

Mary is an occupational therapist who has been hired by the board of a local history museum as consultant. The board is committed to promoting equality, inclusion, and belonging for all their museum visitors. Mary began the collaboration by trying to understand the organization's functioning and desires, needs, and priorities. She met with the director of education, the exhibit design staff, the volunteer coordinator, and the Americans with Disabilities (ADA) Compliance Officer. The Director of Education identified a need for staff and volunteers to develop a greater appreciation for the range of learning needs of museum visitors with an autism spectrum disorder (ASD). They decided to focus first on the field trip program for elementary schools. The occupational therapist then observed the volunteers guiding the school children through the museum and conducted an extensive activity analysis of the features of the program and how various features of the program may impact the experience of visitors with an ASD. This analysis was presented to the staff. Together, the occupational therapist and staff explored images and stereotypes of ASD in the culture and common behaviors associated with an ASD that might be exhibited in a museum context. They collaborated on a list of recommended tips and strategies for promoting inclusive experiences for visitors with an ASD during their museum experience.

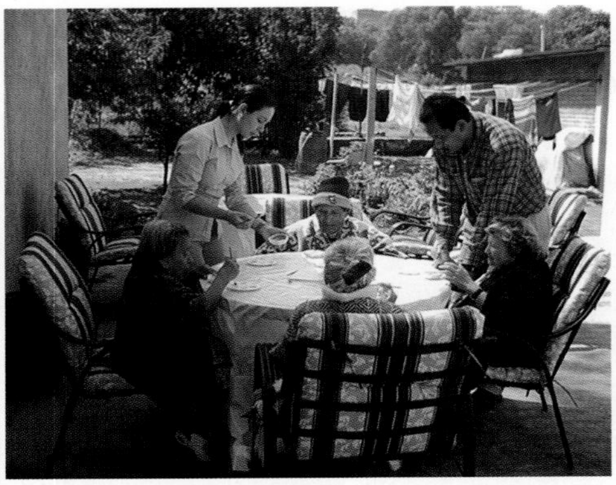

FIGURE 4.2 Occupational therapy students in Mexico City facilitate participation in a home for older adults.

learning to live in his "new body" and cope with the psychological effects of war. And the board members of the history museum want a place that is comfortable to visit for a wide range of people so that it serves to educate all its visitors on the importance of the past.

As these scenarios demonstrate, occupational therapy practitioners provide services to a variety of clients in many settings, from hospitals and schools to community programs and businesses. These services include direct intervention with individuals to programming for groups to consultation within organizations and public advocacy. In all cases, the overarching goal of occupational therapy is to engage people in meaningful and important occupations to support health and to participate as fully as possible in society. See Figure 4.2.

Definition of Occupational Therapy

Occupational therapy is the art and science of helping people do the day-to-day activities that are important and meaningful to their health and well-being through engagement in valued occupations (American Occupational Therapy Association [AOTA], 2008; World Federation of Occupational Therapists [WFOT], 2010c). The *occupation* in occupational therapy comes from an older use of the word, meaning how people use or "occupy" their time. Hasselkus (2006) in her Slagle lecture spoke about everyday occupation as something that is so ordinary and embedded in the every day that we may fail to appreciate its complexity and how our occupations constitute an interwoven network of all we do on a daily basis. Occupation includes the complex network of day-to-day activities that enable people to sustain their health, to meet their needs, to contribute to the life of their families, and to participate in the broader society (AOTA, 2008). Finally, occupational engagement is important because it has the capacity to contribute to health and well-being (Clark et al., 1997; Glass, Mendes de Leon, Marottoli, & Berkman, 1999; Law, Seinwender, & Leclair, 1998). An overview of the concept of occupation is provided in Chapter 1, and aspects of it are more fully described throughout this text.

Occupational therapy draws on the centrality of occupation to daily life. It is concerned with helping clients engage in all of the activities that occupy their time, enable them to construct identity through doing, and provide meaning to their lives (Christiansen, 1999; Zemke, 2004). As the scenarios that opened this chapter illustrate, occupational therapy practitioners provide individual and group interventions as well as consultative services that foster community participation, help restore abilities to engage in life, prevent problems affecting participation, and promote the well-being of individuals and populations in a wide range of settings. The desired outcome of occupational therapy intervention is that people will live their lives engaged in occupations that sustain themselves, support their health, and foster involvement with others in their social world. See Box 4.1.

Occupational Therapy Process

What is the occupational therapy process that supports the provision of services across such a broad array of clients and situations? By understanding occupation and carefully analyzing many factors associated with occupation, practitioners can use this knowledge to turn *occupation* into *therapy*. Occupational therapists must attend to the person or groups doing the occupation, the characteristics of the occupation itself, and the physical and social context in which the occupation occurs. Therapists also appreciate how various occupations interweave and how each support or detract from the other. Therefore, the evaluation process involves careful attention to what the person (or group) wants or needs to do, and how both person factors and contextual factors are affecting actual performance. Intervention then involves very carefully selecting those factors that most affect performance and figuring out ways to tip the balance toward performance. Examples of common approaches include the following:

- Use of actual activities embedded in occupations but in a graded or modified form to promote the development or restoration of performance abilities.
- Changing the physical space and equipment to make performance easier or more effective.
- Changing the social context so that adequate support is provided for effective performance.
- Changing the way an occupation is performed in order to improve performance and compensate for changes in the person's body functions.
- Use of preparatory activities that help the person be able to perform, such as activities and exercises to increase mobility, cognition, and emotional control (AOTA, 2008).

BOX 4.1 Definitions of Occupational Therapy

American Occupational Therapy Association

Excerpts from the AOTA Model Practice Act

The practice of occupational therapy means the therapeutic use of occupations, including everyday life activities with individuals, groups, populations, or organizations to support participation, performance, and function in roles and situations in home, school, workplace, community, and other settings. Occupational therapy services are provided for habilitation, rehabilitation, and the promotion of health and wellness to those who have or are at risk for developing an illness, injury, disease, disorder, condition, impairment, disability, activity limitation, or participation restriction.

Occupational therapy addresses the physical, cognitive, psychosocial, sensory-perceptual, and other aspects of performance in a variety of contexts and environments to support engagement in occupations that affect physical and mental health, well-being, and quality of life (AOTA, 2011a, p. 608).

World Federation of Occupational Therapy

Excerpt from WFOT statement on occupational therapy

Occupational therapy is a client-centred health profession concerned with promoting health and well-being through occupation. The primary goal of occupational therapy is to enable people to participate in the activities of everyday life. Occupational therapists achieve this outcome by working with people and communities to enhance their ability to engage in the occupations they want to, need to, or are expected to do, or by modifying the occupation or the environment to better support their occupational engagement (WFOT, 2010c, p. 1).

In order to use these approaches, occupational therapy practitioners need a wide range of skills related to analyzing and modifying activities, using their own interpersonal skills to encourage and motivate performance, as well as engaging in education, consultation, and advocacy to help clients have desired performance opportunities (AOTA, 2008). Ultimately, improved performance in daily tasks and increased participation in life activities is the goal of all occupational therapy.

Language for Occupational Therapy

As in any profession, occupational therapy uses terminology that has evolved to reflect the specific concerns of the profession. There are broad classifications or **taxonomies** that are useful for understanding the scope of the field and for communication core concerns to wider audiences. Two examples are resources developed by the World Health Organization (WHO) and the AOTA.

World Health Organization International Classifications

The WHO provides several resources for scientists and health care professionals throughout the world. One important document is the International Classification of Diagnosis (ICD), which provides a standard classification of diseases and health problems (WHO, 2010). This resource is most commonly seen in the United States in medical records and on billing sheets where the diagnosis is listed. In recent decades, the WHO recognized that the classification of diseases was not adequate to reflect the concerns of people with disabilities. After extensive development, the *International Classification of Functioning, Disability and Health* (ICF) was developed (WHO, 2001). Refer to Box 4.2 for the WHO's description of the ICF. At the time of this writing, the WHO is in the process of constructing yet another reference entitled the *International Classification of Health Interventions* (ICHI) (WHO, n.d.). It remains to be seen how the profession's approaches will be reflected in the new document. In the meantime, it is important to appreciate that there is worldwide endorsement (in the form of the ICF) of the importance of activities and participation to health. These have long been the core focus of the profession of occupational therapy.

International Classification of Functioning, Disability and Health

The ICF provides an organizing framework in which factors related to persons, their performance, and their performance contexts are clustered. In the most basic sense, health occurs when the person is able to participate in activities due to a good "match" between their health status and the context in which their activities occur. At the person level, individuals have body structures (such as bones and nerves) and body functions (such as muscle endurance or the ability to see). At the whole person level, individuals have the capacity to do activities (ride a bike, make dinner). Their actual participation is affected by physical and social aspects of the performance context (safe space to ride the bike, family member's praise for the meal), and thus, actual participation is a function of both personal capacity and the contextual support. So in the example of Maxine in the beginning of the chapter, her ability to participate declined partly because of her changing cognitive status (body function), but she was able to continue to participate in community activities because of the environmental supports provided (community bus trips and family members driving her). This WHO document thus provides language that occupational therapists can use to explain their services to a broad audience.

BOX 4.2 International Classification of Functioning, Disability and Health

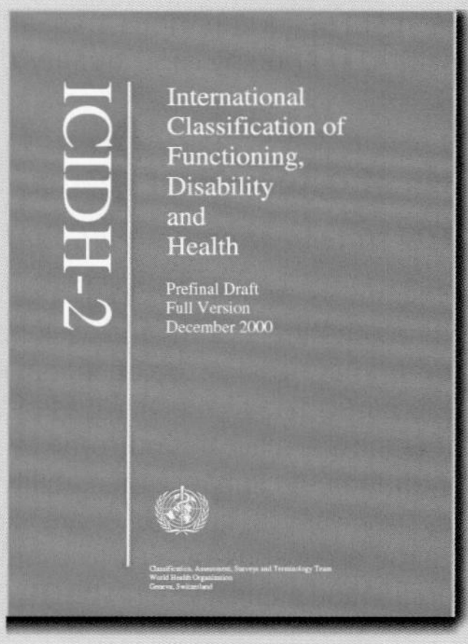

The International Classification of Functioning, Disability and Health, known more commonly as ICF, is a classification of health and health-related domains. These domains are classified from body, individual, and societal perspectives by means of two lists: a list of body functions and structure, and a list of domains of activity and participation. Because an individual's functioning and disability occurs in a context, the ICF also includes a list of environmental factors.

The ICF puts the notions of "health" and "disability" in a new light. It acknowledges that every human being can experience a decrement in health and thereby experience some degree of disability. Disability is not something that only happens to a minority of humanity. The ICF thus "mainstreams" the experience of disability and recognises it as a universal human experience. By shifting the focus from cause to impact it places all health conditions on an equal footing allowing them to be compared using a common metric—the ruler of health and disability. Furthermore, ICF takes into account the social aspects of disability and does not see disability only as a "medical" or "biological" dysfunction. By including contextual factors in which environmental factors are listed ICF allows to records the impact of the environment on the person's functioning. (WHO, 2001, para. 1–2)

Table 4.1 provides a definition of these major classification categories and how each is related to the general functioning. See if you can apply these concepts to each of the scenarios at the beginning of the chapter. Notice the impact each has on performance.

Occupational Therapy Practice Framework

In addition to the WHO, occupational therapy professional organizations also work to provide resources to practitioners. An important one generated by the AOTA is the "Occupational Therapy Practice Framework: Domain and Process (2nd ed.)" (AOTA, 2008). The occupational therapy practice framework (OTPF) presents a "summary of interrelated constructs that define and guide occupational therapy practice" (AOTA, 2008, p. 625). The current edition represents the evolution of a series of documents in which terminology is listed, definitions provided, and the general scope of practice is described. The authors, working on the behalf of the AOTA, attempt to gather commonly agreed-on terms

TABLE 4.1 International Classification of Functioning, Disability and Health Categories with Definitions

Level of Function	ICF Category	Definition
Person's body or body part	Body structures	Anatomical parts of the body such as organs, limbs, and their components
	Body functions	Physiological functions of body systems (including psychological functions)
	Impairments	Problems in body function or structure such as a significant deviation or loss
Whole person	Activity	The execution of a task or action by an individual
	Activity limitations	Difficulties an individual may have in executing activities
Context	Environmental factors	The physical, social, and attitudinal environment in which people live and conduct their lives
Person in context	Participation	Involvement in a life situation
	Participation restrictions	Problems an individual may experience in involvement in life situations

ICF, International Classification of Functioning, Disability and Health

TABLE 4.2 Aspects of Occupational Therapy Domains

Areas of Occupation	Client Factors	Performance Skills	Performance Patterns	Context and Environment	Activity Demands
Activities of daily living (ADL)[a]	Values, beliefs, and spirituality	Sensory-perceptual skills	Habits	Cultural	Objects used and their properties
Rest and sleep	Body functions	Motor and praxis skills	Routines	Personal	Space demands
Education	Structure functions	Emotional regulation skills	Roles	Physical	Social demands
Work		Cognitive skills	Rituals	Social	Sequencing and timing
Play		Communication and social skills		Temporal	Required actions
Leisure				Virtual	Required body functions
Social participation					Required body structures

American Occupational Therapy Association (AOTA) notes that all aspects of the domain transact to support engagement, participation, and health, and no hierarchy is intended (AOTA, 2008, p. 628).

[a]Also referred to as basic activities of daily living (BADL) or personal activities of daily living (PADL). Also includes instrumental activities of daily living (IADL).

Source: American Occupational Therapy Association. (2008). Occupational therapy practice framework: Domain and process, 2nd edition. *American Journal of Occupational Therapy*, p. 628, Figure 4.

and concepts. Having this information in one resource promotes more effective communication among occupational therapy practitioners as well as to the many others, such as those who pay for occupational therapy services and government groups who regulate services. Table 4.2 provides a listing of the major domains that occupational therapy addresses. Note that there is overlap with the WHO's ICF, in that the AOTA adopted some of the same terminology for part of the OTPF (i.e., Body Functions and Structures in the Client Factors list and some of the same categories in Context and Environment). In contrast, careful comparison will show that the AOTA provided a much more nuanced look at the aspects of occupation by including not only major categories or areas of occupation (which are analogous to the WHO's use of the term activities) but also concepts related to the various aspects of occupation and performance (i.e., skills, patterns). This is not surprising because this is the core of the profession's interests. See Figure 4.3, which explores the relationship between the ICF and the OTPF.

In addition to the major domain areas listed, the OTPF goes on to delineate the occupational therapy process and major outcomes of intervention. These are described in more detail in Chapter 23. For now, the important point is to recognize that there is professional language that helps occupational therapists communicate among themselves and with the larger worldwide audience.

Principles That Guide Occupational Therapy Practice

Contemporary occupational therapy practice draws on the historical roots of the profession, filtered through current occupational therapy, health, and human service research and practice. Meyer (1977/1922), for example, in his oft-quoted address to the National Society for the Promotion of Occupational Therapy asserted, "Our role consists in giving opportunities rather than prescriptions. There must be opportunities to work, opportunities to do, to plan and create, and to use material" (p. 641). Engelhardt (1977), and more recently Pörn (1993), asserted that health is measured by an individual's adaptive capacity and engagement in daily activities. In her Eleanor Clarke Slagle Lecture, Yerxa (1967) explained that authentic occupational therapy focuses on clients' humanity and their ability to choose and initiate activities that provide the basis for the discovery of meaning. She further argued that authentic occupational therapy requires that the practitioner "in every professional act defines the profession" and, in doing so, enters into a reciprocal relationship characterized by mutual care and that "to care means to be affected just as surely as it means to affect" (p. 8). Later in her address,

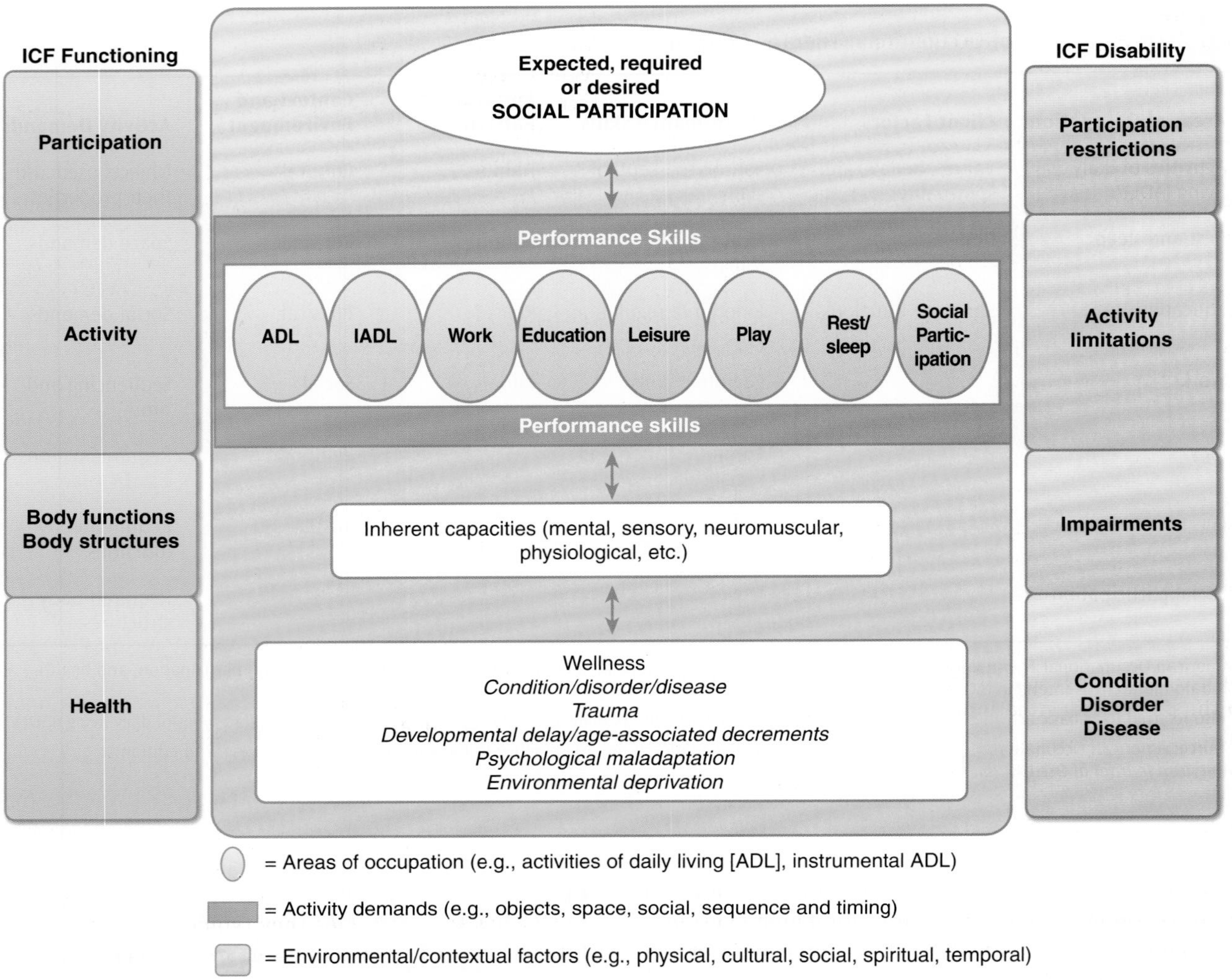

FIGURE 4.3 Connections among the International Classification of Function and the Occupational Therapy Practice Framework. Modified from Rogers, J. C., & Holm, M. B. (2009). The occupational therapy process. In E. B. Crepeau, E. S. Cohn, & B. A. B. Schell (Eds.), *Willard and Spackman's occupational therapy* (11th ed). Philadelphia, PA: Lippincott Williams & Wilkins.

Yerxa called for practitioner engagement in research to promote the development of the knowledge base of the profession. These themes translate into four principles that guide contemporary occupational therapy.

1. Client-centered practice
2. Occupation-centered practice
3. Evidence-based practice
4. Culturally relevant practice

Client-Centered Practice

At the core of occupational therapy is a focus on the client as an active agent seeking to accomplish important day-to-day activities. Occupational therapy practitioners often work with people who are disempowered (Kronenberg & Pollard, 2005; Townsend, 1996). Clients seek care and professional help to "gain mastery over their affairs" (Rappaport, 1987, p. 122). To be client centered, practitioners must be willing to enter the client's world to create a relationship that encourages the other to enhance his or her life in ways that are most meaningful to that person. Practitioners strive to understand the client as a person embedded in a particular context consisting of family and friends, socioeconomic status, culture, and so forth.

In a client-centered model, practitioner and client collaboratively engage in the therapeutic process (Law, 1998). Mattingly (1991) asserted that this process is narrative in nature, which means that the practitioner and client create an understanding of the client's past, present, and future story. Mattingly further asserted that the future story is coconstructed and constantly revised in the midst of therapy. Practitioners strive to understand human feelings and intentions as well as the deeper meaning of people's lives through what Clark (1993) called occupational storytelling. In contrast, occupational storymaking occurs in the midst of therapy. It is that imaginative process through which clients create and then enact new occupational identities (Clark, 1993).

Occupation-Centered Practice

Contemporary occupational therapy emphasizes occupational engagement. Clients seek occupational therapy because they need help engaging in their valued occupations. The emphasis on occupational engagement stems from the profession's beliefs, substantiated by emerging research, that people's occupations are central to their identity and that they can reconstruct themselves through their occupations (Jackson, 1998). Occupations are not isolated activities but are connected in a web of daily activities that help people fulfill their basic needs and contribute to their family, friends, and broader community (Hasselkus, 2006). Occupation-centered practice focuses on meaningful occupations selected by clients and performed in their typical settings (Fisher, 1998; Pierce, 1998). Systematic assessment of clients' occupations and priorities are vital to occupation-centered practice. This information—when coupled with careful analyses of the person's capacities, the task's demands, and the performance context—provides the basis for intervention. Intervention goals are directly connected to the person's occupational concerns, and intervention methods capitalize on the person's occupational interests. In this way, both the means (methods) and the ends (goals) of therapy involve intervention grounded in the occupations of the client (Fisher, 1998; Gray, 1998; Trombly, 1995).

Consistent with client-centered and occupation-based practice, Ann Wilcock and Elizabeth Townsend, leaders in occupational therapy from two different parts of the world, introduced the concept of occupational justice to acknowledge that all people are occupational beings and that meeting all peoples' need for engagement in meaningful occupation is a matter of justice (see Chapter 41). Wilcock and Townsend equate occupational justice with rights, equity, and fairness and argue that every individual has the right to have equal opportunities for and access to occupational participation. To address injustices, occupational therapy practitioners have begun to develop interventions and advocate for people who are disempowered by legislation, war, political upheavals, dictatorships, or natural disasters. Although many of the occupational therapy initiatives to address instances of occupational injustice have been developed in other parts of the world, practitioners in the United States have begun to embrace the ideals of an "occupationally just" world and develop interventions with these goals in mind.

Evidence-Based Practice

One of the important trends in health care is the increasing demand to base intervention decisions on "the conscientious, explicit, and judicious use of current best evidence" (Sackett, Rosenberg, Muir Granny, Haynes, & Richardson, 1996, p. 71). This process, called evidence-based practice, entails being able to integrate research evidence into the professional reasoning process to explain the rationale behind interventions and predict probable outcomes—or, as Gray asserted, "doing the right things right" (as cited in Holm, 2000, p. 576). Beyond "doing the right things right," evidence-based practice involves being able to explain occupational therapy recommendations to clients in a language that the clients will understand (Tickle-Degnen, 2000). Furthermore, intervention based solely on how things have been done in the past no longer meets the ethical requirement that therapists provide therapeutic approaches that are "evidence-based" (AOTA, 2010a, p. 9) and for which the client has been provided with "full disclosure of the benefits, risks, and potential outcomes of any intervention" (p. 11).

The challenge for occupational therapy practitioners is threefold.

- First, in order to practice evidence-based occupational therapy, practitioners must know how to access, evaluate, and interpret relevant research.
- Second, practitioners must have the capacity to synthesize evidence to support their intervention recommendations.
- Third, once practitioners understand the possible interventions and related outcomes, they need to communicate the probable outcomes to clients and/or their care providers so clients can make informed decisions about their participation in occupational therapy.

Not only must practitioners be willing to examine evaluation and intervention practices to see if they are effective but they must also be open to changes in their practice patterns when the evidence suggests more effective approaches than the ones they typically use. There are several sources available to occupational therapy practitioners to begin using and critiquing current evidence as shown in Box 4.3. Chapter 31 provides extensive information on how to effectively use evidence for practice.

Culturally Relevant Practice

As the occupational therapy profession continues to expand around the world, there is increasing recognition that effective occupational therapy practice must fit within the complex social, political, and cultural milieu in which therapy occurs (WFOT, 2010b). Not only are there differences across countries but also within various geographical regions, there are cultural differences that impact the practice of occupational therapy (Jungersen, 1992). For instance, in the United States, there has long been a focus on promoting independence, a prized "American" value deeply embedded in the culture (Brown & Gillespie, 1992). Thus, clients are encouraged to learn to do or to regain the abilities to do things by themselves with as little help as possible. However, within the United States as well as throughout the world, there are cultures that place a greater value on interdependence, and thus, the goal of therapy may be less on the complete independence of the individual and more on helping members of the family or social network understand how to care for the person while still promoting meaningful engagement in valued occupations. This is but one example of how attention to

BOX 4.3 Examples of Resources for Evidence-based Occupational Therapy Practice

OTseeker (http://www.otseeker.com/) is a database that contains abstracts of systematic reviews and randomized controlled trials relevant to occupational therapy. The included trials have been critically appraised and rated to assist the readers in evaluating their validity and interpretability. The ratings can be used by the readers to judge the quality and usefulness of the trials to informing clinical interventions.

OT Search (http://www1.aota.org/otsearch/) is a bibliographic database covering the literature of occupational therapy and related subject areas, such as rehabilitation, education, psychiatry or psychology, and health care delivery or administration.

The McMaster Occupational Therapy Evidence-based Practice Group (http://www.srs-mcmaster.ca/Default.aspx?tabid=630) focuses on research to critically review evidence regarding the effectiveness of occupational therapy interventions and to develop tools for evaluation of occupational therapy programs.

The Cochrane Library (http://www.thecochranelibrary.com/view/0/index.html) is an online collection of databases that brings together, in one place, rigorous and up-to-date research on the effectiveness of health care treatments and interventions including, but not limited to, occupational therapy.

the assumptions that are embedded in our own culture must be carefully examined in light of the client's culture. Effective occupational therapy practice involves recognizing that occupations are inherently shaped by culture, and thus, effective occupational therapy must attend to the culture of the client. See Figure 4.4.

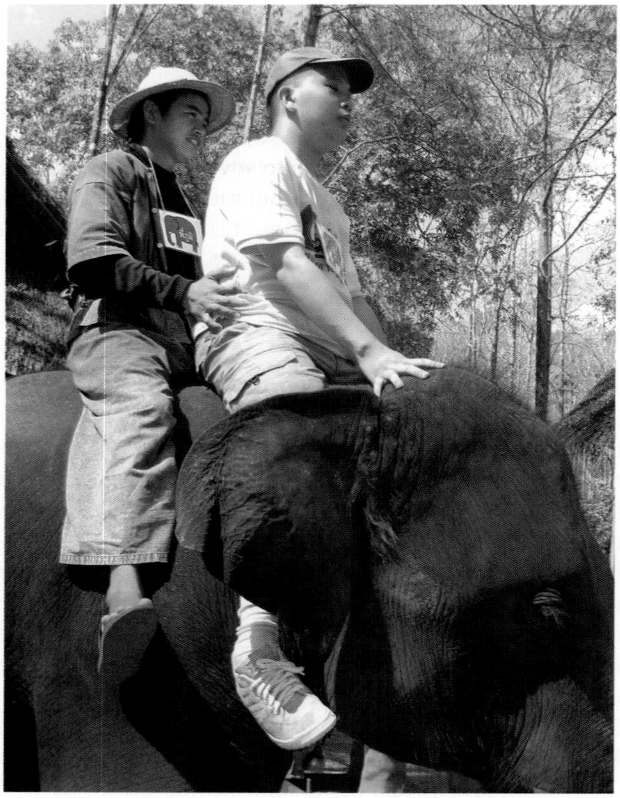

FIGURE 4.4 A child with autism spectrum disorder participates in an elephant camp implemented by occupational therapists in Thailand. Through carefully monitored interactions with the elephants, the outcomes include higher level of adaptive responses and social/communication abilities in the children.

Occupational Therapy Practitioners

Clients are, of course, an essential component of occupational therapy intervention, but occupational therapy practitioners are the other part of the equation. Practitioners use their professional reasoning abilities to actualize their knowledge and skills into therapy actions. Just as clients have an occupational history, so do practitioners. They are also embedded in their own personal, social, and cultural contexts that shape their worldview. Added to this are their preferred theories and intervention techniques, the practical realities of their therapy environment, and the team members with whom they work (Schell, 2008). Chapter 30 provides an overview of general processes associated with professional reasoning.

Occupational Therapy by the Numbers

Occupational therapy practitioners provide services to clients across a wide range of ages, health concerns, and cultures. The WFOT reports affiliations with more than 69 different national or regional occupational therapy professional associations (WFOT, 2011). Denmark and Sweden have the highest number of occupational therapists relative to their populations (Denmark 11:10,000; Sweden 10:10,000). In the United States, the reported ratio is 3:10,000, which is only slightly higher than the worldwide average of 2:10,000 (WFOT, 2010a). In many countries, governmental agencies are the main employers. Throughout the world, women make up an estimated 81% of occupational therapy practitioners; in the United States, the AOTA estimates that about 91.6% of both occupational therapists and occupational therapy assistants are women (AOTA, 2010a).

Practice Areas in the United States

In the United States, most occupational therapy practitioners work in hospitals (26%), schools (22%), or long-term care/skilled nursing facilities (20%) (AOTA, 2010b). Other common practice areas include freestanding outpatient settings (9%), home health (6%), early intervention programs for infants and children (5%), and academic settings (5%). Smaller percentages work in the community, mental health, or other settings. There is a difference between occupational therapists and occupational therapy assistants, in that proportionately more occupational therapy assistants work in long-term care settings.

Vision for the Future

In 2017, the AOTA will celebrate its 100th anniversary. In recognition of this milestone, the AOTA adopted a centennial vision. It states,

> We envision that occupational therapy is a powerful, widely recognized, science-driven, and evidence-based profession with a globally connected and diverse workforce meeting society's occupational needs. (AOTA, 2006, p. 1)

A quick tour of the AOTA webpage (http://www.aota.org) shows the many ways this vision is being enacted.

In countries and regions throughout the world, occupational therapy will continue to grow because of the profession's ability to help solve the problems of daily living. Forces that will affect the profession include the following:

- New systems for organizing and funding care in the United States and countries throughout the world. These systems will occur differently in different parts of the world, reflecting different health care needs, economic challenges, and governmental responses.
- The evidence related to the effectiveness of traditional and emerging intervention strategies. Practitioners will be challenged to identify and justify evaluation and intervention approaches, which clearly lead to valued outcomes (Lin, Murphy, & Robinson, 2010).
- The impact of human genome project on health care approaches and results (Reynolds & Lou, 2009).
- The continued development of occupational justice approaches to respond to social, political, and economic condition that deprive individuals and groups from their rights to engage in occupations (Braveman & Bass-Haugen, 2009; Kronenberg, Pollard, & Sakellariou, 2011).
- The need to respond to community and population level disruptions that occur as a result of natural and man-made disasters (AOTA, 2011b).
- The rapid development of worldwide technologies, including telerehabilitation (AOTA, 2010c), virtual reality, and personal communication devices.

These and many more challenges, yet unseen, will continue to shape the profession.

Conclusion

Occupational therapy is a complex process that involves collaborative interaction between the practitioner and the client embedded in the intervention context. Occupational therapy intervention must be grounded in research and focused on the client as an occupational being. The therapeutic process evolves as the practitioner and client work together to analyze carefully the client's occupations and performance limitations. Because occupational therapy involves doing *with* clients, and not doing *to* them, there is an improvisational aspect of intervention that requires the practitioner and client to coordinate their actions to achieve the client's goal. The rest of this book delineates the various aspects of occupational therapy involved in that process. It emphasizes consistently that best practice involves (1) understanding and respecting clients, (2) collaborating with clients to achieve their occupational goals, (3) using interventions that are supported by research, and (4) tailoring approaches to be consistent with the culture of the client.

As you start your career, our challenge to you is to strive to achieve the ideals of the profession. First, be aware of the influence of your beliefs and your personal and professional contexts and how these influence your actions. Second, consistently challenge yourself to listen to your clients so that you can facilitate their participation in their desired occupations. Third, use the most effective assessment instruments and interventions to support the progress of your clients. Fourth, advocate for your clients so they can obtain the services they need and learn to advocate for themselves. Finally, systematically evaluate your practice to ensure that your client is getting the most effective care. The people whose scenarios opened this chapter remind us that we have the responsibility to live up to the ideals of the profession. Peloquin (2005), one of our philosophers, concluded her 2005 Eleanor Clarke Slagle with the following statement:

> The ethos of occupational therapy restores our clear-sightedness so that we see what is essential: We are pathfinders. We enable occupations that heal. We co-create daily lives. We reach for hearts as well as hands. We are artists and scientists at once. If we discern this in ourselves, if we act on this understanding everyday, we will advance into the future embracing our ethos of engagement. And we will have reclaimed our magnificent heart. (p. 623)

We welcome you to the path of occupational therapy.

References

American Occupational Therapy Association. (2006). *AOTA adopts centennial vision.* Retrieved from http://www.aota.org/News/Media/PR/2006/38538.aspx

American Occupational Therapy Association. (2008). Occupational therapy practice framework: Domain and process, 2nd edition. *American Journal of Occupational Therapy, 62*, 625–683.

American Occupational Therapy Association. (2010a). Occupational therapy code of ethics and ethics standards (2010). *American Journal of Occupational Therapy, 64*(6 Suppl.), S17–S26. doi:10.5014/ajot.2010.64S17

American Occupational Therapy Association. (2010b). *Occupational therapy compensation and workforce study*. Bethesda, MD: AOTA Press.

American Occupational Therapy Association. (2010c). Telerehabilitation. *American Journal of Occupational Therapy, 64*(6 Suppl.), S92–S102. doi:10.5014/ajot.2010.64S92

American Occupational Therapy Association. (2011a). *Association policies: Policy 5.3.1 Definition of occupational therapy practice for state regulation, 65*(6 Suppl.), S81.

American Occupational Therapy Association. (2011b). The role of occupational therapy in disaster preparedness, response and recovery: A concept paper. *American Journal of Occupational Therapy, 65*, S11–S25.

Braveman, B., & Bass-Haugen, J. D. (2009). Social justice and health disparities: An evolving discourse in occupational therapy research and intervention. *American Journal of Occupational Therapy, 63*, 7–12.

Brown, K., & Gillespie, D. (1992). Recovering relationships: A feminist analysis of recovery models. *American Journal of Occupational Therapy, 46*, 1001–1005.

Christiansen, C. H. (1999). Defining lives: Occupation as identity: An essay on competence, coherence, and the creation of meaning. *American Journal of Occupational Therapy, 54*, 547–558.

Clark, F. (1993). The 1993 Eleanor Clarke Slagle Lecture—Occupation embedded in a real life: Interweaving occupational science and occupational therapy. *American Journal of Occupational Therapy, 47*, 1067–1078.

Clark, F., Azen, S. P., Zemke, R., Jackson, J., Carlson, M., Mandel, D., . . . Lipson L. (1997). Occupational therapy for independent-living older adults: A randomized controlled trial. *Journal of the American Medical Association, 278*, 1321–1326.

Engelhardt, H. T. (1977). Defining occupational therapy: The meaning of therapy and the virtues of occupation. *American Journal of Occupational Therapy, 31*, 666–672.

Fisher, A. G. (1998). The 1998 Eleanor Clarke Slagle Lecture—Uniting practice and theory in an occupational framework. *American Journal of Occupational Therapy, 52*, 509–521.

Glass, T. A., Mendes de Leon, C., Marottoli, R. A., & Berkman, L. F. (1999). Population based study of social and productive activities as predictors of survival among elderly Americans. *British Medical Journal, 319*, 478–483.

Gray, J. M. (1998). Putting occupation into practice: Occupation as ends, occupation as means. *American Journal of Occupational Therapy, 52*, 354–364.

Hasselkus, B. R. (2006). The 2006 Eleanor Clarke Slagle Lecture—The world of everyday occupation: Real people, real lives. *American Journal of Occupational Therapy, 60*, 627–640.

Holm, H. B. (2000). The 2000 Eleanor Clarke Slagle Lecture—Our mandate for a new millennium: Evidence-based practice. *American Journal of Occupational Therapy, 54*, 575–585.

Jackson, J. (1998). The value of occupation as the core of treatment: Sandy's experience. *American Journal of Occupational Therapy, 52*, 466–473.

Jungersen, K. (1992). Culture, theory, and practice of occupational therapy in New Zealand/Aotearoa. *American Journal of Occupational Therapy, 46*, 745–750.

Kronenberg, F., & Pollard, N. (2005). Introduction: A beginning. In F. Kronenberg, S. Simo Algado, & N. Pollard (Eds.), *Occupational therapy without borders: Learning from the spirit of survivors* (pp. 1–13). Edinburgh, United Kingdom: Elsevier Churchill Livingstone.

Kronenberg, F., Pollard, N., & Sakellariou, D. (2011). *Occupational therapies without borders: Vol. 2—Towards an ecology of occupation-based practices*. St. Louis, MO: Churchill-Livingston Elsevier.

Law, M. (1998). *Client-centered occupational therapy*. Thorofare, NJ: Slack.

Law, M., Seinwender, S., & Leclair, L. (1998). Occupation, health, and well-being. *Canadian Journal of Occupational Therapy, 65*, 81–91.

Lin, S. H., Murphy, S. L., & Robinson, J. C. (2010). Facilitating evidence-based practice: Process, strategies and resources. *American Journal of Occupational Therapy, 64*, 164–171.

Mattingly, C. (1991). The narrative nature of clinical reasoning. *American Journal of Occupational Therapy, 45*, 979–986.

Meyer, A. (1977). The philosophy of occupational therapy. *American Journal of Occupational Therapy, 31*, 639–642. (Original work published 1922)

Peloquin, S. M. (2005). The 2005 Eleanor Clarke Slagle Lecture—Embracing our ethos, reclaiming our heart. *American Journal of Occupational Therapy, 59*, 611–625.

Pierce, D. (1998). What is the source of occupation's treatment power? *American Journal of Occupational Therapy, 52*, 490–491.

Pörn, I. (1993). Health and adaptedness. *Theoretical Medicine, 14*, 295–303.

Rappaport, J. (1987). Terms of empowerment/exemplars of prevention: Toward a theory for community psychology. *American Journal of Community Psychology, 15*(2), 121–145.

Reynolds, S., & Lou, J. Q. (2009). Occupational therapy in the age of the human genome: Occupational therapists' role in genetics research and its impact on clinical practice. *American Journal of Occupational Therapy, 63*, 511–515.

Sackett, D. L., Rosenberg, W. M. C., Muir Granny, J. A., Haynes, R. B., & Richardson, W. S. (1996). Evidence-based medicine. What it is and what it isn't. *British Medical Journal, 312*, 71–72.

Schell, B. A. B. (2008). Pragmatic reasoning. In B. A. B. Schell & J. W. Schell (Eds.), *Clinical and professional reasoning in occupational therapy* (pp. 169–187). Baltimore, MD: Lippincott Williams & Wilkins.

Tickle-Degnen, L. (2000). Communicating with clients, family members, and colleagues about research evidence. *American Journal of Occupational Therapy, 54*, 341–343.

Townsend, E. (1996). Institutional ethnography: A method for showing how the context shapes practice. *Occupational Therapy Journal of Research, 16*, 179–199.

Trombly, C. A. (1995). The 1995 Eleanor Clarke Slagle Lecture—Purposefulness and meaningfulness as therapeutic mechanisms. *American Journal of Occupational Therapy, 49*, 960–972.

World Federation of Occupational Therapists. (2010a). *Occupational therapy human resources project*. Retrieved from http://www.wfot.org

World Federation of Occupational Therapists. (2010b). *Position statement on diversity and culture*. Retrieved from http://www.wfot.org

World Federation of Occupational Therapists. (2010c). *Statement on occupational therapy. Definitions of occupational therapy from member organizations-Update 3002011*. Retrieved from http://www.wfot.org

World Federation of Occupational Therapists. (2011). *Member organisations of WFOT*. Retrieved from http://www.wfot.org

World Health Organization. (2001). *International Classification of Functioning, Disability and Health*. Retrieved from http://www.who.int/classifications/icf/

World Health Organization. (2010). *International Classification of Diseases* (10th ed.). Retrieved from http://www.who.int/classifications/icd/

World Health Organization. (n.d.). *International Classification of Health Intervention*. Retrieved from http://www.who.int/classifications/ichi/

Yerxa, E. J. (1967). The 1967 Eleanor Clarke Slagle Lecture—Authentic occupational therapy. *American Journal of Occupational Therapy, 21*, 1–9.

Yerxa, E. J., Clark, F., Frank, G., Jackson, J., Parham, D., Pierce, D., . . . Zemke, R. (1989). An introduction to occupational science: The foundation for occupational therapy in the 21st century. *Occupational Therapy in Health Care, 6*(4), 1–17.

Zemke, R. (2004). The 2004 Eleanor Clarke Slagle Lecture—Time, space, and the kaleidoscopes of occupation. *American Journal of Occupational Therapy*, 58, 608–620.

For additional resources on the subjects discussed in this chapter, visit http://thePoint.lww.com/Willard-Spackman12e.

UNIT II

Occupational Nature of Humans

"I believe that the ordinary rhythm of daily living is the deep primordial nourishment of our existence. It is the 'truth'—the primary reality for each one of us. After all, everyday occupation is present in our lives at all *times and in* all *places."*

—Betty Risteen Hasselkus

CHAPTER 5

Transformations of Occupations: A Life Course Perspective

Ruth Humphry, Jenny Womack

OUTLINE

LEARNING OBJECTIVES

After reading this chapter, you will be able to:

1. Apply the principles of a life course perspective to understand how occupational opportunities, people's evaluation of their life situations, and their choices lead to their current pattern of occupations
2. Describe how social institutions create occupational opportunities and create normative expectations for certain occupations
3. Appreciate the process of social participation in occupations through shared engagement and coordinated actions
4. Recognize how occupational performance and experiences of meaning emerge from interconnected elements that make up the occupational situation
5. Discuss how occupations join people with their life situations, enabling them to participate with others during life transitions

Introduction

This chapter is about how people's occupations change over their life course. The ideas presented presume that the reasons people start, change, or discontinue occupations across the life span goes beyond individual preferences or abilities. Rather, these changes represent dynamic transactions among the people, the social and historical context of their time, and their experiences of engaging in the activity itself. As life circumstances change, acquisition of new occupations as well as transformations in what and how things are done are essential for sustained social participation. Thus, these dynamic processes challenge us to think beyond conventional views on human development to understand how these changes occur.

Human Development

Human development is traditionally considered from the standpoint of changes within the individual rather than transformations in what human beings do over time. There are two common ways of thinking reflected in past work on human development: stage theories and life span theories.

Stage Theories

Several stage theories were developed by researchers in the early part of the last century. The original assumptions in these theories framed development as a biological process, dependent on maturation of different body systems. Stage theorists proposed that behavioral development was both universal and predictably sequential. In these models, changing behavior across different age groups or life stages was explained by identifying underlying qualitative changes in an individual's abilities (R. M. Lerner, 2002). For example, R. M. Lerner (2002) describes how Erikson's psychosocial model of development identifies eight stages up to middle adulthood in which life situations require different types of psychosocial adjustment. Because demands change with a person's age, he proposed that each stage is the foundation for the next one. Periods of transitions were often characterized as challenges that the individual needed to work though in order to have positive development or psychological well-being.

Life Span Development Theories

Another traditional group of theorists (primarily psychologists) have embraced the concept of **life span development**, which emerged in the 1970s. Life span theories focused on the continuity and changes in different aspects of personal development (Overton, 2010), such as emotional maturity or ability to make complex judgments. They also recognized that development occurs beyond childhood and lasts throughout one's life. Some theorists focused on the importance of a person's personal motivation or choice as critical to development and negotiation of changing abilities (Brandtsadter & Lerner, 1999).

Stage and life span theorists recognized that interactions with the social and physical environment play a role in development. However, their explanations of changing behaviors were typically described by addressing a single aspect of psychological function such as cognition, self-evaluation, or emotional adjustment only from the individual perspective. By focusing only on a specific subset of psychological factors, these theories neglect to recognize that engagement requires simultaneous integration of different abilities (Humphry, 2002). A second concern about using these theories to explain how occupations change was the assumption that development has a biological base. Although there are biologically based changes over time (such as the onset of puberty), these changes are not sufficient to explain occupational development. If this is the case, then we would be able to assess changes in what a person does and the quality of performance based on chronological age. However, cultural practices influence what occupations, when they appear, and the performance. For instance, in some cultures, women are expected to marry and have children in their early teens; whereas in others, these occupational roles are assumed much later in life.

These theories arising from psychology and biology dominated occupational therapy practice throughout most of the last century and continue to influence some of our clinical approaches. More recent dynamic and contextualized perspectives challenge us to shift the focus toward occupation and the social processes contributing to changing performance and meaning (Humphry 2002, 2005; Humphry & Wakeford, 2006).

The Contextual Nature of Changing Occupations

Before discussing what shapes changes in people's occupations, it is important to think about what it means to acquire a new occupation as well as how that acquisition alters performance and meaning. To explore what this entails, consider Case Study 5.1 on the next page in which three generations engage in yoga.

Consider the historical and social ties evident by the family's engagement in this occupation. Yoga was developed centuries ago in India as an activity for the health of body and mind and is now practiced in many different forms by millions of people worldwide. This family's practice of yoga reflects both continuity of some occupations and a contemporary interest in the activity. When the grandmother was young, exercise for the sake of strengthening and flexibility was not part of her generation's expectations about what young women should do. However, societal values change and Harriet's peer group now considers exercise for the sake of staying active as an important thing to do. Clearly, engagement in occupations is not only an individual decision but is rooted in the past and influenced by changing social values and beliefs of people who are around us.

This family scenario also illustrates that acquisition of new occupations occurs at any point during a lifetime and is not necessarily passed down in a linear fashion from the older to younger generation. It shows us that people may take up the same activity for different reasons and can learn the necessary actions in different ways. Harriet and Lauren learned yoga in a more structured way and share an appreciation of the essential characteristics that define their routine, generating procedural knowledge of how to do the poses. Their sense of why yoga is meaningful as an exercise is also shared. Mariah, on the other hand, was introduced to yoga in infancy as something she did with her mother. As a young preschooler, she mimicked the things adults did based on

CASE STUDY 5.1 A Family Occupation

In Figure 5.1, a grandmother, Harriet; her adult daughter, Lauren; and her granddaughter, Mariah, share a morning exercise routine by doing yoga. Lauren learned the practice of yoga in college from her boyfriend who was attracted to it for the connection between the body/mind and health. After graduation, she took classes and found it a great way to relax and have a good time with friends. When she married the man who introduced her to yoga, they exercised together. After Mariah was born, her mother enrolled her in baby yoga and it became something that mother and daughter did as part of their "special time." When Harriet visited, she watched the yoga class, intrigued by it. The family relocated to be closer to grandparents. Harriet learned from her friends about the importance of an active lifestyle for older adults and agreed to try yoga. Lauren helped her select and practice moves until they became familiar. This picture was taken after Mariah's second birthday when she received stretch pants and her own yoga mat. There was no real effort to teach her what to do because she seemed to just follow along in the routine of her mother and grandmother. Now when Harriet comes over to exercise, Mariah, now age 5, changes her clothes and lays down her mat in the living room to join in the yoga routine.

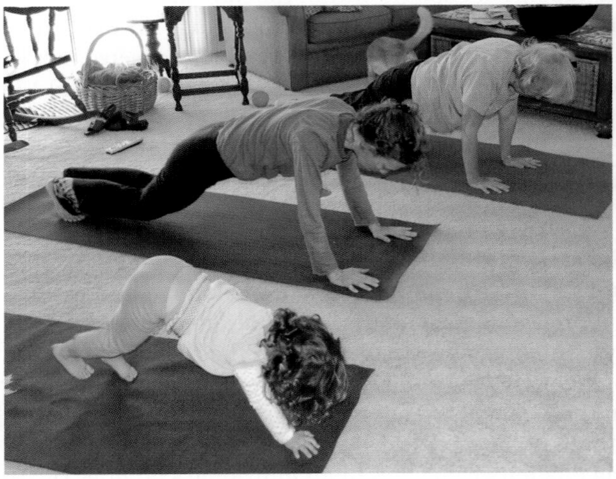

FIGURE 5.1 Engaging in exercise for health and relaxation is an intergenerational occupation for this grandmother, her daughter, and her granddaughter.

her unfolding understanding of the practices of her family. For her, the meaning of doing yoga is one of being part of a family occupation. Her instinctive participation is evidence that acquisition of occupations sometimes is not an individual conscious choice.

One can imagine that performance of all these family members will undergo some changes or transformations over time. For Mariah, her performance unfolds as part of a social process. Subtle transformations in the quality of performance and meaning associated with the occupation can occur within a session as Lauren and Harriet make casual comments about what they are doing. Over weeks and months, Mariah will also gain more skills as she matures and continues to practice yoga. She will also find that there are other things to pay attention to, such as breathing routines and mental practices. This type of learning does not reflect abstract mental change that occurs out of context of the activity but reflects active learning as part of being part of a group or community doing together (Lave & Packer, 2008; Lave & Wenger, 1991). For all the family members, their procedural knowledge of yoga reflects **embodied action**. Embodied action assumes that the mind and body are coupled as an entity that experiences the lived world as a whole rather than in separate and distinct ways (Overton, Muller, & Newman, 2008). The concept of embodied action does not insinuate, however, that habitual practices of doing yoga will appear the same from one session to the next; clearly in the photograph we see all family members engage in a slightly different manner, which reflects different body morphology and understanding of the moves. Variability between people and across repeated actions of the same person reflects the **emergent performance** of their occupations. That is, the physical, mental, sensory, and emotional abilities of each person are integrated with the meanings that they bring to doing yoga at that moment. People master how to coordinate their abilities in doing occupations with their environment (including, in this case, gravity).

Finally, this case study of a family illustrates how people and their occupations are interdependent elements of a larger picture. Focusing on the occupational engagement of one member would lead to an incomplete understanding of how occupations are acquired and performed as a way of joining in something that extends beyond the living room walls. Doing yoga, or any other occupation, is conceptualized as a transactional process where people, the physical space, time, and objects form a functional whole in which the occupation serves to connect people with each other and their life circumstances (Cutchin & Dickie, 2012; Dickie, Cutchin, & Humphry, 2006).

With this background, we return to consider what brings about changes in our occupations. To organize our understanding, we offer the adaptation of different change models—two of which were originally proposed by other disciplines. First, we consider a larger timespan that crosses over years, drawing primarily on the work of sociologists. These ideas are relevant because occupational therapy acknowledges the highly contextualized nature of what people do. Recognizing that lives are situated in time and place, we will consider what brings about changes in occupations as people move between social institutions such as home, school, or workplace, and community organizations and transition between former and new life situations. We will also reflect on changes occurring over shorter time periods, such as changes that might occur in response to an occupational therapy session that takes place after a sudden life transition (Blair, 2000). We draw on work of an interdisciplinary group of activity theorists (Hedegaard, 2009; Lave & Wenger, 1991), which has informed a model for changing occupations (Humphry, 2005). Finally, we discuss moment-to-moment changes in engagement in an occupation (Humphry, 2002).

Life Course Perspective

We propose that the **life course** perspective (Elder & Shanahan, 2006; Johnson, Crosnoe, & Elder, 2011; Mayer, 2009) serves a guiding concept for occupational therapists working with people of all ages to understand how occupations develop and evolve over time as circumstances change. Like life span theorists, life course theorists recognize that systematic changes occur from birth to the end of life but move beyond an emphasis on the physical, mental, social, and emotional changes occurring within the individual (Diewald & Mayer, 2009). Instead, life course theorists emphasize that living is a highly contextualized, socially participatory process in which individuals are part of groups changing social positions and roles across the course of their lives. They recognize that we are born into birth cohorts where the sum effects of the times and the people around us serve to create a trajectory or pathway for our lives. Life transitions such as starting school, first employment, starting a family, and retirement are seen as turning points that can change the trajectory of our lives.

A life course perspective orients us to consider the processes shaping people's lives but does not systematically focus on changing occupations. It links context and individuals in life situations in which we believe occupations occur. Table 5.1 summarizes principles of a life course perspective (Elder & Shanahan, 2006) applied to related concepts about transformations of people's occupations. There are four interdependent reasons that alter circumstances, which in turn shape the pathway or trajectory of a life course. First, we understand that people living in the Western hemisphere typically go through common changes like starting school, moving out of the family home, or retiring from paid employment, which alters their occupations and determines a future pathway of their life course. There are also unanticipated events such as a divorce, diagnosis of a chronic health condition, or the needs of an aging parent that introduce life changes. Circumstances at the societal level also shape people's life course (i.e., the great recession, Afghanistan war, changes in funding for education). Finally, the social and economic circumstances (i.e., gender, ethnicity, age, educational and income levels), which make these societal changes have more or less effect on what people do and the trajectory of their life course. The life course perspective encourages us to acknowledge the intertwined factors leading to the complexity of any one person's occupational engagement.

TABLE 5.1 Principles of a Life Course Perspective Applied to Changing Occupations

Life Course Principle	Example
1. Aging and transformations of occupations are lifelong processes; the accumulated experiences with past occupations impact current forms of engagement.	Childhood experiences, such as helping prepare dinner with a parent, can shape how a young man living on his own cooks and the meal he prepares for his date. Cooking for a family with adolescent children may require changes in what is cooked to meet a busy schedule. Cooking, for the same person, could be altered again with retirement.
2. People live interconnected lives and these networks of relationships shape people's occupations.	A senior that gives up driving stops her volunteer time reading to preschoolers in a Head Start program. The children, who continue to be taught about reading as part of circle time, no longer share a relationship with an adult who models reading for pleasure.
3. Historic times and societal events shape and alter what people do, how they do it, and give it meaning.	Afghanistan war and promises of veterans' educational benefits encouraged a young man to join the army instead of going to the community college as planned. His military experiences made him proud to serve, and he chooses to reenlist instead of going to college.
4. People make choices about their occupations, which reflect their circumstances and perceived occupational opportunities at that particular time.	When farming economy had a downturn, some Iowa farmers took a job in town as well as worked the farm, whereas older farmers tended to sell their farms and move off their land (Elder & Conger, 2000).
5. Antecedents to an event or life transition and the consequences of such events for a person's occupations vary according to timing in the life course.	Working for 11 years before starting a family allowed one parent to save enough money so that she did not have to return to work until her child was a year old. For a 19-year-old starting a family, parenting had to be balanced with the necessity of continued work.

We start by drawing on a life course perspective of occupation that illustrates what people do is simultaneously individual, interpersonal, social, and historical. We turn to consider the case of Wanda and the importance of incorporating a life course perspective of occupation in light of people's lives and the things they choose to do. Wanda's story will be told in parts throughout the remainder of the chapter and here serves to illustrate the relationship of early life experiences to later occupational behavior.

CASE STUDY 5.2 Wanda, *Part I*

Wanda, a 40-year-old patient in a rehabilitation hospital, has heard the young girl in the room next door crying at night. She overhead the 14-year-old say that she is missing the end of her eighth-grade school year while undergoing rehabilitation after having a stroke. Wanda recalls seeing some costumes and masks in the recreation therapy department and asks her therapist if she can borrow a clown mask and wig to cheer up her young neighbor. That same night, she puts on the costume and asks her nurse to help her across the hall to visit her neighbor. Wanda improvises a mime skit about her own disability and soon has her young neighbor laughing. The two of them continue to support one another through the rehabilitation process and say a tearful good-bye when Wanda is discharged. ■

How did Wanda become a human being who, despite her own challenges, reaches out to someone else who is struggling? In this brief introduction to her life, we know only that she is a patient in a rehabilitation hospital, that she is 40 years old and has a disability, and that she has reached out to someone younger in a similar circumstance. This snapshot of her life is lacking, however, in social and historical context. What in her background and experience led her to focus on the needs of her young neighbor while facing her own major life transition? As you continue to read Wanda's story, reflect on how learning about her childhood and family occupations illustrates the value of a life course perspective (Elder & Shanahan, 2006; Johnson et al., 2011) as a lens for understanding the development of occupations.

CASE STUDY 5.2 Wanda, *Part II*

Wanda was born in the early 1950s with spastic quadriplegic cerebral palsy as the only child of parents whom she describes as "loving, encouraging, and protective." The family lived in a small rural community where they were active church and community members, but there were limited services for Wanda's situation. Her parents traveled with her to regional medical centers for treatment when she was young and then sent her at age 8 to attend a boarding school for children with special needs. After 2 years, Wanda and her parents decided she should return to live at home, and she continued living with them through her adult years. Wanda attended the rural public schools when a classroom could accommodate her but primarily received home-based schooling. Wanda had an aptitude for math; and because writing was difficult, her father helped her learn to use an electric typewriter to organize figures into columns to add and subtract. In her 20s, she began helping a friend of her parents to calculate the income from his truck farming operation; once a week he brought Wanda receipts and handwritten notes about his cash income, and she would organize the figures by typing them onto a page, calculating the sums, and returning them to the farmer.

One of Wanda's teenage life experiences was helping her parents as volunteers for the county Meals-on-Wheels program. Her father drove the family around their rural county and Wanda handed meals to her mother from the back seat, who then delivered them to the door. Wanda would wave to the person at the door from the back seat of the car. In time, several recipients came to know the family; and eventually, some met the car at the driveway or mailbox so that they could chat with Wanda rather than simply wave to her.

"It was good for them, too" she said. "It gave them some fresh air and a little exercise. And they depended on us showing up for them every day." ■

Knowing more about Wanda helps to situate her decision to reach out to her young neighbor in the rehabilitation hospital. It had roots in her past experiences when she and her parents entered volunteer roles. Her parents, who valued helping others and including Wanda in their lives, supported Wanda's engagement. When the elderly recipients came out to greet her, volunteering took on additional meaning by connecting her life with theirs. Clearly, this woman's life illustrates the interdependent and situated nature of occupations. Whereas we might, based on a traditional development perspective, have considered a 40-year-old woman with cerebral palsy as never having mastered certain skills, we now see a woman defined not by her disability but by her life experiences, which took place in a given social and historical context.

Wanda's occupations as an informal bookkeeper and volunteer were created not simply by her as an individual but through the relationships within a rural setting and her parents' encouragement. Elements of her circumstance such as the farmer's need for a record of his finances and her father's help in learning to use a typewriter, combined with Wanda's ability to work with numbers, created an occupational opportunity that she readily agreed to do.

The historical time frame in which she was born accounts for differences in services and schooling. Wanda and her parents made the choice not to continue at the residential school for students with special needs. By leaving a school that could accommodate her limited mobility, Wanda and her parents relied more on home schooling, which altered her occupations as a student and likely had consequences for her social occupations with peers. Her limited interactions with age mates also increased her contact with adults. One might argue that the choices disadvantaged Wanda, but her later positive social actions seemed shaped by these experiences.

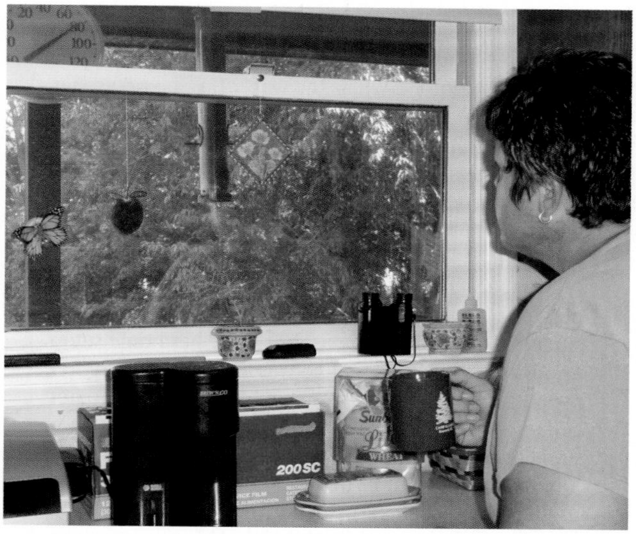

FIGURE 5.2 Patterns of action are shaped over a lifetime as people make choices and develop preferred ways of doing.

A Life Transition and Occupational Therapy

CASE STUDY 5.2 Wanda, *Part III*

At age 40, Wanda wanted to learn to cook and manage the home in which she had lived most of her life. Her mother died when Wanda was 36, and her father passed away 6 months before her 40th birthday. Although Wanda had relatives living nearby who will assist her with household maintenance, she wanted to be able to manage her own life in her home on a day-to-day basis. She and her Medicaid caseworker decided, given Wanda's rural location, that admission into a regional rehabilitation center to maximize her functional skills was the best route to determine her ability to live alone.

The rehabilitation hospital context was a challenge for her as she had to rely on nurses for self-care skills that she has performed independently at home for almost 30 years with the adaptations her parents helped her put in place. Her mobility and speech impairments seemed emphasized in a context where no one was aware of who she was or what she could do. Wanda, however, had two well-developed traits on her side: an outgoing personality that put everyone at ease with her situation and a sense of humor that was soon legendary in the rehabilitation center. Watching her reach out to the young girl crying in the next room made staff aware that Wanda could offer something to her neighbor that staff could not; she was a midlife adult with an understanding of living with disability. Her initiative and actions also brought awareness that Wanda was a person who came into the rehabilitation hospital not to have her disabling condition rehabilitated but to address new challenges brought about by a change in her life situation.

Learning about Wanda's accomplishments throughout her life led her occupational therapist in the rehabilitation center to question why she had never learned to cook or do other things around the house. Wanda laughs when she reports that cooking was one of her mother's favorite things to do, "And she was

(continued)

really good at it! Why would I trade her pot roast for my burned toast?"

Wanda undertook a full range of therapies at the rehabilitation center, but it was in occupational therapy that she identified the activities that had prompted her admission. She grew frustrated when emphasis was placed on trying to reduce tone in her lower extremities or correcting some of her long-preferred speech patterns (which Wanda attributed as much to being Southern as to her dysarthria), but in occupational therapy (OT), she clearly stated her focus on goals that would allow her to stay in her own home.

Wanda had three primary goals related to cooking: to safely use the microwave, to safely make a "real" pot of coffee, and to find ways to effectively open and close food containers. The first and last goals were met within a few weeks using adaptive strategies and creating adaptive tools that she could manage with stabilized gross motor movements. The coffee-making goal became both her greatest challenge and the mark of her stubborn determination.

Although Wanda had better upper extremity control in a seated position, and she used this strategy to manage the microwave, she refused to move her coffee pot to a table or low counter to use it. A home visit and extensive conversation revealed why this was the case. In Wanda's home, the family coffee maker sat right beside the kitchen sink (Figure 5.2). Over the sink was a window, and outside the window were three hanging feeders that Wanda and her father placed there to watch the birds each morning. For longer than she could remember, Wanda woke up smelling coffee that her father had put on to brew, made her way into the kitchen in her pajamas, and stood at the sink watching birds with her father and sipping coffee from a covered mug. She wasn't totally stable in that position—she leaned against the sink counter with her hips and held onto the front of the sink with one hand

(continued)

(continued)

while handling her mug with the other . . . but she was totally content. When she was little, she notes, her mother and father used to have her hold onto the sink in the mornings and stretch out her legs so that she could stand and walk better—sometime in her 20s, the coffee routine was added. Moving the coffee pot from that spot seemed a greater sacrifice than Wanda was willing to make.

In the end, Wanda did successfully make several pots of coffee and pour them into her own mug in a situation simulated to be as much like her home setup as possible. How it happened was a combination of her own bodily stabilization strategies, an adaptation to her coffee pot that allowed her to pivot the canister on a stand rather than lift it to pour, and a stabilizing surface for her mug in front of the pot. Both hospital staff and Wanda's employer participated in crafting the actual modifications she used for this task. Along the way, she also successfully tried a single-cup brewing pot and at the time of discharge was considering asking her aunt for one for her next birthday. ■

Discussion of Wanda's Success

What does Wanda's story have to tell us about the transformation of occupations and life span human development? In traditional developmental models, the biopsychosocial capacities of the human body are often considered prerequisite for action and certainly for skilled performance. How can we then explain the lack of change in Wanda's body relative to an enormous change in her ability to engage in a new occupation? Wanda's spastic movements because of her cerebral palsy did not change during her hospitalization; she did not gain measurable strength or range of motion or endurance beyond that which she had on admission. Yet Wanda's caseworker was satisfied at the time of discharge that with intermittent help from extended family, she could safely manage in her own home on a day-to-day basis. Her ability to do so was evidence of occupational development through a transactional process between her own life experiences with her body, supports in her physical and social environments, and interaction with a therapist who provided safe opportunities for practice and adaptations for success. Recognition of the multitude of factors that influence development of skilled occupational performance and the application of our skills as occupational therapists to draw on all possible sources of transformation lay the foundation for innovative occupation-centered work.

Wanda lived her life as part of various groups recognized and structured by society such as her family, the residential school, church, rural school close to home, and other community organizations including the rehabilitation center. The role of her family and the community organization supporting meal delivery and the occupational therapist who worked with her are part of circumstances that contribute to transformations of occupations. We elaborate on this, illustrating how individuals functioning in social institutions acquire and change their occupations to fulfill the mission of the institution.

Occupations Embedded in Social Institutions

First, social institutions influence the patterns of people's lives and provide structure in the form of opportunities and constraints (Diewald & Mayer, 2009; Elder & Shanahan, 2006). Hedegaard (2009) points out that people moving through their day enter and participate with a variety of these social institutions. Over their life course, people also leave and join new institutions. The timing of joining or leaving a social institution and participation within it are often influenced by both informal and structured age-related **normative expectations.** Within Western society, for example, a family may informally decide when a child is ready to attend a preschool, and programs are available within the social context where many women are employed. On the other hand, leaving the workplace and paid employment to live on retirement cannot occur until a designated age. There is a shared social understanding about what should and should not occur so that opportunities are made available and constraints or consequences put in place. To understand how during the life course we leave and join different social institutions which change our occupations, it helps to consider how they evolve.

Wilcock (2006) proposed that the occupational nature of people evolved simultaneously with sociocultural practices that enabled people to coordinate their actions through their daily occupations for their immediate survival and ultimately sustained survival of the species. It follows that societies create various social institutions to meet needs of different groups of people. Today, institutions such as families, scout troops, senior centers, workplaces, religious organizations, and hospitals draw people together to engage with coordinated, interdependent activities enacting the purpose of the institution. These institutions each have their own cultural practices and values surrounding the occupations and in this way they form communities of practice (Lave & Wenger, 1991). These institutions are structured around social positions or roles that may be formal or informal. To sustain the institutions, there are individuals who fill designated roles as mentors (e.g., teacher, supervisor, older sibling, long-time resident of a retirement community) to orient new members coming to the community. In this way, new members and those less skilled get support in learning to do activities and related practices of the institution. The development of occupations specific to the institution occurs through this process of collaborative engagement.

TABLE 5.2 Proposed Interpersonal Mechanisms Bringing about Change in Occupations

Broad Categories	Proposed Change Mechanisms in Development of an Occupation
Interpersonal influences of occupational engagement	Peripheral participation occurs as novices are part of situations where the occupations occur. As active onlookers, people learn about how things are done, how objects are used, possible outcomes, and what is significant in occupations.
	During co-constructed occupations between two or more people, the performance demands are distributed between participants; people introduce variable situations; and by being engaged with each other, people learn new occupations and alter their understanding about the outcomes and meanings of existing occupation.
	Explicit teaching and scaffolding of the occupation brings a new member's performance to a higher level. The more experienced partner introduces more culturally informed practices and ideas about outcome and meaning.
Engagement in the occupation is transformational for that occupation	Challenges to familiar ways of doing things lead people to try new combinations of their capacities; variations contribute to discovering new performance strategies. Skilled action occurs when people learn to select performance strategies to fit particular situations.
	Altered experiences of outcome and significance of the occupation leads the person to find new performance strategies.
	Performance and capacities are interrelated with reciprocal influences. As a person uses current abilities in occupations, the repeated practice brings about further refinement of abilities and sustains skill—general skill. These changes in turn transform the occupation.

We turn now to elaborate on these social processes that introduce people to new occupations and transforms how they do things. Changes in occupations are not unidirectional; new members with emerging skills of occupational engagement reciprocally define and shape the occupations of other members of their community. To picture this dynamic process, the reader could reflect on ways a practitioner might change occupational situations and support clients in changing their occupations while altering his or her own occupational performance.

Interpersonal Influences Transforming Occupations

As we have seen in the examples of the family engaged in yoga and Wanda's volunteer work with her parents, occupations are co-constructed through coordinated actions of participants within social and historical contexts. Various forces or mechanisms bring about changes in how things are done as people engage with an occupation together (Table 5.2). The changes we address in the remainder of this chapter include not only the acquisition of new occupations but also transformations. These changes include subtle adjustments in performance over time, modifications in performance strategies, and experiences of shared meaning that sustain the occupation as the challenges of new situations are encountered. The cumulative outcome of these changes is notable transformation in occupational performance over time.

Whether young or old, newcomers start as peripheral participants in social institutions, watching other people and gradually joining elements of the occupations (Lave & Wenger, 1991). People who are familiar with the institutional practices expect the novice to watch and acquire the ability to do relevant activities. In this way, learning an occupation is situated where the activity naturally occurs and is carried out by other members of the social institution. In Figure 5.3, as a relatively new member of his family, this toddler is not familiar with various self-care occupations. Once his teeth started to appear, his parents brush his teeth for him as part of their bedtime routine. In this photograph, he is building on past passive experiences by engaging with the object that is part of the occupation. Grasping the toothbrush by the handle and putting the brush in his mouth suggests that he has been an active learner. This does not suggest that he reflects mentally on the functions of oral hygiene or the steps of brushing his

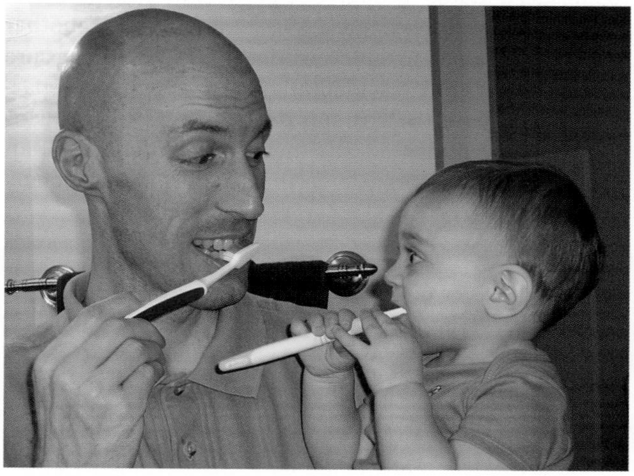

FIGURE 5.3 Father and son's occupation is situated in the bathroom, takes place at certain times of day, and makes use of objects specific to the activity.

own teeth. Rather, his embodied actions lead to his joining with his father by approximating the actions that he has felt and seen. His father's modeling of more refined grip and action on his front teeth may be more specific than the toddler is capable of doing at this time. The child's attention, though, is focused on his father's mouth where the brush is placed. This picture illustrates that the co-construction of occupation takes place at a nonverbal level. Rather, people evolved to read the actions of others as intentional as it unfolds in familiar sociocultural context (Rosenberg, 2008).

A similar pattern of co-construction through embodied actions with objects is seen as an elderly woman with dementia stands looking at a head of cabbage when asked to help chop it for coleslaw. She does not respond to the verbal request but joins in the activity when she sees someone else shredding cabbage at the chopping block. This differential ability can be explained in terms of spared procedural versus semantic or conceptual memory (Vance, Moore, Farr, & Struzick, 2008). The reason the older woman can call on the procedural knowledge is that she has embodied this activity (or a very similar one) in the past. Changes in performance occur through lived bodily experiences of engagement with other people. The point of being able to coordinate actions with the intentional behaviors of others to share an occupation is conceptually important so people of different ages or mental abilities still enter situations where their occupations change.

We return now to the second proposed change mechanism in Table 5.2: the co-construction of occupation that can occur among members of the institution at a similar level of proficiency. A social milieu brought about by doing something together ensures continuity of action while also allowing variability and contributing to the construction of meaning. First, shared engagement means that how-to-do-it knowledge is distributed among two or more people, so if one person forgets how to do something, the intentional acts of another person may serve as a cue or substitute. The important thing is all participants continue to engage, and it is through this participation that further mastery will occur. Second, doing something with another person inevitably introduces variations in how things are done, which stimulates adaptation and challenges all participants to learn to do things differently. Finally, Lawlor (2003) pointed out that at times, the significance of an occupation rests primarily in the sense of being socially engaged. Even when a person might hesitate to do something, the fact someone else is involved will encourage the beginner to try, which in turn may result in him or her potentially embracing a new occupation and experiencing meaning that makes the activity more appealing the next time the occupational opportunity occurs.

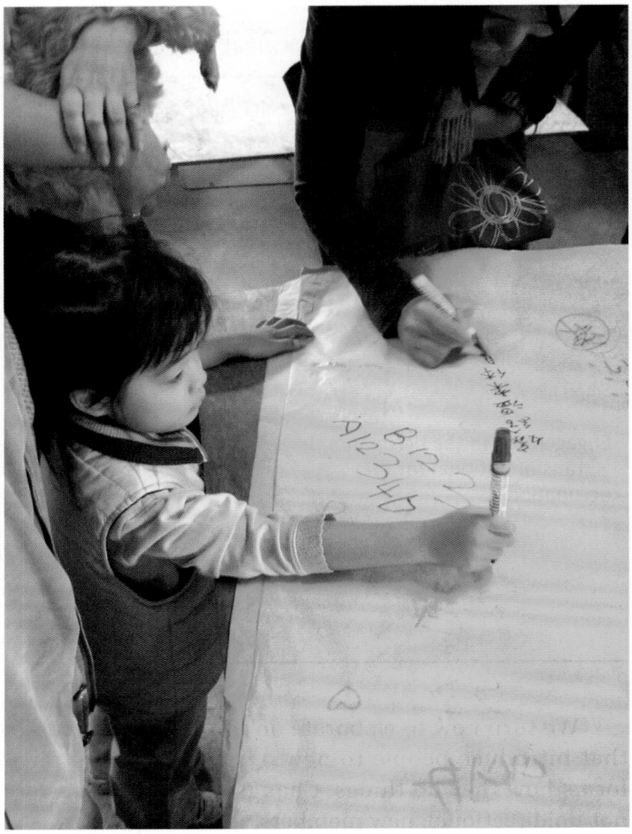

FIGURE 5.4 Social participation enables children to enter situations where they can learn new occupations.

This last point—being drawn into something new for the sake of being socially occupied with someone—illustrates that if new occupations are needed or desired, there are no prerequisites for engagement. In co-constructed occupations, the person with more expertise can fill in missing elements, whereas the beginner experiences participation with occupation at whatever level he or she is able. Figure 5.4 illustrates our final case study.

CASE STUDY 5.3 Participation in a Festival

Shufen is 3 years old and has been watching others engage in the Lantern Festival, a traditional celebration in Taiwan. People write their wishes on the paper that are folded into lanterns and released like a hot air balloon, taking their messages up to the Almighty in the sky. It is customary to include people with various abilities because participants believe that the Almighty has the power and wisdom to understand people's wishes. Shufen has seen her family writing at home and understands many elements of how to write, so she has joined in the tradition despite a lack of formal training in writing Taiwanese characters, which is not introduced until kindergarten.

As you can see, Shufen engaged by writing what she knows; and other people give what she does meaning, writing alongside her in the more traditional characters and regarding her as a cowriter. This suggests that people start being a writer, musician, or playmate by participating with people who write, make music, or play. It also holds true for children with disabilities; engaging in activities that involve writing result in development as a writer, whereas simply addressing underlying skills, like letter recognition, does not lead to the same level of occupational transformation (Hanser, 2010).

Recall from the previous examples that new members of a social institution like a family or workplace have access to experienced members who already know the routines and cultural practices of the institution. When someone new to an occupation has access to more skilled members, the novice often defers to the designated expert. In this way, the power of a shared occupation takes on additional weight as a change process because teaching, scaffolding, or guiding another person's participation becomes part of the situation (Rogoff, 2003). The person with expertise initially adjusts to the situation to be consistent with the novice's understanding (Wertsch, 1999). As everyone involved coordinates his or her actions, facial expressions, words, and actions form the medium for shared meanings. Once a connection is established of doing the occupation together, the expert introduces new definitions of significance and expected outcomes giving more information about what is expected and how things are done. Box 5.1 lists ways in which the experienced person contributes to the development of occupation. The evolving definition of the situation includes a shared sense of the novice gaining expertise, gradually evolving from a beginner to a more experienced participant.

Note that the strategies suggested previously are part of social engagement in an activity, not the formal instruction that might occur in a patient education session or, for example, in the case of a school therapist asking a child to copy letters on a worksheet. Indeed, Lave and Packer (2008) write: "Both 'socialization' and 'formal instruction' involves extensive mythologies about the mechanisms of learning" (p. 29). Socialization without the dynamics of shared engagement leaves the learner in a passive role of being told what is important to do, whereas formal instruction might be a means of transmitting out of context, abstract information. Neither of these forms of learning explains the phenomenon of a novice functioning on the periphery of a social institution where engagement in occupations is central to the continuation of that institution. The authors suggest that this everyday learning takes place in the context of participation when doing accessible parts of the desired occupation and generates an embodied understanding of how to do it.

At this point, we move away from concepts suggested by activity theorists and consider more moment-to-moment transformations in performance. Literature about motor development (Thelen, 2000) and solving problems (Siegler, 2000) inform our discussion. The ideas discussed here continue to rest on ideas about the embodied action, emergent performance, and the situated nature of occupational engagement.

The concept of emergent performance becomes perhaps even clearer when considering occupational transformations in the lives of older adults. If we hold to the premise that maturation of biopsychosocial capacities is a necessary precursor to new performance, it would suggest that either individual capacities are continuing to develop in adult years at a rate similar to childhood or, conversely, that adults reach a static state without much residual capacity for change. In this view, aging would be a predictable process with universal characteristics manifest across all human beings. Although there are relatively evident and predictable biological changes identified throughout the adult life span, many scholars now contend there is more variability than uniformity in aging (Crosnoe & Elder, 2002; Lachman, 2004; Westerhof, Katzko, Dittmann-Kohli, & Hayslip, 2001). We must consider not only the changing capacities of the individual human being but also the social and historical contexts in any given situation as explanations for this variability.

For example, Kaye Tobin is an 81-year-old Californian who travels alone throughout the year—for up to 9 months, at most. She traces her passion for travel to her first trip away from her hometown as a teenager (Lerner, 2011). That we consider Kaye "unusual for her age" is based on our assumptions that a person of 81 would not typically have an intact repertoire of capacities needed for independent travel. Tobin's travel is not with sponsored tours or with others managing her luggage; on the

BOX 5.1 How an Experienced Person Can Support a Novice's Engagement in a Challenging Occupation

1. Create social opportunities to do the activity with another person.
2. Fill in performance gaps, doing difficult parts of the activity.
3. Suggest or model different ways to do the activity.
4. Introduce and model the use of new objects in the activity.
5. Add relevant information about the activity.
6. Elaborate on alternative outcomes.
7. Bring in more culturally shaped meanings regarding why the activity is significant.

contrary, she travels with only a backpack and stays in elder or youth hostels so that she can travel more frequently (Lerner, 2011). The entire significance of Tobin carrying out her passion for travel is not simply that she is defying stereotypes about age. Her independent navigation through new situations speaks to someone with individual capacities that allow her to pursue a favored occupation, but engaging in that occupation in turn helps to maintain those capacities.

Occupations can be transformed also when a person recognizes different outcomes or realizes some new significance in doing it (Humphry, 2002). As discussed earlier, watching other people do things and co-constructing an occupation with others alters the person's experiences about how things are done, what is an expected outcome, and why that matters. People can also discover their own new ideas about their occupations. Even when an occupation seems to be routine, a new meaning changes how it is done or how it is perceived. In U.S. culture, driving becomes routine for many adults, automatic to the point that many of us drive familiar routes without conscious attention to them, or assume that we will be able to drive unless we choose not to do so. For the adult who sustains a traumatic injury or loss of functional ability, however, the inability to either temporarily or permanently operate a vehicle imbues the occupation of driving with new importance. The person who is able to resume driving may drive with heightened appreciation for the ability to do so, whereas the person who cannot resume driving comes to view it as a social status rather than simply a functional ability.

Finally, although maturation of capacities does not completely explain changes in occupational performance, capacities do change with use. In a broad biological sense, development of a person occurs simultaneously at several levels, including genetic activity, body structure, the functions of body systems, capacities, and performance (Gottlieb, 2000). Furthermore, there are reciprocal influences across levels. This means that as people use their capacities, repeated experiences change these levels and directly or indirectly bring their capacities and performance to higher levels of maturity. Subsequently, more mature capacities become available and occupational performance changes. However, the situated and emergent nature of performance in context needs to be remembered.

Conclusion

A colleague once observed that occupations are complex and messy. Using a life course perspective, we recognize a range of factors shaping how occupations are acquired and transformed over months and years. In looking at the family engaged in yoga in which both the grandmother and granddaughter have recently taken up the practice, we saw that age of the individual is not the primary factor in learning to do something new. They also illustrate that there are multiple reasons for choosing to do something. Whereas the grandmother had reflected on the benefits of exercise and saw yoga offering a desired outcome, the granddaughter, without reflection, joined in as a way to be part of the family. In introducing Wanda and her life course, we illustrate how her choice to engage in clowning around to connect with another patient in a rehabilitation center is best understood as a choice that is part of her life course and the experiences she had with her parents. Knowing earlier occupational choices she and her parents made gave her activities in the rehabilitation center some context.

Occupational therapy is indicated when a person is unable to do expected or desired occupations that connect that person with social situations. How occupational therapy practitioners conceptualize the change process determines how they practice. We have presented the importance of taking a contextual view regarding what people do and why they do things. This is reflected in the modified principles of the life course and illustrated with the case of Wanda. How these ideas could be applied to practice with children is discussed elsewhere (Humphry & Wakeford, 2006). In general, we want to emphasize the interconnected elements of the occupational situation and how occupations serve to connect people with their lives (Dickie et al., 2006).

We introduce the idea that people live their lives as members of a variety of different social institutions where occupations with specific cultural practices and routines occur. Whether we enter a new institution as a family member, student, employee, or as a patient following an accident, opportunities are created to learn or transform occupations. Over time, the novice is supported in participating by engaging in occupations that others are already familiar with doing. We see that by being brought into co-constructing occupation, the how-to knowledge and what it means is shared between participants. People's performance changes as they learn the occupational form and experience how it is defined as meaningful by others.

Finally, we suggest that refinement in performance rests on the emergent nature of action where the occupational situation, the person's actual performance, discovery of new strategies, and changing experiences of meaning can all bring about transformations in engagement and understanding about how something is done. Changes in occupational performance and meaning occur over the entire life course and implications of this type of practice for work with people in various life circumstances need further exploration and explication.

References

Blair, S. E. E. (2000). The centrality of occupation during life transitions. *British Journal of Occupational Therapy, 63*, 231–237.

Brandtsadter, J., & Lerner, R. M. (Eds.). (1999). *Action and self-development: Theory and research through the life span.* Thousand Oaks, CA: SAGE.

Crosnoe, R., & Elder, G. H., Jr. (2002). Successful adaptation in the later years: A life course approach to aging. *Social Psychology Quarterly, 65*(4), 309–328.

Cutchin, M., & Dickie, V. A. (2012). Transactionalism: Occupational science and the pragmatic attitude. In G. Whiteford & C. Hocking (Eds.), *Critical perspectives on occupational science: Society, inclusion, participation* (pp. 23–37). London: Wiley Press.

Dickie, V., Cutchin, M. P., & Humphry, R. (2006). Occupation as transactional experience: A critique of individualism in occupational science. *Journal of Occupational Science, 13*, 83–93.

Diewald, M., & Mayer, K. U. (2009). The sociology of the life course and life span psychology: Integrated paradigm or complementing pathways? *Advances in Life Course Research, 14*, 5–14.

Elder, G. H., & Conger, R. D. (2000). *Children of the land: Adversity and success in rural America.* Chicago, IL: The University of Chicago Press.

Elder, G. H., & Shanahan, M. J. (2006). The life course and human development. In R. M. Lerner (Ed.), *Handbook of person psychology* (6th ed., Vol. 1, pp. 665–715). Hoboken, NJ: John Wiley & Sons.

Gottlieb, G. (2000). Understanding genetic activity within a holistic framework. In L. R. Bergman, R. B. Cairns, L. Nilsson, & L. Nystedt (Eds.), *Developmental science and the holistic approach* (pp. 179–201). Mahwah, NJ: Lawrence Erlbaum Associates.

Hanser, G. (2010). Emergent literacy for children with disabilities. *OT Practice, 15*(3), 16–20.

Hedegaard, M. (2009). Children's development from a cultural-historical approach: Children's activity in everyday local settings as foundations for their development. *Mind, Culture and Activity, 16*, 64–81.

Humphry, R. (2002). Young children's occupational behaviors: Explicating the dynamics of developmental processes. *American Journal of Occupational Therapy, 56*, 171–179.

Humphry, R. (2005). Model of processes transforming occupations: Exploring societal and social influences. *Journal of Occupational Science, 12*, 36–41.

Humphry, R., & Wakeford, L. (2006). An occupation-centered discussion of development and implications for practice. *American Journal of Occupational Therapy, 60*, 258–267.

Johnson, M. K., Crosnoe, R., & Elder, G. H. (2011). Insights on adolescence from a life course perspective. *Journal of Research on Adolescence, 21*, 273–280.

Lachman, M. E. (2004). Development in midlife. *Annual Review of Psychology, 55*, 305–331.

Lave, J., & Packer, M. (2008). Towards a social ontology of learning. In K. Nielsen, S. Brinkmann, C. Elmholdt, & G. Kraft (Eds.), *A qualitative stance: In memory of Steinar Kvale, 1938–2008* (pp. 17–47). Denmark: Aarhus University Press.

Lave, J., & Wenger, E. (1991). *Situated learning: Legitimate peripheral participation.* Cambridge, NY: Cambridge Press.

Lawlor, M. (2003). The significance of being occupied: The social construction of childhood occupations. *American Journal of Occupational Therapy, 57*, 424–434.

Lerner, N. (2011). Globetrotting grandma: A woman pursues her dreams on solo trips abroad. *AARP The Magazine, 54*, (4C) 71.

Lerner, R. M. (2002). *Concepts and theories of human development* (3rd ed.). Mahwah, NJ: Lawrence Erlbaum Associates.

Mayer, K. U. (2009). New directions in life course research. *Annual Review of Sociology, 35*, 413–433.

Overton, W. F. (2010). Life-span development: Concepts and issues. In W. F. Overton & R. M. Lerner (Eds.), *The handbook of life-span development: Cognition, biology & methods* (Vol. 1, pp. 1–29). Hoboken, NJ: John Wiley & Sons.

Overton, W. F., Muller, U., & Newman, J. L. (Eds.). (2008). *Developmental perspectives on embodiment and consciousness.* New York, NY: Lawrence Erlbaum Associates.

Rogoff, B. (2003). *The cultural nature of human development.* New York, NY: Oxford University Press.

Rosenberg, A. (2008). *Philosophy of social science* (3rd ed.). Boulder, CO: Westview.

Siegler, R. S. (2000). The rebirth of children's learning. *Child Development, 71*, 26–35.

Thelen, E. (2000). Grounded in the world: Developmental origins of the embodied mind. *Infancy, 1*, 3–28.

Vance, D. E., Moore, B. S., Farr, K. F., & Struzick, T. (2008). Procedural memory and emotional attachement in Alzheimer disease: Implications for meaningful and engaging activities. *Journal of Neuroscience Nursing, 40*, 96–102.

Wertsch, J. V. (1999). The zone of proximal development: Some conceptual issues. In P. Lloyd & C. Fernyhough (Eds.), *Lev Vygotsky: Critical Assessments* (Vol. 3, pp. 67–78). London: Routledge.

Westerhof, G. J., Katzko, M. W., Dittmann-Kohli, F., & Hayslip, B. (2001). Life contexts and health-related selves in old age. *Journal of Aging Studies, 15*, 105.

Wilcock, A. A. (2006). *An occupational perspective of health* (2nd ed.). Thorofare, NJ: SLACK.

For additional resources on the subjects discussed in this chapter, visit http://thePoint.lww.com/Willard-Spackman12e.

CHAPTER 6

Contribution of Occupation to Health and Well-Being

Clare Hocking

OUTLINE

LEARNING OBJECTIVES

After reading this chapter, you will be able to:

1. Describe, in occupational terms, what being healthy means and how that relates to the Ottawa Charter and Healthy People 2020
2. Explore ways that occupation contributes to the health and well-being of all people in terms of meeting biological needs, developing skills, and using capacities
3. Drawing on the international literature, evaluate how occupation influences men's and women's health differently and some workers but not others
4. Describe positive and negative health impacts of people's overall pattern of occupation
5. Analyze how well-being might be influenced by a person's physical, social, and attitudinal environment
6. Evaluate the ways in which people's occupations might be detrimental to health and well-being
7. Analyze how having an impairment might affect well-being, taking environmental barriers into account

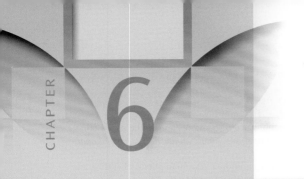

On Monday, I got the lawns cut and got my tomato plants tied up. With this drier weather, there have been a lot of leaves falling, and they were all over the garden. I have got a small leaf rake, which I made out of light reinforcing mesh, and I flicked all the dry leaves to the back along the fence and then I watered them so that they will rot down and make compost. Tidying the garden made my back ache a bit, bending over. It's still a bit wonky. Still, it's only muscular, so it will come right. In the afternoon, I cleaned up a pile of papers; went through and discarded what I didn't want. Sometimes I already know what I will do next, but you never run out of a job unless you're not interested. None of the jobs are a burden. I enjoy doing them and if a job's got to be done, I like to do it properly. It might take me a little bit longer, but I haven't got to do it twice. I just go from one thing to another. Time goes quickly because I have always got something to do. (Frank, aged 97)

(Wright-St. Clair, unpublished data, 2010)

Occupation, Health, and Well-Being

Frank's account of days spent moving from one task to another contains many of the elements that people in Western societies associate with being healthy. Despite his advanced age, Frank's days are full and time goes quickly. He conveys a quiet pride in restoring his garden to order and expects that the muscles made sore by raking leaves will be better in a few days. Frank is interested in the different tasks the seasons bring and finds pleasure in being busy and productive, using tools he made for himself, and doing the job properly (see Figure 6.1). Frank, like most people, does not subscribe to a biomedical view of health, which equates health with the absence of disease (*Health*, 2009). Rather, he perceives himself to be physically and mentally healthy when he is able to engage in his usual occupations (*Healthy People 2010*, n.d.). For Frank, being healthy means maintaining an active lifestyle and being able to do the things that are important to him: keeping his garden productive and tidy, eating homegrown fruits and vegetables, and making sure his personal affairs are in order. Occupational therapists might also note that Frank's **occupations**, meaning all the things he does that occupy his time, are a balance of physically taxing and cognitive tasks, keeping mind and body active.

The relationship between occupation and health is widely recognized; indeed, it is the premise upon which occupational therapy is founded. The link is also recognized by the World Health Organization (WHO). For instance, the WHO's (1986) Ottawa Charter, a key public health policy document that sought to promote broad understandings of the determinants of health, declares that health is a resource that people create in their everyday lives, using their physical capacities and personal and social resources. Although the charter was initially considered idealistic (Larson, 1999), thinking about health as a resource has taken hold and both lay people and health professionals commonly refer to health as "the capacity or ability to engage in various activities, fulfill roles, and meet the demands of daily life" (Williamson & Carr, 2009, p. 108). Accordingly, when present-day researchers set out to establish whether people perceive themselves to be healthy, their experience of participating in occupation is commonly included. For instance, a self-report survey of elderly Sri Lankans undertaken on behalf of the World Bank asked respondents to rate their independence in activities of daily living (eating, dressing, toileting, bathing), instrumental activities of daily living (shopping, preparing a meal, drawing water from a well, sweeping the yard), and social participation (babysitting grandchildren, helping with meals, paid work, etc.). They were also asked about abilities that can be readily interpreted as relating to occupation—being able to hear people speaking at their normal volume and mobility, such as standing from a chair or bowing (Ostbye, Malhotra, & Chan, 2009). Wellness models also typically include a spiritual aspect of health (Larson, 1999), which is enacted through religious observances and other occupations in which people find spiritual meaning.

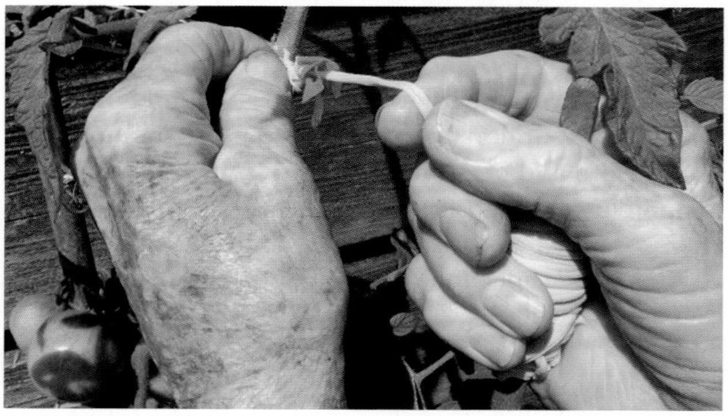

FIGURE 6.1 Frank tying up his tomato plants.

When Frank talks about the ways he fills his days, it is clear that he ascribes to these broad understandings of health as a resource to meet the demands of daily living. He also conveys a sense of **well-being**. Although no definitive description of well-being exists, it is generally understood to be a person's subjective perception of his or her health and encompasses feelings about physical, mental, and social health. In Western societies, in which individualistic values prevail, well-being is commonly associated with self-esteem, happiness, a sense of belonging, and personal growth and having a sense of community (Semenza & Krishnasamy, 2007). Indigenous people generally also include notions of spiritual well-being and connection to the land (Grieves, 2008). Taking an ecological perspective, Wilcock (2006) has also suggested that well-being is inextricably bound to the health of local and global ecosystems, and ecopsychologists support the notion of an implicit link between human health and natural environments (Stevens, 2010).

Feelings of well-being arise from the things people do that provide a sense of vitality, purpose, satisfaction, or fulfillment. Occupational well-being also relates to the things people envision doing in the future. Well-being is expressed in terms of feeling on top of the world; feeling nourished, contented, transformed, at peace, strong, interested, and fully alive; or experiencing intense concentration (Wilcock, 2006). Such views are largely in keeping with the Ottawa Charter, which asserts that to attain complete well-being "an individual or group must be able to identify and to realize aspirations, to satisfy needs, and to change or cope with the environment" (WHO, 1986, p. 1).

Occupational therapists believe that the mechanism by which people achieve these things is through occupation (Kielhofner, 2008; Townsend & Polatajko, 2007), and that certainly seems true of Frank. He adjusts his occupations to the seasons and feels involved in life and competent to look after his plants and solve everyday challenges, such as making a rake that is light enough to use with ease. When he is fully engaged in and enjoying what he is doing, he feels fit and well, an experience that is not diminished by aching muscles. Although his daily routines and occupational choices are different from other times in his life, Frank is generally satisfied with what he achieves and he appears to experience the sense of continuity that has been recognized to be the hallmark of successful aging (Carlson, Clark, & Young, 1998).

Occupation also contributes to the health of people with a health condition. For instance, progressive reengagement in occupation at an intensity they can sustain helps people recovering from mental illness to reintegrate a sense of self and reconnect with the environment. As they progress from the disintegrated experience Sutton (2006) described as non-doing, to half-doing, engaged doing, and, finally, absorbed doing, so they are increasingly able to structure time and space, and future possibilities in the everyday world open up. Knowing that occupation is just as important for the health of people with activity limitations, who are generally less physically active than the rest of us, targeted research programs and interventions are being established. For example, a program to introduce people with spinal cord injury to recreational occupations, including kite flying, handcycling, and sea kayaking, has been reported (Block, Skeels, Keys, & Rimmer, 2005). In addition, targeted research has been recommended, such as studies examining physical fitness programs designed to ameliorate the muscle weakness and poor cardiorespiratory fitness of children with cerebral palsy (Fowler et al., 2007).

As this introduction has shown, the relationship between occupation and well-being is complex. A great number of factors influence the health outcomes of occupation, and knowledge of how the various factors interact is incomplete. To contain the topic and ensure its relevance, priority is given to understandings generated by occupational therapists and occupational scientists. Consistent with those perspectives, the term "occupation" refers to the things people do that they find personally and culturally meaningful, whereas "participation" is used in the more restricted sense of whether a person actually engages in occupation.

To give the discussion depth, evidence reported in the international literature is included. The discussion proceeds by considering some of the ways occupation contributes to health and well-being. That includes what can be learned by its absence, when people are deprived of sufficient occupation. To give a balanced account, there is also discussion of the ways in which occupation can be injurious to health. Contextual factors that act as barriers to achieving good health are also described before concluding with a brief summation of the evidence.

How Occupation Contributes to Health and Well-Being

If we are to assert that **participation** in occupation contributes to keeping good health, we need to understand how that comes about. Ann Wilcock, an eminent occupational scientist, considered that question from a biological perspective. She argued that occupation is essential to individual and species survival, because the basic **biological needs** for sustenance, self-care, shelter, and safety are met through the things people do. In meeting those needs and through other occupations of daily life, people develop "skills, social structures and technology aimed at superiority over predators and the environment" (Wilcock, 1993, p. 20). Those skills include growing and cooking nutritious food and constructing warm clothing and dry houses. Also important, though not always achieved, is the skill of living peacefully with neighbors. Depending on the circumstances, many other skills are also relevant to health. Reading and writing, for example, are important means of conveying information relevant to sustaining health and seeking health care in Western societies. It is also important to note that not everyone needs all the skills that are relevant to survival. Rather, health depends on being part of a family or community of people who together have the skills necessary to survive, and perhaps to flourish, as well as access to the resources to put their skills to use.

Meeting survival needs and becoming skilled are not sufficient to ensure good health; of equal importance is the contribution that occupation makes to developing and exercising personal **capacities** (Wilcock, 1993, 1995). These capacities spring from the biological characteristics shared by all humans: walking upright, opposing thumb and fingers to grasp objects, learning to speak, and so on. People have the capacity to, among other things, carry loads, design new tools and find novel uses for old ones, understand the workings of the universe, accumulate and pass on knowledge, predict what might happen and prepare for the future, form relationships, and express themselves artistically and spiritually. People also have the capacity to play, as Gabbe and her grandfather show us, photographed playing "animals and trains" on the lounge room floor (Figure 6.2).

Each person's capacities reflect this human potential via his or her genetic inheritance, brought into being through the developmental process, and a unique life

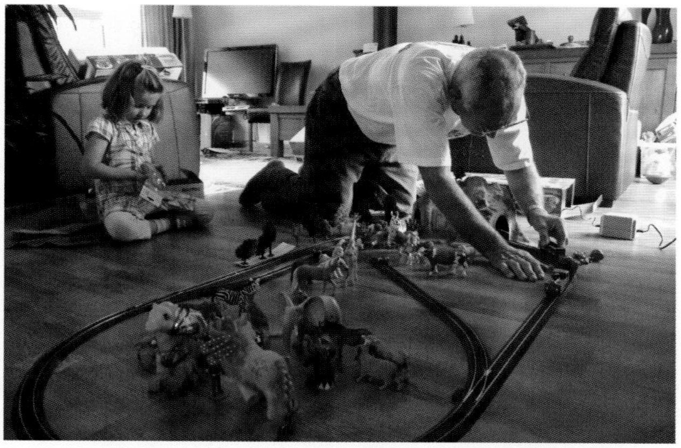

FIGURE 6.2 Gabbe playing "animals and trains" with Granddad.

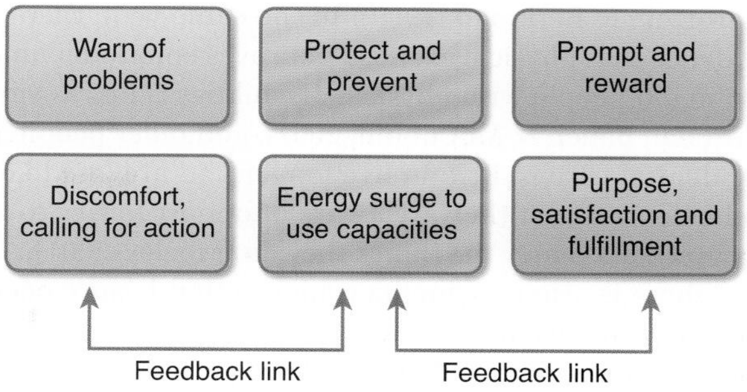

FIGURE 6.3 Biological hierarchy of need for occupation From Wilcock, A. (1993). A theory of the human need for occupation. *Journal of Occupational Science: Australia, 1,* 17–24. doi:10.1080/14427591.1993.9686375

history of occupational opportunities, preferences, and choices. On the basis of their history of doing things and expectations of what they might do in the future, people are generally aware of the capacities they have: whether they are better at sports, art, or music; whether they find schoolwork or practical tasks more congenial; and whether they prefer solitary occupations or mixing socially.

What stimulates people to engage in occupations that enhance their chances of survival, develop skills, and exercise capacities is much debated. One suggestion advanced by Wilcock (1993) is that humans experience biological needs that stimulate occupation, which in turn promotes health. These needs relate, first, to correcting threats to our physiological state, such as being excessively hot or cold or feeling hungry or thirsty. The discomfort of these sensations stimulates us to action: to find some shade, put on more clothing, or seek out food or drink (see Figure 6.3). The second set of needs is protective and preventive, such as the need to develop skills and exercise capacities. These are experienced as a surge of energy that propels us to acquire and practice the skills required to solve problems and plan, interact with others, do whatever generates our livelihood, and so on. In so doing, at least before technology removed many of the physical demands of earlier lifestyles, people exercised their capacity for physical, mental, and social functioning. The third and final set of needs prompts and rewards engagement in occupation. Meeting these needs gives a sense of purpose, satisfaction, and fulfillment (see Box 6.1).

Evidence That Occupation Affects Health and Well-Being

It is widely acknowledged that occupation benefits health, and occupations involving physical activity have been a particular focus. For example, it is known that weight-bearing exercise is important for skeletal development and developing normal bone mass in children and adolescents, and that regular walking contributes to their cardiovascular and psychological health (Ziviani, Scott, & Wadley, 2004). The Healthy People 2020 report prepared for the U.S. government is one of many authoritative sources asserting that physical activity helps maintain healthy weight for people of all ages and strength and agility in older adults. That report also associates good mental health with productive occupations, noting that mental illness often results in people being unable to manage their responsibilities as parents and partners (*Healthy People 2020*, n.d.).

In addition to these physical health benefits, there is evidence that cognitive functioning, psychological health, and positive social networks are maintained by participating in occupations that exercise one's physical, mental, and social capacities. Accordingly, the more older Americans garden, dance, play golf or bowl, swim, cycle, jog, or walk for exercise, the lower the incidence of depression (Vance, Wadley, Ball, Roenker, & Rizzo, 2005). One large-scale study of older Americans is particularly noteworthy. It showed that social and productive occupations decreased their risk of mortality as much as physically demanding occupations did (Glass, de Leon,

BOX 6.1 Biologic Needs Stimulating Occupation (Wilcock, 1993)

1. Correcting threats to physiological state
2. Acquiring skills to protect and prevent
3. Prompt and reward engagement in occupation

Marottoli, & Berkman, 1999). In the same vein, there is evidence that physical exercise improves emotional functioning in people with physical disabilities (Ellis, Kosma, Cardinal, Bauer, & McCubbin, 2007), and older people in residential care in Britain live longer and are less likely to be depressed if they are aware of opportunities to be occupied and enjoy the things they do (Mozley, 2001).

There is also convincing evidence that leisure occupations influence men's and women's health in different ways. A Norwegian study with 50,797 participants found that men who watch sports and attend cultural events and women who actively participate in cultural occupations such as learning a musical instrument, taking art classes, or singing in a group report better health, greater satisfaction with life, and less anxiety and depression than those who do not. What is more, frequent participation is associated with higher levels of well-being than less frequent participation (Cuypers et al., 2011). Some insight into why those leisure pursuits are good for people's health comes from a qualitative study of singing in a choir, which reported the sense of community and accomplishment, stress reduction, and improved mood that choristers experience (Jacob, Guptill, & Sumsion, 2009).

As well as the gender differences noted in relation to leisure, experiencing low work stress has been found to be an important predictor of health for men, whereas women's health is associated with finding meaning in their everyday occupations and having a harmonious repertoire of occupations and effective strategies to manage everyday demands (Håkansson & Ahlborg, 2010; Håkansson, Dahlin-Ivanoff, & Sonn, 2006). The findings of these small-scale studies are supported by evidence that the quality or intensity of engaging in occupation affects its impact on health and well-being. For instance, engaging in occupations that generate flow experiences, those that demand our peak performance and render us oblivious to how much time has passed, is known to have health benefits (Csikszentmihalyi, 1998; Persson, Eklund, & Isacsson, 1999) (see Figure 6.4). The cumulative health benefits of good quality work experiences are evident in population health statistics, which demonstrate that longevity relates to employment, prosperity, and ethnicity; because people who are employed, those with higher incomes, and members of the dominant ethnic group in a society have lower incidences of most chronic diseases and better health care outcomes (Centers for Disease Control and Prevention [CDC], 2005b; Ministry of Health Manatū Hauora, 2005).

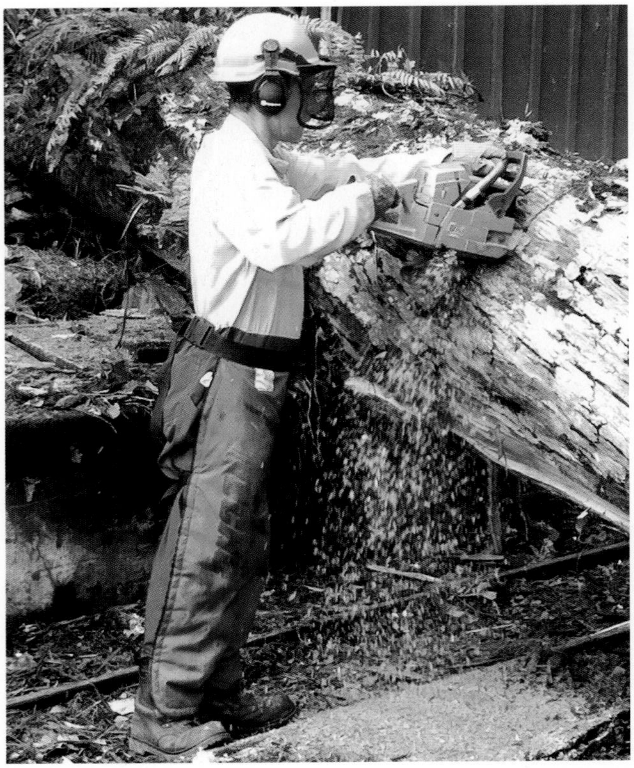

FIGURE 6.4 Good quality work experiences contribute to well-being and longevity.

Health and Patterns of Occupation

The overall pattern of people's occupations is also important. Breaking up active participation in occupation with rest contributes to health, whether that is a short break to stretch before returning to computer work, work-rest schedules to enhance the effects of training, or more prolonged engagement in a restorative leisure occupation. Having a rest confers many benefits, one of which is that it enhances our memory of recent experiences, which explains the value of taking a break when we are trying to study or learn new things (Tambini, Katz, & Davachi, 2010). There is some evidence that taking a break in a natural environment, for example by going for a walk, restores people's ability to focus their attention (Sanders, Yankou, & Andrusyszyn, 2005), and perceptual processing speed is restored by a brief nap but not by resting for an equivalent time (Mednick et al., 2002). Where people go to rest is also important, with natural environments (whether a garden, park, or landscape) thought to have restorative properties.

Whereas rest is associated with good health, two features of modern lifestyles are associated with poor health outcomes. The first is the impact of technologies that have become entrenched social norms but decrease physical activity levels. Examples are people's increasing reliance on their cars, which decreases walking, and passive home entertainment (Schoenberg, Hatcher, & Dignan, 2008). When combined with the consumption of calorie-dense foods, television viewing, computer use, and electronic games are a particularly unhealthy mix for children (Moore & Harré, 2007) (see Figure 6.5). The other health-depleting feature of modern lifestyles is its increasing tempo, which is associated with high workloads, limited access to leisure time pursuits, and increasing levels of stress and stress-related illness (Zuzanek, 1998). Compounding that, because they do not have time to reflect on and experience meaning in living, people with overly busy lives are

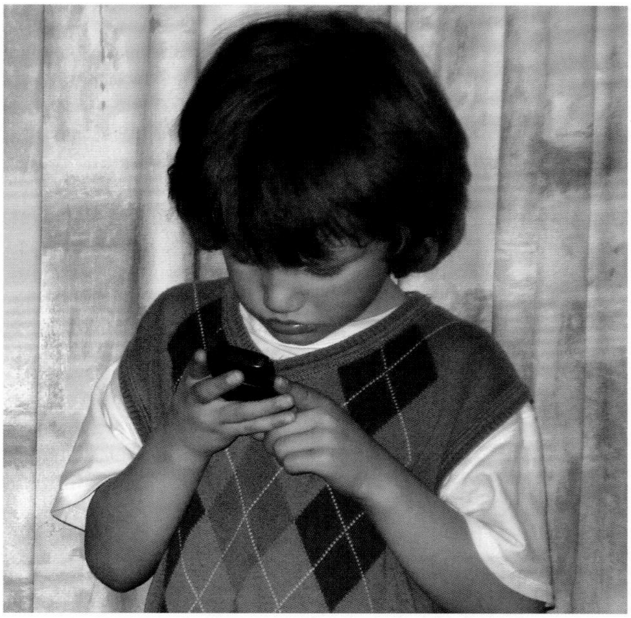

FIGURE 6.5 A feature of modern life: screen time.

channeled toward culturally constructed occupations such as shopping at the mall rather than pastimes they might find more absorbing and rewarding (Clark, 1997). Such lifestyles appear incompatible with high-level well-being, which Erlandsson's (2003) study of 100 Swedish women's time use seems to corroborate. Her study showed that highly complex patterns of occupation characterized by frequent interruptions and changes of task correlate with lower levels of reported well-being than are found in women with less complex occupational patterns. The temporal demands of shift work and female shift workers' practice of sacrificing sleep to fulfill their responsibilities as mothers, caregivers, and homemakers also appear incompatible with well-being (Gallew & Mu, 2004).

Insufficient Occupation Is Detrimental to Health

Occupation's contribution to health is also evident in accounts of the deleterious effects of not doing enough. Again, most attention has been paid to physical exercise. People who do not regularly engage in physically demanding occupations such as gardening, swimming, running, riding a bicycle, playing sport, or cleaning are not maintaining the capacity to exert themselves physically. As well as not being able to sustain physical exertion should they need to, people who have a sedentary lifestyle have increased risk of cardiovascular disease, cancer, diabetes, and osteoporosis, with unfit women having higher mortality risks than unfit men (Hagberg & Lindholm, 2006). Lack of exercise is also associated with the looming crisis of childhood obesity (see the Case Study 6.1).

For those who do not exercise in other ways, walking reasonably quickly for at least 30 minutes a day, 5 days a week, is considered the minimum requirement to maintain health (Wallis, Miranda, & Park, 2005). Estimates of the number of people who achieve this level of activity vary. In the United States, 22.4% of adults engage in vigorous physical activity five times a week; the percent by age range decreases from 31.7% for people aged 18 to 24 to 6.2% for people 75 years and older (CDC, 2005a). In Norway, only 6% of people older than 65 years old meet the exercise guideline (Loland, 2004). Concern over the lower rates of physical activity among older adults is compounded by knowledge of the isolation, loneliness, and depression that results from losing their driver's license and thus access to previous occupations in the community (Classen et al., 2007; Stav, Pierce, Wheatley, & Davis, 2005).

Occupation and Health Threats

Occupational therapists are well aware that having a health condition or impairment can negatively affect occupational performance. Many of the case examples in theory texts, such as those related to the Model of Human Occupation, illustrate that idea. Accordingly, therapeutic processes to enhance people's engagement in occupations that will "support their physical and emotional well-being" are described (Kielhofner, 2008, p. 3). It is also clear that the relationship can work the other way; that occupations might threaten health. Being employed in low quality work, for example, does not guarantee the health benefits accrued from work that is useful and rewarding, carried out in a safe environment, and that allows a balance between work and leisure (Legge, 2007). Thus, people working in sales or customer services rate their health lower than people in managerial and professional roles or in the skilled trades (Lowis, Knight, & Ball, 2010). Additionally, people who experience employment insecurity and decreased wage levels as a consequence of the de-industrialization of Western societies, workers replaced by technology, and those exploited by their employers or exposed to toxic substances have fewer health benefits in the short- or long-term (Legge, 2007). Boredom is another factor to consider. Drawing on her study of young offenders, Farnworth (1998) proposed that boredom is perhaps "endemic in Western industrialized nations" (p. 145). While the short- and long-term impact of boredom on health and well-being is unknown, workplace boredom has been associated with low morale, depression, and engagement in destructive and unauthorized activities (Long, 2004). Other occupations also have inherent health risks. Skateboarding, for instance, caused almost 300,000 medically treated injuries in the United States in 2002 (Haines, Smith, & Baxter, 2010). Driving a motor vehicle can also be risky, with recorded crashes causing 15.6 deaths per 100,000 people in the United States in 1998. There has also been some discussion of substance abuse and alcohol consumption as occupations with well-recognized detrimental effects on health, not just for the addict but also for his or her children (Helbig & McKay, 2003; Vaught & Wittman, 2011).

CASE STUDY 6.1 Do or Die

Dennis is 11 years old and lives in a low socioeconomic level suburb of a large city in Sweden. He likes to watch television, and as he has grown older, has started to play computer games and to surf the Internet. On average, he spends around 3 hours a day on the computer (Magnusson, Hulthén, & Kjellgren, 2005). If he lived in Israel, that figure might have been as high as 4½ or 5 hours per day (Nemet et al., 2005). While he watches, plays games, or surfs, Dennis likes to have a glass of fruit juice or lemonade. Like the other 30% of children in his suburb who are overweight or obese, he also tends to skip breakfast. Despite the health risks adults associate with low levels of physical activity, high calorie intake, and starting the day without food, Dennis does not believe that his lifestyle has any effect on his health (Magnusson et al., 2005).

Is Obesity So Bad?

Were he located in New Zealand, the health risks Dennis faces would be well recognized. If he was one of the 23% of boys of Pacific Island heritage aged 2–14 years who are obese, he would face well-documented risks of joining those already presenting with type 2 diabetes (Ministry of Health Manatū Hauora, 2008). In a few years, he might well contribute to the skyrocketing figures for life-threatening cardiovascular disease and, rather than following the trend of increasing longevity recorded over recent decades, have a substantially reduced life expectancy.

What if Dennis Was American?

If Dennis was part of a low-income American family living in a county with high obesity prevalence, 1 in 7 of the younger children in his neighborhood would also be obese (CDC, 2011). To help Dennis and his family address the issue, his school might have adopted the coordinated approach to childhood obesity promoted by the National Association of State School Boards. That body calls on schools to appoint a school health coordinator, remove food and beverage vending machines, and increase student activity levels by introducing physically active "brain breaks" into school subjects, organizing things to do during recess, and setting up an after-school physical activity program. Safe routes to walk to school might also have been established (Wechsler, McKenna, Lee, & Deitz, 2004).

Dennis's parents would also have a role to play. According to statistics issued by the Henry J. Kaiser Family Foundation, if they took the TV out of his bedroom and set rules about TV watching, playing video games, and computer use, his screen time would decrease by almost 3 hours per day. If even some of that time went into occupations that increased his heart rate and made him breathe harder, he might be more successful in keeping his weight in check (National Heart, Lung, and Blood Institute, n.d.a, n.d.b).

Obesity and Sleep

A meta-analysis of 30 studies examining the relationship between obesity and sleep in adults and children has confirmed a statistically significant link between obesity and curtailed sleep. For children, that means sleeping less than 10 hours per day. The results were consistent across different populations and across all age groups, with a 60% to 80% increase in the likelihood of being obese among short sleepers. A possible explanation is that having fewer hours of sleep is simply a marker of an unhealthy lifestyle. However, one suggestion is that curtailed sleep may trigger a hormonal response that increases appetite, resulting in higher food consumption (Cappuccio et al., 2008). The association between sleep and obesity highlights that occupational therapists need to consider children's occupational pattern across the whole day if they are to be effective in helping them achieve a lifestyle that supports health and well-being.

Questions and Exercises

- Research results cited in this case study identify calorie intake, physical inactivity, ethnicity, and getting enough sleep as factors contributing to childhood obesity and its associated health problems. What other parental, environmental, societal, or legislative factors can you identify as contributing to the problem?
- If you were working with children between 6 and 16 years old, what changes to the home environment would you suggest to limit their access to screen time?

Additionally, other people's occupations can pose health threats. For example, exposure to exhaled tobacco smoke increases the risk of children developing respiratory infections and heart disease (*Healthy People 2010*, n.d.).

Barriers to Healthful Occupation

The discussion to this point has addressed how occupation contributes to health and acknowledged that it is not always beneficial. To bring the discussion to a close, it remains to consider the limitations and barriers that impede access to health promoting occupation. Having an **impairment** associated with a health condition is one thing that can impede participation in occupations that underpin well-being. Consistent with the *International Classification of Functioning, Disability and Health* (WHO, 2001) an impairment is defined as any problem with normal psychological or physiological function or with a body structure such as a joint or organ. The association between impairments and problems with participation is increasingly recognized in documents shaping health policy. For example, low back pain is the second leading cause of lost work time (*Healthy People 2020: Arthritis, Osteoporosis and Chronic Back Conditions*, n.d.) and decreased vision is recognized to hamper driving, "participating in sports, or working with power tools in the yard or around the home. . . [and maintaining] a healthy and active lifestyle well into a person's later years" (*Healthy People 2020: Vision*, n.d.). Impairments can mean that people are not sufficiently strong or flexible, unable to focus their thoughts and attention, or too fatigued to participate in occupations that in other circumstances they would choose to do. People also tend to withdraw from occupation if they are hampered by pain, deformity, breathlessness, malnutrition, despair, or the apathy that comes of boredom or hopelessness.

Reduced participation in occupation due to factors such as these can affect all aspects of well-being. For example, one study of adults with a rapidly advancing neurological disease revealed how they experienced their impairments as losses, evidencing not only diminishing occupational capacity but also loss of valued aspects of identity, inability to access occupational settings that gave variety to life, and an inevitable decline toward dependency and death (Brott, Hocking, & Paddy, 2007; Hocking, Brott, & Paddy, 2006). Expressions of courage, humor, gratitude for remaining abilities, and appreciation for the support received from family and health care workers were overshadowed by fatigue, frustration, distress over loss of the future they had envisaged, and fear of becoming a burden. Each of these has an occupational component:

- Fatigue from basic self-care tasks
- Frustration over declining occupational capacity, barriers to valued occupations, and long hours that were no longer filled with productive activity
- Regret for occupations they had looked forward to and would now not achieve, such as holding a grandchild.

Health conditions can also make occupational demands that undermine a sense of well-being. For instance, people with psoriasis report the extra burden of self-care and housework that comes with the condition, because of the time taken to apply skin crèmes and how frequently they needed to brush, wipe, dust, vacuum, and wash away the flakes of skin they shed. They also experience that some previously enjoyable occupations are spoiled. Shopping for clothes, for example, was no longer fun because they were limited to cotton clothing that did not exacerbate their skin condition and light colors that would not reveal the skin flakes (Hocking, Nayar, Beale, McPherson, & Taylor, 2007). In addition, impairments sometimes impede participation simply because people do not imagine that previously valued occupations are still open to them, albeit in a modified form (Block et al., 2005).

External barriers to occupation are also encountered when the physical, social, or attitudinal context does not support participation in the range of occupations necessary to support health (WHO, 2001). Aesthetically sterile or unsafe urban environments, for example, do not provide spaces for children to be physically active or older residents to develop community networks, disproportionately affecting people on low incomes (Satcher & Higginbotham, 2008; Semenza & Krishnasamy, 2007). Equally, cultural mores that make it unacceptable for Bangladeshi women to walk briskly, the loud music and inappropriate television shows screened at the gym, and their husbands' dislike of them going out alone deter them from exercising (Khanam & Costarelli, 2008). Examples related to disability include inaccessible buildings; the poverty, low levels of educational attainment, and unemployment that are often associated with disability; and the stigma attached to conditions such as AIDS, dementia, and mental illness. Facing these barriers, particularly when they persist, challenges perceptions of well-being. The women in Jakobsen's (2004) study, for instance, battled with the lack of recognition of the additional physical and psychological rigors of self-care and domestic tasks for those who are not able-bodied. They also reported difficulty managing appointments with health care workers, home help, wheelchair maintenance personnel, and care assistants, who were available only during work hours. Despite being highly motivated to work and deriving all the benefits of employment that others report, all three women found participation in work too strenuous and resigned their positions.

Ecological and sociopolitical factors also limit or disrupt access to health-giving occupations. Those recently identified in the occupational therapy and occupational science literature include unemployment (Aldrich & Callanan, 2011), displacement (Frank, 2011), being a refugee or asylum seeker (Burchett & Matheson, 2010), poverty (Beagan, 2007; Pollard, Alsop, & Kronenberg, 2005), and experiences of racism (Beagan & Etowa, 2011). The interdisciplinary literature also recognizes the impact of homelessness, natural disasters such as drought and tornados, lower educational attainment, and displacement.

Conclusion

The things we do meet our biological needs for sustenance and shelter. Occupation keeps us alive, and occupation in natural environments nourishes us. In the longer term, occupation can provide the physical activity, mental stimulation, and social interaction we need to keep our bodies, minds, and communities healthy. In addition, through participation in occupation, we express ourselves, develop skills, experience pleasure and involvement, and achieve the things we believe to be important. In short, we have opportunities for enhanced levels of well-being. However, not all people have equal opportunity to engage in health-giving occupations. People with an impairment can experience limitations in their ability to engage in occupation and are known to have lower levels of engagement in physical exercise. People who live in poverty, are displaced by conflict or devastated by natural disasters, experience unemployment or homelessness, and have lower levels of educational attainment are also likely to experience barriers to participation in occupation that negatively affect health and well-being.

Equally, occupation can threaten or destroy health. Doing too much, doing too little, and doing things that expose us to risk and harm can all have deleterious effects. It is also important to recognize that it is often through having trouble doing things that we become aware of health issues and the full impact of impairments. Furthermore, physical, social, or attitudinal barriers in the environment can exacerbate the impact of a health condition or impairment, sometimes to such an extent that participation in occupation is unsustainable.

References

Aldrich, R. M., & Callanan, Y. (2011). Insights about researching discouraged workers. *Journal of Occupational Science, 18,* 153–166. doi:10.1080/14427591.2011.575756

Beagan, B. L. (2007). Experiences of social class: Learning from occupational therapy students. *Canadian Journal of Occupational Therapy, 74,* 125–133.

Beagan, B. L., & Etowa, J. B. (2011). The meanings and functions of occupations related to spirituality for African Nova Scotian women. *Journal of Occupational Science, 18,* 277–290. doi:10.1080/14427591.2011.594548

Block, P., Skeels, S. E., Keys, C. B., & Rimmer, J. H. (2005). Shake-it-up: Health promotion and capacity building for people with spinal cord injuries and related neurological disabilities. *Disability and Rehabilitation, 27,* 185–190.

Brott, T., Hocking, C., & Paddy, A. (2007). Occupational disruption: Living with motor neurone disease. *British Journal of Occupational Therapy, 70,* 24–31.

Burchett, N., & Matheson, R. (2010). The need for belonging: The impact of restrictions on working on the well-being of an asylum seeker. *Journal of Occupational Science, 17,* 85–91. doi:10.1080/14427591.2010.9686679

Cappuccio, F. P., Taggart, F. M., Kandala, N. B., Currie, A., Peile, E., Stranges, S., & Miller, M. A. (2008). Meta-analysis of short sleep duration and obesity in children and adults. *Sleep, 31,* 619–626.

Carlson, M., Clark, F., & Young, B. (1998). Practical contributions of occupational science to the art of successful ageing: How to sculpt a meaningful life in older adulthood. *Journal of Occupational Science, 5,* 107–118. doi:10.1080/14427591.1998.9686438

Centers for Disease Control and Prevention. (2005a). *Health behaviors of adults: United States, 1999–2000* (Series 10, N. 219, 2003). Washington, DC: U.S. Department of Health and Human Services. Retrieved from http://www.cdc.gov/nchs/products/series/series10.htm

Centers for Disease Control and Prevention. (2005b). *Summary health statistics for the U.S. population: National health interview survey* (Series 10, N. 224, 2003). Washington, DC: U.S. Department of Health and Human Services. Retrieved from http://www.cdc.gov/nchs/products/series/series10.htm

Centers for Disease Control and Prevention. (2011). *Overweight and obesity: Data and statistics.* Atlanta, GA: Author. Retrieved from http://www.cdc.gov/obesity/childhood/data.html

Clark, F. (1997). Reflections on the human as an occupational being: Biological need, tempo and temporality. *Journal of Occupational Science: Australia, 4,* 86–92. doi:10.1080/14427591.1997.9686424

Classen, S., Lopez, E. D. S., Winter, S., Awadzi, K. D., Ferree, N., & Garvan, C. W. (2007). Population-based health promotion perspective for older driver safety: Conceptual framework to intervention plan. *Clinical Interventions in Aging, 2,* 677–693.

Csikszentmihalyi, M. (1998). *Finding flow: The psychology of engagement with everyday life.* New York, NY: Basic Books.

Cuypers, K., Krokstad, S., Holmen, T. L., Knudtsen, M. S., Bygren, L. O., & Holmen, J. (2011). Patterns of receptive and creative cultural activities and their association with perceived health, anxiety, depression and satisfaction with life among adults: The HUNT study, Norway. *Journal of Epidemiological and Community Health,* 1–6. doi:10.1136/jech.2010.113571

Ellis, R., Kosma, M., Cardinal, B. J., Bauer, J. J., & McCubbin, J. A. (2007). Physical activity beliefs and behaviour of adults with physical disabilities. *Disability and Rehabilitation, 29,* 1221–1227.

Erlandsson, L. K. (2003). *101 women's patterns of daily occupations. Characteristics and relationships to health and well-being.* Lund, Sweden: Lund University.

Farnworth, L. (1998). Doing, being, and boredom. *Journal of Occupational Science, 5,* 141–146. doi:10.1080/14427591.1998.9686442

Fowler, E. G., Kolobe, T. H., Damiano, D. L., Thorpe, D. E., Morgan, D. W., Brunstrom, J. E., . . . Stevenson, R. D. (2007). Promotion of physical fitness and prevention of secondary conditions for children with cerebral palsy: Section of Pediatrics Research summit proceedings. *Physical Therapy, 87,* 1495–1510.

Frank, G. (2011). The transactional relationship between occupation and place: Indigenous cultures in the American Southwest. *Journal of Occupational Science, 18,* 3–20. doi:10.1080/14427591.2011.562874

Gallew, H. A., & Mu, K. (2004). An occupational look at temporal adaptation: Night shift nurses. *Journal of Occupational Science, 11,* 23–30. doi:10.1080/14427591.2004.9686528

Glass, T. A., de Leon, C. M., Marottoli, R. A., & Berkman, L. F. (1999). Population based study of social and productive activities as predictors of survival among elderly Americans. *British Medical Journal, 319,* 478–483.

Grieves, V. (2008). Aboriginal spirituality: A baseline for indigenous knowledges development in Australia. *The Canadian Journal of Native Studies, 28,* 363–398.

Hagberg, L. A., & Lindholm, L. (2006). Cost-effectiveness of healthcare-based interventions aimed at improving physical activity. *Scandinavian Journal of Public Health, 34,* 641–653. doi:10.1080/14034940600627853

Haines, C., Smith, T. M., & Baxter, M. F. (2010). Participation in the risk-taking occupation of skateboarding. *Journal of Occupational Science, 17,* 239–245. doi:10.1080/14427591.2010.9686701

Håkansson, C., & Ahlborg, G., Jr. (2010). Perceptions of employment, domestic work, and leisure as predictors of health among men and women. *Journal of Occupational Science, 17,* 150–157. doi:10.1080/14427591.2010.9686689

Håkansson, C., Dahlin-Ivanoff, S., & Sonn, U. (2006). Achieving balance in everyday life. *Journal of Occupational Science, 13,* 74–82. doi:10.1080/14427591.2006.9686572

Health. (2009). In *Mosby's medical dictionary* (8th ed.). Retrieved from http://medical-dictionary.thefreedictionary.com/health

Healthy people 2010: A systematic approach to health improvement. (n.d.). Retrieved from http://www.healthypeople.gov/Document/html/uih/uih_2.htm

Healthy people 2020: Arthritis, osteoporosis and chronic back conditions. (n.d.). Retrieved from http://www.healthypeople.gov/2020/topicsobjectives2020/overview.aspx?topicid=3

Healthy people 2020: Physical activity. (n.d.). Retrieved from http://healthypeople.gov/2020/topicsobjectives2020/overview.aspx?topicid=33

Healthy people 2020: Vision. (n.d.). Retrieved from http://www.healthypeople.gov/2020/topicsobjectives2020/overview.aspx?topicid=42

Helbig, K., & McKay, E. (2003). An exploration of addictive behaviours from an occupational perspective. *Journal of Occupational Science, 10,* 140–145. doi:10.1080/14427591.2003.9686521

Hocking, C., Brott, T., & Paddy, A. (2006). Caring for people with motor neurone disease. *International Journal of Therapy and Rehabilitation, 13,* 351–355.

Hocking, C., Nayar, S., Beale, J., McPherson, K., & Taylor, W. (2007, June). *How occupation matters in life: Critique of the International Classification of Functioning.* Paper presented at the 31st Annual Conference and Exhibition of the College of Occupational Therapists, Manchester, United Kingdom.

Jacob, C., Guptill, C., & Sumsion, T. (2009). Motivation for continuing involvement in a leisure-based choir: The lived experiences of university choir members. *Journal of Occupational Science, 16*, 187–193. doi:10.1080/14427591.2009.9686661

Jakobsen, K. (2004). If work doesn't work: How to enable occupational justice. *Journal of Occupational Science, 11*, 125–134. doi:10.1080/14427591.2004.9686540

Khanam, S., & Costarelli, V. (2008). Attitudes towards health and exercise of overweight women. *The Journal of the Royal Society for the Promotion of Health, 128*, 26–30.

Kielhofner, G. (2008). *Model of human occupation: Theory and application* (4th ed.). Baltimore, MD: Lippincott Williams and Wilkins.

Larson, J. S. (1999). The conceptualization of health. *Medical Care Research and Review, 56*, 123–136.

Legge, D. (2007). Global trade and health promotion. *Health Promotion Journal of Australia, 18*, 92–97.

Loland, N. W. (2004). Exercise, health, and aging. *Journal of Aging and Physical Activity, 12*, 170–184.

Long, C. (2004). On watching paint dry: An exploration of boredom. In M. Molineux (Ed.), *Occupation for occupational therapists* (pp. 78–89). Oxford, United Kingdom: Blackwell.

Lowis, M. J., Knight, J., & Ball, V. (2010). A quantitative analysis of self-rated health and occupational aspects of community-dwelling older adults. *Journal of Occupational Science, 17*, 20–26. doi:10.1080/14427591.2010.9686668

Magnusson, M. B., Hulthén, L., & Kjellgren, K. I. (2005). Obesity, dietary pattern and physical activity among children in a suburb with a high proportion of immigrants. *Journal of Human Nutrition & Dietetics, 18*, 187–194.

Mednick, S. C., Nakayama, K., Cantero, J. L., Atienza, M., Levin, A. A., Pathak, N., & Stickgold, R. (2002). The restorative effect of naps on perceptual deterioration. *Nature Neuroscience, 5*, 677–681.

Ministry of Health Manatū Hauora. (2005). *Decades of disparity II: Socioeconomic mortality trends in New Zealand, 1981–1999*. Wellington, New Zealand: Author.

Ministry of Health Manatū Hauora. (2008). *A portrait of health: Key results of the 2006/07 New Zealand health survey*. Wellington, New Zealand: Author.

Moore, J., & Harré, N. (2007). Eating and activity: The importance of family and environment. *Health Promotion Journal of Australia, 18*, 143–148.

Mozley, C. G. (2001). Exploring the connections between occupation and mental health in care homes for older people. *Journal of Occupational Science, 8*, 14–19.

National Heart, Lung, and Blood Institute. (n.d.a). *Less TV, fewer videos help keep weight in check*. Retrieved from http://www.nhlbi.nih.gov/health/public/heart/obesity/wecan/news-events/matte3.htm

National Heart, Lung, and Blood Institute. (n.d.b). *Reduce screen time*. Retrieved from http://www.nhlbi.nih.gov/health/public/heart/obesity/wecan/reduce-screen-time/index.htm

Nemet, D., Barkan, S., Epstein, Y., Friedland, O., Kowen, G., & Eliakim, A. (2005). Short- and long-term beneficial effects of a combined dietary-behavioral-physical activity intervention for the treatment of childhood obesity. *Pediatrics, 115*, e443–e449.

Ostbye, T., Malhotra, R., & Chan, A. (2009). Thirteen dimensions of health in elderly Sri Lankans: Results of a national Sri Lanka Aging Survey. *Journal of the American Geriatrics Society, 57*, 1376–1387.

Persson, D., Eklund, M., & Isacsson, A. (1999). The experience of everyday occupations and its relation to sense of coherence: A methodological study. *Journal of Occupational Science, 6*, 13–26. doi:10.1080/14427591.1999.9686447

Pollard, N., Alsop, A., & Kronenberg, F. (2005). Reconceptualising occupational therapy. *British Journal of Occupational Therapy, 68*, 524–526.

Sanders, C. M., Yankou, D., & Andrusyszyn, M. A. (2005). Attention and restoration in Post-RN students. *Journal of Continuing Education in Nursing, 36*, 218–225.

Satcher, D., & Higginbotham, E. J. (2008). The public health approach to eliminating disparities in health. *American Journal of Public Health, 98*, 400–403.

Schoenberg, N. E., Hatcher, J., & Dignan, M. B. (2008). Appalachian women's perceptions of their community's health threats. *National Rural Health Association, 24*, 75–83.

Semenza, J. C., & Krishnasamy, P. V. (2007). Design of a health-promoting neighborhood intervention. *Health Promotion Practice, 8*, 243–256.

Stav, W. B., Pierce, S., Wheatley, C. J., & Davis, E. S. (2005). Driving and community mobility. *American Journal of Occupational Therapy, 59*, 666–670.

Stevens, P. (2010). Embedment in the environment: A new paradigm for well-being? *Perspectives in Public Health, 130*, 265–269.

Sutton, D. (2006, July). *The lived experience of occupational performance during recovery from mental illness*. Paper presented at World Federation of Occupational Therapists Congress, Sydney, Australia.

Tambini, A., Katz, N., & Davachi, L. (2010). Enhanced brain correlations during rest are related to memory for recent experiences. *Neurone, 65*, 280–290.

Townsend, E., & Polatajko, H. J. (2007). *Enabling occupation II: Advancing an occupational therapy vision for health, well-being, and justice through occupation*. Ottawa, ON: Canadian Association of Occupational Therapists Publications ACE.

Vance, D. E., Wadley, V. G., Ball, K. K., Roenker, D. L., & Rizzo, M. (2005). The effects of physical activity and sedentary behavior on cognitive health in older adults. *Journal of Aging and Physical Activity, 13*, 294–313.

Vaught, E. L., & Wittman, P. P. (2011). A phenomenological study of the occupational choices of individuals who self identify as adult children of alcoholics. *Journal of Occupational Science, 18*, 356–365. doi:10.1080/14427591.2011.595893

Wallis, C., Miranda, C. A., & Park, A. (2005). Get moving! *Time, 165*, 46–51.

Wechsler, H., McKenna, M. L., Lee, S. M., & Deitz, W. H. (2004). The role of schools in preventing childhood obesity. *The State Education Standard, 5*, 4–12.

Wilcock, A. (1993). A theory of the human need for occupation. *Journal of Occupational Science: Australia, 1*, 17–24. doi:10.1080/14427591.1993.9686375

Wilcock, A. (1995). The occupational brain: A theory of human nature. *Journal of Occupational Science: Australia, 2*, 68–73. doi:10.1080/14427591.1995.9686397

Wilcock, A. A. (2006). *An occupational perspective of health* (2nd ed.). Thorofare, NJ: Slack.

Williamson, D. L., & Carr, J. (2009). Health as a resource for everyday life: Advancing the conceptualization. *Critical Public Health, 19*, 107–122.

World Health Organization. (2001). *International classification of functioning, disability and health: A global model to guide clinical thinking and practice in childhood disability*. Geneva, Switzerland: Author.

World Health Organization, Health and Welfare Canada, Canadian Public Health Association. (1986, November). Ottawa charter for health promotion. In *International Conference on Health Promotion*. Ottawa, Ontario, Canada: Authors.

Ziviani, J., Scott, J., & Wadley, D. (2004). Walking to school: Incidental physical activity in the daily occupations of Australian children. *Occupational Therapy International, 11*, 1–22.

Zuzanek, J. (1998). Time use, time pressure, personal stress, mental health, and life satisfaction from a life cycle perspective. *Journal of Occupational Science, 5*, 26–39. doi:10.1080/14427591.1998.9686432

For additional resources on the subjects discussed in this chapter, visit http://thePoint.lww.com/Willard-Spackman12e.

CHAPTER 7

Occupational Science

The Study of Occupation

Valerie A. Wright-St Clair, Clare Hocking

OUTLINE

LEARNING OBJECTIVES

After reading this chapter, you will be able to:

1. Apply an occupational science evidence-based practice way of thinking about day-to-day practice
2. Interpret the difference between basic and applied occupational science knowledge underpinning practice
3. Analyze the observable and phenomenological aspects of occupations
4. Begin to synthesize occupational science knowledge from diverse studies in order to consider how occupational therapy practice might serve individuals, communities, and society well
5. Evaluate how well your own practice is guided by the existing and emergent basic and applied occupational science knowledge

This chapter explores how occupational science is informing occupational therapy practice. Firstly, the discussion looks at occupational science as a basic science underpinning occupational therapy knowledge, before recent developments in occupational science are showcased as a way of illustrating its growth as an applied science. Along the way, real-world international examples are offered. Each highlights how the "science" of occupational science is guiding evidence-based occupational therapy practice. Each example, in its own way, illustrates occupational science "in play" within the everyday practice worlds of occupational therapists.

Introduction

Logan[1] was 15 when he found out he was going to become a father (**Figure 7.1**). "It was really scary. I didn't know what everyone would

[1]Pseudonym

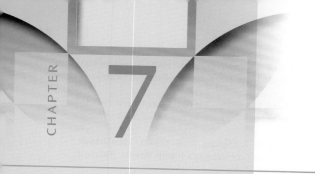

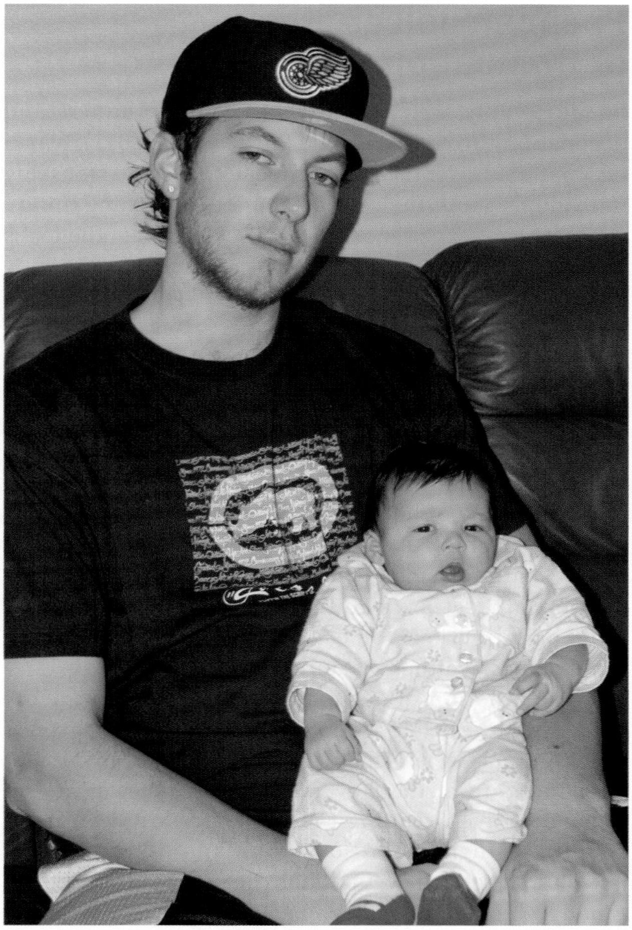

FIGURE 7.1 New father with his daughter. (Photograph taken by Valerie Wright-St Clair.)

think or how I would tell my parents," remembers Logan. "It would have been nice to have someone to talk to before my baby was born." Now 18 years old, Logan is a dedicated full-time dad while his partner pursues her goal of becoming a midwife. At [the community youth center] he's found a place to hang out and says it has given him the confidence to be a better father. "We talk about all sorts—child development, being a good parent, mentoring, just trying to be a better man." The dad's program has also motivated him to build his music skills and consider youth or social work (Ministry of Social Development, 2011, p. 8).

Logan's story reflects what this chapter is about. It reveals how life changes can mean that people, or sometimes communities, need support to learn and successfully engage in new occupations. And it points toward understanding how an in-depth knowledge about humans as occupational beings can inform new ways for occupational therapy to contribute to healthy families and communities. But first, let's go back to the ideas behind this chapter.

Occupational science is a term that many occupational therapists will already recognize. What occupational science is and how it informs occupational therapy practice may be less understood than some of the other sciences occupational therapists have studied, such as the anatomical sciences, like musculoskeletal biology and neuroanatomy; and the social sciences, like sociology and psychology. Occupational science opens up new ways to explore the complexities of human engagement in occupations. As a distinctive field of study, occupational science has its roots as a basic science aimed at building knowledge about the substrates, form, function, and meaning of what people do (Zemke & Clark, 1996) and the occupational nature of being human (Wilcock, 2006). Studying occupation involves building knowledge about its "observable and phenomenological aspects" (Clark & Lawlor, 2009, p. 7). In order to explain the complex ideas behind studying the "observable" and "phenomenological" aspects of occupation, an illustrative tale is offered—Antoine de Saint-Exupéry's (1972) classic story of *The Little Prince*. It opens with the narrator's voice as he reflects back on his boyhood. When only 6 years old, entranced by a picture of a boa constrictor ingesting its prey whole, he produced his first drawing of a boa constrictor having swallowed an elephant. He showed his drawing to the grown-ups and asked if it frightened them. Observing what appeared to be the outline of a hat, the grown-ups said they were not at all frightened. Somewhat puzzled by their response, the boy produced his second drawing. This one left nothing to the imagination; it was a prosection showing the elephant inside the boa constrictor. At this point, the grown-ups advised the boy to give up drawing boa constrictors "whether from the inside or the outside" (de Saint-Exupéry, 1972, p. 8) and concern himself with factual matters in the world. So now he speaks of sensible things such as "bridge, and golf, and politics, and neckties" rather than of fanciful things such as "boa constrictors, or primeval forests, or stars" (de Saint-Exupéry, 1972, p. 9).

In such a simple way, this tale captures the two fundamentally different ways we can study occupation as a basic science. One way is to study its observable aspects. This way of coming to know things is underpinned by the assumption that, like the boy's second drawing of the elephant inside the boa constrictor, the truth about occupations and the occupational nature of humans exists in the world. Therefore, we can come to know it by gathering data gained through our senses (de Poy & Gitlin, 2011). From this view, through quantitative research, truth or reality can be seen, touched, heard, or measured in some objective way. On the other hand, if we accept there is not one but many truths, or multiple realities about occupations and the occupational nature of humans, this opens the way for studying the **phenomenological aspects of occupation** through qualitative research. This way of coming to know about occupation is underpinned by the assumption that, like the boy's first drawing, people experience their own subjective, contextual reality. In essence, "the what," "the whom," and "the why" of occupations can all be studied as units of analysis within occupational science research.

Building a Basic Knowledge of Occupation

Attempting to give an overview of the knowledge occupational scientists are building is a little like swallowing an elephant; there is no agreed way to go about it and, just as an elephant creates a big bulge in a boa constrictor, the breadth of the field and the diverse methodologies employed make it hard to convey its scope within a few paragraphs. Separating observable from phenomenological perspectives gives some structure, and we have also chosen to focus on the recent literature to give a sense of the whole of the science and its likely future directions.

Observable Aspects of Occupation

Comparatively little occupational science research has addressed the **substrates of occupation**, where substrates are the human capacities required to engage in activities that have **form**, **function**, and **meaning**. That is perhaps because many of occupation's substrates are not directly observable, requiring neuroimaging and other technologies to "see" them. One exception in the recent literature is Liew and Aziz-Zadeh's (2011) review of the neuroscientific evidence of linkages between language and action, and the implications that has for understanding interpersonal relationships and the ways language both creates and mediates the meaning of occupation. Another way to "observe" occupation is to synthesize the cross-disciplinary knowledge. For example, Stein, Foran, and Cermak (2011) reviewed literature from psychology, neuroscience, nursing, and other disciplines to investigate one aspect of occupational forms—the patterns apparent in people's occupations. That study revealed that the configuration of daily occupations of parents caring for children with autism impacts the parents' relationships with others, feelings of competence, identity, and the time and energy they invest in meeting personal goals and maintaining their own health.

New understandings of the function of occupation are also observable when an occupational perspective is brought to bear on the cross-disciplinary literature. For example, Smith-Gabai and Ludwig (2011) found that because complying with the Jewish Sabbath requires disengagement from everyday tasks and worries, it functions as an "oasis" of rest and renewal. Aspects of occupation, including its meaning, can also be observed using quantitative measures. Håkansson and Ahlborg (2010), for instance, surveyed over 2,500 Swedish employees about their everyday lives and repeated the measures 2 years later. The researchers established that although both men and women reported experiencing their occupations as meaningful, doing things experienced as meaningful was a good predictor of subjective health for women but not for men.

Phenomenological Aspects of Occupation

Phenomenally, we can study and come to understand occupation through ideas (de Poy & Gitlin, 2011), which occupational scientists have typically accessed by asking individuals about their lived experience of doing things. One aspect of experience that has seldom been the focus of inquiry, however, is the bodily experience of engaging in occupation, even though phenomenology encompasses such understandings and is relevant to developing a science of occupation (Lala & Kinsella, 2011). Nonetheless, insights can be gleaned from studies of participants with physically disabling health conditions and physically challenging occupations. For instance, an older woman who had experienced a stroke is described as "separated from the sense of bodily safety" (Odawara, 2010, p. 16) and an account of skateboarding includes a description of the skillful execution of a trick: "You have to know where your feet are planted . . . to crouch; it's about weight distribution. You can't have too much weight on top" (Haines, Smith, & Baxter, 2010, p. 242).

The function of occupation has also been uncovered by studies that asked people about their experiences. For instance, Canadian women of African descent were found to mediate everyday experiences of racism through prayer, reading the Bible, private devotional activities, singing spiritual songs, and other spiritual and church-related occupations (Beagan & Etowa, 2011). Finally, the meanings occupations hold for particular people in specific contexts are a major theme in the occupational science literature, generated through studies using a wide range of methodologies. One recently published example reports the identity meanings of occupation for "Sam," a former U.S. Marine living with a spinal cord injury (SCI). That study used ethnographic and narrative approaches to uncover Sam's lived experience and, more unusually in occupational science, interpreted his account in relation to broader social discourses (Asaba & Jackson, 2011).

Although we addressed them separately, what is important is not the study of occupation's observable *or* phenomenological aspects but the study of occupation's observable *and* phenomenological aspects. Both dimensions of knowledge are important to studying occupation as a basic science. One informs the other. One exists in accord with the other. It is a synergistic relationship. Beyond these aspects, moral philosophy offers an opportunity to think broadly about living a good life, such as the question of "what counts as an occupationally satisfying life" (Morgan, 2010, p. 217) or, guided by normative ethics, "How ought I practice to enable people to live occupationally satisfying lives?" Such understandings cannot be adequately addressed by observational or phenomenological approaches, but may be addressed as the boundaries of occupational science scholarship extend to include more philosophical concerns.

The Occupational Nature of Being Human

Sitting alongside all the studies of observable and phenomenological aspects of occupation, there is an ongoing thread of discussion about the occupational nature of being human and the extent to which current conceptualizations reflect a normative Western worldview (Hocking, 2012). One challenge to that perspective, which holds that people's engagement in occupation is active, purposeful, **temporal**, and meaningful, drew inspiration from a study of the occupations of inhabitants in a Greek village (Kantartzis & Molineux, 2011). In that more collectivist context, the duration and quality of people's daily occupations are shaped by the belief that periods of hard work should be balanced by adequate rest and relaxation, by free time being less structured and "hanging out" being expected and accepted, and by the needs of the group they are part of and their subjective state. Over time, as occupational scientists encompass understandings that come from diverse socioeconomic, cultural, and historical perspectives, the field will develop knowledge of the occupational nature of humans that better represents the implicit relationship between occupation and well-being.

Occupational Science as an Applied Science

Thus far, we have considered occupational science as a basic science, yet it is more than that; it is emergent as an applied science. Applied sciences like biomechanics, ergonomics, and mental health rehabilitation are already familiar to occupational therapists. As a consequence, therapists will be accustomed to using such applied sciences to guide their day-to-day decisions in practice. Applied sciences provide a knowledge base informing what to do and how to go about practice for a given occupational disruption. Although occupational science may be a new feature within the expansive field of applied sciences, over two decades on from its inception, occupational science's latent potential exists in its capacity to be a "comprehensive translational science" (Clark & Lawlor, 2009, p. 7). Occupational science, as an applied science, is already in the business of transforming rigorous basic science findings into evidence-based occupational therapy. In this way, "occupational science is designed to systematize knowledge about occupation, especially in relation to health and well-being" (Clark & Lawlor, 2009, p. 4). Interpreting this idea further, systematized occupational science knowledge is beginning to guide occupational therapy practice at all levels, from individual health to population health approaches. So let's look more closely at what is meant by the systematizing of knowledge.

Systematizing Occupational Science Knowledge

The origins, or etymology, of the word helps us to make sense of what it means to "systematize" occupational science knowledge. "Systema" in Greek was derived from the root words meaning "together" and to "cause to stand"; in other words, *systema* referred to something that stands as one in an "organized whole" (Harper, 2010). So a process that systematizes occupational science knowledge for occupational therapy is a methodical, rigorous way of developing a disciplined, coherent set of rules or methods for application in practice. Systematizing is about identifying, developing, analyzing, and optimizing knowledge for use. It is a translational process—transforming scientific understandings to practice knowledge. As a **translational science**, occupational science is theory-driven research aimed at resolving real-world concerns (Guerra & Leidy, 2010).

Systematizing occupational science knowledge fits with the international call for health practitioners, including occupational therapists, to use best evidence to guide everyday practice. A methodical way of doing translational occupational science research was put forward by colleagues at the Division of Occupational Science and Occupational Therapy, University of Southern California (USC) in the United States. It is designed as a rigorous way of developing occupational therapy practice knowledge from issues about which little is known but which may have an occupational foundation. Figure 7.2 summarizes the process, which begins with identifying and articulating the practice issue, then gathering a first layer of descriptive evidence from which an intervention is derived. The next layers of evidence come from testing how likely the intervention is to bring about the desired outcome, and still further, by measuring the cost-effectiveness of the intervention if it is successful. These methodical steps might seem enough in themselves, but for this practice knowledge to "stand together" as an organized whole, understanding why the intervention worked is essential. A coherent body of causal evidence then opens the way to build an explanatory theory, bringing together the research observations with interpretive reasoning to explain outcomes of intervention and add to the body of occupation-based knowledge.

Such a rigorous process shows the symbiotic relationship between the practice and research communities (Clark et al., 2006). That is, in the occupational therapy domain, the questions for occupational science research arise from practice-based issues, and the research findings, in return, provide knowledge for practice. Practice and research only exist and thrive together. However, implementing the blueprint for generating new knowledge is not for the fainthearted; it takes years to undertake the multiple studies, and demands significant funding and researcher commitment. The following

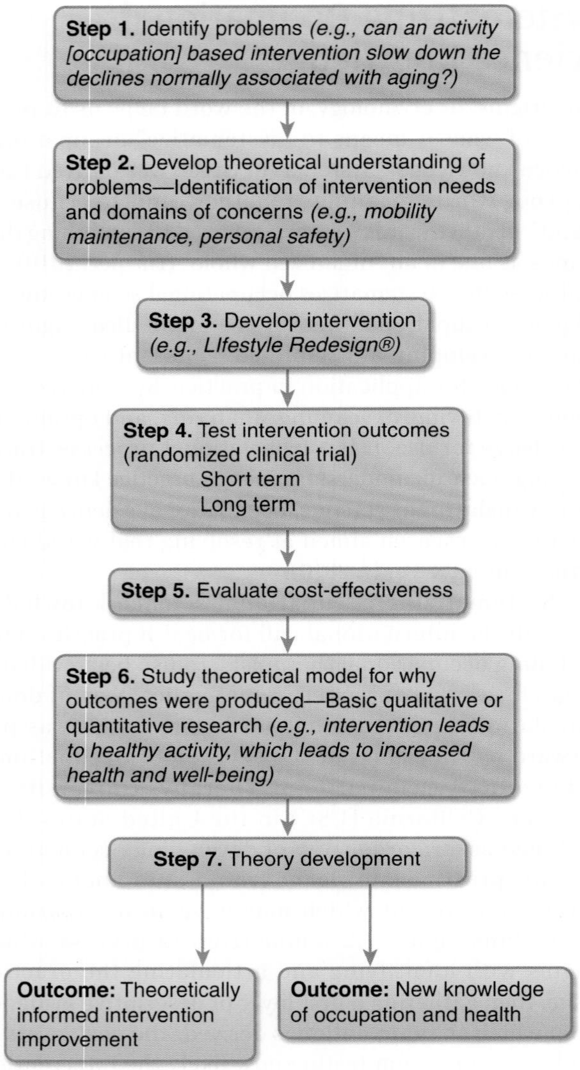
Step 1. Identify problems (e.g., can an activity [occupation] based intervention slow down the declines normally associated with aging?)
Step 2. Develop theoretical understanding of problems—Identification of intervention needs and domains of concerns (e.g., mobility maintenance, personal safety)
Step 3. Develop intervention (e.g., LIfestyle Redesign®)
Step 4. Test intervention outcomes (randomized clinical trial)
Short term
Long term
Step 5. Evaluate cost-effectiveness
Step 6. Study theoretical model for why outcomes were produced—Basic qualitative or quantitative research (e.g., intervention leads to healthy activity, which leads to increased health and well-being)
Step 7. Theory development
Outcome: Theoretically informed intervention improvement
Outcome: New knowledge of occupation and health

FIGURE 7.2 Blueprint for a translational science research program. (Reprinted from Clark, F., & Lawlor, M. C. [2009]. The making and mattering of occupational science. In E. B. Crepeau, E. S. Cohn, & B. A. Schell [Eds.], *Willard & Spackman's occupational therapy* [11th ed., pp. 2–14]. Philadelphia, PA: Lippincott Williams & Wilkins. Permission granted by Wolters Kluwer, http://lww.com.)

examples illustrate how occupational science research can underpin and come to life in the context of occupational therapy practice.

Occupational Science Informing Occupational Therapy

Occupational science informing occupational therapy is an idea whose time has come (Blanche & Henny-Kohler, 2000; Clark, Jackson, & Carlson, 2004; Molineux, 2004; Pierce, 2011). The following three case studies show how scientific understandings about human occupation are informing practice across the international occupational therapy community. Clark and Lawlor's (2009) blueprint for a systematic program of translational science research (Figure 7.2) is used explicitly as a way of illuminating the steps involved.

Conclusion

As is already happening in numerous locations internationally, it is time for occupational science to take center stage as a science informing occupational therapy practice, alongside other more traditional sciences such as neuroanatomy and biomechanics. You might say that knowledge about the occupations people do and their capacities and drive to do them has always informed occupational therapy. At one level, this is true; at a far deeper and expansive level, the work done since the 1980s, beginning with researchers and colleagues at USC, is allowing a more profound philosophical, theoretical, and research knowledge base on humans as occupational beings to take root and to flourish. There is a burgeoning amount of high quality basic science available to practitioners to make sense of in the context of their own practice. Yet, it is occupational science's emergent capacity as a comprehensive applied science informing practice where the future of evidence-based occupational therapy lies.

CASE STUDY 7.1 Occupations and Pressure Ulcer Risk: The USC/Rancho Los Amigos National Rehabilitation Center Pressure Ulcer Prevention Research Program

Step 1: Identify the Practice Problem

In the United States, pressure ulcers are recognized as a common, complex, and costly problem for people with spinal cord injury (SCI). Risk assessment using the existing measurement tools was imprecise. Of particular interest to occupational scientists and therapists was the concern that pressure ulcer occurrence could have an occupational foundation and be a recurrent barrier to adults participating fully in their everyday occupations (Clark et al., 2006). Everyday occupations are not necessarily mundane. For Kerri Morgan (Figure 7.3 & Figure 7.5), training for and racing in Paralympic events are "everyday" occupations.

Step 2: Identify the Intervention Needs

Occupational scientists at USC and their research collaborators designed a holistic ethnographic, qualitative study, now called the Pressure Ulcer Prevention Study I or PUPS I, to explore the

(continued)

CASE STUDY 7.1 Occupations and Pressure Ulcer Risk: The USC/Rancho Los Amigos National Rehabilitation Center Pressure Ulcer Prevention Research Program *(continued)*

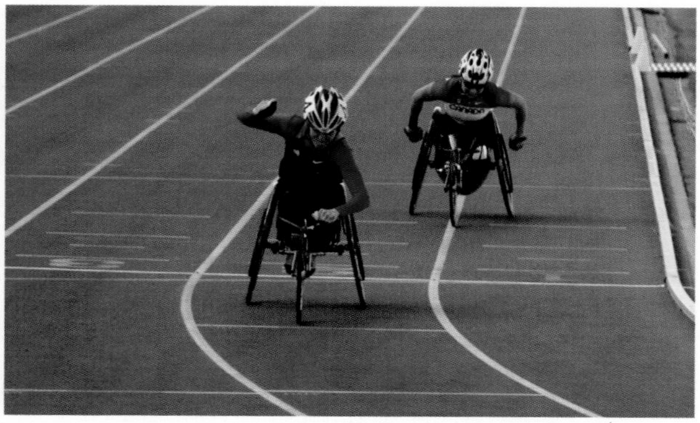
CANADA

FIGURE 7.3 Kerri Morgan, USA, racing in the International Paralympic Committee (IPC) World Athletics Championships in Christchurch, New Zealand. (Photograph taken by Karen Boyle. Reproduced with permission.)

everyday life contexts that contribute to the occurrence of pressure ulcers for men and women from different social backgrounds following SCI (Clark, Sanders, Carlson, Blanche, & Jackson, 2007). Through a prolonged, in-depth process of interviewing the study participants, and observing them as they went about their usual days, the researchers sought to understand how the complex, dynamic mix of daily circumstances played out as risks for pressure ulcers for each person (Clark et al., 2006). For example, Robert's story is highly illustrative of the interplay between his individualized risk profile of tending to overlook his **preventative strategies** in preference for participating in active occupations and the sudden occurrence of a pressure ulcer risk event: "When he was discharged from the rehabilitation facility to a skilled nursing service . . . he started to spend a large amount of time riding around in his wheelchair with two other young men who lived at the facility" (Clark et al., 2006, p. 1519). Robert developed two pressure ulcers as a consequence. Just as the researchers came to understand Robert within his occupational world, an individualized and richly contextualized occupation and risk profile emerged for all the study participants. By interpreting across all of the stories as a whole, the researchers developed a coherent series of pressure ulcer development models, including the dynamic balance of liability and buffering factors, individualized risk profiles, a generalized pressure ulcer event sequence (Figure 7.4), and a long-term pressure ulcer event sequence. Although theoretical in nature, the models are grounded in the richness of the qualitative, occupational science data.

Among other results, the occupational scientists found that pressure ulcers most commonly occurred, and recurred, for those whose historical risk profile was moderately high, in the context of a disruptive health or life event. What the findings highlight is the need for preventative interventions to take account of "the unique constellation of circumstances that comprise a person's everyday life" (Clark et al., 2006, p. 1516). The knowledge gained through this highly iterative process was ready to be further systematized and tested out in an applied study.

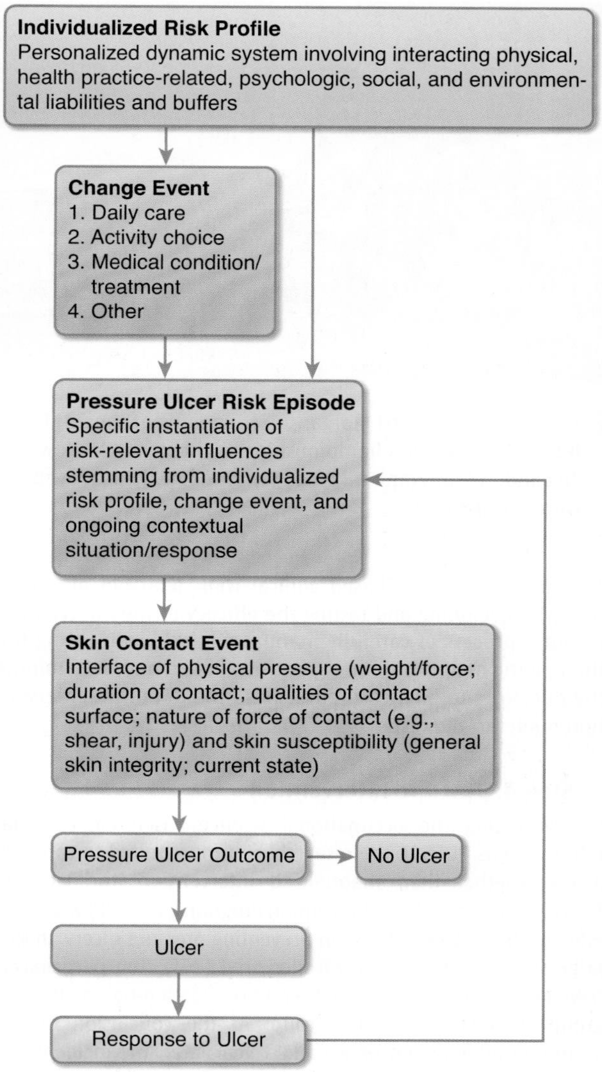
Individualized Risk Profile
Personalized dynamic system involving interacting physical, health practice-related, psychologic, social, and environmental liabilities and buffers
Change Event
1. Daily care
2. Activity choice
3. Medical condition/ treatment
4. Other
Pressure Ulcer Risk Episode
Specific instantiation of risk-relevant influences stemming from individualized risk profile, change event, and ongoing contextual situation/response
Skin Contact Event
Interface of physical pressure (weight/force; duration of contact; qualities of contact surface; nature of force of contact (e.g., shear, injury) and skin susceptibility (general skin integrity; current state)
Pressure Ulcer Outcome
No Ulcer
Ulcer
Response to Ulcer

FIGURE 7.4 Overview of generalized pressure ulcer event sequence. (Reprinted from Clark, F. A., Jackson, J. M., Scott, M. D., Atkins, M. S., Uhles-Tanaka, D., & Rubayi, S. [2006]. Data-based models of how pressure ulcers developing daily-living contexts of adults with spinal cord injury. *Archives of Physical Medicine and Rehabilitation, 87*(11),1516–1525. doi:10.1016/j.apmr.2006.08.329. Copyright [2006], with permission from Elsevier.)

Step 3: Develop the Intervention

Armed with the holistic ethnographic study findings, the occupational scientists understood how pressure ulcer development was a potentially modifiable risk in the occupational lives of people following SCI. Their next step was to thoughtfully apply the basic knowledge to designing a model for occupational therapy intervention to be conducted and tested through an

CASE STUDY 7.1 Occupations and Pressure Ulcer Risk: The USC/Rancho Los Amigos National Rehabilitation Center Pressure Ulcer Prevention Research Program *(continued)*

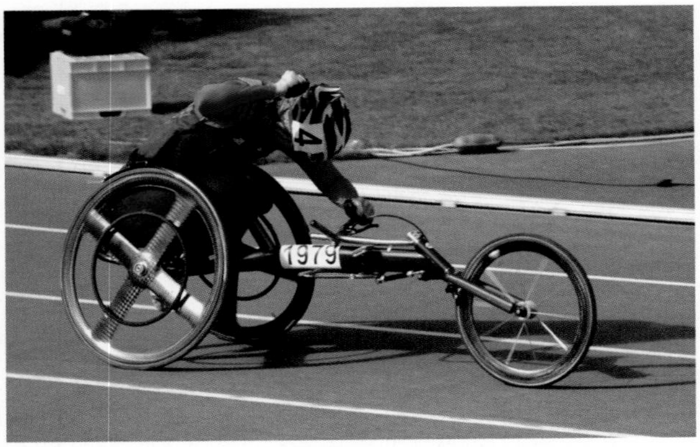

FIGURE 7.5 Kerri Morgan, USA, winning at the 2011 IPC Athletics World Championships in Christchurch, New Zealand. (Photograph taken by Karen Boyle. Reproduced with permission.)

"occupational-science based clinical trial" (Clark et al., 2004, p. 201). Developing and testing the efficacy of the intervention meant a process of carefully manualizing or documenting the therapeutic methods to be rigorously applied and determining the outcomes to be measured. It was time to put the intervention model to the test.

Step 4: Test the Intervention

In conducting the occupational science–based clinical trial referred to as PUPS II, the researchers were required to carefully assess whether their manualized intervention, the Lifestyle Redesign® Pressure Ulcer Prevention Program (LR-PUPP) was more effective than standard care in preventing pressure ulcers. In this large scale, randomized controlled trial (RCT), 160 participants have been randomized into either an occupation-based LR-PUPP group or a standard care group. At the conclusion of the 12-month intervention phase and 1 year later, the incidence of and costs related to the care of pressure ulcers will be compared between the two groups to determine whether statistically significant benefits can be detected for the intervention group.

In addition, as one component of the process of developing the manualized, occupation-based intervention, these occupational scientists generated a comprehensive set of resources that can be employed by occupational therapists (USC/Rancho Lifestyle Redesign® Pressure Ulcer Prevention Project, 2006a), other rehabilitation practitioners (USC/Rancho Lifestyle Redesign® Pressure Ulcer Prevention Project, 2006c), and consumers and their families (USC/Rancho Lifestyle Redesign® Pressure Ulcer Prevention Project, 2006b) to inform programs and best practices related to pressure ulcer prevention. More recently, they have also published a framework that emerged from their data to assist in the development of a comprehensive risk assessment tool (Seip, Carlson, Jackson, & Clark, in press).

Systematizing occupational science knowledge for application by occupational therapists means everyone wins: the clients, their families and friends, the health care funders and providers, the greater community, and of course, the occupational therapists.

Step 5: Evaluate the Cost-Effectiveness

As already specified in step 4, the RCT underway is evaluating the cost-effectiveness of LR-PUPP. On a quarterly basis, the researchers are tracking the costs associated with pressure ulcer care in both the LR-PUPP and standard care groups. Once completed, study results will be able to reveal not only whether the intervention was efficacious but also whether it produced beneficial effects in a cost-effective manner. Because the trial is still in progress and not all participants have completed the intervention phase, the results of the trial have not yet been analyzed.

Step 6: Study Why the Outcomes Were Produced

Finally, within the PUPS II research design, the mechanisms that account for the therapeutic outcomes of LR-PUPP can be examined. For example, as part of the study, it is hypothesized that participants in the study will increase their enactment of prevention behaviors because of increased knowledge, social support, and self-efficacy. This hypothesis will be tested as another key aspect of the study.

Step 7: Develop the Theory

The PUPS research program has already generated considerable theory development. For example, its qualitative arm produced overarching principles of pressure ulcer risk and data-based models therapists can employ to more comprehensively understand the elements that contribute to pressure ulcer risk (Clark et al., 2006; Jackson et al., 2010). However, it is expected that once the RCT is completed, additional theories will be generated on the factors that explain the therapeutic effects. Ultimately, the goal of this research program is to provide occupational therapists with a theoretically guided, scientifically grounded, and evidence-based intervention approach for lessening pressure ulcer risk in their patients with SCI. ■

CASE STUDY 7.2 Participation for Children with Physical Disabilities: The *CanChild* Centre for Childhood Disability Research Program

In a recent position statement to the Canadian Standing Senate Committee on Human Rights, Mary Law (2011) made the case for the exclusion from everyday occupations, such as play (Figure 7.6), and school occupations, such as reading (Figure 7.7) being a human rights issue for young people with physical disabilities. But the capacity to influence good public policy did not start there. It began over a decade ago when the *CanChild* team embarked on a research journey of generating and translating occupational science knowledge for use in occupational therapy practice. As is the case for applied research in occupational therapy, it started with understanding the problem.

Step 1: Identify the Practice Problem

Like many other places, young people with disabilities in Canada make up approximately 5% of the country's population (Law, 2011). Of particular concern to the *CanChild* team was knowledge indicating that these children are often excluded from engaging in age-appropriate occupations, especially leisure and sporting activities (Law, 2011). For example, research with the newly developed Participation and Environment Measure for Children and Youth (PEM-CY) (Coster et al., 2011) indicated that "24% of children and youth with disabilities never take part in unstructured physical activities in the community in comparison to only 2% among their typically developing peers" (Law, 2011, p. 3). As well, in spite of there being quite extensive research on children's play as an occupation, new ideas were emerging about play as a quality of occupational engagement rather than a type of activity (Pollock et al., 1997). Further exploration was warranted.

Step 2: Identify the Intervention Needs

Beginning with a qualitative interview-based study, 10 adolescents with congenital disabilities and 10 age- and gender-matched peers were asked about their play experiences. Both groups said play occupations needed to be self-chosen, and be "playful" or fun in nature. But those with disabilities mentioned more barriers to participation, such as needing to develop the motor skills for engaging, being limited by the physical environment, and feeling different to peers or not belonging (Pollock et al., 1997). Where these qualitative findings hinted at some of the occupational needs faced by young people with disabilities, the *CanChild* longitudinal Participate Study (Law, 2011) provided stronger descriptive evidence. With the aim of determining the factors that enhance participation in childhood occupations for those with physical disabilities, Law and her team observed 427 6- to 16-year-olds over time. Although activity preferences and supportive family relationships were significant contributors, the contextual environment was "one of the most important factors influencing participation of children and youth with disabilities" (Law, 2011, p. 4). The strength of these findings suggested that one approach to improving participation could be by modifying the contextual factors.

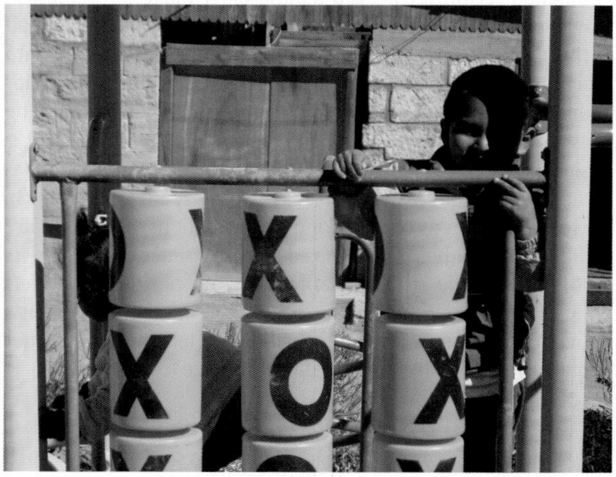

FIGURE 7.6 Young children at play. (Photograph taken by Valerie Wright-St Clair.)

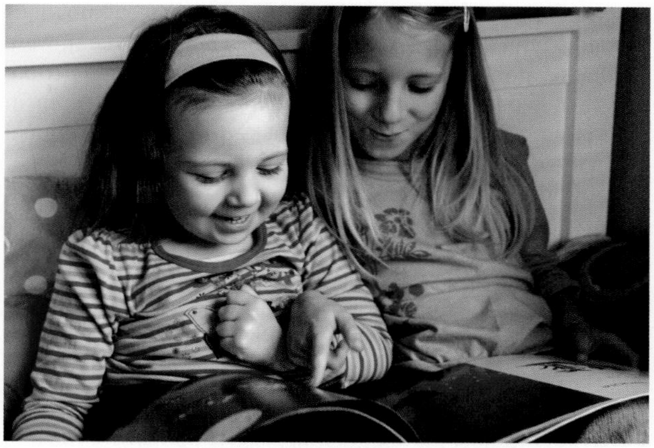

FIGURE 7.7 Children reading together. (Photograph taken by Andrea Casey. Reproduced with permission.)

Step 3: Develop the Intervention

The *CanChild* team partnered with colleagues at the University of Alberta to design a randomized controlled trial to compare the efficacy of two different therapy approaches aimed at promoting children's participation in everyday occupations (Law et al., 2007). One group of children would receive **"context-focused" therapy** aimed at modifying the occupations and environment found to hinder goal-directed participation. The other group would get "child-focused" therapy aimed at identifying and remediating impairments, such as muscle tone, to improve movement patterns and improving a child's skills. By repeating chosen outcome measures over time, the researchers would be able to evaluate the functional gains made between the two intervention groups.

Step 4: Test the Intervention

For the study, 128 children with cerebral palsy received either the context-focused or child-focused weekly intervention for a period of 6 months (Law et al., 2011). Standardized measurements of the children's level of disability, gross motor function,

CASE STUDY 7.2 Participation for Children with Physical Disabilities: The *CanChild* Centre for Childhood Disability Research Program *(continued)*

range of motion, and participation in everyday occupations beyond school activities, as well as family empowerment, were conducted at the beginning and end of the intervention period, and then repeated 3 months later. Interestingly, children in both groups made similar significant gains in their functional and participation outcomes. This important finding means that therapy focusing on changing the occupation and the environment is just as effective as therapy aimed at changing the child's impairments and improving abilities through practice of functional activities.

Step 5: Evaluate the Cost-Effectiveness

Future research can determine the cost-effectiveness of interventions focused on changing the occupation and environment. Observations made during the trial suggest that environmental changes can lead to improved participation very quickly, but this observation needs to be tested.

Step 6: Study Why the Outcomes Were Produced

Both the child-focused and **context-focused** interventions identified goals for therapy intervention. With the child-focused approach, specific problems with performance were identified for intervention. In the context-focused approach, the Canadian Occupational Performance Measure (COPM) (Law et al., 2005) was used to identify individualized child goals. Goal setting has been shown to improve the effectiveness of therapy (Löwing, Bexelius, & Brogren Carlberg, 2009; Ostensjø, Oien, & Fallang, 2008). Through changing the occupation and/or environment, barriers to participation are eliminated to enable the child to perform the occupation using his or her current skills and abilities.

Step 7: Develop the Theory

Thanks to Law's *CanChild* research program focused on children's occupations, therapists have several evidence-based, participation-focused assessment tools to use in practice: the Assessment of Preschool Children's Participation (APCP), the Children's Assessment of Participation and Enjoyment (CAPE), and the Preferences for Activities of Children (PAC) (*CanChild* Centre for Childhood Disability Research, 2011). Therapists can have confidence in shifting their focus from impairments to occupations and the environment in order to promote participation of children with physical disabilities. At the population level, therapists have grounds for promoting public policies that promote "child and youth participation in community settings" (Law, 2011, p. 5). And, by making the research findings and resources available on their Website (http://www.canchild.ca/en/), the *CanChild* Center for Childhood Disability Research ultimately benefits the community as a whole.

CASE STUDY 7.3 Everyday Occupations and Aging Well: The Life and Living in Advanced Age (LiLAC) Cohort study: *Te Puāwaitanga o Ngā Tapuwae Kia Ora Tonu* [Māori translation]

At the School of Population Health, University of Auckland, New Zealand, a multidisciplinary team led by geriatrician Dr. Ngaire Kerse is conducting a prospective cohort study to establish the determinants of aging well for older New Zealanders. In particular, the study aims to understand the relative importance of medical, cultural, functional, activity (occupational), social, and economic factors to relevant health and longevity outcomes. Following a preliminary feasibility study to test an extensive, interview-based questionnaire with 112 participants, 941 older adults were enrolled during 2010 from selected urban and rural regions: 532 non-Māori turning 85, and 409 Māori aged 80 to 90 (extended age criterion to get adequate numbers). At the end of 2011, the first wave of data gathering was complete, the second wave was ready to begin, and a third wave was planned. So, let's look more closely at the occupational science research strand.

Step 1: Identify the Practice Problem

As in most other countries, New Zealand's population is aging. By the late 2030s, one-quarter of the population will be older than 65, compared to 12% in 2005 (Dunstan & Thomson, 2006). Of this population sector, those aged 85 and older make up the fastest growing subgroup, with a predicted 600% increase in the first half of this century. This means many more people will be living into their late 80s and beyond. Accordingly, understanding what helps people age well and live well in advanced age is important. The consensus so far is that engaging in occupations of some sort is positively associated with aging well and longevity (Glass, Mendes de Leon, Marottoli, & Berkman, 1999; Katz, 2000; Menec, 2003). However, findings as to what kind of occupations lead to greater health and well-being are mixed and, at times, inconclusive. Furthermore, little is known about how older New Zealanders prefer to use their time (Figure 7.8). Occupational therapists designing community and individual-level interventions for older adults have little culturally specific knowledge to draw on.

Step 2: Identify the Intervention Needs

Two basic research projects are informing this step of the research program. Initially, a qualitative, hermeneutic phenomenological study was conducted in 2006 to explore how older New Zealanders experience being in their everyday lives. Community-dwelling

(continued)

CASE STUDY 7.3 Everyday Occupations and Aging Well: The Life and Living in Advanced Age (LiLAC) Cohort study: *Te Puāwaitanga o Ngā Tapuwae Kia Ora Tonu* [Māori translation] *(continued)*

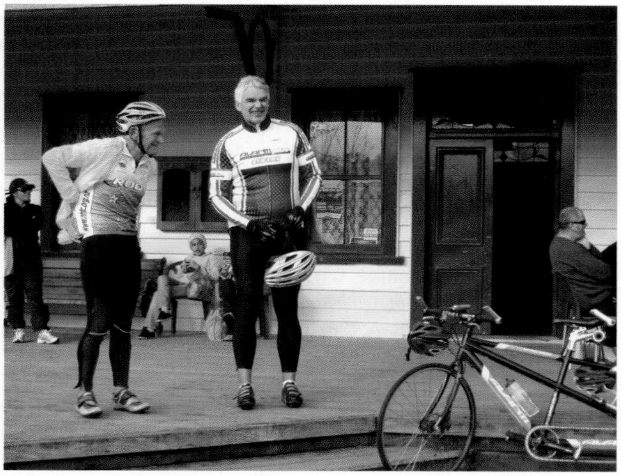

FIGURE 7.8 Leisure time use for Garth Barfoot & Steve Kingdon includes preparing for a club cycle race to the top of the Waitakere Ranges, Auckland, New Zealand, June 2011. (Photograph taken by Valerie Wright-St Clair. Reproduced with permission.)

elder ***Māori*** and non-Māori of European descent, aged 71 to 97 years, were interviewed about their everyday life with a focus on particular events (Wright-St Clair, Kerse, & Smythe, 2011). Several phenomena stood out in the findings. In advanced age, "doing the things ordinarily attended to, in accustomed ways, holds things steady" (Wright-St Clair et al., 2011, p. 93) and keeps things going in the context of getting older. Paradoxically, this accustomed comfortableness in doing things, when it was suddenly lost, revealed potential transition points in life. Such sudden discomforts amid doing usually deeply familiar occupations announced change.

To illustrate, 97-year-old Ferguson, who lived alone with help from his daughter, only came to know his rapidly fading strength when putting his dressing gown on a few days earlier. It was a task usually so easy, so familiar, he ordinarily did not notice doing it. He said he "had a hell of a time. And when I did get it on it was too heavy and yet I have worn it all my life" (Wright-St Clair et al., 2011, p. 92). A few weeks later, Ferguson was admitted to an aged care facility. In addition, the findings suggested that **compelling occupations**, the things that brought a deep purposefulness to being in the everyday, were not only wellness-promoting but essentially different for Māori and non-Māori. Elder Māori spoke more of doing things with and for the collective Māori community. These phenomenological findings justified the case for including an open question about the person's three most important activities and what occupations the person has engaged in over the last 4 weeks within the preliminary feasibility study and wave I, and an additional question about changes to occupations in wave II of the data gathering. Adapted from a study by Häggblom-Kronlöf, Hultberg, Eriksson, and Sonn (2007), participants will be asked whether they have dropped any interests over the last 12 months and, if so, the reasons why.

Although analysis to understand the relative importance of occupations to health and longevity outcomes within the cohort study is yet to begin, descriptive analysis of the feasibility study results offer the promise of what is to come. From the preliminary phase, the occupations nominated as important were coded using the "activities and participation" items in the International Classification of Functioning, Disability and Health (ICF) (World Health Organization [WHO], 2001). Interestingly, "domestic life" occupations showed as being similarly important for Māori, non-Māori, men, and women (26%, 24%, 21%, & 27% respectively). Most commonly, *gardening, cooking, keeping a tidy house,* and *shopping* were mentioned as important (Wright-St Clair et al., 2012). While the men were more likely than the women to nominate interpersonal relationships as being important to them, such as *doing things together with my wife,* the overall occupational patterns were similar for men and women. Differences also showed. Occupations related to "community, social, and civic life" (WHO, 2001) were frequently nominated by elder Māori, including things such as *supporting family, attending [tribal] functions, family gatherings,* or *taking care of mokopuna [grandchildren].* In contrast, a significant number of non-Māori responses revealed "recreation and leisure" (WHO, 2001) activities like *reading newspapers, books* or *magazines, playing cards* or *doing puzzles,* and doing handicrafts like *woodwork, knitting,* or *drawing* as being most important (Wright-St Clair et al., 2012).

A glimpse at the wave I results suggests the elders spend more time doing the things that are important to them. For example, in the last 4 weeks, spending time on a hobby or handicraft every day was something 34% of the elder Māori said they did, compared with 80% of non-Māori; whereas twice as many elder Māori than non-Māori said they visited, or were visited by, family or friends daily. At an interpretive level, the differences may point to spiritual and cultural differences, related to the traditional collective nature of the Māori and the more individualistic focus of non-Māori society.

Step 3: Develop the Intervention

Because this is a longitudinal study, it will be several years before intervention needs for community-dwelling older adults as well as those living in aged care can be fully identified. What is exciting about the occupational thread in New Zealand's largest cohort study of aging well is the potential to explore the predictive qualities of everyday occupations for health, quality of life, and survival outcomes. Several possible applied research projects are envisioned, such as designing and testing an occupation-based screening tool to identify community-based older adults who are at risk of an acute hospital or aged care facility admission; examining whether enabling participation in valued occupations promotes aging well for older New Zealanders; and testing whether an occupational therapy program that enhances participation in occupations that are self-chosen as being important promotes living well for those in aged care facilities. Such questions will only be able to be answered in the context of a systematic program of translational science research.

Acknowledgments

Florence Clark and Mary Law for their commitment to reviewing and contributing essential detail to the case studies.

References

Asaba, E., & Jackson, J. (2011). Social ideologies embedded in everyday life: A narrative analysis about disability, identities, and occupation. *Journal of Occupational Science, 18*, 139–152. doi:10.1080/14427591.2011.579234

Beagan, B. L., & Etowa, J. B. (2011). The meanings and functions of occupations related to spirituality for African Nova Scotian women. *Journal of Occupational Science, 18*, 277–290. doi:10 .1080/14427591.2011.594548

Blanche, E. I., & Henny-Kohler, E. (2000). Philosophy, science and ideology: A proposed relationship for occupational science and occupational therapy. *Occupational Therapy International, 7*, 99–110.

CanChild Centre for Childhood Disability Research. (2011). *Measures of Participation: CAPE & PAC*. Retrieved from http://www.canchild.ca/en/measures/capepac.asp

Clark, F. A., Jackson, J., & Carlson, M. (2004). Occupational science, occupational therapy and evidence-based practice: What the Well Elderly Study has taught us. In M. Molineux (Ed.), *Occupation for occupational therapists* (pp. 200–218). Oxford, United Kingdom: Blackwell.

Clark, F. A., Jackson, J. M., Scott, M. D., Atkins, M. S., Uhles-Tanaka, D., & Rubayi, S. (2006). Data-based models of how pressure ulcers develop in daily-living contexts of adults with spinal cord injury. *Archives of Physical Medicine and Rehabilitation, 87*, 1516–1525. doi:10.1016/j.apmr.2006.08.329

Clark, F., & Lawlor, M. C. (2009). The making and mattering of occupational science. In E. B. Crepeau, E. S. Cohn, & B. A. Schell (Eds.), *Willard & Spackman's occupational therapy* (11th ed., pp. 2–14). Philadelphia, PA: Lippincott Williams & Wilkins.

Clark, F., Sanders, K., Carlson, M., Blanche, E., & Jackson, J. (2007). Synthesis of habit theory. *OTJR: Occupation, Participation and Health, 27*(Suppl 1), 7S–23S.

Coster, W., Bedell, G., Law, M., Khetani, M. A., Teplicky, R., Liljenquist, K., . . . Yao, K. C. (2011). Psychometric evaluation of the Participation and Environment Measure for Children and Youth (PEM-CY). *Developmental Medicine and Child Neurology, 53*, 1030–1037.

de Poy, E., & Gitlin, L. N. (2011). *Introduction to research: Understanding and applying multiple strategies* (4th ed.). St. Louis, MO: Mosby.

de Saint-Exupéry, A. (1972). *The little prince* (K. Woods, Trans.). Harmondsworth, Middlesex: Penguin Books Ltd.

Dunstan, K., & Thomson, N. (2006). *Demographic aspects of New Zealand's ageing population*. Wellington, New Zealand: Statistics New Zealand.

Glass, T. A., Mendes de Leon, C., Marottoli, R. A., & Berkman, L. F. (1999). Population based study of social and productive activities as predictors of survival among elderly Americans. *British Medical Journal, 319*, 478–483.

Guerra, N. G., & Leidy, M. S. (2010). Conducting translational research on child development in community settings: What you need to know and why it is worth the effort. In V. Maholmes & C. G. Lomonaco (Eds.), *Applied research in child and adolescent development: A practical guide* (pp. 155–173). New York, NY: Psychology Press.

Häggblom-Kronlöf, G., Hultberg, J., Eriksson, B. G., & Sonn, U. (2007). Experiences of daily occupations at 99 years of age. *Scandinavian Journal of Occupational Therapy, 14*, 192–200.

Haines, C., Smith, T. M., & Baxter, M. F. (2010). Participation in the risk-taking occupation of skateboarding. *Journal of Occupational Science, 17*, 239–245. doi:10.1080/14427591.2010.9686701

Håkansson, C., & Ahlborg, G., Jr. (2010). Perceptions of employment, domestic work, and leisure as predictors of health among women and men. *Journal of Occupational Science, 17*, 150–157. doi:/10.1080/14427591.2010.9686689

Harper, D. (2010). *Online etymology dictionary*. Retrieved from http://www.etymonline.com/index.php?search=system&searchmode=none

Hocking, C. (2012). Occupations through the looking glass: Reflecting on occupational scientists' ontological assumptions. In G. E. Whiteford & C. Hocking (Eds.), *Society, inclusion, participation: Critical perspectives on occupational science* (pp. 54–68). London, United Kingdom: Oxford Press.

Jackson, J., Carlson, M., Rubayi, S., Scott, M. D., Atkins, M. S., Blanche, E. I., . . . Clark, F. A. (2010). Qualitative study of principles pertaining to lifestyle and pressure ulcer risk in adults with spinal cord injury. *Disability and Rehabilitation, 32*, 567–578.

Kantartzis, S., & Molineux, M. (2011). The influence of Western society's construction of a healthy daily life on the conceptualisation of occupation. *Journal of Occupational Science, 18*, 62–80. doi:10.1080/14427591.2011.566917

Katz, S. (2000). Busy bodies: Activity, aging, and the management of everyday life. *Journal of Aging Studies, 14*, 135–152.

Lala, A. P., & Kinsella, E. A. (2011). Phenomenology and the study of human occupation. *Journal of Occupational Science, 18*, 195–209. doi:10.1080/14427591.2011.581629

Law, M. (2011). *Participation of children and youth with disabilities in recreation and leisure activities*. Hamilton, Ontario: *CanChild* Centre for Childhood Disability Research.

Law, M., Baptiste, S., Carswell, A., McColl, M. A., Polatajko, H., & Pollock, N. (2005). *Canadian Occupational Performance Measure* (Rev. 4th ed.). Ottawa, Ontario: Canadian Association of Occupational Therapists, ACE.

Law, M., Darrah, J., Pollock, N., Rosenbaum, P., Russell, D., Walter, S. D., . . . Wright, V. (2007). Focus on function—A randomized controlled trial comparing two rehabilitation interventions for young people with cerebral palsy. *BMC Pediatrics, 7*, 31. doi:10.1186/1471-2431-7-31

Law, M., Darrah, J., Pollock, N., Wilson, B., Russell, D. J., Walter, S. D., . . . Galuppi, B. (2011). Focus on function: A cluster, randomized controlled trial comparing child- versus context-focused intervention for young people with cerebral palsy. *Developmental Medicine & Child Neurology, 53*, 621–629. doi:10.1111/j.1469-8749.2011.03962.x

Liew, S. L., & Aziz-Zadeh, L. (2011). The neuroscience of language and action in occupations: A review of findings from brain and behavioral sciences. *Journal of Occupational Science, 18*, 97–114. doi:10.1080/14427591.2011.575758

Löwing, K., Bexelius, A., & Brogren Carlberg, E. (2009). Activity focused and goal directed therapy for children with cerebral palsy—Do goals make a difference? *Disability Rehabilitation, 31*, 1808–1816.

Menec, V. H. (2003). The relation between everyday activities and successful aging: A 6-year longitudinal study. *The Journals of Gerontology. Series B, Psychological Sciences and Social Sciences, 58*, S74–S82.

Ministry of Social Development. (2011). Young blokes, good dads. *Rise*, (15), 8–9.

Molineux, M. (Ed.). (2004). *Occupation for occupational therapists*. Oxford, United Kingdom: Blackwell.

Morgan, W. J. (2010). What, exactly, is occupational satisfaction? *Journal of Occupational Science, 17*, 216–223. doi:10.1080/14427591.2010.9686698

Odawara, E. (2010). Occupations for resolving life crises in old age. *Journal of Occupational Science, 17*, 14–19. doi:10.1080/14427591.2010.9686667

Ostensjø, S., Oien, I., & Fallang, B. (2008). Goal-oriented rehabilitation of preschoolers with cerebral palsy—A multi-case study of combined use of the Canadian Occupational Performance Measure (COPM) and the Goal Attainment Scaling (GAS). *Developmental Neurorehabilitation, 11*, 252–259.

Pierce, D. (Ed.). (2011). *Occupational science for occupational therapy*. Thorofare, NJ: Slack.

Pollock, N., Stewart, D., Law, M., Sahagian-Whalen, S., Harvey, S., & Toal, C. (1997). The meaning of play for young people with physical disabilities. *Canadian Journal of Occupational Therapy, 64*, 25–31.

Seip, J., Carlson, M., Jackson, J., & Clark, F. (in press). Pressure ulcer risk assessment in adults with spinal cord injury: The need to incorporate daily lifestyle concerns. *Advances in Skin and Wound Care.*

Smith-Gabai, H., & Ludwig, F. (2011). Observing the Jewish Sabbath: A meaningful restorative ritual for modern times. *Journal of Occupational Science, 18,* 347–355. doi:10.1080/14427591.2011.595891

Stein, L. I., Foran, A. C., & Cermak, S. (2011). Occupational patterns of parents of children with autism spectrum disorder: Revisiting Matuska and Christiansen's model of lifestyle balance. *Journal of Occupational Science, 18,* 115–130. doi:10.1080/14427591.2011.575762

USC/Rancho Lifestyle Redesign® Pressure Ulcer Prevention Project. (2006a). *Lifestyle Redesign® for pressure ulcer prevention.* Unpublished manuscript, USC/Rancho Lifestyle Redesign® Pressure Ulcer Prevention Project. Los Angeles.

USC/Rancho Lifestyle Redesign® Pressure Ulcer Prevention Project. (2006b). *Pressure ulcer prevention project consumer manual online.* Retrieved from http://www.usc.edu/programs/pups

USC/Rancho Lifestyle Redesign® Pressure Ulcer Prevention Project. (2006c). *PUPS study rehabilitation manual.* Unpublished manuscript, USC/Rancho Los Amigos. Los Angeles.

Wilcock, A. A. (2006). *An occupational perspective of health* (2nd ed.). Thorofare, NJ: SLACK.

World Health Organization. (2001). *International classification of functioning, disability and health.* Geneva, Switzerland: Author.

Wright-St Clair, V. A., Kerse, N., & Smythe, L. (2011). Doing everyday occupations both conceals and reveals the phenomenon of being aged. *Australian Occupational Therapy Journal, 58,* 88–94. doi:10.1111/j.1440-1630.2010.00885.x

Wright-St Clair, V. A., Kepa, M., Hoenle, S., Hayman, K., Keeling, S., Connolly, M., . . . Kerse, N. (2012). Doing what's important—Valued activities for elder New Zealand Māori and non-Māori. *Australasian Journal on Ageing.* Retrieved from http://onlinelibrary.wiley.com/journal/10.1111/%28ISSN%291741-6612/earlyview

Zemke, R., & Clark, F. (1996). Preface. In R. Zemke & F. Clark (Eds.), *Occupational science: The evolving discipline* (pp. vii–xviii). Philadelphia, PA: F. A. Davis.

For additional resources on the subjects discussed in this chapter, visit http://thePoint.lww.com/Willard-Spackman12e.

Narrative Perspectives on Occupation and Disability

UNIT III

"A story presumes both a teller and a community of listeners, such that the act of telling the story and responding to it is a reciprocal exercise designed in part to strengthen community bonds."

–Howard Brody

CHAPTER 8

Narrative as a Key to Understanding

Elizabeth Blesedell Crepeau, Ellen S. Cohn

OUTLINE

LEARNING OBJECTIVES

After reading this chapter, you will be able to:

1. Explain the relationship between experience, narrative, and the interpretive process
2. Identify ways to begin to think about narratives and how they may influence clients' experience and occupational therapy intervention
3. Describe the role of narratives in occupational therapy practice
4. Explain why listening to clients' stories is an essential component of occupational therapy practice

Think back over the past few days. How many times have you told a story about an experience you had? How many times have you listened to a story told to you by a friend or family member? We tell stories all the time about the things that we did or that happened to us and to others as a way to share and interpret our experience. In fact, we could be called *Homo narratus* rather than *Homo sapiens* because of the centrality of storytelling to human experience (Fisher, 1984). Some people are better storytellers than others. Good storytellers can infuse their narratives with tension, drama, and suspense; but regardless of how well the story is told, it is human nature to tell or listen to stories (see **Figure 8.1**). The capacity to understand the world through stories can begin early in life. For example, some children learn to listen to stories even before they can speak (see **Figure 8.2**). Consequently, it is not surprising that occupational therapy clients and their family members have stories to tell about their experiences with injury, disease, or disability. This unit is devoted to these stories, written by the people themselves, their family members, or by an occupational therapist who listened to, translated, and interpreted stories of people living with disabilities. Because stories of occupational therapy practitioners are also important to understand, the narrative perspective of practitioners from various practice contexts is included in Unit XIII. That we devote two units to these narratives indicates the importance of

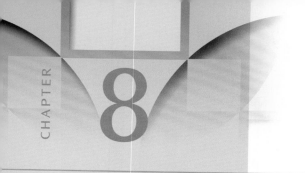

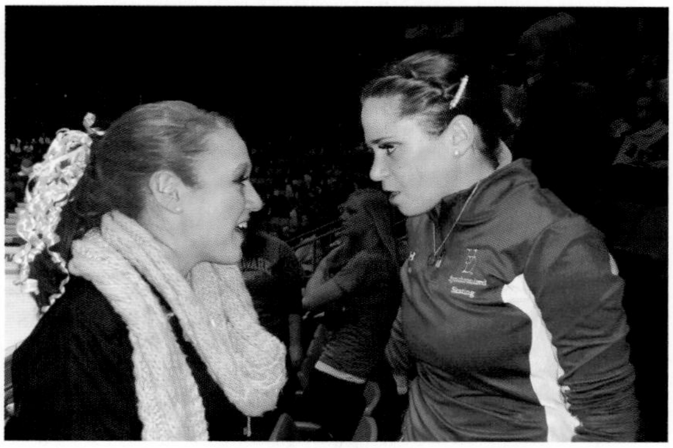

FIGURE 8.1 Stories can be filled with drama and surprise. (Photo courtesy of Ellen S. Cohn.)

the narrative perspectives of the people who seek and provide occupational therapy and how essential narrative is to the entire occupational therapy process.

In the 1980s, social scientists were rediscovering the significance of narrative as a way to understand human experience, and there was a tremendous growth of interest in patients' stories in the health care fields (Clark & Mishler, 1992; Kleinman, 1980; Mishler, 1984; Polkinghorne, 1988). The interest in patients' stories of their experiences living with illness emerged from a "dehumanized" and highly technological approach to health care that lacked sufficient attention to the human aspects of experience. This "narrative turn" in occupational therapy occurred in the mid-1980s when an anthropologist, Cheryl Mattingly, directed the American Occupational Therapy Association (AOTA)/American Occupational Therapy Foundation (AOTF) Clinical Reasoning Study, an ethnographic study of occupational therapists in a large teaching hospital (Mattingly, 1994, 1998; Mattingly & Fleming, 1994). Mattingly and the research team used observation, interviews with therapists and clients, and videotaped occupational therapy sessions to analyze and uncover the stories that emerged during occupational therapy intervention. In her observations of therapists throughout their work day, Mattingly noted that therapists used different forms of talk to discuss their work with clients. Therapists used what Mattingly referred to as "chart talk," a formal reporting register that typically occurred during team meetings and other structured situations to describe the technical and reimbursable aspects of practice. In contrast, therapists told stories during lunch and other times to describe the rich, more interpretive aspects of their meaningful interactions with clients. These stories had all the elements that we have come to expect from a story: a plot, drama, suspense, action, and a moral or lesson.

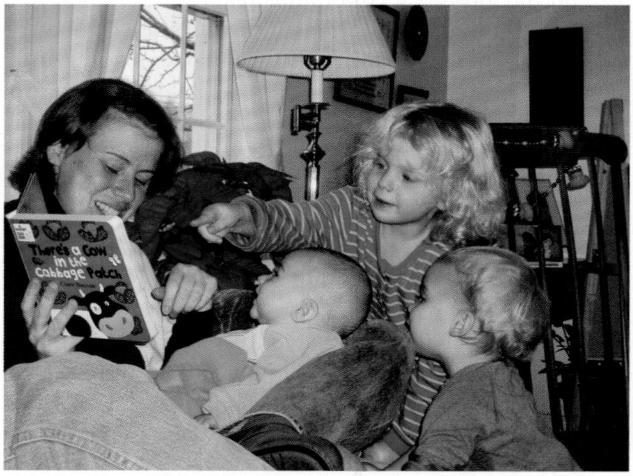

FIGURE 8.2 Reading to children orients them to the power of stories. (Photo courtesy of Elizabeth Blesedell Crepeau.)

Mattingly's work legitimized the telling of stories as an interpretive process that helped therapists to make sense of their experience. This influential work also focused attention on the value of occupational therapy practitioners listening to clients' stories, for it is through storytelling that clients convey the meaning of their experiences. Moving beyond listening and telling stories, Mattingly noted that clients and occupational therapy practitioners collaboratively create new or different "meaningful" life narratives in the context of living with disease or disability. She introduced the idea that occupational therapy intervention involved a "narrative" process in which the therapy involved a dramatic plot transforming therapy into a path of recovery that instilled hope, healing, and a new future (Mattingly, 2010). In addition, the importance of narrative during the occupational therapy assessment process has been recognized (Frank, 1996; Frantis, 2005; Simmons, Crepeau, & White, 2000).

Since then, a significant amount of research in occupational therapy has examined narrative from the perspective of clients (Alsaker & Josephsson, 2010; Braveman & Helfrich, 2001; Price & Miner, 2009), their families (Cohn, 2001; Isaksson, Josephsson, Lexell, & Skär, 2008), and therapists (Labovitz, 2003; Mattingly, 1991). The narrative turn has even influenced research on meetings (Schwartzman, 1989) and team meetings in health care (Atkinson, 1997), how storytelling influences the clinical reasoning of team members (Crepeau, 2000), and alignment of practitioner and client stories (Cohn et al., 2009; Crepeau & Garren, 2011).

Narrative and Story

There are numerous ways to define *narrative* and *story*. In some traditions, particularly literary theory, *narrative* and *story* refer to distinct phenomena. However, in this chapter, we will use *narrative* and *story* equivalently (as do Hamilton 2008; Mattingly & Garro, 2000; Polkinghorne, 1988; Riessman, 2008). In everyday speech, stories are quite common, perhaps so natural that they do not need explaining. Stories are told from the perspective of the speaker. They may be told and retold because they provide a way of understanding and interpreting experience—sharing what is meaningful and important at a particular moment in time rather than a mere accounting of some objective truth (Leight, 2002). Stories are temporally and contextually situated, and although we think a story may be finished, stories are open for new tellings, new interpretations, and new meanings. Consequently, the same story may vary in relation to who tells the story, when the story is told, the sequencing of the story, or the purpose of the story for the intended audience (Bruner, 1990). Although common, stories are incredibly complex and quite difficult to describe. In a very fundamental way, stories concern action and offer a way to make sense of experiences. By linking narrative, act, and consequence, stories offer us windows on social life and human character. Some literary theorists claim that through a chaining of events, stories offer causal explanations of events.

In this chapter, we will draw on Mattingly's definition: "stories are about someone trying to do something, and what happens to her and others as a result" (Mattingly, 1998, p. 7). Consider an excerpt from Alex McIntosh's chapter (see Chapter 10). Alex's story has numerous features that make stories especially appealing for understanding his experiences in living with cerebral palsy. Alex's story is event centered, concerns human action and interaction, and includes the social aspects of human behavior. As the narrator of this story, Alex knows the ending and carefully selects the relevant details to direct our attention to his plot. He narrates the story in a particular way to convey his message and ultimately communicates to the reader that he has an amazing imagination and that walking with crutches is secondary to who he is as a person. His story even has a deeper moral message: Alex's story teaches us that people's ideas about disability are not rationally determined but socially constructed. Alex shows us that a disability is determined by social expectations rather than by diagnostic conditions.

In this story, Alex tells what happened to him and how he and his mother shared an unspoken secret about a naive woman's social construction and understanding of who Alex really is.

> When I was about seven years old, I was firmly convinced that I was a werewolf. I had never actually undergone any physical transformation at the full of the moon, but 7-year-olds are not bothered by such trifles. The crowning touch was that my crutches acted as a second pair of legs, and although when wearing them I could never really manage a wolf-like lope, I made do instead with a sort of galloping skip. Nevertheless, it was fast enough (to me) to reinforce fantasies of running swiftly through the forest on silent paws, seeking unsuspecting prey.
>
> The technical term for the condition of being a werewolf is *lycanthropy,* after the mythical Greek king Lycaon, whom the god Zeus transformed into a wolf as punishment for his tyranny. I knew the word at the age of seven, having read every book on werewolves that I could both find and understand. I was proud to declare myself a lycanthrope to everyone I met.
>
> One day that year, my mother, my younger brother, and I attended a fundraising boat race, the object of which was to allow wealthy yacht owners to raise money for the disabled. I was skipping around the lobby of the yacht club where the event was being held, giving long, mournful, earsplitting howls, as a proper werewolf should. Mom was over in a corner with my brother, trying to pretend that I was someone else's child.
>
> One of the yacht owners saw me, and she said, "Look at you, doing so well. What's your disability, honey?"
>
> "I have lycanthropy!" I said, beaming.
>
> A few minutes later, she was chatting with my mother and said, "I just met your son. What a nice boy. It's so sad that he has lycanthropy."
>
> Mom smirked. "Um, I think there's something you should know . . ."
>
> That is what happens to people who are lacking in disability awareness.

Alex, now a 20-year-old, starts his story by orienting us to the characters and setting, placing himself at a younger age. This particular story serves a referential function. In telling about the things that happened to them and others, people connect their experience to the world beyond themselves and provide a retrospective glance at past events. Alex, a 7-year-old boy, who, using his words "could never really manage" a particular gait, transforms himself into a wolf, "running swiftly through the forest, sneaking up on unsuspecting prey" (the yacht owner) to describe to the reader who he is and what he does in this world. Alex has imaginatively transformed himself from a young boy walking with crutches to a werewolf "skipping" and "howling" around the lobby. He communicates his experience, one in which he is not a child with a disability but a competent and clever young boy playing a trick and perhaps educating an adult who does not understand "disability." Alex draws us into his werewolf fantasy as a means to communicate his experience. Yet, the narrative moment in this story is not even in the story and has no words. We can only imagine the ironic pleasure that Alex and his mother shared in their unspoken words, "If she only knew." Alex's ending creates an experience for us, the audience, and allow us to infer something about what it feels like to be in his world. Alex's story is worth telling because it conveys to the reader a particular outcome that he feels is important for us to understand. We can share in the joy, imagining what it might be like to have some fun while teaching others that Alex is a clever and imaginative child who happens to use crutches.

We have learned a lot about Alex in his story. We know that he has a vivid imagination, that he has loved to read since he was quite young, and that he is an effective storyteller who can incorporate drama, comedy, and irony into his storytelling. By listening to our clients' stories, we can understand their interpretation of their experience and begin to discern who they are as individuals, their illness or disability experience, and how this experience has shaped their daily occupations. The interpretive process of storytelling helps to differentiate our clients from each other, even those with very similar medical and social histories. Although we may work with many clients with the same diagnosis, their lived experience and the stories they tell about their lives will be as important as their particular occupational problems in shaping the way in which we work with them to plan and implement their occupational therapy intervention.

Listening for Meaning

Frank (1995, 2002) argues that in listening to patients' stories, health care practitioners bear witness to suffering as well as to personal strengths and triumphs. Listening to stories of clients opens practitioners to the opportunity to "seeing, feeling, and hearing life differently" (Kirkpatrick, 2008, p. 63). Kirkpatrick urges health care practitioners to listen to and strive to understand narratives at multiple levels, being sensitive to the narrative types from the culture that might frame the stories. Although client narratives are individual representations of experience from the client's experience and current perspective, they are shaped by dominant narratives in the culture (Kirkpatrick, 2008). Consequently, although the same diagnosis may confer similar experiences to individuals, these individuals are quite likely to tell very different stories based on their life history, including their socioeconomic status, ethnicity, religion, and other individual attributes and the cultural narratives available to them. For example, until very recently, the cultural narrative available to girls and young women was very narrow and focused mainly on finding a husband and raising a family (Coontz, 2011; Heilbrun, 1988). This restricted view provided few models for girls to envision a different future. In this section we will describe two ways of interpreting stories. The first focuses on types of illness narratives delineated by Frank. The second takes a more cultural perspective.

Frank (1995) listened to illness and disability stories of others and read personal accounts of illness and disability. Through this process, he identified three types of illness narratives: restitution, chaos, and quest narratives. These narrative types might not be the only types of illness narratives, but Frank reported that they presented themselves in many of the stories he listened to and read. Individuals may use one or more of the types in one story or may shift narrative types depending on the particular standpoint from which they are telling the story.

Clients telling a restitution story are showing how medicine has resolved their problems to return them to health (Frank, 1995). Clients often tell restitution stories retrospectively, but they might also use this story form to project themselves into the future. A plotline might involve a major surgical intervention, such as a joint replacement, followed by rehabilitation and ultimate return to former occupational pursuits. These stories are easy to listen to because they represent the triumph of Western medicine. In contrast, Frank (1995) asserts that chaos narratives are the most difficult to hear because, unlike the restitution narrative, they are not sequenced by a plotline that we are socialized to follow. Chaos narratives represent a life that is out of control with no solutions in sight. They are characterized by events that are connected by phrases such as "and then . . . and then . . . and then. . . ." This lack of causal ordering or plot renders the telling hard to understand because the person is still enmeshed in the experience. Quest narratives, in contrast, show the personal transformation that can occur when clients confront serious illness and disability and, as a result, make fundamental changes in their lives. Simi Linton's book (2006), *My Body Politic: A Memoir*, is an example of a quest narrative. Now, 35 years after a car accident, this disability rights activist recounts her "coming out"—a transformation from early challenges with paraplegia and the marginalization of people with disabilities to promoting the contributions of people with disabilities to society. Her book invites the reader to consider the negative stereotypes attributed to people with disability, particularly its negative representation in society and the arts. This negative representation of people with disabilities is an example of the prejudicial master narrative Kirkpatrick (2008) asserts is so disempowering to those without power.

Master narratives represent the values of a culture, which may reflect the power of the dominant members of society and the prejudices held by them (Kirkpatrick, 2008). These master narratives may become stereotypes, which suppress the individuality of people and convey negative attitudes and prejudices. People who lack power, the poor, disabled, or racial or ethnic minority members are particularly vulnerable to negative narratives that oppress and deprive them of opportunities. Kirkpatrick proposes three levels of narratives: personal stories, community narratives, and dominant cultural narratives. Kirkpatrick, drawing on the work of Clandinin and Connelly (2000), argues that personal stories incorporate (1) individual experience as it is reflected through a temporal lens of past, present, and future; (2) the social interaction that occurs during the storytelling and how this process shapes the story; and (3) place, which provides the social and environmental context containing either opportunities or barriers to the individual. Second, community narratives reflect the communal stories of a group of people. For example, family stories can reflect positive or negative aspects about an individual within the family structure. These stories can be shaped and reshaped over time, both at the level of the family and by the individual. Third, dominant cultural narratives present master narratives of different groups of people. These are stereotypes that provide a shorthand way of characterizing a group. Although master narratives may present those without power in a negative fashion, counter narratives such as Linton's have the power to reshape these negative narratives and provide more positive master narratives for individuals and communities. The recovery movement in mental health has done much to help rewrite the master narrative about mental illness and has provided ways for individuals and programs to use these narratives to foster recovery.

Narrative as an Interpretive Process

Creating stories or narratives is an interpretive process that involves selecting aspects of past experience and representing that experience to others in the present (Bruner, 1986, 1990, 1991). Because storytelling is interpretive, the way in which an individual interprets the past may be strongly influenced by present circumstances (see Figure 8.3). This does not mean that storytelling is a fabrication; rather, stories are constructed to present a coherent interpretation of the past in light of the present. The narratives in this unit tell stories from the perspectives of the authors and offer counterstories to the master narratives about physical disability, mental illness, and caregiving.

Drawing on Riessman's (1993) delineation of the multiple levels of representation of experience in narrative analysis, we propose that the chapters in this unit have several levels of representation. These levels are (1) the author's attention to the experience in the moment, (2) the telling of this experience in the writing of the chapter, (3) the editorial process, and (4) the interpretation derived from reading the chapter. First of all, just as Alex was selective, other storytellers select what is important or meaningful to them at that moment. Second, we asked our chapter authors to tell their story to make it accessible to you. In doing so, they have ordered and interpreted events to create a coherent account that you, as the reader, can understand. Because they were asked to write about their experience for occupational therapy students, their stories are told from that standpoint. Their chapters might have a different focus if they were writing for a different audience. In this sense, the chapters are "constructed" for a certain purpose, to convey their experience to readers who will someday be working with people who might have had similar experiences with illness or disability. Thus, the chapters are positioned to reflect experience from a particular interpretive lens: "Let me tell you my story so that you will understand the experience of your future clients." In fact, some authors end their chapters by addressing you directly as future occupational therapists to be sure that you understand the importance of their message. The third level of the process involves editing the chapter, which may further shape the story. As editors of these chapters, we tried to sustain the perspective of the authors while helping them to bring clarity and order to their writing. This is a delicate process because in editing, we ran the risk of changing the representation of their experience by our shaping of it. Finally, you will bring your own interpretive process to your reading of these chapters based on your own life experience.

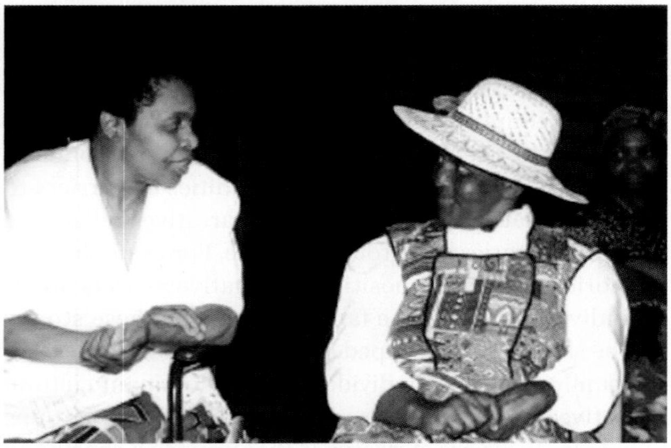

FIGURE 8.3 Storytelling provides a mechanism for shared understanding. (Photo courtesy of Theresa Lorenzo.)

Telling stories is important. We knew this when we decided to have personal narratives in *Willard and Spackman*. But working with the authors of these chapters brought the importance of narratives home to us because the authors reminded us of the value to the authors themselves of writing their narratives. Laurie McIntosh said that the chapter she wrote with her son and husband (Chapter 10) helped them to realize the distinctiveness of their perspectives—being a child with a disability, the child's mother, or the child's father. Writing the chapter provided an opportunity to reflect on their individual experience of raising Alex from the perspective of his departure for college, an important developmental milestone. Should they revise this chapter for the next edition of *Willard and Spackman*, they might interpret Alex's childhood differently because of the events in the intervening years. You will see some of this reinterpretation in Mary Feldhaus-Weber's chapter (Chapter 9) in the sections in which she writes about her brain injury at various times from the accident to the present. The basic elements of Mary's story remain the same, but the passage of time and experience have shifted Mary's interpretation. In working on the chapter for this edition, she said that she felt that she could reveal some of the "darker" aspects of her experience because she no longer felt that it was essential to project a strong image. Mary's artwork, a form of visual narrative, transforms what was previously a private experience to a shared comprehension of the impact of acquired brain injury. Consider all aspects of her paintings, including ambiguity, irony, paradox, or the tone conveyed in the descriptions of the paintings. Don Murray wrote his chapter a year after the death of his wife (see Chapter 12). Although he was a professional writer who wrote frequently about Minnie Mae in his *Boston Globe* column, this chapter provided him with a broader vehicle for integrating and synthesizing the experience of her illness, his caregiving, and her death. He thanked us for this opportunity and said that it helped him to mourn during the year after her death.

Gloria Dickerson's chapter (see Chapter 11) illustrates her exquisite ability to make sense of incredibly painful life experiences and actions that she did not understand as a child. She places her experiences within the context of grand narratives of racism and sexism within our culture and ultimately shows readers how she shapes her future actions by reflecting on her experience to rewrite and live out a new life story. Gloria, in telling her individual story, also illustrates how we may compose stories by adopting the narratives available in our culture. Gloria's story is situated in a paradigm shift within the mental health field over the past two decades. The field has shifted from a focus on pathology to a focus on recovery and living a meaningful life beyond the constraints of illness (Kirkpatrick, 2008). Community or shared narratives within a group of people can influence members' view of themselves. Health care systems or occupational therapy departments, as a form of community narrative, can influence and shape our experience in either empowering or constraining ways. Gloria describes how the community narrative of the Boston University Center for Psychiatric Rehabilitation influenced her recovery by articulating that she had options and held a valued role in life. In this way, the community narrative can be an important element in the change process. In an important and powerfully reciprocal manner, individual stories can impact the community narrative. For example, Gloria's recovery story is a moving account of her recovery and can be instrumental in influencing the community narrative to embrace a strengths-based recovery perspective rather than a disease and deficit-oriented community narrative.

Kate Barrett's translation and interpretation of the stories told to her by people living with disabilities in Ecuador communicates the powerful influence of culture, spirituality, and access to resources in shaping their lives and their stories. How you react to these powerful and inspirational stories will teach you much about how your interpretive lenses influence your worldview.

The Role of Narrative in Occupational Therapy Practice

Storytelling

Occupational therapy practice provides many opportunities to listen to and elicit stories from clients and to tell clients stories as a form of motivation or to help them see themselves in particular kinds of therapeutic plots (Mattingly, 1998). Occupational therapists also tell stories to each other while socializing and during team meetings and other interdisciplinary forms of communication (Crepeau, 2000). They might tell puzzling stories to each other to make sense of what happened or determine how they should proceed with a particular client. They may also use stories to persuade others of a particular point of view or insight about a client. For example, an occupational therapist used a very persuasive account of a patient in a geropsychiatric unit to reformulate the patient's problem from one of refusal to participate in the milieu to one of an inability to participate. The occupational therapist's interpretation of the client's story proved to be a turning point for the team in planning care for this client (Crepeau, 2000). Consequently, the therapist's interpretation of the patient's behavior reconstructed the team's view and plans for her care.

Storymaking

Although this chapter has focused on storytelling as a way to interpret and share experience, stories do not simply look back and interpret past events in light of the present. Mattingly proposed that narratives can shape action and that occupational therapy intervention involves a prospective "therapeutic emplotment" in which clients and therapists create new narratives; that is, new "stories are created in clinical time" (Mattingly, 2000, p. 183). She argued that therapists and clients create a collaborative intervention process to understand and enable clients to move from where or who they are to where or who they want to be (Mattingly, 1991, 1998). Elaborating on Mattingly's argument, Clark (1993) introduced the term *occupational storymaking* to describe how occupational therapists engage people in desired occupations to rewrite, revise, or recreate their life story and imagine new possibilities. As clients engage in desired occupations and experience their potential to participate in desired activities, a new story is enacted in the intervention process. Clark (1993) described her intervention with Penny Richardson, a colleague who experienced a cerebral aneurysm at the age of 47. Because Clark listened to Penny and understood her life story, Clark and Penny were able to identify Penny's challenges to engagement in desired occupations and rewrite potential solutions to occupational problems. In one example of the process, Clark and Penny identified the walker as a constant reminder of Penny's continued balance problems and symbol of disability. Before the aneurysm, Penny enjoyed outdoor activities, was an avid hiker, and pushed herself to be physically competent. Recycling her familiar story lines and attending to her motives to remove stigmatizing barriers, Penny began what she called "cane hiking" to transition herself from walking with a walker to using a cane. This and other redefined occupations enabled Penny to connect her former self to her new self.

Conclusion

Our purpose in writing this chapter is to give you a very brief overview of the importance of narrative to occupational therapy practice. Our hope is that you will read the chapters in this unit and will approach working with others with a respect for the importance of narrative to understand how people interpret their experience and how storytelling and storymaking can be used as part of

BOX 8.1 Narratives: Questions to Consider

1. What is the plot of the chapter and what is the moral of the story?
2. What are major themes represented in the story?
3. What insights have you gained from the stories in these chapters?
4. If you were an occupational therapist for these individuals, how would their narratives shape your work with them?
5. Whose stories get heard?
6. How could the story be told another way?
7. Identify the elements of hope in the story you read and consider how you might integrate hopefulness into your interactions and interventions?

the therapeutic process. By seeking client stories, you will discover the richness of their lives, their fears, and their hopes and dreams. This deeper understanding of their unique perspective will help you create with them a story filled with hope for the future. As you read the following chapters, consider the questions listed in Box 8.1.

References

Alsaker, S., & Josephsson, S. (2010). Occupation and meaning: Narrative in everyday activities of women with chronic rheumatic conditions. *OTJR: Occupation, Participation and Health, 30*, 58–67.

Atkinson, P. (1997). Narrative turn or blind alley? *Qualitative Health Research, 7*(3), 325–344.

Braveman, B., & Helfrich, C. A. (2001). Occupational identity: Exploring the narratives of three men living with AIDS. *Journal of Occupational Science, 8*, 25–31.

Brody, H. (1987). *Stories of sickness*. New Haven, CT: Yale University Press.

Bruner, J. (1986). *Actual minds, possible worlds*. Cambridge, MA: Harvard University Press.

Bruner, J. (1990). *Acts of meaning: Four lectures on mind and culture*. Cambridge, MA: Harvard University Press.

Bruner, J. (1991). The narrative construction of reality. *Critical Inquiry, 18*, 1–21.

Clandinin, D. J., & Connelly, F. M. (2000). *Narrative inquiry: Experience and story in qualitative research*. San Francisco, CA: Jossey-Bass.

Clark, F. (1993). Occupation embedded in a real life: Interweaving occupational science and occupational therapy. 1993 Eleanor Clarke Slagle Lecture. *American Journal of Occupational Therapy, 47*, 1069–1078.

Clark, J. A., & Mishler, E. G. (1992). Attending to patients' stories: Reframing the clinical task. *Sociology of Health & Illness, 14*, 344–372.

Cohn, E. S. (2001). From waiting to relating: Parents' experiences in the waiting room of an occupational therapy clinic. *American Journal of Occupational Therapy, 55*, 168–175.

Cohn, E. S., Cortés, D. E., Hook, J. M., Yinusa-Nyahkoon, L. S., Soloman, J. L., & Bokhour, B. (2009). A narrative of resistance: Presentation of self when parenting children with asthma. *Communication & Medicine, 6*, 27–37.

Coontz, S. (2011). *A strange stirring: The feminine mystique and American women at the dawn of the 1960s*. New York, NY: Basic Books.

Crepeau, E. B. (2000). Reconstructing Gloria: A narrative analysis of team meetings. *Qualitative Health Research, 10*(6), 766–787.

Crepeau, E. B., & Garren, K. (2011). I looked to her as a guide: The therapeutic relationship in hand therapy. *Disability and Rehabilitation, 33*, 872–881.

Fisher, W. R. (1984). Narration as a human communication paradigm: The case of public moral argument. *Communication Monographs, 51*, 1–22.

Frantis, L. E. (2005). Nothing about us without us: Searching for the narrative of disability. *American Journal of Occupational Therapy, 59*, 577–579.

Frank, A. W. (1995). *The wounded storyteller: Body, illness, and ethics*. Chicago, IL: University of Chicago Press.

Frank, A. W. (2002). "How can they act like that?": Clinicians and patients as characters in each other's stories. *Hastings Center Report, 32*, 14–22.

Frank, G. (1996). Life histories in occupational therapy clinical practice. *American Journal of Occupational Therapy, 50*, 251–264.

Hamilton, T. B. (2008). Narrative reasoning. In B. A. Boyt Schell & J. W. Schell (Eds.), *Clinical and professional reasoning in occupational therapy* (pp. 125–126). Baltimore, MD: Lippincott Williams & Wilkins.

Heilbrun, C. G. (1988). *Writing a woman's life*. New York, NY: Ballantine Books.

Isaksson, G., Josephsson, S., Lexell, J., & Skär, L. (2008). Men's experience of giving and taking social support after their wife's spinal cord injury. *Scandinavian Journal of Occupational Therapy, 15*, 236–246.

Kirkpatrick, H. (2008). A narrative framework for understanding experiences of people with severe mental illness. *Archives of Psychiatric Nursing, 22*, 61–68.

Kleinman, A. (1980). *Patients and healers in the context of culture: An exploration of the borderland between anthropology, medicine, and psychiatry*. Berkeley, CA: University of California Press.

Labovitz, D. R. (Ed.). (2003). *Ordinary miracles: True stories about overcoming obstacles and surviving catastrophes*. Thorofare, NJ: SLACK Incorporated.

Leight, S. B. (2002). Starry night: Using story to inform aesthetic knowing in women's health nursing. *Journal of Advanced Nursing, 37*, 108–114.

Linton, S. (2006). *My body politic: A memoir*. Ann Arbor: University of Michigan Press.

Mattingly, C. (1991). The narrative nature of clinical reasoning. *American Journal of Occupational Therapy, 45*, 998–1005.

Mattingly, C. (1994). The narrative nature of clinical reasoning. In R. Mattingly & M. H. Fleming (Eds.), *Clinical reasoning: Forms on inquiry in a therapeutic practice* (pp. 239–269). Philadelphia, PA: F. A. Davis.

Mattingly, C. (1998). *Healing dramas and clinical plots: The narrative structure of experience*. New York, NY: Cambridge University Press.

Mattingly, C. (2000). Emergent narratives. In C. Mattingly & L. C. Garro (Eds.), *Narrative and the cultural construction of illness and healing* (pp. 181–211). Berkeley, CA: University of California Press.

Mattingly, C. (2010). *The anatomy of hope: Journeys through a clinical borderland*. Berkeley, CA: University of California Press.

Mattingly, C., & Fleming, M. H. (1994). *Clinical reasoning: Forms of inquiry in a therapeutic practice*. Philadelphia, PA: F. A. Davis.

Mattingly, C., & Garro, L. C. (2000). *Narrative and the cultural construction of illness and healing*. Berkeley, CA: University of California Press.

Mishler, E. G. (1984). *The discourse of medicine: Dialectics of medical interviews*. Norwood, NJ: Ablex.

Polkinghorne, D. E. (1988). *Narrative knowing and the human sciences*. Albany, NY: State University of New York Press.

Price, M. P., & Miner, S. (2009). Mother becoming: Learning to read Mikala's signs. *Scandinavian Journal of Occupational Therapy, 16*, 68–77.

Riessman, C. K. (1993). *Narrative analysis*. Thousand Oaks, CA: Sage.

Riessman, C. K. (2008). *Narrative methods for the human sciences*. Newbury Park, CA: Sage.

Schwartzman, H. B. (1989). *The meeting: Gatherings in organizations and communities*. New York, NY: Plenum.

Simmons, D. C., Crepeau, E. B., & White, B. P. (2000). The predictive power of narrative data in occupational therapy evaluation. *American Journal of Occupational Therapy, 54*, 471–476.

For additional resources on the subjects discussed in this chapter, visit http://thePoint.lww.com/Willard-Spackman12e.

CHAPTER 9

An Excerpt from *The Book of Sorrows, Book of Dreams*

A First-Person Narrative

Mary Feldhaus-Weber, Sally A. Schreiber-Cohn

OUTLINE

Unit Editor's Prologue

Mary Feldhaus-Weber was in her thirties; lived in Boston; and was a successful playwright, filmmaker, and television producer. She had produced documentaries for the Public Broadcasting System (PBS). Her plays had been produced off-off-Broadway. She had just finished making *Joan Robinson: One Woman's Story*, an award-winning documentary film about her friend's 3-year struggle with and death from ovarian cancer. In December 1979, 3 weeks before this film was to be telecast on PBS, Mary was the passenger in a car that was struck by a drunk driver. Mary was taken from the demolished car and was rushed to a hospital emergency room. Although her head had smashed the car window during the accident, she was released from the hospital that very night. Just 3 days later, Mary began to have seizures. Months later, she was diagnosed as having epilepsy, a seizure disorder, caused by traumatic brain injury. Her brain had been injured when she hit her head during the car accident. She was never hospitalized for this traumatic injury. Her seizures initially were not well controlled with medication. New medication recently has brought them largely under control; however, she has never been able to return to work.

What follows is Mary Feldhaus-Weber's story of her struggle to live with the effects of her brain injury and seizure disorder—in her own words. These excerpts were taken from her book in progress, *The Book of Sorrows, Book of Dreams*. The first part of the story covers the years 1979 to 1981. Mary dictated this part of her story to friends and occupational therapy students who were working with her. Mary was able to write the final three parts of her story by herself. Noted throughout the chapter are references to Mary's paintings.

Note: This narrative was last updated when published in 2009.

1979 to 1981

The Accident

Now let me tell you about this. My friend Sally was driving me home at 3:00 A.M. after working on the Joan Robinson film, getting it ready for its national air date. A large American car, going at a high rate of speed, hit the small foreign car we were in, on the passenger side.

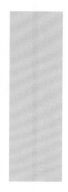

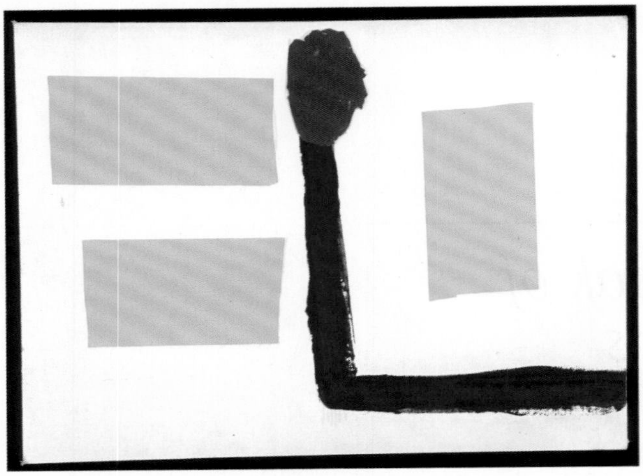

FIGURE 9.1 Intersection: For a long time after the accident, my mind played and replayed the car crash. I finally painted it to get the memory outside of myself. Here was the intersection, and here was the car I was in. Then the collision, the smashing of the car and of me. (Courtesy of Mary Feldhaus-Weber.)

I was the passenger. The car we were in was hit with such intensity that both cars were demolished, totaled (see Figure 9.1, "Intersection"). My head went through the passenger window sideways. The side of my head above the temple totally shattered the glass, hit with such impact that every piece of glass had been knocked out (see Figure 9.2, "The Shattering"). People in the emergency room were astonished that I had no facial cuts. I told them my hard Scandinavian head was harder than glass—like stone or a diamond.

I can remember the car lights coming at us. I can remember the sense that we could not get out of the way. I can remember shouting to my friend, "watch out," and then the impact of the car. But strangely, when the car hit, I had the sense that it had not really hit me or the car I was in, that there had been a buffer that was made of time and space. Eternal. Would not break. A shield.

I was also sure that the driver of my car, my friend Sally Schreiber-Cohn, had reached out at the moment of impact and shielded me with her own body. I was absolutely sure this happened. When we got to the hospital, I asked her. She said, "Oh no, I kept both hands on the wheel, of course." If the other car had hit a few inches further back, I probably would have been decapitated. But it hit where it hit. Sally was bruised and badly shaken up. All the damage has been inside my brain.

One doctor described it as if someone were to have taken Jell-O, the consistency of the brain, and thrown it at a wall as hard as one could. That's how hard the brain hit one side of the skull and then ricocheted back and hit the other side of the skull, leaving me with right- and left-side brain injuries. Even though only one side of my head hit the window, both sides of my brain are damaged (see Figure 9.3, "Damaged Brain").

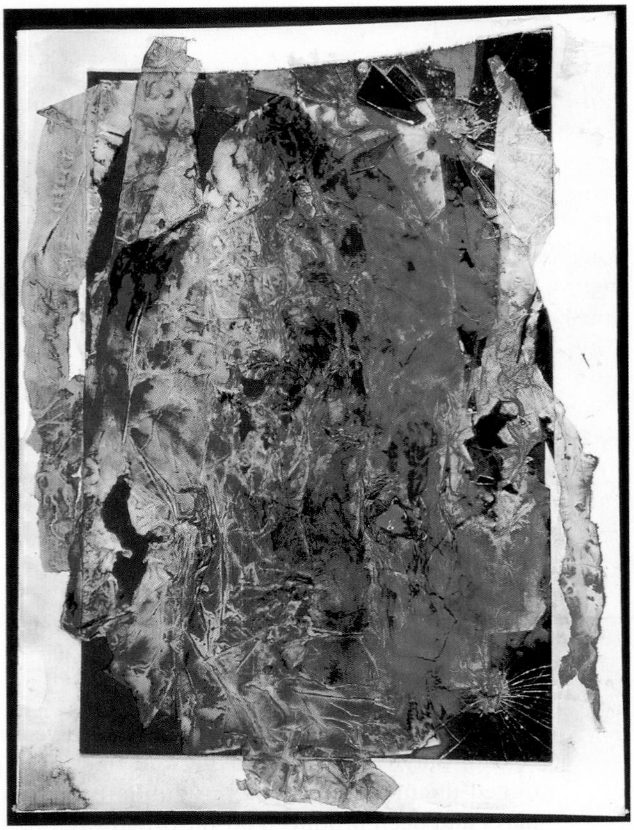

FIGURE 9.2 The Shattering: 11/20/83—I painted this on the fifth anniversary of the accident. I still felt like I was bleeding to death. (Courtesy of Mary Feldhaus-Weber.)

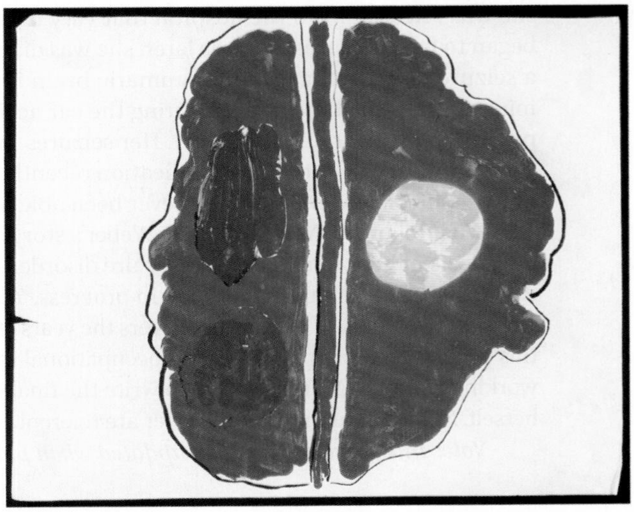

FIGURE 9.3 Damaged Brain: 1981—When I started painting, I painted what I thought my own brain must look like. In this painting I painted a brain that was terribly hurt on both sides—like mine, I thought. Much later, when the doctor ran my CAT scans, indeed my brain was damaged on both sides. (Courtesy of Mary Feldhaus-Weber.)

Six Months after the Accident

Six months after the accident, when I started to have more and more seizures, it became clear that I could no longer live alone, so I had to ask my mother to come from South Dakota to stay with me. I did this with great reluctance because she was 78 and my father wanted her there, taking care of him. When she got here, the thing I remember her saying was that she hadn't realized it had been so bad. Why hadn't I called her sooner? This was the time before the seizures were under any kind of control at all, which is to say, I was very sick.

I sat in the corner day after day, noticing that it was light or dark, noticing that my mother was busy, or sleeping, or crying, noticing that sometimes the phone rang or that it was the day to see the doctor, noticing that sometimes I had pain in my head. My mother said, "I wonder if a cold wet towel on your head would help?" I think we both remembered that if a horse sprains its leg, you wrap its leg in towels. And so Mother would get wet towels from the bathroom and wrap them around my head, my brain becoming like a sprained leg, a muscle that wasn't working. Cramped and tense. Convulsing. Filled with fear.

And then, because things change and time moves on, the pain would stop, and I would become briefly aware that the couch cover was blue, or that the dog had been rolling in the dust, or that Mother wanted to fix soup for lunch. And we discovered that after I had a seizure, or as one doctor called them "spells," I didn't have the coordination, or was too confused, to drink soup or hold a spoon. Because Mother liked soup so much, we seemed to try this many times, larger spoons, smaller spoons, bigger cups, smaller cups. It was decided that tomato soup was the easiest. Why, I'm not sure. Finally, I told Mother I did not like soup and had not for years. Therefore, could we try something else?

At this time, I was having constant seizures. There was no time that I was not either having one, getting ready to have one, feeling "spacey," with a strong metallic taste in my mouth, or feeling confused and disoriented after having had one. I felt like the seizures were a powerful force outside of me that suddenly grabbed my brain, me, the essence of me, and with the kind of fury of winds, blizzards, and driving rain, held me under ice (see Figure 9.4, "Blue Seizure"). While the *me* that was present could breathe the water under the ice, I knew I was caught, forced to be there. I knew if I struggled even slightly, the pain, the terror, became worse. And for the time the active seizure was roaring on inside me, I had to concentrate on total stillness until the fury dissipated and I was released.

All the drive and the tenacity, the ambition, the creativity, all of the things that had made me who I was did not help in this place. I was terrified, and I was alone. I no longer knew the words to ask or tell anyone what I was living through. I could just sense what hurt, and it hurt less to be absolutely still until the force chose to release me. I had no control of when it seized me or when it chose to release me.

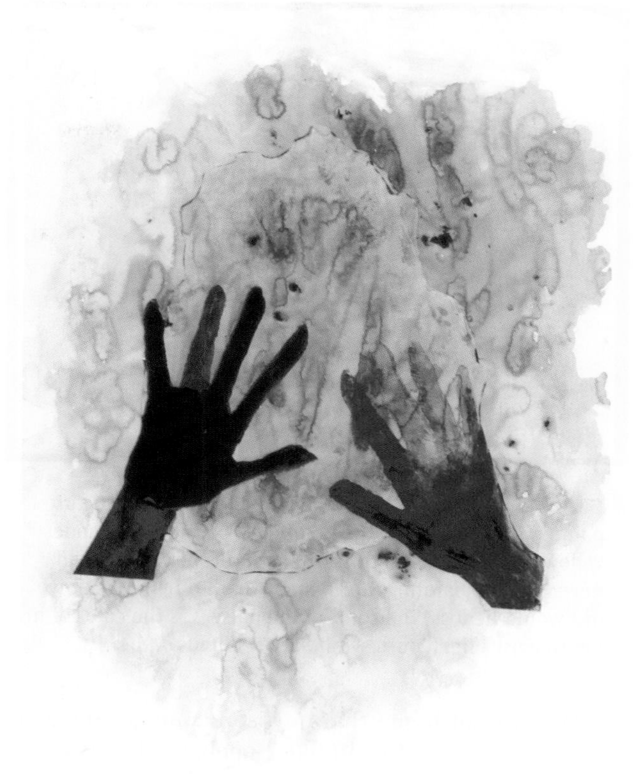

FIGURE 9.4 **Blue Seizure:** Before we discovered an epilepsy medication that worked, I was having constant seizures. This is a picture of what it felt like: a force outside myself (the hands) held my brain under ice. It held me there, terrified, desperate, helpless. Until it chose to release me. One of the fingers was red because I sometimes felt pain during the seizures. This picture broke through to a lot of people. My friend Sally said she had witnessed many of my seizures, but never understood how I felt. This painting, she said, was the only thing that helped her "get it." (Courtesy of Mary Feldhaus-Weber.)

My friend Sally tells me now that looking at me was like watching a candle about to go out. It seemed to her that only 3% of me was left.

I felt that I was being annihilated. The *me* that I had become, lived with, was ceasing to be, over and over and over again. It occurred to me that this was what it felt like to die and, for whatever reason, I was dying again and again.

One Year after the Accident

My mother had to return to South Dakota, so I was living alone. One day at the neurologist's office a year after the accident, still confused and in a deep fog, I noticed the doctor's tie. It was a bright, clear yellow Marimekko tie. I stared at the color yellow. It was the first thing to make sense to me since the accident. I understood what I was seeing. The color yellow. The fog lifted for a minute. I understood something, and I had not had to struggle to understand it. I can remember thinking: I am going to be all right.

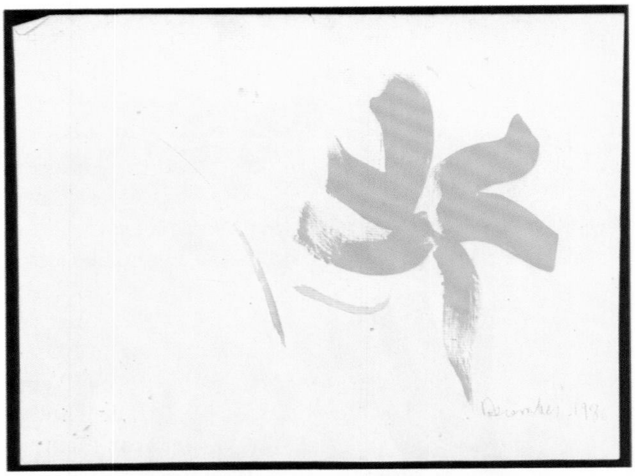

FIGURE 9.5 Daisy: December, 1980—The first picture I painted. One year after the accident, I painted this modest yellow daisy. I came to this with great desperation. I had never studied painting, but I knew I had to fight to survive or I would be lost. The color of the daisy was the color of my neurologist's tie. (Courtesy of Mary Feldhaus-Weber.)

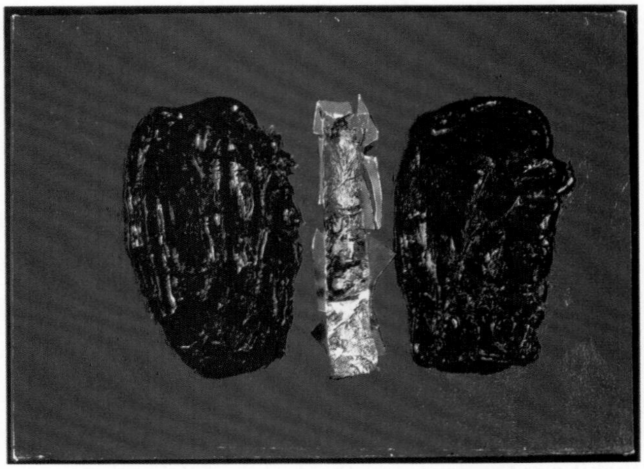

FIGURE 9.6 Hemisphere: Someone told me that for the brain to heal, the two hemispheres of the injured brain had to learn to communicate with each other again—find new pathways that worked. The right side had to take up what the left side used to do. In this picture, I put broken mirrors between the two hemispheres. The idea of my brain ever getting better seemed impossible, painful, exhausting. (Courtesy of Mary Feldhaus-Weber.)

When I got home that day, someone got me a set of poster paints, and I painted a small, bright, vivid, yellow daisy (see Figure 9.5, "Daisy"). And I started painting. When I began painting, I was surprised to find that it didn't turn out so badly, even though I had never painted before. Painting was one thing I could do all by myself, whether anyone was there or not. It didn't matter if I was spacey or sick. I could just lay down the piece of paper I was working on and continue again after the seizure had come and gone.

Some days, I did as many as 10 paintings. Looking back, I realize that I was desperate to understand my situation. I could hear people talk, but nothing made sense. I looked at their faces. I watched their mouths move, but I could not concentrate on what they were telling me. I can remember thinking: I have to try to explain all this to myself—what is happening to me—because I can't understand anyone else. So I painted. The only time I felt like the person I used to be was when I was painting.

I started finger painting with acrylic paint, wet tissue paper, and poster paints. I was drawn to the colors and shapes of things. I started to paint brains. I tried to paint the experience of seizures, which I did over and over again (see Figure 9.6, "Hemisphere"). In a strange kind of way, it was like having an artist's model for myself—not a model I could see, but a model which was myself, an internal experience that I then tried to translate into color. The painting gave me something to talk about other than myself. Something to talk about when people came to the house. It was a relief to have something to show someone, to have them look at pieces of paper, not to look at me. It also gave me a way to try to talk about what I was living through. Part of me hoped that the paintings weren't pitiful, because of all the things I did not want to be, to be pitied seemed the very worst.

I was also aware that I had to start from scratch with painting. I had been at the top of my career in film, and now I had to struggle to squeeze the paint tubes. I had to learn to be patient with myself. I was at the very beginning and grateful to be there.

Two Years after the Accident

I still had no real picture of what happened to my brain, so I spent a great deal of time thinking about it. Trying to think about it (see Figure 9.7, "Dendrites"). I had listened to explanations from doctors, nurses, and social

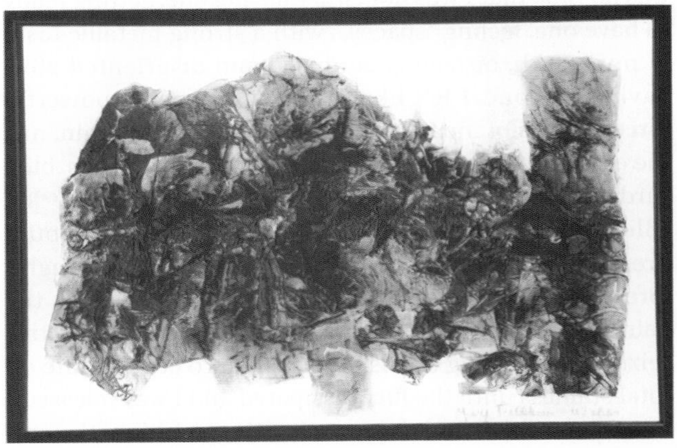

FIGURE 9.7 Dendrites: Painted when I was starting to get better. I began to pick up the jargon of the neurology team I was working with. They explained how parts of the brain communicate. I came home and painted what I thought dendrites might look like. Beautiful and strange. This is one of my favorite paintings. (Courtesy of Susan Mc Ginley.)

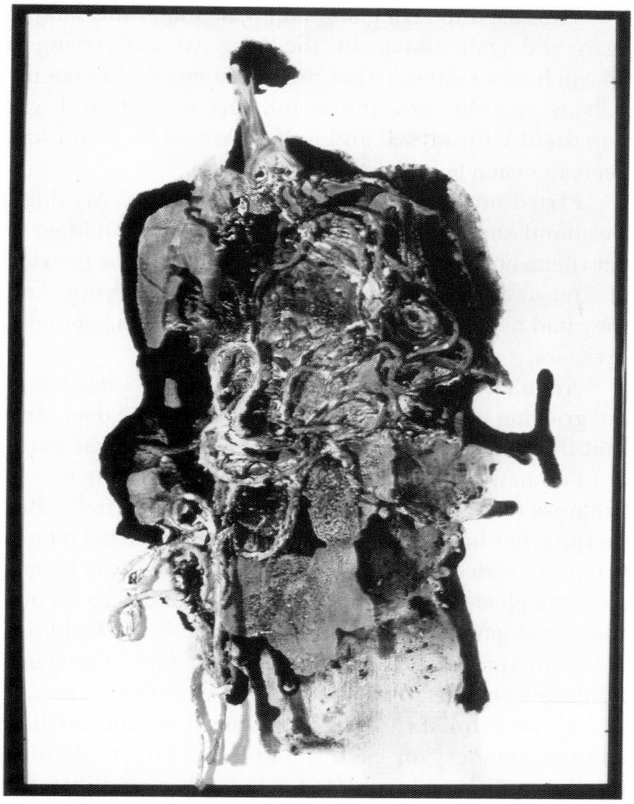

FIGURE 9.8 Self-Portrait: The tiny knob was my head. I felt I had ceased to have intelligence. I was just a confused, tattered body. No part of me worked. (Courtesy of Mary Feldhaus-Weber.)

workers, and none of them had made sense. All I knew was that I was unable to do the simplest thing—make a bed, tell time, count. Add or subtract. Recognize faces. Tell right from left. Read. Understand what people said to me. Remember things. And perhaps worst of all, I did not feel like myself, like *me*. I felt like someone, but not like any one I knew. I was a stranger to myself. I was lost (see Figure 9.8, "Self-Portrait").

On days that I had constant seizures, I had to ask my friend Sally to come and stay with me. It was at these times that we were aware that I was not getting better; in fact, I was barely hanging on.

The everyday litany was long and grim: I fell all the time; I was covered with black and blue marks everywhere. I would come to from a seizure to find that I had bitten the inside of my mouth and was bleeding and had a shard of my broken front tooth sticking out of my bottom lip. Sometimes, I would put my finger in my eyes during a seizure, and the eye would be red and swollen for days. I hit my head. I broke my elbow. It did not seem safe for me to live alone.

I had lost my income when my film company closed after the accident, and I had lost my health insurance with it. Because of these factors, my only option would have been to go on welfare and go into a nursing home. My neurologist felt that if I did that, I would likely never come out. I think he had seen too many people become institutionalized. In other words, they had become helpless and had given up. I still had some small fight left in me; I had been a functional, successful adult. The 3% of me that was left was 3% of a fighter. We were all counting on the fact that I would keep fighting and I would get better. That somehow I would manage. I also knew I desperately needed someone to help me help myself.

Finally, more than 2 years after the accident, we found someone to help me. Sally had called a therapist friend who said that she did know someone who was a gifted occupational therapist and liked dogs. And who was kind. When Sally called the occupational therapist—Anna Deane Scott—she said that she knew very little about head injury. She was a professor at Boston University and the coauthor of a famous occupational therapy textbook, and, yes, she did like dogs. She agreed to come to my house to meet me.

When she first met me, Anna Deane told me later, I was sitting in the dark on a couch, crying. We talked; she admired my dogs and told me about her own dog. After she left, I called her to ask what she thought of the meeting. I was afraid that she might have felt I was beyond help. I asked her how she felt about meeting me. Anna Deane said, "I felt sad." She told me the truth. I knew I could trust her.

Every time Anna Deane came over, we talked about things in the house that were a problem for me. I was afraid of falling in the shower when I was getting spacey from a seizure, so we got a shower chair and a metal bar on the wall and rubber rugs inside the tub and outside the tub. Each one of these areas we worked on took months to identify the problem and with trial and error find the solutions. But in the case of the shower, finally I was able to take a shower, and I was no longer afraid. I was also afraid of burning myself on the flames of my gas stove if I was feeling confused, so we got a large electric hot plate, and I could heat something up without being afraid of lighting myself or my clothes on fire.

I had lost the ability to do things; I knew there were steps to take to do any task, but I had no idea which step came first. I later learned that I had lost the ability to sequence, a loss that sometimes occurs when you have had an injury to the frontal lobe of the brain.

Anna Deane and I set out to discover how to teach me to do things again. She said that there was always another way to do something. First we had to find out how I was still able to learn. You will notice when I speak of Anna Deane and myself, I always say WE did this, WE decided that. Unlike many other health professionals, Anna Deane felt her role was not to tell me what to do, but to work with me, to empower me. She asked me constantly what was important to me. What did I think of something? What did I want to do? And she LISTENED to me. Extraordinary!

One problem in my life was how to unlock my front door. My house has two doors, an outside door and an inner door, and therefore, I have two different keys. If someone would bring me home from the doctor's office, one of the few places that I went, I would often try to get the key in the lock and not be able to. I would try to unlock the door for what felt like hours, over and over again, desperately trying to get into my own house. I asked whoever dropped me off to see that I got into the house before they drove off. Often they would have to open the door for me. I felt stupid, unable to do the simplest thing.

Anna Deane watched me try to get into the house and said she understood what the problem was. She said when I couldn't get in the outside door with one key, that I should try the other key. It had not occurred to me to try the other key. I would stand endlessly with the wrong key doing it over and over again, but when I had this new strategy, it freed me to get into my own house, and each time I opened the door myself, it was such a victory. And I began to feel hope for myself.

Anna Deane and I discovered that it was impossible for me to just follow or understand verbal directions, but if I could also watch someone do a task, listen to the directions, even place my hands on the things at the same time, I could, after a number of tries, do it again myself.

Anna Deane said that we could not be sure which parts of my brain were still working, but we had the best chance for success if we used as many senses as possible, hoping that we could tap into the areas in my brain that still functioned. When Anna Deane first said this, it sounded like the most primitive kind of investigation into unknown territories, all of which were inside me. We were searching for the *me* that was still there. But she was right. With Anna Deane's help, I have learned to do everything (day-to-day, self-maintenance activities) over again—absolutely everything. It is not too strong to say that she gave me my life back.

Another thing that Anna Deane and I worked on was a chart that monitored my daily activities. One of the problems was that I had lost any sense of time. With epilepsy, it is important that you take a certain amount of pills at a certain time every day. It's very simple—if you don't, the seizures come back. You also have to eat and rest regularly in relationship to taking the pills, and before I met Anna Deane, I could not remember whether I had taken a pill, had lunch, let the dogs out; I couldn't tell if it was afternoon or morning or what day it was.

Gradually, over a period of months and many failures, we worked out a chart on a magnetic blackboard that we divided into morning, afternoon, and evening. We used different colored magnets for different parts of the day, as we discovered that I could understand colors better than words. For every victory, such as the discovery that I still remembered colors, there were dozens of defeats. Anna Deane said over and over that there was always another way to do something. We just had to find the other way. And every time we failed, she learned that much more about my brain, what still worked and how it was working. She said there was no such thing as a "failure." She learned something each time we tried something new.

I, on the other hand, felt the failures very keenly. Because I had been quick and life had come easily to me, I was not used to trying and failing at something simple again and again and again. The things we were trying to do, such as a system to get me to remember to take my pills, were both very simple and very important. I was impatient with myself and judged myself by who I had been. For each failure, I shed many tears.

I tried not to cry in front of Anna Deane. My dogs, Desmond and Todd, listened to my crying. I would go to pet them, and their fur would be wet. I would be puzzled at first and then remembered I had been crying. And they had been sitting beside me on the couch, wet with my tears.

Anna Deane said that I was doing what I needed to do, grieving over my losses. I had lost a great deal. And that if one didn't grieve and let the past go, it was harder to do new things. That grief could stand in the way of progress (see Figure 9.9, "The Color of My Grief"). But on the other hand, I also needed to look at the balance of things. I needed to find things that still made me happy, gave me pleasure. It became my job each day to do one thing that gave me pleasure (see Figure 9.10, "Goblin"). This sometimes was as hard to do as the task of grieving. It became obvious to me that the two were connected.

So we refined the magnetic board system further: colored magnets for each time of day, further divided into take pill, have lunch, feed dogs, and so on. When the activity had been completed, I moved the magnet from the not-done category to the done category. The chart is large and colorful, and I can look at it from across the room and tell what I have done and what I haven't done yet and how I'm doing. And so, eventually, time and

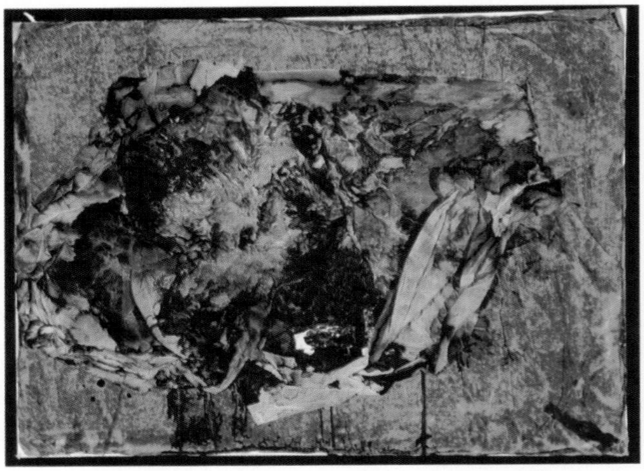

FIGURE 9.9 The Color of My Grief: I connected with a woman in the field of education rehabilitation. With her help I was able to understand the concept of counting again. After several months I was able to count to four. I was thrilled. For some reason I never understood, the agency she was with fired her out of the blue. It was a huge loss to me. Grief upon grief. When you find someone who can help you, they are like gold. I was furious at the people who fired her, and sad beyond words. (Courtesy of Mary Feldhaus-Weber.)

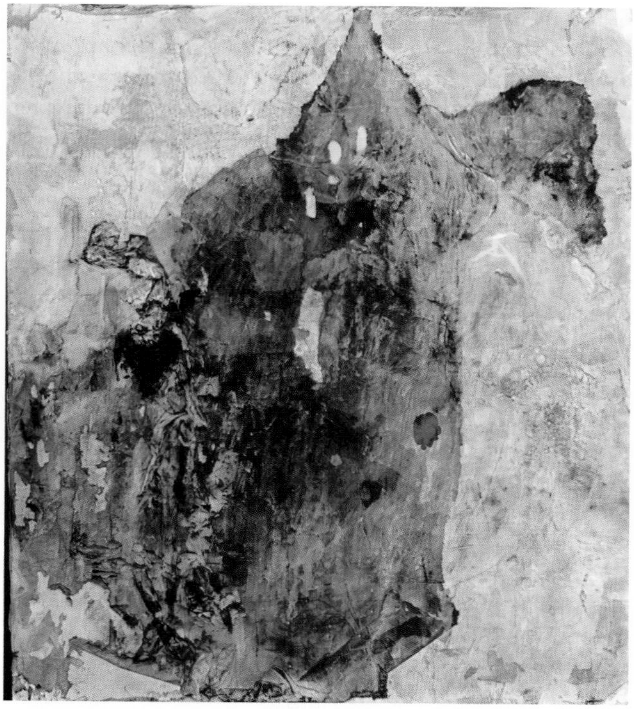

FIGURE 9.10 Goblin: Done for fun. (Courtesy of Mary Feldhaus-Weber.)

memory seemed somewhat under my control again (see Figure 9.11, "Healing Brain").

Anna Deane came to my house every week for an hour, and we talked on the phone a number of times between the visits. In the year that I worked with her, I could see small changes in my life; and as I got greater control over the details of my life again, the person who I had been started to reemerge. I wasn't making films, but I could change the sheets on my bed. I wasn't writing poetry, but I could dress myself. These may seem like small things, but with each skill I regained, I could feel life flowing back into me again.

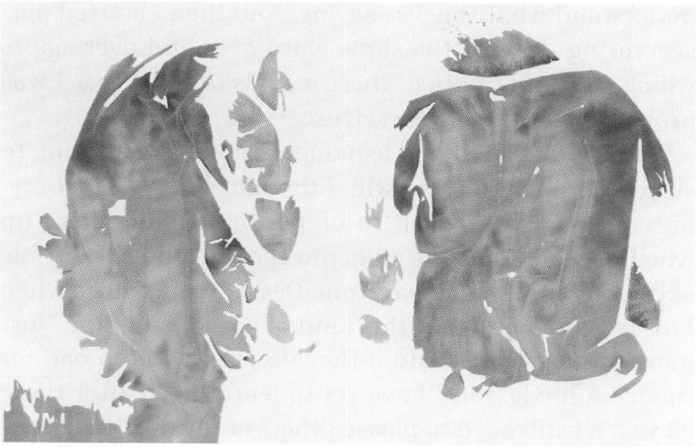

FIGURE 9.11 Healing Brain: Early 1983—This picture shows what I imagined the damaged brain and the healed brain would look like, side by side. (Courtesy of Mary Feldhaus-Weber.)

Another triumph that stands out was the ability to get into and out of buildings. There are many buildings in Boston where you have to buzz the company or office that you are going to, and then they buzz you back and the door opens. I was no more able to decipher this than the Rosetta Stone. It was impossibly complex for me and therefore, overwhelming, and therefore, tear-producing, and therefore, one more thing that I couldn't do.

Anna Deane and I talked about every possible kind of solution and came up with one that worked. The solution was to stand and watch until someone else came along and pushed a button and got in the door, watch how they did it, and either go in with them or do the same thing they did. And it worked.

In large buildings, it's still a problem finding the correct office if I haven't been there before, because in the elevator, I am not able to understand whether 5 is the same as 7 is the same as 9 when the elevator opens. So I have been lost in the best hospitals in Boston. The people who had taken me went to park their car and against their better judgment let me out, me telling them not to worry about it, that I would meet them at the office. And then, 45 minutes later when I did not show up at the office, and it became clear that there was a problem, various people would be sent to find me. For my part, I would be asking people if this was the fourth floor, etc., etc.

Among the least helpful people to give this kind of simple direction are doctors, nurses, or anyone else from "the allied health professions." Among the most helpful, of course, are the other patients and all the cleaning and maintenance people. However, Anna Deane and I have not figured a way around this problem, a way to make me independent, to do it all on my own. It is still, sadly, something that makes me cry.

With Anna Deane's help, I listened to talking books for reading and used a calculator to add and subtract, told time with a digital clock, asked people to take me places and not just give me directions, and used the brightly colored arrows that told me which way to turn the thermostat to heat my house and to turn on the water faucets in the shower. In other words, many victories. And more to come.

Sometimes people ask me what kind of fee Anna Deane charged me for this amount of work and of devotion. The answer is—not one cent. She told me that she did not know enough about brain injury to charge for her services; it was a learning experience for her too. And she did not say it, but I knew she knew that I did not have a cent to my name.

May 1996: Seventeen Years after the Accident

How am I now? I was told that if a function did not come back after a year, it would not come back. They were wrong about this in some cases. I have continued to regain things over a period of 16 years. I can discriminate between right and left again, I am much better at recognizing faces—not perfect, but better. I can understand poetry and most abstractions again. I regained my sense of smell. I can read a bit if the print is big. I can write again.

I still can't count. I still can't do multiplication tables or months of the year. I still see double out of one eye. I still have to sit and think a long time about what steps go into a task such as putting the laundry in the washing machine and what order those steps should take. I still have balance problems. I still have a lot of seizures—several a day most of the time. I have learned to live with these things—the things that are lost to me and the things that have come back but are different.

I had a battery of neuropsychological tests done on me recently, and I still do badly on a number of them. You are reading the writing of someone who now has an IQ still considerably under 100.

I was surprised how many strong feelings I had when I started to answer the simple sounding question—"How are you?" First of all, it is not until I started to get better that I realized how much I had lost. Before that, I was too sick or too overwhelmed to notice, to understand the breadth of the loss. In broad strokes, I lost 10 years of my life where I almost ceased to exist. And I still grieve over that loss; some days it feels like a very big loss, other days it doesn't (see Figure 9.12, "Broken Dreams").

So how am I now? I am doing better without having gotten better. In other words, I learned to do a lot of things in new ways just as Anna Deane Scott, the occupational therapist who worked with me, said I would—tell time with a digital clock, read with talking books, write with a large-screen, large-print computer. I feel like myself again. I am happy most of the time—in fact I seem to be one of the more happy and contented people I know. I have become grateful for things large and small. I am more appreciative of other people. In fact, I think we should all get stars and bluebirds for getting up in the morning. The head injury has forced me to look at myself. Look at all the sad, angry parts of me that I did not consider when I was a hotshot television producer. I was too busy working 18-hour days. Being very busy in a high-visibility job can be seductive. What you are doing seems so important that you can easily push everything else into a corner. But when you are sitting home, day after day, when the phone isn't ringing off the hook, it is less possible to ignore things.

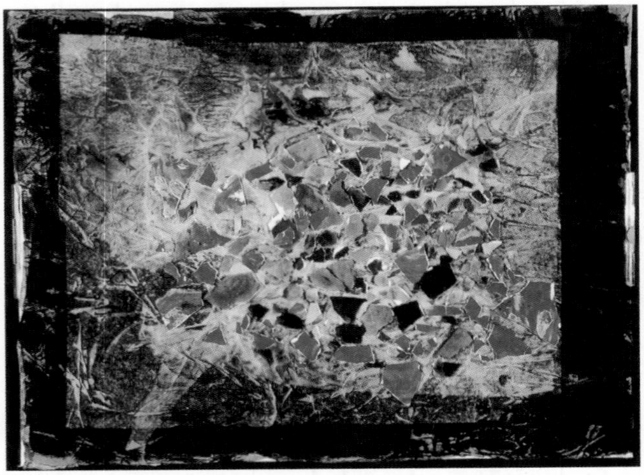

FIGURE 9.12 **Broken Dreams:** I painted this when I saw a friend's film on TV and I realized that the people I worked with in TV production were moving ahead. I, on the other hand, was sitting at home, having seizures and only able to dial the telephone after many tries. (Courtesy of Mary Feldhaus-Weber.)

Being brain injured has given me time to look at who I was, how I got there, and to ask myself what I want to do about my life. Counseling also helped me to survive many assaults on the spirit that can occur when you are forced to endlessly deal with health care providers. Being a patient can be a grueling life. I know that this will seem strange; it seems strange to me even as I write it down. There is a belief that if you have one sense such as sight taken away, your hearing becomes more acute to compensate. To understand my own suffering, I have come to better understand the suffering of others.

I also laugh more, am made happy more easily. I am much more at ease with myself. I feel quite literally that I walked and walked and walked through the valley of the shadow of death, stumbling, crying, falling, breaking bones, and finally came out on the other side. When asked about the brain injury, I tell people I would not wish it on my worst enemy. Yet strangely, I am also grateful for the journey.

July 2001: Twenty-Two Years after the Accident

I continue to live with the physical problems that came from the original injury. And there are still the problems I have because I am who I am. I was on the phone recently with a spit-and-polish person that I don't particularly like. At a point in the conversation, I was not able to understand what she was saying. And then I started perseverating—saying the same word over and over again, which she didn't notice. These signals told me that I was probably about to have a seizure.

I felt frustrated and ashamed. I could do nothing to stop the seizure. Worse still, I thought I might start crying, but I forced myself to be polite. I finally hung up when I began losing the ability to speak. And I felt terrible about myself. I could hear Anne Deane Scott's voice when I used to tell her about this kind of social situation: "Just hang up the phone. And if they don't like it, too bad for them!" A life lesson I have yet to learn. Even after these 22 years, I still need to please others at my own expense.

I have had the best help in the world, so why don't I learn these lessons? I suppose that is because I am a human being and I still carry the same baggage I had before the accident.

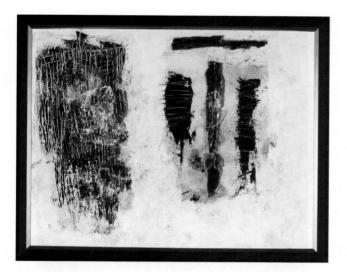

FIGURE 9.13 I Stand By While Good Dogs Die: June, 2001—I have always liked dogs more than anything. I now work as a volunteer with an animal rescue group. I work from home on the telephone when I am able to. Many of the dogs we try to rescue cannot be saved, in spite of our best efforts. There are simply not enough homes to go around. In this picture, I am the figure on the left covered with mica (shiny sheets of mineral), which represents my good intentions. The dogs on the right represent the dogs we cannot save. Their spirits are moving upward toward the shining mica, which represents life beyond life. This is my most recent painting. (Courtesy of Mary Feldhaus-Weber.)

And now I think it is time to tell you about good things.

About 5 years ago, a new antiseizure medicine came on the market that has made a large, positive difference in the quality of my life. At long last, I have fewer seizures and am more clear-headed. I am *me* more of the time. It's wonderful. I have a computer and like it for all the same reasons that everyone else does. Even though I am mostly house-bound, I have the world in front of me.

I have always loved animals, and now I am active with animal rescue and finding homes for abused, homeless animals (see Figure 9.13, "I Stand By While Good Dogs Die"). Because a large part of this can be done on the phone or the Internet, I can do this when I am feeling okay. I have become part of a network of people who care about animals as much as I do. They have no idea that I used to be a filmmaker or even that I was in a terrible accident, although I do tell them about the brain injury if there is a reason to. I never have to fear that anyone will feel sorry for me. I am just one more person who is dedicated to helping animals.

I love this part of my life.

In the 22 years since the accident, I have gone from not being able to read and write at all or to even turn the pages in a book to be able to write what you are reading right now. I write easily now.

Finally, there is something unexpected that I seldom hear discussed by brain-injured survivors or the people who work with them.

The car accident was a crushing, wrenching assault on me. For the first few years after the accident, the question that I asked over and over was this: How could God do this to me?

Before the accident, I had been a spiritual person. I believed in a compassionate, wise God who cared about each sparrow that fell and each lily of the field.

After, it seemed like God cared about everything but me. I was shocked and heartbroken that God let this happen. I thought about it constantly and talked to anyone who would listen. I felt twisted and damaged inside and out (see Figure 9.14, "When I Think of Dying")—and angry. Angry. Angry. You can see this in my paintings (see Figure 9.15, "Pain #2").

The years went by, and I never came to any understanding. After a time, my sorrow blew away like smoke (see Figure 9.16, "White Brain").

I understand now that the greatest damage I experienced was the damage no one can see. It left me feeling afraid of things, not trusting in life, not being able to believe in a kind, loving God. I felt alone.

I have had the best occupational therapy and counseling and profited from them. I have learned to do many of the skills of daily living again. I have changed and grown.

And there is more.

My spirit has been the last to heal.

I am still healing.

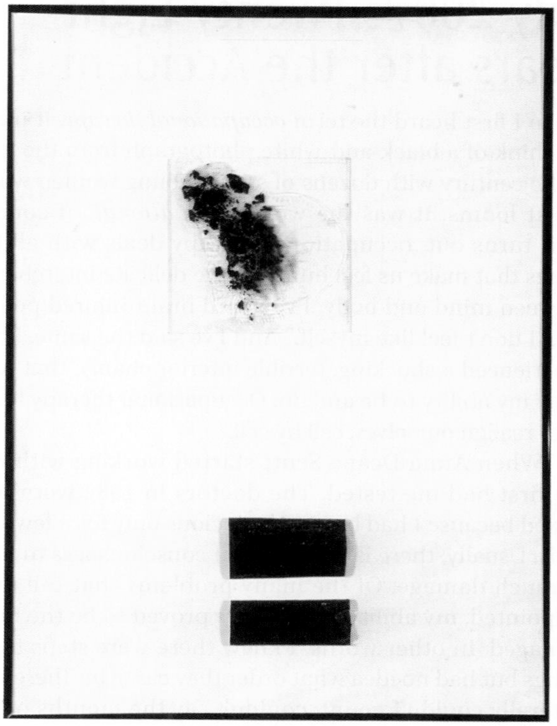

FIGURE 9.14 When I Think of Dying: 10/15/83—As I started to get better, I realized how much I had lost. It was at this time that I thought about suicide. This picture was what I imagined the soul might look like upon leaving the dying body. (Courtesy of Mary Feldhaus-Weber.)

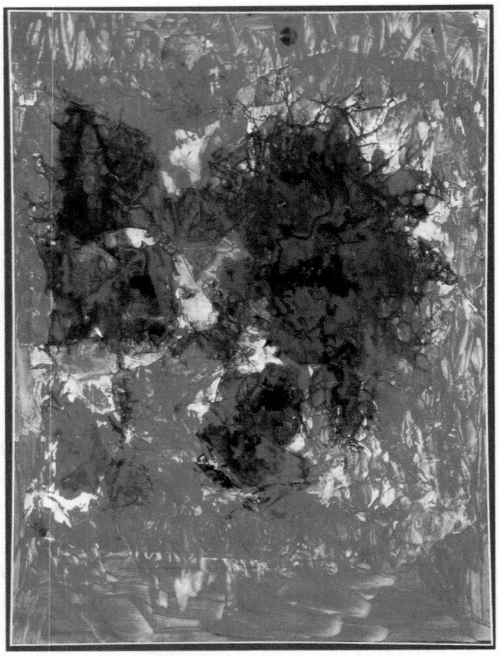

FIGURE 9.15 Pain #2: 1987—More pain, more feeling trapped and desperate. I felt this way a long, long time. My painting was often the only way I had to express it. (Courtesy of Mary Feldhaus-Weber.)

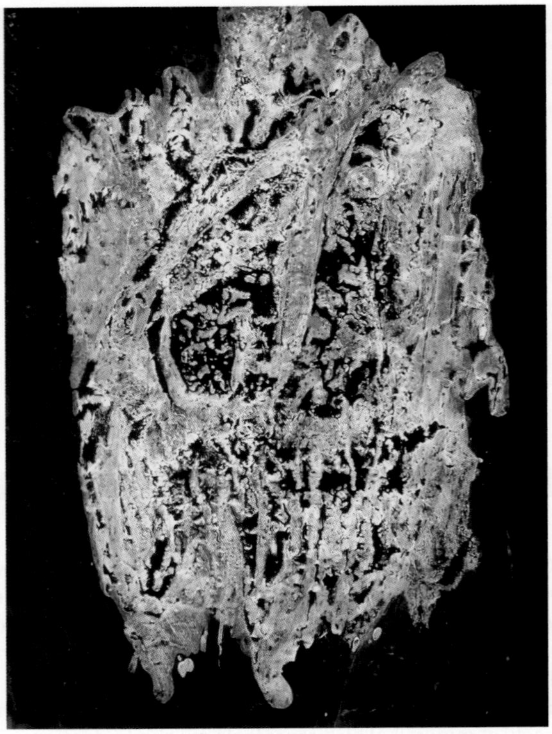

FIGURE 9.16 White Brain: At a certain point, I began to make my brain pictures more "decorative," artistic. I was no longer so obsessed with understanding the damage. I was beginning to integrate my feelings about the head injury. (Courtesy of Mary Feldhaus-Weber.)

July 2007: Twenty-Eight Years after the Accident

When I first heard the term *occupational therapy*, it made me think of a black-and-white photograph from the turn of the century with dozens of sturdy young women working at looms. It was the word *occupational*, of course. As it turns out, occupational therapy deals with all the things that make us feel human—the delicate interchange between mind and body. I've heard brain-injured people say, "I don't feel like myself." And I've said the same. I had experienced a shocking, terrible interior change that took away my ability to be and do. Occupational therapy helps us to realign ourselves, cell by cell.

When Anna Deane Scott started working with me, she first had me tested. The doctors in 1982 were perplexed because I had been unconscious only for a few seconds. Usually, there is more lack of consciousness to have so much damage. Of the many problems that the tests pinpointed, my ability to *sequence* proved to be the most damaged. In other words, I knew there were steps to do things but had no idea what order they came in. Therefore, I literally couldn't count, couldn't say the months of the year, the days of the week. I couldn't tell time. I couldn't read. Unfortunately, the world is made of sequences.

Another problem was an inability at times to find a name for an object or even recognize it. To work with this, Anna Deane said that we should try all of my senses—touch, sound, and so on. One time she put a number of things—lipstick, comb, pencil, spoon—into a sack. I was not able to recognize them with my eyes. When I used my sense of touch, I was able to recognize them, to understand them, and to give them their names with my fingers. I told Anna Dean I felt like Helen Keller when she signed the word WATER for the first time. It was victory for me. It was hope. It was making the undamaged cells take up another function. And they did, even though it has taken years.

Experts in the field of brain injury in 1982 told me that young adult males were most likely to have head injury. And being young, they were quicker to heal. Women my age, on the other hand, statistically did not often suffer brain injury and, being older, did not heal as quickly. These young people hadn't lived very long and therefore, did not have life experience and, because of this, did not have as many life skills as an adult does. I, on the other hand, an older woman—me—had developed a set of work skills. I knew how to do a lot of things. I had been a television producer and filmmaker. To be a successful television producer and filmmaker, you have to have tremendous drive, know how to make things happen, and be a hard worker. The accident had not crushed those parts of me. That and the creative part of me were still there, although at the time, I didn't know this. I was just trying to fill my days, which were also filled with seizures and confusion.

If you look at my paintings, you can see how simply they started. I used finger paint, water, and torn tissue paper. I painted at least 10 paintings a day. Make a painting, lie down, and rest. Make a painting, pet the dogs. Make a painting, cry. Make a painting, stare at the ceiling. And gradually, and with the grace of God, I began healing. There was another plus to my painting. When an artist friend and other friends came over, we often talked about paintings. I had something other than pain and suffering to talk about. Above all, I didn't want people to feel sorry for me.

I have thought so many times that I was lucky to have been born at this time and this place. I was lucky to have lived at a time when people were starting to understand head injury. Head injury—people call it brain injury now. One hundred years ago, if I had this kind of brain injury, I might not have lived through it. Or if I had lived, I would have been tied to a chair in some dreary institution.

On the other side, there were many dark times when I often thought it would have been easier to die. Because life had become an unendurable burden. I didn't feel like myself. I had lost myself. I felt that I would always be caught in this terrible web. It seemed that there was no way out of it. And how could God have done this to me? What did I do to deserve this? I thought of suicide constantly. I didn't talk about this. Not to my parents. Not to Sally. Early on, a man who was educated and sophisticated about the ins and outs of the head injury world visited me. He was kind and reassuring. He also had a brain injury and epilepsy. He told me not to tell anyone you feel suicidal—you would be pink-slipped "for your own good." Meaning you would be put in the insane asylum. Particularly do not tell any of the doctors, he said; and I believed him. You can bet I believed him. That was all I needed, to be in an asylum.

For a time, I was in a discussion group of people with seizures and brain injury. I listened to far too much horrifying "for your own good" that had been done to people. But that is another book.

I am speaking in my own voice right now—not the voice of the overwhelmed, defeated person. In fact, at the time, I was still unable to do the simplest things. And Anna Deane Scott, bless her heart, sent out some of her occupational therapy students to my house to work with me for academic credit. They were wonderful. We all gained. They learned firsthand about brain injury and I learned to do things that I was not able to do on my own. I wanted to write a story about my Jack Russell terrier, Todd. The students wrote down the Todd stories that I was not able to read or write myself. I said the words one by one, and the students wrote them down one by one. The story was named "Todd and the Stars." I was painting and the students went to the store to get yellow paint for me. And they helped me. They were like sunshine coming into a dark room. Anna Deane was so smart. I kept painting. I could see that my pictures were getting better. And though I didn't know it at the time, I was getting better.

I was healing. I lived and went on to tell this story. And I am glad to be alive.

It has been 28 years since the car accident. I had learned to live with my brain injury. For the most part I'm fine at home, with my friends, in familiar places. But I forget that I am not okay in the eyes of the world. I do not do well with new situations. Several years ago, I needed a knee replacement and went to a highly thought-of hospital and rehabilitation facility. After the surgery, I was brought back to my room, groggy, crying, confused, and in pain. The nurse on duty told me that there was a way of controlling my pain—I only had to push a button by my hand and I would receive the right amount of pain meds. She demonstrated it and left. The pain went on and on. My friend Sally could see that I did not understand the sequential steps to make the pain machine work. She called the nurse and told her that I couldn't understand how to use the pain button because I had a brain injury. Sally asked—could she push the pain button for me? The nurse said Sally most certainly could NOT touch the machine and that I had to do it for myself.

A frustrated Sally repeated about my inability to deal with sequences and because of that, I wasn't able to use the pain machine. The nurse told us that everyone is capable of using the pain device—even people 80 years old can do this and "so can you." The nurse left. The pain continued. Sally called for the nurse and again explained about my brain injury. This sequence went on a number of times. I am not sure how it resolved itself, but finally another nurse came in and started to give me shots for the pain. This was the first of many other such episodes. The staff seemed to think that if I was able to talk, I should be able to understand what they wanted me to do.

Next was getting out of bed. There are steps to learn to get out of a bed after knee replacement surgery. A nurse and a nurse's aide told me what to do over and over. I asked over and over and tried to understand what they were telling me. And, worse still, when I struggled to explain something, my speech became garbled and confused. The nurse's aide turned to the nurse and asked what was wrong with me. The nurse looked right at me, put her finger making a circle around her ear—the sign that children use to mean "crazy."

This, even though Sally had told all the nursing staff about my brain injury, had put a sign over the bed to that effect, and had made sure the information was added to my medical file along with my own doctor's evaluation of my situation. Most of the nursing and medical staff were not interested in anything we had to say about my brain injury. They completely dismissed what Sally and I said. Further, alas, they were quick to criticize and say that I wasn't trying hard enough. They talked about me in front of me and others. They talked to me like I was a badly behaved child.

Some of the more frightening situations came up when the rehabilitation people were trying to teach me to do things on my own: go up stairs, get in and out of the bathtub, or walk with the walker. I was frightened because they didn't listen to a word I said. I know how dangerous this situation can be for me. At home, I have fallen and broken bones, broken teeth, bitten the inside of my mouth, and put my fingers in my eyes. These people didn't listen to me about my brain injury. I asked to speak to the supervisor and described the situation I was in. I talked to her about the rehabilitation staff not listening to me. The supervisor said that they must have been tired that day. I talked to my doctor about the same thing. He said to write to the president of the hospital and that no one listened to him either.

Finally, thank God, I got out of that place. It had been a nightmare. All too often this must be how some people—the old, the retarded, the insane, the poor, people who don't speak English—are treated. What they have to endure. And so did I.

Time passed, and I needed to go to a hospital for pneumonia. This new hospital was a far different experience. It is known for its innovative work with brain trauma. The staff took detailed information about my brain injury. They were as interested in it as the other place was not. I sighed with relief. I didn't have to struggle to communicate. When I said I had temporal lobe brain damage, they understood. It was like coming to a different country. And I no longer had to be in a defensive posture. Better than that—they believed me when I described the characteristics, albeit very strange even to me, of my brain injury.

And now on television, I see our men and woman soldiers, damaged, crushed, brought back to many armed services hospitals and rehabilitation facilities where there might be very little or no concept of brain injury or how to deal with it. I would guess that these people coming back from the war and their families are going to run into problems similar to the ones I had and that my friend Sally encountered on my behalf. A recent article in *DISCOVER* Magazine entitled "Dead Men Walking: What Sort of Future Do Brain-Injured Iraq Veterans Face?" by Michael Mason (2007) describes the situation faced by these veterans. When I read this article, it broke my heart because I know brain injury can be a lifelong tragedy.

> In a flash, the blast incinerates air, sprays metal, burns flesh. Milliseconds after an improvised explosive device (IED) detonates, a blink after a mortar shell blows, an overpressurization wave engulfs the human body, and just as quickly, an underpressure wave follows and vanishes. Eardrums burst, bubbles appear in the bloodstream, the heart slows. A soldier or a civilian can survive the blast without a single penetrating wound and still receive the worst diagnosis: traumatic brain injury, or TBI, the signature injury of the Iraq War.
>
> But in the same instant that the blast unleashes chaos, it also activates the most organized and sophisticated trauma care in history. Within a matter of hours, a soldier can be medevaced to a state-of-the-art field hospital, placed on a flying intensive care unit, and receive continuous critical care a sea away. (During Vietnam, it took an average of 15 days to receive that level of treatment. Today the military can deliver it in 13 hours.) Heroic measures may be yielding unprecedented survival rates, but they also carry a grim consequence: No other war has created so many seriously disabled veterans. Soldiers are surviving some brain injuries with only their brain stems unimpaired. (Mason, 2007, para. 1–2)

Later in the article, Mason goes on to write about the rehabilitation possibilities for brain-injured soldiers. When I read this part, I thought about all the things occupational therapists could bring to their suffering. In an interview, Marilyn Price Spivack asserted that

> Men and women in the military will receive excellent care for a time, but eventually, they are going back to their communities. "The military is doing an extraordinary job in saving young soldiers and treating them through the acute rehabilitation phase," says Spivack, who works with the brain-injured population at Spaulding Rehabilitation Hospital in Boston. In the early 1980s she founded the Brain Injury Association, today the foremost advocacy organization for TBI survivors. "Now the government must make a commitment to help them in their recovery, but where are the resources going to come from? As brain-injury professionals, we know that TBI services aren't available in many places across the country, and we are aware of huge holes in the system," she says. "Frankly, I'm frustrated and angry about the government's refusal to give the TBI population the support it desperately needs."
>
> Spivack is not being glib; the giant holes are glaringly apparent. Many states do not have a single brain-injury rehabilitation center, and of the states that do offer some level of TBI treatment, few actually provide enough assistance to acquire even the most basic level of specialized care. At rates that can exceed a thousand dollars a day for postacute TBI rehabilitation, there aren't many American families that can afford a month's worth of treatment, much less the recommended minimum of 90 days.
>
> As recently as mid-July 2006, the VA Office of the Inspector General admitted that patients and families were dealing with major inadequacies. The reality is that a fundamental level of care is simply absent in most states. (Mason, 2007, para. 29–31)

I encourage you to read Mason's powerful article (Mason, 2007). I fear that these veterans will come up against the worst kind of ignorance—people who don't know that they don't know. This is an enormous situation that has no easy answers.

How Am I Now?

I often wonder how things would have been if there hadn't been a car accident. As it is, I have lost many years of my life. Some of those years were complete dropouts, because there are not words for what I went through. I felt that I had fallen into a deep, deep pit. I was alive but not alive. Gradually I have gotten better in many ways.

I have 4 or 5 hours in a day—good hours when I can do things. If I go past that, my speech becomes garbled, my coordination is bad, and I have to worry if I will fall. I have to be SO careful about hanging onto things so I won't fall. I have handles and grab bars all over the house that help me walk. But if I am too exhausted, I have to stay in bed. If I do a small thing that's just too much, my brain becomes frozen, rigid, or like an old car, or a cranky baby. I never know when it will choose to give out. When this happens, I have to be quiet and let it rest.

There are things I wish I could do. I would like to go horseback riding. I'd love to go to movies. I'd like to go to Sweden and see the midnight sun again. I'd like to go to a symphony orchestra again. I'd like to see the cherry blossoms in Washington. And the redwood trees. And animals in Africa. And sit through 5 days of a film festival. And go dancing with a good-looking man—a rascal.

The one movie that I tried to go to, I had to leave and sit in the accessible ladies room because of overload from the pictures and sound. I had to say to the people I was with that I had to go home. It was the *Pirates of the Caribbean*, and I enjoyed the 30 minutes tremendously.

But all that said, I can watch television at home because I can put the sound down if necessary.

And if this fails, I listen to my talking books, which have all kinds of subjects. I can listen to poetry or essays or history with the lights off with my four dogs on the bed, and I am very, very happy.

I'm going to a meeting tomorrow in my wheelchair, and if I have to go to the bathroom, I have to have help, because most restrooms are not accessible for people who have disabilities. I don't talk about the ins and outs of this, but trust me, it's true. People want to think that all of this has changed and the bathrooms are accessible and all of the sidewalks have curb cuts so you don't have to deal with a curb. NOT.

And I don't do as many things as I am able to do because of the complexity of managing the comings and goings.

I live alone and have people who help me. I have my groceries delivered. I have people help me with the housework. I have people who take me to the doctor, if I can make this happen—both coordinating and paying people to take me to the doctor. Many times I can't get someone to take me to the doctor for love or money.

So getting back to more interesting things. Many of my friends and I rescue animals, and we find good homes for them. When we see a dog that has been starved and beaten become a healthy, happy dog, it is a great experience. And I do gardening on my front porch. And like everyone else, I have a computer, and like everyone else, it is my link to the world.

I have most recently started working with people in the inner city. They have been giving Christmas parties for children for years. Last Christmas we got toys, books, and tasty things to eat for 800 children. I was told that these presents might be the only ones the children would receive. This event was wonderful. I sat at a special Christmas gift table with books about animals and toys for the children's pets. I felt I was just exactly where I should be—with children who liked animals as much as I do. One little boy asked if I had any books about snakes, and luckily I did. He was delighted when he opened the present and said, "**SNAKES!!!**" There we were. The child. The snake book. And me. This was one of the happiest moments of my life.

I started to paint again, I laugh with my friends, I am lucky to have come this far.

I had the luck to meet Anna Deane Scott, who had the belief that there was always another way to do something. And indeed that was the case.

I met Maureen Neistadt, who asked me to speak to her OT students and show them my paintings.

I had my beloved trained seizure dog Timmy, who helped me to walk, stopped me from falling, made me feel safe. He was an incredible gift for me when I was frightened and lonely.

In the early years right after the accident, Dr. Thomas Glick, a neurologist, was important to me. He encouraged me, was kind to me, was generous with his time, and listened to my many, many tears. Dr. Glick was a remarkable man.

My mother and father in South Dakota kept me afloat financially and emotionally. They called me day after day. I can't imagine what would have happened to me without their help, when I had next to nothing. They had been so proud of me—of my plays, my films—that had drawn honor and acclaim and added meaning to their lives. I knew what had happened to me had broken their hearts. I could hear it in their voices when they talked to me on the phone.

If I had lived 100 years ago or had been born in the third world, I would never have survived.

Instead, here I am, having the honor of talking to you.

And who am I now? I'm a human being. Just like everyone else.

Postscript: Thoughts for Occupational Therapy Practitioners

I have one final thought that I want to share with you. I have spent a lot of time thinking about what "helps" in the kind of situation I have been in with my brain injury. Why could some people get through to me and not others? Why did some people comfort and heal me and other seemingly well-meaning people shame or humiliate me? In other words: What works? What heals? What helps?

I discovered that power is at the heart of living with an injury, and power is at the heart of getting better. Many of us, particularly women, don't think of ourselves as having power. It is just a word, not something we own or think much about. Yet power is the ability to make things happen.

When I was at my most diminished, it felt as though everyone was more powerful than I was—from the secretary in the doctor's office who had to take the time to push the right elevator button for me to the cab driver I had to trust to give back the correct change because I could not count. The people who had to show me to the restroom when I was not capable of finding it. The doctors who filled out the insurance forms so that I would get disability payments to buy food and pay the rent. It was a very long list, and I was at the bottom. I had to depend on everyone.

Because of the power issues (who has it, who wants it, who needs it, who can share it), I think it is important to check why you are going into the healing professions. Ask yourself tough questions and keep asking them. Questions like "What do I get out of this work?" "How does this situation make me feel about myself?" "Do I need to have things in black and white or can I bear the uncertainty of all the shades of gray that illness and sorrow present us with?" "Can I trust people, however damaged, to know what is best for them?"

So the question I am asking you is this: Can you give over power to another person? Can you honor their own wishes, dreams, abilities? Can you be as interested in their abilities as you are in their disabilities? Can you give them the tools to get their own lives back on track?

And do you listen to people? Do you *hear* what they are telling you? I believe that we are far wiser than we give ourselves or each other credit for. So I am telling you that the two most important things you can do as occupational therapy practitioners are to listen and to empower. The people who helped me the most did both of those things. I continue to bless them and to use what they have taught me every day.

Since I first started occupational therapy with Anna Deane in 1982, books have been written about brain injury, and classes have been given. There are whole hospitals for people with brain injury. Because of the war in Iraq, this is a new time for brain injury, and this is the time when you, as occupational therapy practitioners, are going to have to think new and think large—because there is such a desperate situation. I think it is a disgrace that every injured soldier might not receive occupational therapy. When I read that returning soldiers were not even evaluated for brain injury—it's like the Dark Ages. And so much suffering has been needless.

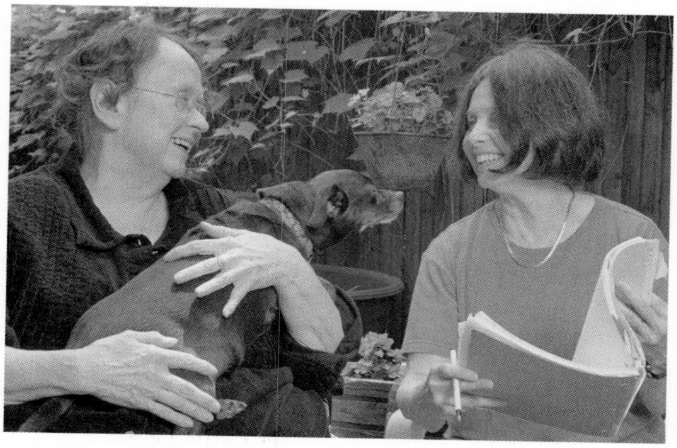

FIGURE 9.17 Mary, Sally, and LaBeam chatting in the garden. (Photo courtesy of L. Nugent, Photographic Services, University of New Hampshire, Durham, NH.)

So then, dear friends who are reading this, I think your calling could be taking care of the soldiers who are coming back from the war. These are times to stand beside the soldiers and to advocate for them.

You have chosen a profession that helps, restores, teaches, and gives comfort. Some of the finest human beings I have ever met are occupational therapy practitioners. You speak for us, the people you serve. You are in our corner. You are needed. Each and every one of you is desperately needed. I am glad that you have chosen this profession. I am proud of you. Bless you. Bless you all.

Acknowledgments

Let me tell you about my friend Sally. Sally Schreiber-Cohn has helped me to make this chapter happen, from taking some of the original dictation when I was too sick to do it myself to bringing me art supplies for my painting. Sally and I were friends before the accident, and she has stayed my friend through these 28 years. Sally, an artist herself, stuck with me on a day-by-day basis, patient, kind, and worked to see that the artist in me did not die. She has always been in my corner.

Sally is a large part of why I came through all this (Figure 9.17).

Reference

Mason, M. (2007, February). Dead men walking: What sort of future do brain-injured Iraq veterans face? *Discover Magazine*. Retrieved from http://discovermagazine.com/2007/mar/dead-men-walking

For additional resources on the subjects discussed in this chapter, visit http://thePoint.lww.com/Willard-Spackman12e.

CHAPTER 10

He's Not Broken—He's Alex: Three Perspectives

Alexander McIntosh, Laurie McIntosh, Lou McIntosh

OUTLINE

In every lifetime, there are directions to take and choices to make. Each one of us carries a vision of our future. When something unexpected happens that takes us down an unfamiliar path, we have to adjust our vision and change our expectations while maintaining our self-identity. When parents discover that their child has a disability, they must adapt to this change and create a new vision for themselves and their child. This is the story of Alex, a person with cerebral palsy, told from three perspectives. Laurie, Alex's mother, begins the chapter. Then comes Lou, Alex's father. Alex has the last word, because it is his story that we want you to remember.

Note: This narrative was written and published in 2009.

Laurie

Before Alex was born, it had been easy to slip into fantasies of his future. I could picture him toddling around the deck of our sailboat. (I would have to remember to look into safety netting.) I would have to be careful to watch him around our home, which was also a boatyard. When he got old enough, we would get him his first toolbox and hand tools. He would bang his little toy hammer side by side with his dad while he worked on boats.

Alex was born 12 weeks before his due date. He weighed 2 pounds and needed all the medical support of the neonatal intensive care unit (NICU) to stay alive. Ten days after his birth, my husband Lou and I were ushered into the conference room near the nurses' station. I remember that the room was darkened. The shades had been drawn against the bright sunlight outside, and no one had turned on the lights. I was surprised to see that the social worker and the neonatologist were joining us—all the players. The neurologist was friendly but somber as he showed us pictures of Alex's latest brain ultrasound. As he used words like *periventricular leukomalacia*, I tried to swim to the surface by putting on my professional hat and being the occupational therapist that I was trained to be. Yes, I knew all about spastic diplegia. He would have trouble moving his arms and legs. Of course, I could help explain this to my husband. Cognition would probably be undamaged. Well, that's something good. Of course, there is always the chance . . . the brain does amazing things. I was in a fog as I left the room, trying to make sense of the news.

Lou and I walked back to Alex's Isolette. We peered in at the uncomfortable little being who was still pulling at his feeding tube and now making a faint mewing sound. I put my hands through the portholes in the side of the box and stroked his arms down away from the tube. I couldn't get myself to talk to him. I stared at him but could not make sense of what I was seeing. Who was this new person? . . . "Spastic diplegia." Would he even walk? I couldn't picture anything. I left the hospital that day with an empty feeling. It was almost as if Alex had died.

However, Alex didn't die. He grew and changed. He developed a unique personality before he even left the NICU. When he finally came home, near the time of his due date, he seemed like a typical baby. I loved showing him off to people and telling them what a miracle baby he was. There were days when I completely forgot about the brain scan and pictured Alex as I had in my dreams before he was born. On other days I would panic over his inability to roll over or sit up. I would imagine him having to use a wheelchair or being unable to get a job. The part of Alex that was his future was completely cloudy to me. All I could do was focus on the Alex that was present.

Throughout Alex's youth, we repeatedly cycled through the stages of grieving. Once, when I was furious with a neurologist, I remembered reading about anger being one of the typical stages, along with denial, bargaining, guilt, and others. In my practice, I frequently heard health professionals scoffing about this parent being in denial or that parent "just going through the anger phase." They sounded so superior, as if they would never handle a situation like this in such an unhealthy manner. Had I been in denial about Alex? Sometimes. Was that a bad thing? Did that make me weak or neurotic? Absolutely not. Professionals who criticize parents for going through the stages of grieving should have a chance to try it themselves. Telling someone that she should not be in denial or not be angry is like trying to tell her to self-actualize. It is just not something that you can do on command.

Our best health professionals were those who listened carefully, recognized where we were coming from on any particular day, and accepted that that was the reality of the day. Some days I was optimistic, and on other days I didn't see how we could possibly manage. Some days I would be full of energy and ask for more exercises or suggestions for activities, and on other days I hid my head in shame because I had not done Alex's stretches faithfully. I was grateful to the professionals who could adapt to my changes and who were patient and knew when to push and when to rest.

As Alex developed into a little person, we began to be able to visualize his future. Our circle of friends began to include other families of children with disabilities. We attended support groups and special activities that were offered through our local agency. Lou began working on some national disabilities issues that brought him into contact with adults with disabilities who were making important changes in legislation. Lou and I were able to get advice from other parents and ask successful adults with disabilities what we should be doing to help Alex. It was this exposure to others in the disability community that allowed us to begin to picture Alex as a successful adult. My training and experience as an occupational therapist helped me to focus on creating a home environment with typical expectations. In my occupational therapy courses, I had learned how a person's habits, routines, attitudes, and values are rooted in the experiences of childhood. I wanted to make sure that Alex grew up with the habits, attitudes, and values that would make him a successful adult.

As Alex became a preschooler, I wanted to give him experiences that were as typical as possible. At this point, he was an incredibly verbal and imaginative child who used a tiny wheelchair. His left hand was nearly typical, but his right hand did not have skilled movements. He needed exercises to strengthen and stretch his legs and to improve his hand use. I found it much easier to embed therapeutic activities into our daily routines than to set aside special times to do "exercises." When I cooked meals, I would give Alex packages to open, mixtures to stir, and food to place in bowls. For example, I would chop green beans and put handfuls of chopped pieces on his tray so that he could place them in the pan. He helped me to fold and sort laundry. His specialty was matching socks. I gave him a radio-frequency remote control switch so that he could control electrical appliances such as the vacuum cleaner, the blender, the radio, or the Christmas tree lights. I supported him in standing at the kitchen sink so that he could "help" with the dishes. He loved washing the car with the hose. This kind of "work" was "play" for Alex. He often pretended to be an adult such as a chef, machine operator, or "car wash guy" as he performed these tasks.

I found out later, while doing research for my master's thesis, that preschoolers have a strong drive to imitate their caregivers. Not only are household chores motivating for young children but they also help children to feel like part of the family. It is one of the first opportunities that children have to contribute and to feel gratified by helping others. By this point, Alex was in grade school, busy with homework and after-school activities and not as interested in helping me around the house. I wanted him to feel a sense of responsibility and to realize that he could be a person on whom other people depended.

Because of his physical limitations, it was difficult to find a task that he could do completely independently. I gave him the job of cleaning the bathroom sink. We soon discovered that he needed to wear an apron for this task to keep the cleanser from getting all over his shirt. He became "Myrtle the Maid." It took several weeks to train him to do all the aspects of cleaning the sink. He had to learn to regulate the amount of cleaning powder that he poured out. He learned to hold the sponge at the correct angle to wipe the sink clean. He learned to work in an organized pattern so that he did not mess up an area that he had just cleaned. When he finished cleaning the sink, he would call me in for the "white glove" test to see whether I approved of his work. Alex was proud of his work, but that pride did not motivate him to clean the sink on his own. When I chose this task for him, I had to commit to never cleaning the sink myself. I needed him to understand that our family depended on him to do it. This was a challenge for me when we had company and I realized that the sink was not clean. I learned to warn Alex when company was coming so that he could clean it before they arrived. Lou and I put Post-it notes addressed to "Myrtle the Maid" on the mirror, asking her to please clean the sink. Alex took his responsibility seriously and, despite complaining, did his job well. After mastering sink cleaning, he moved on to toilet cleaning, dusting, and vacuuming.

Alex always managed to make household chores into something fun, but he did not like his daily living tasks, such as dressing himself. Alex started to realize that I was not really sure how much he could do on his own. He learned that if he had lots of difficulty with a task, I would probably finish it for him. Like any child, he would rather play than work, and putting on his clothes was work. I would watch him struggle with some part of dressing, trying over and over and getting more frustrated by the minute. We were always in a hurry, since everything took a long time for Alex. Inevitably, I would give up and rescue him. The next day, he would not have to struggle as hard to get me to help him because he was unconsciously training me to respond to his frustration and anger. All he had to do was get angry and frustrated sooner. Finally, I caught on to the pattern and decided to pick my battles carefully. On the weekends, when there was plenty of time, I would have him practice some aspect of dressing so that I knew that he could do it. Then, during the week, I would do all the parts of dressing that he had mastered and let him spend the time on the one skill that most needed practice. Some days, I would have him do only the parts of dressing that I knew he could do quickly. Only when there was plenty of time did I ask him to dress himself completely. Eventually, he put it all together and was able to dress himself, although it still took a long time and required lots of patience.

Lou and I knew the power of learned dependence, and we worked hard to create an environment in which Alex felt responsible for himself, even when he needed help with some things. We tried to make sure that he felt the consequences of his choices. Behavior plans became part of our lives. For instance, in the mornings, Alex assumed that we would pack up all of his things, make his bed, put a coat on him, and send him out to the bus. At first, we had to help him with these things because they were physically difficult and time-consuming, but gradually, we tried to fade our assistance. Once we knew that he was capable of doing things on his own, we had to enforce that independence and make it part of his routine. For many years, he had to complete all the tasks on a checklist and get out to the bus on time in order to earn a reward. The reward for Alex was usually a book to read on the bus. Lou and I found that well-thought-out behavior plans worked for us as well as for Alex. We needed constant reminders to let him do things on his own and not jump in to help when things got a little tough.

As parents, we had a fairly good idea of what Alex's capabilities were at any particular time. It was much easier for Alex to take advantage of the well-meaning staff at school. People wanted to help him all the time, especially people in the cafeteria or the bus line. Every year, we had to meet with teachers and staff to explain to them how important it was for Alex to learn to think on his own. One late fall day when Alex was in middle school, I brought him back to school after a dentist appointment. After we checked in at the office, I told Alex to go to class and I would carry his backpack for him. I realized that Alex had no idea how to find his classroom. He had always had an aide or student carry his backpack, and he simply followed them. The next day, he came to school with a backpack on wheels so that he could pull it himself. However, he still had someone with him because there was a policy that a disabled student could not ride the elevator alone. It took a few phone calls to change the policy, and Alex was soon getting around the school completely independently.

Occupational therapy and physical therapy were available to Alex at school, but it was always difficult to balance therapies with academics. Alex was an extremely good student, and he wanted to be in the classroom as much as possible. In elementary school, he was seen outside the classroom for physical therapy, but occupational therapy was done on a consultation basis. Eventually, Alex's physical therapy was changed to a consultation model, which meant that he had to take more responsibility for his own stretching and exercises at home. By the time Alex was in high school, he was switched from an Individual Education Plan to a 504 plan because he did not require special education, merely modifications to regular education. Alex learned to advocate for himself by meeting with his teachers to adjust program requirements as needed. Assistive technology became a necessity in high school. Alex's handwriting and typing were slow, so he used a voice recognition program on the computer that converted his voice to text for taking notes and writing essays. He also found that a digital voice recorder was helpful for taking notes, recording assignments, and remembering tasks that needed to be done.

Recreation activities were another area that required thoughtful planning. My first instinct was to have Alex be involved only in "typical" recreation activities for "typical" children. I did not want him to grow up feeling separate and different from other children. Alex took karate lessons and attended a karate day camp in the summer. He swam at the town pool and attended a theater/puppetry class. He even became a Cub Scout. All these activities were great for him, although they came at a cost. Even though the adults who were in charge of these activities had good intentions, they had difficulty planning the activities with Alex's skills in mind. I became his aide during many activities in order for him to be fully included. Field trips and special activities required special planning to make sure that accessibility was considered and that Alex would be able to stay with the group. We had a few disasters with trips to places that we thought would be accessible but were not or leaders who planned activities that were too physically demanding for him.

It was a great relief to relax my standards and allow Alex to try specialized recreation activities. He participated in adapted horseback riding, handcycling, wheelchair court sports, and adapted skiing (**Figure 10.1**). At these specialized programs, I did not have to worry about making modifications because everything was set up for children with disabilities. Volunteers and program leaders were trained to deal with everything from transfers to helping a child in the bathroom. At many of these programs, parents were able to drop their children off and pick them up 2 hours later. That was a new experience for me! When I did choose to stay, I loved being able to sit back and watch my child having a good time while I stayed on the sidelines and chatted with other parents. It felt so "normal." Alex enjoyed the camaraderie of being with other children who had similar challenges, and many of the friendships that began at these activities have lasted for years.

Preparing for Alex to go to college took a lot of planning and creativity. Alex decided that he wanted to be within a 3-hour drive of home, so we looked at colleges throughout the Northeast. Several of them were willing to accommodate students with disabilities but did not have much experience with this, and the campuses were not fully wheelchair accessible. Alex decided to attend a university near our home. This school had an access office, which coordinated accommodations for students with disabilities. He wanted to live on campus and have a typical college experience, including living on his own in a dorm.

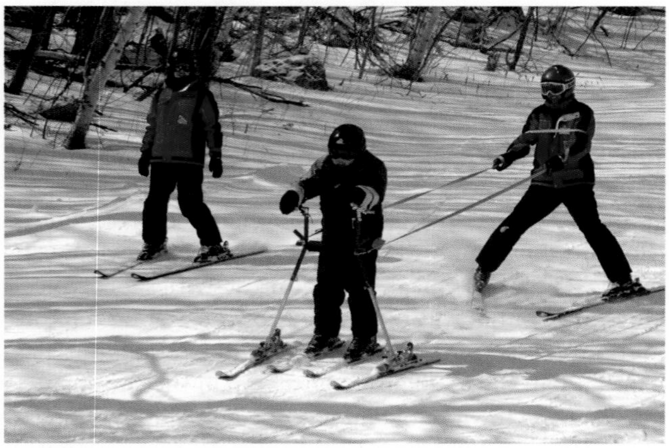

FIGURE 10.1 Alex skiing with the slider. (Photo courtesy of Maine Handicapped Skiing.)

In the summer before he moved on campus, we checked out his dorm room, which had been carefully chosen to meet his needs. He spent several afternoons driving his new three-wheeled scooter around the campus and learning how to get through doors and operate elevators. Alex decided not to hire a personal care attendant even though it was still taking him over an hour to shower and dress in the morning. We carefully set up his room with a special stand for his reacher, sock aid, and dressing stick. We bought a carpet for the room so that he could push his feet into his braces and shoes without having them slide. The dorm already had a fully equipped accessible shower. We purchased special shelves for the closet so that Alex could reach his supplies. We put up several plastic hooks to make it easier for him to hang his bathrobe and coat. A small folding shopping cart doubled as a hamper and a means of getting the laundry down to the laundry room. We practiced washing and folding laundry at a local Laundromat during the summer.

The first few weeks of college were difficult for Lou and me as we waited at home to hear how things were going. Like many college students, Alex was enjoying being on his own and did not feel like calling home. When we finally heard from him, he was doing just fine. There had been a few problems with automatic doors not working, but Alex had contacted the right people to get things fixed. Crossing busy streets in his scooter had been a challenge at first, but he learned to use the crosswalks that were equipped with pedestrian signals. Lou and I were pleased to admit that we had passed the test. Alex was ready to be on his own. We had learned a lot as parents and made many mistakes along the way, but we knew that we had done some things right: Alex grew up feeling like a typical person who happened to have a physical disability. He knew that there were obstacles to overcome, but there were also people to help him when he asked for it. He knew that nothing is impossible and that there is always a way to modify and adapt things for success. He knew that he could help others and contribute to the world. Most of all, he learned that he was in charge of his own life.

Lou

When Alex was born, I suppose I was a typical new father in most respects. I didn't have a clear idea what fatherhood would be like. As far as I knew, dads were supposed to do what they were told by moms, who somehow "just knew" all about babies and young children. I was sure I would be informed of my role when it was time for me to know. My pictures certainly didn't include the possibility that my own child might be born with special needs. I thought I would be playing catch with my 6-year-old in a few years and arguing about access to the car in another few years. I hoped I would be an adequate dad and not let my child down.

So the news that Alex had an abnormal ultrasound scan and probable brain damage was completely outside my experience. I had no idea what to do. I had expected to be less important than Mom, but now I was irrelevant. Mom was an occupational therapist and had professional knowledge about disability. I didn't. There wasn't much that I could contribute to the family except for diaper changes and a paycheck.

I remember feeling utterly marginalized almost from the beginning. Doctors and nurses would talk to Mom, not to me. Mom got the pamphlets and lectures about how to care for Alex. When I went to an appointment with Alex, I was always asked gently whether Mom was planning to arrive later, or . . . ? After all, it was Mom's job to take care of this child, to know about disability, to learn about social services, to make appointments, and to make the decisions about Alex's care. So I began to act the part: I spent less time with my family, had a few too many beers in the evening, and began to hear everything that was said to me as a reproof or insult.

In the years since that time, I have learned that my experience was typical. New dads of children with special needs discover immediately that the world of children's services is focused on the moms. That's unfortunate, because for our own mental health, let alone our ability to support our families emotionally and financially, dads need recognition that their role extends beyond "making sure Mom is listened to" and "pinch hitting." We need recognition that a "dad" is not merely an inferior form of a "mom." (Of course, since so many of the physicians are male, so many of those males are patronizing and condescending, and so many of them seem to know almost nothing about the experience of disability except for the medical part, moms get marginalized in their children's care too and have their own horror stories to share. But I'm telling the dads' story.)

On the other hand, this marginalization can also be very important in allowing dads to think independently about their children's disabilities. One of my memories is about Alex's first pediatrician, who loved babies. When Alex first came home from the hospital, the doctor proudly carried him out and paraded him around the waiting room, exclaiming how perfect he was. But as Alex grew older and his legs and arms didn't work quite the same way as other children's, the doctor seemed to become more and more reluctant to deal with him. He assured Mom and me that our child was "going to be fine! He'll be just fine, you'll see!" When Alex was a year old and unable to roll over, let alone crawl, the doctor warned us that we needed to make sure every part of the house was childproofed. When Alex was 3, still unable to stand up without assistance and able to walk only a few steps on crutches, the doctor lectured us about making sure to hold his hand so that he wouldn't dash out into traffic. The doctor even counseled me, "as one dad to another," that I must "not give up hope" about my son.

At last, during an office visit when Alex was 4 years old, I suddenly realized what was going on. This doctor loved *perfect* babies, but he regarded my "imperfect" son as a failure—a baby he hadn't managed to rescue completely from the results of prematurity, a child he needed to *fix*. I lost my temper and told the doctor that *despite* an inability to run out in traffic, my child was *already* fine, *and* he had cerebral palsy; and that I did not need *hope*, I needed *routine medical advice*. Because Alex wasn't *broken* and didn't need to be *fixed*, I felt that it was time the doctor stopped giving me warnings about dire possibilities that weren't possibilities at all for Alex.

After that experience, I began to notice that the medical and therapeutic worlds have a "broken/fixed" paradigm: "This limb *doesn't work* and we must *restore it to health*." That's fine for rehabilitation situations, but it doesn't fit the facts when we're talking about a child or adult who is *already just fine* and whose legs or arms don't work. As a dad, I certainly want advice and support on how to make my child's movements more functional, but please don't waste my spirit or his self-esteem by trying to tell me he's *broken!* I know better: He is *absolutely fine*, just the way he is.

Families of children with disabilities often claim that our stress levels and divorce rates are higher than those of typical families. The data I have seen tend to suggest, surprisingly, that we're wrong about the divorce rates, but there's no doubt that we're right about the stress levels. The early years of parenting children with disabilities are a very lonely and challenging time for both parents, and dads have very few role models and not much support. It is especially difficult for dads to admit their own weakness. We don't always know how to seek support appropriately, and sometimes our ways of asking are not very clear. Sometimes they're abrupt, and sometimes they're scary. The result is that we antagonize the people from whom we need the most understanding and support. Like many other dads, I slipped into marginalization and irrelevance during Alex's first years of life, and I was very lucky to escape from the trap. The experiences that rescued me were the opportunities I had to contribute in a special way to Alex's life. Those experiences are the most important things I have to share with you, because they transformed my life.

One day when Alex was about 3 years old, his mom and I had our usual fight in which she accused me (correctly) of avoiding the family and spending hour after hour "playing" in the workshop instead of "doing a fair share." At the end, she said something like this:

> I know you're going to just run away again and hide out in that shop; so while you're there, if you actually want to be useful, you could prove it by building something for Alex to sit on. It needs to be some kind of a chair, with a foot rest ten inches below the seat, and a seat depth of eleven inches, and a seat back with a couple of corner pieces to pull his scapulas forward and break up the hyperextension pattern. Oh, yes, and it needs a pommel so he can't arch out of it—and it needs a seat belt—and it would be *really nice* if you could make it light enough so that I could pick it up and move it—you always overbuild everything.

These were fightin' words, but Mom had grown up in a woodshop and was entitled to her opinion even if I didn't agree with it.

So I went out to the workshop, in a very sour mood, and sawed and fitted and fastened for a couple of hours and built a little portable seat with all the dimensions she had given me. It not only was portable, but also could actually be taken apart, and all the loose pieces could be stowed away underneath the chair. I was quite proud of my invention, although of course I was absolutely sure it wouldn't be appreciated.

I brought this creation into the house, and Mom carefully put Alex in the chair and positioned him at the kitchen table with some paper and a couple of crayons. To my utter astonishment, Alex picked up one of the crayons and began to color and draw on his paper independently—skills I had never seen him use before. There must be something good about this "proper positioning" I had been hearing about! Suddenly, I realized that I had actually done something that was directly, obviously related to making Alex successful in overcoming some of the effects of his disability. Perhaps I wasn't as utterly useless as I had thought (Figure 10.2).

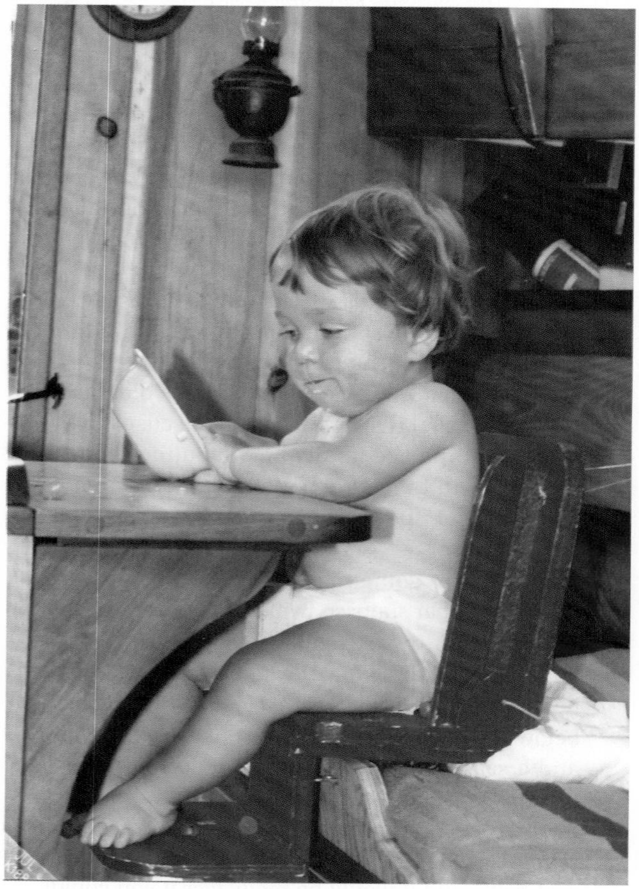

FIGURE 10.2 Alex sitting in his chair on the sailboat. (Photo courtesy of Laurie McIntosh.)

Of course, there is a limit to how many chairs a dad can build before he runs out of baby butts to park in them, so if that was to be my only dad skill, I was still quite a useless fellow. But it was a good start, and I was lucky enough to be able to keep going. Within the next few years, I became an advocate not only for my own family but also for others in the early intervention world. I developed an electronic network for families of special-needs children; I became part of a national committee to oversee early-intervention services for young children across the country; and eventually, I became a professional special education advocate. I know I would not have had any of these experiences if it weren't for that little chair and for the opportunity I was given, as a dad, to contribute to my child's life.

Today, as an advocate, I see moms and dads playing the same stereotyped roles that Alex's mom and I played when he was small. Mom keeps the records, Mom deals with the school folks and the doctors, and Mom goes to the meetings. There is often a feeling that if Dad goes to a meeting, there must be something wrong. Even today, most of the people at educational team meetings are women, and Dad is not likely to feel welcome; in fact, he's often seen as a very scary person who doesn't understand how hard everyone is trying and who doesn't "know how to be reasonable." He is marginalized and excluded, sometimes kindly and sometimes out of fear and hostility, and Mom is left to deal with the child's disability without his assistance.

That is particularly unfortunate because we know from research that it is bad for the children. Longitudinal studies of children with disabilities have shown that family cohesion is one of the best predictors of good outcomes for children with disabilities (Hauser-Cram et al., 1999; Shonkoff & Philips, 2000). Anytime we exclude dads from their children's lives or do anything to diminish dads' importance, we have a direct negative impact on those children's prospects for success in life. If you care about the children, that is unacceptable.

At the same time, I have also learned to remember that Dad's job is to be a parent and Mom's job is also to be a parent. Neither Mom nor Dad needs to be a doctor, therapist, or teacher in order to have credibility. What we bring to the table as "mere parents" is sufficient, because we are the keepers of the dreams and visions for our children, and we will be their advocates and companions long after all their childhood caregivers and teachers have retired. Mom and Dad may *also* be professionals with titles and credentials and lots of education, but the most important hat we will ever wear is the Parent Hat.

Alex

When I was about 7 years old, I was firmly convinced that I was a werewolf. I had never actually undergone any physical transformation at the full of the moon, but 7-year-olds are not bothered by such trifles. The crowning touch was that my crutches acted as a second pair of legs, and although when wearing them I could never really manage a wolf-like lope, I made do instead with a sort of galloping skip. Nevertheless, it was fast enough (to me) to reinforce fantasies of running swiftly through the forest on silent paws, seeking unsuspecting prey.

The technical term for the condition of being a werewolf is *lycanthropy*, after the mythical Greek king Lycaon, whom the god Zeus transformed into a wolf as punishment for his tyranny. I knew the word at the age of 7, having read every book on werewolves that I could both find and understand. I was proud to declare myself a lycanthrope to everyone I met.

One day that year, my mother, my younger brother, and I attended a fund-raising boat race, the object of which was to allow wealthy yacht owners to raise money for the disabled. I was skipping around the lobby of the yacht club where the event was being held, giving long, mournful, earsplitting howls, as a proper werewolf should. Mom was over in a corner with my brother, trying to pretend that I was someone else's child.

One of the yacht owners saw me, and she said, "Look at you, doing so well. What's your disability, honey?"

"I have lycanthropy!" I said, beaming.

A few minutes later, she was chatting with my mother and said, "I just met your son. What a nice boy. It's so sad that he has lycanthropy."

Mom smirked. "Um, I think there's something you should know . . ."

That is what happens to people who are lacking in disability awareness.

When I was about 15, I decided to try my hand at metalwork. My father has a workshop next to the house, and he found me the gloves, jacket, goggles, and apron necessary for working with heated metal. My primary objective during my first experiment was to make a 3-inch-long model sword out of nails.

I learned how to manage a coal fire those first few days and, later, a propane blowtorch. I learned not to leave a nail in the fire for more than a minute or two for fear of burning the metal and that heat dissipates very quickly from a nail after it has been taken out of the fire. I also learned (the hard way) that just because a nail isn't glowing red anymore doesn't mean that it's not hot enough to burn flesh through a glove.

Because I had to strike the nail quickly while the heat was retained, there was a great deal of tension in my hands when I was hammering. My cerebral palsy kept the muscles in my hands rather tight to begin with. Try as I might, I couldn't strike the metal at the right angles to make an even, straight blade or hilt. The nails kept twisting into a corkscrew shape. What I ended up having to do was hammer out the rough shapes as best I could, quench them (dunk them in a bucket of water to cool them), take them out of the vice grips I held them in and clamp them in a vice, then use the vice grips to straighten the twisted parts (Figure 10.3).

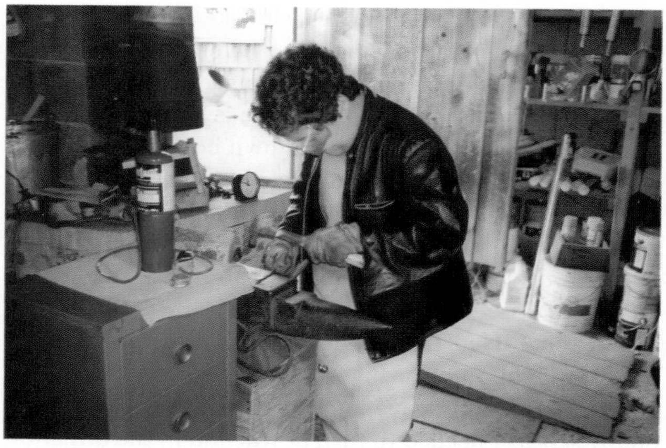

FIGURE 10.3 Alex engaged in metal working. (Photo courtesy of Laurie McIntosh.)

Sometimes the twists were so subtle that I could barely see them. In these instances, I had to make very small, precise movements with my hands, which are difficult enough even for those who don't have cerebral palsy. I often didn't affect the metal at all, and I even more often overshot the mark and twisted it more than it had been originally. I am still learning this skill; I have a long way to go before I can correct subtle flaws in metal.

My father says that the minds of people who have learned to use tools and build things work in a fundamentally different way from other people's minds. Builders' minds have a better combination of practicality and creativity, and they are better able to analyze a problem and come up with a solution. As I become more involved in metalwork, I hope I begin to think this way as well (Figure 10.4).

I have been involved in the Maine Handicapped Skiing Program since I was 6 years old. During most of my time there (twice-monthly lessons from January through March each year), I used normal skis combined with outriggers,

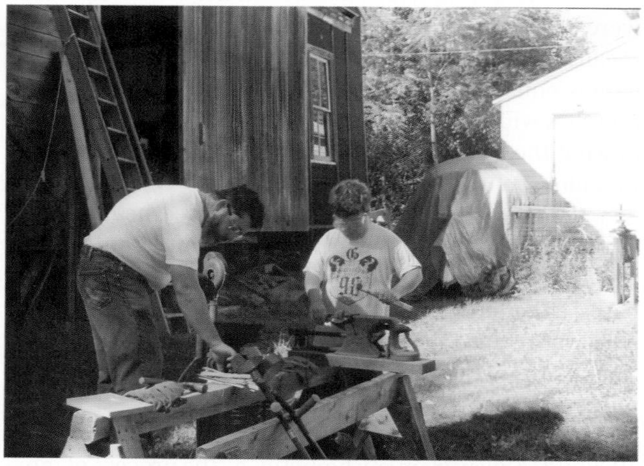

FIGURE 10.4 Alex and his dad doing metal work in the boatyard. (Photo courtesy of Laurie McIntosh.)

devices that resemble crutches with skis attached. I used the same ground for each lesson: the end of a trail right outside the Maine Handicapped Skiing lodge.

I learned very quickly that there is nothing so apt to make one acutely aware of one's own body as the fear of crashing into something. I have learned to use this awareness to judge turns and to move my legs, skis, and outriggers in just the right way to make myself stop. However, in 11 of my 12 years of skiing, my ability to turn came and went.

When I used the outriggers, I had to put a great deal of weight on my arms to hold myself upright on the snow. This did not leave me free to put as much weight on my skis as I needed to turn at will and in the direction I chose. Therefore, my ability to turn on any given day depended largely on how willing I was to take the weight off my arms and, to my mind, increase the risk of falling.

This past year, I tried a new method, using skis and a device called a slider, patterned on the walkers used by the elderly. The slider acts as a support system for my upper body, leaving me free to shift the weight on my legs as needed. I am also tethered to one of my ski instructors, who helps me slow down on especially steep slopes.

With the help of the slider-and-tether system, I am able to travel farther on ski trails than I did in all my 11 previous years of skiing. I can maneuver through rough terrain. In consequence, I believe I am even more in control of my body.

In elementary school and high school, gym class was seldom a productive time for me. This fact hinged on my not being able to run. I used crutches rather than a wheelchair at school. Although the instructor sensibly assigned me the position of flag keeper in games of capture-the-flag, the members of the opposing team who ran past me were always just a little too far away for me to reach out and tag them, which was extremely frustrating. I must admit that sometimes my inability to tag people had more to do with my attention span than my disability.

There were instances in which my teachers came up with creative modifications to such activities, but these were so few and far between that I cannot now clearly recall them. Most of the time, my participation in such games consisted chiefly of my hopping around on my crutches while everyone else ran and making the motions of what the other students were doing. I probably looked ridiculous.

The exception was baseball. I never learned the rules of the game quite as well as my peers, but I could bat as well as anyone in my class. When it came time to run the bases, either I had someone else represent me or my opponent was required to hop on one foot to even the odds.

On the whole, I am glad I no longer have to take physical education courses.

I have recently enrolled at a state university, which is 10 minutes away from my hometown. The process of moving in began with evaluating the accessibility of my dorm: the ease or difficulty of entering and moving around the rooms in an electric scooter and on foot and the accessibility of the bathrooms, laundry room, and lounge areas. Even though we went to the dorm in the summer to see how everything would work, it still took me a while to get used to the new routines once school actually started. I had to remember to grab my little bucket of bathroom supplies before heading down the hall to the bathroom. My schedule now had to include time to get to the dining hall for meals and time to do laundry on the weekends. In short, I had to plan ahead for almost everything.

One of the biggest challenges for me was learning to find my way around the campus. I think that my lack of mobility as a child kept me from learning some fundamental lessons about directions. When I was a young child, I was pushed long distances in a wheelchair, and the distances I walked were very short. I was never left on my own to find my way around because of safety issues. As a teenager, I would go for walks in my neighborhood, but it was a familiar area, and I usually just walked around the block.

The summer before I went to high school, my mother took me to the empty building to practice my routes at least three times before I felt secure. When I arrived on the university campus, I realized that I had a very poor aptitude for map reading. I had no idea how to get from one place to another by looking at a map. Even when I asked people for directions, I would often have to ask several other people along the way before I found my destination.

Since I got my new three-wheeled electric scooter right before school started, I had not had much opportunity to practice driving it. I was not a car driver and had never had a power vehicle. Most of the time, I managed to get places without ruining too much sheetrock or crushing too many toes. Small elevators were a challenge, as was maneuvering in the crowded dining hall without knocking over piles of dishes and spilling drinks. The automatic doors for the buildings on campus usually worked, but there were always a few that were out of commission.

Sometimes I would be lucky enough to find someone to hold the door for me, but I soon learned to hold the door open with one hand while driving the scooter through with the other. Since my door-holding hand is weak, I fear that I may have left some scratches on a few doors. The most difficult problem was parking on the shuttle buses. They were accessible and had lovely ramps, but once inside, I found myself required to parallel park in a specific and confined spot in order for my scooter to be properly tied down. I wished I had had scooter-driving lessons in high school.

My dorm is set up with automatic doors that have remote controls. Students with mobility problems are given small remote control units to attach to our key rings. It gives me such a great sense of power to approach the dorm door at full speed, push the little button and cruise right in without even stopping. Of course, I do this only when there is no one around to run over. Other students stand at the door and fumble for their identification cards in order to run them through the door-opening machine. Most of the other students don't know that I have this remote control device, so I can "magically" open the doors for attractive girls when I'm twenty feet away.

Given that I am late for class more often than I would like (because my morning routine always takes longer than I plan for), I often have to drive my scooter very quickly across the campus. This sometimes proves to be unsafe. At one point, I was racing toward the building in which my class was taking place, and my overfull backpack, hanging on the back of my scooter, caused the scooter to tip sideways. I crashed onto the concrete path, swearing inaudibly but profusely. Fortunately, the noise attracted the attention of two kindhearted passersby, who helped me to my feet and also laboriously got the scooter right side up again. Since that time, I have been more careful to carry less weight in my backpack and take the corners more slowly (Figure 10.5).

The university has been good about making sure that my classes are all held in wheelchair-accessible rooms. There is an access office that coordinates all the services and modifications for students with disabilities. They move classes to accessible rooms for specific students.

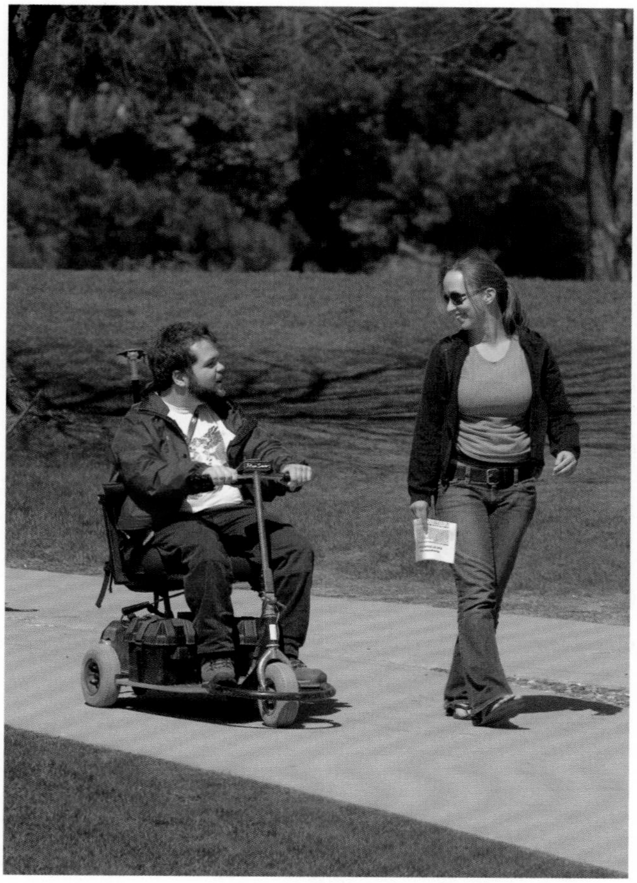

FIGURE 10.5 Alex going to classes on campus. (Photo courtesy of Lisa Nugent, Photographic Services, University of New Hampshire.)

The access office also coordinates student note takers so that students with disabilities can have other students take notes for them. The note takers never know which student in their class is receiving their notes. The note takers deliver the notes to the access office, and the notes are distributed to the students who need them. At this university, the accommodations that are listed on the student's high school Individual Education Plans or 504 plans are respected. For instance, in high school, I was allowed to have extra time to take tests, and I have the same accommodation at the university.

As buildings on campus are renovated, they are made accessible. Unfortunately, the English Department building has not been renovated yet, and since I am majoring in English, this has presented some problems. The department offices, including my advisor's office, are up a flight of stairs. If I need to pick up forms or drop things off, I call on my cell phone, and someone comes downstairs. If I want to see my advisor, I have to e-mail her to set up a specific appointment because I can't just show up during her office hours or drop by to see whether she's in. So far this system seems to work, although it is just one more way in which my life requires more planning.

The teachers and students on campus treat me just like any other student. It is obvious that this school is used to students with disabilities because the community is very accepting. I don't feel patronized or disrespected at all. My teachers expect the same work from me that they would get from someone else except that they are nice enough to give me more time to do it. There are a number of students with various disabilities on the campus, and we all just seem to fit in like anyone else.

Conclusion

Many people, including many new parents of children with disabilities, assume that a disability is like a shadow that hangs over a child's life, forever reminding him or her of things that cannot be done or achieved. As my behavior during the Lycanthropy Incident proved, I couldn't have cared less as a child about my disability in terms of what it prevented me from doing. I was just having fun and living my own life. I was able to do this freely because of what my parents learned, and taught to me, when I was growing up: *I am not broken; I don't need to be fixed.* Knowing this, I was, and am, able to choose who and what to be: werewolf, blacksmith, skier, college student, writer. The list is still being added to.

Questions from Alex

1. What did you expect to find in this chapter? How did it meet, or differ from, your expectations?
2. Can you recall any instance in which the actions of someone with a disability contradicted your assumptions about how that person was going to behave?

3. List some common stereotypes about people with disabilities, and identify information in this chapter that negates those stereotypes.
4. Imagine for a moment that you have been in a horrible accident and your legs have had to be amputated. Brainstorm some modifications to your favorite (physical) recreational activity that will enable you to keep doing it.
5. Research currently available examples of what you came up with in Question 4. What are the similarities and differences between these and your own ideas? Have you come up with something that you think is innovative? If so, why are you still doing this exercise instead of promoting your idea?

Questions from Lou

6. To have a successful and fulfilling role in the life of a child with a disability, each family member needs to have the opportunity to contribute to that child's quality of life. Assigning "homework" is not the same thing and can be very damaging to the family. What is the difference? How can the occupational therapist's intervention support the creation of opportunities instead of the mere assignment of tasks?
7. What can an occupational therapist do to support family cohesion, and why is it important to the child?
8. In this chapter, Alex's father says that "Alex wasn't *broken* and didn't need to be *fixed*." How would you reconcile this perspective with the rehabilitation model of service? Can you reconcile it with the model of human occupation or another occupational therapy model? Why or why not?
9. Parents and siblings of a child with a disability often have no knowledge of occupational therapy and no understanding of why therapeutic interventions are necessary. Yet these "mere parents" bring a vital perspective to the planning process. What is that perspective, and how should the occupational therapist integrate that perspective into the child's treatment plan?

Questions from Laurie

10. Learned dependence can be a more serious disability than cerebral palsy. People who never learn to be responsible for themselves might need assistance for the rest of their lives. How can occupational therapists prevent situations that lead to learned dependence?
11. We used household chores to give Alex a sense of responsibility and an important role in the family. What can occupational therapists do to help parents find useful roles for their children with disabilities?
12. We made sure that all the necessary modifications were in place for Alex to live in a dorm and attend classes at the university. Should some of this have been the responsibility of the high school occupational therapist as part of Alex's transition plan? Why or why not?
13. What was the difference in how Alex felt about himself in physical education classes versus handicapped skiing? How could his physical education classes been set up differently so that he felt better about himself?

Questions from the Editor

14. This chapter presents three perspectives of Alex's life. How do these perspectives differ, and why is it important to have an appreciation of each perspective?

References

Hauser-Cram, P., Warfield, M. E., Shonkoff, J. P., Krauss, M. W., Upshur, C. C., & Sayer, A. (1999). Family influences on adaptive development in young children with Down syndrome. *Child Development, 70,* 979–989.

Shonkoff, J. P., & Philips, D. A. (Eds.). (2000). *From neurons to neighborhoods: The science of early childhood development.* Washington, DC: National Academies Press.

For additional resources on the subjects discussed in this chapter, visit http://thePoint.lww.com/Willard-Spackman12e.

CHAPTER 11

While Focusing on Recovery I Forgot to Get a Life

My Dreams Deferred

Gloria F. Dickerson

Hello! My name is Gloria. I am now a 60-year-old Black woman living in Boston. I first wrote this chapter about six years ago. I was very concerned that my reliance on therapeutic relationships and focus on recovering from trauma led me to forget to "get a life." I realized that I wasn't developing valued relationships in a community of my choice. The focus on my resilience and life hardiness was a substitute for any confidence or plan to make needed changes. This is a legacy of trauma and the resulting lifetime of fears for my safety which led me to cope by living in isolation.

Most of my life, I have meandered along within the bubble of mental health treatment under a variety of designated attributes of being ill. My sole primary and trusted relationships are with providers and colleagues within health services. At age 15, I was introduced to the mental health system as a patient. Now I look back and revisit my journey through a life of treatment in the light of today. From this vantage point, my life seems to have been an initiation into the land of never good enough, never quite arrived, filled with cyclical pain-filled struggles and some rays of sun. My birth seems to have hurled me into a predesignated life sentence of less than and a never-ending journey of repetitive bouts of trying to rise.

In this writing, I am going to tell you about who I am and where I have been. I will attempt to explain how I learned who I was and how this has affected every aspect of my being, from my excess weight to my choices of occupations and even to my dress. My present gifts and my abilities, my pain and my hope, as well as my deficits and despair, can be traced back to events during the first few years of my life. As with everyone on the planet, every event and experience, good or bad, has shaped me and culminated in making me the person that I am. After learning the facts of my life, people who have come to know me are surprised and astonished that I have survived with my intellect and hope intact. After hearing what I have lived through, most people react with jaw-dropping awareness and awe and silence. As people get to know me, they recognize that my life has been filled with extreme horror and that my endurance and survival are amazing.

OUTLINE

The Early Years

I begin with accounts of memories about my family of origin and my early years. My first years in the South as a young girl were riddled with incidents of trauma. I consider myself to be a Southerner because, up to the age of 5, my ancestral roots, my psyche, and consciousness spring from events that occurred within a small town in Alabama. The family relationships and life in this small town caused essential disconnections within myself, with others, and with the world. My experiences include parental abuse resulting in the birth of my daughter, long inpatient stays in mental hospitals, graduation from college, more hospitalizations, suicide attempts, five different postcollege graduate programs, work throughout the human services field, and 39 years of therapy. These are only a few of the most influential and important experiences that dot the course of my life.

For years, I was the only girl child of my parents. My daddy (James) was born in 1925. My ma (Stella) was born in 1927. My brother Andrew is 1 year older and was born in 1949. I was the oldest girl and was born in 1951. My brother Roger was born 11 months later, in 1952. We often joked that this close proximity in our birth made us almost twins. We have always felt closest to each other. My brother Junior was born in July 1953, and he was the baby for many years. My brother Donnie was born in 1955. He died tragically and suddenly, and his existence has been erased from all family accounts. My sister Daisy was born in 1958. Her birth was my dream come true. I always thought she was a personal gift from God. Her choice to become and to remain estranged from me has been one of the greatest losses of my life. My brother George was born in 1962. Amazingly, he still fails to be recognized as a valued and independent person by my family system. My brother David was born in 1967. Although he is nearly 40, his life continues to affirm his status as my mom's "baby." As a Black man with untreated dyslexia, he makes do and escapes all aspects of being an adult, except procreation, and he lives without income on his relationships with others.

As for most of our neighbors, Black and White, life in the South meant Sundays in church, life as a sharecropper, and extremes of joy, violence, calmness, and pain. The residues of lives touched by violent, chaotic nights and the hard-fought-for appearance of calm, peaceful days set the stage for a culture of fear. The minister was pivotal in helping individuals caught in the maze of violence find meaning and maintain hope necessary for endurance. There are at least two types of ministers. Some ministers believe in, are motivated by, and love "God" and all the things that a good "God" stands for. A minister operating from powerful needs to nurture "a loving and hopeful life-affirming world" will make mistakes, but her or his intention is to promote relationships between people that rest on ideals of love and hope. The conscious actions of a good minister start from deep-seated basic beliefs such as "Love your neighbor as you would yourself" and "Do no intentional harm." Other ministers beam out their fears of confronting feelings and thoughts that they deem evil and project negative intentions and motivations onto others. My grandfather was the second type: a fire and brimstone type minister. He could not have designed a better-suited context (the ministry) in which he could hide and insinuate his personal brand of fear and pain. Under the cover of the prevailing myths of goodness, high praise, and quality attributes of a minister, he operated unquestioned. He could do no wrong. His motives were never questioned. His actions were revered. His destruction is immeasurable.

My mother's and my father's children can be understood by looking at my parents' life context. Knowing how we learned to be the people we are is not an excuse for our failures and our deficits. It teaches us how to make meaning and find understanding. The meanings we make tell us how to understand our "self," others, and our relationships in the world. This is the foundation from which we begin to act or not act, choose or not choose, know or not know. We learn what it is to be a human being early. We learn about relationships from those around us. We learn what is important, what our value is, and what is right and what is wrong from our early relationships. They form the lens through which we see and know everything. What follows are some of the experiences that make up my lens. This is my beginning.

My mother was 23 years old and my father 25 years old when I was born. My mother tells a story about my birth and early days of life that has been critical to forming my vision of myself, my character, and my strength that has at different times both supported and diminished my assessment of my worth in my own eyes. I have heard this story since . . . well . . . the beginning. She said,

> When you were born, you weighed 4 pounds and 10 ounces. Your father came to see you. He said you were so small that he was scared to hold you. When he first saw you he looked at you and said, "God, she's so hairy and looks just like a little rat." And while you were in the hospital you lost down to three pounds. Everyone thought you were going to die. You stayed in the hospital for one month in a makeshift incubator. Dr. Everage was so good. He made an incubator from odds and ends and pumped oxygen into it to keep you alive. But you were not gaining weight so they sent you home. I think they thought you were going to die. I was so scared and I put you in a dresser drawer with a hot water bottle. I had to stay up all night with you and I kept pinching you to make you cry because I was so afraid you were going to die. I had to struggle and work so hard to keep you alive. You put me through so much.

My mother has reminded me of this story periodically and with precision throughout my life, reiterating the fact that my father thought I looked like a rat and keeping the wounds of this image alive and potent. Her pronouncements of her great sacrifice and the extreme imposition and burden of my birth have weighed heavily and occasionally tipped the scales in favor of trying to secure my early demise through serious suicide attempts. Often, to make a point during times I "got too big for my britches" or became "too full of myself" by thinking that I was smart or worthy of high praise or love, she would remind me of my botched entrance into the world, reducing me to the reality of her perception that I was "filthy and less than dirt." Her spiel often concluded with pronouncements that the debt I owed her could never be repaid and I was lucky to be alive. The picture my mother painted about how she and my father greeted me and her feelings about me combine with the full weight of subsequent events leave me with profound feelings of guilt and terror and periods of dissociated pain and thoughts that plunged me into depths of despair and my own personal brand of hell all my life.

My mother's family worked as sharecroppers on a farm in Alabama in 1954. My grandfathers on both sides of the family were ministers. As a minister's family, we had some social status among other poor Black families in the area. Yet my grandmother's predicament seemed to be no different from that of other Black women in the area. Most of the women of the South lived as silent subjects in the land of domineering husbands. But Black women that I grew up with had the additional burden of being alternately longed for, sexually desired, while at the same time their essence as beings was despised, sometimes by their husbands and most of the time by all men and women within this slice of society.

I learned at a very early age that a woman's safety depended on the repertoire of defensive maneuvers of women and on the emotional state, whims, and actions of men. Unfortunately for my mom, she grew up with men who became enraged and physically abusive to any woman who dared think and act as if she was as intelligent and entitled to rights as any other human being, particularly a man. My mom tells stories that show her radical insistence on saying what she wanted, when she wanted, relentlessly voicing her opinions, and naming what was unacceptable. To my great despair, her tales of bravery often concluded with epic depictions of her getting "beat down to the ground." Yet to my amazement, she took great delight in the struggle—in the standing up. The defeat seemed to be incidental. The pride she beamed out every time she tossed her head back and recounted her defiance, blow after blow, left its mark on my heart and mind. I resonate with her physical strength and resilience but mostly with her pride of being defiant. This defying of "the beat down" reminds me that I come from a long line of survivors. The need to fight injustice has often thrilled me, motivated me. Overall, my mother's life taught her that she was inferior. She learned that her pain and terror were caused because she was Black and a female. Depending on the context, her Blackness, her womanhood, or both got her mercilessly victimized. She had to endure, cajole her way out of, and fight against rape and verbal and physical assault from early childhood by her father, brother, and other male relatives. Later, as a woman, she entered the world of having to fight off White men in the households where she worked. These are the things that infiltrated my mother's heart, made my mother who she was, and caused her to hate that which came from her: her firstborn girl.

It is as if every time my mother looked at me, she saw a girl with all the qualities and characteristics that she imagined that every person saw that led them to hurt and hate her. My face was a mirror. She looked into my face at 1 week, at 1 year, and for the rest of my life, and she could only see the vile, filthy little girl that got her beat and brutalized and kept her from the life she wanted. I have always felt hated by my mother. I could see that when she looked at me, she felt tremendous hatred and rage. There was no escaping the consequence of my meaning for her. I was everything that she thought others saw that made them hurt her. And I was gonna pay!

The life context in which my family lived overwhelmed their human potential and capacity for being hopeful. In this context, their actions can be understood, though it can never be a justification. The context shows how I learned to make meanings that sustain my life throughout recovery from devastating and unimaginably hurtful events in my life.

Keeping Time in Chaos

The phrase *keeping time in chaos* adequately describes my life during and for years after the emergence of my mental illness. My first 5 years of daily life in the South contained moments of exquisite pleasure, of running through the fields, pulling up peanuts when I wanted, and finding buried treasure by digging deep in the ground and pulling up unsuspecting sweet potatoes or carrots. Sitting by the water at one of the only swimming and fishing areas near our house, I often watched ants. My eyes went back and forth as I followed them as they went scurrying. I remembered wondering what they could possibly be thinking about.

I have always settled for the basic tenets of life, making lemonade out of lemons. Knowing that I missed out on love from a family and from friends, I lacked a viable self that is based on knowing that one is safe and loved. I am left knowing that I substituted therapy for a life and therapeutic relationships for love. My having a mental illness, post-traumatic stress disorder (PTSD) and depression, could not have been avoided. Life circumstances and early relationships made this inevitable. I was lucky and unlucky—lucky because I got mental health treatment. I was unlucky because my disorders are PTSD and dissociative identity disorder (DID). The emergence of DID was a lifesaving technique. I learned that I could live through overwhelming experiences by "turning around inside myself," and soon I had a host of friends and loved ones of my own creations. Having DID allowed me to compartmentalize my life—the tasks, developmental stages, reactions, feelings, thoughts, and reality. I learned to put away what I could not deal with so that I could get through the day and keep functioning with a modicum of sanity. DID, my prize possession, was a great skill. I could, in my mind, change myself to fit any situation, provide for other people's needs, avoid threats, and as for the chameleon, change was a great tool for functioning.

This survival technique, like all maneuvers to change reality, became a double-edged sword. The downside of dissociation, like all actions to change internal states by various techniques of avoidance, was that it took on a life of its own. My style of "functioning" was based on using "magical thinking" and the appearance of functioning well to drift through my life. Changing my state by magical thinking replaces my adult consciousness with a child's-eye view, a child's reactions, and a child's feelings, which are out of place. Yesterday's solution is a barrier now. Along with magical shifts in my consciousness come the pain and horror images, thoughts, and feelings, and my deep immersion in "memory hell." Being in memory hell is like being locked in a closet full of feelings and thought patterns from the most torturous times in my life. Themes of abandonment, terror, humiliation, pain-filled body states, and loss fill my vision and cloud my judgment. I walk through life in a 60-year-old body pretending—pretending so well that even I am not aware of the incongruence between being 60 and acting like I am 5 years old.

As a young adult, I had only a few vague recollections about my past. I never knew when or how my dissociation began. Even a month ago, I did not understand the implication of my trauma reaction and how it affected my perceptions, thoughts, feelings, and daily life. I have great shame and humiliation about being in a 60-year-old body with no ability to monitor lapses in time and no way to place things in chronological order. When asked to remember when an event occurred, confusion and embarrassment erupt, and I usually respond by saying, "Well, I believe it was a couple of weeks ago." Often, I wake up to find that I have been able to justify using an abusive tone and questioning of my allies' commitment, integrity, and moral stance because I was triggered.

The ability to divide my consciousness and convince myself that the shift is real began early in my life. I remember witnessing my brother getting shot by my mother. Later, I saw the rape and brutal murder of my best friend. I experienced sexual abuse and torture at the hands of my mother and father. I witnessed the lynching of my uncle. This all occurred before I turned 6 years old. After my baby brother was killed, before my friend died, and before my uncle was killed, my family left our home in Birmingham. We went to live in my grandfather's home in Alabama. I believe my family was running away from questions about the death of my baby brother.

Starting Over

Life had started over. My brothers, my parents, and I never mentioned the name or existence of my brother again. I became best friends with a little white girl, named Paula. We both knew that we could never be seen together. One day, we were playing in the barn, and Paula, my best friend in the world, was killed. Her slaying was brutal, and today my mother's words still haunt me: "See what happens to your friends." I have come to believe that her death occurred because she was White and a needed target for sexual abuse. After Paula was killed, one night while sleeping, I was awakened by yelling and loud bangs on the door. My family was hauled out into the dark and beaten. I was raped before my family. My uncle was tortured and lynched and eviscerated. My heart was broken as a child. As an adult, I get to relive every gut-wrenching episode, try to metabolize that pain, and free myself from the memory by knowing what it was like through the repetition compulsion and then the frantic attempts to undo that come with hypervigilance.

I believe that the level of trauma my parents experienced and their demoralization are directly responsible for the abuse they heaped on my siblings, on me, and on others in their world. My father and mother gave words to high spiritual values and had a core work ethic that informed them. My father worked in construction, and my mother worked as a presser in a laundry and, in her later life, as a home health aide. My mother demonstrated that maintaining your life is the prime task of life. I am a survivor, and I come from a long line of survivors. We survived physically—some of us with hope and love intact but most often not. Like other victims of racism and genocide, I believed that traumatic and abusive relationships were the only model of how to live. Racism and post-slavery oppression created a caustic environment, showing my parents that hope for a better future and rights of Americans to full citizenship seemed bound to remain a theoretical illusion simply because of the color of their skin. The illusion of freedom and acceptance of all within society made the reality all the harder to bear. Like a knife twisting and distorting their soul, words of freedom, equality, and acceptance remained great high-sounding values that never seemed to make their way into their lives.

No Hope for Safety

I came to Boston when I was approaching my sixth birthday, leaving behind my maternal step-grandmother. On arriving in Boston, I became more immersed in living in my head, because I believed that my step-grandmother was all that stood between my death and me. When I entered school, I lost all hope of being safe in the world. School was terrifying because I was never allowed to be around White people in the South, especially after the murder of my best friend on the farm where my grandfather was a sharecropper. Terror interfered with my functioning as I entered school and I saw my teachers and met the principal. They were all White people, and all the kids were Black.

I was basically nonverbal but had a great imagination. Living in my head created an oasis from chaos, terror, and pain created by adults who were sexually abusive and often enraged for reasons that I could not understand. During September of that year, I heard my birth name, "Gloria," for the first time when my mother took me to kindergarten. On entering kindergarten, I already knew how to write my name. My older brother taught me how to make letters and write my name. He was teaching me that the letters meant something. He would say, "Now Fay," because they all called me "Fay," "make a straight line down, like a pole. Now, make a line on the top of the pole like a hat. That is how you make a 'T.' " I learned to hate messing up because my brother was good at everything. My mother loved everything he did. My father liked what he did. My grandparents thought he was so smart. He was everything to all of them. After all, he was lucky. He was a boy. The difference between how my mother looked at him and how she looked at me made me work harder to overcome my primordial defect of being a girl. So I learned I would have to work extra hard to be liked, to become, to finally deserve to be alive. My prized secrets were that I really was better than my brother and that I could do anything as well as my older brother and any boy or man. This notion that I was deemed inferior by all those I loved was critical to my development. I have lived a life of striving and overcoming. I was going to show everyone that I was as good as a boy. Anyone who stated or indicated in any way that I was inferior to a boy because of my gender could count on my angry protestation. Any authority figure making such accusations could count on my secret retribution for what I felt was a most heinous assault against my very being. I tried to do everything that a boy could do. I rebelled against my lot in life because of the unalterable fact that I happened to be a girl.

As the teacher discovered my skills, she made a decision, and I was placed in first grade. Then the tide turned. The teacher's enthrallment with my gifts was short-lived, and I was demoted and returned to kindergarten. This event precipitated seeds of doubt about my intelligence that has followed me all my life. It is not every child who can say she or he was demoted in first grade. My teacher's explanation was that I was extremely "immature." My persistent hysterical crying, flailing about, and screams for my mother led them to conclude that I was very babyish. This first entry into school began to show that my sorrow and pain were deeply entrenched.

Unprotected Prey

When I was 15, my mother and father fought over money, accusations of extramarital affairs, infidelity, and alcohol-related distress. They also fought over my father's excessive attention and sexual abuse of me. I had been an A student, and up until age 15, I had found school to be a sanctuary. At 15, I became terrified of school. I slept little. During the night, I would literally run out of my house to Boston City Hospital. I would sit in the lounge area with sick people who were waiting to see a doctor. I only went to the hospital because I was aware that as a young girl on the streets of Boston, I was still unprotected prey. Every night for months, I ran away after becoming frightened while trying to sleep. Each night, I envisioned that as soon as I fell asleep, a man would come and stand over me. He would wait until my sleep was deep, and when terror peaked and fear of surprise was imminent, I knew he would spring upon me. I knew as sure as I can see the words on this page that he would end my life in torturous ways. It became safer to stay up all night in the emergency room. I slept during the day. I missed a lot of school. I was able to forge notes from my mom and escaped consequences of unexcused absences for almost a year. My physical and emotional state became unmanageable and my distress apparent. I cried for days. I felt so alone, trapped, and abandoned. There was no one I could tell without getting into trouble. I went to school one day and collapsed on the gym floor. I had a miscarriage. My friend Wanda recently told me that I was curled up in a ball on the floor. I was whispering to her, "Wanda, please don't let them come and get me . . . please . . . please!" She cites this as my introduction to the mental health system. All I know is that in 1966, at age 15, I had my first visit with a psychiatrist.

The Promise of Caring

The psychiatrist was a woman who came from another country. She had a heavy accent. I was too shy to tell her that often I did not understand a word she was saying. I wanted to trust her. I immediately acted as if she loved and cared about me even though I did not really know. I was starved for affection and love. I was so lonely I could die. I wanted someone to trust and love so much that any semblance of trustworthiness and any inquiry into what I wanted passed for love and caring. Simple courtesy and proximity with another human being who asked me questions was soothing. These simple acts of kindness and professionalism were the salve and balm that soothed my wounds emanating from torture, abandonment, and neglect. I learned to glean hope and security from her gestures, pseudo-trust, and questions that I thought were enough for me to prove that she loved me. The professionals became surrogate family with all the attending loyalties and conflicts, and later, therapeutic relationships were enough.

At age 16, I entered a public psychiatric institution and started on my path of receiving professional services in lieu of mutual loving nurturing relationships, with the goal of reducing pain and fear. I was terrified on entering Boston State Hospital, but from the first moment that adults asked me what I thought, what had hurt me, and what I needed, I was hooked on treatment. The focus was on me, and people said they wanted to help me feel better. I have stayed in mental health treatment for 39 years because I settled for the promise of caring. Professional caring was, and still is, the only caring that has felt safe enough for me to allow in my life. This is the only caring that I felt I could get.

My treatment for symptoms of mental illness has been successful in that it allowed me to go to Tufts University and learn from five graduate programs, even though I have not completed a master's degree. I have been able to work and live on the periphery of life, settling for the love of my therapist and an apartment, and substituting work and getting well for getting a life. If appearance was the test of having fully recovered, I often passed with flying colors. As for most of us with a mental illness, recovery is full of relapses and recurrences of illness. The journey of recovery is full of moratoriums and plateaus in between mountains and valleys. The journey becomes less tumultuous for most, but eruptions of symptoms can never be ruled out. Life with mental illness is precarious and a terrible predicament in which to find oneself.

Believe Me

Think of what I have told you about my early life: the accounts of witnessing the death of my brother before age 6, the murder and rape of my best friend, the sexual abuse and torture I experienced, and the lynching of my uncle. Some doctors find my statements unbelievable and preposterous. One doctor even chided me saying, "Now Gloria, think about what you are saying. Don't you believe that the police would have intervened?" I would laugh except I know that his thinking is caused by the fact that most people have forgotten what life was like for Black people in 1955. This lack of historical knowledge, paired with a pervasive need to "not know" the pain of racism and family dysfunction, is extremely prevalent in our society. It always feels like a personal affront when helpers replace my real-life experiences with their theories of what "really" went on. This not being believed simply because what happened to me is out of the experience of my professional friends continually causes me the most pain in my life. The questioning of the truth of my experience occurs because my professional friends believe in the severity of the impact of my trauma and because their training requires them to dissect every statement I make in an attempt to find the errors in my thinking and judgment. This sophisticated way of "nulling" and "voiding" my experience and replacing it with theoretical guessing is really based only on the fantasy in their heads. These interactions always leave me feeling isolated, discriminated against, and demoralized, leaving me hopeless to ever gain credibility when my life experience is diminished because it is so radically different from that of most people.

I realize that once I entered into the contract of therapy and treatment, like a binding contract with the devil—it is perpetual, and its course is certain. It is rare that anyone who enters mental health treatment will ever escape or ever lose the devastating moniker and attributes associated with the status of being a "mental patient." After years of faithful immersion in and commitment to therapeutic treatment, I find myself left feeling tricked, deceived, and abandoned. I believe these feelings are primarily the result of my feelings of being hurt by powerful administrators within the mental health system and worsened when my brother Junior, at age 46, died unnecessarily because of the negligence of staff within a vendor agency of the mental health system.

My interface with medical health providers has added an additional burden to my recovery. I am older and require medical care from doctors who stigmatize and humiliate me because I have been diagnosed as "mentally ill," then react with anger, hostility, and retribution to my complaints about their hurtful behavior. My other professional helpers have not responded to my pleas to help me access basic rights to humane and decent treatment in medical settings. All these factors culminate in leaving me with profound feelings of despair. I missed out on structuring a life that supports and sustains me after the 9-to-5 professional friends go home. My previous therapists all said that my past traumas were too devastating for me ever to marry. Therapy and the psychiatric hospitals have created a cocoon that kept me in isolation, with a fear of living. The stigma of being an older mental patient now fills me with sadness.

My lot in America meant that my life was going to be difficult. The additional burden of abuse, 39 years of mental health treatment, and an active, curious, and generally very fine mind left me disillusioned. With the awareness of what could have been, my losses test my resilience, hope, and faith. I now exist without my many disguises, my alternate selves, and without the benefit of a loving support system. This life of having to make lemonade out of lemons created habitual responses of resilience that now keep me on the planet, however unhappy, and striving for better. My personal existential crisis is how do I endure, do no harm, and wait—after all I have been through? I still have hope in the goodness of people.

An Equal Playing Field

At Boston University Center for Psychiatric Rehabilitation Center, I met people who happened to be professionals. They were outrageously radical professionals. Their theories of how to help were not based on seeking out what is wrong with me. They did not think that it was impossible that I was their equal. They did not label me defective or tell me how sick I was. They spoke of my having options and a valued role in life. They told me that my inability to succeed was caused by barriers. They had requirements and expectations. They made plans based on my needs, wants, and preferences, requiring me to make choices. They believed that I would achieve and grow. They inspired me and sided with my resilience, leaving

BOX 11.1 Effective Therapy

Effective therapy is only as good as the quality of the relationship between the therapist and the consumer, paired with a "goodness of fit" between the need of the consumer and the specific therapeutic tools used. My therapy was effective or "good" only when there was collaboration between my therapist and myself. My most effective therapist knew the difference between her intention to help and my perception of being helped. She understood that my perception of being helped is a subjective state of feeling helped that can be discerned only by me.

My therapist is extremely respectful. She knows that any attempts to help me must be based on my stated wishes, desires, and needs. She allows me to choose, to take risks, and sometimes even to fail. The intention to "help," "being helpful," or "giving help" is only one part of the helping process. ***The "end" of the helping process is achieved when the person being helped feels "helped."***

me feeling energized, ready to act in my own behalf, and hopeful for a better outcome. Dr. Spaniol mentored me and gave me a valued role facilitating recovery groups and co-facilitating statewide workshops. He provided knowledge and skills to increase my competence, and pairing this with doable expectations, he increased my overall life functioning and satisfaction exponentially.

I now have a newly found identity of educator. This was a dream of mine when, as a little girl, I played school with my childhood friends. These experiences allowed me a glimpse into the land of being accepted and well respected. And now, I am forever changed, and giving up is simply harder because of them. Their use of the universal concept that difficulties are caused by barriers took me out of the land of a defective human being failing to function and placed me squarely back in the land of human beings striving to overcome environmental obstacles without judgments about my intellect, character, or motivation. I was on an equal playing field with all others. I was a person who needed help, knowledge, skills, and support. I am not an inferior being treated by superiors. Many of the conflicts and power struggles embedded in traditional therapy are no longer an issue. This subtle and exquisite shift in perspective allows practitioners to have a better chance of greeting a real live person rather than a collection of symptoms.

I am an equal partner with responsibilities to participate to ensure a good outcome. As a partner with the practitioner, I do not sit passively by, awaiting my rescue. The knowledge that my counselors at Boston University cared created a feeling in me that their theories about me, their interventions, and the specific treatment outcomes were never as healing as their personhood, their stated desire and intention. Without their genuine curiosity that allowed them to listen, their respect that kept them from judging, and the high regard for my individualism that allowed them to tolerate me being me, I could not have withstood facing my woundedness and despair. The words "I don't always know how to help but I really want to help you" feel like balm on an open sore and soothe me in ways that I can only approximate by saying, "It healed my soul." This is one of the many supreme gifts of human connection that I have found only in my relationship with my therapist and my counselors at Boston University.

The Phoenix Rising

I have had a lot of experiences that showed me how to "make meaning" and transform injury and devastation into hopeful scenarios. Routinely affirming hopefulness and habitually responding to devastation with resilience are skills that helped me to transform evil and rise from the ashes. "The phoenix rising" is my life metaphor. As life plunges me into the depths of despair, I look inside and find a light of hope to try and live well. I have repeatedly risen from the ashes, and with my faith intact, I can envision no other response. The latest series of life challenges have come in medical treatment settings.

After 10 years of struggle to find a physician who would not attribute my symptoms of shortness of breath and periods of rapid irregular heart beat to PTSD and anxiety, I was able to get medical treatment because of a diagnosis of atrial fibrillation and congestive heart failure. Three brothers have died before the age of 60 years old for similar symptoms. My hope is that one day health care disparities will be non-existent and professionalism is demonstrated routinely in health care settings.

The anonymity of health care providers when they are alone in the room with patients reveals that a great chasm exists between providers who value their role as healers and life-support people and those who are in this position of privilege for all the wrong reasons. My life is a great journey with many challenges, and a huge number of inspiring people who go the extra mile and make every day a welcoming experience for people with histories similar as mine. I have learned to be vigilant, a skeptic and despite all attempts to act counter to fear-based reactions in the presence of others, fear and feeling done too are my default settings. This makes trusting others too fragile. Eventually, even the most trusted individuals in my life have their actions and their motives processed through my feelings of being victimized or potentially hurt. This level of skepticism is very hard on relationships. This default is something I live with and in periods of renewal, I challenge. My dreams of friends, love, and connections that are genuinely felt as reliable and predictable are deferred and hoped for. I don't mind this. My hope springs eternal and is part of my life force that makes the journey more worthwhile than anticipated endpoints. I truly wish

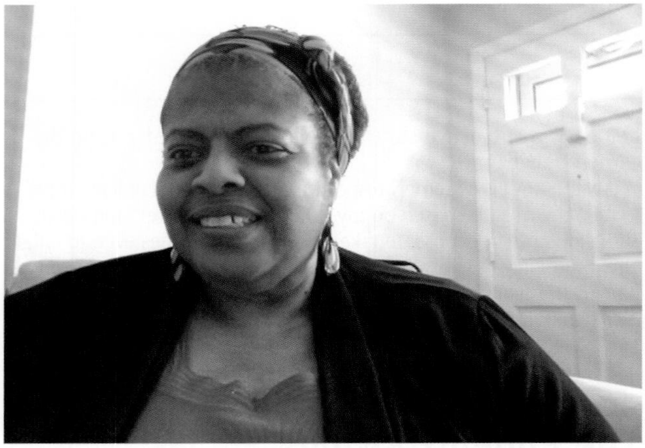

FIGURE 11.1 Gloria Dickerson.

that you can reframe your disappointments in life's lot in ways that keep you on the planet in the pursuit of dreams.

My Life Today

The need for safety still outweighs my desire to make needed changes. This is my lot. I feel resigned and still harbor hope for a miracle, some altered state where relationships do not strike the fear of God in my soul and mind. I hope that I can place my trauma in a context that allows the past to be a foundation, a springboard into my future even at such a late date.

I have endured a life of injustice and mistreatment that was made bearable by my religious upbringing and years of therapy. My religious upbringing was both extremely painful and exquisitely inspiring. The deep, profound hope that is embedded in the words and concepts of the Black Church and Bible gave me a foundation of hope that serves as a compass and, although sorely tested, has never been destroyed. The idea that we are all connected, obligated, and encompassed in a mission greater than each of us gives my life purpose and meaning. I have tried to turn away from my faith and connectedness many times, but life always brought me back to center (Figure 11.1).

The ability to make choices has been critical to my relearning skills of self-reliance and safety when engaging with others. Engagement and building trust have always been elusive concepts. For me, trusting a therapist begins with warm greetings, kindness, and acknowledgment of my rights as an adult. I can endure conflicts, misgivings, errors, hurts, and slights if I feel connected and valued as an adult.

Conclusion

My therapy, though freeing, was very concentrated and focused. Unfortunately for me, all of us forgot one little thing: a therapeutic relationship is an assist to learning to establish other relationships that become a source of primary sustenance. Therapeutic relationships should never become a substitute for intimate, loving family and friends. Life is bigger than the therapy relationship. Stabilization and maintenance are great goals to awaken hurt souls. However, once an individual grasps and mourns the losses and pain that brought her or him into therapy, then what? We need to remember that the primary pain associated with having severe mental illness and trauma often comes out of failed and abusive relationships. My primary "disconnect" emerged over time. Like a stealth bomber, silent at first, it soared in the night and then swooped down, blowing my insides into shards, simply changing the course of my life forever.

In addition to religion, therapy and now sustainable work are primary sources for hope in the goodness of people, for staying alive, and for trying to find a way to live well. Work has become a huge life support. During times of severe depression and feelings of depletion, I rely on my work and my success as the Recovery Specialist at the Center for Social Innovation in Needham to inspire me to embrace my legacy of responding to impending defeat with resilience and tenacious hold on life. I get to create all day long. I write recovery curriculum and Website articles and facilitate national training on moving from consumer involvement to integration and social inclusion. The expert help of my therapist has helped to reduce the effects of parental mistreatment, torture, and sexual and physical abuse.

BOX 11.2 Essential Qualities of Effective Therapists

There are some basic and essential qualities of all effective therapists regardless of theoretical orientation. Therapists must like people, access the ability to personally censor, be curious, respect difference, create a repertoire of skills, and have the ability to maintain commitment over time. Therapists must learn to acknowledge personal biases, avoid harm, and use their personal self-knowledge to educate for change. Skilled therapists use all of their knowledge, skills, and personal gifts and deficits gleaned from their own life journey and operate from the position of being a change agent and healer. It is not enough to be correct theoretically. Therapists must be skilled human beings who care about and like others. The therapists I love have all these qualities.

For additional resources on the subjects discussed in this chapter, visit http://thePoint.lww.com/Willard-Spackman12e.

CHAPTER 12

The Privilege of Giving Care

Donald M. Murray

Note: This narrative was last updated when published in 2009.

"I don't know who he is, but every morning and afternoon, a man comes to see me and he is awfully nice." The woman who said those words was Minnie Mae, my wife of 54 years, and I have lived by those words in the months ever since she broke through her dementia on a Friday afternoon and told the hospice nurse, "No more water. No food. No pills."

Fourteen years earlier, when she was 72, she was given her annual physical. There seemed to be none of the surprises during this exam that had tested Minnie Mae's courage, sense of humor, and ability to survive pain in the past. The doctor's calm and professional "hum's, uh-huh's, mmm's" during the exam reassured us. The doctor studied the lab reports—another comforting "mmm"—and, smiling, our doctor went to the examining room door, turned and told my wife, "You have Parkinson's," stepped out into the corridor, and shut the door behind him.

This not a story of "the elderly" and the global difficulties and pleasures of old age. I have no theories. No statistics. I have not read books, studies, or journal articles on aging. This is simply an account of the final intimacy and love of one couple facing the challenge of Parkinson's, a long-lasting fatal disease for which there is no cure. Like so many of us in our eighties, Minnie Mae was an experienced patient. Before this last illness, she had suffered life-threatening toxemia with our first child, an appendix attack with three separate infections, an emergency hysterectomy, nine—I believe—eye operations, and skin and breast cancer.

We didn't really know what Parkinson's was, but we knew that it wasn't good. There seem to be two types of elderly patients: those who worry and predict and research about what might happen and those like us who simply face each "surprise" with as much acceptance, courage, and toughness as we can summon. We take life a step at a time. Now we had a new challenge: Parkinson's.

We drove immediately to my cardiologist, who referred us to a neurologist. That didn't help as much as we hoped. We wanted to learn how to treat Parkinson's, how it might evolve, how it would affect our daily lives and our future. Instead of answers, we ran into the sort of professional terminology debate that interests doctors but not us.

Our neurologist carried on a debate with himself in front of us. Minnie Mae might have "parkinsonism," or she might have Parkinson's itself. It was never clear what the difference was and how it might affect Minnie

Mae's life. Would Parkinson's or parkinsonism move toward death at a different speed? We were never able to understand the difference, except we were told that a blood pressure drug Minnie Mae had previously used was associated with "parkinsonism" or "Parkinson's" in about 25% of the patients who were prescribed that medication. Minnie Mae (a direct person who like direct answers) asked, "What caused my parkinsonism or Parkinson's, or whatever it is?" The doctor answered, "I'll know when I slice your brain."

Looking back, we seemed remarkably innocent and calm. The unspoken medical message was that aging is tough, but so were we (Figure 12.1).

Wet your pants?

"I have many older patients who have that problem."

Tremor getting worse?

"As you age, you'll have doctors' penmanship."

Stagger?

"That happens. My father was a minister, but when he grew old, he walked like he had two too many."

Bent neck?

"Arthritis. It comes with age."

The neurologist prescribed Sinemet. Minnie Mae took it at lunch and felt better within the hour. The specialist may have been a cold fish, but there was a pill for whatever she had. Our personalities, our genes, and our personal experience with death and illness had taught us not to seek problems. Trouble would come in its time, and we would face it head on. I think this pragmatic stoicism is typical of our Depression and World War II generation, but I also believe that many of my generation develop a passive fatalism together with the belief that the more challenges they face and survive, the stronger they become. There may be something to this. We were stoics, steeling ourselves to confront medical problems and do what was necessary to deal with them. We were not happy with our neurologist's personality, but the pills worked. He must know something even if he didn't know how to relate to his patients. Then he planned, because Minnie Mae was doing so well, to prescribe a new, more powerful drug.

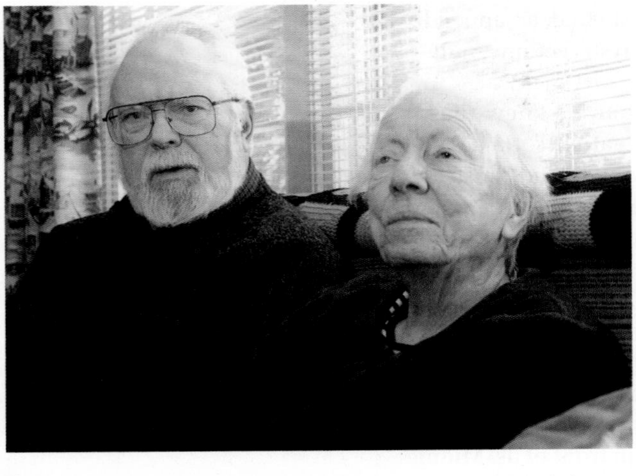

FIGURE 12.1 Don and Minnie Mae Murray in their home. (Courtesy of Donald M. Murray.)

At that moment, we experienced a fortunate coincidence. I was invited to speak at Beth Israel Hospital in Boston because of my *Boston Globe* column on aging. After I spoke, a reader talked to me about the column and mentioned that she was a neurologist. I asked what doctor she would recommend to a member of her family with Parkinson's, and she referred us to a kind doctor who has been called the best neurologist in Boston. He was a listener and an explainer who told us they had tested the new drug our neurologist planned to give Minnie Mae and that it would have irrevocably damaged her brain. We remained his patient until Minnie Mae could no longer make the trip from New Hampshire to Beth Israel.

When we asked him about the future—we prided ourselves on being realists—he explained that each case was so different that there was no way to predict the future. Furthermore, he told us that there was only "treatment." We did not shy away from his diagnosis, ask God why me, search the Internet for miracles, or join one of the therapy groups that help so many. We just did what had to be done hour by hour. I learned new skills, knowing that new demands would be made on those skills in the years ahead.

We learned that the most efficient way to help Minnie Mae up after a fall was to have me plant my size 15 feet on hers to keep her feet from skidding away, then, taking her hands in mine, lift, trying to keep the pressure on each equal. Sometimes it took many attempts to get Minnie Mae on her feet. She used her favorite curse, "Shit fire and save matches," and many times we sat on the floor laughing at our clumsy failures. And when we couldn't get her up, we called for help from a young neighbor.

We survived by our own black humor. "You used to struggle getting my bra off, now you have trouble getting it on." We continued to go out to eat as long as it was possible. We liked The Olive Garden with its sliding chairs. One day, driving to the restaurant, Minnie Mae said, "We should bring a bottle of wine." As she traveled further and further into the confusion of dementia, she kept her humor and I kept mine. She was never a "patient" but the woman I loved.

As the disease inevitably grew worse, we realized that our geography had changed. We avoided stairs without railings, sloping sidewalks, uneven surfaces of grass and sand, and wind that could push Minnie Mae sideways. I still tell people I am with to watch the curb.

The days passed, as a poet said, like a giant water wheel that tumbled slowly, one bucket after another. I never questioned my obligation, and it did not feel like duty. It was another stage in our lives. The most difficult tasks—bladder and bowel accidents, tumbles, falls, getting Minnie Mae to take her pills—became further intimacies in our long life together.

I tried to keep Minnie Mae's life as normal as possible. A friend of mine with good intentions took over all the cooking, shopping, and cleaning. He was caring—too caring. Minnie Mae lost all purpose in her life. She was unneeded, and her mental health suffered.

I helped Minnie Mae with the shopping, but she was in charge. For years, she scooted between the supermarket aisles at full speed with the help of a grocery cart. She had been a great cook, but her meals became ordinary or worse. She knew it, but it was important that she was still in charge of the kitchen. Eating out allowed her to see different people and the beautiful New Hampshire countryside. For a long time, Minnie Mae could still shop for groceries and attend University of New Hampshire hockey games, loudly coaching from the stands far longer than I thought possible. And she would stagger across the lawn with a cane, trying to work in her beloved garden (Figure 12.2).

All the time, I continued to write my column, books, and poetry. I needed to lose myself in the exercise of my craft and its deep concentration. Novelist Bernard Malamud explained, "If it is winter in the book, spring surprises me, when I look up."

It was tragic to see Minnie Mae's world grow small, but neither of us focused on the past. We focused on what could we do now—this morning, this afternoon, this evening. My daughters and I tried to treat Minnie Mae as the acerbic woman with the biting dry humor she had always been.

Many elderly people refuse to allow help to come into their home when they need it. That is a mistake. We were fortunate in having Dot Benson, who came in two or three times a week. She continued to be our cleaning woman, but as the Parkinson's increased, so did Dot's contributions to the quality of our life. She became more friend than employee. She took over the tasks that Minnie Mae could no longer do and I did not have the time to do if I was to continue to be a publishing writer. She also was a therapist, bringing the world to Minnie Mae, whose horizon grew closer and closer. She gave each of us the physical and emotional support we needed. When a couple she was caring for passed away, my psychiatric social worker daughter said, "Grab her. Right now. Get those hours." I resisted, I now recognize, because I didn't want to admit that Minnie Mae was in the early stages of dying. We needed Dot, and I am grateful for my daughter's command.

As Minnie Mae needed more and more care, a daughter, with the best of intentions, hired a team of additional caretakers. That didn't work. They didn't arrive on time or arrived ahead of time, they brought food we didn't need or like, they asked for advances on their pay that they didn't return, and worst of all, they talked to Minnie Mae in baby talk. Dot Benson was just the opposite in every way, and we increased her hours when they became available and then placed her on salary. I was 80 years old when Minnie Mae died. Dot stayed on to help me by taking over my bookkeeping and by providing computer

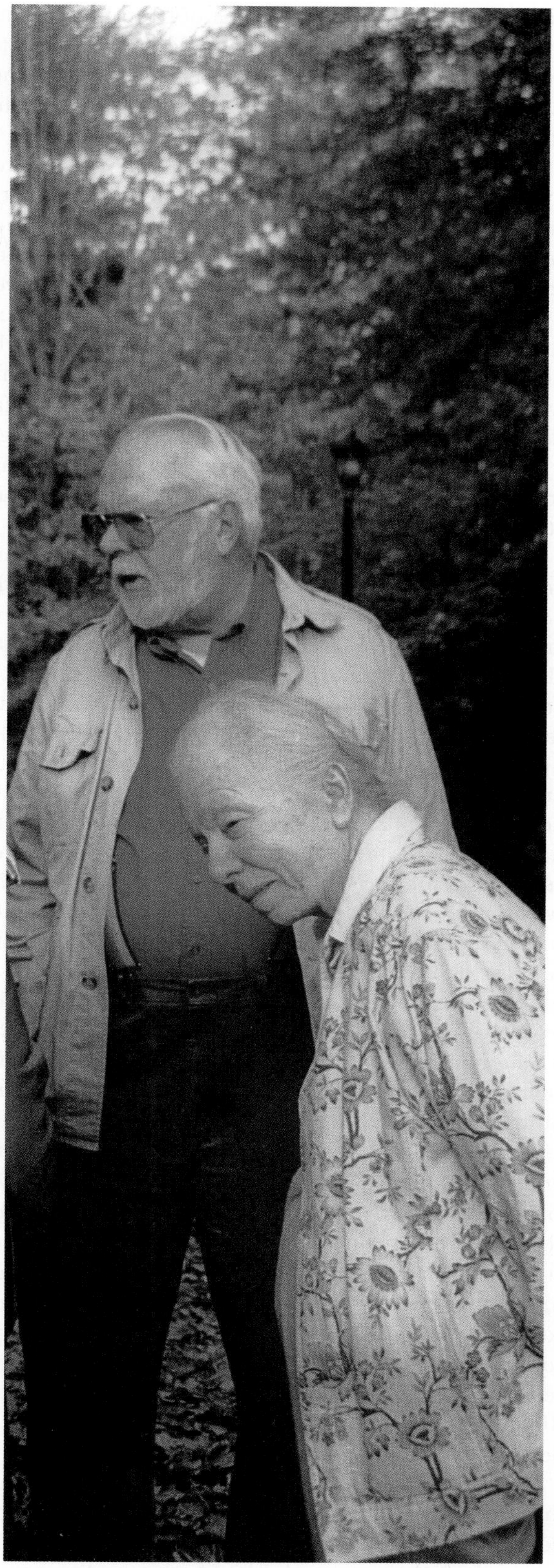

FIGURE 12.2 Don and Minnie Mae Murray in their garden. (Courtesy of Donald M. Murray.)

assistance. She makes an offering of good humor each time she shows up. No cheeriness, no baby talk, just a down-to-earth model in how to live a life with acceptance while making the most of each day. I can't imagine my life before and after Minnie Mae's death without her help.

The years of care became normal and accelerated at the same time. I was uncomfortable with the term *demands*. There were no demands, just the increasing need for closeness and sharing. In my case, the time I had in combat as a paratrooper helped. At the front, you do what needs to be done, no question, no evasion, no excuses. The compliments of friends and neighbors who said how wonderful I was embarrassed and puzzled me. I was not wonderful. I loved Minnie Mae, simple as that. We had enjoyed better, and with the death of our daughter in 1977, we had survived worse. Who else should take care of her but the man who met her when she was a substitute blind date 54 years before?

I was fortunate to be retired from the University and had the time to care for her as I continued to write at home. Caring for someone with Parkinson's and so many other chronic diseases is a matter of small tasks—delivering pills on time, changing clothes, getting to the doctor—that accumulate so slowly that you hardly notice their increase. We had to develop our own tricks for this unplanned new trade of caregiver: how we could brace our feet against each other's so I could lift her efficiently and painlessly after inevitable falls, how a gentle hand under the armpit (developed from a not so gentle hold I learned as a military policeman) could tell Minnie Mae I was there, ready to help if she needed it, how I could wake in the night and watch her blanket so I could tell if she was still breathing.

We were, of course, both patients. She had to learn to protect her feisty, aggressive approach of life. I had to tune my Type A personality to a C while caring for someone who was living in slow motion. I had to learn not to invade her territory and, for example, take over the cooking early on. It became gradually more difficult for her, but cooking was her pride. I could not take it away from her. We had to discover how to calm or sustain each other at moments of terror or despair. When humor or yet another "Law & Order" rerun didn't work, a trip to get a dish of ice cream did. Ginger ice cream was the most therapeutic. Minnie Mae refused to worry about how her more obvious handicaps might disturb people, and we ate out a lot. I should add that everyone, wait staff and fellow customers alike, offered her respect, kindness, good humor, and help when necessary.

I suffered more stress than I felt or admitted. I did what needed to be done, but when my daughters, close friends, and doctors urged me to take care of myself, I shrugged off their counsel. I had had a cardiac bypass years before, and when I felt some heart symptoms, I went to my cardiologist, who examined me and said he would see me in 3 months. The symptoms continued, so a few days later I arranged for Dot to be with Minnie Mae and called 911 at 3 in the morning. Hours after I arrived with flashing lights at the hospital, I had a new cardiologist, and the next day I had six stents placed in the arteries near my heart. There must have been more stress than I realized.

I am surprised to find I miss the caregiving, now it is over, while enjoying the freedom to browse in a bookstore or play my music at top volume. In some way I cannot yet understand, the erotic intimacy of our first years seemed to flow into the intimacy of helping Minnie Mae dress and undress. There was nothing we did not know about each other and no moment when we were not available to the other. My job was to keep Minnie Mae from feeling shame or embarrassment as her body betrayed her. It is what she would have done for me.

The grand landscape of Parkinson's was fearful. But the day-to-day tasks that became essential as we traveled this landscape became intimate and appropriate. These were not years of hope. There are pills that can slow Parkinson's, but there is no cure. We had to accept the reality, but that did not make them dark years. When Minnie Mae started to call her cane a ladder, we laughed. No bother. I didn't correct her but simply brought the cane. Now I realize that dementia had arrived a long time before we admitted it. This was not denial but simply that we kept adapting to the language as we had adjusted to our daughters' first efforts to speak, which only we could understand. I would have expected an incapacitating horror to see the brain of such a smart, quick, opinionated woman change. Of course, it was what we had both feared the most, but it wasn't like that at all.

There are many marriages within a long marriage: no children, three children, moves to new cities and states, promotions and firing, manuscript acceptance and rejection, the children leaving, retirement, and now Parkinson's. Eventually, Minnie Mae's neurologist suggested that she be examined at a psychiatric and geriatric facility at a nearby hospital. As soon as we arrived and I saw Minnie Mae with the nine other patients, I knew we had entered a new territory some time before. Minutes after the chief psychiatrist began what would be a long examination, he turned to me and said I must activate my power of attorney. It was a chilling moment. After days of tests, it was clear that she would not come home. The fear we all have of ending our days filed away in a nursing home had come true for her. They sent her to a nursing home connected with the hospital that was as bad as any I have seen. I was beside Minnie Mae the first day when she was strapped in a chair while two nurses had a fistfight in front of us. She said, "Get me out of here." I answered, "We certainly will."

Dot and I raced from one facility to another in a day and half. Obviously, we should have visited more of them early on, but our "one step at a time" policy kept us from looking too far ahead. Perhaps we were right. Parkinson's varies radically between patients, and neither the doctors nor we could predict the care she would need. Luckily, we found a small assisted living facility—32 patients maximum—7 miles from our home. Minnie Mae had said she would kill herself before she would go to a nursing home, but she moved in without complaint. She seemed, despite the dementia, to know she needed this level of care.

When Minnie Mae was admitted to Kirkwood Corners, an outstanding assisted living facility, a nurse told me that my wife's dementia produced fascinating fantasies. She said Minnie Mae had told the nurse that she had been one of the first people to work in the Pentagon, that she had relayed messages from Secretary of War George Marshall to General Walter Bedell Smith in London, who then told General Dwight D. Eisenhower what to do. My wife added that she was a professional mezzo-soprano who had soloed in Washington, D.C. and Boston. She said she had Q Clearance, the highest possible security status. She added that she might lose that status, since she was, according to the Associated Press, the first person in the country to get people on the sidewalk to sign a petition calling for President Richard Nixon's impeachment.

I told the nurse it was all true, not the product of dementia. The staff got to know her as a woman of accomplishment and not just another patient. "I don't know why these people treat me so well," said my wife, who had promised to kill herself if she had to go to a nursing home. The staff at Kirkwood Corners treated all their patients with respect, but Minnie Mae felt she got special attention.

Understandably, many dedicated doctors, nurses, therapists, aides, and the blessed people from hospice focus on the patient. The care is intense and continual. They are patients, men and woman, who have chronic and terminal illnesses that demand care and love. The Kirkwood Corners staff realized that the patients see themselves not so much as they are but what they were: cabinetmakers, soldiers, parents and grandparents, lawyers, bakers, secretaries, corporate executives, gardeners, researchers, gamblers, teachers, salespeople.

If those who treat the elderly get to know the worlds in which they have been productive, then respect is easy, and all the treatments are given in the context of their entire lives. During my bypass surgery, I was seen as a combat paratrooper who was familiar with pain. It helped me to return, with the staff, to another life.

Minnie Mae's father had been a baker, and when she opened an imaginary bakery in the basement of Kirkwood Corners, the cook discussed recipes as if the business really existed. Staff members took care of Minnie Mae's imaginary pack of strawberry dogs. Office staff helped with flight schedules when she had to fly to London on a secret mission for the CIA. They treated her as if she had Q Clearance. Minnie Mae was obviously happier than at home. She had better care than we could provide, and she was not isolated, as she had become at home. She would watch the daily parade of staff, residents, and visitors with some understanding and a great deal of amusement.

And how did I feel visiting her twice a day? I put aside the larger picture, as I had in combat, and focused entirely on the woman I loved. She recognized me less and less, but when I held her hand, she would give a sudden, tight squeeze, and I knew that somewhere in her clotted brain was an "I love you."

What did I learn from the years of increasing caregiving? There is as much intimacy, caring, and love at the end of a lifetime together as when we first discovered each other and grew our lives together, perhaps more. An elderly couple facing a long struggle with a terminal illness needs a calm, detailed explanation of illness. They do not need evasions. They have lived a long life together

BOX 12.1 Now and Then: Friends Caring and Sharing Show the Way

Donald M. Murray

For those of us who are introspective, life is a continuous exploration into the self, where we hope to find the person we are and the person we may become. Of course, the apple does not fall far from the tree, and we discover we have become a mixed breed of our parents, grandparents, uncles, and aunts. I found this discouraging. I had thought I had made my escape.

Now I accept my genes but imagine I have a tuning dial so that I can adjust their instincts and standards to the life, far different than theirs, I have constructed. This new life has been created by friends who have seen me as I have not yet been able to see myself. With Yankee respect, they have mostly kept their distance, but when they have spoken, or touched a shoulder, or given a smile of encouragement, it has been important to me.

When we lost our daughter, Lee, at 20, it was the subtle but sturdy support of friends that got us through those first years. They saw us as strong when we felt weak. They said we had done more than enough, when we felt we had done far too little. They gave us a future when we thought there was none.

And then came the years of Minnie Mae's Parkinson's. We attended to the hour-by-hour physical demands of living, and then the dementia arrived, and again it was friends who supported and guided me. I often felt like a huge ship being nudged into port by friendly tugs.

These friends and neighbors, too many to name, were there when I began a new life alone. First they eliminated much of the alone with invitations and visits. They approved future relationships before I had imagined them. They suggested small steps of independence and supported me when I took them.

And what have I learned? To pass friendship on. To speak out, to touch, to be there when others need me.

Donald M. Murray, "Now and Then: Friends Caring and Sharing Show the Way." The Boston Globe, December 29, 2006, reprinted with permission.

and are usually tougher than they—or you—think. Truth is better, no matter how hard it is, than the imagination of the patient and gossip about the disease related by friends. What else did I learn?

- Don't yank. Minnie Mae was tugged and painfully hauled up from her falls by many caring passersby. I learned to allow her to do all she could and then be nearby to help if she needed it: hand barely touching her armpit tells her that help is at hand—if SHE needs it.
- Share some of yourself. Minnie Mae was delighted to hear stories about children, grandchildren, and dogs.
- Do not correct someone with dementia, saying, "That didn't happen in Atlanta but Utica." They can't understand, and what difference does it make anyway?

Those of us who find ourselves as caregivers will discover that we have strengths and skills of which we were not aware. What I did and every other caregiver does is done not out of duty, responsibility, and obligation but, above all, love.

Suddenly one Friday afternoon, Minnie Mae's dementia lifted, and she gave the staff clear orders: "No pills. No food. No water." It is what she had wanted, documented in writing, and my daughters and I felt she had the right to die her way, in command to the end. Hospice and the Kirkwood Corner staff were experienced, loving, and professional. Minnie Mae's daughters and I were with her most of the 11 days it took her to sleep away her life. She was treated with dignity, and she suffered no pain. I was holding her hand when she gave one last quick puff of air and was gone.

Afterword

On January 2, 2007, shortly after completing this chapter, Donald M. Murray died while visiting friends. He was an Emeritus Professor of English at the University of New Hampshire. He won the Pulitzer Prize for editorial writing in 1954, and wrote the weekly column "Now and Then" for the *Boston Globe*, which explored his reactions to the process of aging. He also published memoirs, novels, short stories, poetry, and textbooks on the writing process. I asked him to write this chapter because he was a well-known faculty member at the University of New Hampshire. I was acquainted with his work because I had attended several of his writing workshops and knew a number of his former students who revered his contribution to their education and careers. Over the years, I purchased several of his books on writing and his memoirs. Every Tuesday morning I looked for his column, "Now and Then," in the *Boston Globe*.

It was only after his death that I realized how many people he influenced through his teaching, mentorship, and writing. Many of the letters to the editor detailed the personal connection people felt to Don and Minnie Mae from his columns. Many of his former students are newspaper editors, writers, and teachers. He submitted his last column to the *Boston Globe* on December 29th, just a few days before his death. We have reprinted it here as it represents much of his grace and character.

—Elizabeth Crepeau

For additional resources on the subjects discussed in this chapter, visit http://thePoint.lww.com/Willard-Spackman12e.

CHAPTER 13

Experiences with Disability

Stories from Ecuador

Kate Barrett

LEARNING OBJECTIVES

After reading this chapter, you will be able to:

1. Analyze how different aspects of culture influence the experience of disability
2. Explore the potential power of narrative in the context of occupational therapy
3. Explain how context influences the experience of disability

OUTLINE

Gracias

As the listener, interpreter, and translator of these narratives, I would like to begin by expressing my deepest gratitude to Maria, Horacio, Maura, and Don Ulvio for sharing their stories with me. I am in awe of how willing each was to share his or her story in order to contribute to the education of the occupational therapy profession. Each has a moving story; each offers a unique perspective and teaches us something about the experience of living with disability in Ecuador. I traveled to Ecuador to learn from people with disabilities and listen to their stories. These four individuals were chosen because they represent different life stages, different disabilities, and were willing and wanting to share their stories. I listened; wrote what I heard; and, because these are their stories, provided each with an opportunity to provide additions, deletions, and corrections to ensure that these stories honestly and accurately represent their experience. Each narrative below has been read and approved by the person or family described. They are the true authors of this chapter.

Introduction

Statistics about Ecuador

Ecuador is located in South America on the west coast, just north of Peru and south of Colombia (Figure 13.1). With a population of almost 15 million, 38% of the population lives below the national poverty line. Most people speak the official language, Spanish, yet many indigenous also or only

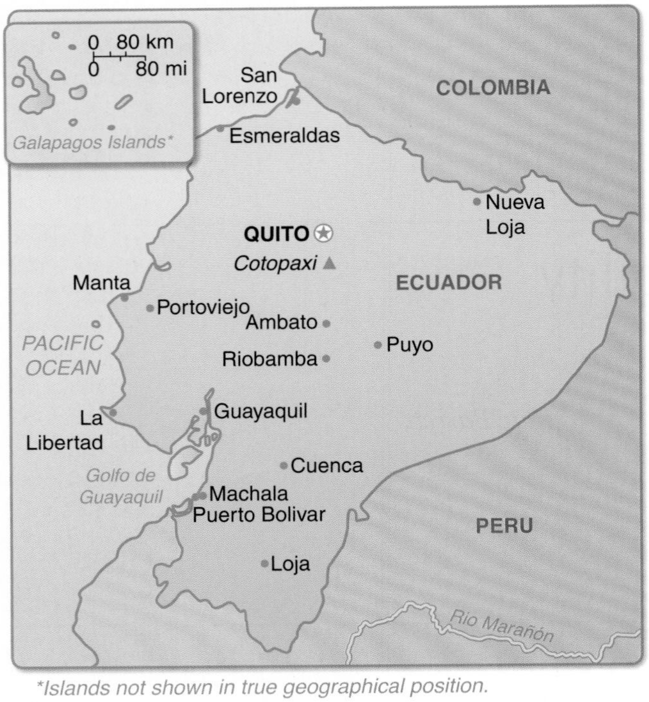

FIGURE 13.1 Map of Ecuador.

speak Quichua, the Ecuadorian dialect of Quechua. The average income for a family is $4,000 per year. The population is made up of a mix of mestizo, indigenous, Afro-Ecuadorian, and European descendants. Sixty percent of the population lives in urban areas. The Amazon tropical forest is sparsely populated, with only 3% of the population living there (U.S. Department of State, 2011).

In the late 1990s, Ecuador moved from using its own money, the sucre, to using the U.S. dollar. This caused an economic crisis, and many Ecuadorians emigrated to the United States and Europe between 2000 and 2001. It is estimated that there are 1 to 2 million Ecuadorians living abroad (U.S. Department of State, 2011).

According to CONADIS (n.d.) (the National Advisory Council for Persons with Disabilities in Ecuador), as many as 13.2% of the total population of Ecuador have some type of disability (as defined by the World Health Organization). Interestingly, Lenin Moreno, Vice President of Ecuador, uses a wheelchair. Ecuador has progressive laws, but enforcement of those laws is lacking. Ecuador has signed several international documents regarding the human rights of persons with disabilities (Table 13.1). Historically, assistance for persons with disabilities was dependent on a charitable model. Slowly, since the 1950s, the models have been shifting away from charity and toward a rights-based model (CONADIS, n.d.).

According to the Center for International Rehabilitation (CIR), as many as 40% of children with disabilities do not attend school in Ecuador. Unemployment for people with disabilities who could be gainfully employed is as high as 70%. Not surprisingly, due to the significant value for family life held in Ecuador, over 90% of persons with disabilities live with their families. Persons with disabilities in Ecuador continue to experience physical, psychological, and sexual abuse. Some people with disabilities are forced to beg on the streets in order to raise money for their families (CIR, n.d.).

Through efforts to improve the quality of life for people with disabilities in Ecuador, the country has established several goals. Businesses who employ 25 or more people are required to have 4% of its employers have disabilities or the business is required to pay a penalty. In addition, a strong emphasis has been placed on access to early intervention for children with disabilities (CONADIS, n.d.). That said, budget allocations prioritize foreign debt over funding for social services. People with disabilities continue to be a vulnerable population in Ecuador.

There is a shortage of occupational therapists in Ecuador. There are two occupational therapy schools across the country. Each graduates approximately 10 to 12 students each year. Students earn a baccalaureate in 3 years and may complete a master's degree in the 4th year of study. Occupational therapists are most typically employed in hospitals, schools, and outpatient settings. The people in the following stories were seen in an outpatient setting. In this setting, clients pay for

TABLE 13.1 Human Rights of Persons with Disabilities in Ecuador

International Policies Signed by Ecuador Regarding Human Rights of Persons with Disabilities in Ecuador	Website
Inter-American Convention on the Elimination of All Forms of Discrimination Against Persons with Disabilities	http://www.unhcr.org/refworld/docid/3de4cb7d4.html
Salamanca Statement on Special Needs Education for Children and Youth	http://www.biceinternational.org/e_upload/pdf/unesco_the_salamanca_statement_and_framework_for_action_on_special_needs_education.pdf
Managua Declaration on Policies for Children and Youth with Disabilities	http://www.inclusion-ia.org/documentos/manadecl-eng.pdf
Cartagena Declaration	http://www.hchr.org.co/ (Go to Documentos Basicos and find Declaracion de Cartagena (English version)

services out of pocket on a sliding fee basis. Clients typically receive services for as long as they can afford them and feel they are beneficial. Occupational therapy services in this setting focus mostly on activities of daily living and functional use of the upper extremity.

I have interpreted the following stories in order to provide a perspective on the experience of disability outside of the United States. I am grateful to the following four individuals who shared their story with me. They provide insight, wisdom, and practical advice to occupational therapy practitioners working with individuals in intercultural settings.

Narratives

Maria: Mother of Samantha

"My daughter is normal, she just happens to have cerebral palsy."

Maria, age 49, is the mother of 11-year-old Samantha. She begins. . . .

My story is long. I come from the Oriente (the rural jungle area of Ecuador). I traveled from the Amazon to get my daughter help. My daughter is my everything, I love my daughter, she was my only child at the time. I had an older daughter, but had lost her to the street. She left home and was running around with men.

My daughter, Samantha, was born healthy. At 9 months she became ill with pneumonia which led to meningitis, which led to seizures. I brought her to the hospital in Tena, the nearest hospital to where we lived in the jungle. She was there for a month, but they were unable to cure her. She continued to have seizures.

I decided to take her to Quito (8 hours by bus). At this point, she was being fed through a nasogastric tube and on oxygen as well. On the way to Quito, Samantha ran out of oxygen and had a seizure. I felt so helpless, I did not know what to do. She could not breathe well on her own and we still had a far way to go. I prayed hard, and I convinced the bus driver to call an ambulance. God got us to Quito in an ambulance. I have never been so sure of His existence and presence in my life.

We arrived at the children's hospital in Quito at 11:00 p.m. at night. By 2:00 in the morning, the doctors told me that Samantha would not live. They told me to leave her to die. But I have a strong character, a very strong character, and I was not going to leave my daughter in a hospital to die. I stayed with her, I did not leave. And then, Samantha did die. I went crazy, I tried to resuscitate her myself. I begged them to give her medicine. I knew that God would not take her from me. The doctors gave me tranquilizers to calm me down, but it did not work. I fought the medicine. I kept blowing into Samantha's mouth, and she came back to life. A mother cannot leave her child, we hold on until the end, until we end up where we end up. Some people do not understand, it is hard to explain, but when you are a mother of a sick child, you understand.

Samantha spent 3 years in the hospital. When she came home I put her in therapy from 8:00 in the morning until 4:00 in the afternoon. I worked while she was in therapy to pay for it. By that point, any money I had was gone; it is expensive to have a child with disabilities. I am a single mother. My husband left me when I was 5 months pregnant with Samantha. He left me with nothing. I was a chef for tourists in the jungle, I made a comfortable living, but when he left me, he took everything, all of our savings, all of my jewelry. In order to pay for Samantha's therapy, I spent no money on myself. I did not buy food or clothing for myself. I would only eat food that was free and wear only clothes that were given to me. All of the money went to Samantha and her therapy; that is what a mother does.

My older daughter, who I lost to the streets, abandoned her two children. I took them in. I take care of them now also, they are ages 6 and 7 (Figure 13.2). We live in a two-room apartment; there is the kitchen, and the bedroom, that is it. The boys have their bed and I sleep with Samantha. She cannot sleep unless I am at her side. We go outside to use the bathroom and bathe. It is what I can afford.

I take care of Samantha, I do everything for her. When she needs to be suctioned, I suction her, when she needs injections, I do that too. I know how to move her, position her, feed her, work with her. I know everything there is to know about her. I manage everything for her, like a doctor. But I don't have a degree, and I don't have a big fancy vocabulary. I get mad when professionals, doctors, nurses, and therapists don't treat me well. When they talk at me like I don't know anything or they know more about Samantha than me. Life has taught me everything I need to know. I don't need a degree to be able to care for Samantha.

I also fight like hell for her. Sometimes, the buses don't want to stop and pick us up because her wheelchair takes up extra room on the bus, or sometimes the bus drivers want to charge me more, but I know my rights

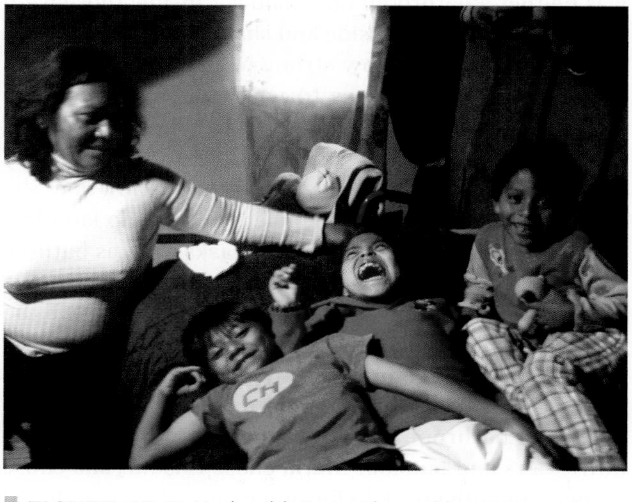

FIGURE 13.2 Maria with Samantha and her two grandsons.

and I know the law. The bus drivers just don't know any better, so it's my job to educate them. I let them know what the law says—Samantha's ticket is half, and mine is discounted. If they continue to treat me poorly, I simply don't pay anything. When they argue with me, I ask to speak with an official who can help me educate the bus drivers. Now they know me, and they know the law. I have quite a reputation with the bus drivers in our community. We need to think and communicate. I used to just fight, but now I understand. We all need to be thinking and communicating with one another about how we collaborate with people with disabilities. As mothers of children with disabilities, it is hard, very very hard, we need to be strong. I ask God for help to be strong every day. I know that nobody else is going to open their eyes up to our children, that it is up to us as mothers. No one knows the life of another. We need to have compassion and work with one another. We should go out of our way to help, rather than discriminate and treat one another as lesser.

I don't know what I will do when she passes. I know she is quite ill, I can hear it when she breathes. We have been through so much together. I can have things planned in my head, but not in my heart. And when I go, what will happen to the boys? Who will feed them? They have suffered alongside me.

My daughter is perfectly normal, she just has cerebral palsy; other than that, she is like the rest of us. Samantha is my fight, she is my purpose, she is my everything.

My Reflection: My Home Visit

I traveled with Maria and Samantha to their home by bus. Maria manages Samantha and her wheelchair up and down the bus stairs. Once on the bus, she puts the brakes on and holds on to the chair. We then walked a few blocks to reach their home, her boys were waiting for us and greeted us with large smiles and they chanted Samantha's name. After climbing the full flight of stairs up to their home, we entered the two-room apartment. It struck me as very clean, organized, and humble. Inside the home, there were beds, a refrigerator, and a stove. There was neither a bathroom nor a shower inside; those were down the stairs and outside and shared with neighbors.

I thought about how strong Maria is, the love and energy she must possess to wake each day, change, bathe, and dress Samantha to travel 1½ hours by bus to get Samantha to therapy on time. In comparison to my challenges to get up and ready for the day . . . How does she change Samantha's diapers? Where do they do laundry? Because of where she lives, simple tasks such as bathing take on a whole new meaning, are more time consuming, require more planning, and take more energy. I have the privilege of doing all of these activities in my own home, and am responsible only for myself. How would I do it with two small children and a third child with disabilities when the bathroom, shower, and laundry are a flight downstairs and outside? Maria chose this life, she chose to love Samantha back to life and care for her abandoned grandchildren. She is incredibly resilient, and is living out what is important to her—love and family.

Horacio: Disability Is Not the Same as Incapacitated

My name is Horacio, I was an engineer. I have congenital spinal stenosis in my cervical spine. The medulla is compressed between C2 through C5. My sickness started 2 years ago with pain in my arms, my stomach, and my back. I then started to have very painful headaches accompanied by a hissing sound between my ears. My pain worsened until I almost could not walk. As the pain worsened, I also became very depressed. I started looking for help; the doctors told me that I would need to have surgery. This worsened my depression because I was convinced that I would die in surgery because of where they would have to operate.

I started to see a psychologist who prescribed antidepressive medication. With the help of the therapy and medicine, my fear of the surgery lessened. I tried alternative medicine such as chiropractics, homeopaths, and herbal medicine. These did not seem to help me. I then visited many different neurologists to help understand if a surgery was indeed the best answer. Finally, I spoke with my wife, and together we agreed to pursue the operation.

I found a neurosurgeon with the best experience and reputation for my surgery. I entered surgery at 3:00 p.m. At 7:00 p.m. that same day, I woke up and the surgeon asked me to try to move an arm or leg. Not only could I not move, I could not feel a thing. I immediately went back into surgery, woke up again, and still there was no movement or sensation whatsoever. I had become a quadriplegic.

I was transferred to a different hospital and they said that they could do nothing for me there because the first surgeon had done so much damage to the medulla. Fifteen days later, a doctor specializing in trauma, agreed to try surgery. After a 5-hour surgery, I woke with a neck collar and IV medicine to decrease the inflammation of the medulla. Again, they put me on antidepressant medication. The doctor told me that I would never walk again. Then they sent me home. My wife looked at the doctors and asked them, "Now what do I do?" The doctor's response was "Go and pray. He will be able to move something eventually." In my mind, this was very poor medical practice regarding my health. I wanted to kill myself, but I couldn't; I couldn't move from the neck down.

After that surgery, my life changed. I went from having all the physical and professional capacity a person can have to nothing. I was 49 years old and my life had changed so definitively. I was no longer the Horacio who only knew life through a materialistic lens and who never did anything to help out someone in need.

When I came home, my wife hired a nurse to help care for me. She would turn me every hour to make sure I did not get bedsores. To calm myself, I needed antidepressants. The experience of being turned like that was very scary. I never knew what was going to happen; I couldn't feel anything.

A week later, my wife hired a therapist to come to the house. My wife was the only one who believed that one day I might be able to move on my own. The therapist spent 4 to 6 hours a day lifting my legs, my arms, moving me, but I did not feel a thing. I didn't want to feel because I was afraid I would feel pain.

Then it dawned on me. I thought about everything I had accomplished in life; nothing had happened to my cognition or intelligence. If I could do what I had done, why could I not rehabilitate? Someone told me that before I could heal, I would have to forgive myself as well as others. I did not know how to do this. I was not familiar with the concept of faith.

I did not have a relationship with my father. When people would ask me about my father, I would respond, "He is dead to me." I knew that in order to heal, I needed to forgive my dad and ask for his forgiveness. I started to forgive myself. My dad forgave me. I put a picture of my dad on my ceiling and would look at it as I did my exercises from my bed. I would ask my dad for the strength I needed to do the exercises.

In the middle of the night, I could not sleep. I found myself praying to God, asking him to give me another opportunity to live, to not just leave me in the bed, unable to move. I promised to help others with disabilities recuperate if I could be healed. I imagined what it would feel like to move. With that, my foot moved, then my body moved. My therapist came the next morning and I told him what had happened. As the therapist started to move me, I could feel the movement; I knew I was on my way to recovery.

Three months after wanting to commit suicide, I stood in a walker. I started to see, feel, and love strength within my body. I promised myself I would never give up on myself, not my mind or my body from that day forward.

Today, I can move all of my limbs (Figure 13.3). I can use the bathroom independently. So far, I still can't write, get up from the floor, or bathe or dress myself, but I think those things will come with time. I am a man that understands what disability means. But disability is not the same as incapable. *Disability does not mean incapacitated.* People with disabilities have the capacity to do things. I accept that I am a person with a disability, and I will learn how to live my life with these added challenges.

I hope to write a book, telling all of my stories about my rehabilitation. I want to serve the society and give an example of how to be patient, consistent, and strong. For now, each day I come to therapy, I try to make it better for my peers. I want to be the center of happiness, strength, and hope for those who arrive to therapy sad, scared, tired, and who are still questioning "why me?" When therapy is done right, people leave feeling better and more hopeful than when they arrived.

On the outside, I appear a clown to help other people feel better, but don't let me fool you; I have a lot of tears on the inside. I still have very hard days, very sad days, I feel a lot of sadness. If you can't recuperate your body, you can recuperate your mind. It is very difficult to understand, but the first thing the mind wants to do is to quit. Every day is a fight to not quit. Only when one is truly dead, is it impossible to live. Every day, I choose to live.

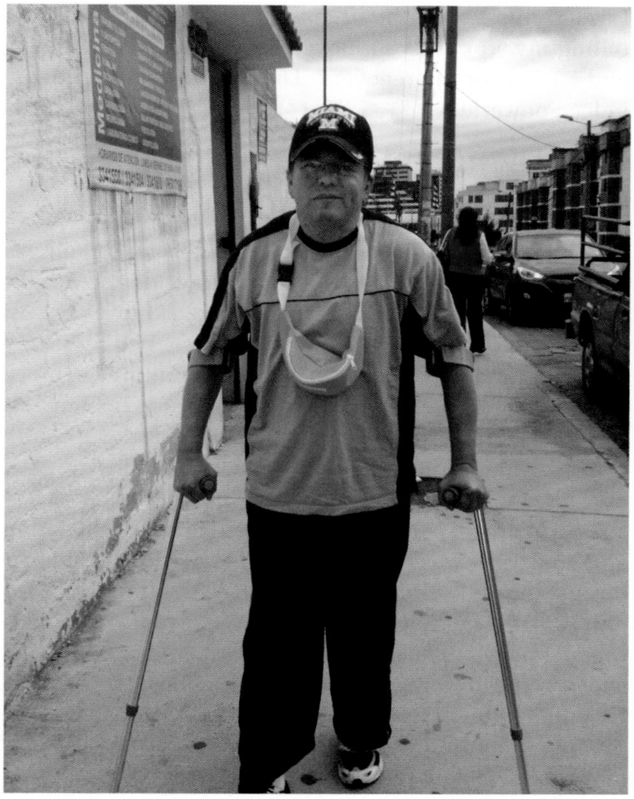

FIGURE 13.3 Horacio.

My Reflection: Walking with Horacio on the Street

When I met Horacio in the clinic, he was telling jokes and laughing with the therapist and other clients in the room. It was clear that everyone thought he was funny and enjoyed his company. I was a bit intimidated by the thought of interviewing him. I wondered if I would understand his use of humor or if he would take the process seriously. When we started the interview, his entire demeanor changed. He spoke slowly and intentionally, he made sure I understood every word. For Horacio, sharing his story with me was very important and serious. I came to understand his sudden change in demeanor as his story unfolded.

After listening to Horacio's story, I walked out to the street with him. He walked very carefully and slowly with two sling crutches. He told me that he wanted to show me something "very big." After crossing over a small incline, Horacio placed both crutches in one hand, and slowly, step-by-step, walked without assistance. He asked me to videotape his walking so that he could appreciate the progress he would make in the next year. The following day Horacio arrived walking with just one crutch. When

I asked him about the other crutch, he replied, "Kate, telling my story to you has given me renewed strength and energy for my recovery. Thank you." Storytelling is indeed powerful.

Don Ulvio Lopez Arquello: The Power of Family and Community

To begin, getting to a life where one can feel tranquility is difficult. I feel like I was close, until the accident. I was hit by a drunk driver, and broke my neck. I can't move my legs; I can move my arms a little, that is getting better. So, my hope for tranquility is gone, but I have to continue to move forward. Medicine will not help me; I have to help myself through therapies. I ask God for help every day. I thank God every day for my family, my beautiful family, my wife, my kids, and everyone who cares for me (Figure 13.4).

The hardest part of being disabled for me is not being able to work. I was a hard worker. I started selling shoes, but I realized I could make shoes to sell, so that is what I did. I started making shoes to sell. They were good shoes too; people could see the quality in them. I would make shoes in the morning; and in the afternoon, I would work on building my house. I built this house, everything you see here, I built. But ultimately, my income was dependent on how many shoes I could sell. My goal was to have a job that paid a salary, a job where I made the same amount of money each month. I wanted a more stable life to provide for my family. So, I started to work for the municipality. They paid a salary; I was very happy with that. Then I decided I wanted to work for myself, so I got a car and started using it as a taxi. I was very contented working for myself. I was a hard worker. Before the accident, I did everything around the house. If the roof needed fixing, I fixed it. I built, I fixed, I did it all. But now, I can do nothing. (He looks at Maura, his daughter-in-law.) She does everything for me now. Sometimes I lose my patience. When I am alone, I start thinking about all of my life. It makes me sad to think that I can't do the things that were so important to me.

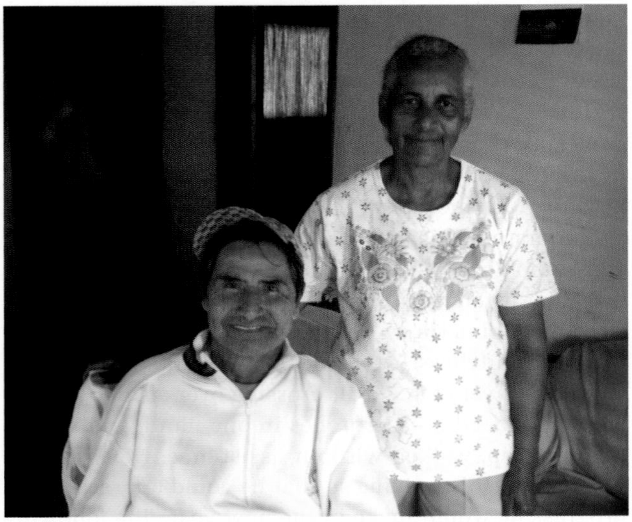

FIGURE 13.4 Don Ulvio and his wife.

I am motivated to keep going by my grandchildren. I want to see them grow up. When I was in the hospital, they were all I could think about. The doctor told me that in order to return home, I needed to be able to breathe and eat on my own. Well, that was all I needed to hear, I would do anything to go home. So, I practiced eating and swallowing until I could do it. Then, we tried to take the oxygen off, and I was OK. I did not want to be on oxygen at home, it is too big and invasive. The only thing I wanted to do when I was in the hospital was to go home and see my children and grandchildren.

When I returned home, I realized that life would never be the same. It was difficult for me to fit into my home in a wheelchair. My neighbors came and made changes to the home so that my family could move me around in it. They also came to visit and brought food with them. I am so blessed. My son is an engineer. He created a pulley system so that my wife can put me to bed by herself (Note: His son created a Hoyer lift in his bedroom). I never knew how many people in my life care about me. In order to pay for my wheelchair and bath chair, I had to sell my chickens and my truck. What if I had had nothing to sell? That is a sad reality for many people. My mind is weak and fragile. I have to remind myself to give God thanks every day for the people who surround me. I feel lucky, I have people in my life to help me organize my life and take care of me. I choose to feel grateful. Everything happens for a reason.

Maura Lucas: Don Ulvio's Caretaker

We live a couple of hours outside of Quito. Don Ulvio was a normal guy. He was a hard worker. He had his own car out of which he worked. His wife also worked in agriculture. He and his wife had four children. They were a poor family but saw to it that their children pursued education and entered a profession. Each child moved to different towns within 2 to 3 hours of home to pursue their careers. Each would return home every 15 days or so to visit their parents. Although Don Ulvio and his wife lived alone, they were happy, they were contented. Although poor, the couple was well known for helping out their neighbors when they were in need.

Just 1 year ago, Don Ulvio was in an accident. He was driving with his son when a drunk driver hit them. Don Ulvio took the impact of the accident, his son was not hurt. Don Ulvio was taken to a hospital, where they found out that he had fractured his cervical spine. All of his children gathered in Quito to discuss the news and support their mother.

Don Ulvio was a smoker, he already had bad lungs. In addition to being paralyzed, he would need to be on oxygen as well. He was also unable to eat independently due to dysphasia, so he had a feeding tube put in. After 3 months in the hospital on oxygen and with a feeding tube, the doctors suggested that we try to take him home without oxygen for a month. If it went well, he could stay home off of oxygen. If it did not go well, he would need oxygen at home.

He came home like a baby, he needed help for everything, he could not move from his neck down. But because he had helped so many people in the past, his neighbors and family all gathered to help support Don Ulvio and his wife. People really came through for us; they came with food, clothes, and their time to help us.

We moved our family to Quito to help with his care. I left my mother, who is on dialysis. It was so hard for me to leave her. When we received the phone call that Don Ulvio had been in a car accident, our entire lives changed. Sometimes I just want to throw in the towel. This is not the life I imagined for myself, taking care of my mother and then my father-in-law and not pursuing my professional career. But where God is, it is immense, and He is here with us. I have to keep going, I have to focus on the positive: he did not lose his mind, his sight, or his hearing. He is still here with us today. We have to grab hold of the love and continue to move forward.

He had his time to enjoy his life, he worked hard to contribute to his community and help those in need. He also put all four children through school and saw to it that they were prepared to become self-sufficient adults. Now is his time to rest and receive care.

For now, this is my life. I visit my mom every month. I care for Don Ulvio. And I take care of my son (4 years old) (**Figure 13.5**). My life is about taking care of delicate people. Sometimes it makes me mad and sad; it is not what I imagined my life to be. I don't have what I want now, but I think God will look down on me one day and see that I am deserving of what I want and He will provide. I ask God for strength and I ask Him for love. We don't have our own home; we live in very tight quarters with my husband's parents. I want to work; I want to be able to send money to my mom. When my son starts school, I hope I can find a job.

My Reflection: Visiting Don Ulvio and Maura in Their Home

I walked out of therapy with Don Ulvio and Maria to the truck in which they had come. They lifted Don Ulvio into the bed of the truck, which was covered overhead and open in the back. Don Ulvio rode in the back of the pickup truck with his wheelchair. They put him on top of a mattress and covered him with blankets. Don Ulvio travels for 2 hours each way to get to therapy.

I asked Don Ulvio if I could visit him in his home, he smiled and invited me along with the three occupational therapists from the center to visit him. We all gratefully accepted the invitation. As we took the 2-hour bus drive, we thought about Don Ulvio making the same trip in the back of the truck. When we arrived, Don Ulvio was outside waiting for us in the sun. As we pulled up to his home, he was grinning from ear to ear. His smile spoke a thousand words. While I was at Don Ulvio's home, his cousin stopped after church for a visit and brought fruit with him for the family. I also was able to see the Hoyer lift that his son made. It was clear that Don Ulvio experienced a lot of family and community support. The occupational therapists and I commented with one another on how positive the experience was for us and how much we enjoyed getting to know Don Ulvio in his home. The occupational therapists commented that they had not met his wife before because she is unable to make the trip to therapy, nor had they appreciated the vast countryside in which he lives. They observed that the amount of community involvement seemed much stronger than what they had seen in the city of Quito. We discussed the role of context in therapy and how the clinical setting can influence how and what we come to know about the people with whom we work.

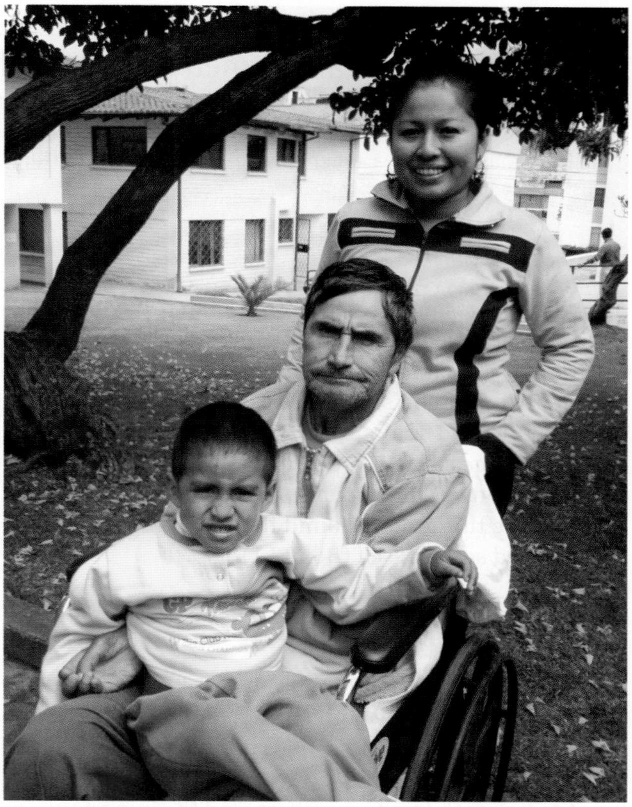

FIGURE 13.5 Maura, Don Ulvio, and Maura's son.

Interpreting Narratives

I have been truly humbled by my experience. When I was initially asked to interpret stories for this chapter, I could not imagine the power, emotion, and tenderness I would find in each story. I experienced the power of storytelling firsthand.

It is clear that there are common threads throughout these narratives that I believe are shared experiences of

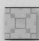

BOX 13.1 Transformed Sense of Self

Think about times in each of the stories in which people experienced and accepted a different and new sense of self and answer the following questions:

- What led to those experiences?
- What or who helped to facilitate the acceptance process?

disability across cultures. The first is that having a disability is very expensive. Maria, Horacio, Don Ulvio, and Maura Lucas each have experienced loss of employment and many extra costs in order to access therapy, care, equipment, and transportation. The second theme throughout the stories is spirituality. Each person turned to a higher power for strength, patience, gratitude, and/or hope. The third theme found in each of the stories is a transformed sense of self (Box 13.1).

Discussion

Each of these stories offers a powerful message. Each also demonstrates how both culture and socioeconomics impact the experience of having a disability. Maria's story teaches us lessons about how to interact with people, how to work with family members, and the importance of respecting the knowledge of the family members. Maria has had negative experiences with health care workers speaking down to her. However, even more powerful is how she has fought for her daughter at every turn. She has gone without food and clothing herself to provide for her children. Without a formal education, she has been an advocate, a nurse, a doctor, a therapist, and a social worker for her daughter.

Horacio's story teaches us about faith. He told a story about forgiveness and hope and how each played an important role in his healing and rehabilitation process. Horacio was so incredibly proud to tell his story, he would sometimes pause to think of the reader and what he wanted them to know. The very act of telling his story was therapeutic for Horacio.

Don Ulvio's story was about the power of love he experienced from family and community after his accident. Don Ulvio's sense of self changed drastically from self-sufficient worker and provider for family to feeling dependent and needing to accept help. His story also teaches us about the significant role that context plays in one's experience of disability. After his accident, it was Don Ulvio's family and friends that were his drive to return home to the countryside, where it is quiet, peaceful, tranquil, and familiar. Maria's story as Don Ulvio's caretaker teaches us about selflessness and family expectations in the Ecuadorian culture.

The four people in these stories are full of warmth and resilience. Their willingness to open up and share their stories of heartbreak, challenge, and acceptance touched something deep inside of me. Reflect on the stories of Maria, Horacio, Don Ulvio, and Maura. Use the following questions to discuss the role of narrative in occupational therapy. As a profession, how can we better understand people's stories?

- How can we take the time to listen, to understand, and to know the people with whom we work?
- How would what we do be different if we knew people's stories?
- How do stories change based on who is telling them, who they are being told to, where they are told, and why they are being told?
- How might we use stories of transformation to understand what it is we do as occupational therapists?

References

Center for International Rehabilitation. (n.d.). *The International Disability Educational Alliance Network*. Retrieved from http://ideanet.org

Consejo Nacional De Discapacidades. (n.d.). Retrieved from http://www.conadis.gob.ec/

For additional resources on the subjects discussed in this chapter, visit http://thePoint.lww.com/Willard-Spackman12e.

UNIT IV

Occupation in Context

"Individuals, families, communities and whole populations engage continuously in a closely bound, interdependent set of occupations on a daily basis. One of the most significant and universal aspects of these daily rounds of occupations is that they always occur in several contexts simultaneously. The relationship is a dynamic one: occupational norms and forms and patterns of engagement are shaped by these contexts and to some extent, these contextual forces in turn are influenced by the net impact of occupations performed both over time and in time."

—Gail Whiteford (2010, p. 135)

CHAPTER 14

Family Perspectives on Occupation, Health, and Disability

Mary C. Lawlor, Cheryl Mattingly

OUTLINE

LEARNING OBJECTIVES

After reading this chapter, you will be able to:

1. Describe characteristics of contemporary family life
2. Identify ways to understand family occupations and the implications for collaborating with families
3. Discuss how family members might experience illness and disability and how these experiences are situated in family life
4. Recognize the expertise that family members have and bring to health care encounters, including occupational therapy sessions
5. Understand the health care encounter as a complex social arena in which perceptions and decisions about care are created, contested, and negotiated by multiple social actors
6. Describe knowledge, skills, and behaviors that facilitate effective "partnering up" and collaboration

Introduction

Many of us have deep understandings of family life drawn from our first hand, experiential knowledge of family whether from family of origin or family created through our engagements in interpersonal worlds. The word *family* itself often evokes a complex array of thoughts, emotions, and embodied actions. The phrase "you are family" marks a belonging to a particular social world. In some ways, it could be said we know family. So how is it that forming effective partnerships with families in our clinical practices can be so complicated?

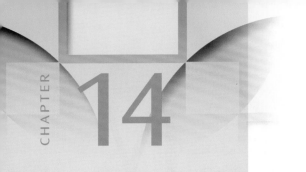

Occupational therapy sessions as well as other health care encounters are key sites for facilitating partnerships, addressing needs and concerns, and supporting family life. Health care encounters are not only specific events but also episodes in the histories of client and family life and, conceivably, also episodes that are embedded in practitioners' lives and institutional cultures. Encounters such as occupational therapy sessions, particularly ones in which significant experiences happen, are events in longer illness and developmental trajectories. Significant moments in therapy sessions may resonate across time to other moments in one's life and across place to the extent that the impact is felt in other contexts, such as life at home, school, or work. Collaborative partnerships with families afford opportunities for salient moments in home and family life to be taken up in ways that influence the happenings that occur in occupational therapy sessions and their mattering in people's lives.

When I (first author) started to study how therapists work with families, I would ask them to tell me a story about a time when they felt they had a particularly successful and positive experience with families and, alternatively, a time when they wished things would have gone very differently. And it probably is not a big surprise that I found that the stories were very similar, revealing the complexity of engagements with families. It is hard to tell a story without some kind of trouble, so even stories of great success often contained reparations, rethinking, changing course, dilemmas, and tensions. These stories, and subsequent research described later in this chapter, also reveal that the mattering of occupational therapy is grounded in family life.

The purpose of this chapter is to provide an overview of family life, introduce family occupations, and discuss how understandings of family experiences related to illnesses and disabilities shape health care encounters including occupational therapy practices. This chapter concludes with a discussion of family-centered care and a case study example to illustrate how occupational therapists collaborate with families. We draw on a longitudinal, urban ethnographic research program entitled Boundary Crossings that we describe later in this chapter and have conducted at the University of Southern California (USC) from 1997 to 2011.[1] The heart of this chapter moves from general considerations of family life to the intricacies, dilemmas, surprises, and riches of therapeutic work that takes seriously the illness and disability experiences of families. Processes related to "partnering up" between practitioners and family members are also examined.

Understanding Family Life

Family life is dynamic, often compelling, complicated, and multifaceted. Although the term *family life* may imply a unitary construct, understanding family life involves the recognition of its heterogeneity and diversity. Family life is situated in broader sociocultural contexts as well as intergenerational and historical contexts. Family life is constituted through an array of cultural and social practices and lived through engagements in occupations (Figure 14.1). The particularities or details of life within families often reveal the relationships, social networks, activities, values, beliefs, priorities, occupations, history, resources, and challenges inherent in families. Family life is enacted through the interplay of the ordinary routines of daily life and the extraordinary experiences of family life, events, and unexpected happenings. The ordinary or everyday occupations reflect the ways that habits and routines give structure and meaning to our lives, but the surface sense of ordinariness often obscures their complexity and particularity in terms of individual and family life (Hasselkus, 2006). For some families who have family members with illnesses or disabilities, the achievement of a sense of routine everydayness or ordinariness can, in fact, be an extraordinary achievement (Mattingly, 2010).

Family life is marked by the interdependency of family members (Bandura, Carprara, Barbaranelli, Regalia, & Scabini, 2011). As Glen Elder (1998) reminds us, lives are *linked* through our engagements in social worlds. Longer life expectancies have contributed to greater opportunities for intergenerational relationships, including those of grandparents and grandchildren, often

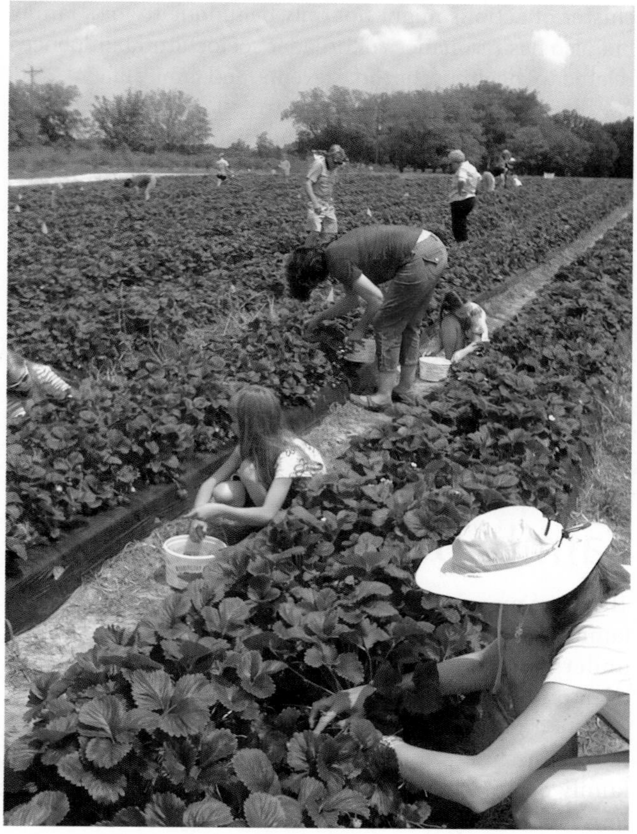

FIGURE 14.1 Families have different activities that they share. Here, cousins and their parents pick strawberries while visiting the grandparents—an annual summer event.

[1]This research program comprised three research grants: MCJ-060745, Maternal and Child Health Program Health and Services Administration Department of Health and Human Services; *Boundary Crossing: A Longitudinal and Ethnographic Study* (#R01 HD 38878); and *Boundary Crossings: Re-Situating Cultural Competence* (#2R01 HD 38878), funded by National Institute of Child Health and Human Development (NICHD), National Institutes of Health (NIH). Pseudonyms are used to provide greater confidentiality.

supported by the parents or middle generation (Swartz, 2009). Relationships with family members permeate our life course and are understood to be both enduring and changing (Swartz, 2009). Families often work to make sure that current family members have an appreciation of family members who are not in proximity due to death, illness, geographic distance, or other factors. Photographs, family stories, naming conventions, and artifacts such as my grandmother's ring or recipes are all cultural resources to infuse contemporary family life with a sense of roots, history, and connectedness. For many, the implicit nature of family culture is revealed when a potentially new family member such as a date, fiancé, partner, or in-home caregiver first enters family life. Such questions as "Is your family always like this?" or comments like "I don't get your family" mark the particularity of family cultures.

Understanding family also involves an appreciation of how culture relates to family life. Families have their own cultures (Fitzgerald, 2004; Lawlor & Elliot, 2012; Lawlor & Mattingly, 2009), and family life is constituted through cultural beliefs practices and occupations that are both particular to any family and illustrative of broader sociocultural influences on family life. For example, birthday parties in Joe's family might always include the cooking of the favorite meal of the celebrant, the wearing of a "Happy Birthday" crown, being seated at the head of the dinner table, and being relieved of any household chores for the day. This cluster of actions might not only be unique to Joe's family but also has resonances of broader sociocultural influences related to mealtime, birthday events, and family life.

Family life also serves as a particularly potent context for learning, particularly for infants and young children. Families constitute the primary social unit by which children first learn about the world and occupations (Fitzgerald, 2004). Learning within the occupations and activities of family life incorporates understandings of a family's beliefs, routines, culture, and cultural practices as well as skill development (Kellegrew, 1998). Harkness et al. (2007) have described how the *developmental niche* is constituted through settings, customs, and what they term as *caregiver psychology*, a construct that includes parental "ethnotheories" or beliefs related to their child, development, or parenting.

Family Occupations

There are many ways to conceptualize occupations within family life. In a general sense, family occupations can be understood as the occupations conducted with more than one family member that contribute to the health, well-being, satisfaction, and interrelationships among family members. Like the occupations of individuals, family occupations represent meaningful engagements in which family members invest energy, skills and talents, and physical and emotional resources to support family life and the ongoing development of family members. These occupations include routine daily practices (e.g., caregiving, cooking, driving children to school) as well as family practices that reflect family culture, intergenerational transmission of values and priorities, and the creation of significant experiences (e.g., orchestration of special events such as a visit from the tooth fairy or maintaining a memento box of the artifacts of childhood).

The term *co-occupation* has been used to describe when more than one person is engaged in an occupation. Other terms to describe occupations that are not individual and are more collective include *shared occupations*, *joint occupations*, and *co-created occupations*. The theoretical basis for these terms is not yet well theorized but reflect recent attempts to develop a more social, dynamic, and transactional approach to understanding occupation (Dickie, Cutchins, & Humphry, 2006; Lawlor, 2003). Other approaches to categorizing family occupations have included designations like mothering, parenting, fathering, and caregiving occupations (e.g., Esdaile & Olson, 2004).

Family Perspectives on Health and Disability

When individuals experience illness or disability, family members also have illness and disability experiences (Lawlor & Mattingly, 2009; Mattingly & Lawlor, 2003). Most people who come to occupational therapy live in social worlds that include families of some kind. Families, in various forms and partnership arrangements, matter for most people who experience illness or disability, no matter what the age, ethnicity, socioeconomic status, or geographical location. Even when people live apart from their families, it is very likely that some family members will be instrumental in healing, recovery, caregiving, and participation in occupations. How clients experience disability and how it affects their functioning in the world often depend heavily on the clients' relationships with family members and other significant people in their social worlds. Family life also influences participation, and family participation and occupations can be affected when one or more family members have disabilities or special health care needs (Law, 2002).

Attempts to understand illness and disability experiences have been facilitated by the "narrative turn" in medicine (Garro & Mattingly, 2000; Hurwitz, Greenhalgh, & Skultans, 2004). Literature in anthropology, particularly medical anthropology, occupational science and therapy, medicine, and other health-related fields are increasingly drawing on narrative approaches to: (1) enhance understanding of illness and disability from the perspectives of the individuals and their families who are living with illnesses or disabilities (e.g., Bluebond-Langer, 1978; A. Frank, 1995; G. Frank, 2000; Kleinman, 1988, 2006; Monks & Frankenberg, 1995; Murphy, 1990), (2) analyze how narrative modes of reasoning or narrative-based ethics influence health and therapeutic practices (e.g., Becker, 1997; Cain, 1991; Charon & Montello, 2002; Fleming & Mattingly,

1994; Hurwitz et al., 2004), and (3) recognize narrative as a structure for creating significant experiences in therapeutic practices (Clark, 1993; Mattingly, 1998).

Occupational therapists have also found it helpful to read and reflect on first-person or family accounts of illness and disability experiences (e.g., Bauby, 1997; Greenfeld, 1978, 1986; Hockenberry, 1995; Jamison, 1996; Park, 1982, 2001; Peete, 2010; Williams, 1992). At times, popular media, including films and television shows, can generate insights that support practitioners' reflections on their clinical practices. Even films or television shows that present portrayals of illnesses or disabilities or health and therapeutic practices that may be disturbing, demeaning, or inaccurate can provide important experiences for clarifying beliefs and philosophies that are critical to the provision of efficacious, collaborative, and compassionate family-centered care.

Family-Centered Care

> So, what I did is, I became very personal with my therapist. She just wasn't a lady I saw once a week; she was adopted into my family. And I brought my family to therapy with me. I brought children. I brought my grandma [*laughs*], so that she could be in on what it is that we would be trying to achieve. What it was that we need my daughter to accomplish. I brought children, aunties, uncles, close neighbors—everybody that was a part of my close daily surroundings, went to therapy. And that's just the way it was. So that the therapy was not just once a week, it was seven days a week. It was from the minute we woke up to the minute we went to bed.

The aforementioned quote is an excerpt from a transcribed interview with a mother who was telling a story about her daughter's occupational therapy program. It is drawn from an ethnographic research study conducted by the authors and an interdisciplinary research team that will be described in more detail later in this chapter. The **family-centered care** movement, cost containment initiatives, and technological advancements in care delivery have fundamentally altered the expectations of families and practitioners, the nature of health care and caregiving practices, and outcomes of interventions. Health care encounters, once characterized by dyadic communication between a patient and doctor, are now complex social arenas in which multiple social actors, including family members, convene. Health care encounters involving family members are sites of intense **boundary crossing** where families and practitioners create, negotiate, contest, and/or modify perceptions, perspectives, and caregiving and treatment practices. Multiple perspectives on health care events are both anticipated and managed within often relatively brief moments of interaction. Some of the interesting dilemmas and opportunities that emerge when practitioners involve families actively in the therapeutic process are highlighted in this chapter.

The implementation of federal initiatives related to providing services for children with special health care needs and their families was documented as early as 1912, with the establishment of the Children's Bureau in Maternal and Child Health (Hanft, 1991) and expanded with the implementation of Title V legislation in 1935 (Colman, 1988). The implementation of P.L. 94-142, Part B, an amendment to the Education for the Handicapped Act (EHA) in 1975, and P.L. 99-457, Part H, an amendment to the EHA in 1986, prompted dramatic changes in the nature of service delivery to children in educational and early childhood settings (Hanft, 1991; Lawlor, 1991). In 1990, EHA was renamed the Individuals with Disabilities Act (Individuals with Disabilities Education Act of 1990). Implementation of these services placed new demands on practitioners to reframe traditional medical models of practice to accommodate to the needs of families as well as the child who was referred for services (American Occupational Therapy Association, 1999). In 2004, IDEA was reauthorized; and although much of the language around family participation has changed, many of the earlier principles have been retained. For example, the new statute still incorporates an Individual Family Service Plan as one of the minimum requirements for a statewide system's provision of services for each infant or toddler with a disability and the family of that child (Individuals with Disabilities Education Improvement Act of 2004).

Although the development of services that center on the needs and values of families began in early childhood programs through family-centered care initiatives (Hanft, 1991; Lawlor & Mattingly, 1998), many of the principles apply to services for people of all ages (Humphry, Gonzales, & Taylor, 1993). As human service systems moved into the community and family members began providing home care, practitioners developed a deeper appreciation of the centrality of families in healing, recovery, and adaptation. Practitioners also recognized that family members often had different perspectives from those of the professionals about the needs, priorities, and strengths. This recognition led to a shift from perceiving family members as people who will carry out the doctors' and practitioners' orders to perceiving family members as people who are most knowledgeable about the client and who are partners in decision making. Family members' perspectives about how the client is doing, what the client needs, what the family needs, and what is most important and meaningful in everyday life have become part of the clinical dialogue.

Family-centered care involves much more than thinking of adding family members into the therapy session; occupational therapy practice is fundamentally altered when family members are brought into the therapeutic process in a central way (Lawlor & Mattingly, 1998). Family members, including parents, often have powerful roles in the creation of significant experiences in therapy (Lawlor, 2009; Mattingly & Lawlor, 2001). The challenge for the occupational therapy practitioner is to collaborate with clients, their families, and other team members in designing a program that builds on strengths and addresses needs. When done successfully, intervention services are individualized to each family and reflect their unique cultural world. Drawing on the work of Dunst, Trivette, and Deal (1988), we have defined *family-centered care* as "an experience that happens when practitioners effectively and compassionately listen to the concerns, address the needs, and support the hopes of people and their families" (Lawlor & Cada, 1993; Lawlor & Mattingly, 1998). Sometimes practitioners can best involve clients and families in the decision-making process by offering multiple options for interventions (Rosen & Granger, 1992). This type of engagement is often described as a means of enabling and empowering families (e.g., Deal, Dunst, & Trivette, 1989).

Family-centered care is enacted through the collaborative efforts of family members and practitioners (Edelman, Greenland, & Mills, 1993; Lawlor & Mattingly, 1998) and typically is provided through multidisciplinary and interdisciplinary team structures. Partnerships are created on the basis of the establishment of trust and rapport as well as respect for family values, beliefs, and routines (Hanft, 1989). Additional elements of successful collaboration include clarity and honesty in communication, mutual agreement on goals, effective information sharing, accessibility, and absence of blame (McGonigel, Kaufmann, & Johnson, 1991). Successful collaboration occurs when practitioners and family members form relationships that foster a shared understanding of the needs, hopes, expectations, and contributions of all partners (Lawlor & Cada, 1993).

The Processes of "Partnering Up" and Collaboration

Occupational therapists draw on both their own life experiences of family as well as professional and theoretical concepts of families when collaborating with families (Fitzgerald, 2004). Collaboration is much more than being "nice" (Lawlor & Mattingly, 1998; Mattingly, 1998). It involves complex interpretative acts in which the practitioner must understand the meanings of interventions, the meanings of illness or disability in a person and family's life, and the feelings that accompany these experiences. Collaboration is also dependent on the development of a quality of interrelatedness that is evident in many therapy sessions that is not merely a question of establishing good rapport, eliciting cooperation, or prompting a client or patient to buy into a particular agenda in order for him or her to perform required tasks (Lawlor, 2003). The central question for practitioners and clients and their families is "How can we come to know enough about each other to effectively partner up?" (Lawlor & Mattingly, 2001). For therapists, the nature of the work in collaboration

> is not merely technical in the sense that a procedure is done or a therapy or other intervention is provided; nor does the work just entail drawing upon clinical expertise. Rather, "partnering-up" requires skilled relational work and involves the drawing upon a range of social skills including, intersubjectivity, communication, engagement, and understanding. (Lawlor, 2004, p. 306)

Assumptions about race, culture, ethnicity, social status, economic level, and education (and frequently the contesting of these assumptions) often powerfully influence the process of partnering up between families and professionals. Family members and practitioners live and operate in a multiplicity of cultural domains that are shaped by their profession, economic class, ethnicity, and community affiliations. When practitioners and family members interact, their values, assumptions, and perceptions about the interaction are shaped by their membership in these cultures.

Partnering up also involves bridging differences, establishing points of common interests and mutuality, and capitalizing on complementarities. This aspect of collaboration is particularly important when family members and practitioners perceive that they come from seemingly differently lived worlds. Mattingly (2006), drawing on reconceptualizations of culture that are prevalent in current anthropology, argues that health care encounters are like border zones, where there is often heightened engagement related to marking differences, finding commonalities, and creating understanding. Families in many ways are the consummate travelers in border zones with the daunting task of coming to understand biomedical, institutional, and practitioner cultural worlds and practices and participating in these practices in such a way that their nonbiomedical conceptualizations of their children, their families, and illness and disability can shape health care encounters.

We have come to conceptualize partnerships with families as grounded in **complementarity** such that all parties contribute expertise, understandings, practical reasoning, desires and hopes, and problem-solving strategies. The most effective partnerships are built on mutual respect and reciprocity but draw on the different perspectives, knowledge, and strengths of all the partners. Like most relationships, collaborative partnerships work best with a degree of differentiation and difference among the partners. In other words, most people who seek advice and care from health care practitioners want the practitioners to offer expertise and decisions that are different from what they already know.

Troublesome Assumptions about Disability, Illness Experiences, and Families

Although over the past 20 years there has been increasing attention toward understanding the ways in which family members participate in health care practices (e.g., Hinojosa, Sproat, Mankhetwit, & Anderson, 2002; Lawlor & Mattingly, 1998), much additional knowledge and reflection are needed (e.g., Cohn, 2001; Ochieng, 2003). Many practitioners who work in multicultural settings recognize the complexity of organizing health care and therapy practices in such a way as to understand and address the specific needs of family members. The following sections illustrate how problematic or flawed assumptions about the illness and disability experiences of family members can affect care.

The Disability Belongs to the Individual

One of the most pervasive assumptions in biomedicine is that the professional's task is to treat the individual who has the illness. Sometimes, this is narrowly interpreted among health professionals as "treating the pathology," but occupational therapy practitioners usually try to remember that they are also treating a person who has a disabling condition. Put differently, practitioners try to treat what anthropologists speak of as *the illness experience* rather than simply the disease (B. Good, 1994; B. Good & M. J. Good, 1994; Kleinman, 1988; Luhrmann, 2000). In the context of occupational therapy, a more accurate term is probably *the disability experience*, for it is certainly possible to have a disability, even one that requires therapy, without being ill. Practitioners try to attend both to the disability as a physiological condition and to the meaning this particular condition carries for the person who has the disability as well as his or her family (Mattingly, 1998, 2000; Mattingly & Fleming, 1994). If a practitioner knows that a client wants to relearn how to drive, dress independently, eat out at restaurants, or continue to work as an auto mechanic, the practitioner may be able to organize therapeutic tasks that aid the client in carrying out these activities. Therapeutic approaches should also situate these goals in an understanding of the family and social worlds that impact on these occupations. This is especially true for goals that concern the client's social world and the connection between functional skills and social relationships. It is artificial to treat only narrowly defined functional skills as though they were unrelated to a client's social world because a key aspect of the meaning of a condition is how it affects an individual's personal relationships, which is one of the trickier aspects of therapeutic work. By contrast, with such goals as learning how to dress oneself and learning wheelchair mobility, goals and concerns that are connected to family relations are much more difficult to define, and they are certainly likely to be hard to measure. Helping a client to reclaim his identity as a good father to his 5-year-old daughter even though he has a spinal cord injury, for example, is harder to translate into discrete, skill-based goals than is learning how to increase upper body strength or learning how to eat independently. However, learning what family members hope for—what they would like to see happen—is critical to the development of collaborative therapy practices with families. As Cohn, Miller, and Tickle-Degnan (2000) found in their qualitative study of parents of children with sensory modulation disorders, skillful listening to parents' perspectives can generate insights that promote therapy that is meaningful in terms of family goals and values.

Family-oriented goals are likely to be tied to outcomes that are diffuse, complex, subtle, and difficult to measure, even when they are deeply significant to the client and family. When a client's goals and concerns are tied to shifting family relationships, these might seem out of professional bounds for the occupational therapy practitioner. Despite the many difficulties in trying to understand a disabling condition as it pertains to a client's role in the family, ignoring this aspect often means being blind to the most significant aspects of the illness (or disability) experience. Ignoring family-oriented goals or the meaning of a disability as it ties to family concerns and family relationships can mean ignoring the person altogether.

There Is Only One Perspective per Family

Although much of the literature on family-centered care presumes that practitioners come to know all members of the family, we have found that often, one member of the family, typically a mother or spouse, serves as the primary contact for the practitioner. It is this individual's perspective that practitioners come to know. However, this might be only one of several perspectives held by family members. Practitioners sometimes get to know other family members; but in many settings, the primary contact is the family member who brings the child to therapy or accompanies an adult or parent to therapy. Often, the family member who comes to the therapy session has a complicated culture-brokering role in which the person needs to both represent home, family, and community life in the clinic world and represent the clinic and institutional world back in home and family life. Such questions as "So, what happened?" are indicative of the information requests that spouses, significant others, grandparents, and other family members might ask.

Family members may also have quite divergent perspectives on the nature of the problem, priorities for intervention, and meanings of illness and disability in daily life (**Figure 14.2**). These within-family differences often generate within-family negotiations and a kind of partnering up within family life that will influence family–practitioner partnerships. The dynamics of these multiple perspectives and within-family negotiations will likely change over time and be influenced by changes in illness trajectories, developmental agendas, household configurations, and constellation of household resources and needs. In addition, illness and disability might only be one subplot or drama in family life, competing with other pressing concerns and needs.

Illness and Disability Generate Only Negative Experiences

There has been, and continues to be, an assumption that all of the effects of illness and disability on a family are negative. This belief leads to the erroneous conclusion

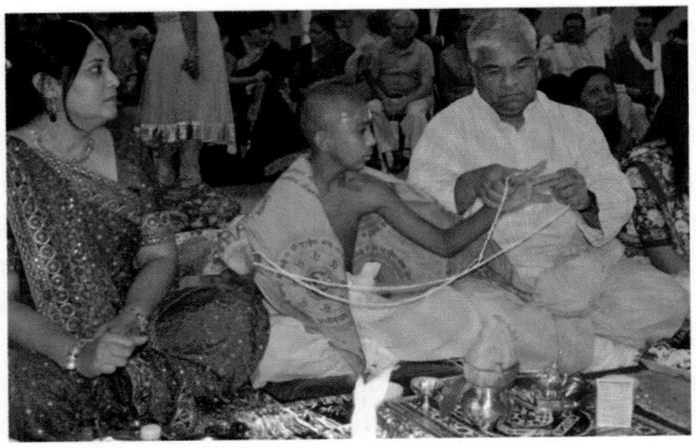

FIGURE 14.2 This boy is engaged in the "Yagnopavit ceremony," a sacred thread ceremony where the concept of Brahman is introduced to a young boy. Traditionally, the ceremony is performed to mark the point at which boys begin their formal education. His mother notes, "It is a joyous event for the family as it marks the first stage of the transition of the youth towards accepting duties" (A. Gajjar, personal communication, June 7, 2012). Note that each family member is likely to have his or her own perspective about important events. Consider the different perspectives that the father, the son, and the mother might each have?

that family reactions to illness and disability are both predictable and shared. In other words, the practitioner might presume to know about the effect of an illness or disability on the family without fully understanding a particular family. These notions get dismissed once one listens to families talk about their experiences. We have been struck by the incredible richness of their stories and the difficulty people have in reducing their complex reactions to a few discrete categories such as stress, grief, or acceptance. Some theorists have also attempted to develop theories based on stages of reactions, but the fixedness of these stages has been criticized (Moses, 1983).

Much of the research that has been conducted that relates to the response of family members to illness or disability has been conducted with parents of children who have special health care needs. Parents and other family members have offered critiques of this body of research (e.g., Lipsky, 1985), citing the failure of researchers to recognize positive outcomes from these experiences. Researchers have tended to measure such predetermined variables as maternal depression and stress. Critics note that personal reports of other effects, including positive changes in family life, have been discounted. Advocates of the family-centered care movement note the failure of many researchers and practitioners to understand the unique features of family adaptation and coping and assert the need for further research that is grounded in the perspectives of family members. Although it is beyond the scope of this chapter to summarize this body of literature, the assumption that the effects of disability are unilateral and negative must be challenged as both simplistic and inadequate.

Practitioners need to seek understanding of the effects of illness and disability on the families of the people who come to them for assistance. These effects will likely change over time, and the perceptions of the relative stress of families will be shaped by other events in the family and the availability of resources. The presumption that the entirety of a family's experience can be summarized as stressful often leads to misunderstandings and lost opportunities to promote any positive aspects and celebrate successes (Lawlor & Cada, 1993; Lawlor & Mattingly, 1998; Mattingly & Lawlor, 2000).

Having a family member with illnesses and/or disabilities can substantially impact family life including participation, routines, priorities, practices and identity (Law, 2002; Werner DeGrace, 2004). Although much of the literature emphasizes potentially negative influences such as stress, decreased economic resources, or excessive time demands, the picture is far more complicated. On the *Boundary Crossings* research program at USC, described briefly later in this chapter, families have worked to make sure that we understand and appreciate the positive elements that having a family member with special needs brings to family life. These include the cultivation of strengths and skills, love, "blessings" and renewed or enhanced spirituality, positive affects on siblings, and adoption of new career paths, advocacy, or social activism. Our intent is not to romanticize family life but rather to point toward the range of possible experiences of families when managing illness or disability trajectories. We have come to understand that strengths and challenges are intimately interrelated and perhaps can best be understood as relational aspects of family experience. Families have often used phrases such as "strengths beget strengths" or "God only gives me what he knows I can handle" to convey their lived experiences of the co-relations of strengths and challenges.

The Professional Is the Expert

Traditionally, Western biomedicine has been concerned with curing people. The notion of the professional as healer is important here. The healer is an expert who can both ascertain what is wrong (assess and diagnose) and identify the correct intervention to cure the ailment (treat) (Biesele & Davis-Floyd, 1996; Davis-Floyd & Sargent, 1997; M. J. Good, 1995). The patient's role has historically been viewed as a submissive one, offering information as requested, submitting to physical examination, and following the expert's directives for treatment. In this view, health care professionals make people healthy by curing disease. The patient's personal history, family situation, and work history might be only of peripheral importance in the healer's task of diagnosing and treating the pathologic condition that is causing the illness. Whereas the hope of medicine has been curing or healing, which implies the ability of the health professional to bring a person from a state of illness to some state of "normalcy" or premorbidity, occupational therapy practitioners are rarely in a position to cure anyone. The people they treat may have rich, full lives, but they are usually living these lives with an impairment or chronic condition that cannot be totally eradicated or fixed.

Practices steeped in Western biomedical traditions frequently adopt professional–client relationships that are based on hierarchical models or expert-driven models. The expert model remains prevalent in early childhood practices despite increasing recognition that elements of this model create barriers to developing collaborative partnerships and understanding family life. The expert model tends to promote dependence within recipients of services, to limit opportunities for families to contribute insights and have their specific concerns and needs addressed, to burden the professional with the unrealistic expectation of always having the expertise to respond to all issues (Cunningham & Davis, 1985), and to organize services in ways that are self-serving to the expert (Howard & Strauss, 1975).

It is not surprising that reliance on expert models fosters relationships between practitioners and family members that incorporate compliance and coercion strategies. This leads to considerable confusion about whether the "story" is one of collaboration, coercion, or compliance (Lawlor & Mattingly, 1998). The issue is not merely a semantics problem. Each approach to working relationships creates distinctly different experiences for all parties. Practitioner judgments that a person is noncompliant, or in the terms used by family members—"bad parent," "bad daughter," and the like, divert energies away from more reflective analysis or direct attempts to understand alternative perspectives (Trostle, 1988). Comments such as "they are just in denial" often indicate a breach in understanding, a dismissal of family or personal perspectives. Families typically have tremendous expertise and knowledge related to their family members, family life, the illness or disability of their family member, and the ways in which treatment recommendations can most likely be implemented in the home. As Bedell, Cohn, and Dumas (2005) note, parents are well situated to promote and support their child's development in home and community life and able to modify or develop effective strategies. Perhaps the most troubling dimension of a hierarchical model of expertise is that family expertise is not acknowledged and taken up in meaningful ways. In fact, in some health care encounters, family expertise remains quite invisible.

Family Experiences and Occupational Therapy Practice

This chapter addresses the need to attend to family perspectives in providing services to people with chronic illnesses or disabilities and the experiences of family members that are related to their participation in occupational therapy services. We have spent many hours watching occupational therapy practices, primarily with children. In addition, we have interviewed many parents and other family members and practitioners. These data have been gathered as part of a longitudinal, urban, ethnographic research project currently entitled *Boundary Crossings: Re-Situating Cultural Competence*. We have followed a cohort of African-American children with illnesses and/or disabilities, their primary caregivers, family members, and the practitioners who serve them for approximately 14 years. This is a multifaceted study that includes analysis of meanings of illness and disability in family and clinical worlds; cross-cultural communication in health care encounters; health care practices including occupational therapy; health disparities; and processes of partnering up and how illness and disability, family life, health care, and development are interrelated (Lawlor, 2003, 2004; Mattingly, 2006). The conceptual framework for the study draws heavily on narrative, interpretive, and phenomenological approaches to understanding human experience.

One of our most striking discoveries is the way in which seemingly casual conversation, brief moments of social engagement, attention to connectedness, and shared moments in the course of therapy sessions can deeply affect the experiences of family members and practitioners and, perhaps most important, the outcomes of therapy. These moments can be quite subtle and appear to be a kind of backdrop to the real work in therapy time or in health care encounters. Their seemingly mundane nature can belie their impact. As is illustrated later in this chapter, there are also times of heightened engagement in which there is intensity around the learning or insights to understanding that are unfolding. There are, of course, other kinds of moments in family-centered care that are also consequential and appear to be marked by conflict, tension, drama, or highly charged emotion. As Laderman and Roseman (1996) remind us, "Medical encounters, no matter how mundane are dramatic events" (p. 1).

In the following passages, we provide examples of family experiences related to illness and disability and their interactions with practitioners, including occupational therapists. Occupational therapists have shared many stories that relate to how they or their practice has been influenced by their experiences with families. We will begin by returning to the quote that was used to introduce family-centered care. In that quote, this mother shared her strategy for ensuring that her family, including extended members, was knowledgeable about her child's therapy program and the clinical world in which therapy takes place. The following passages, excerpted from interviews with the occupational therapist, provide insights into her experiences related to meeting this family and her deep appreciation for lessons learned through this partnership. The occupational therapist credits this mother, whom we will call Leslie, with helping her to learn how to engage with Leslie's daughter, a toddler, who initially would not let the therapist come near her to work with her. As the following quote reveals, this successful partnership began with a rather precarious start:

> And it, it was just such a nice relationship, building of a relationship and then to come back and have her do her therapy with me was a really nice thing. But the first, um, 4 months of therapy I couldn't touch her. And that was interesting. I think that almost was successful because I had to work through Leslie. Leslie did all the therapy and I sort of sat . . . It was really funny [*laughter*]. I wish we could have some videotape, this was so funny. In the room I would sit in the corner. I had . . . I even couldn't approach her (the child) or she would start to cry. And I would sit a certain distance, which got closer and closer each session and I would direct Leslie what to do. And I think that that taught her so much about what she needed to do and gave her that physical, um, experience that just doing something with her daughter and knowing what it was, what the goals were, rather than sitting back and watching it. That might have been . . . I don't know. 'Cause I just see her as so successful with that and I wonder sometimes if that wasn't part of it. . . . 'Cause she had to, to do her daughter's therapy [*laughter*]. I, I couldn't. I couldn't get . . . you know. Then finally, and it was Leslie's idea and my idea, too, to bring her other children in because we couldn't get her to move. She wouldn't . . . she was terrified . . . climb up in things or any normal things that would . . . a normal child would explore. She was terrified. So when you see her today, it's like not the same. It was really, really interesting.

At another time, the therapist elaborated on what she had learned from this mother:

> And so she taught me a lot about that. And she also—what happens when you work with a mother like that, they, they teach you about the power of negotiation and respecting an individual's rights. Because sometimes as a therapist, when the therapist doesn't have children, I can take more of the teacherly role and put my foot down and push through. And, and I can do that. And as a mother, I don't think that works so much in a household. You just get confrontation. You don't have that kind of power over your kids like a teacher. And she has the most incredible way of negotiating with the personality and she actually taught me how to do that with her daughter. So if I, there were situations where I would kinda be more teacherly and put my foot down and this is the rules and here we go. And Leslie would sort of pull me into a more productive understanding of how she raises her kids and that was really helpful.

The therapist, whom we will call Megan, further clarifies how knowledge about family life facilitates the therapeutic process. Leslie's strategy to bring family members into the therapy world not only enabled the family members to understand more about therapy but also provided Megan with information that helped her to picture possibilities of family life. Megan also skillfully incorporated stories into therapy conversations that further illuminated life outside the clinic world. In one interview, she commented,

> But it's not like in Leslie's case where you just get this just fabulous, you know, understanding of what's going on here. And this sort of communication and commitment and feedback about what's happening there in this other world. Like I have such a knowledge of what's happening in Leslie's world. I mean, I feel like I almost have pictures of their family life and I imagine, you know, she'll tell me a story about the Christmas tree and how Kylie's (the child), you know, she's making her put ornaments in this one section high up because then she has to use her arm in that way. And I can just see the family and I, I. . . .

As part of our research, we are trying to understand more about how practitioners and families do come to know and understand enough about each other to effectively partner up and what attributes influence partnerships. Leslie shares her perspective as follows:

> It has nothing whatsoever to do with how much schooling you've had. It's just all from your life experience. And that makes a difference. Because I think my experience that I had with Megan as far as us having to communicate with one another. . . . I don't know a lot—I don't know and I didn't know an awful lot about her personal life. Okay, but I knew enough to know that whatever has happened to her in her life has either made her stronger, or, I don't know if that's what I'm looking for—it gave her a sense of caring about people. Whether it was something that really bad, that she said, "Okay I'm not gonna be like that," or something that was really good because she was brought up in a nurturing environment, it just made her personality care. And, and that made a big difference. 'Cause that's what she brought to the table. You know? And, my strong sense of family, and 'course, that's my baby we're talking about, you know. And you have those two, us two bringing back to the table . . . when we sit down to discuss what

is best for a child. I think that made a big difference. If—if Megan would have been more of just all business, keep it very technical . . . you know, I think the outcome would have been different. And I probably would have told somebody, I don't want her to be my therapist for my baby. You know, I mean 'cause I wouldn't have felt that, that nurturing that's within her. That's needed as far as I'm concerned; to deal with every child, not just mine. But, oh it's, oh, that is so great!

We now want to just briefly describe a portion of an occupational session that illustrates the often subtle but highly effective participation of family members in therapy sessions. The moment that we describe in the case study occurred partway through a session in which an occupational therapist was working with a young boy with a brachial plexus injury. The activity that she planned provided an opportunity to evaluate his sensation, fine motor abilities, and bilateral coordination. This vignette shows the narrative structuring of therapy sessions and the ways in which family members can contribute through both conarration and their participation as social actors in the therapy scene (Lawlor, 2003, 2009; Mattingly, 1998). Even though we are describing only several minutes within a therapy session here, we are excerpting key aspects. Therapy time, particularly sessions with heightened engagement and family participation, is too rich and too complex to provide all the detail and description.

CASE STUDY 14.1 The Magic Box

The therapist, whom we will call Georgia, announces a guessing game and presents a rather elaborately decorated box, approximately 9 in square and 12 in tall. Micah, who is approximately 4 years old; his brother Damian, who is several years older; and his mother, Sheana are all present along with one of the authors who is videotaping. Sheana, who is sitting off to the side, says, "Oooh," with dramatic intonation. Georgia further proclaims that it is a "magic box." The two brothers join her in a fairly tight circle on the floor mat. Georgia instructs Micah that he must reach into the box without peeking and find things (these things are small objects that are buried among beans). By touching his left arm, she cues him that this is the arm she wants him to use. (Micah's brachial plexus injury is on his left side.) "See if you can find anything. Move your arm in there. I'll tell you when you have something. No. [*whispers*] It's a secret box. No, you cannot peek. It's a secret. Find anything in there?" Micah has tried to look under the lid of the box as an adaptive strategy, as he is apparently having trouble feeling the objects buried in the beans. Micah whines a bit in frustration and slips his right hand into the box and quickly retrieves an object. Georgia says, "No, no this hand may not . . ., " and his mother says, "Only lefty can, Micah," thus supporting the therapist's agenda that he use his left arm. Georgia takes the retrieved object and places it in Micah's left hand. She then asks him to show and give the object to his brother, thus smoothly incorporating Micah's older brother into this therapy activity that clearly has potential for further intrigue.

The activity unfolds with continued skillful co-narration and participation of Sheana and Damian. The brothers are highly engaged, and Damian at times seems to scaffold for his brother, thus heightening Micah's potential for success. For example, as Micah reaches into the box, Damian comments, "They might be all the way down," thus facilitating Micah's attempts to move deeper into the box. Sheana, at times, skillfully co-manages the session, seemingly vigilant that Damian does not take over or become too involved, thus disrupting Micah's session or become disengaged in a way that limits his ability to support the therapeutic activity. For example, she calls out Damian's name when she wants him to pull back a bit or, conversely, to pay more attention.

The action that all four of these actors produce is almost seamless, almost choreographed in its fluidity, but also obviously spontaneous and organized in the flow of therapy. The work that the mother, brother, and therapist do to help make this session so effective is not merely related to promoting the desired behavior, although this is important. Both mother and brother skillfully use changes in tone of voice to support Micah's efforts. The transcript of the session is peppered with comments such as "You did it!" and "Oooh," a kind of quieter admiration. They also seem to be heightening the engagement in the doing, making the "guessing game" more appealing, more dramatic. For example, Damian becomes a kind of announcer about the characters that are retrieved from the box. What seemed initially to be a box of farm animals becomes a box with oddities such that Mickey Mouse, lions, and gorillas appear with considerable puzzlement and humor. As Damian comments when Mickey is found, "What's he doing here?"

At other times in this session, Damian was given many of the same tasks as his brother, such as swinging on the trapeze or picking up the beans that had been strewn on the floor while Micah was digging in the "magic box." Damian's inclusion not only helped to make the session more fun but also provided many opportunities for reciprocity, turn taking, and sharing between these two brothers. Sheana's careful attention to the session and her sons' behaviors, as well as her skillful co-narration, further added to the perception that this was a family event.

Near the end of the activity, Sheana comments, "It's a very cute thing." Georgia responds with both a smile and the comment, "It's something you really could enjoy at home." This is a replay of a conversation that occurred partway through the game when Damian had said, "Let's take it home" in the midst of his enjoyment, after his mother's comment "That's a cute little idea—I like that." A brief exchange follows about whether beans or rice would be better. Interspersed throughout this activity had been comments from Georgia related to the ways in which this was a therapeutic activity for Micah. ■

It is always a bit difficult in written text to convey social action among engaged social actors. In the brief passages in the case study, we have attempted to evoke the kinds of animation, attunement, engagement, enjoyment, and joint coordination that marked these moments. These family members and this therapist created a therapeutic experience that addressed Micah's challenging clinical needs while affording an opportunity for engaging moments. These moments were engaging enough that this family was actively designing ways to replicate the experience at home, to recreate this event in the clinic as a family experience at home.

Conclusion

In this chapter, we highlighted many of the challenges that are involved in attempting to respond to the needs of clients and their families. Challenges are coupled with opportunities. As practitioners discover ways of getting to know families and understanding their perspectives, opportunities emerge for practitioners to construct richer, more meaningful experiences. The more meaningful the experience is, the more likely it is that treatment will be efficacious.

We have found that discussions of opportunities must be tempered with specific cautions. Approaches to getting to know families must be noninvasive, sensitive, nonjudgmental, and respectful of the parameters for privacy and disclosure that individuals indicate. Understanding a perspective does not presume that as an occupational therapy practitioner, you are responsible for intervening in every dimension of that perspective. Family-centered care is implemented most effectively in situations in which interdisciplinary efforts are well coordinated and effectively communicated. In situations in which practitioners are working in relative isolation, caution must be exercised to ensure that they are practicing within the bounds of their expertise and appropriately facilitating access to other resources as needed.

One of the greatest challenges for practitioners is to understand how their own lived experience shapes their interactions with family members in the course of providing services. Conceptual models of practice and theory regarding family systems and human development, ethics, and public and institutional policies all contribute to our framework for family-centered interventions. However, practitioners, as the instruments for intervention, bring their own selves and their cultural views of families into clinical interactions.

We intuitively recognize that such things as our ethnicity, nationality, geographical home, and perhaps even religion provide us with powerful cultural worlds. These aspects of our background help to make us who we are, culturally speaking. We are often not fully aware that our profession and our family also offer cultural worlds that shape some of our deepest assumptions, beliefs, and values. This chapter concerns a kind of cultural intersection between the practitioner (acting as a member of a professional culture) and a client (acting as a member of a family culture). Practitioners, of course, have families, and clients often have professions. However, when practitioners and clients meet during occupational therapy intervention, the practitioner's professional and institutional cultures are particularly significant in shaping how the practitioner defines good intervention and a good professional–client relationship.

Occupational therapy practitioners come to their profession with life experiences of being a member of a family. This lived experience of growing up in a family significantly shapes who we are as practitioners, particularly in situations in which practitioners are getting to know a family and seeking to understand their needs, priorities, values, hopes, and resources. These assumptions about family life tend to be quite tacit, and we are often not aware of their influence unless we actively reflect on our actions. Guided reflection through mentorship and supervision as well as discussions with other team members concerning beliefs about specific families are essential components of intervention planning and implementation with clients and their families.

Acknowledgments

This chapter was supported by work related to four research projects. One study was supported by grant MCJ-060745 from the Maternal and Child Health Program (Title V, Social Security Act), Health and Services Administration, Department of Health and Human Services. Appreciation is expressed to the American Occupational Therapy Foundation for their support of pilot work related to that study. Research was also supported by *Boundary Crossing: A Longitudinal and Ethnographic Study* (# R01 HD 38878) and *Boundary Crossings: Re-Situating Cultural Competence* (# 2R01 HD 38878) funded through the National Institute of Child Health and Human Development (NICHD), National Institutes of Health (NIH). The contents of this chapter are solely the responsibility of the authors and do not necessarily represent the official views of any of these agencies. We also would like to express our appreciation to the many children, families, therapists, and practitioners who have participated in these research efforts and who have willingly shared their experiences. We would also like to specifically thank Emily Ochi, Karen Crum, Michelle Elliot, Melissa Park, Beth Crall, Cristine Carrier, Kim Wilkinson, Jesus Diaz, Lisa Hickey, Cynthia Strathmann, Emily Areinoff, Claudia Dunn, and Aaron Bonsall for their contributions and assistance in preparing this chapter.

References

American Occupational Therapy Association. (1999). *Occupational therapy services for children and youth under the Individuals with Disabilities Education Act* (2nd ed.). Bethesda, MD: Author.

Bandura, A., Carprara, G. V., Barbaranelli, C., Regalia, C., & Scabini, E. (2011). Impact of family efficacy beliefs on quality of family functioning and satisfaction with family life. *Applied Psychology: An International Review, 60*(3), 421–448.

Bauby, J. D. (1997). *The diving bell and the butterfly*. New York, NY: Random House.

Becker, G. (1997). *Disrupted lives: How people create meaning in a chaotic world*. Berkeley, CA: University of California Press.

Bedell, G. M., Cohn, E. S., & Dumas, H. M. (2005). Exploring parents' use of strategies to promote social participation of school-age children with acquired brain injuries. *American Journal of Occupational Therapy, 59*(3), 273–284.

Biesele, M., & Davis-Floyd, R. (1996). Dying as a medical performance: The oncologist as Charon. In C. Laderman & M. Roseman (Eds.), *The performance of healing* (pp. 291–321). New York, NY: Routledge.

Bluebond-Langer, M. (1978). *The private worlds of dying children*. Princeton, NJ: Princeton University Press.

Cain, C. (1991). Personal stories: Identity acquisition and self-understanding in Alcoholics Anonymous. *Ethos, 19*, 210–253.

Charon, R., & Montello, M. (2002). *Stories matter: The role of narrative in medical ethics*. New York, NY: Routledge.

Clark, F. (1993). Occupation embedded in real life: Interweaving occupational science and occupational therapy: 1993 Eleanor Clarke Slagle Lecture. *American Journal of Occupational Therapy, 47*(12), 1067–1078.

Cohn, E. S. (2001). From waiting to relating: Parents' experiences in the waiting room of an occupational therapy clinic. *American Journal of Occupational Therapy, 55*, 167–174.

Cohn, E. S., Miller, L. J., & Tickle-Degnan, L. (2000). Parental hopes for therapy outcomes: Children with sensory modulation disorders. *American Journal of Occupational Therapy, 54*(1), 36–43.

Colman, W. (1988). The evolution of occupational therapy in the public schools: The laws mandating practice. *American Journal of Occupational Therapy, 42*, 701–705.

Cunningham, C., & Davis, H. (1985). *Working with parents: Frameworks for collaboration*. Philadelphia, PA: Open University Press.

Davis-Floyd, R., & Sargent, C. (1997). *Childbirth and authoritative knowledge: Cross-cultural perspectives*. Berkeley, CA: University of California Press.

Deal, A., Dunst, C., & Trivette, C. (1989). A flexible and functional approach to developing individualized family support plans. *Infants and Young Children, 1*(4), 32–43.

Dickie, V., Cutchins, M. P., & Humphry, R. (2006). Occupation as transactional experience: A critique of individualism in occupational science. *Journal of Occupational Science, 13*(1), 83–93.

Dunst, C., Trivette, C., & Deal, A. (1988). *Enabling and empowering families: Principles and guidelines for practice*. Cambridge, MA: Brookline.

Edelman, L., Greenland, B., & Mills, B. (1993). *Building parent professional collaboration: Facilitator's guide*. St. Paul, MN: Pathfinder Resources.

Elder, G. (1998). The life course as developmental theory. *Child Development, 69*(1), 1–12.

Esdaile, S., & Olson, J. (Eds.). (2004). *Mothering occupations: Challenge, agency, and participation* (pp. 306–322). Philadelphia, PA: F. A. Davis.

Fitzgerald, M. H. (2004). A dialogue on occupational therapy, culture, and families. *American Journal of Occupational Therapy, 58*, 489–498.

Fleming, M., & Mattingly, C. (1994). *Clinical reasoning: Forms of inquiry in therapeutic practice*. Philadelphia, PA: F. A. Davis.

Frank, A. (1995). *The wounded storyteller: Body, illness, and ethics*. Chicago, IL: University of Chicago Press.

Frank, G. (2000). *Venus on wheels: Two decades of dialogue on disability, biography, and being female in America*. Berkeley, CA: University of California Press.

Garro, L., & Mattingly, C. (2000). Narrative turns. In C. Mattingly & L. C. Garro (Eds.), *Narrative and the cultural construction of illness and healing* (pp. 259–269). Berkeley, CA: University of California Press.

Good, B. (1994). *Medicine, rationality, and experience*. Cambridge, United Kingdom: Cambridge University Press.

Good, B., & Good, M. J. (1994). In the subjunctive mode: Epilepsy narratives in Turkey. *Social Science in Medicine, 38*, 835–842.

Good, M. J. (1995). *American medicine: The quest for competence*. Berkeley, CA: University of California Press.

Greenfeld, J. (1978). *A place for Noah*. New York, NY: Henry Holt.

Greenfeld, J. (1986). *A client called Noah: A family journey continued*. New York, NY: Henry Holt.

Hanft, B. (1989). *Family-centered care: An early intervention resource manual*. Rockville, MD: American Occupational Therapy Association.

Hanft, B. E. (1991). Impact of public policy on pediatric health and education programs. In W. Dunn (Ed.), *Pediatric occupational therapy: Facilitating effective service provision* (pp. 273–284). Thorofare, NJ: Slack.

Harkness, S., Super, C. M., Sutherland, M. A., Blom, M. J. M., Moscardino, U., Marvridas, C. J., & Axia, G. (2007). Culture and the construction of habits in daily life: Implications for the successful development of children with disabilities. *OTJR, 27* (Suppl. 1), S33–S40.

Hasselkus, B. R. (2006). 2006 Eleanor Clarke Slagle Lecture—The world of everyday occupation: Real people, real lives. *American Journal of Occupational Therapy, 60*, 627–640.

Hinojosa, J., Sproat, C. T., Mankhetwit, S., & Anderson, J. (2002). Shifts in parent-therapist partnerships: Twelve years of change. *American Journal of Occupational Therapy, 56*(5), 556–563.

Hockenberry, J. (1995). *Moving violations: War zones, wheelchairs, and declarations of independence*. New York, NY: Hyperion.

Howard, J., & Strauss, A. (1975). *Humanizing health care*. New York, NY: Wiley.

Humphry, R., Gonzales, S., & Taylor, E. (1993). Family involvement in practice: Issues and attitudes. *American Journal of Occupational Therapy, 47*(7), 587–593.

Hurwitz, B., Greenhalgh, T., & Skultans, V. (2004). Introduction. In B. Hurwitz, T. Greenhalgh, & V. Skultans (Eds.), *Narrative research in health and illness* (pp. 1–20). Malden, MA: Blackwell.

Individuals with Disabilities Education Act of 1990, Pub. L. No. 101-476, 104 Stat. 1142 (1990).

Individuals with Disabilities Education Improvement Act of 2004, Pub. L. No. 108-446, 118 Stat. 2647 (2004).

Jamison, K. R. (1996). *An unquiet mid: A memoir of moods and madness*. New York, NY: Vintage Books.

Kellegrew, D. H. (1998). Creating opportunities for occupation: An intervention to promote the self-care independence of young children with special needs. *AJOT, 52*(6), 457–465.

Kleinman, A. (1988). *The illness narratives: Suffering, healing, and the human condition*. New York, NY: Basic Books.

Kleinman, A. (2006). *What really matters: Living a moral life amidst uncertainty and danger*. New York, NY: Oxford University Press.

Laderman, C., & Roseman, M. (Eds.). (1996). Introduction. In *The performance of healing* (pp. 1–16). New York, NY: Routledge.

Law, M. (2002). Participation in the occupations of everyday life. *AJOT, 56*(6), 640–649.

Lawlor, M. C. (1991). Historical and societal influences on school system practice. In A. Bundy (Ed.), *Making a difference: OTs and PTs in public schools* (pp. 1–15). Chicago, IL: University of Illinois.

Lawlor, M. C. (2003). The significance of being occupied: The social construction of childhood occupations. *American Journal of Occupational Therapy, 57*(4), 424–434.

Lawlor, M. C. (2004). Mothering work: Negotiating health care, illness and disability, and development. In S. Esdaille & J. Olson (Eds.), *Mothering occupations: Challenge, agency, and participation* (pp. 306–322). Philadelphia, PA: F. A. Davis.

Lawlor, M. C. (2009). Narrative, development, and engagement: Intersections in therapeutic practices. In U. Jensen & C. Mattingly (Eds.), *Narrative, self, and social practices* (pp. 199–220). Aarhus, Denmark: Philosophia Press, Aarhus University.

Lawlor, M. C., & Cada, E. (1993). Partnerships between therapists, parents, and children. *OSERS News in Print, 5*(4), 27–30.

Lawlor, M. C., & Elliot, M. L. (2012). Physical disability and body image in children. In T. Cash (Ed.), *Encyclopedia of body image and human appearance* (pp. 650–656). Oxford, UK: Elsevier Press.

Lawlor, M. C., & Mattingly, C. (1998). The complexities in family-centered care. *American Journal of Occupational Therapy, 52*, 259–267.

Lawlor, M. C., & Mattingly, C. F. (2001). Beyond the unobtrusive observer. *American Journal of Occupational Therapy, 55*(2), 147–154.

Lawlor, M. C., & Mattingly, C. (2009). Understanding family perspectives on illness and disability experiences. In E. Crepeau, E. Cohn, & B. Schell (Eds.), *Willard & Spackman's occupational therapy* (11th ed., pp. 33–44). Philadelphia, PA: Lippincott Williams & Wilkins.

Lipsky, D. K. (1985). A parental perspective in stress and coping. *American Journal of Orthopsychiatry, 55*, 614–617.

Luhrmann, T. M. (2000). *Of two minds: The growing disorder of American psychiatry*. New York, NY: Knopf.

Mattingly, C. (1998). *Healing dramas and clinical plots: The narrative structure of experience*. Cambridge, United Kingdom: Cambridge University Press.

Mattingly, C. (2000). Emergent narratives. In C. Mattingly & L. C. Garro (Eds.), *Narrative and the cultural construction of healing* (pp. 181–211). Berkeley, CA: University of California Press.

Mattingly, C. (2006). Pocahontas goes to the clinic: Popular culture as lingua franca in a cultural borderland. *American Anthropologist, 106*(3), 494–501.

Mattingly, C. (2010). *The paradox of hope: Travels in clinical borderlands*. Berkeley, CA: University of California Press.

Mattingly, C., & Fleming, M. (1994). *Clinical reasoning: Forms of inquiry in a therapeutic practice*. Philadelphia, PA: F. A. Davis.

Mattingly, C., & Lawlor, M. (2000). Learning from stories: Narrative interviewing in cross-cultural research. *The Scandinavian Journal of Occupational Therapy, 7*, 4–14.

Mattingly, C., & Lawlor, M. (2001). The fragility of healing. *Ethos, 29*(1), 30–57.

Mattingly, C., & Lawlor, M. C. (2003) Disability experience from a family perspective. In E. Crepeau, E. Cohn, & B. Schell (Eds.), *Willard & Spackman's occupational therapy* (10th ed., pp. 69–79). Philadelphia, PA: Lippincott Williams & Wilkins.

McGonigel, M. J., Kaufmann, R. K., & Johnson, B. H. (Eds.). (1991). *Guidelines and recommended practices for the individualized family service plan*. Bethesda, MD: Association for the Care of Children's Health.

Monks, J., & Frankenberg, R. (1995). Being ill and being me: Self, body, and time in multiple sclerosis narratives. In B. Ingstad & S. R. Whyte (Eds.), *Disability and culture* (pp. 107–134). Berkeley, CA: University of California Press.

Moses, K. L. (1983). The impact of initial diagnosis: Mobilizing family resources. In J. Mulick & S. Pueschel (Eds.), *Parent-professional partnerships in developmental disability services* (pp. 11–34). Cambridge, MA: Academic Guild.

Murphy, R. F. (1990). *The body silent*. New York, NY: W. W. Norton.

Ochieng, B. M. N. (2003). Minority ethnic families and family-centered care. *Journal of Child Health Care, 7*(2), 123–132.

Park, C. C. (1982). *The siege: The first eight years of an autistic child*. Boston, MA: Little, Brown.

Park, C. C. (2001). *Exiting Nirvana: A daughter's life with autism*. Boston, MA: Little, Brown.

Peete, R. (2010). *Not my boy: A father, a son and one family's journey with autism*. New York, NY: Hyperion Press.

Rosen, S., & Granger, M. (1992). Early intervention and school programs. In A. Crocker, H. Cohen, & T. Kastner (Eds.), *HIV infection and developmental disabilities: A resource for service providers* (pp. 75–84). Baltimore, MD: Brookes.

Swartz, T. T. (2009). Intergenerational family relations in adulthood: Patterns, variations, and implications in the contemporary United States. *Annual Review of Sociology, 35*, 191–212.

Trostle, J. A. (1988). Medical compliance as an ideology. *Social Sciences in Medicine, 27*, 1299–1308.

Werner DeGrace, B. (2004). The everyday occupation of families with children with autism. *American Journal of Occupational Therapy, 58*, 543–550.

Whiteford, G. (2010). Occupation in context. In M. Curtin, M. Molineux, & J. Supky-Mellson, *Occupational Therapy and Physical Dysfunction: Enabling Occupation* (6th ed., pp. 135–150). London, United Kingdom: Churchill-Livingstone Elsevier.

Williams, D. (1992). *Nobody nowhere: The extraordinary autobiography of an autistic*. New York, NY: Avon Books.

For additional resources on the subjects discussed in this chapter, visit http://thePoint.lww.com/Willard-Spackman12e.

CHAPTER 15

Patterns of Occupation

Kathleen Matuska, Kate Barrett

OUTLINE

LEARNING OBJECTIVES

After reading this chapter, you will be able to:

1. Examine roles, routines, rituals, and habits and their influence on health and well-being
2. Compare/contrast measures of roles, routines, habits, and life balance and their usefulness for occupational therapy assessment
3. Discuss intervention approaches that address problems in occupational patterns
4. Analyze a theoretical model of life balance and its application to occupational therapy

Introduction

This chapter discusses performance patterns and how they contribute to or detract from health and well-being. Other chapters in this book describe occupational therapy assessment and intervention for personal and environmental factors influencing occupational performance (the *what, why,* and *where*), and this chapter explores the patterns of occupations (the *how*) and how those patterns influence health and well-being. The Occupational Therapy Practice Framework: Domain and Process, 2nd Edition (American Occupational Therapy Association [AOTA], 2008) identifies performance patterns as habits, routines, roles, and rituals used in the process of engaging in occupations or activities. This chapter also includes life balance, a holistic view of **occupational patterns** in the context of living.

Roles, habits, routines, rituals, and lifestyles can be healthy or harmful. At the health end of the continuum, patterns of occupation can promote health and well-being and prevent certain diseases, especially those related to lifestyle such as obesity, heart disease, and diabetes.

See **Appendix I, Common Conditions, Resources, and Evidence**, for more information about these conditions.

Certain routines such as engaging in regular exercise or getting adequate sleep can contribute to overall health. For example, occupational therapy addresses the growing epidemic of obesity by helping children build habits and routines, which include engagement in health-promoting activities that influence their weight (AOTA, 2007). At the pathology end of the continuum, habits or routines that are rigid and strong can dominate everyday life (Dunn, 2000). In these cases, people need to complete certain actions or routines before moving on, or they experience discomfort or anxiety. These entrenched habits can be seen in obsessive-compulsive disorder (OCD), autism, and addictions and can impede satisfactory occupational performance. Performance patterns are important to address in occupational therapy across the health pathology continuum.

See **Appendix I, Common Conditions, Resources, and Evidence**, for more information about OCD, autism, and addictions.

Roles

Occupational roles are normative models for behavior shaped by culture and society (Crepeau & Schell, 2009). Examples of roles in life are student, friend, worker, and mother. Roles are dynamic throughout the life course because new roles are learned and old roles are replaced. Individuals experience a sense of purpose, identity, and structure when carrying out roles (Kielhofner, 2009) and are learned through a process of socialization and acculturation.

Roles can be disrupted, altered, or ended by the presence of a disability. For example, a study by Davies Hallet, Zasler, Maurer, and Cash (1992) found that roles change significantly after traumatic brain injury (TBI). The study found that many persons with TBI experienced important role changes such as loss of a worker role, which resulted in feelings of anger, frustration, apprehension, confusion, boredom, and fear. Quigley (1995) studied the impact of spinal cord injury (SCI) on the roles of women. She found that women experienced significant changes in their roles related to how they carried out their daily routines, negotiated their relationships, and navigated new environmental barriers. Role demands are significantly increased for mothers who have children with disabilities (Crowe, VanLeit, Berghmans, & Mann, 1996) and influences how and which roles are performed. Occupational therapists help people to construct or reconstruct their roles when they have experienced a lack of engagement in desired roles or an unexpected/undesired loss or change in their roles.

See **Appendix I, Common Conditions, Resources, and Evidence**, for more information about TBI.

While understanding a person's roles, we must be cautious to not overgeneralize their meaning. Roles do not easily translate from culture to culture and may limit us to singular or normative expectations of behavior and meaning (Jackson, 1998). Expectations of roles change from culture to culture and therefore role assessments cannot always be used across cultures. When considering a person's roles, it is important for the occupational therapy practitioner to listen carefully to the client for his or her own interpretation of the meaning and responsibilities associated with his or her roles.

Assessment of Roles

There are several assessments commonly used in occupational therapy to learn about a client's roles. See Table 15.1 for a review of common role assessments.

Habits

Habits are specific, automatic behaviors; performed repeatedly; relatively automatically; and with little variation. Because they can be performed in different contexts, they are not necessarily performed in exactly the same way each time (Clark, 2000). Habits can be useful, dominating, or impoverished (Clark, 2000) and can be difficult to break.

An example of a useful habit is brushing teeth before bed every night. It is performed consistently without planning, and when barriers arise (such as when stranded overnight at an airport), the loss is noticed but is not incapacitating. Useful habits can help organize time and resources so that less cognitive energy is needed throughout the day. Useful habits increase skill in action because less focus is on the action and more focus on its elaboration. For example, when a habit is created to diligently put car keys on a hook by the door when entering the house, less time and energy is spent trying to find the keys when needed. Or when appointments are immediately recorded on a calendar, the cognitive load to remember the date is reduced. These useful habits reduce fatigue because they require less effort, free attention for other things, and allow novel actions without having to recall or attend to the specific details (Clark as cited in Young, 1988). Simple, useful habits may be developed to manage time and reduce the stress that interferes with daily performance. For example, an occupational therapist may help a client with SCI develop useful habits in the morning routine so that time and energy is not wasted on locating and setting up supplies before going to work.

See **Appendix I, Common Conditions, Resources, and Evidence**, for more information about SCI.

TABLE 15.1 Common Role Assessments

Assessment Tools	Developers	Purpose	Method	Comment
Role Checklist	Oakley, Kielhofner, Barris, and Reichler, 1986	To assess a person's perception of participation in 10 major life roles (i.e., worker, caregiver, volunteer) and the value placed on these roles.	The client identifies and rates the roles that he or she has done in the past, is currently engaged in, as well as roles that he or she would like to have.	It is a relatively easy and quick way to assess how someone feels about the roles that they hold and to see changes in role patterns over time.
The Adolescent Role Assessment	Black, 1976	To assess four domains: developing aspirations, developing interpersonal competencies, developing self-efficacy, and developing autonomy.	A semistructured interview that provides both narrative and quantitative information regarding worker role development.	It is based on the idea that during adolescence one explores interests, assumes increased responsibility, and develops values and goals that influence occupational choice and work attitudes necessary for entering an occupation.
The Role Activity Performance Scale	Good-Ellis, Fine, Spencer, and DiVittis, 1987	To assess a person's role performance in 12 major roles over a period of 18 months. The role activities assessed include work, education, home management, family of origin relationships, extended family relationships, partner/spouse relationship, social relationships, leisure, self-management, hygiene and appearance, and health care.	Interview process that allows for information to be collected from the client as well as other sources including family, medical record, and the health care team.	It is used in mental health settings and is designed to guide intervention planning as well as be used as a research tool to measure intervention outcomes.
The Role Change Assessment	Jackoway, Rogers, and Snow, 1987	To assess the level of engagement and satisfaction experienced in these roles and how they have changed over time.	A semistructured interview format to examine 48 roles in family and social, vocational, self-care, organizational, leisure, and health care categories for older adults.	The interview format allows the occupational therapy practitioner to assess both role stability as well as change.
Worker Role Interview (WRI)	Braveman et al., 2005	To assess psychosocial capacity in injured workers for readiness to return to work. Addresses both psychosocial and environmental factors that impact return to work.	Semistructured interview formats for recently injured workers and persons who are chronically disabled.	The information gathered compliments other work/physical capacity assessments to ensure a well-rounded picture of the client and his or her needs that should be addressed to ensure return to work.

When people have difficulty learning new useful habits because of a dysfunctional internal state, they may have impoverished habits. People with Alzheimer's disease, depression, or attention disorder may not be able to develop new useful habits that help them adjust to their disability (Clark, 2000). Instead, the occupational therapist will consult with the caregivers for ways to modify the environment or the activity for optimal performance. For example, teaching the caregiver to have all lunch supplies available and in one place everyday to cue the individual with Alzheimer's to make a sandwich.

See **Appendix I, Common Conditions, Resources, and Evidence**, for more information about Alzheimer's disease, depression, and attention disorder.

Dominating habits are those that are consistently performed even if they interfere with optimal performance. Over time, some habits can become addicting and affect one's health, such as the need to smoke a cigarette when driving or consuming snacks when watching TV. Occupational therapy intervention may assist individuals to identify and practice alternative habits that are less harmful. Other dominating habits create stress or anxiety if they cannot be performed, such as needing to wash hands after touching anything. The anxiety from performing the hand washing and/or not being able to hand wash make it difficult to carry on with the other tasks in a day. Habit domination can occur with OCD, autism, or other mental health disorders. These can be very difficult to change and are sometimes managed with medication.

Assessment of Habits

The *Assessment of Life Habits* (*LIFE-H*) can be a useful assessment tool for occupational therapy because it was developed to evaluate social participation of people with disabilities and may fit in the International Classification of Functioning, Disability, and Health (ICF) participation domains (Desrosiers et al., 2004). It groups habits into 12 categories (nutrition, fitness, personal care, communication, housing, mobility, responsibility, interpersonal relationships, community, education, employment, and recreation) and documents the extent to which these life habits are carried out. The LIFE-H is either self- or therapist-administered, with response categories for the level of difficulty and the type of assistance required for each life habit. Satisfaction for each item is also reported using a 5-point scale. The long form contains 240 items, whereas the short form contains 77 items. The level of difficulty and the types of assistance are combined and weighted to derive an accomplishment score. Total scores for each life habit category range from 0 to 10 (Spinal Cord Injury Rehabilitation Evidence, 2010). There are no published norms; however, data from various SCI studies provide some basis for comparison (Spinal Cord Injury Rehabilitation Evidence, 2010).

Structured interview with the client, family member, or caregiver is another useful assessment. Questions should address how the individual performs activities of daily living (ADL) and instrumental activities of daily living (IADL) and the specific habits used during performance of each activity. For example, "Describe the steps you take in the morning to get ready for the day." It is important to determine if these habits are a help or hindrance to performance.

Routines

Routines are "a type of higher-order habit that involves sequencing and combining processes, procedures, steps, or occupations and provide a structure for daily life" (Clark, 2000, p. 128S). An example of a health-promoting routine is following a predictable series of stretches and exercises followed by a nutritious breakfast before going to work every day. For someone with a disability, a healthful routine may include taking care of medical equipment and setting up medications for the next day before going to bed. People who have hired caregivers will be most efficient at managing their care if they have a predictable routine to teach their caregiver.

Because routines provide a useful daily structure, the loss of routines can also be disruptive. People who have chronic diseases may find it difficult to maintain a steady routine because managing their disease symptoms is challenging and often unpredictable. Dressing, for example, is typically done in a sequential way with similar steps and procedures used from day to day. However, research on women with rheumatoid arthritis (RA) and diabetes showed they altered their dressing routines because they had much more difficulty performing the steps (Poole & Cordova, 2004). Helping people create high levels of order and routine may be a useful strategy for coping with the unpredictable nature of chronic diseases. Women with fibromyalgia who reported high levels of order and routine in their lives gained greatly from actively coping with their illness compared to women who did not have high levels of routine (Reich, 2000).

Routines can be a very important component of managing one's overall health but can also be damaging (Friese et al., 2002; Segal, 2004). Sometimes, people with chronic diseases avoid making future plans and limit social engagements to minimize potential discomfort. This pattern of avoidance leads to a vicious cycle of less positive social engagements (Zautre, Hamilton, & Yocum, 2000). Long-term patterns of sedentary or isolative behavior such as watching television every night for several hours can have a negative effect on health or well-being.

Performance patterns are disrupted with acute or chronic diseases or conditions. Several diseases have fatigue as one of the primary symptoms; and often, the additional requirement of managing disease symptoms taps into available energy reserves. Occupational therapists address performance patterns and help people create new habits or routines that maximize their available energy. For example, people who had SCI recognized different levels of energy at different times of the day or week and learned to organize their time so that they were doing the most when they felt the best. This type of planning was viewed as a very useful strategy for participating in the activities that were important to them (Chugg & Craik, 2002).

Chronic diseases such as multiple sclerosis, chronic fatigue syndrome, or fibromyalgia include symptoms of severe fatigue that interfere with routines and participation in everyday life.

See **Appendix I, Common Conditions, Resources, and Evidence**, for more information about multiple sclerosis.

Fatigue is often unpredictable and severe, making it difficult to follow desired routines or to make future plans (Matuska & Erickson, 2008). People who experience this type of fatigue are forced to make choices about how they are going to expend their limited energy and make reductions in the number and type of activities in which they participate (Matuska & Erickson, 2008).

Occupational therapists teach principles of energy conservation that address the importance of health-promoting routines in managing fatigue. Common energy conservation strategies include analyzing and modifying activities to reduce energy expenditures, balancing work and rest, delegating some activities, examining and modifying standards and priorities, using the body efficiently, organizing workspaces, and using assistive technologies to conserve energy (Matuska, Mathiowetz, & Finlayson, 2007). All of these strategies create positive changes in daily routines, and when individuals integrate them into their lives, there has been an associated reduced fatigue impact and improved quality of life (Mathiowetz, Finlayson, Matuska, Chen, & Luo, 2005; Mathiowetz, Matuska, & Murphy, 2001).

Family Routines

Family routines are important to address because they have been shown to be important in individual and family well-being (Denham, 2003; Friese et al., 2002; Friese, 2007). Family routines are observable and repetitive patterns involving family members that occur with predictable regularity in family life (Denham, 2002). These routines help define the usual family roles, organize daily life, and reflect family identity (Denham, 2003). Families have health routines associated with dietary practices, sleep and rest patterns, activity, dependent care, avoidance behaviors, medical consultation, and health recovery (Denham, 2002). These health routines are adhered to by family members to support family health and development and communicate with health experts. Routines can help family members arrange everyday life in a way that helps them cope with illness or stress. When families are stressed, interventions are most effective when the new health routines are aligned with family values, are meaningful, applicable to family needs, and when resources were available (Denham, 2002).

Assessment of Routines

Several assessment tools are available to assess routines. See Table 15.2 for a summary of common assessments for routines.

Rituals

Rituals are different from routines in that they include strong elements of symbolism (Crepeau, 1995). Rituals often are a reflection or enactment of one's culture. A strong sense of meaning and identity is experienced when a person feels engaged and included in a ritual. Rituals create a sense of order and an opportunity to carry out one's role. Many people associate the word ritual with religious activities such as a baptism, bar mitzvah, pilgrimage to Mecca, or other religious ceremony. Rituals can also be secular such as a holiday parade, high school graduation, or initiation into a group of people (gang, sorority, fraternity, etc.). Rituals often signify to a community of people a transition from one state of being to another, such as from child to adult, single to married, or student to graduate.

Typically, rituals are performed with more than one person, but one can participate in an individual ritual such as prayer. What makes an occupation a ritual is the symbolism and meaning the individual attaches to it. For example, the goal of going for a run for one person may be to exercise, in this case there is not a strong symbolic or affective component; therefore, it is not a ritual. However, for another person, going for a Sunday run may symbolize the shedding of something weighing him or her down or preparation for the week to come. In this case, there is a symbolic and affective component and could therefore be considered a ritual.

Rituals also exist in the context of families. Family rituals contain symbolic and affective components that serve to construct and affirm family identity (Segal, 2004). Examples of family rituals could include Sunday afternoon picnics, family reunions, or how families greet one another. Rituals occur at regular intervals or on special occasions. They may occur daily (kissing one another hello), weekly (family dinner), annually (reunion), or only once in a lifetime (bar mitzvah). Figure 15.1 shows a group of extended family members making a traditional Irish recipe that brings them together every year.

Rituals offer individuals and groups of people an opportunity to carry out identified roles and to feel a sense of belonging and meaning. Although we do not have a formal way of assessing rituals in occupational therapy, it is important for occupational therapists to be

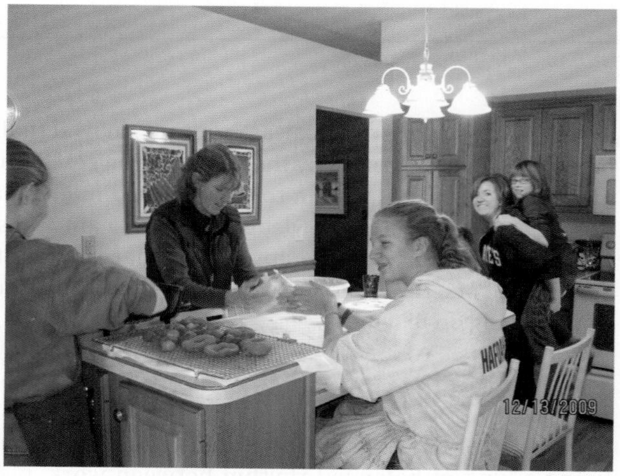

FIGURE 15.1 Extended family members in their annual ritual of making traditional Irish potato donuts.

TABLE 15.2 Assessments of Routines

Assessment Tools	Developers	Purpose	Method	Comment
The Model of Human Occupation Screening Tool (MOHOST) Version 2.0	Kielhofner et al., 2007; Parkinson, Forsyth, and Kielhofner, 2006	Measures the Model of Human Occupation (MOHO) concepts of volition, habituation, communication/interaction skills, motor skills, process skills, and the environment.	One of the six subscales measures performance patterns related to routines, adaptability, roles, and responsibility. Scoring reflects whether the individual's performance patterns facilitate, allow, inhibit, or restrict optimal performance.	The MOHOST has initial validity evidence for use as an overview of occupational performance and for use of the six subscales representing the MOHO concepts.
The Family Routines Inventory	Boyce, Jensen, James, and Peacock, 1983; Jensen, James, Boyce, and Hartnett, 1983	Measures the predictability of routine in the daily life of a family. It measures 28 positive, strength-promoting family routines and has demonstrated validity and reliability.	Scoring is based on the number of routines endorsed by the family (they do the routine), frequency of adherence to the routine (how often they do it), and how important the routine is to them.	Examples of items include "family eats at the same time each night," "each child has some time each day for playing alone," "family regularly visits with the relatives," and "parents and children play together sometime each day."
The Scale of Older Adults' Routine (SOAR)	Zisberg, Young, and Schepp, 2009	Measures stability in activities on a daily and weekly basis for older adults. SOAR provides information about the stability or disruption of routine.	It is administered by in-person interview and includes 42 routine activities in five domains (basic, instrumental, leisure, social, and rest) measured on four dimensions (frequency, timing, duration, and sequence).	This assessment may be useful for occupational therapist in exploring altered routines during transitions such as from home to a retirement community, independent living to assisted living, or a nursing home.
The Social Rhythm Metric (SRM-5)	Monk, Flaherty, Frank, Hoskinson, and Kupfer, 1990; Monk, Frank, Potts, and Kupfer, 2002	To quantify daily lifestyle regularity (routines) with respect to event timing.	Diary-like tool where participants record the timing of five daily events over the course of 1 week; when they get out of bed, have first contact with a person, start of work, school, volunteer or family care, have dinner, and go to bed.	This measure was developed from the theory that social rhythms (i.e., eating and sleeping schedules) are important for structuring individuals' days and for maintaining circadian rhythms, and alterations in these rhythms lead to disentrainment and poor health.

aware that what may appear as "routine" may actually be experienced as a ritual by the person engaged. Rituals may also be thought of as a tool to be used in occupational therapy as we acknowledge the significant transitions one experiences in therapy; from nonacceptance to acceptance of a disability, meeting therapeutic goals, or transitioning off of a unit.

Occupational Balance

Occupational therapy was founded on the idea that practicing a kind of balanced rhythm between work, play, rest, and sleep leads to wholesome living (Meyer, 1977). Occupational therapy is an important profession for addressing lifestyles in both preventative and restorative ways because of the expertise and understanding of occupational patterns. Lifestyles are unique patterns of everyday occupations including roles, habits, routines, and rituals and can lead to an overall life balance or imbalance with long-term consequences on health, well-being, and quality of life. *Occupational balance* refers to a perception that one's patterns of everyday occupations are satisfactory and include a range of meaningful occupations. *Life balance* is similar but uses words more commonly understood outside of the occupational therapy profession (Matuska, 2012b; Matuska & Christiansen, 2009). **Life balance** is defined as "a satisfying pattern of daily activity that is healthful, meaningful, and sustainable to an individual within the context of his or her current life circumstances" (Matuska & Christiansen, 2008, p. 11).

The life balance model (Matuska, 2012b) depicts the relationships between occupational patterns, life outcomes, and the environment (see Box 15.1). Occupational patterns should enable people to meet important needs such as supporting biological health and physical safety (i.e., exercise, rest, medication management), contributing to positive relationships (i.e., friends and family), feeling engaged and challenged (i.e., hobbies, stimulating work), and creating a positive personal identity (i.e., caregiving, volunteering) (Matuska & Christiansen, 2008). The extent people are able to engage in patterns of occupations that address all of these needs, they will perceive their lives as more satisfying, less stressful, and more meaningful, or *balanced*. People also need to have the skill to organize their time and energy in ways that enable them to meet their important personal goals and renewal (Matuska, 2012b). In other words, life balance requires the skill to create a match between how much time one *desires* to engage in activities and *actually* engages in the activities that meet important needs.

It is conceivable that the constraints of the environment could make it difficult to engage in a satisfactory pattern of occupations. Matuska (2012b) found that life balance was lower for people of a racial minority and was negatively affected by employment and having children at home. A highly supportive environment could

BOX 15.1 The Life Balance Model

Figure 15.2 is a visual depiction of the life balance model. The two ovals in the center represent activity configurations. Oval A represents activity configuration *congruence*, which reflects the match between desired and actual time engaged in valued activities. In other words, people are spending the right amount of time doing the things they want. Oval B represents the *equivalence* of satisfaction across the four need-based dimensions in the life balance model (health, relationships, challenge, and identity). The overlap of ovals A and B represents life balance, where people are satisfied with the time spent in activities across the four need areas. Life balance has associated positive outcomes such as lower perceived stress, higher personal well-being, and need satisfaction (Matuska, 2012a). On the other hand, if people are dissatisfied with the amount of time spent in activities or they are not meeting all four need areas, then the model depicts this situation as life imbalance with associated negative health consequences. The model is surrounded by a large oval representing the environment and its influence on life balance.

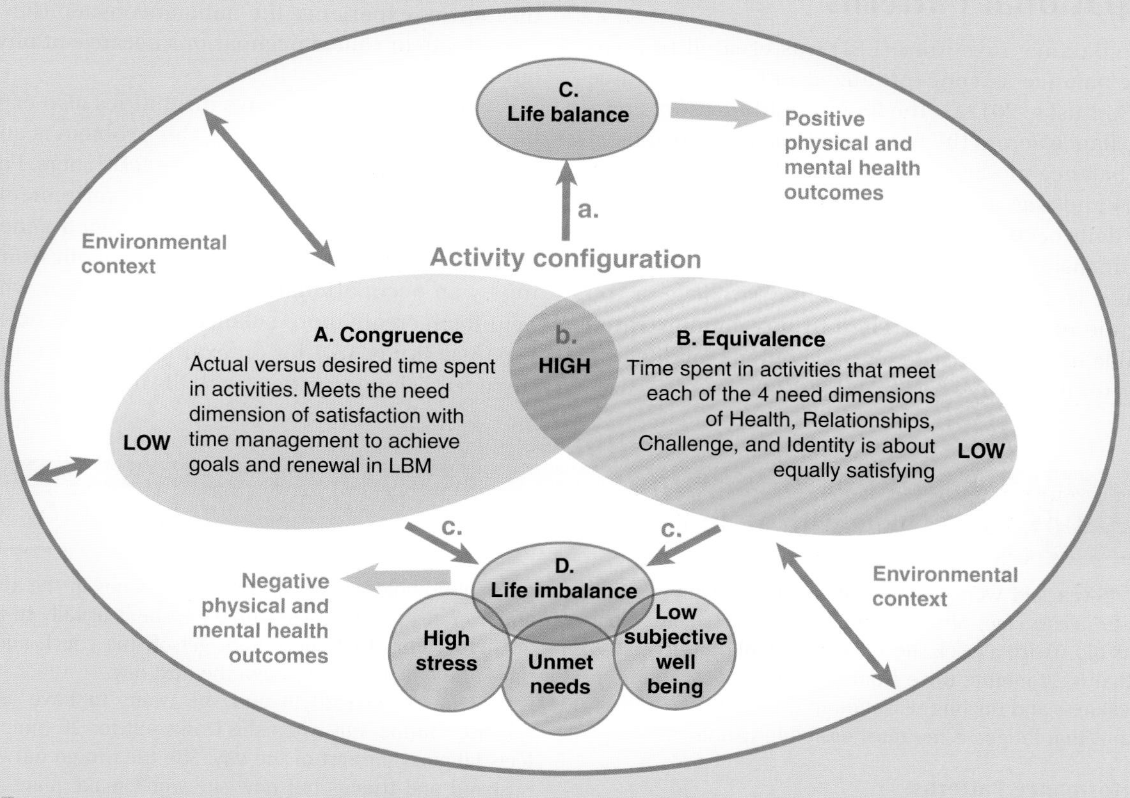

FIGURE 15.2 The Life Balance Model (LBM). (From Matuska, K. [2012b]. Validity evidence for a model and measure of life balance. *Occupational Therapy Journal of Research, 32*[1], 229–237. Copyright 2012 by the American Occupational Therapy Foundation. Reprinted with permission.)

improve life balance. For example, having enough financial security to create a satisfactory life was also viewed as important for life balance among Swedish men and women (Wagman, Håkansson, Matuska, Björklund, & Falkmer, 2011).

Even though there is increasing evidence that life balance is related to lower stress and higher psychological well-being (Matuska, 2012b; Sheldon, Cummins, & Khamble, 2010), creating balanced lives is challenging for most people. It may be even more challenging for people who have chronic illnesses such as multiple sclerosis or parents of children with autism spectrum disorder (Stein, Foran, & Cermak, 2011). These and other chronic health conditions can influence what people are able to do and whether or not they can create a satisfactory balance of occupations in their lives. For example, women with multiple sclerosis expressed how managing their health needs became a major factor in their lives and how they needed to make daily adaptations in order to continue doing things that were important to them (Matuska & Erickson, 2008). Their disease often dictated what their activity options were in a given day. Occupational therapists have an important contribution to fostering life balance in preventative and restorative modes for individuals and families with or without chronic illnesses.

Assessment of Life Balance and Occupational Patterns

The Life Balance Inventory (LBI) was created to measure life balance as conceptualized in the life balance model (Matuska, 2012a). The 53-item LBI measures perceived balance across the four need-based dimensions in the life balance model (health, relationships, challenge, identity) and was designed to allow unique configurations of daily occupations for each person within each of those dimensions. The scoring is based on the idea that imbalance could result from spending too little or too much time in any activity. The LBI has demonstrated acceptable internal consistency and content validity as a measure for life balance (Matuska, 2012a).

The LBI can be accessed online at http://minerva.stkate.edu/LBI.nsf, and the output consists of an overall life balance score and balance scores in each subscale.

Daily activity logs are another method of examining occupational patterns. The purpose of activity logs is to have an accurate record of what occurs in peoples' lives by recording activities at regular intervals. The length of the intervals and what is recorded varies. For example, an activity log could be a 24-hour record divided into 30-minute intervals, and an individual is asked to fill it out for three consecutive 24-hour periods. Individuals could be asked to simply record what they were doing every 30 minutes, or contextual information could be included such as "what I was doing, where it occurred, who I was with, and how I felt." Activity logs help the person to be more aware of how time is spent and can be a first step in making healthy lifestyle changes. Occupational therapy practitioners may coach clients when life imbalances are evident.

Life imbalance is when patterns of daily occupations are perceived to be unsatisfactory (there is not a good match between desired and actual engagement in valued activities), increasing the risk for physical and mental health problems. Life imbalance means that occupational patterns limit or compromise participation in valued relationships; are incongruent for establishing or maintaining physiological health and a satisfactory identity; or are mundane, uninteresting, or unchallenging (Matuska & Christiansen, 2009). People who have disabilities experience life imbalance when they cannot participate in valued occupations because of physical or environmental barriers.

People who do not have disabilities also experience life imbalance, and addressing this problem is an emerging role for occupational therapy practitioners. For example, people who are transitioning into retirement, caring for children and aging parents (sandwich generation), single parents, and workaholics may benefit from coaching by an occupational therapy practitioner who could help them create more balanced patterns of occupation. See Case Study 15.1 for an example of an occupational therapist helping a patient with life imbalance.

CASE STUDY 15.1 Living with Multiple Sclerosis

SJ is a 45-year-old woman who was diagnosed with multiple sclerosis 7 years ago. She is married and has a son who is 14 years old. Twice a week she works as a dental hygienist in a clinic that is 30-minute drive from her home. SJ has intermittent weakness and tingling sensation in her right arm, and she complains that fatigue is her most disabling symptom.

Performance Patterns

SJ has the most energy in the morning and she uses that time to shower, groom, and prepare breakfast for herself and family. After breakfast, she tries to capitalize on her energy by doing other household work. Typically, she crashes in the afternoon and evening, however. On workdays, she is usually so fatigued in the evenings that she cannot get off the couch and sometimes the fatigue lasts through the next day.

SJ has gained 20 lb and she wants to have a regular exercise routine, but when she works out for 20 minutes, she feels fatigued the rest of the day. She used to go out with her husband and friends but now she won't make plans because she doesn't know if she'll feel well enough to go. SJ is very dissatisfied with her life because her fatigue disrupts her social opportunities and fulfilling her roles.

CASE STUDY 15.1 Living with Multiple Sclerosis *(continued)*

Occupational Therapy Assessment

The occupational therapist asked SJ to complete a daily activity log for 1 week where she wrote down what she did every hour and how she felt during that activity, including physical symptoms. Together, they examined the activity log to determine patterns and create an activity plan. SJ discovered that she felt tired after her morning shower but ignored it in order to accomplish more. The 30-minute drive to and from work was also problematic and she noticed much more fatigue on the days after she worked. The occupations that SJ prioritized were continuing to work 2 days a week, doing the laundry, cooking at least two meals a week, working out at least 2 days a week, attending at least one of her son's soccer/basketball games each month, and going out with her husband and friends once or twice each month.

Occupational Therapy Intervention

The occupational therapist discussed with SJ the principles of energy conservation: plan your day; rest before fatigue; spread activities throughout the day; and prioritize, delegate, simplify, and use proper body mechanics.

Morning Routine

She tried showering in the evening right before bed and found that she was less fatigued after her grooming routine in the morning. A 10-minute rest period was built in immediately after breakfast, which helped her feel more energetic the rest of the morning.

Rest throughout the Day

She decided to build a routine of rest into her schedule to prevent the severe disabling fatigue. Every 2 hours, she rested for 15 to 30 minutes. She discussed her fatigue with her employer and she was allowed to bring an easy chair into the back room for resting during her breaks. Instead of doing paperwork over the lunch break, she rests 30 minutes and has more energy at the end of the day to stay a few minutes later to do the paperwork.

Proper Body Mechanics

The occupational therapist discussed principles of body mechanics and restful positioning regarding her 30-minute drive to and from work. SJ repositioned the driver's seat to be more upright and created an armrest out of a shoebox that she placed next to her. She also decided to choose mellow and restful music for the drive home.

Delegate and Simplify

SJ and her occupational therapist discussed the energy conservation strategies with her husband and son. Together, they prioritized the activities where help was needed and ways to simplify activities that SJ wanted to keep. For example, cleaning was delegated to her family, and for SJ to continue doing the laundry, they decided to bring the washer and dryer to the main floor to save energy-draining trips to the basement. SJ agreed to cook dinner on 2 days when she didn't work and to plan the menu ahead so her husband could have the ingredients available. Foods that required less preparation time such as precut vegetables and bag salads would be used regularly. The family planned to rest 10 to 15 minutes after meals before beginning the cleanup. SJ liked this plan because her family spent more time together. ■

Summary

Roles, habits, routines, and rituals create the framework of people's lives and together make up lifestyles that are unique to each person. Life balance should be a consideration in any occupational therapy intervention. Are current lifestyle patterns contributing to a sense of overall well-being or taking away from a sense of well-being? When occupational patterns are dysfunctional, health and well-being are at risk. In turn, adapting or establishing satisfactory roles, habits, routines, and rituals may be used as tools in therapy to help a person improve life balance. Occupational therapy practitioners can use the tools described in this chapter to identify unhealthy patterns of occupation and help their clients create new patterns that are more satisfactory and healthy. The desired outcome for any occupational therapy intervention is life satisfaction and improved quality of life.

References

American Occupational Therapy Association. (2007). Obesity and occupational therapy: Position Paper. *American Journal of Occupational Therapy, 61*(6), 701–703.

American Occupational Therapy Association. (2008). Occupational therapy practice framework: Domain and process, 2nd edition. *American Journal of Occupational Therapy, 62*, 625–683.

Black, M. M. (1976). Adolescent Role Assessment. *American Journal of Occupational Therapy, 30*(2), 73–79.

Boyce, W. T., Jensen, E. W., James, S. A., & Peacock, J. L. (1983). The Family Routines Inventory: Theoretical origins. *Social Sciences Medicine, 17*(4), 193–200.

Braveman, B., Robson, M., Velozo, C., Kielhofner, G., Fisher, G., Forsyth, K., & Kerschbaum, J. (2005). *Model of occupational therapy clearinghouse.* Retrieved from http://www.uic.edu/depts/moho/assess/wri.html

Chugg, A., & Craik, C. (2002). Some factors influencing occupational engagement for people with schizophrenia living in the community. *British Journal of Occupational Therapy, 65*(2), 67–74.

Clark, F. (2000). The concepts of habit and routine: A preliminary synthesis. *The Occupational Therapy Journal of Research, 20*, 123S–137S.

Crepeau, E. B. (1995). Rituals. In C. B. Royeen (Ed.), *The practice of the future: Putting occupation back into therapy* (pp. 5–23). Bethesda, MD: American Occupational Therapy Association.

Crepeau, E. B., & Schell, B. A. B. (2009). Analyzing occupations and activity. In E. B. Crepeau, E. S. Cohn, & B. A. B. Schell (Eds.), *Willard & Spackman's occupational therapy* (11th ed., pp. 359–374). Baltimore, MD: Lippincott Williams & Wilkins.

Crowe, T. K., VanLeit, B., Berghmans, K. K., & Mann, P. (1996). Role perceptions of mothers with young children: The impact of a child's disability. *The American Journal of Occupational Therapy, 51*, 651–661.

Davies Hallet, J., Zasler, N. D., Maurer, P., & Cash, S. (1992). Role change after traumatic brain injury in adults. *The American Journal of Occupational Therapy, 49*, 241–246.

Denham, S. A. (2002). Family routines: A structural perspective for viewing family health. *ANS Advances in Nursing Science, 24*(4), 60–74.

Denham, S. A. (2003). Relationships between family rituals, family routines, and health. *Journal of Family Nursing, 9*, 305–330. doi:10.1177/1074840703255447

Desrosiers, J., Noreau, L., Robichaud, L., Fougeyrollas, P., Rochettel, A., & Viscogliosi, C. (2004). Validity of the assessment of life habits in older adults. *Journal of Rehabilitation Medicine, 36*, 177–182.

Dunn, W. (2000). Habit: What's the brain got to do with it? *Occupational Therapy Journal of Research, 20*, 6S–20S.

Friese, B. H. (2007). Routines and rituals: Opportunities for participation in family health. *OTJR: Occupation, Participation and Health, 27*(Suppl.), 41S–49S.

Friese, B. H., Tomcho, T., Douglas, M., Josephs, K., Poltrock, S., & Baker, T. (2002). A review of 50 years of research on naturally occurring family routines and rituals: Cause for celebration. *Journal of Family Psychology, 16*, 381–390.

Good-Ellis, M. A., Fine, S. B., Spencer, J. H., & DiVittis, A. (1987). Developing a Role Activity Performance Scale. *American Journal of Occupational Therapy, 41*(4), 232–241.

Jackoway, I. S., Rogers, J. C., & Snow, T. L. (1987). The Role Change Assessment: An interview tool for evaluating older adults. *Occupational Therapy in Mental Health, 7*(1), 17–37.

Jackson, J. (1998). Is there a place for role theory in occupational science? *Journal of Occupational Science, 5*, 48–55.

Jensen, E. W., James, S. A., Boyce, T., & Hartnett, S. A. (1983). The Family Routines Inventory: Development and validation. *Social Science Medicine, 17*(4), 201–211.

Kielhofner, G. (2009). *Conceptual foundations of occupational therapy practice* (4th ed.). Bethesda, MD: American Occupational Therapy Association.

Kielhofner, G., Fogg, L., Braveman, B., Forsyth, K., Kramer, J., & Duncan, E. (2007). A factor analytic study of the Model of Human Occupation Screening Tool of hypothesized values. *Occupational Therapy in Mental Health, 25*(2), 127–137.

Mathiowetz, V., Finlayson, M. L., Matuska, K., Chen, H. Y., & Luo, P. (2005). Randomized controlled trial of an energy conservation course for persons with multiple sclerosis. *Multiple Sclerosis, 11*, 592–601.

Mathiowetz, V., Matuska, K., & Murphy, M. (2001). Effectiveness of an energy conservation program for fatigue in multiple sclerosis. *Archives of Physical Medicine and Rehabilitation, 82*, 449–456.

Matuska, K. (2012a). Development of the Life Balance Inventory. *Occupational Therapy Journal of Research, 32*(1), 220–228.

Matuska, K. (2012b). Validity evidence for a model and measure of life balance. *Occupational Therapy Journal of Research, 32*(1), 229–237.

Matuska, K., & Christiansen, C. (2008). A proposed model of lifestyle balance. *Journal of Occupational Science, 15*(1), 9–19.

Matuska, K., & Christiansen, C. (Eds.). (2009). *Life balance: Multidisciplinary theories and research*. Bethesda, MD: American Occupational Therapy Association.

Matuska, K., & Erickson, B. (2008). Lifestyle balance: How it is described and experienced by women with multiple sclerosis? *Journal of Occupational Science, 15*(1), 20–26.

Matuska, K., Mathiowetz, V., & Finlayson, M. (2007). Use and effectiveness of energy conservation strategies for managing multiple sclerosis fatigue. *American Journal of Occupational Therapy, 61*(1), 63–70.

Meyer, A. (1977). The philosophy of occupational therapy. *American Journal of Occupational Therapy, 31*, 639–642.

Monk, T. H., Flaherty, J. F., Frank, E., Hoskinson, K., & Kupfer, D. J. (1990). The Social Rhythm Metric: An instrument to quantify the daily rhythms of life. *The Journal of Nervous and Mental Disease, 178*(2), 120–126.

Monk, T. H., Frank, E., Potts, J. M., & Kupfer, D. J. (2002). A simple way to measure daily lifestyle regularity. *Journal of Sleep Research, 11*, 183–190.

Oakley, F., Kielhofner, G., Barris, R., & Reichler, R. (1986). The Role Checklist: Development and empirical assessment of reliability. *Occupational Therapy Journal of Research, 6*, 157–170.

Parkinson, S., Forsyth, K., & Kielhofner, G. (2006). *The Model of Human Occupation Screening Tool (MOHOST) Version 2.0*. Retrieved from http://www.uic.edu/depts/moho/assess/mohost.htm

Poole, J., & Cordova, J. S. (2004). Dressing routines in women with chronic disease: A pilot study. *New Zealand Journal of Occupational Therapy, 51*(1), 30–35.

Quigley, M. C. (1995). Impact of spinal cord injury on the life roles of women. *American Journal of Occupational Therapy, 49*, 780–786.

Reich, J. W. (2000). Routinization as a factor in the coping and mental health of women with fibromyalgia. *Occupational Therapy Journal of Research, 20*, 41S–51S.

Segal, R. (2004). Family routines and rituals: A context for occupational therapy interventions. *American Journal of Occupational Therapy, 58*, 499–508.

Sheldon, K., Cummins, R., & Khamble, S. (2010). Life balance and well-being: Testing a novel conceptual and measurement approach. *Journal of Personality, 78*(4), 1093–1134.

Spinal Cord Injury Rehabilitation Evidence. (2010). *Assessment of Life Habits Scale (LIFE-H)*. Retrieved from http://www.scireproject.com/outcome-measures/assessment-of-life-habits-scale-life-h

Stein, L., Foran, A., & Cermak, S. (2011). Occupational patterns of parents of children with autism spectrum disorder: Revisiting Matuska and Christiansen's model of lifestyle balance. *Journal of Occupational Science, 18*.

Wagman, P., Håkansson, C., Matuska, K., Björklund, A., & Falkmer, T. (2011). Validating the model of lifestyle balance on a working Swedish population. *Journal of Occupational Science, 4*, 1–9.

Young, M. (1998). *The metronomic society*. Cambridge, MA: Harvard University Press.

Zautre, A. J., Hamilton, N., & Yocum, D. (2000). Patterns of positive social engagement among women with rheumatoid arthritis. *Occupational Therapy Journal of Research, 20*, 21S–40S.

Zisberg, A., Young, H. M., & Schepp, K. (2009). Development and psychometric testing of the Scale of Older Adults' Routine. *Journal of Advanced Nursing, 65*(3), 672–683. doi:10.1111/j.1365-2648.2008.04901.x

For additional resources on the subjects discussed in this chapter, visit http://thePoint.lww.com/Willard-Spackman12e.

CHAPTER 16

Culture, Race, and Ethnicity and the Impact on Occupation and Occupational Performance

Roxie M. Black

"Culture is profoundly and inextricably tied to matters of health and healthcare."

—Jaime Phillip Muñoz (2007)

OUTLINE

LEARNING OBJECTIVES

After reading this chapter, you will be able to:

1. Differentiate between culture, race, and ethnicity
2. Analyze how a client's culture may affect occupational choice and performance
3. Discuss the impact of culture on the occupational therapy evaluation and intervention process
4. Analyze the need for cultural awareness and culturally effective skills in occupational therapy
5. Compare and contrast individualistic and collectivistic cultures

Introduction

Three Practice Dilemmas

Before reading this chapter, please turn to the next page and read the three Practice Dilemmas. Think about answers to the questions in each.

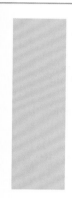

Practice Dilemma

The young, Caucasian occupational therapy (OT) student walked into the clinic of a large urban hospital knowing that the first patient of the day was a 54-year-old African-American man who was a day laborer on the piers. He had recently had hand surgery for a Dupuytren contracture release and needed functional activities to stretch the tendons in the third and fourth fingers of his dominant right hand. She greeted him warmly and then went to the cupboards and pulled out a sand painting kit. She was a technically smart student and knew that pushing the colored sand into the frame to make a small wall hanging would provide the kind of sustained finger stretching that the patient needed.

Following the session, as the student reflected on the activity, she recalled the little shake of the patient's head prior to beginning the task and the sardonic little grin he wore as he seemed to indulge her choice of intervention. "I wonder what that was all about?" she thought.

1. What should the student have considered when choosing an activity for this patient?
2. Even though the student knew the patient's diagnosis and intervention goals, what other information should she have sought from him?
3. Considering this patient's cultural and work history, what other activities might have been more appropriate for this patient?

Practice Dilemma

The OT practitioner was on his first home visit to an older woman who had been discharged from the rehabilitation center following a stroke. He was there to evaluate the home, meet the woman's family, and provide some education about activities of daily living (ADL) techniques. When he arrived, the client introduced the practitioner to her lesbian partner. The practitioner felt uncomfortable in this situation but knew he had to "grin and bear it" and went on to provide the necessary information in a stiff, officious manner.

1. What might the practitioner have done to avoid the "surprise" that awaited him in the client's home?
2. Given his discomfort, what action might the practitioner take to help reflect on his reaction?
3. Because of his discomfort and his concern that he might not be able to provide unbiased and effective therapy, should the practitioner request to be taken off this case?

Practice Dilemma

The young Somali man didn't seem very friendly. He didn't shake the hand of the experienced practitioner and seemed to carry an imperious demeanor. Although the occupational therapist tried many ways to get him to tell her his story and how he understood his mental illness, he finally stood and said that he didn't want to talk to her. He would only discuss this with a man. She wrote in his chart that he was noncompliant.

1. Given the patient's response to her, should the OT practitioner continue to try to work with him or should she ask one of the male therapists to take over this case?
2. What steps should the OT practitioner take to learn more about this patient's culture?
3. If she continues to work with this client, how should she approach him at her next scheduled appointment with him?

What are the similarities among these stories? They are examples of how issues of **culture** and **ethnicity** may impact occupational therapy (OT) practice. Issues of culture, **race**, and ethnicity can all be subsumed under the concept of **diversity**. Being diverse means having "distinct forms and qualities. " (Merriam-Webster, 1995) What is so important about diversity and why should occupational therapists be concerned about these issues? How will knowing about them help one's practice? Muñoz's statement earlier begins to tell the story. These are important questions that frame this chapter.

The world is an ever-changing place, with the demographics of the United States indicating an ever-increasing ethnic diversity in rates that surpass any other generations and improving access to technology that connects us to anyplace else in the world. This is now the world of occupational therapy. Although health care publications in the areas of culture and diversity have proliferated in the past decade (Black & Wells, 2007; Bonder, Martin, & Miracle, 2002; Lattanzi & Purnell, 2006; Srivastava, 2007), a recognition of the need to understand the unique culture of a client was first cited in professional publications in 1968 (Committee on Basic Professional Education, Council on Standards, as cited in Black, 2002). Interestingly, a few of the main reasons that occupational therapists have been concerned about diversity for so long is their belief about the uniqueness of each individual and their emphasis on **client-centered practice** (Law, Baptiste, & Mills, 1995). Client-centered practice focuses on the individual clients with whom we work, attempting to understand their beliefs, values, and dreams in order to collaboratively develop appropriate and meaningful interventions. In order to do this well, OT practitioners must learn about a person's culture as a means of understanding his or her unique characteristics and how that culture impacts the person's occupational choices and behaviors. In the first story earlier, the enthusiastic OT student chose an activity (sand painting) that did achieve the results she wanted (tendon stretching) but had no meaning for the client with whom she was working. As a result, the client would more than likely not repeat this activity outside of the OT clinic. Had the student learned a little of this man's culture and interests, together they may have determined an intervention activity that not only achieved the physical results but would also excite the client in a way that he may choose to repeat it often for its therapeutic and cultural value. Let's begin to further explore this with an examination of culture. A discussion of the other two practice dilemmas will be found in reference to topics later in the chapter.

Culture

Definition of Culture

The stories earlier indicate the importance of the examination of issues of culture for the OT practitioner. Therefore, it is important to understand what we mean by the term. Each person is a cultural being and each has a distinct cultural makeup. *Culture* is a broad term that encompasses many aspects about an individual and has been defined in many ways. Iwama (2004) states that culture is a "slippery concept, taking on a variety of definitions and meanings depending on how it has been socially situated and by whom" (p. 1), yet OT students and practitioners alike must have an understanding of what culture means. Black and Wells (2007) define culture as

> the sum total of a way of living, including values, beliefs, standards, linguistic expression, patterns of thinking, behavioral norms, and styles of communication that influence the behavior(s) of a group of people [and] is transmitted from generation to generation. It includes demographic variables such as age, gender, and place of residence; status variables such as social, educational, and economic levels; and affiliation variables. (p. 5)

One can see by this definition that the concept of culture is all-encompassing and quite complex. It incorporates all those aspects of a person that make him or her unique. Historically, anthropologists and others have determined that a large part of a person's identity is determined by his or her cultural allegiances (La Fontaine, 1985). If identity is determined at some level by one's culture, then it is imperative that OT practitioners learn about a client's culture in order to truly understand that person. Interrelated with the concept of culture are the concepts of race and ethnicity.

Race and Ethnicity

Race

Often, people think of race when asked about culture. Even though the U.S. Census Bureau and many other organizations ask people to check a certain box to indicate their race, scientists today question the validity of the biological concept of race (Haney Lopez, 1994; Marks, 1996). The term *biological race* is used by those who believe that "there exist natural, physical divisions among humans that are hereditary, reflected in morphology, and roughly but correctly captured by terms like Black, White, and Asian" (Haney Lopez, 1994, p. 6). In other words, race is recognized by physical attributes. Marks (1996) believes that dividing the human population among these discrete groupings is "arbitrary, not natural" (p. 124). Additionally, scientists have proven that identifying a group of people by their skin color (which often typifies the concept of race) does not represent a distinct cultural group; rather, "greater genetic variation exists within the populations typically labeled Black and White than between these populations" (Haney Lopez, 1994, p. 13). In contrast to this biological definition, Haney Lopez (1994) believes that race is a social construction and that "terms like Black, White, Asian, and Latino are social groups, not genetically distinct branches of humankind" (p. 14), whereas Relethford (as cited in Nittle, 2011) characterizes race as "a concept of human minds, not of nature." Within each of these social groupings are many different ethnic and cultural groups with different beliefs and values, languages, and behaviors.

What these arbitrary distinctions of race have accomplished is to separate people and support **racism** (Abizadeh, 2001). Racism "is most fundamentally the assessment of individual worth on the basis of real or imputed group characteristics. Its evil lies in the denial of people's right to be judged as individuals, rather than as group members, and in the truncation of opportunities or rights on that basis" (Marks, 1996, p. 131). Racism is a social problem that affects the OT profession. Systematic and institutionalized racism in the United States impacts access to exemplary education to minority populations (Rothenberg, 1998), which, in turn, limits the number of students who are academically prepared for OT education. This results in a limited multicultural workforce, which is a detriment to our profession. Racism also results in health disparities, limiting health access and service to people of color and those otherwise marginalized (Pittz, 2005).

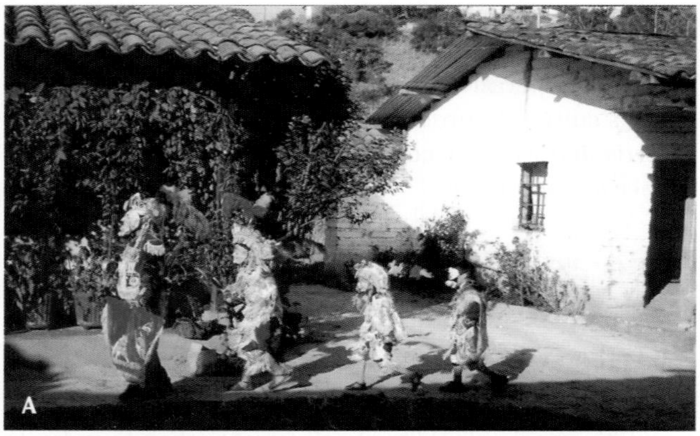

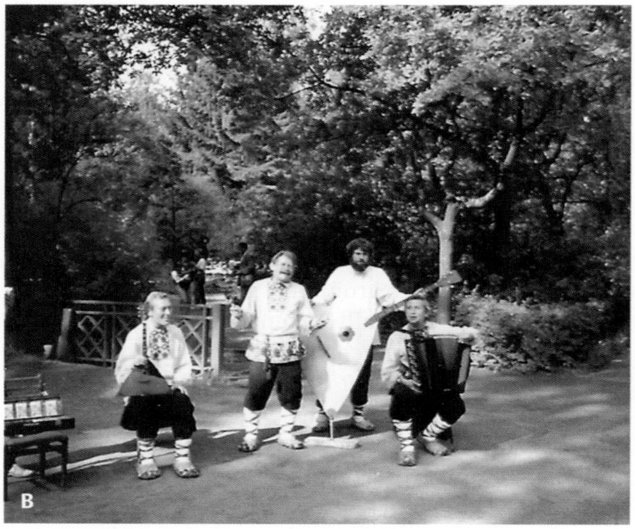

FIGURE 16.1 **A.** Mayan boys in ceremonial dress, Chichicastenango, Guatemala. **B.** Russian folksingers in regional costumes performing outside of Peterhof Palace, Saint Petersburg, Russia. (Photographs courtesy of Virginia Skinger.)

Ethnicity

As with the concept of culture and race, the term *ethnicity* has many definitions, many of which indicate that ethnicity is a social grouping of people who share cultural or national similarities (Figure 16.1). The most common characteristics of an ethnic group include "kinship, family rituals, food preferences, special clothing, and particular celebrations" (Srivastava, 2007, p. 12). Many people who are White or Caucasian living in the United States can identify with an ethnic background such as Italian American, Franco American, or Irish American. People who consider themselves Black or Asian also come from differing ethnic groups, such as Ethiopian or Filipino. Abizadeh (2001) discusses the impact that a common descent has on one's ethnicity. Although he speaks of the myth of common descent, he states, "people share a common ethnicity insofar as they share a myth of common descent—that is, insofar as they *believe* themselves to be descended from common ancestors" (p. 25). Leininger (as cited in Srivastava, 2007, p. 13), however, goes on to remind us that although ethnicity may reflect a shared culture, "the terms 'ethnicity' and 'culture' cannot be used interchangeably." One must remember, however, that as OT students and practitioners, acknowledging the importance of a client's ethnicity and/or culture is a vital aspect and function of client-centered care. Other important client issues are noted subsequently.

Cultural Differences Not Related to Race and Ethnicity

The majority of cultural differences that an OT practitioner may face are not related to race and ethnicity. Some of these include differences in class or socioeconomic status, education, religion, sexual orientation, age, and political views, all of which impact occupational choices and behaviors. Many of these characteristics are personalized by the client and have great meaning to him or her, just as they do for the practitioner. Therefore, these factors are often emotionally laden for both. The inability to recognize and address cultural differences may become problematic in client–practitioner interactions due to of issues of prejudice, stereotyping, and discrimination.

Prejudice and Discrimination

Prejudice

Most OT practitioners in the United States have grown up in a country and culture where racism, sexism, heterosexism, ageism, and many other –isms are prevalent. Most practitioners do not want to characterize people in a negative way, and many may not even be aware that they are doing so; yet, many do. **Prejudice** has been defined as "preconceived ideas and attitudes—usually negative about a particular group of people, often without full examination of the facts" (Black & Wells, 2007, p. 86). Hecht (1998), however, expands that definition by discussing four major metaphors for prejudice: difference as a threat (where prejudice is "a fear of difference or the unknown"), difference as aversive (where prejudice is caused by "a dislike of difference or the unknown"), difference as competition (where prejudice is caused by "competition with difference for scarce resources"), and prejudice as hierarchy (where prejudice is "hierarchical and structured") (p. 3). Looking back at the second story in the introduction of this chapter, one can recognize that the practitioner may be feeling some discomfort because of unrecognized prejudice against people who are homosexual. In that story, his stilted interaction with the couple impacts his client-centered approach, which may result in less than effective intervention planning and implementation. This story may exemplify one of the first two of Hecht's (1998) metaphors (difference as a threat or as aversive). Have you ever noticed prejudice caused by competition or hierarchy, the last two metaphors?

Stereotyping and Ethnocentrism

Prejudice is often the result of stereotyping and ethnocentrism. **Stereotyping** occurs when one attributes certain characteristics to an entire group of people, or what Herbst (1997) defines as "an exaggerated image of their characteristics, without regard to individual attributes" (p. 212). These can be thoughts about people related to age, "race," gender, sexuality, occupation, ethnicity, and physical and mental abilities. Some common stereotypes that have been heard by the author include

All Black people can dance
Obese people are lazy
Feminists are man-haters
Old people are grumpy
Gay men are promiscuous

Many of us have been raised in a society that teaches us stereotypical concepts. Although we often cannot control these thoughts, which may come unbidden to our consciousness, it is important to be aware of them and then choose not to listen to or act on them. This kind of thinking, which negates the importance of recognizing the uniqueness of each individual, may develop into prejudicial beliefs. **Ethnocentrism**, on the other hand, is the "tendency of people to put their own group (*ethnos*) at the center; to see things through the narrow lens of their own culture and use the standards of that culture to judge others" (Herbst, 1997, p. 80). This is a common human response to difference. Instead of looking at someone who is different from oneself as unique, interesting, and someone to learn about and from, a person with an ethnocentric viewpoint would judge the other person to be "less than," not as good as, or inferior to oneself. It is apparent that this combination of stereotyping and ethnocentrism can promote prejudice, and prejudice can lead to discrimination.

Discrimination

If prejudice is related to one's thoughts and beliefs, then discrimination is the action or behavior associated with those beliefs. **Discrimination** "denies equal treatment to people because of their membership in some group" (Herbst, 1997, p. 185) and can occur at many levels including individual, institutional or organizational, and structural (Rothenberg, 1998). Individual discrimination may occur when an immigrant woman is shunned in her community by other residents who believe she is "stealing" welfare support from them. It may also be observed when a Caucasian client or patient refuses to be treated by a practitioner of color. Organizational discrimination reinforces individual discrimination by "instituting rules, policies, and practices that have an adverse effect on nondominant groups such as minorities, women, older people, people with disabilities, and people with varying sexual identities" (Black & Wells, 2007, pp. 88–89). This may be seen in social clubs that disallow women or people of color to join. Another example is the inability of same-sex couples to be married or recognized as family in some states, disallowing partners to have access to one another's insurance coverage for medical care. The highest level of discrimination, structural discrimination, is that which reproduces itself among the fields of employment, education, housing, and government in the following way:

> Discrimination in education denies the credentials to get good jobs. Discrimination in employment denies the economic resources to buy good housing. Discrimination in housing confines minorities to school districts providing inferior education, closing the cycle in the classic form. (Rothenberg, 1998, p. 140)

This systematic level sustains poverty and health disparities, resulting in lack of access to other goods and services to those who are discriminated against. Because of its systematic nature, this level of discrimination is very difficult to change.

Although this discussion of prejudice and discrimination may be somewhat discouraging, there is a brighter side. As OT practitioners, we may not be able to be free of prejudicial thoughts and beliefs, but we can monitor and manage our behaviors. In order to avoid discriminating against others, we must be aware of our beliefs and values. Further discussion of this issue will be found later in this chapter in the section entitled, "Culturally Effective Occupational Therapy Practice."

Culture and Occupational Therapy

Occupational Therapy's Imperative of Culture

To paraphrase the statement by Muñoz (2007) that began this chapter, culture and occupational therapy are inextricably intertwined. Occupational therapy is founded on the recognition of the uniqueness of each individual with whom we work and sustained by a belief in client-centered care. Additional elements that indicate the importance of and mandate the examination of culture for the OT profession include the American Occupational Therapy Association (AOTA) Centennial Vision (AOTA, 2012), the Occupational Therapy Practice Framework (OTPF; AOTA, 2008), AOTA's official document on Occupational Therapy's Commitment to Nondiscrimination and Inclusion (AOTA, 2004), and many occupation-based models of practice.

Client-Centered Care

One of the major tenets of occupational therapy, client-centered or person-centered care, is based on the profession's belief in the worth of and respect for each individual. Client-centered care is rooted in Carl Rogers's (1959/1989) notion of providing clients with "unconditional positive regard." Client-centered care supports the premise that a client is capable of leading the therapy process and making decisions about his or her health care, and that therapy is a collaborative process between the client and the practitioner. This requires the OT practitioner to understand the client's condition through the client's eyes, not his or her own (Sumsion, 1993). Every client who engages in occupational therapy brings his or her own cultural lens and worldview to each session. In order to interact effectively, the OT practitioner must carefully listen to and understand the client's cultural values and beliefs about health and well-being. In other words, as described earlier, effective client-centered care must include an awareness of and knowledge about the client's culture (Black, 2005) and their unique expression of that culture.

AOTA's Centennial Vision

Another aspect of the profession that encourages the examination of culture is the Centennial Vision. In 2006, AOTA's Centennial Vision was presented to the profession in an effort to focus the organization on goals to be met by 2017, AOTA's 100th year anniversary. The Centennial Vision states, "by the year 2017, occupational therapy is a powerful, widely recognized, science-driven, and evidence-based profession with a globally connected and diverse workforce meeting society's occupational needs" (AOTA, 2012, para. 1). Some of the identified drivers of change that led to this statement included the following:

- Aging and longevity
- Diversity of the population
- Changes in lifestyle values and choices (Christiansen, 2005)

These 3 (of 10) indicators are specifically related to issues of culture and diversity and support the Centennial Vision's focus on a "globally connected and diverse workforce." The Centennial Vision can be realized if OT practitioners, educators, researchers, and scientists understand the importance of culture and its impact on occupation and learn how to effectively interact with those who are different from themselves, both locally and globally. One tool that helps an OT practitioner further understand the concept of culture is the OTPF (AOTA, 2008).

Occupational Therapy Practice Framework

In the OTPF (AOTA, 2008), the domain and practice of occupational therapy are described, presenting "a summary of interrelated constructs that define and guide occupational therapy practice" (p. 625). Through this document, the profession identifies and establishes the breadth of OT practice and the ways in which we may work with our clients. One specific area the OTPF identifies as part of the domain of occupational therapy practice is the context and environment within which clients engage in occupation and that influences their occupational performance. The multiple contexts of a person's life identified in the OTPF include cultural, personal, temporal, physical, social, and virtual. A client's cultural context is defined as

> customs, beliefs, activity patterns, behavior standards, and expectations accepted by the society of which the client is a member. [It] includes ethnicity and values as well as political aspects, such as laws that affect access to resources and affirm personal rights. [Cultural context] also includes opportunities for education, employment, and economic support. (AOTA, 2008, p. 645)

This broad-based definition encompasses more than just working with individual clients, providing language and concepts related to working with organizations and populations as well. Because cultural context greatly impacts occupational choice and occupational behaviors based on beliefs, values, and societal expectations, it is necessary and imperative that OT practitioners incorporate cultural knowledge of their clients during their evaluation and intervention planning.

AOTA Official Document on Nondiscrimination and Inclusion

AOTA recognizes the importance and value of a multicultural or pluralistic society. **Multiculturalism** has been defined as "an ideal in which diverse groups in a society coexist amicably, retaining their individual cultural identities" (Herbst, 1997, p. 154). The United States is progressing toward that goal. AOTA's official document on Occupational Therapy's Commitment to Nondiscrimination and Inclusion (AOTA, 2004) clearly speaks to the importance of valuing individuals for all of their unique characteristics and treating everyone fairly and equitably. The authors state, "when we do not discriminate against others and when we include all members of society in our daily lives, we reap the benefits of being with individuals who have different perspectives, opinions, and talents from our own" (AOTA, 2004, p. 668). This very strong statement is a clear mandate to OT practitioners, researchers, and educators for support of diversity, culture, and multiculturalism.

Occupation-Based Models of Practice

Kielhofner and Burke (1980) developed one of the earliest occupation-based models of practice, the *Model of Human Occupation*. From its inception, this model incorporated the analysis of a client's culture and its impact on occupational choice. Subsequently developed models of practice, many of which will be more thoroughly described in Unit IX of this book, also recognize the importance of understanding a client's culture as a necessary focus of analysis in the provision of client-centered care (Baum & Christiansen, 2005; Dunn, Brown, & McGuigan, 1994; Iwama, 2006; Law et al., 1996; Schkade & Schultz, 2003). These practice models provide theoretical and practical approaches for OT intervention, all of which consider the importance of recognizing how a client's culture may impact his or her occupations.

The Impact of Culture on Occupation

Think about all of the activities or occupations you engaged in yesterday. Why did you choose these? **Occupational choice** is determined by one's values, interests and beliefs, social situation, gender, age, sexual identity, and physical, cognitive, and emotional abilities. Many of these factors are characteristics of one's culture. For example, when considering what leisure pursuits to engage in, an African American, 65-year-old educated woman from the northeastern part of the United States may choose activities such as snowshoeing with her grandchildren or meeting friends in a nearby shopping mall for lunch. These activities would meet the expectations of her family, friends, and community and her own beliefs about the appropriate role of women from her society and culture. Across the world, another 65-year-old working-class Chinese woman from a small city in China might choose to exercise on one of the numerous pieces of equipment found in the many small parks near her neighborhood before sharing a cup of tea with a neighbor as they sit together on the stoop of their urban *hutong*. Each of these women has chosen socially and culturally appropriate activities that support her beliefs and lifestyle.

In an OT setting, it is important that occupational choice be focused on the client's interests and values and that the activity hold cultural meaning for him or her. If an older Hispanic man who has had a moderate cerebrovascular accident (CVA) does not want to engage in practicing donning shoes and socks with adaptive equipment in the OT clinic because his wife and his grown daughter will insist on doing it for him when he is back home, should the OT practitioner continue to focus on that activity? What would be a client-centered approach to this issue?

Not only is the choice of occupation determined by one's cultural beliefs and expectations but how one performs an occupation (**occupational performance**) is also influenced by culture. Occupational performance is defined as "the accomplishment of the selected occupation resulting from the dynamic transaction among the client, the context and environment, and the activity" (AOTA, 2008, p. 650). Cultural context certainly impacts one's performance of an activity. For example, eating a meal is an important occupation in many cultures, yet mealtime activities are performed differently all around the world. People in the United States and many other Western countries may sit in chairs at a table at most meals, whereas someone from another culture and place in the world may sit on the ground around an open hearth. Children in most Western cultures are taught to use utensils such as forks, knives, and spoons to eat their food, whereas East Asian children deftly use chopsticks to get their food into their mouths, and many Africans use their hands and fingers to accomplish the same task (Figure 16.2). Family beliefs reflect those of their society's culture and will determine whether everyone eats at the same time, sits around a designated eating space, eats in front of the television and other electronic games, or eats alone in their rooms. Therefore, an OT student or practitioner working with a client on mealtime activities must understand exactly what activities that client engages in during a typical mealtime. One cannot assume that all occupations are performed in the same way at the same time and being sensitive to cultural differences will help a practitioner, in collaboration with the client, to develop appropriate and meaningful interventions. Besides these

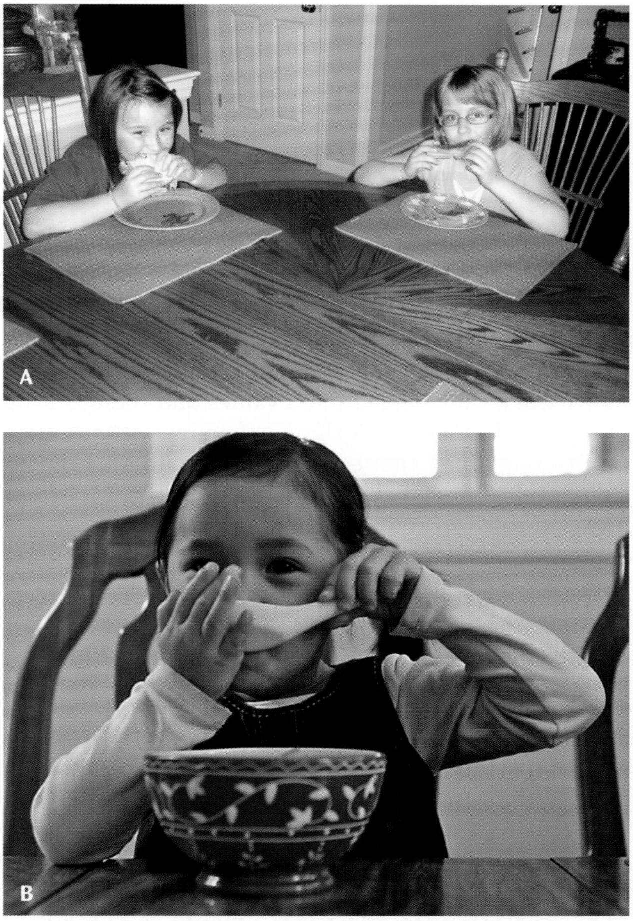

FIGURE 16.2 Diverse mealtime occupational performances. **A.** American children at lunch in York, Pennsylvania, United States. **B.** A Chinese child at lunch. (Photographs courtesy of **[A]** Gretchen Miller and **[B]** Art Hsieh.)

examples, there are many other cultural issues that may impact effective cross-cultural interactions in occupational therapy.

Cultural Issues That May Impact Cross-Cultural Interactions in Occupational Therapy

Cultural differences sometimes result in discord, particularly when they impact one's values and there is little understanding between the participants. It is important to remember that each person within a therapeutic relationship enters that interaction with his or her own cultural lens and worldview, beliefs and values, and preferred behaviors. Therefore, every interaction between an OT practitioner and his or her client could be considered a cross-cultural interaction. There are many specific characteristics of culture that may impact a therapeutic relationship. Issues related to self-concept, perceptions of power and authority, and the beliefs about and use of time have been explored in another publication (Black, 2010). The following are additional examples of issues that may result in discomfort or misunderstanding if the OT practitioner and client are from different cultures.

Beliefs about Health, Well-being, and Illness

Concepts of health, and beliefs about what constitutes well-being and what causes illnesses, or a group's "explanatory model of health and illness" are culturally determined (Kleinman, 1978). One learns about healthy and non-healthy practices from family, peers, and the media (in developed countries). In the United States and many other Western and developed countries, the **biomedical model**, or **allopathic medicine**, prevails. The biomedical model is based on scientific knowledge that "attributes health and illness to physiological, biological, and scientifically explainable changes in one's body" (Lattanzi & Purnell, 2006, p. 137). Typical of an individualistic society (see following section), the biomedical model "emphasizes the treatment of the individual's body and minimizes the links to households, communities or the supernatural" (Lattanzi & Purnell, 2006, p. 138). Health according to this model is the absence of disease, and pharmaceutical intervention is typical, often neglecting the psychological, behavioral, and social dimensions of illness (Srivastava, 2007). However, there has recently been an increased interest in health promotion and wellness and disease prevention in the United States, which shifts the way people view health and illness. Reitz (2010) avers that occupation has been used in multiple cultures to promote well-being and health for centuries. As a result of the current emphasis on health and wellness, many people are more health conscious and are changing their occupational behaviors to support a healthier lifestyle.

There are many groups of people, however, who view health and the cause of illness in a far different manner than the biomedical model. Some may believe that illness is caused by evil and is eradicated through the use of spiritual or magical intervention. One of the most common beliefs is that of the ***evil eye***. The concept of the evil eye is that someone can "project harm by gazing or staring at another's property or person" (Spector, 1985, p. 83). This widespread belief was brought to the United States by immigrants from Southern Europe, the Middle East, and North Africa (Mahoney, 1976) and is still practiced by some of their descendants. Some of the common understandings of the evil eye are that the injury or sickness happens suddenly and the victim may not know the source, and the injury or sickness may be prevented or cured with rituals or symbols (Mahoney, 1976). Someone with a strong belief in the evil eye may not accept medical or OT intervention or follow through on suggested activities but may require a healer from their own culture to provide a ritual before participating in therapy.

Folk Practices

Folk practices are common for many cultures, and it is important for practitioners to be familiar with them. **Folk practices** are traditional home remedies used by certain family, ethnic, and cultural groups to counteract illness and support wellness. In my family, my mother would string a whole nutmeg around my neck when I had the croup as a young child and would pour warm oil in my ears for an earache. I'm not sure that these home remedies actually made me better, but she believed they did. Many of you will be able to recall other practices used in your own family and may chuckle at these approaches, yet how many of us can deny how good chicken soup made us feel when we were sick as children.

Folk practices, however, are very different than health care practices in the United States and have been problematic when immigrants and others have sought out health care. ***Coin rubbing***, for example, is the practice of rubbing a coin, which is sometimes heated or used with oil, vigorously over the body in order to draw out illness. The red welts this causes is evidence to the person doing the rubbing that the sickness has come to the surface of the body. This approach to healing is practiced by many people from Asia, including Cambodians, Chinese, Korean, and Vietnamese (Galanti, 2004; Lattanzi & Purnell, 2006). A similar approach is called ***cupping*** where a heated glass is placed on the back, causing a vacuum that raises and reddens the skin. Users of this practice, including many Asians, Latin Americans, and some Europeans, believe that the hot glass will equalize the coldness in one's body caused by the disease or condition; they also may believe that the cupping will draw out an evil spirit (Galanti, 2004; Lattanzi & Purnell, 2006). Because these practices result in lesions on the skin, health care professionals may misunderstand the cause and may falsely accuse the family of abuse or treat the patient with disrespect. These alternate health occupations and practices must be understood by the OT practitioner in order to provide effective therapy.

Many groups of people who use folk healing also prefer to use a **folk healer** as part of their health care practices. A folk healer is a person who is recognized within the culture who uses traditional magico-religious practices and rituals to help heal the sick. Hispanics may seek out a *curandero* (spiritual healer) or a *yerbera* (herbalist) to treat their symptoms because they believe the U.S. health system alone is insufficient for their needs (Galanti, 2004; Lattanzi & Purnell, 2006; Spector, 1985), whereas a Native American Cherokee woman may search for a shaman or medicine man or woman for adjunctive therapy. Determining how these other health specialists become part of the diverse client's treatment is the job of the intervention team, which may include the OT practitioner.

Gender and Family Roles

Another cultural characteristic that may impact OT practice is the way different cultures determine gender and family roles. Most people have strong personal values and beliefs about gender roles as well as family interactions and expectations. When people with differing beliefs or lifestyles are compelled to interact, such as in a health care setting, these differences may become a barrier to effective communication.

Gender

In North America and much of the Western world, the women's movement began the process to eliminate restrictive gender roles. Although the system is not perfect, women in these societies have moved much closer to equality with men economically and in the areas of education, the workplace, and sometimes the family. However, there are many cultures and societies that do not share this value, and gender roles and expectations are more conservatively practiced. In many traditional cultures, women are seen as mothers, wives, and housekeepers, whereas men continue to hold the power and authority both in public settings and within the family. Men may hold the dominant role in the family, acting as spokesman and decision maker (Galanti, 2004); and in a health care situation, a man may speak and answer for his wife, even if she is the client. Although this kind of interaction may feel uncomfortable for a Western health provider who values a woman's independence, understanding why this occurs and responding appropriately for that culture will facilitate the therapeutic relationship with both the client and her spouse. In many cultures, strict rules are followed regarding public contact between men and women. This is particularly true in some Asian, Middle Eastern, and African communities. If the therapist in the third story at the beginning of the chapter had sought out more information regarding gender role behavior within the Somali culture, where traditional men will not touch a woman outside of his family, she may have understood the young man's refusal to shake her hand rather than labeling him as being noncompliant.

Family Structure

One cannot examine gender roles without understanding the family structure and dynamics within which these roles are enacted. In the United States, a traditional family is composed of a male father, female mother, and their children. However, there are many alternative or nontraditional family structures today. There are increasingly more families with same-sex parents (Lev, 2004), grandparents acting in the parent role (American Association of Retired Persons, n.d.), or one-parent households. Regardless of the structure, however, family cultural issues must be considered in OT practice. Galanti (2004) stated that when nurses were asked what was the most common problem when dealing with non-Anglo ethnic groups, they responded, "Their families!" (p. 76). When an OT practitioner does not understand the cultural values of a particular family and has a difficult time getting the client to say what she expects from therapy until she talks with her father or grandfather, or has trouble effectively treating another client because her room is always filled with extended family members, the OT practitioner might agree with the nurses' sentiment earlier. The U.S. health care system, which naturally reflects Western beliefs and values, is based on the premise that individuals can make their own health care decisions and that independence is a valued goal for all. However, many cultures perceive the family as a unit, and as part of the values of solidarity, responsibility, and harmony, the entire family makes the health care decisions for one of its members (Srivastava, 2007). These cultures, which include traditional Asian (Srivastava, 2007) and many Hispanic families (Galanti, 2004), among others, are considered collectivist societies, whereas the United States and many other Western societies are considered individualistic.

Collectivist versus Individualistic Societies

Despite the rhetoric in the U.S. media about family values and despite the importance placed on their families, in general, U.S. society is considered individualistic in nature. **Individualistic societies**, found in North America, Sweden (Lattanzi & Purnell, 2006), and many other European and Western nations, believe in individual rights, and each person within the family or work unit is viewed as a separate entity. Individualistic societies value self-expression, personal choice, autonomy, individual responsibility, and independence (Srivastava, 2007) and may even expect children to voice their opinions

TABLE 16.1 Aspects of Collectivist and Individualistic Societies

Collectivist	Individualistic
Priority to needs of the group	Focus on needs of individual
Motivated by group norms	Promotion of self-realization
Group-imposed duties	Individual goals and desires
Harmony and cooperation	Competition
Family is primary unit	Individual is primary
Interdependence	Independence
Family makes decisions for children	Children given many options and encouraged to make own decisions
Rarely have advanced directives	Advanced directives are valued
People more important than time constraints	Time constraints are often strictly adhered to

Adapted from Lattanzi, J. B., & Purnell, L. D. (2006). *Developing cultural competence in physical therapy practice.* Philadelphia, PA: F. A. Davis; Srivastava, R. H. (2007). *The healthcare professional's guide to clinical cultural competence.* Toronto, Canada: Mosby Elsevier.

and make simple decisions for themselves. Clients from these societies will share many values with most of their Caucasian, U.S.-born OT practitioners, and may respond best if the therapist

- Recognizes that illness threatens the client's independence,
- Collaborates with the client on all decisions so he or she feels more in control,
- Encourages the client to "work hard" toward his or her recovery and health,
- Respects the client as a unique individual, and
- Sets individual goals toward independence (Black, 2010).

In contrast, people from **collectivist societies** tend to put more value on the family as a unit than on the individual. Interdependence is valued and the focus is on the "we" as opposed to the "I" of individualistic groups. Decisions are made by the family, who considers what is good for the entire group before focusing on the individual. Health may even be measured by how well one can function within the group (Black, 2010). Because these values may differ from those of some U.S. occupational therapists, there may be more chance of misunderstanding or miscommunication. It is important for the OT practitioner who is interacting with someone who has a collectivist worldview to

- Work closely with family and group members when the client needs to make health care decisions,
- Be aware that you may be viewed as an outsider and that you may have to work hard to establish trust with the client and his or her family or group,
- Recognize that the client's family and friends may stay with the client much of the time, and
- Emphasize the team approach for safe and effective care (Black, 2010).

Although not necessarily considered a collectivist society, research indicates that many African-American individuals also rely heavily on closely knit groups of friends and family and are therefore less likely to welcome strangers such as home health care therapists into their homes and health care networks (Gordon, 1995). Table 16.1 outlines aspects of individualistic and collectivist societies.

Having an awareness of gender and family roles and expectations as well as an understanding about where the client falls on the collectivist–individualist continuum will assist the OT student and practitioner in communicating well and providing effective client-centered care with diverse clients. Another cultural characteristic that may impact therapeutic interactions is the use of touch and space.

The Use of Touch and Space (Proxemics)

Touch

Each person has an inherent natural need to touch and be touched. As occupational therapists, we have learned that the tactile (touch) system is the first sensory system to develop in utero (Montagu, 1986), and that touch is one of the main systems used to learn about the environment (Figure 16.3).

CASE STUDY 16.1 Munny

Munny is a 27-year-old Cambodian-American young man who sustained a head injury in a motorcycle accident 2 months ago. He was not wearing a helmet. He is second generation and has assimilated well to his American lifestyle. Before his accident, he contributed much of his time working in the family store. Currently, the client has impaired gross and fine motor coordination, is unable to perform some self-care activities, and has moderate deficits in memory, organization, and judgment. Additionally, he seems depressed. Standard treatment would emphasize Munny's independence in ADL and instrumental ADL (IADL), but he and his family do not seem to agree with this approach.

Jean, the outpatient occupational therapist assigned to Munny's case, was confounded by this attitude, because she believed that he had much more potential than he was showing. She decided to learn more about Cambodian beliefs and values in order to understand Munny and his family better. What she discovered is that Cambodians are considered a collectivist society and that they value interdependence among family members, where the family takes basic responsibility for the care of its members, including decision making. She learned that Cambodians traditionally deal with illness through self-care and self-medication, and traditional or spiritual healers may be sought to restore health. However, they are often reluctant to disclose this practice to Western health care providers because they fear being ridiculed. Although Cambodians will seek out Western medicine if necessary, they expect to receive medications at each visit in order for them to feel like something is being done to alleviate their discomfort.

Armed with this knowledge, Jean decided to more actively include his family in Munny's health care and health decisions. She met with Munny, his father, mother, grandparents, and sisters to discuss his current condition and determine the family's beliefs about his goals and prognosis. She also asked them if they wanted a spiritual healer as part of Munny's health care team. As a result, Jean came to realize that the women in Munny's family would help him with ADL and IADL at home. She subsequently altered her intervention approach to provide educational techniques to the family who would support Munny with these skills. She also worked with Munny's parents and grandfather to make some minor adaptations in the family store and to adjust some of the work activities that Munny typically performed there, so that he could successfully return to work with his family's help. Working toward these goals, incorporating the skills of a spiritual healer, and including a regimen of mild antidepressants also seemed to lessen Munny's depression.

By taking the time to learn about Munny's cultural background and being willing to adjust her goals and approach to therapy based on what she had learned, Jean provided a more culturally effective plan of care for Munny that resulted in successful, if limited, return to life participation. More importantly, this approach increased satisfaction with the results of therapy from both Munny and his family.

Ashley Montagu (1986), the author of the seminal book, *Touching*, states that touching is also "our first medium of communication" (p. 3). Although this may be true, as a child develops, he or she learns the unspoken and overt rules about touch in his or her society; when to touch, how to touch, and who you may touch. The use of touch is culturally determined. Societies may be seen as "high touch" or "low touch" with individuals from each sociocultural group falling somewhere on the continuum between the two. People from **low-touch societies** tend to avoid touch, especially in public, except in prescribed situations such as the handshake during a greeting. For

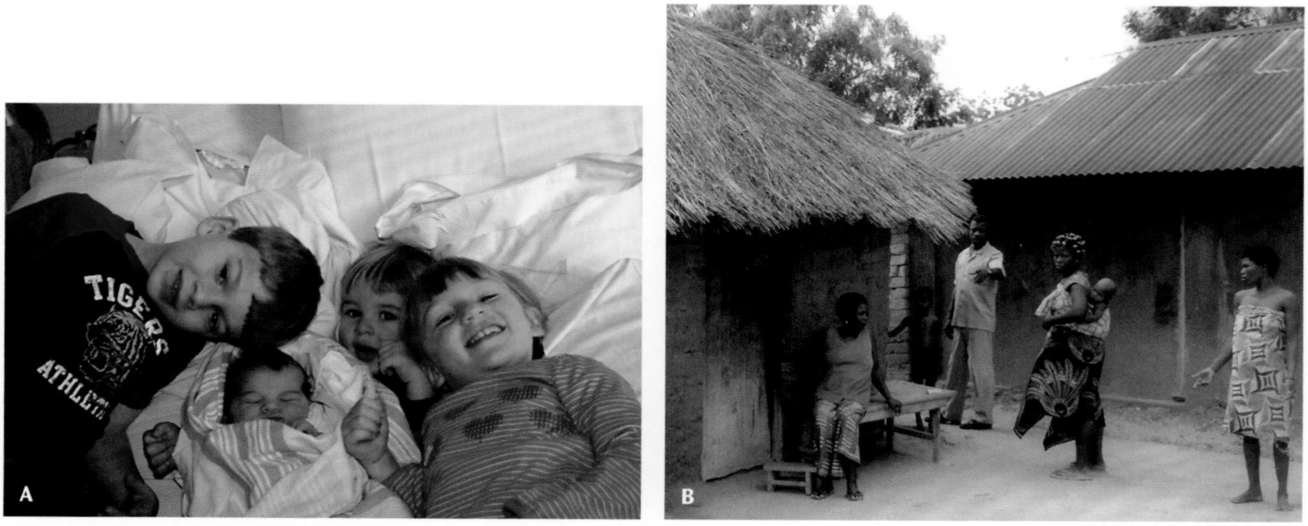

FIGURE 16.3 **A.** The author's grandchildren demonstrating the importance of touch in some cultures. **B.** A mother and baby in South Africa spend much of their time touching. (Photographs courtesy of **[A]** Roxie Black and **[B]** Virginia Skinger.)

many, a casual touch between members of the opposite sex may be interpreted as a sexual overture and should be avoided (Lattanzi & Purnell, 2006). In many Muslim societies, even a handshake between men and women is forbidden. People from **high-touch societies**, however, may seek out touch as a means of communication and are comfortable with casual touch. As OT students or practitioners, we are often expected to touch our clients, but touching may be viewed as personal or intrusive. It is vitally important to understand the meaning of touch for each client and to carefully explain the necessity for touch in the therapeutic intervention process.

Proxemics

Closely associated with touch is the concept of **proxemics**. Anthropologist Edward T. Hall first coined the term in 1966, defining it as "the measureable distance between people as they interact" (p. 114) and addressed how it may affect cross-cultural exchanges. Hall developed the delineation of physical distance as intimate distance (for embracing, touching, or whispering), personal distance (interactions between good friends and family members), social distance (interaction among acquaintances), and public distance (used for public speaking), as shown in Table 16.2 (Hall, 1966/1990).

Various cultures hold different norms about personal space, which they practice unconsciously in order to feel comfortable when interacting with others. For example, people in the United States, Canada, and Great Britain tend to keep about 18 in between themselves when conversing (Lattanzi & Purnell, 2006), whereas some Latinos, who prefer closer contact during conversations, perceive Anglos as being distant and unapproachable (Juckett, 2005).

Additionally, people from Arab countries are more comfortable standing very close to one another when conversing. Their practice of social space is more like North Americans' intimate space (Sheppard, 1996), often resulting in a sense of discomfort for the partner from the United States. I had an opportunity to observe this in a work situation in the United States. I have a Moroccan friend and colleague who often stands very close to others when he speaks, making large gestures as part of his communication style. Several of the women at the facility spoke to me about being nervous or uncomfortable around him and tried to avoid him. One even falsely accused him of sexual harassment. This example indicates how cross-cultural interactions can be negatively impacted if participants do not understand the differences in standards related to proxemics and how important it is to have this knowledge when working with people from diverse cultures. Understanding cultural differences and practicing effective cross-cultural interactions is part of being culturally effective, or culturally competent, an important skill for OT practitioners.

Culturally Effective Occupational Therapy Practice

What is culturally effective practice? Is it **cultural competence**? Can it be called something else? Over the past decade, there has been much published about the need for and importance of cultural awareness and cultural competence in OT practice (Black & Wells, 2007;

TABLE 16.2 Edward T. Hall's Delineation of Physical Distance

Intimate Distance	**For Embracing, Touching, Whispering**
Close phase	Less than 6 in
Far phase	6–18 in
Personal Distance	**For Interactions among Good Friends and Family Members**
Close phase	1.5–2.5 ft
Far phase	2.5–4 ft
Social Distance	**For Interactions among Acquaintances**
Close phase	4–7 ft
Far phase	7–12 ft
Public Distance	**Used for Public Speaking**
Close phase	12–25 ft
Far phase	25 feet or more

Adapted from Hall, E. T. (1990). The hidden dimension. New York, NY: Knopf Doubleday. (Original work published 1966)

Bonder et al., 2002; Mu, Coppard, Bracciano, Doll, & Matthews, 2010; Odawara, 2005; Wells & Black, 2000) as well as the impact of culturally focused curriculum offerings in OT education on the development of cultural competence in OT students and practitioners (Murden et al., 2008; Rasmussen, Lloyd, & Wielandt, 2005; Steed, 2010). Cultural competence is the ability to effectively interact with those who differ from oneself and is often described in the literature as encompassing cultural awareness and attitudes, cultural knowledge of self and others, and cultural skill, which includes effective communication (Black & Wells, 2007; Callister, 2005; Dillard et al., 1992; Saldana, 2001). Developing cultural competency is a somewhat complex process and has been represented as a developing continuum by several theorists (Campinha-Bacote, 2002; Cross, Bazron, Dennis, & Isaacs, 1989; Purnell & Lattanzi, 2006).

Developing the skills and attitudes for cultural competence is not easy, however. Hoops (1979) speaks of the difficulty of moving to cultural competency because of the natural resistance of allowing oneself to be vulnerable and the threat of probing one's identity, which may occur in the process of developing cultural self-awareness. Yet, the importance of developing effective cross-cultural interactions with one's OT clients is essential. Culturally competent care has been found to improve health status among vulnerable populations (Callister, 2005; Lynn-McHale & Deatrick, 2000; Majumdar, Browne, Roberts, & Carpio, 2004) and increase quality and effectiveness of health care as well as decrease costs (Fortier & Bishop, 2004; Suh, 2004). The results of cultural incompetence may be distrust and miscommunication, lack of adherence to therapeutic recommendations, frustration for both the client and the therapist, and decreased quality of intervention and client/therapist interaction.

Although cultural competence has been described as "a journey rather than an end . . . [and] a lifelong process" (Black & Wells, 2007, p. 31), Gupta (2008) states that it "inadvertently implies that a hypothetical end-point exists that can be reached by acquiring the right knowledge and skills and attitudes needed to work with persons of different cultures" (p. 3). Supporting Gupta's words, I've had my own students ask, "How can anyone ever achieve cultural competence? There is so much to learn." Perhaps the terminology itself is a misnomer with the word *competence* misleading people to think that one does have to reach a certain (very high) level in order to achieve this rare state. Other terms used in occupational therapy and other health professions to address cross-cultural interactions include culturally responsive caring, cultural emergent, and cultural congruence. Muñoz (2007) has coined the term "**culturally responsive caring**" which he states "communicates a state of being open to the process of building mutuality with a client and to accepting that the cultural-specific knowledge one has about a group may or may not apply to the client they were currently treating" (p. 274). Bonder, Martin, and Miracle (2004) use the term "**cultural emergent**" to describe a model that "suggests that the symbolic aspects of culture and cultural identity emerge in interaction and are displayed primarily through talk and through action" (p. 162). Bonder and her colleagues believe that culture is uniquely expressed by individuals and that it constantly changes, based on the person's context and experiences. "**Cultural congruence**," a term coined by Leininger and MacFarland (2006), is used to describe how health professionals think and act in ways that fit with a person or group's beliefs and cultural style. This can occur only when one knows and uses in appropriate and meaningful ways the values, expressions, practices, and patterns of various cultural groups. Although the language and meaning of these terms are subtly different, they all encompass basic similarities when talking about effective cross-cultural interactions; one must be culturally self-aware, respect people as individuals, learn about the culture of our diverse clients, and actively engage in the process of developing cultural competence.

Conclusion

Occupational therapy practice is based on the premise that humans are occupational beings and that occupation, or meaningful activities, are necessary for health. The purpose of OT intervention is to achieve "the end-goal of supporting health and participation in life through engagement in occupations" (AOTA, 2008, pp. 646–647). Although occupational therapy's "clients" may include individuals, organizations, and populations, the OT process remains the same: to examine and evaluate the transaction between the client, the environment or context, and the activities in which the client engages in order to collaboratively and effectively choose an intervention plan that supports the client in his or her participation in life activities. Because each person with whom we work is a culturally unique individual, it is vital that therapy practitioners understand how a person's [client's] values, beliefs, and interests influence and impact his or her occupational choices and performance. The profession of occupational therapy has identified the need to examine a client's cultural context, stating that "[c]ultural contexts often influence how occupations are chosen, prioritized, and organized" (AOTA, 2008, p. 646). In fact, the awareness and use of culture in OT theory and practice is ubiquitous and cannot be ignored.

As has been said earlier, every client/therapist interaction can be considered a cross-cultural interaction. Given this statement and the increasing cultural diversity in client populations, providing effective cross-cultural or culturally competent OT care is imperative. Learning to provide this kind of care may be challenging, but it can also leave you impassioned and energized—outstanding traits of highly competent occupational therapists. Although only a brief examination of the importance of culture and culturally effective care is provided in this chapter, there are numerous resources available that can guide you in your quest for further information, both written and online, some of which are included in the reference list at the end of the chapter. I invite and encourage you to examine these and apply what you learn in your professional practice.

References

Abizadeh, A. (2001). Ethnicity, race, and a possible humanity. *World Order, 33*(1), 23–34.

American Association of Retired Persons. (n.d.). *Grandfacts state fact sheet for grandparents, relatives raising grandchildren.* Retrieved from http://www.aarp.org/relationships/friends-family/grandfacts-sheets/?CMP=KNC-360I-GOOGLE-REL FRI&HBX_PK=grandparents_as_parents&utm_source=GOOGLE&utm_medium=cpc&utm_term=grandparents%2Bas%2Bparents&utm_campaign=G_Grandfacts&360cid=SI_308824831_10641909541_1

American Occupational Therapy Association. (2004). AOTA position paper: Occupational therapy's commitment to nondiscrimination and inclusion. *American Journal of Occupational Therapy, 58*, 668.

American Occupational Therapy Association. (2008). Occupational therapy practice framework: Domain and process, 2nd edition. *American Journal of Occupational Therapy, 62*(6), 625–683.

American Occupational Therapy Association. (2012). *AOTA's centennial vision.* Retrieved from http://www.aota.org/News/Centennial.aspx

Baum, C., & Christiansen, C. (2005). Person–environment-occupation-performance: An occupation-based framework for practice. In C. Christiansen & C. Baum (Eds.), *Occupational therapy: Performance, participation and well-being* (pp. 242–267). Thorofare, NJ: Slack.

Black, R. M. (2002). Occupational therapy's dance with diversity. *American Journal of Occupational Therapy, 56*(2), 140–148.

Black, R. M. (2005). Intersections of care: An analysis of culturally competent care, client centered care, and the feminist ethic of care. *Work: A Journal of Prevention, Assessment, and Rehabilitation, 24*(4), 409–422.

Black, R. M. (2010). Culture and meaningful occupation. In K. Sladyk, K. Jacobs, & N. MacRae (Eds.), *Occupational therapy essentials for clinical competence* (pp. 11–22). Thorofare, NJ: Slack.

Black, R. M., & Wells, S. A. (2007). *Culture & occupation: A model of empowerment in occupational therapy.* Bethesda, MD: American Occupation and Therapy Association Press.

Bonder, B., Martin, L., & Miracle, A. (2002). *Culture in clinical care.* Thorofare, NJ: Slack.

Bonder, B., Martin, L., & Miracle, A. (2004). Culture emergent in occupation. *American Journal of Occupational Therapy, 58*(2), 159–168.

Callister, L. C. (2005). What has the literature taught us about culturally competent care of women and children? *American Journal of Maternal/Child Nursing, 30*, 380–388.

Campinha-Bacote, J. (2002). The process of cultural competence in the delivery of health-care services: A model of care. *Journal of Transcultural Nursing, 13*, 181–184.

Christiansen, C. (2005). *Creating a centennial vision: Four possible scenarios.* Retrieved from http://www.aota.org/News?Centennial/Background.36564.aspx

Cross, T. L., Bazron, B. J., Dennis, K. W., & Isaacs, M. R. (1989). *Towards a culturally competent system of care: A monograph on effective services for minority children who are severely emotionally disturbed.* Washington, DC: CASSP Technical Assistance Center, Georgetown University Child Development Center.

Dillard, M., Andonian, L., Flores, O., Lai, L., MacRae, A., & Shakir, M. (1992). Culturally competent occupational therapy in a diversely populated mental health setting. *American Journal of Occupational Therapy, 46*, 721–726.

Diverse. (1995). *The Merriam-Webster dictionary* (10th ed.). Springfield, MA: Merriam-Webster.

Dunn, W., Brown, C., & McGuigan, A. (1994). The ecology of human performance: A framework for considering the effect of context. *American Journal of Occupational Therapy, 48*, 595–607.

Fortier, J. P., & Bishop, D. (2004). *Setting the agenda for research on cultural competence in health care, final report.* Rockville, MD: U.S. Department of Health and Human Services, Office of Minority Health, & Agency for Healthcare Research and Quality. Retrieved from http://www.ahrq.gov/research/cultural.htm

Galanti, G. A. (2004). *Caring for patients from different cultures* (3rd ed.). Philadelphia, PA: University of Pennsylvania Press.

Gordon, A. K. (1995). Deterrents to access and service for blacks and Hispanics: The Medicare Hospice Benefit, healthcare utilization, and cultural barriers. *The Hospice Journal, 10*(2), 65–83.

Gupta, J. (2008). Reflections of one educator on teaching cultural competence. *Education SIS Quarterly, 18*(3), 3.

Hall, E. T. (1990). *The hidden dimension.* New York, NY: Knopf Doubleday. (Original work published 1966)

Haney Lopez, I. F. (1994). The social construction of race: Some observations on illusion, fabrication, and choice. *Harvard Civil Rights-Civil Liberties Law Review, 1*(62), 11–17.

Hecht, M. L. (Ed.). (1998). *Communicating prejudice.* Thousand Oaks, CA: SAGE.

Herbst, P. H. (1997). *The color of words: An encyclopaedic dictionary of ethnic bias in the United States.* Yarmouth, ME: Intercultural Press.

Hoops, D. (1979). Intercultural communication concepts and the psychology of intercultural experiences. In M. Pusch (Ed.), *Multicultural education: A cross-cultural training approach* (pp. 9–38). Yarmouth, ME: Intercultural Press.

Iwama, M. (2004). Meaning and inclusion: Revisiting culture in occupational therapy [Guest Editorial]. *Australian Occupational Therapy Journal, 51*, 1–2.

Iwama, M. (2006). *The KAWA model: Culturally relevant occupational therapy.* Toronto, Canada: Churchill Livingstone.

Juckett, G. (2005). Cross-cultural medicine. *American Family Physician, 72*(11), 2267–2274.

Kielhofner, G., & Burke, J. (1980). A model of human occupation, part one: Conceptual framework and content. *American Journal of Occupational Therapy, 34*, 572–581.

Kleinman, A. (1978). *Patients and healers in the context of culture.* Berkeley, CA: University of California Press.

La Fontaine, J. S. (1985). Person and individual: Some anthropological reflections. In M. Carrithers, S. Collins, & S. Lukes (Eds.), *The category of the person: Anthropology, philosophy, history* (pp. 123–140). Cambridge, United Kingdom: Cambridge University Press.

Lattanzi, J. B., & Purnell, L. D. (2006). *Developing cultural competence in physical therapy practice.* Philadelphia, PA: F. A. Davis.

Law, M., Baptiste, S., & Mills, J. (1995). Client-centred practice: What does it mean and does it make a difference? *Canadian Journal of Occupational Therapy, 62*, 250–257.

Law, M., Cooper, B., Strong, S., Stewart, D., Rigby, P., & Letts, L. (1996). The person-environment-occupation model: A transactive approach to occupational performance. *Canadian Journal of Occupational Therapy, 63*, 9–23.

Leininger, M., & MacFarland, M. R. (2006). *Culture care diversity and universality: A worldwide nursing theory.* Boston, MA: Jones and Bartlett.

Lev, A. I. (2004). *The complete lesbian and gay parenting guide.* New York, NY: Berkley.

Lynn-McHale, D. J., & Deatrick, J. A. (2000). Trust between family and health care providers. *Journal of Family Nursing, 6*, 210–230.

Mahoney, C. (Ed.). (1976). *The evil eye.* New York, NY: Columbia University Press.

Majumdar, B., Browne, G., Roberts, J., & Carpio, B. (2004). Effects of cultural sensitivity training on health care provider attitudes and patient outcomes. *Journal of Nursing Scholarship, 36*, 161–166.

Marks, J. (1996). Science and race. *American Behavioral Scientist, 40*(2), 123–133.

Montagu, A. (1986). *Touching: The human significance of the skin* (3rd ed.). New York, NY: Harper and Row.

Mu, K., Coppard, B. M., Bracciano, A., Doll, J., & Matthews, A. (2010). Fostering cultural competency, clinical reasoning, and leadership through international outreach. *Occupational Therapy in Health Care, 24*(1), 74–85.

Muñoz, J. (2007). Culturally responsive caring in occupational therapy. *Occupational Therapy International, 14*(4), 256–280.

Murden, R., Norman, A., Ross, J., Sturdivant, E., Kedia, M., & Shah, S. (2008). Occupational therapy students' perceptions of their cultural awareness and competency. *Occupational Therapy International, 15*(3), 191–203.

Nittle, N. K. (2011). What is race? Debunking the ideas behind this construct. Retrieved from http://racerelations.about.com/od/understandingrac1/a/WhatIsRace.htm

Odawara, E. (2005). Cultural competency in occupational therapy: Beyond a cross-cultural view of practice. *American Journal of Occupational Therapy, 59*, 325–334.

Pittz, W. (2005). *Closing the gap: Solutions to race-based health disparities.* Applied Research Center and Northwest Federation of Community Organizations. Retrieved from http://www.thepraxisproject.org/tools/ClosingGap.pdf

Purnell, L. D., & Lattanzi, J. B. (2006). Introducing steps to cultural study and cultural competence. In J. B. Lattanzi & L. D. Purnell (Eds.), *Developing cultural competence in physical therapy practice* (pp. 21–37). Philadelphia, PA: F. A. Davis.

Rasmussen, T. M., Lloyd, C., & Wielandt, T. (2005). Cultural awareness among Queensland undergraduate occupational therapy students. *Australian Occupational Therapy Journal, 52*, 302–310.

Reitz, S. M. (2010). Historical and philosophical perspectives of occupational therapy's role in health promotion. In M. E. Scaffa, S. M. Reitz, & M. A. Pizzi (Eds.), *Occupational therapy in the promotion of health and wellness* (pp. 1–21). Philadelphia, PA: F. A. Davis.

Rogers, C. (1989). A theory of therapy, personality, and interpersonal relationships as developed in the client-centered framework. In H. Kirschenbaum & V. Henderson (Eds.), *The Carl Rogers reader* (pp. 236–262). Boston, MA: Houghton Mifflin. (Reprinted from *Psychology: A study of science, Vol. 3. Formulations of the person and the social context*, pp. 184–256, by S. Koch, Ed., 1959, New York, NY: McGraw-Hill.)

Rothenberg, P. S. (1998). *Race, class, and gender in the United States: An integrated study* (4th ed.). New York, NY: St. Martin's Press.

Saldana, D. (2001). *Cultural competency: A practical guide for mental health service providers.* Austin, TX: University of Texas at Austin, Hogg Foundation for Mental Health.

Schkade, J. K., & Schultz, S. (2003). Occupational adaptation. In E. Crepeau, E. Cohn, & B. A. B. Schell (Eds.), *Willard and Spackman's occupational therapy* (10th ed., pp. 200–203). Philadephia, PA: Lippincott Williams & Wilkins.

Sheppard, M. (1996). *Proxemics.* Retrieved from http://www.cs.unm.edu/~sheppard/proxemics.htm

Spector, R. E. (1985). *Cultural diversity in health and illness* (2nd ed.). Norwalk, CT: Appleton-Century-Crofts.

Srivastava, R. H. (2007). *The healthcare professional's guide to clinical cultural competence.* Toronto, Canada: Mosby Elsevier.

Steed, R. (2010). Attitude and beliefs of occupational therapists participating in a cultural competency workshop. *Occupational Therapy International, 17*, 142–151. doi:10.1002/oti.299

Suh, E. E. (2004). The model of cultural competence through an evolutionary concept analysis. *Journal of Transcultural Nursing, 15*, 93–102.

Sumsion, T. (Ed.). (1993). *Client-centered practice in occupational therapy: A guide to implementation.* New York, NY: Churchill Livingstone.

Wells, S. A., & Black, R. M. (2000). *Cultural competency for health professionals.* Bethesda, MD: American Occupational Therapy Association.

For additional resources on the subjects discussed in this chapter, visit http://thePoint.lww.com/Willard-Spackman12e.

CHAPTER 17

Social, Economic, and Political Factors That Influence Occupational Performance

Catherine L. Lysack, Diane E. Adamo

OUTLINE

LEARNING OBJECTIVES

After reading this chapter, you will be able to:

1. Distinguish between socioeconomic status, social class, and social inequalities
2. Discuss how health is related to an individual's position in the social hierarchy
3. Discuss how individual and community level socioeconomic factors impact health
4. Explain how socioeconomic disadvantages experienced in childhood affect the occupational performance of clients as adults
5. Describe three actions that occupational therapy practitioners can take to reduce the negative impact of social inequalities and health disparities in clients' lives

Introduction

The focus of this chapter is on the social and economic forces that affect health and occupational performance across the life course. The bottom line is this—higher socioeconomic status (SES) is associated with better health and more numerous opportunities for engagement in, and benefit from, meaningful occupations. There is an overwhelming preponderance of scientific literature that demonstrates a very robust correlation between SES and health. This correlation suggests that it is not only the poor who tend to be sick when everyone else is healthy but also there is a continual gradient, from the top to the bottom of the SES ladder, relating status to health. Lower SES has been linked to chronic stress, heart disease, ulcers, type 2 diabetes, rheumatoid arthritis, certain types of cancer, and premature aging (Evans, Barer, & Marmor, 1994; U.S. Department of Health and Human Services, Office of Minority Health, 2011; Wilkinson & Marmot, 2003). Although it is true that at very high levels of income health gains become much smaller and incremental, there is no debate that at low, middle, and even upper middle-class income levels this gradient is significant (Lynch et al., 1998).

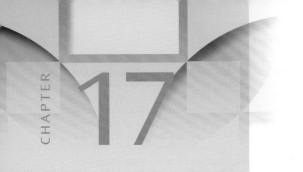

It is not difficult to see how higher education, higher income, and status could be related to better health. In general, well-educated adults tend to get better jobs than those with little or no education. Because health insurance is largely an employment-based benefit, those with paid work are more likely to have health insurance that helps to secure more reliable access to health care services than those working for an hourly wage. People with higher levels of education also have more access to health information and have more ability to interpret it and apply it in their lives. In turn, improved health literacy helps individuals to develop healthy attitudes and healthy behaviors such as eating well and exercising (Evans et al., 1994; Lynch et al., 1998). The challenge that remains is discovering why this occurs and what can be done to change this trend. For occupational therapists, it is important to understand the relationships that exist between SES and health and how this shapes opportunities to participate in and benefit from occupational therapy services.

It is hypothesized that adults with higher SES also experience fewer stressful life events and tend to have more psychological resources (e.g., self-confidence, self-control, delayed gratification) to deal with life's challenges (Kawachi & Berkman, 2003; Schulz et al., 2006; Williams, 1997). Remarkably, there is increasing research that shows that the benefits of higher SES begin even before birth (e.g., a mother's prenatal nutrition, a safe family context), which can influence health even into the final years of life (Barker, 1998; Lynch et al., 1994; Schulz et al., 2006; Shonkoff & Phillips, 2000). Public health research currently underway aims to disentangle the mechanisms beneath these powerful relationships. The remainder of this chapter will explore the consequences of the relationships among social, economic, and political factors and occupational performance across the life course.

Consider the case study of Annie and Desmond and how SES has influenced this family's health. Desmond may have contracted his illness on the job. Living in the inner city, near an industrial area, the entire family may have been exposed to unsafe levels of environmental pollutants that are adversely affecting their health now. How does this compare to the woman that Annie met in hospital? Could Annie's health suffer now because of the social and physical environments of her past? Another important question relates to fairness—why is it that Annie does not qualify for more home support services when she could benefit from those services and others with the same injury (but more money) are receiving them? Another concern is that Annie cannot afford to relocate but her activity level and community participation are being restricted by neighborhood conditions.

Annie is struggling to regain mobility and live safely and independently at home after her fall, but her physical impairments are not the primary barrier that dictates her future. Rather, it is the material and social resources she can muster that matter most now. In this chapter, the focus is on groups of people who are systematically disadvantaged—those rendered most vulnerable by

CASE STUDY 17.1 I Hope the Good Lord Will See Me Through

Annie is 72 years old and spent 2 weeks in the hospital. As Annie described it, she "took a spell" and tumbled down her basement steps. She fractured a hip and two ribs. Annie uses a wheelchair now and hopes it is temporary, but she is worried about managing at home alone. She is also coping with the consequences of a mild stroke 2 years ago. Annie lives in Detroit. Her house has two small bedrooms and a bathroom on the second floor, with laundry facilities in the basement. She is a widow, and her only surviving child, a son, lives in Chicago. For most of her life, Annie stayed home to raise three children while her husband Desmond worked at an automotive supply company. Unfortunately, after 31 years of work, Desmond was laid off, and shortly afterward, he became ill with lung cancer and died. Desmond was a nonsmoker. Des and Annie and other plant workers who lost their family members wondered if their jobs had made them sick. Unfortunately, the plant Des worked for went out of business and this meant Annie lost the small pension she received as a surviving spouse. Now she gets by on her social security check and Medicare. Her income is just over $21,000 per year.

Just before being discharged from the hospital, Annie was assessed by an occupational therapist who gave her recommendations for bathing and dressing and how to manage once she went home. She received information about Dial-a-Ride, a transportation service for older adults and people with disabilities, and the name of a senior center where she could take exercise classes and join in some social activities. Annie was disappointed that she would not receive an in-home evaluation like another woman did. According to Annie, this lady got "a nice solid bathseat and grab bars and even a fancy ramp." Annie's insurance covered none of this—not even the raised toilet seat her therapist told her would help prevent another fall.

After 3 weeks at home, Annie is worried about the slowness of her recovery and her mounting out-of-pocket expenses for medications. Her church friends are dropping in occasionally with a meal and helping with groceries, but Annie is anxious to be more self-sufficient. Still, she doesn't trust her legs "not to buckle out from under me." In a phone call to her son, she also expressed fear about going out in her neighborhood, saying that she felt vulnerable, like "a sitting duck." Annie wonders whether the woman she met weeks ago in the hospital is faring better than she is and how different it would be if she could get more help. Although she calls her friends her "lifeline," she is praying "the good Lord will see [her] through."

underlying social structures and political and economic systems. Disadvantaged groups in this sense include, for example, the elderly, the poor, ethnic and racial minorities, and people with disabilities.

Elsewhere it has been noted that occupational therapy practitioners as a group are overwhelmingly white and middle class (Wells & Black, 2000) and presumably may live more privileged lives than most of their clients. Thus, it is important that competent and ethical practitioners recognize their own social position in relation to their clients. These differences have deep roots that challenge the provision of occupational therapy interventions. Therapists must be aware of these experiential differences and assess their influence in practice. Therapists must take great care to analyze the context and environment of their clients, too, both past and present, to ensure the influences of that context are not overlooked, misunderstood, or minimized.

Defining the Social Causes of Health and Illness

Socioeconomic Status, Class, and Social Mobility

Several terms are used to signal the influence of social and economic factors on health, and each has a different meaning. One of the most familiar terms is **socioeconomic status**. SES refers to the occupational, educational, and income achievements of individuals or groups. Krieger (2001, 2010) has argued that SES may overemphasize social prestige and underemphasize the role of material resources in shaping one's life chances related to health, an idea we will return to in later sections of this chapter.

The term **class** is also used to indicate social differences between groups, as in *lower class*, *working class*, *middle class*, and *upper class*. The Online Dictionary of the Social Sciences (2012) defines class as a group of individuals sharing a common situation within a social structure, usually their shared place in the structure of ownership and control of the means of production. In land-based economies, this means class structures are based on one's relationship to the ownership and control of property. Ownership of property brings with it wealth and power, which means resources are available to be used to achieve better health. It is important to recognize that the degree to which one moves up or down the social ladder of society, something sociologists call **social mobility**, is in large part dictated by class status. Furthermore, there is widespread recognition that one's social class and SES expose a person to conditions that might be good (or bad) for their health (Evans et al., 1994; Link & Phelan, 1995, 2005; Lynch et al., 1994).

Class and SES also affect occupational performance and participation. In 2009, Bass-Haugen reviewed the literature and showed how the activity profiles, home and work environments, experiences in health systems, and outcomes of health care services differ based on SES and class. She concluded that occupational performance deficits are most notable for non-white and low-income Americans through mechanisms related to restricted activity and participation. For example, when neighborhood quality is poor, children find it difficult to find safe places to play, and older adults are denied a walkable environment to exercise and socialize (Schulz et al., 2006; Yen, Michael, & Perdue, 2009). Over time, these disadvantages can accumulate, so that by adulthood the gap between groups who have had rich opportunities to learn, develop, work, and contribute to society and those who have not is wide.

Social Inequalities and Health Disparities

The terms *social inequalities* and *health disparities* come to us from the public health literature and are related to characteristics such as class, gender, age, race, ethnicity, and sexual orientation, among others. **Social inequality** refers to a situation in which individual groups in a society do not have equal social status. Social inequality is linked to racial inequality, gender inequality, and wealth inequality. Social inequality is the portion of the unequal opportunities and rewards that accrue to these subgroups that are *unfair*, *unjust*, *avoidable*, and *unnecessary* (Krieger, 2001, 2010).

A major problem arises when social inequalities lead to problems of access to appropriate medical care and treatment. A **health disparity** is a gap in access to health care, treatment provided, and health outcomes that are unfair and may be the direct result of either underlying social inequalities or improper actions by professionals within the health system (U.S. Department of Health and Human Services [HHS], 2000b). For example, studies have found that even after controlling for symptoms and insurance coverage, U.S. doctors are more likely to offer whites life-preserving treatments, including angioplasty and bypass surgery for cardiac disease, and are more likely to offer minorities various less desirable procedures such as amputations for diabetes (Institute of Medicine [IOM], 2002). This research indicates that clinical encounters between minorities and health care professionals may be the source of additional poor treatment. Stereotyping and institutional racism are widely recognized as unjust forces in the health care environment that must change (Clark, 2004).

The second reason why social inequalities are of great concern to health professionals is that social inequalities put people at risk for poorer health. Life expectancy is shorter and most diseases are more common farther down the social ladder. Decades of research have shown this is true in both rich and poor societies (Marmot & Wilkinson, 1999). In a set of famous studies commonly referred to as the Whitehall studies, Marmot, Shipley, and Rose (1984) studied British civil servants for more than three decades and found that men in the lowest levels of the civil service, office support workers, had a mortality rate four times greater than that of men in the highest administrative jobs. The mechanisms for this are complex, and some researchers point to stress as the fundamental mechanism that explains the relationship between SES and health.

Others draw from the scientific literature in human development and prenatal and early childhood exposures to argue that a range of deleterious environmental exposures, both of a physical nature and a social nature, compounded over time, are the real factors that influence health. Although individuals may experience physiological stress as they experience inequalities and disparities, the most fundamental causes must be examined, too. Addressing and eliminating fundamental causes of health disparities requires confronting the fact that low SES individuals and families have less access to health information, to expensive treatments, and to supportive services that can make life with chronic health problems and disabilities easier. For example, low-income families may not have easy access to affordable and quick transportation. This simple fact makes attending rehabilitation appointments much more difficult and could result in reduced treatment, leading to poorer functional outcomes. This cannot be seen to be the fault of the client, but rather a very real contextual issue of practice that must be part of the therapists' problem-solving process if those with reduced SES are to have the best chance possible to benefit from therapeutic interventions.

Unfortunately, "upward mobility," that is, doing better and having more than our parents, is not happening as much as in the past. As occupational therapists consider the real-life circumstances of their clients each day, it is important to consider how societal trends shaping the patient population and their socioeconomic resources can be deployed to improve occupational performance. Today, persons in the United States are more likely than they were 30 years ago to remain in the same class into which they were born (Bradbury & Katz, 2002). Recent data show that the children of low-income families have only a 1% chance of reaching the top 5% of the income distribution versus children of high-income families who have about a 22% chance (Hertz, 2006). Although the "American dream" of owning a home and earning more than one's parents was only ever accessible to some, the lasting economic recession and housing market collapse has hurt middle-class Americans more than any other group. Many are struggling with the fallout of persistent unemployment and unprecedented levels of debt (Hertz, 2006).

Job stress and home foreclosures do not directly cause poor health but indirectly exert a major negative influence. Bass-Haugen (2009) cites research that documents the link between SES and occupational performance differences in children and adults seen by occupational therapists. She cites research that shows poor adults are two to three times more likely to report that general and specific physical activities are difficult or impossible to perform. Poor adults also had the highest percentage of limitations in activities and need for special equipment as well as the lowest percentage of participation in physical exercise and activities. The living environments and clients matter, too. Non-white children are less likely to report feeling usually or always safe in their neighborhoods and schools or to be living in supportive neighborhoods. For example, 94.2% of White children typically felt safe at school, whereas only 74.6% of Black children and 79.1% of Hispanic children felt this way.

The Intersections of Gender, Ethnicity, Age, Disability, and Sexual Orientation

Other factors that influence health and occupational performance are inextricably linked to the social categories individuals belong to, including gender, ethnic heritage, age, sexual orientation, and whether they are disabled or not (America's Children, 2011; Krieger, 2010; U.S. Department of Health and Human Services, Office of Minority Health, 2011). Individuals often belong to more than one of these categories. As occupational therapists, we must constantly ask ourselves if we make assumptions about our clients based on the social categories they occupy, or do we truly see the person behind the category and practice client-centered occupational therapy?

Gender Inequalities

For some women, the experience of being a woman continues to be one of inequality. For example, women have found it difficult to enter certain professions, such as business, because of gender bias (Kelan, 2009). Others have written about women trapped in roles perceived to be "women's work" (Hesse-Biber & Carter, 2000). In 2005, *The Economist* reported that women account for fewer than 8% of all chief executive officers (CEOs) in the United States even though they constitute 46% of the workforce. Research also confirms a wage gap. Analysis of U.S. Census Bureau data shows that, on average, women's pay is still only 81 cents for every $1 a man earns (Institute for Women's Policy Research, 2011). Although this is partly explained by the types of jobs women have, job classification does not explain the entire difference, and barriers to higher paid job classifications continue to sustain this disparity.

Gender also exerts a strong influence on health. Currently, within much of the Western world, women enjoy a longer average life expectancy than men (Organisation for Economic Co-operation and Development [OECD], 2011). However, once the patterns of illness and disability are examined by gender, the picture is more ambiguous. Although men die earlier than women, women have higher rates of chronic illness at every age. For example, women account for two-thirds of all people diagnosed with arthritis (National Center for Health Statistics [NCHS], 2010). Similarly, depression is nearly twice as common in women as it is in men. Some of these gender differences are accounted for by biological differences between the sexes; others are related to differences in gender roles that may increase stress for women (Adams, Martinez, & Vickerie, 2010). Stress is known to worsen arthritic conditions and depression (HHS, 2000b). Practitioners must recognize that gender differences may lead to health inequalities and unfortunately, sometimes disparities in the treatment women receive.

Ethnic Inequalities

Ethnicity affects life chances for health, but also for a range of other societal opportunities like education and work. The term *ethnicity* is used here rather than *race* to signal cultural rather than biological explanations for differences in social and economic opportunity. Yet, many assume ethnic differences are the cause of these differences when in fact it may be other factors associated with ethnicity that matter much more. For example, on average, poverty rates are higher in ethnic communities than in white communities. However, if there are differences in the educational attainment of children in black neighborhoods versus white neighborhoods, it would be a mistake to assume the cause was the color of the children's skin. It is far more likely to be due to the economic disadvantage of black families.

There is research, however, that suggests poverty cannot explain this entire gap in educational attainment. Roscigno and Ainsworth-Darnell (1999), for example, suggest there may be subtle differences in the treatment of students that account for educational attainment differences based on ethnic group. They cite studies that show teachers may give affluent students more attention, assistance, and higher expectations than their less affluent students (Kau & Thompson, 2003). This is a very subtle mechanism whereby teachers, consciously or not, do not invest time and energy in students if they think the return on their investment will not pay optimal dividends.

Education is a critical factor in life because employment opportunities and income are tied to early educational attainment (Miringoff & Miringoff, 1999; Shonkoff & Phillips, 2000); but neither educational opportunities nor their quality is equally distributed (America's Children, 2011). The U.S. government recognized this fact as early as the 1950s, when it established the Head Start program, a national network of comprehensive child development programs that targeted low-income families and their communities (U.S. Census Bureau, 2003). Poor minority children are at an educational disadvantage because they grow up in poor neighborhoods, which have poorer quality schools, staffed by teachers with fewer resources to enrich the learning environment (Young, 1997). This example highlights the intersection of ethnicity and economic status. Individuals with diminished chances in the early years seldom catch up. A sad fact is that in 2009, 21% of all children ages 0 to 17 (15.5 million) lived in poverty. This is an increase from the low of 16% in 2000 and 2001 (America's Children, 2011).

Poverty affects health directly and so does ethnicity, although the two factors are often found together. Census data show, for example, that the prevalence of hypertension is about 40% higher in African Americans than in non-Hispanic White Americans, and African Americans are 10% less likely to have it under control (U.S. Department of Health and Human Services, Office of Minority Health, 2011). Infant mortality rates indicate a similar pattern. The U.S. average is 6.4 infant deaths per 1,000 live births, but for African Americans the figure is a startling 13.4 infant deaths per 1,000 live births (U.S. Department of Health and Human Services, Office of Minority Health, 2011).

Age Inequalities

Age is another factor that is closely related to health and occupational performance. All societies have some shared cultural expectations of its members based on age. **Ageism** is the term used to describe discrimination based on age (Estes, 2001). Although it is against the law to discriminate in hiring, the 60-year-old who wants or needs to find a new job does not find many open doors regardless of his or her work experience (Wilkinson & Ferraro, 2002). That may change as the full impact of the aging baby boom generation is realized. Baby boomers are healthier, wealthier, better educated, and more politically savvy than previous generations (Soto, 2005). They will exert a considerable influence on what it means to be "old" in the United States. However, a significant number of older adult women, particularly widowed women, remain at high risk for poverty, unemployment, and disability in later life.

Health and aging are tightly intertwined. Not surprisingly, "age is the single most important predictor of mortality and morbidity" (Weitz, 2004, p. 52). Because age and illness are so closely tied, when the average age of the population increases, so does the prevalence of health problems. The U.S. population 65 and older will increase from 35 million in 2000 to 55 million in 2020. By the year 2030, there will be about 72.1 million older persons. People 65 years and older are expected to grow to be 19.3% of the population by 2030 (U.S. Administration on Aging [AoA], 2010). The health problems associated with aging populations and the financial costs of meeting those needs are anticipated to be an enormous financial and political challenge.

Inequalities due to Disability

Disability is associated with disadvantage, regardless of individual skills or financial resources. According to the U.S. Census Bureau (2010), 48.9 million people have a disability. This represents nearly 20% of the population aged 5 years and older living in the community. The opportunities for employment are reduced for all groups of disabled persons as compared to able-bodied persons, but even for those with a disability, there are differences. Of those with mental disabilities, for example, 41% are employed; for wheelchair users, the figure is closer to 22%. The consequences for those who experience multiple inequalities are also noteworthy. Women with disability are sometimes thought to face the cumulative disadvantage or "double jeopardy" of being female and disabled (Chappell & Havens, 1980; Pentland, Tremblay, Spring, & Rosenthal, 1999). Medical and technological advances have enabled people to live longer and be more independent, but full social inclusion and community participation have not been realized. The actions that led to the passage of the Americans with Disabilities Act reflect the long-standing efforts of the disability rights movement and its allies (including occupational therapy practitioners) to improve life conditions for people with disabilities (Colker, 2005; Hurst, 2003).

People with disabilities also have poorer health than nondisabled people. Higher rates of diabetes, depression, elevated blood pressure and blood cholesterol, obesity, and vision and hearing impairments are all reported (HHS, 2000a). Lower rates of positive and recommended health behaviors such as cardiovascular fitness have been found too, as have low rates of patient education and treatment for mental illness.

Inequalities Based on Sexual Orientation

Understanding the inequalities faced by individuals as a function of their sexual orientation is a significant challenge given the tremendous lack of knowledge about the experiences and specific health needs of the lesbian, gay, bisexual, and transgender (LGBT) populations. The IOM (2011), in its report *The Health of Lesbian, Gay, Bisexual, and Transgender People: Building a Foundation for Better Understanding*, has noted that despite the increased visibility of these groups in society, almost nothing is known about their social experiences across the life course, how their health needs may be similar or different from the heterosexual population, and how interventions to address health needs of LGBT individuals should best be tailored.

It must be recognized that the experiences of LGBT individuals are not uniform and are shaped by factors of race, ethnicity, SES, geographical location, and age, any of which can have an effect on health-related concerns and needs (Wilson & Yoshikawa, 2004). Thus, for example, LGBT individuals in same-sex relationships who are also older, or are visible minorities, may face a similar type of "double disadvantage" mentioned earlier. The combined negative effects of occupying two stigmatized statuses may be greater than occupying either status alone (Chappell & Havens, 1980). Although research with visible minorities has documented the deleterious effects of persistent racial discrimination and ensuring chronic stress (Clark, 2004), it is simply not known whether this pattern holds with respect to sexual orientation.

Research is also needed that goes beyond the individual level. LGBT individuals are also in relationships and many have children. When the child in an LGBT family encounters the medical system, how do occupational therapists respond? Many of the same issues arise as in other cases of patient diversity. However, there can be unique challenges that more closely resemble those of new immigrants or migrant workers or even prison populations where a range of legal rights and statuses are relevant to the process of seeking care and being well. For example, children raised in same-sex households may not receive adequate health care if the parents' nontraditional partnership is not recognized as legal. Similarly, children of undocumented immigrants in the United States are facing considerable difficulty enrolling in school, finding a job, and accessing health care services (Vargas, 2011). The 2000 census revealed that same-sex couples are raising children in nearly every U.S. state. Nationwide, 34% of same-sex female partner households and 22% of same-sex male partner households had children younger than the age of 18 living with them (U.S. Census Bureau, 2003), whose needs may be ignored. Yet, despite several resolutions by the American Medical Association targeted to reduce health care disparities based on sexual orientation, legislative challenges persist, particularly in those states banning same-sex civil unions and marriages (Grossberg, 2006). Such restrictions impose health disparities based on sexual orientation that can negatively affect the family at many points across the life course.

The Intersection of Multiple Inequalities

In summary, regardless of our professed beliefs in equal opportunity and despite legislation intended to prevent discrimination, life choices, opportunities, and access to health and meaningful occupations are not equal; they are mediated by an array of powerful social and economic forces that dictate the fate of individuals and ultimately health. These factors are not easily changed or overcome through individual desire and effort, either our own or that of our clients. Much larger forces, including the health system, play an integral role. Previously, we have discussed how inequalities based on gender, age, ethnicity, poverty, and sexual orientation alone shape the activity profiles and occupational experiences of children, working age adults, and the elderly. Also raised was the notion of double jeopardy, that is, the more than additive experience of living with multiple inequalities.

The Political Economy of the Health Care System

To fully appreciate the influence of social and economic factors in the lives of individuals and families, these factors must be set against the backdrop of the U.S. health care system. It is certainly the most expensive system in the world. Health expenditures in the United States in 2009 represented 17.4% of the country's gross domestic product, by far the highest share of any country in the OECD and more than 8% higher than the OECD average of 9.5% (OECD, 2011). The United States spent $7,960 on health per capita in 2009, the most of any single OECD country and two-and-a-half times the OECD average of $3,223 (OECD, 2011). The United States spends more than twice as much per capita on health care as relatively rich European countries such as France and Germany, and as the section that follows highlights, the investment is not providing a strong return.

International Comparisons

Despite the huge amount spent, the United States ranks low on many health indicators (World Health Organization, 2010), and there is mounting evidence that the system is plagued with serious problems at all levels (Moss, 2000; Rylko-Bauer & Farmer, 2002). Life expectancy in the United States stands at 78.2 years, below the average of 79.5 years for the 30 developed countries that belong to the OECD (2011). Japan, Italy, Spain, and Australia all have life expectancies above 81.5 years. Infant mortality in the United States is worse, too: 6.5 deaths per 1,000 live births in 2009, above the OECD average of 4.4. Nordic countries (Iceland, Finland, and Sweden), Japan, Greece, Portugal, and Korea all have lower infant mortality rates than the United States rate, and these countries spend a fraction of what the United States spends on health care (OECD, 2011). This focus on population health outcomes is important because social and environmental context shapes health and opportunities for occupational engagement and participation in society. Preventative care, such as childhood vaccinations and cancer screening, saves lives and significantly reduces the burden of secondary health conditions. In a system where financial resources are the means to access key screening tests as well as expensive medical interventions, then those with low SES are at a distinct disadvantage. Without this care, low SES patients will come to occupational therapy in worse health and with fewer opportunities to benefit from our interventions and recommendations than their high SES counterparts.

The Role of Health Insurance

Health insurance (or, more accurately, medical insurance) is important because access to health care in the mostly private U.S. system requires either a job with health benefits or the financial means to pay out of pocket. A substantial number of U.S. citizens lack both. More than 50.7 million residents are estimated to have no health insurance whatsoever (U.S. Census Bureau, 2009); an equal number are thought to have insufficient coverage (Brouwer, 1998; Cutler, 2004). Ethnic and racial minority groups make up a disproportionate share of the uninsured; African Americans are twice as likely to be uninsured than Whites, and Hispanics are three times more likely than Whites to be uninsured (Adams et al., 2010). Insurance matters because the uninsured and underinsured are in poorer health, have reduced access and less appropriate care, and are more likely to die prematurely (IOM, 2009; Krieger, 1999; U.S. Census Bureau, 2009).

The health disadvantages associated with lack of health insurance are not solely a problem for the unemployed. A report from the Kaiser Family Foundation (2010) found that more than half of all uninsured workers in the United States work in full-time jobs, so the problem is not the lack of jobs that make workers eligible for employer-sponsored health insurance, but rather that fewer middle-class jobs include health benefits. The IOM (2009), in its report *America's Uninsured Crisis*, states, "A severely weakened economy, rising health care and health insurance costs, growing unemployment, and declining employment-based health insurance coverage all provide evidence that the U.S. health insurance system is in a state of crisis" (p. 5). The fallout has been distressing in a variety of ways. For example, a national survey found that 37% of all working persons have trouble paying their medical bills (Doty, Edwards, & Holmgren, 2005). A recent study of bankruptcies in the United States found that 62.1% of all bankruptcies in 2007 were related to medical costs, and 92% of these medical debtors had medical debts over $5,000. More unexpected was the finding that most medical debtors were well educated, owned homes, and had middle-class occupations. Three-quarters of the sample had health insurance. Using identical definitions in 2001 and 2007, the researchers found the share of bankruptcies attributable to medical problems rose by a remarkable 49.6% (Himmelstein, Thorne, Warren, & Woolhandler, 2009).

In government-paid health insurance, such as Medicare and Medicaid, the impact of out-of-pocket expenses is still significant. A recent report from the American Association of Retired Persons Policy Institute (Nonnemaker & Sinclair, 2011) found that Medicare beneficiaries (age 65 and older) spent a median of $3,103 of their own money on health care in 2006. Ten percent of beneficiaries—more than 4 million people—spent more than $8,300 a year. The oldest and poorest beneficiaries spent about one-quarter of their incomes on health care.

In a political effort to improve health care and reduce costs, the *Affordable Care Act* was passed by the Congress and signed by President Obama on March 23, 2010. Effective immediately were measures to reduce out-of-pocket expenses. For example, prescription medication costs for Medicare recipients were offset through rebate checks and discounts. Preventative health services at no cost to the recipient are also part of this initiative and include diabetes screening, mammography screening, annual wellness visits, prostate cancer screening, tobacco cessation counseling, and other services (Affordable Care Act, 2012). Promoting healthy behaviors, given the considerable social and economic burdens associated with chronic diseases (Goode, 2002), has immediate and long-term benefits to the individual and society as a whole. However, people must have the resources to enact healthy behaviors. For example, high-quality, fresh foods are often more expensive than processed foods of lower quality.

There is no question that there is a need to care about the uninsured and rising costs of health care, whether based on social justice or simply as a matter of dollars and cents. Kawachi and Berkman (2003) warn that the least fortunate in society must be cared for, or spillover effects will adversely affect everyone. Wide income disparities lead to stress, family disruption, and mass frustration, which in turn lead to violence and crime. Research shows that the distribution of household income, for example, in the United States is becoming increasingly unequal. In 2007, the top 10% of Americans earned 49.7% of the nation's income (Saez, 2010).

Mechanisms of Disadvantage across the Life Course

There is an untested assumption that health inequalities arise from inadequacies in health care. Of course, there is a gap in this logic. The fact that there are problems with a medical system does not mean that the system caused the problems. So why do differences in health status exist across different groups in society? As a reader of this chapter, you will already appreciate that a significant part of the problem is poverty and income inequality. Figure 17.1 illustrates the many pathways by which SES factors at both the individual and community levels can influence health.

Economic Disadvantage and Health

Poverty is bad for health. The term ***poverty*** refers to the lack of material resources that are necessary for subsistence. Poverty increases exposure to factors that make people sick, and it decreases the chances of having high-quality medical insurance (and thus care) when the person needs it. Children, older adults, new immigrants, persons with disabilities, and members of ethnic minorities are at greatest risk of poverty (U.S. Census Bureau, 2009). An alarming fact is that the poverty rate in the United States in 2009 was 14.3%—up from 13.2% in 2008 and a 26-year low of 11.3% in 2000. In 2009, 43.6 million Americans were living in poverty (U.S. Census Bureau, 2009). This is the largest number in the 51 years the U.S. government has been publishing poverty data.

Economics and health policy experts are asking whether these pronounced levels of income inequality are taking a toll on health and the fabric of society (Wilkinson & Pickett, 2009a). Perhaps this has fueled the entry of two new terms into the popular lexicon: *the working poor* and *the new poor*. The **working poor** are people who work full time but whose wages do not raise them above the poverty line. In 2010, 72.9 million U.S. workers aged 16 and older were paid hourly rates, representing 58.8% of all wage and salary workers. Among those paid by the hour, 1.8 million earned the federal minimum wage of $7.25 an hour (U.S. Department of Labor, 2011). Critics ask how the working poor manage to survive (Ehrenreich, 2001; Shipler, 2005). The **new poor** are those people who have fallen into poverty because of sudden or unexpected circumstances such as serious illness, divorce, or sudden job layoffs.

Money can buy health services, but it also provides safe neighborhoods and pays for better food and for

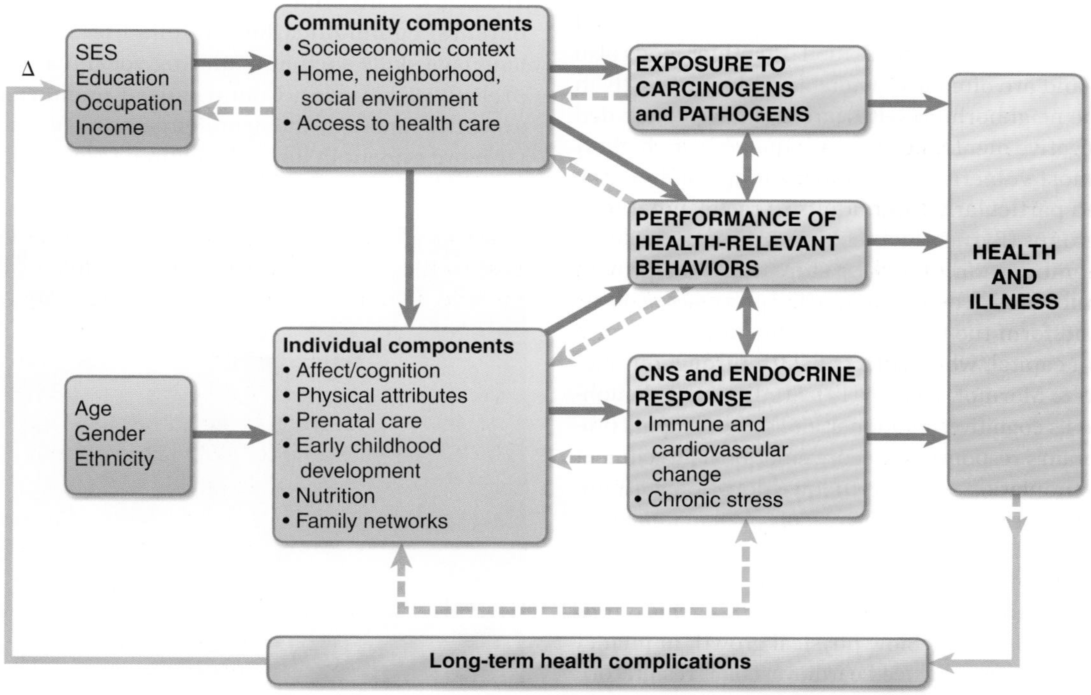

FIGURE 17.1 A model of socioeconomic status (SES) influences and interactions on health.

costs related to participating in sports and staying fit. Money is also necessary to pay college and university tuition fees that will provide the education needed to compete successfully for a well-paid job. In addition, a lack of financial resources can produce prolonged stress, which in turn negatively affects health. Proponents of a "social determinants" or "fundamental causes" perspective argue that to solve these problems will require greater redistribution of wealth (Wilkinson & Pickett, 2009a, 2009b). Health care experts and economists alike are increasingly suggesting that fixing the health care system by addressing disparities in access and medical treatment is only part of the solution (Wilkinson & Pickett, 2009a, 2009b). If improvement in the health of the most disadvantaged in society is desired, reducing the social inequalities that exist in society is imperative. This would need to begin in early childhood and continue throughout life.

Effects over a Lifetime

A plethora of observational research and intervention studies show that the foundations of adult health are laid in early childhood, even before birth (Brown et al., 2004; Hackman, Farah, & Meaney, 2010; Young, 1997). Low SES influences prenatal care and the health of the unborn child/fetus. Compared to women with high SES, women with low SES experience higher levels of stress, higher infection rates, and poorer nutrition during pregnancy that, in turn, lead to low birth weight and premature delivery (Spencer, Bambang, Logan, & Gill, 1999). Increased stress may also lead to poor health practices, such as smoking and choosing foods of low nutritional value (Kramer et al., 2001). Indirectly, but no less importantly, SES determines the access one has to financial resources to purchase adequate food. Healthier foods also cost more and are often less available and more costly in low-income neighborhoods. Researchers have concluded that the negative mental health consequences are highest for those most vulnerable, including young children, the elderly, and particularly older adults in racial and ethnic minority groups (Byrnes, Lichtenberg, & Lysack, 2006).

The combination of a poor start and slow growth "become embedded in biology during the processes of development, and form the basis of the individual's biological and human capital, which affects health throughout life" (Wilkinson & Marmot, 2003, p. 14). Studies have demonstrated that as cognitive, emotional, and sensory inputs program the brain's responses, insecure emotional attachment and poor stimulation can lead to low educational attainment, problem behavior, and the risk of social marginalization in adulthood (Barker, 1998). Higher rates of depression, anxiety, attention problems, and conduct disorders plague children and adolescents from lower SES backgrounds (Merikangas et al., 2010). Slow physical growth in infancy is also associated with reduced cardiovascular, respiratory, pancreatic, and kidney function, which increases the risk of serious illness in adulthood (Shonkoff & Phillips, 2000).

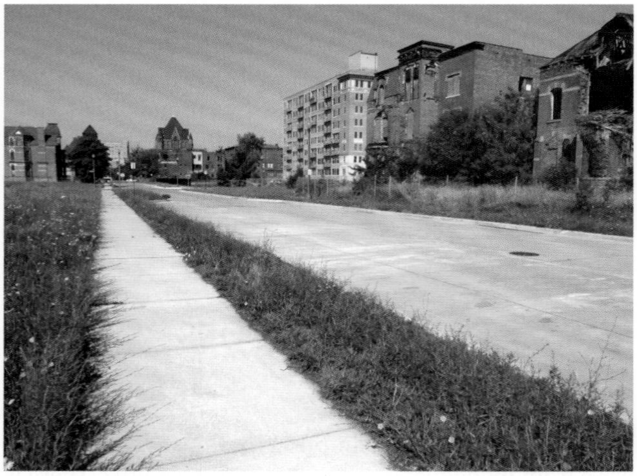

FIGURE 17.2 Unsafe neighborhoods.

Children learn and develop through play. Not only does play help them to learn about themselves as individuals, but it also helps them to acquire their fundamental social interaction and motor and cognitive skills (Case-Smith, 2000). Yet, the playing field is not equal. Kozol (1991, 1995) describes neighborhoods overrun by poverty, crime, and economic neglect. In such neighborhoods, parents are afraid to let their children play outdoors because of high rates of violence and exposure to environmental toxins (Brown et al., 2004; Surkan et al., 2007) that place them at risk for injuries and disease (see Figures 17.2 and 17.3). Living in an impoverished home environment when younger may impede normal development (Martin, McCaughtry, Flory, Murphy, & Wisdom, 2011). The lack of early stimulation from books, computers, and parental communication inhibits the development of language skills such as acquiring vocabulary and interpreting verbal cues. Compromised memory function, executive function, and neural processing of emotions are far more evident in low SES children (Waber et al., 2007),

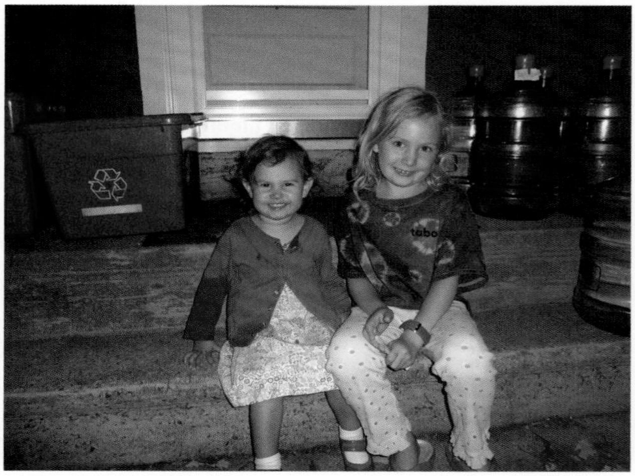

FIGURE 17.3 No place to play.

with far-reaching effects as one grows older. Occupational therapists are trained to identify the smallest opportunities for functional improvement, to facilitate occupational engagement, and to bring tremendous skill in identifying motivational features of the child's interests and environment (Parham & Primeau, 1997).

Social inequalities over the life course contribute to occupational performance deficits in adults as well. This occurs in all areas of occupational performance from social relationships to work. Rates of anxiety, substance abuse, and depression are all higher in populations in which unemployment is high (U.S. Department of Health and Human Services, Office of Minority Health, 2011). For those who are employed, there are other stress-related problems; research has shown that lack of personal autonomy and control in one's work (often characteristic of low-paying, low-skilled jobs) is significantly related to cardiovascular disease (Bosma, Peter, Siegrist, & Marmot, 1998). Chronic stress has deleterious effects on the human body that weaken the immune system and, in turn, place individuals at greater risk for heart disease, stroke, cancer, and other chronic illnesses (Goode, 2002).

Despite clear evidence that stress is bad for health, workers in the U.S. workplace have less and less leisure time for rest and recreation. A recent international travel survey by Expedia.com (2009) found that adults in the United States work the most hours of any affluent country, yet only earn 13 vacation days annually, the fewest of any developed country. This lags behind Canada with 19 days and Germany and France with 27 and 38 vacation days, respectively. The second problem is that the United States is also the only industrialized nation in the world where paid vacation is not mandatory (Expedia.com, 2009). It is estimated that 1 in 4 workers in the United States do not accrue vacation time. Even so, 34% of Americans who are eligible for vacation time do not take all the time they are eligible for, with 19% saying they have cancelled planned vacation time because they are "too busy at work" to get away.

The Role of Occupational Therapy in Addressing Health Disparities

Townsend and Wilcock (2003) asserted that it is an occupational injustice to ignore the social and economic determinants of health and how these, in turn, affect opportunities for and engagement in occupation. Others have called on occupational therapists to address the segregation of groups of people based on lack of meaningful participation in daily life occupations, something that Kronenberg and Pollard (2005) have provocatively called **occupational apartheid**. There is little doubt that social and economic factors are real and exert a powerful influence on health and occupational performance, but what can occupational therapists do in the face of what appears to be intractable problems on a very large scale? After developing greater awareness of the influence of social inequalities on health and the extent of health disparities among the clients occupational therapy practitioners serve, what are the next practical steps?

First, occupational therapists can apply the small but growing body of research evidence available that focused interventions early in a vulnerable child's life can produce meaningful benefits throughout the person's life course. For example, occupational therapy can effectively address sensory motor performance deficits, lack of peer-play relationships (Tanta, Deitz, White, & Billingsley, 2005), and maladaptive family interactions (Bedell, Cohn, & Dumas, 2005), which all may be more prevalent in socioeconomically disadvantaged families. Occupational therapists can also support parents to better understand their children's emotional and cognitive needs and modify school and home environments to facilitate occupational performance (Letts, Rigby, & Stewart, 2003).

Second, occupational therapists are experts at person–environment fit and recognize the centrality of meaningful occupations to facilitate good health. Yet, there are serious gaps in knowledge where more research is needed. For example, little is known about meaningful occupational engagement for chronically unemployed people and what kinds of interventions might be effective. Even less is known about occupational deprivation due to immigration, geographical isolation, and incarceration (Whiteford, 2000). Strong arguments have been advanced to urge occupational therapy to extend its benefits to all marginalized populations that experience occupational disadvantage (Creek, 2011).

Third, a unique strength of the profession is its holistic approach. This does not simply mean that the physical and psychosocial domains are addressed in clients' therapeutic goals. It also means that it is important to learn about clients in the terms of their world, their perceptions, their experiences, and their realities. This is easy to say and much more difficult to do. Purtilo and Haddad (2002) describe many difficulties that arise between practitioners and clients because of socioeconomic and cultural differences. These differences influence how individual occupational therapists feel about clients, including the level of empathy and understanding of clients' lives and daily routines.

Fourth, to act on issues of occupational deprivation and occupational injustice requires that therapists become more educated about economic and other institutional and structural barriers to treatment and fair allocation of rehabilitation services. There is research to show that occupational therapy services are not equally distributed (Neufeld & Lysack, 2004, 2006). Simply put, clients who lack the ability to pay will not access services, or they will receive a lower quality of services unless they are able to access alternative private pay or charitable resources. Therapists

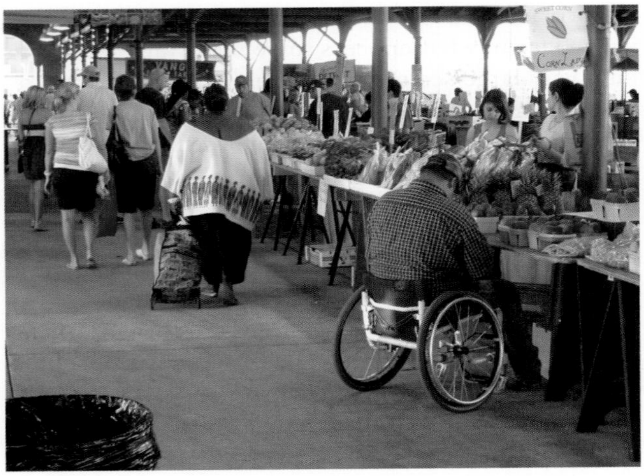

FIGURE 17.4 Farmer's market.

regularly identify socioeconomic barriers in the home that impact occupational performance but may be less attentive to the adequacy of their client's neighborhood and availability of accessible transportation, nutritious foods, and quality housing, for example (see Figure 17.4). As stated earlier in this chapter, occupational therapists must focus some of their therapeutic energies on effecting change at the level of organizations (e.g., schools, hospitals, housing administrators, transportation authorities) and systems (e.g., health insurers, employers).

Finally, occupational therapists must leverage their position in the health care system to reduce the negative consequences of SES and social conditions on their clients' health and occupational performance. For example, therapists can enlighten insurance payers about the needs of their low-income clients by recommending the ideal occupational therapy services for their clients in addition to the documentation required for services currently eligible for reimbursement. Another strategy is to employ the specific rules and language of insurance companies much more strategically so that occupational therapy interventions have the best chance of being accepted by payers (Lohman & Brown, 1997; Uili & Wood, 1995). With persistence, these efforts can be effective and worthwhile because successful changes in policy can benefit thousands of clients.

Conclusion

Client-centered care emphasizes listening, asking the right questions, and truly understanding and empathizing with the client (Law, 1998; Lawlor, 2003; Wood, 1996). Although listening to and learning from individual clients are paramount to effective occupational therapy interventions, this approach individualizes the underlying problems of health disparities and inequalities that are fundamentally social in nature. Occupational therapists who work with socioeconomically disadvantaged clients are well acquainted with this tension. In the occupational therapy literature, Dr. Sandra Galheigo (2011) has spoken boldly about the need to prepare the new generation of occupational therapists to engage in social transformation, not only individual change, and to address issues of invisibility and lack of access to human rights. In her work with orphans in an institutional environment, she has urged therapists to shift their therapeutic attention to working with the children and staff as a collective to create an environment that provides more and better opportunities for occupational engagement.

In a similar vein, Jennifer Creek, in her 2011 Hanneke van Bruggen Lecture, challenges occupational therapists to ask themselves what they are really doing to help their clients. She states,

> We think that we want to hear what the client has to say but, in reality, we fear that we will not be able to understand or cope with a diversity of needs. It is safer to carry out a procedure or fill in a checklist than to confront our own inadequacy in the face of another's distress.

Although some experts have argued that the path forward lies in large-scale professional coalitions aimed at major transformations of the health care system (Cutler, 2004), this takes time to achieve, if it can be achieved at all. In the meantime, occupational therapists must work in a system that is imperfect, knowing fully well that it does not meet many of their clients' most pressing needs.

Recall once more Annie's struggle to recover from a lifetime of social and economic disadvantage. There are many "Annies" who you will meet in occupational therapy practice. To accomplish the true promise of occupational therapy undoubtedly requires better knowledge of the communities from which our clients come and the socioeconomic, historical, and political forces that have shaped their lives and their health. Identifying inequalities and disparities where they exist as well as working to ameliorate them is one of our ethical responsibilities as health care professionals. This is the only way to advance health for all.

References

Adams, P. F., Martinez, M. E., & Vickerie, J. L. (2010). Summary health statistics for the U.S. population: National Health Interview Survey, 2009. *Vital Health Statistics, 10*(248), 1–115.

Affordable Care Act. (2012). *Medicare preventive services*. Retrieved from http://www.healthcare.gov/law/features/65-older/index.html

America's Children. (2011). *Child poverty and family income*. Retrieved from http://www.childstats.gov/americaschildren/eco1.asp

Barker, D. (1998). *Mothers, babies and disease in later life* (2nd ed.). Edinburgh, United Kingdom: Churchill Livingstone.

Bass-Haugen, J. (2009). Health Disparities: Examination of evidence relevant for occupational therapy. *American Journal of Occupational Therapy, 63*(1), 24–34.

Bedell, G. M., Cohn, E. S., & Dumas, H. M. (2005). Exploring parents' use of strategies to promote social participation of school-age children with acquired brain injuries. *American Journal of Occupational Therapy, 59*(3), 273–284.

Bosma, H., Peter, R., Siegrist, J., & Marmot, M. (1998). Two alternative job stress models and risk of coronary heart disease. *American Journal of Public Health, 88*(1), 68–74.

Bradbury, K., & Katz, J. (2002). Women's labor market involvement and family income mobility when marriages end. *New England Economic Review, Q4*, 41–74.

Brouwer, S. (1998). *Sharing the pie: A citizen's guide to wealth and power in America.* New York, NY: Henry Holt.

Brown, B., Bzostek, S., Aufseeser, D., Berry, D., Weitzman, M., Kavanaugh, M., . . . Auinger, P. (Eds.). (2004). *Early child development in social context: A chartbook.* New York, NY: The Commonwealth Fund. Retrieved from http://www.commonwealthfund.org/usr_doc/ChildDevChartbk.pdf

Byrnes, M., Lichtenberg, P., & Lysack, C. (2006). Environmental press, aging in place, and residential satisfaction of urban older adults. *Journal of Applied Sociology, 23*(2), 50–77.

Case-Smith, J. (2000). Effects of occupational therapy services on fine motor and functional performance in preschool children. *American Journal of Occupational Therapy, 54*(4), 372–380.

Chappell, N., & Havens, B. (1980). Old and female: Testing the double jeopardy hypothesis. *The Sociological Quarterly, 21*(2), 157–171.

Clark, R. (2004). Significance of perceived racism: Toward understanding the ethnic group disparities in health, the later years. In N. Anderson, R. Bulato, & B. Cohen (Eds.), *Critical perspectives on racial and ethnic differences in health in late life* (pp. 540–566). Washington, DC: National Academies Press.

Colker, R. (2005). *The disability pendulum: The first decade of the Americans with Disabilities Act.* New York, NY: New York University Press.

Creek, J. (2011, November). 2011 ENOTHE Inaugural Hanneke van Bruggen Lecture "In praise of Diversity." Paper presented at the 2011 annual meeting of the European Network of Occupational Therapy in Higher Education (ENOTHE) in Ghent, Belgium. Retrieved from http://www.enothe.eu/activities/meet/ac11/Appendix3.4.pdf

Cutler, D. (2004). *Your money or your life: Strong medicine for America's health care system.* New York, NY: Oxford University Press.

Doty, M., Edwards, J., & Holmgren, A. (2005). *Seeing red: Americans driven into debt by medical bills.* New York, NY: The Commonwealth Fund. Retrieved from http://www.commonwealthfund.org/Content/Publications/Issue-Briefs/2005/Aug/Seeing-Red—Americans-Driven-into-Debt-by-Medical-Bills.aspx

The Economist. (2005, July 21). *Women in business: The conundrum of the glass ceiling.* Retrieved from http://www.economist.com/node/4197626

Ehrenreich, B. (2001). *Nickel and dimed: On (not) getting by in America.* New York, NY: Henry Holt.

Estes, C. (2001). *Social policy and aging: A critical perspective.* Thousand Oaks, CA: Sage.

Evans, R. G., Barer, M. L., & Marmor, T. L. (Eds.). (1994). *Why are some people healthy and others not? The determinants of health of populations.* New York, NY: Aldine de Gruyter.

Expedia.com. (2009). *Vacation deprivation survey.* Retrieved from http://www.expedia.com/daily/promos/vacations/vacation_deprivation/default.asp

Galheigo, S. M. (2011). What needs to be done? Occupational therapy responsibilities and challenges regarding human rights. *Australian Occupational Therapy Journal, 58*(2), 60–66.

Goode, E. (2002, December 17). The heavy cost of chronic stress. *The New York Times.* Retrieved from http://www.nytimes.com/2002/12/17/science/the-heavy-cost-of-chronic-stress.html?pagewanted=all&src=pm

Grossberg, P. M. (2006). An evidence-based context to address health care for gay and lesbian patients. *Wisconsin Medical Journal, 105*(6), 16–18.

Hackman, D. A., Farah, M. J., & Meany, M. J. (2010). Socioeconomic status and the brain: Mechanistic insights from human and animal research. *Nature Reviews Neuroscience, 11*(9), 651–659.

Hertz, T. (2006). *Understanding mobility in America.* American University. Retrieved from http://www.americanprogress.org/kf/hertz_mobility_analysis.pdf

Hesse-Biber, S., & Carter, G. (2000). *Working women in America: Split dreams.* New York, NY: Oxford University Press.

Himmelstein, D., Thorne, D., Warren, E., & Woolhandler, S. (2009). Medical bankruptcy in the United States, 2007: Results of a national study. *The American Journal of Medicine, 122*(8), 741–746.

Hurst, R. (2003). The international disability rights movement and the ICF. *Disability and Rehabilitation, 25*(11–12), 572–576.

Institute for Women's Policy Research. (2011). *The gender wage gap: 2010.* Retrieved from http://www.iwpr.org/publications/pubs/the-gender-wage-gap-2010-updated-march-2011

Institute of Medicine. (2002). *Unequal treatment: Confronting racial and ethnic disparities in health care.* Washington, DC: National Academies Press.

Institute of Medicine. (2009). *America's uninsured crisis: Consequences for health and health care.* Washington, DC: National Academies Press. Retrieved from http://www.iom.edu/Reports/2009/Americas-Uninsured-Crisis-Consequences-for-Health-and-Health-Care.aspx

Institute of Medicine. (2011). *The health of lesbian, gay, bisexual, and transgender people: Building a foundation for better understanding.* Washington, DC: National Academies Press.

Kaiser Family Foundation. (2010). *Employer health benefits.* Retrieved from http://ehbs.kff.org/pdf/2010/8085.pdf

Kau, G., & Thompson, J. S. (2003). Racial and ethnic stratification of educational achievement and attainment. *Annual Review of Sociology, 29*, 417–442.

Kawachi, I., & Berkman, L. (2003). *Neighborhoods and health.* New York, NY: Oxford University Press.

Kelan, E. K. (2009). *Performing gender at work.* Basingstoke, United Kingdom: Palgrave Macmillan.

Kozol, J. (1991). *Savage inequalities: Children in America's schools.* New York, NY: HarperCollins.

Kozol, J. (1995). *Amazing grace: The lives of children and the conscience of a nation.* New York, NY: Crown.

Kramer, M. S., Goulet, L., Lydon, J., Séquin, L., McNamara, H., Dassa, C., . . . Koren, G. (2001). Socio-economic disparities in preterm birth: Causal pathways and mechanism. *Paediatric Perinatal Epidemiology, 15*(Suppl. 2), 104–123.

Krieger, N. (1999). Embodying inequality: A review of concepts, measures, and methods for studying health consequences of discrimination. *International Journal of Health Services, 29*(2), 295–352.

Krieger, N. (2001). A glossary for social epidemiology. *Journal of Epidemiology and Community Health, 55*(10), 693–700.

Krieger, N. (2010). Social inequalities in health. In J. Olsen, R. Saracci, & D. Trichopolous (Eds.), *Teaching epidemiology: A guide for teachers in epidemiology, public health, and clinical medicine* (3rd ed., pp. 215–239). Oxford, NY: Oxford University Press.

Kronenberg, F., & Pollard, N. (2005). Overcoming occupational apartheid: A preliminary exploration of the political nature of occupational therapy. In F. Kronenberg, S. Algado, & N. Pollard (Eds.), *Occupational therapy without borders: Learning from the spirit of survivors* (pp. 58–86). New York, NY: Elsevier.

Law, M. (1998). *Client-centred occupational therapy.* Thorofare, NJ: Slack.

Lawlor, M. (2003). Gazing anew: The shift from a clinical gaze to an ethnographic lens. *The American Journal of Occupational Therapy, 57*(1), 29–39.

Letts, L., Rigby, P., & Stewart, D. (Eds.). (2003). *Using environments to enable occupational performance.* Thorofare, NJ: Slack.

Link, B., & Phelan, J. (1995). Social conditions as fundamental causes of disease. *Journal of Health and Social Behavior, 35*, 80–94.

Link, B., & Phelan, J. (2005). Fundamental sources of health inequalities. In D. Mechanic, L. Rogut, D. Colby, & J. Knickman (Eds.), *Policy challenges in modern health care* (pp. 71–84). New Brunswick, NJ: Rutgers University Press.

Lohman, H., & Brown, K. (1997). Ethical issues related to managed care: An in-depth discussion of an occupational therapy case study. *Occupational Therapy in Health Care, 10*(4), 1–12.

Lynch, J. W., Kaplan, G. A., Cohen, R. D., Kauhanen, J., Wilson, T. W., Smith, N. L., & Salonen, J. T. (1994). Childhood and adult socioeconomic status as predictors of mortality in Finland. *Lancet*, 343(8896), 524–527.

Lynch, J. W., Kaplan, G. A., Pamuk, E. R., Cohen, R. D., Heck, K. E., Balfour, J. L., & Yen, I. H. (1998). Income inequality and mortality in metropolitan areas of the United States. *American Journal of Public Health, 88*(7), 1074–1080.

Marmot, M., Shipley, M., & Rose, G. (1984). Inequalities in death—specific explanations of a general pattern? *Lancet, 1*(8384), 1003–1006.

Marmot, M., & Wilkinson, R. (Eds.). (1999). *Social determinants of health.* London, United Kingdom: Oxford Press.

Martin, J., McCaughtry, N., Flory, S., Murphy, A., & Wisdom, K. (2011). Using social cognitive theory to predict physical activity and fitness in underserved middle school children. *Research Quarterly for Exercise and Sport, 82*(2), 247–255.

Merikangas K., He, J., Brody, D., Fisher, P., Bourdon, K., & Koretz, D. (2010). Prevalence and treatment of mental disorders among U.S. children in the 2001–2004 NHANES. *Pediatrics, 125*(1), 75–81.

Miringoff, M., & Miringoff, M. (1999). *The social health of the nation: How America is really doing.* New York, NY: Oxford University Press.

Moss, N. (2000). Socioeconomic disparities in health in the US: An agenda for action. *Social Science and Medicine, 51*(11), 1627–1638.

National Center for Health Statistics. (2010). *Health, United States, 2010, with chartbook on trends in the health of Americans.* Hyattsville, MD: Author.

Neufeld, S., & Lysack, C. (2004). Allocation of rehabilitation resources: Who gets a home evaluation. *American Journal of Occupational Therapy, 58*(6), 630–638.

Neufeld, S., & Lysack, C. (2006). Investigating differences among older adults' access to specialized rehabilitation services. *Journal of Aging and Health, 18*(4), 584–603.

Nonnemaker, L., & Sinclair, S. (2011). *Medicare beneficiaries' out-of-pocket spending for health care. Insight on the Issues I48, January 2011.* AARP Public Policy Institute. Retrieved from http://www.aarp.org/health/medicare-insurance/info-02-2011/Insight-I48-oop.html

Online Dictionary of the Social Sciences. (2012). *Online resource.* Retrieved from http://bitbucket.icaap.org

Organisation for Economic Co-operation and Development. (2011). *OECD health data 2011: How does the United States compare.* Retrieved from http://www.oecd.org/dataoecd/46/2/38980580.pdf

Parham, L. D., & Primeau, L. (1997). Play and occupational therapy. In L. D. Parham & L. Fazio (Eds.), *Play in occupational therapy for children* (pp. 2–22). St. Louis, MO: Mosby Year Book.

Pentland, W., Tremblay, M., Spring, K., & Rosenthal, C. (1999). Women with physical disabilities: Occupational impacts of ageing. *Journal of Occupational Science, 6*(3), 111–123.

Purtilo, R., & Haddad, A. (2002). *Health professional and patient interaction* (6th ed.). Philadelphia, PA: Saunders.

Roscigno, V. J., & Ainsworth-Darnell, J. W. (1999). Race, cultural capital, and educational resources: Persistent inequalities and achievement returns. *Sociology of Education, 72,* 158–178.

Rylko-Bauer, B., & Farmer, P. (2002). Managed care or managed inequality? A call for critiques of market-based medicine. *Medical Anthropology Quarterly, 16*(4), 476–502.

Saez, E. (2010). *Striking it richer: The evolution of top incomes in the United States.* Retrieved from http://elsa.berkeley.edu/~saez/

Schulz, A., Israel, B., Zenk, S., Parker, E., Lichtenstein, R., Shellman-Weir, S., & Klem, A. (2006). Psychosocial stress and social support as mediators of relationships between income, length of residence and depressive symptoms among African American women on Detroit's eastside. *Social Science and Medicine, 62*(2), 510–522.

Shipler, D. (2005). *The working poor: Invisible in America.* New York, NY: Knopf.

Shonkoff, J., & Phillips, D. (Eds.). (2000). *From neurons to neighborhoods: The science of early childhood development.* Washington, DC: National Academies Press.

Soto, M. (2005). Will baby boomers drown in debt? *Just the facts on retirement issues,* (15). Boston, MA: Center for Retirement Research at Boston College.

Spencer, N., Bambang, S., Logan, S., & Gill, L. (1999). Socioeconomic status and birth weight: Comparison of an area-based measure with the Registrar General's social class. *Journal of Epidemiology and Community Health, 53*(8), 495–498.

Surkan, P. J., Zhang, A., Trachtenberg, F., Daniel, D. B., Mckinlay, S., & Bellinger, D. C. (2007). Neuropsychological function in children with blood lead levels of <10μg/dl. *NeuroToxicology, 28*(6), 1170–1177.

Tanta, K., Deitz, J., White, O., & Billingsley, F. (2005). The effects of peer-play level on initiations and responses of preschool children with delayed play skills. *American Journal of Occupational Therapy, 59*(4), 437–445.

Townsend, E., & Wilcock, A. (2003). Occupational justice. In C. Christiansen & E. Townsend (Eds.), *Introduction to occupation: The art and science of living* (pp. 243–273). Upper Saddle River, NJ: Prentice Hall.

Uili, R. M., & Wood, R. (1995). The effect of third-party payers on the clinical decision making of physical therapists. *Social Science and Medicine, 40*(7), 873–879.

U.S. Administration on Aging. (2010). *A profile of older Americans: 2010.* Retrieved from http://www.aoa.gov/aoaroot/aging_statistics/Profile/2010/4.aspx

U.S. Census Bureau. (2003). *Same-sex households with children in the United States.* Retrieved from http://www.infoplease.com/us/census/same-sex-households.html

U.S. Census Bureau. (2009). *Income, poverty, and health insurance coverage in the United States: 2009.* Retrieved from http://www.census.gov/prod/2010pubs/p60-238.pdf

U.S. Census Bureau. (2010). *Chartbook on work and disability.* Retrieved from http://www.infouse.com/disabilitydata/workdisability/

U.S. Department of Health and Human Services. (2000a). Disability and secondary conditions. In *Healthy people 2010.* Retrieved from http://fodsupport.org/documents/HealthyPeople2010DisabilityChapter.pdf

U.S. Department of Health and Human Services. (2000b). *Healthy people 2010: Understanding and improving health.* Retrieved from http://www.healthequityks.org/download/Hllthy_People_2010_Improving_Health.pdf

U. S. Department of Health and Human Services, Office of Minority Health. (2011). *Infant mortality and African Americans.* Retrieved from http://minorityhealth.hhs.gov/templates/content.aspx?lvl=2&lvlID=51&ID=3021

U.S. Department of Labor. (2011). *Employment standards administration wage and hour division.* Retrieved from http://www.dol.gov/dol/topic/wages/minimumwage.htm

Vargas, J. (2011, June 22). My life as an undocumented immigrant. *The New York Times.* Retrieved from http://www.nytimes.com/2011/06/26/magazine/my-life-as-an-undocumented-immigrant.html?pagewanted=all

Waber, D., De Moor, C., Forbes, P., Almli, C., Botteron, K., Leonard, G., . . . Rumsey, J. (2007). The NIH MRI study of normal brain development: Performance of a population based sample of healthy children aged 6 to 18 years on a neuropsychological battery. *Journal of the International Neuropsychological Society, 13*(5), 729–746.

Weitz, R. (2004). *The sociology of health, illness, and health care.* Belmont, CA: Wadsworth.

Wells, S., & Black, R. (2000). *Cultural competency for health professionals.* Bethesda, MD: American Occupational Therapy Association.

Whiteford, G. (2000). Occupational deprivation: Global challenge in the new millennium. *British Journal of Occupational Therapy, 63*(5), 200–204.

Wilkinson, J., & Ferraro, K. (2002). Thirty years of ageism research. In T. Nelson (Ed.), *Ageism: Stereotyping and prejudice against older persons* (pp. 339–358). Cambridge, MA: Massachusetts Institute of Technology Press.

Wilkinson, R., & Marmot, M. (Eds.). (2003). *Social determinants of health: The solid facts* (2nd ed.). Copenhagen, Denmark: World Health Organization, Regional Office for Europe.

Wilkinson, R., & Pickett, K. (2009a). Income inequality and social dysfunction. *Annual Review of Sociology, 35,* 493–511.

Wilkinson, R., & Pickett, K. (2009b). *The spirit level: Why equality is better for everyone.* London, United Kingdom: Penguin Books.

Williams, D. R. (1997). Race and health: Basic questions, emerging directions. *Annals of Epidemiology, 7*(5), 322–333.

Wilson, P., & Yoshikawa, H. (2004). Experiences of and responses to social discrimination among Asian and Pacific Islander gay men: Their relationship to HIV risk. *AIDS Education and Prevention, 16*(1), 68–83.

Wood, W. (1996). Delivering occupational therapy's fullest promise: Clinical interpretations of "life domains and adaptive strategies of a group of low-income, well older adults." *American Journal of Occupational Therapy, 50*(2), 109–112.

World Health Organization. (2010). *The world health report 2010.* Geneva, Switzerland: Author.

Yen, I. H., Michael, Y. L., & Perdue, L. (2009). Neighborhood environment in studies of health of older adults: A systematic review. *American Journal of Preventive Medicine, 37*(5), 455–463.

Young, M. E. (1997). *Early childhood development.* Washington, DC: The World Bank Development.

For additional resources on the subjects discussed in this chapter, visit http://thePoint.lww.com/Willard-Spackman12e.

CHAPTER 18

Physical and Virtual Environments

Meaning of Place and Space

David Seamon

OUTLINE

LEARNING OBJECTIVES

After reading this chapter, you will be able to:

1. Explain why and how qualities of the physical environment and place are important dimensions of human life and experience
2. Describe what a phenomenological approach to human experience entails and how it can be used to examine the human experience of environments and places
3. Define place in terms of human experience, using the concepts of insideness and outsideness
4. Define the phenomenological concepts of lived body and environmental embodiment and discuss their relevance for occupational therapy
5. Describe the importance of home and at-homeness in peoples' lives and explain how home and at-homeness can be strengthened or undermined by physical features of dwellings and neighborhoods
6. Explain what virtual worlds and virtual places are and discuss how they might be relevant for the future of occupational therapy and science
7. Explain the critical importance of environment and place for effective occupational therapy practice

Environments, Places, and Occupational Therapy

Since the 1980s, occupational therapists and scientists have given increasing attention to how qualities of physical environments and places contribute to human health, well-being, and productive occupations (Corcoran & Gitlin, 1997; Dunn, Haney McClain, Brown, & Youngstrom, 2003; Gitlin, 2009;

Kielhofner, 1995; Kiernat, 1987; Rowles, 2003; Stewart et al., 2003; Ulrich et al., 2008). In this overview, how human beings *experience* environments, places, and spaces is emphasized; therefore, much of the content is drawn from phenomenological research. Most simply, **phenomenology** is the description and interpretation of human experience (Finlay, 2011; Seamon, 2000; van Manen, 1990). In this chapter, the phenomenological approach is briefly described and four environmental themes important for occupational therapists and scientists are considered including (1) place, (2) environmental embodiment, (3) home and at-homeness, and (4) digital technology and virtual places.

Phenomenology and Occupational Therapy

To study human beings phenomenologically is to study human experiences, behaviors, situations, and meanings as they arise in the world of everyday life. For occupational therapy and science, one significant phenomenological topic is the **lifeworld**—a person or group's everyday world of taken-for-grantedness normally unnoticed and thus hidden as a phenomenon (Finlay, 2011; Seamon, 1979; Toombs, 2001; van Manen, 1990). One aim of phenomenological research is to disclose and describe the various lived structures and dynamics of the lifeworld—for example, the mostly unnoticed but crucial importance of places in peoples' daily lives. An understanding of a client's lifeworld is central for occupational therapists because, typically, the taken-for-grantedness of his or her world has shifted or disappeared, including occupational dimensions (Channine, 2009; Finlay, 1998; Padilla, 2003).

Most of the time in everyday life, the lifeworld is *transparent* in the sense that day-to-day life *just happens*, grounded in spatial-temporal patterns that are more or less regular (Seamon, 1979). An integral part of this lived transparency is good health, which is lived as a kind of tacit attunement normally not given direct attention (Carel, 2008; Gadamer, 1996; Stefanovic, 2008; Svenaeus, 2001; van Manen, 1998). In contrast, illness and disability activate a resistance to the usual lifeworld in that they transform its transparency into awkwardness, unease, or discomfort. Daily life that, before, simply unfolded and happened without the need for self-conscious awareness, is now a continual event to be faced, whether because of pain, inconvenience, or inability to perform as usual. In this sense, one task of occupational therapists is to understand the client's former mode of "being at home" and to locate pathways whereby he or she can reaccess and recover that mode, in the same or related fashion (Svenaeus, 2001, pp. 94–104). As the next sections demonstrate, qualities of places and physical environments can help facilitate this return to "being at home."

Place and Occupational Therapy

One integral dimension of the lifeworld is **place**, which can be defined as any environmental locus that gathers individual or group meanings, intentions, and actions spatially (Casey, 2009; Malpas, 1999; Relph, 1976/2008). A place can range in scale from a furnishing or room to a building, neighborhood, city, or region (Manzo, 2005; Relph, 1976/2008). One of the most accessible phenomenologies of place is geographer Edward Relph's *Place and Placelessness* (Relph, 1976/2008). Relph argued that the existential crux of place experience is *insideness*—in other words, the more deeply a person or group feels themselves inside an environment, the more so does that environment become, existentially, a place. The deepest experience of place attachment and identity is what Relph termed *existential insideness*—a situation where the person or group feel so much at home and at ease in place that they have no self-conscious recognition of its importance in their lives, unless it or people change in some way—for example, one's home is destroyed by flood or one is no longer able to walk because of an auto accident. In one sense, a major aim of occupational therapists is working with a client in ways whereby, as much as possible, they might help him or her reestablish existential insideness.

In his phenomenology of place, Relph described several other modes of place insideness and its lived opposite, *outsideness*—a situation where the person or group feels separate or alienated from place in some way. These modes of place experience (Table 18.1) are useful for the occupational therapist because they provide an accessible language through which can be identified particular place experiences in terms of the intensity of meaning and intention that a person and place hold for each other. Through illness or accident, for example, a person's taken-for-granted sense of existential insideness can be ruptured, and he or she falls into a particular mode of existential outsideness in which the lifeworld as it was before is now different, often strangely or uncomfortably so. Relph's modes of insideness and outsideness offer a flexible means for distinguishing the lived experience of place from its material or assumed qualities. In domestic abuse, for example, the home, typically a place of existential insideness, becomes a place of existential outsideness.

One example of how the themes of place, insideness, and outsideness can offer occupational therapists valuable insights is the research on rural older people conducted by gerontological geographer Graham Rowles (2003). Emphasizing that their lifeworlds typically involve strong emotional attachments to place. Rowles identified three dimensions of place related to Relph's theme of existential insideness: first, *physical insideness*, a sense of being physically entwined with the environment; second, *social insideness*, whereby older people feel an integral part of their community through social relationships and exchanges; and, third, *autobiographical insideness*, the ways in which places and place qualities coalesce into an environmental mosaic relating to and marking out one's personal and communal history in relation to those places (Rowles & Watkins, 2003, pp. 78–79). Rowles (1999) emphasizes that understanding place experience is important for occupational therapists

TABLE 18.1 Modes of Insideness and Outsideness

Mode	Description
Existential insideness	Feeling completely at home and immersed in place, to such a degree the experience is not usually noticed unless the place dramatically changes in some way (e.g., one's home and community are destroyed by natural disaster). The mode of place experience most human beings strive for; typically, the mode of place experience that occupational therapists work toward recovering for their clients.
Existential outsideness	Feeling alienated or separate from place, which may seem oppressive or unreal (e.g., the experience of homesickness or the deep sense of disjunction one feels, having suddenly become disabled because of an accident). The mode of experience that many people fall into after a disabling accident or after becoming ill or leaning they are ill. A major task of the occupational therapist is to help clients shift, as much as possible, out of existential outsideness back toward existential insideness.
Objective outsideness	A dispassionate attitude of separation from place, which becomes an object of study or directed attention (e.g., designing a hospital using measurable criteria like size of potential patient pool, square footage based on functional needs, building layout determined by staff efficiency, and so forth).
Incidental outsideness	The experience in which place is a background or mere setting for activities (e.g., the short-term patient's limited relationship with the hospital environment in which she finds herself temporarily).
Behavioral insideness	A deliberate attending to the appearance of place (e.g., using environmental cues like landmarks and signage to find one's way around a place). The first stage in becoming an insider to a new place (e.g., mastering the layout of a hospital complex where one has just started working).
Empathetic insideness	Being open to place and attempting to understand it more deeply (e.g., the occupational therapist's effort to see and to understand the client's lifeworld as it *really is* and not as the occupational therapist supposes it to be). See Case Study 18.1, "An old woman's lifeworld."
Vicarious insideness	Deeply felt secondhand involvement with place (e.g., learning about worlds of illness or disablement through films, novels, or autobiographical accounts) (e.g., Bauby, 1997; Frank, 2002; Hockenberry, 1995; Hull, 1990; Murphy, 1987). See Case Study 18.1, "An old woman's lifeworld."

From Relph, E. (2008). *Place and placelessness.* London, United Kingdom: Pion Limited. (Original work published 1976)

because it reveals "the role of the person's experienced spatiotemporal environment in conditioning his or her response to dysfunctions and to intervention strategies meant to remedy them" (p. 270).

A second illustrative study drawing on the theme of place is health sociologist Andrew Moore's (2010) case study of the lived process whereby hospice day care patients came to understand the hospice as a place in the context of their illness. Moore identified and documented three stages in the process: first, *drifting*, a situation immediately before and shortly after arrival when patients were uncertain about the hospice and questioned its sustaining value. As patients spent time there, drifting shifted to *sheltering*, a feeling of familiarity and at-homeness. In turn, sheltering set the stage for *venturing*, the patient's seeking out new experiences and situations. Through this process of "place making," patients "found 'home', both within the self and within the world" (A. J. Moore, 2010, p. 160). One important occupational component of the lived shift from drifting to sheltering was the availability to patients of complementary therapies, including massage and aromatherapy, which Moore found significant for helping patients form trusting, embodied relationships with the staff, other patients, and the hospice as a place.

Environmental Embodiment, Home, and At-Homeness

The Lived Body, Body-Subject, and Environmental Embodiment

In exploring human experience, phenomenologists emphasize that humans are *bodily* beings, a lived fact important for occupational therapy's central focus on the well-being of the *whole person*. A phenomenological perspective claims that bodily being is more than physical corporeality: "The body is our basic mode of being in the world, consciousness is embodied consciousness, and a person is embodied being, not just the possessor of a body" (Madjar & Walton, 1999, p. 4). Phenomenologists speak of the

lived body—a body that simultaneously experiences, acts in, and is aware of a world that, normally, responds with immediate pattern, meaning, and contextual presence (Finlay, 2006; Seamon, 2012; Simms, 2008b; Toombs, 2001). The lived body is the primary means of being in, experiencing, and encountering the world. The lived body falls ill, it experiences pain, it fails to heal, it heals badly, it becomes older, it remains impaired, it returns to good health, and it learns new ways to cope with illness or disablement.

In considering the environmental and place dimensions of the lived body, phenomenologists focus on **environmental embodiment**—the various ways, both sensorially and movement wise, that the lived body engages and coordinates with the world at hand, especially its environmental aspects (Gallagher, 1986; Seamon, 2012; Simms, 2008a, 2008b). A key thinker is French phenomenologist Maurice Merleau-Ponty (1962), who emphasized what he termed **body-subject**—the pre-reflective but intelligent awareness of the body manifested through habitual action and typically in sync with the environment in which the action unfolds. Body-subject can incorporate considerable temporal and environmental versatility as expressed in more complex bodily movements and ensembles extending over time and space (Allen, 2004; Cole, 2004; Hill, 1985; Seamon, 1979). One can speak of at least two such ensembles: first, **body routines**—sets of coordinated corporeal actions sustaining a specific task or aim, for example, driving, cooking, or lawn mowing; and second, **time-space routines**—sets of more or less habitual bodily actions that extend through a considerable portion of time, for example, a getting-up routine, a going-to-the-gym routine, or a going-to-church-and-lunch routine (Seamon, 1979, 2002). Clearly, many occupational activities involve such taken-for-granted bodily ensembles.

For teaching occupational therapy, body-subject and its extended habitual patterns are an important dimension of everyday human experience that can be explored through firsthand phenomenological exercises—for example, having occupational therapy students move a thing that has a place in their home to a different place; or setting oneself to go to a destination by a route other than the one he or she normally travels (Seamon, 1979). It is important that students *really see* and understand the significance of the lived presence of body-subject dynamics in their own daily experiences so that they are better able to empathize with the lifeworld changes, distortions, and difficulties that often accompany a client's illness or disablement.

Also useful in facilitating understanding of body-subject are phenomenological studies describing how illness or disability shifts one's sense of environmental embodiment. One striking example is the first-person phenomenological work of philosopher Kay Toombs (2001), who suffers from multiple sclerosis, an incurable, progressively disabling disease of the central nervous system. In her narratives, Toombs elucidated how the illness has affected her ability to see, to hear, to sit, and to stand. Through her perceptive description and interpretation, one realizes the ways in which her lived relationship with space and place has become progressively more limited and more unsettling. For example, Toombs described how her loss of mobility has resulted in a "profound disruption of the lived body" in regard to her everyday environment:

> In the normal course of events, locomotion opens up space, allowing one freely to change position and move towards objects in the world. Loss of mobility anchors one in the Here, engendering a heightened sense of distance between oneself and surrounding things. A location that was formerly regarded as "near" is now experienced as "far." For example, when I could walk, the distance from my office to the classroom (about thirty yards) was unremarkable—as were the stairs I climbed to reach the third floor of the building. As my mobility decreased, the office appeared near to the classroom on the way to the lecture, but far from it on the return journey; the stairs became an obstacle to be avoided, as much as possible, by using the elevator. Today, if I were to be without my wheelchair, the distance from the office to the classroom would appear immense—absolutely beyond my capacity to reach it. And the third floor is unattainable when the elevator malfunctions, leaving me stranded waiting for the repairman. . . .
>
> Loss of mobility illustrates in a concrete way that the subjective experience of space is intimately related to both one's bodily capacities and to the design of the surrounding world. The answer to the question, "Is it too far to go?" has little to do with the distance that can be measured in feet or yards. For the person with mobility problems, the answer depends, in large part, on what is between here and there. Are there obstacles that make it impossible to maneuver with crutches or a cane? Is the terrain suitable for a wheelchair? (Toombs, 2001, p. 249)

See **Appendix A, Common Conditions,** for more information about multiple sclerosis.

Phenomenological explications like Toombs' are important for occupational therapy and science because they provide detailed, experience-grounded depictions of specific modes of illness and disability and how they rupture the lived transparency of the lifeworld, including aspects of environmental embodiment (van Manen, 1998). Related phenomenological studies focus on blindness (Allen, 2004; Hill, 1985), deafness (Finlay & Molano-Fisher, 2007), Alzheimer's disease (Todres & Galvin, 2005), multiple sclerosis (Finlay, 2003), mental illness (Walton, 2001), child and adult motor disabilities (Bjorbaekmo & Engelsrud, 2011; Cole, 2004; Connolly, 2010; Gooberman-Hill, 2007), living with chronic pain (O'Loughlin, 1999), dealing with chronic leg ulcers (Bland, 1999), surviving breast cancer and mastectomy (Shin, 1999), disabled persons' mastering wheelchair use (Standal, 2011), and rehabilitation following flexor tendon surgery (Fitzpatrick & Finlay, 2008).

One exemplary study is movement educator Maureen Connolly's efforts to embed meaningful movement into the everyday school activities of children with ASD—autism spectrum disorder (Connolly, 2010). Recognizing that these children do best when everyday routines and schedules are highly predictable, Connolly aimed, through environmental alterations and movement education, to help children "gradually learn to accept greater levels of variation and unpredictability" (Connolly, 2010, p. 114). For example, Connolly created a classroom environment incorporating subdued lighting; thick, absorptive, unstable surfaces; contrasts in ceiling height; and different places within the classroom for different tasks and functions. These design elements slowed and organized the movements of the children and provided a means, through physical contact, for them to experience a more placid and bodily-grounded engagement with their surroundings.

As Connolly's (2010) teaching efforts suggest, an integral component of environmental embodiment is the physical and spatial environment in which the lived body finds itself. Sometimes drawing on **universal design** (fabricating products and environments that work well for almost everyone), occupational therapists and other professionals have considered how architecture and environmental design can sustain and enhance patients' and clients' lifeworlds (Preiser & Smith, 2011; Rickerson, 2009; Söderback, 2009; Trefler & Hobson, 1997; Ulrich et al., 2008). Brooks and colleagues (2011), for example, examined how patients in assisted-living and rehabilitation settings made use of bedside-table devices and then designed three improved "smart stand" prototypes more efficient in terms of object reach, placement, storage, and mobility. In a study that examined assisted-living residents' walking behaviors, Lu (2010) developed design recommendations to improve residential walkability, including looped indoor and outdoor walkways; hallways with furnished alcoves usable by residents who otherwise might obstruct corridors; and windowed interior walkways that offer residents a visual connection to the world outside, especially the natural environment (Ulrich et al., 2008, pp. 87–91).

Home and Universal Design

Another important aspect of the lifeworld is *home* and *at-homeness* (Blunt & Dowling, 2005; Gitlin, 2003; Mallett, 2004; Manzo, 2003; J. Moore, 2007; Rioux & Werner, 2011; Seamon, 2010). These studies indicate that home has specific physical, personal, social, cultural, and political dimensions but, experientially, is lived as a human and environmental whole that incorporates and facilitates a wide range of existential significances. Home is not only a physical place, but a locus of activities, an anchor of identity, a repository of memories bonding past and present, and a center of stability and continuity (Figure 18.1). This literature also emphasizes that some homes can involve a "shadow side" of discomfort, distress, and trauma—for example, homes of domestic violence (Anthony, 1997; Blunt & Dowling, 2005; Manzo, 2003).

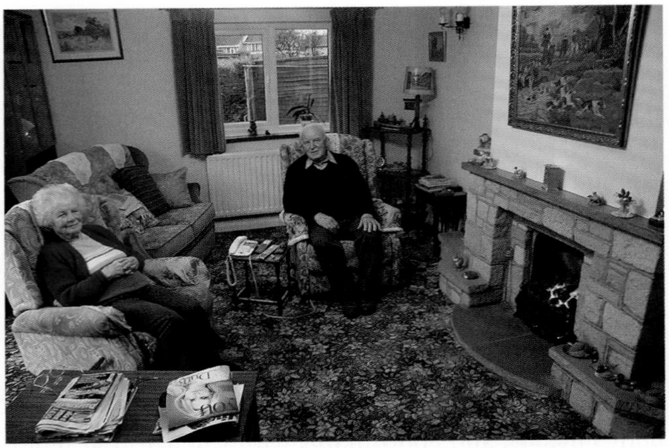

FIGURE 18.1 An older couple at home in their living room in northern England. One's home is not only a physical environment but also a place of activities, an anchor of identity, a repository of memories, and a center of stability and continuity. A major task for the occupational therapist is helping clients to recover as much as possible their sense of home and at-homeness. (Photograph by Walter Lewis and used with permission. © 2011 Walter Lewis.)

For occupational therapy, one key conceptual and lived division is home as a physical environment versus home as a locus of human life and meaning (Rowles, 2006). In studying the former, one considers the home as a dwelling incorporating the equipment, things, and spaces of daily living. One important question is how the dwelling's design and construction sustain or interfere with environmental embodiment, especially if residents are ill, older, or dealing with impairments (Kopec, 2006; Rosenfeld & Chapman, 2008). With regard to aging, for example, research demonstrates that older people typically spend more time in the residence and increasingly centralize their home by setting up "control centers"—for instance, a favorite chair and side table that allow the older person an easy reach to many of his or her daily needs (Rosenfeld & Chapman, 2008; Schaie, Wahl, Mollenkopf, & Oswald, 2003). In addition, older people may rearrange furniture and other home furnishings to remove obstacles to mobility or to provide sturdy anchors so they are less likely to fall when walking (Rowles, 2006).

There is also the question of how, through design, existing houses and dwelling units can be modified to match more closely the lifeworld needs of residents as they age or become ill or less abled (Kopec, 2006). Occupational therapists and other professionals have been actively involved in working out effective ways, through environmental interventions and assistive technology, to make home environments more accommodating—for example, widening doors, installing grab bars, adding entrance ramps, providing intercom systems, and so forth (Cook McCullagh, 2006; Corcoran & Gitlin, 1997; Iwarsson, 2009; Söderback, 2009; Steinfeld & Danford, 1999; Trefler & Hobson, 1997). In some situations, however, environmental interventions and assistive technology in the home can disrupt residents' lives, as Moore, Anderson, Carter, and Coad (2010) demonstrate in their study of the medical equipment and technology that many children with complex needs depend on in their homes: "The home space becomes an appropriated landscape—no longer a family landscape but a landscape of care, 'like a mini hospital', with some parents feeling this particularly keenly" (Moore et al., 2010, p. 4).

Drawing on the principles of universal design, architects and interior designers have made major efforts to envision housing and other environments that accommodate the needs of users, whatever their age or degree of impairment (Cook McCullagh, 2006; Jennings, 2009; Preiser & Smith, 2011; Steinfeld & Danford, 1999; Steinfeld & White, 2010). This work is grounded partly in understanding how people function at different stages of life and in regard to different degrees of ableness and disablement (Kopec, 2006). One aim is homes that support **aging in place**—in other words, dwelling units that residents, if they so choose, can occupy from childhood to old age unless illness or impairment come into play (Rosenfeld & Chapman, 2008; Steinfeld & White, 2010; Young, 2011). As indicated by the dwelling design illustrated in Figure 18.2, this **universal housing** includes such features as stepless entrances with flush thresholds; kitchen and laundry appliances at convenient heights; bathing fixtures allowing multiple bathing options; and clear sight lines and adequate space for wheelchair use, including wide hallways, pocket doors, roll-under sinks, and wheelchair-height fixtures.

Designers developing universal housing emphasize that issues of convenience, mobility, accessibility, and visitability are not limited to the dwelling alone but extend to the realm of the dwelling's immediate surroundings and larger neighborhood (Steinfeld & White, 2010). Research demonstrates that, for a wide range of individuals, gardening is often an important domestic occupation, and one design focus is integrating nature, especially gardens, with the home environment (Ashton-Schaeffer & Constant, 2005; Bhatti, 2006; Cooper Marcus & Barnes, 1999). If a universal dwelling is located in a car-dependent neighborhood, it cannot provide wider-scale accessibility for residents who cannot drive—an increasingly important group as the populations of Western countries age. Many architects and planners today favor compact, human-scaled communities providing easy access to a wide range of functions, services, and activities (Seamon, 2002; Steinfeld & White, 2010). Such walkable, handicap-accessible neighborhoods might motivate residents to be more physically active and thus provide valuable health benefits (Frank, Engelke, & Schmid, 2003). In addition, the higher densities and a more active street life might motivate residents to feel responsible for their neighborhood and be more willing to look out for each other (Gardner, 2011; Klinenberg, 2002; Mehta & Bosson, 2010; Oldenburg, 1999; Rosenbaum, Sweeney, & Windhorst, 2009). The occupational therapist plays a pivotal role in regard to housing needs because he or she has an intimate knowledge of clients' home requirements, restrictions, and possibilities. He or she can serve as an important go-between for helping clients articulate their environmental situation and needs to architects, interior designers, and contractors. Knowing clients' limitations firsthand, the occupational therapist can play a central role in "design teams" that plan aging in place or impairment-accommodating housing and neighborhoods (Gitlin, 2003).

At-Homeness and Occupational Therapy

Besides being a physical dwelling that founds a particular mode of daily living, the home is also a constellation of experiences, meanings, and situations that relates to residents' personal and communal sense of identity and belonging (Manzo, 2003; Percival, 2002; Rowles, 2006; Rowles & Chaudhury, 2005; Stafford, 2009). One phenomenological concept that helps integrate the lived dimensions of home is **at-homeness**, which can be defined as the taken-for-granted situation of feeling completely comfortable and intimately familiar with the world in which one lives his or her everyday life (Oldenburg, 1999, p. 39–41; Seamon, 1979, p. 78). For the clients of occupational therapists, at-homeness has often been disrupted or eroded; a delineation of the lived dimensions of at-homeness provides one means for considering the client's residential needs more precisely and thinking through ways they might be restored or better accommodated.

Table 18.2 depicts the existential structure of at-homeness in terms of five lived qualities that can support or undermine a sense of familiarity and comfort (Seamon, 1979, 2010). First, *rootedness* refers to the quality of at-homeness to organize the habitual, bodily stratum of a person's life and is intimately related to environmental embodiment and body-subject. Literally, the home roots the person spatially, sustaining a physical center for departures and returns. In cases of impairment, illness, or aging, rootedness may be displaced by *disconnectedness*, which can include spatial disorientation, bodily discomfort, or loss of mobility and accessibility. Second, *appropriation* refers to a residents' feeling a sense of autonomy and control in regard to their home and immediate surroundings. At least in the modern Western context, appropriation typically includes a sense of privacy, whereby residents and family can readily be alone. Compromised

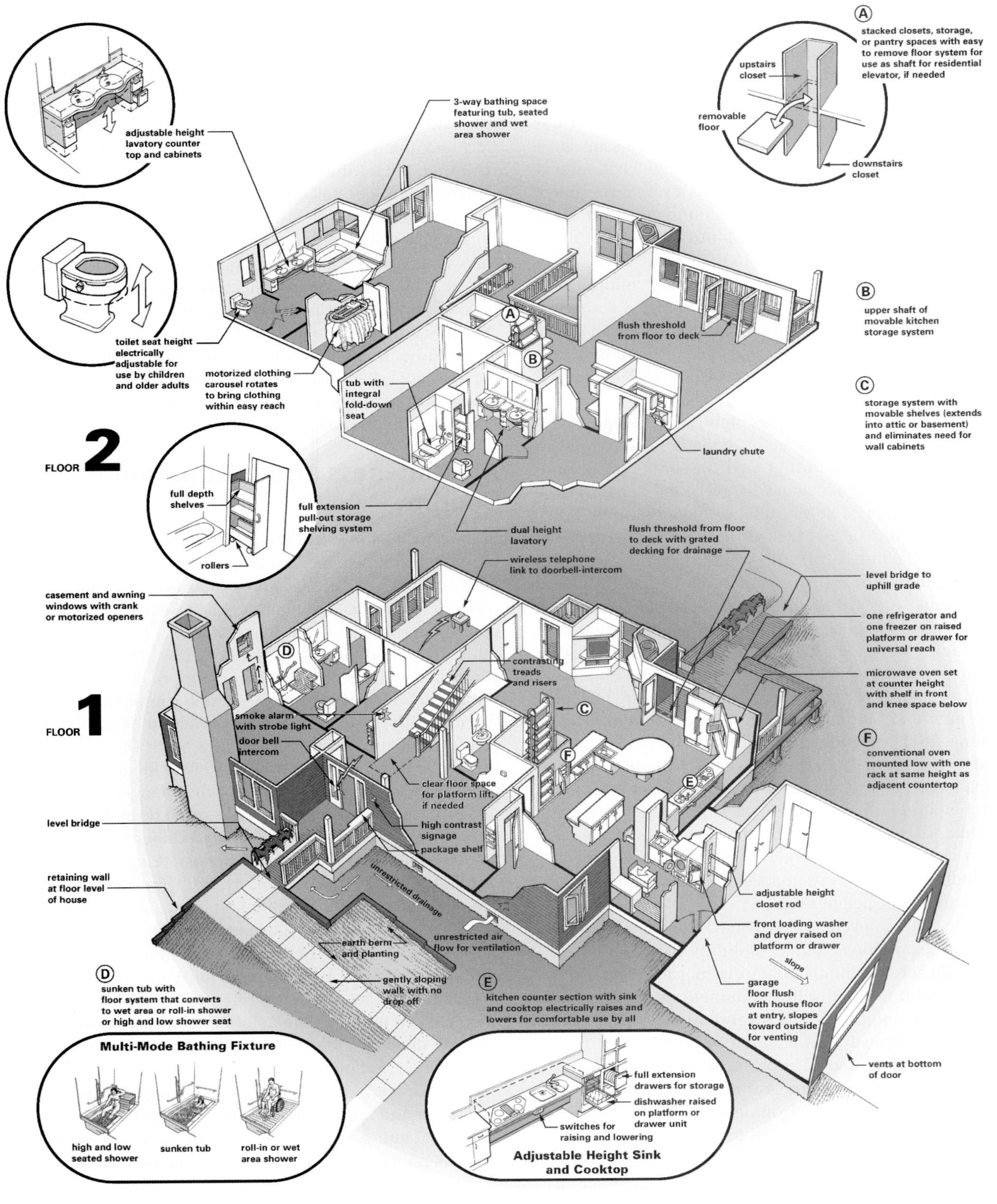

FIGURE 18.2 Two-story universal house. (Source: Preiser, W. F. E., & Smith, K. H. [Eds.]. [2011]. *Universal design handbook* [2nd ed.]. New York, NY: McGraw-Hill, p. 24.6. Illustration by Ron Mace and Rex Pace, Center for Universal Design, North Carolina State University, Raleigh; used with permission of the Center for Universal Design.

TABLE 18.2 Aspects of At-Homeness: Sustaining and Undermining Dimensions

Sustaining Aspect	Description	Spatial Expression	Undermining Aspect	Implications for Occupational Therapy
Rootedness	Organizes the habitual, bodily stratum of a person's life; intimately related to environmental embodiment and body-subject.	Concentrated in places, paths, and points of use, especially favorite places within and around the home; undeveloped in unused portions.	Disconnectedness: Involves spatial disorientation, bodily discomfort, or loss of mobility and accessibility.	Ensure meaningful daily occupations can be maintained through retraining and environmental supports. Focus on the client's bodily "doing" and "being" in and around the home, especially bodily routines and actions.
Appropriation	Involves feeling a sense of autonomy and control in regard to home and immediate surroundings; typically includes a sense of privacy.	Roughly concentric and generally strongest for most important "centers" in the home; intensity in proportion to use and attachment; relates to "centers," paths, places for things, and things themselves.	Imposition: Includes loss of autonomy; dependence on external assistance, whether human, environmental, or technological.	Provide adequate human help and assistive technologies to support personal autonomy and self-worth (e.g., installing appropriate bathing equipment so client can maintain independence).
At-easeness	Involves "freedom to be" and contentment; relates to inner mood and sense of well-being; things and situations that give everyday satisfaction are readily available.	Usually strongest in the home but possible in other places outside the home (i.e., third places) where person feels comfortable and relaxed.	Uneaseness: Involves a situation where comfortableness of lifeworld called into question by personal, social, or environmental changes.	Enable satisfying occupations that can be engaged in alone or with others (e.g., working to maintain client's valued hobbies).
Regeneration	Relates to restorative powers of home and at-homeness; home not only as a site of relaxation and rest but also as a place of psychological recuperation and rejuvenation.	Generally associated with the home, but possible in other places with restorative powers (e.g., the route a person walks his or her dogs each day.	Degeneration: Relates to disruption in rest and regeneration due to personal, social, or environmental changes.	Enable relaxing occupations through environmental modifications (e.g., incorporating more appropriate lighting or changing room use. Consider how such modifications may shift daily activities (e.g., if a living area is converted to a bedroom, where will the client go to relax and engage in leisure?)
Warmth	Relates to supportive ambience of sustenance and well-being; invokes positive emotions like kindness, cheerfulness, good will, and camaraderie.	Most common in interior spaces and expressed by decoration, sense of order, and interpersonal harmony; also present in cared-for outside environments like gardens.	Coldness: Relates to an unpleasant or hostile environmental ambience; spirit of place devolves into raw material space.	Work with client's values and find compromises (e.g., managing a level of cleanliness that is acceptable or de-cluttering a space but preserving what is most meaningful for client).

From Seamon, D. (1979). *A geography of the life world.* New York, NY: St. Martin's Press.

through disablement or illness, appropriation devolves into *imposition*, a situation where the resident is less autonomous and more dependent on external assistance, whether human, environmental, or technological.

A third quality of at-homeness is *at-easeness*, which refers to the "freedom to be." In a situation of at-homeness, residents can be who they most comfortably are and do what they most wish to do, a situation that can shift into *uneasiness* when a lifeworld is upset in some way. Unlike appropriation, which relates more to physical and psychological control of the home, at-easeness relates to inner mood and sense of well-being. To be at ease is to have readily available the things and situations that give one everyday satisfaction and sustain the lifeworld's transparency and taken-for-grantedness. Fourth, *regeneration* refers to the restorative powers of home and at-homeness. Regeneration involves the home not only as a site of relaxation and rest but also as a place of psychological recuperation and rejuvenation. In a disrupted lifeworld, regeneration becomes *degeneration* due to stress, worry, or physical difficulties associated with sleeping and resting. Finally, *warmth* speaks to an intangible atmosphere of sustenance and well-being that often involves positive emotions like joy and happiness. Sometimes the warmth of home life perseveres in times of illness or impairment, or it can disappear or devolve into *coldness*. A sense of place becomes spiritless space.

These five lived qualities of at-homeness are heuristic and broadly diagnostic in that they provide one way to think through a particular client's home situation in terms of daily occupations (Moore et al., 2010, pp. 4–5). Different clients' everyday worlds will involve different combinations and intensities of the five qualities of at-homeness. Their potential value is that each points toward a different set of possibilities and means for transforming a quality's negative pole into its positive opposite. For example, rootedness is grounded in the lived body, and one occupational aim is to find ways, through environmental intervention, assistive technology, and the client's rehabilitation efforts, to return his or her lifeworld to its former taken-for-grantedness in terms of bodily actions and routines. Or, in regard to at-easeness, the occupational therapist works to learn a client's daily pleasures and satisfactions and find ways whereby they might be re-incorporated in his or her everyday life, though sometimes in revised or partial ways. The central aim in using at-homeness as a diagnostic focus is to envision the client's abled and impaired lifeworlds from a multidimensional perspective that might spur creative interventions not imagined otherwise (see Case Study 18.1, "An Old Woman's Lifeworld").

CASE STUDY 18.1 An Old Woman's Lifeworld

The environmental themes discussed in this chapter are illustrated by the lifeworld of 90-year-old indigent Londoner Maudie Fowler, a character rivetingly portrayed in African-British novelist Doris Lessing's *Diaries of Jane Somers* (Lessing, 1984). For students learning to become occupational therapists, this novel can be revelatory because it portrays, in gritty, unflinching detail, the everyday life of Maudie as she struggles as an impoverished older woman living alone in a large, 1980s city. Maudie's life is presented through the eyes of character Janna Somers, a fashionable, middle-aged magazine editor who befriends Maudie after they accidentally meet waiting in line at a local pharmacy. Maudie's world is a life of limitations imposed by circumstances, chance, and age. When Somers first meets encounters Maudie, she sees "a tiny bent-over woman, with a nose nearly meeting her chin, in black heavy dirty clothes . . . [and] a sweet, sour, dusty sort of smell. I saw the grime on her thin old neck, and on her hands" (Lessing, 1984, pp. 12–13). Over time, Somers becomes Maudie's only friend and takes care of her until she dies of stomach cancer several years later.

Lessing's novel provides an unforgettable rendering of place, at-homeness, and environmental embodiment as expressed in Maudie's everyday life (Seamon, 1993). Physically, her world is small spatially and includes her apartment, the street where she lives, and a corner grocery store run by an Indian man with whom she often quarrels because she feels he overcharges. The three-room apartment Maudie has occupied for over 40 years is the center of her world, but Maudie long ago lost interest in housekeeping and maintenance: "I have never," says Somers of her first impression, "seen anything like it outside of condemned houses. . . . The whole place smelled, it smelled awful. . . . It was all so dirty and dingy and grim and awful" (Lessing, 1984, p. 14).

Somers recognizes that, by modern housing standards, Maudie's apartment should be condemned, yet "by any human standard she should stay where she is" (Lessing, 1984, p. 103). She reaches this conclusion because she gradually understands that the decrepit apartment is Maudie's entire world, providing the only reason left for her to live. As she declares to Somers: "'I've never not paid [the rent], not once. Though I've gone without food. No, I learned that early. With your own place you've got everything. Without it, you're a dog. You are nothing. Have you got your own place?'—and when I said yes, she said, nodding fiercely, angrily, 'That's right, and you hold onto it, then nothing can touch you'" (Lessing, 1984, pp. 18–19).

One of the most powerful aspects of Lessing's *Diaries* is getting readers to understand that, in regard to lifeworlds, the seemingly obvious often intimates a much more complex situation. For example, Somers comes to realize that her unpleasant first impression of Maudie's apartment is not because Maudie is slothful but because she has gradually been worn down by the grind of physical upkeep: "What makes poor Maudie labour and groan all through the day [is] the dredge and drag of maintenance" (Lessing, 1984, p. 127). Environmental embodiment

CASE STUDY 18.1 An Old Woman's Lifeworld *(continued)*

for Maudie has become bodily weakness and mobility difficulties that restrict what she can manage. At one point, Somers describes Maudie's typical day, emphasizing the overwhelming difficulties of reaching for an object, shifting rooms, feeding the cat, or going to the toilet—efforts and actions that, for the able person, are taken-for-granted and inconsequential:

> Morning . . . oh, the difficulties of morning, of facing the day . . . each task such a weight to it . . . She sits there, thinking, I have to feed the cat . . . I have to . . . At last, she drags herself up, anxious, because her bowels are threatening again, and, holding on to door handles, chair backs, she gets herself into the kitchen. There is a tin of cat food, half empty. She tries to turn it on to a saucer, it won't come out. It means she has to get a spoon. A long way off, in the sink, are her spoons and forks, she hasn't washed up for days. She winkles out the cat food with her forefinger, her face wrinkled up—is it smelling perhaps? She lets the saucer fall from a small height on to the floor, for bending forward makes her faint. The cats sniffs at it and walks away, with a small miaow. Maudie sees that under the table are saucers, bone dry and empty. The cat needs milk, she needs water. Slowly, slowly, Maudie gets herself to the sink, pulls out of it a dirty saucer which she has not got the energy to wash, runs water into it. Finds a half bottle of milk. Has it gone off? She sniffs. No. She somehow gets the saucer on to the floor, holding on to the table and nearly falling. The cat drinks all the milk, and Maudie knows she is hungry.
>
> Under the table not only the saucers, one, two, three, four, five, but a cat mess. This reminds Maudie she has to let the cat out. She toils to the door, lets out the cat and stands with her back to the door, thinking. A general planning a campaign could not use more cleverness than Maudie does, as she outwits her weakness and her terrible tiredness. She is already at the back door: the toilet is five steps away; if she goes now it will save a journey later . . . Maudie gets herself to the toilet, uses it, remembers there is the commode full of dirt and smell in her room, somehow gets herself along the passage to her room, somehow gets the pot out from under the round top, somehow gets herself and the pot to the toilet (Lessing, 1984, pp. 115–116).

Over time, Somers comes to see the lived ponderousness of Maudie's lifeworld: "I have realized how *heavy* everything is for her" (Lessing, 1984, p. 105). Somers gains her most important insight into Maudie's situation shortly after bathing her for the first time. She understands that the bodily unpleasantness is not really Maudie, who is "still there, alert, very much all there, on guard inside that old witch's appearance. *She* is still there, and everything has collapsed around her, it's too difficult, too much" (Lessing, 1984, p. 55). Somers realizes how physical infirmness can impede a person's actions toward the world:

> I am thinking how Maudie Fowler one day could not trouble herself to clean out her front room, because there was so much junk in it, and then she left it and left it; going in sometimes, thinking, well, it's not so bad. Meanwhile, she was keeping the back room and the kitchen spotless. . . She wasn't feeling well, and didn't bother, once, twice—and then her room was not really cleaned, only the floor in the middle of the room sometimes, and she learned not to look around the edges or under the bed. Her kitchen was last. She scrubbed it and washed shelves, but then things began to slide. But through it all she washed herself, standing at the kitchen table. . . . Then she left longer and longer between washing her hair . . . and then she did not wash her clothes, only took out the cleanest ones there were, putting them back grubby, till they were the cleanest; and so it went on. And at last she was upright in her thick shell of black, her knickers not entirely clean, but not so bad, her neck dirty, but she did not think about it, her scalp unwashed. (Lessing, 1984)

Lessing's account of Maudie's life is significant for occupational therapists because it offers sobering insights into one older person's lifeworld. More so, Lessing's account illustrates a mode of empathetic insideness that is the crux of all effective occupational therapy: Becoming aware of a person's lifeworld in a non-judgmental way and using that awareness to return that person to as much health and well-being as possible. Lessing's frank, brutally realistic account of Maudie Fowler demonstrates that positively changing another person's life is not always possible. If occupational interventions are to work, however, they are best grounded in the kind of sympathetic insight that phenomenological understanding can help facilitate (Finlay, 2011).

Real Places, Virtual Places, and Occupational Therapy

Even in its first decade, there is considerable indication that digital technologies will dramatically reshape human life in the 21st century (Borgmann, 1999; Friesen, 2011; Horan, 2000; Relph, 2007). Currently, we can envision only glimpses of what robotics, virtual realities, and **information and communication technologies (ICT)** might mean for occupations and occupational therapy (Fok, Miller Polgar, Shaw, Luke, & Mandich, 2009; Mihailidis & Davis, 2005). The desire of older and less able individuals to live independently has spurred development of the **smart house**, which incorporates robotics, networked appliances, and other digital devices connecting residents with their home and wider community (van Berlo, 2002). This integration of home services with technology is called **domotics**, which works to "improve safety, security, comfort, communication, and technical management in the home" (Rosenfeld & Chapman, 2008, p. 25). One example is digital lighting that automatically provides residents moving through their home with an illuminated pathway, helping to reduce falls. Also significant are domestic robotic devices that include wheelchairs, "seeing eye dogs," and "robotic assistants," the last of which can provide, among other home services, physical therapy and mental stimulation (Broekens, Heerink, & Rosendal, 2009; Rosenfeld & Chapman, 2008, p. 97). In addition, these robotic devices can monitor health and behaviors and connect residents to health care providers and to friends and relatives living elsewhere (Rosenfeld & Chapman, 2008).

More transformative technological possibilities for occupational activities involve innovations in the **brain-computer interface (BCI),** which allows objects and images to be manipulated via sensory devices registering brain waves or facial movements (Graham-Rowe, 2011). By shifting the eyes or picturing an action or symbol cognitively, the user can direct a robotic assistant, activate networked appliances, or manipulate items on a computer screen (Geng, Gan, & Hu, 2010). For many older and impaired individuals, this technology could well be life changing because one gains the mental and physical autonomy to control computers, wheelchairs, assistive technologies, and other aspects of the person's everyday environment. Perhaps even more compelling is the coupling of BCI with virtual reality technology, which allows people with impairments to generate and participate in online virtual worlds like "Second Life," where users (called "residents") meet other residents, socialize, create virtual homes and other virtual places, offer virtual goods and services, and so forth (Graham-Rowe, 2011).

Currently, there is much controversy as to whether virtual worlds and virtual places will ever be able to comprehensively simulate their lifeworld originals and, if they can, what impact such vicarious simulations might have on those real worlds and places (Borgmann, 1999; Fok et al., 2009; Friesen, 2011; Haythornthwaite & Kendall, 2010; Horan, 2000; Relph, 2007). At this point, the technical and representational possibilities of virtual reality are in their infancy and will probably require a mode of creativity different from traditional creative forms like imaginative literature or film. As Relph (2007) explains,

> Virtual places don't have readers or viewers—they have participants. The original author of a virtual place in some fashion has to anticipate how participation might occur and to provide suitable cues and possibilities for it, though in a fully interactive virtual place, as in a real place, the imaginative involvement of participants will lead to changes that can in no way be anticipated. There are few rules or guidelines for this and the most compelling virtual places might be regarded as continuously changing works of art that reflect the combined imaginations of those who are simultaneously participants and authors. (p. 8)

Whatever form a mature virtual reality eventually takes, it is almost certain that the medium will have a major impact on occupations and occupational therapy because the creative result will be virtual worlds in which a person, no matter how impaired, can participate, whether in firsthand virtual creation or in secondhand virtual involvement. Virtual worlds and virtual places may provide a radically innovative means for occupational therapists to assist clients in recovering and recreating what was called, at the start of this chapter, "being at home." In this sense, occupational therapists will contribute to fabricating virtual places that allow clients to become involved in virtual occupations unlikely or impossible in the clients' real worlds—for example, an older woman's "operating" a virtual café or a wheelchair-bound man's "flying" a virtual airplane. Clearly, virtual realities will entail potential problems, including time wasting, titillation, and addiction. For creating a new world of occupations, however, virtual reality and virtual places will more than likely constitute a remarkable new subfield in occupational therapy and science.

References

Allen, C. (2004). Merleau-Ponty's phenomenology and the body-in-space encounters of visually impaired children. *Environment and Planning D: Society and Space, 22*, 719–735.

Anthony, K. H. (1997). Bitter homes and gardens: The meanings of home to families of divorce. *Journal of Architectural and Planning Research, 14*, 1–19.

Ashton-Schaeffer, C., & Constant, A. (2005). Why do older adults garden? *Activities, Adaptation & Aging, 30*, 1–18.

Bauby, J. D. (1997). *The diving bell and the butterfly* (J. Leggart, Trans.). New York, NY: Vintage International.

Bhatti, M. (2006). "When I'm in the garden I can create my own paradise": Homes and gardens in later life. *The Sociological Review, 54*, 318–341.

Bjorbaekmo, W. S., & Engelsrud, G. H. (2011). "My own way of moving"—Movement improvisation in children's rehabilitation. *Phenomenology & Practice, 5*(1), 27–47.

Bland, M. (1999). On living with chronic leg ulcers. In I. Madjar & J. Walton (Eds.), *Nursing and the experience of illness: Phenomenology in practice* (pp. 33–51). London, United Kingdom: Routledge.

Blunt, A., & Dowling, R. (2005). *Home*. New York, NY: Taylor & Francis.

Borgmann, A. (1999). *Holding on to reality: The nature of information at the turn of the millennium*. Chicago, IL: University of Chicago Press.

Broekens, J., Heerink, M., & Rosendal, H. (2009). Assistive social robots in elderly care: A review. *Gerontechnology, 8*, 94–103.

Brooks, J. O., Smolentzov, L., DeArment, A., Logan, W., Green, K., Walker, I., . . . Yanik, P. (2011). Toward a "smart" nightstand prototype: An examination of nightstand table contents and preferences. *Health Environments Research & Design Journal [HERD], 4*(2), 91–108.

Carel, H. (2008). *Illness: The cry of the flesh*. Stocksfield, United Kingdom: Acumen.

Casey, E. S. (2009). *Getting back into place: Toward a renewed understanding of the place-world* (2nd ed.). Bloomington, IN: Indiana University Press.

Channine, C. (2009). An introduction to interpretative phenomenological analysis: A useful approach for occupational therapy research. *British Journal of Occupational Therapy, 7*, 37–39.

Cole, J. (2004). *Still lives: Narratives of spinal cord injury*. Cambridge, MA: MIT Press.

Connolly, M. (2010). Constructing a curriculum of place: Embedding meaningful movement in mundane activities for children and youth with autism spectrum disorder (ASD). In M. Barber, L. Embree, &

T. J. Nenon (Eds.), *Phenomenology 2010: Vol. 5. Selected essays from North America, Part I* (pp. 107–134). Bucharest, Romania: Zeta Books.

Cook McCullagh, M. (2006). Home modification. *American Journal of Nursing, 106*, 54–63.

Cooper Marcus, C., & Barnes, M. (1999). *Healing gardens: Therapeutic benefits and design recommendations.* New York, NY: Wiley.

Corcoran, M., & Gitlin, L. (1997). The role of the physical environment in occupational performance. In C. Christiansen & C. M. Baum (Eds.), *Occupational therapy: Enabling function and well-being* (pp. 336–360). Thorofare, NJ: SLACK.

Dunn, W., Haney McClain, L., Brown, C., & Youngstrom, M. J. (2003). The ecology of human performance. In E. B. Crepeau, E. S. Cohn, & B. A. Boyt Schell (Eds.), *Willard & Spackman's occupational therapy* (10th ed., pp. 223–227). Philadelphia, PA: Lippincott Williams & Wilkins.

Finlay, L. (1998). *The life world of the occupational therapist: Meaning and motive in an uncertain world.* (Unpublished PhD thesis). Milton Keynes, United Kingdom: The Open University.

Finlay, L. (2003). The intertwining of body, self and world: A phenomenological study of living with recently-diagnosed multiple sclerosis. *Journal of Phenomenological Psychology, 34*, 157–178.

Finlay, L. (2006). The body's disclosure in phenomenological research. *Qualitative Research in Psychology, 3*, 19–30.

Finlay, L. (2009). Debating phenomenological research methods. *Phenomenology & Practice, 3*, 6–25.

Finlay, L. (2011). *Phenomenology for therapists: Researching the lived world.* Chichester, West Sussex: Wiley-Blackwell.

Finlay, L., & Molano-Fisher, P. (2007). "Transforming" self and world: A phenomenological study of a changing lifeworld following a cochlear implant. *Medicine, Health Care, and Philosophy, 11*, 255–267.

Fitzpatrick, N., & Finlay, L. (2008). "Frustrating disability": The lived experience of coping with the rehabilitation phase following flexor tendon surgery. *International Journal of Qualitative Studies on Health and Well-Being, 3*, 143–154.

Fok, D., Miller Polgar, J., Shaw, L., Luke, R., & Mandich. A. (2009). Cyberspace, real place: Thoughts on doing in contemporary occupations. *Journal of Occupational Science, 16*, 38–43.

Frank, A. W. (2002). *At the will of the body: Reflections on illness.* New York, NY: Houghton Mifflin Harcourt.

Frank, L. D., Engelke, P. O., & Schmid, T. L. (2003). *Health and community design: The impact of the built environment on physical activity.* Washington, DC: Island Press.

Friesen, N. (2011). *The place of the classroom and the space of the screen: Relational pedagogy and internet technology.* New York, NY: Peter Lang.

Gadamer, H. G. (1996). *The enigma of health: The art of healing in the scientific age.* Stanford, CA: Stanford University Press.

Gallagher, S. (1986). Lived body and environment. *Research in Phenomenology, 16*, 139–170.

Gardner, P. J. (2011). Natural neighborhood networks—Important social networks in the lives of older adults aging in place. *Journal of Aging Studies, 25*, 263–271.

Geng, T., Gan, J. Q., & Hu, H. (2010). A self-paced BCI for mobile robot control. *International Journal of Advanced Mechatronic Systems, 2*(1–2), 28–35.

Gitlin, L. N. (2003). Conducting research on home environments: Lessons learned and new directions. *The Gerontologist, 43*, 628–637.

Gitlin, L. N. (2009). Environmental adaptations for older adults and their families in the home and community. In I. Söderback (Ed.), *International handbook of occupational therapy interventions* (pp. 53–62). London, United Kingdom: Springer.

Gooberman-Hill, R. (2007). Changing mobility, relationships and space: The experience of difficulty walking in later life. *Viennese Ethnomedicine Newsletter, 9*(2–3), 17–32.

Graham-Rowe, D. (2011, July). Control your home with thought alone: The latest brain-computer interfaces meet smart home technology and virtual gaming. *NewScientist, 2819*, n.p.

Haythornthwaite, C., & Kendall, L. (2010). Internet and community. *American Behavioral Scientist, 53*, 1083–1094.

Hill, M. (1985). Bound to the environment: Towards a phenomenology of sightlessness. In D. Seamon & R. Mugerauer (Eds.), *Dwelling, place and environment: Towards a phenomenology of person and environment* (pp. 99–111). Dordrecht, The Netherlands: Martinus-Nijhof.

Hockenberry, J. (1995). *Moving violations: War zones, wheelchairs, and declarations of independence.* New York, NY: Author.

Horan, T. A. (2000). *Digital places: Building our city of bits.* Washington, DC: Urban Land Institute.

Hull, J. M. (1990). *Touching the rock: An experience of blindness.* New York, NY: Vintage.

Iwarsson, S. (2009). Housing adaptations: Current practices and future challenges. In I. Söderback (Ed.), *International handbook of occupational therapy interventions* (pp. 63–69). London, United Kingdom: Springer.

Jennings, M. B. (2009). Hearing accessibility and assistive technology use by older adults: Application of universal design principles to hearing. In L. Hickson (Ed.), *Proceedings of the second international adult conference: Hearing care for adults 2009—the challenge of aging* (pp. 249–254). Staefa, Switzerland: Phonak AG.

Kielhofner, G. (1995). Environmental influences on occupational behavior. In G. Kielhofner (Ed.), *A model of human occupation: Theory and application* (2nd ed., pp. 91–111). Baltimore, MD: Lippincott Williams & Wilkins.

Kiernat, J. M. (1987). Promoting independence and autonomy through environmental approaches. *Topics in Geriatric Rehabilitation, 3*, 1–6.

Klinenberg, E. (2002). *Heat wave: A social autopsy of disaster in Chicago.* Chicago, IL: University of Chicago Press.

Kopec, D. (2006). *Environmental psychology for design.* New York, NY: Fairchild.

Lessing, D. (1984). *The diaries of Jane Somers.* New York, NY: Random House.

Lu, Z. (2010). Investigating walking environments in and around assisted living facilities: A facility visit study. *Health Environments Research & Design Journal [HERD], 3*(4), 58–74.

Madjar, I., & Walton, J. (Eds.). (1999). *Nursing and the experience of illness: Phenomenology in practice.* London, United Kingdom: Routledge.

Mallett, S. (2004). Understanding home: A critical review of the literature. *The Sociological Review, 52*, 62–89.

Malpas, J. E. (1999). *Place and experience: A philosophical topography.* Cambridge, United Kingdom: Cambridge University Press.

Manzo, L. C. (2003). Beyond house and haven: Toward a revisioning of emotional relationships with place. *Journal of Environmental Psychology, 23*, 47–61.

Manzo, L. C. (2005). For better or worse: Exploring multiple dimensions of place meaning. *Journal of Environmental Psychology, 25*, 67–86.

Mehta, V., & Bosson, J. K. (2009). Third places and the social life of streets. *Environment and Behavior, 42*, 779–805.

Merleau-Ponty, M. (1962). *The phenomenology of perception.* New York, NY: Routledge & Kegan Paul.

Mihailidis, A., & Davis, J. (2005). The potential of intelligent technology as an occupational enabler. *Occupational Therapy Now, 7*(1), 22–23.

Moore, A. J. (2010). *Space, place and home: Lived experiences in hospice day care* (Doctoral dissertation). University of Lancashire, United Kingdom.

Moore, A. J., Anderson, C., Carter, B., & Coad, J. (2010). Appropriated landscapes: The intrusion of technology and equipment into the homes and lives of families with a child of complex needs. *Journal of Child Health Care, 14*, 3–5.

Moore, J. (2007). Polarity or integration? Toward a fuller understanding of home and homelessness. *Journal of Architecture and Planning Research, 24*, 143–159.

Murphy, R. F. (1987). *The body silent: The different world of the disabled.* New York, NY: Henry Holt.

Oldenburg, R. (1999). *The great good place: Café's, coffee shops, bookstores, bars, hair salons, and other hangouts at the heart of a community* (3rd ed.). New York, NY: Marlowe & Company.

O'Loughlin, A. (1999). On living with chronic pain. In I. Madjar & J. Walton (Eds.), *Nursing and the experience of illness: Phenomenology in practice* (pp. 123–144). London, United Kingdom: Routledge.

Padilla, R. (2003). Clara: A phenomenology of disability. *American Journal of Occupational Therapy, 57*, 413–423.

Percival, J. (2002). Domestic spaces: Uses and meanings in the daily lives of older people. *Ageing & Society, 22*, 729–749.

Preiser, W. F. E., & Smith, K. H. (Eds.). (2011). *Universal design handbook* (2nd ed.). New York, NY: McGraw-Hill.

Relph, E. (2008). *Place and placelessness*. London, United Kingdom: Pion Limited. (Original work published 1976)

Relph, E. (2007). Spirit of place and sense of place in virtual realities. *Techné: Research in Philosophy and Technology, 10*(3), 1–8.

Rickerson, N. (2009). Universal design: Principles and practice for people with disabilities. In I. Söderback (Ed.), *International handbook of occupational therapy interventions* (pp. 159–165). London, United Kingdom: Springer Publishing.

Rioux, L., & Werner, C. (2011). Residential satisfaction among aging people living in place. *Journal of Environmental Psychology, 31*, 158–169.

Rosenbaum, M. S., Sweeney, J. C., & Windhorst, C. (2009). The restorative qualities of an activity-based, third place café for seniors: Restoration, social support, and place attachment at Mather's—More than café. *Seniors Housing & Care Journal, 17*(1), 39–54.

Rosenfeld, J. P., & Chapman, W. (2008). *Home design in an aging world*. New York, NY: Fairchild.

Rowles, G. D. (1999). Beyond performance: Being in place as a component of occupational therapy. *American Journal of Occupational Therapy, 45*, 265–271.

Rowles, G. D. (2003). The meaning of place as a component of self. In E. B. Crepeau, E. S. Cohn, & B. A. Boyt Schell (Eds.), *Willard & Spackman's occupational therapy* (10th ed., pp. 111–119). Philadelphia, PA: Lippincott Williams & Wilkins.

Rowles, G. D. (2006). Commentary: A house is not a home: But can it become one? In In H. W. Wahl, H. Brenner, H. Mollenkopf, D. Rothenbacher, & C. Rott (Eds.), *The many faces of health, competence and well-being in old age: Integrating epidemiological, psychological and social perspectives* (pp. 25–32). Dordrecht, The Netherlands: Springer.

Rowles, G. D., & Chaudhury, H. (Eds.). (2005). *Home and identity in late life*. New York, NY: Springer.

Rowles, G. D., & Watkins, F. (2003). History, habit, heart, and hearth: On making spaces into places. In K. W. Schaie, H. W. Wahl, H. Mollenkopf, & F. Oswald (Eds.), *Aging independently: Living arrangements and mobility* (pp. 77–96). New York, NY: Springer.

Schaie, W. K., Wahl, H. W., Mollenkopf, H., & Oswald, F. (Eds.). (2003). *Aging independently: Living arrangements and mobility*. New York, NY: Springer.

Seamon, D. (1979). *A geography of the lifeworld*. New York, NY: St. Martin's Press.

Seamon, D. (1993). Different worlds coming together: A phenomenology of relationship as portrayed in Doris Lessing's *diaries of Jane Somers*. In D. Seamon (Ed.), *Dwelling, seeing, and designing: Toward a phenomenological ecology* (pp. 219–246). Albany, NY: State University of New York Press.

Seamon, D. (2000). A way of seeing people and place: Phenomenology in environment-behavior research. In S. Wapner, J. Demick, T. Yamamoto, & H. Minami (Eds.), *Theoretical perspectives in environment-behavior research–Underlying assumptions, research problems, and methodologies* (pp. 157–178). New York, NY: Plenum.

Seamon, D. (2002). Physical comminglings: Body, habit, and space transformed into place. *OTJR: Occupation, Participation and Health, 22*(Suppl. 1), 42S–51S.

Seamon, D. (2010). Gaston Bachelard's topoanalysis in the 21st century: The lived reciprocity between houses and inhabitants as portrayed by American writer Louis Bromfield. In L. Embree (Ed.), *Phenomenology 2010: Vol. 5. Selected essays from North America, Part I* (pp. 225–243). Bucharest, Romania: Zeta Books.

Seamon, D. (2013). Merleau-Ponty, perception, and environmental embodiment: Implications for architectural and environmental studies. In R. McCann & P. M. Locke (Eds.), *Carnal echoes: Merleau-Ponty and the flesh of architecture*. New York, NY: Routledge.

Shin, K. R. (1999). On surviving breast cancer and mastectomy. In I. Madjar & J. Walton (Eds.), *Nursing and the experience of illness: Phenomenology in practice* (pp. 70–87). London, United Kingdom: Routledge.

Simms, E. (2008a). Children's lived spaces in the inner city: Historical and political aspects of the psychology of place. *The Humanistic Psychologist, 36*(1), 72–89.

Simms, E. (2008b). *The child in the world*. Detroit, MI: Wayne State University Press.

Söderback, I. (2009). Adaptive interventions: Overview. In I. Söderback (Ed.), *International handbook of occupational therapy interventions* (pp. 39–51). London, United Kingdom: Springer.

Stafford, P. B. (2009). *Elderburbia: Aging with a sense of place in America*. Westport, CT: Praeger.

Standal, Ø. F. (2011). "I learned nothing from him . . .": Reflections on problematic issues with peer modeling in rehabilitation. *Phenomenology & Practice, 5*, 48–58.

Stefanovic, I. (2008). Holistic paradigms of health and place: How beneficial are they to environmental policy and practice? In J. Eyles & A. Williams (Eds.) *Sense of place, health and quality of life* (pp. 45–57). Burlington, VT: Ashgate.

Steinfeld, E., & Danford, G. S. (1999). *Enabling environments. Measuring the impact of environment on disability and rehabilitation*. New York, NY: Kluwer Academic.

Steinfeld, E., & White, J. (2010). *Inclusive housing: Design for diversity and equality*. New York, NY: Norton.

Stewart, D., Letts, L., Law, M., Cooper B. A., Strong, S., & Rigby, P. J. (2003). The person-environment occupation model. In E. B. Crepeau, E. S. Cohn, & B. A. Boyt Schell (Eds.), *Willard & Spackman's occupational therapy* (10th ed., pp. 227–233). Philadelphia, PA: Lippincott Williams & Wilkins.

Svenaeus, F. (2001). The phenomenology of health and illness. In S. K. Toombs (Ed.), *Handbook of phenomenology and medicine* (pp. 87–108). Dordrecht, The Netherlands: Kluwer Academic.

Todres, L., & Galvin, K. (2005). Pursuing both breadth and depth in qualitative research: Illustrated by a study of the experience of intimate caring for a loved one with Alzheimer's disease. *International Journal of Qualitative Methods, 4*(2), 1–11.

Toombs, S. K. (Ed.). (2001). *Handbook of phenomenology and medicine*. Dordrecht, The Netherlands: Kluwer Academic.

Trefler, E., & Hobson, D. (1997). Assistive technology. In C. Christiansen & C. M. Baum (Eds.), *Occupational therapy: Enabling function and well being* (pp. 482–506). Thorofare, NJ: SLACK.

Ulrich, R. S., Zimring, C., Zhu, X., DuBose, J., Seo, H., Choi, Y., . . . Joseph, A. (2008). A review of the research literature on evidence-based healthcare design. *Health Environments Research & Design Journal [HERD], 1*(3), 61–125.

van Berlo, A. (2002). Smart home technology: Have older people paved the way? *Gerontechnology, 2*, 77–87.

van Manen, M. (1990). *Researching lived experience: Human science for an action sensitive pedagogy*. Albany, NY: State University of New York Press.

van Manen, M. (1998). Modalities of body experience in illness and health. *Qualitative Health Research, 8*, 7–24.

Walton, J. (2001). The lived experience of mental illness. In S. K. Toombs (Ed.), *Handbook of phenomenology and medicine* (pp. 279–293). Dordrecht, The Netherlands: Kluwer Academic.

Young, L. C. (2011). Universal housing: A critical component of a sustainable community. In W. Preiser & K. H. Smith (Eds.), *Universal design handbook* (2nd ed., pp. 24.3–25.13). New York, NY: McGraw-Hill.

For additional resources on the subjects discussed in this chapter, visit http://thePoint.lww.com/Willard-Spackman12e.

UNIT V

Personal Factors and Occupational Performance

"What we understand the world to be like is determined by many things: our sensory organs, our ability to move and to manipulate objects, the detailed structure of our brain, our culture, and our interactions with the environment. . . ."

—George Lakoff & Mark Johnson

CHAPTER 19

Individual Variance

Body Structures and Functions

Barbara A. Boyt Schell, Glen Gillen, Marjorie E. Scaffa, Ellen S. Cohn

OUTLINE

LEARNING OBJECTIVES

1. Consider how personal characteristics and factors are related to occupations and occupational performance
2. Discuss how knowledge of personal factors is used in occupational therapy evaluation and intervention
3. Identify examples of body functions and structures that are considered in the occupational therapy process

Introduction

Throughout this text, there is recognition that occupation is a function of the individual performing within a specific context. How that occupational performance occurs, then, is a reflection of all the unique characteristics of the person doing the acting as well as the specific context in which the action occurs. In Unit IV, important contextual factors were discussed. In this unit, we examine the personal factors that influence occupational performance.

This chapter provides an overview of the various personal characteristics and factors that affect occupational performance. **Personal factors** is a broad term used here to encompass several aspects of the human condition. Different professional groups, such as the American Occupational Therapy Association (AOTA, 2008) and the World Health Organization (WHO, 2001), organize these descriptors of individuals in different ways. The AOTA Practice Framework uses the term "client factors" (AOTA, 2008, p. 630) to encompass many aspects of the person, the WHO uses the term "body structures and body functions" (WHO, p. 10), and other international models may use the term "performance components" or "occupational performance components" (Chapparo & Ranka, 1997) to refer to many aspects of personal factors.

Regardless of the specific terminology used, occupational therapy requires close attention to the many ways that individuals are unique. Examples include basic information such as the person's age, gender, and ethnicity. People also vary in **body structures**, or anatomical parts, such as bones and organs and **body functions**, or physiological processes of the body, including psychological function (WHO, 2001). For instance, people may vary physically in terms of height, weight, and bodily strength; they may vary in their responses to different sensory experiences such as a preference for spicy food or cold drinks; and they may vary in their emotional responses to specific situations. Furthermore, these differences may or may not impact the person's occupational performance, depending on the demands and challenges the individual experiences in life. See the following case study as an illustration of the many personal factors affecting individual occupational performance. Later in the chapter are tables listing many of the personal factors that may be considered by occupational therapists.

The Whole Is Greater Than the Sum of the Parts

Personal factors do not operate in isolation. Anyone who has tried to maneuver in unfamiliar space in the dark (such as finding the bathroom in a dark hotel room in the middle of the night) can attest to the importance of vision to movement. All bodily factors work synergistically, which is why it is difficult to generate a definitive list of factors to which practitioners should attend. That is the case in this chapter as well, and the selected lists of factors and descriptions are presented to prompt your thinking. The categorizations that are presented here are not, nor can they be, a complete list of all the factors that affect human behavior. They are, at best, suggestions of factors to consider in analyzing occupational performance.

CASE STUDY 19.1 Cynde: Personal Factors Required to Be a Naturalist on a Whale-Watching Boat

Cynde is a naturalist on a whale-watching boat. In this description, some of the personal factors affecting her performance are noted. Refer to Tables 19.1, 19.2, and 19.3 to see if you can pinpoint the specific terms. Additionally, try to match other terms that connect to the many personal factors affecting her performance.

Cynde has been passionate about whales for as long as she can remember, and she is deeply committed to preserving the ocean habitat to ensure their survival (values and beliefs). Her job requires that she orient tourists to the whale boat safety rules, educate tourists about whales, and help them understand what they are seeing when they observe whale surface behavior. Because of her commitment to sustainability, she also tries to explain how personal actions in daily life can impact marine life many miles away from home.

Cynde starts each trip by standing on the dock, going over boat safety rules, and also explaining a bit about whales (Figure 19.1). Note that she has to hold (body function–musculoskeletal) the microphone with one hand (body structure–nervous system, movement-related structures) while demonstrating with another. She had to memorize (body function–long-term memory) what she needs to say (body function–language expression and working memory) and deliver her talk in a certain amount of time (body function–organization, planning, self-monitoring) while the boat is being readied for departure. She demonstrates enthusiasm and humor (body function–range of emotion, appropriate level of excitement) during her presentation. Once on the boat, she has to climb a steep ladder to get to the captain's area, where she will again use the microphone to call attention to the whales and their behavior. She works with the boat captain to detect whales at a long distance, using her visual skills. When she gets closer, she recognizes the distinctive patterns on the whale tails (called flukes), as this is important to tracking individual whales. While she is providing commentary, she is also photographing whales, and supervising science interns as they collect scientific data about whale sightings and surface behavior.

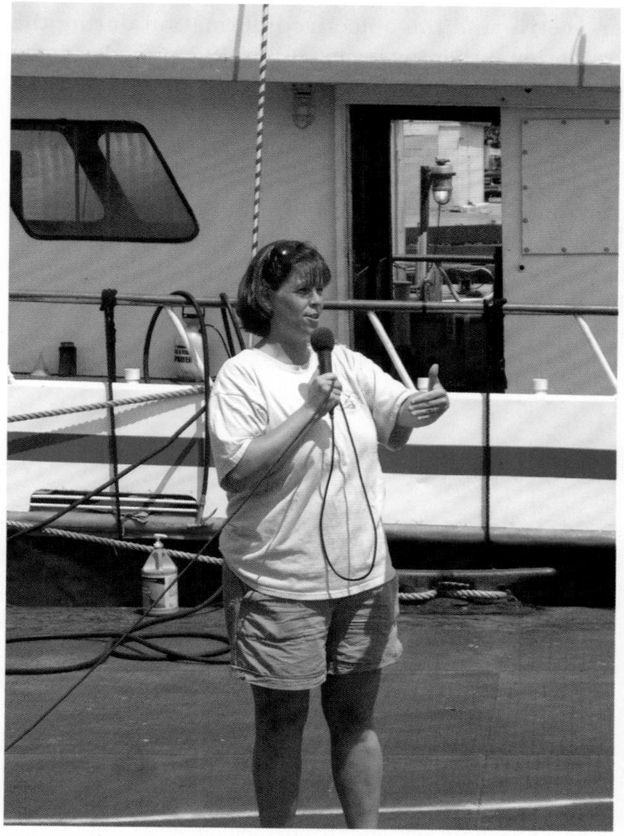

FIGURE 19.1 Cynde is going over boat safety rules and also explaining a bit about whales.

Practitioners can consider all of these factors from an **objective** standpoint or as **subjectively experienced** by the client. When considering personal factors objectively, therapists typically start by carefully observing occupational performance. If more information is needed to understand why the person is acting in a particular way, the therapist may evaluate body functions and structures using standardized approaches that other observers can replicate. Examples include muscle testing, sensory testing, and cognitive testing in relation to occupational performance. Chapters 24 and 25 address the use of objective assessments and the importance of using reliable and valid measures to obtain objective data. Although objective approaches are undeniably useful for informing professional reasoning, the client's subjective experience is also important. For example, objective measurement may indicate impairment; however, the person may not consider this limitation problematic in terms of daily life. Consequently, there may not be a need for intervention. Alternatively, comparison of objective and subjective findings may show that a client is unaware of safety concerns that are observed by the therapist. Therefore, skilled practitioners consider both the client's perspective and the objective information during the occupational therapy process. Box 19.1 provides some examples of objective and subjective reports related to body functions and structures.

Our job as occupational therapy practitioners is twofold. First, we must carefully observe occupational performance so as to understand which personal factors support occupational engagement and which ones are limiting engagement. Additionally, we must go beyond the generic labeling and understandings of diagnostic conditions to a deeper and more personal understanding of how clients perceive and experience their specific situations.

Reasoning about Personal Factors: Occupational Therapy as a Bridge

Occupational therapy practitioners like to say that they treat the whole person. Whereas other professions (such as nursing) legitimately make a similar claim, occupational therapy is unique in its focus on how daily occupations are the synergistic product of the personal factors within the individual and factors that are external to the person in the larger context.

Another way to think about occupational therapy and how we consider the factors under discussion is to contrast occupational therapy with other professions. Think of occupational therapy as a bridge between the medical world and the lifeworld. In the medical world, there are many professions that focus on particular sets of body structures and functions. The field of medicine has obvious examples, with specialties in dermatology, endocrinology, gynecology, psychiatry, ophthalmology, and the list goes on and on. But other professions can also be examples. For instance, nutritionists focus on the digestive system, physical therapists focus on the neuromuscular and musculoskeletal systems, and speech-language pathologists focus primarily on the cognitive and oral-motor systems as they relate to communication. Although all of these professionals are interested in improving an

BOX 19.1 Objective and Subjective Reports of Body Functions and Structures

"I Didn't Have a Clue"

In a study seeking to understand the subjective experience of regaining self-care skills after a stroke or spinal cord injury, Guidetti, Asaba, and Tham (2007) reported numerous examples of what it felt like for the study participants to attempt familiar tasks with various impairments. For instance, one participant who was recovering from a stroke appears to have had what objectively might be documented as a sensory loss, along with neglect of the affected upper extremity. She described her experience this way: "I didn't have a clue where it [her hand] was, it was behind my back and like this, so the first night it could have been anybody's hand" (Guidetti et al., 2007, p. 3).

"When You're Sitting There by Yourself, You're Just Eating"

In a study examining supported socialization for people with mental illness, Davidson and his colleagues (2004) argued that people with persistent mental illness are lonely and isolated, not by choice (or objective impairments) but because of lack of opportunity and encouragement. When viewed solely from an objective perspective, people with persistent mental illness have been described as having impairments in volition, self-awareness, or coping (affective and cognitive impairments) and are thought to no longer desire human connection, with a preference for being alone. In a randomized control trial of supported socialization intervention, Davidson and colleagues found that people with mental illness desire friendships. One participant in the study commented that eating with her friend was better than eating alone at Burger King: "I'm alone. I sit down at the table, I eat a hamburger. But when I go with somebody else, and I'm sitting there at the table and eating it, she'll say 'Oh, is your hamburger good?' Then it becomes, the hamburger becomes noticeable, and then your mind starts to think about the taste. But when you're sitting there by yourself, you're just eating" (Davidson et al., 2001, p. 380).

This woman's description of eating with a friend illustrates the importance of considering clients' subjective experience. Without consideration of the subjective experience, intervention may not address aspects of occupational performance that were meaningful to this woman.

individual's function, their contribution is very specific; and their knowledge about body functions and structures within their specific scope is typically quite extensive.

In contrast, other professions organize themselves around major roles or tasks of life. For instance, vocational evaluators and rehabilitation counselors focus on work-related concerns, educators focus on helping people learn to become productive citizens, recreation professionals focus on play and leisure, and social workers focus on family and community life. These professionals may attend to the impact of personal factors. So, for example, vocational rehabilitation practitioners know a great deal about job demands, employer requirements, and government standards related to work. Special education teachers are particularly aware of the impact of cognitive abilities and limitations for students in the classroom. Similarly, recreation therapists are quite knowledgeable about recreational spaces and places, the value of leisure in life, and the kinds of equipment that individuals might use to pursue leisure interests. However, for the most part, these professionals are very different from those in the medically oriented fields in that they typically have little or no background related to anatomy, physiology, and the specific impact of different health conditions on performance. Additionally, these professions typically are less likely to attend to the full array of social and psychological factors affecting performance. Rather, they have broad working knowledge about the skills and social demands that are required for their area of interest.

Occupational therapists have the education and ability to understand and address the impact of body structures and functions on life roles and tasks. This is done with full appreciation of the interconnected nature of occupations as well as how occupations are learned and change over the life course. In addition, occupational therapy practitioners recognize the transactions among personal factors and the environments in which the person must function (AOTA, 2010). As a result, occupational therapy as a profession provides information that bridges the clients' personal factors with the roles and task competencies required in daily life.

Complexity: An Asset and a Challenge

Occupational therapy is unique as a profession in its willingness to consider all the client's personal factors along with all contextual factors as they shape engagement in the daily activities and routines of life. It is this appreciation of the transactional nature of occupational performance that makes occupational therapy so customized and effective for helping to solve complex problems of daily life. This uniqueness is a tremendous asset. However, for new practitioners and even some experienced ones, it can be challenging not to get absorbed in one aspect and thus lose sight of the larger picture. Practitioners who focus on one area of function may refer to themselves as hand therapists, cognitive therapists, or vision therapists and lose sight of the totality of our work as occupational therapists. Depth of knowledge about the personal factors is very important to expert practice; however, clients are best served when these factors are viewed in relation to the use of occupation as a means for intervention. Further, occupational engagement is the desired outcome, regardless of how individual differences affect the ways in which this outcome is achieved. For example, as opposed to "doing hand therapy," our focus should be stated as "improving occupational performance after a hand injury." Examples of such reasoning are provided through the therapist narratives in Unit XIII. All of the practitioners in Unit XIII indicate a deep understanding of body functions and structures that are relevant to their clients, but they view these factors in relation to occupational performance. Furthermore, occupational therapy practitioners grade their use of interventions in a way that is mindful of each person's individual characteristics, development, impairments, potential for recovery, and/or need for adaptive approaches. Practitioners also are very cognizant of how social and cultural contexts influence their clients' lives. ***Thus, occupational therapy practitioners specialize not in body parts or body functions, but in supporting health and participation in life through engagement in occupation*** (AOTA, 2008).

Intertwining Knowledge and Theories

For occupational therapy practitioners to work effectively with people who have impairments or developmental conditions that affect their performance, practitioners must intertwine knowledge about occupation with knowledge about the client's particular health problems. As noted earlier, this chapter provides only a topical overview of the many person factors that practitioners may consider. Knowing what to do requires in-depth appreciation of relevant theories and research in order to assure effective intervention. Unit XII provides the reader with examples of how theories guide practice to improve occupational performance in the focused areas of motor control, cognition and perception, sensory processing, emotional regulation, and communication/social interaction. The therapists' narratives in Unit XIII provide examples of using different theories to guide practice. Readers are encouraged to look at those chapters for examples of how to integrate theories about body functions and structures into an occupational therapy intervention.

Personal Factors That Are Commonly Considered

In this section, we provide several tables that readers might find helpful to prompt consideration of one or more personal factors (see Tables 19.1, 19.2, 19.3, and 19.4). Readers will likely find the language useful in

TABLE 19.1 Examples of Personal Factors (Excluding Body Functions and Structures) That Are Considered in Occupational Therapy

Factor	Common Categories or Descriptors
Age	Historical cohort (e.g., people who lived through the depression and how that experience affects their worldview) Internalization of societal expectations regarding development and achieving a particular developmental milestone at a given time in the life course Personal expectations about age-related behavior
Gender	Personally adopted social/cultural norms and roles regarding gender
Values	Meanings associated with physical and social spaces Importance of family Standards of conduct Qualities considered desirable Principles considered worthwhile
Beliefs	Knowledge that is held to be truth Beliefs about causes and interventions related to illness Perceived locus of control Cognitive content held as truth
Spirituality	Beliefs about the meaning of life Quest to understand ultimate life questions Religious and sacred beliefs
Family and significant others	Internalized family experiences that shape worldview Internalized expectations about relationships
Socioeconomic status	Financial status Work status Educational attainment
Ethnicity	Internal beliefs about membership in groups of common descent; can include race, culture, language, religion, and politics
Sexual orientation	An individual's sexuality, usually related to an individual's romantic, emotional, and/or sexual attraction to persons of a particular gender

communicating about personal factors. As was discussed earlier, there is no practical way to make a comprehensive list, so we make no claim that the tables are all inclusive. Information for these tables was drawn primarily from the *International Classification of Functioning, Disability and Health* (WHO, 2001), the Occupational Therapy Practice Framework (AOTA, 2008), and topical areas that are addressed in this unit as well as chapters from Unit IV.

Clues to personal factors that could be affecting performance are gained from at least three sources:

- **Reason for referral.** Referral information may contain a medical, psychological, or educational diagnosis and sometimes precautions to consider during intervention. Even when precautions, symptoms, or other descriptors are not included, knowledge about typical body structures and functions that are affected by the condition can guide practitioners regarding factors to consider.

  Example: Diagnosis–Rotator cuff tear. Knowledge of the body structure will lead practitioners to evaluate for the *impact* that pain, weakness, and limited shoulder range of motion may have on identified limitations in occupational performance. Limitations may include inability to perform self-care (e.g., shampooing hair), inability to fulfill a homemaker role (e.g., putting groceries away, washing windows), inability to engage in leisure activities (e.g. fly-fishing), inability to perform job responsibilities (e.g., writing on a blackboard), and/or inability to fulfill child-care responsibilities (e.g., lifting a toddler into a high chair).

- **Client self-report.** Clients themselves, their families, and other key people in their social environments (e.g., teachers, employers, caregivers) often give practitioners information about factors that they believe are affecting client performance.

  Example: A third-grade teacher reports to the occupational therapist that Alicia is highly distractible in class, requires multiple prompts and cues to stay on task, and is falling behind her classmates in reaching educational objectives. Alicia expresses a desire to

TABLE 19.2 Examples of Body Structures Considered in Occupational Therapy

Structure	Common Categories or Descriptors
Nervous system	Brain (cortical, subcortical including brain stem) Spinal cord Spinal nerves Sympathetic and parasympathetic systems
Eye and ear	Eye (retina, cornea, lens) External ocular muscles Ear (inner, middle, outer)
Voice and speech	Mouth (lips, cheek, tongue, teeth, palate) Nose Pharynx (nasal and oral) Larynx (vocal cords)
Cardiovascular, immunological, respiratory	Heart Veins Arteries Lungs Trachea Bronchial tubes Muscles of respiration Lymphatic system
Digestive, metabolic, endocrine	Esophagus Stomach Intestine Many glands
Genitourinary, reproductive	Bladder, ureters, urethra Reproductive structures
Movement-related structures (head/neck, upper and lower extremities, trunk, pelvic region)	Bones Joints Muscles Tendons Ligaments Fascia
Skin and related structures	Skin layers Skin glands Hair Sensing organs in skin

Source: American Occupational Therapy Association. (2008). Occupational therapy practice framework: Domain and process, 2nd edition. *American Journal of Occupational Therapy, 62*(6), 625–683; and World Health Organization. (2001). *International classification of functioning, disability and health (ICF)*. Geneva, Switzerland: Author.

play with other girls during recess but doesn't quite know how to join the group.

- **Observation of client.** Observations of the client engaging in occupations often prompt practitioners to consider one or more factors that are affecting performance.

  Example: During an evaluation of meal preparation skills, the occupational therapy practitioner notes that Mr. Brown is unable to independently complete a task as he did prior to his recent decline in cognitive function. He now requires step-by-step cues to sequence and organize the process of making a soup and salad.

  Example: Coleman attends a residential school for adolescents with traumatic brain injury. Since his accident, Coleman becomes fatigued, withdrawn, and apathetic by mid-afternoon. Every week, six teenage boys plan a Thursday evening community outing to relax and have fun together. The occupational therapist observes that Coleman does not offer suggestions for outings and rarely interacts with his peers during the outing. To accommodate for Coleman's personal factors and engage during a time of day when his performance is optimal, the practitioner plans to change the community outings to Saturday morning.

TABLE 19.3 Examples of Body Functions Considered by Occupational Therapists

ICF	Category	Examples
Global mental functions (affective, cognitive, perceptual)	Consciousness	Alertness, arousal level, continuity of wakeful state
	Orientation	Person Place Time Self Others Past Present
	Intellectual functions	Understanding Integration of cognitive functions
	Psychosocial functions	Interpersonal skills Social interactions
	Temperament/personality	Emotional stability Disposition Confidence
	Energy and drive	Energy level Motivation Impulse control Appetite
	Sleep functions	Amount and onset of sleep Quality Sleep cycle functions
Specific mental functions (affective, cognitive, perceptual)	Attention	Selectivity Sustainability Shifting Divided
	Memory	Short term Long term Working
	Perception	Auditory Visual Olfactory Gustatory Tactile Visuospatial
	Sensory processing	Reception Organization Assimilation Integration
	Thought	Ideation Pace of thought Content
	Higher level cognitive functions	Volition Organization/Planning Purposeful action Self-awareness Self-monitoring Decision making Problem solving Judgment Time management Coping
	Emotional	Behavioral regulation Range of emotion
	Psychomotor functions	Appropriate affect Response time Level of excitement/agitation Speed of behavior
	Mental functions of language	Reception of language (spoken, written, and sign) Expression of language (spoken, written, and sign)
	Mental functions of sequencing complex movement	Praxis

TABLE 19.3 Examples of Body Functions Considered by Occupational Therapists (*Continued*)

ICF	Category	Examples
Sensation and pain	Taste	Quality Intensity
	Smell	Quality Intensity
	Touch	Light Deep pressure
	Temperature	Hot Cold
	Pain	Sharp Stabbing Aching Burning
	Proprioception	Quick Sustained
	Vestibular	Linear Angular
	Visual	Acuity Intensity Contrast
	Auditory	Acuity Intensity Contrast Rhythm
Neuromuscular and movement	Joint mobility	Passive ROM Active ROM
	Muscle strength	Pinch Grip Force
	Muscle tone	Quality
	Voluntary motor control	Coordination (dexterity, gross motor, bilateral integration) Motor execution (mobility)
	Involuntary motor control	Reflexes Unconscious movement
	Posture	Alignment Orientation Stability Control Balance Adaptation
Cardiovascular, immunological, respiratory	Heart rate Blood pressure Respiration	Tension Rate Rhythm Depth

ICF, International Classification of Functioning, Disability and Health; ROM, range of motion.

From American Occupational Therapy Association. (2008). Occupational therapy practice framework: Domain and process, 2nd edition. *American Journal of Occupational Therapy, 62*(6), 625–683; Dunn, W. (2011). *Best practice occupational therapy: In community service with children and families* (2nd ed.). Thorofare, NJ: SLACK.; and World Health Organization. (2001). *International classification of functioning, disability and health (ICF)*. Geneva, Switzerland: Author.

Skillful intervention requires that practitioners respond to these cues and then use credible resources to obtain needed objective information. This information, combined with the subjective data provided by the client, is then synthesized to develop interventions that enable the client's occupational performance. It is important to remember that the "presence or absence of specific body functions and body structures do not necessarily ensure a client's success or difficulty with daily life occupations" (AOTA, 2008, p. 630). A person with memory loss may be able to fully participate in most aspects of life using compensatory strategies such as memory notebooks/diaries, electronic paging systems, written reminder lists posted in the environment, and/or smart phone alarm reminders. Optical aids, text-to-speech translators, and the use of guide dogs can provide a person with vision loss with the ability to live life fully and independently.

TABLE 19.4 Examples of Impaired Body Functions and Potential Impact on Occupational Performance

Impairment of Body Function	Potential Difficulty with Daily Life Occupations
Impaired visuospatial processing	Inability to orient clothing to self Misjudging distance when reaching for a utensil Inability to align car in parking space Spilling juice when pouring from carton into glass Difficulty finding the way in new environments and fear of getting lost results in self-imposed participation restrictions (Árnadóttir, 2011)
Decreased shoulder range of motion	Inability to manage hair care Unable to tuck shirt into back of pants Inability to retrieve book from high shelves at the library Inability to change a light bulb Difficulty holding and playing with one's children or grandchildren Role strain from inability to perform job responsibilities and inability to fulfill role of primary financial provider
Poor emotional regulation	Poor performance at job interview Inability to cope during finals week at college, resulting in poor test performance Social isolation due to inappropriate affect Difficulty initiating, developing, and maintaining interpersonal relationships Inability to make decisions due to overwhelming anxiety
Sensory loss in feet	Increased incidence of falls during community outings Inability to walk on rough terrains (beach, hiking trails, etc.) Inability to drive a car Decreased participation in social/leisure activities due to fear of falling
Decreased attention	Difficulty attending to one conversation at a time at a dinner party Unable to attend to school lectures/lessons Inability to cook toast and tea at the same time Difficulty following verbal and written instructions on the job Experiences of relationship strain as a partner may perceive a lack of interest due to easy distractibility (Gillen, 2009).

Conclusion

Occupational therapy practitioners routinely consider body functions, structures, and other personal factors during intervention. By integrating knowledge and theories about these personal factors with theories that relate to occupation and occupational contexts, practitioners provide a unique contribution to society and to the clients they serve.

References

American Occupational Therapy Association. (2008). Occupational therapy practice framework: Domain and process, 2nd edition. *American Journal of Occupational Therapy, 62*, 625–683.

American Occupational Therapy Association. (2010). Occupational therapy's perspective on the use of environments and contexts to support health and participation in occupations. *American Journal of Occupational Therapy, 64*, S57–S69.

Árnadóttir, G. (2011). Impact of neurobehavioral deficits on activities of daily living. In G. Gillen (Ed.), *Stroke rehabilitation: A function-based approach* (3rd ed., pp. 456–500). St. Louis, MO: Elsevier/Mosby.

Chapparo, C., & Ranka, J. (Eds.). (1997). *Occupational performance model (Australia)* [Monograph 1]. Sydney, Australia: Occupational Performance Network.

Davidson, L., Shahar, G., Stayner, D. A., Chiman, M. J., Rakfeldt, J., & Tebes, J. K. (2004). Supported socialization for people with psychiatric disabilities: Lessons from a randomized control trial. *Journal of Community Psychology, 32*, 453–477.

Davidson, L., Stayner, D. A., Nickou, C., Styron, T. H., Rowe, M., & Chinman, M. L. (2001). "Simply to be let in": Inclusion as a basis for recovery. *Psychiatric Rehabilitation Journal, 24*, 375–388.

Dunn, W. W. (2011). *Best practice occupational therapy: In community service with children and families* (2nd ed.). Thorofare, NJ: SLACK.

Gillen, G. (2009). *Cognitive and perceptual rehabilitation: Optimizing function.* St. Louis, MO: Elsevier/Mosby.

Guidetti, S., Asaba, E., & Tham, K. (2007). The lived experience of recapturing self-care. *American Journal of Occupational Therapy, 61*, 303–310.

World Health Organization. (2001). *International classification of functioning, disability and health (ICF)*. Geneva, Switzerland: Author.

For additional resources on the subjects discussed in this chapter, visit http://thePoint.lww.com/Willard-Spackman12e.

CHAPTER 20

Personal Values, Beliefs, and Spirituality

Christy Billock

"In a way all sacred experience and all journeys of soul lead us to the smallest moment of the most ordinary day."

—Sue Monk Kidd (1996)

OUTLINE

LEARNING OBJECTIVES

After reading this chapter, you will be able to:

1. Develop an understanding of the meaning of personal values, beliefs, and spirituality as related to occupational therapy practice, including definition, related themes, and distinction from religion
2. Recognize the relationship between spirituality, occupation, health, and well-being
3. Identify the relationship of personal beliefs to occupational therapy's history
4. Understand the relevance of individual experiences of spirituality through occupation by examining important factors such as context, reflection and intention, and occupational engagement
5. Describe strategies to integrate personal values, beliefs, and spirituality into occupational therapy practice
6. Explore how personal values, beliefs, spirituality, and occupation might intersect in your own life experiences

Introduction

The profession of occupational therapy thrives on integrating clients' personal experiences of meaning into practice. Understanding the rich interconnections of personal values, beliefs, spirituality, and occupation provides occupational therapy practitioners the opportunity of enhancing the profession's unique holistic approach to health and wellness.

This chapter serves as an introductory resource for understanding personal values, beliefs, and spirituality in occupational therapy practice. This chapter will begin by addressing two fundamental questions:

- How do personal values and beliefs relate to spirituality?
- What is spirituality and how does it relate to occupational therapy?

Second, this chapter will discuss the multiple ways in which spirituality is experienced through occupation. Third, it will provide strategies for integrating personal values, beliefs, and spirituality into occupational therapy practice. Last, this chapter will pose reflective questions that will allow readers to explore their own personal values, beliefs, and views of spirituality.

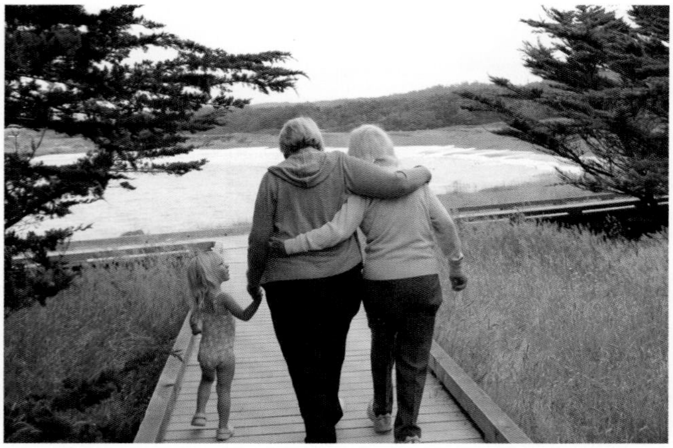

FIGURE 20.1 One facet of spirituality is connectedness to others.

Framing Personal Values, Beliefs, and Spirituality from an Occupational Therapy Perspective

Occupational therapy practice functions within a holistic context of care that involves "addressing both subjective (emotional and psychological) and objective (physically observable) aspects of performance" (American Occupational Therapy Association [AOTA], 2008, p. 628). Subjective aspects of occupational performance often interrelate with a person's values and beliefs. **Values** can be understood as "principles, standards, or qualities considered worthwhile by the client who holds them" (AOTA, 2008, p. 633). The notion of **beliefs** closely relates to values and can be defined as "cognitive content held as true" (AOTA, 2008, p. 633). Both values and beliefs often influence a person's subjective experiences of occupation because of their centrality and individualized nature. Values and beliefs can derive from multiple sources including personal experience, friends and acquaintances, family, culture, religion, and politics, among others. Values and beliefs can also closely relate to spirituality through occupational experience.

To discuss how values, beliefs, and spirituality interconnect calls for defining spirituality, which can prove challenging. The multidimensional and complex nature of spirituality defies simple definition. According to Hasselkus (2010),

> Spirituality cannot be directly observed in the physical sense. We are not even at all sure what behaviors we might identify that represent this phenomenon. We have trouble finding the words to describe what we think we mean when we use the word *spirituality*. Yet we probably all acknowledge the existence of some sort of spiritual nature in ourselves and in the lives of all human beings. (p. 145)

Definitions typically emphasize spirituality as a metaphysical and individually experienced internal phenomenon involving an essential spirit, soul, or essence of a person (Egan & DeLaat, 1994; Hasselkus, 2010; Moore, 1992). Individuals might experience spirituality as a sense of connectedness that relates them to a transcendent being, a belief or value, themselves, others, or the physical world (Figure 20.1). Recurring themes related to spirituality within occupational therapy and other health professions' literature are hope, faith, coping, and self-transcendence (Haase, Britt, Coward, Leidy, & Penn, 1992; Kelly, 2004; Spencer, Davidson, & White, 1997).

Spirituality can be defined as a deep experience of meaning (Urbanowski & Vargo, 1994) brought about by engaging in occupations that involve the enacting of personal values and beliefs, reflection, and intention within a supportive contextual environment (Billock, 2005). Occupational therapy places meaning as a central tenet of the profession; and meaning-making, in its essence, is a spiritual process that seeks expression through occupation (Peloquin, 1997). People often experience spirituality through engagement in everyday activities (Moore, 1992); consequently, occupation creates meaning and helps to answer larger existential questions of the meaning of life (Christiansen, 1997; Frankl, 1959). The AOTA includes spirituality in the practice framework as a client factor and uses Moreira-Almeida and Koenig's (2006) definition that spirituality is

> the personal quest for understanding answers to ultimate questions about life, about meaning and about relationship with the sacred or transcendent, which may (or may not) lead to or arise from the development of religious rituals and the formation of community. (p. 844)

An experiential view of spirituality proves important to understand how values, beliefs, and occupation unfold in a person's life.

Religion is often linked with spirituality and can inform a person's formation of values and beliefs. Religion is defined as an integrated system of beliefs with their attendant practices (Engquist, Short-DeGraff, Gliner, & Oltjenbruns, 1997). As a set of individual and communal practices, religion permeates many people's experiences of spirituality on a daily basis through occupations such as prayer, meditation, reading theological books, and attending religious services. Not only do religions provide followers with practices that directly relate to theological beliefs but also religious beliefs often ascribe spiritual meaning to daily occupations such as food preparation, work, and intimacy, especially if they are "understood as commanded by God" (Frank et al., 1997, p. 201). Although many people use religion as a tool for framing spirituality in their lives, individual spiritual experience is not dependent on religious affiliation or practice.

Spiritual and religious practices can be linked to well-being and health (Low, 1997; Miller & Thoresen, 2003). Spiritual health takes on many definitions but generally connotes being able to experience meaning, fulfillment, and connection with self, others, and a higher power or larger reality (Hawks, Hull, Thalman, & Richins, 1995). These viewpoints also recognize that illness and disease affect the whole person, including the body, mind, and spirit, and all need to be addressed to restore health (do Rozario, 1997). Experiences of occupational alienation (Townsend & Wilcock, 2004), that is, an inability to create meaning and express one's spirit through occupation, demonstrates a lack of spiritual health or well-being for a person (Simo Algado, Mehta, Kronenberg, Cockburn, & Kirsh, 2002).

It is important to address the right of marginalized populations such as people with disabilities, mental illness, and the aged to experience spirituality and practice religion (Eiesland & Saliers, 1998; Koenig, George, & Peterson, 1998; Richards, 1990). These issues of access to occupations as a fundamental human right connect the principles of occupational justice and spirituality (Wilcock, 2001). Additionally, the potential links between religious practice and experiences of coping with disability and caregiving illuminate possibilities for enhanced health and well-being (Michie & Skinner, 2010).

Exploring the historical roots of occupational therapy reveals traces of personal values, beliefs, and spirituality from the profession's founding. Moral treatment influenced the founders of occupational therapy in the early 20th century (Bockoven, 1971). Advocates of moral treatment valued ideals such as holism, humanism, and a recognition that engagement of the mind, body, and spirit through occupation promoted health and brought meaning to life (Meyer, 1922/1977). In the 1920s and 1930s, the medical establishment criticized occupational therapy for its lack of theory grounded in scientific principles (Gritzer & Arluke, 1989). In an attempt to legitimize the profession, occupational therapists adopted reductionistic models through the 1950s, thereby minimizing the emphasis on recognition of the human spirit and subjective experience as expressed in occupation (Yerxa, 1992). In 1962, Reilly expressed concern that the reductionistic view of occupational therapy could not capture the role that occupation could play in facilitating health. Reilly's words proved to be a catalyst for the re-emergence of a holistic perspective valuing spirituality and personal beliefs as a central concept of occupational therapy (Atler, Fisher, Moret, & White, 2000).

In the late 20th century, the Canadian Association of Occupational Therapy (CAOT, 1991, 1997, 2002) explicitly integrated spirituality into theories about client-centered practice and occupational performance, placing spirituality at the center of theoretical constructs of occupation that guide occupational therapy practice (Polatajko, Townsend, & Craik, 2007). In the United States, the AOTA in 1997 devoted an entire issue of the *American Journal of Occupational Therapy* to the topic of spirituality. Spirituality gained inclusion in the "Occupational Therapy Practice Framework" (AOTA, 2002) as a context for occupation, ushering in the official recognition of the importance of spirituality to occupational therapy in the United States. The second edition of the "Occupational Therapy Practice Framework" (AOTA, 2008) shifted its interpretation of spirituality to residing within the person as a client factor.

Experiencing Spirituality through Occupation

People enact personal beliefs and values through occupational engagement, which can yield an experience of spirituality. Although spirituality can be experienced outside of occupation, engaging in occupation is the most common and effective mechanism for these experiences because it is through occupational engagement that spirituality becomes more tangible. Peloquin (1997) refers to occupation as an act of making that represents an extension and animation of the human spirit:

> To see such radical making in the acts that we commonly name *doing* purposeful activities, *performing* life roles and tasks, *adapting* to the environment, *adjusting* to disability, and *achieving* skills or mastery, is to discern the spiritual depth of occupation. (p. 167)

Linking occupation and spirituality together with the notion of "making" implies a fluid and active approach to the phenomenon. In making, a person expresses tangibly the intangible yet vital realities of life. This expression, although invariably interconnected with the social world, is ultimately created and interpreted internally by each individual. These internal representations of values and beliefs about the meaning of reality and the world drive people to orchestrate occupations to express those meanings (Kroeker, 1997).

Trends within Western society signify moving away from practices directed by organized religion and toward personal construction of practices for the foundation of spiritual life (Wuthnow, 1998). McColl (2002) contends that given the erosion of meaning in work from industrialization and the prevalence of secular pluralism in modern society, occupation "may be the most effective medium available through which individuals can affirm their connection with the self, with others, with the cosmos, and with the divine" (p. 352). Orchestration of and engagement in everyday occupation holds the potential of helping people to meet the fundamental need for spiritual expression. For example, the busy executive's attending a yoga class, receiving a massage, or taking a hike might serve the vitally important role of facilitating his or her experiences of spirituality.

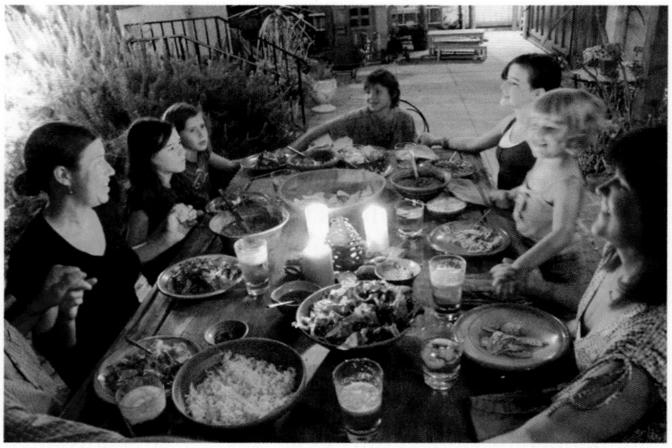

FIGURE 20.2 Gathering to share a meal can be an occupation with spiritual potential.

Contextual Factors

Spiritual experiences through occupation are dependent on and vulnerable to transactions with several contextual factors, including the physical and social world (Billock, 2005). Symbolism is a potent nexus of meaning-making embedded within these contextual factors (Fine, 1999). Places, objects, and communities hold symbolic meanings to individuals that are informed by past history, both individual and communal (Holland, Lachicotte, Skinner, & Cain, 1998).

The physical world can serve to potentially facilitate or block spiritual experiences (Jackson, 1996). Many people communicate experiences of spirituality through occupations in nature such as hiking in the mountains, fly-fishing in a stream, or walking along the beach. Built spaces such as churches, houses, and other structures serve to refine and make more vivid human feeling, perception, and comprehension of reality (Tuan, 1977). Out of experiencing those spaces and the objects within them, a person draws a sense of place that is "an organized world of meaning" (Tuan, 1977, p. 179). For example, a home filled with memories of family gatherings and decorated with special pieces of art and pictures of loved ones can provide support for experiencing spirituality through the occupations that are engaged in within the space. Gathering around a table appointed with grandmother's linens and pottery made by friends, then lighting candles when friends come to share a meal, marks the event as one with special meaning, personal value, and spiritual import (Figure 20.2). Whereas home can support one person's experiences of spirituality, for another person, the home might be a place of strained memories and relationships. For a woman who is physically abused by her husband in the privacy of their home, experiences of occupation within her home may show little potential for spiritual experience.

The social world can significantly influence spiritual experience because meaning is both personally and socially constructed (Hasselkus, 2010). Therefore, attempts to understand spiritual experience involve looking at the doer of the occupation in reference to the social and cultural worlds of engagement. Engaging in occupations with others, or co-occupation (Zemke & Clark, 1996), can potentiate the likelihood of a spiritual experience. Religions recognize the importance of believers practicing their faith with others as a means of mutual support and affirmation of belief (Howard & Howard, 1997). Communal occupations such as attending sporting events, concerts, or political protests as well as family celebrations such as weddings or graduations can be rich environments for spiritual experience and the enacting of personal values and beliefs.

The Centrality of Reflection and Intention

Spiritual experience also relies on personal reflection and intention (Billock, 2005). Reflection refers to the exploration of one's inner world and necessarily involves recognition of feelings, emotions, and motivations to act deriving from personal values and beliefs. Reflection also becomes a tool of interpretation that can lead to a setting apart of spiritual experiences as different from everyday life, something special or transcendent (Bell, 1997). Intention involves a conscious imbuing of meaning or directing occupational experience toward something such as a value, belief, or ideology. Reflection or intention in an occupational experience does not necessarily need to be labeled "spiritual"; rather, it may be sensed as deeply satisfying or meaningful.

Occupations engaging a person's creativity offer the opportunity for deep levels of reflection, intention, and ultimately, spiritual experience (Figure 20.3). Kidd (1996), speaking of creativity and spirituality, says, "My creative life is my greatest prayer" (p. 123). Cameron

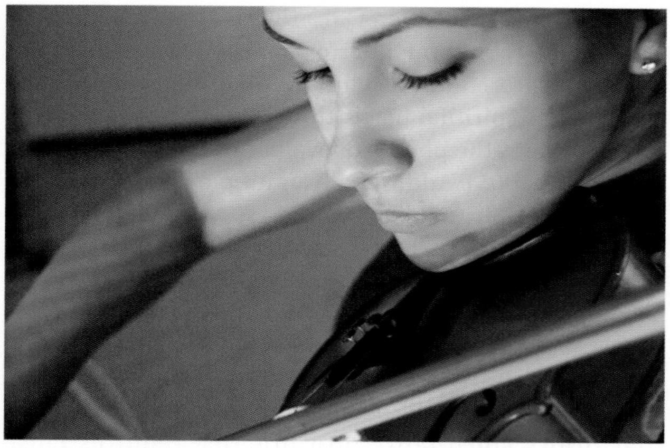

FIGURE 20.3 An occupation that engages creativity can offer the opportunity for a spiritual experience.

(1992) shares a similar view of the intertwining of spirituality and creativity:

> Creativity is an experience—to my eye, a spiritual experience. It does not matter which way you think of it: creativity leading to spirituality or spirituality leading to creativity. In fact, I do not make a distinction between the two. (p. 2)

Infusing occupation with creativity allows for expression of internal states innately spiritual in nature (Simo Algado et al., 2002). Whereas artistic occupations such as painting, making pottery, or writing poetry show high potential for spiritual experience, numerous other everyday occupations can be filled with creativity as well (Hasselkus, 2010). Occupations such as cooking, conversing with others, or planning a party, along with countless others, can be occupations in which creativity is expressed.

Occupational Engagement

Not all occupations are experienced as spiritual, but all occupations hold the potential to be spiritual. Although people often name occupations stemming from religious traditions as spiritual, the lived experience of such occupations might not be spiritual. Everyday occupations such as work, walking the dog, or gardening might be experienced as spiritual but likely would not be named as religious (Howard & Howard, 1997; Unruh, 1997). Occupations that are deeply meaningful to the person, imbued with personal reflection and intention, and carried out within a supportive contextual environment offer the highest potential for spiritual experience (Billock, 2005). Kidd (1996) describes the fleeting nature of spirituality in the midst of the details of a normal morning:

> I rose to make the coffee. I walked to the door and paused. When I looked back, I saw my life shining within every ordinary thing. And I was seized by the same feeling I get whenever I see the ocean—the feeling that it is all too much to behold, too beautiful, too much to bear—and I was filled with an aching love for it. In the next instant the moment was gone, and I was climbing down the stairs, walking into the kitchen, into a day of small, humble, distracting things, and somehow nothing seemed more holy to me than just being there, naturally myself, in the midst of it. Such moments are not as common for me as I might wish. But when they come, they leave me with a willingness to relate to my ordinary space—my work and family and friends and all the mundane duties—more authentically. (p. 222)

The demands of routine activities that must be done often blocks the ability to reflect, be intentional, and find deep meaning in the moment (Norris, 1998).

People frequently experience rituals as spiritual, and throughout history, many ordinary activities such as serving food have been used in ritual (Bell, 1997). Common to understandings of ritual are the notions of repetition, fixedness, and predictability that are usually embedded in the doing of religion (Hasselkus, 2010). Outside of religion, any occupation can take on ritualistic characteristics of formalism, tradition, invariance, sacral symbolization, and performance. It is these characteristics that differentiate sacred experience from the more mundane aspects of life (Bell, 1997). Depending on an individual's engagement, an occupation such as taking a bath could be experienced as spiritual owing to ritualized characteristics. Bell recognizes the importance of ritual-like performances because they "communicate on multiple sensory levels, usually involving highly visual imagery, dramatic sounds, and sometimes even tactile, olfactory, and gustatory stimulation" (p. 160). For example, engagement in the occupations of a holiday celebration with its attendant ritual practices involving food and particular actions offers the possibility of spiritual experience in bringing together personal, familial, social, religious, and cultural aspects of life (Luboshitzky & Gaber, 2001).

Integrating Personal Beliefs, Values, and Spirituality into Occupational Therapy Practice

As a profession rooted in holistic and humanistic values, occupational therapy holds a unique opportunity to help clients restore meaning to their lives, a vitally important and essentially spiritual task. Although most occupational therapy practitioners recognize spirituality as an important aspect of life, integrating a client's personal beliefs, values, and spirituality into occupational therapy practice proves problematic because of ambiguity and the large diversity of practitioners' understanding of the notions (Engquist et al., 1997; Johnston & Mayers, 2005). Also, in light of the drive toward evidence-based practice, inclusion of spirituality in the core of occupational performance has become increasingly controversial (Unruh, Versnel, & Kerr, 2002). These challenges lead to role ambiguity and a lack of confidence in addressing spirituality in practice in spite of a recognized need for its inclusion (Belcham, 2004). As Howard and Howard (1997) indicate, "Occupational therapists need not look beyond the tools, theories, and values of the profession to provide a context for acknowledging the spiritual in the clinic" (p. 185). If spirituality is a deep experience of meaning effectively experienced through occupational engagement, then occupational therapy intervention strategies that uphold holism through occupation-based and client-centered techniques will likely promote clients' spiritual health and well-being.

Recognizing the difficulty of integrating spirituality into practice, Egan and Swedersky (2003) identified four strategies used by occupational therapists who successfully achieve this integration:

- Addressing clients' religious concerns
- Assisting clients in dealing with suffering
- Helping clients to recognize their own worth and efficacy
- Recognizing their own transformations brought about by working with clients

Integrating spirituality into practice starts with the occupational therapy practitioner (Townsend, DeLaat, Egan, Thibeault, & Wright, 1999). Practitioners must consider their own understanding of spirituality and how their spirituality plays out in their occupations and experiences. Additionally, this self-reflective process may lead to the recognition of personal biases, values, or beliefs that could interfere with the crucially needed openness to clients' diverse beliefs and experiences. Self-reflection also aids in the ethically important need for therapeutic interventions to be consistent with the client's spiritual life, not the therapist's (Rosenfeld, 2001). Those who practice therapeutic use of self through active listening, empathy, tolerance, unconditional acceptance, and flexibility toward the client's desires and needs demonstrate a spiritual approach to therapeutic interaction.

Several approaches and tools aid in the integration of spirituality for all the phases of the occupational therapy process. Many consumers of occupational therapy have experienced disruptions to and loss of the occupations through which they experience spirituality and meaning. By honoring the subjective experiences of clients in the evaluation, goal-setting, and intervention planning processes, the practitioner moves toward integrating spirituality into practice and will likely increase the client's motivation (Townsend et al., 1999). Tools such as the Canadian Occupational Performance Measure allow for a client-centered and occupation-based approach that can address spiritual needs through actively integrating the client into the phases of evaluation and intervention (Law et al., 2005). Additionally, multiple health care professions use spiritual history tools as a practical method for including spirituality in practice (Koenig, 2004, 2007). Occupational therapy practitioners have found one such spiritual history, the FICA, practical and convenient for gathering vital information about their clients' spiritual lives (Bouthot, Wells, & Black, 2011).

A client-centered occupational therapy approach that draws spirituality into practice requires close attention to the client's culture (Simo Algado et al., 2002) as well as the form, function, and meaning of the occupations used in intervention (Larson, Wood, & Clark, 2003). Practitioners sometimes feel uncomfortable integrating clients' religious occupations into intervention. If these occupations are important aspects of a client's daily life, religious occupations such as prayer or reading sacred texts can be integrated into intervention sessions as deeply meaningful occupations. Addressing culture might call for learning more about rituals and religious traditions different from the practitioner's own religious experience or exposure. Clergy from the client's religion as well as family members can serve as resources for the practitioner to increase cultural and religious competence (Rosenfeld, 2001). For clients who are dealing with emotional trauma, occupations that encourage reflection and expression of internal states, such as artistic pursuits and storytelling, can provide opportunity for spiritual insight and coping (Simo Algado et al., 2002).

Conclusion

The rich concepts of personal beliefs, values, and spirituality provide occupational therapists with valuable tools for understanding the deep meaning of engaging in occupation. Important to clients' health and well-being, integrating spirituality into occupational therapy practice proves relevant to the profession's goal of providing holistic occupation-based and client-centered care.

References

American Occupational Therapy Association. (2002). Occupational therapy practice framework: Domain and process. *American Journal of Occupational Therapy, 56*, 609–639.

American Occupational Therapy Association. (2008). Occupational therapy practice framework: Domain and process, 2nd edition. *American Journal of Occupational Therapy, 62*, 625–683.

Atler, K., Fisher, C., Moret, S., & White, J. (2000, March). *Combining spirituality and storytelling: Changing lives and enhancing practice.* Paper presented at the annual meeting of the American Occupational Therapy Association, Seattle, WA.

Belcham, C. (2004). Spirituality in occupational therapy: Theory in practice? *British Journal of Occupational Therapy, 67*, 39–46.

Bell, C. (1997). *Ritual: Perspectives and dimensions.* Oxford, United Kingdom: Oxford University Press.

Billock, C. (2005). *Delving into the center: Women's lived experience of spirituality through occupation* (Doctoral dissertation). Retrieved from ProQuest Dissertations and Theses. (Accession Order No. AAT 3219812).

Bockoven, J. S. (1971). Legacy of moral treatment: 1800's to 1910. *American Journal of Occupational Therapy, 25,* 223–226.

Bouthot, J., Wells, T., & Black, R. (2011). Spirituality in practice: Using the FICA spiritual history assessment. *OT Practice, 18*(3), 13–16.

Cameron, J. (1992). *The artist's way: A spiritual path to higher creativity.* New York, NY: Penguin Putnam.

Canadian Association of Occupational Therapy. (1991). *Occupational therapy guidelines for client-centered practice.* Ottawa, Ontario: Author.

Canadian Association of Occupational Therapy. (1997). *Enabling occupation: An occupational perspective.* Ottawa, Ontario: Author.

Canadian Association of Occupational Therapy. (2002). *Occupational therapy guidelines for client-centered practice.* Ottawa, Ontario: Author.

Christiansen, C. (1997). Nationally speaking: Acknowledging a spiritual dimension in occupational therapy practice. *American Journal of Occupational Therapy, 51,* 169–172.

do Rozario, L. A. (1997). Spirituality in the lives of people with disability and chronic illness: A creative paradigm of wholeness and reconstitution. *Disability and Rehabilitation, 19,* 427–434.

Egan, M., & DeLaat, M. D. (1994). Considering spirituality in occupational therapy practice. *Canadian Journal of Occupational Therapy, 61,* 95–101.

Egan, M., & Swedersky, J. (2003). Spirituality as experienced by occupational therapists in practice. *American Journal of Occupational Therapy, 57,* 525–533.

Eiesland, N. L., & Saliers, D. E. (Eds.). (1998). *Human disability and the service of God: Reassessing religious practice.* Nashville, TN: Abingdon.

Engquist, D. E., Short-DeGraff, M., Gliner, J., & Oltjenbruns, K. (1997). Occupational theorists' beliefs and practices with regard to spirituality and therapy. *American Journal of Occupational Therapy, 51,* 173–180.

Fine, S. B. (1999). Symbolization: Making meaning for self and society. In G. Fidler & B. Velde (Eds.), *Activities: Reality and symbol* (pp. 11–25). Thorofare, NJ: Slack.

Frank, G., Bernardo, C. S., Tropper, S., Noguchi, F., Lipman, C., Maulhardt, B., & Weitze, L. (1997). Jewish spirituality through actions in time: Daily occupations of young orthodox Jewish couples in Los Angeles. *American Journal of Occupational Therapy, 51,* 199–206.

Frankl, V. (1959). *Man's search for meaning.* New York, NY: Washington Square Press.

Gritzer, G., & Arluke, A. (1989). *The making of rehabilitation: A political economy of medical specialization* (pp. 1890–1980). Los Angeles, CA: University of California Press.

Haase, J., Britt, T., Coward, D., Leidy, N., & Penn, P. (1992). Simultaneous concept analysis of spiritual perspective, hope, acceptance, and self-transcendence. *IMAGE: Journal of Nursing Scholarship, 24,* 141–147.

Hasselkus, B. R. (2010). *The meaning of everyday occupation* (2nd ed.). Thorofare, NJ: Slack.

Hawks, S. R., Hull, M. L., Thalman, R. L., & Richins, P. M. (1995). Review of spiritual health: Definition, role and intervention strategies in health promotion. *American Journal of Health Promotion, 9,* 371–378.

Holland, D., Lachicotte, W., Skinner, D., & Cain, C. (1998). *Identity and agency in cultural worlds.* Cambridge, MA: Harvard University Press.

Howard, B. S., & Howard, J. R. (1997). Occupation as spiritual activity. *American Journal of Occupational Therapy, 51,* 181–185.

Jackson, J. M. (1996). Living a meaningful existence in old age. In R. Zemke & F. Clark (Eds.), *Occupational science: The evolving discipline* (pp. 339–361). Philadelphia, PA: F. A. Davis.

Johnston, D., & Mayers, C. (2005). Spirituality: A review of how occupational therapists acknowledge, assess, and meet spiritual needs. *British Journal of Occupational Therapy, 68,* 9.

Kelly, J. (2004). Spirituality as a coping mechanism. *Dimensions of Critical Care Nursing, 23*(4), 162–168.

Kidd, S. M. (1996). *Dance of the dissident daughter: A woman's journey from Christian tradition to the sacred feminine.* San Francisco, CA: Harper Collins.

Koenig, H. G. (2004). Taking a spiritual history. *Journal of the American Medical Association, 291,* 2881.

Koenig, H. G. (2007). *Spirituality in patient care: Why, how, when, and what* (2nd ed.). West Conshohocken, PA: Templeton Press.

Koenig, H. G., George, L. K., & Peterson, B. L. (1998). Religiosity and remission of depression in medically ill older patients. *American Journal of Psychiatry, 155,* 536–542.

Kroeker, T. (1997). Spirituality and occupational therapy in a secular culture. *Canadian Journal of Occupational Therapy, 64,* 122–126.

Larson, E., Wood, W., & Clark, F. (2003). Occupational science: Building the science and practice of occupation through an academic discipline. In E. B. Crepeau, E. S. Cohn, & B. A. B. Schell (Eds.), *Willard & Spackman's occupational therapy* (10th ed., pp. 15–26). Philadelphia, PA: Lippincott Williams & Wilkins.

Law, M., Baptiste, S., Carswell, A., McColl, M. A., Polatajko, H., & Pollock, N. (2005). *Canadian Occupational Performance Measure.* Toronto, Canada: CAOT.

Low, J. (1997). Religious orientation and pain management. *American Journal of Occupational Therapy, 51,* 215–219.

Luboshitzky, D., & Gaber, L. B. (2001). Holidays and celebrations as a spiritual occupation. *Australian Occupational Therapy Journal, 48,* 66–74.

McColl, M. A. (2002). Occupation in stressful times. *American Journal of Occupational Therapy, 56,* 350–353.

Meyer, A. (1977). The philosophy of occupation therapy. *American Journal of Occupational Therapy, 31,* 639–642. (Original work published 1922)

Michie, M., & Skinner, D. (2010). Narrating disability, narrating religious practice: Reconciliation and fragile X syndrome. *Journal of Intellectual and Developmental Disability, 48,* 99–111.

Miller, W. R., & Thoresen, C. E. (2003). Spirituality, religion, and health: An emerging research field. *American Psychologist, 58,* 23–35.

Moore, T. (1992). *Care of the soul.* New York, NY: Harper Perennial.

Moreira-Almeida, A., & Koenig, H. (2006). Retaining the meaning of the words religiousness and spirituality: A commentary on the WHOQOL SRPB group's "A cross-cultural study of spirituality, religion, and personal beliefs as components of quality of life" (62, 2005, pp. 1486–1497). *Social Science and Medicine, 63,* 843–845.

Norris, K. (1998). *The quotidian mysteries: Laundry, liturgy, and "women's work."* New York, NY: Paulist Press.

Peloquin, S. M. (1997). Nationally speaking: The spiritual depth of occupation: Making worlds and making lives. *American Journal of Occupational Therapy, 51,* 167–168.

Polatajko, H. J., Townsend, E. A., & Craik, J. (2007). Canadian Model of Occupational Performance and Engagement (CMOP-E). In E. A. Townsend & H. J. Polatajko (Eds.), *Enabling occupation II: Advancing an occupational therapy vision of health, well-being, & justice through occupation* (pp. 22–36). Ottawa, Canada: CAOT ACE.

Reilly, M. (1962). Eleanor Clarke Slagle Lecture: Occupational therapy can be one of the great ideas of 20th century medicine. *American Journal of Occupational Therapy, 16,* 1–9.

Richards, M. (1990). Meeting the spiritual needs of the cognitively impaired. *Generations, 14*(4), 63–64.

Rosenfeld, M. S. (2001). Exploring a spiritual context for care. *OT Practice, 6*(11), 18–26.

Simo Algado, S., Mehta, N., Kronenberg, F., Cockburn, L., & Kirsh, B. (2002). Occupational therapy intervention with children survivors of war. *Canadian Journal of Occupational Therapy, 69,* 205–215.

Spencer, J., Davidson, H., & White, V. (1997). Helping clients develop hopes for the future. *American Journal of Occupational Therapy, 51,* 191–198.

Townsend, E., DeLaat, D., Egan, M., Thibeault, R., & Wright, W. A. (1999). *Spirituality in enabling occupation: A learner-centered workbook.* Ottawa, Canada: CAOT.

Townsend, E., & Wilcock, A. (2004). Occupational justice and client-centered practice: A dialogue in practice. *Canadian Journal of Occupational Therapy, 71,* 75–85.

Tuan, Y. (1977). *Space and place: The perspective of experience.* Minneapolis, MN: University of Minnesota Press.

Unruh, A. M. (1997). Spirituality and occupation: Garden musings and the Himalayan blue poppy. *Canadian Journal of Occupational Therapy, 64*, 156–160.

Unruh, A. M., Versnel, J., & Kerr, N. (2002). Spirituality unplugged: A review of commonalities and contentions, and a resolution. *Canadian Journal of Occupational Therapy, 69*, 5–19.

Urbanowski, R., & Vargo, J. (1994). Spirituality, daily practice and the occupational therapy performance model. *Canadian Journal of Occupational Therapy, 61*, 88–94.

Wilcock, A. (2001). Occupational utopias: Back to the future. *Journal of Occupational Science, 1*, 5–12.

Wuthnow, R. (1998). *After heaven: Spirituality in America since the 1950's.* Los Angeles, CA: University of California Press.

Yerxa, E. J. (1992). Some implications of occupational therapy's history for its epistemology, values, and relation to medicine. *American Journal of Occupational Therapy, 46*, 79–83.

Zemke, R., & Clark, F. (1996). Section V: Co-occupations of mothers and children: Introduction. In R. Zemke & F. Clark (Eds.), *Occupational science: The evolving discipline* (pp. 213–215). Philadelphia, PA: F. A. Davis.

For additional resources on the subjects discussed in this chapter, visit http://thePoint.lww.com/Willard-Spackman12e.

UNIT VI

Analyzing Occupation

"Things that appear simple tend to get complicated, before they get simple again."

–Claudia Allen

CHAPTER 21

Analyzing Occupations and Activity

Elizabeth Blesedell Crepeau, Barbara A. Boyt Schell, Glen Gillen, Marjorie E. Scaffa

OUTLINE

LEARNING OBJECTIVES

After reading this chapter, you will be able to:

1. Describe approaches to analyzing occupations and activities in occupational therapy
2. Describe the similarities and differences between activity analysis and occupational analysis
3. Understand how occupational performance is the result of skilled transactions between the person and the performance context
4. Define occupational orchestration
5. Analyze occupations in order to understand performance strengths and weaknesses
6. Analyze activity in general and as experienced by an individual

Think about all the things you have or will do today as you go about your daily rounds. Perhaps you started your day with a bath or shower. Did you do that? Or do you prefer to bathe at night? Are you someone who prefers to bathe every other day? If you did bathe or shower, did you wash your hair? If you washed your hair, did you shampoo it once or twice? Did you apply a conditioner? Did you wash your hair before or after you washed the rest of your body? Were you standing in a shower, sitting in a tub, or leaning over a sink? How hot was the water? Did your arms get tired? Did you dry your hair with a towel or just comb it and let it dry itself? Or did you style your hair with a hair dryer? Did you use a pick, comb, or brush? What physical functions would you say are critical to doing your hair? What mental functions? Where was the place where you bathed? Did you have to go very far to get to the bathing area? Was it inside or outside? Did you have to carry your supplies or are they stored in the bathing area? Was it a private place or were others bathing at the same time? Were you afraid while you bathed? Now that you think about it, what do you take for granted about bathing? Do you think this is the same for others?

Answering questions such as these are part of the daily thinking processes that occupational therapy practitioners consider when they go about planning and implementing care for their patients and clients. Whether the attention is on self-maintenance activities, such as bathing and hair care, or on work activities, such as driving a bulldozer, practitioners require systematic frameworks to understand exactly what each person wants or needs to do. Application of these systematic frameworks is called **occupational analysis** and **activity analysis**. Occupational analysis refers to systematically analyzing what and how a person or groups of people actually do an activity. Activity analysis refers to considering a more general idea of how things are usually done.

Occupational therapy practitioners analyze activities to understand their component parts, their possible meaning to clients, and their therapeutic potential. For instance, a therapist who sees a lot of clients from a local chicken-processing factory may wish to do an activity analysis to have a good idea of what is usually involved in working in that setting. If the assembly work typically involves reaching up to get the poultry item and then placing it in a container before sending it down the line, then the therapist may wish to create a simulated portion of that activity back in the outpatient clinic using the same sorts of containers at the same work height.

Practitioners analyze the specific occupations of clients as they engage in them to gain an appreciation of specific performance strengths and potential problems clients are encountering and to notice how the context affects the performance. Using the example of the chicken plant, a practitioner may observe a particular worker who is very short to see what specific aspects of the usual factory routine are aggravating a back or hand condition. In a different therapy situation, the therapist may be interested to see how a client manages money. Observing the client while shopping may reveal no problems related to the physical manipulation of money but an inability to calculate money (acalculia). The problems of money management may be worse when the person has no calculator available to compensate. Such a problem can interfere with the occupations of household management, shopping in the mall, or online shopping and banking. Occupational analysis is used to design therapeutic intervention to enable clients to engage or reengage in those occupations that have particular meaning and value.

Practitioners also analyze how clients orchestrate their occupations across a day, week, and longer periods of time. **Occupational orchestration** reflects the capacity of individuals to enact their occupations on a daily basis to meet their own needs and the expectations of the many environments in which they are required to function. This may include attention to habits and routines, and the interface of these with the needs and expectations of others. Orchestration, a musical term, implies a rhythmic, harmonious composition of daily life that has habitual or routine components but is also responsive to changes in demands from day to day (Larson, 2000). Occupational therapy intervention consists of engaging clients in meaningful occupations to enable or improve their ability to meet their goals and participate in daily life. The occupations may be focused, such as taking a shower, or more complex, such as the orchestration of the array of daily occupations necessary to live a full and satisfying life. For example, making up an agenda for the next meeting of the pastoral care committee of the church or cooking dinner for the family may each be very feasible for an individual to perform. Performing these tasks in a timely and effective manner while working full-time and caring for other family needs requires skillful planning and coordination of multiple activities.

The analytic processes practitioners bring to their work are at the core of occupational therapy practice. This chapter describes these processes and links them to professional reasoning as it occurs throughout the therapeutic process.

Two Perspectives on Analysis: Occupation and Activity

Occupational therapy practitioners approach the process of activity analysis from two different perspectives—occupational analysis and activity analysis. In the first approach, practitioners are concerned with understanding the specific situation of the client and therefore must understand the specific **occupations** the client wants or needs to do in the actual context in which these occupations are performed. We refer to this as occupational analysis because the term *occupation* connotes personally experienced performance (Pierce, 2001). This is a customized approach that is embedded in the entire occupational therapy process. Occupational analysis attends carefully to the specific details of the client's occupations within a specific context. Indeed, it is this customized approach that differentiates the occupational therapy perspective from that of many other professions who do activity analysis, such as vocational educators and industrial engineers. In the bathing example provided in the opening paragraph, your answers to how you specifically perform the process of bathing represents part of an occupational analysis in that it helps describe the way that you actually do a particular occupation in your own life. See Box 21.1 for the rationale for the specific terms we are using in this chapter.

The second approach is commonly called activity analysis. In activity analysis, the practitioner considers an activity in the abstract or general sense, as it might typically be done within a given culture (Pierce, 2001). Practitioners do this sort of activity analysis for at least two reasons. First, the practitioner may wish to anticipate possible areas of concern in working with clients

BOX 21.1 Words Matter: Defining Activity and Occupation

Words matter because they shape the way we think and the meanings we ascribe to their underlying concepts (Hymes, 1972). Words also matter because there is an essential link between terminology and theory (Bauerschmidt & Nelson, 2011). Occupational therapy, like many other professions and disciplines, engages in ongoing debates about the meaning of specific terms as they relate to the profession. This debate can become confusing because professional jargon may or may not parallel the way the same words are used in everyday speech (Reed, 2005). Occupation and activity are two such words with everyday meanings and specialized professional meanings. The use of these terms has fluctuated greatly even in our profession's official documents. A recent analysis of 90 years of documents found that "The term occupation appeared dominant in the 1920s, but it appeared to be replaced in whole or in part by the word activity in the 1940s, 1950s, and 1960s. Neither term received much use in the 1970s and 1980s, and the term task, although used to some extent, did not replace them. The use of both occupation and activity—especially occupation—surged in the 2000s" (Bauerschmidt & Nelson, 2011, p. 342). The authors interpreted this shift "to indicate a widespread resurgence in occupational terminology after an extended period during which the term occupation was rarely used" (p. 344). Because these terms are so central to our field, many scholars have attempted to articulate precise meanings. The abundance of these definitions can be confusing, especially to occupational therapy students who are new to the field and seeking to understand it.

Definitions of *occupation* typically include a combination of the following concepts[a]:

- Is personally experienced and goal directed
- Reflects culture and cultural values
- Provides meaning
- Involves pursuits that extend over time
- Involves multiple tasks
- Provides organization and structure to living
- Meets needs of the individual and others in the social world
- Fills/occupies time
- Uses abilities and skills
- May have a physical and/or mental component
- Is recognized by the culture
- Provides pleasure and enjoyment
- Contributes to family and broader community
- Contributes to health and well-being
- Aligns with development of the individual

Definitions of *activity* typically share a mix of the core concepts listed below. Activity is frequently modified with terms such as *purposeful, occupational,* or *functional* to give it more specific meaning. In these cases, the term *activity* itself is not defined but assumed to be common knowledge. The core concepts[b] for most definitions of activity include the following:

- Incorporates small units of behavior
- Includes use of objects
- Involves action
- May or may not result in a product
- Is goal directed
- Is required for development, maturation, and use of sensory-perceptual, motor, social, psychological, and intellectual functions

In contrast, Pierce (2001) has defined activity as

> . . . an idea held in the minds of persons and in their shared cultural language. An activity is a culturally defined and general class of human actions. . . . An activity is not experienced by a specific person; is not observable as an occurrence; and is not located in a fully existent temporal, spatial, and sociocultural context" (p. 139).

For the purpose of this chapter, we have chosen to adopt Pierce's definition of activity because this definition enables us to make the distinction between the general ideas we have about a particular activity for activity analysis—for example, swimming—versus the engagement in swimming as an occupation that is dependent on the way or ways a particular person swims and the meaning he or she ascribes to it. Consequently, throughout the chapter when you read *activity,* you should remember that this reflects the general decontextualized concept and *occupation* is the way a particular person enacts this activity in a specific context. In other chapters in this book you will find terminology used differently. You need to look behind the terminology to understand the intent of the authors in their word choice.

[a]Adapted from Christiansen & Baum, 2005; Clarke et al., 1991; Hinojosa & Kramer, 1997; Law, Polatajko, Baptiste, & Townsend, 1997; Nelson & Jebson-Thomas, 2003; Spear & Crepeau, 2003.
[b]Adapted from Allen, 1987; Cynkin, 1995; Hinojosa & Kramer, 1997; Llorens, 1986; Mosey, 1981; Reed, 2005; Trombly, 1995.

with different kinds of health conditions or occupational performance challenges. Second, practitioners often need to generate **purposeful activities**, "specifically selected activities that allow the client to develop skills that enhance occupational engagement," (American Occupational Therapy Association [AOTA], 2008, p. 653). Examples include practicing transfers in and out of the tub on the rehabilitation unit, practicing shoe tying using one hand, and filling out a mock job application. These activities can be effectively designed or graded to help a client develop, recover from impairment, or learn an adaptive approach. For instance, if a practitioner thinks about what is typically involved in bathing or showering for many people in the United States, then he or she might be able to anticipate possible problems for someone with a partial paralysis (e.g., difficulty stepping over the tub wall, risk of fall, inability to reach the faucets) or difficulty remembering how to sequence activities (e.g., applying soap prior to wetting the body, beginning to dry off before rinsing off soap). Alternatively, while at a toy store or hardware store, the practitioner might notice and mentally consider how various toys or objects lend themselves to helping individuals develop or improve various skills or bodily capacities. For example the practitioner might analyze how the Wii Fit can be used to challenge postural control, eye-hand coordination, motor planning, endurance, self-confidence, and problem solving. Having these ideas in the practitioner's mental "toolbox" makes it easier to generate therapy possibilities for working with clients. Such consideration of activity possibilities is a *decontextualized approach*, because it is an abstract or general idea of what the practitioner thinks typically occurs. It is not what any one particular person actually experiences.

To summarize, the term **activity** is used in this chapter to represent the *general idea* about the kinds of things individuals do and the way they typically do them in a given culture (Pierce, 2001). The term *occupation*(s) is used to denote the *personal activities* that individuals choose or need to engage in and the ways in which each individual actually experiences them. Practitioners must be able to analyze both the general idea of how an activity typically occurs within a culture as well as the actual occupations as they are performed by particular individuals. These perspectives can also be applied to groups of people (e.g., members of a choir or workers in a plant), organizations (e.g., the local recreation center), and populations (e.g., the homeless, middle school students, or elders in a community). This chapter will focus primarily on analysis of activity and occupation at the individual level because the application to groups builds on these core analytic approaches. Other chapters later in the text provide illustrations of how occupational analysis can be used in relation to groups, organizations, and populations.

Performance Contexts and Environments

Occupational performance is by nature embedded within a social and physical environment, situated in a performance context (AOTA, 2008; Dunn, Brown, & Youngstrom, 2003; Pierce, 2001). *Environment* includes the external physical and social environments in which clients perform their occupations. The physical environment includes "the natural and built nonhuman environment including the objects in them. The social environment is constructed by the presence, relationships, and expectations of persons, groups, and organizations with whom the client has contact" (AOTA, 2008, p. 642). **Context** includes the external physical, social, economic, political, and cultural environments in which people function (Kronenberg, Pollard, & Ramugondo, 2011) as well as the internal or personal aspects, such as age, gender, socioeconomic status, education level, and motivation of the person (AOTA, 2008). Additionally, occupations are located in a temporal context in terms of stage of life, the specific amount of time involved, and the history and projected future related to occupation. Finally, some occupations occur in virtual contexts, such as Web-based blogs and spaces, social networking sites, text messaging, and online gaming. Paralleling the distinction just made between activity and occupation, many aspects of the environment and context can be considered in abstract or as the client actually experiences them.

Arenas and Settings

Lave (1988), an anthropologist, makes a distinction between the potential uses of environmental contexts and the ways people actually interact with them. She used the term **arena** to describe the places in which activities occur, such as a library, school, or hospital. In contrast, she used the word **setting** to describe those aspects of the arena to which the person attends. This distinction is useful in that it, once again, illustrates the twin ideas of actual experience versus abstract conceptualizations. For example, a library is an arena, and many of us conjure up an idea of what a library is. In fact, we may even think of a particular library as a physical place in our community and others a virtual place to obtain music and books. Whether physical or virtual, each individual will use the library in different ways and construct different meanings from their experiences. For instance, a man entering a local community library with his young child will most likely go to the children's section to look at colorful picture or chapter books. He is likely to sit on a small chair or a pillow while reading to his child. Later, he may help the child select books to take home. In contrast, another person may go to the computer section in the same library to access online materials. He may finish up a homework assignment for high school. A retired woman may go to the library as a volunteer to help in the gift shop. Thus, while the library as an arena remains the same, the library as a setting differs from person to person. The distinction Lave makes between arena and setting is similar to the distinction made earlier between activity and occupation. Like activity, arena is an abstract or general idea, whereas setting is where the occupational activity is specifically performed.

Roles: Social Constructions versus Personally Enacted

Role theory has had an influence on the development of theory within the profession. For instance, the Model of Human Occupation described in Chapter 39 uses role as a way of articulating how individuals see themselves and the multiple aspects of a person's life. The concept of role is translated into assessments such as the Role Checklist and Worker Role Interview (see Appendix II: Table of Assessments by Title). In sociological and psychological theories, roles are seen as social positions (Jackson, 1998a; Hagendorn, 2000). As Fisher (1998) noted in her Slagle lecture, "the role dimension pertains to the relationship between one's roles and the related collection of task performances that must unfold in a logical, timely, and socially appropriate manner. We must understand the person's perceived roles and any incongruities between his or her role behavior and the role behavior that is expected by society or desired by the person" (p. 544). Thus, roles can be thought of as normative models shaped by the culture. For example, they help articulate expectations for what constitutes being a "good" mother, father, or student, and the activities and occupations people in these positions are supposed to perform. Individuals within roles may adopt these normative expectations or may interpret the expectations to fit their own values and beliefs.

Jackson (1998a, 1998b) argued that our concern should be on the occupations individuals engage in, not their roles, because the concept of role is problematic from several perspectives. First, roles may overlap. For example, it is often impossible to distinguish children's "student" roles from their "friend" roles. When someone is cooking, is it in the role as mother or father, church volunteer, or chef? In both instances, our concern is in the occupation, the person's ability to engage in the occupation, and the meaning the person ascribes to it, not the role to which the occupation connects. Second, although the concept of role provides a shorthand way of understanding the occupational world of an individual, Jackson (1998a) argued that this approach is risky because inherent in the concept of role are the power issues embedded in many cultural models. For example, who decides what a "good mother" is? Who says the mother is the one to do the cooking for the family?

Still, role is not easy to ignore because it is such a widely held concept. For example, Trombly Latham (Trombly, 1995; Trombly Latham, 2008) uses role as an organizing construct; however, she cautions that roles should be considered from the definitional perspective of the individual rather than from the normative expectations of society. But how does one get to this definitional perspective except through understanding the occupations the individual attaches to a particular role? By focusing on occupations people engage in, we can see what people do, what the occupation means to them, how they feel about their performance, and how they organize their occupations to meet their needs and the needs of the people around them. Our analysis begins with occupation and may result, if needed, in clustering these occupations into the individual's personal definition of the occupations associated with the roles. Once again, we see the contrast between the abstract notion of role and the personally experienced situation of the individual, sometimes called **occupational role**.

Jackson's (1998a, 1998b) cautions about the use of roles are important because it is easy to unconsciously slip into normative expectations or use one's personal experience to frame the expectations for others. Practitioners bring unarticulated personal assumptions to the therapy process. Consequently, the concept of role was not chosen as an organizational construct for this chapter because we want to focus on those occupations that are most important to an individual regardless of what role or roles to which that person might be involved. Instead, the orchestration of occupations as they are enfolded and integrated in the course of daily life is examined.

Occupational Analysis and Meaning

Over and over again, practitioners need to remind themselves that meaning is individually constructed and interpreted and is central to human existence (Bruner, 1990; Frankl, 1959; Hasselkus, 2002; Peloquin, 2005, 2007). A practitioner is obligated to understand the meaning of occupations from the client's perspective. Using the library example discussed previously, it is possible if one talked to the father about the meaning of going to the library with his child that he might mention the pleasure he derives from instilling in his child the value and enjoyment of reading and the quiet time they share together. He might recall his childhood and the times he went to the library with one of his parents. Alternatively, he might explain that he never had the opportunity to go to the library with his father because his father had abandoned the family. The latter experience would create an entirely different meaning and motivational structure for **co-occupation** of this father–child dyad. Co-occupation is defined as an occupation that implicitly involves two or more individuals (Zemke & Clark, 1996).

As this example illustrates, the different experiences, values, and beliefs of clients make the interpretation of meaning a particularly complex aspect of practice. This challenge is exacerbated by potential cultural and socioeconomic differences between practitioners and their clients, making it more challenging for practitioners to fully understand the experiences of their clients and the meanings they ascribe to their occupations (Crepeau, 1991; Kielhofner & Barrett, 1998; Payne, DeVol, & Dreussi Smith, 2001; see also Chapters 16, 17, 18, and 20 in this text, which address culture, socioeconomics, place, and spirituality, respectively). It is the practitioner's responsibility to develop therapeutic relationships that foster an understanding of clients and their world (Crepeau & Garren, 2011; Peloquin, 1995; see also Chapter 33, which addresses client-centered collaboration and the therapeutic relationship). Activity analysis and occupational analysis are tools that practitioners can use to achieve this understanding. Table 21.1 provides a quick reference of concepts that are tied to the person's subjective experience versus what terms are more related to practitioners' general understanding of typical demands.

Activity and Occupational Analysis in Practice

Occupational therapy practitioners draw on their education, knowledge of activities, and professional experience

TABLE 21.1 Terms: From the Abstract/General to the Particular/Specific

	Abstract Concept	Real Experience
What is done	Activity	Occupation
Where and with whom	Arena	Setting
How it is organized	Social role	Occupational orchestration

when analyzing activities (Neistadt, McAuley, Zecha, & Shannon, 1993). This analysis may be so automatic that it is often ignored or unappreciated, becoming another aspect of the tacit nature of the reasoning process used by practitioners (Mattingly & Fleming, 1994; Schell & Cervero, 1993). Practitioners analyze activities from the perspective of practice theories to understand problems in performance and intervention strategies appropriate from that theoretical perspective. Their analysis is also based on access to particular activities and the degree to which they are willing to engage in trial and error or experimentation to understand activities more fully (Schell, 2008).

Studies that have attempted to make activity analysis an objective process have demonstrated that the number of variables is so great that the goal of objectivity would be exceedingly difficult to achieve (Llorens, 1986; Neistadt et al., 1993; Trombly, 1995). Adopting the distinction between activity analysis and occupational analysis renders this concern moot. If the outcome of activity analysis is to understand the *potential* demands of an activity, objectivity is not the goal. Rather, identifying the multiple skills typically required and the potential meanings the activity may have enable practitioners to have a deeper understanding of this activity in general.

In contrast to the consideration of activities for their therapeutic implications, occupational analysis is a highly individualized process because it is embedded in the particular perspective of the person, the person's occupational performance, and the performance context. Occupational analysis occurs when attempting to understand the person as an occupational being in concert with identifying occupational performance and barriers to effective performance (Coster, 1998; Fisher & Bray Jones, 2010; Hocking, 2001; Polatajko, Mandich, & Martini, 2000; Trombly, 1995; Trombly Latham, 2008). Client-centered evaluation models examine the ability of a person to engage in a valued occupation and the transaction among actual performance, activity demands, and context (Law, 1998). Box 21.2 provides examples of the various degrees of focus that practitioners use to consider occupations.

Both occupational and activity analysis are required for effective practice. By blending these analytic models, practitioners can gain an understanding of the particular ways in which clients relate to their occupations and can then use their knowledge of activity and practice theories to use those occupational activities for therapeutic purposes. This understanding is achieved through both forms of analysis. Table 21.2 summarizes the questions addressed in both activity and occupational analysis. Box 21.3 shows how practitioners weave analysis of occupational performance throughout the therapy process. Box 21.4 lists some of the ways that these analyses inform practice decisions.

Activity Analysis

Activity analysis is a way of thinking about activities. Practitioners must perform quick analyses while working with clients. In addition, occupational therapy practitioners may also think about activities for their therapeutic potential, for instance by sizing up new games, cooking gadgets, technology, and other objects or activities. Activity analysis addresses the typical demands of an activity, the range of skills involved in its performance, and the various cultural meanings that might be ascribed to it. The goal of activity analysis is to understand as much as possible about an activity, including the particular skills required to do it competently and its relation to participation in the world at large (Cynkin, 1995). It is this knowledge of activities, their properties, and their potential cultural meanings that sensitizes practitioners to the occupations of their clients and helps practitioners know which particular activities to suggest to their clients. Through activity analysis, practitioners gain an understanding of the therapeutic potential of a wide range of activities. Because practitioners routinely analyze activities, they develop the capacity to quickly analyze a wide range of activities for their therapeutic or evaluation potential.

Activity Analysis Format

The activity analysis format shown is based on the organization of the "Occupational Therapy Practice Framework" (AOTA, 2002) and the subsequent edition (AOTA, 2008) as well as information from various chapters within this text. The "Occupational Therapy Practice Framework" is designed to reflect the current practice of occupational therapy and its concern for occupational engagement to support health and participation of people in society. Activity analysis focuses on the identification of activity demands and performance skills. Activity demands include aspects of the activity such as amount of effort, the objects typically used, the space, and social demands of the activity. The analysis

BOX 21.2 Occupational Scale: A Question of Focus

Just as there is little agreement in the field about the definition of activity, there is little agreement about the scope or scale of what actually constitutes an occupation. Hinojosa (Hinojosa, Kramer, Royeen, & Luebben, 2003) captured this dilemma eloquently when he shared his personal reflections about occupation:

> I am uncomfortable with the current trend in the profession to call everything we do as occupation. I personally cannot believe that brushing my teeth or being able to effectively use toilet paper in the bathroom is an occupation. I do believe that they are important purposeful activities. I have come to realize that the combination of these two activities is fundamental to complete personal hygiene occupations. (p. 8)

Hinojosa's concern could be restated as follows:

> Is an occupation a collection of tasks within a broad scope of one's life (cooking) or some of the subtasks within this category (making a meal) or even smaller units (preparing vegetables for the salad)?

Lens	**Example: Cooking**	**Analytical Questions**
Panoramic (Zoom Out)	Making a meal 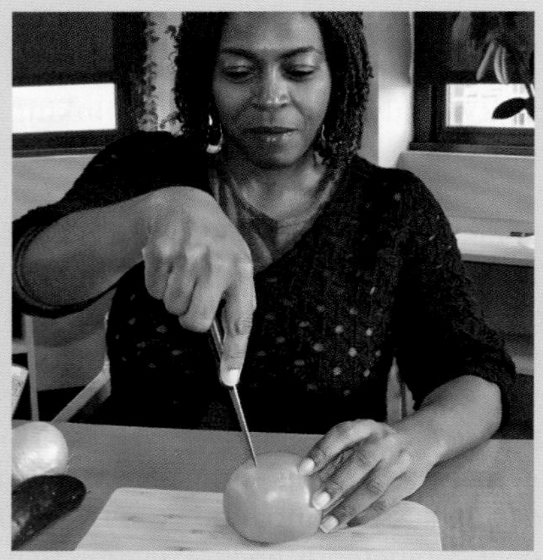	Why does this person cook? What does this person cook? In what settings does the person cook (i.e., home, community center, homeless shelter kitchen)? How often does the person cook? How does it overlap or enfold within other occupations (i.e., is it important in the person's job or to duties to his or her spouse or partner? Can the person do the planning and organization necessary? Does the person have skills to prepare the food? Does the person cook safely? Does the person get each part of the meal done in a timely manner? Is the quality of the result satisfactory to the person and significant others?
	Preparing a salad 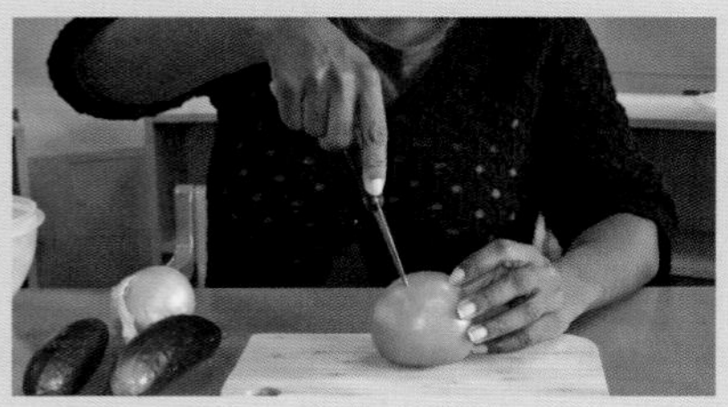	Can the person get the salad ingredients from the refrigerator? Does the person remember to get all of the ingredients and supplies they need? Can the person use a knife safely with different ingredients? Can the person use a knife effectively with all the ingredients? Can the person get the salad to the table? Does the person season it to their own standards and that of those sharing the salad?
Close-Up (Zoom In)	Slicing a tomato 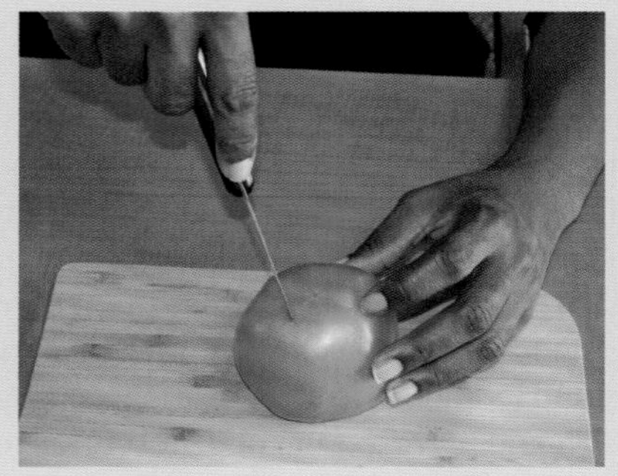	Does the person choose the right utensil to cut the tomato? Can the person grasp the tomato? Does the person hold it too tightly or too loosely? Can the person hold the knife by the handle? Can the person coordinate both hands while holding and cutting the tomato? Does the person know to hold the handle as opposed to the blade? Can the person generate enough force to cut the tomato? Does the person position the knife correctly relative to the tomato? Is the person at risk of being cut? Does the person cut the tomato in the desired shape? Do the tomato slices meet the person's own standards and that of others eating the salad?

BOX 21.2 Occupational Scale: A Question of Focus (*Continued*)

There is little agreement in the field on this issue with scholars proposing a variety of ways to nest the subunits of occupations within the broader category. These include the following:

- Trombly Latham (2008) nests activities within tasks which constitute life roles.
- Polatajko et al (2000) break down occupations into tasks that contain segments, units, and subunits.
- Baum and Christiansen (2005) start with roles, tasks, and actions.
- Fisher (1998) considers the role dimensions of an individual's occupations and places tasks (what the person does) within this category but notes the importance of starting with a person's goals.

The purpose here is to point out the lack of agreement and say that we have no solution to the problem. It is important to recognize that there are varying ways to consider analyzing occupations. Crabtree (1998) uses a metaphor comparing the occupational therapy reasoning process to a camera lens. Sometimes it is important to zoom out to see the big picture and sometimes it is necessary to zoom in to capture the fine details. The depth and scope of analysis is directly related to the client's goals for intervention and the practitioner's reasoning process in responding to these goals, as noted in the example above.

TABLE 21.2 Analysis Format for Activities and Occupations

Scenario: James, a 32-year-old single male, making a sandwich

Activity Analysis	Occupational Analysis	Example of Occupational Analysis
Description		
Describe the activity in one to two sentences.	Briefly describe the occupation. How does the person usually do this occupation and in what settings?	James typically makes a cold cut sandwich with cheese and mayonnaise each weekday morning to bring to work.
Objects used and their properties		
Describe the tools, materials, and equipment typically used. Note the potential symbolism/meaning of the objects in the relevant culture.	Describe the tools, materials, and equipment actually used. Note the symbolism/meaning of the objects to this person.	James uses fresh cold cuts, prepackaged cheese slices, mayonnaise, a store-purchased loaf of bread, a butter knife, a plastic bag, and a paper bag to make and store his lunch. He uses a damp sponge to clean his work space.
Space demands		
Describe the physical environment in which the activity being analyzed is usually performed. Include key aspects, such as the following: • Does this occur in a natural or built environment? • What are the major natural or built structures? • Describe the placement of any furnishings and equipment. • What is the light level? Does it change or is it constant? • Describe the kind and level of noise. How might it impact the activity to be performed? • Describe any other features which may impact the senses (e.g., smell, humidity, texture, temperature) and affect performance. • Is this the typical context for this activity? If not, what other contexts might be appropriate? Briefly describe them, with emphasis on how the other contexts are different.	Describe the actual physical environment in which the occupation will be performed. Consider how the physical environment supports or impedes performance. Include key aspects, such as the following: • Does this occur in a natural or built environment? • What are the major natural or built structures? • How do structures, furnishings and equipment affect the person's performance? • What is the light level and does it change? How does lighting affect performance? • Describe the kind and level of noise, and how it affects performance. • Describe any other features that affect the person's performance (e.g., smell, humidity, texture, temperature). • In addition to the context just described, where else does this person engage in this occupation? Briefly describe all additional contexts, with emphasis on how they are different from the first one described.	James always makes his sandwich in the galley kitchen of his one-bedroom apartment. He keeps the cold cuts and cheese in a bottom left refrigerator drawer and the mayonnaise in the door of the refrigerator. He stores the bread on top of the refrigerator. The knife and storage bags are in adjacent drawers under the counter where he works. The sink including the sponge is directly behind James as he faces his work counter. Due to the small size of his kitchen, all objects are within reach of his countertop work surface. His kitchen is lit by a fluorescent fixture. He keeps the TV on while he does his morning routine to listen to the news.

(*continued*)

TABLE 21.2 Analysis Format for Activities and Occupations (*Continued*)

Activity Analysis	Occupational Analysis	Example of Occupational Analysis
Social demands		
Describe the social and cultural demands or the range of demands that may be required by this activity or elicited by engagement in this activity using the categories listed below. • Describe other people involved in the activity. What is their relationship to each other? What do they expect from each other? • Describe the typical rules, norms, and expectations involved in doing this activity. • Describe the cultural and symbolic meanings typically ascribed to this activity. • Speculate about other social contexts in which the activity might be performed. How might the rules, expectations, and meanings vary from this setting?	Describe the social and cultural demands as the person engages in this occupation using the categories listed below. • Describe other people involved in the occupation. What is their relationship to each other? What do they expect from each other? • Describe the rules, norms, and expectations of this person as he or she engages in this occupation. • Describe the cultural and symbolic meanings that this person and his or her significant others ascribe to this occupation. • Consider all the other social contexts in which the occupation might be performed. How do the rules, expectations, and meanings vary from this setting?	James lives by himself and most typically performs his morning routine alone. Occasionally, a friend may sleep over. On these days, James simultaneously makes a pot of coffee for his guest. If a guest is present, he keeps the TV off so that he can converse with his guest. The kitchen is not conducive to two people working simultaneously, so James takes on full responsibility for the food and drink preparation.
Sequence, timing & patterns		
List the sequential steps (no more than 15) of the activity. Include any timing requirements, such as waiting for glue to dry, bread to rise, etc. • How much flexibility exists in the sequence and timing of the steps of this activity? • Does this activity typically occur or reoccur at a specific time of day? With what frequency? (i.e., daily, weekly, monthly?)	List the sequential steps (no more than 15) of the occupation as the person does it. Include any timing requirements, such as waiting for glue to dry, bread to rise, etc. • How much flexibility exists in the sequence and timing of the steps of this occupation? • Does this occupation typically occur or reoccur at a specific time of day? When and with what frequency? (i.e., daily, weekly, monthly?)	James only makes a lunch sandwich on weekdays because on weekends, he prefers to go out to brunch. Steps include retrieving the bread and placing it on the counter; retrieving the cheese, cold cuts, and mayonnaise from the refrigerator and placing them on the counter; opening the packages and container; retrieving the knife from the drawer; spreading the mayonnaise on both sides of the bread; placing 3 slices of cold cuts and 2 slices of cheese on the bread; folding and cutting the sandwich in half; retrieving the storage bags; placing the sandwich in the plastic bag followed by the paper bag; and restoring and cleaning his workspace by wiping the counter down with a damp sponge.
Required skills (observable actions/performance skills)		
Using the Occupational Therapy Practice Framework, or other published list of skills, identify 5–10 skills critical to activity performance. • Consider skills which demand from the person movement, cognition, sensory and emotional perception as well as communicative and social actions. • Consider skills typically demanded from the applicable environment (physical, social, and virtual).	Using the Occupational Therapy Practice Framework, or other published list of skills, identify 5–10 skills critical to this person's occupational performance. • Consider skills which demand from the person movement, cognition, sensory and emotional perception as well as communicative and social actions. • Consider skills typically demanded from the applicable environment (physical, social, and virtual).	Examples of the skills that James requires include *initiating* the task, *searching for* and *locating* the needed objects, *choosing* the correct objects, *using* the objects appropriately, *bending* and *reaching* for the objects, *manipulating* the objects, *continuing* the task, and knowing when to *terminate* the task.

TABLE 21.2 Analysis Format for Activities and Occupations (*Continued*)

Activity Analysis	Occupational Analysis	Example of Occupational Analysis
Required body structures and functions		
Consider the underlying capacities of the person that are typically required when doing this activity. • Briefly list the body structures (anatomical parts of the body) typically used. • Briefly list the essential body functions (physiological and psychological).	Consider the underlying capacities of the person that are required when doing this occupation in the contexts just identified. • Briefly list the body structures (anatomical parts of the body) the person uses. • Briefly list the essential body functions (physiological and psychological).	Examples of required body structures include all extremities and trunk, including bones, joints, muscle, tendon, eyes, and central and peripheral nervous systems. Examples of body functions include arousal, working memory, sustained attention, praxis, visual acuity, interpreting spatial relationships, problem-solving (e.g.,. if missing an ingredient), tactile feedback, active joint range of motion, muscle strength, and postural alignment and control.
Safety hazards		
List potential safety hazards for this activity. Think especially of children, people with cognitive and judgment problems, people with diminished sensation, etc.	List potential safety hazards for this person as he or she performs this occupation. Consider cognitive and judgment problems, diminished sensation, etc.	Potential hazards include choosing the incorrect knife, using/holding the knife incorrectly (e.g., holding the blade), cutting himself due to poor vision or tactile sensation, falling, leaving the refrigerator open allowing food to spoil, leaving the sink running and having the water overflow.
Adaptability to promote participation		
How much flexibility exists for people to do this activity in different ways? Consider: • Person-based variables (e.g., personal context, impairments) • External contextual variables (physical, social, temporal, virtual, cultural)	How much flexibility exists for this person to do this occupation in different ways? How willing is the person and key stakeholders to consider doing it differently? Consider • Person-based variables (e.g., personal context, impairments) • External contextual variables (physical, social, temporal, virtual, cultural)	James refers to himself as a "creature of habit". His tendency is to make a similar sandwich each day. However, there are days when he does not engage in this occupation but instead buys his lunch on the way to work at his local delicatessen.
Grading		
List three ways to make the task easier in relation to an identified personal or contextual variable.	List three ways to make the occupation easier in relation to an identified personal or contextual variable.	This occupation can be made less challenging regarding organization and sequence skills and/or from an endurance perspective via presetting the work space (e.g.,. placing the bread, knife, and storage bags on the counter prior to beginning the meal preparation, providing James with a list of the necessary steps, labeling the environment, e.g., "silverware drawer").
List three ways to make the task more challenging in relation to an identified personal or contextual variable.	List three ways to make the occupation more challenging in relation to an identified personal or contextual variable.	This occupation can be made more challenging via placing increased demands on balance/postural control, reaching abilities, ideation and organization skills, and selective attentions skills via respectively placing the needed objects out of James's arm span (e.g., paper bags under the sink), placing more objects in the refrigerator to serve as distractors, and providing more environmental stimuli (e.g., turning up the television and discussing current events while James is making the sandwich).

[a]Adapted from American Occupational Therapy Association. (2002). Occupational therapy practice framework: Domain and process. *American Journal of Occupational Therapy, 56,* 609–639; and American Occupational Therapy Association. (2008). Occupational therapy practice framework: Domain and process, 2nd edition. *American Journal of Occupational Therapy, 62*(6), 625–683.

BOX 21.3 Analysis of Occupational Performance

"Occupational performance is the accomplishment of the selected occupation or activity resulting from the dynamic transaction among the client, the context and environment, and the activity."[a] Evaluation of occupational performance involves

- Synthesizing information from the occupational profile to focus on specific areas of occupation and contexts that need to be addressed
- Observing the client's performance in desired occupations and activities, noting effectiveness of the performance skills and performance patterns
- Selecting and using specific assessments to measure performance skills and patterns as appropriate
- Selecting assessments, as needed, to identify and measure more specifically contexts or environments, activity demands, and client factors that are influencing performance skills and performance patterns
- Interpreting the assessment data to identify what supports performance and what hinders performance
- Developing and refining hypotheses about the client's occupational performance strengths and limitations

Following the evaluation of occupational performance, the practitioner then engages in

- Creating goals in collaboration with the client that address the desired outcomes
- Determining procedures to measure the outcomes of intervention
- Delineating potential intervention approach or approaches based on best practice and available evidence

[a]From American Occupational Therapy Association. (2008). Occupational therapy practice framework: Domain and process, 2nd edition. *American Journal of Occupational Therapy,* 62, p. 650.

format also includes consideration of the typically required body structures (e.g., cardiovascular, psychological, and neurological structures) and functions (e.g., attention processes, temperament, joint mobility, gait pattern, emotional regulation) as they relate to the skills often used in the activity. Also included in the analysis are the expected skills that represent the interface between the person and the performance setting (Fisher & Bray Jones, 2010). See Chapter 22 for an in-depth discussion of performance skills.

As part of activity analysis, practitioners may consider the use of the activity as viewed through different theoretical lenses. For instance, a therapist who is working with a population of people with biomechanically related impairments (i.e., hand injuries, back injuries) may analyze activities in terms of the typical strength, range of motion, and endurance required to complete them. Alternatively, someone who is concerned about supporting interpersonal skills in clients with mental illnesses may look primarily at the complexity of social interactions which the activity typically demands (Davidson, 2003). By using the principles of a particular practice theory, occupational therapy practitioners analyze activities as they think about performance strengths and problems addressed by the particular theory. The potential therapeutic intervention should be consistent with the theory and will likely entail the grading and adaptation of the occupations chosen by the client. Table 21.2 presents a format for analysis of activities.

Occupational Analysis

In contrast to activity analysis, occupational analysis *places the person in the foreground* by taking into account the particular person's life experiences, values, interests, and goals. Occupational analysis attends to *the actual* body functions and structures and considers the *actual* performance setting, including physical and social contexts along with the demands of the occupation itself. These considerations shape the practitioner's efforts

BOX 21.4 Ways Activity and Occupational Analysis Inform Practice

Practitioners analyze activity in the abstract for the following reasons:

- To understand the therapeutic potential of a wide range of activities
- To identify activities which lend themselves to
  a. Improving client performance through acquiring new skills or learning adaptive strategies
  b. Restoring a skill or client factor that impacts performance skills
  c. Prevention of future problems by changing or adapting activity demands or performance context

Practitioners analyze the occupations of their clients to

- Evaluate the quality of current performance in valued occupations and the client's effectiveness in orchestrating their occupations
- Determine the impact of personal factors (including health condition) on current performance
- Determine the impact of contextual factors on current performance
- Prognosticate future performance in identified contexts
- Identify ways to grade or adapt occupations to foster improved performance

to help the person reach his or her goals through carefully designed evaluation and intervention. Practitioners vary the scope of the occupational analysis depending on the nature of the client's concerns, occupational performance challenges, health problems, and the nature of the intervention setting.

As discussed earlier, occupational analysis may be focused on a particular occupation, such as using a keyboard on the computer or brushing one's teeth, or it may be focused on a broader scope of how individuals orchestrate numerous aspects of occupational performance into daily life, such as being an effective worker. Two approaches to analyzing occupations which vary by the scope of the client's concerns are illustrated.

- **Occupational analysis:** Analysis of occupations parallels activity analysis, with the important difference that it is examining an actual occupation that the person does in his or her own unique way. Questions used for occupational analysis are found in the middle column of Table 21.2.
- **Analysis of occupational orchestration:** Table 21.3 illustrates ways to consider how individuals engage and manage their multiple occupations.

TABLE 21.3 Analysis of Orchestration of Occupations

Analysis of Orchestration of Occupations	
Occupations	Identify the occupations that are central to the person's identity. List these occupations.
Meaning	• How meaningful are these occupations to the individual? • How central are the occupations to the person's identity? • How important are the occupations to the individual? • How important is the occupation to others in the person's social world (family, friends, coworkers, etc.)?
Purpose	What purpose(s) does each occupation serve in the individual's life? (e.g., self-maintenance, health, support to family, support to friends or others, contribution to community, play or leisure, work).
Level of Skill and Efficiency	For each occupation, does the individual believe that he or she is able to do this occupation at an appropriate level of skill within the expected timelines? • If not, what are the problems/concerns from the individual's perspective? • If not, what are the problems/concerns from the perspective of people in the individual's social world?
Routines	Identify the pattern in which the individual engages in these occupations. • What occupations occur daily? • What occupations occur weekly? • What occupations occur monthly and annually? • Describe a typical day. • Describe a typical week.
Organization of Routines	To what extent is the daily and weekly pattern of occupations routinized (patterns of behavior that are observable, regular, repetitive, and provide structure for daily life. Routines and occupations with established sequences)? • Is the individual satisfied with this level of organization? If not, why not? • To what extent do these routines meet the expectations of family, friends, and coworkers? • Are these expectations reasonable given the person's physical and emotional capacities, and expectations from the context, family, friends, and employers? • Describe the degree to which these routines are disorganized, stable, or hyperstable.
Adaptability to Promote Participation	To what extent are the occupations and/or routines flexible based on: • Individual-based variables: personal context, impairments, openness to change? • Expectations from social environment (family, friends, coworkers)? • Environmental adaptability (potential to change physical environment to promote increased participation)?
Needs	Describe the extent to which the occupational routine is sufficient to meet the person's needs and the needs of those in his or her social world. This might include attention to occupational deprivation or overload. Describe the changes required to meet the individual's needs: • Changes in the individual (skill development) • Changes in the social environment (expectations for performance) • Changes in the occupation (adapting or grading to promote more effective performance)

TABLE 21.4 Analysis of Personal Factors That May Support or Impede Performance

Activity to be analyzed: *Morning Self-Care*

Body Function	Support For Effective and Efficient Occupational Performance	Impairment of Body Function Resulting in Occupational Error
Praxis	Understands the concept of a morning routine, knows how to use tools (comb, razor, socks, etc.), is able to organize and sequence the steps of the task and to plan movements.	Apraxia: Uses the comb to brush teeth; improperly sequences the steps of dressing (socks on top of shoes); unable to plan movements related to donning pants, resulting in clumsy and inefficient movements.
Visuospatial processing	Judges depth and distance, orients clothing properly to body, differentiates foreground from background such as finding a bar of white soap on a white sink.	Spatial relations impairment: Spills toothpaste when attempting to squeeze it on to the brush, dons shirt backwards, unable to differentiate sleeves from the body of shirt.
Arousal/attention	Alert, stays on task, disregards irrelevant environmental stimuli, attends to stimuli in both the right and left attentional fields.	Arousal/attention deficits: Falls asleep, gets distracted by television and stops dressing before completing the task, does not attend to clothing hanging on the left side of the closet.
Motor control	Controls posture to stand at the sink, bends to retrieve shoes from the floor, reaches into the closet for a tie, coordinates movements to brush teeth.	Impaired motor control: Leans to the left while standing at the sink, loses balance while bending or reaching for clothing, trembles while reaching for brush, can't reverse movements for efficient tooth brushing.
Affect	Motivated to engage in tasks, able to tolerate frustrations that arise, show affect appropriate to situation and task.	Affective disturbance: requires coaxing and encouragement to participate in and continue morning care, easily frustrated and terminates task, moods shift rapidly during performance.

Data from Árnadóttir, G. (1990). *The brain and behavior: Assessing cortical dysfunction through activities of daily living.* St. Louis, MO: Elsevier/Mosby; and Árnadóttir, G. (2011). Impact of neurobehavioral deficits on activities of daily living. In G. Gillen (Ed.), Stroke rehabilitation: A function-based approach (3rd ed., pp. 456-500). St. Louis, MO: Elsevier/Mosby.

Analysis of Occupational Performance Skills

Occupational therapy practitioners apply the analytic processes just described when observing individuals as they engage in their desired occupations. This may range from observing a student in the classroom or on the playground, a person working in an office or factory, an older adult in a leisure setting or an assisted living facility, or a homeless person at a shelter. In all these situations, the practitioner's attention is on the dynamic transaction of the person's occupational performance within the performance environment and context. Although the practitioner must be concerned with the quality of the results, the major focus is on the process of engagement. Thus, practitioners become adept at carefully observing skills associated with occupational performance. These performance skills are the smallest observable units of occupational performance; goal-directed actions a person carries out one by one during naturalistic and relevant daily life task performances (Fisher & Bray Jones, 2010). See Chapter 22 for an in-depth discussion of performance skills.

Analysis of Personal Factors That Impede or Support Performance

Occupational therapy practitioners may also analyze chosen occupations from a micro perspective in terms of how the presence, absence, or impairment of body functions support or limit occupational performance. Árnadóttir (2011) suggests that the therapist can use occupational analysis to detect occupational errors via skilled observation of occupational performance. She further states that these errors may indicate the effect of neurobehavioral deficits on task performance. Subsequently, the therapist can hypothesize about the impaired body functions that caused the error. "Therapists can benefit from detecting errors in occupational performance while observing activities of daily living and thereby gain an understanding of the impairments affecting the patient's activity limitation. Therapists can use the information based on observed task performance in a systematic way as a structure for clinical reasoning to help them assess functional independence related to the performance and to subsequently detect impaired neurologic body functions" (p. 462). The approach suggested by Árnadóttir can be expanded to include musculoskeletal impairments, psychological impairments, and so forth (see Table 21.4). See Chapter 19 for in-depth discussion of personal factors.

Conclusion

This chapter describes two types of analyses: activity analysis and occupational analysis. Use of these analyses requires practitioners to understand the following:

- The general properties and demands of activities as they are customarily performed in given arenas and cultures

- How to select activities that are occupationally relevant to clients
- How to use occupations valued by clients to achieve their goals as occupational beings

These core skills are critical for effective occupational therapy evaluation and intervention. Both processes ultimately center on occupation and its capacity to motivate people to act and to create meaning in their lives. Brockelman (1980), a philosopher, recognized the importance of occupation in the following statement: "The tools of our minds and the tools of our hands are of meaningless use without deep and personal reasons of the heart to set their purpose and guide their use" (p. 24). It is through practitioners' deep understanding of people as occupational beings that effective occupational therapy intervention occurs.

References

Allen, C. K. (1987). Activity, occupational therapy's treatment method. 1987 Eleanor Clarke Slagle lecture. *American Journal of Occupational Therapy, 41*, 563–575.

American Occupational Therapy Association. (2002). Occupational therapy practice framework: Domain and process. *American Journal of Occupational Therapy, 56*, 609–639.

American Occupational Therapy Association. (2008). Occupational therapy practice framework: Domain and process, 2nd edition. *American Journal of Occupational Therapy, 62*, 625–683.

Árnadóttir, G. (1990). *The brain and behavior: Assessing cortical dysfunction through activities of daily living.* St. Louis, MO: Elsevier/Mosby.

Árnadóttir, G. (2011). Impact of neurobehavioral deficits on activities of daily living. In G. Gillen (Ed.), *Stroke rehabilitation: A function-based approach* (3rd ed., pp. 456–500). St. Louis, MO: Elsevier/Mosby.

Bauerschmidt, B., & Nelson, D. L. (2011). The terms occupation and activity over the history of official occupational therapy publications. *American Journal of Occupational Therapy, 65*, 338–345.

Baum, C. M., & Christiansen, C. H. (2005). Person-environment-occupation-performance: An occupation-based framework for practice. In C. H. Christiansen, C. M. Baum, & J. Bass-Haugen (Eds.), *Occupational therapy: Performance, participation, and well-being* (3rd ed., pp. 243–266). Thorofare, NJ: SLACK Incorporated.

Brockelman, P. T. (1980). *Existential phenomenology and the world of ordinary experience: An introduction.* Lanham, MD: University Press of America.

Bruner, J. (1990). *Acts of meaning.* Cambridge, MA: Harvard University Press.

Christiansen, C. H., & Baum, C. M. (2005). The complexity of human occupation. In C. H. Christiansen, C. M. Baum, & J. Bass-Haugen (Eds.). *Occupational therapy: Performance, participation, and well-being* (3rd ed., pp. 4–23). Thorofare, NJ: SLACK Incorporated.

Clarke, F. A., Parham, D., Carlson, M. E., Frank, G., Jackson, J., Pierce, D., . . . Zemke, R. (1991). Occupational science: Academic innovation in the service of occupational therapy's future. *American Journal of Occupational Therapy, 45*, 300–310.

Coster, W. (1998). Occupation-centered assessment of children. *American Journal of Occupational Therapy, 52*, 337–344.

Crabtree, M. (1998). Images of reasoning: A literature review. *Australian Occupational Therapy Journal, 45*, 113–123.

Crepeau, E. B. (1991). Achieving intersubjective understanding: Examples from an occupational therapy treatment session. *American Journal of Occupational Therapy, 45*, 1016–1025.

Crepeau, E. B., & Garren, K. R. (2011). I looked to her as a guide: The therapeutic relationship in hand therapy. *Disability and Rehabilitation, 33*, 872–881.

Cynkin, S. (1995). Activities. In C. B. Royeen (Ed.), *AOTA self-study series: The practice of the future: Putting occupation back into therapy* (Module 7; pp. 1–52). Rockville, MD: American Occupational Therapy Association.

Davidson, L. (2003). *Living outside mental illness: Qualitative studies of recovery in schizophrenia.* New York, NY: New York University Press.

Dunn, W., Brown, C., & Youngstrom, M. J. (2003). Ecological model of occupation. In P. Kramer, J. Hinojosa, & C. B. Royeen (Eds.). *Perspectives in human occupation: Participation in life* (pp. 222–263). Philadelphia, PA: Lippincott Williams & Wilkins.

Fisher, A. G. (1998). Uniting practice and theory in an occupational framework. 1998 Eleanor Clarke Slagle Lecture. *American Journal of Occupational Therapy, 52*, 509–521.

Fisher, A. G., & Bray Jones, K. (2010). *Assessment of Motor and Process Skills. Vol. 1: Development, standardization, and administration manual* (7th ed.). Fort Collins, CO: Three Star Press.

Frankl, V. E. (1959). *Man's search for meaning: An introduction to logotherapy.* New York, NY: Pocket Books.

Hagendorn, R. (2000). Glossary. In R. Hagendorn (Ed.), *Tools for practice in occupational therapy: A structured approach to core skills and processes* (pp. 307–312). Edinburgh, United Kingdom: Churchill Livingstone.

Hasselkus, B. R. (2002). *The meaning of everyday occupation.* Thorofare, NJ: SLACK Incorporated.

Hinojosa, J., & Kramer, P. (1997). Statement—Fundamental concepts of occupational therapy: Occupation, purposeful activity, and function. *American Journal of Occupational Therapy, 51*, 864–866.

Hinojosa, J., Kramer, P., Royeen, C. B., & Luebben, A. J. (2003). Core concept of occupation. In P. Kramer, J. Hinojosa, & C. B. Royeen (Eds.). *Perspectives in human occupation* (pp. 1–17). Philadelphia, PA: Lippincott Williams & Wilkins.

Hocking, C. (2001). Implementing occupation-based assessment. *American Journal of Occupational Therapy, 55*, 463–469.

Hymes, D. (1972). Toward ethnographies of communication: The analysis of communicative events. In P. P. Giglioli (Ed.), *Language and social context* (pp. 21–44). New York, NY: Pelican.

Jackson, J. (1998a). Contemporary criticisms of role theory. *Journal of Occupational Science, 5*, 49–55.

Jackson, J. (1998b). Is there a place for role theory in occupational science? *Journal of Occupational Science, 5*, 56–65.

Kielhofner, G., & Barrett, L. (1998). Meaning and misunderstanding in occupational forms: A study of therapeutic goal setting. *American Journal of Occupational Therapy, 52*, 345–353.

Kronenberg, F., Pollard, N., & Ramugondo, E. (2011). Introduction: Courage to dance politics. In F. Kronenberg, N. Pollard, & Sakellariou, D. (Eds.), *Occupational therapies without borders – Vol. 2: Towards an ecology of occupation-based practices* (pp. 1–16). New York, NY: Churchill-Livingstone Elsevier.

Larson, E. A. (2000). The orchestration of occupation: The dance of mothers. *American Journal of Occupational Therapy, 54*, 269–280.

Lave, J. (1988). *Cognition in practice: Mind, mathematics and culture in everyday life.* Cambridge, United Kingdom: Cambridge University Press.

Law, M. (Ed.). (1998). *Client-centered occupational therapy.* Thorofare, NJ: SLACK Incorporated.

Law, M., Polatajko, H., Baptiste, W., & Townsend, E. (1997). Core concepts in occupational therapy. In E. Townsend (Ed.), *Enabling occupation: An occupational therapy perspective* (pp. 29–56). Ottawa, ON: Canadian Association of Occupational Therapists.

Llorens, L. A. (1986). Activity analysis: Agreement among factors in a sensory processing model. *American Journal of Occupational Therapy, 40*, 103–110.

Mattingly, C., & Fleming, M. H. (1994). *Clinical reasoning: Forms of inquiry in a therapeutic practice.* Philadelphia, PA: F. A. Davis.

Mosey, A. C. (1981). *Occupational therapy: Configuration of a profession.* New York, NY: Raven Press.

Neistadt, M. E., McAuley, D., Zecha, D., & Shannon, R. (1993). An analysis of a board game as a treatment activity. *American Journal of Occupational Therapy, 47*, 154–160.

Nelson, D. J., & Jebson-Thomas, J. (2003). Occupational form, occupational performance, and a conceptual framework for therapeutic occupation. In P. Kramer, J. Hinojosa, & C. Brasic Royeen (Eds.), *Perspectives in human occupation: Participation in life* (pp. 87–155). Philadelphia, PA: Lippincott Williams & Wilkins.

Payne, R. K., DeVol, P., & Dreussi Smith, T. (2001). *Bridges out of poverty: Strategies for Professionals and Communities* (Rev. ed.). Highland, TX: Aha Process.

Peloquin, S. M. (1995). The fullness of empathy: Reflections and illustrations. *American Journal of Occupational Therapy, 49*, 24–31.

Peloquin, S. M. (2005). Embracing our ethos: Reclaiming our heart. The 2005 Eleanor Clarke Slagle Lecture. *American Journal of Occupational Therapy, 59*, 611–625.

Peloquin, S. M. (2007). The issue is: A reconsideration of occupational therapy's core values. *American Journal of Occupational Therapy, 61*, 474–478.

Pierce, D. (2001). Untangling occupation and activity. *American Journal of Occupational Therapy, 55*, 138–146.

Polatajko, H. J., Mandich, A., & Martini, R. (2000). Dynamic performance analysis: A framework for understanding occupational performance. *American Journal of Occupational Therapy, 54*, 65–72.

Reed, K. L. (2005). An annotated history of the concepts used in occupational therapy. In C. H. Christiansen, C. M. Baum, and J. Bass-Haugen (Eds.), *Occupational therapy: Performance, participation, and well-being* (3rd ed., pp. 567–626). Thorofare, NJ: SLACK Incorporated.

Schell, B. A. (2008). Pragmatic reasoning. In B. A. B. Schell & J. W. Schell (Eds.), *Clinical and professional reasoning in occupational therapy* (pp. 169–187). Philadelphia, PA: Lippincott Williams & Wilkins.

Schell, B. A., & Cervero, R. M. (1993). Clinical reasoning in occupational therapy: An integrative review. *American Journal of Occupational Therapy, 47*, 605–610.

Spear, P. S., & Crepeau, E. B. (2003). Glossary. In E. B. Crepeau, E. S. Cohn, & B. A. Boyt Schell (Eds.), *Willard & Spackman's occupational therapy* (10th ed., pp. 1025–1035). Philadelphia, PA: Lippincott Williams & Wilkins.

Trombly, C. A. (1995). Occupation, purposefulness and meaningfulness as therapeutic mechanisms. 1995 Eleanor Clarke Slagle Lecture. *American Journal of Occupational Therapy, 49*, 960–972.

Trombly Latham, C. A. (2008). Conceptual foundations for practice. In M. V. Radomski & C. A. Trombly Latham (Eds.), *Occupational therapy for physical dysfunction* (6th ed., pp. 1–20). Baltimore, MD: Lippincott Williams & Wilkins.

Zemke R., & Clark, F. (1996). *Occupational science: The evolving discipline*. Philadelphia, PA: F. A. Davis.

For additional resources on the subjects discussed in this chapter, visit http://thePoint.lww.com/Willard-Spackman12e.

CHAPTER 22

Performance Skills

Implementing Performance Analyses to Evaluate Quality of Occupational Performance

Anne G. Fisher, Lou Ann Griswold

LEARNING OBJECTIVES

After reading this chapter, you will be able to:

1. Describe the difference between (1) performance skills and (2) body functions
2. Implement an analysis of performance skills (performance analysis) and document a person's baseline quality of occupational performance
3. Describe how the results of a performance analysis are used to collaboratively establish client-centered goals

OUTLINE

Introduction to Performance Skills

Performance skills are the smallest observable actions or units of occupational performance that we can observe as a person carries out his or her daily life tasks. Noting the degree of performance skill that can be observed is critical for evaluating the quality of a person's occupational performance. Consider, for example, what Karla observes as she watches Maurice perform daily life tasks (see Case Study 22.1).

In Case Study 22.1, Karla evaluated the quality of Maurice's occupational performance by observing the small goal-directed actions Maurice enacted one by one as he engaged in relevant and meaningful daily life task performances. More specifically, she observed the quality of his occupational **performance skills** (Fisher, 2009; Fisher & Kielhofner, 1995; Kielhofner, 2008). Kielhofner (2008) referred to these observable performance skills as "discrete purposeful actions [that] can be discerned" (p. 103). Performance skills are links in a larger chain of actions, which link by link, action by action, become the whole chain—the task performance (Fisher, 2009) (see Figure 22.1).

The term *performance skills* has been used to refer to these smallest observable units of occupational performance because each person we evaluate demonstrates more or less occupational skill when he or she completes (i.e., "constructs") a daily life task performance. These small units of observable actions were first conceptualized in the mid-1980s

CASE STUDY 22.1 Performance Skills—Observable Chains of Goal-directed Actions

Karla, Maurice's occupational therapist, observes him as he is engaged in preparing himself a glass of orange juice and a bowl of cereal. As she observes his occupational performance **motor skills**, she observes that he momentarily props (*stabilizes*) on the kitchen counter as he *walks* to the refrigerator. He then *bends* forward, *reaches* out, and grasps (*grips*) the handle on the door of the refrigerator without any evidence of clumsiness or increased physical effort. When he attempts to open the door of the refrigerator (*moves*), he does not pull hard enough (*calibrates*)—the door does not open. She then observes him as he pulls again (*moves, calibrates*) on the handle of the refrigerator door and, this time, she sees the refrigerator door open. Karla then observes that Maurice effectively *reaches* in, *grips* a container of orange juice, *lifts* it, and takes it out of the refrigerator, but that he is somewhat unstable (*stabilizes*) when he *walks* and *transports* the container of juice over to the counter where he has placed a glass.

As Karla observes Maurice as he is engaged in preparing his breakfast, she also observes his occupational performance **process skills**. For example, Karla observes that although Maurice *initiates* most task actions without a delay, he pauses momentarily before reaching for the handle of the refrigerator door. She also sees that he *continues* each action through to completion without any unnecessary pauses (e.g., continuing pulling on the refrigerator door until it is open, continuing walking until the orange juice is transported to the counter). As Maurice *initiates* pouring orange juice into the glass on the counter, he again pauses. Moreover, Karla observes that he does not *terminate* pouring the orange juice before some orange juice spills over the rim of the glass. She also observes that Maurice performs task actions in a logical order (*sequences*). For example, she observes that he opens the lid of the orange juice container and then pours juice into the glass and not vice versa. Finally, she observes Maurice as he *searches* for and *locates* the orange juice container in the refrigerator, *chooses* orange juice, *gathers* the orange juice container to the same workspace where he has placed the glass, and *organizes* his workspace effectively—not too crowded, not too spread out.

Later, as Karla observes Maurice as he is engaged in a social exchange with his care provider, Joyce—planning the weekly meals and making a shopping list—she observes Maurice's **social interaction skills**. More specifically, she observes that he readily *approaches* his social partner and *starts* a conversation. As he does so, and throughout the social exchange, Maurice *turns toward*, but frequently does not *look* at his social partner when they are talking to each other. As Maurice is talking, she observes that he *produces speech* that is clearly audible and that he *gesticulates* by nodding his head and smiling in a manner that is socially appropriate. She also observes that Maurice often stammers and pauses during his spoken messages (*speaks fluently*), and that he occasionally starts messages but leaves them "hanging in the air" and never finishes them (*times duration*). When Joyce asks Maurice questions (e.g., "What would you like to eat this week?"), he frequently *replies* with messages that are markedly irrelevant to the ongoing conversation (e.g., "My son called me last night."). Finally, Karla observes Maurice as he *takes turns* with his social partner, and that he frequently "talks over" and interrupts his social partner (*times response*).

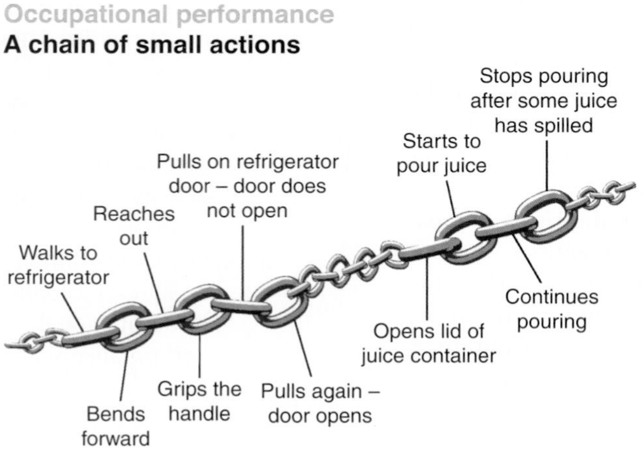

FIGURE 22.1 Performance skills: Smallest observable units of occupational performance—links in a chain of ongoing actions that a person performs one by one as he or she "constructs" the overall daily life task performance. (Adapted from Fisher, A. G. [2009]. *Occupational Therapy Intervention Process Model: A model for planning and implementing top–down, client-centered, and occupation-based interventions.* Fort Collins, CO: Three Star Press. Reprinted with permission.)

(Fisher, 2006), and they have now been incorporated into major occupational therapy models of practice, including the Model of Human Occupation (Kielhofner, 1995, 2008) and the Occupational Therapy Intervention Process Model (Fisher, 1998, 2009). They were also included in the first edition of the Occupational Therapy Practice Framework (American Occupational Therapy Association [AOTA], 2002). The smallest observable actions of occupational performance have been variously referred to as *performance skills* (AOTA, 2002; Fisher, 2006; Fisher & Kielhofner, 1995), *performance units* (Hagedorn, 2000), *units* or *subunits of occupational performance* (Fisher, 2006; Polatajko, Mandich, & Martini, 2000), *occupational skill* (Kielhofner, 2008), and *actions of performance* (Fisher, 1998). Within the *International Classification of Functioning, Disability, and Health* (ICF) (World Health Organization [WHO], 2001), performance skills are analogous to the smaller discrete actions that are part of larger task performances defined within the "Activities and Participation" domains. In all of these instances, performance skills have been clearly differentiated from underlying body functions.

Differentiation between Performance Skills and Body Functions

Body functions pertain to *what the person's body systems do* (see Chapter 19). Examples of body functions include memory, motor planning and praxis skill, perceptual skill, joint mobility, muscle power, fine motor coordination, and emotional regulation. In contrast, performance skills pertain to *what the person does* as he or she interacts with task objects (e.g., *swing* a baseball bat and *hit* a baseball, *jump* rope, *choose* a pencil and *use* it to *write*) in the context of engagement in meaningful occupation (playing baseball with friends, jumping rope with classmates, completing a schoolwork task) (see Figure 22.2). When a person is engaged in occupation that includes social interaction with others, it also becomes possible to observe social interaction skills (*greet* one's friends, *laugh* at a friend's joke) (see the "Commentary on the Evidence" box).

As shown in Figure 22.2, person factors and body functions are not the same thing as performance skills. Although body functions (as well as task and environmental demands) can support or hinder quality of occupational performance, body functions and performance skills represent different constructs. Swinging a bat and hitting a ball may be supported by the person having strength and coordination, but being strong and coordinated does not mean that the person can skillfully swing a bat and hit a ball. Moreover, people can demonstrate occupational skill despite having impairments of their body functions.

Origin of Performance Skills

The concept of performance skills—the goal-directed actions a person carries out one by one during

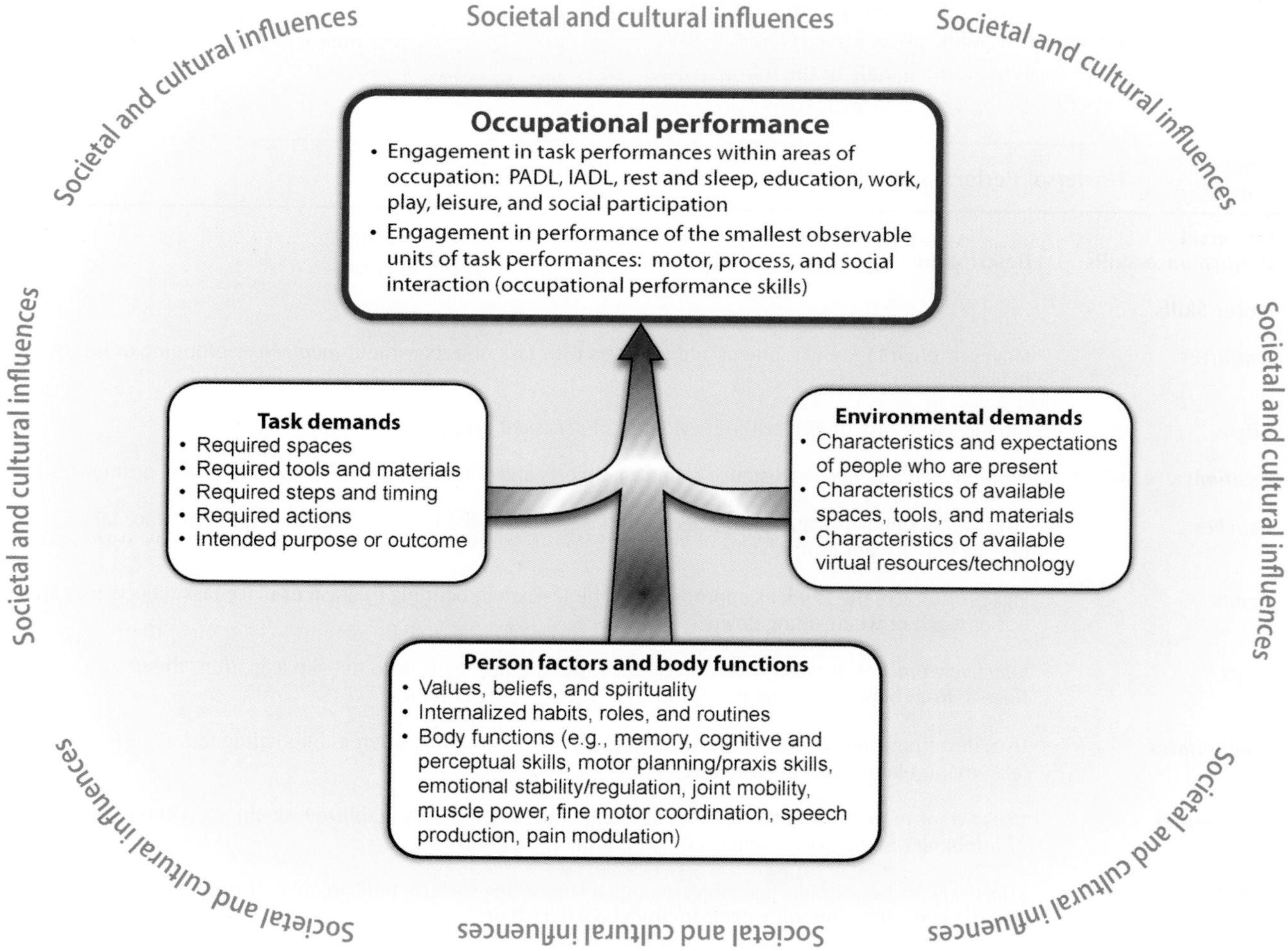

FIGURE 22.2 Schematic representation of occupational performance unfolding as a transaction among person factors and body functions, task demands, environmental demands, and societal and cultural influences. *IADL*, instrumental activities of daily living; *PADL*, personal activities of daily living. (Adapted from Fisher, A. G. [2009]. *Occupational Therapy Intervention Process Model: A model for planning and implementing top–down, client-centered, and occupation-based interventions.* Fort Collins, CO: Three Star Press. Reprinted with permission.)

Commentary on the Evidence

Performance Skills Cannot Be Equated with Body Functions

Many respected authors within occupational therapy equate performance skills with body functions. That is, (1) process skills are sometimes referred to as cognitive skills; and/or (2) motor planning, executive functions, and perceptual skills are considered to be performance skills. One such example is the second edition of the Occupational Therapy Practice Framework (AOTA, 2008). Within the framework, performance skills are described as including motor and praxis skills, sensory-perceptual skills, emotional regulation skills, cognitive skills, and communication and social skills. When compared to Figure 22.2, one can readily see a discrepancy. In both Figure 22.2 and within the ICF (WHO, 2001), praxis skill (i.e., motor planning), perceptual skill, cognitive skill, and emotional regulation are viewed as underlying body functions, not performance skills.

What is the evidence to support the differentiation between performance skills and these underlying body functions? One such resource comes from Rexroth, Fisher, Merritt, and Gliner (2005) who implemented a study where they compared the level of motor and process skill between 1,939 persons with right hemispheric strokes and 1,939 persons with left hemispheric strokes. If we compare these two groups, persons who have had right hemispheric strokes are much more likely to demonstrate visual perceptual impairments and unilateral neglect, whereas persons who have had left hemispheric strokes are much more likely to demonstrate aphasia and apraxia (Bartels, Duffy, & Beland, 2011). These are impairments of body functions.

If performance skills, specifically motor and process skills, are to be equated with praxis and perceptual skill, it should follow that persons with right versus left hemispheric stroke will differ significantly in terms of their levels of motor and/or process skill. Yet, Rexroth et al. (2005) found that there was no significant difference between the two groups in any of the 36 motor and process skills studied. These results indicate that performance analysis, focused on performance skill (i.e., the person's observed quality of doing), is very different from assessment methods focused on underlying body functions (see **Table 22.1** for a list of the 36 performance skills they compared).

TABLE 22.1 Universal Performance Skills

Universal Performance Skills	Description
Motor Skills	
Stabilizes	Moves through task environment and interacts with task objects without *momentary* propping or loss of balance
Aligns	Interacts with task objects without evidence of *persistent* propping or *persistent* leaning
Positions	Positions self an effective distance from task objects and without evidence of awkward body positions
Reaches	Effectively extends the arm and, when appropriate, bends the trunk to effectively grasp or place task objects that are out of reach
Bends	Flexes or rotates the trunk as appropriate to the task when bending to grasp or place task objects that are out of reach or when sitting down
Grips	Effectively pinches or grasps task objects such that the task objects do not slip (e.g., from the person's fingers, from between the teeth)
Manipulates	Uses dexterous finger movements, without evidence of fumbling, when manipulating task objects (e.g., manipulating buttons when buttoning)
Coordinates	Uses two or more body parts together to manipulate, hold, and/or stabilize task objects without evidence of fumbling task objects or objects slipping from one's grasp
Moves	Effectively pushes or pulls task objects along a supporting surface, pulls to open or pushes to close doors and drawers, or pushes on wheels to propel a wheelchair
Lifts	Effectively raises or lifts task objects without evidence of increased effort
Walks	During the task performance, ambulates on level surfaces without shuffling the feet, instability, propping, or use of assistive devices
Transports	Carries task objects from one place to another while walking or moving in a wheelchair

TABLE 22.1 Universal Performance Skills (*Continued*)

Universal Performance Skills	Description
Calibrates	Uses movements of appropriate force, speed, or extent when interacting with task objects (e.g., not crushing task objects, pushing a door with enough force that it closes)
Flows	Uses smooth and fluid arm and wrist movements when interacting with task objects
Endures	Persists and completes the task without *obvious* evidence of physical fatigue, pausing to rest, or stopping to "catch one's breath"
Paces	Maintains a consistent and effective rate or tempo of performance throughout the entire task
Process Skills	
Paces	Maintains a consistent and effective rate or tempo of performance throughout the entire task
Attends	Does not look away from what he or she is doing, thus interrupting the ongoing task progression
Heeds	Carries out and completes the task originally agreed on or specified by another
Chooses	Selects necessary and appropriate type and number of tools and materials for the task, including the tools and materials that the person was directed to use or specified he or she would use
Uses	Employs tools and materials as they are intended (e.g., using a pencil sharpener to sharpen a pencil, but not to sharpen a crayon) and in a hygienic fashion
Handles	Supports or stabilizes tools and materials in an appropriate manner, protecting them from damage, slipping, moving, or falling
Inquires	(1) Seeks needed verbal or written information by asking questions or reading directions or labels and (2) does *not* ask for information in situations where the person had been fully oriented to the task and environment and had immediate prior awareness of the answer
Initiates	Starts or begins *the next* action or step without hesitation
Continues	Performs single actions or steps without interruptions, such that once an action or task step is initiated, the individual continues on without pauses or delays until the action or step is completed
Sequences	Performs steps in an effective or logical order and with an absence of (1) randomness or lack of logic in the ordering and/or (2) inappropriate repetition of steps
Terminates	Brings to completion *single actions* or *single steps* without inappropriate persistence or premature cessation
Searches/Locates	Looks for and locates tools and materials in a logical manner, both within and beyond the immediate environment
Gathers	Collects together *related* tools and materials into the same workspace and "regathers" tools or materials that have spilled, fallen, or been misplaced
Organizes	Logically positions or spatially arranges tools and materials in an orderly fashion within a single workspace and between multiple appropriate workspaces, such that the workspace is not too spread out or too crowded
Restores	Puts away tools and materials in appropriate places and ensures that the immediate workspace is restored to its original condition
Navigates	Moves the arm, body, or wheelchair without bumping into obstacles when moving in the task environment or interacting with task objects
Notices/Responds	Responds appropriately to (1) nonverbal task-related cues (e.g., heat, movement), (2) the spatial arrangement and alignment of task objects to one another, and (3) cupboard doors or drawers that have been left open during the task performance
Adjusts	Effectively (1) goes to new workspaces; (2) moves tools and materials out of the current workspace; and (3) adjusts knobs, dials, or water taps to overcome problems with ongoing task performance
Accommodates	Prevents ineffective task performance
Benefits	Prevents problems with task performance from recurring or persisting

(*continued*)

TABLE 22.1 Universal Performance Skills (*Continued*)

Universal Performance Skills	Description
Social Interaction Skills	
Approaches/Starts	Approaches and/or initiates interaction with the social partner in a manner that is socially appropriate
Concludes/ Disengages	Effectively terminates the conversation or social interaction, brings to closure the topic under discussion, and disengages or says goodbye
Produces speech	Produces spoken, signed, or augmentative (i.e., computer generated) messages that are audible and clearly articulated
Gesticulates	Uses socially appropriate gestures to communicate or support a message
Speaks fluently	Speaks in a fluent and continuous manner, with an even flow (not too fast, not too slow), and without pauses or delays *during* the message being sent
Turns toward	Actively positions or turns the body and the face toward the social partner or the person who is speaking
Looks	Makes eye contact with the social partner
Places self	Places oneself at an appropriate distance from the social partner during the social interaction
Touches	Responds to and uses touch or bodily contact with the social partner in a manner that is socially appropriate
Regulates	Does not demonstrate irrelevant, repetitive, or impulsive behaviors that are not part of social interaction
Questions	Requests relevant facts and information and asks questions that support the intended purpose of the social interaction (e.g., asking about the social partner's opinions)
Replies	Keeps conversation going by replying appropriately to questions and comments
Discloses	Reveals opinions, feelings, and private information *about oneself* or *others* in a manner that is socially appropriate
Expresses emotion	Displays affect and emotions in a way that is socially appropriate
Disagrees	Expresses differences of opinion in a socially appropriate manner
Thanks	Uses appropriate words and gestures to acknowledge receipt of services, gifts, and/or compliments
Transitions	Smoothly transitions the conversation and/or changes the topic without disrupting the ongoing conversation
Times response	Replies to social messages without delay or hesitation and without interrupting the social partner
Times duration	Speaks for reasonable time periods given the complexity of the message sent
Takes turns	Takes one's turn and gives the social partner the freedom to take his or her turn
Matches language	Uses a tone of voice, dialect, and level of language that is socially appropriate and matched to the social partner's abilities and level of understanding
Clarifies	Responds to gestures or verbal messages signaling that the social partner does not comprehend or understand a message and ensures that the social partner is "following" the conversation
Acknowledges/ Encourages	Acknowledges receipt of messages, encourages the social partner to continue interaction, and encourages all social partners to participate in social interaction
Empathizes	Expresses a supportive attitude toward the social partner by agreeing with, empathizing with, or expressing understanding of the social partner's feelings and experiences
Heeds	Uses goal-directed social interactions that are focused toward carrying out and completing the intended purpose of the social interaction
Accommodates	Prevents ineffective or socially inappropriate social interaction
Benefits	Prevents problems with ineffective or socially inappropriate social interaction from recurring or persisting

Adapted from Fisher, A. G. (2009). *Occupational Therapy Intervention Process Model: A model for planning and implementing top–down, client-centered, and occupation-based interventions*. Fort Collins, CO: Three Star Press. Reprinted with permission.

naturalistic and relevant daily life task performances—emerged as a result of an ongoing dialog between persons from different occupational therapy traditions who were struggling to better understand the difference between underlying body functions and performance skills. One of those persons was Gary Kielhofner who came from a background within the occupational behavior tradition. The other was Anne Fisher, the first author of this chapter, an occupational therapist with a background in sensory integration, neuropsychological disorders, neurological disorders, and motor control theories.

The focus of their struggle was to understand if motor and process skills were small units of occupation, something the person does, or underlying body functions, something within the person that the person's brain–body does. In the end, Kielhofner (1995) and Fisher (1998) concluded that performance skills are the smallest observable units of occupational performance, not body functions. What enabled Kielhofner and Fisher to come to this conclusion was the realization that as occupational therapists, we often think we can observe impairments of underlying body functions, but what we actually observe are "errors" of occupational performance. These occupational performance errors, however, reflect diminished occupational performance skill, not impairments of body functions.

For example, in Case Study 22.1, we note that when Karla observed Maurice as he attempted to open the refrigerator door, he did not pull hard enough and the door did not open. From the perspective of occupational performance (what Maurice did), Karla observed that Maurice did not pull with enough force to open the refrigerator door. When Karla began to reason as to why Maurice might not have pulled with enough force to open the door, her first thought was that he might have diminished strength in his upper limb.

In such instances, occupational therapists may think they "see" decreased strength, but in fact, they do not. Rather, they observe the person to perform some action that has an underlying demand for strength and therefore reason that diminished strength is the cause of the occupational performance problem observed. But Karla has not observed diminished strength because strength cannot be directly observed, nor was diminished strength necessarily the reason Maurice did not open the refrigerator door.

When Karla reasoned as to why did Maurice not open the door on his first attempt, she actually considered many possibilities besides diminished upper limb strength, such as "Is the seal on the refrigerator door unusually tight?" "Is he unfamiliar with this particular refrigerator and more familiar with one that opens more easily?" She could not determine the answer based solely on what she had observed. She needed to use her professional reasoning skills to speculate about possible reasons or causes for Maurice's observed problem with occupational performance and then evaluate further to determine why Maurice did not open the door on his first attempt. Karla also was aware that the reasons or causes may be related not only to body functions but also to person factors, task demands, environmental demands, and/or societal and cultural influences (see Figure 22.2).

Universal versus Task-specific Performance Skills

Universal Performance Skills

Performance skills can be viewed as being *universal* or more *task specific*. The brief definitions of universal motor, process, and social interaction performance skills included in Table 22.1 are based on the operational definitions of each skill within three standardized tests of occupational performance skill: the *Assessment of Motor and Process Skills* (AMPS) (Fisher & Jones, 2011a, 2011b), the *School Version of the Assessment of Motor and Process Skills* (School AMPS) (Fisher, Bryze, Hume, & Griswold, 2007), and the *Evaluation of Social Interaction* (ESI) (Fisher & Griswold, 2010). They are considered to be universal because they can be observed in virtually any daily life task performance and, in the case of social interaction skills, virtually any daily life task performance involving social interaction. As we will discuss next, these universal performance skills can be complemented by an endless number of task-specific occupational performance skills.

Using the AMPS as an example, Figure 22.3 helps to clarify the concept of *universal skills*. As the AMPS is a test of a person's ability to perform personal activities of daily living (PADL) tasks and instrumental activities of daily living (IADL) tasks (collectively, activities of daily living [ADL]), the motor and process performance skills included in the AMPS are referred to as ADL skills. There are more than 120 standardized ADL tasks in the current edition of the AMPS (Fisher & Jones, 2011b). No matter which of these ADL tasks a person is observed performing, the occupational therapist can observe the person's degree of occupational performance skill as the person *lifts* tasks objects, *moves* objects, *walks* within the task environment, *chooses* needed tools and materials, *initiates* task actions, and so on. Moreover, when performing ADL tasks, easier performance skills (e.g., *Endures, Lifts, Uses, Chooses*) are likely to be easier actions to perform in a skilled manner no matter which ADL task the person performs. Which ADL motor and ADL process skills are harder or easier and the extent to which the challenge of an ADL task can affect the degree of observed occupational performance skill has been based on a many-facet Rasch analysis of more than 148,000 people who are currently included in the international standardization sample of the AMPS (Fisher &

Easier ADL tasks*

Eating a snack with utensil
Brushing or combing hair
Upper body dressing – garment within reach
Shaving the face using an electric razor
Feeding a cat – dry cat food and water
Loading and starting a washing machine
Setting a table for two persons
Hand washing dishes
Ironing a shirt – ironing board already set up
Heating a precooked meal or dessert in a microwave
Presliced meat or cheese sandwich
Showering
Sweeping outside
Changing standard sheets on a bed
Hot cereal and beverage
Mopping the floor
Weeding
Pasta with meat sauce, and beverage
Cleaning a bathroom

Harder ADL tasks

Easier ADL motor items**

Endures
Lifts
Aligns
Moves
Transports
Flows
Grips
Reaches
Bends
Manipulates
Walks
Stabilizes
Coordinates
Paces
Calibrates
Positions

Harder ADL motor items

Easier ADL process items**

Uses
Chooses
Sequences
Searches/Locates
Attends
Inquires
Gathers
Heeds
Terminates
Navigates
Handles
Adjusts
Continues
Restores
Initiates
Organizes
Paces
Notices/Responds
Benefits
Accommodates

Harder ADL process items

* Each person evaluated using the AMPS chooses to perform, from among over 120 ADL tasks included in the AMPS manual, two ADL tasks that are meaningful, perceived as presenting a challenge, and prioritized for intervention.

** The 16 ADL motor and 20 ADL process items (universal performance skills) that can be observed during any ADL task performance and are scored based on the person's quality of performance of each of the two chosen ADL tasks.

FIGURE 22.3 Selected standardized tasks included in the Assessment of Motor and Process Skills (AMPS) and each of the activities of daily living (ADL) motor and ADL process items (task actions, performance skills) that are scored based on the person's quality of performance of each ADL task action (degree of skill as indicated by lack of observable clumsiness or physical effort, inefficiency, safety risk, and/or need for assistance).

Jones, 2011a). These same principles also apply to the school motor and school process skills included in the School AMPS and the social interaction skills included in the ESI.

Task-specific Performance Skills

Although the occupational therapist can use the existing taxonomies of universal motor, process, and social interaction skills listed in Table 22.1 in either a standardized or a nonstandardized manner, the occupational therapist is never restricted to these taxonomies. Rather, the occupational therapist may observe and evaluate the quality of any motor, process, or social action that is part of the observed occupational performance (i.e., the observable links in the chain of task actions). Moreover, many daily life task performances involve the performance of motor, process, and social actions that are more unique to the particular task performed. For example, when Michaela watches José as he is playing baseball, she observes him *throw* the ball to the first baseman, and she observes the first baseman *catch* the ball. Later, when José is up to bat, she observes him *swing* the bat, *drop* the bat, *run*, and *slide* into first base. Finally, she observes José's mother *smile* and the audience *cheer*.

A Rationale for Implementing Performance Analyses

There are several interrelated advantages of implementing a **performance analysis**, either standardized or nonstandardized. The first is that by implementing performance analyses, we, as occupational therapists, focus our evaluation on occupational performance, not person factors and body functions or environmental demands that may underlie or cause the ineffective performance (see Figure 22.2). The second advantage is that we make explicit which performance skills the person performed effectively and which were performed ineffectively (i.e., errors of occupational performance). The result is that we become better able to differentiate between occupational performance skill and underlying body functions and describe to others—including the client, team members, and third-party payers—using "everyday language," the person's observed problems of occupational performance. The final two advantages may be the ones that are most important. That is, if we use "everyday language" in describing quality of occupational performance, the result will be that we more readily

(1) work collaboratively with the client to establish occupation-focused goals and plan and implement occupation-based interventions and (2) use "occupation-first" language in our documentation and in our communication with others. The advantage is that people will better understand that occupation is the important focus of our profession.

Advantages and Disadvantages of Standardized and Nonstandardized Performance Analyses

Although standardized performance analyses such as the AMPS, School AMPS, and ESI have several advantages, they also have a number of disadvantages. One major advantage is that the use of standardized performance analyses allows the trained occupational therapist to generate an objective linearized measure (Bond & Fox, 2007) of the person's quality of occupational performance that can be used to document outcomes and implement evidence-based practice. The second advantage is that evaluation practices become more consistent, which promotes the ability to compare results across occupational therapists, clients, and settings (e.g., hospital vs. community). Another important advantage is that the person's linear performance measure can be compared to established criterion measures and normative values that enable the interpretation of the person's results from a criterion-referenced and a norm-referenced perspective. The final advantage is that formal training in standardized performance analysis methods facilitates the occupational therapist's ability to perform nonstandardized performance analyses and avoid common misperceptions that performance skills can be likened to body functions.

An important disadvantage of existing standardized performance analyses is that formal training and rater calibration often is required. Another disadvantage is that standardized assessments sometimes lack the flexibility needed to observe virtually any daily life task performance. For example, the AMPS is a test of ADL, and the School AMPS is a test of schoolwork task performance (e.g., cutting, writing, drawing, computing). Neither can be used to assess the quality of task performance in the areas of work or play.

Obviously, the major advantage of nonstandardized performance analyses is their flexibility. That is, the occupational therapist can implement an informal evaluation of performance skills based on the observation of performance of any daily life task. The only requirements are that the occupational therapist and the person observed must have a clear idea of what the person plans to do, or, if directed by another, what the person has been directed to do. For example, if the occupational therapist plans to observe a child in a classroom setting, he or she must know what the teacher has asked the students to do and what tools and materials they are expected to use. Then, after observing the person's performance, the occupational therapist must systematically rate each universal or task-specific motor skill, process skill, and (when relevant) social interaction skill observed. For example, the occupational therapist can subjectively judge whether the observed actions were skilled, and if not, if the actions (i.e., performance skills) were mildly, moderately, or markedly ineffective. The occupational therapist can also note the frequency or duration of any observed occupational performance errors (Fisher, 2009).

Differentiating Performance Analyses from Task, Activity, and Occupational Analyses

Performance analysis should not be confused with **task analysis** or **activity analysis**, which are intended for purposes of identifying (1) the underlying impairments of body functions as well as other person-related, environmental, task-related, and/or societal and cultural factors that underlie or cause the person's observed problems with occupational performance or (2) the inherent therapeutic value of a task for remediating underlying impairments, respectively (AOTA, 1993; Hagedorn, 1995; Llorens, 1993; Mosey, 1986; Trombly Latham, 2008; Watson, 1997) (see Table 22.2). An example of a standardized *task analysis* is the Neurobehavioral (NB) scale of the ADL-focused Occupation-based Neurobehavioral Evaluation (A-ONE; formerly, Árnadóttir OT-ADL Neurobehavioral Evaluation) (Árnadóttir, 1990, 2011; Árnadóttir, Fisher, & Löfgren, 2009). The NB scale of the A-ONE was designed to be used to evaluate the underlying neurobehavioral impairments that cause diminished ADL task performance based on direct observation within the natural context of those ADL task performances. More specifically, scoring of the A-ONE requires that the trained occupational therapist use the operational definitions of the NB items, combined with his or her professional reasoning skills and knowledge of neurology and neuropsychology, to formulate hypotheses related to interpreting the observed errors of ADL task performance. The goal is to identify what underlying neurobehavioral impairments are speculated to be the cause of the person's diminished occupational performance (Árnadóttir, 2011; Árnadóttir et al., 2009; Árnadóttir, Löfgren, & Fisher, 2010).

Standardized task analyses such as the NB scale of the A-ONE; Kitchen Task Assessment (KTA) (Baum & Edwards, 1993); Children's Kitchen Task Assessment (CKTA) (Rocke, Hays, Edwards, & Berg, 2008); Executive Function Performance Test (EFPT) (Baum et al., 2008; Baum, Morrison, Hahn, & Edwards, 2008/2010); the Perceive, Recall, Plan, and Perform (PRPP) System of Task Analysis (Aubin, Chapparo, Gélinas, Stip, & Rainville, 2009; Nott, Chapparo, & Heard, 2009); and the visual motor, fine motor, and gross motor scales of the Miller

TABLE 22.2 Comparison among Performance Analyses, Task Analyses, and Activity Analyses

Type of Analysis	Based on Observation of Doing?	Level of Analysis	Interpretation
Performance analyses	Yes	Performance skills	Quality of occupational performance—the degree of occupational skill observed during naturalistic daily life task performance
Task analyses	Yes	Person factors and body functions, task demands, environmental demands, and/or societal and cultural influences	Reason for or cause of the person's occupational performance problems—why the person can/cannot perform a task well
Activity analysis	No; analysis of activity in the abstract	Person factors and body functions, task demands, environmental demands, and/or societal and cultural influences	What is typically required in a given culture to successfully perform a task and how to modify a task to design therapeutic occupation

Adapted from Fisher, A. G. (2009). *Occupational Therapy Intervention Process Model: A model for planning and implementing top–down, client-centered, and occupation-based interventions*. Fort Collins CO: Three Star Press. Reprinted with permission.

Function and Participation Scales (M-FUN) (Miller, 2006) were all designed to fulfill an important need within occupational therapy for more ecologically relevant assessments of underlying body functions (e.g., cognition, including executive functions and information processing; gross and fine motor coordination; motor planning; visual motor skills) based on professional reasoning about the causes of observed occupational performance errors. They fulfill, however, an important need that is very different from the one that is filled by standardized or nonstandardized performance analyses. Performance analyses are used at the stages of the occupational therapy intervention process where the occupational therapist (1) observes the person perform prioritized daily life tasks and (2) identifies what task actions (performance skills) the person performed effectively or ineffectively. In contrast, task analyses are used to help the occupational therapist clarify the cause of the ineffective actions (see Figure 22.4).

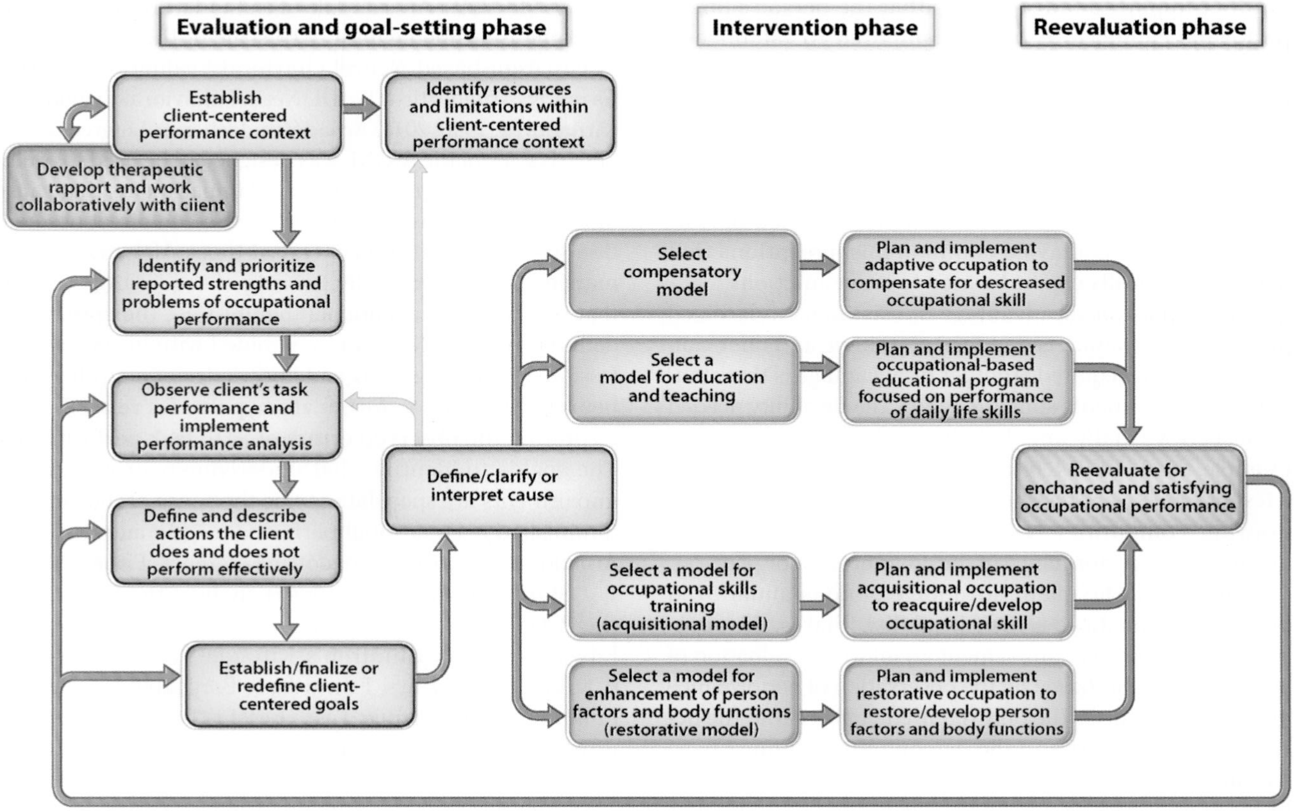

FIGURE 22.4 Schematic representation of the occupational therapy intervention process. (Adapted from Fisher, A. G. [2009]. *Occupational Therapy Intervention Process Model: A model for planning and implementing top–down, client-centered, and occupation-based interventions.* Fort Collins, CO: Three Star Press. Reprinted with permission.)

Performance analyses also should not be confused with the term **occupational analysis** as described in Chapter 21. An occupational analysis includes steps in the occupational therapy intervention process that precede as well as follow the actual performance analysis. Thus, performance analysis can be viewed as one part of the more global occupational analysis.

Implementing Performance Analyses: Evaluations of Occupational Performance Skill

With this background information related to performance skills and performance analysis, we will turn to discussing in more detail how an occupational therapist implements a performance analysis. Our focus, and the case example, will be on implementing nonstandardized performance analyses.

When an occupational therapist implements a performance analysis, the evaluation always occurs within the context of observing the person as he or she is engaged in the performance of a prioritized task. That is, each task performance observed should be one that the client has identified as a concern and prioritized as a potential target for intervention. Which tasks to observe are typically determined based on a thorough occupational therapy interview where the occupational therapist comes to understand the client from the client's perspective, what resources and limitations exist within the context of the client's task performances, and what task performances the client views as occupational strengths or problems of occupational performance (see Figure 22.4).

Once the client and the occupational therapist have collaboratively determined which task performances to prioritize, the occupational therapist introduces the idea of observing the person perform prioritized tasks and initiates one or more performance analyses. Each performance analysis progresses over four steps:

- **Step 1:** Observe the person perform a chosen and prioritized daily life task in his or her usual manner and take observational notes of observed occupational performance errors.
- **Step 2:** Rate the person's observed level of occupational performance skill. Either the universal performance motor, process, and social interaction skills shown in Table 22.1, or more task-specific motor, process, and social interaction skills can be evaluated. Each performance skill is rated in terms of ease (physical effort and/or clumsiness), efficiency (time and space organization), safety (risk of harm to person or damage to task objects), independence, or, in the case of social interaction skills, social appropriateness. The occupational therapist can use standardized scoring criteria outlined in the respective test manual or he or she can use a nonstandardized qualitative scale (e.g., no problem, mild problem, moderate problem, or severe problem) to rate the observed quality of each performance skill (Fisher, 2009).
- **Step 3:** Make a list of all of the ineffective performance skills observed and select up to 10 motor and process skills and/or 10 social interaction skills that best capture the person's diminished quality of occupational performance. In a similar manner, the motor, process, and/or social interaction skills that best capture the person's strengths of occupational performance also should be identified.
- **Step 4:** Create clusters of interrelated performance skills and write summary statements that can be used to document the person's quality of occupational performance.

In Figure 22.4, step 1 is shown as *Observe client's task performance and implement performance analysis.* Steps 2 through 4 are all part of the phase in the occupational therapy process where the occupational therapist is to *define and describe actions the client does and does not perform effectively.*

Once the occupational therapist has completed the performance analysis and determined which performance skills most reflect and best describe the person's quality of occupational performance, the occupational therapist has progressed to the phase in the occupational therapy intervention process where he or she and the client work collaboratively to establish and document client-centered goals (see Figure 22.4). The summary statements developed in step 4 of the performance analysis represent the person's baseline level of occupational performance. They provide the foundation for collaboratively developing observable and measurable client-centered and occupation-focused goals.

Finally, the occupational therapist considers the reasons or "causes" for the person's diminished quality of occupational performance (see Figure 22.4). The various factors that may be contributing to and influencing the quality of the person's occupational performance are the internal and external factors that comprise the context of the observed occupational performance: person factors and body functions, task demands, environmental demands, and/or more overarching societal or cultural influences (see Figure 22.2). This phase most often involves the implementation of standardized or nonstandardized task analyses. The process of implementing a performance analysis, preceded by a thorough occupational therapy interview and followed by establishing client-centered goals, is illustrated in Case Study 22.2.

CASE STUDY 22.2 Implementing Nonstandardized Performance Analyses

Background: Referral and Occupational Therapy Interview

Maurice is 78 years of age and lives in his own home. Until recently, Maurice was considered a healthy aging adult; but over the past 6 months, he has fallen on several occasions and was hospitalized for observation and treatment of severe lacerations on the back of his head. These falls and hospitalizations have taken their toll; Maurice has become increasingly frail. His doctor has spoken to Maurice and his family, and he has recommended that they consider some form of alternative housing for Maurice, somewhere where he would have 24-hour supervision.

Maurice, however, is determined to continue living at home. He already pays for a woman, Joyce, to come in each day and help him with his daily chores. Because his family wants to support Maurice's wishes, they have requested an occupational therapy evaluation to ensure Maurice's safety, particularly during the time that Joyce is not with him. When they contacted Karla, the occupational therapist, they mentioned not only Maurice's recent falls, but also that he often seems to be "a bit confused." They feel that his confusion, combined with moderate hearing loss, has led to increasing challenges when they are trying to communicate with him. They expressed concern that Maurice and Joyce may also be having similar problems when discussing his desires and needs.

With this background information gathered during the referral process, Karla contacted Maurice and made arrangements for a visit. Karla began her occupational therapy interview by introducing herself and telling Maurice that she was an occupational therapist and that her role was to help him do the things that he wanted to do, such as dressing, doing activities around the house, going out in the community, and engaging in leisure activities. She then transitioned to asking Maurice to tell her about what he currently does during a typical day, what he would like to do, and what are his concerns and priorities.

During this occupational therapy interview, Karla learned that Maurice is satisfied overall with his current living situation. He has a supportive family with whom he has daily telephone contact and biweekly visits. He explained that Joyce comes in 8 hours a day, 6 days a week to prepare his lunch and dinner, clean, take him on errands, and spend time with him. Maurice has daily routines that include getting dressed, preparing his breakfast, and reading the newspaper, all of which he performs before Joyce comes for the day. He also showers twice each week before Joyce arrives. During the day, he watches television, uses his computer, talks to family on the phone, and reads. He likes to go to town two or three times a week to go to the bank, post office, and grocery store. Joyce drives him to town and accompanies him, but Maurice takes care of his own errands. He has had his bathroom adapted to include grab bars, a raised toilet seat, and a shower bench, enabling him to remain independent in personal activities of daily living.

As the interview progressed, Karla guided the discussion to learn about tasks that Maurice currently does that are challenging for him and to hear about other tasks that Maurice does not currently do but might want to do. Maurice stated that he is satisfied with most of the tasks he is doing and does not have others that he wants to do at this time. He said that he is having difficulty putting on his shoes and socks. He also said that preparing his breakfast (orange juice and cold cereal) has gradually become more difficult and that he wants to be able to keep doing that for himself each morning. When she focused in on other aspects of dressing and showering, tasks Karla reasoned also were likely to be challenging, Maurice denied any problems.

Desiring to maintain a client-centered focus and to ensure that Maurice is safe in doing the two tasks that he identified as more challenging and important to him, Karla and Maurice decided that she would observe him perform these. She told Maurice that after she observed his performance she would be able to make suggestions to help him do these tasks more easily. As Maurice had also acknowledged that he does not always "follow conversations" when he is interacting with others, he also agreed that Karla could observe him when he and Joyce would be deciding on meals for the week and writing a shopping list for the grocery store.

Implementing a Performance Analysis: Step 1—Observe the Person Perform Chosen Daily Life Tasks

When Karla observed Maurice perform the two activities of daily living (ADL) tasks and the social interaction with Joyce, she ensured that he performed each task in his usual manner and she remained an unobtrusive observer. During each of his task performances, she took notes of any occupational performance errors that reflected diminished quality of Maurice's occupational performance.

Implementing a Performance Analysis: Step 2—Rating the Person's Quality of Performance

After Karla had observed Maurice perform the two ADL tasks and engage in social interaction with Joyce, she proceeded to rate Maurice's quality of performance in relation to each of the motor, process, and social interaction skills shown in Table 22.1. When she did her rating, she used a four-category qualitative scale: no problem, mild problem, moderate problem, and marked problem.

Implementing a Performance Analysis: Step 3—Defining the Actions of Performance That Were Effective/Ineffective

After scoring both of the observed ADL tasks and the social exchange, Karla transitioned to making a list of all of the motor and process skills and all of the social interaction skills that she had observed to be ineffective. When she did this, she first listed each performance skill and then she made note of what behavior she had observed that led to her rating. Finally, Karla put a check mark (√) by those performance skills that she reasoned best captured Maurice's diminished quality of occupational performance (Tables 22.3 and 22.4 show Karla's lists for *Putting on socks and shoes* and *Planning the weekly meals and making a shopping list*). As she also wanted to capture Maurice's relative strengths, she made similar lists of the motor, process, and social interaction skills that most supported his occupational performance.

CASE STUDY 22.2 Implementing Nonstandardized Performance Analyses (*Continued*)

TABLE 22.3 Maurice's Motor and Process Skills That Most Reflected His Diminished Quality of ADL Task Performance—Putting On His Socks and Shoes

ADL Motor Skills	Behavior Observed	Rating
√ Stabilizes	• Risk of a fall—standing and bending down to get shoes	• Marked
√ Reaches	• Increased effort and risk for fall—reaching down to get shoes • Increased effort and audible shortness of breath—reaching forward to pull leg up over opposite knee	• Marked • Moderate
√ Bends	• Increased effort and risk of a fall—bending down to get shoes • Increased effort and audible shortness of breath—bending forward to pull leg up over opposite knee	• Marked • Moderate
Grips	• Grip slips from socks when pulling them up	• Mild
Manipulates	• Fumbles shoelaces	• Mild
√ Moves	• Increased effort and audible shortness of breath—pulling leg up over opposite knee and pulling up socks	• Moderate
√ Lifts	• Increased effort and risk of a fall—lifting shoes from the floor	• Marked
Walks	• Walks using a walker	• Mild
√ Endures	• Audible shortness of breath	• Moderate
ADL Process Skills	**Behavior Observed**	**Rating**
Initiates	• Occasional short pauses before initiating task steps	• Mild
Continues	• Starts to pull up sock, pauses, returns to pulling up sock	• Mild
√ Accommodates	• Demonstrates risk of a fall (Reaches, Bends, Lifts); he did not prevent his problems	• Marked
√ Benefits	• Audible shortness of breath persisted (Reaches, Bends, Moves, Endures)	• Moderate

ADL, activities of daily living.

Implementing a Performance Analysis: Step 4—Identifying Clusters of Interrelated Skills and Writing Summary Statements for Use in Documentation

Karla's next step was to create clusters of performance skills that she judged to be interrelated. Once she created each cluster, she wrote a summary statement that she used to document Maurice's baseline level of occupational performance. For example, she created three clusters of motor and process skills related to the task of *Putting on shoes and socks* and four clusters related to social interaction skills. Those clusters and her summary statements were as follows:

Putting On Socks and Shoes

- ***Stabilizes, Reaches, Bends, Lifts:*** *Maurice demonstrated marked fall risk when standing and bending to reach down and lift his shoes up from the floor.*
- ***Reaches, Bends, Moves, Endures:*** *He also demonstrated moderate increase in effort and audible shortness of breath when reaching forward to pull his leg up over his opposite knee and when pulling up his socks.*
- ***Accommodates, Benefits:*** *Maurice did not anticipate and prevent problems from occurring, and his problems persisted throughout the task performance.*

Planning Weekly Meals and Making a Shopping List together with Care Provider

- ***Looks, Regulates:*** *He frequently looked down and away from his social partner and occasionally "fidgeted" with task objects (e.g., pencil and note pad).*
- ***Speaks Fluently, Times Duration:*** *More importantly, he frequently paused "mid-message." On two occasions, these pauses were 3 to 4 seconds in length; and on two additional occasions, he began but never finished sending his messages.*
- ***Replies, Transitions, Clarifies, Heeds:*** *Moreover, on two occasions, his replies were markedly irrelevant to the intended purpose of the social exchange.*
- ***Accommodates, Benefits:*** *Finally, Maurice did not modify his social interactions to prevent these problems from occurring, and his problems often reoccurred during the ongoing social exchange.*

(*continued*)

CASE STUDY 22.2 Implementing Nonstandardized Performance Analyses (*Continued*)

TABLE 22.4 Maurice's Social Interaction Skills That Most Reflected His Ineffective Quality of Social Interaction—Planning Weekly Meals and Making a Shopping List Together with Joyce

Social Interaction Skills	Behavior Observed	Rating
√ ***Concludes/Disengages***	• J starts to bring discussion to a close, but M continues to talk about what he will eat	• Mild
Speaks fluently	• Speaks in a hesitant manner, with short pauses and stammering, "I think w-we . . . should . . . buy some apples" • On two occasions, M pauses 3–4 seconds in the middle of a message	• Mild • Moderate
√ ***Looks***	• Frequently looks down and away from J	• Mild
√ ***Regulates***	• Occasionally fidgets with pencil and notepad used for shopping list	• Mild
√ ***Replies***	• Replies with markedly irrelevant responses (e.g., when asked what he wants to eat, he replies, "My son called")	• Marked
√ ***Transitions***	• Transitions to a markedly irrelevant topic (e.g., abruptly changes topic to getting a phone call from his son)	• Marked
√ ***Times response***	• M interrupts J as she is speaking; occasionally delays before replying to J's questions	• Moderate
√ ***Times duration***	• Starts messages, but leaves two messages "hanging in the air"	• Moderate
√ ***Clarifies***	• J asks M to clarify what he meant, "Let's buy some scapple"; he does not clarify; his reply is markedly irrelevant, "I need to make a doctor's appointment"	• Marked
√ ***Heeds***	• When engaged in a social interaction with an intended purpose of making a shopping list, M begins to discuss his son and a doctor's appointment	• Moderate
√ ***Accommodates***	• Demonstrated markedly inappropriate Replies, Transitions, and Clarifies skill; he did not prevent his problems	• Marked
√ ***Benefits***	• Several of M's moderately inappropriate social interaction skill deficits persisted	• Moderate

When Karla actually documented Maurice's baseline level of occupational performance, she wanted to place her summary statements in the context of her overall observation. Therefore, she began with an introductory phrase to clarify what it was that Maurice had done (e.g., put on his socks and shoes) and incorporated into that a global baseline statement that would document his overall quality of ADL task performance. Then, she added her summary statements so as to document his specific baseline. For example, her final documentation for *Putting on socks and shoes* was as follows:

> *While Maurice was independent when putting on his shoes and socks, he demonstrated marked safety risk and moderate increase in physical effort. More specifically, Maurice demonstrated marked fall risk when standing and bending to reach down and lift his shoes up from the floor. He also demonstrated moderate increase in effort and audible shortness of breath when reaching forward to pull his leg up over his opposite knee and when pulling up his socks. Maurice did not anticipate and prevent problems from occurring, and his problems persisted throughout the task performance.*

Progressing from Implementing a Performance Analysis to Establishing Client-centered Goals

When Karla documented his baseline level of occupational performance, she also discussed with Maurice her observations and engaged him in a discussion of how he felt about his performance and what might be his desired outcomes of occupational therapy services. For example, she pointed out to Maurice that even though he was holding onto his rollator, he almost fell when he bent down and picked up his shoes from the floor. Maurice acknowledged that falling has been a major issue and is one of the reasons his doctor does not want him living at home anymore. Maurice indicated that he wanted to be able to perform tasks without fall risk.

Karla, therefore, discussed with him his baseline statement related to putting on socks and shoes—***marked** fall risk when standing and bending to reach down and lift his shoes up from the floor*—and engaged Maurice in determining what was his desired goal. As Maurice specified that he did not want to have a fall risk, Karla and Maurice decided that his goal would be *no fall risk when putting on socks and shoes*. Karla did not refer to Maurice's standing, bending down, or lifting his shoes as she wanted to leave open the option for introducing compensatory

CASE STUDY 22.2 Implementing Nonstandardized Performance Analyses (*Continued*)

strategies that would enable Maurice to avoid fall risk. Karla engaged Maurice in similar collaborative discussions related to his obvious increased physical effort and shortness of breath when putting on his socks and shoes as well as the challenges he faced with preparing his breakfast and engaging in social interaction with his care provider.

Questions to Prompt Professional Reasoning

1. Given that Maurice likely has problems with balance, would you have been inclined to use a different assessment approach than was described in this chapter?
2. How would your evaluation process have differed from the evaluation process described in this chapter?
3. How might intervention have changed had Karla focused on evaluating body functions rather than analyzing performance skills observed during desired task performances?
4. What was the benefit of Karla's separately describing the quality of each of Maurice's task performances, based on her analysis of his observed level of occupational performance skill, when she wrote her documentation?
5. Three visits from occupational therapy are not many. Karla decided to use one visit for evaluation, leaving her with only two more visits. Discuss the benefit of spending time doing a performance analysis for Maurice.

References

American Occupational Therapy Association. (1993). Position paper: Purposeful activity. *American Journal of Occupational Therapy, 47,* 1081–1082.

American Occupational Therapy Association. (2002). Occupational therapy practice framework: Domain and process. *American Journal of Occupational Therapy, 56,* 609–639.

American Occupational Therapy Association. (2008). Occupational therapy practice framework: Domain and process, 2nd edition. *American Journal of Occupational Therapy, 62,* 625–683.

Árnadóttir, G. (1990). *The brain and behavior: Assessing cortical dysfunction through activities of daily living.* St. Louis, MO: Mosby Elsevier.

Árnadóttir, G. (2011). Impact of neurobehavioral deficits on activities of daily living. In G. Gillen (Ed.), *Stroke rehabilitation: A function-based approach* (3rd ed., pp. 456–500). St. Louis, MO: Mosby Elsevier.

Árnadóttir, G., Fisher, A. G., & Löfgren, B. (2009). Dimensionality of nonmotor neurobehavioral impairments when observed in the natural contexts of ADL task performance. *Neurorehabilitation & Neural Repair, 23,* 579–586.

Árnadóttir, G., Löfgren, B., & Fisher, A. G. (2010). Difference in impact of neurobehavioural dysfunction on activities of daily living performance between right and left hemispheric stroke. *Journal of Rehabilitation Medicine, 42,* 903–907.

Aubin, G., Chapparo, C., Gélinas, I., Stip, E., & Rainville, C. (2009). Use of the Perceive, Recall, Plan, and Perform System of Task Analysis for persons with schizophrenia: A preliminary study. *Australian Occupational Therapy Journal, 56,* 189–199.

Bartels, M. N., Duffy, C. A., & Beland, H. E. (2011). Pathophysiology, medical management, and acute rehabilitation of stroke survivors. In G. Gillen (Ed.), *Stroke rehabilitation: A function-based approach* (3rd ed., pp. 1–48). St. Louis, MO: Mosby Elsevier.

Baum, C. M., Connor, L. T., Morrison, T., Hahn, M., Dromerick, A. W., & Edwards, D. F. (2008). Reliability, validity, and clinical utility of the Executive Function Performance Test: A measure of executive function in a sample of people with stroke. *American Journal of Occupational Therapy, 62,* 446–455.

Baum, C. M., & Edwards, D. F. (1993). Cognitive performance in senile dementia of the Alzheimer's type: The Kitchen Task Assessment. *American Journal of Occupational Therapy, 47,* 431–436.

Baum, C. M., Morrison, T., Hahn, M., & Edwards, D. F. (2008/2010). *Test protocol booklet: Executive Function Performance Test.* Program in Occupational Therapy. St. Louis, MO: Washington University School of Medicine.

Bond, T. G., & Fox, C. M. (2007). *Applying the Rasch model: Fundamental measurement in the human sciences* (2nd ed.). Mahwah, NJ: Lawrence Erlbaum Associates.

Fisher, A. G. (1998). Uniting practice and theory in an occupational framework: 1998 Eleanor Clarke Slagle Lecture. *American Journal of Occupational Therapy, 52,* 509–521.

Fisher, A. G. (2006). Overview of performance skills and client factors. In H. M. Pendleton, & W. Schultz-Krohn (Eds.), *Pedretti's occupational therapy: Practice skills for physical dysfunction* (6th ed., pp. 372–402). St. Louis, MO: Mosby Elsevier.

Fisher, A. G. (2009). *Occupational Therapy Intervention Process Model: A model for planning and implementing top–down, client-centered, and occupation-based interventions.* Fort Collins, CO: Three Star Press.

Fisher, A. G., Bryze, K., Hume, V., & Griswold, L. A. (2007). *School AMPS: School Version of the Assessment of Motor and Process Skills* (2nd ed.). Fort Collins, CO: Three Star Press.

Fisher, A. G., & Griswold, L. A. (2010). *Evaluation of social interaction* (2nd ed.). Fort Collins, CO: Three Star Press.

Fisher, A. G., & Jones, K. B. (2011a). *Assessment of Motor and Process Skills: Development, standardization, and administration manual* (7th ed. Rev.). Fort Collins, CO: Three Star Press.

Fisher, A. G., & Jones, K. B. (2011b). *Assessment of Motor and Process Skills: User manual* (7th ed. Rev.). Fort Collins, CO: Three Star Press.

Fisher, A. G., & Kielhofner, G. (1995). Skill in occupational performance. In G. Kielhofner (Ed.), *A model of human occupation: Theory and application* (2nd ed., pp. 113–137). Baltimore, MD: Williams & Wilkins.

Hagedorn, R. (1995). *Occupational therapy: Perspectives and processes.* Edinburgh, United Kingdom: Churchill Livingstone.

Hagedorn, R. (2000). *Tools for practice in occupational therapy: A structured approach to core skills and processes.* Edinburgh, United Kingdom: Churchill Livingstone.

Kielhofner, G. (1995). *A model of human occupation: Theory and application* (2nd ed.). Baltimore, MD: Williams & Wilkins.

Kielhofner, G. (2008). *Model of Human Occupation: Theory and application* (4th ed.). Baltimore, MD: Lippincott Williams & Wilkins.

Llorens, L. A. (1993). Activity analysis: Agreement between participants and observers on perceived factors in occupation components. *Occupational Therapy Journal of Research, 13,* 198–211.

Miller, L. J. (2006). *Miller Function and Participation Scales.* San Antonio, TX: PsychCorp.

Mosey, A. C. (1986). *Psychosocial components of occupational therapy.* New York, NY: Raven Press.

Nott, M. T., Chapparo, C., & Heard, R. (2009). Reliability of the Perceive, Recall, Plan and Perform System of Task Analysis: A criterion-referenced assessment. *Australian Occupational Therapy Journal, 56*, 307–314.

Polatajko, H. J., Mandich, A., & Martini, R. (2000). Dynamic performance analysis: A framework for understanding occupational performance. *American Journal of Occupational Therapy, 54*, 65–72.

Rexroth, P., Fisher, A. G., Merritt, B. K., & Gliner, J. (2005). Ability differences in persons with unilateral hemispheric stroke. *Canadian Journal of Occupational Therapy, 72*, 212–221.

Rocke, K., Hays, P., Edwards, D., & Berg, C. (2008). Development of a performance assessment of executive function: The Children's Kitchen Task Assessment. *American Journal of Occupational Therapy, 62*, 528–537.

Trombly Latham, C. A. (2008). Occupation as therapy: Selection, gradation, analysis, and adaptation. In M. V. Radomski & C. A. Trombly Latham (Eds.), *Occupational therapy for physical dysfunction* (6th ed., pp. 358–401). Philadelphia, PA: Lippincott Williams & Wilkins.

Watson, D. E. (1997). *Task analysis: An occupational performance approach*. Bethesda, MD: American Occupational Therapy Association.

World Health Organization. (2001). *International classification of functioning, disability and health: ICF*. Geneva, Switzerland: Author.

For additional resources on the subjects discussed in this chapter, visit http://thePoint.lww.com/Willard-Spackman12e.

Occupational Therapy Process

UNIT VII

"Therapists work to create significant experiences for their patients because if therapy is to be effective, the therapeutic process must matter to the patient."

—Cheryl Mattingly

CHAPTER 23

Overview of the Occupational Therapy Process and Outcomes

Denise Chisholm, Barbara A. Boyt Schell

OUTLINE

LEARNING OBJECTIVES

After reading this chapter, you will be able to:

1. Describe the components of the occupational therapy process
2. Discuss how evidence from research and practice is integrated in the occupational therapy process
3. Explain the professional reasoning typically associated with components of the occupational therapy process
4. Apply the occupational therapy process to client cases

Introduction

This chapter provides an overview of the occupational therapy process in preparation for understanding the more detailed information regarding assessing client needs as well as the provision of intervention services presented in the following chapters in this unit. First, we will describe the general process of service delivery and its relationship with occupational therapy. In the second section of this chapter, an illustration or "map" of the occupational therapy process is provided to assist you in visualizing the essential components and their dynamic and interactive relationships. Each component of the occupational therapy process—evaluation, intervention, reevaluation, and continuation/discontinuation of services based on client outcomes—will be expanded on in subsequent sections. Our hope is that the occupational therapy process map will direct the services you provide as an occupational therapy practitioner. Evidence and professional reasoning have been embedded in the process map as essential markers to assure accuracy in planning the most effective occupational therapy services. Case studies have been woven throughout this chapter to give you the opportunity to apply the occupational therapy process map.

Occupational Therapy as a Process

Occupation is the central focus of occupational therapy services. The general process used in the delivery of occupational therapy services parallels the process used by other health-related professionals (e.g., nurses, physical therapists, physicians, dieticians). It provides a structure for practitioners to employ therapeutic professional reasoning based on evidence in order to address the client's health-related problems. The process is neither condition- (i.e., diagnosis, condition, disorder) nor age-specific and can be applied in any practice setting—hospital, outpatient clinic, school, workplace, or client's home. Occupational therapy practitioners customize the process with the end goal of supporting the client's health and participation through engagement in occupations (American Occupational Therapy Association [AOTA], 2008). Occupational therapy services incorporate the therapeutic use of occupation as a primary means for promoting the client's engagement in and performance of his or her preferred daily activities. The use of occupation as both an end goal and a means to achieve the goal is occupational therapy's unique application of the service delivery process. Occupational therapy practitioners must deliver services that are occupation centered. In the words of Fisher (2009), if we are to practice as *occupational* therapy practitioners, we must use *occupation* as our primary form of therapy; that is, we must implement occupational therapy (p. 10).

The Occupational Therapy Process Map

Embarking on a trip without a map increases the risk of getting lost, which in turn results in confusion and frustration. This is analogous to what can occur when an occupational therapy practitioner provides therapy services without the guidance of a process "map." Just as when someone takes a trip, occupational therapy practitioners need a clear diagram illustrating the road for traveling from the starting point—that is, evaluation—to the final destination or outcome of the therapy journey. We need to become competent in reading the markers that provide us with the evidence that supports taking the best route in both the evaluation and intervention portions of the trip. Our competency in "map reading" is reliant on our professional reasoning, which is used to calculate and recalculate or problem-solve the best route options, assuring sound therapy decisions. With a thorough understanding of the process map, you can effectively educate your client about his or her occupational therapy services. When clients "know where they are going," they can actively and collaboratively participate in the process to support their health and participation in life through engagement in occupation.

There are many different interpretations and illustrations of the occupational therapy process (AOTA, 2008; Christiansen & Baum, 1997; Christiansen, Baum, & Bass-Haugen, 2005; Fearing, Law, & Clark, 1997; Fisher, 1998, 2009; Law, Baum, & Dunn, 2005; Reed & Sanderson, 1999; Rogers & Holm, 1989, 2009). Our occupational therapy process map (Figure 23.1) is an adaptation of the

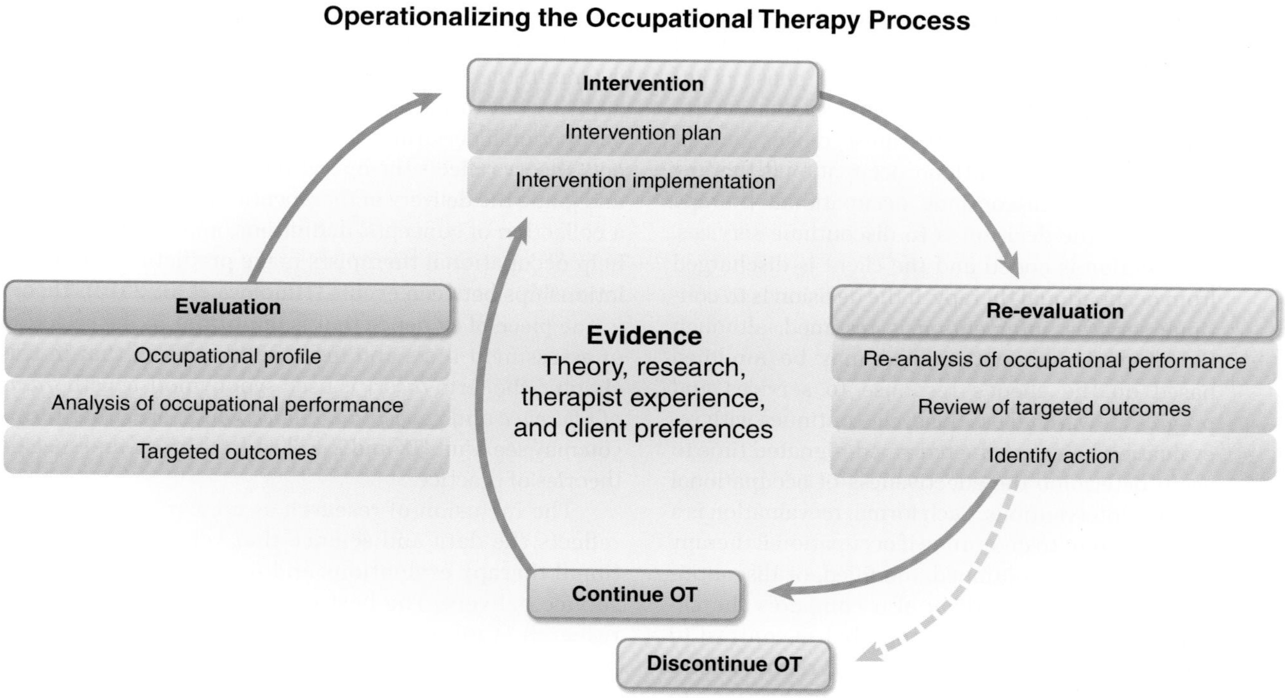

FIGURE 23.1 The occupational therapy process. OT, occupational therapy.

process outlined in the "Occupational Therapy Practice Framework" (AOTA, 2008).

Although the occupational therapy process is highly dynamic and cyclical, it does have a definitive starting point and important milestones along the way. These are evaluation, intervention, reevaluation, and therapy outcomes.

- **Evaluation** is the systematic collection and analysis of data needed to make decisions. Occupational therapy practitioners use the evaluation results and conclusions to plan and implement interventions to assist clients in positively changing their occupational performance. Sometimes the terms *evaluation* and *assessment* are used interchangeably; however, consistently using these terms based on distinct definitions can increase occupational therapy's efficacy (Hinojosa, Kramer, & Crist, 2010). We will delineate the terms as follows: evaluation is the comprehensive process of obtaining and interpreting data necessary to understand the person, system, or situation for intervention (AOTA, 2010, p. 2); and assessment refers to specific tools, instruments, or systematic interactions (e.g., observation, interview protocol) used during the evaluation process (AOTA, 2010, p. 2).
- **Intervention** is the implementation of actions directed at facilitating the client's engagement in his or her occupations. In order to determine the effectiveness of occupational therapy interventions, another evaluation or reevaluation must be conducted.
- **Reevaluation** can be conducted both *formally* and *informally*. *Formal reevaluation* compares the client's occupational performance data obtained during evaluation with the client's occupational performance after having received a phase of intervention. Based on the formal reevaluation results, the occupational therapist makes one of two decisions—to continue occupational therapy services or to discontinue occupational therapy services. If the decision is to discontinue services, intervention is ended and the client is discharged from occupational therapy. If the decision is to continue services, intervention is resumed, although the original intervention plan may be modified based on the client's response to services and progress toward goals. The cycle continues with reevaluation being conducted at a designated time to again determine the effectiveness of occupational therapy interventions. Each formal reevaluation is a decision point to determine if occupational therapy services will be continued, modified, or discontinued. *Informal reevaluation* also compares the client's occupational performance; but in contrast to formal reevaluation, during informal reevaluations, the occupational therapist is making decisions to continue or discontinue select interventions based on the client's response to the intervention, progress toward goals, and attainment of outcomes. The subsections for each component (evaluation, intervention, reevaluation, and outcomes) of the process will be described in more detail later in this chapter.

The consideration of **outcomes** is inherent in every phase of the process. Outcomes are specifically identified results of planned therapy intervention (AOTA, 2008). In occupational therapy, outcomes include improved occupational performance and participation in a full range of desired and meaningful occupations as well as increased abilities to adapt to occupational challenges. Additional outcomes include engaging in activities designed to prevent future limitation or to promote health and wellness. Improved quality of life, competence in occupational roles, and the ability to self-advocate are additional outcomes. Anticipated outcomes serve as goals to guide the therapy process. As benchmarks, they help both the client and the therapist decide if occupational therapy is effective, completed, or needs to be modified in some way to either achieve different or additional outcomes or to see if different occupational therapy approaches will be more successful in reaching desired outcomes.

Evidence provides the background that supports the occupational therapy process map. The components of the process are influenced and guided by a collection of evidence that includes theory, research, the therapist's experience, and the client's preferences (AOTA, 2008). This facilitates evidence-based practice, which is a process that combines the current best-published evidence with practitioner expertise and client preferences (Law & Baum, 1998; Sackett, Straus, Richardson, Rosenberg, & Haynes, 2000). Chapter 31 in Unit VIII specifically addresses evidence-based practice.

Occupational therapy, like most health professions, is a multi-theory profession with occupational therapists applying one or more theories to examine and explain the occupational performance strengths and needs of each client. Theory reflects the operating assumptions that direct and guide the delivery of therapeutic services. Theories are a collection of concepts, definitions, and hypotheses that help occupational therapists make predictions about relationships between events (Hinojosa et al., 2010). Theory is one piece of evidence that is important in the selection of assessment tools and interventions. Note that in this chapter, the term *theory* is used synonymously with *frame of reference* and *conceptual model*, which are other terms you may see. Units IX and X will address broad and specific theories of practice.

The inclusion of research as an aspect of evidence reflects the data and science that verifies the occupational therapy evaluations and interventions we use in service delivery. The best quantitative and qualitative research is information obtained from peer-reviewed journals. Occupational therapy practitioners need research to establish validity for evaluation and intervention decisions. In addition to theory and research, both the therapist's experience and the client's preferences are important sources of evidence. Your experience as an occupational therapy practitioner—including your knowledge, training, and competencies—supports your implementation of the occupational therapy process. The experience of the occupational therapy practitioner provides evidence that the right professional is providing the right service in the right way, in the right place, and at the right time, which should then result in the right result (Graham, 1996; Gray, 1997; Holm, 2000; Sackett et al., 2000; Silverman, 1998).

The occupational therapy process is accomplished through a collaborative relationship between clients and practitioners. Note that the term *client* can be an individual or a group (AOTA, 2008). For individuals, the term includes not only the individual with the occupational performance problem but also includes their advocates (e.g., family members, significant others, caregivers, care managers, community members). Examples of groups that are clients are organizations (e.g., businesses, industries, or agencies) and populations (or groups of people) within a community (e.g., veterans, people with mental illness). The client's preferences are based on his or her life experiences, values, choices, needs, and priorities and are an integral piece of evidence supporting the occupational therapy process. Occupational therapists need to consciously and systematically integrate the client's preferences into all components of the occupational therapy process because they can significantly influence the outcomes. The best available evidence, including theory, research, therapist experience, and client preferences, must be used to achieve the best outcomes. Of significance is the choice of the word *and* in the previous sentence versus *or*. *All* available aspects of evidence must be used versus only using theory or only using the practitioner's experience combined with research. A disconnect between the evidence, including the client's preferences and the components of the process, can reduce the support needed for the client to gain maximum therapeutic benefit from occupational therapy services (Holm, 2000; Law, 1998; Lee & Miller, 2003).

Just as each component is supported by evidence, each component of the occupational therapy process requires professional reasoning. Professional reasoning, sometimes referred to as clinical reasoning, includes therapy decisions and problem solving. Chapter 30 discusses the nature of professional reasoning. In this chapter, in addition to taking a closer look at the details of the occupational therapy process, we describe the professional reasoning and evidence focus for each component. Subsequent chapters in this unit will provide further and more in-depth examination of evaluation and intervention and factors that connect with and shape the occupational therapy process.

Evaluation

Evaluation is the beginning of the occupational therapy process journey (Figure 23.2). The data occupational therapists collect and analyze is information about the client's occupational performance—strengths and problems. The occupational therapist is responsible for evaluating the client; however, the occupational therapy assistant can contribute to the evaluation. For example, the occupational therapy assistant, under the supervision of the occupational therapist, may administer a standardized assessment, perform an activities of daily living (ADL) evaluation, or other elements of the evaluation that do not require the professional judgment or skills of an occupational therapist. There are professional guidelines to assist occupational therapists in determining when it is appropriate to delegate to occupational therapy assistants (see Chapters 67 and 72 for further discussion of these).

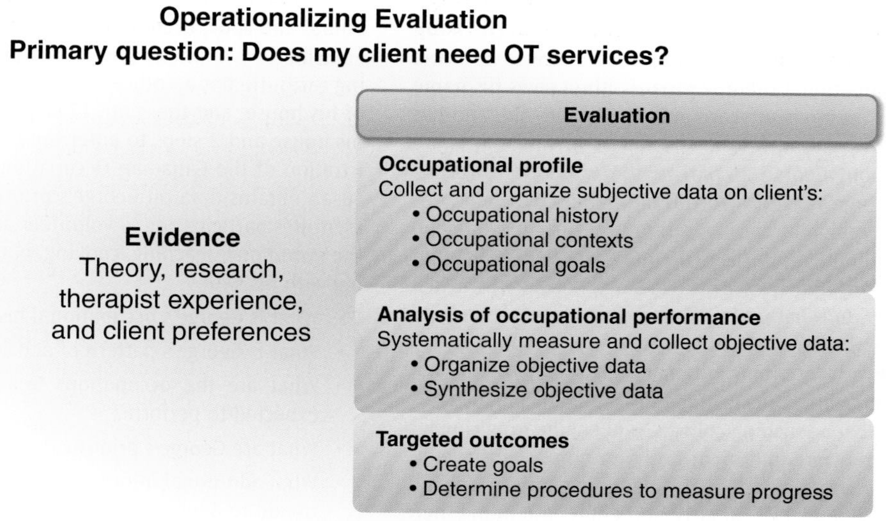
Operationalizing Evaluation
Primary question: Does my client need OT services?
Evaluation
Occupational profile
Collect and organize subjective data on client's:
• Occupational history
• Occupational contexts
• Occupational goals
Evidence
Theory, research, therapist experience, and client preferences
Analysis of occupational performance
Systematically measure and collect objective data:
• Organize objective data
• Synthesize objective data
Targeted outcomes
• Create goals
• Determine procedures to measure progress

FIGURE 23.2 Operationalizing evaluation. OT, occupational therapy.

The primary question or therapy decision the occupational therapist has to make during evaluation is "Who is my client and does my client need occupational therapy services?" In order to make the therapeutic decision about the need for occupational therapy services, we must first obtain information that will assist us in problem solving answers to several secondary questions. These include but are not limited to the following:

- What is the client's occupational history and experience?
- What is the client's pattern of ADL?
- What are the occupations the client needs, wants, and is expected to perform?
- What is/are the client's problem(s)?
- Can occupational therapy assist in resolving the client's problem(s)?
- What are the client's priorities?
- What are the client's environmental issues?
- What occupations is the client able to and unable to perform?
- What occupations, skills, patterns, and aspects of the environment affect the client's performance?
- What measurable and objective goals can address the client's targeted outcomes?

In order to effectively problem solve the answers, we need to complete the occupational profile, perform an analysis of occupational performance, and identify targeted outcomes.

Occupational Profile

A profile provides a description and includes a summary of information related to the client's history, resources, and performance. Because the focus of our services is on occupation, we want to create an occupational profile of our clients in order to better understand and describe their occupational performance. In order to establish an occupational profile, we collect and organize data on the client's occupational history, occupational contexts, and occupational goals (AOTA, 2008). We gather the client's perceptions about his or her occupations and related performance strengths and concerns. This information may or may not be consistent with what others might say who observe the client's performance. It is important to get the client's own view of the situation. Remember also that the client may include not only the person with an occupational performance concern but also others important in the client's life, such as spouses or partners, family members, caregivers, as well as those who are concerned about the client's performance, such as employers or teachers.

The historical information collected from and about clients' needs to relate to the performance of their life activities, that is, ADL, instrumental ADL, rest and sleep, education and work, play and leisure, and social participation (AOTA, 2008). The contextual information collected needs to describe the physical and social environments where the client performs his or her preferred occupations and illustrate cultural issues relevant to the client. The occupational profile also needs to include information related to the client's occupational goals. Occupational therapists need to know why their clients are seeking services; what their occupational performance concerns are; and what daily occupations they need, want, and are expected to perform. And finally, it is imperative that we know the outcomes the client wants and expects to attain through occupational therapy. Refer to Case Study 23.1 to see how an occupational profile emerges during the evaluation process.

CASE STUDY 23.1 Occupational Profile: Who Is George?

Susan, an occupational therapist, receives a new client on her caseload. Based on the information she received with the referral for occupational therapy services, she knows his name is George, he is on the acute care unit, is 62 years old, and has multiple sclerosis. Susan knows she needs to find out more information about George as part of the evaluation process. She reviews George's medical record and learns that George is married, has three children, is a semiretired teacher, has had recent falls without injury, uses a cane, has type 2 diabetes and hypertension, and lives in a two-story house with a first floor bedroom and bathroom. Susan introduces herself to George and describes occupational therapy (refer to Box 23.1 to see approaches to describing occupational therapy). Through discussion with George, Susan finds out he is an engineer by profession, has been teaching college-level engineering courses for the past 15 years, and is currently an adjunct instructor, co-teaching two courses each year. George has four grandchildren (ages 4, 7, 8, and 11—all girls) and enjoys attending their school and sport events. He plays the violin and volunteers as an usher for symphony events. George enjoys cooking and playing cards. He has an office and music room on the second floor of his house, and there are 12 steps to enter the front door of his house and 2 steps to enter the back door. Through administration of the Canadian Occupational Performance Measure, Susan obtains data on George's priority daily activities. George identifies participating in volunteer activities at his church and the symphony, teaching, cooking, bathing, and ballroom dancing with his wife.

- What is George's occupational history and experience?
- What is George's pattern of activities of daily living?
- What are the occupations George needs, wants, and is expected to perform?
- What are George's priorities?
- What additional information would be beneficial for Susan to add to George's occupational profile?

As a reminder, the occupational profile is a "summary" of information; so although there is a wide range of data options, the occupational therapist collects what is most relevant to the specific client's occupational performance. Additionally, although we collect much of the data during the first session with the client, we also add to the data over sessions while working with the client.

Occupational Performance Analysis

Whereas the occupational profile addresses the collection and organization of primarily *subjective data* based on the client's perceptions, the analysis of occupational performance addresses the collection, organization, and synthesis of primarily *objective data* regarding the client's occupational performance (AOTA, 2008). Objective data are descriptions that can be easily replicated by others observing the same phenomenon. In order to collect objective data, we need to have the client perform selected activities important to his or her occupations. These typically include activities that the client wants or needs to perform or activities that others expect him or her to perform. Ideally, the client performs the priority occupations in his or her usual manner, with the objects and equipment they usually use, in the setting or settings in which they typically perform the occupation (Rogers & Holm, 2009). The ideal performance situation reflects the client's real-life situation. However, attainment of the real-life or ideal performance situation is dependent on the practice setting and may not always be feasible. In that case, the practitioner attempts to replicate the real-life performance context as closely as possible given the constraints of the practice setting. Therapists need to understand that in the contrived performance setting of the occupational therapy clinic, the performance demands are different and thus may not fully reflect actual performance in the natural context. Dr. Joan Rogers, well known for her research in task performance, highlights this issue well when she would challenge participants in her workshops by saying "If you want to understand the importance of context, try going home and making dinner in your neighbor's kitchen . . . see how much longer it takes and whether you are able to do things as well."

In order to collect objective data, therapists need to rely on valid and reliable assessment tools specifically designed to measure factors that support and restrict occupational performance. Chapters 24 and 25 provide in-depth discussions about the importance of effective assessment tools. Performance may be impacted by the person's body structures and functions, by the context of the performance, or by the transaction among them in the form of skills and patterns of performance. Therefore, depending on the client's needs, assessment tools may be used to measure client factors, contexts and environments, activity demands, performance skills, and performance patterns in one or more areas of occupation (AOTA, 2008). As a reminder, although the occupational profile and analysis of occupational performance are presented sequentially, they are dynamic in nature and are typically integrated when evaluating a client. Data, both objective and subjective, should be collected about the client's strengths as well as limitations. See Case Study 23.2 to apply the concepts about evaluation discussed so far.

CASE STUDY 23.2 Evaluation: Does Nicholas Need Occupational Therapy Services?

Nicholas is 7 years old and was referred for school-based occupational therapy services because he has sloppy handwriting, difficulty sitting still in class, and easily becomes frustrated. Gina, the school occupational therapist, meets with Nicholas's first grade teacher, his father, and Nicholas to describe occupational therapy services (see Box 23.1, describing occupational therapy) and to obtain information for Nicholas's occupational profile. Gina finds out the following information: Nicholas has recently been diagnosed with attention deficit/hyperactivity disorder; his father and mother wish to try behavior strategies before considering medications; he has three older teenage siblings and a 5-month-old brother; he has difficulty following rules at home and in the classroom; enjoys gym class; he takes swimming lessons and is a cub scout; and he is slow to complete schoolwork, dress himself, and do his chores. Gina analyzed Nicholas's occupational performance by observing him in the classroom, administering standardized assessment tools to Nicholas, and requesting his parents and teacher to complete standardized questionnaires. The data indicated that Nicholas had problems with fine motor skills (difficulty holding and manipulating everyday objects—pencil, fork, toothbrush), dressing (difficulty fastening and adjusting clothes, unable to tie shoes), cognitive skills (difficulty following directions and organizing himself and his environment and limited attention span). The data also indicated that Nicholas had strengths in gross motor activities (swimming, running, and kicking and throwing balls), motivation (wanted to do well in school and at home and please his parents and teacher), and social skills (got along well with his siblings and peers).

- What are Nicholas's problems?
- Do Nicholas's problems relate to his occupational performance?
- What outcomes would be appropriate for Gina to target in occupational therapy services in the school setting?
- Can occupational therapy assist in resolving Nicholas's problems?
- What goals can address Nicholas's targeted outcomes?

BOX 23.1 Describing Occupational Therapy

Each occupational therapy practitioner has his or her own individual therapeutic style when describing the occupational therapy process to a client. Additionally, the description is tailored to make it relevant to the client. Although there is not a cookbook for what to say to your client, the following are some helpful hints when describing occupational therapy.

- Say occupational therapy, occupational therapist, and occupational therapy assistant versus "OT."

  Hello George. My name is Susan. I am your occupational therapist. My job as your occupational therapist is to help you do the things that you need and want to do throughout your day.

- Use examples of relevant daily occupations based on what you know about your client.

  Examples for George might include *safely getting dressed and showered, doing activities in your home such as making meals and yard work,* and *visiting with family and friends.*

  Examples for Nicholas might include *tying shoes, using a pencil, throwing a ball, organizing his desk and backpack,* and *playing board games.*

- Engage your client in a dialogue—ask questions and follow up on responses by asking additional questions to obtain more information

  Have you ever heard of occupational therapy or known someone who had occupational therapy? If the person says, "yes," ask them to tell you about the experience to determine if it is similar to or different from the services they will have.

  Ask the person about his or her daily routine:
  Describe your daily routine to me.
  Tell me about what you do at home.
  Tell me about what you do at school.
  Tell me about what you do at work.
  Tell me about the daily activities you need or want to do.
  Ask your client if they have questions.

- Clients need reinforcement of learning—orient or educate your client on an ongoing basis throughout the occupational therapy process.

  Sometimes occupational therapy practitioners complain about having to "always explain what we do." Think of orienting clients as continuing throughout the occupational therapy process, that is, it does not just occur when you meet the client for the first time or during the evaluation session. Practitioners need to orient or educate the client on an ongoing basis throughout the occupational therapy process.

  Have your client describe what they do in occupational therapy to a new client—it is a great way to see how effective you were in orienting the client to occupational therapy.

- Don't use medical or health care buzzwords, acronyms, or abbreviations—they are likely meaningless to your client and can be confusing.

- Emphasize that the occupational therapy process is collaborative.

  George, we are going to work together to help you get back to your volunteer activities at church and the symphony.
  Nicholas, you and I are a team; together we are going to make your school activities easier and more fun.

- Practice makes perfect. Practice describing occupational therapy . . . to your family, friends, colleagues, and to your clients. What did you say? Did you use person-centered communication? Did you address occupation? Did you customize your comments? How did you engage the person in the collaborative process?

Targeted Outcomes

Once the data are collected and organized, the final task is to synthesize the data in order to define the performance problems that occupational therapy interventions can appropriately target. As part of the synthesis, the occupational therapist develops hypotheses about the client's occupational performance (Rogers & Holm, 1989, 2009). The hypotheses explain why the problem is occurring based on the subjective and objective data. It is important to be highly specific in identifying occupational performance problems and hypotheses. Well-defined problem statements and hypotheses are needed to develop relevant targeted outcomes. Creating short-term (i.e., goals achieved in the near future—in a few days, week, or month) and long-term goals (i.e., ones achieved over a longer period of time—in 2 months to a year) and determining procedures to measure progress toward attainment of goals are in the final aspect of evaluation—targeted outcomes (AOTA, 2008).

Goal establishment is done in collaboration with the client and needs to address the targeted outcomes that reflect occupational performance problems relevant to the client's discharge needs. Goals need to be written as objective, measurable statements with an identifiable time frame and predetermined objective methods to measure progress. Even if the problem limiting the client's ability to perform his or her daily occupations is related to a client factor, performance skill or pattern, or the environment, the goal statement needs to be connected with an area of occupation in addition to addressing the specific occupational performance problem. In practice, short-term goals typically address performance skills or body functions such as strength, movement, actions, or behaviors, and long-term goals reflect performance of the client's meaningful and important daily occupations. The targeted outcomes, including both the long- and short-term goals, help us envision and predict what the client will achieve through occupational therapy intervention.

Evidence Focus during Evaluation

The evidence focus for evaluation requires the therapist to use evidence-based information that supports the acquisition of information needed for the occupational profile, analysis of occupational performance, and targeted outcomes. For evaluation, we need to consider what theory or operating assumptions are most relevant for the client and clinical setting. We need to identify and integrate the available *research* regarding the validity and reliability of appropriate assessment tools. Examples of relevant evidence for evaluation includes studies addressing the use of a theoretical perspective with clients similar to your client and studies reporting the reliability of assessment tools appropriate to use with your client. The *therapist experience* is an essential consideration. The occupational therapist needs to reflect on the following questions: "What is my experience in evaluating this type of client?" and "What is my experience in administering the appropriate assessment tools?" Your responses to these questions are important in determining what your needs are in order to best evaluate your client. And finally, but very important in conducting the evaluation, is the evidence related to the *client's preferences*. Your client is central to the occupational therapy process, so the evidence indicating his or her preferred occupations has to be systematically and meticulously collected because it provides the foundation for a client-centered, occupation-centered evaluation. The therapist must reason in a manner that considers

- The client's preferred occupational outcomes,
- The therapist's analysis of the factors affecting performance, and
- The agreed-upon target outcomes.

The results of the therapist's professional reasoning in turn affect the transition into the next component of the occupational therapy process—intervention.

Intervention

Intervention follows evaluation in the occupational therapy process (Figure 23.3). The data collected and analyzed about the client's occupational performance during the evaluation provide navigational information for determining the best therapeutic route for the planning and implementation of intervention services. The primary question or therapy decision the occupational therapy practitioner has to make during intervention is "What occupational therapy interventions can best help my client?" In order to decide the appropriate intervention course, we must consider information obtained from problem-solving answers to secondary questions relevant to intervention planning and implementation. These include but are not limited to the following:

- What is the range of appropriate interventions based on the evidence?
- Which interventions would the client prefer performing?
- Which interventions are most effective?
- Which interventions can be implemented given the environment parameters of the therapeutic setting?
- How does the client respond to the interventions?
- Are the interventions addressing the client's occupational performance problems?
- Are the interventions promoting the client's engagement in and performance of his or her preferred daily activities?

Occupational therapy practitioners need to repeatedly ask themselves these questions throughout the intervention phase of the occupational therapy process. Discussing possible answers with colleagues can

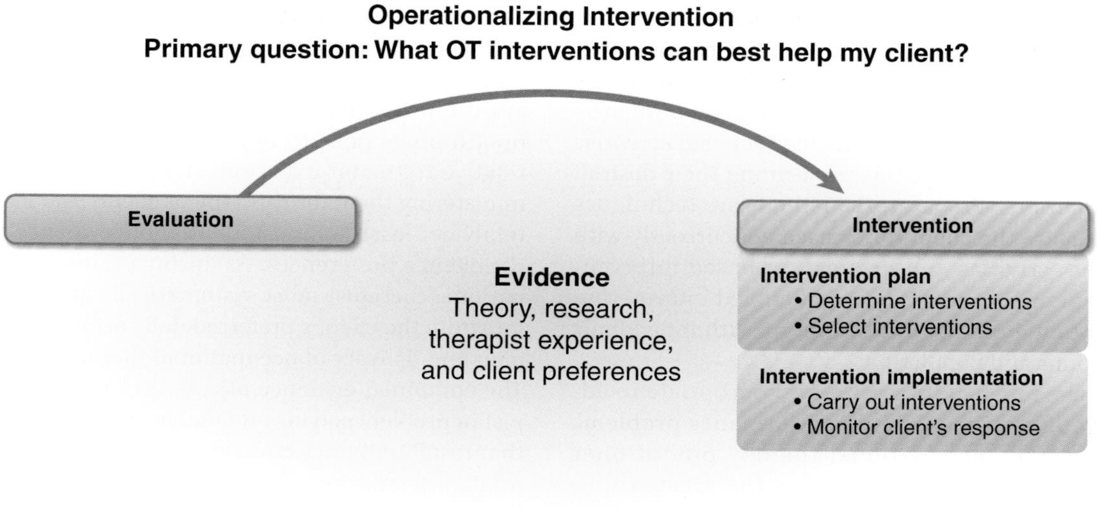

FIGURE 23.3 Operationalizing intervention. OT, occupational therapy.

assist in increasing the breadth and depth of one's professional reasoning. Think of these questions as road markers or billboard announcements directing you toward your destination of occupational therapy interventions that best help your client. Making therapy decisions based on answers to these questions will help focus your interventions on your clients' occupational performance needs.

The **intervention** component of the occupational therapy process includes the intervention plan and intervention implementation (AOTA, 2008). In order to develop an intervention plan, we need to consider the client's current occupational performance and envision what the client will achieve through occupational therapy interventions. The results of the client's occupational profile and analysis of occupational performance provide subjective and objective information about the client's current occupational performance, and the targeted outcomes predict what the client will achieve through occupational therapy interventions. Therefore, although intervention is a separate component in the occupational therapy process, it is fully dependent on and explicitly interconnected with evaluation.

Intervention Plan

The intervention plan determines the selection of specific occupational therapy activities used to address the client's targeted outcomes (AOTA, 2008). The intervention plan is developed in collaboration with the client. Although the occupational therapist is responsible for the development of the plan, it is the *client's* intervention plan, not the occupational therapist's intervention plan. The first step in developing the plan is to determine the range of interventions appropriate to address the client's occupational performance problems. Occupational therapy interventions can be categorized as an occupation-based intervention, purposeful activity, or preparatory method (AOTA, 2008). Occupation-based interventions focus on the client engaging in client-directed occupations that match the client's targeted outcomes. Purposeful activities are specifically selected activities that allow clients to develop skills that enhance occupational performance. These interventions engage clients in practicing activities related to occupations versus performing their desired daily occupations. Preparatory methods are techniques used to prepare the client for or used concurrently with purposeful activities and occupation-based interventions. Chapters 26 and 27 provide detailed information on occupational therapy interventions with individuals and for groups and populations.

Once the range of interventions appropriate to address the client's occupational performance problems is identified, the occupational therapy practitioner selects the interventions that have the greatest potential to improve performance and that are the best match with the client's occupational profile. The final decision to include a selected intervention is made in collaboration with the client. Doing so maximizes the client's understanding of the relationship between the selected interventions and his or her preferred daily occupations.

Intervention Implementation

Once the plan is established, the next step is to put the plan into action. Intervention implementation includes the process of carrying out the interventions and monitoring the client's response (AOTA, 2008). The interventions clients engage in need to be appropriate to address their targeted outcomes related to their occupational performance problems. Although monitoring of the client's response to his or her performance of interventions is listed separate from carrying out the interventions, both occur concurrently. The occupational therapy practitioner is observing and examining the client's performance while the client engages in the intervention. The practitioner adjusts aspects of the intervention as needed to better accommodate or challenge the client's occupational performance in order to achieve the targeted outcomes. Monitoring the client's response is part of the informal reevaluation described earlier in the chapter. See Case Study 23.3 for a clinical example of the intervention component of the occupational therapy process.

Evidence Focus during Intervention

Theory, research, the therapist's experience, and the client's preferences influence and guide intervention as much as they do evaluation but with a different focus. The focus for evidence to support intervention is on planning and implementation of intervention services. Examples of relevant information would be studies about the relative benefits of one approach versus another, studies about common occupational challenges for clients in a similar place in their life, and medical or educational information about the client's condition. Occupational therapists need to consider how each intervention identified within the range of interventions relates to the theory or operating assumptions most relevant for the client and the clinical setting. In addition, practitioners need to reflect on personal competencies relative to the intervention, along with experiences administering them for this type of client. And last but certainly not least, we must identify the evidence related to the client's preferences. As during evaluation, the occupational therapist must systematically and meticulously integrate the client's preferred daily occupations into the plan and delivery of occupational therapy interventions. The combined evidence assists the occupational therapist in problem solving and making therapeutic decisions that result in the selection and implementation of appropriate interventions. These therapeutic decisions reflect informal aspects of the next component of the occupational therapy process—reevaluation. The occupational therapist informally reevaluates the client's response to

CASE STUDY 23.3 Intervention: What Occupational Therapy Interventions Can Best Help Rosa?

John, an occupational therapy assistant on an orthopedic rehabilitation unit, is assigned a new client, Rosa, on his caseload by the occupational therapist he works with. Rosa is 72 years old and was just transferred from the acute care unit where she had surgery to replace her hip. She is a widow; lives in an apartment building with elevator access; uses the public bus system; enjoys gardening; plays bingo at the local senior citizen center three nights a week; and does all her own shopping, cooking, laundry, and cleaning of her apartment. The laundry facilities are in the basement of her apartment building; her bathroom has a tub with a shower—she prefers baths; she has season tickets to the local theater with her sister; she is an avid reader of mystery novels, retired as a bank teller 7 years ago, and loves to travel—she and her sister have plans to go on a cruise to Alaska in a month. Rosa is currently using a walker; however, she anticipates only needing a cane when she is discharged. Her upper extremity strength is limited and she fatigues easily. Rosa has some pain in her hip and is fearful of falling. Rosa's priority is to be able to go on the cruise with her sister.

- What is the range of appropriate interventions John might include in Rosa's intervention plan?
- Which interventions do you think Rosa will prefer performing?
- Which interventions would be most effective for Rosa?
- How do the interventions promote Rosa's engagement in and performance of her preferred daily activities?
- How do you think Rosa will respond to the interventions?

each intervention and effectiveness in assisting the client in achieving his or her goals.

Reevaluation

The third component of the occupational therapy process is reevaluation (Figure 23.4). The formal reevaluation is basically a return to the evaluation component of the process. Data about the client's occupational performance is again collected and analyzed. As with evaluation, reevaluation provides navigational information for determining the best therapeutic route for the planning and implementation of intervention services. During reevaluation, the targeted outcomes established during evaluation are assessed using the same measures employed during the original or initial evaluation. Ultimately, the occupational therapist is determining if the best therapeutic intervention route was taken previously along with identifying the best therapeutic route to take from this point forward.

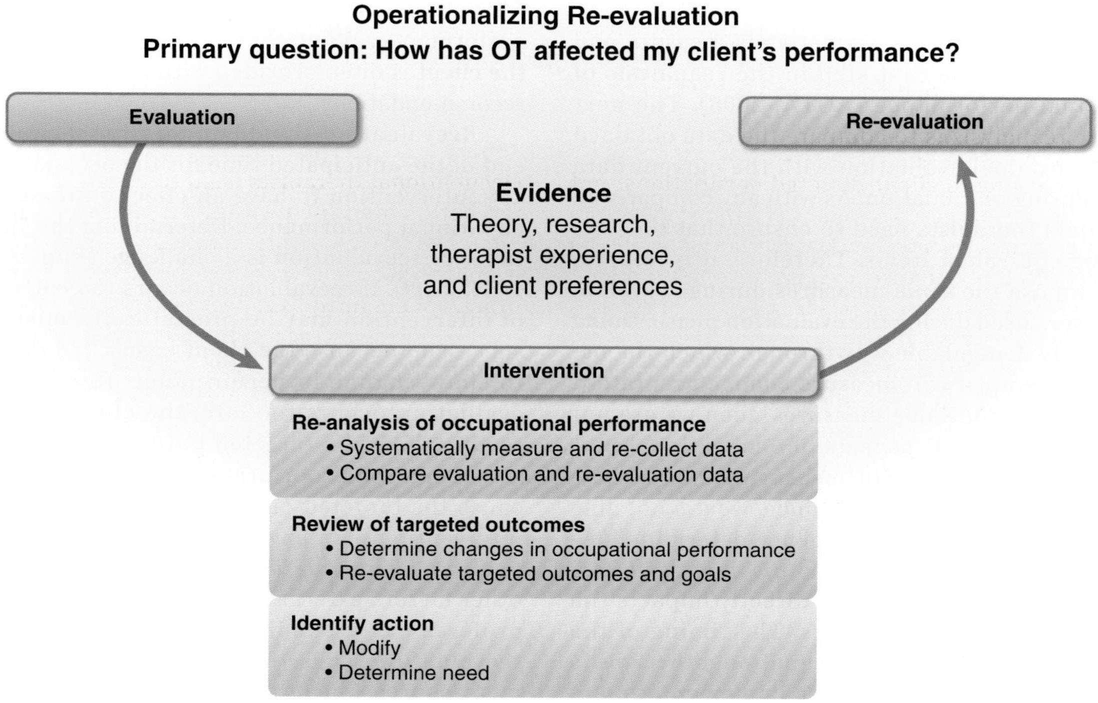

FIGURE 23.4 Operationalizing reevaluation. OT, occupational therapy.

The primary question or therapy decision the occupational therapist has to make during reevaluation is "How has occupational therapy affected my client's occupational performance?" As with the other components of the occupational therapy process, in order to make the therapeutic decision about the continued need for services, we must first obtain information that will assist us in problem solving answers to the following secondary questions. These include but are not limited to the following:

- Based on the assessment tools administered at evaluation, how has the client's occupational performance changed?
- What occupations are the client now able to perform?
- What occupations are the client still unable to perform?
- Can occupational therapy continue to assist in resolving the client's occupational performance problem(s)?
- How do the client's measurable and objective goals need to be modified to address the client's targeted outcomes?

In order to effectively problem solve the answers, we need to reanalyze the client's occupational performance, review the client's targeted outcomes, and identify the appropriate action to take regarding the continuation of occupational therapy services.

Reanalysis of Occupational Performance

Occupational therapists systematically measure and re-collect data as the first step in the reanalysis of occupational performance (AOTA, 2008). The next step in the reanalysis is to compare the data obtained during the original evaluation with the current data obtained during reevaluation. As with any comparison, occupational therapists need to ensure that they are comparing equivalent items. Therefore, it is imperative that we use the same measures during reevaluation that were used during the evaluation phase. Doing so is the only dependable way through which the occupational therapist can measure change accurately. If we do not use the same measures, then we are not measuring comparable aspects of occupational performance. And if we are not measuring comparable aspects of occupational performance, we are not able to accurately and with valid evidence determine how occupational therapy has affected the client's performance. The comparison of data directly impacts the review of the targeted outcomes. The timing of the reevaluation is based on the occupational therapist's prediction of how long it will take implementation of the occupational therapy interventions to achieve the client's targeted outcomes.

Review of Targeted Outcomes

Changes in occupational performance are used to determine whether occupational therapy interventions achieved the intended targeted outcomes through goal attainment. Review of the targeted outcomes requires the occupational therapist to determine change in the client's occupational performance relevant to the measureable goals established during evaluation (AOTA, 2008). The degree of goal attainment can be determined by comparing the client's performance measured at evaluation with performance measured at reevaluation. The targeted outcomes and goals are then reviewed and reevaluated in order to identify the appropriate action (AOTA, 2008).

Action Identification

After reevaluation, the therapist considers whether to continue therapy, refer the client to another service or specialty, or discontinue services. Continuation of services is justified if the client is making progress toward the overall goals or if there is reason to believe alternate approaches might work to improve progress. Additionally, new or altered targeted outcomes and goals may emerge as a result of the therapy process. In some cases, it may be apparent that the client could benefit from the services of other professionals, in addition to occupational therapy, or that a different specialty intervention within occupational therapy is warranted. In those cases, the occupational therapist refers the client to the appropriate resources. Services are terminated when the client has reached targeted outcomes or there is evidence to suggest that further intervention will not substantially improve occupational performance. When therapy services are terminated, the client is often provided with aftercare or follow-up recommendations.

Reevaluation should be ideally scheduled at the end of the anticipated time for the occupational therapy intervention to have an effect on the client's occupational performance. Determining the "just right" time for reevaluation is a challenge (Rogers & Holm, 1989, 2009). If reevaluation occurs too early, a course of intervention may be prematurely considered unsuccessful because the client hasn't had enough time to show change in performance. In contrast, if reevaluation occurs too late, the client may have already achieved a targeted outcome and progression in occupational performance is not continuing because the targeted outcomes, measurable goals, and intervention plan have not been appropriately modified to accommodate the positive change. There are other factors external to the occupational therapist's professional reasoning that determine the time for reevaluation. These factors include third party payment sources, health organization policies and procedures, and practice guidelines. The evidence focus for reevaluation requires occupational therapists to

CASE STUDY 23.4 Reevaluation: How Has Occupational Therapy Affected Tim's Occupational Performance?

Tim is 24 years old and sustained a traumatic brain injury 2 months ago due to a car accident. One month ago, he was discharged from the hospital and referred for occupational therapy at the outpatient center. The data Mark, Tim's occupational therapist, collected during the evaluation indicated that Tim requires moderate physical assistance for putting on lower and upper body clothing due to decreased right arm strength and sequencing problems; Tim needed moderate physical and cognitive assistance to perform money management and meal preparation tasks; he required constant supervision for safety when performing tasks due to impulsivity; and he easily became frustrated, exhibiting angry outbursts. Mark predicted that it would take 4 weeks to achieve the goals addressing the targeted outcomes he and Tim identified. Mark administered the same measures to Tim during the formal reevaluation that he had administered to him during the initial evaluation in order to accurately compare his past and current occupational performance and to determine progress. The following is Tim's current occupational performance: his right arm strength is now adequate for him to put on and off his clothing; however, he is unable to fasten his clothing (buttons/zippers); Tim is able to independently sequence dressing tasks with the use of written outline; he requires minimal assistance to physically perform money management and meal preparation tasks; however, he continues to require moderate cognitive assistance and supervision for safety in the kitchen environment; and Tim is now able to ask Mark for assistance when he becomes frustrated without display of anger.

- How has Tim's occupational performance changed since evaluation?
- What occupations is Tim now able to perform?
- What occupations is Tim still unable to perform?
- Can occupational therapy continue to assist in resolving Tim's occupational performance problems?
- How do Tim's goals need to be modified to address his targeted outcomes?

consider the available research regarding reevaluation for the specific type of client and the assessment tools administered at evaluation. Evidence for reevaluation combines relevant information from studies supporting evaluation decisions with those addressing intervention options. Although we would hope that the external factors impacting decisions regarding reevaluation are based on evidence, occupational therapists need to be aware that this is not always the case. We need to be advocates for the use of evidence-based decisions regarding all aspects of occupational therapy services, including reevaluation. See Case Study 23.4 for a clinical example of the reevaluation component of the occupational therapy process.

Outcomes: Continue or Discontinue

Outcomes are integrated throughout the occupational therapy process (Figure 23.5). As previously stated, "supporting health and participation in life through engagement in occupation" is the all-encompassing goal of the occupational therapy services (AOTA, 2008). Occupational therapy's unique focus on occupation is a primary focus in this inclusive outcome. As previously addressed in evaluation, targeted outcomes are identified that reflect the client's occupational performance problems. Measurable goals with an identifiable time frame and predetermined objective method to measure progress are essential in determining the attainment of targeted outcomes. The occupational therapist carefully considers the client's targeted outcomes when developing an intervention plan and implementing interventions. The targeted outcomes are revisited formally during reevaluation to address progress.

The primary question the occupational therapist must answer is "Does my client continue to need occupational therapy services?" As with all previous aspects of the process, the occupational therapist must obtain information to problem-solve secondary questions. These include the following:

- Has occupational therapy positively impacted the client's ability to perform daily occupations?
- Can occupational therapy continue to assist in resolving the client's occupational performance problems?
- Has the client achieved as much benefit as possible from occupational therapy services?
- Does the client want to continue receiving occupational therapy services?
- Is there sufficient justification for continuing occupational therapy services?

The occupational therapist uses information from evaluation, intervention, and reevaluation to determine the answers in order to conclude if occupational therapy services should be continued or discontinued.

As with all other aspects of the occupational therapy process, evidence provides the foundation for determining whether the client needs continued

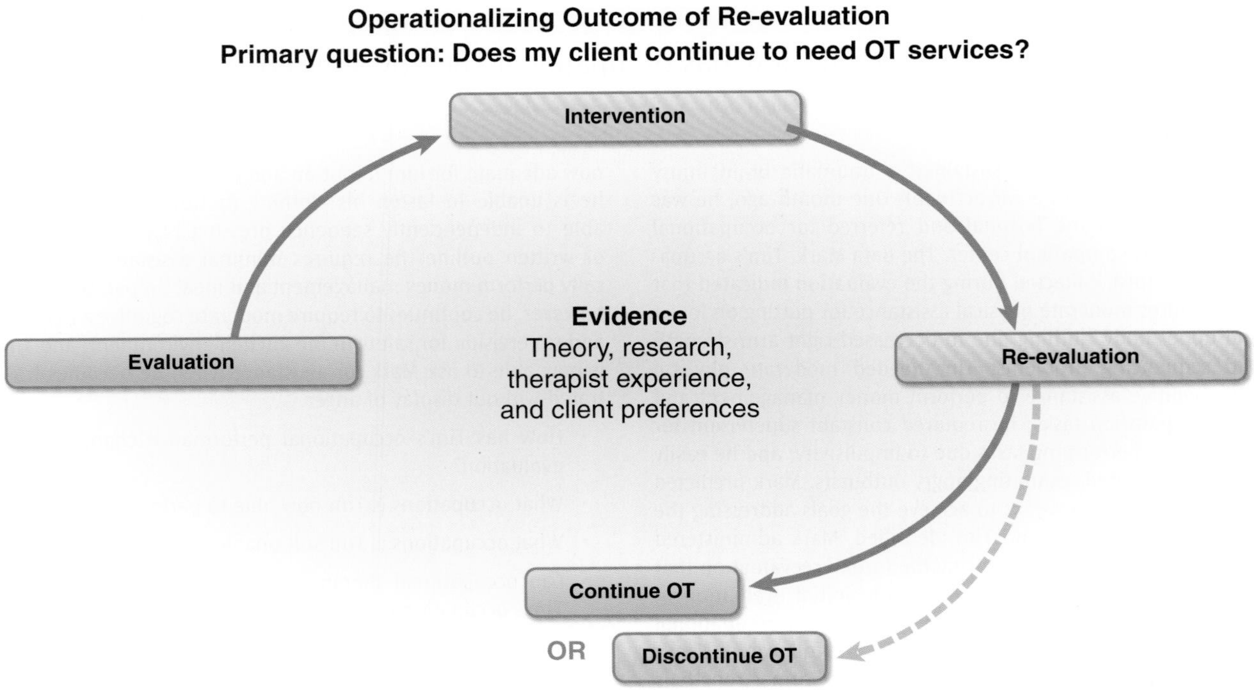

FIGURE 23.5 Operationalizing outcome of reevaluation. OT, occupational therapy.

occupational therapy services. The *evidence focus* requires the identification of the available research regarding the duration of services for this type of client based on evaluation and reevaluation results. Additionally, theoretical perspectives, the therapist's experience with the intervention route and attainment of targeted outcomes for similar clients, and the specific client's preferences in addition to his or her evaluation and reevaluation data must be considered when making the therapy decision. If the evidence supports that the client would benefit from continued occupational therapy services, then the targeted outcomes, goals, and intervention plan are modified as needed and intervention is resumed. At

CASE STUDY 23.5 Outcomes: Does Margaret Continue to Need Occupational Therapy Services?

Margaret is 57 years old and sustained a right wrist fracture. She has been receiving occupational therapy services at an outpatient center since her cast was removed 3 weeks ago. When Pam, her occupational therapist, completed her initial evaluation, she had limited range of motion in her left wrist; decreased strength; experienced increased pain with movement; and reported difficulty performing her work activities (typing, mouse use, filing), opening doors, washing dishes, unloading/loading the washer/dryer, lifting objects (pots, bags of groceries), driving, and engaging in leisure activities (needlepoint, tennis). Upon reevaluation, Margaret's range of motion is within functional limits; her strength has increased and she is able to lift medium-weight objects—prefers using two hands for heavy objects; Margaret is able to perform her work activities using the strategies that Pam taught her—taking breaks, performing stretching exercises, varying her activities, etc.; she is able to open doors and drive; she has resumed doing her needlepoint for short periods of time and just yesterday started practicing hitting the tennis ball. Margaret reports minimal pain and only when lifting heavy objects. Margaret is able to perform her home activity and exercise program independently and is able to use the strategies that Pam instructed her in to upgrade her activities and exercises. Margaret reports that she feels that her wrist has improved and that she is able to do almost all of her daily activities.

- Has occupational therapy positively impacted Margaret's ability to perform her daily occupations?
- Can occupational therapy continue to assist in resolving Margaret's occupational performance problems?
- Has Margaret achieved as much benefit as possible from occupational therapy services?
- Does Margaret want to continue receiving occupational therapy services?
- Is there sufficient justification for continuing Margaret's occupational therapy services?

CASE STUDY 23.6 Outcomes: Does Cheng Continue to Need Occupational Therapy Services?

Cheng is 26 years old with schizophrenia. He currently lives in a group home. Cheng's most recent hospitalization was 6 months ago; and since that time, he has been working with Bonnie, his occupational therapist, one time a week. His occupational therapy sessions have primarily focused on his work-related goal to maintain a part-time job. Cheng's occupational therapy interventions have addressed appropriate grooming and hygiene for the work setting; interpersonal skills with coworkers and customers; time management; work skills and patterns; initiation, sustaining, and completing work tasks; and compliance with work norms and procedures. Cheng recently began working part-time at a local grocery store stocking shelves in the evening. Bonnie has continued seeing Cheng for occupational therapy sessions to assure continuation of his work performance; however, because he has achieved his goal, he may be appropriate for discharge in the next few weeks. During Cheng's last session, he said that because he is now working and has an income that he would like to pursue living in his own apartment.

- Has occpational therapy positively impacted Cheng's ability to perform his daily occupations?
- Can occupational therapy continue to assist in resolving Cheng's occupational performance problems?
- Has Cheng achieved as much benefit as possible from occupational therapy services?
- Does Cheng want to continue receiving occupational therapy services?
- Is there sufficient justification for continuing Cheng's occupational therapy services?

a predetermined time, another reevaluation is completed to systematically measure and to re-collect data using the previously administered assessment tools. Based on the new reevaluation results, a therapeutic decision is made based on the evidence—both prior and new evidence—that either supports the continuation or discontinuation of occupational therapy services; and intervention and reevaluation is repeated until ideally, the targeted outcomes are attained and the evidence supports the discontinuation of occupational therapy services. The more frequently the process is navigated, the more observant we are of the markers directing us to the evidence that supports our professional reasoning throughout all aspects of the occupational therapy process. See Case Studies 23.5 and 23.6 for clinical examples of the outcomes component of the occupational therapy process.

Summary

Occupation is fundamental to the occupational therapy process and is embedded with both the best available and comprehensive evidence and the individual occupational therapist's professional reasoning. In this chapter, we have provided a map of the primary components of the occupational therapy process—evaluation, intervention, reevaluation, and continuation/discontinuation of services—to assist you in successfully navigating the occupational therapy services you provide to your clients. As you gain experience in map reading and navigation, we are confident that your use of the evidence and professional reasoning will correspondingly develop, assuring sound therapy decisions and successful outcomes in the therapy journey you take with your clients.

References

American Occupational Therapy Association. (2008). Occupational therapy practice framework: Domain and process, 2nd edition. *American Journal of Occupational Therapy, 62*, 625–683.

American Occupational Therapy Association. (2010). Standards of practice for occupational therapy. *American Journal of Occupational Therapy, 64*, S106–S111. doi:10.5014/ajot.2010.64S106-64S111

Christiansen, C. H., & Baum, C. M. (Eds.). (1997). *Occupational therapy: Enabling function and well-being*. Thorofare, NJ: Slack.

Christiansen, C. H., Baum, C. M., & Bass-Haugen, J. (Eds.). (2005). *Occupational therapy: Performance, participation, and well-being*. Thorofare, NJ: Slack.

Fearing, G., Law, M., & Clark, J. (1997). An occupational performance process model: Fostering client and therapist alliances. *Canadian Journal of Occupational Therapy, 64*, 7–15.

Fisher, A. G. (1998). The 1998 Eleanor Clarke Slagle lecture. Uniting practice and theory in an occupational framework. *American Journal of Occupational Therapy, 52*, 509–521.

Fisher, A. G. (2009). *Occupational therapy intervention process model: A model for planning and implementing, top-down, client-centered, and occupation-based interventions*. Fort Collins, CO: Three Star Press.

Graham, G. (1996, June). Clinical effective medicine in a rational health service. *Health Director*, 11–12.

Gray, J. A. M. (1997). *Evidence-based healthcare: How to make health policy and management decisions*. New York, NY: Churchill Livingstone.

Hinojosa, J., Kramer, P., & Crist, P. (Eds.). (2010). Evaluation: Where do we begin? In *Evaluation: Obtaining and interpreting data* (3rd ed., pp. 1–20). Rockville, MD: AOTA Press.

Holm, M. B. (2000). The 2000 Eleanor Clarke Slagle lecture. Our mandate for the new millennium: Evidence-based practice. *American Journal of Occupational Therapy, 54*, 575–585.

Law, M. (1998). *Client-centered occupational therapy*. Thorofare, NJ: Slack.

Law, M., & Baum, C. M. (1998). Evidence-based occupational therapy. *Canadian Journal of Occupational Therapy, 65*, 131–135.

Law, M., Baum, C. M., & Dunn, W. (2005). *Measuring occupational performance: Supporting best practice in occupational therapy* (2nd ed.). Thorofare, NJ: Slack.

Lee, C. J., & Miller, L. T. (2003). The process of evidence-based clinical decision making in occupational therapy. *American Journal of Occupational Therapy, 56*, 344–349.

Reed, K. L., & Sanderson, S. N. (1999). *Concepts of occupational therapy* (4th ed.). Baltimore, MD: Lippincott Williams & Wilkins.

Rogers, J. C., & Holm, M. B. (1989). The therapist's thinking behind functional assessment. In C. Royeen (Ed.), *Assessment of function: An action guide* (pp. 1–29). Rockville, MD: American Occupational Therapy Association.

Rogers, J. C., & Holm, M. B. (2009). The occupational therapy process. In E. B. Crepeau, E. S. Cohn, & B. A. B. Schell (Eds.), *Willard & Spackman's occupational therapy* (11th ed., pp. 478–518). Baltimore, MD: Lippincott Williams & Wilkins.

Sackett, D. L., Straus, S. E., Richardson, W. S., Rosenberg, W., & Haynes, R. B. (2000). *Evidence-based medicine: How to practice and teach EBM* (2nd ed.). New York, NY: Churchill Livingstone.

Silverman, W. A. (1998). *Where's the evidence? Debates in modern medicine.* New York, NY: Oxford University Press.

For additional resources on the subjects discussed in this chapter, visit http://thePoint.lww.com/Willard-Spackman12e.

CHAPTER 24

Evaluating Clients

Mary P. Shotwell

LEARNING OBJECTIVES

After reading this chapter, you will be able to:

1. Understand the differences between screening, assessment, and evaluation
2. Apply the Occupational Therapy Practice Framework to the evaluation process
3. Identify strategies for interviewing about, observing, and assessing occupational performance
4. Discuss personal and contextual factors that influence the evaluation process

OUTLINE

Introduction

This chapter reviews the process of client evaluation. The first section of the chapter defines terminology and discusses components of the evaluation process, including review of documentation/referral, interview and occupational profile, specific assessment measures, interpretation and findings, and recommendations for intervention. The second part of this chapter will explore models that might be used to guide client-centered evaluation, including the Occupational Therapy Intervention Process Model (Fisher, 2009) and the use of the "Occupational Therapy Practice Framework, 2nd Edition" (American Occupational Therapy Association [AOTA], 2008) as a guide for the evaluation process. The third part of this chapter considers factors that influence the evaluation process such as practice environment, therapist experience, tools and documentation used in the evaluation process, and ethical issues in evaluation.

Terms Relevant to Evaluation

In a discussion of the evaluation process, it is important to clarify relevant terms such as *screening*, *evaluation*, and *assessment* because they each have specific meaning as used in this chapter and common professional documents in the United States.

Screening

Screening is often the first part of the occupational therapy (OT) process and consists of a quick review of the client's situation to determine if an OT evaluation is warranted. It may occur when a referral is made or may be a routine activity that a therapist does any time a new client enters a given practice setting. For example, in long-term care settings, it is a routine practice for newly admitted residents to be screened for potential to benefit from OT services. Once the therapist determines that the client might be a candidate for OT and it is agreed that the client will use the service, the evaluation process begins.

Evaluation

Evaluation is the term used for the whole process of obtaining and interpreting information needed for intervention planning and effectiveness review. This includes planning for and documenting both the evaluation process and the results (AOTA, 2008, 2010b). Niestadt (2000) posited that "Occupational therapy evaluation is both a set of procedures and a thought process" (p. 1). The procedural part of the OT evaluation can consist of performing interviews, observations, assessments, and hands-on strategies to understand the client's strengths and challenges in occupational performance. In reality, it is not possible to ever fully separate evaluation from intervention, because practitioners maintain an evaluative view of clients throughout the OT process (screening to discharge). The thought process of evaluation uses all types of professional and clinical reasoning as the therapist considers medical, social, and/or educational diagnoses; contextual factors in the client's world; and pragmatic factors that influence the client and the intervention process (Hinojosa et al., 2010). Closely related to evaluation, **reevaluation** is "the process of critical analysis of client response to intervention" (AOTA, 2010b, p. 2). As discussed in Chapter 23, reevaluation enables the therapist to assess the client's response to intervention and to collaborate with the client to determine changes to the intervention plan.

Assessment

As part of the evaluation, therapists may need to gather specific information via the use of assessment tools. Hinojosa et al. (2010) describe an **assessment** as " . . . a specific tool, instrument or systematic interaction used to collect occupational profile and occupational performance areas during the evaluation process" (p. 3). An assessment can be informal in that the therapist uses a given situation to obtain data or it may involve using a standardized interview or observation tool. Standardized assessments typically involve a process in which the client performs specific actions that are graded or rated by the therapist according to a predetermined set of criteria. Assessments can be *criterion-referenced* where the client is graded in terms of some behavioral standard or *norm-referenced* where the client is compared to a group of other people who have taken the same measure. In today's practice environment, it is often not practical to perform numerous assessments; therefore, it is critical that therapists carefully choose assessment tools when measuring occupational performance. Chapter 25 provides guidance about factors to consider in choosing tools to assess client performance.

Professional Standards Related to Evaluation

Because the occupational therapist is educated at the professional level, he or she is responsible for all aspects of the evaluation process (AOTA, 2010b). In addition to gathering and interpreting information, evaluation includes making recommendations for OT intervention and/or referral to other services from which the client might benefit. Occupational therapists may ask occupational therapy assistants (OTAs) to contribute to the evaluation process. Under the supervision of an occupational therapist, OTAs may perform and report findings from selected assessments for which they have service competency (AOTA, 2009). Chapter 67 provides more information about the process of establishing competence, and Chapter 72 discusses the overall differences in practice roles between the professionally educated occupational therapist and the technically educated OTA.

In addition to following professional guidelines, OT practitioners must respond to referrals and procedures in a manner that complies with regulatory, financial, and ethical requirements. Verbal and/or written communication of evaluation findings should be provided within time frames as specified by practice settings, legal/regulatory, accreditation, and payer requirements. All communication regarding clients should be conducted within boundaries of ethics related to client confidentiality (AOTA, 2010a).

Occupational Therapy Evaluation as Choreography

The practice of OT, like that of many service professions, is an art as well as a science. The science is evident in the methodical processes used by therapists as they explore client challenges and collaborate with the client to develop strategies for dealing with problems in daily living. The artistry in OT comes from the relationship or the connectedness with the client and his or her situation in order to generate individualized and creative solutions to help enhance the client's quality of life. Part of the artistry in practicing OT is the ongoing dance that happens between evaluation and intervention throughout the OT process. Typically, throughout the evaluation phase, the therapist may be incorporating intervention strategies. Similarly, when implementing intervention, therapists gather data to evaluate the client's response and modify therapy accordingly. Evaluation does not only happen at the beginning and at the end of intervention; it should be happening throughout the OT process to explore effectiveness of intervention (AOTA, 2008).

The metaphor of dance provides a helpful way to examine the process; because in order to provide effective client-centered services, occupational therapists must choreograph the whole OT process (Figure 24.1). The process of choreography includes several components such as sources of inspiration, collaboration with others, entering the studio, elements of creation, making movement, composing the piece, and performing the piece (Canadian National Centre for the Arts, n.d.). Table 24.1 demonstrates parallels between choreographing a dance and the OT process.

Throughout the process of composing a dance, the choreographer must always keep in mind the "end product," which is the dance that will be performed before an audience. The choreographer considers all elements such as use of space, costume, set, and lighting, for example. Similarly, the occupational therapist must simultaneously consider evaluation, intervention, and discharge planning in light of client and contextual factors. Skilled practitioners carefully choose interview and assessment strategies that will help gather the most valuable information to guide intervention. Novice therapists might not consider discharge planning until they are well into the intervention process, but more experienced practitioners know to treat each client visit as though it might be the last visit before discharge or transfer to another setting. The OT evaluation typically follows a sequence that includes screening and referral, document review, interview and occupational profile, specific assessment measures, interpretation and findings, and recommendations for intervention.

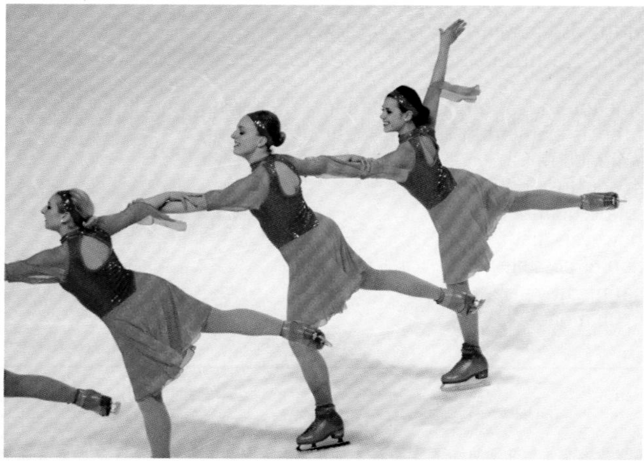

FIGURE 24.1 Just as these world class synchronized skaters must attend carefully to each other in order to create an effective performance, occupational therapists must work with their clients to choreograph an evaluation that results in effective intervention. (Photo courtesy of Ellen Cohn.)

Much like a beginning dancer, the novice OT practitioner is often somewhat clumsy and mechanical in interviewing, observing client performance, and in administering standardized assessments. Inexperienced therapists may be so concerned with their own performance (especially when being closely supervised) that they have limited ability to engage or enjoy the artistry of their practice. Focusing on the mechanics of performing an evaluation may result in limited mental reserves available for interpretation, synthesis, and documentation of findings. An expert occupational therapist seems to effortlessly flow through the dance of evaluation as he or she carefully chooses interview questions and observes relevant performance factors. The seasoned therapist can demonstrate skilled reasoning to select appropriate assessment tools, seemingly knowing what questions to ask, what assessment tools to use, and when the evaluation is completed. Taking the metaphor of determining client needs as choreography a little further, foundational texts on choreography will tell us that in order to compose a dance, there are factors that influence the outcome. These elements will be our guide for the rest of this chapter.

Screening and Referral: Prelude to the Dance

In many practice settings, screening for services often occurs prior to referral for OT. In some settings, occupational therapists screen new clients as a matter of course, whereas in other settings, occupational therapists only screen clients as requested by other professionals such as nurses or teachers. In many long-term care settings, for example, all new residents are screened for their potential to benefit from therapy services as a way of potentially helping the client to transition to this new living environment. In school system practice, the therapist often engages with the teacher or a support team to screen students (often via observation or work samples) and makes recommendations (often in the form of adaptations) that the teacher might implement to see if problems can be abated. Should the child not respond to the support team recommendations, there is often a referral for an OT evaluation.

Screening involves gathering preliminary data about a client's challenges in occupational performance and determining whether or not the client may benefit from skilled OT services or perhaps referral(s) to other professionals. Screening is viewed as a "hands-off"

TABLE 24.1 Comparing Choreography of Dance to Occupational Therapy Process

Element of Choreography in Dance	Related Concept in the Occupational Therapy Process	Pragmatics with Clients in Occupational Therapy
Collaboration Even the solo performer is dependent on stage people to adjust environmental factors including lighting, music, and costumes. The end product is a collaboration between the dancer and many other people.	Working "with" the client rather than "doing for" the client. Occupation therapists should also be aware of practitioners in other disciplines who might be working with the client and ensure collaboration in the best interest of the client.	Occupational therapist must ask the client what he or she wants to accomplish. Client must participate in goal setting rather than merely agree with goals you generate.
Studio The place where the dance is crafted, but the ultimate test is to perform the dance on a stage in front of an audience.	The place where you do therapy (which may not be the place in which the skill is generalized).	Occupational therapist must provide opportunities for skills to generalize to different settings, times, social situations, etc.
Elements The who, what, and where of the dance. What is the story the dance is trying to tell? Where will the dance be performed? What will the backdrop look like? What costumes will be worn?	Clients come with a multitude of factors that influence occupational performance. Similarly, therapists have their context that they bring to the OT process.	Occupational therapist's job is to figure out what needs to be emphasized during the OT process.
Making movement Deciding at what point in the music the dance will begin. Dancers must consider elements of timing, space, and props.	Typically, time must be spent on developing therapeutic rapport with the client, especially when dealing with sensitive or personal information. Therapists need to have some degree of logical flow through an assessment or an intervention session. In medicine, the physical assessment begins at the head and ends with private parts so as not to invade one's most intimate area at the beginning of the assessment.	Occupational therapist must consider time, tools, and therapist skills available for assessment.
Composition How does the piece flow from beginning to end? Are there "movements" in the piece that signify "chapters" in the story?	The more smoothly the assessment process flows, the more confidence the client has in the therapeutic relationship and in the potential outcomes of intervention. There needs to be some degree of transparency in the assessment process.	Occupational therapist must use time during an assessment wisely, often intertwining interviewing with other assessment measures.
Final step Any composition needs closure that signifies the conclusion and interpretation of the piece.	Clients typically expect some interpretation to be made at the end of the assessment session. Therapists are cautioned not to be too quick to make firm conclusions about the client's source of occupational performance problems; however, they should give some indication of possible sources and thus goals that might be used to address the occupational challenge.	Occupational therapist has to know when to close the assessment.

CASE STUDY 24.1 Amanda: Screening an Adolescent in an Alternative School

When I started working in a residential and alternative school setting for adolescents, I was asked to screen each of the students. For a week, I went into the facility and met each of the adolescents one at a time, getting to know them and performing screenings and requesting occupational therapy (OT) evaluation orders where appropriate. Amanda was a resident who I began "screening" the first day I started working at this facility. The first thing one of the staff said was, "I don't know whether or not you can help her (Amanda), but she needs something . . ." Amanda noted that I hadn't "picked her" yet and yelled across the day room: "Hey OT lady, aren't you going to work with me? . . . Probably not, they say I'm too much trouble".

Throughout my few days there, I had noticed that Amanda seemed to seek attention from staff and from male students. She seemed to impose herself on groups during unstructured time; and according to the staff, she often "stirred up trouble" between students, particularly if two girls were interested in one boy. Upon reviewing her records, I noted that she had been in three different residential facilities in the past year and a half. Apparently, she was discharged from these facilities due to fighting with other female students. Without more information, I wasn't sure what I might be able to do with her; but it seemed clear that she was having some occupational performance concerns, so I asked for an OT order to evaluate the student.

approach where there is limited interaction between the client and the therapist, often taking the form of consulting with staff members or reviewing intake information on clients who are new to a facility or an agency. ***The key things that the occupational therapist should look for in intake information are recent changes in living environment, health status, or occupational performance.*** For example, in a long-term care environment, the client's records might be screened for recent history of falls or declines in performance of activities of daily living (ADL). In school system settings, screenings often take place after the student support team has recommended that the occupational therapist observe a student in a classroom and has given suggestions for the teacher to implement to enhance a child's classroom performance.

The mere presence of a diagnosis or clinical condition should not dictate whether a client is screened for or receives OT services; clients should be screened when he or she is experiencing challenges in occupational performance. When dealing with caregivers, organizations, or populations, screening can be done by using results of surveys, incident reports, and population statistics that might influence occupational performance. Some examples of documents that might be used for determining if OT screenings might be needed for a group or population might be the number of falls in a facility, the causes of back injuries to staff members, or national health statistics about secondary disability in a population of people with spinal cord injury.

Once it is determined that an OT evaluation is warranted, the therapist receives the appropriate written referral as per agency policies and procedures. For example, in most medical settings, a physician order is necessary for an OT evaluation. In a school system setting, the referral for an OT evaluation usually comes from the student support team, the special education staff, or the school psychologist. Occupational therapists in the United States typically have the legal ability to enter a case without a referral from another professional, so clients can self-refer for OT services and they can self-pay; however, more often, agency or payment requirements and mere pragmatics often supersede self-referral or self-payment. See Case Study 24.1 for an example of how a screening might result in a referral.

Clients: The Source of Inspiration

In the arts, there are many sources of inspiration. In OT, the client is the source. Fisher (2009) categorizes the client in three ways: (1) the "client" can be a "person" who seeks or is referred for OT services; (2) a "client constellation" that includes both the individual who seeks or was referred for services and others who are closely connected to that individual; and (3) a "client group" that includes people who share similar problems in occupational performance (p. 3). Table 24.2 gives examples of terms and strategies for assessing different types of clients.

Regardless of the way in which we define the term *client*, a collaborative focus on occupation is critical in the OT process. This is true even when the therapist feels the client goals are unrealistic. Consider Adam in Case Study 24.2.

Document Review: Understanding the Backdrop for the Dance

In many settings, there are client records that can provide useful information, such as demographic information, and often some type of history about the recent events or challenges experienced by the client. For example, in a medical or long-term care environment, the patient's record will discuss the reason for coming to the facility, procedures performed, and results of tests. In the educational setting, the student records may have reports from

TABLE 24.2 Terms and Assessment Strategies for Working with Different Types of Clients

	Client	Client Constellation	Client Group/Population
Terms used to describe	• Patient • Student • Consumer • Resident • Member • Customer	• Family members • Caregiving staff • Teachers • Church groups • Support circle	• Class • Support group • Community • Staff • Organization or agency
Strategies for assessing needs	• Interview • Observation • Performance measures	• Interview • Self-efficacy surveys • Observation of performance	• Focus groups • Surveys • Reports • Performance measures
Considerations	• Must be able to articulate needs	• Being a caregiver does not necessitate OT involvement; caregivers must face challenges in their caregiving role to warrant intervention.	• Individual or group making the OT referral may have different opinions about the occupational performance challenges than do the individuals with whom you are directly working.

OT, occupational therapy.

various professionals, results of educational testing, and an Individualized Education Plan (IEP) or a 504 Plan (student accommodations in educational settings) where appropriate. In the case of groups or populations, documents may include personnel files, incident reports, survey results, and statistics about a concern or health condition. For new practitioners, as well as those new to a particular practice area, it can be difficult to identify which documents and what information should be the focus of the record review. Table 24.3 gives suggestions of potentially important documents to review by practice setting.

In medical settings, records will contain a history and physical, which reviews the systems in the body and the past medical history and provides consultation reports. The medical report, specialist consultation reports, progress notes, and results of testing can provide information vital to the OT evaluation, such as reason for admission (i.e., stroke or admission for a surgical procedure); and it provides information about body systems/functions that might have an impact on occupational performance. A key understanding of the results of a history and physical can guide the therapist's choice of evaluation strategies

CASE STUDY 24.2 Adam: A Man with a Mission (Part1)

While working in a rehabilitation facility, I encountered Adam, a 46-year-old man who was diagnosed with Guillain-Barré syndrome after being ill with a flu-like illness for about 2 weeks prior to admission. In my prior experience, I had worked with people who had made rapid recovery from this condition, so I expected a similar situation. When I went in Adam's room and asked him what he would like to accomplish, he stated that his main goal was to return to work as a project manager for a defense agency. He stated, "I don't care about getting dressed, just figure out a way that I can use my computer from my bed."

My initial bedside evaluation revealed that Adam had no cognitive or perceptual difficulties, but he had severe pain that limited my ability to perform sensory or motor testing. When I moved his extremities to check passive range of motion (he was quadriplegic at this point), he screamed out in pain. He told me to stop moving him and to reposition him so he was comfortable. This activity took about 20 minutes as we could not find the right spot for his pillow where he was comfortable for me to leave the room. At this point, he was completely dependent in all self-care and mobility. How could I help him use his computer if he couldn't even move his body?

1. Consider what else you might want to know?
2. Read through to the chapter to see options to consider.

Note: Case continues at the end.

TABLE 24.3 Types of Documents Helpful in the Records Review Process

Setting	Medical	Long-Term Care/ Skilled Nursing Facility	Educational	Outpatient/Home Health	Mental Health	Group/ Organization	Population
Types of documents available	• Demographic sheet • Doctors' orders/ precautions • Consultation reports • Daily progress notes	• Demographic sheet • Doctors' orders • MDS/RUGs • Therapy plan of care • Daily notes	• Demographic sheet • Educational testing • Specialist reports • IEP/RtI (individualized education plan/ response to intervention in public school systems)	• Demographic sheet • Discharge notes from medical setting • Initial evaluation from intake coordinator • Therapy plan of care • IFSP (early intervention) • Progress notes	• Demographic sheet • Doctors' orders • Consultation • Reports • Care plan	• Reports of prior intervention • Incident reports • In-service logs • Meeting minutes • Survey or observation results	• Request for proposal • Health statistics or community data
Important notes	• Nurses • Specialist notes • PT/SLP notes	• Nurses • Specialist notes • PT/SLP notes	• Teacher reports • Psychologist reports • Educational testing	• Nurses • Specialist notes • PT/SLP notes	• Psychiatrist • Neuropsychology • Nursing • Mental health technician • Behavioral specialist	Must know who is requesting OT intervention. If the recipients are not the same people who requested the service, they may have a mistrust that the organization is employing an OT to find problems with individuals or groups.	
Tests and lab results	• X-rays • Blood work • Cardiac/ respiratory	• X-rays • Blood work • Cardiac/ respiratory	• Hearing and vision screening • Psychological evaluation • Standardized testing	• X-rays	• Blood work (may be important to determine therapeutic levels of medications)	Tests and lab results may be reported for groups and population, but these are typically reported by means and standard deviations and may not always be valuable in planning a group- or population-based intervention.	

IFSP, Individual Family Service Plan; MDS, minimum data set; OT, occupational therapy; PT, physical therapy; RUGs, resource utilization groups; SLP, speech-language pathologists.

as well as guide intervention. For example, a history and physical that lists sensory awareness as impaired would guide the therapist to interview and observe performance related to safety in the home environment. The history and physical, as well as sections regarding orders and test results, may guide the therapist to a particular action or precaution that may be indicated for a specific client. For example, when test results are indicative of a blood clot, the client may be on bed rest; or when electrolytes are imbalanced, the therapist might notice the client to be mentally confused. When in doubt about anything in a client's records, the clinician should seek clarification prior to working with a client.

The first thing that the OT practitioner should review is the reason for the OT referral. Often, the referral will read, "OT eval and treat," which is short for "perform an evaluation and treat per OT guidelines." On the one hand, this open-ended language is good for our profession in that we have opportunity to be client-centered; but for the novice practitioner, it provides little guidance about why the referral source believes this individual or group may need the services of an occupational therapist. The occupational therapist is cautioned against merely assuming that the diagnosis is the reason for the referral. For example, a client might be admitted to the hospital for a hip fracture but have a former diagnosis of a left hemiplegia due to a stroke that might be impeding use of a walker, which in turn may affect self-care. In this case, the occupational therapist may need to assist the client to compensate for inability to use their left upper extremity.

Once the clinician reviews the reason for the referral, the next step is to understand basic demographic information about the client. In many contexts in which individual services occur, there is a *face sheet* or some other introductory information sheet about the client that includes name, age, address, names of family members or guardians, diagnosis(es), education level or grade in school, and, in some settings, religious or spiritual preferences. This information can be used to more efficiently get to know the client by providing a starting point in the OT interview questions. For example, the client's *demographic sheet* in a medical setting might say that she is a retired teacher who lives with her sister in a large metropolitan area. These demographic characteristics might be used to ask the client about the sister's ability to help in the home or the availability of public transportation when the client returns home. In educational settings, there are often reports of the student's progress along with testing that also might be used to interview the student, teacher, or family member(s) about the student's strengths and challenges in the educational setting. In this way, the occupational therapist can begin to build an occupational profile of the client as well as anticipate possible occupational performance needs and challenges.

After reviewing the demographic information, the therapist then focuses on important data within a client's documentation that might be pertinent to the client, the setting, and the OT process. Particular attention should be paid to issues related to client safety that might include factors such as unstable medical status (vital signs, blood chemistry, seizures, presence of an infection, precautions, response to medication, etc.), history of falls or other injuries, unpredictable behavioral changes, and response to intervention thus far. ***In short, the therapist wants to know what to expect with regard to potential adverse events that might influence evaluation and intervention.*** The therapist might also use information about medical status to anticipate any potential communication difficulties in interviewing the client. For example, if the client is on a ventilator, it may be difficult or at least time consuming to obtain verbal responses. Similarly, if the record says that the client has unpredictable behavioral changes, the therapist might want to modulate the initial interview so as not to agitate the client.

Understanding Client Precautions: Dancing Safely

The therapist should review and note any precautions in the physician's order or documentation that should be attended to during evaluation and intervention. Precautions may include those related to diet and swallowing, neurological and orthopedic conditions (such as a lack of sensation or motion and weight-bearing restrictions), seizures, behavioral or cognitive impairments (particularly nighttime confusion in elderly clients), infection control (particularly important with clients who are immunosuppressed), open wounds or surgical sites, precautions related to medical devices, general cautions related to medications or blood chemistry (such as patients taking blood thinners need to take extra caution when shaving), and preparation for a procedure (such as restriction of water or food prior to testing).

Critical Pathways: Script for the Dance

In many rehabilitation settings, therapists employ the use of interdisciplinary critical pathways as a guide for evaluation and intervention. Commonly used in settings with patient populations who have orthopedic impairments or strokes, rehabilitation teams generate typical pathways or "care maps" that guide clinicians about what evaluation and intervention activities should be done by each clinical discipline for each day or week of care. Novalis, Messenger, and Morris (2000) reviewed data across multiple organizations that used care plans for clients with hip fractures finding that OT practitioners were most commonly involved in evaluation and intervention for self-care activities as well as transfers and mobility. For example, a care plan for an elderly woman with a hip fracture in an acute care setting might include tasks

TABLE 24.4 Sample of Occupational Therapy (OT) Aspects of a Care Plan

	OT Assessment and Intervention
Day 1	**1.** OT assessment completed within 24 hours after admission. **a.** Assessment includes measurement of ROM and strength in UE. **b.** Assessment of BADL. **c.** Interview regarding discharge plan and home environment.
Day 2	**2.** Client will sit up in chair. **3.** Client will engage in and demonstrate use of long-handled equipment for dressing. **4.** Client will be able to ambulate into bathroom with walker and transfer on and off commode with minimum assist.
Day 3	**1.** Preparation for discharge home. **2.** Reassessment of neuromusculoskeletal factors, areas of occupation. **3.** Client will be able to perform transfers to and from toilet and tub bench with SBA. **4.** Client will adhere to orthopedic precautions while performing mobility and ADL tasks.

ADL, activities of daily living; BADL, basic activities of daily living; ROM, range of motion; SBA, stand by assist; UE, upper extremities.

to be accomplished on each day for the 3 days after an open reduction and internal fixation. Table 24.4 gives a sample of what might be included in the OT portion of a care plan.

Interview and Occupational Profile: Collaborating in the Dance

Once the "preparation" for the evaluation is completed, the therapist then meets the client and performs an interview to ascertain the client's perspective. Brown (2009) states, "The usefulness of interview and observation should not go unmentioned. . . . An interview can be invaluable in determining underlying factors that are interfering with performance" (p. 164). Depending on the practice setting, the interview may take many different forms. It can be structured in terms of using a standard agency-based form in which therapists ask questions and fills out a form. Conversely, there may be no guidance for the interview, and the therapist follows the client conversation to guide the interview questions. Just as we might learn about a dance partner while dancing with him or her, the interview is often interspersed with occupation-based assessment strategies. Regardless of the interview format, the therapist must ascertain some degree of information regarding the client's perceptions about occupational performance.

Depending on the practice setting, therapists often find key questions that help them understand the occupational life of the client. Table 24.5 gives some typical questions asked in various practice settings along with typical spaces in which evaluations occur. A question such as "Tell me about a typical day?" often elicits information about what the client needs, wants, or is expected to do. The client response guides the therapist in knowing the occupations in which the client typically engages. To understand more about occupational challenges, therapists can ask the question: "What is the most stressful/least stressful time of day?" That may help the therapist know about activities that have different levels of demand for the client. Depending on the client's response to this question, the therapist may wish to probe further about why the client sees this time of day or a particular activity as challenging. For example, if you were to ask me the two times of day that I find particularly challenging, I would say (1) getting myself and my two adolescent children out of the house each morning and (2) coming home and deciding what to fix for dinner. My response might lead you to generate several hypotheses about my occupational challenges, which might include home or time management as well as caring for my children, not to mention cooking.

A skilled therapist can quickly ascertain multiple patient factors while asking the patient simple interview questions. The interview is an excellent opportunity to discover what the patient needs or wants to do when he or she leaves the hospital setting. The therapist gathers information about typical activities in which the client engages as well as the client's "home" environment and potential support the patient has, which may be critical factors in discharge planning. The interview is an excellent tool for gaining an overall picture of the patient's cognitive status (and is frequently the best and only method required, thus limiting embedding a cognitive evaluation). Finally and most important, the interview helps establish rapport with clients. ***A word of caution is advised about interviewing clients with cognitive impairment who may not have accurate insights about their performance or needs. In this case, the clinician may also interview family, friends, or staff who can offer insights***

TABLE 24.5 Potential Assessment Strategies in Various Practice Settings

	Occupational Profile Questions	Focused Questions that may Elicit Rich Responses to Guide the OT Process	Observation Environments/Items Needed	Common Assessment Tools	Key Forms of Documentation	Important Considerations for this Setting
Acute care medical setting	• Before you came to the hospital, what was your typical day like? • What do you think a typical day will be like during the weeks after you are discharged from here?	What things might hinder you from going home?	Client's bed/ chair and bathroom Wash basin, toothbrush, comb, etc.	• COPM • ROM • MMT • BADL	• Standard evaluation form • Critical pathway • Daily progress notes	• Medical stability and necessary precautions. • Relationships with medical/ nursing personnel.
Adult rehabilitation/ long-term care setting	Tell me about a typical day for you. What do you need, want, or are required to do? In your home? In the community?	What things might hinder you from going home?	Client's bed/chair and bathroom, therapy area, ADL suite	• COPM • ROM/MMT • FIM • Cognitive-perceptual • BADL/IADL	• Standard evaluation form/plan of care • Daily/weekly progress notes	Medicare Part A requirements for clients' ability to tolerate therapy hours appropriate to the setting.
Home health	Tell me about a typical day for you. What do you need, want, or are required to do?	What do you need to be able to do to continue living at home?	Client's living, dining, and bedroom as well as kitchen BP cuff, gait belt, adaptive ADL equipment as needed	• COPM • BADL/IADL	• Standard evaluation form/plan of care • Daily/weekly progress notes	With Medicare funding, occupational therapists may not have permission to "open" a case; must be opened by nurse or physical therapist.
Community mental health	Tell me about a typical day for you. What do you need, want, or are required to do? In your home or at work/ school?	Tell me about your daily chores. Do you cook? Clean? Do laundry, etc.? With whom do you eat and/or socialize? Tell me about your work/transportation situation. . . .	Home, group/day treatment setting; work environment Pencil, paper, IADL activities (e.g., making a grocery list; steps to do laundry)	• COPM • Cognitive-perceptual • BADL/IADL • Prevocational or career assessments	• Documentation may not be standardized.	May have to educate agency on potential services of OT.

School system	To teacher: What is the student expected to do? To student: What kinds of things do you have to do at school? Like to do?	What subject is your (most/least) favorite? Who do you play with at recess? What games do you play at recess?	Classroom, playground, cafeteria, bathroom Pencil, paper, seating adaptations, visual and fine motor activities	• School function assessment • Quick neurological screening test	• IEP; RtI • Daily or weekly progress notes • 6-month or annual reports • Handwriting assessment tools • Visual perceptual and visual-motor assessment tools	OT services are related and must be educationally relevant to educator-generated IEP goals.
Private pediatric setting	To parent: Tell me about your child and their role in your family. What things do you want them to be able to do?	For the parent: What is the worst/best time of day for you with your child? Tell me about your child's friends. Child: If you could do any play activity right now, what would it be?	Clinic, suspended equipment, table top activities, floor mobility activities, fine motor manipulatives	• Sensory Integration and Praxis Tests • Peabody Developmental Motor Scales • Bruininks-Oseretsky Test of Motor skills • Sensory Profile	• Initial evaluation report • Plan of care • Daily/weekly progress notes	Services often require prior authorization, therefore therapists must estimate number of visits requested.
Work-based setting	Tell me about your job. Tell me about your responsibilities at home. What do you do in your free time since you haven't been able to work?	What did you like best/least about your job? Your coworkers? Your boss? What do you see needing to happen in order for you to return to work or be retrained for another job? If you had a choice, would you return to your job or train for another job?	Actual or simulated work environment; work hardening setting/clinic	• Career interest inventories • Career aptitude measures • Focus on barriers to work performance, environment, body functions, performance skills	• Initial evaluation report • Plan of care • Daily/weekly progress notes	In order to delineate OT from other services, focus on the interaction of person-task-environment. Significant interaction with case managers.

ADL, activities of daily living; BADL, basic activities of daily living; COPM, Canadian Occupational Performance Measure; FIM, Functional Independence Measure; IADL, instrumental activities of daily living; IEP, Individualized Education Plan; MMT, manual muscle testing; OT, occupational therapy; ROM, range of motion; RtI, response to intervention.

about the client's occupational challenges. At the same time, one should still obtain the client's perspective, because the presence of cognitive impairment doesn't negate the need to understand and respond to the client's concerns.

In order to facilitate occupation-based practice, the therapist should begin with a client-centered interview. Chisholm, Dolhi, and Schreiber (2004) state that "putting occupation into your practice is often easier said than done" (p. 5). They recommend doing a client-centered interview by asking a client to list five occupations in three key areas—(1) occupations I need to do, (2) occupations I want to do, and (3) occupations I am expected to do—and then having the client circle the five most important occupations that they want to address. Once these five important occupations are identified, the performance factors contributing to these occupations would be further evaluated. This occupational performance analysis helps the therapist target the appropriate behaviors the client needs to perform desired occupations.

The Canadian Occupational Performance Measure (COPM) (Law et al., 2005) is a standardized semi-structured client-centered interview to explore the client's perceptions about his or her current level of function in self-care, productivity, and leisure. The client is asked to identify the five most important problems in occupational performance. Using a visual analog scale ranging from one to ten, the patient is then asked to take each of these five problems and rate the importance and level of satisfaction with activity performance. The value in using the COPM is that patient's perception can be used as an objective measure of progress, which may be particularly valuable when progress is slower than expected or in cases where a client seems to be "higher functioning" but is having quality of life concerns.

Roberts and colleagues (2008) used the COPM throughout the United Kingdom and found that there was an increase in mean scores of satisfaction with occupational performance. This same study found that both clients and physicians were more satisfied with the services of OT after implementing the use of the COPM. Roberts et al. (2008) saw patterns of responses when using the COPM, whereby older adults reported more concerns with regard to self-care and younger people tended to report more difficulties with productivity, which confirms that a "one-size-for-all" approach to evaluation may not be appropriate. It is therefore critical to ascertain each client's concern about his or her occupational performance.

Therapists often intersperse observation of occupational performance or client factors with the interview. The most difficult part of this "dance" is knowing what questions to ask and when to ask them, because clients may not be able to focus on action and answering questions at the same time. It is also helpful to the client if the interview questions relate to the actions being performed. For example, the therapist may be asking the client to sit at the edge of the bed, and while the client is moving or resting after performing this action, the therapist may ask an interview question about anticipated difficulties getting in and out of bed when they go home. Brown (2009) notes that where possible, observation of a client in their natural environment can yield valuable information about the client's method of doing a particular occupation and can also help identify barriers to performing an occupation.

The Occupational Therapy Practice Framework: Backdrop for the Dance

The "Occupational Therapy Practice Framework" (OTPF) (AOTA, 2008) notes the interview and occupational performance analysis to be effective tools to identify factors such as body functions that may be influencing occupational performance. During the interview, the therapist should ask clients about

- Performance patterns, including habits, roles, and routines;
- Contexts for occupational performance that include cultural, personal, physical, social, temporal, or virtual; and
- Activity demands that take into account objects used, space demands, social demands, sequencing, required actions, and body functions or structures that the patient typically performs in his or her daily life activities.

Occupational therapists from the Cardinal Hill Healthcare System (Skubik-Peplaski, Paris, Boyle, & Culpert, 2006) attempted to operationalize the 2002 version of the OTPF and worked across all practice areas in their organization to incorporate occupation into services and OT documentation. Using the framework, they developed forms and structured interview protocols to be able to understand the client's occupational needs. Interview protocols that they developed typically ask clients about a typical day and about activity demands, objects, space, and timing of daily life occupations. They assert that therapists should ask clients about areas beyond basic self-care, such as work and leisure. They also advocate asking interview questions about context, particularly social support. The online resources listed on the Willard and Spackman Website provide a sample evaluation form, which is adapted from a sample evaluation by Robinson and Shotwell (2010) containing ideas similar to those in the Cardinal Hill application of the OTPF.

Strategies for Assessment: Adding Elements to the Dance

Tables 24.6 to 24.13 provide examples of how a practitioner might incorporate concepts described in the OTPF. The evaluation should begin with the client's perception of his or her own performance in areas of occupation. Clients should be asked about a typical day to understand the areas of occupation in which the client engages.

In addition to interview and understanding client perceptions, the evaluation should also include the use of standardized assessment tools for areas in which the therapist seeks further information. The use of standardized assessment tools also contributes to the goal of our profession to provide evidence to support our practice.

In evaluating the areas of occupations, the therapist is trying to find out about basic or personal activities of daily living (BADL or PADL) as well as instrumental activities of daily living (IADL) that are necessary to "run our lives." Some of the IADL occupations include managing one's finances, cleaning one's home, shopping for goods and services, and so forth. Therapists need to ascertain if the client is having difficulties with sleep, rest, work, school, or participation in leisure activities. In acute medical situations, clients may not think about ADL or functional performance and may assume that these skills will immediately return once the body functions or body structures are restored to health. Although this may be true in some cases, occupational therapists can often ease the process and reduce the time that it takes a client to engage in desired occupations. In many cases, this can alleviate the need to stay in a congregate care facility (e.g., hospital, nursing home, or assisted living facility) and help to enhance the individual's quality of life. In institutional environments, it may be difficult to have the client engage in some of the IADL tasks during the evaluation process; so many times, information is gathered via interview rather than actual occupational performance. Table 24.6 gives some strategies for assessment of areas of occupation.

Assessing Overlapping Occupational Concerns: Composition of the Dance

To say that occupation is complex seems to be an understatement. Many times, it is not one occupation that is problematic, but, often, the interface among various occupational demands may be causing difficulty in occupational performance. This orchestration of various occupational demands can be challenging just as it can be challenging for dancers to combine different dance elements. For example, I am quite capable of cooking and cleaning, but my role of worker and of parent often supersede my engagement (or motivation) to engage in these tasks necessary for the "job of living." Case Study 24.3 provides an example of an individual who was working in a sheltered workshop setting. Although this client was successful in performing work-related tasks, the client had difficulty transitioning from sheltered to community-based employment because of occupational performance concerns regarding hygiene and clothing management.

After understanding the client's areas of occupational engagement, the therapist begins to try to

TABLE 24.6 Strategies for Evaluation of Areas of Occupation

	Examples of Standardized Measures	Interview/Observational Strategies
Areas of occupation	• Canadian Occupational Performance Measure (COPM) • Occupational Performance History Interview II	• Ask client about a typical day.
Basic activities of daily living (BADL)	• Functional Independence Measure (FIM/WeeFim)	• Observe client dressing, bathing, feeding, etc.
Instrumental activities of daily living (IADL)	• Kohlman Evaluation of Living Skills • Milwaukee Evaluation of Daily Living Skills	• Observe client doing a shopping, budgeting, or cooking task.
Education/work	• School Function Assessment • School Assessment of Motor and Process Skills • Worker Role Interview	• Observe client doing a work-related or school-related task.
Play/leisure	• Transdisciplinary Play-Based Assessment • Leisure Assessment Inventory	• Observe child on the playground.
Social participation	• Social Interaction Scale of the Bay Area Functional Performance Evaluation (BaFPE)	• Note interaction during interview. • Ask client about his or her social life. • Observe in structured and nonstructured social environments.
Rest/sleep	• National Institutes of Health Activity Record	• Do you have difficulty with sleeping?

CASE STUDY 24.3 Allen: Combining Work and Self-care for Effective Participation

Allen was a 47-year-old man who I encountered while working in a vocational program that included community placements as well as "sheltered workshop" employment. The goal of the agency was that all clients eventually be employed in community-based settings; but the staff was concerned about Allen, not because of his work skills but more because of his hygiene. Allen had been involved with this agency for the past 2 years, and the staff reported that he was capable of learning new jobs and could perform simple one- to two-step work tasks such as placing labels on boxes or repackaging materials for store display. The staff was concerned that they could not move Allen into a community-based position because he needed constant cueing to brush his teeth and take a shower. When picking Allen up on the facility bus each morning, the bus driver stated that at least once or twice a month, she did not allow Allen to get on the bus because of his poor personal hygiene (which is a requirement for participating in the program). When told that he needed to go back into his home to shower, Allen would do so, but he seemed to have limited insight regarding why personal hygiene was necessary for successful work performance.

Questions:

1. Why do you think that Allen has difficulty with his habits of self-care?
2. What environmental factors might be influencing Allen's difficulties in self-care?

understand various factors that may facilitate or hinder occupational performance. Client factors include values, beliefs, and spirituality; body functions; and body structures. In many settings, the focus of OT evaluation and intervention is on body functions, such as cognition, sensory, and neuromusculoskeletal functions; but therapists are cautioned to recognize the importance of values, beliefs, and spirituality on both the therapeutic relationship and the whole OT process.

A point worth mentioning in terms of client factors is that the term *spirituality* is meant in the broadest sense rather than religiosity. Although religion may provide a sense of spirituality, people may have many factors that influence their sense of inner peace and focus. When I interview a client, I sometimes ask what activities give them a sense of peace and calm, and client responses are often indicative of spirituality. Typical answers from clients might be "prayer"; "meditation"; "being out in nature"; "petting my dog"; and "being with family." Table 24.7 lists some possible measures and questions a therapist might attend to with regard to values, beliefs, and spirituality.

In many practice settings, the focus of evaluation and intervention is on client factors such as the body functions of cognitive, sensory processing, or neuromusculoskeletal factors that influence occupational performance. Body functions can be evaluated via the use of standardized assessment tools or through interview and observation. In medical or rehabilitation settings, typically, body functions such as sensory functions and neuromusculoskeletal functions are emphasized, but the therapist should always keep in mind that impairments in these functions do not necessitate dysfunction in occupation. Table 24.8 gives potential strategies for evaluating body functions.

CASE STUDY 24.2 Adam: A Man with a Mission (*Continued*)

When working with Adam (Man on a Mission), I was working in a rehabilitation setting that placed a high value on the use of the Functional Independence Measure (FIM) (Uniform Data System, 2010) as one of the main outcome tools to determine whether a "patient" was making adequate progress. Given that Adam had severe pain and discomfort along with requiring total assistance for ADL, I initially viewed him as an inappropriate candidate for rehabilitation because he only wanted to do therapy while he was in his hospital bed. By being hyperfocused on the FIM scale, I couldn't see that being independent in self-care was not nearly as important to this client as was his returning to productive employment.

Adam taught me that if I was to be an effective practitioner, I had to listen to my clients and to trust, rather than question, their wishes and desires. Instead of focusing on his performance of BADL, I eventually began to explore his level of pain and possible strategies to reduce pain. Additionally, because of his strong desire to return to using a computer, I realized that I could use computer use as a valued occupation to promote movement and pain reduction. I was able to figure out how to use a sip and puff interface for Adam to be able to use his computer. We started slowly by just playing solitaire to learn the mechanics of operating a computer in a new way. After one day of using the computer, Adam was able to reduce his pain level and he began to have the desire to sit up for longer periods and to learn to transfer to a wheelchair to attend therapy sessions. I used his strong values of "work" as being critical to his identity and used as a motivator to guide therapeutic intervention.

TABLE 24.7 Strategies for Evaluation of Client Factors—Values, Beliefs, and Spirituality

	Examples of Standardized Measures	Interview/Observational Strategies
Values, beliefs, spirituality	• Canadian Occupational Performance Measure (COPM) • Quality of Life Inventory • Health-Related Quality of Life	• Tell me about your life . . . Family? Work? Social? • Do you engage in any practices that enhance your spirituality? • What is the most important (occupation) for you to be able to do?

TABLE 24.8 Strategies for Evaluation of Client Factors—Body Functions

Body Functions	Examples of Standardized Measures	Interview/Observational Strategies
• Specific mental functions	• Allen Cognitive Level Screen • Toglia Category Assessment	• Have you noticed a change in your ability to remember, to pay attention, or to follow directions?
• Global mental functions	• Mini-Mental State Examination • Cognitive Assessment of Minnesota	• Have you noticed a change in your mental abilities?
• Sensory functions and pain	• Sensory Profile (all ages) • McGill Pain Questionnaire • Vision or hearing screening	• Do you have numbness or tingling anywhere in your body? • Do you have pain? Where? Type? Duration? What makes it better? • Do you have difficulty tuning out specific sensory things in the environment (noise, visual distractions, and things next to your body)? • Do you have difficulty getting aroused or calmed down?
Neuromusculoskeletal and movement-related functions	• Quick Neurological Screening • Range of motion or manual muscle testing • Berg Balance Scale	• Notice coordination, strength (effort), or difficulty moving. • If you notice difficulty in the above you might ask this: • Do you have a history of falls? • Do you have difficulty bending, reaching, or grasping?
Voice and speech functions	• Usually done by observation rather than formal assessment, which is typically done by a speech-language pathologist.	• During the interview, note particularly soft or loud voice, ability to articulate words, or difficulties in expressive or receptive language. • Ask client to talk after eating or drinking (a "wet" sounding voice may be indicative of swallowing problems).
Organ system function (cardiovascular, respiratory, hematological, immunological, digestive, metabolic, endocrine, genitourinary and reproductive functions)	• Pulse oximetry, blood pressure; pulmonary function test. Occupational therapists may be involved in a modified barium swallow study, which is designed to view the swallowing functions or they may administer the Swallowing Ability and Function Evaluation (SAFE)	• When working with clients who are on digital monitor, therapist can note changes in these numbers during the occupational therapy (OT) session. For example, a client may be comatose but have changes in heart rate or blood pressure when the therapist moves an extremity during fabrication of a splint. OT practitioners should be keenly aware by looking, feeling, and listening to changes in body functions as evidenced by changes in sweating, color of skin, respiration patterns, and so forth, because these may be signs of organ system changes.

In addition to understanding the client's body functions, therapists must have some appreciation for body structures that might have potential to influence occupational performance. Although these are not typically evaluated in a formal manner, therapists (particularly those working with clients with more acute medical concerns) must have awareness of these areas. Information about body structures can be gathered via test results such as the laboratory reports or X-rays. Many of the diagnostic procedures performed by medical specialists are designed to evaluate body structures. Table 24.9 lists potential strategies for evaluation of body structures.

Ultimately, it is the goal of OT to help a client enhance occupational performance. Therapists must assess how clients use body functions and structures to perform given skills that comprise occupations. In other words, I could have the body "structures" necessary to see and to move my fingers to type this chapter and I could have the body "functions" such as global and specific mental functions necessary to organize my thoughts for ideas to write this chapter, but I could have great difficulty in enacting this occupation of "professional writing." My difficulties could be in performance skills (initiating, attending, or problem solving to find good references) or with performance patterns (e.g., not making the time to write or conflicting roles between that of writer and parent). Tables 24.10 and 24.11 give potential strategies for how a therapist might evaluate occupational performance skills and performance patterns that may include both standardized assessment tools as well as interview.

Our job as therapists is to identify which components of occupation (client factors, performance skills, performance patterns, or context) are causing the greatest challenge and to remediate or compensate for these challenges to enable performance.

Assessing the Environment and the Demands: The Setting for the Dance

The choreographer must know the setting for the dance and the type of dance to be performed. If the stage has a different type of flooring or lighting on which the dancers are not familiar, the rehearsal period may need to be extended. Additionally, if a dance requires a high degree of lifting or athleticism, the choreographer or director will choose dancers who excel in strength and endurance because of the demands of the piece to be performed. Similarly, the occupational therapist needs to understand the context in which occupations are performed and how those tasks are typically performed. When it is not possible to be in the real environment, the therapist asks questions about the environment and the ways in which the client typically performs tasks. This may include asking questions about location, surfaces, heights of various objects or surfaces, tools used, and social or cognitive aspects of task performance.

Table 24.12 gives strategies for evaluation of context and environment. Although many occupational therapists tend to focus on the physical environment, one must also consider the other aspects of the environment that can influence occupational performance. Consider the case of Alfonso who was gainfully employed but underproductive in his work environment. In this case, my main interest was in a contextual evaluation of his work area(s), tools, tasks, and social and cultural aspects involved in productive employment as a grocery store employee.

TABLE 24.9 Strategies for Evaluation of Client Factors—Body Structures

Body Structures	Evaluation Method	Interview/Observational Strategies
Nervous system Eyes, ear, and related structures Structures involved in voice/speech Structures related to movement Skin and related structures Organ system structures (cardiovascular, respiratory, immunological, digestive, metabolic, endocrine, genitourinary, and reproductive systems)	Not typically evaluated by an occupational therapist because occupational therapists do not evaluate structures independent of a functional/purposeful activity. Many of the diagnostic procedures that physicians request would be used to assess body structures. An example might be an X-ray, an angiogram, or a magnetic resonance imaging, which are all designed to view structures and any potential abnormalities.	Much of this information can be found in clients' records. Look for history and physical that details prior injuries, procedures, and tests that the client may have undergone. Although the questions below are not necessarily indicative of a structural problem, positive client responses may be indicative of potential difficulties with body structures (and certainly warrant further evaluation and/or referral). • Do you have numbness, tingling, or difficulty moving? • Do you have any trouble with your eyes or hearing? • Do you have any wounds right now? Difficulty with skin healing? • Have you had any procedures for your heart, lungs, stomach, or reproductive system? Why?

TABLE 24.10 Strategies for Evaluation of Performance Skills

Performance Skills	Examples of Standardized Measures	Interview/Observational Strategies
Overall performance	• Assessment of Motor and Process Skills	Watch a client engage in an activities of daily living (ADL) that involves neuromusculoskeletal, cognitive, and social interaction, which may give some overall picture of performance.
Sensory/ perceptual	• Test of Visual-Motor Skills • Motor-Free Visual Perception Test	Observe client as he or she engages in tasks in his or her environment. Does client tend to miss things on one side of his or her world? Does client have evidence of poor visual acuity?
Motor/praxis	• Jebsen Hand Function Test • Peabody Developmental Motor Scales	Observe client as he or she engages in occupational tasks. Does he or she have a tremor? Slowness or problems with speed of movement? Is the accuracy of movement impaired? Does the client seem to have difficulty executing movements necessary for functional tasks?
Emotional regulation	• Coping Inventory/Early Coping Inventory • Tennessee Self-Concept Scale	When presented with a task that challenges a client's competence, does he or she become frustrated or defeated? Is the client's response to his or her situation proportional to the magnitude of client's challenges?
Cognitive	• Routine Task Inventory • Performance Assessment of Self-Care Skills	Does the client seem to have difficulty initiating, sequencing, terminating, problem solving, and so forth, during occupational performance?
Communication/social skills	• Assessment of Communication and Social Interaction • Vineland Adaptive Behavior Scales	Is the client able to communicate his or her needs, wants, desires?

In order to provide a "complete" picture of a client's occupational performance, the therapist must also have understanding of activity demands. Table 24.13 lists some possible strategies for exploration of activity demands. In reviewing the "activity demands" of Alfonso's position at this grocery store, I reviewed the job description used for all people in his same position. Job descriptions can provide some guidance about the tools, space, and body functions required for a specific job. In the workplace, this may be easy as locating job descriptions, which often have lists of "essential functions"; however, for many other occupations, such as homemaking or hobbies, the activity demands are evaluated by interviewing the client about the task demands. For example, one client may do laundry by going to a commercial laundry facility, whereas another client has to go to the basement in his or her home to do

TABLE 24.11 Strategies for Evaluation of Performance Patterns

Performance Patterns	Examples of Standardized Measures	Interview/Observational Strategies
• Habits • Roles • Routines/rituals	• Role Checklist • Adolescent Role Assessment • Self-Discovery Tapestry • Worker Role Interview • National Institutes of Health Activity Record • OPHI; OCAIRS	• Tell me about a typical day for you. • May have to structure questions into categories for self-care, homemaking, work/school, social/leisure activities.

OCAIRS, Occupational Circumstances Assessment-Interview Rating Scale; OPHI, Occupational Performance History Interview.

TABLE 24.12 Strategies for Evaluation of Context and Environment

	Examples of Standardized Measures	Interview/Observational Strategies
Cultural	• Many of the tools used in occupational therapy tend to emphasize physical environment to address physical safety; however, when used in a client's home/work, the therapist will typically also observe for cultural, social, temporal, and virtual environmental factors. • Work Environment Impact Scale • Safety Assessment of Function and the Environment for Rehabilitation (SAFER) • School Setting Interview	• Where do you live? Work? Engage in leisure? With whom?
Personal	◦	• Are there special rituals, foods, practices in which you engage?
Physical	◦	• Do you prefer to do things alone or with others?
Social	◦	• Tell me about your home. . . . Try to identify potential barriers/strengths.
Temporal	◦	• With whom do you live? Other sources of social support?
Virtual	◦ ◦	• What is the best/worst time of day for you or your family? • Do you use the Internet, e-mail, cell phone, etc.? ◦ If so, for what purpose(s)?

laundry (see Figure 24.2). The fact that the demand for one person may require driving or walking a distance to access a laundry facility may be a barrier for the first client, whereas ascending and descending steps to do laundry may provide a barrier for the second individual.

Typically, after the client has identified their top five valued activities, the therapist can probe further about the activity demands of these tasks because people vary greatly in task demands based on all of the other factors involved in analysis of occupation. Therapists are cautioned about making judgments about the "right or wrong" way to perform an occupation. If we are to help clients with occupational performance, we need to help them learn or resume occupations in ways that they are most comfortable, rather than using our preferred method of occupational engagement.

Another strategy for understanding the activity demands is to observe a client engaging in his or her valued occupation. The ability to see the client actually performing a task in his or her own environment using his or her own tools and space is most optimal, although this may not be possible in clinical settings. Therapists are encouraged to try to simulate occupational performance to best analyze the fit between the "person" (client factors, performance

CASE STUDY 24.4 Alfonso: Contextual and Activity Demands

As I observed Alfonso in the grocery store, I noticed that the store had several employees with disabilities of varying types. Additionally, there were posters around the break room that supported the company's efforts to promote diversity, which might be indicative that the cultural context of this organization was to support diversity practices including the hiring of people with disabilities. I noticed that all of the associates took time to speak with each other, particularly the employees with disabilities to "make them feel special." Although this culture of social acceptance of people with disabilities was desirable, I also noticed that there seemed to be "lower" expectations of the employees with disabilities, that is, until Alfonso's manager noticed and questioned that his productivity and accuracy was not consistent with nondisabled employees in the same position. I observed him take at least 15 minutes to empty one trash can, and he took 30 minutes to sweep a small area near the pharmacy section. I also noticed that most workers seemed to be hurried about their work and that the temporal context of the workplace was to enable customers to get out of the store as efficiently as possible. Alfonso's slowness in work performance was not consistent with the temporal demands of the environment. ■

TABLE 24.13 Strategies for Evaluation of Activity Demands

Activity Demand	Interview/Observational Strategies
Objects used and their properties	• Do you have all of the tools needed to do the activity? • Weight, size, amount of resistance of various objects/tools.
Space demands	• Environmental considerations (social, cultural, physical, etc.). • Organization of space and materials.
Social demands	• Do you "have" to do this task or "want" to do it? • Is this a task that you enjoy? If not, have you tried to get someone else to help you with the task?
Sequencing and timing	• Frequency; repetitions and duration of a task/subtask. • Temporal components of the task (speed, sequencing, flow). • Is this a task that could be broken up into parts? Do all the steps of the task need to be done in one time period?
Required body functions	• **Neuromusculoskeletal:** difficulty in bending, reaching, gripping, stiff or effortful movement; apparent lack of awareness of body in space. • Does it involve climbing, stooping, and frequent bending or prolonged body position? • **Perceptual/cognitive:** missing one aspect of the visual field on a consistent basis; forgetting the steps to a task; doing the task inaccurately or incorrect sequence; forget what you were doing during this or other tasks? • Do you lose your tools/objects or forget what you were doing while engaging in this activity? • **Social/emotional:** easily frustrated; tends to work alone; does not share materials; becomes easily discouraged; seeks constant reinforcement or never asks for help; passive; disinterested; hyperfocused; and lack of ability to transition.
Required body structures	• Required strength, joint mobility, respiratory status, etc.? • Do you need to sit or rest during this activity? Do you become short of breath or fatigued?

skills, performance patterns), the "environment" (cultural, physical, temporal, social, etc.), and the "task" (activity demands). In the case of Alfonso, I wanted Alfonso to stay gainfully employed; however, I questioned the match between the person, the task, and the environment. My report and my recommendations for intervention would have to take person, task, and environment into account if I was to help Alfonso be successful in his employment.

Factors Influencing the Evaluation Process

Just as the choreographer may be influenced by the potential audience, the space, the budget, and the artistic desires of various stakeholders, so, too, is the occupational therapist influenced by ethics, reimbursement, organizational factors, and requirements for documentation. First is the Occupational Therapy Code of Ethics, in which all principles seem to apply to evaluation and intervention. Beneficence and nonmaleficence apply to safety and doing what is in the best interest of the client. Autonomy and confidentiality related to respecting the rights and privacy of clients throughout the OT process. The ethical principle of duty relates to maintaining professional competence and using the best evidence available to provide client care. Procedural justice relates to evaluation and intervention in that the occupational therapist must comply with laws and policies guiding the OT profession.

In terms of complying with laws and policies, occupational therapists speak to many audiences in their communication regarding evaluation and intervention. Not only do facilities have specific requirements for what should be included in evaluation and progress reports but accreditation agencies as well as funding organizations often require specific factors be attended to in OT practice. This being said, occupation therapists need to be mindful in preventing non-OT personnel dictating what should be included in OT evaluation and intervention planning as well as documentation. In order to advocate for OT, practitioners are advised to keep abreast of laws, policies, and the professional evidence regarding our practice.

Interpretation and Intervention Planning: Doing the Dance

Practitioners use their professional reasoning to interpret results of interview, observation, and assessment(s). Typically, the interpretation involves making some

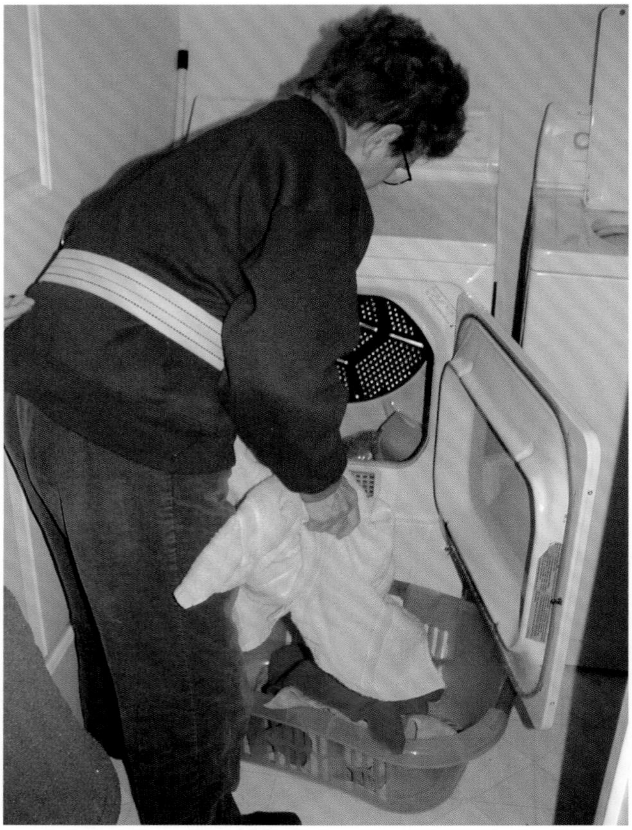

FIGURE 24.2 As part of the evaluation process, clients are observed performing tasks that are important to their daily routines. This requires attention to safety as well as the quality of performance. This client is wearing a gait belt because she has problems with balance when she bends over. In this way, the therapist can observe her routine performance but be ready to support her if needed.(Photo courtesy of Mary Shotwell.)

judgment about the client's strengths and challenges with regard to occupational performance. The therapist makes a statement about the client's ability to benefit from therapy and predicts the duration, frequency, and type of intervention strategies that will likely be used. In some organizations, the use of a "critical pathway" may guide these decisions; however, one must keep in mind that critical pathways are based on statistical means and may not apply to all individuals.

Once the therapist determines that the client may benefit from OT services, long- and short-term goals are formulated in collaboration with the client. Long-term goals may be accomplished in days, weeks, or months depending on the intervention context. Therapists must estimate the number of visits that a client will require so they must have some idea about typical lengths of stay or the number of visits that a client might need for their specific concerns. In the acute care setting, the length of stay can be as short as one day, so the evaluation, intervention, and discharge plan may all occur within the same day. For example, a client with an orthopedic condition may have an evaluation, receive adaptive equipment and education in its use, and be ready to go home. In this situation, the therapist may believe that the client will need follow-up OT services in his or her own home.

Client goals should be behaviorally oriented in terms of what the client will do. For example, the goal might read, "Client will participate in education regarding . . ." rather than "therapist will educate client about . . ." Goals should be timed and measureable, which is often a challenge for the novice therapist who has little experience knowing how long it will take a client to achieve a goal; let alone being able to identify the benchmark for successful outcome(s) of services. When generating individualized goals and intervention plans, the therapist must consider person, task, and environment. Intervention plans typically consider a multitude of factors such as medical stability of the client, home environment, available social support, and task/activity demands.

Summary

In this chapter, we have reviewed the OT process of determining client needs. The therapist must be good at interspersing interviews with assessment and maximizing the time allotted to complete an evaluation in order to best reflect the client's concerns regarding occupational performance. Like well-planned choreography, effective evaluation requires attention to multiple factors. When done well, the "dance" of therapy flows from evaluation into intervention. In this process, the clinician is challenged to consider contextual factors of the client as well as the practice setting and to incorporate the use of interviews, observation, and standardized assessment tools where possible. Using guides for evaluation such as the AOTA Practice Framework (AOTA, 2008) and *The Guide to Occupational Therapy Practice* (Moyers & Dale, 2009) may aid the occupational therapists' reasoning by providing the range of factors affecting occupational performance.

References

American Occupational Therapy Association. (2008). Occupational therapy practice framework: Domain and process, 2nd edition. *American Journal of Occupational Therapy, 62*, 625–683.

American Occupational Therapy Association. (2009). Guidelines for supervision, roles, and responsibilities during the delivery of occupational therapy services. *American Journal of Occupational Therapy, 63*, 173–179.

American Occupational Therapy Association. (2010a). Occupational therapy code of ethics and ethics standards. *American Journal of Occupational Therapy, 64*(Suppl.), S17–S26.

American Occupational Therapy Association. (2010b). Standards of practice for occupational therapy. *American Journal of Occupational Therapy, 64*(Suppl.), S10–S11.

Brown, C. (2009). Functional assessment and intervention in occupational therapy. *Psychiatric Rehabilitation Journal, 32* 162–170.

Canadian National Centre for the Arts. (n.d.). *The choreographic process.* Retrieved from http://artsalive.ca/en/dan/make/process/chprocess.asp

Chisholm, D., Dolhi, C., & Schreiber, J. (2004). *Occupational therapy intervention resource manual: A guide for occupation-based practice.* Clifton Park, NY: Delmar Learning.

Fisher, A. G. (2009). *Occupational therapy intervention process model: A model for planning and implementing top-down, client-centered, and occupation-based interventions.* Fort Collins, CO: Three Star Press.

Hinojosa, J., Kramer, P., & Crist, P. (2005). *Evaluation: Obtaining and interpreting data.* Bethesda, MD: AOTA Press.

Law, M., Baptiste, S., Carswell, A., McColl, M. A., Polatajko, H., & Pollock, N. (2005). *The Canadian Occupational Performance Measure* (4th ed.). Ottawa, Canada: CAOT.

Moyers, P. A., & Dale, L. M. (2007). *The guide to occupational therapy practice* (2nd ed.). Bethesda, MD: AOTA Press.

Niestadt, M. E. (2000). *Occupational therapy evaluation for adults: A pocket guide.* Philadelphia, PA: Lippincott Williams & Wilkins.

Novalis, S. D., Messenger, M. J., & Morris, L. (2000). Occupational therapy benchmarks within orthopedic (hip) critical pathways. *American Journal of Occupational Therapy,54*(2),155–158.

Roberts, A. E. K., James, A., Drew, J., Moreton, S., Thompson, R., & Dickson, M. (2008). Measuring occupational performance and client priorities in the community: The COPM. *International Journal of Therapy and Rehabilitation, 15*(1),22–29.

Robinson, K., & Shotwell, M. (2010). Evaluation in acute care occupational therapy. In H. Gabai (Ed.), *Acute care occupational therapy.* Bethesda, MD: AOTA Press.

Skubik-Peplaski, C., Paris, C., Boyle, D., & Culpert, A. (2006). *Applying the occupational therapy practice framework: The Cardinal Hill occupational participation process.* Bethesda, MD: American Occupational Therapy Association.

Uniform Data System. (2010). *About the FIM system.* Retrieved from http://www.udsmr.org/WebModules/FIM/Fim_About.aspx

For additional resources on the subjects discussed in this chapter, visit http://thePoint.lww.com/Willard-Spackman12e.

CHAPTER 25

Critiquing Assessments

Sherrilene Classen, Craig A. Velozo

OUTLINE

LEARNING OBJECTIVES

After reading this chapter, you will be able to:

1. Discuss the application and importance of measurement theory relative to occupational therapy assessment
2. Describe traditional versus modern testing approaches as they relate to occupational therapy practice
3. Describe and apply a framework to evaluate assessments by type and structure
4. Recognize the uses of standardized versus nonstandardized tests
5. Define and apply the concepts of reliability to occupational therapy assessments
6. Identify the components of validity and apply that knowledge to assessments
7. Describe the basic components of item response theory (IRT)
8. Discuss factors important in critiquing IRT-based assessments

Introduction

This chapter provides students and occupational therapy practitioners with the basic knowledge necessary for critiquing assessment tools used in practice. As noted in Chapter 24, the use of assessment tools is inherent in the occupational therapy evaluation process because they are important sources of evidence to inform effective decision making for both therapists and clients. Additionally, the prediction and measurement of occupational performance is a cornerstone for developing evidence to enhance therapy services. Therapists must critically evaluate which assessments are best to use in a given situation, and this in turn requires an understanding of the concepts of measurement and the process of using assessment tools. Key information covered includes the concepts of measurement theory, how to evaluate potential assessment tools and their psychometric properties (including reliability, internal consistency, and validity), information on the implications of using standardized versus nonstandardized assessments, and the need to be aware if any cut points exist to understand the sensitivity and specificity of measures used. To help readers apply this information, an ongoing case study is provided featuring an occupational therapist, Karen, as she seeks to evaluate a client who is at risk in terms of driving safety.

CASE STUDY 25.1 Karen Evaluates a Client for Driving

Karen is an occupational therapist working in a regional medical center. She needs to evaluate Mr. Patel, a patient with Parkinson's disease (PD). One concern is whether Mr. Patel should continue driving. For many individuals in the United States and similar countries, the ability to drive has a far-reaching impact on community participation. Thus, Karen has to carefully select and administer the best possible assessments in order for her to make an informed recommendation to Mr. Patel, his family, and the appropriate medical and legal authorities. ■

Foundational to understanding measurement issues is an understanding of classical test theory (CTT) as well as generalizability theory approaches, which are part of traditional measurement. However, because measurement theory is advancing, Karen should also appreciate a more "revolutionary" way to think about assessing and more specifically "measuring" her client. Traditional measurement approaches continue to have a prominent role in our understanding of assessment, but modern approaches are having a significant impact on how Karen and others will assess clients, especially in the future. Therefore, this chapter includes information on both classical and modern approaches to critiquing assessments. The more modern approaches include presentations of a comparison of item response theory (IRT) to traditional test theory, advantages of IRT (efficiency and precision), linking assessments, computerized adaptive testing, and a modern approach to psychometric assessment. In this way, the chapter provides foundational information for occupational therapists to critique assessments used in everyday practice.

Traditional Approach to Critiquing Assessments

Measurement, in its simplest form, is defined as the rules for quantifying a classification of certain attributes or characteristics (Law, 1987). For example, occupational therapists use measures to reflect a child's performance in school tasks or an adult's ability to perform self-care or community living skills. The assignment of a number makes it possible to mathematically evaluate the attributes that are being measured in a standardized way. This allows comparisons about performance or capacity across individuals or groups of individuals. It also provides a way to document how an individual's performance has changed over time and across performance contexts. Because occupational therapists make judgments that affect the lives of our clients, it is an ethical responsibility to understand the strengths and limitations of any measure used as part of the evaluation process. The occupational therapy practitioner must understand aspects related to the types of assessments; their structural characteristics; and basics about construction, standardization, reliability, and validity.

Nonstandardized versus Standardized Assessments

As noted in Chapter 24, many occupational therapy evaluations include a blend of standardized and nonstandardized assessments. Although standardized assessments bring confidence in validity and reliability when used appropriately, nonstandardized assessments were, are, and will continue to be an important source of information gathering during the occupational therapy process. Luebben and Royeen argue that "every standardized assessment begins its life as a non-standardized test" and that "a new assessment moves along non-standardized continuum toward the standardize end as a result of rigorous development . . ." (as cited in Hinojosa, Kramer, & Crist, 2005, p. 125).

Nonstandardized assessments, as the name implies, do not follow a standard approach or protocol. For instance, they may not involve a consistent set of questions, directions, or conditions for administration, testing, or scoring. Such assessments may contain data collected from observations or interviews (e.g., with the referring physician, the client, or the family member) as well as during the occupational therapy evaluation via questionnaires (e.g., demographic, health, or medication) and observation of performance. Data obtained from this method are most effective when they reflect attention to the issues raised in Box 25.1 (Hinojosa et al., 2005). Additionally, this data is most useful when combined with the following approaches.

A **standardized assessment** is developed using prescribed procedures. It is administered and scored in a consistent manner under the same conditions and test directions. The standardization of test questions, directions related to performance, conditions of testing, and scoring is needed to make test scores comparable and to assure, as much as possible, that clients have equal, unbiased opportunities to demonstrate what they know and can do (Association of American Publishers, n.d.). Standardized assessments have typically undergone

BOX 25.1 Questions to Ask in Critiquing Nonstandardized Assessments

- Is it guided by theoretical frameworks and/or models of practice?
- Does it inform further clinical reasoning and decision making?
- Is it client centered?
- Is it a means to an end and not an end in itself?
- Is it based on having a good rapport with the client?
- Does it acknowledge the diversity of clients?

extensive development. Usually, the developers of such assessments provide a user manual detailing the process of development, protocol for administration, procedure for scoring, rules for interpretation, criteria or norms for performance, and the psychometric properties of the assessment. Research on the development of the assessment should be available in peer-reviewed journals to demonstrate that the quality of the assessment has been critically appraised. Box 25.2 provides a list of the different aspects of a standardized test that need to be considered in choosing an assessment, each of which is defined in the sections the follow, along issues to consider regarding each of these factors.

Types of Assessments

Generally, assessments can be classified as descriptive, evaluative, or predictive. An assessment can be used to meet the demands of both a descriptive and an evaluative tool, for example; but for illustrative purposes, we will provide examples of each type.

Descriptive Assessments

Descriptive assessments use items to describe individuals within groups and to characterize the differences between individuals on the attribute being measured. This information can be used by the therapist to assess the specific characteristics of an individual to determine if and what type of intervention is needed. An example of a descriptive assessment is the Dementia Rating Scale, a clinical staging assessment for dementia (Morris, 1993). Broadly, it characterizes six domains of cognitive and functional performance: memory, orientation, judgment and problem solving, community affairs, home and hobbies, and personal care. The information to make each rating is obtained through a semistructured interview with a client and a reliable collateral source, such as a caregiver or family member. The Dementia Rating Scale table provides descriptors that guide the clinician in making appropriate ratings based on interview data and clinical judgment. In addition to ratings on a 5-point scale for each domain (except personal care, which is rated on a 4-point scale), an overall Dementia Rating Scale score is derived. This score is useful for globally staging the level of impairment: 0 = no impairment, 0.5 = very mild dementia, 1 = mild dementia, 2 = moderate dementia, and 3 = severe dementia (Morris, 1993).

Evaluative Assessments

Evaluative assessments use criteria or items to measure an individual's trait or attribute over time. The most appropriate characteristics included in an evaluative assessment are those that can be sensitive to change within an individual. The Simulator Sickness Questionnaire (SSQ) (Kennedy, Lane, Berbaum, & Lilienthal, 1993), used to quantify simulator sickness symptoms as a result of being exposed to a driving simulator, is an example of an evaluative measure. The SSQ can be administered at

CASE STUDY 25.2 Assessing Mr. Patel's Driving Performance—Nonstandardized Assessment

Before selecting assessments to measure Mr. Patel's driving ability, Karen first wants to know a little more about him. Karen reviews the personal and medical history available from his chart and decides that her first step is to interview Mr. Patel to get his self-report on potential problems that may impact his driving ability. Karen also interviews his wife, asking her about his driving performance to form a more comprehensive approach of his driving abilities. As a result of her nonstandardized assessments (chart review and interviews), she finds that Mr. Patel is a 72-year-old man who is retired from business and lives in the community with his wife. He has some college after high school graduation. Mr. Patel has had PD for 17 years and is on antiparkinsonian drugs. He also has arthritis in his knees and neck and wears trifocals to see well. He was referred by a neurologist from a movement disorders center with a concern about his continued safe driving. Mr. Patel tells Karen that he feels sleepy during the day, and she notes that he demonstrates a flat affect during the interview. He has a driver's license, drives about 3 to 4 days per week, mainly with his wife. His wife adds that he has had two citations in the last 3 years and a fender bender. Karen is now ready to think through which standardized evaluations she wishes to use to complete her initial evaluation.

BOX 25.2 Components to Consider When Critiquing Standardized Assessments

1. Type
   a. Descriptive
   b. Evaluative
   c. Predictive
2. Structural
   a. Format
   b. Cost
   c. Orientation
   d. Clinical utility
3. Construction
   a. Levels of measurement
      i. Nominal
      ii. Ordinal
      iii. Interval
      iv. Ratio
4. Psychometric evaluation
   a. Reliability (classical test theory versus generalizability theory)
      i. Measurement error
         1. Random
         2. Systematic
         3. Sources
      ii. Type
         1. Test–retest
         2. Rater (interrater and intrarater)
         3. Internal consistency (split half, Cronbach's alpha, Kuder-Richardson formulas)
   b. Validity (evidence to support the construct)
      i. What the instrument looks like
         1. Face
         2. Content
      ii. How the instrument acts
         1. Construct (convergent, discriminant)
         2. Criterion (concurrent, predicitve)
   c. Screening
      i. Sensitivity
      ii. Specificity
      iii. Positive predicitve value
      iv. Negative predicitve value
   d. Item Response Theory
      i. Unidimensionality (fit statistics/factor analysis)
      ii. Local independence
      iii. Precision
      iv. Person-item match
5. Summary of strengths and weaknesses of the assessment

various time points during the simulator drive so that comparisons can be made to assess whether simulator sickness symptoms are increasing. This is important clinically to determine whether the client will be able to tolerate use of the simulator without becoming ill. Essentially, the SSQ rates 16 symptoms across three domains, which include the oculomotor, disorientation, and nausea domains. Clients report the degree to which they experience each symptoms on a scale from 0 to 3, with 0 = none, 1 = slight, 2 = moderate, 3 = severe. The total SSQ score is derived by using a weighted scale and a standard algorithm (a step-by-step procedure for calculations). By

CASE STUDY 25.3 Assessing Mr. Patel's Driving Performance—Selecting Standardized Assessments

Knowing that advanced stages of PD can also affect cognition, especially the executive functions, Karen decides that she will have to assess Mr. Patel's general cognition. Recently, she has also read in one of her journals that divided attention, a critical important function for driving, may be affected in people with neurological disorders. Thus, Karen decides to use the Mini-Mental State Examination (MMSE) (Folstein, Folstein, & McHugh, 1975) to assess Mr. Patel's general cognition and the Trail Making Test Part B (Trails B) (Reitan, 1958) to assess Mr. Patel's divided attention, which is also known as set shifting. She is also concerned about visual changes that may have occurred as a result of the chronic neurological progression of PD as well as his impaired range of motion (ROM) due to the arthritis in his neck and trunk. Karen decides to also include a comprehensive visual battery using the Optec 2500 visual analyzer (Registered trademark of Stereo Optical Co., Inc. that measures visual acuity, peripheral vision, contrast sensitivity, depth perception, lateral and vertical phorias, and color discrimination). Finally, she used her knowledge of ROM and manual muscle strength testing to assess the corresponding functions in Mr. Patel's neck and trunk. All of these assessments are considered standardized, but Karen is aware that she must delve a bit deeper into the published literature as well as the assessment manuals to be sure that she has identified good measures that she is justified in using to make a reasonable fitness-to-drive recommendation for Mr. Patel.

CASE STUDY 25.4 Descriptive, Predictive, and Evaluative Assessments

After reviewing the nature of the assessments she has selected, Karen is convinced that the Trails B is a *predictive assessment*, especially after reading in a recent article that Trails B was highly correlated with passing/failing an on-road test in people with PD (Classen et al., 2009). In the same study, Karen also read that the MMSE was moderately correlated to on-road outcomes. She is not sure if the MMSE is sufficiently predictive or not. Knowing that using the Optec 2500 visual analyzer to determine Mr. Patel's visual function can characterize his visual acuity, peripheral visual fields, contrast sensitivity, ocular movements, and depth perception, Karen decides that these assessments fit the *descriptive* criteria well. Certainly, the ROM tests as well as the manual muscle strength tests can be considered *evaluative tools*, especially because Karen can expect changes (improvements) in Mr. Patel's measures based on interventions to improve his neck and trunk mobility and strength.

comparing the scores after the first 5 minutes of driving with the scores obtained after 15 minutes of driving, the occupational therapy practitioner may be able to intervene with clients who show an increase in simulator sickness symptoms. For a description of the use of the SSQ and clinical application with returning combat veterans with mild traumatic brain injury (TBI), please see Classen and Owens (2011).

Predictive Assessments

Predictive assessments use criteria to classify individuals to predict a certain trait in comparison to set criteria. For example, a predictive tool can measure skills underlying driving performance to predict whether an older adult will be able to successfully return to driving. The Useful Field of View (UFOV), a computer-based assessment of visual attention (subtest 1), divided attention (subtest 2), and selective attention (subtest 3), is an example of a predictive assessment (Edwards et al., 2006). The first UFOV subtest involves identifying a single object (either a car or a truck) presented centrally on the touch screen. Subtest 2 (divided attention) required the client to identify a peripheral target while still attempting to correctly identify the central target (car or truck). Subtest 3 (selective attention) involves the same procedure as subtest 2, with the exception of distracter triangles being present surrounding the peripheral target. After completion, threshold scores are provided as well as a risk index (low, moderate, and high) for all tasks. Higher scores indicate longer times to process the information and thus, poorer performance. The UFOV is one of the best predictors of crash involvement and poor on-road performance for drivers with Alzheimer's disease (Owsley & McGwin, 1999). The divided attention component (subtest 2) is rated as the best predictor of (at-fault) crash involvement among older adults (Owsley, McGwin, & Ball, 1998).

Structure of Assessments

The previous section introduced the reader to the types of assessments. We will next discuss the structure of the assessments as it pertains to its characteristics, clinical utility, and basic information on constructing items. Characteristics of the assessments may include the format, cost, and orientation of the test.

Format

Assessments may appear in a paper-and-pencil format, for example, the Mini-Mental State Examination (MMSE); or as a computerized test, for example, the UFOV. Paper-and-pencil tests are very common in state, national, and international organizations, but computer-based testing (CBT) is gaining ground quickly. Some advantages of CBT include reduced administration time, fewer data entry errors, worldwide testing via the Web, and quick results (Kraut et al., 2004; Streiner & Norman, 2008a). However, limitations of CBT include questionable reliability and validity, apprehension for individuals not skilled with computers, and security of test materials.

Cost

Cost of the assessment is an important consideration because some assessment tools may be available free of charge, for example, the Craig Handicap Assessment and Reporting Technique (CHART) (Whiteneck et al., 1998). Others, such as a driving simulator, may be very expensive in terms of equipment and training costs.

Orientation

Knowledge about the *orientation*, whether the assessment is invasive or not and insight into how much cooperation from the client and/or other stakeholders is needed, must be considered. Therefore, the occupational therapy practitioner must also consider the *clinical utility* of the test.

Clinical Utility

Clinical utility refers to how *acceptable* the assessment will be among occupational therapy practitioners when used in the clinic. As such, acceptability may be influenced by the clinical applicability of the assessment (usefulness of the assessment for making interpretations to facilitate interventions), time demands (time to

CASE STUDY 25.5 Karen Considers Assessment Characteristics

Karen knows that the assessment tools she has selected use paper-and-pencil method for scoring (MMSE, Trails B), with the exception of Optec 2500 visual analyzer, which is computer based. The cost of all the assessments, with the exception of the Optec 2500 visual analyzer machine, is reasonably low. Luckily, Karen's facility has invested in the Optec to measure the visual function of the low-vision clients; thus, no further financial expenses are incurred for her to use this assessment. She also realizes that the ROM and MMSE may be a little invasive because they require hands-on testing, but it is important to assess whether such functions are impaired in Mr. Patel because they are important for neck and trunk movement during driving, especially during backup functions. She doesn't think that it will pose a problem and thus is satisfied that she has identified tools that are feasible to use in her setting.

Karen is confident that all the assessments that she has chosen will help her clinical reasoning to assess Mr. Patel's abilities important for driving performance. She has calculated that it will take her about 28 minutes to assess Mr. Patel's visual (15 minutes with the Optec), cognitive (5 minutes for the MMSE and 3 minutes for Trails B), and physical abilities (MMSE and ROM for 3 minutes). True to following a client-centered approach, she discusses the type of assessments with Mr. Patel, and he concurs to participate as she conducts this part of her evaluation. ■

complete the assessment, time allocated to scoring of the test, and time required to be trained to administer the assessment), and acceptability of the assessment to the clients (Rudman & Hannah, 1998).

In general, occupational therapy practitioners need to make decisions regarding which test to use (descriptive, evaluative, or predictive) based on the specific purpose of the assessment, characteristics of the assessment, and clinical utility of the tool, including the practical steps in administering the tool.

Construction

Construction of a test pertains to devising or writing the items in such a way that they will match the purpose of the assessment. For a more detailed discussion on aspects of construction, please go to http://thePoint.lww.com/Willard-Spackman12e and see the document entitled "Constructing Assessments". Items can be constructed to include different levels of measurement, discussed next in detail. Refer to Box 25.3 for a summary of measurement

BOX 25.3 Scales of Measurement

Assigning numbers to traits results in measurement scales. The four scales of measurement are nominal, ordinal, interval, and ratio (Portney & Watkins, 2009).

- ***Nominal.*** The nominal scale represents the first level of measurement. This involves mutually exclusive categories (e.g., female versus male, driving versus nondriving). Assigned numbers are simply used as labels or means of identification with no attempt to quantify or order the differences.
- ***Ordinal.*** A second level is the ordinal scale. In this scale, the numbers represent the relative rank order of the trait under investigation. For example, driving evaluators often use a Global Rating Scale, indicating whether a client who has taken an on-road test should fail = 1, fail with options for remediation = 2, pass with recommendations = 3, or pass = 4 (Justiss, Mann, Stav, & Velozo, 2006). The assigned numbers merely indicate the rank order; they do not represent absolute quantities, and the intervals between the ranks cannot be presumed equal. In this example, someone who is passing the on-road test is not twice as competent as someone who is passing with recommendations. Thus, no inference can be made about the magnitude of the difference between scores.
- ***Interval.*** The interval scales represent the third level. The intervals between scores are equal so that comparisons can be made between individuals. Also, characteristic of an interval scale is that there is no true zero value. An example of an interval scale that is commonly used in occupational therapy surveys is the bipolar (goes in both directions) Likert scale (e.g., 0 = strongly disagree, 1 = disagree, 2 = agree, 3 = strongly agree) and the unipolar (goes in one direction) adjectival scale, (e.g., 0 = cannot do, 1 = very difficult, 2 = somewhat difficult, 3 = a little difficult, 4 = not difficult).[a] Although a client can get the lowest value (a zero) on a driving assessment that uses the adjectival scale, there is no true "absence of driving safety." Although not having an absolute zero limits some mathematical operations, most psychometric operations such as calculations of means and standard deviations are commonly performed on interval scales.
- ***Ratio.*** The ratio scales reflect the fourth and highest level scale in measurement. It has equal distances but, in addition, has a meaningful zero point. The zero point indicates a total absence of whatever trait is being measured. To use these scales, absence of the attribute being measured must be meaningful. ROM measurements assessed by a trained clinician with standardized equipment, such as a goniometer, will yield ratio data. All mathematical operations can be accomplished with a ratio scale data (addition, subtraction, multiplication, division) and statistical (means, standard deviations, and standard errors) calculations. In this case, it is correct to indicate that a person has gained twice as much movement between measurements of 20 degrees elbow flexion and 40 degrees elbow flexion.

[a]Some measurement experts believe that Likert scales are not interval scales. Although Likert scales look like they are interval in nature, for example, the distance between a value of one to two and two to three are equal, we cannot be assured that there are equal distances between the qualifiers that these numbers represent (e.g., maximum assistance, moderate assistance, and minimum assistance) (Bond & Fox, 2007).

levels and scales. These are important because they dictate the kinds of statistical analyses that can be done using the assessment results across clients. It is helpful to realize that measurement exists on different levels and that the scale itself limits or determines the analysis of the data. For example, if ordinal data are to be analyzed, then the scale from which these data are derived must contain defined ranks and intervals to approximate rank order. Moreover, critiquing measures must be pursued with knowledge of its rules, the nature of the trait being measured, and a consideration of the purpose of measuring.

In addition to how a test is constructed, a psychometric evaluation or an empirical way to evaluate the quality of the assessment tool must include testing related to **reliability** (Does the test yield the same or similar scores consistently?), **external validity** (Can generalizations be made to the general population?), **internal validity** (Does the assessment measure what it is supposed to measure, i.e., a specific trait, behavior, construct, or performance?), **sensitivity** (predictor test's ability to obtain a positive test when the condition really exists), and **specificity** (predictor test's ability to obtain a negative test when the condition does not exist). Each of these components of the psychometric evaluation will be discussed next.

Reliability—Traditional Approaches

Reliability pertains to the reproducibility of test results and the amount of variation measured that is real and not due to error. Reliability, generally, is based on a correlation coefficient or a measure of agreement and referred to as a reliability coefficient, which can range from 0 to ±1 (0 = no reliability and 1 = perfect reliability). Two theoretical concepts related to reliability are CTT and generalizability theory.

Classical test theory, also called classical reliability theory, centers around the notion that each observation or test score has a single true score and yields a single reliability coefficient (Nunnally & Bernstein, 1994). CTT postulates that a test score has two components: the true score and the measurement error score. Although many sources of error exist, only one source (e.g., either the rater or the assessment itself) is estimated; meaning that the difference therefore between the observed score and the true score is due to random error (Portney & Watkins, 2009). This model is overly restrictive and often unrealistic in situations where there may be multiple sources of error. Examples of multiple error sources include differences among raters (see interrater reliability) and differences in testing context (e.g., driving assessed in one's own car or driving assessed in an evaluator's car). Additionally, measures themselves are heterogeneous (e.g., driving can be operationalized, and therefore measured, in various ways such as driving awareness, driving behaviors, driving confidence, driving habits, driving fitness, driving performance and/or driving safety).

Generalizability theory provides a framework for conceptualizing, investigating, and designing reliable observations. It was originally introduced by Cronbach and colleagues (Cronbach, Gleser, Nanda, & Rajaratnam, 1972; Cronbach, Nageswari, & Gleser, 1963) in response to the limitations of CTT. Generalizability theory recognizes different sources of error and attempts to quantify the sources from those various errors. So, not all variations in the administration of an assessment are attributed to random error. Relevant testing conditions that may influence test scores are identified (e.g., time of day such as driving in the midmorning versus driving in peak traffic where there are many more demands from the driving environment). In identifying the different sources of error, one may be better able to identify why an assessment score changes and thus provide additional explanations beyond the assumption of random error (Portney & Watkins, 2009).

Measurement Error

Measurement error arises when there is a difference between the true value, such as one's absolute weight measured with a precise scale (e.g., an electronic scale in a doctor's office), and the observed value (e.g., weight as measured by a spring-based bathroom scale). The observed value (X) is therefore a function of two components: a true score (T) and an error component (E), expressed as

$$\text{Observed Score} = \text{True Score} \pm \text{Error}$$
$$X = T \pm E$$

Error can appear as random error or systematic error. *Random error* is represented by inconsistencies that cannot be predicted, for example, fatigue or mechanical inaccuracy of the measurement assessment, causing the error. *Systematic error* refers to predictable fluctuations occurring during measurement. Systematic error may occur in design flaws such as subject selection, for example, recruiting from a pool of clients that includes individuals only from low socioeconomic backgrounds. Usually, systematic errors occur in one direction and consistently overestimate or underestimate the true score. When the error is identified, it may be easier to manage or correct the systematic error compared to when random error occurs as outlined in Box 25.4.

Types of Reliability

There are several different types of reliability that reported related to assessments. See Table 25.1 for a synopsis of reliability testing.

Test–Retest Reliability

The test–retest method estimates the reliability or stability of measurements when the same test is given to the same people after a period of time. One obtains a correlation between scores on the two administrations of the same test. It is presumed that responses to the test will correlate because they reflect the same true score;

BOX 25.4 Sources of Systematic Measurement Error

- The individual taking the measurements (e.g., raters or evaluators that are biased in expecting the client to have improved due to driving training)
- The measurement assessment (e.g., poorly calibrated mechanical parts of a driving simulator)
- The variability of the characteristics being measured (e.g., ROM when measured early in the morning may be different than when measured late in the day)

however, the correlation of measurements across time will be less than perfect. This may occur because of *instability* of measurements taken over various time points. For example, a client may be distracted, have a bad (or a good) day, or be influenced by the test administrator (Carmines & Zeller, 1979; Portney & Watkins, 2009). Other factors that can influence (increase or decrease) test–retest reliability are the following:

- *A construct may change*, such as a driver's perception about safe driving before and after the driver takes a driver's refresher course.
- *Reactivity*, or change in the measured trait or behavior occurring as a result of the testing. For example, drivers may alter their performance due to their awareness of being observed. Therefore, drivers may perform more optimally when driving with a driving evaluator than when they drive by themselves under natural conditions.
- *Overestimation or underestimation*. It is well known in the driving literature that older drivers (as most other drivers as well) overestimate their driving ability as they report that they are better

TABLE 25.1 Reliability by Type, Use, Source or Error, and Method of Testing

Type	Use	Sources of Error	Method to Test
Test–retest reliability	Test is given to the same people after a period of time.	The effect of time, changes in the construct, reactivity, over or underestimation	Intraclass correlation coefficient (ICC)[a]
Rater reliability	To illustrate the stability of data collected.		ICC or kappa[a]
• ***Intrarater reliability***	To illustrate the stability of data collected by one rater on two or more trials over time.	Tool administration procedures, calibration of instrument, untrained rater, recall, or other forms of bias	ICC or kappa[a]
• ***Interrater reliability***	To determine rater variability between two or more raters who measure the same clients.	The effect of time, rater interaction with the client, or variables that may influence observation skills of the raters	ICC or kappa[a]
Internal consistency	To determine the degree of agreement between the items in a test that measure an underlying trait or construct.		Cronbach's coefficient alpha[a]
• ***Alternate form***	Tests the same group of people on two separate occasions using two distinct but parallel forms of the test.	Length of the test	ICC[a]
• ***Split-halves***	The same group of people partakes in the test where the total set of items in the test is divided in half.	Method of splitting	Spearman-Brown Prophecy statistic
• ***Cronbach's alpha or Kuder-Richardson formulas***	To estimate the reliability of scales or commonality of one item in a test with other items in a test.	Consistency of content of test	Cronbach's coefficient alpha[a]

[a]A perfect correlation is indicated by a correlation coefficient expressed as $r = 1.0$, $p \leq .05$. A strong correlation is indicated if $r \geq 0.75$, a moderate correlation if $r \geq 0.50$ but <0.75, and weaker correlation if $r = <0.50$ when $p \leq .05$. Also note that acceptability of correlation strength may vary according to the purpose for reliability testing. For example, one may tolerate lower reliability estimates to indicate differences/similarities of groups, but values required for making accurate predictions in terms of diagnoses will need to have a high correlation coefficient. Correlations can be conducted with various methods, such as kappa and intraclass correlation coefficient (ICC) through Cronbach's coefficient alpha (Portney & Watkins, 2009).

drivers than what they really are when compared to their performance on a road test. Similarly, older drivers may underestimate number of citations received when their self-report data are compared to official citation records.

Rater Reliability

Intrarater reliability refers to the stability of data collected by one rater on two or more trials over time. The objective nature of scientific inquiry demands that even when experts are used, that intrarater reliability should be tested. Error in this type of reliability can be reduced by training the rater in the use of the tool(s), using the tool administration procedures, calibrating measurement assessments, training rater skills to avoid deterioration over time, and assessing the rater for bias based on memory, training, views, and/or assumptions. Developing objective grading criteria may be conducive to limiting measurement error occurring as a result of intrarater reliability (Hinojosa et al., 2005; Portney & Watkins, 2009).

Interrater reliability concerns detecting rater variability between two or more raters who measure the same clients (Portney & Watkins, 2009). To establish interrater reliability, it is best for the raters to view the same clients at the same point in time. In driving research, for example, the use of a driving simulator, which allows for video playback versus on-road testing, is particularly helpful for raters to rate a subject and useful for researchers to establish interrater reliability. Not only can one include a wide variety of raters with this testing method but also disagreements among the raters may be resolved through consensus and rewatching the video. Should the raters test the client during an on-road driving test, their scores may be influenced by their seating position in the vehicle as well as the interaction of the evaluator with the tester. For example, the optimal seating position for the driving evaluator is the right front seat and the worst seating position is the back left seat because observation of many driver responses, such as eye movements or positioning of the vehicle, may be restricted as a result of the seating position. Likewise, the evaluator that is providing travel directions to the driver may rate the driver differently than the raters without any interaction with the driver.

Internal Consistency

Internal consistency determines the degree of agreement between the items in a test that measure an underlying trait or construct. It is essentially an estimation of the *homogeneity* of the test. Ways to test for internal consistency are alternate form, split-halves, Cronbach's alpha, or Kuder-Richardson formulas.

- *Alternate form* tests the same group of people on two separate occasions using two distinct but parallel forms of the test. Although more expensive and time consuming, because two forms of the test need to be developed, this method is obviously superior to test–retest method. Specifically, it reduces the effect to which the individual's memory can bias the results (i.e., result in improved score due to recall of the test questions) and therefore also the strength of the correlation.
- In contrast to the alternate form method, the *split-halves method* can be conducted in one time period. Specifically, the same group of people partakes in the test wherein the total set of items in the test is divided in half. The scores on the halves are then correlated to obtain an estimate of reliability. One limitation is that the manner in which the items are subdivided will affect the reliability coefficient (Carmines & Zeller, 1979; Portney & Watkins, 2009; Streiner & Norman, 2008b). The Spearman-Brown Prophecy formula, a statistical method, can be used to correct for such incongruent results (Carmines & Zeller, 1979).
- *Cronbach's alpha* (also referred to as *coefficient alpha)* and *Kuder-Richardson formulas* are used to estimate the reliability of scales or commonality of one item in a test with other items in a test. The difference is that Cronbach's alpha is used when the test scale is composed of *nondichotomous* responses (i.e., rating scale), whereas the Kuder-Richardson formula is used for *dichotomously* scored items (e.g., correct/incorrect). Essentially, the purpose of applying these formulas is to identify the items that do not contribute to the overall construct that are being measured and therefore, such items may be lowering a test's reliability. The reader is referred to select references (Carmines & Zeller, 1979; Portney & Watkins, 2009; Streiner & Norman, 2008a) for more information on these methods.

Validity—Traditional Approaches

Validity is defined as the extent to which any assessment measures what it is intended to measure. The definition of validity is straightforward, but it is imperative to realize that although an assessment may yield valid data when being used to measure certain population traits under certain conditions, the same assessment may not be replicated if traits of a different population are being measured. Likewise, the same assessment may not be replicated if the same population is being measured under different conditions. For example, the Driving Habits Questionnaire has been developed and tested psychometrically for use among older adults in a research setting (Owsley, Stalvey, Wells, & Sloane, 1999). As such, if this tool is being used in a group of novice drivers (different population), or used to record the history of night driving in older drivers (different conditions), the validity may be

TABLE 25.2 Validity by Type, Use, and Method to Test and Strength of Estimate

Type	Use	Method to Test	Strength of Estimate
Face validity	Is the measure testing what it is supposed to measure? Are the items plausible?	Peer review	No statistical inference testing
Content validity	Does the measurement instrument reflect a specific domain of content?	Content validity index (CVI)	CVI ≥80%
Construct validity	Does the assessment measure a construct and the theoretical components underlying the construct?	Tests of correlation	Higher correlation coefficients are better, thus $r = \geq 0.80$, $p \leq .05$
• ***Convergent validity***	Is the level of agreement between two tests that are being used to measure the same construct acceptable?	Tests of correlation	Higher correlation coefficients are better, thus $r = \geq 0.80$, $p \leq .05$
• ***Discriminant validity***	Is the level of disagreement (poor or zero correlation) when two tests measure a trait, behavior, or characteristic acceptable?	Tests of correlation	Higher correlation coefficients are better, thus $r \geq 0.80$, $p \leq .05$
Criterion validity	Can the outcome of one assessment be used as a substitute test to the established *gold standard criterion* test?	Prediction methods	See below
• ***Concurrent validity***	Do the results of a criterion measure and a target test, given at the same relative time point, concur with one another?	Receiver operating characteristics (ROC) curves	Area under the curve (AUC) ≥0.70, with $p \leq .05$
• ***Predictive validity***	Does the outcome of a target test predict a future criterion score or outcome?	Prediction methods, for example, regression analyses	The higher the R^2 in the prediction model, the better the validity

Note. The above statistical tests are examples to illustrate the points raised. To evaluate validity, other methods may be explored with biostatistician or psychometrician colleagues because the reader gets more accomplished in applying principles of validity testing.

impacted. The question then becomes not if the assessment is valid, but *if the assessment is valid for making the decisions for which the practitioner is using it.*

To determine the accuracy of a measurement tool, one may ask what the assessment *looks* like and also how it *acts*. The "look" pertains to whether the assessment has *face validity* (e.g., Does it overall look like the assessment is measuring what it is supposed to measure?) and/or *content validity* (e.g., Do expert raters rate the items in that they are comprehensively represent the content area?). The "act" pertains to a more rigorous process in assessment development that includes *construct validity*, or how the assessment compares to other assessments measuring the same construct (*convergent*) or different (*divergent*) constructs; as well as *criterion validity*, which may be *concurrent* (measured at the same point in time) or *predictive* (measured at some point in future). See Table 25.2 for a synopsis of validity.

Face Validity

Face validity indicates that a measure is testing what it is supposed to and that the items are viewed as plausible. No statistical manipulation of the data is involved in this process, and the measure is peer reviewed (i.e., reviewed by experts in the field) to determine plausibility of the items. For example, in the development of the items of the Safe Driving Behavioral Measure (SDBM), face validity was tested by asking a group of doctoral students and researchers to evaluate the chosen items based on ease of reading, content, clarity, appropriateness, and time that it took to answer the items. Recommendations from the peer review were followed in refining the items prior to content validity testing (Classen et al., 2010).

Content Validity

Fundamentally, **content validity** depends on the extent to which an empirical measurement reflects a specific domain of content. Following the guidelines of Lynn (1986), Classen and colleagues (2010) invited four expert raters to complete a *content validity index* (CVI)—an index of consensus related to the relevance of the items—on each of the items in the SDBM. Apart from rating each SDBM item on a 4-point Likert scale (1 = not relevant, 2 = relevant with major revisions, 3 = relevant with minor revisions, and 4 = very relevant), the experts also gave feedback on item accuracy, purpose, organization, clarity, appearance, understandability, and adequacy (Grant & Davis, 1997). Usually, content validity can be claimed if the rater agreement on the item relevance is 80% or higher (House, House, & Campbell, 1981).

Construct Validity

Construct validity establishes whether the assessment measures a construct and the theoretical components underlying the construct. A construct is an abstract idea that we cannot observe directly. Many, if not all, occupational assessments measure abstract ideas that we can only indirectly observe through behaviors. For example, we cannot directly observe job satisfaction but can indirectly assess it by direct observation (e.g., watching an individual in a job situation) or through questionnaires (e.g., asking the client his or her satisfaction with different aspects of his or her job). Two different types of construct validity can be established, *convergent* and *discriminant.*

- ***Convergent validity*** is the level of agreement between two tests that are being used to measure the same construct. For example, if one wants to determine if *lane maintenance* is challenging for a novice driver, one may test the driver on a driving simulator and on the road. Should there be a high correlation between lane maintenance under these two testing conditions (simulator and on road), one may infer construct validity pertaining to the lane maintenance aspect of driving.
- ***Discriminant validity*** is the level of disagreement (poor or zero correlation) when two tests measure a trait, behavior, or characteristic. Let's assume that community-dwelling older drivers are screened before taking an on-road test. The driving rehabilitation specialist will administer an MMSE to assess cognitive functioning and a visual acuity test to assess distant vision before participating in an on-road test (Folstein et al., 1975; Folstein, Folstein, White, & Messer, 2010). A successful evaluation of discriminant validity will show that the test of cognition (MMSE) is poorly correlated with a test of visual acuity because these tests are designed to measure different concepts.

The process of establishing construct validity involves at least three steps (Carmines & Zeller, 1979):

1. Determine the theoretical relationship between the concepts themselves.
2. Determine the empirical relationship between the measures of the concepts.
3. Interpret the empirical evidence to clarify the construct validity of a measure.

This is a challenge to researchers as a construct, for example, safe driving is an *abstract* idea and is *multidimensional* (e.g., includes aspects of the driver, the vehicle, and the environment). Testing the construct is an ongoing process, and statistical methods used may include factor analysis or hypothesis testing, next described.

- ***Factor analysis*** is based on the idea that a construct contains one or more dimensions or theoretical components. As such, thinking about safe driving, one may assume that at least three dimensions are involved to execute a driving maneuver such as exiting a ramp and merging with traffic. Those are the person dimension (e.g., vision, cognition, and motor functions), the environment dimension (e.g., highway ramp, lanes on highway, traffic, weather, light), and the vehicle dimension (e.g., roadworthiness of vehicle and working status of all vehicle controls). Factor analysis helps to tease out the underlying dimensions of an assessment by grouping variables or items that correlate highly with one another.
- ***Hypothesis testing*** can be used to determine if an assessment can distinguish between people at different levels of safe driving. For example, one may postulate that older women who resume driving after the death of a spouse may have a greater number of errors related to driving skills when compared to older men who are the primary drivers in a family. If the assessment is able to detect such differences and affirm the hypothesis, one may infer construct validity pertaining to the population for the given test conditions.

Criterion Validity

Criterion validity implies that the outcome of one assessment can be used as a substitute test for the established gold standard criterion test. Criterion validity can be tested as concurrent validity or predictive validity.

- ***Concurrent validity*** is inferred when two measures, the criterion measure and a target test, are given at relatively the same point in time and the results of the two tests concur with one another. Most often, when proven more efficient and/or cost-effective than the criterion test, the target test may be used as a substitute for the gold standard test. Currently, a comprehensive driving evaluation (CDE) conducted by a driving rehabilitation specialist is considered the industry or gold standard to determine driving ability (Di Stefano & Macdonald, 2005). However, the CDE is expensive, time consuming, offers limited access (i.e., presently, there is a shortage of driving rehabilitation specialists), and invites an element of risk because it is conducted in the real world. To overcome many of these challenges, researchers are investigating the concurrent validity between the driving simulator and the CDE (Allen, Classen, & Cook, in press; Bédard, Parkkari, Weaver, Riendeau, & Dahlquist, 2010; Shechtman, Classen, Awadzi, & Mann, 2009).
- ***Predictive validity*** establishes that the outcome of a target test can be used to predict a future criterion score or outcome. For example, in a review of vision impairment and driving, the UFOV was shown to be one of the best predictors of crash involvement

as tested in a simulator and on road (gold standard criterion) in drivers with Alzheimer's disease (Owsley et al., 1998). Thus, one may infer that the UFOV has predictive validity with the criterion (on-road testing) for the population under study.

Ecological Validity

Ecological validity implies that the outcome of an assessment can "hold up" in the real-world circumstances. For example, if Mr. Patel, our case study participant, is deemed to be able to drive based on the findings of an assessment, one must ask if that assessment outcome will also hold true in the real world. If so, one can infer ecological validity.

Screening Tools

Many assessments are specifically developed for the purposes of being used as a *screening* tool. A screening is a brief measure that tests the presence or absence of a disease, condition, or an outcome. Because screening tools are often used by clinicians to determine if a client will require further treatment, it is very important to verify their validity (see Box 25.5 for an example).

Sensitivity and Specificity

Sensitivity is defined as the predictor test's ability to obtain a positive test when the condition really exists (a true positive). For example, when a predictor test

CASE STUDY 25.6 Karen Critiques Her Assessments and Completes Her Evaluation

Karen is ready to critique her assessments. She has developed a matrix displayed in Table 25.3 and included information from the published studies that she has read to assess if she is on the right track.

Karen has chosen assessments with a structure that is conducive to Mr. Patel's needs. All five of the assessments provide interval-level data. Even though not all the components of reliability and validity are known (through the publications that she has read), the overall psychometrics of the tools are acceptable and suggesting that Karen's decision to use these tools is evidence based.

Karen proceeds to assess Mr. Patel using the MMSE and Trails B. She also assesses his vision with the Optec 2500 along with selected ROM and Manual Muscle Testing (MMT) pertinent to driving. From these results, she finds that he is demonstrating some mild difficulty with divided attention, impaired contrast sensitivity, and limitations in his neck and trunk mobility. All these impairments may affect Mr. Patel's ability to continue to drive. Based on these results, she recommends an on-road driving evaluation to be conducted by a certified driving rehabilitation specialist, both to determine a baseline for his driving performance and to make recommendations for any modifications, adaptations, compensatory strategies, or referrals (e.g., to an ophthalmologist) needed to assure appropriate fitness-to-drive abilities.

TABLE 25.3 Matrix to Critique Assessments

Assessment	Structure				Level of Measurement	Psychometrics: Reliability		Psychometrics: Validity				
	Format	Cost	Orientation	Clinical utility	Nominal Ordinal Ratio Interval	Test–Retest	Rater reliability	Internal Consistency	Face	Content	Construct	Criterion
MMSE	x	x	x	x	I	x	x	?	x	x	x	x
Trails B	x	x	x	x	I	x	x	x	x	x	x	x
Vision	x	x	x	x	I	x	?	?	x	x	x	x
ROM	x	x	x	x	R	x	x	?	x	x	x	?
MMT	x	x	x	x	O	x	x	?	x	x	x	?

Note. The "x" indicates a positive response to reflect that the component of the assessment that is being rated is acceptable. The "?" indicates that the component of the assessment being rated is not known. I, interval; R, ratio; O, ordinal; MMSE, Mini-Mental State Examination; MMT, Manual Muscle Testing; ROM, range of motion.

BOX 25.5 Using Evidence to Evaluate Screening Tools: An Example from the Literature

Occupational therapists are encouraged to make decisions regarding screening tools by examining the evidence that the tool is effective to predict the relevant criterion outcome. For example, in a pilot study with 19 drivers with Parkinson's disease (PD) who underwent a clinical battery of tests and an on-road driving test, the researchers wanted to determine which of the screening tests were most predictive of those clients who failed the on-road test. Figure 25.1 demonstrates how to calculate sensitivity, specificity, positive predictive value, and negative predictive value for the Useful Field of View (UFOV) Risk Index is 3 points cutoff value (N = 19 drivers with PD). The researchers determined that the sensitivity (true positives or those drivers with PD who really failed the road test and who were predicted to fail by the UFOV) was 87%. The specificity (true negative or those drivers with PD who really passed the road test and who were predicted to pass by the UFOV) was 82%. The positive predictive value (probability of the driver with PD, given a cut point of 3 on the UFOV Risk Index to fail the on-road test) was 78%. The negative predictive value (probability of the PD drivers, given a cut point of 3 on the UFOV Risk Index to pass the on-road test) was 90%. In this study, the authors concluded that among this sample of drivers with PD tested and compared to other clinical measures of disease, cognition, and vision, the UFOV was a superior screening measure for predicting on-road outcomes (Classen et al., 2009).

UFOV risk index	Global rating scale (fail/pass): + (FAIL)	Global rating scale (fail/pass): – (PASS)
+ (UFOV ≥3)	*a* true-positives (hits) [n=7]	*b* false-positives (misses) [n=2]
– (UFOV ≤3)	*c* false-negatives (false alarms) [n=1]	*d* true-negatives (correct rejections) [n=9]

FIGURE 25.1 Calculating sensitivity, specificity, positive predictive value, negative predictive value, and error for the Useful Field of View (UFOV) Risk Index value of 3 (N = 19 drivers with Parkinson's disease). Sensitivity = $a/(a + c)$ [7/(7 + 1) = 0.87]; Specificity = $d/(b + d)$ [9/(2 + 9) = 0.82]; Positive predictive value = $a/(a + b)$ [7/(7 + 2) = 0.78]; Negative predictive value = $d/(c + d)$ [9/(1 + 10) = 0.90]; total error = 1 − Sensitivity + 1 − Specificity [0.13 + 0.18 = 0.31].

suggests that the client will fail an on-road test, and this prediction is then verified by the actual outcome of the on-road test, sensitivity is evident. **Specificity** is defined as the predictor test's ability to obtain a negative result when the condition is really absent (a true negative). An example here is if the predictor test suggests that the client should pass, and this result is then verified by the client passing the on-road test (Portney & Watkins, 2009).

Positive and Negative Predictive Value

Positive predictive value is the probability of the client, given a certain cut point on the predictor test to fail in the actual situation (e.g., the on-road test). **Negative predictive value** is the probability of the client, given a cut point on the predictor test, to pass (in this case to pass the on-road test). It is important to note that the number of false positives (those who receive a failing score but pass the road test) and false negatives (those who receive a passing score but fail the road test) and thus the sensitivity and specificity values, change with the cutoff value. Ultimately, one wants the false positives and false negatives to be as close to zero as possible. The formulas for calculating these values are well described in many of the texts cited in this chapter.

Modern Approaches to Critiquing Assessments

Although most occupational therapy clinicians and researchers have been trained on traditional psychometric methods (CTT and generalizability theory), unfortunately, these approaches have several shortcomings. First, traditional assessments generate *scores* versus *measures*. Scores are simply the sum of the frequency of answers marked as "correct" or if using a Likert or adjectival scale, the sum of the ratings of each item. Although our scores on our assessments may look more sophisticated when converted into a percentage of the total score, in essence, they still simply reflect a frequency count. Second, the traditional analyses are specific to the sample from which they were derived. That is, although most researchers report on the reliability and validity of an assessment as if it is a stable characteristic, it is not. Reliability and validity are *sample dependent*. That is, reliability and validity values are unique to the particular sample from which they were derived. Although impractical, every time we use an assessment for a clinical population or research study, we should reevaluate the reliability of that assessment.

Third, scores are *test dependent*. That is, a score on one assessment cannot be readily translated to a score on a second assessment. For example, a score of 50 on one road test does not carry the same meaning as a score of a 50 on any other road test. Test scores are dependent on the difficulty of the items (tasks or questions) of the assessment. An individual with a particular level of ability (e.g., who can drive well only in his or her home town) will get a low score on a challenging driving assessment (e.g., one that only involves complex driving situations such as negotiating traffic in peak traffic hours) and a high score on an easy driving assessment

BOX 25.6 Examples of Occupational Therapy Assessments Using Item Response Theory Methods

Assessment of Motor and Process Skills (AMPS) (A. G. Fisher, 1993)
School AMPS (Munkholm, Löfgren, & Fisher, 2012)
Safe Driving Behavior Measure (Classen et al., 2012a; Classen et al., 2012b)
Occupational Performance History Interview (Kielhofner, Dobria, Forsyth, & Basu, 2005)
Pediatric Evaluation of Disability Inventory (Haley, Ludlow, & Coster, 1993)
School Function Assessment (Coster, Deeney, Haltiwanger, & Haley, 1998).
DriveSafe and DriveAware (Kay, Bundy & Clemson, 2009)

(e.g., one that only involves simple driving situations such as putting the car in gear and pulling out of the driveway). Finally, in most cases, traditional assessments require the client to take all items of the assessment. Obviously, if a client takes fewer of the items and the items are summed for a total score, he or she will get a lower score on the assessment, even though his or her ability has not changed.

In recent years, there have been dramatic advances in measurement theory in health care. Modern Test Theory (MTT), more commonly referred to as IRT and Rasch measurement theory, which emerged from the field of education, has had dramatic impact on clinical assessments in occupational therapy and health care (Cella & Chang, 2000). For purposes of this chapter, we will use the term *item response theory*. Several occupational therapy assessments have been developed using IRT methods, as shown in Box 25.6. The purpose of this part of the chapter is to introduce IRT or Rasch measurement theory and its applications in critiquing occupational therapy assessments.

Item Response Theory

In contrast to traditional psychometrics that focuses on the entire "test," IRT, as the name implies, focuses on the items of the test. As a measurement theory, IRT addresses many limitations of traditional test theory. First, IRT is *sample free*. That is, one should expect that the results from an IRT analysis should be the same no matter what sample is chosen from a population. Second, IRT is *test free*. The basis of an assessment being test free is that in IRT, the items of an assessment measure a latent trait. A *latent trait* is a hypothesized construct or attribute that is not directly observed but is inferred from responses on an assessment (Smith, 2000). For example, driving, as assessed by a specific driving assessment, is represented by the particular items from that assessment. Tasks such as stopping at stop lights, turning at an intersection, and passing another vehicle on a highway only represent a small sample of the almost infinite number of driving tasks that can represent the latent trait of driving. Finally, in contrast to scores (frequency counts) generated from traditional assessments that are only ordinal in nature, the measures generated for some IRT models are interval in nature. Note that we are using the term *scores* to refer to the numbers obtained from traditional assessments and the term *measures* for values derived from IRT-based assessments. That is, measures have equal intervals between their values (i.e., there are equal "distances" between a one and two, two and three, etc.). Interval-level data are necessary for any level of mathematics, from the simplest addition of two numbers to complicated statistical analyses.

The aforementioned unique characteristics of IRT offer advantages of measurement that have not been achievable with traditional psychometric approaches. First, because IRT is sample free, norms are not *necessary* for measurement. That does not mean that norms are unimportant in occupational therapy. On the contrary, for example, developmental norms are extremely important in determining if a client is within the range of what is "normal" or "typical," as for instance, for a developing child. But norms are not necessary for measurement (i.e., norms are not necessary to determine if you have more or less of something). Because IRT is sample free, an assessment should perform the same way for every sample from a particular population. That is, the relative challenge of the items on an instrument should have the same difficulty for every sample taken from a population. For example, for the population of elder drivers, predriving skills (e.g., opening a car door, inserting a key into the ignition) will always be easier than on-the-road driving skills (e.g., taking left-hand turns against traffic, merging onto a highway), independent of whether they have low or high driving ability. When using IRT, one should be confident that measures are replicable across different samples.

Advantages of Item Response Theory

Because IRT is test free, two important advantages arise. First, it is unnecessary to use all the items from an assessment to measure a client. Although typically, when using traditional assessments, one sums the responses on all the items of the assessment to determine the "ability" of the client, with IRT, instead of using all the items or an assessment, one can use only the most relevant items to measure a particular client. This can be exemplified in the area of motor

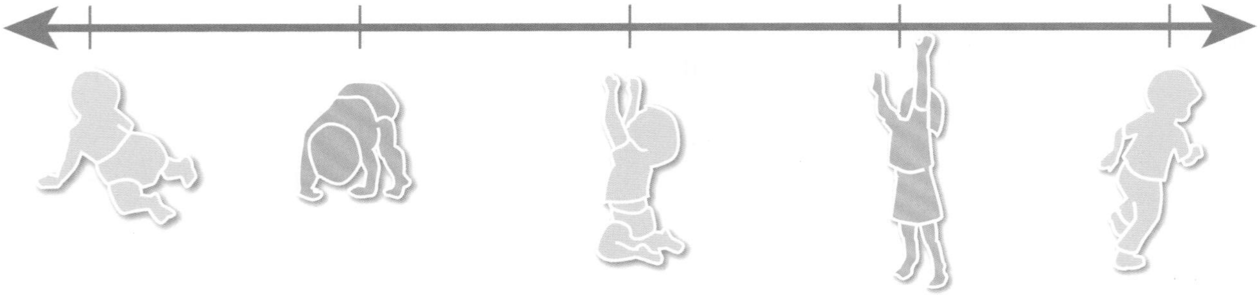

FIGURE 25.2 Proposed scale of motor development.

development. Figure 25.2 shows pictures from a typical motor development assessment. To the far left are easy tasks such as crawling and attempting to stand. To the far right are challenging tasks such as standing/reaching and running. Based on typical development, it would be irrational to assess a child for standing and running if he or she can only crawl (see Figure 25.2). This individualized type of testing, which is common in motor development, can be applied with other latent traits (e.g., driving, activities of daily living [ADL], cognitive ability). For example, if an individual is capable of driving on a highway in stormy weather, he or she is very likely to be capable of driving on streets nearby home. If a client is successful at a more challenging task, it is unnecessary to test them on a very easy task. This feature of IRT provides considerable efficiency for both the client and therapist. Clients do not have to be burdened by taking all the items of an assessment, and therapists can save time by only assessing items that are most relevant to a client.

The second advantage of the test-free nature of IRT is communication between assessments. With traditional assessments, the scores generated from one assessment are not readily comparable to the scores generated from another assessment. For example, even though most ADL assessments have similar items (e.g., eating, grooming, dressing, bathing), the scores generated from each assessment carry different meanings (i.e., a score of 50 on the Functional Independence Measure [FIM™] has a different meaning than a 50 on the Barthel ADL Index). When using an IRT-based assessment, the concept of the individual assessment fades. Instead, all assessments measuring a particular latent trait represent subsets of the "infinite" number of items that can represent that latent trait. If specific assessments represent subsets of items from the same latent trait (e.g., ADL), then measures from one assessment should be readily translatable to another assessment. Fisher and colleagues used this principle to translate measures between two ADL scales, the FIM and the Patient Evaluation Conference System (PECS) (W. P. Fisher, 1995). Velozo, Byers, and Joseph (2007) have also used this principle to translate measures between the FIM and the ADL items of the Minimum Data Set (MDS). Because different assessments are often used in different facilities (e.g., FIM in inpatient rehabilitation facilities and MDS in skilled nursing facilities), linking assessments provides the capability of monitoring a client's progress as he or she move from facility to facility even when those facilities use different assessments.

Basic Formula Underlying Item Response Theory

As noted previously, there are several IRT models with the most basic IRT models being the one-parameter Rasch model. In spite of their complexity, all IRT models compare *person ability* to *item difficulty*. If it is a math test, it is whether or not the student (person ability) can pass the question (item), "8 + 8 = ?" If the person is more able than the question, he or she gets it correct; but if the person is less able than the question, he or she gets it wrong. This basic principle works for all assessment situations, even the assessment of clients in occupational therapy. If someone is assessed on driving, the critical question is whether the client (person) can pass the driving task (item). For example, is the client successful in taking a left-hand turn against traffic? If the client is more able than the task, he or she passes the task; but if the client is less able than the task, he or she fails the task.

A basic statistical formula that expresses this comparison of person ability and item difficulty is the one-parameter IRT or Rasch formula (Figure 25.3). The left side of the formula represents the probability of the person passing a specific item (P_{ni}) divided by the person failing an item ($1\text{-}P_{ni}$). The right side of the equation represents the comparison of person ability versus item difficulty ($B_n\text{-}D_i$).

$$\log [P_{ni}/1\text{-}P_{ni}] = B_n - D_i$$

P_{ni} = probability of person n passing item i
$1\text{-} P_{ni}$ = probability of person n failing item i
B_n = ability of person n
D_i = difficulty of item in i

FIGURE 25.3 Rasch one-parameter item response theory formula.

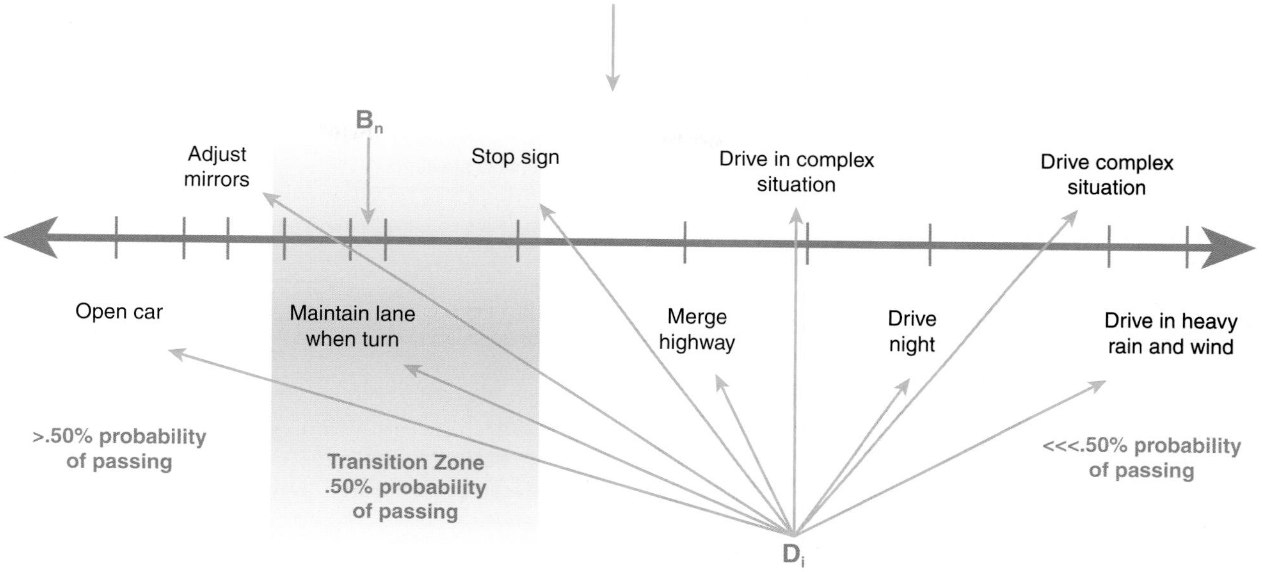

FIGURE 25.4 Comparison of person ability (B_n) to item difficulty (D_i) for a driving assessment.

Figure 25.4 presents how this formula "works" when assessing someone on a driving assessment. B_n from the formula is represented by B_1, a person with a "low" driving ability level. D_i from the formula is represented by nine driving items of different difficulty levels. To the far left are easy items, represented by predriving activities such as opening a car door and adjusting mirrors. To the far right are difficult items, such as driving at night, driving in complex situations, and driving in heavy rain and wind. The client B_1 will have a higher than .50 probability of passing the easy items such as opening a car door and a much lower than .50 probability of passing the difficult items such as driving in heavy rain and wind. But for the items that are close to his or her ability level (e.g., staying in the proper lane when turning), he or she will have a .50 probability of passing. These items are at "just the right" challenge for the individual.

This IRT model of relating a person's ability to item difficulty can be applied to assessing any client on any assessment. If we can think of our assessments as a series of items or tasks that have different challenges, we would expect that our client would have a high probability of being successful with items that were "below" his or her ability (the easiest items). These items could be "easy" ADL tasks such as eating and grooming, easy motor development items such as being able to roll from prone to supine, or easy upper extremity movement tasks such as moving one's arm in a gravity-eliminated position. We would expect that our client would have a low probability of being successful on items that were above his or her ability level. Challenging ADL tasks could be bathing or walking up the stairs, challenging motor development items could be running and jumping, and challenging upper extremity movement tasks can be lifting one's arm while extended holding a 10-lb object. As an occupational therapist, a major interest is determining the ability of a client. From a clinical perspective, IRT can be described as finding the "just right" challenge for a client. That is, not what is too easy or too hard, but the tasks that are appropriately challenging for a client.

One of the advantages of an IRT perspective for critiquing an assessment is that it provides solutions to increasing assessment efficiency (reducing respondent burden) and maximizing assessment precision. Because one acquires the most information from an assessment by using items that match a client's ability, it is logical that all of the items of an assessment are not necessary. Items that are too easy or too hard provide fairly little information about a client. This leads to the concept of "efficiency," assessing clients on only the most relevant items. This has the advantage of reducing respondent (client) burden and therapist assessment time. The IRT perspective also allows for maximizing measurement precision. A client's improvement can be measured by including items that he or she can do now but could not do previously. For example, referring to Figure 25.4, if prior to rehabilitation, a client could only accomplish predriving activities (e.g., opening car door and adjusting mirrors) but through rehabilitation can now do some basic driving skills (e.g., maintain lane when turning, stop at stop sign), improvement will be detected by including these basic driving tasks. This logic can also be used to eliminate floor effects (the inability of the assessment to discriminate among clients of low ability) and ceiling effects (the inability of the assessment to discriminate among clients of high ability). To remove a floor effect, easy items can be administered (e.g., more predriving tasks), and to remove a ceiling effect, hard items can be administered (e.g., challenging driving tasks). Although this approach is logical, the obvious question is, "How do I find the most relevant assessment items for an individual?" If an assessment has a logical hierarchy in terms of the difficulty of items, such as a motor development test, this can be quite easy to find the most appropriate items. This can be accomplished by starting with easy items and progressively administering more difficult items until the client fails several items (e.g., DENVER II, previously known as the Denver Developmental Screening Test; Frankenburg et al., 1992).

IRT-based assessments are also effectively designed for goal setting and treatment planning. As indicated in Figure 25.4, the client ability measure (B_n) is associated with the client having a .50 probability of being successful with items at his or her ability level (e.g., maintaining a lane when turning), and he or she has a lower probability of being successful for items above his or her ability level (e.g., stopping at a stop sign, merging on the highway, driving in a complex situation). Logical short-term goals would be to increase the client's success on items at his or her ability level, and logical longer-term goals would be to increase the client's success on items above his or her ability level. Treatment plans can be designed that involve activities that have similar challenge to those at the client's ability level, and activities can be graded in difficulty so that the client eventually achieves activities of challenge above his or her ability level. Coster and colleagues (1998) show how "item maps," which include the item ratings on the School Function Assessment, can be used to set realistic goals (e.g., moving from a rating of a "3," inconsistent performance, to "4," consistent performance, on more challenging items). Velozo and Woodbury (2011) have used similar maps of the Fugl-Meyer Assessment of upper extremity to suggest short- and long-term goals for clients recovering from upper extremity movement impairments following stroke.

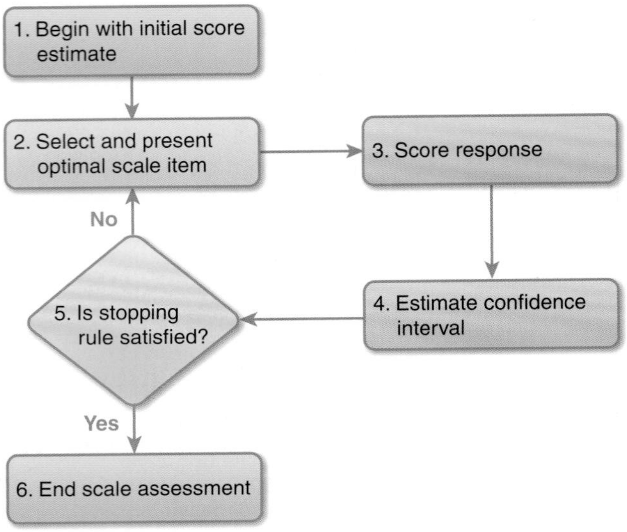

FIGURE 25.5 Computer adaptive test algorithm. (Adapted from Wainer, H., Dorans, N. J., Eignor, D., Flaugher, R., Green, B., Mislevy, R. J., . . . Thissen, D. [2000]. *Computerized adaptive testing: A primer* (2nd ed.). Mahwah, NJ: Lawrence Erlbaum Associates.)

Computerized Adaptive Testing

For assessments in which we do not have a clear item difficulty order, paper-and-pencil administration techniques may be ineffective. We would have to search through our assessment for the most appropriate items for our client. For example, if we find our client failing items, we would have to locate easier items. Similarly, if we found our client passing items, we would have to locate harder items. Unfortunately, for many of our assessments, the item difficulty order is not clear, thus making the selection of the most relevant items for a client even more challenging. In those cases, computer technology provides the solution. Computer software programs can be programmed to select items, even from hundreds of items (often referred to as an item bank), to administer the most relevant items to a client.

IRT, in combination with computer application of assessment items, can be used to automate both efficiency and precision in measurement. Computers can be programmed with algorithms (i.e., sets of rules) to direct only the most appropriate items to the client to maximize efficiency (use the fewest number of items) and maximize precision (use those items that differentiate one client from another or differentiate a client from one stage of progress to another) (see Figure 25.5). In general, computerized adaptive testing involves presenting questions to a client until a desired level of precision (reduced error) is reached. At the beginning of the assessment, before we present any items, we have little idea of the client's ability (e.g., he or she could be a poor driver or could be an excellent driver), our error is large, and we have a large confidence interval. But every time we assess the client on an item or task, we get more information on the client, reduce our error of measurement, and get a smaller confidence interval. A simple computerized adaptive testing algorithm can be described in six steps (see Figure 25.5). At the beginning of an assessment, we have little idea of the client's ability (ADL, driving, depression, etc); therefore, we typically estimate the client's ability to be at the "middle difficulty" of the items. Steps 2 through 5 represent the item administration process. The computer presents the item that most closely matches the client's initial ability estimate and/or the item that provides the most information about a client (e.g., "Do you stop at stop signs?") (step 2), and the client is scored on the item (step 3). That is, they either pass or fail (successfully stop or fail to stop) or get a particular rating (1 = failed to stop, 2 = partially stopped, 3 = stopped completely). After answering each question, the computer algorithm estimates a confidence interval or amount of precision we have in our measurement of a client (step 4). Upon answering each question, we get a smaller confidence interval and more precision. The computer continues to administer questions until we have reduced the confidence interval to a designated level (step 5); we then end the assessment and provide the client with a final assessment measure (step 6).

Presently, there are no specific occupational therapy computerized adaptive tests available for clinical use. This is probably because most assessments in occupational therapy are performance-based and computerized adaptive tests are typically self-report (often referred to as patient-reported) or proxy-report assessments. Patient-reported outcomes (PROs) are gaining considerable attention in health care area and several of these measures exist in the broader area of rehabilitation (e.g., Activity Measure for Post Acute Care [AM-PAC], Computer Adaptive Measure of Functional Cognition for Traumatic Brain Injury [CAMFC-TBI]) (Donovan et al., 2011; Haley et al., 2006). The National Institutes of Health invested in several PRO computerized adaptive measures for chronic disease, including the Patient Reported Outcomes System (PROMIS) and Neuro-QoL (Cella et al., 2007; Cella et al., 2012). As these assessments become readily available via the Web, occupational therapists and other rehabilitation professionals are likely to incorporate these assessments in clinical practice.

Critiquing IRT-Based Assessments

IRT, being a different psychometric theory than CTT and generalizability theory, demands a different set of methods for evaluation. IRT is based on a set of strong psychometric assumptions or requirements. Although most of these methods are beyond the scope of the masters-level occupational therapist practice, we will generally describe them here. There are four general areas in which IRT is typically critiqued: unidimensionality, local independence, precision, and person-item match.

Unidimensionality

Unidimensionality is the determination of whether an assessment measures a single trait. Although it is often argued that human beings are multidimensional, assessing multiple dimensions at the same time often leads to confusion. For example, ADL assessments often involve both physical function and cognitive items when evaluating a total score on the assessment; it is difficult to know what combination of attributes makes up that total score. Does the score reflect equal amounts of physical function and cognition items? Does the score represent a person with a lot of physical function ability and little cognitive ability or a lot of cognitive ability and little physical function ability? This becomes more complex interpretation following treatment of the client. Let's say that a client improves in his or her overall ADL score from admission to discharge. Has he or she improved in both physical and cognitive functioning? Improved just in physical functioning or improved just in cognitive functioning? Measuring a single or unidimensional trait is less confusing.

There are several psychometric methods to determine unidimensionality. One method is "item fit." This statistic determines how well items fit the IRT model. Items that do not fit the IRT model may be measuring a second trait (Bond & Fox, 2007). A second, more preferred method of determining unidimensionality is factor analysis. In general, factor analysis groups items that correlate with each other. An indication of unidimensionality is when all assessment items show a high correlation, or "load" on a single factor (e.g., all load on physical functioning). An indication of multidimensionality is when items load on separate factors (e.g., physical functioning and cognitive functioning).

Local Independence

Local independence is an indication of whether the items of an assessment independently contribute to the measurement of a particular trait. That is, are some items redundant or not adding anything new to the measuring of a particular trait? This can be a particularly confusing concept and may seem in conflict with an objective of assessing a client. For example, from a *qualitative* perspective, one would want to know every aspect of a client's driving ability (e.g., can he or she insert a key into the ignition, open the window, and press the gas pedal?). But some of these items may be redundant in terms of measuring driving ability. For example, pressing the gas pedal may be essentially equivalent to pressing the break or doing some other lower extremity activity. Turning a key may be essentially equivalent to adjusting a car mirror. If this is the case, then one can remove items that are redundant. Fairly sophisticated analyses, such as polychloric correlations or the correlation of item residuals, identify that items are redundant and can be removed from an assessment (Reeve et al., 2007).

Precision

Precision of an assessment is a critical feature of measurement in IRT. Obviously, we would like to have assessments that are as precise as possible; because we would expect that the more precise assessment will be more effective in differentiating our patients from one another and, more importantly, be effective in detecting change in our clients following occupational therapy intervention. There are several indices of precision used in IRT. Two important indicators of precision are error and information. Although in traditional testing, one gets only one value of error for an assessment in IRT, error can be plotted across the range of an assessment (across easy to hard items). Typically, we find that the error of an assessment increases at the extremes of the assessment. That is, there is usually more error at the easy and hard items of an assessment. Information is the reciprocal or inverse of error; therefore, the more information provided by an assessment, the more precise it is.

Person-Item Match

Person-item match, as noted earlier, characteristic of all IRT models is the comparison of person ability to item difficulty. This relationship can tell us how well the items of our assessment match the abilities of the clients under study. This can be exemplified by ceiling and floor effects in our assessments. Ceilings effects are when an assessment cannot differentiate the most able clients (i.e., clients are more able than what our assessment can assess), and floor effect are when an assessment cannot differentiate the least able clients that (i.e., clients are less able than what our assessment can assess). Based on IRT models, this is related to whether or not we have items that match a client's ability. For ceiling effects, we do not have items that differentiate the most able clients. For example, if we have good drivers in our sample and our hardest item is driving in our hometown, it is likely that all of these clients will get "perfect" measures on our assessment. The reality may be that if we tested these clients on more challenging items, for example, merging onto a highway, we would then be able to differentiate these clients of high ability. Similarly, a floor effect suggests that we do not have items that differentiate the lowest ability-level clients and likely indicates that we do not have easy enough items to differentiate these clients. For example, if we do not have predriving tasks on our assessment, we may not be able to differentiate those individuals who cannot do on-the-road driving. If one has a good conceptual model for an assessment, that is, an understanding of the relative challenge of the items of our assessment, resolving these problems can be easy. Ceiling effects can be eliminated by creating more challenging items, and floor effects can be eliminated by creating easy items.

Summary

The purpose of this chapter was to provide an overview on the many methods used to critique assessments. As evident by the number of areas covered in this chapter, critiquing assessments is not an easy task. It requires both clinical knowledge of one's specialty area and statistical knowledge on reliability and validity. Critiquing assessments becomes more daunting with the addition of new measurement theories such as IRT and new test administration methods such as computerized adaptive testing. Obviously, the practicing therapist cannot be up to date on all occupational therapy assessments. But as a practicing occupational therapist, it is essential that one is able to critique the assessments that one uses in daily practice.

References

Allen, W. R., Classen, S., & Cook, M. (in press). Driving simulator applications in research and clinical practice. *Advances in Transportation Studies: An International Journal.*

Association of American Publishers. (n.d.). *Standardized assessment: A primer* (Rev. ed.). Washington, DC: Author.

Bédard, M., Parkkari, M., Weaver, B., Riendeau, J., & Dahlquist, M. (2010). Assessment of driving performance using a simulator protocol: Validity and reproducibility. *American Journal of Occupational Therapy, 64*(2), 336–340.

Bond, T. G., & Fox, C. M. (2007). *Applying the Rasch model: Fundamental measurement in the human sciences.* Mahwah, NJ: Lawrence Erlbaum Associates.

Carmines, E. G., & Zeller, R. (Eds.). (1979). *Reliability and validity assessment.* Thousand Oaks, CA: Sage.

Cella, D., & Chang, C. H. (2000). A discussion of item response theory and its applications in health status assessment. *Medical Care, 38*(9, Suppl.), II66–72.

Cella, D., Lai, J. S., Nowinski, C. J., Victorson, D., Peterman, A., Miller, D., . . . Moy, C. (2012). Neuro-QOL: Brief measures of health-related quality of life for clinical research in neurology. *Neurology, 78*(23), 1860–1867

Cella, D., Yount, S., Rothrock, N., Gershon, R., Cook, K., Reeve, B., . . . Rose, M. (2007). The patient-reported outcomes measurement information system (PROMIS): Progress of an NIH roadmap cooperative group during its first two years. *Medical Care, 45*(5, Suppl. 1), S3–S11.

Classen, S., McCarthy, D. P., Shechtman, O., Awadzi, K. D., Lanford, D. N., Okun, M. S., . . . Fernandez, H. H. (2009). Useful field of view as a reliable screening measure of driving performance in people with Parkinson's disease: Results of a pilot study. *Traffic Injury Prevention, 10*(6), 593–598.

Classen, S., & Owens, A. B. (2011). Simulator sickness among returning combat veterans with mild traumatic brain injury and/or post-traumatic stress disorder (2010 Special Issue). *Advances in Transportation Studies: An International Journal,* 45–52.

Classen, S., Wen, P. S., Velozo, C. A., Bédard, M., Winter, S. M., Brumback, B. A., & Lanford, D. N. (2012a). Psychometrics of the self-report Safe Driving Behavior Measure for older adults. *American Journal of Occupational Therapy, 66*(2), 233–241.

Classen, S., Wen, P. S., Velozo, C. A., Bédard, M., Winter, S. M., Brumback, B. A., & Lanford, D. N. (2012b). Rater reliability and rater effects of the Safe Driving Behavior Measure. *American Journal of Occupational Therapy, 66*(1), 69–77.

Classen, S., Winter, S. M., Velozo, C. A., Bédard, M., Lanford, D., Brumback, B. A., & Lutz, B. J. (2010). Item development and validity testing for a Safe Driving Behavior Measure. *American Journal of Occupational Therapy, 64*(2), 296–305.

Coster, W., Deeney, T., Haltiwanger, J., & Haley, S. (1998). *School Function Assessment user manual.* San Antonio, TX: Psychological Corporation.

Cronbach, L. J., Gleser, G. C., Nanda, H., & Rajaratnam, N. (1972). *The dependability of behavioral measurements: Theory of generalizability for scores and profiles.* New York, NY: Wiley.

Cronbach, L. J., Nageswari, R., & Gleser, G. C. (1963). Theory of generalizability: A liberation of reliability theory. *The British Journal of Statistical Psychology, 16,* 137–163.

Di Stefano, M., & Macdonald, W. (2005). On-the-road evaluation of driving performance. In J. M. Pellerito (Ed.), *Driver rehabilitation and community principles and practice* (pp. 255–274). St Louis, MO: Elsevier Mosby.

Donovan, N. J., Heaton, S. C., Kimberg, C. I., Wen, P. S., Waid-Ebbs, J. K., Coster, W., . . . Velozo, C. A. (2011). Conceptualizing functional cognition in traumatic brain injury rehabilitation. *Brain Injury, 25*(4), 348–364.

Edwards, J. D., Ross, L. A., Wadley, V. G., Clay, O. J., Crowe, M., Roenker, D. L., & Ball, K. K. (2006). The Useful Field of View test: Normative data for older adults. *Archives of Clinical Neuropsychology, 21*(4), 275–286.

Fisher, A. G. (1993). The assessment of IADL motor skills: An application of many-faceted Rasch analysis. *American Journal of Occupational Therapy, 47*(4), 319–329.

Fisher, W. P., Jr. (1995). Rehabits: A common language of functional assessment. *Archives of Physical Medicine & Rehabiliation, 76*(2), 113–122.

Folstein, M. F., Folstein, S. E., & McHugh, P. R. (1975). "Mini-mental state." A practical method for grading the cognitive state of patients for the clinician. *Journal of Psychiatric Research, 12*(3), 189–198.

Folstein, M. F., Folstein, S. E., White, T., & Messer, M. A. (2010). *Mini-mental state exam, user's guide* (2nd ed.). Lutz, FL: PAR.

Frankenburg, W. K., Doods, J., Archer, P., Bresnick, B., Maschka, P., Edelman, N., & Shapiro, H. (1992). *DENVER II training manual.* Denver, CO: Denver Developmental Materials.

Grant, J. S., & Davis, L. L. (1997). Selection and use of content experts for instrument development. *Research in Nursing & Health, 20*(3), 269–274.

Haley, S. M., Ludlow, L. H., & Coster, W. J. (1993). Pediatric evaluation of disability inventory: Clinical interpretation of summary scores using Rasch rating scale methodology. *Physical Medicine and Rehabilation Clinics of North America, 4*, 529–540.

Haley, S. M., Siebens, H., Coster, W. J., Tao, W., Black-Schaffer, R. M., Gandek, B., . . . Ni, P. (2006). Computerized adaptive testing for follow-up after discharge from inpatient rehabilitation: I. Activity outcomes. *Archives of Physical Medicine & Rehabiliation, 87*(8), 1033–1042.

Hinojosa, J., Kramer, P., & Crist, P. (Eds.). (2005). *Evaluation: Obtaining and interpreting data* (2nd ed). Bethesda, MD: AOTA Press.

House, A. E., House, B. J., & Campbell, M. B. (1981). Measures of interobserver agreement: Calculation formulas and distribution effects. *Journal of Behavioral Assessment, 3*(1), 37–57.

Justiss, M. D., Mann, W. C., Stav, W., & Velozo, C. (2006). Development of a behind-the-wheel driving performance assessment for older adults. *Topics in Geriatric Rehabilitation, 22*(2), 121–128.

Kay, L., Bundy, A., & Clemson, L. (2009). Predicting fitness to drive in people with cognitive impairments by using DriveSafe and DriveAware. *Archives of Physical Medicine & Rehabilitation, 90*(9), 1514–1522. doi:10.1016/j.apmr.2009.03.0118

Kennedy, R. S., Lane, N. E., Berbaum, K. S., & Lilienthal, M. G. (1993). Simulator Sickness questionnaire: An enhanced method for quantifying simulator sickness. *The International Journal of Aviation Psychology, 3*(3), 203–220.

Kielhofner, G., Dobria, L., Forsyth, K., & Basu, S. (2005). The construction of keyforms for obtaining instantaneous measures from the occupational performance history interview rating scales: Empirical quantitative study. *OTJR: Occupation, Participation and Health, 25*(1), 23–32.

Kraut, R., Olson, J., Banaji, M., Bruckman, A., Cohen, J., & Couper, M. (2004). Psychological research online: Report of Board of Scientific Affairs' Advisory Group on the Conduct of Research on the Internet. *American Psychologist, 59*(2), 105–117.

Law, M. (1987). Measurement in occupational therapy: Scientific criteria for evaluation. *Canadian Journal of Occupational Therapy, 54*(3), 133–138.

Lynn, M. R. (1986). Determination and quantification of content validity. *Nursing Research, 35*(6), 382–385.

Morris, J. C. (1993). The clinical dementia rating (CDR): Current version and scoring rules. *Neurology, 43*(11), 2412–2414.

Munkholm, M., Löfgren, B., & Fisher, A. G. (2012). Reliability of the school AMPS measures. *Scandinavian Journal Of Occupational Therapy, 19*(1), 2–8. doi:10.3109/11038128.2010.525721

Nunnally, J. C., & Bernstein, I. H. (1994). *Psychometric theory* (3rd ed.). New York, NY: McGraw Hill.

Owsley, C., Ball, K. K., McGwin, G., Sloane, M. E., Roenker, D. L., White, M. F., & Overley, E. T. (1998). Visual processing impairment and risk of motor vehicle crash among older adults. *Journal of the American Medical Association, 279*(14), 1083–1088.

Owsley, C., & McGwin, G., Jr. (1999). Vision impairment and driving. *Survey of Ophthalmology, 43*(6), 535–550.

Owsley, C., McGwin, G., Jr., & Ball, K. K. (1998). Vision impairment, eye disease, and injurious motor vehicle crashes in the elderly. *Ophthalmic Epidemiology, 5*(2), 101–113.

Owsley, C., Stalvey, B. T., Wells, J., & Sloane, M. E. (1999). Older drivers and cataract: Driving habits and crash risk. *Journal of Gerontology: Series A: Biological Sciences & Medical Sciences, 54*(4), M203–M211.

Portney, L., & Watkins, M. P. (2009). *Foundations of clinical research: Applications to practice* (3nd ed.). Upper Saddle River, NJ: Prentice Hall Health.

Reeve, B. B., Hays, R. D., Bjorner, J. B., Cook, K. F., Crane, P. K., Teresi, J. A., . . . Cella, D. (2007). Psychometric evaluation and calibration of health-related quality of life item banks: Plans for the patient-reported outcomes measurement information system (PROMIS). *Medical Care, 45*(5, Suppl. 1), S22–31.

Reitan, R. M. (1958). Validity of the Trail Making test as an indicator of organic brain damage. *Perceptual and Motor Skills, 8*, 271–276.

Rudman, D., & Hannah, S. (1998). An instrument evaluation framework: Description and application to assessments of hand function. *Journal of Hand Therapy, 11*, 266–277.

Shechtman, O., Classen, S., Awadzi, K. D., & Mann, W. (2009). Comparison of driving errors between on-the-road and simulated driving assessment: A validation study. *Traffic Injury Prevention, 10* (4), 379–385.

Smith, R. (2000). Fit analysis in latent trait measurement models. *Journal of Applied Measurement, 1*(2), 199–218.

Streiner, D. L., & Norman, G. R. (Eds.). (2008a). Devising the items. In *Health measurement scales: A practical guide to their development and use* (4th ed., pp. 17–36). Oxford, NY: Oxford University Press.

Streiner, D. L., & Norman, G. R. (Eds.). (2008b). *Health measurement scales: A practical guide to their development and use* (4th ed.). Oxford, NY: Oxford University Press

Velozo, C. A., Byers, K., & Joseph, B. (2007). Translating measures across the continuum of care: Using Rasch analysis to create a crosswalk between the functional independence measure and the minimum data set. *Journal of Rehabilitation Research and Development, 44*(3), 467.

Velozo, C. A., & Woodbury, M. L. (2011). Translating measurement findings into rehabilitation practice: An example using Fugl-Meyer assessment-upper extremity with patients following stroke. *Journal of Rehabilitation Research and Development, 48*(10), 1211–1222.

Wainer, H., Dorans, N. J., Eignor, D., Flaugher, R., Green, B., Mislevy, R. J., . . . Thissen, D. (2000). *Computerized adaptive testing: A primer* (2nd ed.). Mahwah, NJ: Lawrence Erlbaum Associates.

Whiteneck, G., Brooks, C. A., Charlifue, S., Gerhart, K. A., Mellick, D., Overholser, D., & Richardson, G. N. (1998). *Craig Handicap Assessment and Reporting Technique 1998*. Retrieved from http://www.craighospital.org/repository/documents/Research%20Instruments/CHART%20Manual.pdf

For additional resources on the subjects discussed in this chapter, visit http://thePoint.lww.com/Willard-Spackman12e.

CHAPTER 26

Occupational Therapy Interventions for Individuals

Glen Gillen

OUTLINE

LEARNING OBJECTIVES

After reading this chapter, you will be able to:

1. Understand the overarching themes that occupational therapists embrace when choosing interventions for their clients
2. Differentiate between interventions that are categorized as "occupation as ends" and "occupation as means"
3. Develop and choose interventions for clients that combine the principles of occupation as ends and occupation as means
4. Compare and contrast a variety of specific intervention approaches that are used for clients receiving occupational therapy services
5. Begin to understand when to choose one type of intervention over another, combine interventions, and/or switch the intervention plan
6. Understand the concept of grading interventions

Introduction

When developing intervention plans for clients, occupational therapists work under the guidance of three overarching and interrelated themes. Interventions must be client centered, evidence based, and chosen based on sound professional reasoning. The term *client-centered practice* has been defined as

> an approach to providing occupational therapy, which embraces a philosophy of respect for and partnership with people receiving services. It recognizes the autonomy of individuals, the need for client choice in making decisions about occupational needs, the strengths clients bring to an occupational therapy encounter and the benefits of client-therapist partnership and the need to ensure that services are accessible and fit the context in which a client lives. (Law, Baptiste, & Mills, 1995, p. 253)

Sumsion and Law (2006) have reviewed and analyzed subsequent definitions of client-centered practice and concluded that the various definitions share many similar components including "... a strong emphasis on a collaborative approach or partnership, respect for the client, facilitating choice and involving the client in determining the occupational goals that emerge from his or her choices" (p. 154). The reader is referred to Chapter 33 for a further discussion on this topic.

Sumsion and Law (2006) further point out that development of the literature regarding client-centered practice parallels the development of our understanding of evidence-based practice. Sackett, Strauss, Richardson, Rosenberg, and Haynes (2000) define evidence-based practice as "the integration of best research evidence with clinical expertise and patient values" (p. 1). Client values include "the unique preferences, concerns and expectations each patient brings to a clinical encounter" (p. 1). A major component of evidence-based practice is the clear message that we, as occupational therapists, must use evidence to inform our intervention choices (Bennett et al., 2003). Bennett and Bennett (2000) summarize that the research literature can provide guidance concerning the effectiveness and choices of OT interventions, the way in which interventions are best implemented, and whether there are any associated difficulties related to the intervention. They conclude that "occupational therapists can use this sort of research evidence to help clients understand, plan and cope with their situation" (p. 173). See Chapter 31 for more detail regarding evidence-based practice.

The literature regarding evidence-based decision making has consistently emphasized that research evidence alone is not adequate to guide the choice of interventions. Rather, clinicians must apply their clinical expertise and professional reasoning to assess the patient's deficits while at the same time incorporating the research evidence (Haynes, Devereaux, & Guyatt, 2002). Bennett and Bennett (2000) also stress that evidence needs to be integrated with clinical expertise and reasoning so that the practitioner can decide if valid and potentially useful results from a research study can apply to the individual that he or she is working with. They proposed the following questions to guide the application of evidence:

1. "Do these results apply to my client? (i.e., is my client so different from those in the study that its results cannot help me?)
2. Does the treatment fit in with my client's values and preferences?
3. Are there resources available to implement the treatment?" (p. 177)

In addition to these questions, the occupational therapist must consider how/if the evidence relates to our profession's underlying assumptions and philosophy (American Occupational Therapy Association [AOTA], 2008). It is important to remember that just because an intervention is deemed effective does not automatically mean that it is an appropriate occupational therapy (OT) intervention. The reader is further referred to Chapter 30 for detailed information regarding the professional reasoning process. Case Study 26.1 was developed to provide the reader with insight into the OT intervention process that will be described in detail in this chapter. As you read, note that the various interventions were developed based on the clients' needs and desire to maintain access to their community. The interventions were planned based on the findings of a variety of evaluation techniques. Finally, note that the combinations of interventions were used to meet client-centered goals. More case studies are provided at the end of this chapter to further illustrate intervention processes.

Occupation as Therapy

As occupational therapists, our outcomes are focused on improving occupational performance. We achieve this goal by using occupation as a therapeutic change agent. Therefore, we believe in the therapeutic value of occupational engagement and that engagement in occupations is also the ultimate goal of therapy (AOTA, 2011a). The therapeutic occupations we use are ideally both *meaningful* and *purposeful*. Meaningful suggests that the task at hand is motivating and has some level of significance (Trombly, 1995). The task may be something the person wants to do, has to do, or needs to do throughout the day. The purposeful component may serve to organize and enhance performance as it pertains to the client's aim, reason for doing, or personal goal (Fisher, 1998; Trombly, 1995). Interventions may involve changing occupations in ways that either foster development or improvement in desired performance or allow for participation in spite of limitations. Based on the intervention choices that are outlined in the following discussion, occupations can be graded to create "just the right challenge." The term **grading** refers to systematically increasing the demands of an occupation to stimulate improved function or reducing the demands to respond to client difficulties in performance.

When grading, the OT practitioner increases the demands of the task at hand to potentially reduce an underlying impairment or performance skill deficit. In other cases, the OT practitioner may downgrade the demands so that the task can be achieved despite a client's limitations. A person who is recovering from cardiac transplant surgery that was preceded by a long period of bed rest may be engaged in occupations that are systematically graded to improve strength and endurance as to foster participation in meaningful occupations. The therapist may grade therapeutic occupations based on the posture assumed while performing tasks (standing as opposed to sitting), duration of the task, number of rest breaks, use of adaptive equipment, and vanishing physical assistance by the therapist to complete the task. Occupational therapists may also downgrade demands and modify the task or the environment so that a client can still participate

CASE STUDY 26.1 Benjamin: A Married Older Man Whose Family Is Concerned about His Driving Abilities

Occupational Profile

Benjamin is a 79-year-old male who lives with his wife Bess in a retirement community. Benjamin and Bess have always enjoyed visiting their children and grandchildren who live in neighboring towns. Benjamin had a myocardial infarction about 7 years ago and underwent bypass surgery. Although Benjamin remains independent in his basic activities of daily living, plays cards with his longtime buddies, and enjoys walks about the community's gardens, he can get short of breath with exertion. One year ago, Bess experienced a mild/moderate stroke with residual left-sided weakness and a visual field cut. She has not driven since the stroke, needs assistance with transfers, and uses a scooter except for short distances, thus making road trips more stressful due to mobility and vision issues. Up until a year ago, Benjamin and Bess shared driving responsibilities, functioning as a team for navigation. Since Benjamin assumed full responsibility for driving and navigation, Bess has reported several "near misses" while driving, but Benjamin is quick to report that these incidents were the fault of other drivers. Recently, they both were upset after a "fender bender" that Benjamin insisted was the fault of a driver who "came out of nowhere." Bess tearfully admits that she struggles to assist in navigation and there have been some tense moments as they struggled to find their way home when returning from a trip to see their grandchildren. She relies on her husband for transportation, so she waffles back and forth with her concerns. The adult children are now worried for both of their parents' safety and discussed the issue with Benjamin and Bess's physician. The physician referred Bess to a general practice occupational therapist to address her mobility issues, and Benjamin was referred to an occupational therapist who is a driver rehabilitation specialist for a comprehensive driving evaluation.

Assessment Findings

Benjamin, Bess, and their adult children were interviewed by the driver rehabilitation specialist to review Benjamin's medical and driving history as well as to understand the environmental context for community mobility resources. The occupational therapist reviewed Benjamin's medications and cardiac history and administered an array of clinical assessments to cover his cognitive, motor, and visual abilities. Specifically, assessments included (1) functional range of motion and strength of the neck, arms, and legs; (2) visual acuity; (3) contrast sensitivity; (4) visual fields and tracking; (5) Short Blessed cognitive exam; (6) Trail-Making Test A and B; (7) the Useful Field of View (UFOV) (computer-based screen for selective attention); (8) clock drawing; (9) brake reaction timer; and the occupational therapist observed Benjamin making a meat and cheese sandwich and coffee. Benjamin wore his glasses for the vision testing and demonstrated very poor contrast sensitivity and vision that was 20/70. When asked, Benjamin had not had a vision evaluation for more than 10 years. There were no field cuts or difficulty tracking visually. Benjamin's cognitive abilities did not show any sign of significant dementia, but his processing speeds were slow with the Trail-Making Test, UFOV, and brake reaction timer. He also had some range of motion restrictions with his neck. The behind the wheel (BTW) evaluation was delayed until Benjamin was able to see an optometrist. After the optometrist evaluated Benjamin's vision and prescribed new glasses, his visual acuity increased to 20/30. However, the contrast sensitivity remained poor, not unusual for his age. The BTW assessment demonstrated that Benjamin follows the rules of the road, did not make any significant errors, but was slow in making decisions at unprotected turns and drove significantly slower than other traffic on the highway component of the evaluation.

Goal

Several goals were established: (1) Their automobile would be modified with a swing front seat for improved transfer for Bess; (2) Benjamin would remain independent in driving with a recommended restricted license; and (3) Benjamin, Bess, and their children would make plans for alternative transportation when needed and eventual driving retirement.

Intervention

Bess was seen by an occupational therapist generalist who recommended that their motor vehicle be modified with a scooter lift as well as a swing-out seat for ease of transfers from the scooter to the front passenger seat to decrease the physical toll when using their automobile (*adaptation*). Both Benjamin and Bess would be *educated* on the proper use. The therapist also evaluated Bess's instrumental activities of daily living (IADL) in the home and assisted her in modifying the kitchen and bathroom to improve her independence (*environmental modifications*).

Using a *prevention* approach, the driver rehabilitation specialist made the recommendation to restrict Benjamin's license to daytime driving only due to the poor contrast sensitivity because evidence demonstrates the relationship of contrast sensitivity and crashes (Owsley & McGwin, 1999; Owsley, Sekuler, & Siemsen, 1983; Owsley, Stalvey, Wells, & Sloane, 1999). The therapist also recommended that highway driving be eliminated as well as planning local routes to avoid unprotected turns or yield signs because evidence shows that risk of crashes of these types of intersections increase significantly with slowed processing (Stutts, Martell, & Staplin, 2009). The driving rehabilitation specialist reviewed Benjamin and Bess's community mobility needs and planned routes that posed less risk for crashes, including right-hand turns and intersections with signals. Meeting with the adult children, Benjamin, and Bess, alternative transportation plans included the children picking up their parents when an activity might involve nighttime driving and the grandchildren would alternate in picking their grandparents up for a visit. Both began to use the retirement community's transportation for some events. Three months later, Bess and Benjamin indicated that traveling had become much easier with the scooter lift and transfer seat. No further "close calls" were reported and Benjamin and Bess reported it was sometimes delightful to be chauffeured by their grandchildren.

despite persistent impairments. A therapist may work with an adult who is living with schizophrenia to circumvent daily life problems by teaching use of a daily planner to help organize and complete home and work tasks. The therapist may grade the number of verbal cues required for organization and sequencing when teaching the client to use the planner to create a grocery list.

Fisher (1998) describes occupation as a "noun of action" that has the power to enable people "to perform the actions they need and want to perform so that they can engage in and 'do' the familiar, ordinary, goal directed activities of every day in a manner that brings meaning and personal satisfaction" (p. 511). She further outlines groups of activities and their attributes that can be implemented as OT (see Table 26.1).

Occupation as Ends as Intervention

In her Eleanor Clarke Slagle Lecture, Catherine Trombly (1995) described **occupation as ends** as being "not only purposeful but also meaningful because it is the performance of activities or tasks that a person sees as

TABLE 26.1 Intervention Methods Potentially Used by Occupational Therapy Practitioners

Activity Type	Examples	Focus of Therapy	Source of Meaning and Purpose	How Real or Natural	OT Practice Framework Classification
Exercise: rote exercise or practice	Elastic bands, weight lifting, practice line drawing for eye–hand coordination	Remediation of impairments	Practitioner-chosen for therapy benefits Client expected to "comply"	Contrived—typically only done in therapy situation	Preparatory method
Contrived occupation: exercise with added purpose and occupation with a contrived component	Practice picking up balls from the floor and placing them in a bucket, placing cones on a shelf pretending they are dishes, hammering nails into wood, throwing bean bags at a target	Remediation of impairments or skill development	Practitioner-chosen for therapy benefits Client expected to "comply"	Contrived, therapy using culturally common objects	Purposeful activity
*Therapeutic occupation: graded occupations to treat impairments, direct intervention of impairments in the context of occupation	Challenging balance skills via organizing library book shelves for a client who loves to read, working on social skills during a group focused on adolescents making a cake for one of their mothers, using a favorite card game to improve attention	Remediation of impairments or skill development	Chosen collaboratively for meaning to client and therapy potential	More naturalistic, uses authentic aspects of occupation (tools, context)	Occupation-based intervention
*Adaptive/compensatory occupation: assistive devices, teach compensatory strategies, modify physical or social environments	Adapting a shopping task to compensate for poor endurance Learning to drive again after an orthopedic injury Working in a job for person with developmental disabilities	Improved occupational performance	Chosen collaboratively based on occupations, with therapy processes selected to support performance	Naturalistic activity in natural contexts	Occupation-based intervention

Note that current trends in the field suggest that occupation-based approaches (indicated by *) are often most effective and provide a clearer external reflection of occupational therapy profession's contribution to health care. Additionally, interventions may involve a mix of methods in order to both minimize effects of impairment and promote occupational functioning.

Data from Fisher, A. G. (1998). Uniting practice and theory in an occupational therapy framework, 1998 Eleanor Clarke Slagle lecture. *American Journal of Occupational Therapy, 52*, 509–522.

BOX 26.1 Examples of Using Occupation as Ends

- Teaching a person who has just had a hip replacement adapted positions so that sexual activities can be engaged in safely.
- Practice of one-handed shoe tying after stroke or upper limb amputation.
- Repetitive practice of components of meal preparation.
- Teaching a child living with developmental delays to use an augmentative communication device.
- Recommending magnifying devices so that a person living with macular degeneration can read the newspaper.
- Recommending and training with vehicular hand controls so that a person who does not have use of his or her lower extremities after a spinal cord injury can drive again.
- Teaching an adult living with schizophrenia a new leisure activity, such as photography.
- Task-specific practice of handwriting, such as writing out a weekly grocery list.
- Teaching a person who has survived a stroke how to propel a wheelchair using an arm and leg for functional mobility within the home.
- Demonstrating and teaching the use of bilateral upper limb prostheses to eat a meal after upper limb amputations.
- Demonstrating and teaching an adaptive swallowing technique to promote independent and safe self-feeding.

important" (p. 963). Occupation as ends refers to engaging your client in occupations that constitute the end product of therapy (i.e., the occupations to be learned or relearned). Occupation as ends has been described by Trombly (1995) as the following:

- Directly teaching the activity or task
- Using whatever abilities a client has at his or her disposal to learn a task
- Providing adaptations to learn a task or activity
- A rehabilitative approach
- A skills training approach
- An approach in which the therapist serves as teacher or adaptor of a task
- Influenced by learning and cognitive information-processing theories regarding the therapeutic principle behind this approach
- *Not* being used to make a therapeutic change of underlying capabilities such as strength or memory

Using occupation as ends as an intervention serves as the goal to be learned or achieved. For example, Peter, who is undergoing inpatient rehabilitation after a spinal cord injury (SCI) left him paraplegic, may have a goal to independently transfer from his wheelchair to his car or to his bathtub. If you were to watch the therapist and Peter in action, they would be engaged in specifically chosen areas of occupation and you may observe actual practice of these mobility skills: the therapist teaching Peter how to use a sliding board to move from surface to surface, the therapist suggesting environmental modifications such as a tub bench and nonslip bath mats, and/or the therapist gradually decreasing the amount of physical, cognitive, and emotional support required to perform the task as the client becomes more independent. The occupations chosen are based on the occupations that the client wants to, needs to, or has to resume or continue in his or her various life roles. Using occupation as ends as an intervention approach makes the focus of OT quite clear, particularly when a collaborative approach to intervention planning is used (see Box 26.1).

Occupation as Means as Intervention

Occupation as means refers to "the occupation acting as the therapeutic change agent to remediate impaired abilities or capacities" (Trombly, 1995, p. 964). Also referred to by some authors as purposeful activity (Hinojosa & Kramer, 1997), Trombly (1995) further describes occupation as means as follows:

- Including a variety of interventions, such as arts and crafts, games, sports, and specifically chosen daily activities
- Requiring more constrained responses as compared to occupation as ends
- Chosen based on both client interest and potential to remediate an underlying impairment
- Providing a challenge that is slightly beyond what the client can easily achieve. This concept has also been described as finding "just the right challenge"

An assumption inherent in this intervention approach is "that acquisition or reacquisition of motor, cognitive, and psychological skills will ultimately result in successful performance of activities of daily living" (Weinstock-Zlotnick & Hinojosa, 2004, p. 594). Box 26.2 provides examples of using occupation as means as an intervention. Unlike occupation as ends, simply observing a client engaged in occupation as means may not provide the observer with a clear understanding of why the intervention was chosen. In many cases, this understanding emerges after a discussion with the OT practitioner as to the rationale for the choice of the intervention. Teaching someone a new board game may be considered

BOX 26.2 Examples of Using Occupation as Means

- Rolling out dough to strengthen an older adult's upper limbs so that he or she can regain independence in homemaking tasks such as washing dishes.
- Engaging a child in a playground climbing activity to promote body awareness and motor planning so that he or she can engage in age-appropriate play such as bike riding.
- Playing a game of Connect Four with game pieces placed on the left side to promote spatial awareness so that a person may be able to locate grooming items placed on the left side of the sink.
- Using arts and crafts activities to improve self-esteem and/or lessen anxiety so that a person feels more confident when socializing with others.
- Leading a group of adults in a session of water aerobics to promote joint flexibility so that they can maintain independence in home activities such as putting away groceries.
- Engaging in a gardening task to develop reach and coordination skills that may then be used during self-care activities.
- Engaging a client in a challenging occupation such as money management to promote awareness of cognitive deficits. This improved awareness may then result in the client understanding that he or she requires adaptive cognitive strategies to manage at home.

occupation as ends if the client's goals include expanding their repertoire of leisure-based occupations. A board game may also be chosen as a therapeutic mechanism for a variety of reasons that may classify the intervention choice as occupation as means. Examples include using manipulation of game pieces to acquire or reacquire dexterity, placing game pieces out of reach to promote postural control, using the game to develop social skills such as turn taking, grading how long the client plays the game to improve sustained attention skills, and using the game to enhance self-efficacy or lessen anxiety. When this approach is used, the therapist *must* clearly link the potential change in underlying skills and client factors to improveed occupational performance. Improved dexterity would not be considered the end product of OT. However, regaining the ability to manipulate fasteners to independently dress, independently finger feed, or be able to manipulate scissors while making holiday cards in school would all be considered examples of desired outcomes depending on client preference and the context of therapy.

When using occupation as means as the intervention, it is particularly important that the OT practitioner choose occupations that have meaning and that the rationale for the intervention is made explicit. Otherwise, clients may find it difficult to understand the focus of OT. It is important that clients do not leave a session simply thinking "we played cards in OT today."

Combining Occupation as Means and as Ends

It is possible to combine aspects of occupation as ends and occupation as means. Using this method, a collaborative approach is used to determine goals and to understand a client's interests. The OT practitioner then uses his or her skills of occupational analysis to determine which underlying performance skills and/or client factors may need to be challenged. In her discussion of combining occupation as ends and means, Gray (1998) states,

> Rather than completing an assessment and using problem areas (components) to decide which activities to use for treatment (e.g., macrame is great for coordination, parquetry puzzles are assumed to help visual perceptual deficits), the occupational therapist has the added challenge of looking into the client's occupational history and selecting activities related to the client's occupations and interests that can be modified and structured to improve coordination and visual perception. Perhaps that particular client enjoyed waxing the car, making fried chicken, or playing with his or her nieces. The occupational therapist could, with a little creativity and ingenuity, tailor those occupations to treat the very same coordination or visual perceptual deficits. (p. 358)

To be successful, this approach requires that the OT practitioner has mastered the skill of occupational analysis. See Chapter 21 for detailed information on occupational analysis. In summary, occupation is always the ends and is the most frequent means with the addition of purposeful and preparatory methods as needed. See Table 26.2 for examples of combining occupation as ends and means.

Specific Intervention Approaches

OT practitioners

> address the interaction among client factors, performance skills, performance patterns, contexts and environments, and activity demands

TABLE 26.2 Combining Occupation as Means and Occupation as Ends

Goal: Independently manage/navigate a subway system in order to attend Alcoholics Anonymous meetings.	Goal: Independent in toileting.
Occupation as ends: Task-specific training of the occupation using graded physical and verbal cues for difficult aspects of the task such as interpreting a subway map. Helping the client perform parts of the task that are difficult (e.g., money management) so that the task can be completed. Adapting the task so that it can be completed (e.g., providing a prepaid fare card so that the client does not need to manage money).	*Occupation as ends*: Task-specific training of the occupation using graded physical and verbal cues for difficult aspects of the task such as maneuvering from a wheelchair to the commode. Helping the client perform parts of the task that are difficult (e.g., clothing management) so that the task can be completed. Adapting the task so that it can be completed (e.g., providing grab bars or a raised toilet seat).
Occupation as means: Managing and navigating the subway is used to challenge a variety of underlying skills and factors such as the following: – Manipulation of money – Way finding in new environments – Social skills development such as appropriately waiting in line for the attendant – Problem solving if there is a schedule or service change – Calculation of change after money exchange – Maintaining balance when the train is in motion – Endurance for ambulation, stair climbing, and standing tolerance	*Occupation as means*: Using aspects of toileting to challenge a variety of underlying skills and factors such as the following: – Postural control when transitioning from sitting to standing – Motor planning during manipulation of toilet paper – Sequencing the steps of the toileting task – Promoting safety awareness in reference to locking brakes and manipulating footplates out of the way – Challenging sitting balance – Manipulation skills when fastening pants – Awareness of body position in space when transitioning from chair to commode – Lower extremity strength and control to transition from sit to stand and stand to sit

> that influence occupational performance within those occupations the person needs and wants to do. The intervention focus is on modifying the environment/contexts and activity demands or patterns, promoting health, establishing or restoring and maintaining occupational performance, and preventing further disability and occupational performance problems. (AOTA, 2008, p. 652)

A variety of intervention approaches are available. In some cases, only one category of intervention is used to meet client goals. Other clinical situations require the use of several categories of intervention or a change in intervention choice based on a poor response, reimbursement issues, or a change in client status. Practitioners base their choice of interventions on a variety of factors including client choice (see Chapter 33), interpretation of assessment findings (see Chapter 24), evidence (see Chapter 31), clinical experience and professional reasoning (see Chapter 30), knowledge of disease and disability (see Appendix I, Common Conditions, Resources, and Evidence), setting (see Chapter 59), length of stay, and reimbursement (see Chapter 71) . The following paragraphs will describe the specific approaches, give examples of evidence that support the approaches, and provide further examples in Table 26.3.

Preparatory Interventions

Preparatory interventions have been defined as "methods and techniques that prepare the client for occupational performance" (AOTA, 2008, p. 653). Indeed, a recent systematic review (Amini, 2011) of OT for individuals with work-related injuries and illnesses as summarized by Arbesman, Lieberman, and Thomas (2011) documented

> the effectiveness of several preparatory activities such as exercise, the use of the thermal modality of heat, and early mobilization after fractures and acute trauma. Other preparatory methods have been found to be effective for specific clinical conditions, including splinting for osteoarthritis and carpal tunnel syndrome; scar massage to prevent hypertrophic scarring and promote extensibility; the use of sensory focusing, a cognitive pain control technique during burn dressing changes; and the use of pressure garment work gloves after burns. (p. 14)

These interventions are only used in preparation for or concurrently with occupation-based interventions (see Box 26.3).

Remediation or Restoration of Client Factors, Performance Skills, and/or Performance Patterns to Improve Occupational Performance

The **remediation** or restoration approach is used to enhance client factors (body functions and body structures) such as range of motion, strength, endurance,

TABLE 26.3 Examples of Specific Intervention Approaches

Intervention Approach	Examples
Remediation or restoration of personal factors, performance skills, and/or performance patterns to improve occupational performance	– Therapeutic exercise to strengthen a muscle. – Use of a video game to improve sustained attention. – Goal-oriented reaching to improve upper limb function. – Constraint-induced movement therapy to improve upper limb control. – Mall walking program to improve endurance. – Using homemaking tasks to challenge cognitive functions such as safety and judgment. – Sensory integration techniques.
Occupational skill acquisition	– Teaching meal preparation skills. – Task-specific practice of handwriting. – Mental practice of IADL. – Teaching adaptive coping skills. – Using motor learning principles such as random practice schedules to learn or relearn self-care skills. – Teaching a recently widowed woman how to manage monthly bills (which her husband had previously taken care of). – Developing crawling ability in a nonambulatory child with developmental delays.
Adaptation/compensation approach to improve occupational performance	– Using a wrist extension orthosis to allow keyboarding. – Using a checklist system to perform assigned tasks in a supported employment program. – Using a tub seat, handheld shower, and long-handled sponge to enable bathing. – Using lightweight cookware during meal preparation. – Using built-up handles on school supplies. – Using a power scooter during grocery shopping. – Using an augmentative communication device to interact with other students.
Environmental modifications to improve occupational performance	– Performing a home visit and suggesting removing throw rugs, sliding shower doors, and unnecessary furniture to promote wheelchair access. – Recommending appropriate playground equipment for children with varying skills. – Recommending minimizing environmental stimuli (e.g., television on in the background, many people talking at once) for those who are easily distracted. – Providing specific information re: the gradient for a wheelchair ramp. – Removing trip hazards in a home or work setting to decrease fall risks. – Setting up a bathroom so that needed grooming and hygiene items are placed on the right for those who do not attend to the left. – Assisting a family in developing a caretaker schedule for a loved one with a disability. – Assisting parents in understanding the type and timing of verbal cues required for their child to focus on homework. – Demonstrating how the ground floor of a two-story dwelling can be set up so that a nonambulatory person can live independently on one floor. – Providing sensory input such as music to improve alertness during a therapy session.
Educational approach to improve occupational performance	– Instructing caretakers on proper transfer techniques. – Informing a person as to the signs and symptoms of emerging depression. – Leading a stroke education group focused on community resources and leisure opportunities. – Providing information about alternative community access after a driver's license is lost due to visual impairment. – Instructing a client or caregiver on skin inspection techniques and the signs of skin breakdown.
Prevention approach to maintain occupational performance	– Instructing a stock person in a retail store on proper lifting techniques. – Instructing nursing staff on an appropriate in-bed turning schedule to prevent the development of decubitus ulcers. – Educating a person who types most of the day on proper posture, rest breaks, etc. to prevent carpal tunnel syndrome. – Preventing social isolation by suggesting appropriate leisure-based after-work activities such as a bowling league, participation in a chorus, etc.
Palliative approaches	– Prescribing positioning equipment that allows more time out of bed. – Engaging in reminiscence activities. – Engage in activities related to leaving a legacy such as finally writing down and sharing a secret recipe, engagement in creative arts, scrapbooking, etc. – Physical agent modalities, positioning, edema management, and fabricating an orthosis to reduce pain. – Teaching caregivers handling techniques for bed mobility assist as the client's physical status declines.
Therapeutic use of self	– Developing rapport. – Appropriate use of humor. – Maintaining open communication. – Being empathetic. – Establishing trust. – Being motivational. – Maintaining a caring attitude. – Active listening.

IADL, instrumental activities of daily living.

BOX 26.3 Examples of Preparatory Methods and Interventions Used in Conjunction with or Preparation for Engagement in Occupation

- Applying a therapeutic hot pack to and stretching both shoulders prior to a remediation session that uses reaching into kitchen cabinets as a means to improve shoulder range of motion.
- Teaching a person with an anxiety disorder to use deep breathing and guided imagery to promote relaxation prior to interviewing for a new job.
- Teaching a morning flexibility program to be completed after a warm morning shower to prepare for a variety of morning activities such as making breakfast.
- Having a hospitalized child who survived a burn interact with a therapy dog to decrease anxiety prior to a potentially painful therapy session.
- Suggesting morning yoga as a method of promoting mental focus prior to facing the day.
- Using biofeedback to manage increased muscle tone and maximize the use of an involved limb after traumatic brain injury.
- Massaging edema out of a swollen hand to improve finger range of motion with the goal of enabling coin manipulation.

thoughts, feelings, cognitive processing, etc. with the goal of improving occupational performance. The approach is also used to enhance performance skills and patterns in order to support occupational performance. It is imperative that clinicians link potential changes in underlying abilities to changes in occupational performance. For example, an objective improvement in strength on a manual muscle test or improved cognitive testing without a resultant change in performance may reveal that this is the incorrect intervention approach for a client or that underlying impairment being treated was incorrectly chosen. Although some impairments are not amenable to remediation (e.g., severe memory loss, denervated muscles, endurance impairments that emerge during the end stages of disease), others are amenable but require substantial time, motivation, and commitment to achieve a positive outcome. These factors must be considered carefully when choosing this approach. See Figure 26.1 for an example of using pet therapy as part of an intervention designed to remediate coordination problems.

Therapists working with stroke survivors frequently (although not exclusively) use a variety of methods to remediate motor control and cognitive-perceptual processing to enhance occupational performance (see Chapters 54 and 55). A systematic review examined the effects of OT for persons with stroke, specifically examining remediation of impairments (Ma & Trombly, 2002). The authors found that homemaking tasks resulted in greater improvement of cognitive ability than paper-and-pencil drills and that tasks that forced awareness of neglected space, including movement of the opposite limb into that space, improved unilateral neglect. In terms of improving motor capacities after stroke, they found that coordinated movement improved under these conditions: (1) following written and illustrated guides for movement exercises, (2) using meaningful goal objects as targets, (3) practicing movements with specific goals, (4) moving both arms simultaneously but independently, and (5) imagining functional use of the affected limb.

A remediation approach called sensory integration may also be adopted when working with children who have varying abilities related to processing incoming sensory information (see Chapter 56). A recent systematic review of the evidence examined the effectiveness of interventions using a sensory integrative approach for children. The authors examined 27 studies on the effectiveness of sensory integration intervention on the ability of children with difficulty processing and integrating sensory information to engage in desired occupations. The authors concluded that this remediation approach may result in positive outcomes in sensorimotor skills

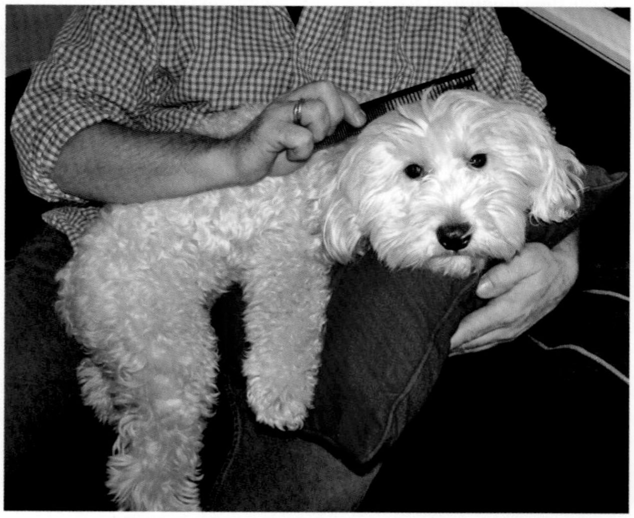

FIGURE 26.1 Occupation as means. Pet therapy can be used to increase range of motion, develop motor planning skills, improve coordination, or lessen anxiety. If the client was a pet owner with the goal of resuming care for his pet, this intervention may be considered occupation as ends.

and motor planning; socialization, attention, and behavioral regulation; reading-related skills; participation in active play; and achievement of individualized goals (May-Benson & Koomar, 2010).

Occupational Skill Acquisition (Development and Restoration of Occupational Performance)

Interventions that focus specifically on skill development (**occupational skill acquisition**) are frequently used in OT. "Skills for the job of living" is a phrase frequently associated with OT. Skills may include those that were previously developed and are now limited or lost. This situation may occur, for example, with an adolescent or adult who sustains a trauma. It is also an appropriate approach to develop skills for those with developmental delays such as a young adult with intellectual delay or a child with developmental coordination disorder. Lastly, it is appropriate for those who are required to learn new skills based on a change in their role. An example is that of a recent widow who depended on her husband for transportation because she had never learned to drive and is now required to learn to drive or use public transportation (see Figure 26.2).

Social skills training is an example of this intervention, and evidence supports the use of this intervention for particular populations (see Chapter 58). A recent study compared the daily living skills of children with and without attention deficit/hyperactivity disorder (ADHD) and the influence of a social skills training group on these skills. Children in the group with ADHD were randomly selected to attend group treatment that focused on social skills training through meaningful occupations such as art, games, and cooking. The children were evaluated at the beginning of group treatment and after 10 sessions using the Assessment of Motor and Process Skills (AMPS). Ten children without ADHD were evaluated at similar intervals. Children with ADHD initially achieved significantly lower scores on the AMPS in all process skills and in the coordination motor subtest than children without ADHD. Children with ADHD significantly improved from the first to the second evaluation and no longer differed from the children without ADHD after treatment. The authors concluded that the results emphasize the need for a focus on occupation in assessment and treatment of children with ADHD (Goll & Jarus, 2005).

Community reintegration training also serves as an example of this intervention. A recent experiment was carried out to examine the effect of an OT intervention focused on improving community skills after a lower extremity major joint replacement. One hundred and seven subjects, status-post total hip or total knee replacement, were examined pre- and post-community reintegration intervention involving practice of community skills in a natural environment. Skills included safely transferring out of the vehicle, managing outdoor obstacles such as uneven surfaces, ambulating throughout the destination, and appropriately transferring back into the car. Participants reported significantly higher scores postintervention on measures of satisfaction, performance, and confidence related to community living skills. Self-reported scores were significantly higher for individual community skills as well as the overall score (Gillen et al., 2007).

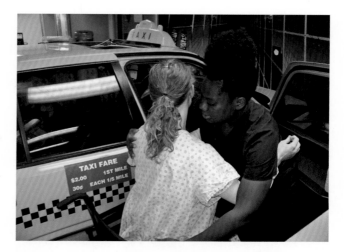

FIGURE 26.2 Occupation as ends. The therapist is using physical assist during a session focused on functional retraining of mobility using an adaptive transfer technique.

Adaptation/Compensation Approach to Improve Occupational Performance

The **adaptation** or compensation approach is used in a variety of situations. These include when a disability is considered permanent (e.g., after the amputation of a limb), underlying client factors or performance skills are not expected to improve (e.g., prolonged and severe short-term memory loss or severe and persistent lower limb weakness after an SCI), limited access to therapy prevents engagement in a remediation program, and/or clients and their families prefer this approach. This intervention is frequently combined with environmental modifications, which will be described next. Many times, this approach is also used in conjunction with a remediation approach. A person who is recovering from the resection of a brain tumor may use adaptive activities of daily living (ADL) methods while they are undergoing motor control remediation interventions. Specific areas of occupation are the focus of this approach, with an emphasis on modifying the demands of the task and using adaptive equipment/assistive devices (see Figure 26.3).

Mann, Ottenbacher, Fraas, Tomita, and Granger (1999) examined a total of 104 home-based frail elderly

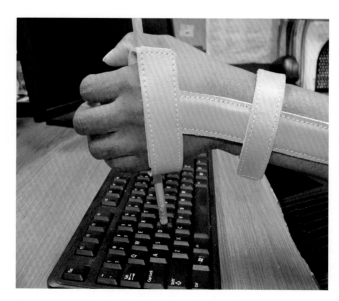

FIGURE 26.3 Adaptive device used to promote independence in typing, writing, feeding, etc. for those with wrist and hand weakness.

persons living in western New York that were assigned to 1 of 2 groups (52 treatment, 52 control). All participants underwent a comprehensive functional assessment as well as an evaluation of their home environment. Participants in the treatment group received assistive technology and home environmental interventions (see later). Examples of assistive devices used in this study include devices to compensate for motor impairment such as devices to support participation in bathing, meal preparation, dressing, leisure, and telephone use; devices to compensate for fine motor impairment such as adapted scissors, door handles, bag handles, car door openers, and faucet extenders; devices to compensate for low vision such as magnifying glasses, lamps, low-vision watches; and electronic devices with larger buttons or dials were also prescribed in this study. The results of the study indicated that the rate of functional decline can be slowed, and institutional and certain in-home personnel costs can be reduced through a systematic approach to providing assistive technology and home environmental interventions.

This approach can also be useful within the cognitive rehabilitation domain. Another example of evidence to support the use of this approach is a study that examined the effect of cognitive adaptation training (CAT) on a sample of people living with schizophrenia who had been in the community at least 3 months. CAT is a series of adaptive supports and environmental modifications (see later) designed to compensate for deficits in cognitive functioning. Examples of supports include signs, alarms, labels, and organization of belongings to cue and sequence adaptive behavior in the client's home and work environments. Forty-five participants were randomly assigned to one of three conditions: (1) CAT, (2) a condition that controlled for therapist time and provided environmental changes unrelated to cognitive deficits or, (3) follow-up only. Results of repeated measures indicated that those participating in CAT had better adaptive function and quality of life and fewer positive symptoms than those in the two non-CAT conditions. The authors concluded that compensatory strategies may improve various outcomes in those living with schizophrenia (Velligan et al., 2002).

Environmental Modifications to Improve Occupational Performance

Modifying the environment (**environmental modification**) is also considered an adaptive approach as described earlier. It includes modifying both the physical environment that includes the natural (geographic terrain, sensory qualities of the environment, plants and animals) and built nonhuman environment (buildings, furniture, etc.) as well as the social environment (relationships and expectations of persons, organizations, populations) (AOTA, 2008). Physical environment modifications may include incorporating aspects of barrier free and universal design into intervention plans. An example of social environment modifications would be teaching caregivers the most efficient cuing method to assure that the person living with dementia can continue to participate in family meals.

The Mann et al. (1999) study cited earlier also included home environmental interventions. These interventions consisted of kitchen modifications, bathroom repair, modifying lighting, adding ceiling fans and air conditioners, redirecting wires, adding a ramp, widening or replacing doors, modifying the kitchen, adding hand rails, etc.

A variety of sources of evidence for the efficacy of environment-based interventions on the affect, behavior, and performance of people with Alzheimer's disease and related dementias exists. Environmental modifications such as ambient music or aromatherapy may be used to reduce agitation and visually complex environments that give the illusion of barriers deter people from wandering to unsafe places. There is also preliminary evidence that bright light therapy can aid in regulating mood and the sleep–wake cycle and thus help people remain awake during the day (Padilla, 2011).

Another study examined the short-term effects of a home environmental intervention on self-efficacy and upset in caregivers and daily function of dementia patients. One hundred and seventy-one families were examined and were randomized to intervention or usual care control group. The intervention involved five 90-minute home visits by occupational therapists who provided education and physical and social environmental modifications. The intervention involved the following:

- Educating caregivers about the impact of the environment on dementia-related behaviors.

- Helping caregivers simplify objects in the home (e.g., remove clutter), break down tasks (e.g., one- or two-step commands, lay out clothing in the order in which it is to be donned).
- Involving other members of the family network or formal supports in daily caregiving tasks.

The authors demonstrated that, as compared with controls, intervention caregivers reported fewer declines in patients' instrumental activities of daily living (IADL), less decline in self-care, and fewer behavior problems in patients. The intervention spouses reported reduced upset, women reported enhanced self-efficacy in managing behaviors, and women and minorities reported enhanced self-efficacy in managing functional dependency. The authors concluded that the environmental program appeared to have a modest effect on those with dementia IADL dependence as well as improve self-efficacy and reduce upset in specific areas of caregiving (Gitlin, Corcoran, Winter, Boyce, & Hauck, 2001).

Educational Approach to Improve Occupational Performance

OT practitioners frequently take on the role of teacher and use an education-based approach when working with clients. Education approaches may be used in both individual and group settings. This approach may be aimed directly at the clients, their caregivers, significant others, employers, etc.

Teaching joint protection techniques would serve as an example of this approach. Researchers have assessed the effects on pain, disability, and health status of an educational joint protection program in a group of people with moderate-to-severe rheumatoid arthritis (RA). Eighty-five subjects were enrolled into the study and randomized into either an experimental group or a control group. The intervention consisted of four educational meetings. These included information on pathophysiology and evolution of RA, joint protection during ADL, suggestions on how to adapt the surrounding environment, and self-learning exercises to perform at home. The study showed that 8 months after attending an educational joint protection program, subjects with moderate-to-severe RA presented with less pain and disability and thus an enhanced health status (Masiero et al., 2007).

Teaching those with fatigue issues how to manage and conserve their energy throughout the day would also fall under this category of intervention. A randomized controlled trial of an energy conservation program examining 169 persons with multiple sclerosis was conducted and published. This education program addressed the importance of rest throughout the day, positive and effective communication, proper body mechanics, ergonomic principles, modification of the environment, priority setting, activity analysis and modification, and living a balanced lifestyle. The format of this education program consisted of lectures, discussions, long- and short-term goal setting, activity stations, and homework activities to teach participants to integrate the energy conservation principles into their performance of everyday tasks. Participants were randomly assigned to an immediate intervention group or a delayed control group using a crossover design. The outcome measures (Fatigue Impact Scale and SF-36 Health Survey, a quality of life measure) were administered four times before and after courses. Results showed that the beneficial effects were maintained 1-year post course compared with immediate post course. The authors concluded that the results provided strong evidence that the beneficial effects of the energy conservation course taught by occupational therapists were maintained up to 1-year post course (Mathiowetz, Matuska, Finlayson, Luo, & Chen, 2007).

Prevention Approach to Maintain Occupational Performance

The **prevention** intervention approach can be used for those living with or without a disability but who are at risk for developing limitations in occupational performance (AOTA, 2008). It can also be used to prevent secondary impairments that may limit occupational performance such as pain, contracture, skin breakdown, depression, etc.

An ongoing clinical trial (the Lifestyle Redesign® for pressure ulcer prevention in SCI) falls under this approach. The specific aim of this program is to test a lifestyle intervention that promises to significantly reduce pressure ulcers in the population of adults with SCI. The intervention was developed based on the results of a qualitative investigation of lifestyle and ulcer risk among adults with SCI (Clark et al., 2006). The aims of the ongoing 5-year trial include (1) assess the Lifestyle Redesign® intervention's ability to reduce medically serious (stage 3 or 4) pressure ulcers and associated surgeries in adults with SCI, (2) assess the cost-effectiveness and potential cost savings of the intervention, (3) examine the intervention's effects on participants' quality of life, and (4) model the intervening process mechanisms that mediate the effects of the intervention. The investigators have identified the long-term objective of this project as to identify an intervention option that can enhance the health and life quality of the population of adults with SCI while simultaneously diminishing the heavy health care burden that results from the problem of SCI-related pressure ulcers (USC/Rancho Lifestyle Redesign® Pressure Ulcer Prevention Project, 2006).

Cumming et al. (1999) examined 530 participants to determine if a home visit by an occupational therapist prevented falls. The intervention was a home visit by an experienced occupational therapist who assessed the home for environmental hazards and facilitated any necessary home modifications. The primary study outcome was falls, ascertained over a 12-month follow-up period using a monthly falls calendar. The authors concluded that home visits by occupational therapists can prevent falls among older people who are at increased risk of falling. They also noted that the effect may not be caused by home modifications alone, because home visits by occupational therapists may also lead to changes in behavior that enable older people to live more safely in both the home and the external environment.

Palliative Approaches

The **palliative** approach focuses on providing clients with relief from the symptoms, pain, and stress of a serious illness regardless of the diagnosis. The goal is to improve quality of life for both the client and their family. Unlike hospice care (end-of-life care), it can be carried out throughout the disease course and not just during the last months of life. Curative care interventions also may be considered under the umbrellas of the palliative approach; however, curative services are not provided when a client is receiving hospice care (AOTA, 2011b).

AOTA (2011b) defines the role of OT in this context as

> occupational therapy practitioners help clients find relief from pain and suffering and improve their quality of life by supporting their engagement in daily life occupations that clients find meaningful and purposeful. The occupational therapy practitioner considers environmental and contextual factors (e.g., caregiver training, accessibility of objects or places in the environment, social contacts available to prevent isolation), as well as personal factors (e.g., decreased endurance, increased anxiety) that may be limiting a client's abilities and satisfaction when performing desired occupations. The occupational therapy practitioner collaborates with the client and family members throughout the occupational therapy process to identify occupations that are especially meaningful and to incorporate strategies that support occupational engagement. (p. 2)

Home-based OT is a typical context in which palliative care is delivered. A recent study examined OT for patients in the palliative stage of cancer care from the perspective of the patients and carers. This study defined the palliative stage of cancer care as the point from which the patient is no longer responsive to curative treatment until death. The study examined 30 clients and their primary informal carers via a structured interview. The results suggested that both patients and their carers valued the service provided and report high levels of satisfaction, although there were gaps identified in service provision. The authors concluded that there is a need to build on the good work being done by home-based occupational therapists in the area of palliative cancer care and increase education and resources to ensure that a client-centered, holistic approach to care is used, addressing both the needs of the patient and their carers (Kealey & Mcintyre, 2005).

Therapeutic Use of Self

Therapeutic use of self, a component of the therapeutic relationship, should not be considered a separate intervention but should instead influence and inform all of the aforementioned intervention approaches. Although there is no consensus on a definition, therapeutic use of self has been defined as the "planned use of his or her personality, insights, perceptions, and judgments as part of the therapeutic process" (Punwar & Peloquin, 2000, p. 285). This term is also used to refer to therapists' conscious efforts to optimize their interactions with clients (Punwar & Peloquin, 2000).

Although this area of clinical practice can benefit from further research emphasis and attention in education programs (Taylor, Lee, Kielhofner, & Ketkar 2009), it is a foundation of practice. A survey of 129 occupational therapists practicing in various areas found that therapists strongly emphasized empathy, rapport, and open communication as being important in the therapeutic relationship. Participants also perceived the therapeutic relationship as critical to therapy outcomes (Cole & McLean, 2003).

Eklund and Hallberg (2001) reported the results from a survey investigating psychiatric occupational therapists' (n = 292) use of verbal interaction on a regular basis with their clients. Among predefined areas, verbal interaction, routine occupations, self-image, and ego-strengthening interventions were among the most frequently given alternatives. The content analysis indicated that the occupational therapists used verbal interaction to

- Enhance the therapeutic relationship. This was expressed as efforts to make contact, to stimulate motivation in the patient, or to enhance mutuality and make the patient participate actively.
- Give the patients opportunities to reflect on and articulate feelings and experiences (e.g., formulate feelings and opinions; make their own thoughts, feelings, and actions clear; have the patient reflect on his or her behavior in the OT sessions).
- Make assessments (i.e., to assess capacities, resources, functions, liabilities, problems, and motivation).
- Make treatment plans to arrive at an appropriate treatment plan together with the patient and set goals.
- Provide interventions in order to reach certain goals. The intention of acting to remedy problems and give support in order to reach certain goals.
- Evaluate and follow up their practice.

See Table 26.2 for specific examples of interventions.

Case Vignettes

One may note that the aforementioned approaches are not mutually exclusive. As described earlier, you may use an *education*-based approach to *prevent* joint destruction and further decline in occupational performance for those living with arthritis. A therapist involved in *palliative* care with a client with a non-operable brain tumor may use *adaptive* seating in a wheelchair to decrease back pain. In many cases, therapists use a variety of approaches with the same client, whereas in other cases may focus on one approach. The following case vignettes will highlight this point. Cases will include an **occupational profile**, relevant assessment findings, goals, and intervention choices.

CASE STUDY 26.2 James: A Married Banker Who Survived a Stroke

Occupational Profile

James is 62-year-old banker. He lives in a two-story house in a suburban town with his wife Carla and Max, the family dog. James was in his usual state of health (hypertension and type 2 diabetes mellitus) when he woke up on the floor, unable to move his left limbs, drooling, and slurring his words when yelling for help. He was admitted to the neurology unit of the local hospital. After a 3-day stay, he was transferred to the inpatient rehabilitation unit. Upon initial meeting with his occupational therapist, Dan, the therapist learned that James has been looking forward to retiring soon to "spend time with my wife, fish in the lake, read classic novels, and get to know my children and grandchildren again." He reports that he is a workaholic and regrets "missing out" on key family functions. He states that he is "fiercely independent and mortified about the help he needs with basic hygiene." He also reports that he is "very left handed" and frustrated by the lack of motor output in his left limbs.

Assessment Findings

Dan first administered the Canadian Occupational Performance Measure (COPM), a self-report measure of occupational performance. James identified toileting, using his tablet computer to access work and personal e-mail, performing grooming using both hands, reading work documents, and holding his new grandchild as initial areas of focus. He rated his performance of these tasks as between 2 and 4 on a 1 to 10 scale. He rated his satisfaction with his performance as 2/10 for all five of the identified tasks. The Functional Independence Measure (FIM™) was used to objectively document his self-care and mobility skills. James required moderate assist for all aspects of self-care except that he was able to feed himself with minimal assist. James also required moderate assist for ambulation and all transfers. Based on behaviors noted during the FIM administration, Dan was concerned about the presence of left neglect. Left neglect is a neurologic phenomenon in which a client will overfocus on the right side of the environment and pay less attention to (i.e., neglect) the left side. Some behaviors that were noted included spending the majority of time brushing the right side of the mouth, leaving the left arm behind when rolling in bed, and multiple left-sided collisions when propelling his wheelchair. To document the impact of left neglect on daily function, the therapist administered the Catherine Bergego Scale (CBS). This scale is based on observation of ADL, mobility, and social interaction to objectify the quantity and quality of left-sided errors. James scored 17/30, with low scores indicating less impairment. Based on some statements James was making in therapy (e.g., "Why can't I read? It is my arm and leg that are weak. There is nothing wrong with my eyes!"), Dan decided to ask James to score himself on the client report version of the CBS. James scored himself as 5/30, indicating that James was overestimating his level of function and underestimating his level of impairment (i.e., the impact of the left neglect). Finally, James was quite concerned about using his limbs again. A manual muscle test revealed that his left limbs fell into the 1/5 to 2/5 range, with 5 indicating normal strength. Sensation was preserved.

Goals

Based on the occupational profile, the COPM results, and the analysis of occupational performance, James's initial short goals were set as (1) James will perform toilet transfers with minimal assistance, (2) James will perform grooming using both hands with minimal assist, and (3) James will read the daily weather report accurately with tactile and verbal cues four out of five times.

Interventions

Dan developed an intervention plan that combined *acquisition*, *adaptive*, *remediation*, and *environmental modification* approaches. As James stated multiple times that he was concerned and "embarrassed" about being helped with hygiene, Dan worked with James twice per day and the morning session was focused on these tasks. Because of James's significant weakness, Dan first *modified the environment* by providing a raised toilet seat. Dan also checked that the already placed grab bars were secure. James was encouraged to use his left arm as a stabilizer on the grab bar (*remediation* of motor control). Dan also had to *adapt* the method in which James would perform the task. It was decided that James would use a stand-pivot technique to move from his wheelchair to the toilet. Once the method was decided, Dan worked with James to learn and *acquire* the skill. Dan used a variety of motor learning principles (see Chapter 54) to assist James in acquiring this skill. These included blocked practice at first followed by random practice, providing James with feedback about his performance, demonstrating the task for James, and decreasing the number of verbal and physical cues as James's performance improved. Several of the cues that were provided were related to using his left limbs (*remediation*) as able ("Push up with your left arm"; "Straighten your left knee"). This session demonstrates the use of a combined *occupation as ends/means* approach. That is, the focus is toileting the "goal to be learned," and toileting is being used as a therapeutic change agent to remediate left-sided motor control and left-sided awareness.

CASE STUDY 26.2 James: A Married Banker Who Survived a Stroke *(Continued)*

In the grooming domain, both James's motor status and his left neglect limited his occupational performance. Dan first *modified the environment* by placing a colored piece of tape on the far left side of the sink and the left edge of the mirror. This "perceptual anchor" was used as an environmental cue to scan to the left (Gillen, 2009). Dan attempted to *remediate* his haphazard scanning ability. Prior to starting the task, Dan worked with James to find all of the objects required for the task by systematically scanning the workspace. He was taught to scan to the left until he saw the blue tape, scan back right, and so on. Although James is left handed, the therapist began to *remediate* James's left limb by showing him how to use his left hand as a nondominant assist. He was able to stabilize the toothpaste with the left hand and use his right hand to guide his left to control the faucets. Similar to the earlier discussion, a variety of cues and methods of feedback were used to help James *acquire* the skill of oral care. Again, using a combined *occupation as ends/means* approach, oral care is the goal to be learned, whereas grooming is also being used to improve scanning, left-sided attention, and left-sided motor control (see Figure 26.4).

In terms of reading, Dan was concerned that James was not aware of the reason that he could not read (i.e., his left neglect). Because reading was a critical aspect of both his work and planned leisure pursuits, Dan decided that starting with reading training proper would probably result in failure based on the assessment findings. Dan was concerned that failure may result in the possible development of anxiety/depression. Instead, Dan decided to use an *occupation as means* approach to begin with using activities on James's tablet computer as the therapeutic change agent. Dan first used the *adaptive* settings to enlarge the screen, and James was encouraged to hold the tablet vertically. It came up in casual conversation that James enjoyed playing solitaire. Dan decided to use this game as the method to begin to teach James, further scanning strategies (*remediation*) and begin introducing reading preparation (pre-skill *acquisition*). After the solitaire application loaded the cards, Dan asked James to read the initial seven cards dealt. James initially only read the five cards biased toward the right. When this pointed out, James became

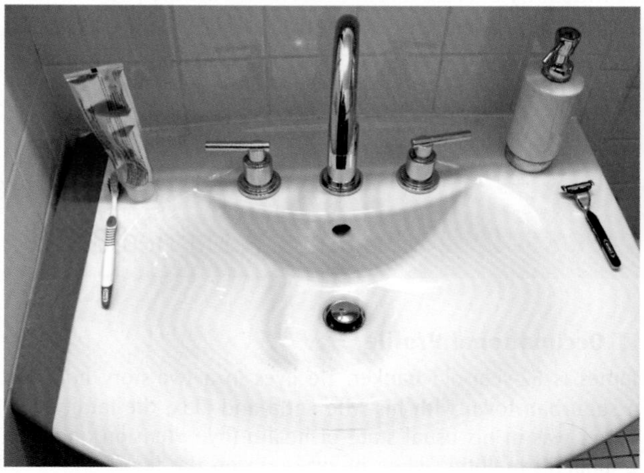

FIGURE 26.4 Environmental modification. A colored strip of tape on the sink used as a perceptual anchor to improve awareness to the left side of the environment.

concerned. Dan began to use this discussion as a way to *remediate* awareness regarding his neglect. It was pointed out that when he missed cards, they were always on the left. Dan made connections to the mistakes made during this game to other behaviors such as having difficulty finding objects on the left side of the sink, etc. Dan asked James to hold the tablet in both hands (*remediation* of motor function) and to use his left hand as the perceptual anchor (*adaptation*) to know when he has scanned far enough to the left. Dan then continued to use more complex games (e.g., word search) that required left to right scanning and reading skills. Dan continued these interventions until James became more proficient in using these skills and strategies. Dan then found Websites that had one to two line descriptors of the daily weather. Using the enlarged print command (*adaptation*) and the newly *acquired* scanning skills, James met his short-term goal.

CASE STUDY 26.3 Sahar: An 8-Year-Old Girl Living with Cerebral Palsy

Occupational Profile

Sahar is an 8-year-old girl who attends a mainstream school. Sahar receives occupational, physical, and speech therapy in school to manage her spastic cerebral palsy. She has an attendant with her at all times. Sahar enjoys art, pop music, playing with her dog, and, until recently, school. Until the recent past, she particularly enjoyed spelling and English classes. She recently started to make comments to her parents that she "does not fit in," is "tired of being teased," "does not want to feel different," and that she "is a bad friend." Her parents are concerned about her self-esteem and her new disinterest in school. They are getting reports from her teacher that she is "falling behind" and seems "disinterested."

Assessment Findings

Sahar recently started working with a new occupational therapist. His assessment findings included the following:

- Environmental: Sahar's power wheelchair was ill fitting. Her seating system was not providing enough support and

CASE STUDY 26.3 Sahar: An 8-Year-Old Girl Living with Cerebral Palsy *(Continued)*

she tended to lean to the left and sit with a flexed spine and neck. This position limited her eye contact, which resulted in difficulty seeing the teacher and information written on the blackboard. In addition, she has recently started to drool occasionally because of her neck position. The wheelchair was too high to pull up to the desks and tables in the classroom so she was always positioned behind the class with her aide, which also added to her difficulty interacting with peers and seeing her teacher. Finally, due to her poor seated position, she was having trouble controlling the wheelchair, and her aide was now assisting her in navigating the school.

- Children's Assessment of Participation and Enjoyment (CAPE): The CAPE was used to measure Sahar's participation in activities outside of school. Sahar presented with overall low participation in activities. Specifically, she reported low participation in recreational, physical, and social activities. Many activities were engaged in alone and many were confined to her bedroom.
- School Function Assessment (SFA): Sahar scored 2 (participation in a few activities) for most items on the participation scale; 1 or 2 (moderate-to-extensive assistance and adaptions) for most items on the task supports scale; and 1 or 2 (does not perform or partial performance) for most items on the activity performance scale.
- Evaluation of Social Interaction (ESI): Sahar's score on the ESI was indicative of problematic social interactions severe enough to limit interactions with others (moderately to markedly ineffective and/or immature social interaction skills). Particular items that were difficult for Sahar included not approaching/starting interactions, physical difficulties not supporting interaction (looks, turns toward), not replying, and at times not taking turns.
- Vision: Sahar has worn glasses since she was 3. The therapist found that Sahar's acuity was decreased (20/60) for far vision using a Snellen chart.

Goals

(1) Sahar will navigate her school in a power wheelchair with distant supervision. (2) Sahar will answer two questions per day during teaching lessons. (3) Sahar will improve her overall academic performance as indicated by her quarterly report card. (4) Sahar will initiate two conversations per day with peers during recess or other group activities.

Interventions

Sahar's new therapist took the lead in terms of managing this change in Sahar's function. He focused on maximizing her social and academic participation in school, making Sahar feel more comfortable about fitting in with peers, and improving her self-esteem. He used a variety of approaches including *environmental modifications* and *adaptive* and *acquisition* approaches. In addition, he referred Sahar to an eye care specialist to change the prescription in her glasses. Sahar's occupational therapist first collaborated with a wheelchair vendor to update the chair that she has outgrown and update her seating system. An *adapted* wheelchair frame that has the ability to tilt in space was ordered. A tilt system changed Sahar's orientation in space while maintaining fixed hip, knee, and ankle angles. This tilt helped to promote proper alignment including an extended spine. A head rest was provided to maintain Sahar's head in extension, expand her field of vision, and decrease the tendency to drool. Lateral supports were added to the system to further help maintain Sahar's posture. A removable lap tray was provided so that Sahar could use it as a work/play space when not at a table or desk. The occupational therapist ordered an *adapted* joystick with a "t-bar" to compensate for Sahar's poor hand function and promote independent mobility. The occupational therapist spent time with Sahar teaching her to *acquire* the skill of controlling the wheelchair both indoors and outdoors. Time was spent learning how to navigate doorways, ramps, and curb cuts. Particular attention was spent teaching Sahar how to safely navigate the playground and recess areas.

The occupational therapist collaborated with Sahar's teacher to *modify the environment*. Desks/tables were rearranged to assure that Sahar's chair could easily navigate the classroom. The therapist placed table risers on one table so that Sahar's wheelchair could fit underneath it. With these modifications, Sahar was able to navigate the classroom and sit with other students. This also served to facilitate her interactions with peers and her teacher during lesson plans.

Although these changes resulted in Sahar making statements that reflect improved esteem, the occupational therapist and Sahar's parents were concerned about her feeling socially isolated. The therapist then shifted back to an *acquisition* approach focused on social skills training. The therapist tapped into Sahar's love of art and collaborated with Sahar's teacher to integrate an arts and crafts lesson once a week. The focus of the lesson was for the students to make seasonal decorations for a bulletin board. The therapist provided *adaptive* art supplies such as a loop scissor mounted on the table and a paint brush that was built up with foam. As Sahar's physical participation began to improve, the therapist used the arts and crafts sessions to encourage Sahar to initiate conversations, maintain eye contact, and answer appropriately when spoken to. Because Sahar had limited manipulation abilities, as her confidence grew, she took on the primary role of deciding the overall theme and design of the bulletin board while her peers took main responsibility for the implementation of the design. The interventions in total helped Sahar reach her goals.

CASE STUDY 26.4 Lois: An Adult with Schizophrenia Living at Home

Occupational Profile

Lois is a 32-year-old who is currently living with her parents in an apartment in a large city. Lois was diagnosed with schizophrenia in college when she began to develop delusions that her roommate was following her all over campus and that all the teachers "wanted me to fail." Her behavior became more erratic and disorganized, causing her to drop out of school. She was soon admitted to an inpatient unit for medical stabilization of her symptoms. Over the years, Lois has been inconsistent with her medications and has required at least two other hospitalizations. Her parents are concerned about her recent lack of structure secondary to quitting her job. They feel that when she lacks structure, her symptoms begin to worsen. They have noticed that she is not paying attention to personal hygiene and reports that she sits on the couch all day. Lois reports that she is just "busy." Her parents want her to contribute to household chores and make herself "useful."

Assessment Findings

An informal interview was conducted with Lois along with her parents. Lois agreed that it would be helpful if her parents were part of the therapy process. The occupational therapist, Nadia, inquired as to how Lois spent her days. Lois was able to describe her morning care routine and eating meals with her family but described little else in terms of active participation. Her parents corroborated that most of her day is spent watching television. Her parents then again articulated their concerns about Lois not contributing to the household management. Nadia asked Lois if she would be willing to take on household responsibilities. Reluctantly, Lois agreed to contribute to shopping and cooking simple meals such as lunch. Nadia first administered the Assessment of Motor and Process Skills (AMPS). The AMPS is an observational assessment that is used to measure the quality of a person's ADL. The quality of the person's ADL performance is assessed by rating the effort, efficiency, safety, and independence of 16 ADL motor and 20 ADL process skill items while the person is doing chosen, familiar, and life-relevant ADL tasks. Nadia observed three AMPS tasks including making canned soup, making a luncheon meat sandwich, and sweeping the floor. Skill items that were considered ineffective or markedly deficient included paces, chooses, search/locate, inquires, sequences, calibrates, benefits, adjusts, and accommodates. The Test of Grocery Shopping Skills (TOGGS) was also administered. The TOGGS is a performance-based assessment that measures how accurately and efficiently clients can locate items in a grocery store. Scales include accuracy (finding the correct item, correct size, and lowest price), time to locate the items, and redundancy (e.g., returning to the same aisle). Lois scored 17 out of a possible 30 on this measure.

Goals

Based on the interview with Lois and her parents as well as the standardized measures outlined earlier, two goals were set for Lois. (1) Lois will prepare grilled cheese safely and efficiently with distant supervision and verbal cues for sequencing and locating items. (2) Lois will successfully grocery shop for 10 items with 85% accuracy in less than 35 minutes.

Interventions

Acquisition, *adaptive*, *therapeutic use of self*, and *environmental modification* approaches were used to help Lois meet these goals. The intervention for teaching Lois grocery shopping skills was based on an evidence-based protocol (Brown, Rempfer, & Hamera, 2002). This intervention is designed to compensate (*adaptation*) for cognitive impairments by providing strategies that organize/simplify the task (*adaptation*) and environment (*environmental modifications*). During all sessions, Nadia used encouragement, positive feedback, and open communication to keep Lois motivated (*therapeutic use of self*). Based on the protocol, Nadia worked with Lois for nine sessions on *acquiring* this skill. The authors of the protocol integrated strategies from several learning theories to help clients acquire this skill. Examples of strategies that were used include repeated practice, structured feedback, motivational incentives, scripting of the process, situated cognitive approaches, and cuing (Brown et al., 2002). Training the skill was based on a script of three questions with corresponding strategies. These questions helped Lois sequence the task. The three aspects of training included "Where is it?" "Is this what I am looking for?" and "Is this the lowest price?" Examples of strategies for the Where is it? step include use overhead signs, know the store layout or use a map, and ask for help (Brown et al., 2002).

Based on the work of Duncombe (2004), Nadia assisted Lois in learning the skills of cooking using an *acquisition* approach. The first lesson emphasized the aspects of cooking required for a simple stove top task (making pudding). Lois was given a guideline that listed 10 steps necessary for cooking simple foods (*adaptive*). The list included skills such as washing hands prior to cooking, clearing a space to work, gathering equipment and ingredients, safety, etc. Nadia hung these guidelines in Lois's kitchen. During the next two sessions, Nadia had Lois cook meals that were similar in the number of steps but differed in ingredients. The rationale was to help Lois begin to generalize and transfer the skills she was learning. During session 2, Lois made a sandwich, emphasizing 7 of the 10 cooking guidelines. During the next session, the task was upgraded to preparing soup during which all 10 of the guidelines were followed (Duncombe, 2004). The combined intervention approaches allowed Lois to meet her goals.

CASE STUDY 26.5 Shirley: Receiving Home Hospice with End-stage Amyotrophic Lateral Sclerosis

Occupational Profile

Shirley is a 60-year-old woman who was diagnosed with amyotrophic lateral sclerosis (ALS) 1 year ago. The occupational therapist on this case, Yin, first met Shirley when she was diagnosed and monitored her functional status during monthly clinic visits. Shirley is now homebound and receiving end-of-life care via home hospice. Shirley was a homemaker; and her pride and joy are her two children and, more recently, her three grandchildren, all younger than 3 years old. Occupational therapy was ordered for three to four home visits to implement *palliative* and *prevention* interventions and maximize the family's ability to care for her using both *adaptive* and *education* approaches, with an overarching theme of *therapeutic use of self* during this difficult time.

Assessment Findings

Prior to the home visit, Yin reviewed Shirley's medical record. Her last documented ALS Functional Rating Scale-Revised was 15. This tool estimates degree of functional impairment. The scores range from 0 to 48 (best). An informal interview indicated that the family was most concerned about keeping Shirley pain free as she recently started to wince when they were assisting her to move in bed, transfer, and dress. Shirley's husband, Tom, reported that he wanted to be very hands on with her care despite having the hospice team. He reported that his low back has been hurting him ever since Shirley developed a substantial loss of strength in her legs and trunk. Before this latest decline in status, Shirley had been typing letters to her three young grandchildren. Her plan was to give these letters to her children in a sealed envelope to be given to the grandchildren when they turned 16. Tom reported that Shirley was devastated that she would not see them grow up and she wanted to be remembered by them. Shirley was not able to talk despite being grossly cognitively intact. Yin established a yes/no system of responses using eye movements (one blink indicated "yes," two "no," and wide eyes indicated "pain"). Through this blinking system, Shirley was able to indicate that she was highly motivated to finish the letters and that it was painful in her low back, shoulders, and hips when she was being assisted with ADL/mobility. The Caregiver Burden Scale was administered to Tom. Findings suggested that Tom felt quite burdened in all five domains (general strain, isolation, disappointment, emotional involvement, and environment). In addition, Yin observed Tom assisting Shirley in and out of bed and from her bed to her wheelchair. Tom was noted to hold Shirley tightly under her arms during transfers and demonstrated poor body mechanics (twisting his back) during the transfer.

Goals

Based on Shirley and her family's concerns, the following goals were established: (1) Tom will demonstrate proper body mechanics and safe technique when transferring Shirley to her wheelchair with supervision; (2) Shirley will, with supervision, complete writing three letters with assistive devices; and (3) Tom will independently and safely position Shirley in bed.

Interventions

The first intervention was *education based* to *prevent* injury to Tom's back as well as to *prevent* Shirley from becoming injured during transfers and mobility. Yin demonstrated and discussed proper body mechanics and demonstrated proper transfer techniques. As Tom was still having difficulty, Yin further *adapted* the transfer method and showed Tom how to use a sliding board to assist Shirley from her bed to the wheelchair. Tom reported that he felt more secure with this technique. Continuing with an *education* approach, Yin demonstrated proper positioning in bed to keep Shirley's joints in neutral as to *prevent* contractures and pain. While Shirley was in bed, Yin additionally taught Tom to perform gentle passive range of motion following the application of heating pads on Shirley's shoulders and hips to help control pain (*palliative* approach). Yin told Tom that the heat could be used two to three times per day for 20 minutes to help control Shirley's pain.

At the next home-based session, Yin observed that Shirley was in a much better position in her bed. Yin asked to observe Tom transfer Shirley to her wheelchair. He transferred her safely and effectively. Yin borrowed three pieces of equipment from the ALS clinic to allow Shirley to complete her letters using an *adaptive* approach. Yin applied a static wrist orthosis to Shirley's right wrist for stability and applied a universal cuff to her right hand (refer back to Figure 26.3). The cuff is designed to give persons with limited grip or dexterity controlled use of items such as eating utensils and writing tools. A pencil was inserted into the universal cuff with the eraser side facing down. Next, Yin attached an overhead suspension sling to Shirley's wheelchair. Using this device, Shirley's arm was supported by a sling and suspended by an overhead rod. This device is used for people presenting with proximal weakness, with muscle grades in the 1/5 to 3/5 range. The sling acts to unweight Shirley's weak arm to allow her to use her remaining muscle strength to guide her hand to the proper letters on the keyboard. Using these adaptations, Shirley was able to complete her letters, albeit slowly.

Conclusion

OT practitioners have a variety of intervention approaches available to choose from and combine. The correct choices of interventions are based on a variety of data including client choice, knowledge of disease/disability, assessment findings, clinical experience, and professional reasoning. No matter which approach is chosen, occupation is always the end and is the most frequent means with the addition of purposeful and preparatory methods as needed.

Acknowledgments

The author would like to acknowledge the contributions of Anne E. Dickerson, PhD, OTR/L, FAOTA and Elin Schold Davis, OTR/L, CDRS for contributing the driving vignette. He would also like to acknowledge Emily Raphael-Greenfield, EdD, OTR/L and Debra Tupé, PhD OTR for useful feedback.

References

American Occupational Therapy Association. (2008). Occupational therapy practice framework: Domain and process, 2nd edition. *American Journal of Occupational Therapy, 62*, 625–683.

American Occupational Therapy Association. (2011a). The philosophical base of occupational therapy. *American Journal of Occupational Therapy, 65*(Suppl. 6), S65.

American Occupational Therapy Association. (2011b). The role of occupational therapy in end-of-life care. *American Journal of Occupational Therapy, 65*, S66–S75.

Amini, D. (2011). Occupational therapy interventions for work-related injuries and conditions of the forearm, wrist, and hand: A systematic review. *American Journal of Occupational Therapy, 65*, 29–36.

Arbesman, M., Lieberman, D., & Thomas, V. J. (2011). Methodology for the systematic reviews on occupational therapy for individuals with work-related injuries and illnesses. *American Journal of Occupational Therapy, 65*, 10–15.

Bennett, S., & Bennett J. W. (2000). The process of evidence-based practice in occupational therapy: Informing clinical decisions. *Australian Occupational Therapy Journal, 47*, 171–180.

Bennett, S., Hoffmann, T., McCluskey, A., McKenna, K., Strong, J., & Tooth, L. (2003). Evidence-based practice forum. Introducing OTseeker (Occupational Therapy Systematic Evaluation of Evidence): A new evidence database for occupational therapists. *American Journal of Occupational Therapy, 57*, 635–638.

Brown, C., Rempfer, M., & Hamera, E. (2002). Teaching grocery shopping skills to people with schizophrenia. *Occupational Therapy journal of Research, 22*(S), 90S–91S.

Clark, F. A., Jackson, J. M., Scott, M. D., Carlson, M. E., Atkins, M. S., Uhles-Tanaka, D., & Rubayi. S. (2006). Data-based models of how pressure ulcers develop in daily-living contexts of adults with spinal cord injury. *Archives of Physical Medicine and Rehabilitation, 87*, 1516–1525.

Cole, B., & McLean, V. (2003). Therapeutic relationships re-defined. *Occupational Therapy in Mental Health, 19*, 33–56.

Cumming, R. G., Thomas, M., Szonyi, G., Salkeld, G., O'Neill, E., Westbury, C., et al. (1999). Home visits by an occupational therapist for assessment and modification of environmental hazards: A randomized trial of falls prevention. *Journal of the American Geriatrics Society, 47*(12),1397–1402.

Duncombe, L. W. (2004). Comparing learning of cooking in home and clinic for people with schizophrenia. *American Journal of Occupational Therapy, 58*, 272–278.

Eklund, M., & Hallberg, I. R. (2001). Psychiatric occupational therapists' verbal interaction with their clients. *Occupational Therapy International, 8*, 1–16.

Fisher, A. G. (1998). Uniting practice and theory in an occupational therapy framework, 1998 Eleanor Clarke Slagle lecture. *American Journal of Occupational Therapy, 52*, 509–522.

Gillen, G. (2009). *Cognitive and perceptual rehabilitation: Optimizing function*. St. Louis, MO: Elsevier/Mosby.

Gillen, G., Berger, S., Lotia, S., Morreale, J., Siber, M., & Trudo, W. (2007). Improving community skills after lower extremity joint replacement. *Physical and Occupational Therapy in Geriatrics, 25*, 41–54.

Gitlin, L. N., Corcoran, M., Winter, L., Boyce, A., & Hauck, W. W. (2001). A randomized, controlled trial of a home environmental intervention: Effect on efficacy and upset in caregivers and on daily function of persons with dementia. *Gerontologist, 41*, 4–14.

Goll, D., & Jarus, T. (2005). Effect of a social skills training group on everyday activities of children with attention deficit–hyperactivity disorder. *Developmental Medicine & Child Neurology, 47*, 539–545.

Gray, J. M. (1998). Putting occupation into practice: Occupation as ends, occupation as means. *American Journal of Occupational Therapy, 52*, 354–364.

Haynes, R. B., Devereaux, P. J., & Guyatt, G. H. (2002). Clinical expertise in the era of evidence-based medicine and patient choice. *ACP Journal Club, 136*, A11–A14.

Hinojosa, J., & Kramer, P. (1997). Fundamental concepts of occupational therapy: Occupation, purposeful activity, and function [Statement]. *American Journal of Occupational Therapy, 51*, 864–866.

Kealey, P., & Mcintyre, I. (2005). An evaluation of the domiciliary occupational therapy service in palliative cancer care in a community trust: A patient and carers perspective. *European Journal of Cancer Care, 14*, 232–243.

Law, M., Baptiste, S., & Mills, J. (1995). Client-centred practice: What does it mean and does it make a difference? *Canadian Journal of Occupational Therapy, 62*, 250–257.

Ma, H., & Trombly, C. A. (2002). A synthesis of the effects of occupational therapy for persons with stroke, part II: Remediation of impairments. *American Journal of Occupational Therapy, 56*, 260–274.

Mann, W. C., Ottenbacher, K. J., Fraas, L., Tomita, M., & Granger, C. V. (1999). Independence and reducing home care costs for the frail elderly. *Archives of Family Medicine, 8*, 210–217.

Masiero, S., Boniolo, A., Wassermann, L., Machiedo, H., Volante, D., & Punzi, L. (2007). Effects of an educational-behavioral joint protection program on people with moderate to severe rheumatoid arthritis: A randomized controlled triai. *Clinical Rheumatology, 26*, 2043–2050.

Mathiowetz, V. G., Matuska, K. M., Finlayson, M. L., Luo, P., & Chen, H. Y. (2007). One-year follow-up to a randomized controlled trial of an energy conservation course for persons with multiple sclerosis. *International Journal of Rehabilitation Research, 30*, 305–313.

May-Benson, T. A., & Koomar, J. A. (2010). Systematic review of the research evidence examining the effectiveness of interventions using a sensory integrative approach for children. *American Journal of Occupational Therapy, 64*, 403–414.

Owsley, C., & McGwin, G. (1999). Vision impairment and driving. *Survey Ophthalmology, 43*, 535–550.

Owsley, C., Sekuler, R., & Siemsen, D. (1983). Contrast sensitivity throughout adulthood. *Vision Research, 23*, 689–699.

Owsley, C., Stalvey, B. T., Wells, J., & Sloane, M. E. (1999). Older drivers and cataract: Driving habits and crash risk. *The Journals of Gerontology. Series A, Biological Sciences and Medical Sciences, 54*, M203–M211.

Padilla, R. (2011). Effectiveness of environment-based interventions for people with Alzheimer's disease and related dementias. *American Journal of Occupational Therapy, 65*, 514–522.

Punwar, J., & Peloquin, M. (2000). *Occupational therapy: Principles and practice* (pp. 42–98). Philadelphia, PA: Lippincott.

Sackett, D. L., Strauss S. E., Richardson, W. S., Rosenberg, W., & Haynes, R. B. (2000). *Evidenced-based medicine: How to practice and teach*. Edinburgh, United Kingdom: Churchill Livingstone.

Stutts, J., Martell, C., & Staplin, L. (2009). *Identifying behaviors and situations associated with increased crash risk for older drivers* (Report No. DOT HS 811 09). Washington, DC: National Highway Traffic Safety Administration.

Sumsion, T., & Law, M. (2006). A review of evidence on the conceptual elements informing client-centred practice. *Canadian Journal of Occupational Therapy. Revue Canadienne d'Ergotherapie, 73,* 153–162.

Taylor, R. R., Lee, S. W., Kielhofner, G., & Ketkar, M. (2009). Therapeutic use of self: A nationwide survey of practitioners' attitudes and experiences. *American Journal of Occupational Therapy, 63,* 198–207.

Trombly, C. A. (1995). Occupation: Purposefulness and meaningfulness as therapeutic mechanisms. 1995 Eleanor Clarke Slagle Lecture. *American Journal of Occupational Therapy, 49,* 960–972.

USC/Rancho Lifestyle Redesign® Pressure Ulcer Prevention Project. (2006). Retrieved from http://www.usc.edu/programs/pups/

Velligan, D. I., Prihoda, T. J., Ritch, J. L., Maples, N., Bow-Thomas, C. C., & Dassori, A. (2002). A randomized single-blind pilot study of compensatory strategies in schizophrenia outpatients. *Schizophrenia Bulletin, 28,* 283–292.

Weinstock-Zlotnick, G., & Hinojosa, J. (2004). The issue is: Bottom-up or top-down evaluation: Is one better than the other? *American Journal of Occupational Therapy, 58,* 594–598.

For additional resources on the subjects discussed in this chapter, visit http://thePoint.lww.com/Willard-Spackman12e.

CHAPTER 27

Occupational Therapy Interventions for Organizations, Communities, and Populations

Marjorie E. Scaffa

OUTLINE

LEARNING OBJECTIVES

After reading this chapter, you will be able to:

1. Identify client factors and performance patterns that apply to organizations, communities, and populations
2. Discuss the application of client-centered, evidence-based, and occupation-based interventions to organizations, communities, and populations
3. Describe potential outcomes of occupational therapy intervention for organizations, communities, and populations
4. Compare and contrast a variety of specific intervention approaches that are used for organizations, communities, and populations receiving occupational therapy services

Introduction

In many settings where occupational therapy is practiced, the term *client* refers to an individual who is receiving services. However, occupational therapy clients may be families, organizations, worksites, communities, or populations. In the *Occupational Therapy Practice Framework*, clients are categorized as persons, organizations, and populations (American Occupational Therapy Association [AOTA], 2008b). *Persons* include individuals, families, caregivers, teachers, and employers, among others, who may receive occupational therapy services. *Organizations* include businesses, agencies, schools, clubs, and associations. **Communities** can be defined as collectives of "people identified by common values and mutual concern for the development and well-being of their group or geographical area" (Green & Kreuter, 1991, p. 504). **Populations** refer to groups of people within a community who share common characteristics; for example, homeless persons, veterans, refugees, and people with chronic mental and/or physical disabilities (AOTA, 2008b). The terms *communities* and *populations* are sometimes used interchangeably. However, typically, there may be a variety of populations within one community. For example, within my community, there are populations of students, professionals, persons who are homeless, veterans, and immigrants, among others.

Communities and populations, like individuals, may experience various challenges to engagement in occupations, including occupational delays, disparities, interruptions, and/or imbalances and therefore may benefit from occupational therapy intervention (Bass-Haugen, Henderson, Larson, & Matuska, 2005). Bass-Haugen (2009) identified several health disparities among children and adults across racial, ethnic, and socioeconomic groups that are appropriate for occupational therapy intervention. These include disparities in health behavior characteristics, activity profiles, home and work environments, and experiences and outcomes of health care services, which can ultimately impact occupational performance and participation. Organization-based, community-based, and population-based services address the "needs of a group of individuals as a whole rather than the specific needs of an individual" (Moyers, 1999, p. 263).

The previous chapter described occupational therapy interventions for individuals receiving services. This chapter focuses on interventions for organizations, communities, and populations. The occupational therapy intervention process "consists of the skilled actions taken by occupational therapy practitioners in collaboration with the client to facilitate engagement in occupation related to health and participation" (AOTA, 2008b, p. 652). Interventions addressing the needs of organizations, communities, and populations are sometimes referred to as **programs**. Programs are "systematic efforts to achieve preplanned objectives such as changes in knowledge, attitudes, skills, and behaviors to maintain or improve function and/or health" (Brownson, 2001, p. 96).

According to Youngstrom and Brown (2005), occupational therapy interventions, whether designed for individuals, organizations, communities, or populations, are "grounded in basic principles that guide the planning and implementation process" (p. 937). Occupational therapy interventions are client centered, context driven, occupation based, and evidence based (Youngstrom & Brown, 2005) and address "the interaction among client factors, performance skills, performance patterns, contexts and environments, and activity demands that influence occupational performance" (AOTA, 2008b, p. 652). The outcomes of occupational therapy intervention for organizations, communities, and populations may include improved occupational performance, increased occupational participation, enhanced well-being and quality of life, prevention of occupational performance problems, and occupational justice for individuals and for the collective.

Designing and implementing occupational therapy intervention for organizations, communities, and populations require an understanding of the (1) people (lifestyles, health status, risk and resiliency factors, and performance patterns), (2) occupation and activity demands, and (3) environments in which these occupations occur (Watson & Wilson, 2003). The following sections describe client-centered, context-driven, evidence-based, and occupation-based approaches to intervention for organizations, communities, and populations.

Client-Centered Approaches for Organizations, Communities, and Populations

Regardless of whether the client is an individual, group, organization, community, or population, occupational therapy practitioners provide client-centered care. This means ongoing collaboration and incorporation of the aggregate needs, priorities, and choices of the organization, community, or population in the intervention. Client-centered intervention or program development for organizations, communities, and populations is based on two main principles: (1) the principle of relevance and (2) the principle of participation. The principle of relevance refers to starting "where the people are" and addressing the perceived needs of the program participants rather than those of the intervention planners. The principle of participation emphasizes the importance of involving clients in the intervention planning, implementation, and evaluation processes. Research has shown that participation in intervention planning itself is health enhancing and that clients meet their goals more effectively and efficiently when they are actively involved in the planning process (Baker & Brownson, 1998).

In order to be truly client centered, the intervention must address occupations the client finds meaningful and be focused on the client's interests, needs, and priorities. This is accomplished, in part, through the development of an occupational profile and the process of occupational analysis. An occupational profile includes "information that describes the client's occupational history and experiences, patterns of daily living, interests, values and needs" (AOTA, 2008b, p. 649). When the client is an organization, the occupational analysis involves the identification of variations in levels of occupational participation and the degree of lifestyle and/or occupational balance among its members. *Lifestyle balance* has been defined by Christiansen and Matuska (2006) as "a consistent pattern of occupations that results in reduced stress and improved health and well-being" (p. 50). Lifestyle imbalance can result in emotional disturbances, sleep deprivation, insufficient time for leisure and social participation, lack of need fulfillment, and inability to meet role demands. Lifestyle imbalance is not only a function of individual behavior but also of conditions in the organization or larger community (Christiansen & Matuska, 2006).

When the client is a population, the occupational analysis involves profiling participation rates and barriers and facilitating factors for occupational performance and occupational participation. Occupational performance analysis focuses on client factors and occupational performance patterns. The characteristics of interest for populations include

- "Health indicators;
- The lifestyles of the community or cohort of people;
- Sociocultural values;
- Prevalence, incidence, and temporal trends in impairments, conditions, and risk behaviors, and
- Commitment to and preparedness for change" (Watson & Wilson, 2003, p. 30).

In addition, it is important to profile organizational, community, and/or population strengths and assets. **Assets** are the "inherent attributes and available resources of populations that might be used in attaining target outcomes" (Watson & Wilson, 2003, p. 37). Assets may be economic, educational, environmental, religious, political, social, and/or cultural. An occupational therapist might ascertain community assets by gathering data on the number of options in the community for healthy leisure activity (parks, recreation centers, youth organizations, public swimming pools, etc.) and on the number and variety of healthy food outlets (grocery stores, fresh food markets, local produce, etc.) and public transportation to and from these venues (see Figure 27.1).

Client Factors and Occupational Performance Patterns

Interventions for organizations and populations may be designed to address client factors and/or performance patterns. *Client factors* are "specific abilities, characteristics, or beliefs that reside within the client and may affect performance in areas of occupation" (AOTA, 2008b, p. 630). Client factors related to organizations include values and beliefs as evidenced in the organization or agency's vision and mission statements and code of ethics; functions such as planning, goal setting, coordinating, and producing; and structures, for example, departments, management, titles, and job descriptions. Client factors related to communities and populations include values and beliefs as evidenced by culture and religious traditions; functions such as economic, educational, political, and social; and structure, for example, similarities across individuals based on health-related conditions, genetics, and risk factors, among others (AOTA, 2008b).

Performance patterns are those habits, routines, rituals, and roles that support or hinder occupational performance. Clients may have the performance skills necessary for effective occupational participation; however, if performance patterns are lacking, the healthy enactment of occupations may be negatively affected. Performance patterns associated with organizations include

- Rituals or social events, such as birthdays, celebrations of accomplishment, fundraising, retreats, among others;
- Roles, for example, of departments within the organization, leadership and management roles in the organizational hierarchy, and roles of the organization in the community and in society; and
- Routines, such as regularly scheduled meetings, documentation practices, communication channels, dress codes, and safety procedures.

Performance patterns associated with communities and populations include

- Rituals and social customs such as national, religious, and cultural holiday celebrations;
- Roles, for example, community leadership roles, roles of agencies within the community, and role of the community/population vis-à-vis other communities and populations; and
- Routines, such as regular health practices, annual community events, and seasonal work practices.

Client-centered interventions address the unique client factors and occupational performance patterns of the organization, community, or population served.

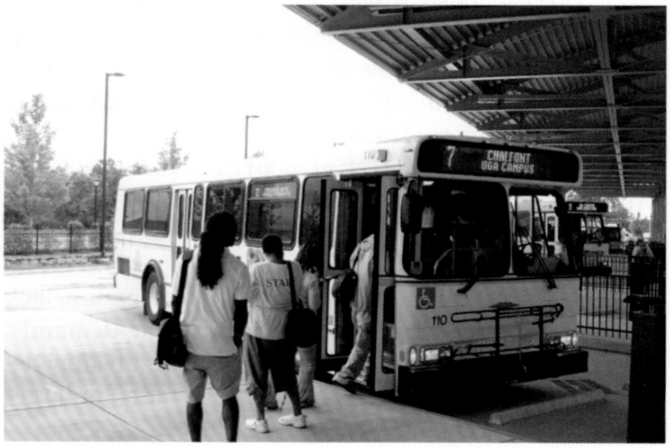

FIGURE 27.1 Accessible transportation is a valuable community asset. (Photo courtesy of J. Schell)

Context-Driven Approaches for Organizations, Communities, and Populations

In addition to client factors and occupational performance patterns, occupational performance analysis requires identification of environmental and contextual factors that support or hinder occupational performance and participation. In the *Occupational Therapy Practice Framework*, *environment* refers to the external physical and social setting or milieu within which occupations occur; and *context*

TABLE 27.1 Examples of Environments and Contexts Associated with Organizations, Communities, and Populations

Environment or Context	Examples
Physical	
Organization	Office building, factory, school building, hospital complex
Community/population	Public transportation system, city parks, natural resources
Social	
Organization	Committees, advisory board, volunteers
Community/population	City government, nonprofit agencies, chamber of commerce
Cultural	
Organization	Dress codes, interaction patterns, and behavioral expectations within the organization
Community/population	National and religious holiday celebrations
Temporal	
Organization	Annual fundraising events, seasonal activities
Community/population	Cultural routines such as siestas, afternoon tea, religious holidays
Virtual	
Organization	Video conferencing, instant messaging, telephone conference calls
Community/population	Virtual community of gamers, Internet social networks

refers to cultural, temporal, and virtual conditions surrounding the client (AOTA, 2008b). Table 27.1 provides some examples of contexts and environments associated with organizations, communities, and populations.

All interventions occur within a specific environment and context, which influences the design, implementation, and effectiveness of the intervention. For example, the physical and social environments in which they are located would significantly impact the development and implementation of interventions for immigrant women and children. A program for homeless immigrant women and children living in temporary shelters would be much different than a church-based program for immigrant women and children hosted by foster families. Similarly, contextual factors also impact interventions for organizations, communities, and populations. Cultural contexts, in particular, must be considered for population-based interventions to be effective. The incorporation of cultural values, beliefs, activity patterns, behavioral standards, and expectations in the intervention significantly enhance the likelihood of success.

The environment and/or context are often the primary features addressed in interventions for organizations, communities, and populations (Youngstrom & Brown, 2005). Each environment or context provides unique barriers and supports to occupational performance. Therefore, modification of the environment and/or context can impact the occupational performance and participation of all members of an organization, community, or population. Interventions focused on environmental factors are typically based on socioenvironmental and ecological models (ecological models are described in more detail in Chapter 38). For populations, interventions focus on the broad determinants of health through community-centered change. The World Health Organization (1986) has identified the fundamental conditions and resources for population health, which include food, shelter, education, income, a stable ecosystem, sustainable resources, peace, equity, and social justice. The lack of these resources for health produces stress, impairment, health problems, and occupational injustices that are amenable to occupational therapy intervention (Kronenberg & Pollard, 2006). For example, Blakeney and Marshall (2009) identified occupational imbalance, deprivation, and alienation among residents of a rural Kentucky community due to watershed pollution that resulted from specific coal mining practices. This three-phase study demonstrated how occupational therapy researchers and practitioners could assist communities discover factors that impact occupational performance and participation and recommend interventions.

Evidence-Based Approaches for Organizations, Communities, and Populations

As in all areas of practice, interventions provided to organizations, communities, and populations should be based on the best available evidence. Although evidence on occupational therapy interventions for organizations, communities, and populations specifically is not plentiful, some strong evidence exists in other disciplines that can guide the development of occupational therapy interventions (see "Commentary on the Evidence" box). Occupational therapy practice guidelines and official documents also can be useful in this regard. Examples of useful documents relevant to providing interventions for

Commentary on the Evidence

Evidence to support occupational therapy interventions at the organizational, community, and population levels is limited at present. However, evidence from health education, health promotion, and public health can guide the design and evaluation of occupational therapy interventions. Evidence-based techniques vary depending on the desired outcomes and level of intervention. A few studies from occupational therapy and other disciplines providing evidence for the efficacy of interventions for organizations, communities, and populations are briefly described here.

Occupational therapy interventions for individuals typically focus on the intrapersonal level and occasionally incorporate the interpersonal level. However, interventions for organizations, communities, and populations require a broader focus and the incorporation of multiple levels of intervention. Obesity, particularly childhood obesity, is an example of a public health problem that has captured the attention of occupational therapy practitioners (AOTA, 2007; Kugel, 2010; Lau, 2011). It has become obvious that this epidemic must be addressed not only on the individual and family levels but also on the organizational, community, and population levels. Table 27.2 provides an example of addressing childhood obesity at several levels of intervention. Potential roles for occupational therapy are provided based on the *Occupational Therapy Practice Framework: Domain and Process, 2nd Edition* (AOTA, 2008b). Although none of these roles are unique to occupational therapy, the pervasiveness of this public health problem invites the participation of occupational therapists and occupational therapy assistants.

Authors	Findings
Classen et al. (2007)	Identified 11 factors in three categories (behavioral, health, and environmental) related to safe driving for older adults that can be used as elements of a population-based health promotion intervention.
Guoping, Yanchun, Yingjie, & Gongxiang (2010)	In a study of middle-aged and older adults, a Tai Chi intervention improved physical and mental health and quality of life. Muscle tone, body weight, balance, and flexibility were superior in the intervention group as compared to the control group.
Maller, Townsend, Pryor, Brown, & St. Leger (2006)	Presents empirical and theoretical evidence of the importance contact with nature plays in human health and well-being and describes public health strategies to optimize the health-promoting effects of nature-based interventions.
Lamontagne, Keegel, Louie, Ostry, & Landsbergis (2007)	A systematic review indicated the efficacy of organizational-level primary prevention strategies addressing the causes and consequences of workplace stress in improving work productivity and decreasing job stress.
Hutchison, Steginga, & Dunn (2006)	Describes a community-based psychosocial intervention using a tiered model for persons affected by cancer.
McClure et al. (2005)	An evidence-based review of the characteristics of effective population-based approaches to the prevention of falls among older people.
Dehghan, Akhtar-Danesh, & Merchant (2005)	A review of intervention strategies for the prevention of childhood obesity including school-based interventions to increase physical activity.
Webb, Joseph, Yardley, & Michie (2010)	An investigation of the characteristics of effective Internet-based health promotion interventions. The use of theory, multiple behavior change techniques, and various methods for interacting with participants were deemed to be significant factors.

TABLE 27.2 Addressing Childhood Obesity at Multiple Levels of Intervention

Level of Intervention	Potential Occupational Therapy Role (terminology from Occupational Therapy Framework; AOTA, 2008b)
Intrapersonal/individual	Facilitate regular physical activity through engagement in meaningful and enjoyable occupations (leisure participation, health management and maintenance)
Interpersonal	Teach children and their parents how to develop and implement healthy meal plans for the family (meal preparation)
Organizational	Consult with local agencies to provide developmentally appropriate after-school active play or leisure activities for children (play exploration and play participation) (see Figure 27.2)
Community	Advocate for accessible and safe walking and biking paths for persons of diverse abilities (safety and emergency maintenance, community mobility)
Public policy/government	Lobby for improvements in the nutritional value of school lunches and vending machine snacks (health management and maintenance)

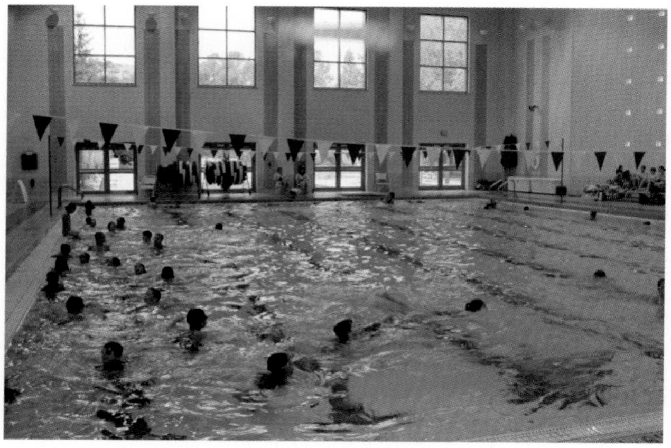

FIGURE 27.2 Providing healthy after-school and summer leisure activities that are developmentally appropriate. (Photo courtesy of J. Schell)

organizations, communities, and populations include, but are not limited to, the *Occupational Therapy Practice Framework: Domain and Process, 2nd Edition* (AOTA, 2008b); *Occupational Therapy in the Promotion of Health and the Prevention of Disease and Disability* (AOTA, 2008a); and *The Role of Occupational Therapy in Disaster Preparedness, Response, and Recovery* (AOTA, 2011).

Evidence in health education, health promotion, and public health suggests that interventions for organizations, communities, and populations based on ecological models are most effective (Kok, Gottlieb, Commers & Smerecnik, 2008; Sallis, Owen, & Fisher, 2008). Ecologically based interventions address multiple levels and include multiple approaches to achieve their goals and objectives. According to Brownson (2001), the levels addressed include

- **Intrapersonal level**: characteristics of individuals within the organization or population that influence behavior and impact occupational performance, participation, and health;
- **Interpersonal level**: relationships among family, friends, peers, and groups that provide support, identity, and role definition and facilitate or constrain occupational performance and/or participation and impact health;
- **Organizational level**: rules, regulations, policies, procedures, programs, and resources within agencies and organizations that impact occupational performance and/or participation and impact health;
- **Community level**: social networks, norms, trends, and standards that facilitate or constrain desired occupational performance and/or participation and impact health; and
- **Public policy level**: local, state and federal policies, laws, and programs that regulate, support, or constrain desired occupational performance and/or participation and impact health.

In addition, effective interventions for organizations, communities, and populations appear to adhere to certain core evidence-based principles (Davis, Schwartz, Wheeler, & Lancaster, 1998; Freudenberg et al., 1995). These interventions

- Are tailored to the expressed needs of a particular organization, community, or population in a specific setting;
- Involve the participants in all phases of the intervention including planning, implementation, and evaluation;
- Incorporate intervention strategies at multiple levels;
- Improve client health, well-being, and quality of life by addressing various life concerns;
- Build on client strengths and cultural norms;
- Use existing resources;
- Advocate for needed policy and resource changes to achieve objectives; and
- Prepare clients to become effective self-managers and self-advocates.

Occupation-Based Approaches for Organizations, Communities, and Populations

Occupation-based interventions are designed to enable the client to enact occupational performance effectively and to participate in desired occupations fully. As described in Chapter 26, occupational performance and occupational participation are the end goals and outcomes of occupational therapy for individuals and frequently the means or process of achieving those goals as well. These are also the end goals and outcomes of occupational therapy interventions for organizations, communities, and populations.

Various intervention approaches may be used with organizations, communities, and populations depending on the desired change and goals to be achieved. Some intervention approaches are designed to influence change in the client (restoration and skill acquisition training); others to modify the task, environment, or context (adaptation, compensation); and others to proffer the best client-environment fit (Youngstrom & Brown, 2005). Often, a combination of approaches produces the best results. The following paragraphs will describe the specific approaches and their application to organizations, communities, and/or populations and provide further examples in Table 27.3. These categories of intervention approaches are not mutually exclusive. Some interventions may fit into multiple categories depending on the goal and level addressed.

Restoration approaches are designed to enhance performance capacities and/or reduce or eliminate performance constraints. Restoration interventions for populations may

TABLE 27.3 Examples of Specific Intervention Approaches

Intervention Approach	Intervention Level	Examples
Remediation or restoration approach: using occupations and purposeful activities to improve occupational performance	Intrapersonal	Establishing a walking program at a local shopping mall for older adults to improve endurance
	Interpersonal	Providing social and occupation-based activities for young, single mothers to facilitate interpersonal support
	Organizational	Using a school facility after hours for a drop-in program for homeless adolescents focusing on healthy leisure occupations and assistance with school assignments
Skill acquisition or training approach: providing information, training, and practice to enhance a skill or process	Intrapersonal	Teaching occupation-based adaptive coping skills to clients in a substance abuse treatment program.
	Interpersonal	Training adolescents in conflict resolution skills to improve relationships with parents, teachers, and peers and improve social participation
	Organizational	Incorporating regular training for police, firefighters, and emergency medical personnel regarding responding to the needs of persons with mental disorders
Adaptation or compensation approach: modifying tasks or using devices or equipment to enable occupational participation	Intrapersonal	Modifying home environments in order to facilitate aging in place
	Organizational	Adapting the policies and procedures of a worksite to address the needs of persons with mental disorders
	Community	Providing motorized scooters in public facilities for persons with mobility impairments
Environmental modifications approach: changing the physical and/or social environment and modifying contexts	Organizational	Providing specific information regarding the gradient for a wheelchair ramp to accommodate a newly hired employee
	Community	Addressing the stigma against mental disorders by modifying the social context through social media campaigns
	Public policy	Recommending the development and implementation of driver's license restrictions for older adults based on driving assessments
Educational approach: providing information and employing methods, strategies, and tools that facilitate learning to improve knowledge, attitudes, and behaviors	Intrapersonal	Leading a stroke education group focused on community resources and leisure opportunities
	Interpersonal	Educating family caregivers on strategies for keeping persons with dementia mentally and physically active though adapted occupational activities
	Organizational	Teaching staff at a group home for adjudicated youth how to manage difficult behaviors during chores
	Public policy	Educating policymakers regarding the need for funding to build or modify housing that is accessible for persons with disabilities
Prevention or health promotion approach: combining educational, social, and environmental intervention strategies to enhance health and prevent injury, disease, and disability	Intrapersonal	Providing occupation-based mental health services in a school following a traumatic event
	Organizational	Preventing compassion fatigue in health care workers by designing and creating a safe and comfortable space for emotional decompression and collegial support
	Community	Offering a chronic disease self-management program at a local church
Consultation approach: using the knowledge and skill of an expert to assist clients make better decisions or deal more effectively with situations	Organizational	Advising an organization that responds to disaster on how best to meet the needs of persons with disabilities in shelters
	Community	Advising local government officials regarding the integration of persons with mental disorders into the community after discharge from the state psychiatric hospital
	Public policy	Counseling state government agencies in establishing polices related to best practices for intervention for children with autism and their families
Advocacy approach: using the power of persuasion to alter opinions and mobilize resources	Organizational	Persuading management to modify the work environment to reduce the incidence of repetitive strain injuries
	Community	Advocating for the hiring of returning soldiers with disabilities to local businesses
	Public policy	Advocating for the establishment of policies that facilitate full participation of persons with disabilities in public recreational facilities

take the form of developing a program to enhance balance, endurance, and strength for residents of an assisted living facility in order to prevent falls or providing training in work simplification and energy conservation for cancer survivors.

Occupational skill acquisition or training approaches are designed to develop or enhance an occupational performance skill or process. Occupational skill acquisition or training interventions for populations may take the form of developing and implementing an after-school anger management program for adolescents to enhance emotional regulation skills and reduce bullying or a parenting program to address the special needs of parents of children with disabilities.

Adaptation and compensation approaches are designed to diminish constraints by modifying contexts or activity demands in order to support occupational performance and occupational participation in natural contexts. Adaptation and compensation interventions for populations may take the form of adapting a task or providing special equipment in order to facilitate the participation of children with disabilities in a summer day camp or providing adaptive equipment and mobility devices in an emergency shelter to accommodate the needs of persons with disabilities.

The environmental modification approach is designed to reduce natural, built, and social environmental barriers to occupational performance and occupational participation. Environmental modification interventions for populations may take the form of designing accessible playgrounds based on universal design principles to enhance the development of children of all abilities or adapting the environment of senior housing to facilitate the safety of older adults with low vision.

Prevention and health promotion approaches are designed to avert the occurrence of illness, injury, and disability and enhance well-being and quality of life by reducing risk factors and enhancing protective and resiliency factors (Scaffa & Brownson, 2005). The World Health Organization (1986) defined *health promotion* as a "process of enabling people to increase control over and to improve their health" and the "science and art of helping people change their lifestyle to move toward a state of optimal health" and "enhance awareness, change behavior and create environments that support good health practices" (p. iii). The Well Elderly Study by Clark et al. (2001) and Clark et al. (1997), a classic randomized controlled trial, demonstrated the effectiveness of a population-based health promotion occupational therapy intervention for community-dwelling older adults. In comparison to subjects who participated in social activities and those who received no treatment, individuals who received occupational therapy services demonstrated improved vitality, physical and social functioning, life satisfaction, and general mental health. Other prevention and health promotion interventions for populations may take the form of adapting computer workstations at a nonprofit organization in order to prevent repetitive motion injuries or providing community-based programs on chronic disease self-management that have been shown to prevent the development of secondary conditions that limit occupational performance (Arbesman & Mosley, 2012).

Educational approaches are designed to facilitate positive changes in knowledge, attitudes, and behaviors that support health, occupational performance, and occupational participation. Educational interventions for populations may take the form of teaching safe lifting techniques at a factory to avoid back injuries among workers or teaching staff at a long-term care facility how best to facilitate the occupational engagement of patients with dementia.

Consultation approaches are designed to enable the client to solve occupation-related problems independently. Consultation involves establishing a collaborative relationship with the client in order to define the occupational concern to be addressed, identify potential solutions, and develop implementation strategies. However, the actual implementation of the intervention is the responsibility of the client. Consultation interventions for populations may take the form of designing a wheelchair basketball program for a local Boys and Girls Club or making recommendations for improving Ticket to Work services for persons with disabilities.

Advocacy approaches are designed to impact decision making within political, economic, and social systems and institutions to "promote occupational justice and empower clients to seek and obtain resources to fully participate in their daily life occupations" (AOTA, 2008b, p. 654). Advocacy interventions for populations may take the form of collaborating with mental health agencies to increase public awareness of stigma and discrimination or serving on boards of community nonprofit organizations to secure funding for programs.

Regardless of the intervention approach used, therapeutic use of self and establishing a therapeutic alliance with the client are critical to the success of any intervention with an organization, community, or population. *Therapeutic use of self* is defined as "an occupational therapy practitioner's use of his or her personality, insights, perceptions, and judgments as part of the therapeutic process" (AOTA, 2008b, p. 653). Developing rapport, communicating effectively, displaying empathy, establishing trust, providing motivation, listening actively, and maintaining a caring attitude are prerequisite to effectively interacting with any client.

Case Vignettes

The following case vignettes provide examples of occupational therapy interventions for an organization, a community, and a population. As can be seen, multiple intervention approaches are incorporated in each scenario. Each case includes an occupational profile, occupational performance analysis findings, goals, and intervention approaches used.

Organization-Based Case

An elementary school in Pensacola, Florida has a significantly higher enrollment of children with parents on military deployment than other schools in the area. This is due in part to its location near multiple military bases. Approximately 40% of children attending the school have one or both parents deployed in the Middle East conflict zone. Many of these children are being cared for by grandparents or other relatives.

Over the past 6 months, teachers have noted increased absences, decreased classroom participation, reduced social interaction with peers, and falling grades among this group of children. The principal has asked Danielle, the school-based occupational therapist, to work with the school counselor to identify and address the needs of these children.

The school counselor administered a depression inventory and noted that approximately 70% of these children scored in the mild-to-moderate range for depressive symptoms. Teachers completed the Child Behavior Checklist (CBCL) (Achenbach, 2009). The scores on the CBCL indicated that the children had elevated scores on both the internalizing and externalizing scales. Internalizing behaviors include emotional reactivity, anxiety, depression, withdrawal, and somatic complaints. Externalizing behaviors include attention deficits and aggression.

The occupational therapist administered the Children's Assessment of Participation and Enjoyment (CAPE) (King et al., 2004), the Social Skills Rating System (SSRS) (Gresham & Elliott, 2007), School Function Assessment (SFA) (Coster, Deeney, Haltiwanger, & Haley, 1998), and the Perceived Efficacy and Goal Setting System (PEGS) (Missiuna, Pollock, & Law, 2004) to children with deployed parents whom the teachers identified as at risk for academic failure. Results from the CAPE indicated a low level of social participation and a low level of enjoyment of activity participation among 65% of the children tested. The SSRS supported the results of the CBCL and indicated high levels of internalizing and externalizing behaviors including anxiety, sadness, and poor anger management. In addition, the SSRS indicated a high level of hyperactivity and impulsivity among a small number of the children.

The SFA (participation and activity performance sections only) data was collected by interviewing the classroom teachers. The children demonstrated low scores on playground/recess and social behaviors during transitions. They had few problems in physical tasks but demonstrated deficits in compliance with adult directives and school rules, task behavior/completion, positive interaction, and behavior regulation. Each child and caregiver completed the PEGS with the following results:

1. Children perceived self-efficacy and competence in self-care and leisure activities but lower levels of competence in school-related activities.
2. Caregivers perceived competence in the child for self-care activities but lower levels of competence in school-related activities and leisure activities. Caregivers were concerned with the lack of active leisure and social withdrawal on the part of the children.

One of the strategies recommended (consultation) by the occupational therapist was to develop a mentoring program pairing a same gender high school student who has experienced parental deployments with an elementary school student with a currently deployed parent (interpersonal level). The program would be designed to increase play/leisure participation, improve academic performance, and enhance social participation. The pairs would meet once a week to play games, complete homework, take walks, and eat together.

In addition, the occupational therapist created an expressive arts program that teachers could incorporate into the regular classroom curriculum. These activities would provide an opportunity for children with deployed parents to have an outlet for nonverbal emotional expression and to socially interact with peers (interpersonal level). Danielle was careful to develop expressive art activities that were age appropriate for each grade level. Activities in the expressive arts program included, but were not limited to, arts and crafts, puppetry, drama, music activities, fairy tale enactments, dance and movement activities, and bibliotherapy (remediation or restoration approach). These activities were chosen based on research reported by Jackson and Arbesman (2005) that indicated the efficacy of creative art activities for emotional expression.

A program for parents and other caregivers was also developed by the occupational therapist and offered online via the school's Website (educational approach, organizational level). Topics included preparing children for a parent's deployment, identifying signs and responding to emotional distress, managing difficult behaviors, and preparing children for a parent's return (interpersonal level). Other topics to meet the parents' personal needs included stress management, occupational balance, routines and rituals, social support, and community resources.

Last, the occupational therapist and school counselor began researching and developing a grant proposal to establish an after-school program for children in military families regardless of deployment status. They also requested that the school board provide an additional school counselor and more hours of occupational therapy time for this particular school (advocacy approach).

Community-Based Case

Due to the closing of a state psychiatric facility, there has been a significant increase in the number of men with mental disorders who are homeless and wandering the streets. The local mental health services agency has an inadequate number of group homes to accommodate this sudden influx of persons needing housing. The executive director of the mental health agency has contacted the occupational therapy department at the local university and requested assistance in addressing the needs of persons with mental disorders who are homeless (consultation approach, organizational level).

In order to determine the needs and assets of the community, Michael, the occupational therapist, conducted a focus group consisting of five homeless men with mental health problems and key informant interviews with staff of current group homes and members of the housing board. The staff of the group homes stated that a significant problem is the lack of life skills assessment of adults with mental disorders prior to placement in community housing. This leads to clients being placed in group homes who lack the basic skills for community living. As a result, these clients often "bounce back" to the inpatient psychiatric facilities or come to the hospital emergency room in psychiatric crisis. The members of the housing board were in consensus regarding the need for additional housing but stated that they did not have money to build housing or to provide support staff for the group homes.

After meeting with the stakeholders involved including the housing board, the mental health agency, the homeless coalition, and local elected officials, the occupational therapist facilitated a collaborative effort to address the problem (advocacy approach, public policy level). An old hotel that was no longer being used could be purchased and renovated by the housing board, the mental health agency would provide staffing, and the homeless coalition would provide basic furnishings. The local elected officials lobbied for funding from the State Department of Mental Health for support services and from the U.S. Department of Housing and Urban Development (HUD) for renovations to the site. Occupational therapy students at the university would be involved in administering screening and assessment tools and providing an independent living skills program (skill acquisition) for the residents based on an intervention developed by occupational therapy practitioners Helfrich, Chan, and Sabol (2011) and incorporating the evidence-based permanent supportive housing model (Substance Abuse and Mental Health Services Administration, 2010). Level I fieldwork students would assist mental health staff in the delivery of services.

Population-Based Case

A large hospital in a metropolitan area is designated as a transplant center. Individuals in need of transplants and their families often move from distant parts of the country to live near the transplant center. Currently, the hospital does not have services for families awaiting transplants or for those actively involved in the transplant process.

Courtney, an occupational therapist at a home care agency in the same city has recently been receiving an influx of patients posttransplantation for evaluation and intervention. Many of the problems experienced by transplant recipients stem from physical deconditioning and emotional stress. The family members, especially the caregivers, also report high levels of fatigue and nervous tension.

The occupational therapist works with the transplant recipients to increase endurance and strength by working on activities of daily living. She is also teaching the patients energy conservation and work simplification techniques as well as providing assistive devices as needed. Initially, the occupational therapist included family members in the interventions so they could learn energy conservation and work simplification techniques themselves. In addition, the occupational therapist provided caregiver training that included the importance of good body mechanics and occupational balance in one's lifestyle (health promotion/prevention approach, intrapersonal and interpersonal levels).

After several months of working with these families, the occupational therapist approached the management of the home care agency about initiating a support group for families of persons awaiting transplantation and families of transplant recipients (advocacy approach, organizational level). Such a support group would assist family members in arranging, supervising, and providing care for their loved ones. The home care agency met with hospital staff, and the hospital agreed to provide the space and some funding for the support group. The occupational therapist and social worker began to collaboratively develop a 6-week group protocol to meet the needs of this population. The group would address psychosocial concerns especially stress management and provide practical occupation-based strategies for everyday living (educational approach, population level).

Conclusion

Occupational therapy practice is based on the premise that participation in meaningful occupations can improve occupational performance and overall health. If one agrees that occupation is a determinant of health, then it is not difficult to recognize the role of occupational therapy practitioners in developing, implementing, and evaluating occupation-based interventions for organizations, communities, and populations. The profession of occupational therapy has unprecedented opportunity to respond to and help resolve various social problems that impact health and occupational participation including violence and abuse, homelessness, poverty, unintentional injury, joblessness, and social discrimination (Baum & Law, 1998). These social problems are best addressed through interventions designed to impact organizations, communities, and populations. Collaboration with existing agencies and the development of funding streams will be vital to the successful participation of occupational therapy in these endeavors.

References

Achenbach, T. M. (2009). *The Achenbach System of Empirically Based Assessment (ASEBA): Development, findings, theory, and applications.* Burlington, VT: University of Vermont Research Center for Children, Youth and Families. Retrieved from http://www.aseba.org/schoolage.html

American Occupational Therapy Association. (2007). Obesity and occupational therapy: Position paper. *American Journal of Occupational Therapy, 61,* 701–703.

American Occupational Therapy Association. (2008a). Occupational therapy in the promotion of health and the prevention of disease and disability. *American Journal of Occupational Therapy, 62,* 694–703.

American Occupational Therapy Association. (2008b). Occupational therapy practice framework: Domain and process, 2nd edition. *American Journal of Occupational Therapy, 62,* 625–683.

American Occupational Therapy Association. (2011). The role of occupational therapy in disaster preparedness, response and recovery. *American Journal of Occupational Therapy, 65*(6, Suppl.), S11–S25.

Arbesman M., & Mosley, L. J. (2012). Systematic review of occupation- and activity-based health management and maintenance interventions for community-dwelling older adults. *American Journal of Occupational Therapy, 66*, 277–283.

Baker, E. A., & Brownson, C. A. (1998). Defining characteristics of community-based health promotion programs. *Journal of Public Health Management and Practice, 4*(2), 1–9.

Bass-Haugen, J. (2009). Health disparities: Examination of evidence relevant for occupational therapy. *American Journal of Occupational Therapy, 63*, 24–34.

Bass-Haugen, J., Henderson, M. L., Larson, B. A., & Matuska, K. (2005). Occupational issues of concern in populations. In C. H. Christiansen, C. M. Baum, & J. Bass-Haugen (Eds.), *Occupational therapy: Performance, participation, and well-being* (3rd ed., pp. 166–187). Thorofare, NJ: Slack.

Baum, C., & Law, M. (1998). Community health: A responsibility, an opportunity, and a fit for occupational therapy. *American Journal of Occupational Therapy, 52*, 7–10.

Blakeney, A. B., & Marshall, A. (2009). Water quality, health, and human occupations. *American Journal of Occupational Therapy, 63*, 46–57.

Brownson, C. A. (2001). Program development for community health: Planning, implementation and evaluation strategies. In M. Scaffa (Ed.), *Occupational therapy in community-based practice settings.* Philadelphia, PA: F. A. Davis.

Christiansen, C. H., & Matuska, K. M. (2006). Lifestyle balance: A review of concepts and research. *Journal of Occupational Science, 13*(1), 49–61.

Clark, F., Azen, S. P., Carlson, M., Mandel, D., LaBree, L., Hay, J., . . . Lipson, L. (2001). Embedding health-promoting changes into the daily lives of independent-living older adults: Long-term follow-up of occupational therapy intervention. *Journal of Gerontology: Psychological Sciences, 56*(1), 60–63.

Clark, F., Azen, S. P., Zemke, R., Jackson, J., Carlson, M., Mandel, D., . . . Lipson, L. (1997). Occupational therapy for independent-living older adults: A randomized controlled trial. *Journal of the American Medical Association, 278*, 1321–1326.

Classen, S., Lopez, E., Winter, S., Awadzi, K. D., Ferree, N. & Garvan, C. W. (2007). Population-based health promotion perspective for older driver safety: Conceptual framework to intervention plan. *Clinical Interventions in Aging, 2*, 677–693.

Coster, W., Deeney, T., Haltiwanger, J., & Haley, S. (1998). *School Function Assessment (SFA).* Retrieved from http://www.pearsonassessments.com/HAIWEB/Cultures/en-us/Productdetail.htm?Pid=076-1615-709&Mode=summary

Davis, J. R., Schwartz, R., Wheeler, F., & Lancaster, B. (1998). Intervention methods for chronic disease control. In R. C. Brownson, P. L. Remington, & J. R. Davis (Eds.), *Chronic disease epidemiology and control* (2nd ed., pp. 77–116). Washington, DC: American Public Health Association.

Dehghan, M., Akhtar-Danesh, N., & Merchant, A. T. (2005). Childhood obesity, prevalence, and prevention. *Nutrition Journal, 4*(24). doi:10.1186/1475-2891-4-24

Freudenberg, N., Eng, E., Flay, B., Parcel, G., Rogers, T., & Wallerstein, N. (1995). Strengthening individual and community capacity to prevent disease and promote health: In search of relevant theories and principles. *Health Education Quarterly, 22*, 290–306.

Green, L. W., & Kreuter, M. W. (1991). *Health promotion planning: An educational and environmental approach* (2nd ed.). Mountainview, CA: Mayfield.

Gresham, F. M., & Elliott, S. N. (2007). *Social skills rating system.* Los Angeles, CA: Western Psychological Services.

Guoping, L., Yanchun, F., Yingjie, Z., & Gongxiang, D. (2010). Effect of Tai Chi on physical and mental health of middle-aged and elderly population. Retrieved from http://en.cnki.com.cn/Article_en/CJFDTOTAL-HLXZ201003003.htm

Helfrich, C. A., Chan, D. V., & Sabol, P. (2011). Cognitive predictors of life skill intervention outcomes for adults with mental illness at risk for homelessness. *American Journal of Occupational Therapy, 65*, 277–286.

Hutchison, S. D., Steginga, S. K., & Dunn, J. (2006). The tiered model of psychosocial intervention in cancer: A community based approach. *Psycho-Oncology, 15*, 541–546.

Jackson, L. L., & Arbesman, M. (2005). *Occupational therapy practice guidelines for children with behavioral and psychosocial needs.* Bethesda, MD: AOTA Press.

King, G., Law, M., King, S., Hurley, P., Hanna, S., Kertoy, M., . . . Young, K. (2004). *Children's Assessment of Participation and Enjoyment (CAPE) and Preferences for Activities of Children (PAC).* San Antonio, TX: Harcourt Assessment.

Kok, G., Gottlieb, N. H., Commers, M., & Smerecnik, C. (2008). The ecological approach in health promotion programs: A decade later. *American Journal of Health Promotion, 22*, 437–442.

Kronenberg, F., & Pollard, N. (2006). Political dimensions of occupation and the role of occupational therapy. *American Journal of Occupational Therapy, 60*, 617–626.

Kugel, J. (2010). Combating childhood obesity through community practice. *OT Practice, 15*(15), 17–18.

Lamontagne, A. D., Keegel, T., Louie, A. M., Ostry, A., & Landsbergis, P. A. (2007). A systematic review of the job-stress intervention evaluation literature, 1990–2005. *International Journal of Occupational and Environmental Health, 13*, 268–280.

Lau, C. (2011). Food & fun for kids: Preventing childhood obesity through OT. *OT Practice, 16*(6), 11–17.

Maller, C., Townsend, M., Pryor, A., Brown, P., & St. Leger, L. (2006). Healthy nature healthy people: 'contact with nature' as an upstream health promotion intervention for populations. *Health Promotion International, 21*, 45–54.

McClure, R. J., Turner, C., Peel, N., Spinks, A., Eakin, E., & Hughes, K. (2005). Population-based interventions for the prevention of fall-related injuries in older people. *Cochrane Database of Systematic Reviews* 2005, (1), CD004441. doi:10.1002/14651858.CD004441.pub2

Missiuna, C., Pollock, N., & Law, M. (2004). *The perceived efficacy and goal setting system.* San Antonio, TX: Harcourt Assessment.

Moyers, P. A. (1999). Guide to occupational therapy practice. *American Journal of Occupational Therapy, 53*, 248–322.

Sallis, J. F., Owen, N., & Fisher, E. B. (2008). Ecological models of health behavior. In K. Glanz, B. K. Rimer, & K. Viswanath (Eds.), *Health behavior and health education: Theory, research, and practice* (4th ed.). San Francisco, CA: Jossey-Bass.

Scaffa, M. E., & Brownson, C. A. (2005). Occupational therapy interventions: Community health approaches. In C. H. Christiansen, C. M. Baum, & J. Bass-Haugen (Eds.), *Occupational therapy: Performance, participation, and well-being* (3rd ed.). Thorofare, NJ: Slack.

Substance Abuse and Mental Health Services Administration. (2010). *Permanent supportive housing evidence-based practices kit.* Retrieved from http://store.samhsa.gov/product/Permanent-Supportive-Housing-Evidence-Based-Practices-EBP-KIT/SMA10-4510

Watson, D. E., & Wilson, S. A. (2003). *Task analysis: An individual and population approach* (2nd ed.). Bethesda, MD: AOTA Press.

Webb, T. L., Joseph, J., Yardley, L., & Michie, S. (2010). Using the Internet to promote health behavior change: A systematic review and meta-analysis on the impact of theoretical basis, use of behavior change techniques, and mode of delivery on efficacy. *Journal of Medical Internet Research, 12*(1), e4. doi:10.2196/jmir.1376

World Health Organization. (1986). *The Ottawa charter for health promotion.* Retrieved from http://www.who.int/hpr/NPH/docs/ottawa_charter_hp.pdf

Youngstrom, M. J., & Brown, C. (2005). Categories and principles of interventions. In C. H. Christiansen, C. M. Baum, & J. Bass-Haugen (Eds.), *Occupational therapy: Performance, participation, and well-being* (3rd ed., pp. 396–419). Thorofare, NJ: Slack.

For additional resources on the subjects discussed in this chapter, visit http://thePoint.lww.com/Willard-Spackman12e.

CHAPTER 28

Educating Clients

Sue Berger

"What we say doesn't matter as much as what patients understand, remember, and do. If their understanding is incorrect or incomplete, we did not find the right way to reach them."

—Regina Benjamin

LEARNING OBJECTIVES

After reading this chapter, you will be able to:

1. Understand key factors that contribute to effective client education
2. Understand the importance of health literacy throughout all types of client education
3. Choose and/or develop appropriate client education materials

OUTLINE

Introduction

As health care professionals, occupational therapy (OT) practitioners are educators. We teach our clients the knowledge and skills they need to enhance their well-being and live as safely as possible (Figure 28.1). Not surprisingly, Sharry, McKenna, and Tooth (2002) found that client education was frequently used as a core intervention approach by occupational therapists. To be effective clinicians, we must know what specific strategies to teach our clients, and we need to know *how* to teach our clients. We need to know the various ways to stabilize a bowl for mixing when one has the use of only one arm, but we also need to know how to teach clients so they will remember the strategy, be successful with the strategy, and be able to generalize the strategy to all environments where they might cook. Therefore, this chapter focuses on specific education strategies and how to effectively use them. Chapter 45 provides additional theoretical background related to teaching and learning.

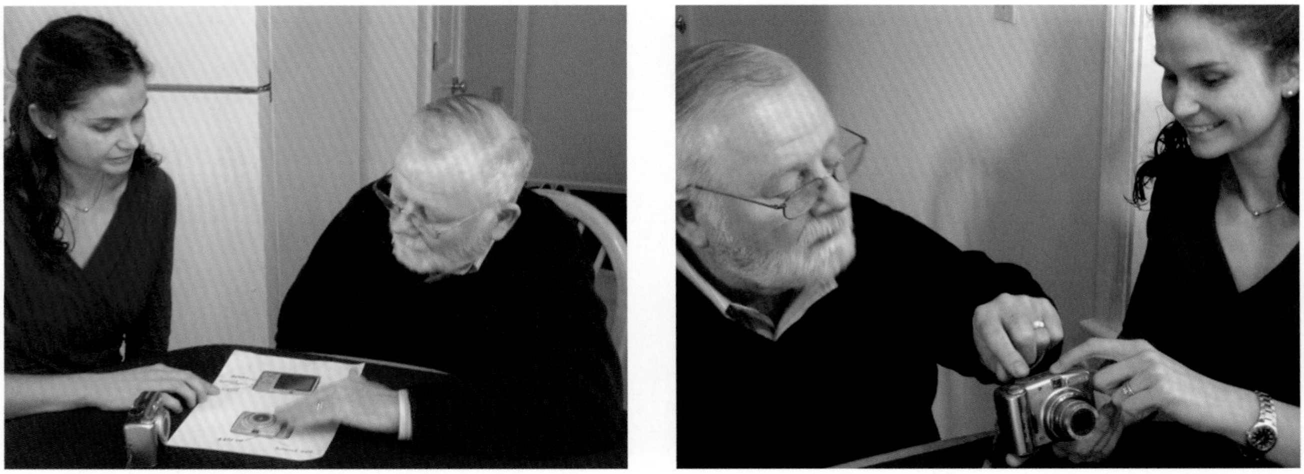

FIGURE 28.1 Reinforcing verbal directions in use of a digital camera, with a handout that includes a simple, clearly labeled photo.

When educating clients, OT practitioners must consider the following questions:

- *Why* does the information need to be communicated?
- *Who* needs to know the information?
- *What* information needs to be conveyed?
- *Where* is the best place to communicate the information?
- *When* is the best time to communicate the information?
- *How* is the best way to communicate the information?

Why Does the Information Need To Be Communicated?

Educating clients decreases anxiety, builds trust, and leads to better outcomes (van Servellen, 2009). Client education can shorten hospital stays and decrease costs of health care, especially for those living with chronic conditions (Dreeben, 2010). When individuals become ill, those who are educated about the illness and treatment stay motivated and adhere to recommendations (Drench, Noonan, Sharby, & Hallenborg, 2007). Client education maximizes an individual's ability to participate in daily activities. For all of this to occur, OT practitioners need to communicate information clearly, and, more importantly, they need to ensure that clients understand the material conveyed.

Client education is more than telling someone what to do; rather, it is a complex yet important concept that includes careful consideration of teaching and learning strategies that ultimately will affect client outcomes in the clinic and at home (Dreeben, 2010). Effective client education is at the core of quality care.

Who Needs to Know the Information?

Just as the profession of OT uses the term *clients* to broadly refer to individuals, organizations, or populations who receive service (American Occupational Therapy Association [AOTA], 2008; Moyers & Dale, 2007), the term *clients* in this chapter includes families, caregivers, teachers, employers, and relevant others. It is important to consider the unique learning needs of all clients that we work with. In addition, it is important to note that the learning needs of one client, for example, an individual living with a stroke, may be different than those of his wife, daughter, or home health aide. OT practitioners must learn to effectively communicate with the different individuals and groups relevant to each case.

As with all intervention, knowing the client and his or her strengths, limitations, culture, values, interests, age, primary language, and auditory ability is fundamental. Knowing the client's literacy skills is also important. Although the definition of literacy focuses on reading and writing, it also affects one's ability to comprehend oral information (Dreeben, 2010; van Servellen, 2009).

Literacy

Health literacy is defined as "the degree to which individuals have the capacity to obtain, process, and understand basic health information and services needed to make appropriate health decisions" (Institute of Medicine [IOM], 2004, para. 1). Therefore, being health literate involves more than reading and writing; one also needs to have effective speaking and listening skills. Because technology has emerged as an important way to communicate and share information—especially health information—one also needs to be computer literate. Finally, motivation, cognitive ability, and social skills influence one's ability to gather, understand, and use health information (Berkman, Davis, & McCormack, 2010). Other definitions of health literacy include the interaction between an individual's skills and the demands of the environment (i.e., health care system), and this implies that an individual's health literacy changes depending on the clarity of the health-related materials (Berkman et al., 2010; IOM, 2004). It is our responsibility as health care practitioners to assure that our clients are functioning at their highest literacy abilities by providing educational information in a way that they can effectively use it.

The 2003 National Adult Literacy Survey (NALS) found that approximately one in three Americans is **functionally illiterate**, defined as reading below the fifth-grade level. This number increases to one in two people who struggle with reading when those with only marginally better reading skills are included (Kutner, Greenberg, Jin, & Paulsen, 2006). Of these people, 5% reported having a learning disability. Only 15% were born outside the United States; most of those who cannot read are native-born Americans (American Medical Association [AMA], 1999). Older adults, those with less than a high school diploma, and those who are Black and Hispanic have the lowest literacy scores (Kutner et al., 2006).

Good observation skills can provide a great deal of information about **reading level**. When giving any written material to a client, one should note whether the client states something similar to "I'll read this later so I can discuss it with my husband," "I left my glasses at home," or "I'll remember what you say—no need to write it down." Does the client appear to read something but then is unable to follow the instructions? Although there are standardized reading level assessments such as the Rapid Estimate of Adult Literacy in Medicine (REALM; Davis et al., 1991) and the Test of Functional Health Literacy in Adults (TOFHLA; Parker, Baker, Williams, & Nurss, 1995), they can be time consuming to administer and embarrassing for clients. Sometimes, a simple question such as "How confident are you in filling out medical forms?" can identify persons with limited health literacy as accurately (and quicker) than the TOFHLA (Sarkar, Schillinger, Lopez, & Sudore, 2011).

Culture

Knowing the culture of an individual is critical to providing effective education. Terminology, topics, and ideas should all be relevant to the intended audience. When possible, communication should be in the person's primary language. Native speaker, professional interpreters are best to prevent miscommunication and ensure privacy (Centers for Disease Control and Prevention [CDC], 2009; Rankin, Stallings, & London, 2005). However, this is not always possible; and family members might be the only available interpreters. Caution should be used in this situation, as family members' own opinions and reactions are often conveyed as well or instead of the client's (Osborne, 2005).

Being culturally sensitive involves more than speaking in the client's primary language. One should consider the meaning of personal space and time within the client's culture, be careful about making judgments or interpretations without checking this out with the person, and use culturally relevant scenarios (Dreeben, 2010; van Servellen, 2009). For example, when addressing nutrition, discuss food and habits that are culturally appropriate for the client (e.g., soy sauce or ketchup; use of utensils or hands). Being cognizant of cultural differences and beliefs in health and wellness is the first step toward effective communication with individuals of cultures other than one's own.

Caregivers

There is extensive evidence that the educational needs of caregivers are unmet (Washington, Meadows, Elliott, & Koopman, 2011). Caregivers want more information about the health condition, prognosis, general treatment options, and community services available. Along with this general information, caregivers also want educational information tailored to their specific needs (e.g., how to help their spouse get into the shower safely) (Hafsteinsdóttir, Vergunst, Lindeman, & Schuurmans, 2011; Washington et al., 2011). Several studies of caregiver education discussed the importance of accessible information. It is important to explain information instead of just handing out a brochure and to avoid medical jargon (Allison, Evans, Kilbride, & Campbell, 2008; Nikoletti, Kristjanson, Tataryn, McPhee, & Burt, 2003; O'Connell, Baker, & Prosser, 2003). As OT practitioners, we strive to provide effective education to all clients and must remember that each client has unique needs. Caregivers, in particular, require educational strategies and materials focused on their specific needs.

What Information Needs to Be Conveyed?

Several studies have found large discrepancies between what clients want to know and what health professionals believe is most important. Davis et al. (1998) found that low-income, low-literacy, minority women were most interested in learning about cost of procedures, something that was rarely addressed. Reid et al. (1995) learned that many people wanted information about treatment and prognosis, yet this was often not addressed.

As OT practitioners, we teach our clients strategies to help them participate in daily life. We teach individuals strategies for using community transportation. We teach parents strategies to help their children participate in play activities. We teach mental health workers strategies

Practice Dilemma

Helping Mr. Cervero Learn to Dress Himself

Mr. Cervero is an 85-year-old man who came to the United States from Spain many years ago. He has aphasia; and although he struggles to read, he understands most of what is being said. Although he was fluent in English prior to his stroke 3 weeks ago, his native language is Spanish. He went to school in Spain through sixth grade and then began working at his family's store.

His goal is to be able to do his own self-care because his wife's emphysema is getting worse, and she needs to cut down on the assistance she provides for him. Currently, he is working on one-handed dressing. Although he can put on his sweater in the clinic with visual and verbal cues, you want to send home instructions for reminders so that he can practice in-between sessions when dressing at home.

As you read the remaining sections of this chapter, think about the following questions:

1. What are some strategies to use to make this handout user friendly for Mr. Cervero?
2. Are there other strategies to use besides print material to reinforce at home what is learned in the clinic?

to adapt the environment to best meet the needs of their patients. The list is endless. The key for all client education is to limit the objectives, focusing on information that clients want or need to know. Although something that is nice to know might seem valuable to include, *more* is often not *better* (Weiss, 2007). Remember to prioritize information by what is important to the client, not what you believe is important for the client to know.

Where Is the Best Place to Communicate the Information?

The environment in which client education occurs can influence comprehension and recall. Information should be shared in a shame-free environment (Osborne, 2005; Weiss, 2007), a setting in which the client feels free to ask questions, admit lack of understanding, or ask for repetition. A quiet space with no distractions provides an environment where clients can focus on the topic being discussed (Caress, 2003). For example, ask for permission to turn off the television or radio, or find a better time if a favorite show is playing. Find a private room or corner. If the client is reading material, be sure there is adequate lighting with little or no glare.

When Is the Best Time to Communicate the Information?

Internal distractions such as pain, anxiety, hunger, or need to use the bathroom affect one's ability to absorb and understand information. When possible, resolve these distractions prior to client education. Because some people are "morning people" and others are more alert and receptive to information in the evening, consider the timing of all client education. When working in schools, schedule evening hours to provide parent education. Parents who need to take time off from work to attend a meeting may arrive frustrated and angry and will be less open to hearing new information.

It is important to consider timing of information over the course of care. In a systematic review of educational needs of patients with stroke and their caregivers, researchers found that educational needs change over time (Hafsteinsdóttir et al., 2011). For example, educational needs in the acute phase of health care differ from those during rehabilitation. Timing of client education needs to be considered related to both time of day and time in the recovery process.

How Is the Best Way to Communicate the Information?

Recall of information depends on how the information is presented. Organization of content presented helps clients understand and apply information. Although this is especially true for individuals with low literacy, all people—especially those who are in a new environment, are learning new information, are in pain, or are anxious—will benefit when material is presented clearly and in an organized manner. Therefore, plan the information to be conveyed before talking and remember to sequence your information logically (Weiss, 2007). For example, if you are working with a group of children to help them lighten their backpacks, begin by stating, "First, decide what needs to go in; second, put heavy books at the back of the pack; and third, put lighter objects in the front of the pack." In both speaking and developing written materials, present essential information by itself and first; and when using numbers to represent quality, the higher number should always convey better quality (Berkman et al., 2011). Information that is given as specific suggestions is recalled more often than general suggestions (Bradshaw, Ley, & Kincey, 1975). For example, "Walk briskly for 30 minutes three times a week" would be recalled more often than "Exercise several times a week."

BOX 28.1 Multiple Methods to Consider When Educating Clients

Explain
Provide written or audio instructions
Demonstrate, when possible (by practitioner)
- Perform activity
- Use model
- Show pictures
- Show video
- Use multimedia

Teach-back technique (by client)
- Return demonstration
- Re-explain in own words
- Teach a peer

Using demonstrations, models, and pictures along with oral communication also helps people to understand information (Berkman et al., 2011; Rudd & Anderson, 2006; Weiss, 2007). When teaching clients about the importance of eliminating clutter for safety, show before and after pictures of a kitchen and point out safety hazards and ways they were resolved. When teaching use of adaptive equipment, explain and demonstrate. Use multiple teaching methods, especially when working with groups of individuals, because different people learn differently. Even when working with one client, multiple teaching methods help to emphasize key information and facilitate comprehension and memory (see Box 28.1).

Finally, one must verify understanding. The practitioner might believe that he or she was clear, organized, and consistent; but if the client did not understand the message, the practitioner was not successful. The individual who is passive or constantly nodding in agreement might not fully understand or adhere to the recommendations. Therefore, whenever possible, employ the "teach-back technique," having clients return demonstration, repeat in their own words, or explain a concept using a different example (Doak, Doak, & Root, 1996; Weiss, 2007). This technique is effective in making sure that clients understand the information and, more importantly, in improving health outcomes (Schillinger et al., 2003). If appropriate, ask one client to demonstrate or to teach other clients. Clients are more likely to ask questions and admit lack of understanding with a peer than with a therapist.

In their extensive systematic review, Berkman et al. (2011) summarized key principles to consider for all forms of client education to improve health outcomes, including repetition, pilot testing of material, and emphasis on skill building. In general, there are three ways to communicate with clients: orally, in writing, and via media (including video, audio, and ***multimedia***).

Communicating Orally

Evidence suggests that communicating with clients face to face is most effective because it provides the opportunity to use conversational style speaking, provides nonverbal cues for acknowledgement, and allows for interpretation of nonverbal cues to determine comprehension (Qualls, Harris, & Rogers, 2002). Face-to-face communication is also often interactive because clients are able to demonstrate understanding through answering questions or performing the task (Doak et al., 1996). Oral communication also provides opportunity to develop rapport and trust, which ultimately can lead to better therapeutic outcomes (van Servellen, 2009).

In communicating verbally with someone with low literacy skills, it is helpful to be consistent with word choice. During a session on feeding skills, for example, the word *silverware* should be used throughout instead of alternating with *utensil.* Unusual or challenging words used in conversation should be defined, and acronyms should be explained (CDC, 2009). Words such as *assessment* or *intervention* should be defined, or more common words should be used. Acronyms such as *ROM* and *ADL* should be used only after they are fully explained; even then, be sure to verify comprehension. If you are unsure of word choice, ask the client what word he or she uses to describe an item, and use that word consistently. For example, you might ask a girl or a woman whether she refers to her top as her *shirt* or *blouse.*

Communicating with clients who are hard of hearing poses other challenges. It is helpful to choose an environment that is quiet and free of distractions, get the client's attention before speaking, and position oneself directly in front of the client (Osborne, 2005). Often, a client hears better from one side than the other, so take the time to find this out and position oneself on the side which is better. If the person wears hearing aids, make sure they are in place and working. If hearing is severely impaired, use other methods of communication along with, or instead of, speaking.

Communicating in Writing

Most people forget up to 80% of what they are told during a patient–physician interaction; and almost half of what they believe they remember, they remember incorrectly (Kessels, 2003). Reinforcing oral communication with print material can help recall and comprehension. Written forms of communication reinforce what is said, provide a record of what is said, and provide reminders of what is conveyed.

BOX 28.2 Simplified Measure of Gobbledygook Readability Activity

Try to determine the readability level of this chapter. Using the Simplified Measure of Gobbledygook formula, determine the number of words with three or more syllables in the following sentences: first 10 sentences of the chapter, last 10 sentences of the chapter, first 10 sentences of the section "Reading Level of the Material." Take that number, find the nearest perfect square (e.g., if there are 67 words with 3 or more syllables, the nearest perfect square is 64), take the square root of that (i.e., 8), and then add a constant of 3 (i.e., 11). This number equals the approximate grade/reading level of the material.

The ability to understand verbal information differs from the ability to understand written information because the reader can control the pace of obtaining written information and can review it as often as needed (Wilson & Wolf, 2009). If it is worth the time to write down information, it is important to ensure that the reader can use the material. To effectively communicate in writing, one needs to consider the reading level and presentation of the material (CDC, 2009; National Cancer Institute [NCI], 2003; Weiss, 2007).

Reading Level of the Material

Public information, such as newspapers, is often written at the 10th-grade level or higher; but many people read at a much lower level. In a study reviewing OT written educational materials, Griffin, McKenna, and Tooth (2006) found that the materials were written at a 9th- or 10th-grade level, whereas the clients mean reading ability was at a 7th- to 8th-grade level. In a large randomized controlled study about polio immunization information, Davis et al. (1998) found that comprehension increased with written material at a 4th- to 6th-grade level for all individuals. The study also showed that the simpler form did not insult those with higher education and higher income. Use of a low reading level in written materials meets the needs of a large number of people.

There are numerous assessments to determine the reading level of written material such as the FRY formula (Fry, 1968) and the Gunning Fog index scale (Gunning & Kallan, 1994) along with computer-generated readability scores (Microsoft Office Online, 2010). The Simplified Measure of Gobbledygook (SMOG) formula is shown in Box 28.2. In general, however, using short sentences and one- or two-syllable words is a simple strategy that will keep the reading level low (Rudd & Anderson, 2006; Weiss, 2007).

In addition to reading level, other factors influence the readability of printed material. For example, the use of all capital letters is more challenging to read than is a combination of uppercase and lowercase letters because readers use the shapes of words to help read. For example, when typed in all capitals, *AND* looks like a rectangle and is visually very similar to *FOR*, *THE*, or any other three-letter word. If typed with lowercase letters, *and*, *for*, and *the* all have different shapes, and it is therefore easier to quickly determine the word (Doak et al., 1996; Weiss, 2007). Box 28.3 provides examples of easy and difficult to use layouts and fonts.

To make written information readable, use active rather than passive wording and use positive terminology (CDC, 2009; Executive Secretariat, 2003; Weiss, 2007). For example, write, "Put your right arm in first when getting dressed" instead of "Your right arm should be put in first when getting dressed," and state, "Raise your arm slowly" instead of "Do not raise your arm quickly."

Similar to oral communication, use of common words in writing makes reading easier (Executive Secretariat, 2003; Osborne, 2005; Rudd & Anderson, 2006; Weiss, 2007). Using the word *doctor* instead of *physician* is often appropriate. Most people understand the phrase *thinking skills* better than they do *cognition*. If it is important to use the term *cognition*, define it and use it consistently. Use of descriptions that are simple to visualize is another helpful strategy. In encouraging someone to lift only small items, the commonly used expression "no bigger than a bread box" is easier to understand than "no bigger than 2 ft by 1 ft by 1 ft."

Presentation of the Material

The overall presentation of all written communication is important. Presentation includes, but is not limited to, the type of paper used, the color of paper and print, font size and style, visuals, and organization. These factors affect one's ability to see the material, read the material, and understand the material as well as one's motivation to read the material.

BOX 28.3 Examples of Easy versus Difficult to Read Fonts and Layout

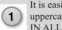

1. It is easier to read material that is written using a combination of uppercase and lowercase letters THAN MATERIAL WRITTEN IN ALL CAPITALS.
2. It is easier to read print in Times New Roman, a font with serif than to read material printed in Arial, a sans serif font.
3. It is easier to read material that uses a 12-point font than material that uses a 9-point font.
4. It is easier to read the material written above that is single-spaced than what you are reading right now, which is less than single space. Remember that spacing and allowing for white space are important.

Font and Paper. To ensure that most people can see the written material, it should be typed in a font with serifs (the small lines at the end of characters) and a font size of 12 points (CDC, 2009). Font size of 14 or greater should be used for readers with low vision (Osborne, 2005) (see Box 28.3). These authors also recommend limiting the use of fancy fonts or italics. In general, the same font style should be used throughout a document.

Matte paper should be used because glossy paper can cause glare and make reading difficult. Black print on white paper is often most effective for contrast (Osborne, 2005). However, if color is desired, it is important to use opposing colors from the color wheel. For example, if yellow paper is used, the font should be blue (opposite yellow) rather than orange (next to yellow).

Organization. The organization of the material affects readability. Highlighting key information by making it bold or underlining it adds focus to important information. Headings are helpful to group information. Including white space, rather than filling up all the paper with words and pictures, facilitates self-efficacy (CDC, 2009; Weiss, 2007). Looking at a brochure that is unappealing and crammed with information will be discouraging for clients, regardless of the information in the brochure (see Figure 28.2). Include key information first or last because readers remember this information best (CDC, 2009; NCI, 2003).

Spacing is important for visual cues. Leave more space above headings and subheadings than below. This ties information together at a quick visual glance. Consider using simple questions as headers, such as "What is energy conservation?" and "What are the key principles of energy conservation?" Chunking information into five or fewer categories facilitates recall. Information can be divided by rooms in a house (for a handout on environmental adaptations), by senses (for a handout on sensory processing), or according to any categorization that is appropriate for the topic (see Box 28.4).

When possible, the material should be personalized. This can be done simply by writing the user's name at the top of the material or by leaving blank space for individualizing exercises or adding suggestions. Using terminology such as "your exercise program" rather than "the exercise program" has been shown to make a difference in both recall and satisfaction with the material (Wagner, Davis, & Handelsman, 1998).

Visuals. The old saying "A picture is worth a thousand words" is true only if the picture is clear and relevant. Several studies have shown that written materials that used both text and visuals were better received than were materials with text alone (Bernardini, Ambrogi, Fardella, Perioli, & Grandolini, 2001; Katz, Kripalani, & Weiss, 2006). Health literacy literature emphasizes the importance of visuals that are culturally appropriate, easy to understand, and used with simple captions (CDC, 2009; NCI, 2003). Use shapes with simple words that are universally recognized. For example, use a picture of a stop sign to reinforce the importance of stopping activity before pain occurs. Visuals, like words, should convey the positive. For example, include pictures of healthy foods rather than a picture of chips and cookies with a line through it. Some visuals can be confusing rather than helpful. For example, pictures with many arrows or bus schedules with small font and many columns are difficult to use. The purpose of using visuals is to facilitate comprehension. Pictures as decorations can detract from the message (CDC, 2009). All pictures that are included should convey an idea, enhancing the message in the text.

Assessing Print Material. The best way to develop effective printed material is to engage members of the intended audience in the development of the material, ask potential users for feedback of a draft and revise accordingly (Weiss, 2007). The Suitability Assessment of Materials (SAM) (Doak et al., 1996) is one of several published assessments that can be used to ensure that written materials are developed well. The SAM takes approximately 30 minutes, and the result is a numerical score, with a higher score indicating better suitability of the material for a given audience. Box 28.5 provides a quick checklist to consider in developing or choosing print material to use with clients.

Communicating with Media

Audio, video, and multimedia are other strategies that can be used to communicate information to clients. Theoretically, these modes of communication have several advantages, including being cost-efficient (i.e., once developed, they can be used over and over again) (Keulers, Welters, Spauwen, & Houpt, 2007) and effective for those with limited literacy (Weiss, 2007). Individuals with low literacy skills may benefit from listening to and viewing information if it is developed in a fun, interactive, and appropriate way. However, using media is not a panacea for those with low literacy skills. Although possibly having average or above average intelligence, individuals who struggle to read often process information differently and might have limited vocabulary and a limited attention span (Doak et al., 1996). Everyone has a different learning style. Some learn best by reading, others by listening, and others by seeing. For many, learning information in multiple forms reinforces the information and assists with recall.

Audio and Video

In choosing or developing audio or video materials, similar considerations should be used as for written materials. For instance, limiting objectives is important for all client education; the message should be 5 minutes or less for audio and 8 minutes or less for video unless breaks are incorporated (Doak et al., 1996). For printed material, information included at the beginning and

LOW VISION TIPS

1. Improve the lighting
- Direct light onto the surface of reading or writing material.
- Bring light closer to surface.
- Turn on overhead light along with task light.
- Make sure all lights have working bulbs and be sure to turn them on.
- Keep on a nightlight or keep a flashlight by the bed.

2. Increase the contrast
- Consider painting walls "opposite" colors of the carpeting.
- Add high contrast throw pillows or afghan to chairs and couches.
- Use colored towels and floor mat to provide high contrast to bathroom walls.
- Use black marker on white paper.
- Choose hard covered books, which provide more contrast than paperbacks.

3. Decrease the glare
- Make sure the light bulb is fully covered by the shade.
- Wear baseball caps inside and outside.
- Wear wraparound filters when outside.
- Use low gloss or no gloss floor and table polish or use table cloths to cover shiny surfaces.

4. Increase the size
- Label items with large print, high contrast lettering.
- Borrow large print books from the library.
- Change the font on the computer to a

A

LOW VISION TIPS

IMPROVE THE LIGHTING

Direct light onto the surface of reading or writing material
Bring light closer to surface
Turn on overhead light along with task light
Make sure all lights have working bulbs and be sure to turn them on.
Keep on a nightlight or keep a flashlight by the bed.

INCREASE THE CONTRAST

Consider painting walls "opposite" colors of the carpeting.
Add high contrast throw pillows or afghan to chairs and couches.
Use colored towels and floor mat to provide high contrast to bathroom walls.
Use black marker on white paper.
Choose hard covered books, which provide more contrast than paperbacks

DECREASE THE GLARE

Make sure the light bulb is fully covered by the shade
Wear baseball caps inside and outside
Wear wraparound filters when outside
Use low gloss or no gloss floor and table polish or use table cloths to cover shiny surfaces

INCREASE THE SIZE

Label items with large print, high contrast lettering
Borrow large print books from the library
Change the font on the computer to a larger font
Purchase commercially available large print items (e.g., large print playing cards; large print wall clock, large print calendar)

USE YOUR OTHER SENSES

Mark items such as the stove and telephone with raised dots or bright colored stickers.
Purchase commercially available talking items (e.g., talking clock)
Smell certain items in refrigerator before eating to make sure they haven't gone bad.

B

FIGURE 28.2 **A.** Well-designed brochure that is easy to read. **B.** Poorly designed brochure (with the same content as part A) that would discourage the reader.

BOX 28.4 Examples of Difficult-to-Read versus Easy-to-Read Formats

Bedroom
– Put a light on the bed table
– Keep a telephone next to the bed

Bathroom
– Keep a nightlight on at night
– Put nonskid decals in the tub

- **Bedroom**
– Put a light on the bed table
– Keep a telephone next to the bed

- **Bathroom**
– Keep a nightlight on at night
– Put nonskid decals in the tub

at the end of the material is most often remembered; whereas with audio and video, the information presented at the end is recalled most often (Doak et al., 1996). For audio, when possible, use voices of people like the intended audience; and for video, be sure that images are of people like the intended audience. Whenever possible, these tools should be used in an interactive format.

There are mixed results regarding the effectiveness of using video for educating clients. In a study exploring the comprehension of video media messages related to cancer, Mazor et al. (2010) found that the information presented was frequently misunderstood. Haines et al. (2009), in a study exploring the effectiveness of a video-based exercise program to reduce falls of older adults, found no significant differences between the control group who received usual care and the group that received a video exercise program in addition to usual care. Other studies, however, have found use of video to be effective (Janda, Stanek, Newman, Obermair, & Trimmel, 2002; Pignone, Harris, & Kinsinger, 2000), and Weiss (2007) emphasizes that client education through videos can be effective if the videos are made keeping health literacy principles in mind.

Multimedia

There are a myriad of new and innovative communication techniques that can be used to facilitate positive health outcomes. For example, embodied conversation agents are computer-animated characters that simulate

BOX 28.5 Checklist of Things to Consider in Developing or Choosing Printed Materials

Characteristics of the user

___ Was the age of the user considered?
___ Was the education and/or reading level of the user considered?
___ Were the values, beliefs, and interests of the user considered?

Information included

___ Is the information what the user might want to know?
___ Is the information what the user might need to know?
___ Is information limited to a few key objectives?

Reading level of the material

___ Is there a limited number of long and/or compound sentences?
___ Are there only a few three or more syllable words? Are the majority of these common, everyday words?
___ Are unusual words defined? Are all other words common, everyday words?
___ Is the same term used consistently?
___ Are common descriptions used to assist with visualization?
___ Is active terminology used?
___ Is terminology phrased in the positive?

Presentation of the material

___ Is a font style with serif used?
___ Is the font size at least 12 points (greater for people with low vision)?
___ Is there a strong contrast between color of print and color of paper?
___ Is matte paper used?
___ Is bold or underlining used for emphasis?
___ Are headings and subheadings used to chunk information and for layout?
___ Is adequate white space used?
___ Is key information included first or last?
___ Is information personalized?

Visuals

___ Are visuals culturally appropriate?
___ Are simple captions included for each visual?
___ Are visuals conveyed in the positive?
___ Do the visuals convey information (not just for decoration)?
___ Are the visuals clearly sequenced?

Cultural relevance

___ Is the material relevant to the intended audience?
___ Is the terminology culturally appropriate?
___ Was the material reviewed with the intended audience prior to distribution?
___ Is the material available in the user's primary language?

face-to-face conversation and can convey nonverbal behaviors. Information can be provided in a consistent, repetitive manner in an environment with no time pressure and has been shown to be effective with clients of all levels of literacy (Bickmore et al., 2010).

Computer games and software that require touch screen interaction (with the response generating the next question) are often fun, motivating, and effective in conveying information (Rankin et al., 2005; Weiss, 2007). A review of the literature showed that computer-based education in addition to face-to-face education is more effective than face to face alone (Wofford, Smith, & Miller, 2005) because clients receive extra information and attention (Beranova & Sykes, 2007). In a systematic review of the influence of computer-generated patient education materials on clinical practice, a small, positive effect was found (Treweek, Glenton, Oxman, & Penrose, 2002).

Although there is increased research over the past 15 years regarding the use of computers in health education, the potential has not been realized because of the lack of accessibility and usability. The intent and hope of increased use of technology for client education was that it would help increase comprehension by those with limited health literacy and decrease health disparities; however, currently, there is concern that the use of computer technology may be exacerbating health disparities because many with low literacy are unable to access or use the technology (Bickmore et al., 2010; Sarkar et al., 2010; van Servellen, 2009). If using computer technology for client education, be sure to consider the client's information technology knowledge, motivation and interest, the usability and functionality of the application, the costs of implementation and use, and the infrastructure and support (Ammenwerth, Iller, & Mahler, 2006).

Communicating through video, audio, or multimedia can be effective; but it is more expensive to produce and more time consuming to develop than written materials. Although there are numerous ways, as discussed earlier, to make written material user-friendly and increase readability, many people cannot understand print materials alone no matter how well developed they are (Atkinson, 2003). For the client who struggles to read, the use of media as an alternative might be worth the expense and time (Rankin et al., 2005).

Conclusion

No one method of client education is effective for all individuals (van Servellen, 2009). Some material and learning are better suited for certain methods of teaching, and some individuals learn best via certain teaching strategies. "One size fits all" is not an effective motto for educating clients. Although more research is needed to determine the best ways to provide client education, considering multiple modes of communication and the specific needs of the individual or groups of individuals will help to convey valuable information to clients.

References

Allison, R., Evans, P. H., Kilbride, C., & Campbell, J. L. (2008). Secondary prevention of stroke: Using the experiences of patients and carers to inform the development of an educational resource. *Family Practice, 25*, 355–361. doi:10.1093/fampra/cmn048

American Medical Association. (1999). Health literacy: Report of the council on scientific affairs. *Journal of the American Medical Association, 281*, 552–557.

American Occupational Therapy Association. (2008). Occupational therapy practice framework: Domain and process, 2nd edition. *American Journal of Occupational Therapy, 62*, 625–683. doi:10.5014/ajot.62.6.625

Ammenwerth, E., Iller, C., & Mahler, C. (2006). IT-adoption and the interaction of task, technology and individuals: A fit framework and a case study. *BMC Medical Informatics and Decision Making, 6*, 3. Retrieved from http://www.biomedcentral.com/content/pdf/1472-6947-6-3.pdf

Atkinson, T. (2003). Plain language and patient education: A summary of current research. *Research Briefs on Health Communication.* The Centre for Literacy. Retrieved from http://www.centreforliteracy.qc.ca/health/briefs/no1/no1.pdf

Beranova, E., & Sykes, C. (2007). A systematic review of computer-based softwares for educating patients with coronary heart disease. *Patient Education and Counseling, 66*, 21–28. doi:10.1016/j.pec.2006.09.006

Berkman, N. D., Davis, T. C., & McCormack, L. (2010). Health literacy: What is it? *Journal of Health Communication, 15*(Suppl. 2), 9–19. doi: 0.1080/10810730.2010.499985

Berkman, N. D., Sheridan, S. L., Donahue, K. E., Halpern, D. J., Viera, A., Crotty, K., . . . Viswanathan, M. (2011). *Health Literacy Interventions and Outcomes: An updated systematic review* (Evidence Report/ Technology Assessment, 199. AHRQ Pub. No. 11-E006). Rockville, MD: Agency for Healthcare Research and Quality.

Bernardini, C., Ambrogi, V., Fardella, G., Perioli, L., & Grandolini, G. (2001). How to improve the readability of the patient package leaflet: A survey on the use of colour, print size, and layout. *Pharmacological Research, 43*(5), 437–444. doi:10.1006/phrs.2001.0798

Bickmore, T. W., Pfeifer, L. M., Byron, D., Forsythe, S., Henault, L. E., Jack, B. W., . . . Paasche-Orlow, M. K. (2010). Usability of conversational agents by patients with inadequate health literacy: Evidence from two clinical trials. *Journal of Health Communication, 15*(Suppl. 2), 197–210. doi: 10.1080/10810730.2010.499991

Bradshaw, P. W., Ley, P., & Kincey, J. A. (1975). Recall of medical advice: Comprehensibility and specificity. *The British Journal of Social and Clinical Psychology, 14*, 55–62.

Caress, A. L. (2003). Giving information to patients. *Nursing Standard, 17*(43), 47–54.

Centers for Disease Control and Prevention. (2009). *Simply put: A guide for creating easy-to-understand materials* (3rd ed.). Atlanta, GA: Author. Retrieved from http://www.cdc.gov/healthcommunication/ToolsTemplates/Simply_Put_082010.pdf

Davis, T. C., Crouch, M. A., Long, S. W., Jackson, R. H., Bates, P., George, R. B., & Bairnsfather, L. E. (1991). Rapid assessment of literacy levels of adult primary care patients. *Family Medicine, 23*, 433–435.

Davis, T. C., Fredrickson, D. D., Arnold, C., Murphy, P. W., Herbst, M., & Bocchini, J. A. (1998). A polio immunization pamphlet with increased appeal and simplified language does not improve comprehension to an acceptable level. *Patient and Education and Counseling, 33*, 25–37.

Doak, C. C., Doak, L. G., & Root, J. H. (1996). *Teaching patients with low literacy skills* (2nd ed.). Philadelphia, PA: J. B. Lippincott.

Dreeben, O. (2010). *Patient education in rehabilitation.* Boston, MA: Jones and Bartlett.

Drench, M. E., Noonan, A. C., Sharby, N., & Hallenborg, V. S. (2007). *Psychosocial aspects of health care* (2nd ed.). Upper Saddle River, NJ: Pearson Education.

Executive Secretariat. (2003). *The plain language initiative.* Retrieved from http://execsec.od.nih.gov/plainlang/guidelines/index.html

Fry, E. (1968). A readability formula that saves time. *Journal of Reading, 11*, 513–516.

Griffin, J., McKenna, K., & Tooth, L. (2006). Discrepancy between older clients' ability to read and comprehend and the reading level of written educational materials used by occupational therapists. *American Journal of Occupational Therapy, 60*, 70–80.

Gunning, R., & Kallan, R. (1994). *How to take the fog out of business writing.* Chicago, IL: Dartnell.

Hafsteinsdóttir, T. B., Vergunst, M., Lindeman, E., & Schuurmans, M. (2011). Education needs of patients with a stroke and their caregivers: A systematic review of the literature. *Patient Education and Counseling*, 85(1), 14–25. doi:10.1016/j.pec.2010.07.046

Haines, T. P., Russell, T., Brauer, S. G., Erwin, S., Lane, P., Urry, S., . . . Condie, P. (2009). Effectiveness of a video-based exercise programme to reduce falls and improve health-related quality of life among older adults discharged from hospital: A pilot randomized controlled trial. *Clinical Rehabilitation, 23*, 973–985. doi: 10.1177/0269215509338998

Institute of Medicine. (2004). *Health literacy: A prescription to end confusion* (Report Brief). Washington, DC: The National Academies Press. Retrieved from http://www.iom.edu/Reports/2004/Health-Literacy-A-Prescription-to-End-Confusion.aspx

Janda, M., Stanek, C., Newman, B., Obermair, A., & Trimmel, M. (2002). Impact of videotaped information on frequency and confidence of breast self-examination. *Breast Cancer Research and Treatment, 73*, 37–43.

Katz, M., Kripalani, S., & Weiss, B. D. (2006). Use of pictorial aids in medication instructions: A review of the literature. *American Journal of Health-System Pharmacy, 63*, 2391–2397. doi:10.2146/ajhp060162

Kessels, R. P. C. (2003). Patients' memory for medical information. *Journal of the Royal Society of Medicine, 96*, 219–222.

Keulers, B. J., Welters, C. F. M., Spauwen, P. H. M., & Houpt, P. (2007). Can face-to-face patient education be replaced by computer-based patient education? A randomised trial. *Patient Education and Counseling, 67*, 176–182. doi:10.1016/j.pec.2007.03.012

Kutner, M., Greenberg, E., Jin, Y., & Paulsen, C. (2006). *The Health Literacy of America's Adults: Results from the 2003 national assessment of adult literacy* (NCES 2006–483). U.S. Department of Education. Washington, DC: National Center for Education Statistics.

Mazor, K. M., Calvi, J., Cowan, R., Costanza, M. E., Han, P. K. J., Greene, S. M., . . . Williams, A. (2010). Media messages about cancer: What do people understand? *Journal of Health Communication, 15*(Suppl. 2), 126–145. doi:10.1080/10810730.2010.499983

Microsoft Office Online. (2010). *Test your documents readability.* Retrieved from http://office.microsoft.com

Moyers, P. A., & Dale, L. M. (2007). *The guide to occupational therapy practice* (2nd ed.). Bethesda, MD: AOTA Press.

National Cancer Institute. (2003). *Clear and simple: Developing effective print materials for low-literate readers.* Retrieved from http://www.cancer.gov/cancertopics/cancerlibrary/clear-and-simple/page1

Nikoletti, S., Kristjanson, L. J., Tataryn, D., McPhee, I., & Burt, L. (2003). Information needs and coping styles of primary family caregivers of women following breast cancer surgery. *Oncology Nursing Forum, 30*, 987–996. doi:10.1188/03.ONF.987–996

O'Connell, B., Baker, L., & Prosser, A. (2003). The educational needs of caregivers of stroke survivors in acute and community settings. *The Journal of Neuroscience Nursing, 35*, 21–28.

Osborne, H. (2005). *Health literacy from A to Z: Practical ways to communicate your health message.* Sudbury, MA: Jones and Bartlett.

Parker, R. M., Baker, D. W., Williams, M. V., & Nurss, J. R. (1995). The test of functional health literacy in adults: A new instrument for measuring patients' literacy skills. *Journal of General Internal Medicine, 10*, 537–541.

Pignone, M., Harris, R., & Kinsinger, L. (2000). Videotape-based decision aid for colon cancer screening. A randomized, controlled trial. *Annals of Internal Medicine, 133*(10), 761–769.

Qualls, C., Harris, J., & Rogers, W. (2002). Cognitive-linguistic aging: Considerations for home health care environments. In W. Rogers & A. Fisk (Eds.), *Human factors interventions for the health care of older adults* (pp. 47–67). Mahwah, NJ: Lawrence Erlbaum.

Rankin, S. H., Stallings, K. D., & London, F. (2005). *Patient education in health and illness* (5th ed.). Philadelphia, PA: Lippincott.

Reid, J. C., Klachko, D. M., Kardash, C. A. M., Robinson, R. D., Scholes, R., & Howard, D. (1995). Why people don't learn from diabetes literature: Influence of text and reader characteristics. *Patient Education and Counseling, 25*, 31–38.

Rudd, R. E., & Anderson, J. E. (2006). *The health literacy environment of hospitals and health centers. Partners for action: Making your health care facility literacy-friendly.* Boston, MA: Harvard School of Public Health. Retrieved from http://www.hsph.harvard.edu/healthliteracy/files/healthliteracyenvironment.pdf

Sarkar, U., Karter, A. J., Liu, J. Y., Adler, N. E., Nguyen, R., Lopez, A., & Schillinger, D. (2010). The literacy divide: Health literacy and the use of an internet-based patient portal in an integrated health system-results from the diabetes study of northern California. *Journal of Health Communication, 15*(Suppl. 2), 183–196. doi:10.1080/10810730.2010.499988

Sarkar, U., Schillinger, D., López, A., & Sudore, R. (2011). Validation of self-reported health literacy questions among diverse English and Spanish-speaking populations. *Journal of General Internal Medicine, 26*(3), 265–271. doi:10.1007/s11606-010-1552-1

Schillinger, D., Piette, J., Grumbach, K., Wang, F., Wilson, C., Daher, C., . . . Bindman, A. B. (2003). Closing the loop: Physician communication with diabetic patients who have low health literacy. *Archives of Internal Medicine, 163*, 83–90.

Sharry, R., McKenna, K., & Tooth, L. (2002). Occupational therapists' use and perceptions of written client education materials. *The American Journal of Occupational Therapy, 56*, 573–576.

Treweek, S. P., Glenton, C., Oxman, A. D., & Penrose, A. (2002). Computer-generated patient education materials: Do they affect professional practice? A systematic review. *Journal of the American Medical Informatics Association, 9*, 346–358. doi:10.1197/jamia.M1070

van Servellen, G. (2009). *Communication skills for the health care professional: Concepts, practice, and evidence* (2nd ed.). Sudbury, MA: Jones and Bartlett.

Wagner, L., Davis, S., & Handelsman, M. M. (1998). In search of the abominable consent form: The impact of readability and personalization. *Journal of Clinical Psychology, 54*(1), 115–120.

Washington, K. T., Meadows, S. E., Elliott, S. G., & Koopman, R. J. (2011). Information needs of informal caregivers of older adults with chronic health conditions. *Patient Education and Counseling, 83*, 37–44. doi:10.1016.j.pec.2010.04.017

Weiss, B. D. (2007). *Health literacy and patient safety: Help patients understand* (2nd ed.). Chicago, IL: American Medical Association Foundation. Retrieved from http://www.ama-assn.org/ama1/pub/upload/mm/367/healthlitclinicians.pdf

Wilson, E. A., & Wolf, M. S. (2009). Working memory and the design of health materials: A cognitive factors perspective. *Patient Education and Counseling, 74*(3), 318–322. doi:10.1016/j.pec.2008.11.005

Wofford, J. L., Smith, E. D., & Miller, D. P. (2005). The multimedia computer for office-based patient education: a systematic review. *Patient Education and Counseling, 59*, 148–157. doi:10.1016/j.pec.2004.10.011

For additional resources on the subjects discussed in this chapter, visit http://thePoint.lww.com/Willard-Spackman12e.

CHAPTER 29

Modifying Performance Contexts

Patricia Rigby, Barry Trentham, Lori Letts

OUTLINE

LEARNING OBJECTIVES

After reading this chapter, you will be able to:

1. Describe why occupational therapists view occupation in context
2. Analyze how environmental factors contribute to performance context
3. Describe interventions that can be applied in various contexts across the life course in clients' homes, workplaces, schools, and communities
4. Critically reflect on how contextual factors may influence your practice as an occupational therapist
5. Examine the evidence supporting specific environmental intervention approaches

Introduction: The Role of Environment and Context in Occupational Therapy Practice

Each human lives in a life space that is built on a system of environments. Occupational therapists recognize that environmental factors have an important influence on their clients' engagement in and performance of occupations (American Occupational Therapy Association [AOTA], 2008; Townsend & Polatajko, 2007). The environment features prominently in numerous models of occupational behavior, performance, and engagement (e.g., Dunn, Brown, & McGuigan, 1994; Kielhofner, 2008; Law et al., 1996; Townsend & Polatajko, 2007). These models view environment broadly, and some emphasize the transactional person-environment-occupation (PEO) relationship. Conceptually, the outcome of a congruent PEO relationship or good PEO fit is optimal occupational performance and engagement (Law et al., 1996). When there is less congruence or a poor PEO fit, modifying the environment becomes an important strategy to improve fit and occupational performance and engagement.

Environments, as described in the *International Classification System for Functioning, Disability and Health* (ICF) (World Health Organization [WHO], 2001), can include physical elements (products and technology and natural environment and human-made changes to the environment); social elements (social support and relationships); attitudes (arising from customs, practices, ideologies, values, norms, and beliefs); and services, systems, and policies. These are described more fully in Box 29.1. The ICF also notes that **context** is the interconnection of personal factors such as gender, race, age, lifestyle, social background, education, occupation, and psychological characteristics with environmental factors (WHO, 2001).

The environment also plays an important role in shaping human experience and behavior over time. A person's values and beliefs are shaped by social and cultural elements of the environment. At the same time, people actively shape and influence the environments in which they live, work, and play. Occupations occur within a context that is unique to each person's circumstances. Consequently, the meaning attached to that occupation and to the place or environment in which the occupation takes place will influence a person's engagement in any given occupation, and this may vary across time. Thus, it is critical that we understand that our clients' occupational experiences cannot be separated from ***contextual influences*** (AOTA, 2008). In Chapter 18, the meaning of place and space was explored and explained. Those concepts and recommendations for occupational therapy practice are critically important when considering interventions to modify the context for occupational performance and engagement.

Occupational therapists routinely modify environments to enable clients to engage in occupations. These modifications can enhance performance and engagement in occupations, plus the safety and comfort of the client, caregivers, and others. Environmental modifications may also affect others in a setting, not just our clients. Thus, we must consider what is most appropriate for all who use or could use the setting.

Environmental settings can afford people with possibilities for actions, which, depending on an individual's previous and current experiences, can be viewed as opportunities and resources or demands and barriers. For example, a retired couple moved from their house in the suburbs to a condominium in a high-rise building in the center of their city, which was connected to a large shopping mall with shops, businesses, theatres, and access to the public transit system. They anticipated using the many resources in the mall and being actively engaged in the many leisure opportunities available to them. However, they found it difficult to find their way around the mall, the doors were heavy and difficult to open, and the crowds made them nervous. As a result, environmental features initially viewed as supportive became barriers to participation and engagement in occupations.

There is a growing body of evidence that demonstrates the efficacy of modifying context to enable occupational performance and engagement. For example, home modifications and assistive technologies (ATs) for the home, together with caregiver training and education, help improve clients' activities of daily living (ADL), prevent falls, and reduce injuries (Gosman-Hedstrom, Claesson, & Blomstrand, 2002; Niva & Skar, 2006; Stark, 2004). Participation in social and community-based occupations is enabled when environmental barriers are removed (Lysack, Komanecky, Kabel, Cross, & Neufeld, 2007; Ward, Mitchell, & Price, 2007). Furthermore, occupational therapists agree that modifying performance contexts can

BOX 29.1 Environment Factors of the ICF

1. ***Products and technology***: The natural or human-made products or systems of products, equipment, and technology in an individual's immediate environment that are gathered, created, produced, or manufactured. Examples include wheelchairs and speech-generating devices.
2. ***Natural environment and human-made changes to environment:*** Animate and inanimate elements of the natural or physical environment and components of that environment that have been modified by people as well as characteristics of the population in that environment. Examples include sound, temperature, and lighting.
3. ***Support and relationships***: People or animals that provide practical physical or emotional support, nurturing, protection and assistance, and relationships to other persons in the home, place of work, school, at play, or in other aspects of their daily activities. Examples include family members, friends, and personal care workers.
4. ***Attitudes:*** Attitudes are the observable consequences of customs, practices, ideologies, values, norms, factual beliefs, and religious beliefs. The attitudes classified are those of people external to the person whose situation is being described, not of the person himself or herself. Examples include individual attitudes of family and professionals, societal attitudes, and social norms.
5. ***Services, systems, and policies***: *Services* comprise structured programs, operations, and services—public, private, or voluntary—established at a local, community, regional, national, or international level by employers, associations, organizations, agencies, or government in order to meet the needs of individuals and includes the persons who provide these services. *Systems* and *policies* respectively comprise the administrative control and monitoring mechanisms and rules, regulations, and standards established by local, regional, national, and international government or other recognized authorities, which organize services, programs, and other infrastructural activities in various sectors of society. Examples include availability of and policies for accessible transportation and housing.

be easier to achieve and have more immediate enabling effects than using interventions that try to "fix the person" (Egilson & Traustadottir, 2009; Rigby & Letts, 2003; Stark, 2004). The evidence to support modifying contexts is described in greater detail at the end of this chapter.

Terminology Use in This Chapter

Throughout this chapter, the term *client* may refer to individuals, groups, organizations, or communities regardless of their health or functional status. Although occupational therapists, for the most part, work with individual clients who live with physical or mental health conditions or disabilities, the authors of this chapter assume that clients may include anyone who experiences barriers to occupational performance or engagement. So, for example, people who are not disabled with respect to activity limitations may indeed still face barriers to occupational participation due to restrictive or discriminatory societal attitudes or life course occupational transition difficulties and could therefore benefit from the expertise of an occupational therapist.

Human Rights and the Rights to an Inclusive and Accessible Environment

The Universal Declaration of Human Rights (U.S. Department of State, 1948) outlines the rights and freedoms to which all humans are entitled regardless of their status, including race, color, sex, social origins, or other status. From this, various legislation has been developed across the world, bridging the gap from international treaties to state-level, municipal, or organizational policies. They all shape how social groups or individuals are included or not in the public domain. These laws and policies reflect cultural values, from the more individualist North American cultures to those of more collectivist societies in Africa and Asia, where values placed on the common good are reflected in the development and access to public spaces and institutions.

Antidiscrimination laws have been developed in many jurisdictions to ensure ***inclusion*** of all minority groups, including peoples of minority ethnic, religious, or sexual identities. For example, the Canadian Human Rights Act (1976) prohibits discrimination based on race, national or ethnic origin, color, religion, age, sex, sexual orientation, disability, and other status. Many of these policies were hard-won achievements and, like the American Civil Rights Act of 1964, came at the expense of tremendous committed effort and even the lives of people dedicated to making the world a more socially inclusive place for all people to participate. At an organizational level, companies and public institutions develop employment equity policies that ideally prevent discrimination. These laws and policies serve to ensure that all people have access to housing, work, education, and other publicly and privately funded opportunities. In essence, they enable or disable occupational engagement.

The rights of people with disabilities are typically protected in developed countries through human or civil rights laws. For example, the Americans with Disabilities Act (ADA; 1990) was designed to create equal opportunity and equal access to public environments, services, employment, accommodations, telecommunications, and transportation across the United States. The ADA Amendments Act of 2008 provides a revised definition of "disability" to more broadly encompass impairments that substantially limit a major life activity, such as going to work. The ADA Standards for Accessible Design outline how both public and private sector services, programs, and facilities must comply with and implement accessibility requirements (U.S. Department of Justice, 2010). Accessibility guidelines have also been developed for play areas, public rights of way, and outdoor recreation areas (U.S. Access Board, 2005, 2007). The focus of the ADA and of similar legislation in many countries is to enable people with disabilities to achieve social inclusion and independent living. Chapter 70 provides additional insight about these issues. Occupational therapists should become familiar with the policies and laws that influence marginalized populations and persons with disabilities because this knowledge will affect their practice.

These social policies undergo ongoing revision and development and provide a space for occupational therapists to promote equitable access to occupational engagement for all social groups. Indeed, many leaders in the field have called on occupational therapists as potential leaders themselves to become more involved in building healthy public policy (Clark, 2010; Letts, 2009; Scaffa & Bonder, 2009; Townsend & Polatajko, 2007) within whatever environmental contexts they potentially have influence. Many occupational therapy and occupational science researchers actively use their research to promote the creation of public policy that fosters socially and physically inclusive environments. In short, to become leaders in society, occupational therapists must go beyond acting as gatekeepers and implementers of existing public policy to becoming active in the development and creation of inclusive social policy.

Framing Interventions to Modify Performance Context

While the ICF is useful in rehabilitation because it classifies environmental factors and illustrates the complex relationship between disability, participation, and environment (WHO, 2001), the authors of this chapter feel it is also useful to view the environment from the perspective of Bronfenbrenner's (2005) bioecological model. His model describes the interrelationships between the various levels of environment. Although this model is primarily concerned with human development over time, the manner in which it conceptualizes the dynamic interplay of environmental systems is particularly relevant for occupational therapy's focus on occupational engagement and performance.

The model is composed of five systems: the *microsystem*, *mesosystem*, *exosystem*, *macrosystem*, and *chronosystem*, as shown in Figure 29.1. The nested systems interact and fuse with each other. The microsystem is where individuals have the most direct involvement and includes home, neighborhoods, places of worship, or schools. The mesosystem represents the interaction of various microsystems. For example, a child's family relationships in the home environment will impact how he or she performs within the school microsystem. The exosystem is a sphere that people have less involvement with but nevertheless impacts their occupational engagement. For example, government policies that define funding opportunities for assistive technologies (ATs) impact how an individual functions within any given microsystem. The macrosystem includes the cultural and social structures within which all people live. The values and traditions that guide how people interact with one another are examples of the contextual features of this system. One might consider how the values associated with the culturally dominant Western ways of thinking within a North American context shape shared understandings of the therapeutic process and how these interact with the many diverse cultural contexts within which therapists work. Finally, the chronosystem is concerned with the important element of time and history and how changing contexts over time impact on and interact with the life course transitions of individuals.

Importantly, Bonfrenbrenner's model recognizes that people engage within these environmental systems by taking on changing roles at different times throughout their lives. As well, as noted earlier, occupational therapists interact in different ways across these systems in order to enable the occupational performance of their clients. The case study of Gary Lau in this chapter illustrates how occupational therapists might engage with individuals within the home microsystem to improve physical access while **advocating** at the level of the exosystem for greater access to funding for home renovations and ATs. The case study also shows how both the client's and the therapist's cultural values interact at a macrosystem level, which influences the therapeutic relationship.

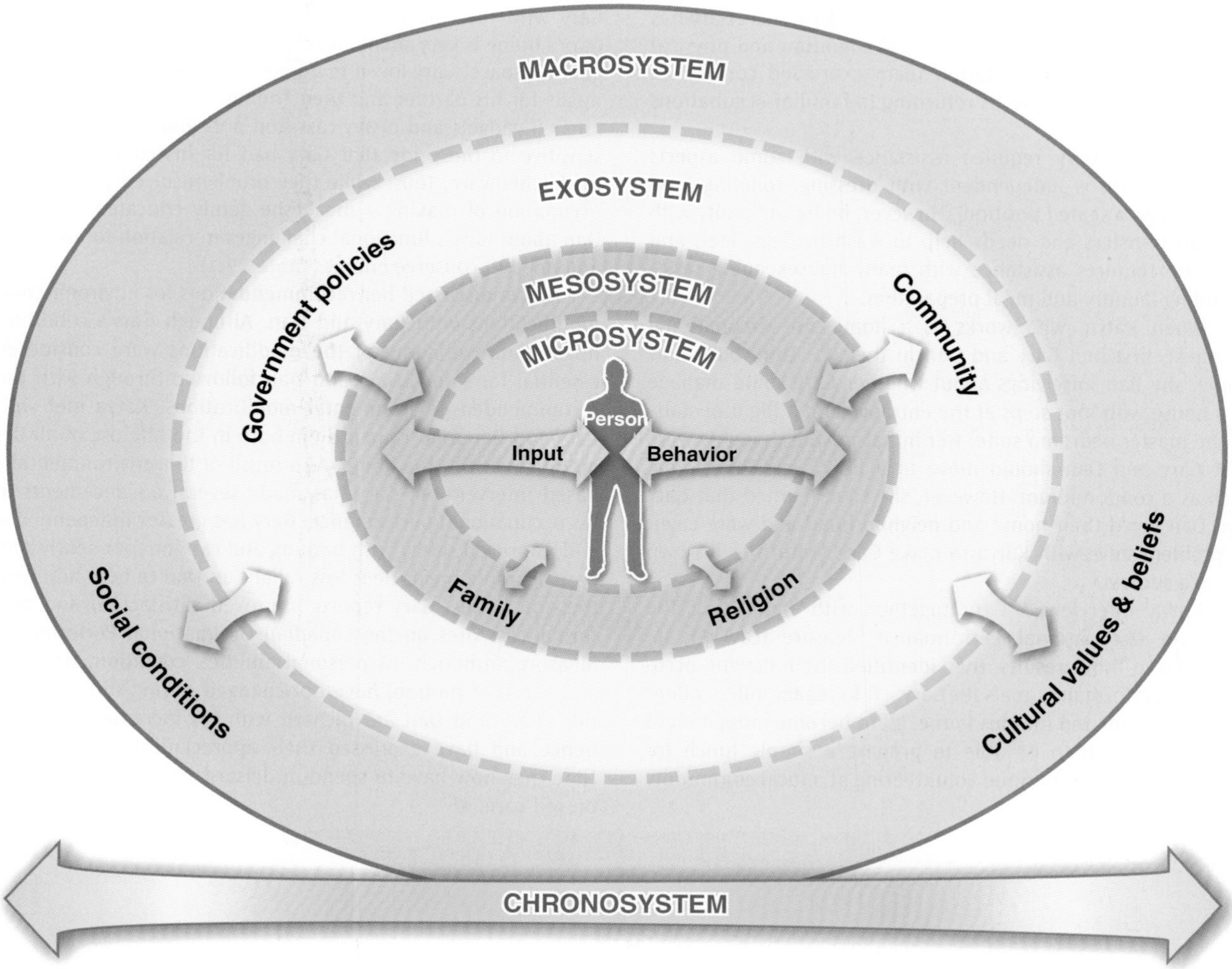

FIGURE 29.1 The dynamic interplay between levels of the environment as demonstrated by Bronfenbrenner's bioecological model.

CASE STUDY 29.1 Part One: Gary Lau Readjusting to Home Life Following an Acquired Brain Injury

Gary Lau is a 52-year-old man who sustained a closed brain injury with diffuse axonal injury as the result of a motor vehicle accident (see Appendix I, Common Conditions, for more information about acquired brain injury). Before his brain injury, Gary worked full time as a mechanical engineer. He lives with his partner, Dan; they have no children. In the past, he enjoyed participating in social activities with family and friends, community volunteering, playing sports, and many outdoor activities. Gary perceives himself to be very independent, a risk taker, and stubborn at times.

The brain injury resulted in both cognitive and physical impairments. Following 5 months of intensive therapy, Gary was discharged home. Gary has left hemiplegia, decreased balance, and an unsteady gait; he uses a quad cane (a cane with four prongs) for walking. He has no voluntary spontaneous movement in his left hand and cannot grasp things with that hand. In addition to impairments to his short-term memory, he has limitations in his executive function, including difficulty initiating tasks, poor organization, and poor judgment and safety. He demonstrates decreased insight; although aware of his deficits, he does not fully appreciate how his deficits affect his occupational performance. Gary has made appreciable gains in recovery of cognition and physical abilities, and the rehabilitation team expressed confidence that he will recover more by returning to familiar occupations in familiar settings.

Currently, Gary requires assistance with some aspects of self-care. He is independent with dressing, toileting, and grooming (in a seated position). However, he has difficulty with bathtub transfers and needs help to wash his legs, feet, and back. He requires assistance with many housekeeping tasks, including laundry and meal preparation.

When Katya, who works as a home-care occupational therapist, first met Gary and Dan in their 1½ story bungalow home, she had misgivings about whether Gary could manage in a house with four steps at the entrance and a flight of stairs to the master bedroom suite. Her initial private thoughts were that Gary and Dan should move to a fully accessible home, such as a condominium. However, she soon learned that Gary and Dan loved their home and neighborhood and were eager to problem-solve with Katya to make Gary's return to his own home a success.

Katya interviewed Gary together with Dan using the Canadian Occupational Performance Measure (Law et al., 2005). From those results, they identified the following occupational performance goals for Gary: (1) to regain independent mobility within and into his home, (2) to become independent with bathing, (3) to be able to prepare a simple lunch for himself, and (4) to continue volunteering at a local community center.

The first priority for Gary and Dan was accessibility in the home. A ramp was installed at the side entrance to the house and a stair lift was installed to enable Gary to access the second floor. Katya helped access funding for these renovations through Gary's private health insurance.

Katya's initial assessment of the bathroom and the kitchen revealed numerous barriers. Katya then analyzed the accessibility of the bathroom in relation to Gary's occupational performance needs. This analysis led her to recommend several minor modifications using ATs, which included installing a bath transfer bench with a back, plus a clamp-on bar at the side of the tub and a vertical grab bar on the wall beside the tub. She also recommended he use a nonslip bath mat in the tub to reduce his chances of slipping and falling and a handheld shower, which will allow him to control the shower spray and provide him greater independence with bathing.

Gary presents with decreased safety and independence with meal preparation secondary to both cognitive and physical impairments. On assessing the kitchen environment, Katya could see that some physical features were not a good fit for Gary with his current functional limitations. The kitchen in Gary's home is very small and cluttered, and it has very limited counter space. Gary loved to do gourmet cooking and to make meals for his partner and their friends. He has many modern kitchen gadgets and heavy cast iron pots and pans. Katya was sensitive to the pride that Gary had for his cooking and for his kitchenware; thus, while they problem-solved through the occupation of making a meal, she gently educated Gary and Dan about Gary's functional challenges in relation to his safety and need to conserve energy (Table 29.1).

Katya discussed her recommendations for environmental modifications with Gary and Dan. Although Gary's condition might improve, some of the modifications were considered essential for safety. Gary and Dan followed through with the recommended environmental modifications. Katya met with Gary and Dan and trained them both in the safe use of all the modifications in the home. As a result of this environmentally based intervention, Gary has made several advancements in his occupational performance. Gary has greater independence and improved safety with bathing and can independently prepare a simple meal. He is less reliant on Dan to help him with these activities. Gary reports improved satisfaction and performance scores on the Canadian Occupational Performance Measure, although his personal abilities (cognition, strength, and range of motion) have not changed during this intervention. Gary and Dan are pleased with his increased independence and have expressed their appreciation for the extra time they now have to spend on leisure activities rather than on self-care. ■

CASE STUDY 29.1 Part One: Gary Lau Readjusting to Home Life Following an Acquired Brain Injury *(Continued)*

TABLE 29.1 Modifications to Gary Lau's Kitchen to Address the Occupational Performance Goal of Preparing a Simple Meal

Occupational Performance	Intervention Recommendations	Rationale for Intervention
Meal Preparation • Mobility: Gary is ambulating around the kitchen with a quad cane, and he has impaired left hand function. He finds it difficult to transfer heavier items such as foods and plates.	• Recommend that Gary use a four-wheeled walker (rollator) with a tray/basket or a tea trolley. • Consider purchasing lightweight pots, pans, and plates.	• Enable him to independently and safely transfer items to and from counter, stove, and refrigerator to the table. • Enable him to safely lift and use items while conserving energy.
• Cupboards are installed high on walls, with dishes stored on the top shelves. Gary's ability to engage in overhead reaching is limited by poor balance and impaired fine and gross motor coordination.	• Lower the height of the cupboards. • Relocate items in the cupboards so the items that are most frequently used are in easy-to-reach places. • A long-handled reacher can be used for overhead reaching of light items.	• Allow Gary to have easy access and promote safe reaching. • Avoid unnecessary bending and reaching. • Reduce risk of falls due to overreaching (which can contribute to loss of balance).
• Deficits in short-term memory and executive function • Gary sometimes forgets and needs to be reminded to turn off the stove.	• Place written sign above stove that reads "TURN OFF STOVE." • Use a timer for reminder; when the timer sounds, that acts as a cue to turn off the stove. • When preparing a meal while home alone, prepare something that does not require use of the stove.	• Use compensatory strategies to enhance independence and safety.
• Deficits in short-term memory and executive function	• Group ingredients, tools, and items that Gary uses most frequently together in one area (in cupboard, in the refrigerator). • Label drawers and cupboards so that Gary knows exactly where to look to retrieve the cooking utensils and ingredients that he needs. • Gary and Dan could generate step-by-step instructions for commonly prepared items and place these in clear plastic jackets so that Gary can use an erasable marker to tick off steps as they are completed.	• Compensates for short-term memory deficits and increases independence.

Importantly, therapists need to be aware of how their own micro, meso, exo, macro, and chronological contexts shape their interactions with their clients. This requires a ***reflexive*** and critically self-aware stance.

Interventions

When the assessment process is complete, interventions focusing on the client's identified targeted occupational goals are developed using a systematic approach such as the Occupational Therapy Practice Framework (AOTA, 2008) or the Canadian Practice Process Framework (Craik, Davis, & Polatajko, 2007). The goal of enabling occupational performance and engagement guides the development of the intervention plan.

In this section, we first present design approaches and technologies that support occupational performance and engagement and then describe various intervention strategies for the home, school, workplace, and community settings. Some interventions can be applied at the microsystem and mesosystem level with individual clients, and others can be applied at the broader exosystem and macrosystem levels with groups and communities or at a societal level. Those interventions applied at the microsystem and mesosystems level are typically client centered and take into account the clients' specific needs and their situations, whereas interventions from the group or population perspective should be based on knowledge of the common and diverse challenges, expectations, and/or needs of that population (Iwarsson & Ståhl, 2003).

Interventions directed at modifying physical context involve making architectural changes to places and spaces and the provision of ATs. Modifying the social context can involve developing and mobilizing social resources, plus training and educating these resources about how best to support the occupational performance and engagement of our clients. Modifying social and cultural context can involve advocacy, consultation, education, and policy development at the mesosystem, macrosystem, and exosystem to broaden awareness, change attitudes and views, and support programs and services for our clients. Occupational therapists typically employ several of these strategies in concert. Throughout this chapter, examples from the case study of Gary Lau are used to illustrate various strategies for modifying the performance context, including those that use several strategies in concert.

Design Strategies and Technologies to Support Occupational Performance

Universal Design

Universal design (UD) is a way to create products and environments that are more usable by everyone, regardless of age or ability (Mace, 1985; Ostrof, 2001). UD involves thinking about a range of human abilities before the environment is built. The seven principles of UD developed by the Center for Universal Design (1997) integrate accessibility and usability features in design. Today, UD is considered across most settings, including housing, office buildings, airports, restaurants, and parks. It recognizes human differences in shapes, sizes, ages, abilities, and cultures and promotes inclusion and ergonomic design for all people. For example, the level entrance and power sliding doors at the entrance to a grocery store makes the store accessible to everyone. In this case, the entrance design accommodates people who are pushing the grocery carts, those pushing baby carriages, or those moving large objects on a cart as well as those using wheelchairs or mobility devices.

Accessible Design

Accessible design, also referred to as barrier-free design, adds accessibility to otherwise inaccessible buildings, products, and services to enable persons with disabilities to function independently (Iwarsson & Ståhl, 2003). For example, braille can be added to elevator keypads to enable persons with visual impairments to select the floor number they want. Often, accessible design responds to specific requirements and standards as laid out in legislation, such as the ADA and in building codes. It can be applied to make buildings, products, and services accessible to special populations. Accessible design can also be applied at the microsystem level with changes made to specific aspect of the environment in the home, school, or workplace to achieve PEO fit for individual clients. Occupational therapists routinely apply their knowledge about accessible design in their daily practice.

Assistive Technologies

Assistive technologies are devices, adaptive equipment, or products that are designed to enable persons with disabilities to engage in daily occupations within their homes, schools, workplaces, and communities. (Cook & Polgar, 2008). They fall into the products and technology category within the environmental factors domain of the ICF (WHO, 2001). As will be shown throughout this chapter, ATs are routinely prescribed by occupational therapists to address specific occupational performance goals of their clients, including those for ADL, mobility, and communication. These technologies range from simple devices such as grab bars and raised toilet seats to more complex devices such as powered wheelchairs and speech-generating devices (Figure 29.2).

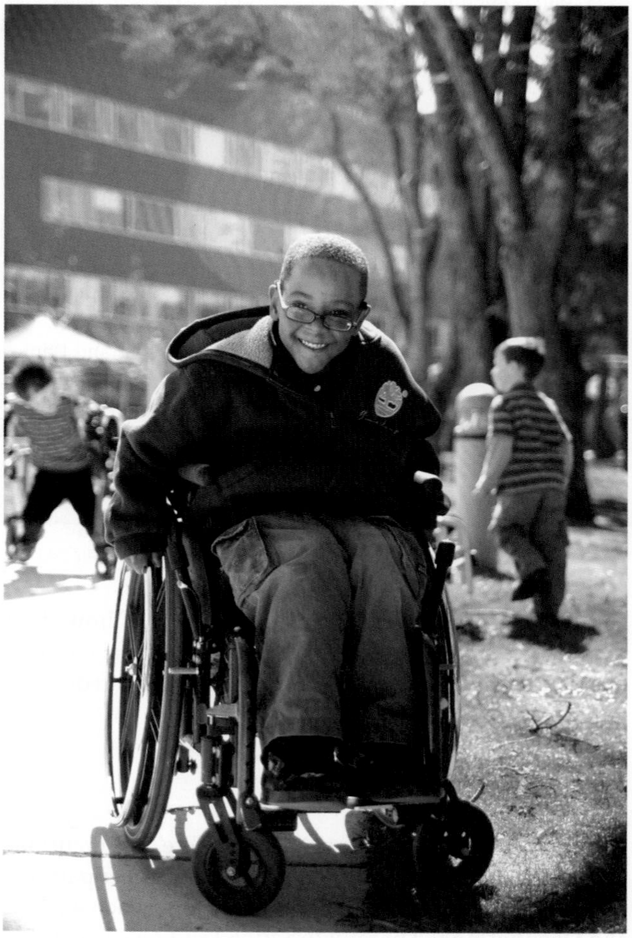

FIGURE 29.2 Wheelchairs are a commonly used assistive technology for mobility and enable participation in daily life.

ATs have undergone dramatic innovation over the past 20 years, and the availability and quality of the technologies have greatly improved (Cook & Polgar, 2008; Fuhrer, Jutai, Scherer, & DeRuyter, 2003). ATs are widely used by persons with disabilities. For example, in 2006, nearly two-thirds of the 2.7 million Canadians with a disability who were 15 years and older used ATs to help them perform one or more daily occupations (Statistics Canada, 2006). In the mid-1990s, in the United States, there were 1.6 million wheelchair users living in the community (Kaye, Kang, & LaPlante, 2000). There is growing evidence that ATs can improve occupational performance (e.g., Rigby, Ryan, & Campbell, 2009; Ripat, 2006), enhance quality of life (e.g., Chan & Chan, 2007; Rigby, Ryan, & Campbell, 2011), and reduce caregiver burden (e.g., Agree, Freedman, Cornman, Wolf, & Marcotee, 2005; Chen, Mann, Tomita, & Nochajski, 2000).

Smart Technologies

Computers and smart technologies are transforming how people live their lives and perform their daily occupations. Smart phones and mobile computers are rapidly developing and many have been developed using UD principles, making them very user friendly and accessible. For example, many have easy to use and see LCD touch screens, enlarged keyboards, and menu-driven software. It is becoming common to see many people, from children through older adults, using smart phones, computer tablets, and laptop computers in public spaces. Occupational therapists find many features and new applications made for these technologies helpful for enabling their clients' occupational performance. For example, persons with memory impairments can use the schedule reminder on their smart phone to organize their day, and persons with motor impairments can use voice commands to operate their phone.

Smart home technologies are also becoming more common and range from simple forms of home automation like the X-10 system that allows the remote control of multiple electronic switches in the home such as lights and appliances, to innovative new systems that use sophisticated artificial intelligence to provide persons with cognitive impairments with reminders and guidance through their daily routines (Mihailidis, Boger, Hoey, & Jiancaro, 2011).

Web-Based Technologies

Web-based technologies are rapidly changing and have changed the structure of communities (Figure 29.3). We are now a networked society in which we have multiple links to various work, community, and friendship networks. Social support as experienced through online communities has been shown to have correlates with ratings on mental health and well-being, life satisfaction, engagement in social activities, and sense of community (Aguilar, Boerema, & Harrison, 2010; Erickson & Johnson, 2011; Sum, Mathews, Pourghasem, & Hughes, 2009). Networked communities have been shown to support community development (CD) initiatives where neighborhood and interest group linkages have enabled groups to collectively advocate for shared interests, and lobby companies or government officials for proposed changes (Hampton & Wellman, 2003).

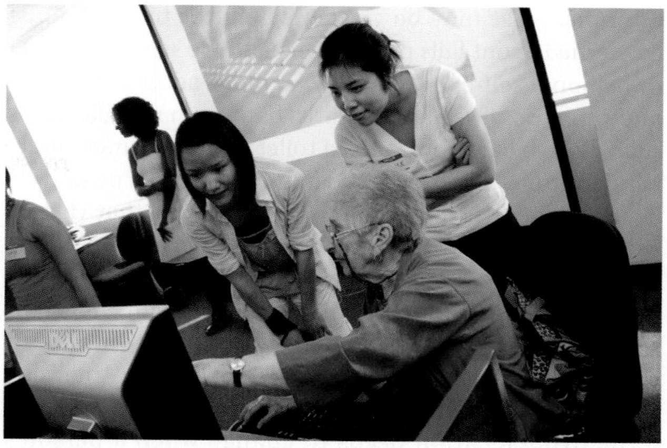

FIGURE 29.3 Occupational therapy students collaborating with an older adult on the use of Web-based, social media.

Disabled and isolated older adults stand to benefit in particular from online community engagement because they are no longer limited by physical access barriers, geographic distances, or perhaps even ageist attitudes that disrupt information sharing. Enabling online participation is now an important consideration for occupational therapists. Much has been written about the potential barriers faced by people living with disabilities as well as the unique design features that should be considered when developing accessible Web spaces and online community formats. Examples include poor vision, diminished fine-motor control and coordination, as well as, for older adults, the possibility for changes to learning speed and accuracy (Snyder, 2002).

Occupational therapists can play a vital role in assisting their clients to access and learn how to use these various technologies in their daily lives. It is important that occupational therapists stay abreast of new developments and be open to their potential for enabling occupation.

Modifying the Home Environment

Home is the context for a broad range of occupations, from basic ADL like bathing to social events and celebrations with family. Home is a multidimensional concept, which includes a physical space within a geographic location but has emotional, cultural, and personal elements (Mitty & Flores, 2009). Home is frequently one of the most cherished environments in people's lives, and people make meaning out of their life events through their homes (Cristoforetti, Gennai, & Rodeschini, 2011). The home has been described as having three elements: physical, social, and personal (Tanner, Tilse, & deJonge, 2008). The implications of modifications to a physical aspect of a home should be considered in light of these other elements. For example, what may be viewed as clutter to a therapist concerned about falls prevention could be seen as a threat to personal self-expression by an older adult with many important possessions. Similarly, bathroom modifications such as grab bars and a raised toilet seat to promote independent toileting for a client might be viewed negatively by the client if the bathroom is the main one that visitors would use. Chapter 18 provides more information on the meaning of place and space in daily life.

Often, the primary goal of clients in an inpatient setting is to go home; the goal of older adults with chronic conditions is to be able to stay home (American Association of Retired Persons, 2000). However, even if the living location needs to change when a person's health or social situation requires support in a congregate living environment, that new home can be given meaning with personal objects (Cipriani et al., 2009).

Beyond considering the home as a physical space and the need for modifications of the physical environment within clients' homes, therapists need to be attentive to the nature of home as a social sphere, which might also be modified to support clients' return to or remaining home. **Social supports** at home can sometimes be implemented as an environmental intervention that can overcome physical barriers associated with the home environment. The elements of the social and personal meanings of home may help therapists and others understand the importance of home beyond its physical layout and features. This is illustrated in the case study of Gary Lau.

When dealing with clients' homes, a number of intervention strategies can be considered in the environment to maximize the person's ability to engage in his or her occupations. These can range from building a new home following a catastrophic injury to making minor changes to the living space like rearranging furniture. Modifications can also incorporate formal or informal supports, ranging from personal care workers to help with bathing to family assistance with meal preparations.

Occupational therapists should also keep in mind that any modifications to different types of homes, whether they are situated in suburban neighborhoods, urban apartments or condominiums, or within congregate living arrangements such as group homes or retirement homes, are contingent on different regulations and processes. Prior to making recommendations, therapists should inform themselves of the various policy and legal considerations and guidelines that apply to the various housing types. In addition, therapists must be aware of how home modifications will impact other residents. This is particularly an issue when working in congregate living settings.

Ideal Features of an Accessible Home

For people requiring accessible housing, ideal features vary depending on their needs. Most frequently, accessible housing is sought when people have issues related to mobility, requiring use of a mobility device such as a walker or manual or power wheelchair. Box 29.2 includes a number of the key features that can make a home accessible for someone with mobility impairments

ATs can be incorporated to improve accessibility. For example, electronic aids to daily living, which enable a person to electronically control the physical environment, can be installed (e.g., for locking and unlocking entrances, opening and closing blinds, and manipulating home electronics such as the television).

Occupational therapists may provide consultation to clients if accessible housing is being sought or built. This may occur following an acquired disability resulting from an incident causing spinal cord injury or acquired brain injury. In these situations, it is important to work with the client and family to identify the most important accessibility features required.

Major Home Modifications

Not all clients are able to find accessible housing. Other clients are reluctant to move away from their family home. Both of these situations may result in a need to consider modifying the physical environment of the home in which the client is currently residing. The two most common areas of the home that require modifications are the entrance to the home and bathrooms.

Entrances are most frequently modified with the installation of either ramps or porch lifts. A major consideration in recommending these relates to the height from the ground level to the entrance. Because a ramp requires a minimum of 12 in of length for each inch of rise, there

BOX 29.2 Physical Features of an Accessible Home

- Exterior walkway smooth and graded
- Level entrance
- Lever handles on all doors
- Inside doorway widths sufficient for mobility device
- Adequate turning space in bathrooms/entry
- Access to home systems (e.g., electrical panel, furnace)
- Ample lighting
- Cabinet heights in kitchen and bathroom allow seated access
- Furniture arrangements allow mobility
- Floor surface levels allow mobility
- Structural supports for equipment such as ceiling tracks
- Access to environmental controls (e.g., light switches) and appliances
- Emergency exit available

are occasions when a ramp is simply not feasible. When they are possible, a front or side door is typically designated for access.

In circumstances when the height from the ground to the entrance is too high to make a ramp feasible, the most common alternative used is a porch lift. In addition, some clients are unwilling to install a ramp because of concerns related to aesthetics, and they choose a lift because it can be more discreetly installed. Some considerations in the selection of lifts include back-up electrical or manual systems in case of power failures and a need to consider the climate in which the home is located. Ideally, there will be more than one entrance/exit accessible to the client so that in case of an emergency such as a fire, at least one exit is available. If there is only one accessible entrance, escape plans in case of emergencies are advised. In the case study of Gary Lau, the occupational therapist helped Gary and his partner consider the various options for making the entrance to his home accessible; and in his case, a ramp to the side entrance to his home was considered the best solution.

Bathrooms often require major modification because they are typically small, making mobility within the space challenging. In addition, transferring to and from a toilet and bath/shower can present challenges. Although minor modifications such as grab bars and handheld showers might be adequate in some circumstances, other clients require major modifications in the bathroom. These can range from moving or removing fixtures to installation of new fixtures such as roll-in shower stalls, higher toilets, and sink and tap fixtures that can be readily managed.

Because major modifications at the entrance and bathroom are costly, it is important for the therapist to work closely with the client and family to consider current as well as possible future needs.

Minor Home Modifications

Major modifications to the physical environment of a client's home are not always required. There are many times when minor modifications provide solutions to challenges experienced in the home. ATs such as a bath bench and handheld shower for someone who is unable to enter and stand for a shower is a common minor modification that occupational therapists provide. Therapists also recommend off-the-shelf products that support performance such as adding a handrail to the wall for stairs to the basement or an automatic shut-off kettle for someone with early cognitive decline.

Occupational therapists can also suggest that clients modify the way they use the physical environment. For example, they can teach individuals to make use of features of their existing environment in ways that make it safer or easier to perform daily activities. This may mean rearranging items in kitchen cupboards, organizing items in a basket to be carried up and down stairs, or programming the telephone to make use of autodial functions to make it easy for someone with memory issues to contact family.

Supports from others are often also important to consider. Sometimes, help from others can make it possible for someone to remain in his or her home environment. For example, having a neighbor collect mail from a community mailbox can not only overcome challenges with outdoor mobility but can also provide a social connection for an older adult living alone. Having a personal support worker assist with bathing can be an alternative to installing assistive devices.

Considerations to Implementing Home Modifications

By focusing on the goals of the client, the therapist can generate several possible environmental strategies that can be implemented. There is often more than one environmental solution available to address an occupational issue. For example, in the case study for Gary Lau, modifications to the bathroom could be avoided if Gary were to receive personal assistance for transfers in and out of the bathtub and bathing (either from Gary's partner Dan or from a paid support worker). Another strategy would be to make major modifications to Gary and Dan's bathroom to replace the traditional tub and shower space with a walk-in shower with a modular seat. In the end, the occupational therapist, Gary, and Dan chose to use a combination of minor modifications (grab bars) and simple off-the-shelf products (bath mat, hand held shower). It is important to review with a client the range of environmental modifications that might address his or her goals and work together to consider current and future needs, the needs of others living in or using the home environment, costs, and complexity of each modification in order to support the client to choose the solution that is optimal.

Funding of home modifications is an important factor and can sometimes present a barrier to implementation of the optimal solution. Renovations can be expensive, and, depending on the client's circumstances, insurance companies may not provide financial supports. People often rely on personal resources or social service agencies to fund the modifications. Occupational therapists should be familiar with their local social service agencies that provide for such modifications and may need to work collaboratively with the client to apply for funding supports. Occupational therapists have an important duty to help justify the need for home modifications to payers (whether insurers, social service agencies, or other funding bodies). Although home renovations are costly, paid support workers are also expensive. Justification for modifications to the physical environment may in part be that the increased independence of the client will decrease costs associated with paid support workers.

A final consideration related to home modifications is the relationship between the various parties involved in any renovations. Although occupational therapists may recommend major or minor modifications to the physical environment, the implementation of any modifications is completed by others and should be overseen by the client or family. The AT vendor or a skilled family member can sometimes do minor modifications, such as installing grab bars. Major modifications or home renovations involve a complex team that might include an architect, contractor, trades people, AT vendors, or even builders in the case of a new home. However, occupational therapists can advise clients on strategies to consult and collaborate with all parties to oversee modifications to the home environment.

Modifying the School Context

Occupational therapists play a critical role in enabling students with various conditions and disabilities to succeed in school settings and to participate in classroom, playground, and extracurricular activities (Mu & Royeen, 2004; Reid, Chu, Sinclair, Wehrmann, & Nazeer, 2006). Researchers describe how various environmental factors can help or hinder students' participation in school-based occupations and urge occupational therapists to modify school contexts to support students at school (Egilson & Traustadottir, 2009; Heah, Case, McGuire, & Law, 2007; Law, Petrenchik, King, & Hurley, 2007; Villeneuve, 2009). Examples provided subsequently demonstrate how therapists can modify the school context from the microsystem through exosystem levels. Further information about school-based practice is provided in Chapter 48.

Although it is now common to find legislation and policies that support the inclusion of students with ***disabling*** conditions in their local schools, inclusion can be challenging to achieve due to many environmental obstacles. Physical barriers, such as heavy doors, raised thresholds at doors, and absence of elevators in multilevel schools are still common. School culture and attitudes of teachers and classmates can also create barriers to inclusion. For example, a teacher may misunderstand the classroom behaviors and performance of a student with a learning disability and react in a manner that exacerbates the student's distress, and classmates might make fun of and exclude this same student. The participation and inclusion of students with disabilities cannot succeed until adequate resources and supports are put into place to address these barriers.

Modifying the performance context in schools can take many forms. The most common approach is to modify the physical environment by modifying and adapting furniture and educational materials, accessing ATs, and making architectural modifications to schools. Occupational therapists also use strategies to modify the social, cultural, and organizational environments of schools to support students' inclusion and participation. Examples include sensitivity education for school staff and students, advocating for social supports in the classroom (e.g., teaching assistants or peer mentors) and collaborating with teachers to modify and adapt curriculum to support students' learning.

Modifications to the physical environment can happen at the microsystem level for individual students and at the exosystem level to make schools accessible for persons with disabilities. For example, therapists can consult about and advocate for architectural accessibility and the use of universal design principles within schools. They can also consult with individual schools or school boards to prepare annual accessibility plans or to assist in the design and planning of new schools and planning for major renovations to make schools more accessible. Examples of specific modifications using ATs can include installing electronic door openers, lever-style taps at sinks, and grab bars in the toilet stall.

Classroom environments can have high levels of sensory stimuli in terms of noise, visual clutter, and the physical activity of a classroom full of students, which can have a disorganizing effect for children with sensory-processing problems. Occupational therapists assess the classroom environment to identify the sensory features that either facilitate or hinder students' ability to complete schoolwork and recommend modifying the space to better fit students' sensory-processing needs. For example, sound-absorbing partitions and low lighting can enable some students to focus their attention while working on individual assignments. The therapist might recommend setting up a quiet space in the classroom where a student with autism can use a rocking chair to seek calming sensory input and put on a headset to listen to music or a taped story.

Abend's (2001) guide, *Planning and Designing for Students with Disabilities*, provides useful design principles that are applicable to students with various disabling conditions, including physical, sensory, attention, and/or learning impairments. For example, Abend suggests that modular furniture can be combined or separated to support a variety of activities, such as individual and group work, and can include accessible desks and computer workstations to accommodate students who use wheelchairs or who need writing aids such as laptop computers.

The occupational therapist should become familiar with the conditions and terms for funding environmental modifications and special or adapted furniture and ATs for schools. Some environmental modifications can be made at little expense, whereas others will be costly and involve applying to the school board or a government agency for special funding.

Modifying the Workplace

For many people, the ability to work is a primary occupational performance goal. However, the workplace can contribute to illness and injury and can pose barriers to those with various chronic conditions and disabilities who wish to enter the workforce or return to work. The scope for occupational therapy in the workplace is broad; the focus can be on health promotion and wellness, injury prevention, or return to work. All of these areas involve making modifications to the work environment and can range from microsystem to exosystem levels and address physical, social, cultural, and organizational factors. The role of the occupational therapist in the workplace is explored in detail in Chapter 49. This chapter focuses on modifications to the workplace to enable individuals with occupational performance challenges to enter or return to work and successfully perform their jobs.

The ADA and similar human rights legislation in many countries support the individual's right to work by prohibiting discrimination against people with disabilities. In the United States, when people with disabilities can perform the essential functions of a job with accommodations, they are allowed to apply for and maintain a job. Under the ADA Section 101, an employer is responsible for providing the reasonable accommodations necessary for a qualified individual to perform the job. The ADA, in relation to work, is described more fully in Chapter 49.

When **job accommodations** are necessary, the occupational therapist can lead a team to identify the environmental resources and barriers that influence an employee's ability to work and help to access resources and/or remove these barriers. In addition to the occupational therapist, the team members typically include the employer, key employees, and the group that is responsible for implementing the environmental modifications. Reasonable accommodations are more likely to succeed with an appropriate balance of the following four goals for interventions: ensure accessibility, create an enabling environment, reduce or contain disability, and minimize risk (Pigini, Andrich, Liverani, Bucciarelli, & Occhipinti, 2010).

The Job Accommodation Network Website (see http://askjan.org/) provides an excellent resource for therapists, employers, and employees with disabilities to identify possible workplace modifications in relation to specific work performance challenges. Examples are provided in Box 29.3. Architectural changes to the environment, such as installing electronic door openers and modifying a bathroom, can make the workplace accessible for employees and others who use mobility aids such as a wheelchair. ATs are commonly prescribed, particularly for workers with motor weakness and/or impairments like Gary Lau in our case study. For example, because Gary has hemiplegia and is not able to use his left hand functionally, he can be enabled to use a computer with a one-handed keyboard with a reduced number of keys to depress when typing and/or speech recognition software that enters data to the computer via voice command. The social, cultural, and organizational aspects of the workplace can also be modified to support and enable workers to perform their job. For example, in order to accommodate Gary's cognitive impairments with organizational skills and short-term memory, his employer could assign him a peer mentor to assist Gary to break down daily tasks into achievable steps, create daily to-do lists, and provide him with daily guidance. His employer could also provide sensitivity training to coworkers

Changing the physical environment can be expensive and complicated to implement. Under the ADA, workers are permitted "reasonable accommodations" as long as these do not cause "undue hardship" to the employer. A small company that has a very small profit margin might not be required to pay for an elevator if it would cause the company bankruptcy, but the employer might be required to move the office of an employee with a mobility impairment to the first floor if space was available. The outcome of the job accommodation should be evaluated, and the continued success of the accommodations should be monitored over time to ensure the best worker-job-environment fit.

Modifying Community Contexts

The exosystem level of the environment contains spaces in which most people visit on a less frequent basis than the work or home environment. Examples include government agencies, cultural venues, shopping complexes, and stores. Although people often spend less time in

BOX 29.3 Examples of Job Accommodations for Specific Work Challenges

Work Performance Challenge: Gripping or Pinching Tools or Objects

People have physical limitations that result in difficulty gripping or pinching objects. Accommodations may involve the office, industrial, service, and medical industries and can extend to personal needs. Options for the office include the following:

- Providing alternative telephone access: auto-dialers, gooseneck telephone holders, hands-free telephones, and computer-telephone integration
- Offering filing modifications such as modified filing trays, Lazy-Susan carousels, and automated filing systems
- Providing grip aids such as reachers and door knob grips
- Providing page turners and book holders

Work Performance Challenge: Working at Full Production

People may have physical limitations that result in difficulty working at full production levels. Accommodations may include the following:

- Reducing or eliminating physical exertion and workplace stress
- Scheduling periodic rest breaks away from the workstation
- Implementing ergonomic workstation design with ergonomic equipment (e.g., copy holders, electric hole punches, electric stapler, foot rests, forearm supports, headsets, etc.)
- Providing adjustable/ergonomic chairs or stand/lean stools
- Providing compact lifting devices
- Providing anti-fatigue matting and anti-vibration materials
- Providing a scooter or other mobility aid if walking cannot be reduced

Source: Job Accommodation Network. (n.d.) *Job accommodation network searchable online accommodation resource.* Retrieved from http://askjan.org

these spaces, they serve as links between more private spaces such as work and home; and they contain critical goods and services necessary for successful participation in community life. Community contexts are important for socialization, recreation, and civic and social engagement. Socially exclusive environments with poor accessibility can negatively affect the community participation of people with disabilities and other marginalized groups.

Communities are important venues for social and physical change interventions. Communities can be fostered, developed, enabled, built, enhanced, created, or organized with the aim to enhance the wellness of their members. Scaffa and Bonder (2009) view wellness as distinct from health and use Gallup's (1999) definition of wellness as an individual's perception of physical and psychological well-being characterized by adequate physical capacity for accomplishment of desired activities, coupled with overall satisfaction with one's life situation. With this in mind, in the case example of Gary Lau, the occupational therapist saw it as her role to influence both the ***social structures*** and physical access concerns of Gary's community center. The concepts of **community**, **community participation**, and **community development** are outlined subsequently and provide a basis from which therapists can bring about social and physical change.

CASE STUDY 29.1 Part Two: Gary Lau and Community Reintegration *(Continued)*

Once the home-based physical accessibility issues were worked out, Katya met further with Gary to discuss his interest in reengaging with his local community. She spent time exploring his past leisure interests using the Occupational Performance History Interview-Second Version (OPHI-II) (Kielhofner et al., 2004), his values, culture, and spirituality. It became clear that volunteering is consistent with his past interests and the importance he and his partner place on being part of a community. Although neither Gary nor his partner identified with any religious community, it became clear that the values and traditions they now hold were influenced by their parents' Buddhist cultural roots (Gary is a third-generation American) as well as mainstream American values related to being neighborly and helping others out.

Once Gary and Katya identified a number of possible volunteering roles, she accompanied him to a local community center to assess any accessibility issues that he might experience. She suggested that Gary call the center prior to their visit to inquire about accessibility. They were assured that the center was fully accessible. Once there, an enthusiastic volunteer coordinator greeted them and quickly outlined the various volunteer opportunities available. Throughout the interview, the coordinator directed her comments and responses to Katya even when Gary asked the question. Katya noticed this and attempted on several occasions to redirect the coordinator's attention to Gary. At some point, Gary asked to use the toilet. Returning some time later, he pointed out to Katya that he had difficulty getting up from the toilet as there were no grab bars. Katya asked the coordinator if anything could be done to improve the accessibility of the bathrooms. The coordinator replied politely that she would check into it but that the center was not designed for crippled or mentally retarded people and that perhaps they should seek out other community programs.

Katya tactfully informed the coordinator that Gary did not label himself as crippled nor mentally retarded and that they were under the impression that public spaces such as this were to be fully accessible under the Americans with Disabilities Act guidelines. She asked if there was someone at the center whom she could talk to about accessibility and accommodation options. The coordinator gave her a name and number and encouraged her to call. Although it was clear that there were a number of opportunities available at the center that Gary was interested in and could likely manage, both he and Katya were turned off by the polite brush-off that they felt from the coordinator.

Afterward, Katya discussed with Gary and his partner their interest in pursuing volunteer opportunities at this location. She offered to follow up with the contact given to her by the coordinator and to see what could be done regarding the center's approach to social inclusion of people with disabilities. They were both agreeable to this plan.

Katya was also aware of several other clients who lived in this area who could benefit from the opportunities available at this center. She was, however, reluctant to suggest this center given her experience. In keeping with Katya's knowledge and appreciation for the occupational therapy role in advocating for socially inclusive environments, Katya recognized the importance of doing something about the center's social barriers to people with disabilities. She considered how she might go about dealing with that at a broader level.

Fortunately, a component of Katya's position allowed her to work with community agencies on issues related to disability and inclusion. She set up a meeting with the community agency's executive director and identified her concerns about the attitudes conveyed by some of the staff regarding accessibility issues at the center. She informed the director that there were several people she worked with who, although living with some type of disability, would benefit from their participation in the community center if it were accessible not only in terms of the physical requirements but also the social attitudes conveyed by the staff. Katya offered her support to work with the center to develop this and suggested starting with an accessibility and social inclusion audit of the various programs at the center. Katya agreed also to provide education on relevant legislation and policies that organizations such as this one must adhere to. Katya had experience with working with design teams and running stakeholder focus groups for other community organizations. She emphasized the importance of including people living with disabilities on the design team and also as part of relevant focus groups. She suggested including several of her clients to assist in the development of education sessions aimed at informing the community center staff around issues of stigma and accessibility. Dilemmas faced by occupational therapists within the social environment are presented in the Practice Dilemma box. ■

Practice Dilemma

Addressing Diversity Issues

Gary Lau's narrative presents several key dilemmas that occupational therapists may be faced with, particularly with respect to interventions aimed at the social environment.

As a social resource herself, Katya, the occupational therapist, can be considered a part of Gary's social environment. The ethnocultural values and social attitudes that she brings to Gary's situation can influence how she works with him and could determine how effective she will be in enabling his preferred occupations. The degree to which the therapist is aware of her own cultural values and attitudes and how they shape her therapeutic interactions will be of primary importance. Beyond her own self-awareness of the cross-cultural nature of this particular therapeutic relationship, her awareness of the social resources available to Gary and his partner will be crucial. Social attitudinal barriers and discrimination faced by many gay or lesbian people have been well documented (Hammack & Cohler, 2009; Kirsh, Trentham, & Cole, 2006) and have impacts on their use of mainstream services. How open will Gary be to participating in any community organizations that might present such barriers? Similarly, a lack of knowledge about lesbian, gay, bisexual, and transgender (LGBT) culture, communities, and social and recreational resources limits the effectiveness of the therapist in supporting Gary's efforts to reintegrate into the community. A similar scenario can be imagined for any client who identifies with a culture, religion, or community that is different from that of the therapist. How well informed is the therapist to respond to these types of cross-cultural interactions?

Questions for Consideration:

1. Consider a situation where your cultural or religious values conflict with those of your client. How might you reconcile your need to enable the occupations of choice of your client while being true to your own values?
2. To what extent do you feel occupational therapists are obliged to become familiar with the cultural practices and health and social resources of their clients?
3. How might the therapist in this situation navigate the cross-cultural interaction?

The concept of community is often linked to ideas about human connection, social cohesiveness, or support. Less discussed are the less positive aspects of community that can also be associated with exclusivity as illustrated, for example, in the commonly used acronym NIMBYism (not in my backyard). And so, communities can, as often, serve to keep people out as to bring people together. Communities can offer opportunities for occupational engagement through the manner in which occupational roles are created, delegated, acknowledged, and made accessible. They can as likely create barriers to occupational engagement by creating inaccessible physical environments or by fostering discriminatory and stigmatizing social attitudes that alienate, segregate, and limit the participation of particular groups including people living with disabilities. At its most basic, however, community can refer to people living within a particular geographic area who share common services and/or to a group of people who simply share a common identity, for example, older people with disabilities.

In summary, despite the potential restrictive and constraining aspects of community, ideally, community can be a space where the unique value of each person can develop and through which individual needs for integration, participation, and relationship with others is realized. The view that communities serve as a forum for shared identity development, social occupational participation, and expression reflects a desire to understand community as a context for occupational role development and enablement. How then do occupational therapists enable community participation?

Enabling Community Participation

In this chapter, *participation* refers to active participation of individuals who both benefit and contribute to the community through their actions, ideas, knowledge, or skills. Community participation is about relating to others; to be in some sort of relationship with them. Communities or, at the very least, a sense of community can be fostered by the social spaces that occupational therapists work within, such as congregate living environments or neighborhoods. So, how then can communities be developed and how can occupational therapists be involved?

Community Development

Hoffman and Duponte (1992) state, "community development is about . . . helping people to develop the skills they need, and removing the structural barriers that prevent them from achieving their full potential as members of the community" (p. 21). CD strategies aim to create supportive environments and strengthen the capacity of communities to respond to health problems (WHO, 1986).

Rothman and Tropman's (1987) classic taxonomy of three CD approaches can be helpful for occupational therapists considering this type of work. A *locality development* approach views the change process as involving many people, most often within one geographic community, in determining goals and action. Emphasis is placed on process components and on strengthening the connections among community members. Neighborhood safety committees use this approach. *Social planning* uses a top-down process where a governing body typically defines issues and solutions. Finally, *social action* demands a critical social analysis based on class, gender, ability, and race to create change and views problems as rooted within inequitable power structures (Alinsky, 1971); thus, efforts are directed at changing power structures.

Social action approaches share many assumptions with what occupational therapists and occupational scientists refer to as occupational justice. Its growing discourse (Townsend & Polatajko, 2007; Townsend & Wilcock, 2004) highlights the need for practitioners to become aware of the impacts of occupational injustice as experienced through occupational alienation, occupational marginalization, occupational imbalance (Townsend & Wilcock, 2004), or occupational deprivation (Whiteford, 2005). From this perspective, individuals and groups (e.g., cultural minorities) may be alienated from meaningful occupations and roles, prevented from access to decision making, may be over or underemployed, or may be deprived of opportunities for meaningful occupational engagement. Chapter 41 is devoted to exploring occupational justice.

In one particularly illustrative example of CD strategies, occupational therapists working at a community health center in Canada articulated their role within an occupational approach (Trentham, Cockburn, & Shin, 2007). In response to a community needs survey that identified physical inaccessibility and social isolation of older adults, they invited older adults and others living with disabilities as members of an urban neighborhood to help create a more physically accessible and socially supportive neighborhood. Facilitated activities helped the participants envision the possibilities for a "senior-friendly" neighborhood.

The group began with achievable, less complex projects because the successful completion of smaller projects could help build the confidence of the working group while making meaningful change. The provision of optimal structure, group facilitation techniques, shared storytelling, active listening, and environmental adaptations helped to work toward a more supportive and accessible community. Examples of the group's action outcomes included the creation of a grocery delivery guide for homebound seniors, an increased number of sidewalk curb cuts in the local area, and installation of street benches in strategic positions for seniors with less physical tolerance.

After working together for some time and gaining knowledge about advocacy approaches at the municipal level, the group became aware of the larger policy issues that impact on their lives. They shifted from using a locality development approach to a social action approach by focusing on broader level change directed at underlying inequities.

Such CD strategies provide a means to collaborate with clients to bring about both physical and social changes. Very often, however, the therapist may be working from a consultative framework rather than a facilitative approach and is charged with the task of providing recommendations to improve community accessibility. Knowledge of both the enabling and *disabling* aspects of both the physical and social environment is important and further discussed subsequently.

Enabling Community Participation—Modifying Physical Access in Public and Community Spaces

Public spaces are typically designed to meet the needs of average individuals and are based on general guidelines such as the ADA-Architectural Barriers Act (ABA) Accessibility Guidelines (U.S. Access Board, 2004) and building codes in Canada. Greater accessibility can be achieved by working directly with clients, by working with community property owners or consultants, and by working as advocates in the community. For example, people with activity or participation restrictions may face barriers navigating public transportation systems, an important component of occupational performance. Iwarsson, Ståhl, and Carlsson (2003) described collaborative work between occupational therapy, traffic planning, and engineering in an initiative to understand the accessibility of transportation systems.

Barrier removal might not always be possible. In some cases, without regulatory incentives in place (e.g., mandatory accessibility guidelines), it might not be possible to make changes. It is the occupational therapist's role, however, to understand current legislation and minimum standards and to help clients advocate for change. It is also possible to identify barriers through the assessment process to help clients make decisions about how they could access and use spaces. In this case, understanding the physical environment is the goal, even though modification might not be possible.

Conclusions and Future Considerations

Physical, social, cultural, institutional, and technological aspects of environment can create barriers or provide resources and supports toward enabling optimal occupational performance and engagement. Occupational therapists have considerable experience and have demonstrated leadership and success with modifying home, school, work, and community contexts to support the participation of their clients in their daily pursuits. Today, more people who have previously been marginalized, excluded, or discriminated against are able to live with greater autonomy, go to school, return to work, and actively participate in their communities through efforts made by occupational therapists to reduce environmental barriers and harness environmental resources. To provide this leadership, it is critical that occupational therapists maintain a strong working knowledge about applicable policies and legislation, building codes, and accessibility guidelines that can improve the overall

Commentary on the Evidence

The Effectiveness of Environmental Modifications

Environmental modifications can be applied in many contexts and for a wide variety of purposes. For this review, two common occupational therapy interventions are discussed: modifying the physical environment to prevent falls and modifying environments to reduce caregiver burden.

Falls Prevention through Environmental Modifications

Falls prevention interventions for older adults can include many components that address physical performance of the person (e.g., through strengthening or balance exercises), medication reviews, group education, and assessment and modification of the home environment, often with a focus on home hazards. Sometimes, these are provided singly; in other work, a multicomponent intervention approach is used. Falls prevention research has included a large number of randomized controlled trials and subsequent systematic reviews and meta-analyses of the data from these studies (Law, Di Rezze, & Bradley, 2010). Although not always provided as a single intervention, several reviews have examined the effectiveness of modifications of the physical environment as a strategy to prevent falls.

In a systematic review of falls prevention interventions for older adults living in community settings, Gillespie et al. (2009) found that home safety interventions were effective in reducing falls in people with visual impairments and those with high risk of falling; but the intervention was not effective in reducing the number of falls in the general population of older adults (relative risk 0.89, 95% confidence interval 0.80 to 1.00). Similarly, Clemson, Mackenzie, Ballinger, Close, and Cumming (2008) conducted a meta-analysis and estimated that environmental interventions for older adults at high risk for falls reduced the risk of falls by 39%, compared to a more modest reduction of 21% in a more general sample of older adults. Similar findings are reported in other reviews of falls prevention interventions (Costello & Edelstein, 2008; Tse, 2005).

Reducing Caregiver Burden

Much of the literature about the effectiveness of environmental modifications to reduce caregiver burden focuses on caregivers of people with dementia. Interventions that focus on the environment have used caregiver education and training to deal with challenging behaviors, selecting activities to match capabilities, and adapting to changing activities of daily living (Schaber & Lieberman, 2010).

In one study, environmental skill–building included six occupational therapy visits that resulted in improved skills in caregivers, decreased need for assistance from people with dementia, and fewer challenging behaviors (Gitlin, Corcoran, Winter, Boyce & Hauck, 2001). In a similar intervention conducted in the Netherlands, caregivers received 10 occupational therapy visits that focused on compensatory and environmental interventions, with significant improvements in function of people with dementia and reductions in caregiver burden (Graff et al., 2006). A less intense occupational therapy intervention reported by Dooley and Hinojosa (2004) had a focus on meeting with caregivers to review occupational therapy recommendations (compared to mailing the report and recommendations). Although brief, caregivers in the intervention group reported higher quality of life and positive affect. Finally, an intervention focusing on teaching caregivers to select and tailor activities for the person with dementia to suit his or her capabilities resulted in increased activity engagement and few problem behaviors (Gitlin, et al., 2009).

These interventions focus on the caregiver managing their own actions (as part of the social environment of the person with dementia) as well as the physical environment to address challenges in managing people with dementia at home. Together, the results of these four studies demonstrate that occupational therapy can result in positive effects for both the caregiver and the person with dementia by focusing on combinations of physical and social aspects of the environment.

participation and empowerment of their clients. Beyond this awareness, however, as enablers of occupation, therapists can serve their clients by boldly participating in efforts to shape more inclusive social and public policies and to join the efforts of others, including their clients, in creating the spaces and opportunities that foster meaningful participation in life for all.

References

Abend, A. (2001). *Planning and designing for students with disabilities.* Washington, DC: National Clearinghouse for Educational Facilities. Retrieved from http://www.ncef.org/pubs/disabilities.pdf

Agree, E. M., Freedman, V. A., Cornman, J. C., Wolf, D. A., & Marcotte, J. E. (2005). Reconsidering substitution in long-term care: When does assistive technology take the place of personal care? *Psychological Sciences and Social Sciences, 60,* S272–S280.

Aguilar, A., Boerema, C., & Harrison, J. (2010). Meanings attributed by older adults to computer use. *Journal of Occupational Science, 17*(1), 27–33.

Alinsky, S. D. (1971). *Rules for radicals: A practical primer for realistic radicals.* New York, NY: Vintage Books.

American Association of Retired Persons. (2000). *Fixing to stay: A national survey on housing and home modification issues—Executive summary.* Washington, DC: Author.

American Civil Rights Act of 1964, Pub. L. No. 88-352, § 78, Stat. 241 (1964). Retrieved from http://www.archives.gov/education/lessons/civil-rights-act/

American Occupational Therapy Association. (2008). Occupational therapy practice framework: Domain and process, 2nd edition. *American Journal of Occupational Therapy, 62,* 625–683.

American with Disabilities Act of 1990, Pub. L. No. 101-336, 42 U.S.C. § 12101 (1990). Retrieved from http://www.ada.gov/

American with Disabilities Act Amendments of 2008, Pub. L. No. 110-325 (2008). Retrieved from http://www.ada.gov/pubs/ada.htm

Bronfenbrenner, U. (2005). *Making human beings human: Bioecological perspectives on human development.* Thousand Oaks, CA: Sage.

Canadian Human Rights Act of 1976, R.S.C. §§ 33-1 (1976). Retrieved from http://laws-lois.justice.gc.ca/eng/acts/h-6/page-1.html#h-2

Center for Universal Design. (1997). *A blueprint for action: A resource for promoting home modifications.* Raleigh, NC: North Carolina State University.

Chan, S. C., & Chan, A. P. (2007). User satisfaction, community participation and quality of life among Chinese wheelchair users with spinal cord injury: A preliminary study. *Occupational Therapy International, 14,* 123–143.

Chen, T. Y., Mann, W. C., Tomita, M., & Nochajski, S. (2000). Caregiver involvement in the use of assistive devices by frail elderly persons. *Occupational Therapy Journal of Research, 20,* 179–199.

Cipriani, J., Kreider, M., Sapulak, K., Jacobson, M., Skrypski, M., & Sprau, K. (2009). Understanding object attachment and meaning for nursing home residents: An exploratory study, including implications for occupational therapy. *Physical and Occupational Therapy in Geriatrics, 27,* 405–422.

Clark, F. A. (2010). Power and confidence in professions: Lessons for occupational therapy. *Canadian Journal of Occupational Therapy, 77*(5), 264–269.

Clemson, L., Mackenzie, L., Ballinger, C., Close, J. C., & Cumming, R. G. (2008). Environmental interventions to prevent falls in community-dwelling older people: A meta-analysis of randomized trials. *Journal of Aging & Health, 20,* 954–971.

Cook, A. M., & Polgar, J. M. (2008). *Cook and Hussey's assistive technology: Principles and practice.* Toronto, Canada: Elsevier.

Costello, E., & Edelstein, J. E. (2008). Update on falls prevention for community-dwelling older adults: Review of single and multifactorial intervention programs. *Journal of Rehabilitation Research & Development, 45,* 1135–1152.

Craik, J., Davis, J., & Polatajko, H. J. (2007). Introducing the Canadian Practice Process Framework (CPPF): Amplifying the context. In E. A. Townsend & H. J. Polatajko (Eds.), *Enabling occupation II: Advancing an occupational therapy vision for health, well-being, and justice through occupation* (pp. 229–246). Ottawa, Canada: Canadian Association of Occupational Therapists.

Cristoforetti, A., Gennai, F., & Rodeschini, G. (2011). Home sweet home: The emotional construction of places. *Journal of Aging Studies, 25,* 225–232.

Dooley, N. R., & Hinojosa, J. (2004). Improving quality of life for persons with Alzheimer's disease and their family caregivers: Brief occupational therapy intervention. *American Journal of Occupational Therapy, 58,* 561–569.

Dunn, W., Brown, C., & McGuigan, A. (1994). The ecology of human performance: A framework for considering the effect of context. *American Journal of Occupational Therapy, 48,* 595–607.

Egilson, S. T., & Traustadottir, R. (2009). Participation of students with physical disabilities in the school environment. *American Journal of Occupational Therapy, 63,* 264–272.

Erickson, J., & Johnson, G. (2011). Internet use and psychological well-ness during late adulthood. *Canadian Journal on Aging, 30*(2), 197–209.

Fuhrer, M. J., Jutai, J. W., Scherer, M. J., & DeRuyter, F. (2003). A framework for the conceptual modeling of assistive technology outcomes. *Disability and Rehabilitation, 25,* 1243–1251.

Gallup, J. W. (1999). Wellness centers: A guide for the design professional. New York, NY: Wiley.

Gillespie, L. D., Robertson, M. C., Gillespie, W. J., Lamb, S. E., Gates, S., Cumming, R. G., & Rowe, B. H. (2009). Interventions for preventing falls in older people living in the community. *Cochrane Database of Systematic Reviews,* (2), CD007146. doi:10.1002/14651858.CD007146.pub2

Gitlin, L. N., Corcoran, M., Winter, L., Boyce, A., & Huack, W. W. (2001). A randomized, controlled trial of a home environmental intervention: Effect on efficacy and upset in caregivers and on daily function. *The Gerontologist, 41,* 4–14.

Gitlin, L. N., Winter, L., Earland, T. V., Herge, E. A., Chernett, N. L., Piersol, C. V., & Burke, J. P. (2009). The tailored activity program to reduce behavioral symptoms in individuals with dementia: Feasibility, acceptability, and replication potential. *The Gerontologist, 49,* 428–439.

Gosman-Hedstrom, G., Claesson, L., & Blomstrand, C. (2002). Assistive devices in elderly people after stroke: A longitudinal, randomized study—The Goteborg stroke study. *Scandinavian Journal of Occupational Therapy, 9,* 109–118.

Graff, M. J. L., Vernooij-Dassen, M. J. M., Thijssen, M., Dekker, J., Hoefnagels, W. H. L., & Rikkert, M. G. M. (2006). Community-based occupational therapy for patients with dementia and their caregivers: Randomized controlled trial. *British Medical Journal, 333,* 1196–1201.

Hammack, P. L., & Cohler, B. J. (Eds.). (2009). *The story of sexual identity: Narrative perspectives on the gay and lesbian life course.* New York, NY: Oxford University Press.

Hampton, K., & Wellman, B. (2003). Neighboring in Netville: How the internet supports community and social capital in a wired suburb. *City and Community, 2*(4), 277–311.

Heah, T., Case, T., McGuire, B., & Law, M. (2007). Successful participation: The lived experience among children with disabilities. *Canadian Journal of Occupational Therapy, 74,* 38–47.

Hoffman, K., & Duponte, J. (1992). *Community health centres and community development.* Ottawa, Canada: Health and Welfare Canada.

Iwarsson, S., & Ståhl, A. (2003). Accessibility, usability and universal design—Positioning and definition of concepts describing person-environment relationships. *Disability and Rehabilitation, 25,* 57–66.

Iwarsson, S., Ståhl, A., & Carlsson, G. (2003). Accessible transportation: Novel occupational therapy perspectives. In L. Letts, P. Rigby, & D. Stewart (Eds.), *Using environments to enable occupational performance* (pp. 235–251). Thorofare, NJ: Slack.

Job Accommodation Network. (n.d.). *Job accommodation network searchable online accommodation resource.* Retrieved from http://askjan.org

Kaye, H. S., Kang, T., & LaPlante, M. P. (2000). *Mobility use in the United States. Disability Statistics Report 14.* Washington, DC: U.S. Department of Education, National Institute of Disability and Rehabilitation Research.

Kielhofner, G. (2008). *Model of human occupation: Theory and application.* Philadelphia, PA: Lippincott Wilkins & Williams.

Kielhofner, G., Mallinson, T., Crawford, C., Nowak, M., Rigby, M., Henry, A., & Walens, D. (2004). *Occupational performance history interview II (OPHI-II) Version 2.1.* Chicago, IL: MOHO Clearinghouse.

Kirsh, B., Trentham, B., & Cole, S. (2006). Diversity in occupational therapy: Experiences of consumers who identify themselves as minority group members. *Australian Occupational Therapy Journal, 53*(4), 302–313.

Law, M., Baptiste, S., Carswell, A., McColl, M., Polatajko, H., & Pollock, N. (2005). *Canadian Occupational Performance Measure* (4th ed.). Ottawa, Canada: Canadian Association of Occupational Therapists.

Law, M., Cooper, B., Strong, S., Stewart, D., Rigby, P., & Letts, L. (1996). The person-environment-occupation model: A transactive approach to occupational performance. *Canadian Journal of Occupational Therapy, 63*(1), 9–23.

Law, M., Di Rezze, B., & Bradley, L. (2010). Environmental change to improve outcomes. In M. Law & M. A. McColl (Eds.), *Interventions, effects and outcomes in occupational therapy: Adults and older adults* (pp. 155–182). Thorofare, NJ: Slack.

Law, M., Petrenchik, T., King, G., & Hurley, P. (2007). Perceived environmental barriers to recreational, community, and school participation for children and youth with physical disabilities. *Archives of Physical Medicine & Rehabilitation, 88,* 1636–1642.

Letts, L. (2009). Health promotion. In E. B. Crepeau, E. S. Cohn, & B. A. Boyt Schell (Eds.), *Willard & Spackman's occupational therapy* (11th ed.). New York, NY: Lippincott Williams & Wilkins.

Lysack, C., Komanecky, M., Kabel, A., Cross, K., & Neufeld, S. (2007). Environmental factors and their role in community integration after spinal cord injury. *Canadian Journal of Occupational Therapy, 74*(2), 243–254.

Mace, R. (1985). Universal design: Barrier-free environments for everyone. *Designer West, 3,* 147–152.

Mihailidis, A., Boger, J., Hoey, J., & Jiancaro, T. (2011). Zero effort technologies: Considerations, challenges and use in health, wellness, and rehabilitation. In R. M. Baecker (Ed.), *Synthesis lectures on assistive, rehabilitative, and health-preserving technologies.* San Rafael, CA: Morgan & Claypool.

Mitty, E., & Flores, S. (2009). There's no place like home. *Geriatric Nursing, 30,* 126–129.

Mu, K., & Royeen, C. (2004). Facilitating participation of students with severe disabilities: Aligning school-based occupational therapy practice with best practices in severe disabilities. *Physical and Occupational Therapy in Pediatrics, 24,* 5–21.

Niva, B., & Skar, L. (2006). A pilot study of the activity patterns of five elderly persons after a housing adaptation. *Occupational Therapy International, 13,* 21–28.

Ostrof, E. (2001). Universal design: the new paradigm. In W. F. E. Preiser & E. Ostrof (Eds.), *Universal design handbook.* New York, NY: McGraw-Hill.

Pigini, L., Andrich, R., Liverani, G., Bucciarelli, P., & Occhipinti, E. (2010). Designing reasonable accommodation of the workplace: A new methodology based on risk assessment. *Disability and Rehabilitation: Assistive Technology, 5,* 184–198.

Reid, D., Chu, T., Sinclair, G., Wehrmann, S., & Nazeer, Z. (2006). Evaluation of occupational therapy school-based consultation service for students with fine-motor difficulties. *Canadian Journal of Occupational Therapy, 73,* 215–224.

Rigby, P., & Letts, L. (2003). Environment and occupational performance: Theoretical considerations. In L. Letts, P. Rigby, & D. Stewart (Eds.), *Using environments to enable occupational performance* (pp. 17–32). Thorofare, NJ: Slack.

Rigby, P., Ryan, S. E., & Campbell, K. A. (2009). Effect of adaptive seating devices on the activity performance of children with cerebral palsy. *Archives of Physical Medicine & Rehabilitation, 90,* 1389–1395.

Rigby, P., Ryan, S. E., & Campbell, K. (2011). Electronic aids to daily living and quality of life for persons with tetraplegia. *Disability and Rehabilitation: Assistive Technology, 6,* 260–267.

Ripat, J. (2006). Function and impact of electronic aids to daily living for experienced users. *Technology & Disability, 18,* 79–87.

Rothman, J., & Tropman, J. E. (1987). Models of community organization and macro practice perspectives. In F. M. Cox, J. L. Erlich, J. Rothman, & J. E. Tropman (Eds.), *Strategies of community organization* (4th ed., pp. 26–63). Itasca, IL: Peacock.

Scaffa, M., & Bonder, B. (2009). Health promotion and wellness. In B. Bonder & V. Dal Bello-Haas (Eds.), *Functional performance in older adults* (3rd ed., pp. 449–467). Philadelphia, PA: F. A. Davis.

Schaber, P., & Lieberman, D. (2010). *Occupational therapy practice guidelines for adults with Alzheimer's disease and related disorders.* Bethesda, MD: American Occupational Therapy Association.

Snyder, M. M. (2002). The design of online learning communities for older adults. *Journal of Instruction Delivery Systems, 16*(3), 27–33.

Stark, S. (2004). Removing environmental barriers in the homes of older adults with disabilities improves occupational performance. *Occupational Therapy Journal of Research, 24*(1), 32–39.

Statistics Canada. (2006). *Participation and activity limitation survey: A profile of assistive technology for people with disabilities.* Ottawa, Canada: Government of Canada Social and Aboriginal Statistics Department.

Sum, S., Mathews, R. M., Pourghasem, M., & Hughes, I. (2009). Internet use as a predictor of sense of community in older people. *CyberPsychology & Behavior, 12*(2), 235–239.

Tanner, B., Tilse, C., & deJonge, D. (2008). Restoring and sustaining home: The impact of home modifications on the meaning of home for older people. *Journal of Housing for the Elderly, 22,* 195–215.

Townsend, E. A., & Polatajko, H. J. (2007). *Enabling occupation II: Advancing an occupational therapy vision for health, well-being, and justice through occupation.* Ottawa, Canada: Canadian Association of Occupational Therapists.

Townsend, E., & Wilcock, A. (2004). Occupational justice. In C. H. Christiansen & E. A. Townsend (Eds.), *Introduction to occupation, the art and science of living* (pp. 243–273). Upper Saddle River, NJ: Prentice Hall.

Trentham, B., Cockburn, L., & Shin, J. (2007). Health promotion and community development: An application of occupational therapy in primary health care. *Canadian Journal of Community Mental Health, 26,* 53–70.

Tse, T. (2005). The environment and falls prevention: Do environmental modifications make a difference? *Australian Occupational Therapy Journal, 52,* 271–281.

U.S. Access Board. (2004). *ADA and Architectural Barriers Act (ABA) Accessibility Guidelines.* Retrieved from http://www.access-board.gov/ada-aba/final.pdf

U.S. Access Board. (2005). *Accessible play areas: A summary of accessibility guidelines for play areas.* Retrieved from http://www.access-board.gov/play/guide/guide.pdf

U.S. Access Board. (2007). *Proposed ABA Accessibility Guidelines for Outdoor Developed Areas.* Retrieved from http://www.access-board.gov/outdoor/nprm/

U.S. Department of Justice. (2010). *ADA Standards for Accessible Design.* Retrieved from http://www.ada.gov/2010ADAstandards_index.htm

U.S. Department of State. (2008). *Appendix A: Universal declaration of human rights.* Retrieved from http://www.state.gov/g/drl/rls/irf/2008/108544.htm

Villeneuve, M. A. (2009). Critical examination of school-based occupational therapy collaborative consultation. *Canadian Journal of Occupational Therapy, 76,* 206–218.

Ward, K., Mitchell, J., & Price, P. (2007). Occupation-based practice and its relationship to social and occupational participation in adults with spinal cord injury. *OTJR Occupation, Participation and Health, 27*(4), 149–156.

Whiteford, G. (2005). Understanding the occupational deprivation of refugees: A case study from Kosovo. *Canadian Journal of Occupational Therapy, 72*(2), 78–88.

World Health Organization. (1986). Ottawa charter for health promotion. *Health Promotion, 1,* iii–v.

World Health Organization. (2001). *International classification of functioning, disability and health.* Geneva, Switzerland: Author. Retrieved from http://www.who.int/classification/icf/

Resources

American Printing House for the Blind (provides materials, alternative media, tools, and resources for individuals who are blind or visually impaired): http://www.aph.org/

Americans with Disabilities Act: http://www.ada.gov/

Center for Inclusive Design and Universal Access (IDeA): http://www.ap.buffalo.edu/idea/Home/index.asp

Center for Universal Design at North Carolina State University: http://www.ncsu.edu/project/design-projects/udi/

Centre for Accessible Environments, United Kingdom: http://www.cae.org.uk/

Home Modification Information Clearing House in Australia: http://www.homemods.info/

Institute for Human Centered Design: http://www.adaptenv.org/

Job Accommodation Network (JAN): http://askjan.org/

National Centre on Accessibility (promotes access for people with disabilities in recreation): http://www.ncaonline.org

Services for People with Disabilities from Services Canada: http://www.servicecanada.gc.ca/eng/audiences/disabilities/employment.shtml

U.S. Architectural and Transportation Barriers Compliance Board (a federal agency committed to accessible design): www.access-board.gov/

U.S. Equal Employment Opportunity Commission: http://www.eeoc.gov/

For additional resources on the subjects discussed in this chapter, visit http://thePoint.lww.com/Willard-Spackman12e.

UNIT

VIII

Core Concepts and Skills

"Happiness comes when we test our skills towards some meaningful purpose."

—John Stossel

CHAPTER 30

Professional Reasoning in Practice

Barbara A. Boyt Schell

OUTLINE

LEARNING OBJECTIVES

After reading this chapter, you will be able to:

1. Analyze important aspects of reasoning in occupational therapy practice
2. Discuss how the reasoning process is embedded in the transactions that occur among the practitioner, the client, and the practice context
3. Identify the different facets of professional reasoning based on personal reflection, practitioners' descriptions, and case studies
4. Describe the process of developing expertise and discuss characteristic reasoning processes along a continuum of expertise

Introduction

Professional reasoning is the process that practitioners use to plan, direct, perform, and reflect on client care. It is typically performed quickly because the practitioner has to act on that reasoning right away. It is a complex and multifaceted process, and it has been called by several different names. In the past, many authors referred to it as ***clinical reasoning*** (Mattingly & Fleming, 1994; Rogers, 1983; Schell & Cervero, 1993); but terms such as **professional reasoning** (Schell & Schell, 2007) and ***therapeutic reasoning*** (Kielhofner & Forsyth, 2002) have surfaced in an attempt to find a word that is not so closely aligned with medicine because occupational therapy practices not only in medical settings but also in many educational and community settings as well. When using these labels, authors are talking about how therapists *actually think* when they are engaged in practice. This requires **metacognitive** analysis or, in simple terms, *thinking about thinking*. This is important because newcomers to the field might incorrectly understand professional reasoning as something that practitioners "choose to do" or confuse it with the many occupational therapy intervention theories.

It is neither of those things. Whenever you are thinking about or doing occupational therapy for an identified individual or group, you are engaged in professional reasoning. It is not a question of whether you are doing it, only a question of how well. Furthermore, many practice theories are discussed throughout this text that will inform your reasoning and help you to think about your clients. However, the theories about reasoning that are discussed in this chapter are theories about how you as an occupational therapy practitioner are likely to think as you engage in therapy. Thus, the focus is on the therapist, not on the client, although obviously, therapists do this thinking in the service of client care. Keep in mind these important distinctions as you become mindful of your own reasoning processes.

This chapter examines professional reasoning from several perspectives. To help you see real examples of the material discussed, the following Case Study 30.1, which is adapted with name changes from an actual situation, provides an example of an encounter between an occupational therapist, Terry and her client Mrs. Munro. Read this case study before continuing with the text, paying special attention to the different kinds of issues and problems that the occupational therapy practitioner has to address. Then keep referring back to it as you read about the nature of professional reasoning.

CASE STUDY 30.1 Terry and Mrs. Munro: Determining Appropriate Recommendations

Terry, an occupational therapist, goes up to a client's room in the neurology unit of a regional medical center. Along the way, she shares her thoughts with Barb, a researcher who is observing Terry's practice. Terry fills Barb in on the client they are about to see. The client, Mrs. Munro, is a widow who lives alone in a house in town. A couple of days earlier, she had a stroke—a right cerebrovascular accident—and was brought by a neighbor to the hospital. Mrs. Munro has made a rapid recovery and demonstrates good return of her motor skills. She still has some left-sided weakness and incoordination, along with some cognitive problems. She is a delightful, pleasant older woman and is anxious to return home.

Terry is seeing this client for the third time, and her primary concern is to assess whether Mrs. Munro has any residual cognitive effects from her stroke that would put her at serious risk if she returned home alone. Terry plans to do some more in-depth activities of daily living with Mrs. Munro to see how well she demonstrates safety awareness. Terry thinks that she will probably have Mrs. Munro get out of bed, obtain her clothing and hygiene supplies, perform her morning hygiene routines at the sink, and then get dressed. Terry wants to see the degree to which Mrs. Munro is spontaneously able to manage these tasks as well as how good her judgment appears to be. Terry's thought is that if she can engage Mrs. Munro in several multistep activities that also require her to perform in different positions, Terry should be able to detect any cognitive and motor problems that pose a serious safety threat.

When Terry arrives at the room, she greets Mrs. Munro who says, "I am so excited. The doctor says I can go home today."

Terry turns to Barb and raises her eyebrows as if to say, "I told you so." On the way to the room, Terry had told Barb that she was worried that the physician who was managing Mrs. Munro's case tended to think that as soon as clients could physically get up, they should go home. Terry went on to defend the physician by saying that in today's cost-conscious environment, doctors were under a lot of pressure not to keep clients in the hospital.

As Terry converses with Mrs. Munro about generalities, she notices that Mrs. Munro is already dressed in her housecoat. When she talks to Mrs. Munro about doing some self-care activities, it becomes apparent that Mrs. Munro has already completed her bathing and dressing routines, with help from a nurse. When Terry suggests that she perhaps brush her teeth and comb her hair, Mrs. Munro is happy to get up out of bed but notes that her neighbor never did bring in her dentures. Mrs. Munro sits on the edge of the bed and, after a reminder from Terry, puts on her slippers. She then stands and walks to the nearby sink, finds her comb, and combs her hair. While she is doing this, Terry looks around for some other ideas about what to do because Mrs. Munro has already completed the self-care tasks Terry had planned to do with her.

Terry's eyes light on some wilted flowers by the bed. She suggests to Mrs. Munro that she might want to dispose of the flowers and clean the vase so that it will be ready to pack when it is time to go home. Mrs. Munro agrees and proceeds to walk somewhat unsteadily over to the vase. Picking it up, she carries it to the sink, where she pulls out the dead flowers. Terry follows her, staying slightly behind and within reach of Mrs. Munro. When Mrs. Munro stops after removing the flowers, Terry suggests that she rinse out the vase, which she does. She then dries it and returns the vase to the bedside table. Terry reminds her to throw out the dead flowers. While Mrs. Munro does this, they talk some more about her plans to return home.

Mrs. Munro tells Terry that she has lived in her home for 40 years, and even though her husband died more than 10 years ago, she still feels his presence there. He used to love her cooking, and she still cooks three meals a day for herself. Mrs. Munro starts to cry when they talk about cooking but then cheers up. Terry tells her that it might be safer if she had someone around the house for a few weeks until she recovers a bit more from her stroke. Mrs. Munro thinks that she can get some help from her neighbor. Terry says she is also going to suggest some home care therapy, just to make sure Mrs. Munro is safe in the kitchen, bathroom, and so on, noting, "We sure don't want to see you have a bad fall just when you are doing so well after your stroke."

After reviewing some coordination exercises for Mrs. Munro's left hand, Terry says good-bye. Terry and Barb leave the room. Terry stops at the nurses' station to note in the chart that Mrs. Munro demonstrated good safety awareness in familiar tasks at her bedside but did require cueing to complete multistep tasks. Terry also notes some motor instability in task performance

(continued)

CASE STUDY 30.1 Terry and Mrs. Munro: Determining Appropriate Recommendations *(Continued)*

during ambulation. Terry recommends a referral to a home health occupational therapy practitioner "to assess safety and equipment needs during bathroom activities, meal preparation, and routine homemaking tasks." Terry comments to Barb, as they walk off the unit, that she thinks Mrs. Munro did pretty well; but Terry remains concerned about the risks once Mrs. Munro goes home, particularly when she is tired. Terry wants someone to monitor Mrs. Munro in a familiar setting to see whether she handles her daily routines adequately. Terry would really like to see Mrs. Munro start to consider a more supported living environment, but the client doesn't have either long-term care insurance or the personal finances to support that. Terry believes that she might at least be able to get one home care visit to evaluate home safety, particularly fall prevention. Staying in her own home seems to be Mrs. Munro's major goal, and Terry is going to do what she can to try to help her attain that goal. Terry will catch up with the social worker later to discuss the need for Mrs. Munro to have good support from any neighbors, friends, or relatives.

Questions and Exercises

1. How did Terry develop her concerns about Mrs. Munro?
2. How did Terry know what to do when her initial plans did not work out?
3. What factors seem to guide Terry's recommendations at the end?

Reasoning in Practice: A Whole-body Process

With the case study in mind, let's explore the nature of reasoning during practice. Perhaps one of the first things to note is that professional reasoning is a *whole-body* process. That is one reason why it is a different experience to read a case study than to be the practitioner in the situation. Some professional reasoning involves straightforward thinking processes that the practitioner can easily describe. Examples include assessing occupational performance, such as daily living skills and work behaviors. Occupational therapy practitioners use their observations and theoretical knowledge to identify relevant client factors that contribute to occupational performance problems. Practitioners also attend to the contextual factors that affect performance. For instance, Terry was able to describe her concerns about Mrs. Munro's safety in returning home. In particular, Terry was addressing self-care and homemaking activities. She had analyzed relevant contextual factors about the home setting and Mrs. Munro's social and financial situation. Terry had identified some impairments in cognition and motor control that were affecting her client's occupational performance skills. This was all information that Terry could readily share with Barb. However, there was more knowledge from the therapy session that Terry either did not or could not put into words.

Part of Terry's professional reasoning involved body-based knowledge that she gained from her senses. For instance, Terry used her sense of touch to feel the muscle tension (or lack of tension) in Mrs. Munro's affected arm when she was doing an activity. During her evaluation, Terry did some quick stretches to Mrs. Munro's elbow and wrist to determine whether she could feel evidence of spasticity, an abnormal reflex response that is commonly found in individuals who are recovering from a stroke. When Mrs. Munro stood up, Terry gauged the distance she stood from Mrs. Munro, because Mrs. Munro was at some risk of falling. Terry was careful to stand not so close that she crowded or overprotected Mrs. Munro but close enough to protect her should she lose her balance. While close to Mrs. Munro, Terry could smell her, gaining a quick sense of possible hygiene or continence problems. Terry used her voice quality to display encouragement and support. Terry watched and listened carefully for clues about the nature of Mrs. Munro's emotional state. In particular, she watched facial expressions and listened for evidence of fear or insecurity during Mrs. Munro's performance of activities. All of these sensations contributed to an image of Mrs. Munro that influenced Terry's practice.

There are other aspects of reasoning during therapy that are even harder to describe. Fleming (1994c) described this as "knowing more than we can tell" (p. 24). She explained that much of the profession's knowledge is practical knowledge, which is "seldom discussed and rarely described" (p. 25). This tacit knowledge, combined with the rich sensory aspects of actual practice, helps to explain why reading about therapy and doing therapy are such different experiences. In her exploration of therapists who provided services to children, Harris (2005) concluded that each therapist's individual bodily differences and preferences may subtly shape therapy, in that some therapists might avoid situations that they find physically uncomfortable (e.g., if they are intolerant of certain smells), and others might engage in therapy practices that they themselves find comforting (e.g., applying deep pressure, much like what one gets when being hugged). Hooper (1997, 2008) has also noted the importance of how our own values, beliefs, and assumptions underpin each practitioner's grasp of the therapy process. So keep in mind that therapy always happens in the real world with real people, and you will see variations because each therapist is different.

Theory and Practice

There has been a long-standing discussion in many professions about the role of theory in professional practice (Kessels & Korthagen, 1996). Theories help practitioners to make decisions, although Cohn (1989) noted that the problems of practice rarely present themselves in the straightforward manner described in textbook theories. Professional reasoning involves the naming and framing of problems on the basis of a personal understanding of the client's situation (Schön, 1983). In problem identification and problem solution, practitioners blend theories with their own personal and practice experiences to guide their actions. Theoretical knowledge helps the practitioner to avoid unjustified assumptions or the use of ineffective therapy techniques and to reflect on how his or her own experiences in therapy are similar to or different from theoretical understandings (Parham, 1987). In Chapter 37, you will find more information about how theories inform practice as well as how our underlying assumptions shape our therapy actions. The point here is that although practice can (and should) be informed by theories, it is ultimately a result of how each therapist interprets each therapy situation and then acts on that understanding.

Cognitive Processes Underlying Professional Reasoning

In the case study, Terry had to remember, obtain, and manage a great deal of information quickly to provide effective and efficient intervention. How did she do it? Research findings from the field of cognitive psychology help to explain how practitioners think and how experience combined with reflection fosters increasing expertise. Individuals receive, store, and organize information in *frames* or *scripts*, which are complex representations of phenomena (Bruning, Schraw, & Ronning, 1999; Carr & Shotwell, 2007). This process involves both working memory and long-term memory. Working memory can hold very few thoughts at a time, which is one reason that one sometimes has to look at the phone book two or three times in order to correctly recall a number that one is dialing. Similarly, students and new practitioners find it challenging to try to keep all the important considerations in mind when dealing with a client. Practitioners with extensive experience have this information organized and stored in their long-term memories and thus do not have to actively juggle all the details. For example, in school, Terry probably learned many of the common problems associated with someone who has had a stroke. She also has seen perhaps 100 people with strokes over the past several years. She has built up a general representation in her mind of what to expect when she receives a referral for someone who has had a stroke. She anticipates that many of these individuals will have extensive medical charts because they almost always have prior medical problems, such as diabetes and high blood pressure. She will not be surprised if the person is overweight. She expects to see impairments in cognition that often affect the person's ability to do everyday tasks, such as dressing, cooking, and driving. As part of her frame, Terry has built-in mental rules that help her to categorize and detect differences. For instance, although she knows that many people who have strokes have movement impairments, she knows that not all do. Furthermore, when movement is impaired, she expects individuals with a left cerebrovascular accident (CVA) to have right-sided weakness and those with a right CVA to have left-sided weakness. Additionally, she knows that a person's social support system is critical for promoting an adaptive response to disability. She may use certain cues, such as the presence or absence of frequent family visits, to prompt her to categorize a family as supportive or non-supportive.

In addition to framing or "chunking" information, Terry also creates and uses scripts or procedural rules that guide her thinking (Bruning et al., 1999; Carr & Shotwell, 2007). Just as her mental frames help her to organize and retrieve her knowledge about common aspects of stroke, scripts help her to organize common occurrences or events. For instance, she understands that her role involves responding to the referral by seeing the client, writing her findings on the correct form, providing interventions, communicating verbally with the other team members, and developing discharge plans. Terry likely has scripts about the implications for clients with supportive families and those without. In her experience, a supportive family cares for its family member at home, regardless of the family's financial resources. Alternatively, clients with little family support are more likely to face institutional care. Again, these scripts are formed by Terry's observations and experiences over time and serve the purpose of helping her to anticipate likely events.

The mind appears to use frames and scripts to support effective processing of information by providing efficient mental frameworks for handling complex information (Carr & Shotwell, 2007). Each person individually constructs them. It is no surprise that students and new practitioners often struggle to retain and effectively use their therapy knowledge. It takes time and repetition of experiences to develop effective reasoning based on efficient storage in long-term memory allowing for targeted use of short-term memory as therapy happens. Important aspects of the process are as follows (Roberts, 1996):

- *Cue acquisition:* Searching for the helpful and targeted information through observation and questioning.
- *Pattern recognition:* Noticing similarities and differences among situations.
- *Limiting the problem space:* Using patterns to help focus cue acquisition and knowledge application on the most fruitful areas.

- *Problem formulation:* Developing an explanation of what is going on, why it is going on, and what a better situation or outcome might be.
- *Problem solution:* Identifying courses of action based on the problem formulation.

These cognitive processes are interactive and rarely occur in a linear fashion. Rather, the mind jumps around between the information at hand and that which has been stored up from prior learning while attempting to make sense of the situation. Now that we have a better understanding of the basic systems our mind uses to support our professional reasoning, we turn our attention to research on the different aspects of professional reasoning that have surfaced from research on occupational therapists.

Aspects of Professional Reasoning

Although there appear to be common processes underlying reasoning in practice, the focus of that mental activity appears to vary with the demands of the problems to be addressed. Fleming (1991) was the first within occupational therapy to describe how occupational therapists seemed to use different thinking approaches, depending on the nature of the clinical problem they were addressing. She referred to this process as the "therapist with the three-track mind" (p. 1007). Since that time, others have examined the different aspects of occupational therapy professional reasoning. Most of this research has been done with occupational therapists, although at least one case study (Lyons & Crepeau, 2001) suggests there is some application for occupational therapy assistants as well. These aspects of professional reasoning are listed in Table 30.1, along with the typical focus clues for recognizing when that sort of reasoning is occurring.

Scientific Reasoning

Scientific reasoning is used to understand the condition that is affecting an individual and to decide on interventions that are in the client's best interest. It is a logical process that parallels scientific inquiry. Forms of scientific reasoning that are described in occupational therapy are diagnostic reasoning (Rogers & Holm, 1991) and procedural reasoning (Fleming, 1991, 1994b) in addition to the general use of hypothetical-deductive reasoning (Tomlin, 2008). Scientific reasoning is also referred to as treatment planning (Pelland, 1987) in which the therapist uses selected theories both to identify problems and to guide decision making.

Diagnostic reasoning is concerned with clinical problem sensing and problem definition. The process

TABLE 30.1 Aspects of Reasoning in Occupational Therapy

Reasoning Aspect	Clues for Recognizing in Therapist Discussions	Examples of the Therapy Problems or Questions which Draw Out This Reasoning
Scientific Reasoning involving the use of applied logical and scientific methods, such as hypothesis testing, pattern recognition, theory-based decision making, and statistical evidence.	Impersonal, focused on the diagnosis, condition, guiding theory, evidence from research, or what "typically" happens with clients like the one being considered.	What is the nature of the illness, injury, or development problem? What are the common impairments or disabilities resulting from this condition? What are the typical contextual factors that affect performance? What theories and research are available to guide assessment and intervention?
Diagnostic Investigative reasoning and analysis of cause or nature of conditions requiring occupational therapy intervention can be considered one component of scientific reasoning.	Uses both personal and impersonal information. Therapists attempt to explain why client is experiencing problems using a blend of science- and client-based information.	What are the occupational performance problems this client has or may have in the future? What are the factors contributing to this problem (impairments, performance context)? How are these problems manifest (skills, habits, routines, occupational roles)?
Procedural Reasoning in which therapist considers and uses intervention routines for identified conditions. May be science based or may reflect the habits and culture of the intervention setting.	Characterized by therapist using therapy regimes or routines thought to be effective with problems identified and that are typically used with clients in that setting.	What evaluation and intervention protocols are applicable to this person's situation? How are clients like this usually handled in my setting?

TABLE 30.1 Aspects of Reasoning in Occupational Therapy *(Continued)*

Reasoning Aspect	Clues for Recognizing in Therapist Discussions	Examples of the Therapy Problems or Questions which Draw Out This Reasoning
Narrative Reasoning process used to make sense of people's particular circumstances; prospectively imagine the effect of illness, disability, or occupational performance problems on their daily lives; and create a collaborative story that is enacted with clients and families through intervention.	Personal, focused on the client, including past, present, and anticipated future. Involves an appreciation of client culture as the basis for understanding client narrative. Relates to the "so what" of the condition for the person's life.	What is this person's life story? What is the nature of this person as an occupational being? How has the health condition affected the person's life story or ability to continue his or her life story? What occupational activities are most important to this person? What occupational activities are both meaningful to this person and useful for meeting therapy goals?
Pragmatic Practical reasoning that is used to fit therapy possibilities into the current realities of service delivery, such as scheduling options, payment for services, equipment availability, therapists' skills, management directives, and the personal situation of the therapist.	Generally not focused on client or client's condition but rather on all the physical and social "stuff" that surrounds the therapy encounter, as well as the therapist's internal sense of what he or she is capable of and has the time and energy to complete.	Who referred this person and why? Who is paying for services, and what are their rules? What family or caregiver resources are there to support intervention? What are the expectations of my supervisor and workplace? How much time do I have to see this person? What therapy space and equipment are available? What are my practice competencies?
Ethical Reasoning directed toward analyzing an ethical dilemma, generating alternative solutions, and determining actions to be taken. Systematic approach to moral conflict.	Tension is often evident as therapist attempts to determine what is the "right" thing to do particularly when faced with dilemmas in therapy competing principles, risks, and benefits.	Are the benefits of therapy worth the cost? Are the risks of therapy worth the benefits? How should I prioritize my caseload? What are the limits of how I change my documentation to maximize payment? What should I do when other members of the treatment team are operating in ways that I feel conflict with the goals of the person receiving services?
Interactive Thinking directed toward building positive interpersonal relationships with clients, permitting collaborative problem identification and problem solving.	Therapist is concerned with what client likes or does not like. Use of praise, empathetic comments, and nonverbal behaviors to encourage and support client's cooperation.	How can I best relate to this person? How can I put this person at ease? What is the best way for me to encourage this person? What nonverbal strategies should I use in this situation? Where should I place myself relative to this person so that I support him or her but do not "invade" the person? What cultural factors do I need to consider as I engage with the person?
Conditional A blending of all forms of reasoning for the purposes of flexibly responding to changing conditions or predicting possible client futures.	Typically found with more experienced therapists who can "see" multiple futures based on the therapist's past experiences and current information.	Where is this person going? How will the various therapy options play out, given this person's health condition, social situation, economic status, and culture? Given these future possible trajectories, what is the best action I can take now?

For more additional summaries of these aspects, refer to Carrier, Levasseur, Bédard, & Desrosiers, J. 2010; Schell & Schell, 2007; and Unsworth, 2011.

starts in advance of seeing a client. Occupational therapy practitioners, because of their domains of concern, look primarily for occupational performance problems. Furthermore, the nature of the problems they expect to find is influenced by the information in the requests for services. Some of Terry's diagnostic reasoning, described earlier, included information about the typical symptoms associated with having a stroke.

Procedural reasoning occurs when practitioners are "thinking about the disease or disability and deciding which intervention activities (procedures) they might employ to remediate the person's functional performance problems" (Fleming, 1991, p. 1008). This may involve an interview, an observation of the person engaged in a task, or formal evaluations using standardized measures. Although one hopes that procedural reasoning is science based, Tomlin makes the important observation that procedural reasoning can become an unquestioned implementation of therapy protocols, in which case it becomes less scientific in nature (Tomlin, 2008). That is why there is such an emphasis on evidence-based practice, which challenges the practitioner to routinely evaluate customary therapy approaches based on of the best information currently available (Holm, 2000; Law & MacDermid, 2008; Tickle-Degnen, 2000). Chapter 31 speaks on the importance of evidence-based practice, and all of the chapters in this text, along with many other occupational therapy texts, include evidence that can help guide practice.

In the case study, Terry used a combination of interview and observation, both of which were guided by her working hypothesis that Mrs. Munro had cognitive problems that might affect her safe performance at home. She was likely operating on the basis of her understanding of cognitive theories (such as those described in Chapter 55) as well as her own experience with similar clients. As intervention begins, more data are collected, and the occupational therapy practitioner gains a sharper clinical image. This clinical image is the result of the interplay between what the occupational therapy practitioner expects to see (such as the usual course of the disease) and the client's actual performance. In the case study, there was congruence between Mrs. Munro's abilities and problems in performing activities of daily living and Terry's expectations of someone making a good recovery from a stroke.

Mattingly (1994b) made the point that occupational therapists have a "two-body practice" (p. 37). By that, she meant that occupational therapy practitioners view a person in two ways: the body as a machine, in which parts may be broken, and the person as a life, filled with personal meanings and hopes. Much of the procedural reasoning in occupational therapy addresses issues related to the body as machine, although current theories in the field do place much more emphasis on the need to understand the client as an open system, responsive to and acting upon the environment. The next form of reasoning, narrative reasoning, provides the occupational therapy practitioner with a way to understand a person's illness experience.

Narrative Reasoning

Understanding the meaning that a disease, illness, or disability has to an individual is a task that goes beyond the scientific understanding of disease processes and organ systems. Rather, it requires that practitioners find a way to understand the meaning of this experience from the client's perspective. Mattingly (1994a) suggested that practitioners do this through a form of reasoning called narrative reasoning. Narrative reasoning is so named because it involves thinking in story form. It is not uncommon for an occupational therapy practitioner who is preparing to substitute for another with a client to ask the other practitioner, "So what is the client's story?"

In the case study, part of Terry's reasoning was concerned with making decisions in light of what was important to Mrs. Munro. This process of collaboration and empathy has been described as "building a communal horizon of understanding" (Clark, Ennevor, & Richardson, 1996, p. 376). Terry gained understanding by listening attentively to Mrs. Munro's stories about her husband and how he loved her cooking. It is apparent from this session that Mrs. Munro's home is more than just a house. It is the place in which she lived with her husband, where he died, and where she still felt his presence. Part of Mrs. Munro's story is that going home is going back to her husband. If this stroke were to prevent that, Mrs. Munro would lose more than her independence; she would lose symbolic connections to her husband. Although a logical case might be made that Mrs. Munro should start considering a more supportive living environment, Terry understands that for Mrs. Munro, this would not be an acceptable ending. Consequently, Terry worked hard to obtain the support systems that would be necessary for Mrs. Munro to function in her chosen environment, where she will continue her life story.

Often, occupational therapy practitioners work with individuals whose life stories are so severely disrupted that they cannot imagine what their future will look like. Mattingly (1994a) believed that in these situations, skillful practitioners help their clients to invent new life stories. More recently this has been referred to as helping client's "recraft" their "occupational narratives" (Auzmendia, de las Heras, Kielhofner, & Miranda, 2008, p. 313). To some degree, these stories become visible as the occupational therapy practitioner and the client develop goals together. The use of life stories is also apparent when activities are selected for both their healing potential and their particular significance to the person. To do this, one must first solicit occupational stories from the individual (Clark et al., 1996, Hamilton, 2008). With an understanding of clients' past occupational stories, practitioners can help individuals to create new stories and new futures for themselves. If Mrs. Munro's symptoms were more severe and she was in a more extended therapy process, Terry might explore

Mrs. Munro's interest in cooking as an activity that she liked and that would offer many therapeutic opportunities. Furthermore, Mrs. Munro might find that she could express her pleasure in cooking for others by making special treats, first for other clients and then perhaps for neighbors in exchange for their help with chores. During this process, Mrs. Munro would not only be regaining coordination and dexterity but also she would be regaining her sense of self as a productive person. This narrative aspect of clinical reasoning, which ultimately focuses on the person as an occupational being, provides a link between the founding values of the profession and current practice demands (Gray, 1998).

Pragmatic Reasoning

Pragmatic reasoning is yet another strand of reasoning that goes beyond the practitioner–client relationship and addresses the world in which therapy occurs (Schell, 2007; Schell & Cervero,1993). This world is considered from two perspectives: the practice context and the personal context. Because reasoning during therapy is a practical activity, a number of everyday issues have been identified over the years that affect the therapy process. These include resources for intervention, organizational culture, power relationships among team members, reimbursement practices, and practice trends in the profession (Barris, 1987; Howard, 1991; Neuhaus, 1988; Rogers & Holm, 1991). Studies examining clinical reasoning have confirmed that occupational therapy practitioners both actively consider and are influenced by their practice contexts (Creighton, Dijkers, Bennett, & Brown, 1995; Schell, 1994; Strong, Gilbert, Cassidy, & Bennett, 1995, Unsworth, 2005). An example of pragmatic reasoning in the case study was Terry's use of immediate resources (the flower vase) in Mrs. Munro's room as a therapy tool. Although Terry had thought of appropriate activities related to self-care, she had to identify practical alternatives quickly when it turned out that Mrs. Munro was already dressed. Practical constraints for Terry included (1) the time it would take to move Mrs. Munro to the clinic, where there might be more resources; (2) the need to get the required information on that day because Mrs. Munro was going home; and (3) the physical constraints of what was available within the room. Terry's invention of a feasible alternative was a product of both her therapeutic imagination and the cues that were provided within her practice setting.

Terry's attention to the influence of team members demonstrates pragmatic reasoning directed to interpersonal and group issues. She knew that the physician had the power to make discharge decisions. She was aware of the pressures on the physician by third-party payers to discharge clients as quickly as possible. Practice requires that practitioners' reason about negotiating their clients' interests within the practice culture.

The practitioner's personal situation also is part of the pragmatic reasoning process. Although less readily identified in research, Unsworth (2005) surfaced some examples in her research in which therapists "weighed their own therapy skills against the therapeutic needs of the clients" (p. 36) in order to decide whether to refer to others with more expertise. A person's clinical competencies, preferences, commitment to the profession, and life role demands outside of work all affect the therapy choices that are considered and thus enter into the reasoning process. For instance, if a practitioner does not feel safe helping a client stand or transfer to a bed, the therapist is more likely to use tabletop activities in which the client can participate from a wheelchair. Another occupational therapy practitioner might feel uncomfortable interacting with individuals who have depression and, therefore, might be quick to suggest that such clients are not motivated for therapy. A practitioner who has a young family to go home to might opt not to schedule clients late in the day so as to get home as early as possible. These simple personal issues result in clinical decisions that affect the scope and timing of therapy services. Hooper (1997, 2008) suggested that fundamental issues, such as a practitioner's values and general worldview, strongly affect the way in which an individual constructs his or her reasoning. Such worldviews play an important role in the next kind of reasoning: ethical reasoning.

Ethical Reasoning

All of the forms of reasoning that have been described so far help the practitioner to respond to the following questions: What is this person's current occupational situation? What can be done to enhance the person's situation? Ethical reasoning goes one step further and asks: What should be done? Rogers (1983) framed these three questions (here paraphrased) in her Eleanor Clark Slagle Lecture and went on to state, "The clinical reasoning process terminates in an ethical decision, rather than a scientific one, and the ethical nature of the goal of clinical reasoning projects itself over the entire sequence" (p. 602). In the case study, Terry's ethical dilemma is to understand Mrs. Munro's personal wishes and to honor them when developing a therapy plan that realistically addresses Mrs. Munro's limitations. This can be particularly challenging when the pressures of financial realities (such as Mrs. Munro's limited income and the lack of insurance for supported living) affect available options. A number of occupational therapy authors have addressed the ethical aspect of professional reasoning (Fondiller, Rosage, & Neuhaus, 1990; Howard, 1991; Neuhaus, 1988; Peloquin, 1993), and Chapter 32 of this text is devoted to the issue of the ethics of the profession. The purpose here is to introduce ethical reasoning as yet another of the components of professional reasoning in occupational therapy.

Interactive Reasoning

The provision of therapy is inherently a communicative process (Schwartzberg, 2002). In occupational therapy, practitioners must gain the trust of their clients and of people who are important in the clients' world. This is because occupational therapy involves "doing with" as opposed to "doing to" clients (Mattingly & Fleming, 1994, p. 178). A therapist gains this trust by entering the client's life world (Crepeau, 1991) and by using several interpersonal strategies that are designed to motivate clients, such as those discussed in Chapter 33. Once they are in the client's life world, occupational therapy practitioners can better understand how to help the individuals resolve performance problems.

It is likely that some reasoning focused on interaction is conscious, as when a practitioner remembers that "I need to be sure to praise the client often because he gets discouraged so easily." Other interpersonal acts might be quite automatic, such as when a therapist touches a person's arm to convey sympathy. It is sometimes easiest to detect the importance of effective interactive reasoning when the therapist makes a mistake or gets an unexpected reaction and is forced to regroup and rebuild the therapy relationship.

A Process of Synthesis in Shared Activity

The preceding section described the aspects of professional reasoning separately to illustrate the different parts of the process. Table 30.1 includes examples of the kinds of questions that practitioners seek to answer with the different aspects of professional reasoning. However, these facets of reasoning are not separate or parallel processes; rather, the opposite appears to be the case. Virtually all the research about reasoning in practice suggests that these different forms interact and overlap with each other (Carrier et al., 2010; Mitchell & Unsworth, 2005). Furthermore, Toth-Cohen (2008) makes the point that the "shared activity" that occurs during the therapy process is an "integral part" of the reasoning process (p. 82).

Reasoning to Solve Problems

Scientific, narrative, pragmatic, ethical, and interactive reasoning processes are intertwined throughout the therapy process. Indeed, each perspective informs the other. In the case study, Terry's understanding of medical science helped her to know what might be the potential impairments and performance problems, but her narrative reasoning helped her to understand the importance to Mrs. Munro of returning home. Put together, these two forms of reasoning help Terry to reach an unspoken understanding that there would be a high risk for depression (which could worsen her client's medical condition) if Mrs. Munro did not return to her home, which means so much to her. Furthermore, the practical constraints associated with the setting and Mrs. Munro's reimbursement prompted Terry to reason about the ethics of suggesting that she return home alone (where she might not be safe), consider more alternative supported living (which she may not want and probably can't afford), and finally of allowing her to return home with the support of home health care and neighbors.

Conditional Process

Not only must practitioners blend different aspects of reasoning in order to interact effectively with their clients, but they must also flexibly modify interventions in response to changing conditions and to the context in which the therapy is occurring. Terry showed her flexibility by inventing an activity with the flower vase when her plan to work with Mrs. Munro on bathing and dressing did not pan out. Creighton and colleagues (1995) noticed that occupational therapy practitioners preplanned interventions in a hierarchical manner. They observed that practitioners typically brought several sets of supplies to an intervention session. One set would be directed to the expected level of performance, the others to a stage higher and a stage lower than the expected performance. As an example, one practitioner, in preparation for a writing activity with a client who had a spinal cord injury, brought a short writing splint and unlined paper. This practitioner also brought a longer splint to provide wrist support (in case the client's hand control was worse than expected) and lined paper, which required more precision (in case the hand control was better than expected). This practitioner blended scientific and pragmatic concerns in a way that anticipated several possible situations that might occur.

On a larger scale, Fleming (1994a) described the ability of skilled occupational therapy practitioners to "form an image of future life possibilities for the person" (p. 234). The ability to form these images (or schemata, to use a cognitive terms) seems to require a blend of all the forms of clinical reasoning, along with sufficient clinical experience to have seen various different outcomes with former clients. These images help practitioners to select therapeutic activities on a day-to-day basis. For instance, the writing activity for the client who had a spinal cord injury not only is a good activity for increasing coordination but also presages occupations that will enable the client to regain control of his or her life through writing his or her own checks, signing his or her name on legal documents, and using various forms of technology for work and play. If this client were an accountant, these would be powerful images. Conversely, if the client were a professional athlete, the occupational therapy practitioner might have to create different activities to allow the client to develop a vision of himself as a future coach or teacher. The activities that are used in occupational therapy can help to meet specific short-term goals and shape long-term expectations. It is in this way that practitioners help individuals to reengage in their lives through the use of meaningful occupations.

Ecological View of Professional Reasoning

In Units I, II, and IV, several chapters discuss how occupational performance is the result of a complex transaction among a person's inherent capacities, the person's prior experiences, and the demands of the performance context. Similarly, the professional reasoning process and the resulting therapy actions represent transactions that occur among the practitioner, the client, the therapy context, and the actual therapy activity (Schell, Unsworth, & Schell, 2008; Toth-Cohen, 2008).

The practitioner's reasoning is shaped by both personal and professional perspectives as shown in Figure 30.1. Each practitioner brings to the therapy situation knowledge and skills that are grounded in life experiences, including personal characteristics such as physical capacities, personality, values, and beliefs. These form a *personal* self that consists of the person's embodied characteristics (Lakoff & Johnson, 1999) along with their interpretation of the experiences or worldview (Hooper, 2008). These personal factors shape each person's perception and interpretation of all life activities, and thus act as a *personal lens* through which each practitioner views all life events. Layered over or entwined with this personal self is the *professional self*, which includes the therapist's professional knowledge from education, experiences from prior clients, and beliefs about what is important to do in therapy along with knowledge of specific technical skills and therapy routines available for use in the practice context. Thus, a therapist views therapy situations through both a personal and *professional lens*, which over time likely merge into the therapist's customary ways of viewing the therapy process. The personal and professional selves act in concert to respond to various problems of practice.

Just as with the therapist, the client comes to therapy with his or her own life experiences and personal characteristics, life situation, and performance problems that prompted the need for therapy. The client may also come with his or her own theories about what is causing the performance

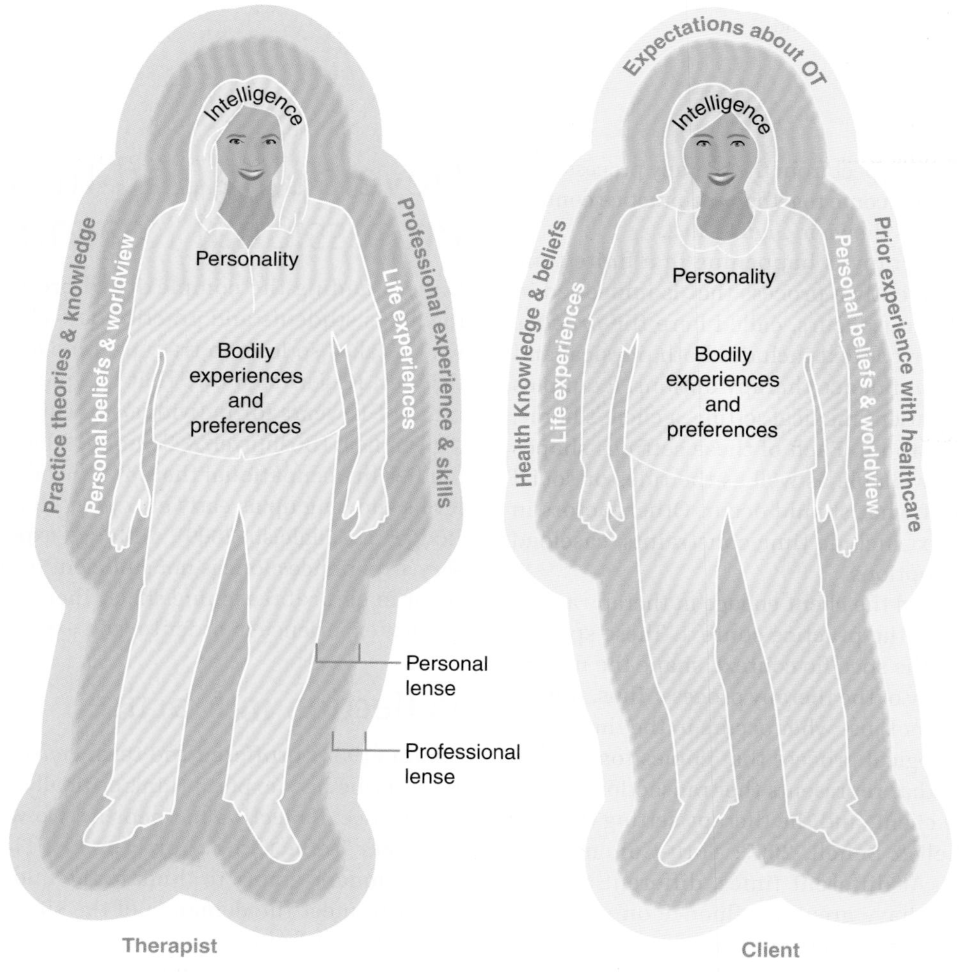

FIGURE 30.1 Personal and professional lenses shape occupational therapists' professional reasoning.

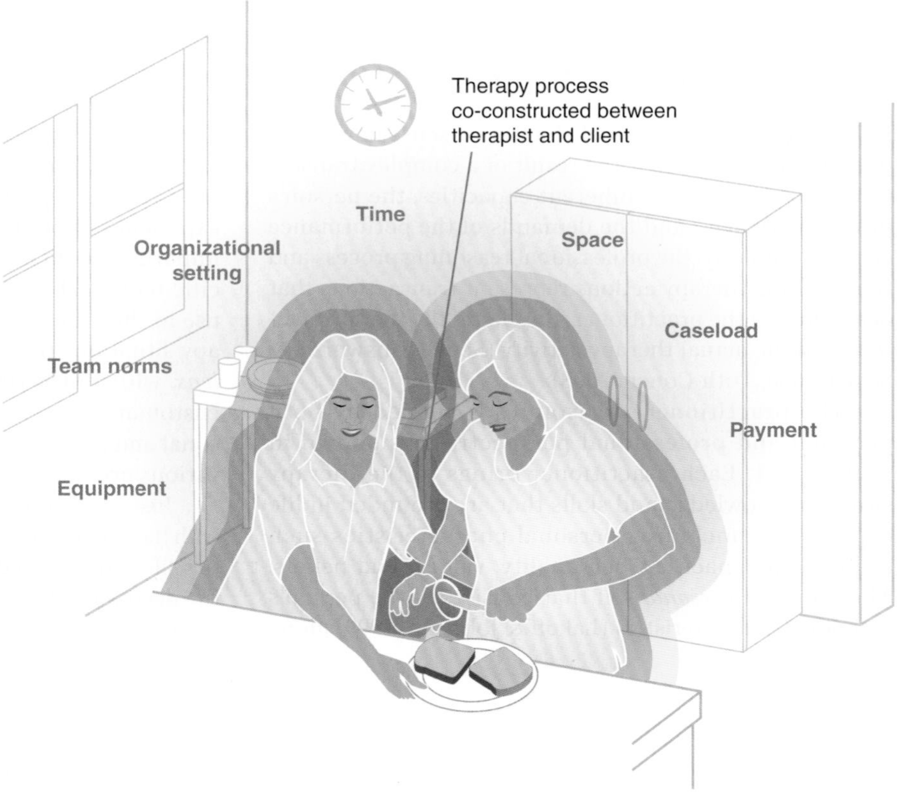

FIGURE 30.2 Schell's Ecological Model of Professional Reasoning. Professional reasoning is an ecological process in which the therapist and the client engage in therapy activities in a specific setting. All of these components transact to shape therapist reasoning, resulting actions with the client, and ultimately, therapy outcomes.

problems and what to expect from the therapy process. The therapist and the client come together in a practice context to engage in therapy, as shown in Figure 30.2.

Because this therapy is happening in a finite time and place, it is inherently a process that is imbedded in the setting in which it occurs, called here the *practice context*. The practice context includes both physical and social aspects that influence therapy options. Examples might include outpatient medical setting, a client's home, or a student's classroom. Each of these settings shapes the therapy tools available as well as the rules or social expectations about what should occur. Other factors in the practice context include time constraints, caseload size, and payment options.

The therapist and the client engage in therapy activities together within the practice context. These specific actors, working in the specific context, shape the nature, scope, and trajectory of the therapy process. Thus, professional reasoning is not just what occurs in the therapist's mind; it is an ecological process that comes together in a therapy activity that represents the transaction among the therapist, the client, and the therapy setting (Carrier et al., 2010; Schell & Schell, 2007; Toth-Cohen, 2008; Unsworth, 2011). At different times, different aspects of this system will have greater influence on what will occur. Reflective therapists are encouraged to be mindful of all these factors and their influence on their reasoning and associated therapy actions and therapy outcomes.

Developing and Improving Professional Reasoning

Understanding the complexity of professional reasoning helps students and practitioners alike to appreciate why it takes so long to truly become an excellent practitioner. Research shows that it typically takes a minimum of 10 years for individuals to gain expertise within a given field (Boshuizen & Schmidt, 2000), although some studies in occupational therapy show differing expertise levels showing up as early as 5 years (Rassafiani, Ziviani, Rodger, & Dalgleish, 2009). Although experience is necessary, experience alone is not sufficient to ensure advancement in clinical reasoning skills. Therapists must reflect on that experience in order to gain expertise.

Reflection in Practice

Schön (1983) proffered the term *reflective practitioner* to describe how experts think critically about their own experience. Reflection happens in two ways. First, practitioners "reflect in action" (p. 49). This involves the practitioners' ability to think in the midst of action and adapt to meet the demands of the situation. Reflection in action most often occurs when the usual approaches are not working. "Reflection on action" (p. 61) is the term Schön uses for critical thinking that occurs after the fact.

TABLE 30.2 Professional Reasoning Continuum and Characteristics

Category & Reflective Experience	Characteristics
Novice (No experience in practice area)	• No experience in situation of practice; depends on theory to guide practice. • Uses rule-based procedural reasoning to guide actions but does not recognize contextual cues; not skillful in adapting rules to fit situation. • Narrative reasoning is used to establish social relationships but does not significantly inform practice. • Pragmatic reasoning is stressed in terms of job survival skills. • Recognizes overt ethical issues.
Advanced beginner (<1 yr)	• Begins to incorporate contextual information into rule-based thinking. • Recognizes differences between theoretical expectations and presenting problems. • Limited experience impedes recognition of patterns and salient cues; does not prioritize well. • Relies on external guides so as forms to guide reasoning. • Gaining skill in pragmatic and narrative reasoning. • Begins to recognize more subtle ethical issues.
Competent (1–3 yr)	• Automatically performs more therapeutic skills and attends to more issues. • Is able to develop communal horizon with people receiving service. • Is able to sort relevant data and prioritize intervention goals related to desired outcomes. • Planning is deliberate, efficient, and responsive to contextual issues. • Uses conditional reasoning to modify intervention but lacks flexibility. • Recognizes ethical dilemmas posed by practice setting.
Proficient (3–5 yr)	• Perceives situations as wholes. • Reflects on expanded range of experiences, permitting more focused evaluation and more flexibility in intervention. • Creatively combines different diagnostic and procedural approaches. • More attentive to occupational stories and relevance for intervention. • More skillful in negotiating resources to meet patient/client needs. • Increased sophistication in recognizing situational nature of ethical reasoning.
Expert (5–10 yr)	• Clinical reasoning becomes a quick intuitive process. • Procedural and pragmatic reasoning more detailed. • Able to flow conversation and action smoothly. • Use understanding of client and client's perspective to determine intervention. • Relies on internal guides or images to support actions.

From Benner, 1984; Clark et al., 1996; Creighton et al., 1995; Dreyfus & Dreyfus, 1986; Mattingly & Fleming, 1994; Rassafiani et al., 2009; Slater & Cohn, 1991; Strong et al., 1995, Unsworth, 2001; Unsworth & Mitchell, 2005

Reflection about practice, identifying what worked and what did not, and being open to alternative conceptions are necessary to support the learning associated with advancing expertise. As described in Chapters 31 and 37, the use of research evidence to support practice and the application of formal theories along with systematic observation and data collection are important to reflection and, thus, to expert professional reasoning.

Expertise Continuum

There is a slowly growing body of evidence about the nature of professional reasoning in occupational therapy. Dreyfus and Dreyfus' (1986) conceptualization of professional expertise has been applied to occupational therapy (Slater & Cohn, 1991) and elaborated on over time by a number of researchers, although often, the research dichotomizes beginners or novices from experts. Table 30.2 summarizes changes that have surfaced in research about the reasoning of occupational therapists as they develop expertise. Although the changes that are listed in Table 30.2 are associated with typical years of experience, it is important to recognize that development is dynamic and influenced by many factors beyond just the years of experience. One important consideration is the familiarity of the task and the context. Expertise is a function of how consistently a person is effective within a given context (Benner, 1984; Rassafiani et al, 2009; Toth-Cohen, 2008). Someone who demonstrates expertise at providing services in a school setting might be just minimally competent in a nursing home setting. Additionally, active reflection about one's experiences is critical to becoming an expert (Benner, 1984; Gambrill, 2005; Slater & Cohn, 1991). Refer to Chapter 67 for more discussion about professional development, continuing competence, and expertise.

Conclusion

Professional reasoning is the process that practitioners use to plan, direct, perform, and reflect on client care. It is a whole-body and multisensory process that requires complex cognitive activity. Practitioners develop cognitive frames and scripts as they gain experience, forming the basis of professional knowledge and action. Professional reasoning is multifaceted and enables practitioners to understand client issues from different perspectives. Practitioners use the logical processes associated with scientific reasoning to understand the client's impairments, disabilities, and performance contexts and to predict the impact these have on occupational performance. Narrative reasoning helps practitioners to appreciate the meaning of occupational performance limitations to the client, thus supporting client-centered care. Practitioners use pragmatic reasoning when they address the practical realities associated with service delivery. All of these forms of reasoning lead to an ethical reasoning process by which practitioners select the best therapy action to respond to the client's occupational performance needs. The process of professional reasoning involves a transaction among the practitioner's personal and professional perspectives, the client's perspectives, and the demands of the practice context that unfolds in therapy activities. Expertise develops as the practitioner gains experience and reflects on that experience for deeper understanding.

References

Auzmendia, A. L., de las Heras, C. G., Kielhofner, G., & Miranda, C. (2008). Recrafting occupational narratives. In G. Kielhofner (Ed.), *Model of human occupation* (4th ed., pp. 313–336). Baltimore, MD: Lippincott Williams & Wilkins.

Barris, R. (1987). Clinical reasoning in psychosocial occupational therapy: The evaluation process. *Occupational Therapy Journal of Research, 7*, 147–162.

Benner, P. (1984). *From novice to expert.* Menlo Park, CA: Addison-Wesley.

Boshuizen, H. P. A., & Schmidt, H. G. (2000). The development of clinical reasoning expertise. In J. Higgs & M. Jones (Eds.), *Clinical reasoning in the health professions* (2nd ed., pp. 15–22). Boston, MA: Butterworth Heinemann.

Bruning, R. H., Schraw, G. J., & Ronning, R. R. (1999). *Cognitive psychology and instruction* (3rd ed.). Upper Saddle River, NJ: Merrill.

Carr, M., & Shotwell, M. (2007). Information processing and clinical reasoning. In B. A. B. Schell & J. W. Schell (Eds.), *Clinical and professional reasoning in occupational therapy.* Baltimore, MD: Lippincott Williams & Wilkins.

Carrier, A., Levasseur, M., Bédard, D., & Desrosiers, J. (2010). Community occupational therapists' clinical reasoning: Identifying tacit knowledge. *Australian Occupational Therapy Journal, 57*, 356–365.

Clark, F., Ennevor, B. L., & Richardson, P. L. (1996). A grounded theory of techniques for occupational storytelling and occupational story making. In R. Zemke & F. Clark (Eds.), *Occupational science: The evolving discipline* (pp. 373–392). Philadelphia, PA: F. A. Davis.

Cohn, E. S. (1989). Fieldwork education: Shaping a foundation for clinical reasoning. *American Journal of Occupational Therapy, 43*, 240–244.

Creighton, C., Dijkers, M., Bennett, N., & Brown, K. (1995). Reasoning and the art of therapy for spinal cord injury. *American Journal of Occupational Therapy, 49*, 311–317.

Crepeau, E. B. (1991). Achieving intersubjective understanding: Examples from an occupational therapy treatment session. *American Journal of Occupational Therapy, 44*, 1016–1024.

Dreyfus, H. L., & Dreyfus, S. E. (1986). *Mind over machine: The power of human intuition and expertise in the era of the computer.* New York, NY: Free Press.

Fleming, M. H. (1991). The therapist with the three-track mind. *American Journal of Occupational Therapy, 45*, 1007–1014.

Fleming, M. H. (1994a). Conditional reasoning: Creating meaningful experiences. In C. Mattingly & M. H. Fleming (Eds.), *Clinical reasoning-forms of inquiry in a therapeutic practice* (pp. 197–235). Philadelphia, PA: F. A. Davis.

Fleming, M. H. (1994b). Procedural reasoning: Addressing functional limitations. In C. Mattingly & M. H. Fleming (Eds.), *Clinical reasoning: Forms of inquiry in a therapeutic practice* (pp. 137–177). Philadelphia, PA: F. A. Davis.

Fleming, M. H. (1994c). The search for tacit knowledge. In C. Mattingly & M. H. Fleming (Eds.), *Clinical reasoning: Forms of inquiry in a therapeutic practice* (pp. 22–33). Philadelphia, PA: F. A. Davis.

Fondiller, E. D., Rosage, L. J., & Neuhaus, B. E. (1990). Values influencing clinical reasoning in occupational therapy: An exploratory study. *Occupational Therapy Journal of Research, 10*, 41–55.

Gambrill, E. (2005). *Critical thinking in clinical practice: Improving the quality of judgments and decisions* (2nd ed.). Hoboken, NJ: Wiley & Sons.

Gray, J. M. (1998). Putting occupation in practice: Occupation as ends, occupation as means. *American Journal of Occupational Therapy, 52*, 354–364.

Hamilton, T. B. (2008). Narrative reasoning. In B. A. B. Schell & J. W. Schell (Eds.), *Clinical and professional reasoning in occupational therapy.* Baltimore, MD: Lippincott Williams & Wilkins.

Harris, D. L. (2005). *Therapist's sensory processing and its influence upon occupational therapy interventions in children with autism* (Unpublished master's thesis). Brenau University, Gainesville, GA.

Holm, M. B. (2000). Our mandate for the new millennium: Evidence-based practice. The 2000 Eleanor Clarke Slagle Lecture. *American Journal of Occupational Therapy, 54*, 575–585.

Hooper, B. (1997). The relationship between pretheoretical assumptions and clinical reasoning. *American Journal of Occupational Therapy, 51*, 328–338.

Hooper, B. (2008). Therapists' assumptions as a dimension of professional reasoning. In B. A. B. Schell & J. W. Schell (Eds.), *Clinical and professional reasoning in occupational therapy.* Baltimore, MD: Lippincott Williams & Wilkins.

Howard, B. S. (1991). How high do we jump?: The effect of reimbursement on occupational therapy. *American Journal of Occupational Therapy, 45*, 875–881.

Kessels, J. P. A. M., & Korthagen, F. A. (1996). The relationship between theory and practice: Back to the classics. *Educational Researcher, 25*(32), 17–22.

Kielhofner, G., & Forsyth, K. (2002). Thinking with theory: A framework for therapeutic reasoning. In G. Kielhofner (Ed.), *A model of human occupation: Theory and application* (3rd ed., pp. 162–178). Baltimore, MD: Lippincott Williams & Wilkins.

Lakoff, G., & Johnson, M. (1999). *Philosophy in the flesh: The embodied mind and its challenge to Western thought.* New York, NY: Basic Books.

Law, M., & MacDermid, J. (Ed.). (2008). *Evidence-based rehabilitation: A guide to practice* (2nd ed.). Thorofare, NJ: Slack.

Lyons, K. D., & Crepeau, E. B. (2001). Case report: The clinical reasoning of a certified occupational therapy assistant. *American Journal of Occupational Therapy, 55*, 577–581.

Mattingly, C. (1994a). The narrative nature of clinical reasoning. In C. Mattingly & M. H. Fleming (Eds.), *Clinical reasoning: Forms of inquiry in a therapeutic practice* (pp. 239–269). Philadelphia, PA: F. A. Davis.

Mattingly, C. (1994b). Occupational therapy as a two body practice: Body as machine. In C. Mattingly & M. H. Fleming (Eds.), *Clinical reasoning: Forms of inquiry in a therapeutic practice* (pp. 37–63). Philadelphia, PA: F. A. Davis.

Mattingly, C., & Fleming, M. H. (1994). Interactive reasoning: Collaborating with the person. In C. Mattingly & M. H. Fleming (Eds.),

Clinical reasoning: Forms of inquiry in a therapeutic practice (pp. 178–196). Philadelphia, PA: F. A. Davis.

Mitchell, R., & Unsworth, C. A. (2005). Clinical reasoning during community health home visits: Expert and novice differences. *British Journal of Occupational Therapy, 68*, 215–223.

Neuhaus, B. E. (1988). Ethical considerations in clinical reasoning: The impact of technology and cost containment. *American Journal of Occupational Therapy, 42*, 288–294.

Parham, D. (1987). Nationally speaking—toward professionalism: The reflective occupational therapy practitioner. *American Journal of Occupational Therapy, 41*, 555–561.

Pelland, M. J. (1987). A conceptual model for the instruction and supervision of treatment planning. *American Journal of Occupational Therapy, 41*, 351–359.

Peloquin, S. M. (1993). The depersonalization of patients: A profile gleaned from narratives. *American Journal of Occupational Therapy, 49*, 830–837.

Rassafiani, M., Ziviani, J., Rodger, S., & Dalgleish, L. (2009). Identification of occupational therapy clinical expertise: Decision-making characteristics. *Australian Journal of Occupational Therapy, 56*, 156–166.

Roberts, A. E. (1996). Clinical reasoning in occupational therapy: Idiosyncrasies in content and process. *British Journal of Occupational Therapy, 59*, 372–376.

Rogers, J. C. (1983). Clinical reasoning: The ethics, science, and art. *American Journal of Occupational Therapy, 37*, 601–616.

Rogers, J. C., & Holm, M. B. (1991). Occupational therapy diagnostic reasoning: A component of clinical reasoning. *American Journal of Occupational Therapy, 45*, 1045–1053.

Schell, B. A. B. (1994). The effect of practice context on occupational therapy practitioner's clinical reasoning (Doctoral dissertation, University of Georgia, 1994). *Dissertation Abstracts International*, AAT 9507243.

Schell, B. A. B. (2007). Pragmatic reasoning. In B. A. B. Schell & J. W. Schell (Eds.), *Clinical and professional reasoning in occupational therapy*. Baltimore, MD: Lippincott Williams & Wilkins.

Schell, B. A., & Cervero, R. M. (1993). Clinical reasoning in occupational therapy: An integrative review. *American Journal of Occupational Therapy, 47*, 605–610.

Schell, B. A. B., & Schell, J. W. (2007). *Clinical and professional reasoning in occupational therapy*. Baltimore, MD: Lippincott Williams & Wilkins.

Schell, B. A. B., Unsworth, C., & Schell, J. (2008). Theory and practice: New directions for research in professional reasoning. In B. A. B. Schell & J. W. Schell (Eds.), *Clinical and professional reasoning in occupational therapy*. Baltimore, MD: Lippincott Williams & Wilkins.

Schön, D. A. (1983). *The reflective practitioner: How professionals think in action*. New York, NY: Basic.

Schwartzberg, S. (2002). *Interactive reasoning in the practice of occupational therapy*. Upper Saddle River, NJ: Prentice Hall.

Slater, D. Y., & Cohn, E. S. (1991). Staff development through analysis of practice. *American Journal of Occupational Therapy, 45*, 1038–1044.

Strong, J., Gilbert, J., Cassidy, S., & Bennett, S. (1995). Expert clinicians and student view on clinical reasoning in occupational therapy. *British Journal of Occupational Therapy, 58*, 119–123.

Tickle-Degnen, L. (2000). Evidence-based practice forum: Gathering current research evidence to enhance clinical reasoning. *American Journal of Occupational Therapy, 54*, 102–105.

Tomlin, G. (2008). Scientific reasoning. In B. A. B. Schell & J. W. Schell (Eds.), *Clinical and professional reasoning in occupational therapy*. Baltimore, MD: Lippincott Williams & Wilkins.

Toth-Cohen, S. (2008). Using cultural-historical activity theory to study clinical reasoning in context. *Scandinavian Journal of Occupational Therapy, 15*, 82–94.

Unsworth, C. A. (2005). Using a head-mounted video camera to explore current conceptualizations of clinical reasoning in occupational therapy. *American Journal of Occupational Therapy, 59*, 31–40.

Unsworth, C. A. (2011). The evolving theory of clinical reasoning. In E. A. S. Duncan (Ed.), *Foundations for practice in occupational therapy* (5th ed.). New York, NY: Elsevier.

For additional resources on the subjects discussed in this chapter, visit http://thePoint.lww.com/Willard-Spackman12e.

CHAPTER 31

Evidence-Based Practice

Integrating Evidence to Inform Practice

Nancy Baker, Linda Tickle-Degnen

OUTLINE

LEARNING OBJECTIVES

After reading this chapter, you will be able to:

1. Define evidence-based practice and how it is integrated into clinical practice
2. Describe how to organize evidence around clinical tasks
3. Name the basic steps of evidence-based practice
4. Write answerable questions for different clinical tasks
5. Identify key methods for searching research literature effectively
6. Describe how to appraise the clinical relevance and trustworthiness of a research report
7. Describe how to interpret the results of a study for generalizability and clinical importance
8. Describe qualities of effective communication about evidence

Introduction

Imagine that you are going to work with a new client tomorrow. What do you do? How do you decide what this client needs and how you might help the client to achieve occupational goals? Let's imagine a hypothetical occupational therapy student, Rhonda, as she prepares to meet a new client on her first fieldwork. Rhonda's fieldwork supervisor has assigned her to work with Judy, a middle-aged woman with rheumatoid arthritis (RA). Judy is not only a new client to Rhonda but also her first client in a busy, fast-paced, outpatient clinic and one with an unfamiliar diagnosis.

In preparation, Rhonda discusses Judy with her supervisor to receive expert guidance and then looks over Judy's medical chart to orient herself to the nature of Judy's medical problem and current interventions. Judy has had RA for 2 years; she has recently experienced a decline in function and increase in hand pain. Judy's rheumatologist has sent her for occupational therapy to address functional issues. Rhonda completes a biomechanical assessment of Judy's impairments and talks with her about her goals. She identifies that Judy has mild structural deformities of the hand that limit occupational

Practice Dilemma

Occupational therapy practitioners are very busy and rarely have enough time to complete a reflective, systematic, and thorough review of the literature to guide their clinical tasks with a single client. In a clinical setting that does not provide organizational support for evidence-based practice, what strategies would you develop to support your evidence-based practice?

tasks requiring intensive hand use such as typing (Judy is a secretary) and housework. Judy has decreased hand strength and is reporting that pain is increasingly problematic. Rhonda identifies goals related to reducing pain, increasing hand strength, and improving activities of daily living (ADL) performance. She initiates a strengthening and pain management program but feels frustrated about identifying methods to teach techniques that will enable Judy and others like her to continue progressing at home. None of her colleagues have any suggestions of an educational program that may be effective post therapy.

This chapter will demonstrate how **evidence-based practice** might create a different scenario for working with a client like Judy (Shin, Randolph, & Rauch, 2010; Straus, Richardson, Glasziou, & Haynes, 2005). Rhonda recognized that she needed information or evidence to guide her provision of occupational therapy services to Judy. The forms of evidence that she used to inform her work with Judy were expert opinion, medical records about tests and interventions conducted with Judy, information from Judy herself, and direct observation of Judy's wrist function. Rhonda did not seek out or use evidence from research studies to inform her practice with Judy, the type of evidence meant in the term *evidence-based practice*. This chapter describes how evidence from research studies can be put into practice consistently and in a manner that enriches the contributions of occupational therapy and the outcomes of clients.

The Evidence-Based Practitioner

Implementing evidence-based practice is a priority within occupational therapy practice (Lin, Murphy, & Robinson, 2010). Because evidence-based practice has been associated with better outcomes (Shin et al., 2010), it has already started to affect daily practice, reimbursement, and policy. The shift to evidence-based practice started in the early 1990s. Health care practitioners realized that traditional information sources used in practice (textbooks, experts, and continuing education) were often out of date, ineffective, or just plain wrong (Straus et al., 2005). In its earliest years, evidence-based practice focused on finding experimental studies and analyzing them to determine their credibility based on the validity of the study design and scientific rigor. If the experimental evidence was credible, "best evidence," it was used to determine practice. Practitioners placed little emphasis on clinical decision making (Shin et al., 2010). This original definition was predicated on the idea that the evidence was undeniably applicable to a medical situation, so that the translation from the evidence to the real world of the clinic was relatively straightforward. However, as clinicians have struggled with using evidence to make appropriate decisions for individual patients, a more pragmatic definition of evidence-based practice has emerged (Shin et al., 2010). This pragmatic approach uses evidence as part of a clinical decision-making process that also takes into consideration the relevance of the evidence to the treatment environment and the individual clients' values and circumstances (Mayer, 2010). These latter two areas are as important as the evidence in the decision-making process. Although evidence may support a treatment, if the environment lacks resources for the therapist and client to engage in that treatment, the treatment remains nonviable. In a like manner, even if the evidence supports a treatment but does not match a client's values and circumstances, it will not constitute client-centered practice—a cornerstone of occupational therapy. Thus, evidence-based practice is composed of three equal core components: (1) the current best evidence, (2) the treatment environment, and (3) each client's values and circumstances (Shin et al., 2010), which, in combination with a clinician's expertise, aid in clinical decision making. Figure 31.1 provides a schematic

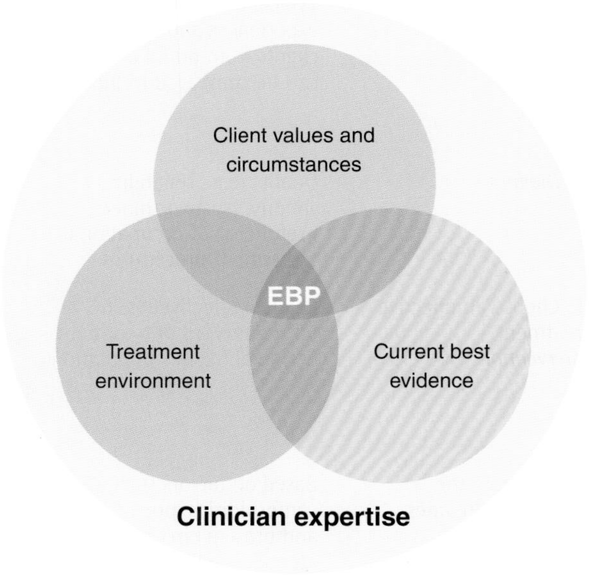

FIGURE 31.1 Interaction between the elements of clinical decision making in evidence-based practice.

of the interaction between client, clinician, evidence, and environment representative of the current thinking about evidence-based practice (Mayer, 2010; Shin et al., 2010). Although it is generally understood that occupational therapists are skilled in providing clinical expertise, understanding their clinical environment, and identifying client values and circumstances, their skill is more likely to be deficient in identifying "current best evidence."

Organizing Evidence around Central Clinical Tasks

Imagine yourself just about to meet the Judy of Rhonda's clinical experience. As an evidence-based practitioner, you would use scientific reasoning along with the current best evidence from research studies to support central clinical tasks, such as the selection of appropriate and valid assessment procedures, interventions, and procedures for monitoring clinical progress (Law & MacDermid, 2008; Straus et al., 2005). It is important to understand that in evidence-based practice, research evidence does not replace reasoning that is informed by clinical experience, theory, core values of practice, and ethics. Nor does the use of research evidence replace the clinical use of information derived from observing clients and talking with their family members or from consulting with experts and peers. Evidence-based clinical reasoning involves the use of all forms of evidence in the pursuit of optimal client outcomes. It is the integration of scientific reasoning with reasoning that has been matured by clinical experience, validated practice theory, and client-centered values and ethics (Egan, Dubouloz, von Zweck, & Vallerand, 1998; Lee & Miller, 2003; Rappolt, 2003).

Table 31.1 shows how, you, the evidence-based practitioner, could organize the search for and interpret evidence around central clinical tasks, in general, and, specifically, with respect to Judy. One of the first clinical tasks that the practitioner faces in working with a client is *getting to know the client.* One aspect of getting to know a client is obtaining *background knowledge* about the client's disorder. Background knowledge provides the basic information on the clinical nature of a disease (Mayer, 2010). It is often knowledge that has been in existence for many years and, therefore, "current best evidence" may be readily available in textbooks or on credible Websites. The task of getting to know a client also involves gathering evidence that is descriptive of the experiences and needs of clients with the disorder in general (e.g., clients who have been research participants in published studies). Expert clinicians who have treated many people with a specific diagnosis may choose to forgo obtaining specific background information because their clinical expertise will already include pertinent information, but a novice clinician, such as Rhonda, should obtain background information before seeing a client. Research designs that would be relevant to this aspect of getting to know the client are **descriptive research**, such as **qualitative studies** and **case series**, and **exploratory research**, such as **cross-sectional studies** and **cohort studies**.

TABLE 31.1 Organizing Evidence around Clinical Tasks with Judy

Central Clinical Task	Research Evidence	Relevant Research Designs	Use of Evidence for Judy's Case
I. Get to know a client *a. Background*	Typical occupational experiences and needs of clients from populations who can be compared to Judy	Descriptive and exploratory research 1. Qualitative studies 2. Case series 3. Cohort studies 4. Cross-sectional studies	Generate a discussion with Judy about her own occupational experiences and needs in comparison with the research samples'.
b. Diagnosis	Quality (e.g., reliability, validity, trustworthiness, usefulness) of occupational assessment procedures	Exploratory research that evaluate assessment tools 1. Cross-sectional studies 2. Case-control studies	Select the best assessment method to identify Judy's unique occupational experiences and needs.
II. Choose an effective treatment *Intervention*	Relative effectiveness of different types of treatments designed for this population	Experimental and exploratory research 1. Randomized clinical trials 2. Quasi-experimental studies 3. *N* of 1 studies 4. Cohort studies	Select, ideally in collaboration with Judy, potentially beneficial interventions.
III. Estimate the probable outcomes *Prognosis*	Based on factors such as comorbidities, previous and present circumstances identify the outcomes most commonly occurring for these populations	Exploratory and descriptive research 1. Cohort studies 2. Case-control studies 3. Case Series	Assists with planning for discharge, training, and support services necessary for Judy.

Background knowledge provides the foundation from which to develop treatment strategies, but it must be tempered with information coming from the specific client. **Diagnosis**, assessing the presence and degree of disorders and their effect on a client's current status with respect to occupational needs and status, is an important part of getting to know a client (Fritz & Wainner, 2001; Straus et al., 2005). Research on diagnostic studies tests the quality of assessment procedures for determining an individual client's unique experiences and needs. High quality evidence on diagnostic tools ensures that services are relevant and beneficial, specifically for that person. Research designs that would be relevant to this task are exploratory research, such as cross-sectional studies and **case-control studies** (Oxford Centre for Evidence-Based Medicine Levels of Evidence Working Group, 2011).

With respect to Judy, descriptions of the occupational lives of women with RA or similar disorders that can affect the structural integrity of the hands could enhance your understanding of possible issues that Judy might face in her own life and could generate a discussion with Judy about her own life. Such a discussion might identify what specific types of in-depth information about Judy you want to learn in the assessment procedures. After targeting key areas to assess, you could go back to the research literature to find evidence about the **reliability** and **validity** of methods to select the most valuable methods for assessing those areas.

Another central clinical task is that of *choosing an effective treatment* approach and procedure for addressing the client's specific needs and goals. The research evidence that would be relevant to this task includes findings about the relative effectiveness of different types of interventions designed for individuals with a particular type of personal characteristic or health care condition. The task of choosing an effective intervention for a client involves gathering evidence that evaluates the **effectiveness** or **efficacy** of a type of intervention in comparison to alternative interventions or no intervention at all. Effectiveness evidence is published in studies that used an intervention or treatment research design or procedure. The most relevant research designs are **experimental research**, such as **randomized clinical trials (RCTs)**, **quasi-experimental studies**, and ***N* of 1 studies**, or exploratory research such as cohort studies (Oxford Centre for Evidence-Based Medicine Levels of Evidence Working Group, 2011). With respect to Judy, you could use **effectiveness evidence** about interventions designed for individuals with RA and similar disorders to select an appropriate intervention. In a client-centered approach, this selection would involve collaboration with Judy (Tickle-Degnen, 2002a).

A third central clinical task is that of *estimating the probable outcomes* for the patient based on variables such as the client age, history, comorbidities, symptoms, and response to treatment, often referred to as **prognosis** (Moons, Royston, Vergouwe, Grobbee, & Altman, 2009). This task assists the occupational therapist and patient to engage in long-range treatment planning as well as discharge planning, including additional therapies, home programs, education and training, and accessing resources. Relevant evidence tracks people over time and looks for relationships between baseline and long-term outcomes. The most relevant research designs are exploratory research, such as cohort studies and case-control studies, or descriptive research, such as case series (Oxford Centre for Evidence-Based Medicine Levels of Evidence Working Group, 2011).

For Judy, it would be important to identify the general prognosis of clients with RA. Prognosis in RA has actually changed in the last 10 years. Current prognostic evidence suggests that people with RA treated aggressively with disease-modifying antirheumatic drugs (DMARDs) and the appropriate biologic therapies, such as etanercept or adalimumab, are much less likely to experience the severe fixed deformities and significant joint degeneration experienced by previous generations of people with RA (Cush, Weinblatt, & Kavanaugh, 2008). This shift in outcome makes it even more imperative that recent literature rather than textbooks or clinical experience be used to estimate prognosis.

The Steps of Evidence-Based Practice

Evidence-based practitioners systematically integrate research evidence into practice by carrying out a series of steps (Lin et al., 2010; Mayer, 2010; Straus et al., 2005).

1. Writing an answerable clinical question
2. Gathering current published evidence that might answer the question
3. Appraising the gathered evidence to determine what is the "best" evidence for answering the question
4. Using the evidence to guide practice for individual clients by collaboratively communicating the results to patients

Step 1: Writing an Answerable Clinical Question

The first systematic step, writing an answerable question, helps the practitioner to focus on the specific type of evidence that would help a clinical task. The question must be written by using key words and terminology that tap into a general body of research literature that may hold an answer to the question and that locates evidence that is relevant to performing a particular clinical task with a specific client. There are two types of questions: **background questions** and **foreground questions** (Mayer, 2010; Straus et al., 2005).

Background questions identify descriptive research that is used to better understand the nature of the problem. There are two elements to a background question: a

TABLE 31.2 Examples of Answerable Questions for Each Type of Clinical Task

	Get to Know a Client		*Choose an Effective Treatment*	*Estimate the Probable Outcomes*
	Background	**Diagnosis**	**Intervention**	**Prognosis**
Example: Answerable questions	Root: How common Verb and problem: are hand structural deformities in RA?	P: 44-year-old woman with RA I: Reliable and valid test to evaluate hand dysfunction O: Identify changes in hand function.	P: 44-year-old woman with RA I: Behavioral-based joint protection program C: Standard education program O: Increase occupational performance and grip strength and reduce pain.	P: 44-year-old woman with RA I: On methotrexate & adalimumab O: Remain employed for 10 years following diagnosis
	How common are hand structural deformities in RA?	What is a valid and reliable test to identify changes in hand function in a middle-aged woman with RA?	Will a behaviorally based joint protection program cause greater increases in occupational performance and grip strength and greater reductions in pain than a standard education program for a middle-aged woman with RA?	How likely is it for a middle-aged woman with RA on methotrexate and adalimumab to remain employed for 10 years after diagnosis?
Example: Key terms (*MeSH terms*)	RA (*arthritis; rheumatic diseases; autoimmune diseases*) Hand structural deformities (*hand deformities, acquired*)	RA (*arthritis; rheumatic diseases; autoimmune diseases*) Test (*evaluation*) Hand function reliable or valid (*psychometrics*)	RA (*arthritis; rheumatic diseases; autoimmune diseases*) Joint protection program (*educational program; self-management program; health education; patient education*) Occupational performance (*Activities of daily living, work, participation*) Pain (*discomfort*) Grip (*grasp*)	RA (*arthritis; rheumatic diseases; autoimmune diseases*) Employment (*work; occupation*) Methotrexate or adalimumab (*biologics; TNF-inhibitors*)

C, comparison; I, intervention; MeSH, Medical Subject Headings; O, outcome; P, patient, population, or problem; RA, rheumatoid arthritis; TNF, tumor necrosis factor.

question's root (e.g., who, what, when, where) combined with a verb and a disorder, problem, or some aspect of patient care (Mayer, 2010; Straus et al., 2005). A background question for Judy is provided in Table 31.2.

Foreground questions are about current knowledge related to best practice treatment of a specific patient. They focus on recent interventions, diagnostic tests, potential patient outcomes, and theories about causation (Mayer, 2010). There are three to four elements to an answerable foreground intervention research question (Lou & Durando, 2008; Mayer, 2010; Straus et al., 2005):

- The *patient, population, or problem* (P). The element identifies features of the client population of interest, such as the client's clinical condition or diagnosis, gender, ethnicity, age group, and socioeconomic status. Defining the patient, population, or problems establishes the acceptable characteristics of the sample of any research study. Important features are those that identify populations or subpopulations of which the client is a member, ensuring that retrieved evidence will be relevant to the client.
- The *intervention* of interest (I). This can be a specific technique or a general type of treatment.
- The *comparison* treatment (C). The best intervention studies are experimental and examine the effectiveness of one treatment in comparison to some other treatment. The "some other treatment" does not necessarily have to be specified in the answerable question, particularly if the clinician is not particularly interested if one treatment is better than another, only if the treatment works. Therefore, the comparison treatment may be omitted.
- The desired *outcomes* (O). These should be concrete results that are directly applicable to occupational performance. Variables of interest are attributes of clients that are addressed in occupational therapy, such as their physical or psychosocial functioning, occupational performance, or satisfaction with outcomes. Models and theories of occupation and occupational therapy, such as the Person-Environment-Occupation Model (Law et al., 1996), as well as more general models of health that encompass an occupational therapy

perspective, such as the *International Classification of Functioning, Disability, and Health* (World Health Organization, 2005), provide the language needed to identify occupational variables.

The foreground question is often referred to as a *PICO* question (the acronym of the first letters of each element). The PICO type question has to be modified when looking for diagnostic or prognostic evidence. For diagnostic/assessment questions, the *intervention* will become a diagnostic tool, whereas the **outcome** will be the ability of the tool to accurately identify the degree of the problem, distinguish a diagnosis, or the psychometrics of the tool. Prognosis, too, requires modifications in the standard PICO question with the intervention becoming **predictor variables** that are expected to alter outcomes, and the outcomes tending to focus on long-term participation, health and wellness, and quality of life. Table 31.2 provides examples of answerable questions for each type of clinical task.

Step 2: Gathering Current Published Evidence

Once a clinical question has been written, the practitioner draws on the elements of the question to search for and gather evidence to answer the question. Relevant research is published in various fields: occupational therapy, medicine, nursing, physical therapy, education, psychology, sociology, anthropology, and so on. Consequently, search strategies should tap into the research literature of different disciplines.

Each element of an answerable clinical question contains one or more *key terms* for searching the literature. A whole body of literature can be excluded inadvertently simply because the key terms that are used in the search do not match terminology used by the researchers or the cataloguers of the research literature. Some of the important terms that occupational therapy practitioners use to identify clinical conditions (e.g., sensory integrative disorder) or occupational variables (e.g., occupational performance) are not the most typical terms used to describe or catalogue research studies in the broader literature. Therefore, it is important to generate a list of synonyms for each key term in each element of the question before beginning the search.

One list of terms that is used by the national databases PubMed and Medline to structure the citations of over 5,400 of the leading biomedical journals is the U.S. National Medical Libraries *Medical Subject Headings (MeSH)* terminology (U.S. National Library of Medicine, 2010). MeSH is a controlled vocabulary thesaurus, arranged in a 12-level hierarchy with broader, more encompassing terms connected to progressively more specific terms. MeSH is designed to link multiple terms to its overall hierarchy and provides a good starting point for identifying common terminology. Freely accessible literature search services such as PubMed (National Center for Biotechnology Information, 2011) provide online tutorials so that evidence-based practitioners can learn how to more effectively search the literature with MeSH terms.

Table 31.2 shows examples of questions that you could write with respect to Judy for each of the clinical tasks. Possible key terms and alternatives that are synonyms and terms that are broader or more specific are listed. For diagnosis ("What is a valid and reliable test to document and identify changes in hand function in a middle aged woman with RA?"), a combination of *hand function*, *rheumatoid arthritis*, *reliable*, and *test* yield six citations of various hand function tests using PubMed, suggesting that this search strategy is effective.

There are numerous free search engines available online for searching the literature as well as clearinghouses for summaries, systematic reviews, and other useful sources of evidence (Lin et al., 2010). One source available to all practitioners is Google Scholar (http://scholar.google.com/), which provides links to full text articles if they are available.

Step 3: Appraising the Evidence

The term *best evidence* is often used in relationship to evidence-based practice. Practitioners are encouraged to use the best evidence to guide practice. As should be apparent, the best evidence is not one type of study design or one type of source; it is dependent on the type of question being asked as well as the access to that evidence. Even after a research study has been identified and acquired, it must be appraised to determine if the study is best evidence for the clinical problem on hand. Evidence that is clinically useful and valuable (1) is relevant to the clinical task, (2) is trustworthy, (3) has **generalizability**, and (4) has clinically important results (Carter, Lubinsky, & Domholdt, 2011) (Figure 31.2). There are

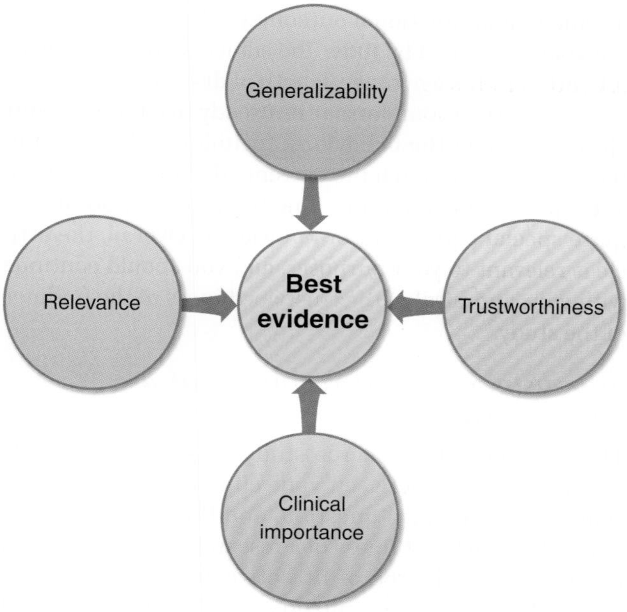

FIGURE 31.2 Elements of best evidence.

many excellent resources for guiding the appraisal of research evidence (e.g., Law & MacDermid, 2008; Straus et al., 2005).

Appraising the Relevance of a Research Study

The **relevance** of a research study is determined by the degree to which it answers the clinical question and how well its methods fit within the constraints and resources of the practitioner's context of practice (Tickle-Degnen, 2001, 2002b). Rarely will the search for evidence locate a study or set of studies that directly answers the clinical question. Studies are designed to answer the authors' research questions, not your clinical question. The most relevant research study is one that (1) investigates a variable that is the occupational variable of interest or one highly related to that variable, (2) includes research participants who are members of your client's population, and (3) offers clinical methods that are suitable to your context of practice.

To illustrate the process of examining relevance, we return to the citation retrieved in response to the intervention question in Table 31.2, "Will a behaviorally based joint protection program cause greater increases in occupational performance and grip strength and greater reductions in pain than a standard education program for a middle-aged woman with RA?" One citation was for a paper by Hammond and Freeman (2001), which can be retrieved in full text from *Rheumatology*.

Table 31.3 provides the aim and general methods of Hammond and Freeman's (2001) research study as applied to determining best evidence. The study tested the efficacy of a group focused on acquiring joint protection behaviors through behavioral training methods to reduce pain, impairment, and dysfunction at 1 year in comparison to a group focused on general, didactic education about managing RA. The researchers addressed pain, impairment, and functional outcomes, which are similar to the goals identified by Judy. The subjects are people with RA within Judy's age range, length of disease, and severity of disease. The group format is already used within your clinic, although the behavioral techniques described in the study do not match the current educational methods. They are feasible for your clinic because they do not require special equipment or knowledge. Overall, the article is relevant to your purposes, and you should continue with your appraisal of the trustworthiness of the findings of the study.

Appraising the Trustworthiness of a Research Study

The relevance of a research study is assessed primarily as a degree of fit between your clinical need, as represented in the clinical question, and the methods of the study. The trustworthiness of a research study is assessed primarily as a degree of fit between the researcher's research question, or purpose, and the methods of the study. A trustworthy study is one for which the conclusions are defensible with respect to the methods of the study, and there are few, if any, **alternative plausible explanations**—scientific explanations for the findings beyond the conclusions drawn from the study and its researchers (Carter et al., 2011). Trustworthiness is enhanced when the researcher carefully and rigorously maintains standards of discovery, description, and explanation (Carpenter & Hammell, 2000).

The most trustworthy research study is one that (1) uses a study design that will achieve the stated purpose and (2) provides various methods to enhance trustworthiness within the study design with respect to standards of science. The evidence-based practitioner attempts to evaluate the degree to which a descriptive study provides a defensible description of a client or clinical population; the degree to which an assessment study provides a strong test of the reliability, validity, or usefulness of an assessment procedure; or the degree to which an intervention effectiveness study supports the conclusion that client outcomes were caused by the intervention and not by other factors.

The first area to assess to determine the trustworthiness of a study is to ensure that the best design was used to answer the research question. Over many decades of trial and error, a set of basic study designs have evolved. Table 31.4 provides the most common types of study designs and their trustworthiness for different clinical tasks. Each type of study is best used for different types of questions; for example, randomized clinical trials and other experimental research are the strongest design for answering intervention questions because they are most suited to determining cause and effect. Cross-sectional studies are the strongest design diagnosis because they capture subjects at a single point of time in the diagnostic continuum, allowing for an accurate determination if the instrument can accurately identify a problem or disease. Hierarchies of evidence have been developed to rank the trustworthiness of different study designs. Table 31.5 provides a hierarchy of evidence for the categories of diagnostic, intervention effectiveness, and prognosis evidence.

The second area to assess to determine the trustworthiness of a study is the use of methods to reduce **bias** and enhance validity. All studies have some form of bias (see Hartman, Forsen, Wallace, & Neely, 2002, for an excellent discussion of bias); nonetheless, some studies provide stronger evidence with respect to trustworthiness than others because they have attempted to carefully and rigorously address these and other potential limitations (Carter et al., 2011). There are numerous scales to assess trustworthiness (e.g., Hempel et al., 2011; Higgins & Green, 2011; Jadad et al., 1996; Mahar, Sherrington, Herbert, Mosely, & Elkins, 2003). Table 31.6 provides one set of assessment criteria (Straus et al., 2005) that can identify studies that have the minimum controls to ensure truthful outcomes.

With respect to the study done by Hammond and Freeman (2001), the type of design is a randomized

TABLE 31.3 Evaluation of Hammond and Freeman (2001) as "Best Evidence"

	Criteria	Hammond and Freeman (2001)	
Aim of study	"To evaluate whether joint protection can reduce pain and local inflammation and maintain the integrity of joint structures and functional ability of people with RA 1 year after attending an educational-behavioral joint protection program." (p. 1045)		
Relevance	Investigates an occupational variable of interest	Outcome variables included adherence with joint protection techniques (Joint Protection Behavior Assessment), ADL performance (Arthritis Impact Measurement Scale for ADL), hand pain experienced during moderate activity (100 mm VAS) and grip strength (kg).	
	Study participants are members of your client's population	Inclusion criteria: diagnosed with RA within the last 5 years (mean disease duration ~19.4 months); age 18–65 years (mean age ~51 years); both genders; hand pain on activity; no other medical conditions affecting hand function; history of wrist and/or metacarpophalangeal (MCP) joint pain/inflammation; mild to severe disease rating	
	Clinical methods suitable to your context of practice	Educational-behavioral joint protection program (intervention): Educators used multiple methods (educational, behavioral, motor learning, and self-efficacy enhancing strategies) to educate and practice joint protection techniques. Subjects developed goals for home implementation of joint protection techniques and problem-solved as a group. Subjects also received education on RA and drug therapy. Group size: 3–6 people with RA and partners standard education program (control). Short talks from health professionals on RA, drug treatments, alternate therapies, diet, exercise, rest, energy conservation, joint protection, assistive devices, splinting, pain, and relaxation. Some practice time was included for topics such as joint protection. Group size was 6–10 people with RA and partners. Duration for both groups: 8 hours (four 2-hour sessions)	
Trustworthiness	Type of design that will achieve the stated purpose	Randomized control study—considered to be the strongest evidence for an intervention study.	
	Methods to enhance trustworthiness (Table 3)	**1.** Random assignment—Yes **2.** Concealed random allocation—Yes (allocation sequence preloaded in envelopes) **3.** Similar groups at study baseline—Yes (Table 1) **4.** Follow-up of subjects sufficiently long and complete—Yes (1 year) **5.** Subjects results analyzed in the groups to which they were allocated—Yes (Table 2) **6.** Subjects/study personnel blinded—Yes (independent assessor of outcome measures) **7.** Groups treated equally apart from the experimental intervention—Yes **8.** Attrition less than 20%—Yes (2%; Table 2)	
Generalizability	p value < .05 (significance)	Statistical tests: unpaired t tests, Mann-Whitney U test, and chi-square tests. Significant between group differences at 1 year favoring the treatment group for using joint protection behaviors during activities ($p = .001$), hand pain ($p = .02$), and ADL ($p = .04$). Nonsignificant differences between groups at 1 year favoring the treatment group for grip strength ($p = .83$).	
Clinical importance	Effect size	**Between Treatment and Control Groups** Joint Protection Behavior Assessment = large effect (Cohen's d = 0.79) Hand pain = small effect (Cohen's d = −0.33) ADL = negligible effect (Cohen's d = −0.13) Grip strength = negligible effect (Cohen's d = 0.18)	**Within Treatment Group (Baseline to 1 Year)** Joint Protection Behavior Assessment = large effect (Cohen's d = 0.93) Hand pain = small effect (Cohen's d = −0.21) ADL = negligible effect (Cohen's d = −0.15) Grip strength = small effect (Cohen's d = 0.27)
	MCID	VAS hand pain MCID is 2. The difference between 1 year VAS and baseline VAS was 0.56	

ADL, activities of daily living; MCID, minimal clinically important difference; RA, rheumatoid arthritis; VAS, visual analogue scale.

TABLE 31.4 Common Research Study Designs

Study Design	Definition
Experimental (test hypotheses, identify cause and effect)	
Randomized controlled trials (RCT)	An intervention study in which subjects are randomly assigned to the experimental treatment group or the control group.
Quasi-experimental	An intervention study in which subjects are non–randomly assigned to the experimental treatment group or the control group.
N of 1	An intervention study in which a **single subject** is the total population of the study. This subject receives several treatment periods; one period involves the experimental treatment, and the others, alternative or placebo treatments. Usually the subject receives multiple baseline measurements and multiple outcome measurements to determine if the intervention causes change.
Associative (identify risk factors or possible causes; hypothesis generating)	
Cohort	A study in which subjects who represent a particular population are measured on suspected risk factors or predictors of outcome(s) of interest and are followed over time to determine (1) the incidence or natural history of the outcome and (2) the relationship between the predictors and the outcome(s).
Case-control	A retrospective study in which subjects with the outcome of interest (cases) are selected and matched to subjects without the outcome of interest (controls). The presence of risk factors or predictors is determined through self-report or chart review, and the relationship between these retrospective predictors and the outcome of interest is determined.
Cross-sectional	A study in which subjects who represent a particular population are measured simultaneously for suspected risk factors or predictors and outcome(s) of interest to determine (1) the prevalence of the outcome and (2) the relationship between the predictors and the outcome(s).
Descriptive (describe problem)	
Qualitative	A research paradigm based on the assumption that there are multiple constructed realities and that the purpose of research is to describe and analyze these realities to facilitate the understanding of the phenomena.
Case series (case study)	A study that tracks several patients over the course of a disease. The results are not aggregated and detailed information on the diagnosis, treatment, and outcomes is provided for each individual patient (a case study tracks a single patient in a like manner).

TABLE 31.5 Hierarchy of Trustworthiness of Study Designs

Diagnosis	Intervention	Prognosis
I: SR of cross-sectional studies with consistently applied **reference standards** and **blinding**.	**I:** SR of RCT or *N* of 1 studies	**I:** SR of inception cohort studies
II: Cross-sectional study with consistently applied reference standards and blinding.	**II:** RCT or **observational study** with dramatic effect	**II:** **Inception cohort study**
III: **Nonconsecutive** cross-sectional study or studies without consistently applied reference standards	**III:** Non–randomized controlled cohort study	**III:** Cohort study or **control arm** of RCT
IV: Case-control study	**IV:** Case-series, case-control study, or **historically controlled study**	**IV:** Case-series, case-control study, or poor quality prognostic cohort study
V: **Mechanism-based reasoning**	**V:** Mechanism-based reasoning	**V:** n/a

Hierarchy is represented by the Roman numerals from I (*strongest design*) to V (*weakest design*).

RCT, randomized controlled trial; SR, systematic review.

Adapted with permission from the Oxford Centre for Evidence-Based Medicine Levels of Evidence Working Group. (2011). *The Oxford Centre for evidence-based medicine 2011 levels of evidence*. Retrieved from http://www.cebm.net/index.aspx?o=5653

TABLE 31.6 Criteria for Determining Trustworthiness

Diagnosis	Intervention	Prognosis
1. Independent, blind comparison of the new diagnostic test to a reference standard 2. Evaluation of the new diagnostic test on a full spectrum of patients 3. Both reference standard and new diagnostic test obtained on all study subjects	1. Random assignment 2. **Concealed random allocation** 3. Similar groups at study baseline 4. Follow-up of subjects sufficiently long and complete 5. Subjects results analyzed in the groups to which they were allocated 6. Subjects/study personnel blinded 7. Groups treated equally apart from the experimental intervention 8. **Attrition** less than 20%	1. Baseline data obtained on a defined, representative sample at a common point in their treatment 2. Follow-up of subjects sufficiently long and complete 3. Objective outcome measures applied at follow-up by blinded assessors 4. Adjustments for important prognostic **covariates** for subgroups with different prognostic outcomes 5. **Validation study** completed

Data from Straus, S. E., Richardson, W. S., Glasziou, P., & Haynes, R. B. (2005). *Evidence-based medicine* (3rd ed.). New York, NY: Churchill Livingstone.

clinical trial. The clinical task is one of identifying intervention effectiveness, and a randomized clinical trial is the best choice for determining cause and effect (see Table 31.4). A review of the study using the eight criteria proposed for an intervention study in Table 31.6 suggests that this study has excellent general validity and therefore the results are probably trustworthy (see Table 31.4).

Interpreting the Results of a Study: Generalizability and Clinical Importance

Now that you have completed a basic evaluation of the relevance and trustworthiness of the evidence from the study, it is time to examine the results in terms of whether they can help answer the clinical question. First, the results must be generalizable from the sample to the population; and second, they must be clinically important (see Figure 31.2).

A hallmark of the quantitative paradigm of research and the scientific method is the aim of understanding general, population-centered truths rather than individual outcomes (Babbie, 1990). However, clinical research cannot be completed on a population because it is not feasible to access every person with the characteristics of interest and study them. Therefore, research is performed on a sample of people who are assumed to be representative of the whole population. Research studies describe the characteristics of the sample (inclusion/exclusion criteria and demographics) so that readers can determine how well the sample of a study matches a population and how well their clients match the sample. All data generated from a study, therefore, is sample specific and represents the sample participants, but may or may not represent the larger population from which the sample was taken. If the study is trustworthy, then the results are considered to provide a good representation of actual sample outcomes. How do we know that these trustworthy, sample-specific results can translate to the population? **Inferential statistics** allow us to determine how confident we should be that sample results can be applied or generalized to the client population. In other words, they allow for generalizability. The statistic that is commonly used to estimate the confidence that sample results can be generalized is the ***p* value**. By an arbitrary convention, the threshold to distinguish between statistically significant results that inspire higher confidence about generalizability versus nonsignificant results that inspire lower confidence is generally set at $p \leq .05$. Essentially, a $p \leq .05$ states, "the probability that the results in this study are due to chance is less than 1 in 20, and based on this low probability, we feel somewhat confident that we can generalize the results to the population." Many methodologists have suggested that **confidence intervals** replace or augment the use of the p value statistic for interpretation of study results (Cohen, 1990; Cummings & Finch, 2005). Whereas the p value provides a probability value related to chance findings, the confidence interval indicates the range of possible results that are likely to be found in the larger population. The p value and confidence interval are statistically related to one another in that the higher the p value, the larger the confidence interval around the average finding; that is, the larger the range of possible results in the population.

Inferential statistics are applied to understanding all forms of evidence, yet for purposes of demonstrating the meaning of p values and confidence intervals, we provide an example of an intervention effectiveness study. Imagine a study in which participants in an occupational therapy intervention condition scored an average of five points higher on a postintervention function test than participants in the control condition, and the difference was statistically significant at $p < .05$. Let's say that the confidence interval around the average difference was found to range from one to nine points. This finding suggests that in the population as a whole, we would be somewhat confident that the average postintervention function score would be one to nine points higher in individuals receiving the intervention, and that the probability was low that the average difference between the two conditions was due to chance alone.

An intervention study finding in which a p value is statistically nonsignificant (e.g., $p > .05$) indicates that we should not feel as confident in generalizing the sample results to the population and that the range of possible responses to the intervention is large. This nonsignificant finding does not tell us that the intervention is ineffective. Rather, it tells us that we cannot be sure that the intervention would or would not be effective. We must use caution in generalizing nonsignificant results to the population and to our client.

Note that inferential statistics, whether they yield statistically significant or nonsignificant results, tell us only about general tendencies in the population and not about our particular client's responses. However, the results of inferential statistics aid us in our clinical reasoning as we work with the client. We are more likely to feel confident in applying statistically significant results to our client's situation than nonsignificant results.

The results of Hammond and Freeman's (2001) study indicated that people in the **treatment group** did statistically significantly better than people in the control group at 1 year for joint protection behaviors, hand pain, and ADL performance. Grip strength, however, was not statistically significantly different (see Table 31.3). The authors reported p values but no confidence intervals. The p values associated with the results suggest that improvements in joint protection behaviors, hand pain, and ADL performance would also be seen on the average in the population and therefore, we might expect Judy to show improvement with this type of intervention.

Separate from statistical significance is the concept of clinical importance. Statistical significance focuses on the ability to generalize the results from the sample to the population, regardless of how effective those results are. Statistical significance is strongly tied to sample size because it examines the probability that the results represent a true effect. Thus, with a large enough sample, *any* result can be statistically significant and represent a true effect, as long as the study was highly controlled and used trustworthy, reliable, and valid assessment procedures. However, this true effect may not be large enough to affect clients in any meaningful way. Recognizing that just providing whether or not a result is significant may not ultimately be useful for clinical practice; recent best practice guidelines for reporting research results have identified the inclusion of effect sizes as a key aspect of good reporting (Moher et al., 2010). It is important to know that small sample sizes that produce a nonsignificant result may actually have produced an effect that would generalize to the population if the study were to be replicated with a larger sample size. The study's sample size might be too small to detect that the effect would generalize to the population (i.e., it does not provide us with enough confidence in the generalizability of the findings).

An **effect size** describes the magnitude of the difference between two treatment effects or the magnitude of the relationship between two variables using some form of a standardized score (Ferguson, 2009). The standardized score eliminates the scale of the original instrument used to measure the variable, which allows effects sizes to be compared between instruments or between studies. There are many different forms of effect sizes, and the most appropriate type depends on the type of data being evaluated and the statistical analyses performed (Table 31.7). Often, the numerical effect size is translated into a verbal interpretation, such as "small," "moderate," or "large," to assist clinicians in estimating the magnitude of the effect on treatment (Ferguson, 2009; Portney & Watkins, 2009; Tickle-Degnen, 2001).

Another way to determine clinical effectiveness is the **minimal clinically important difference (MCID)**. The MCID is the smallest change in an outcome that will lead to some perceived clinically beneficial improvement. For example, Salaffi, Stancati, Silvestri, Ciapetti, and Grassi (2004) identified the MCID for pain for people with chronic musculoskeletal pain due to arthritis after a 3-month period using a numerical rating scale (NRS). They found that a mean change of two corresponded with a report of "much better" improvement. Thus, a study that reported a change of approximately two on a NRS would suggest that the intervention had a clinically important effect on pain for the average client. More and more studies are examining the percentage of subjects who achieve an MCID during the study as one measure of outcome. The biggest barrier to using MCID in clinical practice is that clinicians must know the MCID for different outcome measures, and these are not always readily available. Clinicians should collect MCID for outcomes that are important to them to facilitate interpreting the clinical importance of different studies.

The effect sizes calculated for the Hammond and Freeman's (2001) study suggest that although the educational program had a large effect in altering joint protection behaviors (see Table 31.3) in the treatment group, these changes in behaviors only had a small corresponding effect on impairment and function. Overall, people in the treatment group had only small improvements in function in comparison to the control group, and even when the effect within the treatment group alone was evaluated from baseline to posttest at 1 year, the results remained negligible to small. The MCID for hand pain also suggests that the changes were not enough to affect clinical performance. Therefore, although the results are generalizable from the sample to the population (significance), they are not necessarily clinically important.

The small effect sizes from this study require the use of clinical reasoning for understanding their implications for Judy and other clients like her. On one hand, the results suggest minimal benefit. However, these results are 1-year postintervention on a disease process that routinely causes continued deterioration of abilities. The fact that the participants in this study not only did not get worse but also improved in comparison to a group

TABLE 31.7 Effect Sizes

Effect Size	Clinical Task	Definition	Citations
Sensitivity	Diagnosis	Proportion of people with the target disorder who have a positive result on the diagnostic test.	Fritz & Wainner, 2001 Portney & Watkins, 2009, pp. 619–634 Straus et al., 2005, pp. 73–77
Specificity	Diagnosis	Proportion of people without the target disorder who have a negative result on the diagnostic test	
Positive predictive value	Diagnosis	Proportion of people with a positive diagnostic test who have the target disorder.	
Negative predictive value	Diagnosis	Proportion of people with a negative diagnostic test who do not have the target disorder.	
Likelihood ratios	Diagnosis	The likelihood that a specific test result would be seen in a person with the target disorder.	
Kappa	Diagnosis	A reliability coefficient that identifies the degree of agreement between two measure made by two observers measuring the same item while controlling for chance agreement.	Portney & Watkins, 2009, pp. 598–605
Intraclass correlation coefficients (ICC)	Diagnosis	A reliability coefficient that evaluates the consistency of two measures made by observers measuring the same item.	Portney & Watkins, 2009, pp. 588–598
Cohen's *d*, Hedge's *g*, Glass's Δ	Intervention	Measures the magnitude of the difference between two means in standard deviation units (each cited measure uses a different variation of standard deviation units).	Lipsey & Wilson, 2001, pp. 34–71 Tickle-Degnen, 2001
r	Intervention	The degree of shared variance between two measures.	
Number needed to treat (NNT)	Intervention	The number of patients who would need to receive treatment to produce a positive outcome in one patient who otherwise would have had a negative outcome.	Dalton & Keating, 2000 Straus et al., 2005, pp. 73–77
Odds ratio; risk ratio	Intervention; prognosis	Estimate of the difference in the risk for a particular outcome between two or more groups.	Portney & Watkins, 2009, pp. 667–670

of similar individuals suggests that this treatment may be more beneficial than the effect sizes indicate. We do not know how Judy would respond herself to this type of intervention. This clinical conundrum demonstrates the importance of clinician expertise and client input into the decision-making process.

Thus, best evidence is a combination of the relevance of the results to the clinician's practice, the trustworthiness of the research design in obtaining "true" sample results for the study sample, the ability to generalize the results from the sample to the population, and results that are not only "significant" but clinically important as well. Finally, best evidence should demonstrate replication; numerous studies should show similar results related to treatment, diagnoses, or prognoses. **Systematic reviews** are frequently cited as the best "best evidence" because they synthesize the results from multiple studies (Lin et al., 2010; Oxford Centre for Evidence Based Medicine Levels of Evidence Working Group, 2011). A meta-analysis, a form of systematic review that includes statistical techniques to combine the results of multiple studies into a single effect size, provides one of the best overall reviews of evidence. The Cochrane Collaboration is one group that has provided numerous high-quality systematic reviews on various topics (Cochrane Collaboration, 2010) including occupational therapy for RA (Steultjens et al., 2004), problems in ADL after stroke (Hoffmann, Bennett, Koh, & McKenna, 2010), and multiple sclerosis (Steultjens et al., 2003). Although systematic reviews provide overall evidence of the efficacy of a treatment, it may be limited in its use for individual clients. Often, the summaries address a heterogeneous group of subjects or broad treatment plans which reduce their relevance to day-to-day practice. Systematic reviews are best when a topic is well established. They are less effective for new and emerging practices where they may underestimate the effect due to small sample sizes or unreliable assessment procedures or overestimate it due to poorly controlled studies with biased assessment procedures. Systematic reviews are excellent sources of articles that deal with a specific sample or treatment topic; evidence-based practitioners can use the reviews to identify and obtain more specific articles for treatments that show an overall effectiveness.

There is one other consideration regarding best evidence. The best evidence is the best that can be found and not best in the sense of meeting all of the standards. The possible answer this best evidence delivers may be one about which you can feel a high, moderate, or low degree of confidence. You might not have enough time to gather and evaluate enough evidence to form a confident opinion, which is very likely, given, in this scenario, how busy you are as a practitioner in an outpatient clinic. Even with little research evidence about which you feel a modicum of confidence, you may go to the next step of evidence-based practice: communication about the evidence with the client, in this case, Judy, and other individuals who are important to the client.

Step 4: Using the Evidence to Guide Practice

By appraising the relevance of the evidence, you will have identified that a study can potentially be applied to your client; it matches his or her general characteristics and it is feasible within your clinical setting. You will also know from your appraisal that the study results are generally trustworthy and demonstrate potentially generalizable and important results. This study can now be used as a tool to help develop and implement treatment. However, before you decide to use the results of a study, you must determine if they truly match the values and circumstances of your client (see Figure 31.1). This is done by communicating the evidence to the client to inform the process of decision making about treatment.

As has been put forward in this chapter, evidence-based practice emerges from the core values and ethics of occupational therapy (American Occupational Therapy Association, 2010; Christiansen & Lou, 2001). Evidence-based practice occurs in a respectful, truthful, and collaborative relationship with the client and with those acting on the client's behalf. Clients are viewed as active contributors to the planning and intervention process of therapy rather than as passive recipients of information or services (Law, Baptiste, & Mills, 1995). To be active rather than passive, that is, to act with as much autonomy as possible and the least amount of dependency, clients and those acting on their behalf must be informed rather than uninformed or misinformed. To be an informed client means to know the meaning of one's occupational status in relationship to one's quality of life, to know the nature and quality of possible occupational therapy assessments to be undertaken, to know the quality and probable outcomes of relevant interventions, and to have the means to assess one's own progress toward meaningful outcomes. Once informed, clients and those acting on their behalf can reason and act with the degree of autonomy of which they are capable.

The main goal of communicating about evidence is to inform the process of decision making (Tickle-Degnen, 2000, 2002b). Wise decisions are ones that are likely to benefit the client and family members and are embraced by client, family members, you (the occupational therapy practitioner), and others of importance to the client, such as other practitioners. Communication that achieves these types of decisions (1) has content that accurately represents the research evidence, including its strengths and weaknesses related to relevance and trustworthiness; (2) involves language that is mutually understandable to all participants; and (3) encourages an open and mutual discussion of information and ideas rather than a closed-ended or unidirectional delivery of information from one individual to another. Even a small amount of evidence in which you have a small degree of confidence can be helpful in decision making if it is presented with these qualities in mind.

Communication with Judy about the joint protection program might be as follows: "Generally, clients' hand pain improves with behavioral joint protection programs. However, some improve more than others. Would you be interested in participating in a joint protection group?" In this communication, the findings are accurately portrayed in the past rather than present tense, and the pertinent relevance issue is addressed, enabling Judy to assess the evidence herself.

One implication of autonomous reasoning and action is that clients can choose to participate or not participate in occupational therapy assessments and interventions. Likewise, family members or other health practitioners may decide to encourage or discourage client participation. Evidence-based practice is not about the imposition of the will of one individual on the will of the other but rather is a mutual search for and discussion about information that will aid informed, wise decision making. The practitioner's responsibility is to provide information in such a manner that reasoned decision making is maximized.

Summary

Evidence-based practice has become an integral part of occupational therapy practice. In combination with the treatment environment and client values and circumstances, evidence forms a strong base from which to achieve best practice clinical decision making. To best inform the process of decision making, evidence can be clustered into three types of clinical tasks: getting to know the client, or diagnosis; choosing an effective treatment, or intervention; and estimating probable outcomes, or prognosis. Occupational therapists must develop the skills to identify answerable clinical questions, find and critically appraise research to identify the best evidence for each of the clinical tasks, use their clinical expertise to integrate this best evidence with their clients' values and needs, and implement it within their treatment environment. Critically appraising the evidence involves identifying the relevance, trustworthiness, generalizability, and clinical importance of research. Once best evidence is determined, occupational therapists must be able to communicate the evidence to clients to ensure collaborative and informed treatment decisions. Without skills in evidence-based practice, an occupational therapist will not be competitive in today's health care system. Evidence-based practice takes time and energy; the skills needed are acquired through active learning and practice. Throughout your career as an occupational therapist, you will refine and improve your skills and ensure that you use the best evidence to provide the best treatment for all of your clients.

References

American Occupational Therapy Association. (2010). Occupational therapy code of ethics and ethics standards. *American Journal of Occupational Therapy, 64*, 151–160. Retrieved from http://www.aota.org/Pubs/AJOT_1.aspx

Babbie, E. (1990). *Survey research methods* (2nd ed.). Belmont, CA: Wadsworth.

Carpenter, C., & Hammell, K. (2000). Evaluating qualitative research. In K. W. Hammell, C. Carpenter, & I. Dyck (Eds.), *Using qualitative research: A practical introduction for occupational and physical therapists*. Edinburgh, United Kingdom: Churchill Livingstone.

Carter, R. E., Lubinsky, J., & Domholdt, E. (2011). *Rehabilitation research: Principles and applications* (4th ed.). St. Louis, MO: Elsevier Saunders.

Christiansen, C., & Lou, J. Q. (2001). Ethical considerations related to evidence-based practice. *American Journal of Occupational Therapy, 55*, 345–349. Retrieved from http://www.aota.org/Pubs/AJOT_1.aspx

Cochrane Collaboration. (2010). *The Cochrane collaboration*. Retrieved from http://www.cochrane.org/

Cohen, J. (1990). Things I have learned (so far). *American Psychologist, 45*, 1304–1312. Retrieved from http://www.apa.org/pubs/journals/amp/index.aspx

Cummings, G., & Finch, S. (2005). Inference by eye: Confidence intervals and how to read pictures of data. *American Psychologist, 60*, 170–180. doi:10.1037/0003-066X.60.2.170

Cush, J. J., Weinblatt, M. E., & Kavanaugh, A. (2008). *Rheumatoid arthritis: Early diagnosis and treatment* (2nd ed.). West Islip, NY: Professional Communications.

Dalton, G. W., & Keating, J. L. (2000). Number needed to treat: A statistic relevant for physical therapists. *Physical Therapy, 80*, 1214–1219. Retrieved from http://ptjournal.apta.org/content/80/12/1214.long

Egan, M., Dubouloz, C. J., von Zweck, C., & Vallerand, J. (1998). The client-centered evidence-based practice of occupational therapy. *Canadian Journal of Occupational Therapy, 65*, 136–143. Retrieved from http://www.cmaj.ca/

Ferguson, C. J. (2009). An effect size primer: A guide for clinicians and researchers. *Professional Psychology: Research and Practice, 40*, 532–538. doi:10.1037/a0015808

Fritz, J. M., & Wainner, R. S. (2001). Examining diagnostic tests: An evidence-based perspective. *Physical Therapy, 81*, 1546–1564. Retrieved from http://ptjournal.apta.org/

Hammond, A., & Freeman, K. (2001). One-year outcomes of a randomized controlled trial of an educational-behavioural joint protection programme for people with rheumatoid arthritis. *Rheumatology, 40*, 1044–1051. doi:10.1093/rheumatology/40.9.1044

Hartman, J. M., Forsen, J. W., Wallace, M. S., & Neely, J. G. (2002). Tutorials in clinical research: Part IV. Recognizing and controlling bias. *The Laryngoscope, 112*, 23–31. doi:10.1097/00005537-200201000-00005

Hempel, S., Suttorp, M. J., Miles, J. N. V., Wang, Z., Maglione, M., Morton, S., . . . Shekelle, P. G. (2011). *Empirical evidence of associations between trial quality and effect sizes*. Rockville, MD: Agency for Healthcare Research and Quality.

Higgins, J. P. T., & Green, S. (Eds.). (2011). *Cochrane handbook for systematic reviews of interventions version 5.1.0 [updated March 2011]. The Cochrane Collaboration, 2011*. Retrieved from http://www.cochrane-handbook.org

Hoffmann, T., Bennett, S., Koh, C. L., & McKenna, K. T. (2010). Occupational therapy for cognitive impairment in stroke patients. *Cochrane Database of Systematic Reviews*, (9), CD006430. doi:10.1002/14651858.CD006430.pub2

Jadad, A. R., Moore, R. A., Carroll, D., Jenkinson, C., Reynolds, D. J. M., Gavaghan, D. J., & McQuay, H. J. (1996). Assessing the quality of reports of randomized clinical trials: Is blinding necessary? *Controlled Clinical Trials, 17*, 1–12. Retrieved from http://www.sciencedirect.com/science/journal/01972456

Law, M., Baptiste, S., & Mills, J. (1995). Client-centered practice: What does it mean and does it make a difference? *Canadian Journal of Occupational Therapy, 62*, 250–257. Retrieved from http://www.cmaj.ca/

Law, M., Cooper, B., Strong, S., Stewart, D., Rigby, P., & Letts, L. (1996). The person-environment-occupation model: A transactive approach to occupational performance. *Canadian Journal of Occupational Therapy, 63*, 9–23. Retrieved from http://www.cmaj.ca/

Law, M., & MacDermid, J. (Eds.). (2008). *Evidence-based rehabilitation: A guide to practice* (2nd ed.). Thorofare, NJ: Slack.

Lee, C. J., & Miller, L. T. (2003). The process of evidence-based clinical decision making in occupational therapy. *American Journal of Occupational Therapy, 57*, 473–477. Retrieved from http://www.aota.org/Pubs/AJOT_1.aspx

Lin, S. H., Murphy, S. L., & Robinson, J. C. (2010). Facilitating evidence-based practice: Process, strategies and resources. *American Journal of Occupational Therapy, 64*, 164–171. Retrieved from http://www.aota.org/Pubs/AJOT_1.aspx

Lipsey, M. W., & Wilson, D. B. (2001). *Practical meta-analysis*. Thousand Oaks, CA: Sage.

Lou, J. Q., & Durando, P. (2008). Asking clinical questions and searching for the evidence. In M. Law & J. MacDermid (Eds.), *Evidence-based rehabilitation* (2nd ed., pp. 95–117). Thorofare, NJ: Slack.

Mahar, C. G., Sherrington, C., Herbert, R. D., Mosely, A. M., & Elkins, M. (2003). Reliability of the PEDro scale for rating quality of randomized controlled trials. *Physical Therapy, 83*, 713–721. Retrieved from http://ptjournal.apta.org/

Mayer, D. (2010). *Essential evidence-based medicine* (2nd ed.). New York, NY: Cambridge University Press.

Moher, D., Hopewell, S., Schulz, K. F., Montori, V., Gotzsche, P. C., Devereaux, P. J., . . . Altman, D. G. (2010). CONSORT 2010 explanation and elaboration: Updated guidelines for reporting parallel group randomised trials. *Journal of Clinical Epidemiology, 63*, e1–e37. doi:10.1016/j.jclinepi.2010.03.004

Moons, K. G. M., Royston, P., Vergouwe, Y., Grobbee, D., & Altman, D. G. (2009). Prognosis and prognostic research: What, why, and how. *BMJ, 338*, 1317–1320. doi:10.1136/bmj.b375

National Center for Biotechnology Information. (2011). *PubMed*. Retrieved from http://www.ncbi.nlm.nih.gov/pubmed/

Oxford Centre for Evidence-Based Medicine Levels of Evidence Working Group. (2011). *The Oxford Centre for evidence-based medicine 2011 levels of evidence*. Retrieved from http://www.cebm.net/index.aspx?o=5653

Portney, L. G., & Watkins, M. P. (2009). *Foundations of clinical research: Applications to practice* (3rd ed.). Upper Saddle River, NJ: Pearson Education.

Rappolt, S. (2003). The role of professional expertise in evidence-based occupational therapy. *American Journal of Occupational Therapy, 57*, 589–593. Retrieved from http://www.aota.org/Pubs/AJOT_1.aspx

Salaffi, F., Stancati, A., Silvestri, C. A., Ciapetti, A., & Grassi, W. (2004). Minimal clinically important changes in chronic musculoskeletal pain intensity measured on a numerical rating scale. *European Journal of Pain, 8*, 283–291. doi:10.1016/j.ejpain.2003.09.004

Shin, J., Randolph, G. W., & Rauch, S. D. (2010). Evidence-based medicine in otolaryngology, part 1: The multiple faces of evidence-based medicine. *Otolaryngology—Head and Neck Surgery, 142*, 637–646. doi:10.1016/j.otohns.2010.01.018

Steultjens, E. E. M. J., Dekker, J. J., Bouter, L. M., Cardol, M. M., Van den Ende, E. C. H. M., & van de Nes, J. (2003). Occupational therapy for multiple sclerosis. *Cochrane Database of Systematic Reviews*, (3), CD003608. doi:10.1002/14651858.CD003608

Steultjens, E. E. M. J., Dekker, J. J., Bouter, L. M., Schaardenburg, D. D., Kuyk, M. A. M. A. H., & Van den Ende, E. C. H. M. (2004). Occupational therapy for rheumatoid arthritis. *Cochrane Database of Systematic Reviews*, (1), CD003114. doi:10.1002/14651858.CD003114.pub2

Straus, S. E., Richardson, W. S., Glasziou, P., & Haynes, R. B. (2005). *Evidence-based medicine* (3rd ed.). New York, NY: Churchill Livingstone.

Tickle-Degnen, L. (2000). Communicating with clients, family members, and colleagues about research evidence. *American Journal of Occupational Therapy*, *54*, 341–343. Retrieved from http://www.aota.org/Pubs/AJOT_1.aspx

Tickle-Degnen, L. (2001). From the general to the specific: Using meta-analytic reports in clinical decision making. *Evaluation & The Health Professions*, *24*, 308–326. doi:10.1177/01632780122034939

Tickle-Degnen, L. (2002a). Client-centered practice, therapeutic relationship, and the use of research evidence. *American Journal of Occupational Therapy*, *56*, 470–473. Retrieved from http://www.aota.org/Pubs/AJOT_1.aspx

Tickle-Degnen, L. (2002b). Communicating evidence to clients, managers, and funders. In M. Law (Ed.), *Evidence-based rehabilitation: A guide to practice* (pp. 221–254). Thorofare, NJ: Slack.

U.S. National Library of Medicine. (2010). *Medical subject headings (MeSH)*. Retrieved from http://www.nlm.nih.gov/mesh/meshhome.html

World Health Organization. (2005). *International classification of functioning, disability, and health*. Retrieved from http://www3.who.int/icf/onlinebrowser/icf.cfm

For additional resources on the subjects discussed in this chapter, visit http://thePoint.lww.com/Willard-Spackman12e.

CHAPTER 32

Ethical Practice

Regina F. Doherty

"Practitioners must be grounded not only by a moral conscience to do what is right, but also by the courage to proceed and ensure the best interests of the patient."

—BRANDT & HOMENKO (2011)

LEARNING OBJECTIVES

After reading this chapter, you will be able to:

1. Recognize the ethical issues that occupational therapy practitioners encounter in professional practice
2. Identify the virtues of health care professionals
3. Understand basic ethics problems, ethical theories, and approaches to ethics
4. Understand and apply an ethical decision-making guide for case analysis
5. Understand and apply ethical reasoning as a construct within the decision-making process
6. Identify and know how to access ethics resources
7. Understand effective communication strategies for difficult conversations

OUTLINE

Why Ethics?

Ask yourself the following questions:

- What would I say to a patient in a mental health setting who asked me if I could be his "Facebook friend" while he is undergoing active treatment on the unit where I practice?
- What would I say to a colleague who asked me to change my documentation to indicate that a client is worse than he really is so that the client can qualify for additional services?

- How would I feel if the family of a client with autism told me they were discontinuing his occupational therapy services because they had no means to pay for his continued care?

Ethical questions like these often arise for occupational therapy practitioners in their day-to-day practice. These questions must be attended to so that normal care delivery is not disrupted and best practice is achieved. This requires practitioners to recognize ethical situations and to have both the capacity and the willingness to address these situations systematically. In this chapter, ethical issues that arise in occupational therapy practice are discussed. This serves as a foundation to aid the reader in understanding, recognizing, and reasoning through ethical issues.

Occupational therapy practitioners in all professional roles will encounter ethical problems. Ethics is about reflecting, thinking, critically reasoning, justifying, acting on, and evaluating decisions. Ethical problems are often dynamic and complex, requiring additional knowledge and consultation with various resources. Consequently, knowledge and understanding of ethical reasoning and ethical decision making are essential for competent occupational therapy practice.

Ethics, Morality, and Moral Reasoning

The terms *ethical* and *moral* are often used interchangeably in professional practice, and although related, they have slightly different meanings. The term *ethic*s stems from the Greek word *ethos*, meaning "character." Ethics is a branch of philosophy that involves systemic study and reflection providing language, methods, and guidelines to study and reflect on morality (Purtilo & Doherty, 2011). In contrast, the term *morality* refers to social conventions about right and wrong human conduct and sets the stage for ethical behavior. Values, duty, and moral character guide reasoning and inform ethical decisions (Beauchamp & Childress, 2008). Values are the beliefs or objects a person holds dear (e.g., life). Duties describe an action that is required (e.g., provide food and shelter to care for one's family). Moral character describes traits or dispositions that facilitate trust and human flourishing (e.g., compassion, honesty) (Purtilo & Doherty, 2011).

There are three types of morality: personal or individual, group or organizational, and societal (Glaser, 2005). Personal morality includes individual beliefs and values. Acting in accordance with these values preserves one's integrity. Group morality is the morality of the profession or organization to which an individual belongs. A professional organization, such as the American Occupational Therapy Association (AOTA), maintains collective values that guide group decisions. For occupational therapists (OTs), this might be the emphasis on collaborative practice and occupation. Societal morality is the morality of society as a whole. Societal values may change over time, and different communities may fight for the protection of different values and rights. Tension often exists between these three realms of morality. It is important to reflect on how these different moralities interrelate because in a pluralistic society, no single vision of morality prevails, making ethical decision making challenging.

Moral reasoning is a term used to describe the process of reflecting on ethical issues. Moral reasoning is about norms and values, ideas of right and wrong, and how practitioners make decisions in professional work (Barnitt, 1993; Purtilo & Doherty, 2011). Moral reasoning is a reflective process that leads to ethically supported actions. It is a manifestation of moral character and mindful reflection (Slater, 2010). We use our moral reasoning to think critically about the meaning and values of a variety of situations including, but not limited to, the therapeutic relationship; the context of practice situations; and the institutional, cultural, and societal influences on the provision of health care (Delany, Edwards, Jensen, & Skinner, 2010). Consequently, effective moral reasoning and ethical decision making are closely linked to effective practice (Bebeau, 2002; Hartwell, 1995; Sisola, 2000).

Ethical Implications of Trends in Health Care and Occupational Therapy Practice

Health care systems are increasingly complex. Demographic and epidemiologic forces will continue to change the delivery of health care services. New technologies, including those used in intensive care, life-sustaining treatment, reproductive medicine, organ/tissue transplantation, robotics, and genomic medicine have created ethical questions for health care professionals. Improved lifestyle choices, managed care, and changes in health care policy and legislation also complicate the delivery of care, increasing the likelihood of encountering moral distress. **Moral distress** is an ethical problem that occurs when practitioners know the right thing to do but cannot achieve it because of external barriers or uncertainty about the outcome (Purtilo & Doherty, 2011). Common ethical concerns that occupational therapy practitioners encounter in practice are highlighted in Box 32.1. Issues that cause moral distress in occupational therapy practice with high frequency include those surrounding reimbursement, maintaining confidentiality, agreeing on goal setting, and balancing institutional needs versus what is best for the client (Doherty et al., 2012; Foye et al., 2002; Slater & Brandt, 2011).

BOX 32.1 Common Causes of Moral Distress

Common causes of moral distress in occupational therapy practice include the following:

- Confidentiality and disclosure
- Issues related to quality of life
- Issues related to client decision-making capacity and participation
- Professional boundaries
- Conflicts with organizational policies
- Resource allocation and priorities in treatment
- Cultural, religious, and family considerations
- Balancing benefits and burdens in care
- Reimbursement
- Difficult client behaviors
- Conflicting values surrounding goals of care

(From Barnitt, 1998; Doherty, Dellinger, Gately, Pullo, & Sullivan, 2012; Foye, Kirschner, Wagner, Stocking, & Siegler, 2002; Kassberg & Skar, 2008; Kinsella, Park, Appiagyei, Chang, & Chow, 2008; Purtilo & Doherty, 2011; Slater & Brandt, 2011.)

Virtues of Health Care Professionals

Health care professionals hold a unique societal role because the public expects them to uphold particular virtues. These include the virtues of integrity, benevolence, competence, kindness, trustworthiness, fairness, conscientiousness, caring, and compassion (Beauchamp & Childress, 2008; Devettere, 2009; Gawande, 2002; Pellegrino, 1995, 2002; Purtilo, 2004; Purtilo & Doherty, 2011). First and foremost, occupational therapy practitioners (OTs and occupational therapy assistants) must be benevolent and focus on what is best for the client. Second, the practitioner must be competent. All practitioners are responsible for achieving and maintaining competence in their area of occupational therapy practice. They must use evidence to guide practice decisions and engage in continuing education. Third, practitioners must be caring. Care enhances comfort and recovery and is an essential feature of professional practice (Fry & Veatch, 2000; Purtilo & Doherty, 2011). Although most practitioners recognize that caring is inherent in the health care professional's role, there are times when professionals must deal with difficult clients or families. There may be lack of reciprocity and mutuality caused by the condition itself, such as combativeness resulting from a head injury, which can erode the caring relationship. Erosions in care relationships also can occur when the complexity of patient/client needs increases and staffing diminishes (Maupin, 1995). Finally, practitioners must be compassionate. Compassion is the ability to enter into the experience of illness with the client (Pellegrino, 1982). Compassion is being kind, understanding, genuine, empathetic, caring, considerate, and professional in carrying out a task or duty. From time to time, every health care provider will experience complex situations and conflicting demands. It is during these times that practitioners must call on both character and conduct to provide compassionate care.

Distinguishing among Clinical, Legal, and Ethical Problems in Practice

Practitioners must learn to distinguish ethical questions from other questions that they encounter in the care of clients. Many times, what might appear to be an ethical issue is in fact something else, such as a miscommunication or a clinical or legal issue. For example, a clinical question would be "Can clients with severe dysphagia due to end-stage amyotrophic lateral sclerosis (ALS) eat?" This is a clinical question because there is a diagnostic answer to it. Clients who pass a bedside swallowing evaluation and modified barium swallow (MBS) test are clinically able to eat. If they fail this test but want to continue eating orally, an ethical question could arise. The ethical question would be "Should clients with end-stage ALS who fail an MBS test eat?" This is an ethical question because it raises questions relative to quality of life and the risks and benefits of eating with diminished swallowing capacity.

Legal questions may also arise in patient care decision making. Law and ethics are related fields; however, they have different goals and sanctions. Both rely on analytical processes and ground rules for good decision making; however, laws are legislated and are legally enforceable (Horner, 2003). Laws prescribe what we cannot do. What may be permitted legally might not be justified ethically and vice versa. In the case of clients with ALS, a legal question would be "Do competent clients have the right to refuse medical advice and continue eating orally despite the recommendation of the team?" This example highlights the importance of distinguishing and interpreting the type of question to more critically reason through the problem. Interpretation is a critical step in professional reasoning because how the practitioner or team understands the situation has great influence on how they will respond to it (Sullivan & Rosin, 2008).

CASE STUDY 32.1 Considering Virtues

Victoria is an occupational therapy student completing her second Level II fieldwork affiliation in an inpatient rehabilitation setting. She is 8 weeks into her placement and has been enjoying the increased independence and confidence that comes with practice experience and mentorship. Victoria has been primarily assigned to the neurology unit but is working with Tara this week, a covering clinical instructor who practices on the orthopedic unit. She has enjoyed the change of pace and exposure to new diagnoses while working on this unit. Tara and Victoria receive a referral for a newly admitted client named Joe. Joe was injured in a motor vehicle collision 10 days prior to his admission to the rehab facility. His injuries include open ulna and radius fractures, s/p open reduction and internal fixation with skin grafting to cover a soft tissue deficit, a tibia fracture, and a mild concussion.

See **Appendix I, Common Conditions Resources, and Evidence**, for more information about fractures and traumatic brain injury.

Tara is excited to treat Joe. The medical team told her about his upper extremity reconstruction in rounds this morning, requesting a splint to immobilize his forearm. Tara and Victoria go in together to meet Joe. He is sedated and very groggy. Tara introduces herself to Joe and tells him that she needs to make him a splint to protect his forearm where the surgery took place. Joe replies, "I'm too tired." Tara knows that Joe must have this fitted today so that the graft is protected and so he can begin daily dressing changes to advance his soft tissue healing. Tara communicates the need for the procedure to happen today and tells Joe he can just "chill out" and she and Victoria will do all the work. Joe agrees to the session stating, "Ok I trust you girls, just get it done and try not to hurt me."

Tara and Victoria begin the splint fabrication, and Victoria is so pleased that she is the student assisting in this intervention session. She has not seen any grafts on her fieldwork experiences so far and finds them a fascinating way to achieve soft tissue closure. Joe tolerates the session surprisingly well, with very little pain or discomfort at the operative site. When Joe's dressing is removed, Tara turns to Victoria and says, "Wow this is the best graft I have seen! Hold his arm up Victoria I want to take a picture of it on my phone. It's perfect for my blog." Victoria holds Joe's arm but is immediately uncomfortable with this as Joe is sedated and not aware that the photo is being taken. She feels her uneasiness rise as Tara goes on to take several photos of Joe without his knowledge. She knows that she has a responsibility to do something but is unsure what to do. She broaches the subject by saying, "I know on the neurology unit, we have to get written consent for all photos we take of our clients. Don't you guys have the same policy on this unit?" Tara responds by saying, "Yeah, but he's out of it. No harm done. I'll ask him another time. I'm sure he won't mind. Now can you rotate his arm a little? I want to get a few more images." Victoria is frustrated and her mind is awhirl thinking of what she should do next.

The case of Victoria highlights the need to call on both character and conduct in professional practice. It also highlights how quickly demands are placed on our reasoning in the practice environment, necessitating us to use our skills of discernment and moral reasoning.

- What are the virtues that should guide Victoria in this situation?
- Victoria is no doubt feeling vulnerable and is at a power differential with Tara. What are the consequences of speaking up versus staying silent in this scenario?
- How can Victoria best advocate for Joe and uphold the virtue of professional integrity?

Reflection and Ethical Practice

Recognizing the morally significant features of a situation is one of the first steps in ethical reflection. **Reflection** is a form of self-assessment that can be used to improve practice. Developing reflective capacity is a critical element in professional development and competence (Jensen & Richert, 2005). When reflecting on ethical aspects of practice, practitioners must consider their own values and how those values might influence their work. A value is a belief or an ideal to which an individual is committed (Kanny, 1993). Clarifying values and opinions allows practitioners to see elements of a situation that they did not see before, allowing for better appreciation of the complexity of decisions. For a values clarification exercise, see Exercise 32.A on the Willard and Spackman Website.

Another form of reflection is mindfulness. Mindfulness is a way of tuning in to what is happening in and around us (Schoeberlein & Sheth, 2009). Mindful practice enables practitioners to listen more attentively to clients' distress, recognize their own errors, refine their technical skills, make evidence-based decisions, and recognize the values necessary to act with compassion, competence, presence, and insight (Epstein, 1999).

Use of narratives, both written and oral, is another form of reflection. Telling stories allows therapists to reason through the moral features of a situation and develop a judgment about what ought to be done (Mattingly, 1998). Guided narrative review with a mentor is an effective way to infuse ethical reasoning into occupational therapy practice.

Identifying Different Types of Ethical Problems

When reflecting on an ethical issue, it is important to distinguish among the different types of ethical problems that occur in practice. An ***ethical problem*** is a situation that is believed to have negative implications regarding cherished moral values and duties *and* that will pose an extremely difficult choice to an individual or group of individuals (Purtilo & Doherty, 2011). It may be manifested by an emotional reaction such as discomfort, anxiety, or anger and is often captured when the practitioner says, "This just doesn't feel right." This "not right" feeling is an emotional response that serves as a trigger to initiate ethical reflection. These feelings are often moral challenges and must be worked out beyond gut feelings to reasoned alternatives and actions.

Moral Distress

Moral distress (as defined earlier) results from the conflict of knowing the right thing to do, but not being able to achieve it. This cognitive discomfort helps the practitioner realize the potential threat to ethical integrity. Often, multiple stakeholders are involved in the care of the client (e.g., the primary care physician, consulting specialists, rehabilitation practitioners, the organizational administrator, the private insurer, the family). Moral distress can occur when stakeholders hold different opinions regarding the goals of care, leaving practitioners with no clear course of action.

When conflict arises in the care of patients, the paramount goal should always be patient's welfare. Moral distress must be worked through so that this goal can be achieved. An example of moral distress can be found in the case of Etta Jorani.

Ethical Dilemma

An ethical dilemma is slightly different from a moral distress. A dilemma exists when the individual has obligations to do both X and Y but cannot do both (Horner, 2003). In a true dilemma, there is a strong persuasive argument both for and against a "right" course of action. Each choice, or course of action presented to the moral agent, is morally acceptable in some respects and morally unacceptable in others (Beauchamp & Childress, 2008). In other words, each choice has an element of right and wrong posing a moral conflict. Ethical dilemmas are more complex problems as they often pit values and cherished moral principles against each other (Wells, 2003).

The case of Victoria presented earlier in this chapter is an ethical dilemma. As you will recall, Victoria is the student working with Joe, the client status post upper extremity reconstruction who was being photographed by Tara, his primary therapist, without his knowledge or consent. It is easy to see that Victoria is experiencing moral distress; however, she also has an ethical dilemma.

Victoria has dual obligations. She has a loyalty to her supervising therapist (and the organization) under whom she is practicing. Tara is a well-respected clinician and has been a resource to Victoria throughout her student affiliation. Victoria wants to honor the student–mentor relationship they have developed. At the same time, she questions whether honoring this relationship is supported because it would disregard the promise she made on entering the occupational therapy profession—to above all respect the rights of individuals and refrain from any actions that cause harm (AOTA, 2010a). Victoria knows that she also has an obligation to treat her supervisor with respect and discretion. Tara states that she will obtain consent from Joe later. Victoria wonders—does this meet the intent of consent and adequately protect Joe from harm? Can she trust this will happen? Victoria may also be thinking—I am just a student so technically

CASE STUDY 32.2 Experiencing Moral Distress

Etta is a 72-year-old woman who was visiting her daughter in New York City from her home in the Philippines. During her visit, Etta suffered a left middle cerebral artery (MCA) cerebrovascular accident (CVA) with severe right-sided hemiplegia.

See **Appendix I, Common Conditions Resources, and Evidence**, for more information on CVA/stroke.

She requires moderate assistance with all activities of daily living (ADL) and is motivated to work with occupational therapist despite her limited English skills. The neurologist caring for Etta lets the team know that she is medically ready for discharge. The occupational therapist (OT), physical therapist (PT), and speech-language pathologist (SLP) all recommend inpatient rehabilitation; however, because Etta is not a U.S. citizen, she is not covered by insurance for this level of care in the United States. The case manager who coordinates the discharge services lets Etta know that she will not be eligible for rehabilitation care in the United States. Etta is visibly upset and says, "What do you mean? Where am I supposed to go? My daughter works and takes care of her own kids in a one-bedroom apartment. I can't stay with her and there is no way I can get back to the Philippines like this. I don't understand; you saved me only to leave me alone and helpless." The OT and the interprofessional team caring for Etta feel terrible. They do not want Etta to mistook the limitations in her resources as noncaring on the part of the providers. They are experiencing moral distress. They know the right thing to do (transfer Etta to an inpatient rehabilitation hospital for continued intense treatment), but a barrier (the lack of insurance) stands in the way. They all want the best outcome for Etta but are limited by the context and the constraints of her situation. They must work together to problem-solve through this moral distress so Etta and her family achieve the best outcome. ■

I could just let this go. After all, what if there were repercussions for continuing to insist that Tara not take photos (and delete the ones she has already taken)? Upon reflection, Victoria also realizes that by holding Joe's arm she was an active participant in the session and may be responsible for any consequences of this action. She wonders if she could lose her student affiliation for this. She is feeling angry, anxious, and vulnerable.

Victoria weighs possible courses of action. One option would be to continue to trust Tara's supervisory guidance, allowing her to take the photos and obtain consent from Joe once he is awake. Perhaps Tara is right; Joe won't mind (and may even be flattered) knowing the photos will be used to educate other therapists. Victoria justifies this action thinking—that would be a "good outcome"—no harm would be done and perhaps even some good would come out of it. By not objecting and deferring to Tara's judgment, Victoria avoids conflict and does not place her student affiliation at risk by bringing the incident to the attention of others.

Victoria then reasons through another option. In this option, she continues to advocate for Joe and insists that Tara not photograph Joe without his consent. In this way, Victoria upholds her professional responsibility by being both responsive (to the patient's well-being) and by sharing what she knows with her supervisor who is accountable for the action. This action takes both character and courage on Victoria's part as it may cause conflict within the student–mentor relationship. Tara may be upset. She may dismiss Victoria from the case, or Tara may be pleased and she may commend Victoria for her advocacy skills. Either way, if Victoria refrains from further participation in the session, she highlights for Tara that taking photographs without consent is a wrong act (both ethically and legally). This option ensures safety for the client, but it runs the risk of eroding the mentoring relationship, something Victoria greatly values. It also has potential professional repercussions for both Victoria and Tara. The fact is that Victoria cannot choose both options. She must act on one or the other. She has an ethical dilemma.

Ethical Theories and Principles That Apply to Occupational Therapy Practice

Theories provide support for ethical decision making. Ethical theories and principles provide a language for diagnosing, communicating, and problem-solving ethical questions. Ethical theories are well-developed, systematic frameworks of rules and principles (Nash, 2002). They provide reasons and ideals for ethical standards. Many ethical approaches and theories serve as a reference point for guiding decision making. The most commonly used ethical approaches in health care are principle-based approaches, virtue- and character-based ethics, utilitarianism, and deontology.

Principle-Based Approach

A principle-based approach to ethics relies on ordinary shared moral beliefs as theoretical content. Principles are duties, rights, or other moral guidelines that provide a logical approach to analyzing ethical issues for a given situation. In case analysis, principles are identified, applied, and compared to weigh one principle against another in deciding a course of action. The following principles are commonly used in health care:

- *Autonomy*. Autonomy is the ability to act freely and independently on one's own decisions (Beauchamp & Childress, 2008). It is often called the principle of self-determination.
- *Beneficence*. Beneficence refers to actions done on or for the benefit of others.
- *Nonmaleficence*. Nonmaleficence is the duty not to harm others.
- *Fidelity*. Fidelity means being faithful to one's promises or commitments.
- *Justice*. Justice refers to equal treatment. It deals with the proper distribution of benefits, burdens, and resources. Procedural justice is often used to reflect impartial decision-making procedures. Distributive justice refers to the equitable allocation of societal resources such as health care (Horner, 2003).
- *Veracity*. Veracity refers to telling the truth.
- *Paternalism (or parentalism)*. Paternalism occurs when a health professional, or other individual, assumes to know what is best and limits the client's autonomy by making decisions for the client rather than with the client (Purtilo & Doherty, 2011).

Virtue and Character-Based Ethics

Virtues are dispositions of character and conduct that motivate and enable practitioners to provide good care (Fletcher, Miller, & Spencer, 1997). Virtue ethics, derived from Aristotle and Thomas Aquinas, focuses on moral agents and their good character. Using this approach, moral goodness is achieved when behaviors are chosen for the sake of virtue (caring and kindness) rather than obligation.

Utilitarianism

Utilitarianism, derived from the work of Jeremy Bentham and John Stuart Mill, is concerned with actions that maximize good consequences and minimize bad consequences. From this perspective, morally right acts produce the best overall results; that is, the ends justify the means. The ethical action is one whose outcome brings about the most good or the least harm overall (Purtilo & Doherty, 2011). Utilitarianism is often used in public policy development.

Deontology

Deontology is a duty-based moral theory that is based primarily on the work of Immanuel Kant. In this theory, moral rules are universal and never to be broken; consequently, doing one's duty is considered primary, regardless of the consequences. For example, truthfulness is an unconditional Kantian duty. A practitioner would never keep the truth from a client even if the truth would harm the client in some way. From a Kantian perspective, respect for people is a moral imperative; therefore, withholding the truth disrespects the client's right to know.

The Ethical Decision-Making Process

The ethical decision-making process aids the occupational therapy practitioner in reasoning through a problem in a structured and systematic way. This process provides a structure for practitioners to give due consideration to issues, reflect on them, formulate possible alternatives, and make thoughtful choices. It guides client-centered care with an emphasis on moral conduct (Purtilo & Doherty, 2011). There are many ethical decision-making models available to practitioners. Common aspects of all ethical decision-making models are the need for the practitioners to do the following:

1. Recognize and define the ethical question
2. Gather the relevant data
3. Formulate a moral diagnosis and analyze the problem using ethics theory/principles
4. Problem-solve practical alternatives and decide on an action
5. Act on a morally acceptable choice
6. Evaluate and reflect on the process/action/results

(Bailey & Schwartzberg, 2003; Gervais, 2005; Hansen & Kyler-Hutchison, 1989; Purtilo & Doherty, 2011; Scanlon & Glover, 1995; Swisher, Arslanian, & Davis, 2005)

Ethical Resources and Jurisdiction

Resources

Practitioners who face ethical issues must be knowledgeable about the resources that exist to support them in this dimension of their clinical reasoning. Resources are crucial for dealing with the uncertainties related to ethical issues that practitioners encounter at all levels of practice.

Ethics Committees

Ethics committees support practitioners who need assistance in reasoning about ethical dimensions of care. The three primary roles of ethics committees are consultation, education, and policy review and development. Accrediting agencies, such as the Joint Commission, require that all health care organizations have a process to address ethical issues involving patient care and organizational ethics. Ethics committees provide an environment for safe and open discussion of basic moral questions, ease the feelings of staff, provide knowledgeable resources, and empower practitioners and families to make morally justified decisions.

Effective ethics committees are interdisciplinary and have strong institutional support. They analyze cases from many different perspectives to ensure the best outcome for clients. Occupational therapy practitioners who are either interested novices or experts in ethics should serve as members of ethics committees because they can bring broad perspectives to ethics discussions, are resources for topics related to values clarification and quality of life, and are skilled in group facilitation. Practitioners in settings without ethics committees should use their mentors, managers, administrative supports, and professional organizations for assistance with ethical issues. Other organizational resources such as the office of patient care advocacy (also known as the ombudsman), office of social work, chaplaincy service, and office of legal counsel can also provide guidance with ethical issues.

Institutional Review Boards

Increased impetus for research and attention to evidence-based practice have resulted in an increase in the number of occupational therapy practitioners involved in research. All practitioners who are involved in research activity have a moral obligation to familiarize themselves with the rules, regulations, and ethical obligations of conducting responsible research. There are many ethical considerations in research (e.g., data integrity, conflict of interest, authorship), but the most compelling pertains to human subjects as research participants.

To ensure an objective review of ethical issues related to human subject research, any institution that receives federal funding is required to have an **institutional review board (IRB)**. An IRB is a panel of diverse individuals, including organization staff and at least one community member, who are responsible for reviewing all research proposals and grants to ensure that adequate protections for research participants are in place. These protections include informed consent, research design and methodology, recruitment, the balance of risks and benefits, and confidentiality. The three fundamental principles that guide the ethical conduct of research involving human participants are respect for persons (autonomy), beneficence, and justice (National Commission for the Protection of Human Subjects of Biomedical and Behavioral Research, 1979). Occupational therapy practitioners should refer to their organization's specific policies and regulations regarding oversight and training in the ethical conduct of research.

CASE STUDY 32.3 Applying the Ethical Decision-Making Process

Nicole is an occupational therapist working in an early intervention setting. She has been working with an interprofessional team of practitioners treating the Suarez family. Their client, Gabriella Suarez, is a 2-and-a-half-year-old female s/p embolic cerebrovascular accident (CVA).

See **Appendix I, Common Conditions Resources, and Evidence**, for more information on CVA.

Gabriella spent more than 3 months in the acute rehabilitation setting because she had lost her ability to perform all ADL's, including her ability to speak, eat, and play. The loss of these previously achieved developmental milestones was traumatic to the family who surrounded this outgoing and loving toddler, with support and encouragement throughout her rehabilitation. After weeks of occupational therapy and speech therapy, it was determined that Gabriella was ready to be transitioned back to taking food by mouth (since her stroke, she had been receiving nourishment through a gastric tube because she was unable to swallow without aspirating). She was awaiting a modified barium swallow test as the final step in this transition.

One afternoon, Nicole arrived to find Gabriella's mother feeding her daughter a cookie. Her initial reaction of joy at the fact that the child was able to enjoy a cookie for the first time in months was quickly overwhelmed by her sobering realization that she had not yet been cleared to eat solid foods. Over the last month, Nicole had become very close to both the child and her mother who were thrilled with this victory. Gabriella smiled, an expression of emotion that Nicole had never seen her exhibit before. This gave the mother great hope, something she had been without for many weeks. Nicole then realized that she was in a tough place when the mother then asked her to "please, please not tell anyone" that she had given her daughter the cookie.

To ensure a professional and caring response to this situation, Nicole must analyze the situation using an ethical decision-making process. This will help guide her thinking and her actions.

Identify the Ethical Question

First, Nicole must identify and reflect on the ethical questions that emerged in the case. This often begins with the question, "What should I do?" In the case of Gabriella and her mother, some questions would be the following: Should Nicole tell the team that the client's mother fed her the cookie? Should she honor the mother's request not to report the action, knowing that this may cause harm to the child? How can Nicole balance her obligations to the child, the mother, and the early intervention (EI) agency?

Gather the Relevant Data

The next step in ethical analysis is to gather the relevant data, identifying the known facts and beliefs about the case. It is important to distinguish between the two. Facts are needed to make judicious decisions. Facts regarding medical information and factors such as family context, client preferences, social and cultural issues, institutional factors, and provider considerations should be confirmed for accuracy. Additional information should be sought if needed. Take a moment and think about the facts and beliefs in this case.

Formulate a Moral Diagnosis and Apply Ethics Principles/Theory to the Case

Once the information has been gathered, a moral diagnosis must be formulated by identifying the type of ethical problem and the ethical principles that apply to the case. If there is more than one problem, they should be ranked in order of importance.

Having considered the ethical questions in the case of Gabriella, Nicole must decide whether the ethical problem is moral distress or ethical dilemma. She decides that she is facing moral distress. Nicole knows the correct course of action requires her to tell the team that the mother has fed the child prior to medical clearance. The relationship that she had with the child and her mother, and the mother's emotional plea for her not to tell, was a barrier to that disclosure. She was torn with how to best care for Gabriella and show care and concern to the mother. Key ethical principles that relate to this moral distress are beneficence and nonmaleficence. There are other principles and theories that apply, think about which ones as you continue to reason through the case.

Problem-Solve Practical Alternatives and Decide on a Course of Action

Now Nicole must begin to identify practical alternatives and decide what do. She must ask herself, "What is the good or right thing to do?" She would be wise to seek out resources in her facility and to ask her mentors for guidance in this ethical analysis. She might consult with various stakeholders, such as the interprofessional team, to identify strategies to best educate the family and ensure Gabriella's safety. She also could refer to the AOTA "Occupational Therapy Code of Ethics and Ethics Standards" (2010a). Generating a list of alternatives enables evaluation of the positive and negative consequences. Once the alternatives have been identified, ethical theory should be applied to support and justify the proposed action.

Nicole brainstormed a list of possible alternatives:

- Ask the mother why she gave Gabriella the cookie and why she does not want other members of the EI team to know. This is an important piece of information to explore. What were the motivating factors behind the mother's decision to give Gabriella the cookie? Did she want to be the first person to reintroduce food to her child? What are the cultural expectations and the meaning of food for the Suarez family?
- Offer support to the mother. She may fear judgment of others or may feel that if the information is revealed, her daughter may suffer consequences of her action causing a delay in her progress.
- Deny the mother's request and inform the team.
- Say nothing to the mother but document the observation in the record. (It is important to note that this alternative is not one that has moral grounding, as it has the potential to cause more harm to all parties involved. It fractures the therapeutic relationship with the family; and although it may alleviate Nicole's anxiety, will only do so temporarily, creating possible future distress).

CASE STUDY 32.3 Applying the Ethical Decision-Making Process *(Continued)*

- Talk with the mother about the concerns Nicole has related to Gabriella's safety. In a supportive way, this allows the mother to gain better insight into the seriousness of her actions. This conversation may even lead to a joint discussion with other members of the team regarding the mother's understanding of the process for transitioning back to oral feeding.
- Describe the situation with the EI nurse without identifying which family was involved.
- Tell the mother that she will not tell the team as long as the mother agrees to not give Gabriella any more food by mouth until medically cleared.

Nicole will need to reason through the alternatives, apply ethical theory to support her actions, and come to a judgment on the best approach. Having virtue, sensitivity to ethical issues, and a process for analyzing ethical questions are important elements in ethical decision making. If you were Nicole, which alternative would you choose?

Act on a Morally Acceptable Choice

Now that Nicole has decided on the course of action, she must act on the decision, bridging the gap between knowing what she ought to do and actually doing it. This is where the Aristotelian notion of practical wisdom and moral argument join together with clinical judgment for action. Often, this is the most difficult step because it requires calling on moral courage to take positions that are unpopular or contrary to the interest of others (Aulisio, Arnold, & Younger, 2000). Moral courage is a skill. It involves facing and overcoming fear to uphold an ultimate good.

Nicole will need courage to talk with Gabriella's mother. She will need to be attentive to the interests and emotions of the mother and remember the ultimate goal, which is to ensure the best care for Gabriella.

Evaluate and Reflect on the Process/Action/Results

Finally, Nicole must evaluate the results of her action. Evaluation includes both current and retrospective analysis. This reflection can guide future action by either avoiding or preventing a similar situation, or knowing how to act should a similar situation arise in the future. Questions Nicole might ask are as follows:

- What was the most challenging aspect of this situation?
- What have I learned from this case to help improve future patient care?
- What did I learn from the family/team regarding my course of action?
- What have I learned that will contribute to my own moral life and to my virtues as a practitioner?
- How has this case affected me as a care provider? What would I do differently if faced with the same situation again?

Evaluation of the decision-making process in cases such as this one has the potential to change practice, policies, education, or service delivery systems. Evaluation provides the opportunity for personal and professional reflection that can lead to further professional development and greater confidence to respond to future moral distress. Nicole could also work with her colleagues and the EI agency to propose policies and staff education so that similar confusion does not occur in the future. Nicole should also consider how those she consulted with contributed to the case and should critique her own decision-making process to improve her future practice.

Codes of Ethics

Codes of ethics are written documents produced by professional associations, organizations, or regulatory bodies that state the commitment to a service ideal, core purpose, or standard of conduct. Ethical codes ensure public trust and safeguard the reputation of a profession. Codes of ethics are often aspirational, educational, and regulatory in nature (Banks, 2004). The values articulated in the ethical code serve to guide professional practice.

The "Occupational Therapy Code of Ethics and Ethics Standards" (AOTA, 2010a) serves as a guide for professional conduct. Along with the "Standards of Practice for Occupational Therapy" (AOTA, 2010b), this document serves as resource to all occupational therapy practitioners, educators, students, and researchers encouraging them to attain the highest level of professional behavior. The purpose of the "Occupational Therapy Code of Ethics and Ethics Standards" (AOTA, 2010a) is to

1. Identify and describe the principles supported by the occupational therapy profession;
2. Educate the general public and members regarding established principles to which occupational therapy personnel are accountable;
3. Socialize occupational therapy personnel to expected standards of conduct; and
4. Assist occupational therapy personnel in recognition and resolution of ethical dilemmas (AOTA, 2010a, p. 152).

Additional information about the code and related documents and the AOTA Ethics Commission can be found at http://www.aota.org.

Regulatory Agencies

Three organizations provide oversight for occupational therapy practice: the AOTA, the National Board for Certification in Occupational Therapy (NBCOT), and state regulatory boards (SRBs). Each has distinct concerns, sanctions, and jurisdiction, but one commonality is their concern for ethical practice.

The American Occupational Therapy Association

AOTA, the professional association for occupational therapy, is the primary vehicle for influencing, promoting, and developing the profession's services to society (Doherty, Peterson, & Braveman, 2006). The AOTA develops standards of practice for all occupational therapy practitioners. These standards are an essential resource for practitioners, students, educators, and researchers.

Within AOTA, the Ethics Commission reviews the AOTA Occupational Therapy Code of Ethics every 5 years. Its primary responsibility is to recommend the ethics standards for the profession. It also educates members and consumers regarding ethics standards. Ethics Commission members and staff of the AOTA Ethics Program are resources for students, practitioners, educators, and consumers. They provide assistance with the interpretation of relevant ethical principles via advisory opinions, consultation, articles, and presentations. Finally, the Ethics Commission is responsible for the process of developing and implementing the enforcement procedures for the code. Disciplinary actions apply to members of AOTA and include reprimand, censure, probation, suspension, and permanent revocation of membership.

National Board for Certification in Occupational Therapy

The NBCOT is a credentialing agency that provides certification for the occupational therapy profession. Its mission is to serve the public interest by ensuring the competency of all certified occupational therapy practitioners (NBCOT, 2010). The NBCOT establishes minimum standards for certification to enter practice and ongoing recertification standards, including continuing competency through professional development. The NBCOT Certificant Code of Conduct outlines professional responsibilities for certified occupational therapy practitioners. As in many organizational codes of conduct, the NBCOT Certificant Code of Conduct includes ethics-related principles such as integrity, responsibility, honesty, fairness, and technical competence. Violation of this code of conduct is grounds for sanction, which may entail reprimand, probation, or suspension or revocation of certification. Suspension or revocation of certification prohibits sanctioned individuals from practicing occupational therapy.

The NBCOT Qualifications and Compliance Review Committee oversees certification violation issues such as breaches of ethics and unprofessional practice. The NBCOT notifies SRBs and the public of any complaints it receives and the disciplinary action it takes in response to these complaints. Additional information about NBCOT and the NBCOT Certificant Code of Conduct can be found at http://www.nbcot.org.

State Regulatory Boards

SRBs or licensing boards safeguard and promote the public welfare by ensuring that qualifications and standards for professional practice are properly evaluated, applied, and enforced (Doherty et al., 2006). They ensure the health and safety of citizens in their respective states. Occupational therapy is regulated in all 50 states and in three U.S. territories. The level of regulation varies; therefore, all occupational therapy practitioners must be aware of the specific provisions and statutes for the state in which they work. Most states use professional licensure to regulate practice, but several states have certification, registration, or title protection. Licensure is a means of defining a lawful scope of practice. It ensures patient protections and legally articulates the domain of practice for the profession. Licensure also prevents nonqualified individuals from practicing occupational therapy or using the title "occupational therapist" or "occupational therapy assistant." Many states include codes of ethics statements (most adopt the AOTA code and ethics standards) in their licensure law or regulations. SRBs have the authority by state law to discipline occupational therapy practitioners who violate regulations, including the state's code of ethics. Practitioners have the responsibility to understand the regulations under which they work and the procedure for processing a complaint.

Difficult Conversations

The cases of Etta, Victoria and Gabriella highlight how practitioners must engage in difficult conversations. Some of these are with clients, some with families, and some with colleagues. Although these conversations may be uncomfortable and awkward, through development of effective listening and communication strategies, practitioners can become more skillful and confident in meeting this challenge. Communication is a fundamental aspect of therapeutic relationships, interprofessional practice, and client-centered care.

Empathetic listening is relevant in ethical decision making because it can help practitioners appreciate the experience of those who seek their care. However difficult ethical problems and client communications might be, clients also face difficult paths and difficult choices. Developing the ability to evaluate a client or family's behavior requires practitioners to appreciate and accept a different perspective and different choices (Cohen, 2004). This is the first step in demonstrating moral sensitivity.

Open communication and empathy are key components to the delivery of compassionate care. The following are suggestions for effective communication:

1. **Be present.** Always respect others. Try to minimize interruptions and ensure that the environment is as free of distractions as possible. Choose an appropriate communication style for the situation. Establish rapport by making good eye contact and show interest, care, warmth, and responsiveness. These factors are predictive of effective client communication (Levetown, 2008).
2. **Use open-ended communication and listen quietly.** Health care practitioners often say too

much, which does not allow time for the other person to speak. Talk less and listen more. Phrases such as "go on" can encourage the person to examine issues at a deeper level (Cameron, 2004).

3. **Remain focused on the person and the goals of intervention.** Strive to understand the client's story. What is his or her perspective? What are the connections between the circumstances, beliefs, values, and resources in the client narrative? Are the goals appropriate and achievable? Do they maximize benefit and minimize burden?
4. **Be contrite and humble.** If you do not know the answer to a question, say so and assure the person that you will find the answer. Then find the answer and follow up with the person. Share your uncertainty about the case or prognosis.
5. **Legitimize the losses that the person is experiencing.** It is important to acknowledge the person's experience. Many clients are not prepared to cope with their newly diagnosed condition. They never expected to be in a compromised state, and their family might not be able to cope with the personal or financial implications of this change. Denial, depression, and anger are common responses to disease and disability. Practitioners need to acknowledge these emotions openly by stating, "What I am hearing you say is that you are angry that you can no longer live alone" or "Let me see if I can summarize what your daughter is trying to say . . . Is that correct?"
6. **Ensure shared decision making.** Questions surrounding new disability, quality-of-life, and end-of-life issues can be especially complex. Clients experience biographical disruption when confronted with illness challenging their fundamental values and autonomy (Mars, Kempen, Widdershoven, Janssen, & van Eijk, 2008). Occupational therapy practitioners who have established relationships with their clients are obligated to fully inform clients of the likelihood of the success or failure of therapeutic interventions. It is important to engage clients in shared decision making. Shared decision making is a process in which information is exchanged between the professional and the client (Purtilo & Doherty, 2011). Practitioners should keep questions straightforward, listen carefully to answers, and follow the person's lead by asking focused follow-up questions using the person's own words. Asking questions such as "What are your most important hopes?" and "What are your biggest fears?" can assist both practitioner and client in setting appropriate goals for care (Quill, 2000).
7. **Make a team effort.** In today's complex health care environments, teams of professionals have a moral obligation to work together to deliver the best care. Ethical approaches must focus on interprofessional teamwork because it is unreasonable to expect that individuals can resolve complex situations and moral distress alone (Carpenter, 2010). Effective interprofessional working relationships are foundational to collaborative care delivery. Effective interprofessional teams respect and value each other's contribution to client care, listen attentively, use understandable communication, provide feedback to others, respond to feedback from others, and address interprofessional conflict (Interprofessional Education Collaborative Expert Panel, 2011).

Conclusion

Ethical issues are ever-present in professional practice and will continue to challenge occupational therapy practitioners as the fields of medicine, technology, and health care delivery evolve. OTs must recognize, critically reason, act, and reflect on ethical issues that arise in their professional roles. Occupational therapy practitioners who are reflective and knowledgeable in ethical decision-making processes are best prepared to successfully address ethical aspects of practice. Ethical behavior is the responsibility of all occupational therapy professionals.

> *"The tools of ethical decision making include developing 'habits of thought' for reflection on complex, changing situations that are part of everyday practice."*
>
> —Jensen (2005)

References

American Occupational Therapy Association. (2010a). Occupational therapy code of ethics and ethics standards. *American Journal of Occupational Therapy, 64*, 151–160.

American Occupational Therapy Association. (2010b). Standards of practice for occupational therapy. *American Journal of Occupational Therapy, 64*, 415–420.

Aulisio, M. P., Arnold, R. M., & Younger, S. J. (2000). Health care ethics consultation: Nature, goals, and competencies: A position paper from the Society for Health and Human Values-Society for Bioethics Consultation Task Force on Standards for Bioethics Consultation. *Annals of Internal Medicine, 133*, 59–69.

Bailey, D. M., & Schwartzberg, S. L. (Eds.). (2003). *Ethical and legal dilemmas in occupational therapy* (2nd ed.). Philadelphia, PA: F. A. Davis.

Banks, S. (2004). *Ethics, accountability, and the social professions*. New York, NY: Palgrave Macmillan.

Barnitt, R. E. (1993). Deeply troubling questions: The teaching of ethics in undergraduate courses. *British Journal of Occupational Therapy, 56*, 401–406.

Barnitt, R. (1998). Ethical dilemmas in occupational therapy and physical therapy: A survey of practitioners in the UK National Health Service. *Journal of Medical Ethics, 24*, 193–199.

Beauchamp, T. L., & Childress, J. F. (2008). *Principles of biomedical ethics* (6th ed.). New York, NY: Oxford University Press.

Bebeau, M. J. (2002). The Defining Issues Test and the four component model: Contributions to professional education. *Journal of Moral Education, 31*, 271–293.

Brandt, L. C., & Homenko, D. F. (2011). Balancing patient rights and practitioner values. In D. Y. Slater (Ed.), *Reference guide to the occupational therapy code of ethics and ethics standards* 2010 Edition (pp. 123–126). Bethesda, MD: AOTA Press.

Cameron, M. (2004). Ethical listening as therapy. *Journal of Professional Nursing, 20*, 141–142.

Carpenter, C. (2010). Moral distress in physical therapy practice. *Physiotherapy Theory and Practice, 26*(2), 69–78.

Cohen, S. (2004). *The nature of moral reasoning: The framework and activities of ethical deliberation, argument and decision making.* New York, NY: Oxford University Press.

Delany, C. M., Edwards, I., Jensen, G. M., & Skinner, E. (2010). Closing the gap between ethics knowledge and practice through active engagement: An applied model of physical therapy ethics. *Physical Therapy, 90*, 1068–1078.

Devettere, R. J. (2009). *Practical decision making in health care ethics: Cases and concepts* (3rd ed.). Washington, DC: Georgetown University Press.

Doherty, R., Dellinger, A., Gately, M., Pullo, R., & Sullivan, S. (2012, April). *Ethical issues in occupational therapy: A survey of practitioners.* Paper presented at the American Occupational Therapy Association 2012 Annual Conference, Indianapolis, IN.

Doherty, R., Peterson, E. W., & Braveman, B. (2006). Responsible participation in a profession. In B. Braveman (Ed.), *Leading and managing occupational therapy services: An evidence-based approach.* Philadelphia, PA: F. A. Davis.

Epstein, R. M. (1999). Mindful practice. *Journal of the American Medical Association, 282*, 833–839.

Fletcher, J. C., Miller, F. G., & Spencer, E. M. (1997). Clinical ethics: History, content and resources. In J. C. Fletcher, P. A. Lombardo, M. F. Marshall, & F. G. Miller (Eds.), *Introduction to clinical ethics* (2nd ed., pp. 3–20). Hagerstown, MD: University Publishing Group.

Foye, S. J., Kirschner, K. L., Wagner, L. C. B., Stocking, C., & Siegler, M. (2002). Ethics in practice: Ethical issues in rehabilitation: A qualitative analysis of dilemmas identified by occupational therapists. *Topics in Stroke Rehabilitation, 9*(3), 89–101.

Fry, S. T., & Veatch, R. M. (2000). *Case studies in nursing ethics.* Sudbury, MA: Jones & Bartlett.

Gawande, A. (2002). *Complications: A surgeon's notes on an imperfect science.* New York, NY: Picador.

Gervais, K. G. (2005). A model for ethical decision making to inform the ethics education of future professionals. In R. Purtilo, G. M. Jensen, & C. B. Royeen (Eds.), *Educating for moral action: A sourcebook in health and rehabilitation ethics* (pp. 185–190). Philadelphia, PA: F. A. Davis.

Glaser, J. W. (2005). Three realms of ethics: An integrating map of ethics for the future. In R. Purtilo, G. M. Jensen, & C. B. Royeen (Eds.), *Educating for moral action: A sourcebook in health and rehabilitation ethics* (pp. 169–184). Philadelphia, PA: F. A. Davis.

Hansen, R., & Kyler-Hutchison, P. (1989, April). *Light at the end of the tunnel.* Workshop presented at the annual conference of the American Occupational Therapy Association, Baltimore, MD.

Hartwell, S. (1995). Promoting moral development through experiential teaching. *Clinical Law Review, 1*, 505–539.

Horner, J. (2003). Morality, ethics and law: Introductory concepts. *Seminars in Speech and Language, 24*, 263–274.

Interprofessional Education Collaborative Expert Panel. (2011). *Core competencies for interprofessional collaborative practice: Report of an expert panel.* Washington, DC: Interprofessional Education Collaborative.

Jensen, G. M. (2005). Mindfulness: Applications for teaching and learning in ethics education. In R. Purtilo, G. M. Jensen, & C. B. Royeen (Eds.), *Educating for moral action: A sourcebook in health and rehabilitation ethics* (pp. 191–202). Philadelphia, PA: F. A. Davis.

Jensen, G. M., & Richert, A. E. (2005). Reflection on the teaching of ethics in physical therapist education: Integrating cases, theory, and learning. *Journal of Physical Therapy Education, 19*(3), 78–85.

Kanny, E. (1993). Core values and attitudes of occupational therapy practice. *American Journal of Occupational Therapy, 47*, 1085–1086.

Kassberg, A. C., & Skar, L. (2008). Ethical dilemmas in rehabilitation: Swedish occupational therapists' perspectives. *Scandinavian Journal of Occupational Therapy, 15*, 204–211.

Kinsella, E. A., Park, A. J., Appiagyei, J., Chang, E., & Chow, D. (2008). Through the eyes of students: Ethical tensions in occupational therapy practice. *Canadian Journal of Occupational Therapy, 75*, 176–183.

Levetown, M. (2008). Communicating with children and families: From everyday interactions to skill in conveying distressing information. *Pediatrics, 121*, 1441–1460.

Mars, G. M. J., Kempen, G., Widdershoven, G., Janssen, P., & van Eijk, J. (2008). Conceptualizing autonomy in the context of chronic physical illness: relating philosophical theories to social scientific perspectives. *Health, 12*, 333–348.

Mattingly, C. (1998). In search of the good: Narrative reasoning in clinical practice. *Medical Anthropology Quarterly, 12*, 273–297.

Maupin, C. R. (1995). The potential for noncaring when dealing with difficult patients: Strategies for making moral decisions. *Journal of Cardiovascular Nursing, 9*, 11–12.

Nash, R. J. (2002). *Real world ethics: Frameworks for educators and human service professionals* (2nd ed.). New York, NY: Teachers College Press.

National Board for Certification of Occupational Therapy. (2010). *About us.* Retrieved from http://www.NBCOT.org

National Commission for the Protection of Human Subjects of Biomedical and Behavioral Research. (1979). *The Belmont report.* Retrieved from http://www.hhs.gov/ ohrp/humansubjects/guidance/belmont.htm

Pellegrino, E. D. (1982). Being ill and being healed: Some reflections on the grounding of medical morality. In V. Kestenbaum (Ed.), *The humanity of the ill: Phenomenological perspectives* (pp. 157–166). Knoxville, TN: University of Tennessee Press.

Pellegrino, E. D. (1995). Toward a virtue-based normative ethics for the health professions. *Kennedy Institute of Ethics Journal, 5*, 253–277.

Pellegrino, E. D. (2002). Professionalism, profession and the virtues of the good physician. *The Mount Sinai Journal of Medicine, 69*, 378–384.

Purtilo, R. (2004). Professional–patient relationship: III. Ethical issues. In S.G. Post (Ed.), *Encyclopedia of Bioethics* (3rd ed., pp. 2150–2158). New York, NY: Macmillan Reference.

Purtilo, R. B., & Doherty, R. F. (2011). *Ethical dimensions in the health professions* (5th ed.). St. Louis, MO: Elsevier Saunders.

Quill, T. E. (2000). Initiating end of life discussions with seriously ill patients: Addressing the "elephant in the room." *Journal of the American Medical Association, 284*, 2502–2507.

Scanlon, C., & Glover, J. (1995). Ethical issues: A professional code of ethics: Providing a moral compass for turbulent times. *Oncology Nursing Forum, 10*, 1515–1521.

Schoeberlein, D., & Sheth, S. (2009). *Mindful teaching and teaching mindfulness.* Boston, MA: Wisdom.

Sisola, S. W. (2000). Moral reasoning as a predictor of clinical practice: The development of physical therapy students across the professional curriculum. *Journal of Physical Therapy Education, 14*(3), 26–34.

Slater, D. Y. (2010). *Reference guide to the occupational therapy code of ethic and ethics standards.* Bethesda, MD: AOTA Press.

Slater, D. Y., & Brandt, L. C. (2011). Combating moral distress. In D. Y. Slater (Ed.), *Reference guide to the occupational therapy code of ethics and ethics standards, 2010 edition* (pp. 107–113). Bethesda, MD: AOTA Press.

Sullivan, W. M., & Rosin, M. S. (2008). *A new agenda for higher education: Shaping a life of the mind for practice.* San Francisco, CA: Jossey-Bass.

Swisher, L., Arslanian, L. E., & Davis, C. M. (2005). The Realm-Individual-Process-Situation (RIPS) model of ethical decision making. *HPA Resource – Official publication of the American Physical Therapy Association Section on Health Policy and Administration, 5*(3), 3–18.

Wells, B. G. (2003). Leadership for ethical decision making. *American journal of Pharmaceutical Education, 67*, 5–8.

For additional resources on the subjects discussed in this chapter, visit http://thePoint.lww.com/Willard-Spackman12e.

CHAPTER 33

Therapeutic Relationship and Client Collaboration

Applying the Intentional Relationship Model

Renée R. Taylor

LEARNING OBJECTIVES

After reading this chapter, you will be able to:

1. Discuss the evidence supporting therapeutic use of self in occupational therapy
2. Describe the components of the Intentional Relationship Model
3. Define and give examples of interpersonal events that can occur during the therapy process
4. Describe the strengths and weaknesses of each of the six interpersonal modes
5. Apply the interpersonal reasoning process, including the six modes to clinical scenarios and case examples

OUTLINE

Introduction: The Nature of the Therapeutic Relationship in Occupational Therapy

Many therapists enter the field of occupational therapy because they anticipate a technically challenging and emotionally fulfilling career of service to individuals with various kinds of illnesses and impairments. What many do not anticipate is that the daily experience of clinical care is often complicated by the anxiety, demoralization, and anger that clients naturally experience as they undergo treatment. Immediately and over time, the impairment experience affects all aspects of life, including daily routines, levels of independence in physical and cognitive functioning, employment, friendships, intimate relationships, parenting, and emotional well-being. During rehabilitation, clients are faced with fatigue, pain, economic expense, loss, and uncertainty about the future. These experiences can lead to feelings of disorientation or confusion, helplessness, isolation, abandonment, stigma, despair, and anxiety even in the highest functioning individuals (Johnson & Webster, 2002; Moorey & Greer, 2002).

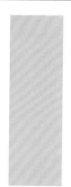

When problems arise, many therapists tend to focus on functional impairments and environmental barriers to the exclusion of the internal psychological and interpersonal aspects. To address these problems, some therapists apply personal intuition, past experience, or other atheoretical, popular psychology strategies. Although some of these strategies may work in the short term, they are insufficient in the face of more complex and intractable interpersonal dynamics. Many therapists tend to view higher level complexities that may emerge during the therapeutic relationship as being outside of their roles, expertise, and scope of practice as occupational therapists. The ***Intentional Relationship Model (IRM)*** seeks to address all of these challenges by providing a concrete skill set and an interpersonal reasoning approach that can guide this understudied yet important area of practice.

Biopsychosocial Issues and Psychiatric Overlay

Beyond the usual range of negative emotions that clients experience lies a level of interpersonal complexity that is introduced by clients with **psychiatric overlay** or coexisting mental health diagnoses. It has been estimated that roughly 15% to 39% of individuals with chronic illness or impairments also have clinically significant psychiatric overlay (Guthrie, 1996). Depending on the diagnosis, psychiatric overlay can introduce a host of challenges to the therapeutic relationship, ranging from behaviors that are often labeled as "noncompliance" or "resistance" to manipulative behaviors or excessive demands on the therapist's time and energy. An individual's personality and premorbid psychological history can play significant roles in adjustment to impairment because the impairment itself inevitably functions as an additional source of stress (S. E. Taylor & Aspinwall, 1990). Those with prior histories of trauma and psychopathology may be more vulnerable to developing an exaggerated emotional response to the impairment or to engaging in maladaptive health behaviors (White, 2001).

A recent study found that therapists reported remarkably high rates of difficult client emotions, behaviors, and interpersonal problems in a predominantly nonpsychiatric sample of occupational therapy clients (R. R. Taylor, Lee, Kielhofner, & Ketkar, 2009). Therapists from a wide range of practice settings and disciplines, treating clients ranging in age from neonates to older adults, found that between 20% and 30% of their clients frequently exhibited behaviors characterized as manipulative, demanding, or dependent. A further 10% to 16% described their clients as frequently hostile, oppositional, resistive, passive, self-denigrating, and unrealistic about treatment or in denial about their impairments. Surprisingly, between 2% and 9% of therapists described their clients as frequently exhibiting hostility, questioning their knowledge or criticizing their approach, uninvested in therapy, resisting feedback and suggestions, and having difficulties with rapport and trust.

From a psychological perspective, it can be argued that all of these behaviors can be attenuated or exacerbated within the therapeutic relationship depending on the experience and skill level of the therapist. Importantly, the way these behaviors are managed (or ignored) within the relationship has lasting consequences for occupational therapy outcomes—both immediately and in the long term.

When these and other psychosocial issues are not adequately addressed in therapy, clients may feel unsupported or alone in the process. Inattention to psychosocial aspects may intensify maladaptive coping or other psychological difficulties that can accompany chronic illness and disability. Additionally, psychosocial issues have been found to affect the cause, course, and prognosis of the chronic illness or impairment itself (S. E. Taylor & Aspinwall, 1990). Any unwitting exacerbation of these issues due to poor or unskilled management of the therapeutic relationship may have a domino effect on the client's physical health and functioning.

Whereas some therapists feel comfortable addressing the challenging client attitudes and behaviors that sometimes manifest within the relationship, many wish they had more information and training. Interestingly, in a survey by R. R. Taylor and colleagues (2009), less than 5% of therapists reported having taken a course solely dedicated to developing skills to enhance the therapeutic relationship during their training to become an occupational therapist. Fewer than 30% felt there was sufficient knowledge about this area in the field of occupational therapy, and only 51% reported feeling adequately trained upon graduating from occupational therapy school (R. R. Taylor et al., 2009). The IRM (R. R. Taylor, 2008) was developed to guide students and therapists in navigating the complex challenges involved in interacting with clients (and particularly those with psychiatric overlay and other psychosocial difficulties). This model will be discussed in detail later in this chapter.

Background and Evidence Base

As a well-established health care discipline, occupational therapy traditionally emphasizes the value and importance of therapists' interactions with their clients. One of the most common terms used to refer to therapist–client interactions is the **therapeutic relationship** (Anderson & Hinojosa, 1984; Cole & McLean, 2003; Eklund, 1996; Rosa & Hasselkus, 1996). Literature and dialogue about the therapeutic relationship commonly address topics such as rapport building, communication, conflict resolution, emotional sharing, collaboration, and partnership between therapists and clients. **Therapeutic use of self** is a popular term used in occupational therapy to refer to the therapists' deliberate efforts to enhance their interactions with clients (Cole & McLean, 2003; Punwar, 2000).

Although there have been varied definitions and emphases on how therapists are expected to optimize their interactions with clients throughout the history of the field, the most widely cited reference describes therapeutic use of self as a therapist's "planned use of his or her personality, insights, perceptions, and judgments as part of the therapeutic process" (American Occupational Therapy Association, 2008; Punwar, 2000, p. 285). Because therapeutic use of self explains how a therapist is expected to reason and behave within the therapeutic relationship, both terms (the broader reference to the relationship, and the more specific reference to what the therapist does within that relationship) will be used to refer to similar ideas and topics throughout this chapter.

Collaboration is a critical element in **client-centered care**. Collaboration refers to the process of mutual participation on the part of client and therapist (Jenkins, Mallett, O'Neill, McFadden, & Baird, 1994). It also includes providing choice, involving clients in decision making, and encouraging clients to actively contribute and to set their own goals for therapy (Kielhofner, 2009; Palmadottir, 2006) Theoretically, all of this should occur within the context of an egalitarian relationship (Norrby & Bellner, 1995). One of the primary approaches to collaboration involves educating clients about all aspects of the treatment process and providing them with information about the purpose and relevance of any procedure or treatment approach. Providing a rationale at each session increases the likelihood of client involvement in therapy (Peloquin, 1988).

Relative to the vast conceptual literature on this topic, a smaller number of empirical studies have focused on examining the role of the therapeutic relationship, collaboration, or aspects of therapeutic use of self in occupational therapy. One study specifically examined the interpersonal strategies that occupational therapists use to respond to clients' interpersonal needs and characteristics (R. R. Taylor, Lee, & Kielhofner, 2011). Findings from 563 practitioners revealed that therapists most preferred to encourage their clients by reminding them of their strengths, providing positive reinforcement, and by instilling hope and confidence. The second most preferred approach involved collaborating with clients by encouraging them to make more decisions during the therapy process, by supporting their perspectives, by gathering feedback from the client before selecting or recommending an activity, and by asking the client to recommend his or her own goals for therapy. Other approaches involving problem solving, empathizing, and instructing clients were less frequently used. Interestingly, these findings did not differ based on the age group of the clients being treated.

In a Swedish study, Eklund and Hallberg (2001) investigated the extent of use of verbal communication during occupational therapy in a psychiatric setting. In a sample of 292 occupational therapists, verbal interaction was used during assessment, intervention, treatment planning, and posttreatment evaluation. Verbal communication was deemed a significant component of the therapeutic relationship. Findings emphasized the need to study and develop the verbal as well as the doing aspect of occupational therapy.

Cole and McLean (2003) conducted another survey study that focused on approaches to communication among 129 practicing occupational therapists from various practice areas. They found that therapists strongly emphasized rapport, open communication, and empathy as important roles in the therapist/patient relationship. They also found that therapists perceived the therapeutic relationship as critical to therapy outcomes.

In a qualitative study that used focus groups as the main data source, Allison and Strong (1994) examined the use of verbal interaction among 23 occupational therapists in an adult general rehabilitation setting. They concluded that good clinical communicators accommodated their interactions to clients' needs. Similarly, Jenkins et al. (1994) systematically observed the communication patterns of eight practitioners in a geriatric setting. Therapists with more experience achieved more mutual participation in the therapy process than those with less experience.

Palmadottir's (2006) qualitative study (as cited in R. R. Taylor et al., 2009) explored adult clients' perceptions of the therapy relationship in a rehabilitation setting. Based on interviews with 20 adult clients, she recommended the following: Therapists needed to pay more attention to their clients' occupational issues and needs, involve them more in a goal-directed therapy process, and have more awareness of how their own attitudes are communicated and acted out in therapy.

Rosa and Hasselkaus (1996) interviewed 83 occupational therapists who were practicing nationwide. Their qualitative analysis concluded that therapists' personal identities seemed to be merged with their professional identities. They concluded that it is important to have a sense of "connecting" with clients in terms of helping and caring.

Guidetti and Tham (2002; as cited in R. R. Taylor et al., 2009) interviewed 12 occupational therapy practitioners who worked on self-care training with clients with either stroke or spinal cord injury. Their study identified interpersonal strategies used by practitioners. They included relationship-building, trust, motivating clients, and providing an enabling occupational experience.

Eklund (1996) investigated whether the therapeutic relationship was related to outcomes in mental health practice. In an observational study of 20 patients and 5 occupational therapists, she found that both therapists and clients perceived their working relationship as good. Although, no consistent relationships with outcomes were found using a measure of the quality of the working relationship, both clients' and therapists' perceptions of the extent of client participation in the treatment process were related to outcomes.

These studies form a beginning knowledge base concerning current attitudes and behaviors that comprise the therapeutic relationship in occupational therapy. They provide preliminary evidence to suggest that a wide range of interpersonal skills are necessary to sustain a productive therapeutic relationship. There is a clear need for increased self awareness, empathy, and power-sharing within the therapeutic relationship. Moreover, confidence, self-awareness, and an orientation toward the client's intepersonal needs may lead to improved therapeutic outcomes.

The Intentional Relationship Model

Today's practice environment requires a therapist to skillfully navigate a client's interpersonal challenges while simultaneously facilitating occupational engagement (R. R. Taylor, 2008). The IRM provides a practical skill set and an interpersonal reasoning approach that presents different approaches to communication that are necessary to sustain a positive working relationship with a client. According to IRM, it is the therapist's responsibility to work to develop a predictable and trusting relationship with the client irrespective of any interpersonal difficulties or misgivings that the client may bring into the therapy process (R. R. Taylor, 2008). This does not assume that the therapist will always be successful at building such a relationship. However, it does assume the therapist recognizes it is his or her responsibility to establish and maintain this relationship.

The IRM focuses on four main components of the therapist–client relationship. These include the client, the interpersonal events that occur during therapy, the therapist's use of self, and the occupation. The IRM asks therapists to observe and understand their clients from an interpersonal perspective, to be prepared to respond therapeutically to rifts and other significant interpersonal events, and to communicate within a **mode** that matches the client's interpersonal needs of the moment (R. R. Taylor, 2008). This model, which is diagramed in Figure 33.1, provides a theoretical framework for attempting to understand the meaning of the communication and interpersonal behavior that occurs during therapy. It also provides guidance about how to therapeutically respond in a manner that best serves the client. Each of the central components of the model will be described in the following pages, and more extensive information is presented in Taylor.

Client Interpersonal Characteristics

Individuals react to chronic conditions with tremendous variability. Recognizing and responding appropriately to psychological heterogeneity within and between clients is vital to a successful therapy outcome. Fear, anxiety, sadness, hopelessness, anger, and rage are inevitable emotions that any client with a chronic condition faces during the course of his or her experience. However, the duration and degree to which these emotions become entrenched and affect overall psychological, interpersonal, occupational, and health-related behavior and functioning varies considerably within and between individuals. For example, studies have shown that individuals with the same chronic condition can vary widely in terms of psychological response (Bombardier, D'Amico, & Jordan, 1990; Lacroix, Martin, Avendano, & Goldstein, 1991). Beck (1996) has acknowledged that there is a significant diversity in terms of the intensity of individuals' reactions to specific life circumstances over time, and there is also variation in terms of individuals' non-pathological psychological reactions to life events.

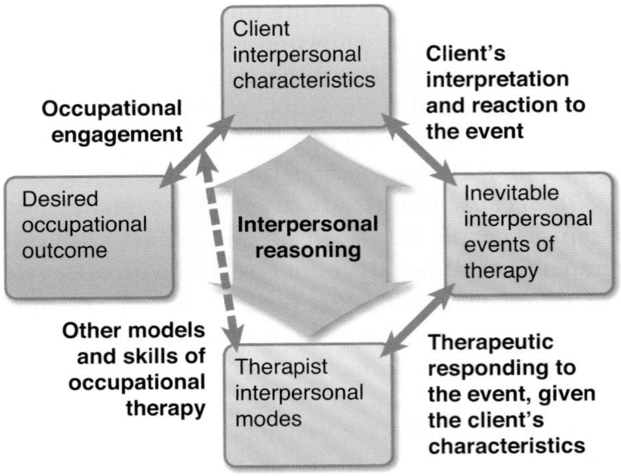

FIGURE 33.1 A Model of the Intentional Relationship in Occupational Therapy

For these reasons, the IRM emphasizes the need for every therapist to gain an understanding of each client's interpersonal characteristics. This is typically accomplished by maintaining a mental (or written, if first beginning) list of features of a client's personality that represent strengths and weaknesses. For example, if a client has a heightened need for control, this will become clear the moment he or she asks what seems to be an unnecessary question for the third time. A client's reluctance to engage in an activity may become apparent when he or she appears not to have heard a given instruction. One quickly learns of a client's limited capacity to assert his or her needs when he or she is found lying on a mat without a means to get up, not having asked anyone for help. Although these are common characteristics of clients in everyday practice, they are not traditionally discussed as fundamental aspects of occupational therapy care plans or documented in a client's chart notes. Understanding the more challenging aspects of a client's interpersonal characteristics from an objective but empathic perspective will assist a therapist to act in a way that is intentional and facilitating of occupational engagement.

TABLE 33.1 Client Interpersonal Characteristics

Interpersonal Characteristic	Practice Example
Communication style	Ana is a reluctant communicator. She tends to be quiet during therapy and only provides information when responding to a question. This makes it difficult for the therapist to read and understand her needs and it limits the spontaneity of the interaction. This style causes the therapist to over-function by asking Ana more questions than she would otherwise ask a client during therapy. This style was present from the first moment of therapy and has not changed.
Capacity for trust	Ana has a low capacity for trust. She demonstrates hesitancy in attempting new activities despite encouragement. She recoils from eye contact and does not look at the therapist often. She is guarded and will not share her thoughts, feelings, and reactions with the therapist.
Need for control	Ana is highly passive during therapy and has a low need for control. She is cooperative, but the therapist is unable to read what activities are more or less important and enjoyable for her. She appears to respond to every activity, particularly new ones, in the same hesitant but compliant manner.
Capacity to assert needs	Ana lacks the capacity to assert her needs in therapy. On one occasion, she wore her splint for a longer period than necessary because a fieldwork student had forgotten to have her take it off. Ana did not seem to care or react, despite any inconvenience or discomfort associated with wearing the splint.
Response to change and challenge	Unable to locate a regularly used paring knife for a baking activity, Ana gives up early and waits for the therapist to take control. When prompted to come up with an alternative solution, Ana remains puzzled and frozen.
Affect	Ana's affect vacillates between being flat and showing a slightly sad facial expression. In response to praise, she is either indifferent or displays a weak and almost pleading type of smile.
Predisposition to giving feedback	Ana never provides the therapist with unsolicited feedback about her experience in therapy. When the therapist asks for feedback, she frequently responds that everything is "fine" or weakly says "I'm good."
Capacity to receive feedback	Ana responds well, almost robotically, to corrective feedback. She occasionally offers a weak smile but is generally indifferent to praise or reinforcement.
Response to human diversity	Ana does seem to show slightly more interest and enthusiasm when working with the physical therapist who is a male. Her occupational therapist is a female. It is not clear why this is the case.
Orientation toward relating	Ana shows a need to remain safely distant from the therapist and all others on the unit. She is unwilling to disclose information, including even superficial thoughts, feelings, and reactions in the moment. She appears indifferent to any personal disclosures or expressions of empathy made by the therapist and recoils from eye contact.
Preference for touch	Ana never initiates touch but does not flinch when the therapist does. At this time, it is unclear what Ana's preference for touch is, so the therapist tends to limit touch to that which is necessary to complete the more impairment-focused tasks of therapy.
Capacity for reciprocity	Ana does not appear interested in the therapist as a person and does not show any appreciation of therapy or expressions of gratitude. This appears consistent with her reactions to other providers on the unit.

IRM defines the essential interpersonal characteristics of a client in terms of 12 categories, presented in Table 33.1.

Communication style refers to a client's ability to communicate in a clear, well-paced, and detailed yet succinct manner that is appropriate to his or her developmental level and cognitive ability. Reticence to communicate or, by contrast, excessive loquaciousness, will undoubtedly affect the therapeutic dynamic and the quality of occupational engagement that might otherwise be possible to achieve. Therefore, the IRM calls for therapists to consider communication difficulties such as these in building the therapeutic alliance, selecting an approach to communication, and ultimately, in establishing the occupational therapy care plan. The same approach applies to the remaining categories of **client characteristics.** ***Capacity for trust*** refers to a client's ability to trust that the therapist has his or her best interests in mind and that every effort will be made to ensure his or her physical safety and emotional well-being.

Need for control is defined as the degree to which a client takes an active versus passive role within the relationship and in determining the course of therapy. ***Capacity to assert needs*** defines a client's approach to expressing his or her wishes and needs for support, information, resources, or other requests within the therapeutic relationship. **Response to change and challenge** refers to a client's ability to adapt to changes in the therapy plan or environment and his or her approach to occupational therapy tasks and situations that are new or challenging. **Affect** is defined as a client's general emotional expression during therapy, ranging from appropriately buoyant for the situation (flexible) to flat (absence of expression) to heightened (intensely emotional) to labile (fluctuating anywhere between elation, anger, angst, and despair). **Predisposition to giving feedback** involves a client's ability to provide the therapist with appropriate negative or positive comments about his or her reactions to the therapist and experience of therapy as either helpful or unhelpful. ***Capacity to receive feedback*** describes a client's ability to maintain perspective when receiving praise from the therapist or when receiving correction during performance, limits on behavior, or information about his or her strengths and weaknesses.

Response to human diversity is defined by a client's reaction to ways in which he or she may be the same or different from the therapist in terms of observable sociodemographic characteristics (e.g., race, ethnicity, gender, age) and other interpretations of outward appearance or perceived worldview. Some clients have more difficulty than others relating to a therapist whom they perceive as differing from them in fundamental ways. **Orientation toward relating** defines a client's need for interpersonal closeness versus professional distance within the therapeutic relationship. Difficulties may occur when the client's expectations about the relationship differ from those of the therapist. **Preference for touch** involves a client's observed comfort or discomfort with or expressed reaction to any type of physical touch, whether it be a necessary part of treatment or an expression of caring. ***Capacity for reciprocity*** refers to a client's ability to engage fully in the therapy process and/or show appreciation toward the therapist as a separate but connected partner within the therapy process. Some clients may be so focused on their own situations that they may lack this capacity, whereas others may function in an active and mutual way within the relationship. Regardless of the outcome, a client's capacity for reciprocity is always felt by the therapist and must be managed accordingly.

In summary, understanding client interpersonal characteristics is fundamental to planning how to respond during therapeutic interactions. This becomes particularly important when clients present with more difficult or challenging interpersonal characteristics or when a therapist has a negative or apprehensive feeling about a client's personality. An extensive discussion of client characteristics may be found in R. R. Taylor (2008).

The Inevitable Interpersonal Events of Therapy

Similar to client characteristics, uncomfortable or emotionally laden situations that occur during therapy are a normal part of everyday practice for the experienced therapist. However, knowing how to anticipate and respond to them in a deliberate and therapeutic way is not necessarily an assumed, universal skill. According to IRM, an **interpersonal event** is a naturally occurring communication, reaction, process, task, or general circumstance that occurs during therapy and that has the potential to fortify or weaken the therapeutic relationship, depending on how it is handled (R. R. Taylor, 2008). The 11 categories of interpersonal events, their definitions, and practice examples are presented in Table 33.2.

When interpersonal events occur, their interpretation by the client is a product of the client's unique set of interpersonal characteristics and mood. Sometimes the event may have a significant effect upon the client, and other times a client will be unaffected or minimally affected. When such events occur, it is important that the therapist be aware that the event has occurred and take responsibility for assessing the client's response and responding appropriately. According to R. R. Taylor (2008), interpersonal events are inevitable during the course of therapy and ripe with both threat and opportunity. Similar to our everyday relationships with coworkers, friends, and loved ones, when something significant happens, how we respond to that event typically has a lasting impact on that relationship. Interpersonal events are part of the constant give and take that occurs during therapy. If these events go unnoticed, are deliberately ignored, or are responded to without intentionality, these events can threaten both the therapeutic relationship and the client's occupational engagement. When optimally responded to, these events can provide opportunities for positive client learning or change and for solidifying the therapeutic relationship. Because they are unavoidable in any therapeutic interaction, one of the primary tasks of a therapist is to respond to these inevitable events in a way that leads to repair and strengthening of the therapeutic relationship (R. R. Taylor, 2008).

The Therapist's Use of Self: The Six Modes

According to IRM, effective use of self requires therapists to recognize and cultivate strengths within their personalities and develop less used aspects of their personalities

TABLE 33.2 The Inevitable Interpersonal Events of Occupational Therapy

Interpersonal Event	Definition	Practice Example
Expression of strong emotion	Observable manifestations of internal feelings that occur with a higher-than-usual level of intensity given a client's cultural context and norms. Can be positive or negative expressions.	Carl, a client in the neurosurgical intensive care unit, is justifiably angry because he is uncomfortable and the nursing staff is not responding to his calls. He proceeds to rip the vital sign monitors off his body so that a distress signal will be emitted and he will receive care.
Intimate self-disclosures	Statements or stories that reveal something personal or sensitive about the person making a disclosure. These can be stories about oneself or about close others.	During inpatient rehabilitation, Carl confides in the therapist that he intends to continue smoking when he returns home, despite what his wife will think or do about it.
Power dilemmas	Feelings of stress or conflict that emerge when the client and therapist disagree about something. Power dilemmas can manifest overtly or covertly during therapy. They are more likely to occur when clients feel a lack or loss of control over their lives (which is a common feeling when undergoing rehabilitation).	Carl decides that he does not want to clean up the sawdust and woodworking tools after a therapy activity. Instead, he stands and watches while the therapist does it. The same behavior repeats itself during the following session. When the therapist says something about it, Carl tells her that he is the one paying her bill.
Nonverbal cues	Communications that do not involve the use of formal language. Some examples of these are facial expressions, movement patterns, body posture, and eye contact.	Carl stares at the therapist with anger in his eyes when he feels that a therapy task is pointless or undesirable.
Crisis points	Unanticipated, stressful events that cause clients to become absent or distracted from therapy. Examples include major weather disasters, a change in the client's health status, or an emergency involving a client's family member.	Carl collapses and experiences an unanticipated grand mal seizure while attempting to walk to the therapy room with the therapist.
Resistance and reluctance	Resistance is a client's passive or active refusal to participate in some or all aspects of therapy for reasons linked to the therapeutic relationship (e.g., unexpressed anger toward the therapist or situation). Reluctance is disinclination toward some aspect of therapy for reasons outside the therapeutic relationship, such as client anxiety about task difficulty or other concerns about performance.	Carl ignores the therapist's directions when he does not want to engage in a task or activity.
Boundary testing	A client behavior that violates or asks the therapist to disclose something or act in ways that the therapist is not comfortable with or that are outside the definition of a professional relationship.	At the beginning of therapy, Carl asks the therapist a series of questions about her educational and employment history as well as what her qualifications are to treat him. Although these questions are within the parameters of the therapeutic relationship, they cause the therapist to feel that Carl has prejudices about her competence as a professional.
Empathic breaks	Any action initiated by the therapist, or something a therapist fails to notice or acknowledge, that results in a client feeling disappointed, disillusioned, insignificant, or emotionally injured.	Carl asks the therapist to compare his progress with others with the same diagnosis, and the therapist tells him that she feels his progress would improve if he exerted more effort during sessions. Carl's facial expression appears deflated.
Emotionally charged therapy tasks and situations	Activities or circumstances that the client feels strongly about due to a past experience, a high level of value for the activity, or due to something embarrassing about the activity.	During a physically challenging activity, Carl experiences increased oral secretions that he is unable to control. He immediately discontinues the activity with a shameful look on his face.
Limitations of therapy	Restrictions on the available or possible services, time, resources, or nature of the desired relationship with the therapist.	Close to the time of discharge, Carl and the therapist review his accomplishments in therapy and his goals for the future. Carl asks the therapist if he could pay her out-of-pocket to continue home visits with him. The therapist informs Carl that she already works a 60-h workweek and that she does not have the time to honor his request.
Contextual inconsistencies	Any aspect of a client's interpersonal or physical environment that changes during the course of therapy.	When Carl is moved from intensive care into the step-down neurorehabilitation unit, he is initially nervous because of the decreased intensity of services provided.

TABLE 33.3 The Six Therapeutic Modes

Mode	Definition	Practice Example
Advocating	Ensuring that the client's rights are enforced and resources are secured. May require the therapist to serve as a mediator, facilitator, negotiator, enforcer, or other type of advocate with external persons and agencies.	Upon discharge, the occupational therapist discusses with Carl's wife the possibilities of continuing to work on established goals for therapy and educates her on how she can support and encourage his continued efforts toward those goals.
Collaborating	Expecting the client to be an active and equal participant in therapy. Ensuring choice, freedom, and autonomy to the greatest extent possible.	The therapist shows respect and value for Carl's knowledge about his own medical condition and often asks him to provide his perspective regarding the objectives and tasks of therapy.
Empathizing	Ongoing striving to understand the client's thoughts, feelings, and behaviors while suspending any judgment. Ensuring that the client verifies and experiences the therapist's understanding as truthful and validating.	When Carl shares how he ripped the leads off his chest to attract the attention of the nursing staff when in pain during the night, the therapist summarizes and validates his feelings of desperation and anger in attempting to communicate and express his needs to staff.
Encouraging	Seizing the opportunity to instill hope in a client. Celebrating a client's thinking or behavior through positive reinforcement. Conveying an attitude of joyfulness, playfulness, and confidence.	When working in the kitchen, the therapist often jokes with Carl that he can cook better than she does. Carl appears to enjoy this banter.
Instructing	Carefully structuring therapy activities and being explicit with clients about the plan, sequence, and events of therapy. Providing clear instruction and feedback about performance. Setting limits on a client's requests or behavior.	The therapist typically prepares on certain evenings before sessions with Carl if she knows that they will be discussing some of his questions about assistive technologies or his functioning at work. During therapy, the therapist often cites empirical evidence and provides information about these technologies.
Problem solving	Facilitating pragmatic thinking and solving dilemmas by outlining choices, posing strategic questions, and providing opportunities for comparative or analytical thinking.	When Carl presents the therapist with complex questions for which there are no right or wrong answers, the therapist often responds by asking him for his opinion or by helping him create a list of options and weigh pros and cons.

through honest appraisal of the effects of their behavior on clients (R. R. Taylor, 2008). The first step in accomplishing this is through an understanding of the six therapist interpersonal modes. A **therapeutic mode** is a specific way of relating to a client. The IRM identifies six therapeutic modes:

1. **Advocating**
2. **Collaborating**
3. **Empathizing**
4. **Encouraging**
5. **Instructing**
6. **Problem solving**

A brief definition of each mode and an example of its use in a therapy situation is provided in Table 33.3.

Therapists naturally use therapeutic modes that are consistent with their fundamental personality characteristics. For example, a person who feels most confident and comfortable with others when teaching and sharing information with them would likely use instructing as a primary therapeutic mode in therapy. Therapists vary widely in terms of the range and flexibility with which they use modes in relating to clients. Some therapists relate to clients in one or two primary ways, whereas others draw upon multiple therapeutic modes depending upon the interpersonal characteristics of the client and the situation, or inevitable interpersonal events, at hand. One of the goals in using IRM is to become increasingly comfortable using any of six of the modes flexibly and interchangeably depending upon the client's needs. A therapeutic mode or set of modes define a therapist's general **interpersonal style** when interacting with a client. Therapists able to use all six of the modes flexibly and comfortably and match those modes to the client and the situation are described as having a **multimodal** interpersonal style.

According to the IRM, a therapist's choice and application of a particular therapeutic mode or set of modes should depend largely on the interpersonal characteristics of the client and his or her reaction to any

TABLE 33.4 The Six Steps of the Interpersonal Reasoning Process

Step of Interpersonal Reasoning	Definition
1. Anticipate	Based on your observations, information from others who have had experience with the client, and any experience you have had with the client, anticipate the likely interpersonal events that may occur during therapy and the modes that might work best. If you have met the client previously, be certain to incorporate your knowledge of the client's interpersonal characteristics in predicting events that might occur and modes that might work best.
2. Identify and cope	Use Intentional Relationship Model language to label a difficult client characteristic or interpersonal event when it occurs. Do what it takes to collect yourself and get emotional perspective on the situation. Remind yourself not to take it personally.
3. Determine if a mode shift is required	Ask yourself the following questions to determine whether a mode shift is required: What mode am I currently using with this client, if any? What are the effects of the mode on the client? Would another mode better serve the interpersonal needs of this client at this moment?
4. Choose a response mode or mode sequence	Interact within the mode or modes that you think the client prefers/needs at this moment. Think about a sequence of modes that you might use to accommodate changes in what the client might need from moment to moment.
5. Draw upon any relevant interpersonal skills associated with the mode(s)	Think about other communication, rapport building, and/or conflict resolution skills that you might draw upon in association with your mode use.
6. Gather feedback	Gather nonverbal or verbal feedback from the client as to whether or not he or she feels comfortable with the way you approached the event or difficulty.

interpersonal events that may be occurring. Although a client may prefer that the therapist use one or two central modes, certain interpersonal events in therapy may call for a mode shift. A **mode shift** is a conscious change in one's way of relating to a client.

For example, if a client perceives a therapist's attempts at problem solving to be insensitive or off the mark, a therapist would be wise to switch from the **problem solving mode** to an ***empathizing mode*** so that he or she can get a better understanding of the client's reaction and the root of the dilemma. An **interpersonal reasoning** process, described in the following section, can be used to guide the therapist in deciding when a mode shift might be required and determining which alternative mode to select. Because the interpersonal aspects of occupational therapy practice are complex and require a therapist to possess a highly adaptive therapeutic personality, the intentional relationship model recommends that therapists learn to draw upon all six of the therapeutic modes in a flexible manner according to the different interpersonal needs of each client and the unique demands of each clinical situation. See the Case Study for an example of how the interpersonal reasoning process and the six modes may be used during occupational therapy.

Interpersonal Reasoning

According to IRM, an important competency to develop as a therapist is the capacity to engage in an ongoing interpersonal reasoning process during therapy. This is particularly important when an interpersonal dilemma presents itself in therapy. Interpersonal reasoning is a step-wise process by which a therapist decides what to say, do, or express in reaction to a client's interpersonal characteristics or behavior. It includes developing a mental vigilance toward the interpersonal aspects of therapy in anticipation that a dilemma might occur and a means of reviewing and evaluating options for responding. The six steps of interpersonal reasoning and their definitions are presented in Table 33.4. An extensive description and discussion of these steps can be found in R. R. Taylor (2008). The following case study is a partially fictionalized extraction from an actual consultation provided to an occupational therapist by the author. Demographic information of the client has been changed to protect the client's anonymity.

Conclusion

In this chapter, we reviewed evidence that supports therapeutic use of self in occupational therapy. We learned about the field's emphasis on collaboration and about how the IRM can support that emphasis. The IRM is a conceptual practice model that explains how therapists can apply an interpersonal reasoning process to understand and respond supportively to clients in difficult or awkward moments. The model requires therapists to take responsibility for the emotional well-being of their clients during the therapy interaction by understanding the client's unique interpersonal characteristics and adjusting their therapeutic personalities accordingly. The model articulates six therapist interpersonal modes that represent different facets of the therapeutic personality. Learning how to change those modes depending on each individual client's needs is a dynamic, lifelong process. Occupational therapists should strive to understand each client interpersonally, putting one's personal and emotional reactions to clients to productive use without prejudice or judgment.

CASE STUDY 33.1 Cynthia: A Woman with a Rotator Cuff Injury and Comorbid Posttraumatic Stress Disorder

Cynthia is a 26-year-old woman who recently graduated with an associate degree to become a small-animal veterinary technician. She moved to Chicago from Madison, Wisconsin, where she had grown up and attended school. She is new to the large, fast-paced, and sometimes dangerous lifestyle of urban Chicago. On the way to take her certification exam for licensure, she was physically assaulted by an adolescent male on a metro platform in return for her wallet, ID card holder, and cell phone. In an attempt to keep her items, she engaged in a physical battle with the assailant and experienced facial abrasions, tooth breakage, and a complete rotator cuff injury requiring surgical repair. She presented to occupational therapy in the outpatient rehabilitation unit to address her shoulder issues. A review of her records revealed the presence of psychiatric overlay involving symptoms of posttraumatic stress disorder (PTSD).

Applying principles of Intentional Relationship Model (IRM) (R.R. Taylor, 2008), the treating occupational therapist immediately began the process of interpersonal reasoning before meeting with the client. Applying her knowledge of PTSD from a prior fieldwork experience, she reviewed its primary symptoms by referencing the *Diagnostic and Statistical Manual of Mental Disorders* and discussed typical features of the diagnosis during a brief consultation with a psychiatry resident in the cafeteria. Knowing that Cynthia is new to Chicago, likes animals, and engaged physically with her assailant gave her some preliminary data to anticipate the interpersonal events that might occur during therapy and some of the client interpersonal characteristics that might become important to watch in Cynthia's case.

In terms of client characteristics, the therapist prepared herself to assess Cynthia's need for control because she may have feelings of lost control due to the assault. For example, Cynthia may feel out of control when experiencing PTSD symptoms such as flashbacks and visceral reexperiencing of sights, sounds, smells, and sensations that trigger memories of the trauma. She may react to these feelings by exhibiting an abnormally high or abnormally low need for control during the therapy process. A second important characteristic to watch would be Cynthia's affect and how it may change in response to the different demands and activities of therapy, particularly when certain practices might induce pain or discomfort. A third important characteristic to watch for would be Cynthia's preference for touch, because individuals with PTSD tend to be hypervigilant and have an exaggerated startle response if approached unexpectedly.

With respect to inevitable interpersonal events, it would be important to look for power dilemmas to occur, particularly if Cynthia exhibits a high need for control during therapy. Additionally, it would be important to watch for nonverbal cues signaling her discomfort with aspects of the therapy process. Finally, it would be important to anticipate therapy tasks or recommendations that might be emotionally charged for Cynthia, such as those involving using public transportation within the city of Chicago or those involving work with or care for animals, because animals appear to be important in her life.

During her consultation with Cynthia, many of the therapist's hypotheses about the interpersonal characteristics and events were confirmed. The therapist experienced Cynthia as a self-assured but traumatized young woman who had a fair amount of medical knowledge and a high need to express her knowledge and make decisions during therapy. The therapist deliberately avoided potential power dilemmas with Cynthia by selecting the ***collaborating mode*** as her primary mode, followed by the **instructing mode** when Cynthia's affect appeared anxious. The problem-solving mode was used when other nonverbal cues indicated that she was irritable and insecure.

The therapist was very careful to forewarn Cynthia each time she needed to help her partially disrobe and touch her shoulder. Each time, she was careful to use the instructing mode to explain the nature of the touch and why it was required to range, manipulate, or otherwise touch her shoulder in that particular way. When Cynthia's nonverbal cues and affect indicated that she was anticipating or experiencing discomfort, the therapist relied upon the empathizing mode to validate Cynthia's reactions. Using the instructing mode, the therapist also mentioned to Cynthia that sometimes touch can trigger symptoms of PTSD, and if that was the case, to be sure to let her know so that she can stop and be of support to her.

Although brief, what could have been an uncomfortable therapy process was optimized by the therapist's application of the interpersonal reasoning process to anticipate, select, and shift modes according to Cynthia's needs.

Now that you have read the case study and basic overview of the IRM, review the practice dilemma and questions. Can you see differences between the way the therapist managed the interpersonal dynamics with Cynthia versus the way she managed them with George? (See the Practice Dilemma.)

Practice Dilemma

Gayle and George

George is a 54-year-old biomedical engineer who endured a mild traumatic brain injury and several bone fractures from a motor scooter accident. Following surgery on his pelvis, he was referred to Gayle, a newly licensed occupational therapist working in the inpatient rehabilitation unit of a major metropolitan teaching hospital. In passing, a nurse from the acute care unit informed Gayle that George has been causing a lot of disruption on the unit. He had made a series of complaints to the head of nursing about the lack of timeliness and intensity of his nursing care. Additionally, he had made excessive demands for incidental items such as specific newspapers and brand name toiletries that the hospital does not routinely provide.

Having graduated from occupational therapy school with a high grade point average and an award for her outstanding performance in fieldwork, Gayle was not deterred by this information. Instead, she was determined to do everything she could to ensure that George was satisfied with the quality of care that she would provide him in therapy. Because she knew that George was highly educated and of high income, she decided to begin therapy by giving her best explanation of what occupational therapy is and by asking him what his goals were. In her mind, she thought she was taking a client-centered approach. She was immediately disillusioned by his condescending tone of voice and sarcastic response: "My goal is to make sure my Vespa is salvageable and to be back on the road as soon as possible."

In an equally sarcastic tone, she immediately reacted by asking him if he planned to wear a helmet this time. She thought maybe he would find the comment humorous and that it might break the ice. Instead, the remainder of the session was occupied an air of tension. Gayle initiated passive range of motion exercises and made numerous futile attempts to make conversation by asking George about his job and hobbies.

Following the session, George contacted the director of services at the hospital to file a complaint about Gayle. He reported that her attitude was arrogant and unprofessional during the session and that he felt she did not have the experience or maturity required to be of any help to him. He requested to be seen by a different therapist in the future. Upon hearing this news from her supervisor, Gayle was devastated and could figure out what she could have done differently with this challenging client.

Questions

After introducing herself and describing occupational therapy, which of the six modes did Gayle use to begin the session? Was this mode successful with George? Why or why not?

1. Did an empathic break occur during the session?
2. Is there anything that Gayle could have done differently during the session to prevent the complaint that George made about her?

References

Allison, H., & Strong, J. (1994). Verbal strategies used by occupational therapists in direct client encounters. *Occupational Therapy Journal of Research, 14*, 112–129.

American Occupational Therapy Association. (2008). Occupational therapy practice framework: Domain and process, 2nd edition. *American Journal of Occupational Therapy, 62*, 625–683.

Anderson, J., & Hinojosa, J. (1984). Parents and therapists in a professional partnership. *American Journal of Occupational Therapy, 38*, 452–461.

Beck, A. T. (1996). Beyond belief: A theory of modes, personality, and psychopathology. In P. M. Salkovskis (Ed.), *Frontiers of cognitive therapy* (pp. 1–25). New York, NY: Guilford Press.

Bombardier, C. H., D'Amico, C., & Jordan, J. S. (1990). The relationship of appraisal and coping to chronic illness adjustment. *Behavior Research and Therapy, 28*, 297–304.

Cole, M. B., & McLean, V. (2003). Therapeutic relationships re-defined. *Occupational Therapy in Mental Health, 19*, 33–56.

Eklund, M. (1996). Working relationship, participation and outcome in a psychiatric day care unit based on occupational therapy. *Scandinavian Journal of Occupational Therapy, 3*, 106–113.

Eklund, M., & Hallberg, I. R. (2001). Psychiatric occupational therapists' verbal interaction with their clients. *Occupational Therapy International, 8*, 1–16.

Guidetti, S., & Tham, K. (2002). Therapeutic strategies used by occupational therapists in self-care training: A qualitative study. *Occupational Therapy International, 9*, 257–276.

Guthrie, E. (1996). Emotional disorder in chronic illness: Psychotherapeutic interventions. *British Journal of Psychiatry, 168*, 265–273.

Jenkins, M., Mallett, J., O'Neill, C., McFadden, M., & Baird, H. (1994). Insights into "practice" communication: An interactional approach. *British Journal of Occupational Therapy, 57*, 297–302.

Johnson, C., & Webster, D. (2002). *Recrafting a life: Solutions for chronic pain and illness.* New York, NY: Psychology Press.

Kielhofner, G. (2009). *Conceptual Foundations of Occupational Therapy* (4th ed.). Philadelphia, PA: F.A. Davis.

Lacroix, J. M., Martin, B., Avendano, M., & Goldstein, R. (1991). Symptom schema in chronic respiratory patients. *Health Psychology, 10*, 268–273.

Moorey, S., & Greer, S. (2002). *Cognitive behaviour therapy for people with cancer.* Oxford, United Kingdom: Oxford University Press.

Norrby, E., & Bellner, A. L. (1995). The helping encounter–Occupational therapists' perception of therapeutic relationships. *Scandinavian Journal of Caring Science, 9*, 41–46.

Palmadottir, G. (2006). Client-therapist relationships: Experiences of occupational therapy clients in rehabilitation. *British Journal of Occupational Therapy, 69*, 394–401.

Peloquin, S. M. (1988). Linking purpose to procedure during interactions with patients. *American Journal of Occupational Therapy, 42*, 775–781.

Punwar, A. J. (2000). The art and science of practice. In A. J. Punwar & S. Peloquin (Eds.), *Occupational therapy: Principles and practice* (3rd ed.). Philadelphia, PA: Lippincott Williams & Wilkins.

Rosa, S. A., & Hasselkus, B. R. (1996). Connecting with patients: The personal experience of professional helping. *Occupational Therapy Journal of Research, 16*, 245–260.

Taylor, R. R. (2008). *The intentional relationship: Occupational therapy and use of self.* Philadelphia, PA: F. A. Davis.

Taylor, R. R., Lee, S. W., & Kielhofner, G. (2011). Practitioners' use of interpersonal modes within the therapeutic relationship: Results from a nationwide study. *OTJR: Occupation, Participation and Health, 31*, 6–14.

Taylor, R. R., Lee, S. W., Kielhofner, G., & Ketkar, M. (2009). Therapeutic use of self: A nationwide survey of practitioners' attitudes and experiences. *American Journal of Occupational Therapy, 63*, 198–207.

Taylor, S. E., & Aspinwall, L. G. (1990). Psychosocial aspects of chronic illness. In P. T. Costa & G. R. Vanden Bos (Eds.), *Psychosocial aspects of serious illness: Chronic conditions, fatal diseases, and clinical care. Master lectures in psychology* (pp. 3–60). Washington, DC: American Psychological Association.

White, C. A. (2001). *Cognitive behaviour therapy for chronic medical problems: A guide to assessment and treatment in practice.* West Sussex, United Kingdom: John Wiley & Sons.

For additional resources on the subjects discussed in this chapter, visit http://thePoint.lww.com/Willard-Spackman12e.

CHAPTER 34

Group Process and Group Intervention

Marjorie E. Scaffa

LEARNING OBJECTIVES

After reading this chapter, you will be able to:

1. Appreciate the complexity and value of small groups in occupational therapy
2. Understand factors influencing group process dynamics
3. Discuss the characteristics of effective group leadership
4. Describe various types of occupational therapy intervention groups
5. Identify the basic components of a group intervention protocol
6. Identify group members' behaviors that indicate occupational performance deficits

OUTLINE

Introduction

A **group** is an aggregate of people who share a common purpose that can only be achieved through collaboration. Groups are organized systems of interrelated, interactive, and interdependent individuals. Occupational therapists provide intervention in groups in various settings, including schools, hospitals, skilled nursing facilities, psychiatric services, day care programs, independent living centers, and community social service agencies, to name a few. The age range of members of these groups is very broad, from children to older adults. Group interventions in occupational therapy provide opportunities to develop task skills and interpersonal interaction skills (Mosey, 1973). Change occurs in individuals and in the group as a whole as a result of the interactions and feedback among group members (see Figure 34.1).

Although group work can be quite challenging, there are many benefits to be derived from developing and implementing group interventions. Based on years of research, Yalom (1995) developed a classification of "curative factors" or therapeutic factors that make group interventions particularly effective (see Box 34.1). A therapeutic factor is "an element occurring in group therapy that contributes to improvement in a patient's condition and is a function of the actions of a group therapist, the patient, or fellow group members" (Bloch, 1986, p. 679).

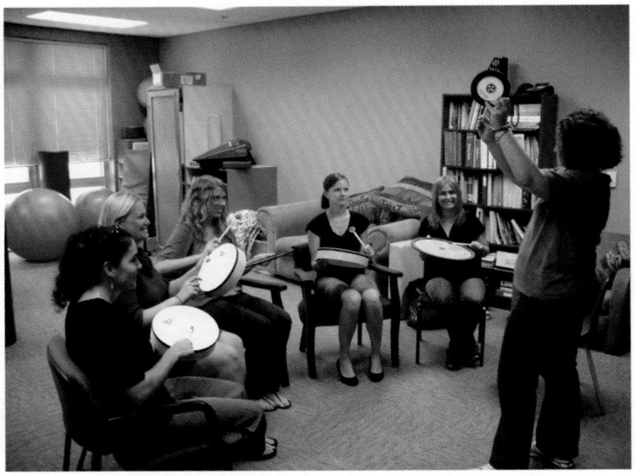

FIGURE 34.1 Occupational therapy often occurs within a group format. (Photo courtesy of Elizabeth Alford, MS, OTR.)

Groups used in occupational therapy intervention are typically determined and planned based on the purpose or goal of the group and include energy conservation groups, psychoeducational groups, social skills groups, activities of daily living groups, reminiscence groups, leisure groups, and sensorimotor groups, among others (see Table 34.1).

Group interventions are cost-effective and versatile, build social relationships, provide a context for social support, and can be designed to achieve multiple goals simultaneously. In addition, group interventions

- "Enhance communication and self-expression,"
- "Provide an atmosphere of nonjudgmental acceptance,"
- "Offer multiple opportunities to share learning," and
- "Facilitate client participation" and provide a context for problem solving in relationships (Cole, 2012, p. 70).

In this chapter, basic group processes will be described, including various characteristics of intervention groups, and stages of group development. In addition, types of occupational therapy group interventions will be discussed and the development and implementation of occupational therapy group interventions will be explored.

Group Process

There are sets of constantly changing dynamics that operate in small groups regardless of setting. The interrelationships and interactions between members, leaders, and the group as a whole are called **group process**. Group process "is the here-and-now experience in the group that describes how the group is functioning, the quality of relationships between and among group members and with the leader, the emotional experiences and reactions of the group, and the group's strongest desires and fears" (Brown, 2003, p. 228). The moment-to-moment interaction between leaders and members makes up the here-and-now process of a group. At a minimum, as an interdependent system, interaction operates simultaneously in six ways: (1) member to member, (2) leader to member and member to leader, (3) subgroups, (4) group as a whole, (5) engagement in occupation, and (6) the culture or environment. In a system-centered model, the group is viewed as an organized body of mutually dependent interacting parts. "It is the interactive system that changes through the developmental stages, not the individual group members" (Howe & Schwartzberg, 2001, p. 22).

Characteristics of Groups

Intervention groups have the following characteristics:

- Group context and climate
- Boundaries/membership
- Roles
- Group cohesiveness
- Group norms
- Group goals

BOX 34.1 Yalom's Primary Therapeutic Factors of Groups

- Altruism: sharing with others, reaching out to others, giving of oneself to help others
- Catharsis: sharing feelings and experiences, expressing and releasing emotions
- Cohesiveness: sense of belonging, developing relationships based on trust, support, and caring
- Imitative behavior: observing the behaviors of others and then experimenting and applying positive behaviors modeled by other group members and the group leader to one's own life
- Imparting information: learning about one's health, illness, or disability through discussion with other group members
- Instillation of hope: receiving reassurance, experiencing optimism and positive expectations based on observation of improvement in others
- Interpersonal learning: learning about and from others in the group, developing an awareness of others, correcting past misinterpretations about others
- Self-understanding: discovering and accepting previously unknown aspects of the self, developing insight
- Socializing techniques: learning, practicing, and developing social skills
- Universality: recognizing shared feelings, developing an awareness that one is not alone and that others have similar problems and experiences

From Yalom, I. D. (1995). *The theory and practice of group psychotherapy* (4th ed.). New York, NY: Basic Books; Yalom, I. D., & Leszcz, M. (2005). *The theory and practice of group psychotherapy* (5th ed.). New York, NY: Basic Books.

TABLE 34.1 Examples of Occupational Therapy Intervention Groups

Occupational Therapy Intervention Group Type and Purpose	Occupational Therapy Practice Example
Psychoeducational Group Educates clients regarding health concerns that impact occupational performance, participation, and well-being; enhances the client's capacity for health management and maintenance. Psychoeducational groups typically have a cognitive behavioral element embedded in the intervention.	A group of soldiers who are recovering from posttraumatic stress disorder (PTSD) attend occupational therapy sessions one night per week at an outpatient mental health facility to learn stress management strategies and how to incorporate them during their daily occupations.
Social Skills Group Provides opportunities for the development, establishment, and remediation of skills needed for social participation. Creating a situation where group members are socially connected allows members to develop social interaction skills and learn from one another.	In an outpatient program for substance dependence, an occupational therapist provides group sessions that incorporate role-playing various social situations, which are generated based on concerns clients have expressed. The members help each other gain insight regarding how they are perceived by others and provide/receive social support.
Activities of Daily Living (ADL)Group Designed to establish, remediate, or restore ADL & instrumental ADL (IADL) skills. Group members gain awareness, knowledge, and skills necessary for mastery of occupational performance. Improved functional outcomes are realized through intervention focused on skill development and adaptations.	An occupational therapist facilitates an ADL group for persons with low vision at the local senior center. The members explore the strategies and adaptations suggested by the occupational therapist and by individuals who are successfully participating in home-management and self-care activities.
Reminiscence Group The goal is to support, maintain, protect, or preserve a person's current occupational interests and abilities by participating in meaningful activities from their past.	An occupational therapy assistant leads a recreation group for persons in the middle stages of dementia, all of whom like to play cards. She plays a matching game using picture cards placed face up on the table. This parallel activity requires only simple recognition, which enhances the client's potential for success.
Leisure Group Provides opportunities to explore and participate in various leisure activities in order to achieve and maintain occupational balance.	An occupational therapist is hired to develop community reintegration plans with members of a clubhouse program that incorporate activities offered by the local parks and recreation department.
Sensorimotor Group Designed to facilitate adaptation; activities are generally dependent on the developmental level of the group. It is common for sensorimotor groups to address neurological or cognitive dysfunction in a thematic format.	At a recreational group for adolescents with mild traumatic brain injury, an occupational therapist uses a parachute activity to help the members move to various types of music and rhythms.
Energy Conservation Group Group members participate in activities that focus on health promotion to reduce the incidence of a disease or disorder or to prevent secondary conditions in cases of progressive or degenerative diseases.	An occupational therapist who visits a continuing care retirement community (CCRC) develops a group to teach the principles of energy conservation to seniors with arthritis and to help them incorporate these techniques into their daily occupational routines.

Groups are systems that exist within larger systems and occur within historical, social, and environmental contexts. These contexts impact the internal functioning of the group and its relationships with other systems. According to Schwartzberg, Howe, and Barnes (2008), "group climate refers to the physical and interpersonal or emotional environment affecting the group" (p. 8). An inviting physical environment and a safe, accepting interpersonal climate enhances group function.

Group boundaries may be flexible, rigid, or have variable degrees of permeability. Typically, intervention groups have inclusion and exclusion criteria for membership. Groups can be closed, with no new members added, or open with changing membership. Members can be selected to be similar to one another or heterogeneous. Small groups can range in size from 3 members to 10 or even 12 members. Group size influences group methods, leader strategies, and outcomes (Howe & Schwartzberg, 2001).

People take on various roles in intervention groups. A **role** is a set of socially agreed on behavioral expectations, rights, and responsibilities for a specific position or status in a group or in society. Roles may be related to task accomplishment or to the social/emotional needs of group members, both of which are critical to the effective functioning of the group. A list of task and social emotional roles is provided in Box 34.2 (Benne & Sheats, 1978). The performance of roles within a group mirrors role expectations in all areas of life and provides an opportunity for the development of role competence. There may be a mismatch between the roles members take on and the demands of a situation. If everyone offers emotional support and no one carries out actions such

BOX 34.2 Task and Social Emotional Roles in Intervention Groups

Task Roles

- Initiator/contributor
- Information seeker/information giver
- Opinion seeker/opinion giver
- Elaborator
- Coordinator
- Orienter
- Evaluator/critic
- Energizer (prods group to action)
- Procedural technician (performs routine tasks)

Social-Emotional Roles

- Encourager
- Harmonizer (mediates differences among group members)
- Compromiser (changes own behavior to maintain group harmony)
- Gatekeeper
- Standard setter
- Group observer (provides feedback on group process)
- Follower

as offering suggestions, the group falters. Conversely, if the group focuses only on getting the job done, the members will feel emotionally dissatisfied and isolated. Group cohesion results when the member roles are congruent with the task.

Group cohesiveness refers to the degree of understanding, acceptance, and feelings of closeness group members have toward each other and the value they place on the group. It is the group members' sense of liking, their trust and desire to work together, a feeling of togetherness, and sense of security. Group cohesiveness facilitates group function and individual development. Group cohesiveness can be enhanced through frequent group meetings, emphasizing similarities among group members, competition against other groups, and consensus regarding the group's norms and goals.

Group norms reflect the value system of the group—what members believe are appropriate ways of thinking, feeling, and behaving. Norms provide a safety net, and expectations of the individual and group are clear. Norms can be explicit or implicit and change over time as the group develops and matures. Some groups have specific written rules or contracts that govern attendance, expectations, roles, and interpersonal interactions (Schwartzberg et al., 2008).

Group goals are a future state toward which most group members' efforts are directed. Goals determine the group's focus and may be explicit or implicit. Goals give the group identity and provide meaning; goals are the standards by which the individual's and group's activities may be judged. Groups function better when members are clear about and invest in the group's purpose and goals (Schwartzberg et al., 2008).

Group Leadership

Leadership implies a relationship between an individual and a group built around some common interest. A leader is "a person who can influence others to be more effective in working to achieve their mutual goals and maintain effective working relationships among members" (Johnson & Johnson, 2006, p. 168). Leadership styles include directive, facilitative, and advisory (see Box 34.3 for descriptions). There are advantages and disadvantages of each leadership style. Therefore, it is best to use the approach that is most appropriate for a given situation, level of client functioning, and stage of group development. For example, directive leadership is necessary for lower functioning clients who may not have adequate safety awareness and therefore may be at risk for injury during activity. The facilitative leadership style is most likely to lead to group cohesiveness, and the advisory leadership style is most appropriate for working with caregivers, families, and community organizations in a

BOX 34.3 Leadership Styles

Directive: Leader defines the group, selects activities, and structures the group for therapeutic purposes.
Facilitative: Facilitator earns the support of the members, members make decisions with leader's guidance, and the therapist serves as a resource person and educator.

Advisory: Leader offers expertise as needed or requested but does not provide structure or goals; motivation comes from within the group.

Data from Cole, M. B. (2012). *Group dynamics in occupational therapy: The theoretical basis and practice application of group intervention* (4th ed.). Thorofare, NJ: Slack.

consultative role. For this reason, effective leaders have all three styles as part of their repertoire (Cole, 2012).

A leader "helps members learn new behaviors that will increase their ability to balance the task and social-emotional aspects of the group" and "members learn to effectively and appropriately meet other members' needs while achieving group goals" (Schwartzberg et al., 2008, p. 59). In order to effectively facilitate this learning process, the leader employs the skills of interactive reasoning, including establishing rapport through empathic listening, building alliances, giving and receiving information and feedback, validating success, sharing personal stories, and reflective responding (Mattingly & Fleming, 1994).

Research indicates that there are four functions of leadership that are important to group members (Yalom & Leszcz, 2005):

- Emotional activation (eliciting feelings, facilitating emotional expression, challenging, and confronting as necessary)
- Caring (offering support, concern, acceptance, etc.)
- Meaning attribution (providing clarification, explanation, interpretation, etc.)
- Executive function (managing time, setting limits, recommending strategies and procedures)

Kouzes and Posner (2007) describe five practices of exemplary leadership. These include modeling the way, inspiring a shared vision, challenging the process, enabling others to act, and encouraging the heart. Modeling the way involves setting an example by clarifying, affirming, and acting on values shared by the group. Inspiring a shared vision based on collective aspirations builds commitment to action among group members. Challenging the process promotes initiative, creativity, and innovation among group members. Enabling others to act fosters relationship building, collaboration based on trust, and the development of individual and group competence. Encouraging the heart demonstrates appreciation for group members' contributions and creates a spirit of community in the group.

Group Development

Intervention groups can be short term (crisis intervention) or long term (recovery). Whether they are short term or long term, groups change over time. Various interpersonal concerns emerge as groups evolve. The phases of group development provide a conceptual model of the evolution of group issues. Tuckman (1965) identified four stages of group development: (1) forming (uncertainty of one's role in the group, purpose, and procedures of group), (2) storming (conflict and rebellion in group because members resist group influence), (3) norming (group discovers ways to work together, set norms to enable cohesiveness), and (4) performing (group is flexible in ways of working together to achieve aims). Gazda (1989) provided an updated description (see Box 34.4). The phases or stages of group development often do not occur in a predictable, linear sequence but rather in a fluctuating, cyclical pattern. Groups may plateau or revert to earlier stages during times of stress and renegotiate norms, goals, and strategies in order to grow in a more positive direction.

Managing Disruptive Behaviors in Groups

One of the challenges of facilitating effective intervention groups is managing the disruptive and difficult behaviors

BOX 34.4 Gazda's (1989) Stages of Group Development

Exploratory Stage

- Set ground rules/norms for the group
- Clarify goals
- Inform participants of their responsibilities
- Leader centered
- Getting acquainted
- Establishing roles/functions in the group

Transition Stage

- Conflict and polarization
- Resistance to group influence
- Emotional responses
- Insecurity
- Defensiveness and frustration
- Problems seem insurmountable
- Group survival is in question

Action Stage

- Work/task focus
- Resistance is overcome
- Trust and cohesiveness is developed
- Increased self-disclosure
- Increased spontaneity
- Decreased reliance on the leader
- Problems are easily resolved

Termination Stage

- Usually short duration
- Decreased self-disclosure
- Attempts at closure
- Need to say good-bye and move on

TABLE 34.2 Managing Disruptive Behaviors in Groups

Problem Behavior	Possible Therapeutic Modes to Employ	Example
Hallucinations and delusions	Instructing	Provide reality-based orientation; keep activity structured.
Akathisia	Empathizing & Problem-solving	Allow freedom of movement if needed, plan for movement-oriented breaks, select gross motor activities, or adapt fine motor activities.
Storming out of the group	Collaborating & Problem-solving	Determine the reason for the behavior and collaborate in addressing the client's concerns.
Demonstrating inappropriate sexual behavior	Instructing & Empathizing	Explain in clear terms that the behavior is inappropriate and unacceptable. Help the person find appropriate ways to show affection or request attention.
Interrupting other members, excessive talking, or monopolizing discussions and leader's time	Instructing	Design structured activities. Ask questions that require answers from all members of the group. Teach and model methods of taking turns in a conversation, redirect the client's attention to group goals, activities, or discussions.
Using offensive language Displaying escalating or aggressive behavior	Instructing & Problem-solving	Actively listen, use a calm tone of voice, address problem behavior immediately, and adhere to boundaries, referring often to established group rules.
Excessive or inappropriate approval seeking	Collaborating	Ensure choice and autonomy, expect client to be an active participant and decision maker.
Lack of participation in group activity and/or interactions	Encouraging	Provide positive reinforcement for participation, celebrate accomplishments, and instill hopefulness.

of group members. These behaviors may indicate anxiety, frustration, boredom, fear, or symptom exacerbation on the part of the client. Disruptive behaviors may be the client's way of alerting the occupational therapist that he or she needs or wants more structure, guidance, or reassurance. When difficult situations that arise during group interventions are handled effectively, client learning and growth is facilitated; and the therapeutic alliance with the therapist is enhanced. If handled poorly, these events can undermine the efficacy of the group intervention and harm relationships within the group.

Understanding the underlying cause or motivation for the behavior will help the occupational therapist determine the best response or therapeutic mode to employ. Therapeutic modes are described in more detail in Chapter 33. Some common problem behaviors and management strategies are outlined in Table 34.2.

Using Groups to Assess Function

Occupational performance is the product of the interaction between the client, the occupation, and the environment. As a result, groups can be a useful context for evaluating certain client factors, performance skills, and performance patterns. Although various client factors can be assessed during group activities, specific and global mental functions that are readily apparent in group situations include attention, memory, perception, thought, temperament and personality, energy, and drive.

Performance skills, particularly cognitive, emotional regulation, and communication and social skills, are easily assessed during group activities. Cognitive skills such as judging, selecting, organizing, sequencing, prioritizing, and problem solving are evident when a client is planning and managing the performance of an occupation or activity in the group context and while interacting with other group members. Observing clients during craft activities, such as those included in the *Allen Diagnostic Module*, may be useful to evaluate cognitive skills during group task sessions. The Comprehensive Occupational Therapy Evaluation (COTE) can also be used to assess task-related behaviors and skills.

Emotional regulation skills are those "actions or behaviors a client uses to identify, manage, and express feelings while engaging in activities or interacting with others" (American Occupational Therapy Association, 2008, p. 640). These behaviors include managing frustration and anger, empathizing and responding to the feelings of others, displaying emotions appropriately, and coping with stressful situations. Dialectical Behavioral Therapy (DBT) diary cards are useful for clients to monitor their emotional reactions and their use of emotional regulation skills. By tracking emotions and behaviors on a daily basis, problematic patterns become apparent and can be addressed. An electronic version of the DBT diary card is available as an iPhone application (The DBT iPhone App, 2012).

Practice Dilemma

Just One of Those Days . . .

In a busy urban hospital outpatient behavioral health unit, an occupational therapist and a certified occupational therapy assistant (COTA) are responsible for the provision of a social skills group for clients recovering from traumatic brain injuries (TBIs). The group has five members not including the leaders. Martin is a 55-year-old former high school basketball coach who was involved in a serious car accident 5 months ago. He has frequent emotional outbursts and a tendency toward disruptive behaviors that escalate. Joanna is a 36-year-old mother of two children. She was involved in an accident at her job with the power company. She fell from a bucket truck while on the job, which resulted in a TBI. Joanna frequently displays manic behaviors and at times is sexually inappropriate toward other group members.

Louis is a 60-year-old street musician who was hit by an oncoming car when the driver lost control and ran up onto the sidewalk of a busy city square. Louis is quiet and mild mannered but often withdraws from the group activity or refuses to participate. He also experiences hallucinations. Marcella and Elaine are 22-year-old twins who were diagnosed with juvenile onset Huntington's disease. Their frequent jerky movements and limited cognitive abilities are often complained about by other group members.

In order to develop and practice communication and social skills, the group is working on completion of a group collage requiring collaborative decision making and planning. Within the first 15 minutes of the session, the occupational therapist notes that Louis begins to have active hallucinations. About this time, a nurse, who had arrived to deliver medication, hurried through the door to the occupational therapy room, creating a draft that blew all of the magazine pictures to be used for the collage onto the floor. Martin, with his voice raised, shouted at the nurse, calling her stupid for knocking over all of the pictures.

Although this was a difficult project for Elaine and Marcella because of their decreased fine motor abilities, the occupational therapist had constructed larger, foam board pictures of various foods for the twins to use to contribute to the collage. Even with this adaptation, the clients were expressing frustration by talking loudly and abandoning the group activity. Joanna's akathisia and inappropriate sexual behavior seemed to be disrupting task completion and social interaction among group members.

The occupational therapist and the COTA discussed the group session later while preparing the documentation, analyzing the tremendous impact clients' problem behaviors had had on their group in a 1-hour session on a single day. The occupational therapist looked at the COTA, and concluded, "Oh, well, I guess it is all in a day's work, and it was just one of THOSE days!"

Questions

1. Which of the disruptive behaviors in the practice dilemma would be the most difficult for you to address? Why?
2. What strategies or therapeutic modes might you employ in the practice scenario to manage each client's disruptive behaviors?
3. How might you have prevented these problems from occurring beforehand?

Communication and social skills are nearly impossible to evaluate outside of the group context. The skills that can be observed during group interaction include maintaining eye contact, initiating conversations, responding to questions, taking turns, sharing limited supplies, respecting the perspectives and beliefs of others, and use of appropriate interpersonal distance. There are many useful occupational therapy assessments for communication and social skills, including the Assessment of Communication and Interaction Skills (ACIS) based on the Model of Human Occupation, the Social Interaction Scale (SIS) of the Bay Area Functional Performance Evaluation (BaFPE), and the COTE.

Intervention Groups in Occupational Therapy

Schwartzberg et al. (2008) provide several important reasons why occupational therapy practitioners should incorporate group interventions in their practice, including the following:

- "Groups provide an occupation-based experience that is reality-oriented and that promotes adaptation."
- "Groups are a natural environment that can provide feedback and support for individual and social needs."
- "Through participating in group activities that promote growth and change, members can learn and practice skills to master and achieve competence in activities required for daily life."
- "When groups provide an opportunity for dealing with real-life issues and objects, people can maintain, improve or enhance their occupational nature to fulfill social demand" (p. 39).

Occupational therapy intervention groups may take many forms, for example, client-centered groups, developmental groups, task-oriented groups, and functional groups. Each of these will be described briefly. However, it is important to realize that these forms of group intervention are frequently combined into hybrid forms and rarely used singularly.

Client-Centered Groups

A client-centered approach has become one of the major foundational underpinnings of occupational therapy practice and applies to planning and implementing group interventions as well as individual interventions. Client-centered practice is based primarily on the humanistic approach to mental health care. The client-centered intervention approach is based on the following principles that are incorporated into the group process:

- Clients know what they want from therapy and what they need to reach their optimum level of occupational performance.
- The only relevant frame of reference or vantage point for therapy is that of the client.
- The therapist cannot actually promote change; he or she can only create an environment that facilitates change.
- Respect for clients and their families and the choices they make is central to therapist–client interactions.
- Clients and families have the ultimate responsibility for decisions about daily occupations and occupational therapy services.
- Client participation is to be facilitated in all aspects of occupational therapy service.
- Occupational therapy service delivery should be flexible and individualized to the client's needs.
- The goal is to enable and empower clients to address their occupational performance issues.
- Intervention has a focus on the person-environment-occupation relationship (Law, 1998).

Client-centered groups facilitate client self-expression, identification of strengths and weaknesses, prioritization of problem areas, identification of goals, awareness of options and choice, and exploration of the impact of context on occupational performance and participation (Cole, 2012). Incorporating client-centered practice principles in group interventions can take many forms, including values clarification exercises, group and individual goal setting and action planning, information seeking and sharing, role playing, and occupational exploration. However, the primary client-centered intervention is the development of a therapeutic relationship with the client through therapeutic use of self.

Developmental Groups

Mosey (1970) was the first occupational therapist to describe the nature of developmental groups and postulated that group interaction skills develop in a specific sequence from parallel group participation, through project group, egocentric cooperative group, to cooperative group, and, finally, to mature group participation. This represents a continuum from leader-dependent to member-driven groups. Mature, adaptive group interaction skills are required to effectively function in various groups. Effective group functioning is satisfying to oneself and to other group members and meets the demands of the social environment.

Developmental groups are not age specific but rather a reflection of the group's level of functioning. Group experiences and activities are graded to facilitate the client's development of appropriate group interaction skills. Developmental groups represent simulations of groups typically encountered in the normal developmental process and are used in intervention as modalities for planned change. A few of the strategies that can be implemented to facilitate the development of group interaction skills are (1) encouraging clients to imitate the behaviors of the therapist or other group members, (2) encouraging clients to experiment with various behavioral responses within the safety of the group, (3) providing encouragement and positive feedback for engaging in productive group interactions, and (4) discussing and role-playing possible behavioral options to various social situations (Mosey, 1970). Donohue (2010) updated Mosey's work on developmental groups and described five levels of social participation (see Box 34.5). In addition, Cole and Donohue (2011) developed and validated the Social Profile, an assessment designed to measure three categories of social participation: group membership, group interaction, and group activity behavior. Results from the Social Profile can be used to guide the planning and implementation of therapeutic group interventions.

Task-Oriented Groups

Task-oriented groups provide an opportunity for active involvement in occupation in natural contexts. A *task* is defined as any activity or process that produces an end product or provides service for the group as a whole or for persons not in the group (Fidler, 1969). The group members work together to accomplish a task. In this way, task groups resemble demands persons encounter in community living.

Mosey (1981) believed that task group interventions facilitate the development of adaptive skills, including sensory integration skills, cognitive skills, dyadic interaction skills, group interaction skills, self-identity skills, and sexual identity skills. Task-oriented group interventions provide a shared work experience that facilitates the integration of thinking, feeling, and behavior and provides structure for interaction, as well as opportunities for problem solving and skill development (Fidler, 1969). Task-oriented groups require collaboration, clear communication, interdependence, and shared decision making in real-life scenarios, thus enhancing the learning needed for functioning in home, school, work, and community contexts. Various task skills can be learned in a group setting (see Box 34.6).

Choosing an appropriate activity for a task-oriented group requires the occupational therapist to analyze the activity demands and the level and types of skills required to successfully complete the task. Tasks chosen should provide the "just right challenge" for group members; tasks that are too easy or too difficult will not provide an experience conducive to skill development.

BOX 34.5 Donohue's (2010) Five Levels of Social Participation

Parallel Participation

- Carrying out activities in the presence of others in a supportive manner
- Working side by side
- Members show awareness of others
- With minimal verbal or nonverbal interaction between group members

Associative Participation

- Brief verbal and nonverbal interactions, for example, greetings, short conversations
- Evidence of some beginning cooperation and competition
- Focus is on the task, minimal interaction outside the task
- Can give and receive minimal assistance with the task

Basic Cooperative Participation

- Joint tasks carried out over time, emphasis is on completion of the project
- Members jointly select, implement, and execute activity
- Members begin to express ideas and try to meet the needs of others
- Mutual interest in the task, activity, or goal
- Members respect each others' rights and follow group rules

Supportive Cooperative Participation

- Emphasizes camaraderie and emotional sharing around a task
- Members of the group are typically homogeneous
- Aim to fulfill each other's needs and derive mutual satisfaction from the activity
- Task is considered secondary to emotional support
- Feelings are frequently expressed, members grow in personal and interpersonal insight

Mature Participation

- Combines the skills of the basic and supportive cooperative participation levels
- Group members are often heterogeneous
- Members take turns in various complementary roles—teaching, learning, experimenting, and mentoring
- Goal is to complete the activity harmoniously and efficiently while enjoying the process
- Members balance task accomplishment with meeting social-emotional needs of group members

Functional Groups

The goal of a **functional group** is to promote adaptation and health through group action and engagement in occupation (Schwartzberg et al., 2008). *Adaptation* refers to the process by which a person adjusts to his or her environment and life circumstances. The four types of actions that are characteristic of a functional group include (1) purposeful action, (2) **self-initiated action**, (3) **spontaneous action** or here-and-now action, and (4) **group-centered action** (see Box 34.7). According to Schwartzberg et al. (2008), "It is through the dynamic interaction of these four types of action . . . that the group matures and members develop their ability to function" (p. 95).

Functional groups are experiential in nature; they are designed to motivate group members to meaningful action in order to facilitate independent or interdependent function. Functional groups are activity based and make use of the human and nonhuman environments for therapeutic purposes. In functional groups, "objects guide action" and "talking is used to clarify doing." The goal is not the product of the activity but rather the learning that occurs through group participation.

Activities chosen for use in functional groups may be school, work, play, leisure, or social in nature. In selecting activities to use for intervention, Schwartzberg et al. (2008) recommend considering the following:

- The activity goals should be meaningful to the clients.
- Clients should have input in the choice of activities.
- The demands of the activity should be congruent with the clients' ability to participate.
- Clients should be able to interact with the environment at a subcortical level.
- Activities should be chosen that are compatible with the clients' ages, skills, and performance levels.

BOX 34.6 Task Skills That Can Be Learned in a Group Setting

- A fairly normal rate of performance
- Appropriate use of tools and materials
- Willingness to engage in doing tasks
- Sustained interest in a task
- Ability to follow demonstrated, oral, and written directions
- An acceptable level of neatness
- Appropriate attention to detail
- The ability to solve problems that arise in performing a task
- Ability to organize tasks in a logical manner

BOX 34.7 Howe and Schwartzberg's (2001) Functional Group Actions

- **Purposeful action:** Meaningful for individuals and group as a whole.
- **Self-initiated action:** Member takes initiative verbally or nonverbally.
- **Spontaneous action:** Action occurs in the here and now.
- **Group-centered action:** Member actions are interdependent.

CASE STUDY 34.1 Marcus

Marcus is 32-year-old sergeant in the U.S. Army. He is serving in his third deployment with the Airborne Ranger sniper team and is the current leader of his reconnaissance platoon. During his first deployment, Marcus sustained a blast injury to his right side in combat, which required extensive occupational therapy rehabilitation intervention. During this combat, he also witnessed the death of two members of his platoon. Although the death of his colleagues could not have been prevented, his injury had prevented him from employing a rescue attempt. For this, he suffered frequent nightmares and flashbacks. His right upper extremity, although functional, continued to be weak. The weakness of his dominant right upper extremity led to a repetitive use injury in his left shoulder that required him to be on pain medication.

The mission commander referred Marcus to the Combat and Operational Stress Control unit (COSC) because of growing concern that he was consuming an excessive amount of pain medication and potentially becoming drug dependent. It was also noted by his superiors, as well as his subordinates, that he was making critical decisions too quickly; reacting impulsively and sometimes explosively during mission planning and debriefing meetings. The sergeant was in danger of losing his position as the platoon leader.

The COSC prevention team, consisting of a U.S. Army occupational therapist, a physician extender, and a psychiatrist, performed a mental health evaluation. The evaluation revealed a history of substance and alcohol abuse, chronic pain related to an injury sustained in an automobile accident as a child, and posttraumatic stress disorder (PTSD) and major depressive disorder that had not been formerly diagnosed or treated. Marcus' treatment plan consisted of a planned reduction of pain medication dependence through incorporation of an individualized physical fitness program to include daily stretching and strengthening exercises.

See **Appendix I, Common Conditions Resources, and Evidence**, for more information on PTSD (included in anxiety disorders), depression (included with mood disorders), and substance abuse.

A cognitive behavioral program was designed for Marcus to address his frequent expressions of distorted thinking, impulsivity, and verbally explosive outbursts to his supervisor and his subordinates. The cognitive behavioral module was delivered through group therapy. The format of the group allowed soldiers to come together and discuss traumatic events. The U.S. Army occupational therapist, who led the group as a facilitator, gave the soldiers new opportunities to discuss events with a group of peers who had experienced similar traumas. The group leader used projective art techniques, leisure activities, pet therapy, stress reduction, and anger management strategies.

The group sessions were often saturated with strong emotions like anger, resentment, guilt, and grief. During a final session, Marcus shared an insight.

> Sometimes I just get so angry, and I don't even know what the anger is about. Jonathon, our group leader, asked me a question about something I said in our group and I got mad at him, really laid into him. The other members just stared at me. I told him that I didn't have to explain anything to him. But I realize now, it wasn't about his question or even about the group. What I learned is that I didn't want to answer questions because I was afraid I'd get it wrong and fail like I failed my soldiers when I didn't rescue them.

The occupational therapist used a facilitative approach and provided a format for progressive relaxation, diaphragmatic breathing, and mindfulness meditation at the close of each group session. The short-term goal and outcome for the group was to provide a sense of relief and closure that would facilitate gradual behavioral changes resulting in improved mental health. The long-term goal was to normalize traumatic events that are unfortunately associated with combat, to teach coping skills, and to educate soldiers about warning signs of posttraumatic stress. Perhaps the most important advantage for use of a therapeutic group in this case was the unmistakable peer support shown for one another. Peer support is a protective factor for mental health and facilitates resiliency in the face of danger and the physical and psychosocial effects of traumatic events.

Source: Case Study courtesy of Courtney Sasse, MS, OTR, used with permission.

Implementing Intervention Groups in Occupational Therapy

Regardless of whether the group is client centered, developmental, task oriented, or functional in nature, the occupational therapy intervention group format is significantly different from verbal psychotherapy groups conducted by other mental health professionals. Cole (2012) has provided an excellent framework for implementing occupational therapy intervention groups that consists of a seven-step process (see Box 34.8). A description of this process follows.

Step 1: Introduction

The introduction step is always included regardless of frame of reference or type of group. It is important for group members to learn each other's names and the name of the group leader. The warm-up exercise is designed to capture the group's attention, relax group members, and prepare them to participate in the activity. The warm-up exercise should be challenging but not beyond the group members' capabilities and can be formal or informal in nature. Examples of warm-up exercises include a feelings check-in, review of a previous session, or team-building activity. It is important during the introduction step to set the mood for the group session using the environment and verbal and nonverbal communication. The group leader communicates what is expected of group members and serves as a role model. The purpose of the group should be explained clearly; understanding leads to increased motivation and participation. The group leader describes the structure and processes to be used in the session, including how long the activity will last, what will be done after the activity, and who will keep any products of the activity.

Step 2: Activity

It is critical that the group leader is adequately prepared to lead the group, understands the therapeutic goals, and is aware of the physical and mental capabilities of the group members. The group leader must be knowledgeable in conducting the group activity and skilled in modifying and adapting the activity to meet client needs

BOX 34.8 Cole's (2012) Seven Step Group Process

Step 1: Introduction

- Introduce self (name, title, name of the group)
- Have group members introduce themselves
- Warm-up exercise
- Communicate expectations of group members
- Explain purpose of the group clearly
- Brief outline of the session/structure of the group

Step 2: Activity

- Timing—not more than 1/3 of group session, simple, short activity
- Consider the therapeutic goals—what is to be accomplished by the activity?
- Consider the physical and mental capabilities of the group members
- Modify/adapt to suit client needs and goals
- Present instructions clearly, provide example or demonstration as appropriate
- Get feedback from group members to be sure they understand the directions
- Have materials and supplies ready but out of view
- After activity, collect supplies

Step 3: Sharing

- Members share their work or experience with the group
- Role model sharing for group members
- Make sure each group member has an opportunity to share
- Acknowledge each person's contribution verbally or nonverbally

Step 4: Processing

- Members share their feelings (about each other, about the experience, about the leader) with the group
- Role model sharing for group members
- Make sure each group member has an opportunity to share
- Acknowledge each person's contribution verbally or nonverbally

Step 5: Generalizing

- Sum up the group experience in a few general principles
- Point out like or similar responses
- Point out contrasts or differences
- State one or two principles learned from the experience

Step 6: Application

- Verbalize the meaning or significance of the experience
- Discuss how principles learned in the group can be applied to everyday life
- Relate the experience to issues/problems of members
- Use concrete examples

Step 7: Summary

- Emphasize the most important aspects of the group
- Review goals, content, and process of the group
- Verbally reinforce group's learning (interpersonal, emotional, & cognitive)
- Thank members for their participation
- End group on time

and goals. Instructions for the activity can be presented verbally, as written directions and/or through demonstration. It is important to get feedback from group members to be sure they understand the directions. This can be accomplished simply by asking group members to repeat the instructions back to you in their own words. It is a good idea to have the materials and supplies for the activity ready but out of view. This will help to decrease distractions while providing instructions.

Step 3: Sharing

The sharing step is designed to facilitate interpersonal learning as group members share their work or experience with the group. It is best to ask for a volunteer and not force anyone to share who is reticent. Role modeling how you want group members to share their activity experience facilitates the learning process. Make sure each group member has the opportunity to share and acknowledge each person's contribution to the group, either verbally ("thank you for sharing") or nonverbally (nodding and making eye contact).

Step 4: Processing

The processing step is designed to facilitate emotional learning as group members share their feelings (about each other, about the experience, about the leader) with the group. In this step, as in the sharing phase, it is best to ask for volunteers, model appropriate responses, provide an opportunity for all who desire to share, and acknowledge each person's contribution. During the processing step, the group leader may discuss nonverbal aspects of the group, for example, struggles for power and control, scapegoating, conflict, attraction, and avoidance. This is done in order to help the group understand its own processes.

Step 5: Generalizing

The generalizing step is designed to facilitate cognitive learning. Cognitive learning is facilitated when the group leader sums up the group experience in a few general principles. These principles are derived directly from the lived experience of the group members and are not preplanned. These principles should relate to the group goals whenever possible. One way to derive these general principles from the group experience is to look for patterns in responses (similarities, differences). Another way is to observe group energy levels (what energized the group, what subdued the group) and present these observations as general principles to be learned by the group experience.

Step 6: Application

The application step is designed to facilitate the application of the principles learned in the group to everyday life. This is accomplished when the group leader and group members verbalize the meaning or significance of the experience to their problems and personal lives. This may take the form of group problem solving. The best examples of application are simple, concrete, and specific. The group leader may provide examples of how they use the principles in their personal and professional life.

Step 7: Summary

The summary step is designed to reinforce the group's interpersonal, emotional, and cognitive learning. The group leader emphasizes the most important aspects of the group, reviews the goals, content, and process of the group, and thanks group members for their participation. Ending the group on time demonstrates respect for group members' time and other obligations.

Developing Group Protocols

Occupational therapy group interventions involve the processes of observation, evaluation, planning, analyzing, responding, and documenting. Group protocols are one method for coordinating this process. Evaluating client needs is the first step in developing a group intervention. The identification of clients' specific occupational concerns and priorities guides the selection of group goals, activities, structure, and process. The basic process of developing and implementing a group intervention involves

1. Identifying and evaluating the client population,
2. Selecting a model or theory or frame of reference to use in the design of the group intervention,
3. Determining a focus area or problem for intervention,
4. Searching for evidence that can be applied to the group intervention,
5. Writing a group intervention outline,
6. Developing individual group sessions,
7. Implementing the group intervention, and
8. Evaluating the effectiveness of the group intervention.

A **group protocol** is basically an intervention plan for a specific client population. Most groups consist of several sessions and the group protocol outlines the overall goals of the group and the objectives for each session. Each session is outlined in detail including

- Group membership and size;
- Session format;
- Areas of occupation, performance patterns, or performance skills addressed;
- Intervention approach;
- Time and place;
- A step-by-step description of the therapeutic activity to be used;

BOX 34.9 Theories Commonly Used in the Development of Group Interventions

- **Cognitive Disabilities**: focuses on cognitive processes, functional behavior, and problem solving; incorporates cueing, environmental adaptation, and task modification
- **Cognitive Behavioral**: focuses on social learning, cognitive distortions, and self-regulation; incorporates cognitive restructuring, role modeling, and behavioral techniques
- **Psychodynamic**: focuses on self-identity, interpersonal relationships, and spirituality; incorporates the symbolic and metaphorical meanings of activity
- **Model of Human Occupation (MOHO):** focuses on occupational performance, participation and adaptation, performance patterns, and skills; incorporates systems theory, contextual factors, and occupational choice, exploration, and mastery
- **Developmental**: focuses on normal developmental tasks, performance patterns, and life transitions; incorporates developmentally appropriate activities and emphasizes the application of learning to everyday life
- **Sensorimotor**: focuses on sensory, motor, and perceptual processes and the learning or relearning of motor skills; incorporates sensory stimulation, purposeful movement, and real-life tasks

Data from Cole, M. B. (2012). *Group dynamics in occupational therapy: The theoretical basis and practice application of group intervention* (4th ed.). Thorofare, NJ: Slack.

- The role of the group leader;
- Supplies and costs;
- Environmental set-up;
- Potential safety issues;
- Grading and adapting the activity; and
- Evaluation strategies (Cole, 2012).

Group protocols should be theory based and use the best available evidence on group interventions. Common theories used in developing group interventions are briefly described in Box 34.9.

Special Considerations

Working with groups has many challenges and specific ethical and legal issues to be considered. Group leaders/therapists have a "dual responsibility (a) to protect the welfare of each individual group member and (b) to ensure that the group as a whole functions in a way that benefits everyone involved" (Herlihy & Flowers, 2010, p. 191). All of the ethical concerns related to occupational therapy services for individuals also apply to group work. In addition, due to the differences in the treatment approaches, there are some special considerations that must be addressed when providing group interventions. Confidentiality, managing group boundaries, transference, and documentation issues will be briefly described here.

Confidentiality concerns are multiplied when providing group interventions because participants not only disclose personal information to the therapist but also to the group as a whole. It is incumbent on the group leader to emphasize the importance of confidentiality to group members. The leader must address violations of confidentiality or trust will be diminished and the boundaries of the group will be weakened.

Managing group boundaries is another challenge. This means not only the professional boundaries between therapist and client but also the boundaries among group members and boundaries between group members and nonmembers. Social relationships outside of the clinical setting between therapist and group members are discouraged. The boundaries between group members and nonmembers must be clear enough to prevent outside intrusion and to provide a sense of security for group members (Herlihy & Flowers, 2010).

Another concern relates to transference and countertransference in group situations. Transference occurs when clients transfer feelings, expectations, and impressions about a person in their past onto the therapist or other group members. For example, the therapist (or other group member) may remind a client of his or her parent or spouse and the client may interact in a way that recreates that former relationship (Haley & Carrier, 2010). Countertransference, where the therapist experiences transference with the client, is also possible. For example, when the group leader has positive or negative feelings toward a specific group member, it may be because the therapist is recreating a relationship with someone in his or her past.

Documentation of group interventions must conform to third-party payors, state, and federal requirements. In order for group interventions to be billable, the therapist must be an active participant in the process, and most of the group session should involve interaction between the participants and the therapist. Typically, each client's progress is documented following each group session, and notes are kept on the group's function as a whole. In addition, outcome measures may be used to determine the effectiveness of the group intervention in meeting client goals.

Conclusion

Occupational therapy intervention groups have the potential to incorporate many, if not all, of Yalom's (1995) therapeutic factors. One study indicated that psychiatric clients in four occupational therapy intervention groups most valued the therapeutic factors of cohesiveness, instillation of hope, and interpersonal learning (Falk-Kessler, Momich, & Perel, 1991). Occupation-based groups may be particularly effective in promoting hopefulness because occupational exploration facilitates the development of competence and achievement. Hopefulness and a sense of belonging are key affective motivators for learning, change, and growth. Falk-Kessler et al. (1991) propose, "activities can be used to facilitate the development of helpful therapeutic factors and therapeutic factors can be used to maximize the inherent or prescribed therapeutic effect of the activities" (p. 65). The "Commentary on the Evidence" box outlines additional evidence of the efficacy of group interventions. It is therefore important to incorporate these therapeutic factors in the design and implementation of occupation-based group interventions regardless of the population served or the setting in which the intervention occurs.

Commentary on the Evidence

Evidence to support the use of group interventions comes from various disciplines, including counseling, psychology, social work, and occupational therapy. Research suggests that occupational therapy–related intervention in groups is effective in addressing outcomes in body function (e.g., mental functions) and occupational performance areas and skills such as social participation and communication/interaction skills (Howe & Schwartzberg, 2001). Evidence-based techniques vary depending on the desired outcomes and client problem. Intervention for performance areas and skills conducted in a group setting may result in greater client satisfaction and compliance with intervention regimes (Howe & Schwartzberg, 2001). Because the range of skills addressed is so varied, it is best to examine the literature specific to the client factor and outcome in question. There is a need to expand the evidence in all areas of occupational therapy intervention in which group process is applied to specific client problems.

A few studies providing evidence for the efficacy of group work are briefly described here.

Authors	Findings
Klyczek & Mann (1986)	In a psychiatric day treatment program, clients in an activity group as compared to a verbal group demonstrated greater symptom reduction, increased self-esteem, and improved decision making.
Lundgren & Persechino (1986)	In a study of adults with head injury, Mosey's developmental groups demonstrated improvements in memory and social interaction skills.
Clark et al., (1997)	Group intervention for elderly living independently in the community demonstrated improvements in vitality, health, function, occupational participation, and quality of life.
Eklund (1999)	A comparison of an outpatient occupational therapy group in a psychiatric setting to a matched group receiving verbal therapy found that the occupational therapy group had greater improvement in global mental health and reduced psychiatric symptoms.
Glass, Mendes de Leon, & Berkman (1999)	Thirteen-year study of older adults identified the importance of social engagement and productive activity in reducing mortality.
Bober, McLellan, McBee, & Westreich (2002)	An art-based activity group for persons with Alzheimer's disease was effective in improving participants' ability to identify emotions and socialize with other group members.
Peterson (2003)	A randomized controlled trial designed to evaluate the efficacy of an eight-session, group-based fall prevention program for older adults demonstrated increased social participation and improved community mobility.
Boisvert (2004)	A client-centered occupational therapy group (based on the Model of Human Occupation) for persons with substance dependence demonstrated significant improvement in participants' self-esteem.
Capasso, Gorman, & Blick (2010)	A study of persons with cerebrovascular accident and resultant hemiparesis demonstrated improved upper extremity function as a result of participation in a social breakfast group intervention as an alternative to repetitive exercise.

References

American Occupational Therapy Association. (2008). Occupational therapy practice framework: Domain and process, 2nd edition. *American Journal of Occupational Therapy, 62*, 625–683.

Benne, K. D., & Sheats, P. (1978). Functional roles of group members. In L. P. Bradford (Ed.), *Group development*, (2nd ed., pp. 52–61). LaJolla, CA: University Associates.

Bloch, S. (1986). Therapeutic factors in group psychotherapy. In A.J. Frances & R.E. Hales (Eds.), *Annual review* (Vol. 5, pp. 678–698). Washington, DC: American Psychiatric Press.

Bober, S. J., McLellan, E., McBee, L., & Westreich, L. (2002). The feelings art group: A vehicle for personal expression in skilled nursing home residents with dementia. *Journal of Social Work in Long Term Care, 1*(4), 73–87.

Boisvert, R. A. (2004). Enhancing substance dependence intervention. *Occupational Therapy Practice, 9*(10), 11–16.

Brown, N. W. (2003). Conceptualizing process. *International Journal of Group Psychotherapy, 53*, 225–244.

Capasso, N., Gorman, A., & Blick, C. (2010). Breakfast group in an acute rehabilitation setting: A restorative program for incorporating client's hemiparetic upper extremities for function. *Occupational Therapy Practice, 5*(8), 14–18.

Clark, F., Azen, S., Zemke, R., Jackson, J., Carlson, M., Mandel, D., . . . Lipson, L. (1997). Occupational therapy for independent-living older adults: A randomized controlled trial. *Journal of the American Medical Association, 278*, 1321–1326.

Cole, M. B. (2012). *Group dynamics in occupational therapy: The theoretical basis and practice application of group intervention* (4th ed.). Thorofare, NJ: Slack.

Cole, M. B., & Donohue, M. (2011). *Social participation in occupational contexts: In schools, clinics and communities.* Thorofare, NJ: Slack.

The DBT iPhone App. (2012). *DBT diary card.* Retrieved from http://www.diarycard.net/

Donohue, M. (2010). *Five levels of social participation.* Retrieved from http://www.social-profile.com/social_levels.html

Eklund, M. (1999). Outcome of occupational therapy in a psychiatric day care unit for long-term mentally ill patients. *Occupational Therapy in Mental Health, 14*(4), 21–45.

Falk-Kessler, J., Momich, C., & Perel, S. (1991). Therapeutic factors in occupational therapy groups. *American Journal of Occupational Therapy, 45*, 59–66.

Fidler, G. S. (1969). The task-oriented group as a context for treatment. *American Journal of Occupational Therapy, 23*, 43–48.

Gazda, G. M. (1989). *Group counseling: A developmental approach* (4th ed.). Boston, MA: Allyn & Bacon.

Glass, T. A., Mendes de Leon, C., & Berkman, L. F. (1999). Population-based study of social and productive activities as predictors of survival among elderly Americans. *British Medical Journal, 319*, 478–483.

Haley, M., & Carrier, J. W. (2010). Psychotherapy groups. In D. Capuzzi, D. R. Gross, & M. D. Stauffer (Eds.), *Introduction to group work* (5th ed.). Denver, CO: Love.

Herlihy, B. R., & Flowers, L. (2010). Group work: Ethical and legal considerations. In D. Capuzzi, D. R. Gross, & M. D. Stauffer (Eds.), *Introduction to group work* (5th ed.). Denver, CO: Love.

Howe, M. C., & Schwartzberg, S. L. (2001). *A functional approach to group work in occupational therapy* (3rd ed.). Philadelphia, PA: Lippincott Williams & Wilkins.

Johnson, D. W., & Johnson, F. P. (2006). *Joining together: Group theory and group skills* (9th ed.). Boston, MA: Pearson.

Klyczek, J. P., & Mann, W. C. (1986). Therapeutic modality comparisons in day treatment. *American Journal of Occupational Therapy, 40*, 606–611.

Kouzes, J., & Posner, B. (2007). *The leadership challenge* (4th ed.). San Francisco, CA: Jossey-Bass.

Law, M. (1998). *Client-centered occupational therapy.* Thorofare, NJ: Slack.

Lundgren, C. C., & Persechino, E. L. (1986). Cognitive group: A treatment program for head-injured adults. *American Journal of Occupational Therapy, 40*, 397–401.

Mattingly, C., & Fleming, M. H. (1994). *Clinical reasoning: Forms of inquiry in a therapeutic practice.* Philadelphia, PA: F. A. Davis.

Mosey, A. C. (1970). The concept and use of developmental groups. *American Journal of Occupational Therapy, 24*, 272–275.

Mosey, A. C. (1973). *Activities therapy.* New York, NY: Raven Press.

Mosey, A. C. (1981). *Occupational therapy: Configuration of a profession.* New York, NY: Raven Press.

Peterson, E. W. (2003). Evidence-based practice case example: A matter of balance. *Occupational Therapy Practice, 8*(3), 12–14.

Schwartzberg, S. L., Howe, M., & Barnes, M. (2008). *Groups: Applying the functional group model.* Philadelphia, PA: F. A. Davis.

Tuckman, B. W. (1965). Developmental sequence in small groups. *Psychological Bulletin, 63*, 384–399.

Yalom, I. D. (1995). *The theory and practice of group psychotherapy* (4th ed.). New York, NY: Basic Books.

Yalom, I. D., & Leszcz, M. (2005). *The theory and practice of group psychotherapy* (5th ed.). New York, NY: Basic Books.

For additional resources on the subjects discussed in this chapter, visit http://thePoint.lww.com/Willard-Spackman12e.

CHAPTER 35

Professionalism, Communication, and Teamwork

Janet Falk-Kessler

OUTLINE

LEARNING OBJECTIVES

After reading this chapter, you will be able to:

1. Understand what it means to be a professional
2. Understand what types of behaviors are viewed as professional and as unprofessional, and why
3. Understand the value of teamwork
4. Be able to distinguish between different types of teams and how they function
5. Be able to describe the "do's and don't's" of social media participation

Introduction

The purpose of this chapter is to review professionalism and collaborative behavior. In this chapter, professionalism encompasses how one presents oneself as a professional and the individual's responsibilities and obligations as a professional and to one's profession.

Professionalism is a concept that has many attributes. It includes behaviors that are on public display; knowledge and skill-based competencies that are continually sought and demonstrated; and overall responsibilities to one's clients, colleagues, profession, and society (Monrouxe, Reese, & Hu, 2011). Becoming a professional is a process—one that begins by learning what a professional is and does, enacting the professional role by meeting expectations, and eventually embodying and internalizing professional qualities. Implicit and explicit guidelines, rules, and expectations within social contexts contribute to professional development (Clouder, 2003; Monrouxe et al., 2011).

Professionalism reflects the person as well as one's profession. Within medically related professions, professionalism includes subordinating self-interest; being mindful of the needs of patients/clients, their families, and society; exhibiting values that are humanistic in nature; being accountable to self and others; adhering to ethical principles and values; contributing to the advancement of one's profession; and pursuing excellence (Swick, 2000; Wynia, Latham, Kao, Berg, & Emanuel, 1999). These characteristics echo how professionalism in occupational therapy has been described (Glennon & Van

Oss, 2010; Wood, 2004) and serve as the foundation for one's behaviors, commitments, collaboration, and teamwork. As one's professionalism develops, one's role as a contributing member of the health care team and the occupational therapy profession is strengthened. This chapter will review professionalism as it relates to each of these areas.

Professionalism has been garnering a vast amount of attention in both the public and professional media. Demonstrating professionalism has become a focus within many academic settings, including academic medical centers (Wear & Kuczewski, 2004; Wynia et al., 1999). The development of values, attitudes, and behaviors that mirror one's profession is a process that continually evolves throughout one's career and is in part reflective of a contract between one's discipline and society in general (Cruess & Cruess, 2009; Kurlander, Morin, & Wynia, 2004). Maintaining standards of practice, which include maintaining competency, demonstrating **evidence-based practice**, using appropriate judgment, and abiding by our profession's ethical code, is a professional responsibility (American Occupational Therapy Association [AOTA], 2010a, 2010b; Paterson & Higgs, 2008).

Participating in local, state, and national organizations that work to market occupational therapy services to various stakeholders—including consumers, third-party payers, and policy makers—and that sponsor continuing education opportunities, provide members with a range of literature, and inform members of legislation as well as other concerns of interest is part of one's professional responsibility. A shared vision to promote one's profession, as articulated in AOTA's Centennial Vision, is generated by these responsibilities and is testimony to the importance of professionalism.

Although historically, the transmission of professionalism relied on immersion in a professional environment, it is now viewed as something to be taught, with the attributes of professionalism internalized over time (Cruess & Cruess, 2006; Johnson, 2006; Krinn, 2011; Monrouxe et al., 2011). These obligations and responsibilities are depicted in Figure 35.1.

Workplace Professionalism and Behavior

In the last few decades, many medical professionals have emphasized and embraced their long-held, traditional values. This is certainly the case within occupational therapy, as the AOTA's Centennial Vision has centralized professional emphasis on values that reflect humanism, holism, and science—the same values that were present since the beginnings of our profession (Schwartz, 2009). The "Occupational Therapy Practice Framework" (AOTA, 2008), with its emphasis on occupational engagement, similarly reminds therapists of the roots of professional practice and the professional responsibility to use terminology that reflects these values (Youngstrom, 2002). It has been suggested that "nostalgic professionalism" within medical fields has emerged as a result of the values diverting a profession from its core principles—values that may lead to the emergence of unprofessional behavior (Hafferty, 2009). These values range from materialism to personal entitlement.

Regardless of situation or interaction (e.g., a professor, supervisor, client and/or the client's family, a team meeting, or conference presentation), professionalism is expected. Professional behavior has become so important that it is included in academic accreditation standards for all levels of occupational therapy education (Accreditation Council for Occupational Therapy Education, 2010) and is an integral part of the *Fieldwork Performance Evaluation for the Occupational Therapy Student* (AOTA, 2002).

Among the many characteristics that shape professionals are values about work, roles, and service recipients. Many believe that values, especially those that revolve around work ethic, cause conflict in academic and employment environments. In recent decades, attention has been paid to differences in work values and expectation that is generationally linked (Lancaster & Stillman, 2002). How one behaves is rooted in the cultural and societal norms

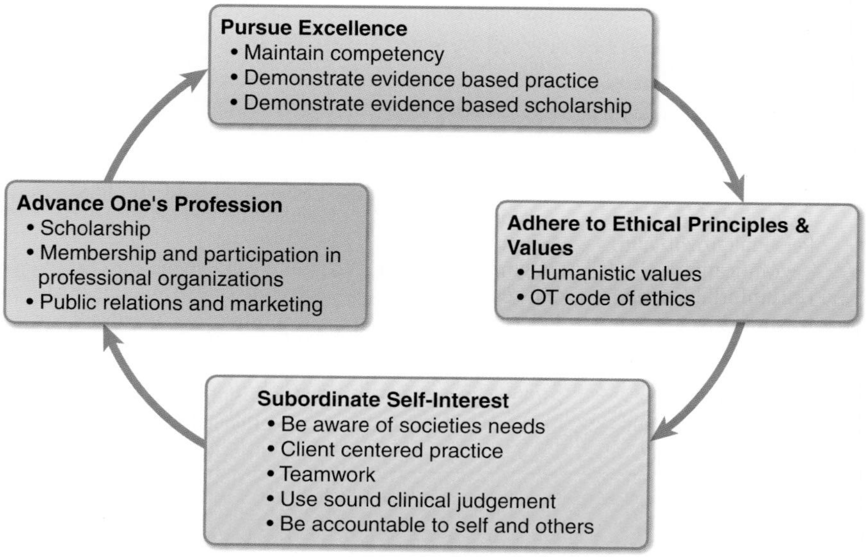

FIGURE 35.1 Professionalism and occupational therapy practitioners.

and expectations in which one was raised. For example, the most recent "generation" that is entering the health care workforce has been described as technologically savvy, adept at multitasking, civic-minded, and diverse (Johnson & Romanello, 2005; Lancaster & Stillman, 2002; Twenge, 2006). They have also been described as lazy (Rampell, 2011), lacking empathy (Konrath, O'Brien, & Hsing, 2011), entitled (Alsop, 2008), and self-important (Twenge, 2006; Twenge & Campbell, 2009). Furthermore, it has been argued that today's society, which serves as the context of the health care culture, may have contributed to the unraveling of professionalism (Coulehan, 2005; Glennon & Van Oss, 2010).

Historically, as each generation enters the workforce, characteristics are identified that distinguish them from previous generations (Lancaster & Stillman, 2002; Zemke, 2000). This is certainly the case with the "Millennials," those most recently acculturated into the work environment (Glennon, 2009; Lower, 2008). These generational differences may also promote conflict (Johnson, 2006) because there are varying perspectives on what constitutes professional and unprofessional behavior. Often, an individual may acknowledge what is considered unprofessional behavior but can rationalize this behavior as not unprofessional when they themselves display it (Aurora, Wayne, Anderson, Didwania, & Humphrey, 2008). Generally, the individual displaying such behavior has no idea that he or she is perceived as inappropriate, unreasonable, and even disrespectful. It has been suggested that these behaviors reflect how individuals perceive and understand rules and their expectations of and for themselves (Lake, 2009). As an example, those individuals of the more recent generations grew up within home, school, and societal environments that promoted self-esteem, emphasized individualism, and placed little emphasis on social rules. This can result in the expectation of entitlements (Twenge, 2006). The previous generations grew up with a respect for authority and the notion that achievement is based on what one has actually accomplished. Table 35.1 presents the comparison of generations.

TABLE 35.1 Generational Comparisons

	Veterans	Baby Boomers	Gen Xers	Millennials
Also known as ...	Traditionalists Silent generation (or "Silents")	Sandwich generation	Slacker generation Me generation	Gen Y Nexters Trophy kids Echo boomers
Birth years	before 1946	1946–1964	1965–1980	1981–2002
Descriptors	Loyal, formal	Optimistic, tactful	Skeptical, blunt	Pragmatic, Polite
Learning styles	Process oriented	Personal experiences Caring environment Handouts Note-taking	Efficient Only study what is personally useful Own pace, own time Detailed review & study guides Like technology	Collaborative Technology is necessary Experiential Immediate feedback Want it right the first time
Career goals and rewards	To "build a legacy" Feel a personal responsibility for their organization Doing a good job is personally satisfying	"Build a stellar career" Achievement, recognition, financial remuneration	"Build a portable career" (career security vs. job security), Freedom	"Build parallel careers" Multitask at work; multiple careers in life Seek personally meaningful work
Workplace values and ethics	Loyalty, dedication, and sacrifice Hard work Respect for authority Respect for hierarchy, elders Adhere to rules Duty first Conformity Responds to directive leadership	Dedication Respect authority Want "face time" Team oriented Personal growth and gratification Uncomfortable with conflict Can be overly sensitive to feedback Can be judgmental Responds to directive leadership	Work–life balance Want autonomy, flexibility, and informality Accept diversity Pragmatic/practical Self-reliant Reject rules Mistrust institutions Use technology Multitaskers	Need feedback and recognition Nurtured Seek fulfillment and fun Celebrate diversity Optimistic Self-inventive Rewrite rules Institutions are irrelevant Not awed by hierarchy, elders Expect technology Multitask fast Have difficulty dealing with "difficult people" issues

Information compiled from the following sources: Fogg (2008); Johnson and Romanello (2005); Lancaster and Stillman (2002); Mohr, Moreno-Walton, Mills, Brunett, & Promes (2011); Tulgan (2009); and Zemke (2000).

TABLE 35.2 Student Behaviors

Generational Factor (Lake, 2009)	Behavior
Rules "have trouble understanding rules as guides for their behavior, unless particularized to them"	A student refused to go to her fieldwork assignment because ADL sessions started at 7:30 a.m., and she isn't "a morning person." A student is ½ hour late for an exam and asks for extra time to finish it. A student did not attend a Monday class because it interfered with her long weekend plans. She asked the professor to go over what she missed.
Rewards "have grown up constantly rewarded, not punished"	A student earned a 94 on a case study. She made an appointment with her professor to complain because she felt she deserved a higher grade. A student complained to the administration that faculty won't let them redo assignments for a better grade. A student complained that he didn't get a higher grade in the course. After all, he attended all of the classes.
Avoidance "When confronted with rules . . . instinctively respond with avoidance behaviors . . . or find a way around it "	A student was absent from a fieldwork assignment and asked a friend to inform her supervisor. A professor asked a student to make an appointment with him. The student never followed through. After doing a literature search, many of the references that emerged were not available online but were available in the school's library. The student only used what he accessed online.
Decision makers "often make their decisions in close connection with family members and friends."	A student's parents advised him to change his level 2 fieldwork placement because he had no intention of seeking a job with the client population to which he was assigned. A student expressed concern over a requirement she didn't know existed. She never visited the school or spoke with anyone from the school prior to attending. She relied on information she received from a friend who graduated 4 years earlier.

Differences in how one perceives work/career values and rewards lead to conflict (Lancaster & Stillman, 2002). When one considers that professionalism within academia and health care is typically defined by those from the veteran or baby boomer generations, it is not surprising that those from the more recent generations are unaware that their attitudes and behaviors are viewed as unprofessional. These attitudes and behaviors may be the cause for fieldwork/workplace difficulties and failure (Fischer, 2005). Student scenarios provided by academic and clinical colleagues across the country are presented in Table 35.2. Each example demonstrates behavior that has been considered unprofessional.

To further illustrate differences in how individuals from different generations perceive professionalism, consider Case Study 35.1.

What indeed is the underlying issue portrayed in the case study? Individuals from two different generations perceive behaviors in very different ways. These perceptions come from experiences specific to their "generational culture." Political and societal events shape perception just as experience does. Being from different generational cultures is not an excuse to maintain behaviors and expectations that are viewed by many as unprofessional nor to hold on to behaviors and expectations that might no longer be appropriate. Although the supervisor in this case example is frustrated by what she sees as disrespectful behaviors, the younger therapist believes in efficiency and transparency and likes to "tell it like it is." Both are coming from their own generational context. However, in practice settings, one must remember that the client's needs come first and that most likely, there are generational differences between therapist and client as well. Therefore, those joining the workforce will succeed if they are aware of how they are perceived and learn to demonstrate professionalism that will garner them respect from the multigenerational contexts. Their supervisors will similarly have more satisfying relationships with those they oversee if they, too, understand how to adapt their supervisory styles in order to help the new therapists adapt and to not blame their supervisees for behaviors shaped by their culture.

Professionalism and Teamwork

Interprofessional teamwork is ubiquitous. Thus, an important feature of professionalism is one's ability to be an effective team member. **Teamwork** as applied in the health care environment is, simply put, "the ability to recognize and respect the expertise of others and work with them in the patient's best interest" (Cruess, Cruess, & Steinert, 2009, p. 286). Interprofessional teams in particular benefit client safety and care and are based on the premise that no one person has all the skills and

CASE STUDY 35.1 Lee-Ann at Work

Lee-Ann Gold, just shy of her 26th birthday and having graduated from occupational therapy school 1 year earlier, is on her second occupational therapy position. She resigned from her initial place of employment after working for 10 months because she felt it wasn't an ideal match. She enjoyed the clinical work but felt she was expected to act more "formally" than she was used to. For example, she used informal salutations (e.g., "Hey" instead of "Hello"; first name instead of last) and abbreviations ("u r" instead of "you are") in her emails to colleagues. She assumed that if she came into work a few minutes late, it didn't matter; and if she was an hour late, she could simply make up the time at her convenience. She also would exchange days off with a peer without clearing this with her supervisor.

At her new job, she interacted with her supervisor regularly and received informal feedback on her performance. After her first 2 months in this new job, her supervisor Dana Beck requested a more formal meeting to review her overall performance. Dana, who was also the department head, had over 20 years of occupational therapy experience plus several specialty certifications and was on her second job as well. She has been at the current site for 7 years. Lee-Ann was looking forward to this meeting, as she was confident in her performance. She also thought this would be a good time to present some of her ideas about how the department should be run. She had thoughts on how to improve scheduling, rotations, weekend coverage, and office space assignment.

At the meeting, Lee-Ann was told that her assessment and intervention skills were good and that she brought a vibrant approach to their team. Lee-Ann was also told that when she worked with someone with a condition she was not that familiar with, she was expected to use resources to learn about it as well as research evidence-based intervention approaches. She would probably need to use break time or evenings for this because the workday is typically filled with assignments. Lee-Ann was also told that although patients liked her, they commented that she was always looking at her cell phone during intervention sessions. Staff members similarly commented that she would read and respond to texts during meetings. The final area of feedback related to her timeliness when getting to her meetings. Lee-Ann knew she was sometimes a bit late, but the office she was in was a 6-minute walk to the conference rooms where team meetings were held. She noted that when she first arrived at that hospital, she anticipated a "late" attendance and suggested that the staff therapists switch offices with the supervisors who did not attend the same meetings and whose offices were in a more central location.

Lee-Ann Gold and her supervisor Dana Beck have the same perspective of Lee-Ann's clinical skills, which appropriately display competence and confidence, but they have very different perceptions of Lee-Ann's work ethic and professionalism. Lee-Ann sees herself as hard working and pragmatic. Her supervisor, while praising her practice skills, sees Lee-Ann as entitled and unprofessional. The following summarizes their respective perceptions:

Lee-Ann Gold

Lee-Ann wondered why people were making a "big deal" over everything. She used her cell phone to check the time because she didn't want to wear a watch, she was able to multitask at meetings while paying attention, and again thought about how formal everything seemed. In this new setting, she had to make appointments when seeking discussion time with colleagues rather than simply talking to them in the hallway when she saw them. Expecting to follow the organization's hierarchy and abide by the policies of the institution, even when the rules and regulations imposed by the department and institution were neither logical nor practical, was emblematic of what she called the "antiquated system." She was surprised when told that she should not automatically refer to a superior, especially one in a different department, by first name. Because Lee-Ann isn't impressed by titles and pays more attention to what one does, she thought this was an example of posturing. Finally, as she was no longer a student, Lee-Ann felt all work-related activities should be done at work and even suggested to her supervisor that her schedule should be revised to accommodate this. Lee-Ann had never before received feedback that wasn't all positive and thought her supervisor was overreacting.

Dana Beck

After 20 years of experience, she wondered what has happened to this new generation of therapists. Even though they seem to know what to do clinically and they talk about client-centered care, they don't seem to really understand that the entire work environment is about their clients and not about themselves. Furthermore, they do not seem to show respect for their more experienced colleagues. They believe they know more. Lee-Ann and others her age interrupt someone's conversation if they want something but are resentful if asked to do something during their lunch break. They assume that they are entitled to make their own decisions without understanding how these decisions fit with the working environment. They don't seem to know how to communicate professionally. Everything starts with, "Hey," "I want . . ." or "This will only take a minute." And when they send an e-mail, it is filled with spelling mistakes, abbreviations, and rarely signed. They don't understand that they need to keep their private life at home because they seem to be always looking at or texting on their cell phones. They even ignore our rule that phones must be "off," not even on vibrate, when with clients. They want to be spoon-fed information or able to find it immediately on the Internet and resent having to do a little research on their own and on their own time. They don't even want to use proper search engines on the Internet but would rather rely on Wikipedia or Google (or its equivalent) and refuse to go to a library. They don't seem to want to put "extra" effort into anything. Finally, they expect to be praised simply for showing up.

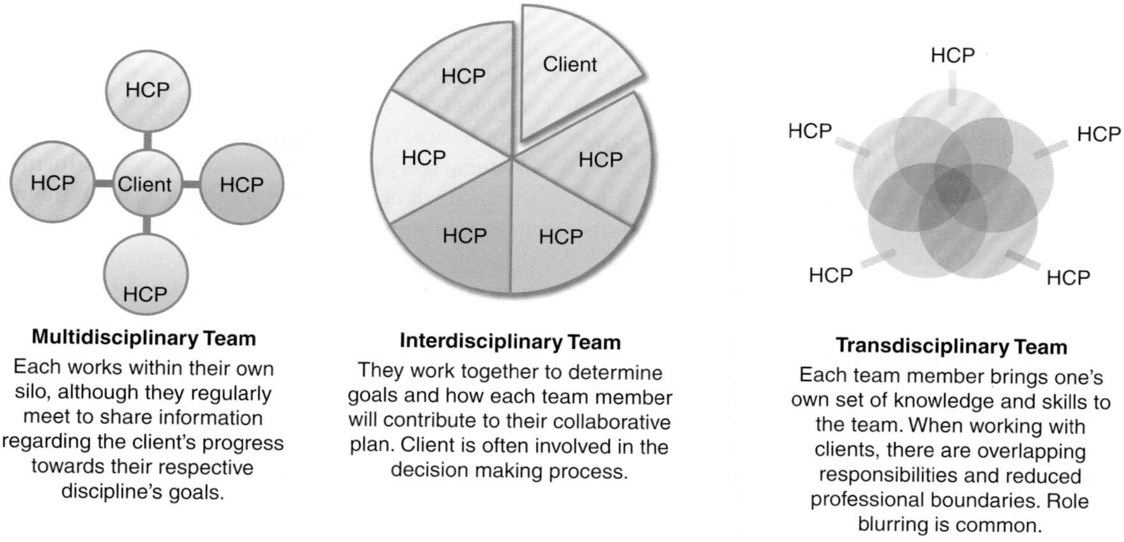

HCP
HCP
Client
HCP
HCP
Multidisciplinary Team
Each works within their own silo, although they regularly meet to share information regarding the client's progress towards their respective discipline's goals.
HCP
Client
HCP
HCP
HCP
HCP
Interdisciplinary Team
They work together to determine goals and how each team member will contribute to their collaborative plan. Client is often involved in the decision making process.
HCP
HCP
HCP
HCP
HCP
Transdisciplinary Team
Each team member brings one's own set of knowledge and skills to the team. When working with clients, there are overlapping responsibilities and reduced professional boundaries. Role blurring is common.

FIGURE 35.2 Interprofessional collaboration of health care practitioners (HCP).

knowledge to meet the client's goals. One's role as a professional includes an understanding that respect of, communication with, and appreciation for what each can contribute to their clients is paramount (Dillon, 2001).

It has been well documented that effective teamwork is linked with improved client outcomes (Zwarenstein, Goldman, & Reeves, 2009), including outcomes in rehabilitation settings (Sinclair, Lingard, & Mohabeer, 2009) and improved client safety (Kohn, Corrigan, & Donaldson, 2000; Salas, Rosen, & King, 2007). Failures related to the environment's culture and to interpersonal communication can result in treatment errors (Deering, Johnston, & Colacchio, 2011; Salas et al., 2007). Improving health care is a direct result of improving communication and collaboration (Zwarenstein et al., 2009).

Interprofessional health care teams can be traced to the World War II era, although some professionals were calling out for teamwork well before then in order to gain professional recognition. Teams that comprised members from different disciplines were first formed for clinical efficiency purposes but soon demonstrated enhanced communication, improved quality of health care, and cost containment. Enhanced patient compliance as well as patient satisfaction has also been documented (Baldwin, 2007).

Teams are an outgrowth of the knowledge that an individual who functions alone is not as helpful to the client as a team that works well together. The reasoning process, when done in a group, is more effective than when done in isolation (Mercier & Sperber, 2011). This reduces the risk of ignoring information that does not fit within one's belief system and increases access to information from others, which helps decision making.

Effective teams, whether they be made up by two individuals such as an occupational therapist and an occupational therapy assistant or representing a group of various health care professionals, are all characterized by communication and collaboration, formal and informal learning opportunities, and, above all, trust (Cartmill, Soklaridis, & Cassidy, 2011; Dillon, 2001; Jones & Jones, 2011; Kalisch, Lee, & Rochman, 2010.). These attributes are developed through group cohesion, shared mental models, and objective leadership and often result in increased job satisfaction (Kalisch et al., 2010). In addition, the explicit importance of team meetings, the role of shared objectives in conflict management, and the value of autonomy within the team (Jones & Jones, 2011) are further examples of effective interprofessional teams.

There are three categories of interprofessional teams that exist in health care: multidisciplinary, interdisciplinary, and transdisciplinary (see Figure 35.2). Each is composed of individuals from various professional backgrounds, and each is focused on a common client. It is helpful to consider these teams as a continuum of interprofessional cooperation. Multidisciplinary teams emerged first, with other forms of teams developing as team objectives changed.

Multidisciplinary Teams

Coordination of care is essential if a patient is to benefit from multiple health care services provided by various health care professionals (Zwarenstein et al., 2009). The **multidisciplinary team**, like all interprofessional teams, is composed of individuals representing professional disciplines that serve the client. In the multidisciplinary team, each professional is responsible for identifying and carrying out one's own discipline-related evaluation and intervention. Multidisciplinary teams generally have access to each other's written record, as each typically contributes to chart notes, etc. If they meet as a group, which is often the case, they share information about their client's progress relative to the discipline specific goals, and they may coordinate their efforts. For example, they may arrange intervention sessions to be on the same day. Multidisciplinary teams can also provide an opportunity for its members to learn from each other. The objective, however, is coordination and cooperation, not necessarily to share goals with a common outcome. Although the expectation is that knowledge of the expertise of other team members will promote cooperation and communication that ultimately benefits the client; each team member functions in a parallel fashion and maintains professional autonomy (Jessup, 2007).

The multidisciplinary team can be seen in various settings, from inpatient and community settings to global crisis intervention and management. Consider the intervention plan for an individual with vision loss secondary to diabetes. The physician oversees medical care. The ophthalmologist and optometrist monitor and manage diabetic retinopathy. The occupational therapist addresses the individual's functional ability and safety in light of vision loss and peripheral neuropathy (see AOTA, 2011, for the specific role and function of an occupational therapist in diabetes management). The nurse addresses wound care, blood glucose monitoring, and prevention of complications, and the nutritionist monitors and educates about diet. Although each of these professionals has a focused role, the client benefits because these professionals share their knowledge and progress with each other.

Interdisciplinary Teams

The **interdisciplinary team** is distinct from the multidisciplinary team. Although similarly composed of members representing and using knowledge and skills of their respective discipline, the team members identify goals and plan intervention collaboratively. They also discuss with each other how their intervention plans will be implemented. Although their skills may complement each other, team members become interdependent as they work toward improving health outcomes for their clients. It is common for interdisciplinary teams to meet as a group with the client, the client's family, etc. This type of team is further distinguished from the multidisciplinary team in that some interventions may be jointly carried out, and the client is often involved in the decision-making process (Cartmill et al., 2011; Jessup, 2007).

The benefits of interdisciplinary teams are many (Jessup, 2007; Zwarenstein et al., 2009). It is client centered, giving the client a role in his or her care. Team members share their knowledge, which leads to respecting the roles and functions of each other. Because team members share a great deal with each other about how they implement intervention, a synergy develops in how different disciplines address common and complementary goals. Intervention plans for clients are developed holistically and cost-effectively. Job satisfaction is increased. Ultimately, client care and outcomes are enhanced.

There are several potential problems that can also emerge in the functioning of an interdisciplinary team. An overly assertive team member can dominate the meetings, thereby pushing an agenda that was not collaboratively agreed upon. A silent or unassertive team member can easily be ignored, assuming his or her silence means compliance. If a hierarchy develops, decision making can be negatively affected (Jessup, 2007). If norms develop that restrict equal participation of its team members, creative and innovative thinking can be inhibited. Many of these issues can be handled or even avoided if nonjudgmental, process-oriented discussions that focus on each member's experience and input are valued (Miller, 1989). The very important attribute of trust is key in ensuring effective teamwork.

Interdisciplinary teams are seen in many settings. In fact, settings have designed specific models of interdisciplinary teams that are deemed effective (Deering et al., 2011; Medlock, McKee, Feinstein, Bell, & Tracy, 2011). Consider, as an example, a day hospital setting serving those with major mental illnesses. An interdisciplinary team may decide that for a particular client with schizophrenia, the goal is to have him be able to live in a group home and participate in chores and be able to attend a sheltered workshop that prepares packages for shipment. Team members also are aware that he can become noncompliant with medication, has sensory processing issues, has difficulty with following instructions and making decisions, and complains about not seeing his brother often enough. In this team, different professionals address the same objectives and goals collaboratively. For example, the psychiatrist and nurse monitor his medication while the occupational therapist is able to observe if any medication side effects are interfering with function. The occupational therapist is addressing sensory and cognitive impairment while having the recreational therapist monitor changes in leisure function. The social worker is addressing family issues, with the occupational therapist and the nurse attending to activities of daily living (ADL) issues raised by the brother.

Transdisciplinary Teams

The **transdisciplinary team** is one that functions without discipline-centered boundaries. Members in these types of teams appear to have blurred roles because many of their role-related functions become interchangeable. As distinguished from interdisciplinary teams, the expertise related to discipline-specific tasks is shared and result in the taking on of each other's responsibilities (Cartmill et al., 2011). This type of team is the most efficient and may be cost-effective because in some examples, fewer professionals interact with a specific client (King, Tucker, Desserud, & Shillington, 2009).

It has been suggested that there are three key elements for successful and responsible transdiscipinary teamwork. The first is overall assessment conducted by one professional but observed by all. This type of arena assessment allows each to provide information based on their unique base of knowledge and skill. Next is ongoing interaction between team members so that each can continuously contribute their knowledge to the plan of care. Perhaps most critical is the third element, which is role release. This allows interprofessional intervention to be carried out by one individual. Ideally and responsibly, this should be done under the direction of and continuous consultation from those responsible for what is being implemented (King et al., 2009).

The transdisciplinary team can be highly effective if used with the right population and in the right manner. A noncompetitive and nonhierarchical environment is important in order to allow for effective intervention. These teams are especially helpful in situations where interprofessional intervention is required, yet it is in the best interest of the client to have only one individual interact. A very good example of effective transdisciplinary teamwork can be seen in a report of a home visiting program for infants in which the family benefits from the expertise of many professionals but interacts with only one (King et al., 2009). As described by these authors, a home-visiting program for infants with developmental disabilities is established, with the objectives of promoting child development along a series of domains. Rather than overwhelm the caregiver with various visiting professionals, one individual is assigned to each family. Team members learn theories and techniques from each other in order to provide service that spans disciplinary boundaries. The team is responsible for continually appraising and providing input to the professional who visits.

The transdisciplinary team approach is also useful in settings that can benefit from a system-wide approach, in settings with limited resources that do not have access to different professionals, in remote settings where access is limited, or following a crisis or natural disaster. The use of technology can support the functioning of transdisciplinary teams, ensuring a high level of competency.

Paramount for the success of transdisciplinary teams are the same elements identified for interdisciplinary teams: trust, communication, and respect. One concern of transdisciplinary teamwork is that when the "agent" for the team is not as skilled or knowledgeable as the team members being represented, the effectiveness of the intervention may be compromised. Furthermore, if an individual professional providing intervention ceases to obtain ongoing input from fellow team members, the client is at risk for adverse events.

Transdisciplinary approaches have additional concerns. As described in an AOTA report on the "Promotion of Occupational Therapy in Mental Health Systems" (Pitts et al., 2005), role blurring has a long history in community-based and some inpatient mental health settings. However, when disciplinary roles appear to merge, professional identity as well as discipline-specific expertise may be weakened. Furthermore, assuming responsibilities of other professionals gives rise to regulatory violations and scope of practice concerns. This is not the case when there is overlap in assessment and intervention modalities or techniques. Each team member has a responsibility to provide service within his or her scope of practice and request the provision of direct service from another team member when it is necessary to provide service outside of one's scope of practice.

Research Teams

Although much of this section has focused on interprofessional teams in practice settings, there are two important arenas in which interprofessional teams are critical for their success. The first that warrants mention is the research team.

In medically related research, for example, discipline-specific investigators focusing primarily on basic science have carried out investigations. Having one discipline central to a study can result in outcomes in which knowledge gaps are prevalent (Metzger & Zare, 1999). The advantages of interdisciplinary research include being able to better address the complex issues involved in research, allow for innovative approaches, and translate results into effective interventions (Rashid et al., 2009) that are functionally and clinically relevant. Interdisciplinary research identifies problems and solutions that are more easily adopted by an interdisciplinary practice environment (Logan & Graham, 1998). The federal government has placed increased emphasis on interdisciplinary collaborative research and has set up structures to support the translation and application of basic research to practice-related outcomes (Bear-Lehman, 2011; Rashid et al., 2009). It is critical that occupational science and occupational therapy researchers are part of these efforts (Bear-Lehman, 2011).

Health Care Policy Teams

Another area that warrants mention is health care policy development. Just as research and intervention addresses complex needs, health care policy deals with issues that are also multifaceted. From setting health care agendas to outlining their implementation in order to improve health service delivery, policymakers need to collaborate on teams to be effective. To ensure this, an interprofessional approach to policy development, just as with clinical care and with research, allows for access to varied sources of information and promotes perspectives that represent different areas of expertise. It has also been suggested that interprofessional team-based learning opportunities facilitate collaboration and enhances the development of effective health care policy (Rider, Brashers, & Costanza, 2008).

Scholarship: Presentations and Publications

More than a decade ago, Margo B. Holm (2000), in her Eleanor Clarke Slagle Lecture, called for occupational therapists to acquire evidence to support occupational therapy services and to practice based on that evidence

Practice Dilemma

You are an occupational therapist with 2 years of experience. You have been educated and trained in the use of physical agent modalities and have used these in your practice as part of preparatory procedures to enhance occupational performance. You have recently moved to another state that restricts your use of physical agent modalities. Your new place of employment uses transdisciplinary teams. You are the "lead" on your team with a particular client for whom the team determined the use of deep thermal modalities. It is expected by the team that you provide this service because they are aware of your abilities in this area.

As a new employee skilled in the use of such modalities, what do you do?

(see Table 35.3 for steps to become an evidence-based practitioner). Using evidence in practice, however, is challenging because it requires time and effort to identify evidence that addresses a particular practice situation. Despite this, it is critical for professionals to use as well as generate outcome studies that have met standards of scientific rigor in order to justify occupational therapy interventions.

Two of the many reasons to be an evidence-based practitioner are competency and currency. As scientific knowledge continues to amass in an ever-changing health care environment, practitioners, and educators alike need to embrace and be proficient in interventions proven to be efficacious and cost-effective. Learning from those with a proven scholarly record, such as individuals whose work has appeared in peer-reviewed journals or who are presenting research at conferences or workshops under organizations and/or companies that have met requirements for continuing education, such as AOTA Approved Provider of Continuing Education, is important. The information learned must be reliable, accurate, and evidence based. It is also incumbent on researchers to address questions pertinent to the practice of occupational therapy so that the services provided can be both efficacious and cost-effective. Thus, it is the responsibility of all occupational therapy practitioners to participate in learning opportunities based on the most recent knowledge that can be applied to practice.

Presenting and publishing is part of the professional role and provides another venue for sharing information (see Table 35.4). When one has an opportunity to present or to publish, it is similarly important to consider the context in which one chooses to present and publish. Again, presenting under the auspices of an approved provider of continuing education enhances its credibility. Presentations take many forms. Within clinical settings, one presents in a team meeting, at a grand rounds, and at in-service training. Some of these settings may appear informal, but the presenter must remember that his or her style of presenting will reflect his or her credibility and professionalism. In conference type settings, one might present a poster or platform presentation in which key points along with graphics are printed on a poster that is usually mounted to a bulletin board. A poster session, which typically lasts 2 hours, allows the presenter to discuss points of interest to those who review the poster. A paper presentation, which can be anywhere from 20 minutes to 2 hours, is a formal presentation to an audience and typically includes audiovisual technology. Workshop presentations, which are somewhat modeled after a classroom setting, also include audiovisual technology and can be in a half-day format or as long as a 5-day format. Panel presentations consist of several experts on a single topic in which brief presentations are made to

TABLE 35.3 Steps for Being an Evidence-Based Practitioner

Six Steps for Evidence-Based Practice
1. Identify the clinical question.
2. Search for evidence.
3. Evaluate the evidence for validity and utility.
4. Incorporate your assessment of the evidence with your clinical experience and expertise and from a client-centered perspective.
5. After implementing a change based on the evidence, think about its effectiveness and ease of putting into practice.
6. Share what you have learned.

Source: Lin, S. H., Murphy, S. L., & Robinson, J. (2010). The issue is—Facilitating evidence-based practice: Process, strategies, and resources. *American Journal of Occupational Therapy, 64*, 164–171. doi:10.5014/ajot.64.1.164

TABLE 35.4 A Sample of Venues for Disseminating Knowledge

Presentations		Publications	
Professional Venues	**Consumer Venues**	**Peer Reviewed**	**Non-Peer Reviewed**
Team meeting	Community event	Practice-oriented periodicals[a]	Trade magazines
In-service presentation	Consumer organization	Journals	Practice-oriented periodicals[a]
Grand rounds		Book chapters[a]	Newsletters
Poster session		Websites[a]	News periodicals
Panel discussion			Book chapters[a]
Platform sessions			Self-published books
Workshops			Blogs
Courses			Websites[a]

[a]These venues may or may not be peer reviewed.

facilitate discussion with the audience. Although each of these types of presentations allow for the dissemination of information, it is equally important to be sure that one's manner of presenting is professional. There are many guidelines available electronically and in libraries that one can refer to on *how* to present (e.g., Eggleston, n.d.), guidelines that remind one to be articulate, focus on the question at hand, and engage the audience, no matter how big or how small. These guidelines also include attention to eye contact; avoiding the use of filler words such as "um," "you know," and "like"; and maintenance of proper posture.

Similarly, there are various types of publications, each with varying levels of review and rigor. These not only target different audiences but may also have varying levels of perceived value as well. Publications fall into two general categories: peer-reviewed and non-peer reviewed. **Peer review** simply refers to a procedure in which a manuscript, once submitted for publication, is reviewed by experts in the field who provide feedback and contribute to the decision of whether or not the manuscript meets the criteria for publication. Peer review provides a layer of critical evaluation to the publishing process (Fletcher & Fletcher, 2003; Jacobs, 2009) and is often a more challenging route of publication for the writer. Peer-reviewed articles are typically in scientific journals. ***Non-peer review*** refers to manuscripts that are submitted or invited to be published in books, periodicals, or trade magazines and might be reviewed by an editor rather than go through a longer, more critical process (Jacobs, 2009). Non–peer reviewed articles are in news or practice-oriented periodicals and trade publications. Non-peer review also includes self-publication, such as blogs and personal Websites as well as self-published books. Publishing in peer-reviewed or non–peer reviewed media may carry different perceived value as a result of the review process. Electronic databases may even limit their searches of journal articles to those in selected peer-reviewed journals (ProQuest, 2004).

Professionalism and Social Media: Opportunities and Pitfalls

There is a great deal of dependency on and use of social media. Whether used as a way to network professionally or personally, **social media** is becoming a tool that enables one to communicate quickly and to a very wide audience. As more and more consumers use Internet

Ethical Dilemma

You decided to attend a continuing education workshop on treating cognitive deficits because the location and timing of this was convenient. Although the program was not being offered by an approved provider of continuing education, you knew that you could tally the hours spent and record these as professional development units. At the workshop, you received copies of the slideshow but no reference list. During the presentation, you realized that you had seen some of these slides at another workshop taught by a reputable scholar in the field. There was no mention of this scholar's name during the presentation. In addition, many of the examples given were anecdotal, with little or no evidence to support it. Finally, the only places you could find references to some of the facts that were given were in an online discussion board and in a therapist's blog.

Have any ethics been violated, and if so, which one(s)? What degree of scholarship was demonstrated by the presenter? What responsibility do you have to the other attendees or potential attendees? How might you handle your concerns without violating your ethical principles?

sites including social media sites to gain and share information about health care, a responsibility exists to ensure that this information is factual and evidence based. As stated in a recent PEW report (Fox, 2011), 75% of all adults in the United States use the Internet, 60% of all adults have used the Internet to access medical information, and between 7% and 11% have used social media sites to either gain medical information or to follow someone with a medical condition. These numbers are likely to increase.

Reasons for using such sites include obtaining information and seeking social connectedness. The use of social media is also on the rise for hospitals and professional practices, which are turning to this technology in order to provide information related to medical updates and health information to their patients and the general public (Ficarra, 2011). Social media sites are actively used by occupational therapists (Kashani, Burwash, & Hamilton, 2010).

Relationships and communication are often nurtured through social networks (Bahk, Sheil, Rohm, & Lin, 2010), yet behavior on these networks has come under scrutiny. Indeed, attention is being paid to how social media and other forms of electronic communications (e.g., e-mail, voice mail) are and have been used in education (Gerlich, Browning, & Westermann, 2010), health care (Chretien, Greysen, Chretien, & Kind, 2009), and corporate (Woodbury, 2000) contexts. The prevailing concern revolves around the individual's right to privacy and one's commitment to his or her professional environment.

Professionalism in the use of social media is important. Professionalism in part stems from a contract between one's discipline and society, and therefore, how one behaves is a reflection of his or her professionalism. It has been argued that because social media has such a widespread audience and that behavior on social media sites can reflect negatively on one's place of work and on one's profession, policies and guidelines are needed (Greysen, Kind, & Chretien, 2010).

Many have claimed that what one does on one's own time is an issue of individual rights and of privacy. Yet, by virtue of being on an Internet site, the information that is posted can be accessed by third parties (Barnes, 2006). There are reports of how universities, potential employers, and medical centers have all accessed sites for information or have launched investigations, as a result of what was shared (Anonymous, 2008; Resmer, 2006; "When No Patient," 2011). The Internet has not only allowed for efficient communication but has also widened the net with whom one communicates. As a result, professionals have an obligation to understand that their postings on any site can be viewed by unlimited numbers of individuals without restriction. Once information is posted, one can no longer control its intended audience.

There is mounting evidence of the misuse of social media sites by some professionals. News reports are filled with examples of employees improperly posting the following: disrespectful comments about their colleagues, clients, and place of work; photos and videos of work-related activities and people; and photos and videos of themselves or their friends engaged in compromising activities. Many of these types of postings have resulted in a wide range of disciplinary actions (Anonymous, 2008; Clark, 2011; "Facebook Can Ruin," 2008). There have been similar reports of health care students and professionals inappropriately posting (Chretien et al., 2009; Greysen et al., 2010; Lago, Kaufman, Asch, & Armstrong, 2008; Thompson, Dawson, Ferdig, & Black, 2008) with a call for stressing their awareness of professionalism when on the Internet (Chretien, Greysen, & Kind, 2010; Farnan, Reddy, & Arora, 2010; Jenssen & Klein, 2010). In addition to potential violations of Health Insurance Portability and Accountability Act (HIPAA) and Family and Educational Rights and Privacy Act (FERPA) legislation, ethical concerns have been raised. "Friending" patients and clients on Facebook, for example, may impact the therapeutic relationship (Guseh, Brendel, & Brendel, 2009). As stated earlier, inappropriate behaviors, even if subjectively inappropriate, can negatively impact the professional expectations held by the public.

Social media, however, can be an important tool in promoting one's profession. Just as it can be used to enhance learning opportunities at the college level (Gerlich et al., 2010), social media has and can be used to share relevant information with peers and to provide learning opportunities about health and wellness to the public (Greysen et al., 2010; McNab, 2009). Possible uses of social media include using blogs to teach persons with multiple sclerosis about energy conservation or fall prevention strategies to the elderly and providing tips on identifying cognitive impairment in daily activities or ways to identify the beginning signs of driving impairment. Using a Facebook site to promote a professional practice, sharing videos on sites such as YouTube that demonstrate an assessment or intervention technique, tweeting about opportunities for community participation, and connecting with professionals to promote evidence-based research collaboration on a specific topic are also possible uses of social media.

When producing content electronically, it is helpful to remember the "do's and don't's." Table 35.5 provides a checklist for proper online content and conduct.

Summary

The professional role carries with it a great deal of responsibility. Professionals, whose responsibilities are to one's clients, one's profession, and to society, are ambassadors for their field. Whether or not one is at work, with friends, or in the virtual world, how one is perceived as a person may be a reflection of who one is as a professional.

TABLE 35.5 Social Media and E-mail Checklist for the Professional

YES	NO	For Social Media Sites, such as Facebook, LinkedIn, Twitter, as well as Personal Websites and Blogs; for E-mails and Texts.
❑	❑	Did you target the correct audience for your posts?
❑	❑	Is the information you posted factual and backed up by evidence?
❑	❑	Are you in compliance with HIPAA and/or FERPA regulations?
❑	❑	Are you in compliance with your workplace's policies?
❑	❑	Are your remarks (and/or status updates) respectful (i.e., Did you avoid making comments that someone might find offensive or hurtful?)?
❑	❑	Did you use proper spelling, grammar, and punctuation in your professional postings? Did you avoid using "text" abbreviations, such as "u" or "r," on sites not limited in character number?
❑	❑	Did you avoid posting photographs or videos of yourself or others that can be considered improper, even if these photographs were taken and posted in non–work related venues (i.e., Would you want your family, your professors, your boss, or your clients to see these)?
❑	❑	If you posted a photo or video, does it comply with HIPAA, FERPA, and/or additional workplace policies?
❑	❑	Did you send a communication to a colleague that is grammatically and structurally correct?
❑	❑	Did you remember to sign your name on all e-mails so that the recipient can identify you?
❑	❑	Did you remember that whatever you post will be accessible forever, in spite of privacy assurances from Websites?
❑	❑	Did you avoid overuse of punctuation marks, all capital letters, and boldface in your e-mail? These may cause the reader to misinterpret your intent or make it difficult to read.
❑	❑	Does your e-mail reflect the appropriate level of formality? For example, did you avoid using the greeting "Hey" in a message to a colleague?

The world of occupational therapy is an exciting one. Our science is growing, our practice areas are expanding, and our presence is ubiquitous. As an occupational therapy professional, you have an opportunity to not only participate in this wonderful profession, but also to contribute to its development.

Ethical Dilemma

You are working in a mental health setting. A member of your interdisciplinary team, who often takes client groups to events in your community, has "friended" you on Facebook. You also socialize with this colleague after work hours.

You check your Facebook newsfeed and see that your coworker/friend has posted a photograph of the backs of a few of the clients under the marquee of a show they are about to see. The status update with this photo is "fun at work." You also see a photo posted of her at a bar, holding up two beer bottles. The status update on this photo is "just getting started."

What action do you take after seeing these posts? Do both posts warrant a response, as one was work related and one was not? What responsibility, if any, do you have to your employer?

References

Accreditation Council for Occupational Therapy Education. (2010). *Accreditation council for occupational therapy education (ACOTE) Standards and Interpretive Guidelines.* Bethesda, MD: American Occupational Therapy Association.

Alsop, R. (2008, Oct 21). The trophy kids go to work. *The Wall Street Journal*, p. D1.

American Occupational Therapy Association. (2002). *Fieldwork performance evaluation for the occupational therapy student.* Bethesda, MD: Author.

American Occupational Therapy Association. (2008). Occupational therapy practice framework: Domain and process, 2nd edition. *American Journal of Occupational Therapy, 62*, 625–683.

American Occupational Therapy Association. (2010a). Occupational therapy code of ethics and ethics standards. *American Journal of Occupational Therapy*, 64:S17–S267.

American Occupational Therapy Association. (2010b). Standards of practice for occupational therapy. *American Journal of Occupational Therapy, 64*(6 Suppl.), S10–S11. doi:10.5014/ajot.2010.64.

American Occupational Therapy Association. (2011). *Occupational therapy's role in diabetes self-management.* Retrieved from http://www.aota.org/Practitioners/PracticeAreas/Aging/Tools/Diabetes.aspx?FT=.pdf

Anonymous. (2008). NC school employee fired over Facebook posting. *Spartanburg Herald- Journal.* Retrieved from http://ezproxy.cul.columbia.edu/login?url=http://search.proquest.com/docview/370252926?accountid=10226./

Aurora, V., Wayne, D., Anderson, R., Didwania, A., & Humphrey, H. (2008). Unprofessional behavior of interns. *Journal of the American Medical Association, 300*, 1132–1134.

Bahk, C. M., Sheil, A., Rohm, C. E., & Lin, F. (2010). Digital media dependency, relational orientation and social networking. *Communications of the IIMA*, *10*(3), 69–78.

Baldwin, D. C., Jr. (2007). Some historical notes on interdisciplinary and interprofessional education and practice in health care in the USA. *Journal of Interprofessional Care*, *21*(s1), 23–37. (Reprinted from *Journal of Interprofessional Care*, 1996, *10*, 173–187).

Barnes, S. (2006). A privacy paradox: Social networking in the United States. *First Monday*, *11*(9). Retrieved from http://firstmonday.org/htbin/cgiwrap/bin/ojs/index.php/fm/article/view/1394/1312

Bear-Lehman, J. (2011). The NIH Roadmap: An opportunity for occupational therapy. *OTJR: Occupation, Participation, and Health*, *31*, 106–107.

Cartmill, C., Soklaridis, S., & Cassidy, J. D. (2011). Transdisciplinary teamwork: The experience of clinicians. *Journal of Occupational Rehabilitation*, *21*, 1–8.

Chretien, K. C., Greysen, S. R., Chretien, J., & Kind, T. (2009). Online posting of unprofessional content by medical students. *Journal of the American Medical Association*, *302*, 1309–1315.

Chretien, K. C., Greysen, S. R., & Kind, T. (2010). Medical students and unprofessional online content [Letter to the editor]. *Journal of the American Medical Association*, *303*, 329.

Clark, A. (2011). Watch what you post: Your boss also is watching. *Gainesville Sun*. Retrieved fron http://www.gainesville.com/article/20110218/ARTICLES/110219428

Clouder, L. (2003). Becoming professional: Exploring the complexities of professional socialization in health and social care. *Learning in Health & Social Care*, *2*, 213–222.

Coulehan, J. (2005). Viewpoint: Today's professionalism: Engaging the mind but not the heart. *Academic Medicine*, *80*, 892–898.

Cruess, R., & Cruess, S. (2006). Teaching professionalism: General principles. *Medical Teacher*, *28*, 205–208.

Cruess, R., & Cruess, S. (2009). Cognitive base of professionalism. In R. Cruess, S. Cruess, & Y. Steinert (Eds.), *Teaching medical professionalism* (pp. 7–30). New York, NY: Cambridge University Press.

Cruess, R., Cruess, S., & Steinert, Y. (Eds.) (2009). Core attributes of professionalism. *Teaching medical professionalism* (pp. 285–286). New York, NY: Cambridge University Press.

Deering, S. J., Johnston, L. C., & Colacchio, K. (2011). Multidisciplinary teamwork and communication training. *Seminars in Perinatology*, *35*, 89–96.

Dillon, T. (2001). Practitioner perspectives: Effective intraprofessional relationships in occupational therapy. *Occupational Therapy in Health Care*, *14*, 1–15.

Eggleston, S. (n.d.). *Key steps to an effective presentation*. Retrieved from http://www.theegglestongroup.com/writing/keystep1.php

Facebook can ruin your life. And so can MySpace, Bebo . . . : People will post just about anything on social networking sites. (2008). *Belfast Telegraph*. Retrieved from http://www.belfasttelegraph.co.uk/lifestyle/technology-gadgets/facebook-can-ruin-your-life-and-so-can-myspace-bebo-13384229.html

Farnan, J. M., Reddy, S. T., & Arora, V. M. (2010). Medical students and unprofessional online content [Letter to the editor]. *Journal of the American Medical Association*, *303*, 328.

Ficarra, B. (2011). *Social media: Medical social networking—Part 2*. Retrieved from http://healthin30.com/2011/03/social-media-medical-social-networking-part-2/

Fischer, K. (2005). Professional behaviors as a foundation for fieldwork. *Occupational Therapy Practice*, *11*(4), 10–12.

Fletcher, R. H., & Fletcher, S. W. (2003). The effectiveness of journal peer review. In F. A. Godlee (Ed.), *Peer review in health sciences* (2nd ed., pp. 62–75). London, United Kingdom: BMJ Books.

Fogg, P. (2008, July 18). When generations collide. *The Chronical of Higher Education*, *54*(45), p. B18.

Fox, S. (2011). *The social life of health information, 2011*. Retrieved from http://pewinternet.org/Reports/2011/Social-Life-of-Health-Info.aspx

Gerlich, R. N., Browning, L., & Westermann, L. (2010). The Social Media Affinity Scale: Implications for education. *Contemporary Issues in Education Research*, *3*, 35–41.

Glennon, T. (2009). Millennials in the workforce: Implications for managers. *Special Interest Section Quarterly: Administration and Management*, *25*(1), 1–4.

Glennon, T., & Van Oss, T. (2010). Identifying and promoting professional behavior: Best practices for establishing, maintaining, and improving professional behavior by occupational therapy practitioners. *Occupational Therapy Practice*, *15*(17), 13–16.

Greysen, S. R., Kind, T., & Chretien, K. C. (2010). Online professionalism and the mirror of social media. *Journal of General Internal Medicine*, *25*, 1227–1229.

Guseh, J. S., II, Brendel, R., & Brendel, D. H. (2009). Medical professionalism in the age of online social networking. *Journal of Medical Ethics*, *35*, 584–586.

Hafferty, F. (2009). Professionalism and the socialization of medical students. In R. Cruess, S. Cruess, & Y. Steinert (Eds.), *Teaching medical professionalism* (pp. 53–70). New York, NY: Cambridge University Press.

Holm, M. B. (2000). The 2000 Eleanor Clarke Slagle Lecture. Our mandate for the new millennium: Evidence-based practice. *American Journal of Occupational Therapy*, *54*, 575–585.

Jacobs, K. (2009). Professional presentations and publications. In E. B. Crepeau, E. S. Cohn, & B. A. Schell (Eds.), *Willard and Spackman's occupational therapy* (11th ed., pp. 411–417). Philadelphia, PA: Lippincott Williams & Wilkins.

Jenssen, B. P., & Klein, J. D. (2010). Medical students and unprofessional online content [Letter to the editor]. *Journal of the American Medical Association*, *303*, 328.

Jessup, R. L. (2007). Interdisciplinary versus multidisciplinary care teams: Do we understand the difference? *Australian Health Review*. Retrieved from http://findarticles.com/p/articles/mi_6800/is_3_31/ai_n28446050

Johnson, S. (2006). See one, do one, teach one: Developing professionalism across the generations. *Clinical Orthopaedics and Related Research*, (449), 186–192.

Johnson, S. A., & Romanello, M. L. (2005). Generational diversity: Teaching and learning approaches. *Nurse Educator*, *30*, 212–216.

Jones, A., & Jones, D. (2011). Improving teamwork, trust, and safety: An ethnographic study of an interprofessional initiative. *Journal of Interprofessional Care*, *25*, 175–181.

Kalisch, B. J., Lee, H., & Rochman, M. (2010). Nursing staff teamwork and job satisfaction. *Journal of Nursing Management*, *18*, 938–947.

Kashani, R. M., Burwash, S., & Hamilton, A. (2010). To be or not to be on Facebook: That is the question. *Occupational Therapy Now*, *12*(6), 19–22.

King, G., Tucker, M., Desserud, S., & Shillington, M. (2009). The application of a transdisciplinary model for early intervention services. *Infants & Young Children*, *22*, 211–223.

Kohn, L., Corrigan, J., & Donaldson, M. (Eds.). (2000). *To err is human: Building a safer health system*. Retrieved from http://www.nap.edu/catalog/9728.html

Konrath, S. H., O'Brien, E. H., & Hsing, C. (2011). Changes in dispositional empathy in American college students over time: A meta-analysis. *Personality and Social Psychology Review*, *15*, 180–198.

Krinn, K. (2011). What is professionalism? *Journal of Environmental Health*, *73*, 4–5.

Kurlander, M., Morin, J., & Wynia, K. (2004). The social-contract model of professionalism: Baby or bath water? *American Journal of Bioethics*, *4*, 33–36.

Lago, T., Kaufman, E. J., Asch, D. A., & Armstrong, K. (2008). Content of weblogs written by health professionals. *Journal of General Internal Medicine*, *23*, 1642–1646.

Lake, P. (2009, April 17). Student discipline: The case against legalistic approaches. *The Chronicle of Higher Education*, *55*(32), pp. A31–A32.

Lancaster, L., & Stillman, D. (2002). *When generations collide*. New York, NY: Harper Collins.

Lin, S. H., Murphy, S. L., & Robinson, J. (2010). The issue is—Facilitating evidence-based practice: Process, strategies, and resources. *American Journal of Occupational Therapy*, *64*, 164–171. doi:10.5014/ajot.64.1.164

Logan, J., & Graham, I. (1998). Toward a comprehensive interdisciplinary model of health care research use. *Science Communication*, *20*(2), 227–246. doi:10.1177/1075547098020002004

Lower, J. (2008). Brace yourself here comes generation Y. *Critical Care Nurse, 28*, 80–85.

McNab, C. (2009). What social media offers to health professionals and citizens. *Bulletin of the World Health Organization, 87*, 566–567.

Medlock, A., McKee, E., Feinstein, J., Bell, S. H., & Tracy, C. S. (2011). Applying an innovative model of interprofessional team practice: The view from occupational therapy. *Occupational Therapy Now, 13*(3), 7–9.

Mercier, H., & Sperber, D. (2011). Why do humans reason? Arguments for an argumentative theory. *Behavioral and Brain Sciences, 34*, 57–111. doi:10.1017/S0140525X10000968

Metzger, N., & Zare, R. (1999). Interdisciplinary research: From belief to reality. *Science, 283*, 642–643. doi:10.1126/science.283.5402.642

Miller, P. A. (1989). Teaching process: Its importance in geriatric teamwork. *Physical and Occupational Therapy in Geriatrics, 6*(3–4), 121–132. doi:10.1080/J148V06N03_07

Mohr, N., Moreno-Walton, L., Mills, A. M., Brunett, P. H., & Promes, S. B. (2011). Generational influences in academic emergency medicine: Teaching and learning, mentoring, and technology (Part I). *Academic Emergency Medicine, 18*, 190–199.

Monrouxe, L., Reese, C. E., & Hu, W. (2011). Professionalism. *Medical Education, 45*, 585–602.

Paterson, M., & Higgs, J. (2008). Professional practice judgement artistry. In J. Higgs, M. A. Jones, S. Loftus, & N. Christensen (Eds.), *Clinical reasoning in the health professions* (pp. 181–189). Philadelphia, PA: Elsevier.

Pitts, D. B., Lamb, A., Ramsay, D., Learnard, L., Clark, F., Scheinholtz, M., . . . Nanoff, T. (2005). *Promotion of occupational therapy in mental health systems.* Retrieved from http://www.aota.org/News/Centennial/Background/AdHoc/41327/41347.aspx?FT=.pdf

ProQuest. (2004). *Scholarly journals, trade publications, and popular magazines.* Retrieved from http://training.proquest.com/trc/training/en/peervsscholarly.pdf

Rampell, C. (2011). Are young college grads too lazy to work? *Economix: Explaining the Science of Everyday Life.* Retrieved from http://economix.blogs.nytimes.com/2011/05/19/are-young-college-grads-too-lazy-to-work/?pag

Rashid, J., Spengler, R., Wagne, R., Melanson, C., Skillen, E., Mays, R. J., Jr., . . . Long, J. (2009). Eliminating health disparities through transdisciplinary research, cross-agency collaboration, and public participation. *American Journal of Public Health, 99*, 1955–1961. doi:10.2105/AJPH.2009.167932

Resmer, C. (2006, April 26). UVM students pay for Facebook faux pas. *Seven Days, 11*, p. 13A.

Rider, E. A., Brashers, V. L., & Costanza, M. E. (2008). Using interprofessional team-based learning to develop health care policy. *Medical Education, 42*, 519–520.

Salas, E., Rosen, M. A., & King, H. (2007). Managing teams managing crises: Principles of teamwork to improve patient safety in the emergency room and beyond. *Theoretical Issues in Ergonomics, 8*, 381–394.

Schwartz, K. B. (2009). Reclaiming our heritage: Connecting the founding vision to the centennial vision [Eleanor Clarke Slagle Lecture]. *American Journal of Occupational Therapy, 63*, 681–690.

Sinclair, L. B., Lingard, L. A., & Mohabeer, R. N. (2009). What's so great about rehabilitation teams? An ethnographic study of interprofessional collaboration in a rehabilitation unit. *Archives of Physical Medicine and Rehabilitation, 90*, 1196–1201.

Swick, H. (2000). Toward a normative definition of medical professionalism. *Academic Medicine, 75*, 612–616.

Thompson, L. A., Dawson, K., Ferdig, R., & Black, E. W. (2008). The intersection of online social networking with medical professionalism. *Journal of General Internal Medicine, 23*, 954–957.

Tulgan, B. (2009). *Not everyone gets a trophy.* San Francisco, CA: Jossey-Bass.

Twenge, J. M. (2006). *Generation me: Why today's young Americans are more confident, assertive, entitled—And more miserable than ever before.* New York, NY: Free Press.

Twenge, J. M., & Campbell, W. K. (2009). *The narcissism epidemic: Living in the age of entitlement.* New York, NY: Free Press.

Wear, D., & Kuczewski, M. (2004). The professionalism movement: Can we pause? *The American Journal of Bioethics, 4*, 1–10.

When no patient privacy interests were implicated, court enjoined nursing college's suspension of student who posted medical photos on facebook. (2011). *The Computer & Internet Lawyer, 28*(4), 19–20.

Wood, W. (2004). The heart, mind, and soul of professionalism in occupational therapy. *American Journal of Occupational Therapy, 58*, 249–257.

Woodbury, M. (2000). Email, voicemail, and privacy: What policy is ethical? *Science and Engineering Ethics, 6*, 235–244.

Wynia, M. K., Latham, S. R., Kao, A. C., Berg, J. W., & Emanuel, L. L. (1999). Medical professionalism in society. *The New England Journal of Medicine, 341*, 1612–1616.

Youngstrom, M. (2002). The occupational therapy practice framework: The evolution of our professional language. *American Journal of Occupational Therapy, 56*, 607–608.

Zemke, R. R. (2000). *Generations at work—Managing the clash of veterans, boomers, xers and nexters in your workplace.* New York, NY: AMA Publications.

Zwarenstein, M., Goldman, J., & Reeves, S. (2009). Interprofessinal collaboration: Effects of practice-based interventions n professional practice and healthcare outcomes. *Cochrane Database of Systematic Reviews*, (3), CD000072. doi:10.1002/14651858.CD000072.pub2

For additional resources on the subjects discussed in this chapter, visit http://thePoint.lww.com/Willard-Spackman12e.

CHAPTER 36

Documentation in Practice

Karen M. Sames

OUTLINE

"It's not what you tell them . . . it's what they hear."

—RED AUERBACH

LEARNING OBJECTIVES

After reading this chapter, you will be able to:

1. Identify the primary reasons for documentation of occupational therapy services
2. Describe the types of clinical, educational, and administrative documentation used in occupational therapy practice
3. Compare and contrast the key features of occupational therapy documentation in clinical and educational settings
4. Identify the components of well-written goals
5. Write a SOAP note
6. Discuss ethical issues in documentation

Introduction

Occupational therapy practitioners communicate with many different types of people on a daily basis. They provide instructions for home programs to clients and their caregivers. They inform other professionals on the care team about the client's progress in occupational therapy. They write letters to foundations seeking funding for new programs. This chapter will address the various audiences and types of documentation that occupational therapy practitioners may use at some point during their careers.

Audience

How one documents depends greatly on who will read it—one's audience. Writers must understand the reader's background and motives (Oliu, Brausaw, & Alred, 1995). How a letter to an insurance company is worded might be very different from the way a letter to a parent or physician is worded. Documentation that is read by members of the clinical care team might use more precise anatomical and technical words than would an Individualized Family Service Plan (IFSP) that is shared with the parents of a 2-year-old. Knowing who will read what is being communicated is an important aspect of effective documentation.

The potential audiences for occupational therapy documentation include the following:

- Medical professionals (medical doctors, nurses, psychologists, physical therapists, speech-language pathologists, social workers, case managers, quality management staff, etc.)
- Education professionals (teachers, principals, etc.)
- Lawyers, judges, and juries
- Accreditation agencies (the Joint Commission, Commission on Accreditation of Rehabilitation Facilities [CARF], Department of Education, etc.)
- Payers (health maintenance organizations, Medicare contractors, Medicaid reviewers, etc.)
- The client or the client's guardian

Each audience reads documentation through a different lens, depending on practice setting, educational level, motivation, and cultural background (Sames, 2010).

Communicating with medical professionals requires the writer to be very precise. A physician, for example, would not be satisfied with a diagnosis of "stroke" for a client with whom the occupational therapy practitioner is working. The physician might want to know whether the stroke was affecting the right or left side, whether it was mild or severe, and how long it has been since the stroke. Nurses need to know more than that the patient needs assistance with dressing; they need to know how much assistance and the nature of the assistance.

When one is communicating in a school setting, there is a need to focus on the educational relevance of the information. The entire team working with the child might not understand medical jargon, so educational terms are more appropriate.

Occupational therapy practitioners need to communicate with each other and with other professionals. The word choices and the tone of the writing or speech used in professional, or formal, communication are very different from those used in informal communication between friends. Professional communication requires a level of respect and formality that is not found in informal communication.

Professional communication uses complete sentences and avoids slang or emotionally charged words. Informal communication often uses slang and emotionally charged words and is usually directed toward someone known by the speaker or writer. When writing appeal letters, official memos, or progress notes, the writer might or might not know the person on the receiving end of the communication. Professional titles, rather than first names, are used in professional communication. This is where first impressions count.

Formal documentation often requires compliance with specific standards. For example, the Individuals with Disabilities Education Act (IDEA) requires that specific items be included on the Individualized Education Program (IEP), and Medicare requires specific documentation elements for outpatient therapy reimbursement. The Joint Commission requires that certain abbreviations be avoided to minimize the likelihood of medical errors due to abbreviations that are remarkably close in appearance (The Joint Commission, 2012). In addition, employers might have policies or procedures that further direct the method (electronic or paper and pen), timing, placement, and word choices of the documentation. Box 36.1 contains some documentation tips that apply to all documentation.

Two important considerations for all documentation are the following:

1. People form an impression of your professionalism and intelligence by reading what you write.
2. What you write can be used as evidence in a court proceeding, whether you are on trial or not (Sames, 2010).

Legal and Ethical Considerations

Health records are legal documents. Health records can be entered as evidence in any type of legal proceeding involving **malpractice**, **fraud**, **negligence**, or **incompetence**. Occupational therapy documentation can be called into

BOX 36.1 Documentation Tips

- Use correct
  - Grammar
  - Spelling
  - Syntax
  - Word choice
  - Literacy level for the reader(s)
- Read spell-checker and grammar checker recommendations carefully; sometimes it is better to click "Ignore" than to use what they recommend.
- Follow directions carefully.
- Have a dictionary and a writing manual handy.
- Write legibly.
- Proofread, proofread, and proofread again (Sames, 2010).

court, with or without the occupational therapist being there to explain the documentation, even years after the services were provided. What was written at or near the actual time the event or events in question occurred is stronger evidence than what a person can recall months or years after the event. To remain mindful that all documentation is legal evidence, some people mentally preface their documentation by saying to themselves "Ladies and gentlemen of the jury . . ." before putting pen to paper (Sames, 2010).

Medicare and other government payers can review clinical documentation and client charge (billing) records at any time to determine whether fraud has been committed. If documentation is not adequate to support the charges, Medicare (and other payers) can refuse to pay for the services; and the occupational therapist responsible for documenting the services could face both civil and criminal penalties, as well as loss of certification and licensure (Centers for Medicare & Medicaid Services [CMS], 2012; Fremgen, 2002; Kornblau & Starling, 2000; Liang, 2000).

In addition to legal issues of documentation, there are ethical concerns. The American Occupational Therapy Association (AOTA) Code of Ethics and Ethical Standards (2010) states in Principle 3.H that occupational therapy practitioners shall "maintain the confidentiality of all verbal, written, electronic, augmentative, and non-verbal communications, including compliance with HIPAA regulations" (p. 6). The document goes on to say in Principles 6.C and D that occupational therapy practitioners shall "record and report in an accurate and timely manner, and in accordance with applicable regulations, all information related to professional activities" and "ensure that documentation for reimbursement purposes is done in accordance with applicable laws, guidelines, and regulations" (p. 9). Thus, the key ethical issues in documentation include confidentiality, accuracy, timeliness, and compliance.

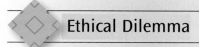

Ethical Dilemma

Documentation Standards

You work for a company that provides on-call occupational therapy personnel to hospitals and long-term care facilities in a large metropolitan area. You have been asked to work at a large, long-term care facility that normally has a part-time occupational therapist and a full-time occupational therapy assistant. The occupational therapist went into labor early, and the temporary person who was hired to take her place during her maternity leave cannot start for at least 3 weeks. You have never worked in this facility before, but you have worked in other long-term care facilities and are familiar with the documentation requirements for Medicare and Medicaid.

On your first day there, you open the file for your patients and see that a few patients should have had 90-day intervention plans (renewals) written last week; but you can find no evidence that this was done. You ask the occupational therapy assistant whether the documentation could be somewhere else, and he says no. You find some progress notes on these patients, but they are irregular and inconsistent. Mostly, they just list some activities the patients worked on and say that the patients continue to progress toward their goals. Ten minutes later, you get a call from the medical records director saying that there are five patients for whom she cannot find a discontinuation summary and that the discontinuation summaries are needed for reimbursement. She asks you to write them, even though you have never seen the patients and the patients were discharged from the facility over a week ago. You know that the documentation must be done in order for the facility to get paid, but you feel uncomfortable documenting the care of patients you have never seen. The occupational therapy assistant says that he cannot help you because he is too busy with his own patients and he did not pay a lot of attention to the patients the occupational therapist was working with. What do you do?

Documentation in Clinical Settings

In hospitals, rehabilitation facilities, outpatient clinics, long-term care, mental health centers, home health, and related settings, similar types of documentation are used, although the frequency of documentation may vary. Clinical documentation generally involves reporting and interpreting the clients' responses on assessments and to interventions in a clinical record. Clinical documentation is important for the following reasons:

- Continuity of care within the department
- Communication across shifts, disciplines
- Chronological record of care
- Legal record
- Reimbursement requirements (Sames, 2010)

It is critical that the objective information reported in the documentation be clearly differentiated from the subjective information. Both are important. If a practitioner states that a client appeared depressed, that is a subjective statement. It is a conclusion drawn from the practitioner's observations. To make an objective statement, the practitioner should describe what was seen or heard that would logically lead to the conclusion that the client appeared depressed. For example, the practitioner could say, "Client stared at the floor for the entire session. She slouched forward in her chair, responded to questions with one syllable words, and did not initiate any conversations with peers."

All clinical documentation must be done in compliance with the standards of the setting and the payers as well as standards set by the profession. For example, every entry in the clinical record must be dated (AOTA, 2008a). With electronic documentation, the date and time are automatically recorded by the system. If the documentation is handwritten, the date must be put either at the top of the documentation or at the bottom, by the signature, whichever is the standard at the facility. The essential features of all clinical documentation are as follows (items with an * are automatic in an electronic health record):

- *Date of completion of report
- *Full signature and **credentials**
- *Type of document
- *Client name and case number
- Acceptable abbreviations as determined by the facility
- Acceptable terminology as determined by the facility
- Record storage and disposal that complies with federal and state laws and facility procedures
- Protections of confidentiality (AOTA, 2008a; Sames, 2010)

In addition, if the documentation is handwritten, the following essential features apply:

- Corrections made with a single line through the error and initials of person who made the error are written above
- No use of an eraser or correction tape or fluid
- Black or blue ink, never pencil (Sames, 2010; AOTA, 2008a)

The occupational therapy practitioner's rationale—the reasons behind the intervention—should be made clear in the documentation. For example, clients with mental health challenges might have problems in living that are not as visible as physical challenges. Whereas people who use wheelchairs might have difficulty with grocery shopping because they cannot reach all the shelves or push the cart while seated in a wheelchair, people with bipolar disorder might have difficulty shopping because of an inability to control impulses to buy everything and talk to everyone in the store. Simply saying a client is working on shopping is not sufficient; the rationale for working on this occupation must be made clear.

Documentation of the Initiation of Occupational Therapy Services

The first type of clinical documentation reflects the first steps in the clinician–client interaction. In some settings, such as in a long-term care facility, the first step is a **screening** of all new admissions to the facility. A screening is used to determine whether or not the person would benefit from an occupational therapy evaluation. In other settings, the first step might be an introduction, or it might be the beginning of the evaluation process.

If the client is seen for a screening or introduction prior to an **evaluation**, a short note is usually written in the health record summarizing the conversation and/or results of the screening. The occupational therapist or occupational therapy assistant writes a short summary and indicates the next step in the intervention process.

Evaluation reports are written by occupational therapists to document the starting point of occupational therapy intervention. Occupational therapy assistants may contribute to the evaluation, but the responsibility for writing the evaluation report rests with the occupational therapist (AOTA, 2010). Evaluation reports contain factual data collected during the evaluation process and an interpretation of the evaluation findings. The need for occupational therapy services must be documented before interventions can be implemented. The report must show which occupations are limited or at risk of being limited. Often, there will be an initial **plan of care** (also called care plan, treatment plan, or intervention plan) embedded in the evaluation report. This plan includes measurable, functional, and time-limited goals for the client (Borcherding, 2000; Sames, 2010).

The AOTA (2008a) guidelines for documentation identify content needed for an evaluation. The evaluation report content is based on the "Occupational Therapy Practice Framework: Domain and Process, 2nd Edition" (AOTA, 2008b). In an acute care setting, especially for short stay clients, a complete evaluation might not be conducted. Although AOTA recommends that a complete evaluation be conducted and documented for each client, the time constraints of certain settings might require that the occupational therapist abbreviate the evaluation process.

Because payers often make decisions about whether or not to pay for occupational therapy on the basis of the evaluation report, it must show the need for skilled occupational therapy intervention (Lemke, 2004). The documentation must contain enough information to communicate that occupational therapy is the appropriate discipline to provide the needed intervention, it meets a medical need, requires the skills of an occupational therapist or occupational therapy assistant under the supervision of an occupational therapist, and that intervention will result in change in the client's function (Lemke, 2004).

Typically, the evaluation report contains the following:

- Identifying information and background information (e.g., client's name, age, diagnosis or condition, date of referral, date of report, **precautions**, and **contraindications**)
- Referral information (date, time, who referred the client, and why)
- Evaluation procedures and/or tests used
- **Occupational profile**
- Findings or results of the evaluation process (**occupational analysis**)
- An interpretation of the meaning of the findings or results that reflects the occupational needs of the client
- A plan, including goals, frequency, duration, and location of intervention
- Signature and credentials of the occupational therapist (AOTA, 2008a; Sames, 2010)

The occupational profile (AOTA, 2008b) summarizes the client's "occupational history and experiences, patterns of daily living, interests, values, and needs" (p. 649). This information is gathered primarily through interviewing the client (or client's surrogate). It will help the occupational therapist understand the client's concerns and goals and be useful in selecting outcome measures

The occupational analysis is the process of selecting and administering appropriate assessment tools, and then using this information, along with the information gathered from the occupational profile, to develop a hypothesis about what is going on with the client and set goals to help the client achieve desired outcomes (AOTA, 2008b).

The initial plan of care is based on the occupational profile and occupational analysis. The initial plan of care sets long- (outcome) and short-term goals, and describes the types of interventions that will be used to help the client achieve his or her goals.

The occupational therapist, with input from the occupational therapy assistant, and in collaboration with the client, sets short- and long-term goals. Long-term goals describe what the client will do by the time of discharge from occupational therapy—the outcome of occupational therapy interventions. Short-term goals describe what the client will do in the next 1 to 30 days. If the client will receive occupational therapy services for just a couple days, only one set of goals may be developed rather than separate long- and short-term goals. All goals must address performance in areas of occupation, describe observable behavior, be measureable, and be time limited (state target date for when the goal will be met) (Sames, 2010). See Table 36.1 for examples of poorly written goals and how to improve them.

The goals and interventions will help the client create or promote health, establish (habilitate) or restore (rehabilitate or remediate) function, maintain or preserve occupational performance, modify (compensate or adapt) contexts or activity demands, or prevent barriers to performance (AOTA, 2008b).

Documentation of Continuing Occupational Therapy Services

In clinical settings, **progress notes**, or clinical notes, are usually written after each intervention session. The occupational therapy practitioner who provided the service writes the progress note. Although Medicare does not require that progress notes written by an occupational therapy assistant be cosigned by the occupational therapist, state licensure laws may dictate whether or not a progress note needs to be cosigned (Sames, 2010). Progress notes may be written in a narrative or SOAP format or on a flow sheet (Sames, 2010). Regardless of the format, this documentation must show what the client did in occupational therapy and describe the client's reaction to the intervention that was provided. The progress note should include more than a list of the activities the client engaged in during the session. A reader will want to know how client's performance has changed since the last intervention session, any functional improvements, adaptive equipment provided, and client or caregiver understanding of any instructions (Lemke, 2004; Sames, 2010).

One of the most common forms of documenting the client's progress is called a **SOAP note**. This note writing format is used by many medical disciplines, a practice

TABLE 36.1 Examples of Poorly Written Goals and Improved Goals

Examples of Poorly Written Goals	Examples of Improved Goals	Why the Improved Goal is Better
Improve elbow range of motion	By June 1, 2012, Maria will use elbow flexion and extension to fold three t-shirts.	It specifies by when the goal will be met and describes performance in an area of occupation.
Jamal will dress himself independently.	Jamal will consistently dress himself, including shoes and socks, independently by discharge.	It is more specific about what is included in "dressing himself" and specifies by when the goal will be achieved.
Tsoyushi will use an adapted pencil to write legibly by the end of the year.	By June 15, 2012, Tsoyushi will write two complete, legible sentences within 5 minutes.	It is more specific about the length of the goal, it includes a measurement (2 legible sentences within 5 minutes).
By September 13, 2012, Agnes will make toast and tea.	By September 13, 2012, Agnes will prepare toast and tea with no more than one verbal cue.	It includes a measurement.
Jenny will put six golf tees in each bag, completing each bag in 2 minutes or less, with 90% accuracy on 75% of trials on 3 consecutive days within 2 weeks.	By August 8, 2012 Jenny will package golf tees accurately on 75% of trials.	It is clearer—the original goal had too many measurements, and providing an end date for the goal is clearer than saying within 2 weeks.

Information compiled from the following sources: Humphry, 2006; Crosnoe, 2011; Packer, 2008.

that strengthens communication among professionals. Dr. Lawrence Weed developed the SOAP note format in the 1960s as part of a Problem-Oriented Medical Record (Borcherding, 2000; Sames, 2010). Each letter of the word SOAP represents a different component of the note (Borcherding, 2000; Sames, 2010):

S = Subjective: the subjective experience of the client, what the client says
O = Objective: the clinician's objective observations and measurements
A = Assessment: the clinician's interpretation of the meaning of the "O" section
P = Plan: description of what will happen next (frequency, duration, location)

The most difficult part of writing a SOAP note is separating the objective information from the interpretation of it (assessment). Every statement in the "A" section needs to be supported with evidence in the "S" and the "O" sections (Sames, 2010). Box 36.2 shows an example of a SOAP note.

A progress report is written to document progress over a period of time. The required frequency of progress notes may be dictated by third-party payers. For example, Medicare has specific documentation requirements for long-term care settings that change over time. The CMS (CMS.gov) is the best source of up-to-date information regarding these documentation requirements. The progress report must be written by the occupational therapist, but an occupational therapy assistant may contribute to the report (CMS, 2008).

An updated plan of care is written in settings in which clients are seen for an extended period of time (up to 90 calendar days, depending on the setting). This documents the progress that has occurred since the last plan of care was written (or an explanation for lack of progress); updates the short-term goals and sets new ones; and verifies the frequency, duration, and location of continued intervention (AOTA, 2008a; Sames 2010). The long-term goal, the outcome goal, usually remains the same.

Documentation of Termination of Occupational Therapy Services

Once clients have met their long- and short-term goals or other circumstances require that occupational therapy services end, a **discontinuation summary** (discharge summary) is written (AOTA, 2008a; Sames 2010). This summary includes the following:

- Client identification and background information
- Summary of the client's functional status at the initiation of occupational therapy services
- Summary of change in functional status at the close of occupational therapy services
- Results of outcome measures
- Recommendations for follow-up
- Signature, credentials, and date

According to AOTA (2008b), outcomes of occupational therapy intervention can include "occupational performance, adaptation, health and wellness, participation, prevention, self-advocacy, quality of life, and occupational justice" (p. 661). Outcomes are reflected in subjective and objective data gathered at the end of occupational therapy interventions. Subjective data would be based on client reports, and objective data would come from standardized or non-standardized testing (AOTA, 2008b).

Electronic Health Records

Electronic health records are replacing paper charts in many practice settings. Electronic health records require health care providers to enter clinical data into a computerized system. These systems may use desktop, laptop, or tablet computers; smartphones; or other handheld devices (Figure 36.1). Because these systems are electronic, special precautions need to be taken to assure the security and confidentiality of each client's health record. These systems allow nearly instant access to

BOX 36.2 SOAP Note

S: "It hurts to reach items on the second shelf. No way could I reach the top shelf. I can't even put my hair in a ponytail. It just hurts too much."

O: Client reached items on the second shelf of the kitchen cabinet with her right hand, expressing discomfort throughout the range. Client did not attempt to reach items on the top shelf. Client pointed to the anterior aspect of the glenoid fossa when asked where it hurt. Scapular elevation and trunk rotation substituted for part of shoulder flexion and abduction; she never raised her arm above 80 degrees. Client used internal rotation to place items retrieved from the shelf on the counter with no complaints. Client did not use external rotation in replacing objects on shelf, reporting severe pain using that kind of motion. She rated her pain a 9 on a 0–10 point scale.

A: Right shoulder range of motion is severely limited and very painful. Limited range of motion interferes with meal preparation, dressing, hygiene, and grooming.

P: OT 2×/wk, for 30 min outpatient sessions to instruct client in use of reacher, discuss environmental adaptation principles related to placement of objects within comfort zone, and develop a home program to facilitate regaining pain-free range of motion.

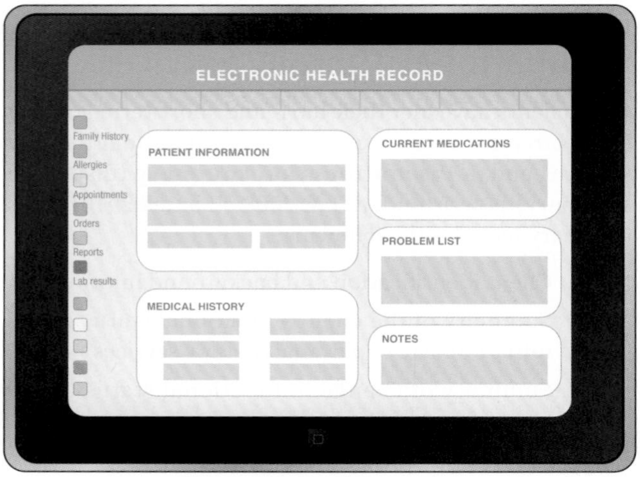

FIGURE 36.1 Electronic health records require health care providers to enter clinical data into a computerized system.

updated information about the client's health care, test results, medications, and consultation reports.

Occupational therapy practitioners (and all other health care providers) need to log in and log out of the system even if they are going to be away from their computer (or other device) for a minute or two. No computer can be left unattended while a client's health record is open. When you are logged in, every client record you access, every note you write, and every error you make and correct, is recorded under your "signature."

Access to any client's health record has to be limited to those who have a need to know what is in that record. Recently, 32 employees of a health system in Minnesota were fired because they looked at the health records of people involved in a highly publicized case (several teens overdosed at a party) when they were not involved in the care of any of teens. They were caught because of routine audits that check to see who has viewed selected health records (Lauritsen, 2011).

Before using an electronic health record, employees receive extensive training in the use of the system, policies to protect client confidentiality, and system security. Each electronic health record system has its quirks, strengths, and weaknesses. Table 36.2 lists the pros and cons of electronic documentation systems.

Documentation in School Settings

Documentation in educational settings can be very different from clinical documentation, but the same documentation principles apply. Documentation in school systems can be divided into three main categories: notice and consent forms, **Individualized Family Service Plans**, and **Individualized Education Programs** (AOTA, 1999; Sames, 2010).

Documentation of Notice and Consent

According to the IDEA, notice and consent forms are required to communicate with parents or guardians of children being served by the school district. Documents may include notices of team meetings, notice and consent for evaluation or reevaluation, referral for an initial evaluation, procedural safeguards, and a report of an IFSP or IEP meeting (Sames, 2010).

Documentation of Services from Birth through Age 2 Years

Services for infants and toddlers are described in Part C of IDEA (AOTA, 1999). IFSPs are written to address

TABLE 36.2 Advantages and Disadvantages of Electronic Documentation Systems

Advantages	Disadvantages
Legibility	Less flexibility in content
Speed (one click may enter a full sentence)	Investment in time and money
Automatic entry of client information	Learning curve required to develop proficiency in the system
Increased availability of health information from remote sites	Concerns about confidentiality and security of medical information
Increased storage capacity for longer periods of time	Reduced patient interaction due to need to sit at a computer to complete documentation tasks
Accessible by anyone on the team	Need for staff training and continuous software updates
Improved organization of the medical record	
Immediate retrieval of information	

Sources: Greiver, M., Barnsley, J., Glazier, R. H., Moineddin, R., & Harvey, B. J. (2011). Implementation of electronic medical records: Theory-informed qualitative study. *Canadian Family Physician, 57*, e390–e397; Embi, P. J., Yackel, T. R., Logan, J. R., Bowen, J. L., Cooney, T. G., & Gorman, P. N. (2004). Impacts of computerized physician documentation in a teaching hospital: Perceptions of faculty and resident physicians. *Journal of the American Medical Informatics Association, 11*, 300–309; and Sullivan, C. (2001). Electronic documentation: The process of facility-wide implementation. *Administration and Management Special Interest Section Quarterly, 17*(3), 1–3.

these services. Each state designates a lead agency (education, health, or human services) to serve the needs of infants and toddlers with special needs to help ready them for school. The lead agency is responsible for creating an IFSP for each child served that is tailored to the specific needs of the child and the child's family. Occupational therapists can serve as **service coordinators** (case managers) for IFSPs. The service coordinator is responsible for ensuring that the proper documentation is completed and scheduling team meetings as needed or required by IDEA. An IFSP includes the following:

- A summary of the child's present level of performance (physical, cognitive, communicative, social or emotional, and adaptive development)
- Identification of the family's concerns, priorities, and resources
- A summary of expected outcomes (measurable goals)
- Identification of early intervention services needed, including frequency, intensity, and service delivery method
- Identification of the child's natural environment (where services will be delivered)
- Date services will start and the anticipated length of services
- Identification of a service coordinator for the child
- Identification of the steps that will be taken to help the toddler transition to the preschool setting (IDEA, 2004).

Documentation of Services from Age 3 to 21 Years

The IEP is the document that guides services for a child with disabilities between the ages of 3 and 21 years. The requirements for IEPs are described in Part B of IDEA. IEP services may include both **special education** and **related services.** For the purposes of the IEP, occupational therapy services are considered related services. As a related service provider, the occupational therapist would not serve as a service coordinator for children with IEPs but would contribute to the process of writing and revising the IEP. The IEP is written every year and reviewed every 6 months.

An IEP must contain the following elements:

- Present level of educational performance
- Annual goals
- Special education and related services
- Participation with nondisabled children
- Participation in statewide and districtwide tests
- Starting date and location of services
- Transition services (for children aged 14 years and older transitioning to adult programs or work settings)
- Measurement of progress (IDEA, 2004)

The fundamental difference between the IFSP and the IEP is that the IFSP is more holistic; it can address a broader range of needs (AOTA, 1999). An IEP must be educationally related. Each state or each school district within a state may establish its own forms for these documents; the federal regulations do not require use of specific forms. The federal regulations mandate the timetables for completing the documents and the content of the documents (Sames, 2010).

Documentation in Emerging Practice Settings

Occupational therapy practitioners are now working in community-based programs such as homeless shelters, prisons, Welfare-to-Work programs, home hospice, and summer camps. In some cases, occupational therapy programs are new to these settings. The clinical approach to documentation might not be appropriate, especially if there is no health record in which to enter occupational therapy documentation. If the occupational therapy practitioner is working with individuals in the new program, it is advisable to develop evaluation, intervention plan, progress, and discontinuation reports that are consistent with the AOTA documentation guidelines (2008a) to the greatest extent possible. However, if the occupational therapy practitioners are providing services at a community or population level, they may simply provide the agency with periodic consultation reports with a less structured format. Most consultation reports are narrative descriptions of the needs assessment, plan, implementation, and/or outcomes of the occupational therapy program.

Because occupational therapy practitioners in emerging practice settings are demonstrating the value of occupational therapy in new ways, they may use their documentation as a mechanism to demonstrate successful outcomes and benefits of occupational therapy services.

Administrative Documentation

Occupational therapists in any setting may have to write an incident report, a letter of appeal to a payer source, a grant proposal, or **policies** and **procedures.** These types of documentation are administrative because they are necessary for the ongoing administration of occupational therapy services. For example, to be paid for delivering

BOX 36.3 Writing for an Evaluation Report Compared to a Prior Authorization Request Letter

Tatiana is a 16-month-old girl from a Midwestern city. Three weeks ago, while under the care of her mother's boyfriend, she was allegedly shaken violently. Her mother brought her to the hospital 2 days later because the baby was sleepier than normal, did not seem to want to eat or drink, did not hold her head up, and did not engage in any play activities or smile at her mother.

Excerpt from Evaluation Report:

Tatiana did not focus on or visually track any objects in any direction. She did not reach for any toys that were quietly placed in front of her, but she did turn her head to localize sounds and flailed her hands in reaction to sound. Her fingers closed around a rattle placed in the palm of her hand. Passive range of motion was within normal limits in all extremities. Muscle tone was generally low. She rubbed her face or arm in response to light touch. When placed on her stomach, she rolled her head from side to side but did not lift her head. When placed in a sitting position, she was unable to hold her head up or maintain sitting unassisted. Tatiana made no attempts to roll over or bear weight on her arms. She is fed through a nasogastric tube; therefore, chewing and swallowing were not evaluated at this time. She cried and made other noises but did not form any words. Tatiana will need adaptive seating with head support and occupational therapy intervention to maximize her abilities to actively interact with people and her environment.

Excerpt from Prior Authorization Letter:

This 16-month-old girl was diagnosed with shaken baby syndrome resulting in severe head trauma. She has low muscle tone and cannot assume or maintain a seated position unassisted. This child will need adaptive seating and positioning devices to ensure proper positioning of her trunk and limbs and to prevent deformities. Proper positioning is also important for her cognitive, social, and physical development. Her vision is severely limited; she is functionally blind. In a seated position, she will better be able to localize sound, use her arms and hands, and begin to engage in social interactions. Please refer to the attached list of recommended adaptive positioning devices and their respective costs. In addition, I recommend occupational therapy intervention twice a week for 3 months (24 visits) to work on developing the movement, social, and cognitive skills needed to enable participation in daily life activities of typical toddlers. A list of measurable goals is included.

occupational therapy services, occupational therapy practitioners may need to write letters to request funding or to respond to a denial of a payment. Policies and procedures must be written clearly so that all employees of the department understand and follow the departmental standards, ensuring that the department functions well. To effectively do their jobs, aides—who may be high school graduates with some on-the-job training—as well as professional staff must understand policies and procedures.

Administrative documentation requires the use of terminology that anyone can understand; people who have limited understanding of occupational therapy jargon or medical terms may read these documents. Often, the first person who reads an appeal letter will be someone who is trained to interpret insurance company standards but who might not have a medical background.

Box 36.3 shows an example of a section of an evaluation report written for a medical record and how it might be translated in a letter to an insurance company requesting authorization for services.

Conclusion

Although occupational therapy documentation across settings has some typical features, it is important to recognize that individual agencies may opt to develop or purchase their own documentation formats. However, it is critical that whatever documentation formats are chosen conform to federal and state laws as well as the requirements of reimbursement sources. In addition, occupational therapy documentation should adhere to professional ethical guidelines and practice standards. It is the occupational therapy practitioner's responsibility to be aware of and comply with all documentation requirements.

References

American Occupational Therapy Association. (1999). *Occupational therapy services for children and youth under the Individuals with Disabilities Education Act* (2nd ed.). Bethesda, MD: Author.

American Occupational Therapy Association. (2008a). Guidelines for documentation of occupational therapy. *American Journal of Occupational Therapy, 62*(6), 684–690.

American Occupational Therapy Association. (2008b). Occupational therapy practice framework: Domain and process, 2nd edition. *American Journal of Occupational Therapy, 62*, 625–683.

American Occupational Therapy Association. (2010). *Occupational therapy code of ethics and ethical standards.* Retrieved from http://www.aota.org/Practitioners/Official/Ethics/40611.aspx?FT=.pdf

Borcherding, S. (2000). *Documentation manual for writing SOAP notes in occupational therapy.* Thorofare, NJ: SLACK Incorporated.

Centers for Medicare and Medicaid Services. (2008). *Pub100-02 Medicare benefit policy: Transmittal 88.* Retrieved from http://www.cms.hhs.gov/transmittals/downloads/R88BP.pdf

Centers for Medicare and Medicaid Services. (2012). *Medicare fraud and abuse: Detection, prevention, and reporting.* Retrieved from http://www.jointcommission.org/topics/patient_safety.aspx

Embi, P. J., Yackel, T. R., Logan, J. R., Bowen, J. L., Cooney, T. G., & Gorman, P. N. (2004). Impacts of computerized physician documentation in a teaching hospital: Perceptions of faculty and resident physicians. *Journal of the American Medical Informatics Association, 11*, 300–309.

Fremgen, B. F. (2002). *Medical law and ethics.* Upper Saddle River, NJ: Prentice Hall.

Greiver, M., Barnsley, J., Glazier, R. H., Moineddin, R., & Harvey, B. J. (2011). Implementation of electronic medical records: Theory-informed qualitative study. *Canadian Family Physician, 57*, e390–e397.
Individuals with Disabilities Education Act of 2004, 20 U.S.C. § 1414. Retrieved from http://www.gpo.gov/fdsys/pkg/PLAW-108publ446/html/PLAW-108publ446.htm
Individuals with Disabilities Education Act of 2004, 20 U.S.C. § 1436 [d] [1–8]. Retrieved from http://www.gpo.gov/fdsys/pkg/PLAW-108publ446/html/PLAW-108publ446.htm
The Joint Commission. (2012). *Facts about the official "Do not use" list of abbreviations.* Retrieved from http://www.jointcommission.org/topics/patient_safety.aspx
Kornblau, B. L., & Starling, S. P. (2000). *Ethics in rehabilitation: A clinical perspective.* Thorofare, NJ: SLACK Incorporated.
Lauritsen, J. (2011, May 6). *Allina fires 32 employees for snooping at patient records.* Retrieved from http://minnesota.cbslocal.com/2011/05/06/allina-fires-32-employees-for-snooping-at-patient-records/
Lemke, L. (2004). Defensive documentation: Managing Medicare denials. *OT Practice, 9*(16), 8–12.
Liang, B. A. (2000). *Health law & policy: A survival guide to medicolegal issues for practitioners.* Woburn, MA: Butterworth-Heinemann.
Oliu, W. E., Brusaw, C. T., & Alred, G. J. (1995). *Writing that works: How to write effectively on the job* (5th ed.). New York, NY: St. Martin's Press.
Sames, K. M. (2010). *Documenting occupational therapy practice* (2nd ed.). Upper Saddle River, NJ: Pearson Prentice Hall.
Sullivan, C. (2001). Electronic documentation: The process of facility-wide implementation. *Administration and Management Special Interest Section Quarterly, 17*(3), 1–3.

For additional resources on the subjects discussed in this chapter, visit http://thePoint.lww.com/Willard-Spackman12e.

Occupational Performance Theories of Practice

UNIT IX

"A theory is a good theory if it satisfies two requirements: It must accurately describe a large class of observation on the basis of a model that contains only a few arbitrary elements, and it must make definite predictions about the results of future observation."

—Stephen W. Hawking

CHAPTER 37

Unpacking Our Theoretical Reasoning

Theory and Practice in Occupational Therapy

Ellen S. Cohn, Wendy J. Coster

OUTLINE

"In theory there is no difference between theory and practice. In practice there is."

—YOGI BERRA

LEARNING OBJECTIVES

After reading this chapter, you will be able to:

1. Explain the distinction between personal and formal theories
2. Explain the distinction between tacit and explicit knowledge
3. Identify assumptions and propositions guiding practice
4. Critically examine theory to identify assumptions and propositions of theory

When occupational therapy (OT) practitioners meet a client[1] for the first time, they must quickly figure out why the client has come for intervention, what is important to the client, what might be helping or interfering with his or her desired occupations, and what might be the best possible intervention to enable the client to achieve his or her goals. Figuring out what to do requires complex professional reasoning processes that involve ongoing analysis and reflection on our knowledge, observations, and understanding of the lives of clients and what matters to them.

In order to enable clients to achieve their occupational performance goals, OT practitioners must decide which interventions are most likely to achieve these goals. When we propose an intervention that involves particular actions or steps, our reasoning about what to do is guided by our ideas of how change might occur. These ideas include theoretical assumptions and propositions that guide us in what to observe and

[1]The entity that receives occupational therapy services. Clients may include (1) individuals and other persons relevant to the individual's life, including family, caregivers, teachers, employers, and others who also may help or be served indirectly; (2) organizations such as business, industries, or agencies; and (3) populations within a community (American Occupational Therapy Association, 2008).

CASE STUDY 37.1 Alex

Alex, a 9-year-old child, has been referred to you, an occupational therapy student completing your Level II fieldwork experience in an outpatient private practice for children. Alex is reluctant to try new activities, is beginning to have difficulty keeping up with his peers in school, wanders around the periphery of the playground during recess, and refuses to participate in gym class. The other children have begun to tease Alex, and he has not developed friendships. After observing Alex struggle to complete a variety of fine and gross motor activities, you conduct formal assessments and document delays in both fine and gross motor development. You also complete the Perceived Efficacy and Goal Setting System (PEGS) with Alex to gain insight into his perspectives and concerns. The PEGS is a standardized system designed to enable young children with disabilities to self-report their perceived competence in everyday activities and to set goals for intervention. Alex wants to be able to play baseball, shuffle playing cards, and type on the computer. You are now clear about the outcomes Alex hopes to achieve but need to determine how to best intervene to help Alex achieve his goals in an effective and efficient manner. Your supervisor asks you to explain the "theoretical rationale" of the intervention you propose for Alex. Your supervisor wants to know what you think the "mechanisms of action" are for the intervention.

Before reading further, take a moment to think about and write down your ideas about:

1. Why might Alex have trouble developing friendships?
2. Why might Alex be reluctant to try new activities?

how to describe, explain, or predict outcomes from the interventions we might use. That is, in addition to our experience and available research evidence, we are guided by personal and formal theories. The theories that guide professional reasoning are both personal and formal and both tacit and explicit. Whatever their form, theories help practitioners reason about what to assess, how to understand occupational performance problems, how to intervene, and what to expect from the intervention. Often, we need to articulate our reasoning process to others (clients, other professionals, peers, supervisors, third party payers, etc.) to communicate what they may expect from OT intervention.

The purpose of this chapter is to provide a structure to help OT practitioners "unpack" or critically examine the theories they use to understand the problems clients present and to guide intervention. Our goal is to help practitioners clarify and evaluate the assumptions and propositions that guide their practice. This analysis is important for several reasons. First, it helps us to determine whether our professional reasoning is sound. Then, based on whether we conclude that it is sound or not, we may need to modify our reasoning and potentially the services we provide. Finally, examining our thinking helps us to articulate our professional reasoning to others so we can explain why we are using the assessments we have chosen, how the intervention we are providing works, and what outcomes we expect. The scenario in Case Study 37.1 illustrates a common challenge many OT students confront during their fieldwork experience.

Propositions and Assumptions

To begin our discussion, we make a distinction between two types of ideas that are part of most theories: **propositions** and **assumptions**. *Propositions* are formal statements about causes and effects or the nature of relationships among features of the world. Their distinguishing feature is that it is possible (hypothetically at least) to test them and therefore to prove them false—a characteristic that is referred to in philosophy of science as "falsifiability" (Popper, 1959). Sometimes, it is possible to test a proposition directly; for example, to test the proposition that a virus causes a particular illness. Other times, evidence accumulates from various sources that eventually makes clear that the "old" ideas about the world do not fit with the data as, for example, when scientists challenged the proposition that the sun revolved around the earth. Modern science is built around the posing and testing of hypotheses, which are propositions about how the world "works." In order to make the proposed relationships among the factors explicit, it can be helpful to formulate propositions as "if/then" statements. Table 37.1 presents some examples of propositions, their corresponding if/then statements, and how they might be tested.

In contrast, *assumptions* are ideas we "believe to be true." This term is used a little differently in everyday language and in the language of science. In everyday language, we use the term to refer to a wide variety of situations where we have drawn a conclusion without having definite evidence. For example, we might tell our friend we "assume" that Mary took her book because she was the last person we saw reading it. In this situation, although we don't have the evidence on hand to prove our statement, we could readily gather evidence by asking Mary if she has the book. In other words, our conclusion is "falsifiable" and thus more like a proposition. In the language of science, the term "assumption" is applied much more specifically to ideas that really cannot be definitively proven true or false, for example, the idea that people have an inherent drive for mastery of their environment. Evidence can be judged to be more or less consistent with a particular assumption like this, but there is no way to obtain definitive proof.

TABLE 37.1 Examples of Propositions with If/Then Statements

Proposition	If/Then Statement	How It Would Be Tested
Practice of a skill in the context in which it will typically be applied leads to more effective long-term mastery.	If a person practices a skill in the natural context in which it is typically performed, then he or she will achieve more effective long-term mastery than if the skill is practiced in a contrived context.	A controlled comparison of the transfer of a skill learned under two different conditions: in typical context and in a laboratory context.
Organization of movement is different when reaching toward a desired object (i.e., a goal) than when simply reaching into space.	If a person reaches toward a goal, then his or her movement is organized differently than when he or she reaches into space without a goal.	Kinematic analysis of specific characteristics of reaching movements by the same person under the two different conditions.
Sensory defensiveness is a defining characteristic of children with autism.	If a child has autism, then he or she will display sensory defensiveness.	Use of a structured protocol to examine responses to sensory stimuli in a large sample of children with autism. Calculate prevalence of sensory defensiveness and compare this rate to that of a sample with a different diagnosis.

Because assumptions are so completely accepted, it can be hard at first to recognize when a particular idea is an assumption rather than a proposition that is well supported by evidence. Our assumptions may derive from different sources. Some may have been learned during formal education, for example, from study of the theories of an academic discipline. Others reflect our personal theories and our assumptions derived from our culture and individual experience. The distinction between personal and "academic" assumptions is not always clear-cut; often, our preference for a particular formal theory is based on its compatibility with our personal assumptions. For example, we may find it easier to accept theories that emphasize personal control over outcomes because we have a personal assumption that "people are in control of their fates." Table 37.2 gives some examples of how personal and theory-based assumptions might be expressed in the literature or in a person's statements regarding his or her observations.

Our assumptions about the nature of human behavior and corresponding views of reality may shape what we attend to when planning the evaluation process and developing intervention strategies with clients. Our day-to-day practices are rooted in both assumptions and propositions (Hooper, 1997). Often, propositions and assumptions are confounded, viewed as the same things, or confused with each other. Making a distinction between them helps us to identify them more easily, to reflect on how they may influence our reasoning about evaluation and intervention, and to evaluate whether they make sense. If we distinguish our propositions and assumptions, we can then search for relevant evidence to evaluate the propositions, evaluate whether our assumptions are logical and consistent with current knowledge, and reflect on how both the assumptions and propositions are influencing our reasoning and expectations for intervention outcomes.

Note that some of the examples in Table 37.2 have elements that could be tested or checked for their consistency with the evidence. However, the *broader* assumptions would be hard to prove or disprove. For example, how would one *prove* that all people want to be as independent as possible? This is one reason why it is important to evaluate the evidence supporting your ideas about how to intervene with a client. If you cannot find any evidence, that is one clue that you may be basing your approach on assumptions.

It is important to keep in mind that we all make assumptions; they provide answers to important fundamental questions such as "what is the nature of the person?" or "am I in control of my fate?" It is not really possible to construct theories without them. However, because assumptions cannot be fully disproved, we need to be cautious in applying them as guides for practice. The propositions of a theory, on the other hand, can be tested so that we can determine whether or not they are accurate guides for achieving desired changes. This systematic testing is what leads to new discoveries and therefore more effective practice.

CASE STUDY 37.1 Alex *(Continued)*

Go back and review your explanations for why Alex might have trouble developing friendships and be reluctant to try new activities.

1. Which ideas are testable (i.e., are propositions)?
2. How might you test the propositions?
3. Which are more like assumptions?
4. Can you identify the sources of some of your assumptions?

TABLE 37.2 Examples of How Personal and Theory-Based Assumptions Might be Expressed

Types of Assumptions	Examples of Assumptions	How the Assumption Might Be Expressed in a Formal Theory	How the Assumption Might Be Expressed in a Personal Theory
Assumptions about causes	People are largely in control of their own behavior.	A theory proposes that behavior is directed by commitment to personal goals.	"If she really wanted to, she could change that bad habit."
	Behavior is largely controlled by external social influences.	A theory proposes that negative social influences (e.g., unsafe neighborhood, low socioeconomic status) explain poor outcomes among youth.	"You can't blame him, given the kind of neighborhood he grew up in."
	Behavior is largely controlled by unconscious motives and conflicts.	A theory proposes that unconscious conflicts stemming from early experiences explain a person's current behavior.	"She's doing that because she's in denial about what happened."
Assumptions about the nature of the person	People are largely aware of and can report accurately on the reasons for their behavior.	A theory proposes that information gained through self-report on motives and goals accurately reflects the real causes of their behavior.	"Once we have talked with her, we should have a much better idea of what caused her to do that."
	People have an inherent drive to experience sensory stimulation.	A theory proposes that the experiences derived from sensory input are highly rewarding.	"Providing rich sensory experiences for his or her child is one of the most important things a parent can do."
	People have an inherent drive to make sense of their experience.	A theory proposes that people automatically formulate explanations of their experience without being taught to do so.	"There must be a reason why this happened to me."
	People are inherently rational.	A theory proposes that given adequate information, people will choose their actions based on an accurate weighing of the pros and cons of various options.	"I don't get it: I explained the importance of doing this, but he's still resisting!"
	All people desire to be independent as much as possible.	A theory proposes that being able to do things without the support of others is the greatest indication of success.	"Even though he says he likes living in the group home, I'm sure he really wants to live on his own."
Assumptions about human development	There is a universal, optimal sequence to developing competence.	A theory proposes that failure to follow a standard sequence for mastering skills will result in less optimal functioning.	"If we don't focus on building stronger component abilities first, then he'll always be relying on less effective splinter skills."
	There is a timetable of experiences required for optimal development that is universal across cultures.	A theory proposes that if a child does not have certain experiences at a particular time, he or she will not achieve the same skills as his or her peers.	"It is important to make sure you talk to your baby to develop his attention and listening skills for school."
Assumptions about knowledge and learning	The essence of learning is acquiring more information.	A theory proposes that lack of accurate or sufficiently detailed information explains why people act ineffectively.	"We have a lot of parents who aren't providing the right kind of experiences for their child. We should offer a presentation about typical motor development."
	The essence of learning is changing the way we think about something.	A theory proposes that people must integrate new information into their existing personal system of knowledge before they can organize new ways to act.	"An interactive teaching session observing how their child solves movement 'problems' will help parents change their approach to supporting their child."

Tacit and Explicit

Sometimes our reasoning is **tacit**; that is, implicit or based on information or experiences that we cannot easily put into language. Experienced practitioners have an implicit or tacit understanding of what they do in practice and will make adjustments to the intervention to address the subtle and complex cues observed in the process of intervention. For example, through experience, a therapist might determine that the strength of a muscle "just doesn't seem right" and the therapist then automatically adjusts the activity to compensate for the person's limited strength. Another therapist might instinctively sing a calming, gentle song to soothe a young child who is screaming and agitated. The philosopher Polanyi (1966/2009, p. 4) eloquently summarized this process when he noted, "We can know more than we can tell." Tacit reasoning is important to our practice because it allows us to work quickly and effectively in the moment. However, in order to evaluate whether the approach was effective (and if we should continue to use it), we need to be able to translate our tacit or implicit reasoning into clear ***explicit*** propositions about what we think promoted the desired change for the client. In order to evaluate whether our model of change is logical and is supported by evidence, we need to describe the exact mechanism that we think caused the change. For example, on reflection, we may realize that we asked a client to repeat the same movement numerous times as we increased the task demands because we hypothesized, based on motor learning theory, that "repetition under condition of ever-increasing task demands" will promote change in the movement (Plautz, Milliken, & Nudo, 2000). Then, we could review whether the evidence supports this theoretical proposition.

Theories Vary in Specificity

In OT, authors have used many different terms to define similar concepts (theory, conceptual foundation, frame of reference, paradigm, practice model). Different authors may provide very different definitions of the same terms, which can be confusing. Rather than try to clarify the subtle distinctions across these definitions, this chapter takes a different approach. We suggest that theories can be located along a continuum that reflects their degree of specificity.

Broad

One definition of a theory (2010) is "a plausible or scientifically acceptable general principle or body of principles offered to explain phenomena." This definition is **broad**, global, and explanatory. A broad theory serves as an "overarching model that helps to explain a large set of findings or observations" (Whyte, 2006, p. 100). A broad or global theory provides a way of organizing or systematizing the elements of the phenomena being observed and helps us focus our observations and decide what cues to attend to. A broad theory specifies how concepts or factors are related and gives a name to a set of elements that share something in common. However, propositions about change are not specified in precise detail in broad theories. For example, ecological theory tells us to pay attention to the person–environment interaction, but it does not tell us how to intervene to enable the client to participate more satisfactorily in desired occupations. Therefore, broad theories do not provide precise information on how we can intervene to enable change.

In OT, we often use ecological and systems theories[2], which propose a transactional relation between the mind, body, and the environment. We consider the context or environment in its broadest sense (including culture and social aspects) and assume that humans have an innate drive to explore and be competent in their environments. Some broad ecological theories explain the influence of the environment in greater detail than others. These broad theories commonly suggest that in order to explore and be competent in our environments, people need skills and abilities; and we judge our competence by the feedback we receive from the environment. Consequently, in this example, the broad theories help us focus our initial observations of human behavior on the complex transactions among mind, body, and environment.

Several ecological theorists in the field of human development have offered explanations of the transactional relationship between person and environment. Bronfenbrenner (1979), a social scientist, proposed an ecological theory to explain how a person's biology and interactions among ever-changing and multilevel environments are key to human development. Bronfenbrenner proposed that social factors such as families, friends, communities, or institutions can enhance or inhibit development. Gibson's (1979) concept of affordances describes the idea that people's perception of the relationship between objects in the environment and their own personal capabilities enables action. Lawton (1986) proposed the concept of press to explain the idea that the demands of the environment or task impact human performance and suggested that "goodness of fit" between a person's abilities and the demands of the task influences human performance. Numerous theories proposed by occupational therapists (Ecology of Human Performance [Dunn, Brown, & McGuian, 1994], Person-Environment-Occupation [Law et al., 1996], Person-Environment-Occupation Performance [Baum & Christiansen, 2005], and Model of Human Occupation [Kielhofner, 2008; Kielhofner & Burke, 1980]) are based on these ecological principles. When observing occupational performance, ideas drawn from these ecological theories direct the occupational therapist to focus his or her observations on the person, the environment, and the occupation and how these elements influence each other.

---

[2]For a thorough description of these theories, see primary sources.

BOX 37.1 Characteristics of Broad and Discrete Theories

Broad →	Discrete
• Global • Explanatory: help explain a large set of findings or observations • Map out the elements of phenomena being observed • Specify what is related to what and gives a name to a set of elements that share something in common • Help us focus our initial observations (i.e., what is important to attend to rather than what to do)	• Testable specific postulates about causal relationships • Specify how to behave in intervention, what to say or do, under what conditions changes will occur • Explanatory: help explain how intervention works • Predictive: specify what might happen or what to expect as a result of intervention • Each particular proposition of the theory is supported by evidence and specified so you can anticipate what the outcome is likely to be

Discrete

Another definition of a theory (2010) is a "hypothesis assumed for the sake of argument or investigation". This definition describes discrete theories, which often draw on the ideas of broad theories and describe specific causal relationships. These theories may be efforts to identify the specific causes of a problem or may propose how an aspect of intervention leads to therapeutic change. Because discrete theories identify ways in which a phenomenon can be changed or controlled, they help us determine what to do or say in providing interventions and they inform our treatment or intervention theories. A treatment theory helps to narrow the scope of possibilities for change and states how a specific intervention is believed to act. By clearly specifying the "**mechanisms of action**,[3]" that is, how specific intervention strategies lead to particular outcomes, treatment theories explicate how change proceeds and the particular conditions under which an intervention achieves the desired results. Consequently, treatment or intervention theories also help us determine what types of clients might benefit from the intervention, how the intervention is best delivered, and what outcomes we might expect.

Broad and discrete theories both make claims about hypothesized relationships. However, these theories are on a continuum in terms of the degree of development and specificity regarding how to intervene, clarity about the essential features, or element of the intervention and evidence to support their propositions. One way to determine where a theory may be on the broad to discrete continuum is to examine the degree to which each causal relationship proposed in the theory is supported by sound evidence. Theories with more developed propositions include clear assertions of the effects of an intervention, the mechanism through which the intervention is believed to exert these effects, and identification of the components of the intervention that are most responsible for the effects. Because research is conducted to test the hypothesized relationships, theories become more refined and we gain greater clarity about the effectiveness of the various components of an intervention. Box 37.1 provides a simple schematic of the continuum from broad to discrete theories.

Where Do Theories Come From?

What prompts someone to propose a new or a revised theory? Recall that theories are an effort to *explain* a particular phenomenon or process and to *organize* information about that phenomenon. Thus, theories, particularly clinical or practice theories, are often developed in response to an observation or experience that the person cannot adequately account for using existing explanations. For example, when Jean Ayres (1972) was working with children in the 1970s, she found that the accepted theories about learning difficulties did not adequately account for the full range of difficulties that she saw in the children she worked with and didn't offer useful guidance for how to intervene. Eventually, this experience led her to develop sensory integration theory and develop a new approach to intervention based on this theory. Sometimes, theory or research in a related field suggests new ways to understand or intervene with clinical problems. For example, Taub, Uswatte, and Pidikiti (1999) developed constraint-induced movement therapy for people with stroke after observing what he termed "learned non-use" in monkeys who had central nervous system (CNS) damage.

Clinical theories are based on the knowledge available at the time they are first developed. Over time, more

[3] You may also see the term "mechanism of change" used in the literature to describe ideas about how change happens during intervention. These terms are essentially equivalent.

evidence will become available about whether or not the propositions of the theory are correct or whether they need to be modified. For example, evidence may show that a specific feature of the intervention is particularly effective in achieving the desired change and that other features of the intervention may not be necessary. Therefore, it is important for practitioners to remain current in the research related to the theories they are applying in practice.

CASE STUDY 37.1 Alex *(Continued)*

Before reading further, take another moment to think about this question:

Are your ideas about Alex's challenges with friendships and new activities based on personal theories or some formal theories that you may have learned in your studies to date?

1. Identify in writing the personal theories that guided your reasoning about Alex.
2. Identify in writing the formal theories (either broad or discrete) that guided your reasoning about Alex.

Cognitive Orientation to Daily Occupational Performance (CO-OP)

After a thorough review of interventions to address the needs of children with motor coordination challenges, we discover the Cognitive Orientation to Daily Occupational Performance (CO-OP) intervention developed by occupational therapists Polatajko et al. (2001). The CO-OP approach was developed because various intervention approaches offered to children with mild-to-moderate movement difficulties were primarily deficit oriented, focusing on remediating underlying deficits thought to interfere with functional performance (Mandich, Polatajko, Macnab, & Miller, 2001). Dissatisfied with the lack of generalization to skilled action, occupational therapists Helene Polatajko and Angela Mandich turned to literature about growing understanding of motor control and skill learning to develop a highly individualized metacognitive approach to help children master motor skills. The CO-OP is a client-centered, metacognitive, performance-based intervention that combines motor learning principles with other theories that emphasize the role of cognitive processes and goal setting in developing movement skills. CO-OP is an example of a theory-based intervention informed by multiple theoretical perspectives from a range of disciplines, including behavioral and cognitive psychology, human movement science, and OT. The purpose of the intervention is to teach children to use strategies that support skill acquisition through a process of guided discovery. The CO-OP intervention might be an effective approach to help Alex achieve his goals to play baseball, shuffle playing cards, and type on the computer. The overarching broad assumption of CO-OP is that successful participation in everyday occupation is essential to health and well-being. Figure 37.1 provides a general overview of the key theoretical propositions and features of the CO-OP intervention. Table 37.3 presents the if/then statements for the key theoretical propositions.

Based on principles of motor learning and goal setting, the therapist would help Alex to identify goals and discover the relevant aspects of the task, examine how he is currently performing the task, identify where he is getting "stuck," and generate alternative solutions. Bandura (1997) noted that children's actual experiences performing an activity contribute to their self-perceptions, and that when children set their own goals, they feel more empowered to work toward achieving their goals. A global strategy is used to provide a consistent framework in which task-specific strategies are discovered by Alex. This structure was based on the problem-solving structure first described by Luria (1976), who drew from Vygotsky's (1967) observation of problem-solving attempts of children, and then further developed by Meichenbaum (1977). In addition to the global problem-solving strategy proposed by Meichenbaum, occupational therapist Angela Mandich (Mandich, Polatajko, Missiuna, & Miller, 2001), who was a graduate student at the time Polatajko and her colleagues were developing the CO-OP intervention, identified eight specific strategies directly related to specific task performance problems. Mandich proposed that task knowledge and cognitive strategies specific to the performance challenges were necessary "mechanisms of action" to support children's competence in their desired occupations. Informed by principles of mediated learning described by educators Feuerstein, Hoffman, Jensen, Tzuriel, and Hoffman (1986) and Haywood (1988), the therapist structures the environment by asking probing questions to facilitate Alex's awareness and reflection on his performance. Once Alex identifies a helpful strategy, the therapist uses questions to help Alex think about how he might apply or generalize the strategy to other situations.

Figure 37.2 provides a conceptual mapping of what the practitioner actually does to implement the intervention in a way that reflects the theoretical propositions. We could actually test the propositions of the theory by observing the therapist's actions and Alex's responses. For example, to test the proposition related to goal setting, we could observe the therapist asking Alex to identity three skills that he needs, wants, or is expected to do at school, home, or when playing. We could determine whether Alex increases his efforts to catch a small ball after setting a goal focused on ball catching.

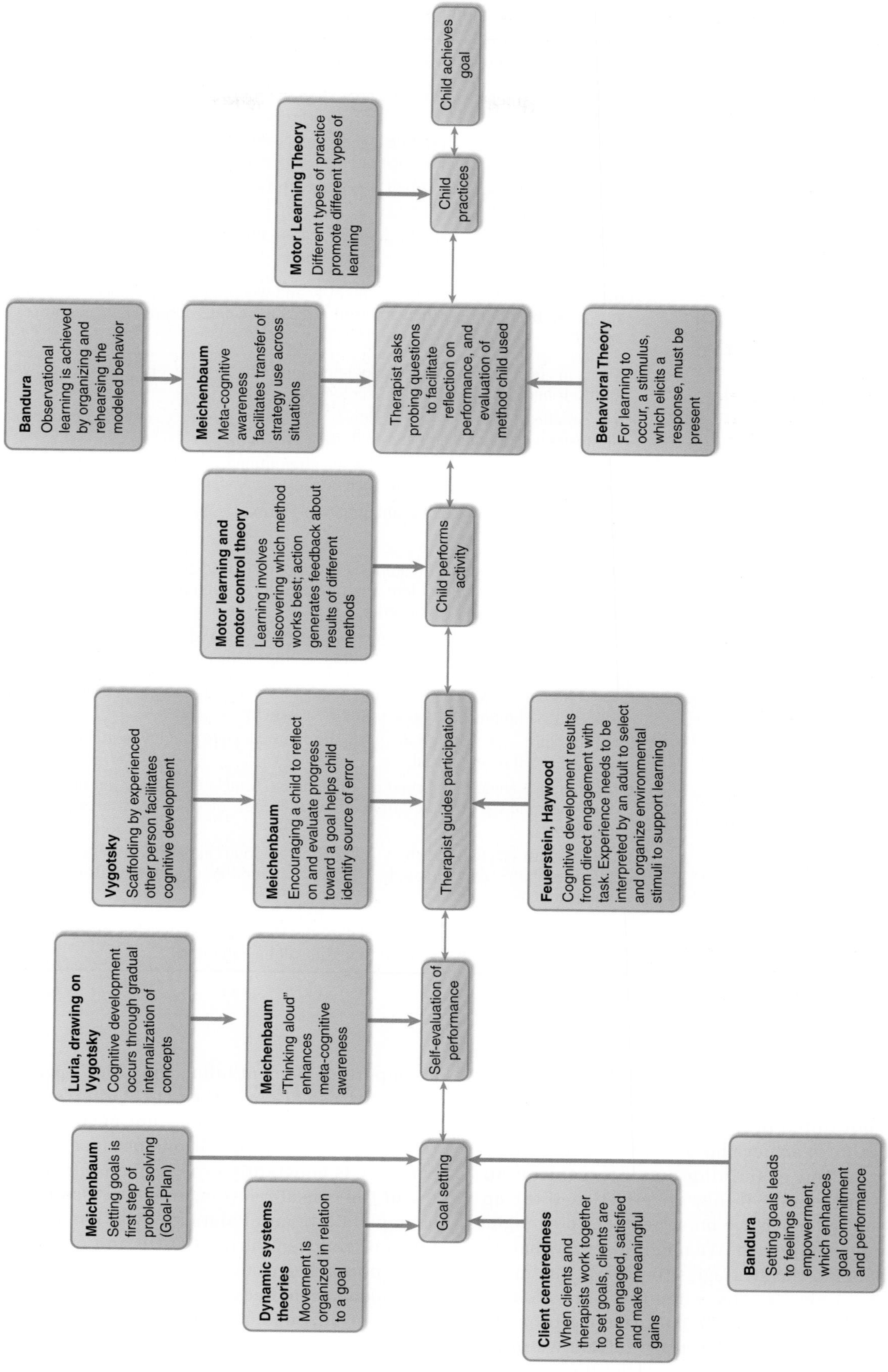

FIGURE 37.1 Theoretical propositions and key features of the CO-OP intervention. *CO-OP*, Cognitive Orientation to Daily Occupational Performance.

TABLE 37.3 Theoretical Propositions and If/Then Statements of the CO-OP Intervention

Intervention Feature	If/Then Statements from Key Theories
Goal setting: client-chosen goals	If a movement is directed toward a goal, then that movement will be organized uniquely in relation to that goal. If the person is engaged in setting a goal, then his or her problem-solving process in relation to that goal will be facilitated. If the person is engaged in setting a goal, then he or she will experience an increased feeling of self-efficacy. If the person's feeling of self-efficacy is increased, then his or her motivation and commitment to the goal will be enhanced.
Dynamic performance analysis	If the dimension of performance complexity and where the performance is breaking down can be identified, then a person can assist in determining possible sources of error.
Cognitive strategy use	If a person engages in talking aloud while attempting to solve a problem, then awareness of his or her performance will be enhanced. If a person develops strategies to address the challenges/sources of error, then using the strategies will enable competence in desired activity. If a person engages in talking aloud while attempting to solve a problem, then the problem-solving process will be facilitated. If a person is engaged in self-evaluation of performance, his or her sense of self-efficacy will be enhanced.
Guided discovery	If a more experienced person guides and supports (scaffolds) a learner who is attempting to solve a problem, then the learner's problem-solving capacity (cognitive development) will be enhanced. If an adult models the thinking process to be mastered and if the child repeats the steps of that process aloud, then the child's learning of the process will be enhanced.
Enabling principles based on learning and motor behavior	If the child performs an activity, then he or she will receive meaningful feedback about the results of a particular approach to the activity. If the therapist asks appropriate questions, then the child's ability to identify effective strategies will be enhanced. If the therapist engages the child in "thinking out loud" about his or her performance, then the child's ability to evaluate the effectiveness of his or her strategies will be enhanced. If the therapist engages the child in "thinking out loud" about his or her performance, then the child's ability to apply strategies across different situations (transfer) will be enhanced.
Child practice	If the child practices a developing skill in the way that best matches his or her current stage of learning the skill, then that skill will be enhanced.

The intervention process is dynamic and continuously changes over time as we learn more and reflect on our initial propositions. As we continue to work with Alex to achieve his goals, we are constantly reflecting on and examining our intervention approaches to determine if they are effective. If the approach is not effective, we must be open to changing or adapting the approach. We might discover that, for Alex, verbalizing the strategies to prompt the motor movement is only effective when there are no other distracters in the immediate context. Based on this ongoing examination of the intervention, we might modify the context as distracting stimuli emerged as an important element influencing Alex's performance. We might also discover the CO-OP intervention works well with Alex, but that does not mean that we stop reflecting on the propositions because the research evidence is constantly evolving and our understanding of the causal relationships may also change. For example, Batte and Polatajko (2006) analyzed videotapes of children during CO-OP and other intervention approaches to determine the role of practice in skill acquisition. Because CO-OP is a cognitive-based intervention, the children who received the CO-OP intervention spent more intervention time discussing performance. The children who received other

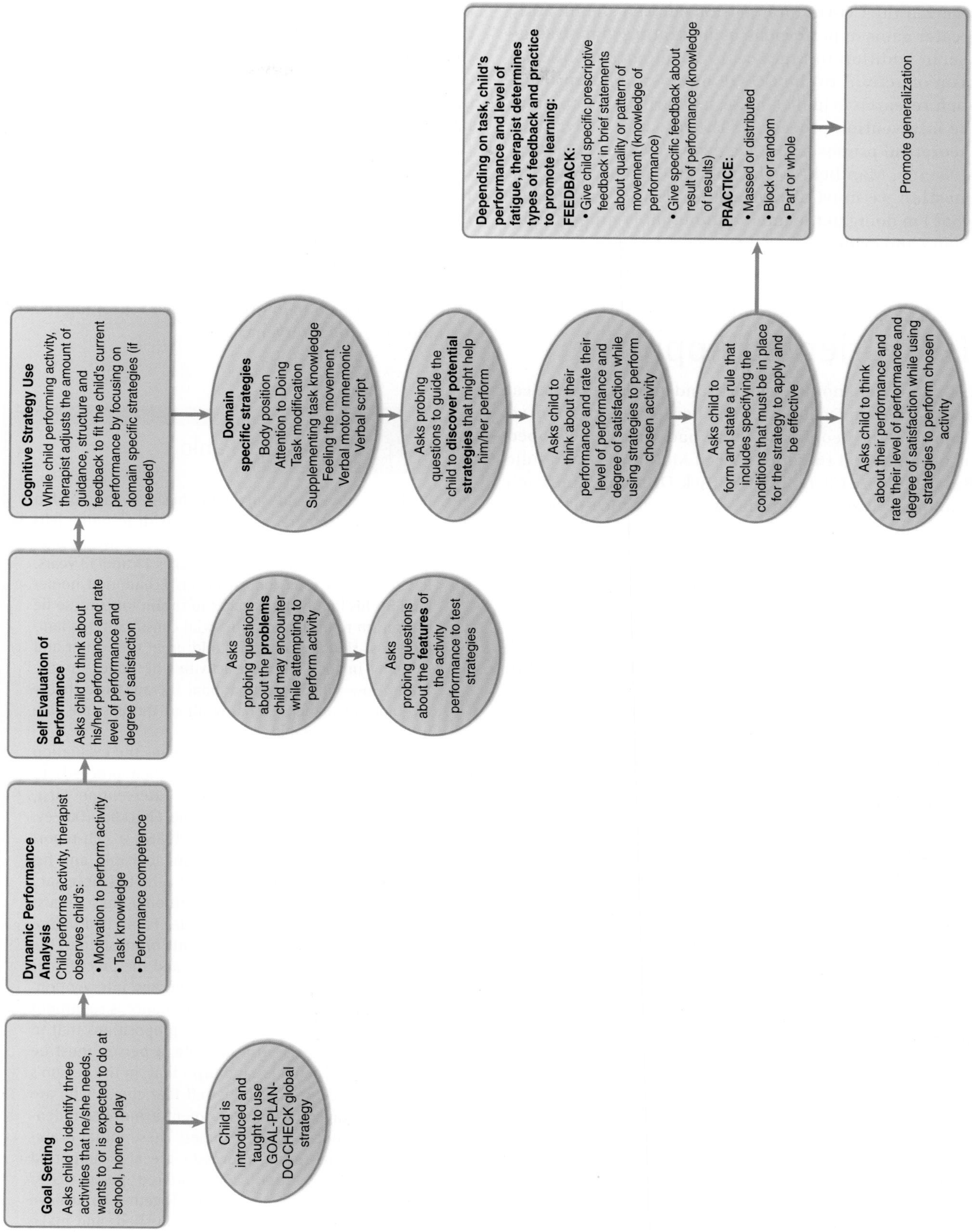

FIGURE 37.2 Conceptual mapping of practitioner's actions.

interventions had more practice time than the children receiving the CO-OP approach. Yet, the children who received the CO-OP intervention showed significantly greater gains in performance, illustrating that strategy use, in addition to practice, is an important "mechanism of action" in the CO-OP intervention approach. Such research evidence helps us clarify what to do in the intervention process. As the research evolves, the theoretical propositions also evolve (Miller, Polatajko, Missiuna, Mandich, & Macnab, 2001). Therefore, the question we must always ask is, "Is there a basis to what I'm doing in the intervention that is supported by theory and evidence?"

Occupational Therapy Task-Oriented Approach

Let's consider another scenario and another theoretical approach, the Occupational Therapy Task-Oriented Approach for people who have had stroke, developed by occupational therapists Virgil Mathiowetz and Julie Bass-Haugen (1994). The OT Task-Oriented Approach is another example of a theory and evidence-based intervention informed by multiple theoretical perspectives from a range of disciplines. During the early 1990s, many researchers began to question the assumptions and propositions of theories of motor development (Thelen & Ulrich, 1991) and motor behavior change (Jongbloed, Stacey, & Brighton, 1989; Sabari, 1991). Therapists were using interventions based on assumptions such as: 1) the CNS is hierarchically organized, 2) normal movement can be facilitated by providing specific patterns of sensory input, and 3) recovery from brain damage follows a predictable sequence. Clients were not making desired changes and practitioners were searching for new understandings of the challenges clients presented. Therapists and clients were particularly dissatisfied that retraining of normal movement patterns did not result in carry over to functional daily living skills.

The OT Task-Oriented Approach includes assumptions and propositions from broad OT theories, a systems model of motor control, an ecological approach to perception, and action and dynamic systems theory. This multidisciplinary approach represents understanding of motor control and learning from the neuropsychological, biomechanical, and behavioral sciences. An overarching assumption of the OT Task-Oriented Approach is that movement is organized around a goal and influenced by the environment. Movement emerges as an interaction among many systems, each contributing to motor control.

The term *task-oriented approach* was first proposed by a physical therapist at a professional conference focused on contemporary management of motor control problems (Horak, 1991). Occupational therapists revised the task-oriented approach to consider task performance in relation to a person's valued life roles. The inclusion of role performance in the OT Task-Oriented Approach is based on Trombly's (1995) proposition that to engage satisfactorily in a life role, a person must be able to do the activities and tasks that, in the person's opinion, make up that role. As research and theories have evolved, the OT Task-Oriented Approach continues to evolve and become more discrete as new research helps us refine the specific mechanisms of action (Bass-Haugen, Mathiowetz, & Flinn, 2008; Mathiowetz, 2011; Preissner, 2010).

As we examine the OT Task-Oriented Approach, consider Case Study 37.2 and how a practitioner working with Pablo following a stroke might adopt the OT Task-Oriented Approach to inform his or her reasoning related to evaluation and intervention.

CASE STUDY 37.2 Pablo

Pablo, a 52-year-old successful businessman, had a right middle cerebral artery stroke with resulting left-sided weakness and decreased balance 3 weeks ago. He lives with his wife and 2 sons, ages 11 and 13 years. Pablo loves to cook food from his Ecuadorian homeland for his family. He is eager to regain function so he can return to his job as a financial consultant. His family enjoys sledding with his children in the winter and camping in the summer—activities he hopes to continue. How will the occupational therapist use theory to guide his or her reasoning about the best possible intervention for Pablo?

The occupational therapist begins the evaluation by focusing on Pablo's roles and then proceeds to identify his priorities and goals for intervention. First, the therapist administers the Role Checklist (Oakley, Kielhofner, Barris, & Reichler, 1986), a self-report measure to assess roles significant to Pablo and his motivation to engage in tasks or activities necessary to fulfill valued roles. The practitioner may discuss with Pablo and his wife which roles Pablo had before his stroke and which roles he wants or must do in the future. Together, Pablo, his wife, and the practitioner identify goals for occupational therapy intervention. The initial emphasis on role performance is congruent with Trombly's (1995) theoretical propositions that to satisfactorily engage in a life role, a person must be able to do the activities and tasks that, in the person's opinion, make up that role, and that clients who are actively engaged in their treatment achieve self-identified goals and better outcomes. These initial evaluation and goal-setting processes are also supported by propositions from client-centered perspectives: when clients and therapist work together to achieve goals, clients are more engaged, satisfied, and make meaningful gains.

(continued)

(continued)

After discussing Pablo's important life roles and his goals for occupational therapy, Pablo and the occupational therapist decide to try making a fruit drink in the occupational therapy department kitchen in the rehabilitation hospital. As Pablo cuts a papaya, the occupational therapist notices that Pablo places his left arm on the table to stabilize the bowl as he puts the cut-up pieces of papaya in the bowl. When cued to use his left hand, he tries to pick up a mango; but the mango drops to the floor because Pablo's grasp is too weak to hold the mango. The therapist then completes performance-based assessments to determine if Pablo has the necessary performance skills to complete desired tasks.

The OT practitioner also uses the OT Task-Oriented Approach to guide Pablo's intervention. The emphasis of intervention is on enabling clients to successfully engage in tasks and activities associated with the roles and occupations clients are expected to, need to, or want to fulfill; purposeful and meaningful tasks are the primary intervention modality. The practitioner believes that the OT Task-Oriented Approach might be an effective intervention to help Pablo achieve his goals to cook, return to work, and enjoy outdoor activities with his family. The overarching assumptions of the OT Task-Oriented Approach are presented in Box 37.2.

Figure 37.3 provides a general overview of the key theoretical propositions and features of the OT Task-Oriented Approach. Table 37.4 presents if/then statements for the key theoretical propositions outlined in Figure 37.3.

Following an assessment of Pablo's performance in relation to desired tasks and activities, the therapist and Pablo will consider whether to develop compensatory approaches for challenging tasks or attempt to remediate skills necessary for successful task completion. Based on dynamical systems theory, the therapist continuously analyzes the critical control parameters—personal and environmental variables that may have potential to impact task performance. A review of available evidence will support the practitioner's reasoning regarding the probability of changing a control parameter to support performance. The dynamic systems perspective that proposes that movement is organized in relation to a goal echoes the propositions informed by other theoretical perspectives. Together, these theoretical perspectives inform the practitioner's actions with Pablo. It is possible to test these propositions, and numerous researchers have conducted studies to demonstrate support for these propositions (for one example, see Trombly, Radomski, & Davis, 1998).

At first glance, the CO-OP and the OT Task-Oriented Approach appear quite similar because both approaches are based on the proposition that if a person is engaged in the process of setting goals for intervention based on his or her values and preferences, he or she will engage in more effective problem solving and be more motivated to engage in the intervention activities. Guided practice with specific feedback is another common feature of the two approaches. Yet, the CO-OP approach is informed by metacognitive theories, whereas the OT Task-Oriented Approach is derived from motor learning and behavioral control theories, thus, the discrete propositions are different; intervention strategies and the resulting therapist actions might differ. Baking cookies and a cake provides a useful metaphor for capturing this distinction. We might use the ingredients of flour, sugar, and butter in preparing both cake and cookies. Yet, in order to achieve our goal or desired outcome, we need to use the appropriate amount or dose of ingredients, perhaps select among different forms of the ingredients, add other unique ingredients, and introduce the ingredients in a particular order or sequence. In contrast to baking, OT is a complex and dynamic process; and the outcome being sought is unique to each client. This complexity requires a unique approach for each client that is constructed and continually revised through application of the therapist's professional reasoning. In order to ensure that one's intervention is optimally suited to the client's capacities and effective to achieve the client's goals, the therapist must continually articulate and examine the

BOX 37.2 Assumptions of OT Task-Oriented Approach

- Personal and environmental systems, including the CNS, are heterarchically organized.
- Functional tasks help organize behavior.
- Occupational performance emerges from the interaction of persons and their environment.
- Experimentation with various strategies leads to optimal solutions to motor problems.
- Recovery is variable because patient factors and environmental contexts are unique.
- Behavioral changes reflect attempt to compensate to achieve task performance.

CNS, central nervous system; OT, occupational therapy.
From Mathiowetz, V. (2011). Task-oriented approach to stroke rehabilitation. In G. Gillen (Ed.), *Stroke rehabilitation* (pp. 80–99). St. Louis, MO: Elsevier Mosby.

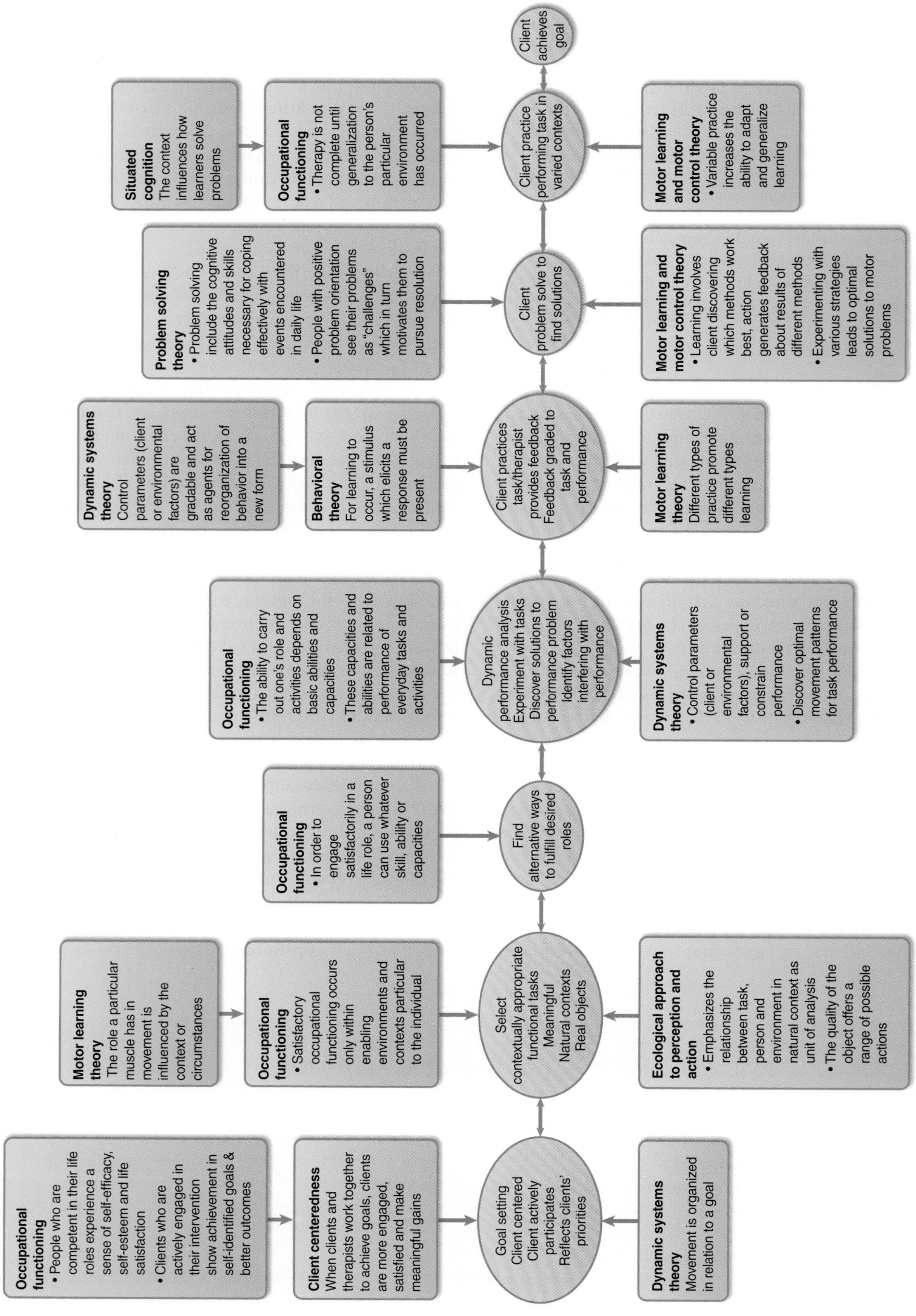

Occupational functioning
• People who are competent in their life roles experience a sense of self-efficacy, self-esteem and life satisfaction
• Clients who are actively engaged in their intervention show achievement in self-identified goals & better outcomes
Client centeredness
When clients and therapists work together to achieve goals, clients are more engaged, satisfied and make meaningful gains
Goal setting
Client centered
Client actively participates
Reflects clients' priorities
Dynamic systems theory
Movement is organized in relation to a goal
Motor learning theory
The role a particular muscle has in movement is influenced by the context or circumstances
Occupational functioning
• Satisfactory occupational functioning occurs only within enabling environments and contexts particular to the individual
Select contextually appropriate functional tasks
Meaningful
Natural contexts
Real objects
Ecological approach to perception and action
• Emphasizes the relationship between task, person and environment in natural context as unit of analysis
• The quality of the object offers a range of possible actions
Occupational functioning
• In order to engage satisfactorily in a life role, a person can use whatever skill, ability or capacities
Find alternative ways to fulfill desired roles
Occupational functioning
• The ability to carry out one's role and activities depends on basic abilities and capacities
• These capacities and abilities are related to performance of everyday tasks and activities
Dynamic performance analysis
Experiment with tasks
Discover solutions to performance problem
Identify factors interfering with performance
Dynamic systems theory
• Control parameters (client or environmental factors), support or constrain performance
• Discover optimal movement patterns for task performance
Dynamic systems theory
Control parameters (client or environmental factors) are gradable and act as agents for reorganization of behavior into a new form
Behavioral theory
For learning to occur, a stimulus which elicits a response must be present
Client practices task/therapist provides feedback
Feedback graded to task and performance
Motor learning theory
Different types of practice promote different types learning
Problem solving theory
• Problem solving include the cognitive attitudes and skills necessary for coping effectively with events encountered in daily life
• People with positive problem orientation see their problems as "challenges" which in turn motivates them to pursue resolution
Client problem solve to find solutions
Motor learning and motor control theory
• Learning involves client discovering which methods work best, action generates feedback about results of different methods
• Experimenting with various strategies leads to optimal solutions to motor problems
Situated cognition
The context influences how learners solve problems
Occupational functioning
• Therapy is not complete until generalization to the person's particular environment has occurred
Client practice performing task in varied contexts
Motor learning and motor control theory
• Variable practice increases the ability to adapt and generalize learning
Client achieves goal

FIGURE 37.3 General overview of Occupational Therapy Task-Oriented Approach.

TABLE 37.4 Theoretical Propositions and If/Then Statements of the Occupational Therapy Task-Oriented Approach

Intervention Feature	If/Then Statements from Key Theories	Evidence to Support Proposition
Goal setting: client guides selection of tasks for intervention • Client centered • Intervention reflects client's priorities • Elicit active participation of client	If the client sets goals for intervention, then he or she will be more engaged in intervention and achieve desired outcomes.	Law, Babtiste, and Mills (1995) Law and Mills (1998) Siegert and Taylor (2004) Trombly (1995)
Functional and meaningful tasks	If the task is functional and meaningful to the client, then quality of movement will be better.	Lin, Wu, Tickle-Degnen, and Coster (1997) Wu, Wong, Lin, and Chen (2001)
Natural context (if rehabilitation setting, should simulate real-life setting as much as possible)	If the intervention is provided in natural context, then clients will develop more flexible movement patterns for the task and context.	Bernstein (1967) Burgess (1989) Gillen and Wasserman (2004)
Real objects	If a person uses real objects, rather than rote exercise without objects, then quality of movement will be better.	Nelson et al. (1996) Wu, Trombly, Lin, and Tickle-Degnen (2000) Mathiowetz and Wade (1995)
Help clients adjust to role and task performance limitations	If clients can find alternative ways to fulfill roles or perform associated tasks, then they will be able to continue desired roles.	Trombly (1995)
Dynamic performance analysis • Experiment with functional tasks to discover efficient strategies for optimal solutions to performance problems • Identify salient client or environmental factors interfering with effective and efficient task performance	If the client experiments with functional activities, then he or she will discover the most effective and efficient way to perform task. If the client factor (e.g., strength, sensation) is critical to occupational performance of desired task and the client has potential to change, then remedial techniques should be used. • If a client, after a stroke, has active wrist and finger extension in the involved extremity, then the client is likely to benefit from constraint-induced movement therapy (CIMT). – If a client has active extension of the wrist >10 degrees starting at neutral, some active abduction of the carpometacarpal (CMC) joint of thumb, and 10 degrees of active extension in elbow flexion, then the client is likely to befit from modified constraint-induced therapy (mCIT). If remediation is unlikely, then adaptive and compensatory approaches should be used.	Van Peppen et al. (2004) Flinn (1995) Bonaiuti, Rebasti, and Sioli (2007) Gillen (2002)
Adapt task to promote optimal performance	Changing task and environmental characteristics can elicit changes in the client's movement forms and patterns.	Davis and Burton (1991)
Client practices task and therapist provides feedback to facilitate learning • Feedback graded to task and performance	If the therapist provides graded feedback for the type of task and client performance, then the client will learn the task. If the feedback is gradually tapered, then the client will learn how to use his or her own feedback mechanisms to monitor and evaluate his or her own performance.	Crutchfield and Barnes (1993)
Problem-solve with client	If the client can break down task and problem-solve on his or her own, then he or she will be more likely to generate solutions in other contexts and environments.	Elliott (1999) D'Zurilla & Nezu (2007)
Practice performing tasks outside of therapy context • Follow-up	If the client uses abilities discovered in therapy in varied contexts, then abilities will become more automatic.	Gillen and Wasserman (2004) Trombly (1995)

assumptions and propositions underlying his or her actions and be prepared to revise his or her approach when desired outcomes are not achieved or the evidence does not support the reasoning.

Conclusion

Within OT, some of our interventions and treatment theories are more developed than others. As we develop a more refined understanding of the causal relationships represented in our intervention theories and deconstruct how the intervention works, we can be more precise in our intervention. We can also articulate the basis of what we are doing more clearly to others. Thus, for example, we can explain to Pablo how the activities he is engaging in during an intervention session relate to achieving the goal he has set for himself or explain to the supervisor why we expect CO-OP to be more effective for Alex than simple practice of desired skills with feedback. It is our professional responsibility to continually examine the assumptions and theoretical propositions guiding our intervention approaches so that we can improve practice and achieve desired outcomes for clients.

References

American Occupational Therapy Association. (2008). Occupational therapy practice framework: Domain and process, 2nd edition. *American Journal of Occupational Therapy, 62*, 625–683.

Ayres, A. J. (1972). *Sensory integration and learning disorders.* Los Angeles, CA: Western Psychological Services.

Bandura, A. (1997). *Self-efficacy: The exercise of control.* New York, NY: W. H. Freeman.

Bass-Haugen, J., Mathiowetz, V., & Flinn, N. (2008). Optimizing motor behavior using the occupational therapy task-oriented approach. In M. V. Radomski & C. A. T. Latham (Eds.), *Occupational therapy for physical dysfunction* (6th ed., pp. 598–617). Philadelphia, PA: Lippincott Williams & Wilkins.

Batte, M., & Polatajko, H. J. (2006). *CO-OP vs. practice for children with Developmental Coordination Disorder: A question of strategy* (Unpublished dissertation). University of Toronto, Canada:.

Baum, C. M., & Christiansen, C. H. (2005). Person-environment-occupation-performance: An occupation-based framework for practice. In C. H. Christiansen, C. M. Baum, & J. Bass-Haugen (Eds.), *Occupational therapy: Performance, participation, and well-being* (pp. 242–266). Thorofare, NJ: Slack.

Bernstein, N. (1967). *The coordination and regulation of movements.* Elmsford, NY: Pergamon Press.

Bonaiuti, D., Rebasti, L., & Sioli, P. (2007). The constraint induced movement therapy: A systematic review of randomized controlled trials on the adult stroke patients. *Eura Medicophys, 43*, 139–146.

Bronfenbrenner, U. (1979). *The ecology of human development: Experiments by nature and design.* Cambridge, MA: Harvard University Press.

Burgess, M. K. (1989). Motor control and the role of occupational therapy: Past, present, and future. *American Journal of Occupational Therapy, 43*, 345–348.

Crutchfield, C. A., & Barnes, M. R. (1993). *Motor control and motor learning in rehabilitation.* Atlanta, GA: Stokesville.

Davis, W. E., & Burton, A. W. (1991). Ecological task analysis: Behavior theory into practice. *Adapted Physical Activity Quarterly, 8*, 154–177.

Dunn, W., Brown, C., & McGuian, M. (1994). The ecology of human performance: A framework for considering the effect of context. *American Journal of Occupational Therapy, 48*, 595–607.

D'Zurilla, T., & Nezu, A. (2007). *Problem-solving therapy: A positive approach to clinical intervention* (3rd ed.). New York, NY: Springer Publishing.

Elliott, T. R. (1999). Social problem-solving abilities and adjustment to recent-onset spinal cord injury. *Rehabilitation Psychology, 44*, 315–332.

Feuerstein, R., Hoffman, M., Jensen, M., Tzuriel, D., & Hoffman, D. (1986). Learning to learn: Mediated learning experiences and instrumental enrichment. *Special Services in Schools, 3*, 48–82.

Flinn, N. (1995). A task-oriented approach to the treatment of a client with hemiplegia. *American Journal of Occupational Therapy, 49*, 560–569.

Gibson, J. J. (1979). *The ecological approach to visual perception.* Boston, MA: Houghton Mifflin.

Gillen, G. (2002). Improving mobility and community access in an adult with ataxia. *American Journal of Occupational Therapy, 56*, 462–466.

Gillen, G., & Wasserman, M. (2004). Mobility: Examining the impact of environment on transfer performance. *Physical and Occupational Therapy in Geriatrics, 22*, 21–29.

Haywood, H. C. (1988). Bridging: A special technique of mediation. *The Thinking Teacher, 4*, 4–5.

Hooper, B. (1997). The relationship between pretheoretical assumptions and clinical reasoning. *American Journal of Occupational Therapy, 51*, 328–338.

Horak, F. B. (1991). Assumptions underlying motor control for neurologic rehabilitation. In M. J. Lister (Ed.), *Contemporary management of motor control problems: Proceeding of the II STEP conference* (pp. 11–27). Alexandria, VA: Foundation for Physical Therapy.

Jongbloed, L., Stacey, S., & Brighton, C. (1989). Stroke rehabilitation: Sensorimotor integrative treatment versus functional treatment. *American Journal of Occupational Therapy, 43*, 391–397.

Kielhofner, G. (2008). *The model of human occupation: Theory and application* (4th ed.). Philadelphia, PA: Lippincott Williams & Wilkins.

Kielhofner, G., & Burke, J. P. (1980). A model of human occupation, part 1. Conceptual framework and content. *American Journal of Occupational Therapy, 54*, 572–581.

Law, M., Babtiste, S., & Mills, J. (1995). Client-centered practice: What does it mean and does it make a difference? *Canadian Journal of Occupational Therapy, 62*, 250–257.

Law, M., Cooper, B., Strong, S., Stewart, D., Rigby, P., & Letts, L. (1996). The person-environment-occupational model: A transactive approach to occupational performance. *Canadian Journal of Occupational Therapy, 63*, 9–23.

Law, M., & Mills, J. (1998). Client-centered occupational therapy. In M. Law (Ed.), *Client-centered occupational therapy* (pp. 1–18). Thorofare, NJ: Slack.

Lawton, M. P. (1986). *Environment and aging* (2nd ed.). Albany, NY: Plenum Press.

Lin, K., Wu, C., Tickle-Degnen, L., & Coster, W. (1997). Enhancing occupational performance through occupationally embedded exercise: A meta-analytic review. *Occupational Therapy Journal of Research, 17*, 25–47.

Luria, A. R. (1976). *Cognitive development: Its cultural and social foundations.* Cambridge, MA: Harvard University Press.

Mandich, A., Polatajko, H. J., Macnab, J. J., & Miller, L. T. (2001). Treatment of children with developmental coordination disorder: What is the evidence? *Physical and Occupational Therapy in Pediatrics, 20*, 51–68.

Mandich, A. D., Polatajko, H. J., Missiuna, C., & Miller, L. T. (2001). Cognitive strategies and motor performance in children with developmental coordination disorder. *Physical and Occupational Therapy in Pediatrics, 20*(2/3), 125–143.

Mathiowetz, V. (2011). Task-oriented approach to stroke rehabilitation. In G. Gillen (Ed.), *Stroke rehabilitation* (pp. 80–99). St. Louis, MO: Elsevier Mosby.

Mathiowetz, V., & Bass-Haugen, J. (1994). Motor behavior research: Implications for therapeutic approaches to CND dysfunction. *American Journal of Occupational Therapy, 48*, 733–745.

Mathiowetz, V. G., & Wade, M. (1995). Task constraints and functional motor performance of individuals with and without multiple sclerosis. *Ecological Psychology, 7*, 99–123.

Meichenbaum, D. (1977). *Cognitive behaviour modification.* New York, NY: Plenum Press.

Miller, L. T., Polatajko, H. J., Missiuna, C., Mandich, A. D., & Macnab, J. J. (2001). A pilot trial of a cognitive treatment for children with developmental coordination disorder. *Human Movement Science, 20,* 183–210.

Nelson, D. L., Konosky, K., Fleharty, K., Webb, R., Newer, K., Hazboun, V. P., . . . Licht, B. C. (1996). The effects of an occupationally embedded exercise on bilaterally assisted supination in persons with hemiplegia. *American Journal of Occupational Therapy, 50,* 639–646.

Oakley, F., Kielhofner, G., Barris, R., & Reichler, R. (1986). The Role Checklist: Development and empirical assessment of reliability. *Occupational Therapy Journal of Research, 6,* 157–170.

Plautz, E. J., Milliken, G. W., & Nudo, R. J. (2000). Effects of repetitive motor training on movement representations in adult squirrel monkeys: Role of use versus learning. *Neurobiology of Learning and Memory, 74,* 27–55.

Polanyi, M. (2009). *The tacit dimension.* Chicago, IL: University of Chicago Press. (Original work published 1966)

Polatajko, H. J., Mandich, A. D., Missiuna, C., Miller, L. T., Macnab, J. J., Malloy-Miller, T., & Kinsella, E. A. (2001). Cognitive orientation to daily occupational performance (CO-OP): Part III–The protocol in brief. In C. Missiuna (Ed.), *Children with developmental coordination disorder: Strategies for success* (pp. 107–123). New York, NY: Haworth Press.

Popper, K. (1959). *The logic of scientific discovery.* Oxford, United Kingdom: Basic Books.

Preissner, K. (2010). Use of the occupational therapy task-oriented approach to optimize the motor performance of a client with cognitive limitations. *American Journal of Occupational Therapy, 64,* 727–734. doi:10.5014/ajot.2010.08026

Sabari, J. S. (1991). Motor learning concepts applied to activity-based intervention with adults with hemiplegia. *American Journal of Occupational Therapy, 45,* 523–530.

Siegert, R. J., & Taylor, W. J. (2004). Theoretical aspects of goal-setting and motivation in rehabilitation. *Disability & Rehabilitation, 26*(1), 1–8.

Taub, E., Uswatte, G., & Pidikiti, R. (1999). Constraint-induced movement therapy: A new family of techniques with broad application to physical rehabilitation. *Journal of Rehabilitation Research and Development, 6,* 237–251.

Thelen, E., & Ulrich, B. D. (1991). Hidden skills. *Monographs of the Society for Research in Child Development, 56,* 1–98.

Theory. (2010). In *Merriam-Webster Online Dictionary.* Retrieved from http://www.merriam-webster.com/dictionary/theory

Trombly, C. A. (1995). Occupation: Purposefulness and meaningfulness as therapeutic mechanisms. *American Journal of Occupational Therapy, 49,* 960–972.

Trombly, C., Radomski, M. V., & Davis, E. S. (1998). Achievement of self-identified goals by adults with traumatic brain injury: Phase I. *American Journal of Occupational Therapy, 52,* 810–818.

Van Peppen, R. P., Kwakkel, G., Wood-Dauphinee, S., Hendriks, H. J., Van der Wees, P. J., & Dekker, J. (2004). The impact of physical therapy on functional outcomes after stroke: What's the evidence? *Clinical Rehabilitation, 18,* 833–862.

Vygotsky, L. S. (1967). Play and its role in the mental development of the child. *Soviet Psychology, 5,* 6–18.

Whyte, J. (2006). Using treatment theories to refine the designs of brain injury rehabilitation treatment effectiveness studies. *Journal of Head Trauma Rehabilitation, 21,* 99–106.

Wu, C., Trombly, C. A., Lin, K., & Tickle-Degnen, L. (2000). A kinematic study of contextual effects on reaching performance in persons with and without stroke: Influences of object availability. *Archives of Physical Medicine and Rehabilitation, 81,* 95–101.

Wu, C., Wong, M., Lin, K., & Chen, H. (2001). Effects of task goal and personal preference on seated reaching kinematics after stroke. *Stroke, 32,* 70–76.

For additional resources on the subjects discussed in this chapter, visit http://thePoint.lww.com/Willard-Spackman12e.

CHAPTER 38

Ecological Models in Occupational Therapy

Catana E. Brown

OUTLINE

LEARNING OBJECTIVES

After reading this chapter, you will be able to:

1. Describe the historical foundations of ecological models and how these concepts contributed to the development of occupational therapy ecological models
2. Evaluate the role of the environment in understanding occupational performance
3. Identify the similarities and differences among the three ecological models described in the chapter (Ecology of Human Performance, Person-Environment-Occupation, and Person-Environment-Occupational-Performance)
4. Analyze and apply the ecological models (Ecology of Human Performance, Person-Environment-Occupation, and Person-Environment-Occupational-Performance) and their concepts to occupational therapy practice
5. Distinguish the five intervention strategies: establish/restore, adapt/modify, alter, prevent, and create

Introduction

In the 1990s, three groups of occupational therapists working independently created three separate models that emphasized the importance of considering the environment in occupational therapy practice. The three models—the Ecology of Human Performance model (EHP) (Dunn, Brown, & McGuigan, 1994), the Person-Environment-Occupational-Performance model (PEOP) (Christiansen & Baum, 1997), and the Person-Environment-Occupation Model (PEO) (Law et al., 1996)—share many similarities and a few distinctions. The three dynamic models consider occupational (task) performance as the primary outcome of interest to occupational therapists. In addition, all of the models indicate that occupational performance is determined by the person, environment (context), and occupation (task). However, of the constructs of person, environment, and occupation, there was a concern by the developers of the models that the environment was the construct not receiving adequate attention. There is a tendency for occupational therapists and practitioners from other disciplines to focus on person factors and neglect the influence of the environment on occupational performance. Therefore, the ecological models were developed so that along with consideration for the person and occupation, occupational therapy practice includes assessments and interventions that focus on the environment. When the distinct characteristics of the person, environment, and task are taken together, the uniqueness of each situation is more fully appreciated. The differences in the models lie primarily in their definitions, components, and structures, which will be discussed further in the sections that follow.

Intellectual Heritage

The ecological models were built on social science theory, earlier occupational therapy models, and the disability movement. Each of the ecological models draws heavily on social science theories that describe person–environment interactions. Bronfenbrenner (1979) developed an ecological model that explored the influence of social factors on development. This nested model has the individual at the center of a system that is influenced by family, friends, communities, and institutions. These interactions can either enhance or inhibit development. For example, changes in economic systems and the increased numbers of women working have had a major influence on the family and child development.

Gibson's (1979) concept of affordances is applied primarily to the physical environment. People perceive objects in the environment as having specific characteristics that result in action or meaning. People do not consciously think about affordances, but people's perceptions determine how they interact with objects. For example, the flat surface of a table affords such activities as eating a meal or writing a note.

Lawton (1986) developed the concept of environmental press. **Press** is described as the demands of the environment. A good fit occurs when the person's adaptive behavior and affect match the environmental press; a poor fit occurs when the person cannot meet the demands of the environment. When curb cuts are available, the environmental press is more adaptive for a wheelchair user; however, other environmental features, such as a sidewalk with a steep grade or the presence of snow, can create demands that make performance impossible. Another goodness-of-fit model is based on the concept of flow (Csikszentmihalyi, 1990). A flow experience occurs when the person's skills and abilities match the challenges of the activity. However, flow is more than a good match; when in flow, the person is at one with the occupation and so completely absorbed that the passage of time goes unnoticed. The EHP, PEO, and PEOP models are based on the idea of goodness of fit. Occupational performance is optimal when the environment and the person's skills and abilities match the demands of the occupation (task). A disruption in any area of person, environment, or occupation will interfere with performance.

Earlier models of occupational therapy that take account of the environment contributed to the conceptualization of the EHP, PEO, and PEOP models. In the Model of Human Occupation (Kielhofner, 2004), environmental impact refers to the unique influence of the environment on the person. Environments are sources of opportunities and resources as well as demands and constraints. David Nelson (1988) addresses the environment by making a distinction between the terms *occupational performance* and *occupational form*. *Performance* is the doing of an occupation. *Form* is the context in which the doing takes place and includes the physical and sociocultural circumstances that are external to the person. Occupational form contributes to the personal meaning and purpose that the individual attributes to an occupation. The theory of Occupational Adaptation (Schkade & Schultz, 1992) proposes that the person desires mastery and the occupational environment demands mastery. Therefore, the interaction of the person and environment combine in a press for mastery resulting in an adaptive response.

Finally, the ecological models in occupational therapy were influenced by the disability civil rights movement. Health care practice is dominated by a focus on impairment in the person and interventions that are designed to fix that impairment. Individuals with disabilities have challenged this perspective. People in the independent living movement have pointed out that environmental barriers are typically the greatest impediment to a successful and satisfying life (DeJong, 1979; Shapiro, 1994). Furthermore, individuals with psychiatric disabilities have revealed that the power of stigma and subsequent discrimination interfere with full participation in community life (Chamberlin, 1990; Deegan, 1993).

The disability movements advocated for civil rights for individuals with disabilities and promoted self-determination and empowerment. The ecological models embrace the values of the disability movement. This is reflected in both the emphasis on the environment as a significant barrier and facilitator of occupational performance and the adoption of principles of client-centered practice.

Definitions

Person

The EHP, PEO, and PEOP models have similar definitions of the ***person***. The holistic view of the person acknowledges the mind, body, and spirit. Variables associated with the person include values and interests, skills and abilities, and life experiences. Values and interests help to determine what is important, meaningful, and enjoyable to the person. Skills and abilities include cognitive, social, emotional, and sensorimotor skills as well as abilities such as reading and knowing how to balance a checkbook. Life experiences form the person's history and personal narrative. The person influences and is influenced by the environment. For example, a person's family and friends contribute to the development of particular values and interests. A child might develop a love of reading because of the availability of books in the home and parents who read to the child, whereas having a child in the home might cause the parents to be more concerned about having healthy foods at home and creating a safe physical environment.

Environment

The **environment** is also described similarly across the three models. The environment is where occupational performance takes place and consists of physical, cultural, and social components. The EHP model also includes the temporal environment. The physical environment is the most tangible. It includes built and natural features, large elements such as the terrain or buildings, and small objects such as tools. The cultural environment is based on shared experiences that determine values, beliefs, and customs. The cultural environment includes, but is not limited to, ethnicity, religion, and national identity. For example, individuals may also adopt values and beliefs from the culture of their family, profession, organizations or clubs, and peer group.

The social environment is made up of many layers. It includes close interpersonal relationships such as family and friends. Another layer includes work groups or social organizations to which the individual belongs. A larger layer consists of political and economic systems, which can have a profound effect on the daily life of people with disabilities. These systems make decisions related to the rights of people with disabilities, availability of services, and financial benefits, such as social security disability and health insurance. The temporal environment is made up of time-oriented factors associated with the person (developmental and life stage) and the task (when it takes place, how often, and for how long).

Occupational performance cannot be understood outside of the context or environment. The environment can both create barriers to performance and enhance occupational performance. For example, a well-organized and familiar grocery store that provides foods that are culturally familiar and consistent with the person's likes might be described as an adaptive environment. Conversely, the grocery store might be a barrier if the person is overwhelmed by many choices, cannot find the items he or she is looking for, and is anxious when there are too many people around.

Occupation or Task

The biggest difference in the three models is found in the concepts related to **occupations** or ***tasks***. PEO and PEOP use the term *occupation*, whereas EHP uses *task*. The developers of EHP were intentional about the selection of the term *task* because a primary purpose of the model was to facilitate interdisciplinary collaboration. It was felt that the term *task* would be more accessible to other disciplines. Tasks are defined as objective representations of all possible activities available in the universe. Although this was not explicitly expressed in the early writings of EHP, occupations exist when the person and context factors come together to give meaning to tasks (Dunn, McClain, Brown, & Youngstrom, 2003). The PEO and PEOP models describe a series of nested concepts that make up occupations.

In PEO, activities are the basic units of tasks. Tasks are purposeful activities, and occupations are self-directed tasks that a person engages in over the life course. The PEOP model involves actions, which are observable behaviors; tasks, which are combinations of actions with a common purpose; and occupations, which are goal-directed, meaningful pursuits that typically extend over time. For example, chopping vegetables might be the observable behavior or activity, embedded within the task of preparing soup, which falls under the larger occupation of cooking dinner for the family. See Table 38.1 for a comparison of definitions of the ecological models.

TABLE 38.1 Definitions of Task, Activity, and Occupation Used by Ecological Models

	PEO	PEOP	EHP	Example
Activity	Recognizable and observable behavior	Basic units of tasks	Tasks and activities are not differentiated. Tasks are the objective set of behaviors necessary to achieve a goal.	Chopping vegetables
Task	Purposeful activities recognized by the task performer	Combinations of actions with a common purpose		Cooking a meal
Occupation	Self-directed tasks that a person engages in over the life course	Goal-directed, meaningful pursuits that extend over time	Tasks that acquire meaning through the person–environment interaction	Making dinner for the family

EHP, Ecology of Human Performance; PEO, Person-Environment-Occupation; PEOP, Person-Environment-Occupational-Performance.

Occupational Performance

Occupational performance is the outcome that is associated with the confluence of the person, environment, and occupation factors. The degree to which occupational performance is possible depends on the goodness of fit of these factors. The structures of the models are depicted in slightly different ways. In PEO, a Venn diagram is used to illustrate the meeting of person, environment, and occupation variables (Figure 38.1). The space in which the three circles come together is occupational performance. PEOP is similar; however, there are four circles instead of three (Figure 38.2). Person and environment touch but do not overlap. Occupation and performance are two separate circles that overlay person and environment. These circles come together to form occupational performance and participation. In EHP, the person is embedded inside the context, with tasks floating all around (Figure 38.3). The performance range includes the tasks that are available to the person because of the existing environment supports and his or her own skills, abilities, and experiences.

In all of the models, the performance range or occupational performance area is constantly changing as the other variables change. The area of occupational performance increases or the performance range expands when the person acquires new skills. Likewise, expansion occurs when stigma is decreased, physical barriers are removed, additional social supports are acquired, or schedules are accommodating. Unfortunately, people with disabilities are often faced with limited personal capacities and multiple environmental barriers. The role of the occupational therapist is to change this dynamic so that more occupations are available to the person.

Intervention Strategies

Additional terms that are included in the EHP model are five different intervention strategies: (1) *establish/restore*, (2) *adapt/modify*, (3) *alter*, (4) *prevent*, and (5) *create*. These interventions were spelled out so that occupational therapists would consider the full range of options. In particular, the enumeration of intervention choices was designed to encourage occupational therapists to use more interventions directed at the environment.

- **Establish/restore interventions** target the person and are aimed at developing and improving skills and abilities so that the person can perform tasks (occupations) in context. Increasing range of motion so that an individual can better manage self-care tasks and teaching someone how to use a microwave oven for meal preparation involve establish/restore strategies.
- **Adapt/modify interventions** change the environment or task to increase the individual's performance range. Using assistive devices such as an adapted car for driving or a built-up handled spoon for eating are interventions that change the typical environment. Changes to the physical environments are most common in occupational therapy; however, it is important to consider interventions that target the social and cultural environment as well. Adapt/modify strategies can include providing education about disabilities to students in an elementary school classroom so that the child with special needs will be more accepted. This is an adapt/modify strategy because the social environment is being changed. Other adapt/modify interventions could include providing social support for someone who is fearful of riding the bus or changing the work schedule for someone with endurance problems so that physically demanding tasks are spread throughout the day.
- **Alter interventions** do not change the person, task, or environment but are designed to make a better fit. Occupational therapists may overlook

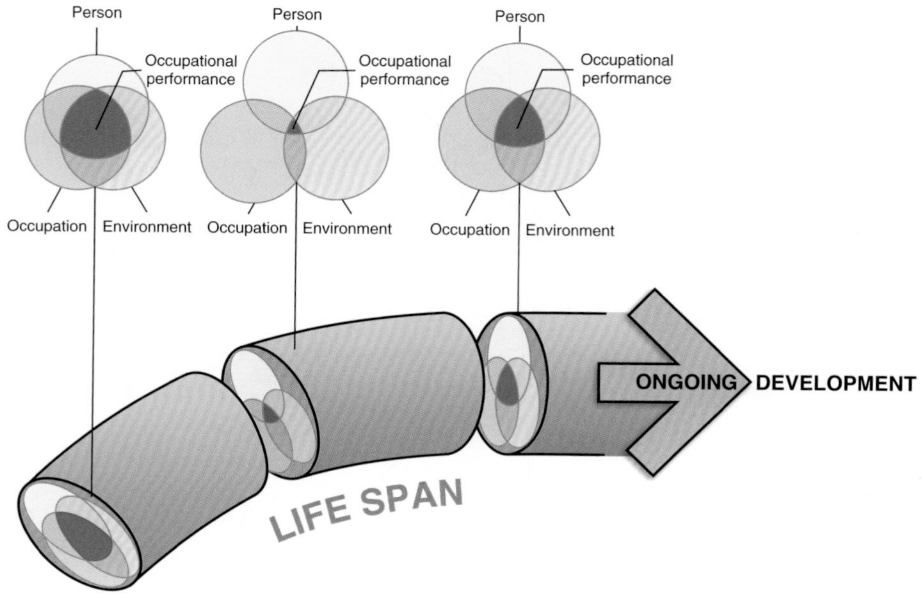

FIGURE 38.1 Person-Environment-Occupation Model. (Reprinted with permission from Law, M., Cooper, B., Strong, S., Stewart, D., Rigby, P., & Letts, L. [1996]. The person-environment-occupation model: A transactive approach to occupational performance. *Canadian Journal of Occupational Therapy, 63*, 9–23.)

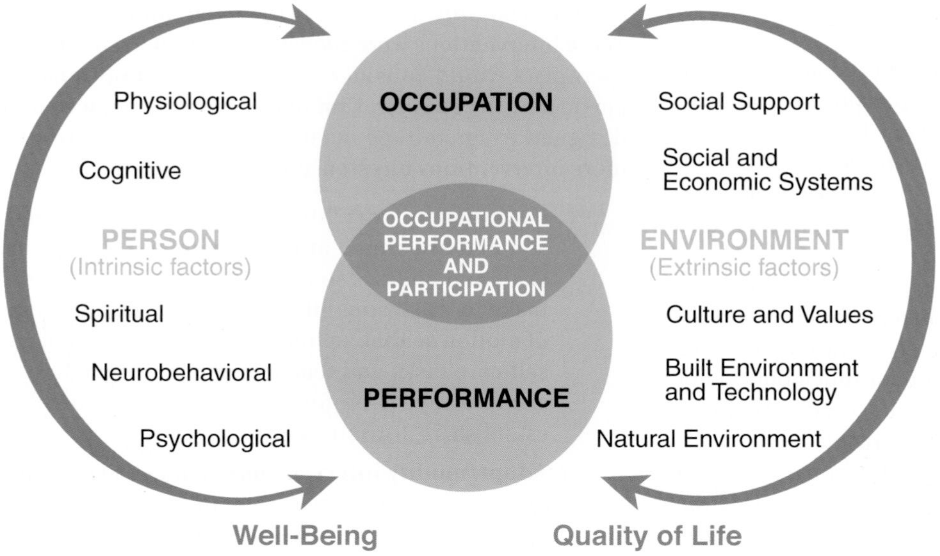

FIGURE 38.2 Person-Environment-Occupation-Performance model. (Reprinted with permission from Christiansen, C., Baum, C., & Bass-Haugen, J., [Eds.]. [2005]. *Occupational therapy: Performance, participation, and well-being* [3rd ed.]. Thorofare, NJ: Slack.)

alter interventions because it does not appear that they are "doing" anything. However, alter interventions can be very effective because they take advantage of what is already naturally occurring. Making a good match requires that the occupational therapist have strong skills in activity analysis and environmental assessment. Moving from a two-story house with stairs to a ranch home would be an alter intervention for someone with limited endurance. Helping an individual to find a club or organization to join based on his or her values and beliefs and matching the person's skills with a particular job are examples of alter interventions.

- **Prevent interventions** are implemented to change the course of events when a negative outcome is predicted. Prevention can use interventions that change the person (establish/restore), change the environment (adapt/modify), or make a better match (alter); but these occur before the problem develops. Teaching at-risk parents skills in facilitating developmentally appropriate play is an example of a prevent strategy, as is using a special cushion in a wheelchair to prevent decubitus or pressure ulcers.
- **Create interventions** do not assume that a problem has occurred or will occur but are designed to promote performance in context. These interventions enrich occupational performance in context. Like the prevent strategies, create interventions can use establish/restore, adapt, or alter approaches.

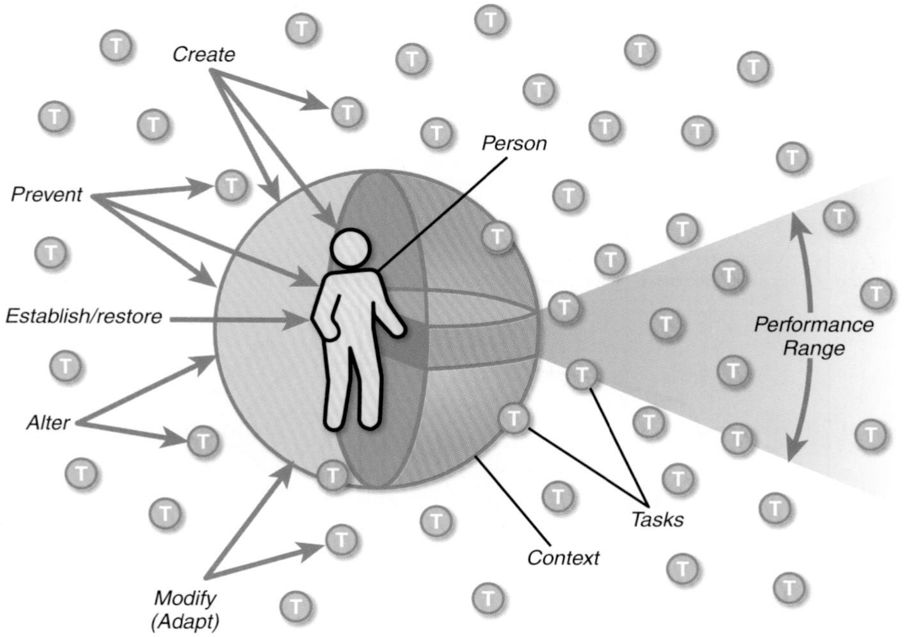

FIGURE 38.3 Ecology of Human Performance model. (Reprinted with permission from Dunn, W.,McClain, L. H., Brown, C., & Youngstrom, M. J. [2003]. The ecology of human performance. In E. B. Crepeau, E. S. Cohn, & B. A. B. Schell [Eds.], *Willard & Spackman's occupational therapy* [10th ed., pp. 223–226]. Philadelphia, PA: Lippincott William & Wilkins.)

Setting up a study space within a quiet area with adequate lighting, finding a good roommate, and practicing interview skills prior to an actual job interview are examples of create interventions.

Assumptions of the Ecological Models

- The relationships between people, environments, and occupations are dynamic and unique. They interact continually and across time and space. Therefore, occupational therapists should approach each situation as ever changing and distinct.
- The environment is a major factor in the prediction of successful and satisfying occupational performance. Environments can either facilitate or inhibit occupational performance. All aspects of the environment (physical, social, cultural, and temporal) should be evaluated to determine relevant environmental influences.
- Rather than exclusively using interventions that change the person, it is often more efficient and effective to change the environment or find a person–environment match.
- Occupational performance is determined by the confluence of person, environment, and occupation factors. People, environments, and occupations are constantly changing; and as these factors change, so does occupational performance.
- Occupational therapy practice begins by identifying what occupations the person wants or needs to perform. Using a top-down approach, the targeted area of occupational performance is identified first by the client or family. This is followed by an assessment of barriers and facilitators within the person, environment, and occupation that affect occupational performance.
- Occupational therapy practice involves promoting self-determination and the inclusion of people with disabilities in all environments. The person or system that is the service recipient is the primary decision maker in the occupational therapy process. Occupational therapists should act as advocates for people with disabilities and should support their clients in self-advocacy.

Application to Practice

The ecological models provide a framework for thinking about occupational therapy practice but do not delineate specific assessments or techniques. Using an ecological model requires an intentional effort on the part of the occupational therapist to consider the environment as extensively as he or she considers the person. An overarching value of the ecological models is a client-centered approach to practice. The person and occupational therapist collaborate throughout all stages of the occupational therapy process, and the process begins by identifying what the person wants or needs to do in his or her life (see Box 38.1). Consequently, the stage is set so that assessment and intervention are not driven by the therapist but are framed in terms of what is most important to the person. The person is not viewed in isolation but instead is considered in terms of the environment in which occupational performance takes place. The dynamic interrelationships of person, environment, and occupation compel the therapist to appreciate the uniqueness of each situation. This means that practice is not an unyielding protocol applied to everyone with the same diagnosis but a thoughtful, reasoned, and collaborative process of evaluation and intervention tailored to each individual.

Once the person identifies the relevant area(s) of occupational performance, the evaluation process determines what features of the person, environment, and occupation support or interfere with occupational performance. Therefore, occupational therapy assessment must be comprehensive and include measures that consider the person, environment, and occupation. Occupational therapists are most familiar with measures of person factors and are skilled at complex task analysis. Environmental assessment is an area that has received less attention, although there are several good resources describing numerous environmental measures (Cooper, Letts, Rigby, Stewart, & Strong, 2001; Letts et al., 1994; Letts, Rigby, & Stewart, 2003).

Some standardized assessments such as the Performance Assessment of Self-Care Skills (Holm & Rogers, 2008) and the Test of Grocery Shopping Skills (Brown, Rempfer, & Hamera, 2009) are designed to assess occupational performance in the natural environment, whereas other assessments such as the In-Home Occupational Performance Evaluation (Stark, Somerville, & Morris, 2010) specifically measure the impact of the environment on performance. When standardized assessments do not exist, occupational therapists may consider using skilled observation of the identified area of occupation in the relevant environment. Therapists will need to bring in more specific practice models to guide the selection of assessments and later the intervention plan.

Ecological models provide a framework for practice but do not provide specific guidelines or theory about specific assessments or intervention techniques. However, the selection of practice models should be faithful to the values of the ecological models. Mostly, this means that the practice models that are used to guide assessment and intervention cannot be limited to person and occupational factors but must address the environment as well. The dynamic nature of the ecological models acknowledges that situations are constantly changing, indicating that regular reevaluation should occur.

The five intervention options proposed by the EHP model require occupational therapists to use a wide

BOX 38.1 Clinical Questions Related to Constructs of the Ecological Models

Person

Skills (cognitive, social, psychological, sensory, motor)
- What are the person's inherent strengths?
- What are potential areas of cognitive, social, or sensorimotor impairment?

Life skills
- What life skills has the person learned and what skills has the person not learned?
- What life skills has the person mastered and what skills are problematic?

Interests
- What does the person like to do?

Experiences
- What are the life experiences that contribute to or interfere with occupational performance?
- What are the major life events for the person?
- What are themes in the person's life story?

Environment/Context

Culture
- What cultural groups does the person identify with?
- What values does the person derive from these cultural groups?
- Are the beliefs and expectations of these cultural groups accepting of the person?

Social
- Are friends and family available to provide support?
- What providers are involved?
- How does public policy influence the person's ability to engage in tasks or occupations?

Physical
- Does the built environment or the natural environment create barriers to performance?
- Does the person have access to objects that facilitate performance?

Temporal
- Is the person able to engage in occupations that are consistent with the person's developmental or life phases?
- Does the person have too much time or not enough time to perform important tasks or occupations?

Occupation or Tasks

- What does the person want or need to do?
- What occupations or tasks come together to create roles or identity for the person?
- What occupations or tasks give meaning to the person's life?

Performance or Performance Range

- Which tasks or occupations fall inside or outside of the performance range?
- Are there factors related to the person, environment/context, or occupation that interfere with performance?

Therapeutic Intervention

- What intervention approach would be the most efficient and have the most desirable outcomes?
- Is there evidence to support the intervention approach?
- Which intervention approach does the service recipient want?

range of intervention approaches. Intervention can take many directions, and those interventions that target the environment should always be considered as one option. Furthermore, occupational therapy practice is not limited to existing problems but includes enhancing occupational performance and prevention of occupational performance problems. The association of ecological models with disability rights means that occupational therapists should also be involved at the systems level, supporting policy that promotes full participation in all aspects of community life. The case study on The Asbury Café demonstrates the ecological model in practice.

CASE STUDY 38.1 The Asbury Café

The Asbury Café is an employment program developed by the author. The Asbury Café operates every Wednesday night at a local church. Five individuals with serious mental illness are employees of the café. A meal is served at a reasonable cost for church members, neighbors, and friends. An occupational therapist oversees the running of the café, assisted by volunteers and college students. It is an example of a program that uses the principles of the ecological models to promote work performance for people with psychiatric disabilities. However, that is just one of the aims of the program, which on a larger scale aspires to make changes in social and cultural environments to reduce the stigma associated with serious mental illness. People with serious mental illness are frequently depicted in the media as dangerous, peculiar, and in need of care and protection. Although serious mental illness is not uncommon, many people do not disclose their diagnosis because of the associated stigma. The Asbury Café provides an opportunity for people with and without mental illness to come together and interact in a positive environment (Figure 38.4).

The first aim of the program is to provide employment to individuals with psychiatric disabilities. Individuals who are referred by the vocational team to this worksite are typically individuals who have less work experience, have more overt symptomatology,

CASE STUDY 38.1 The Asbury Café (*Continued*)

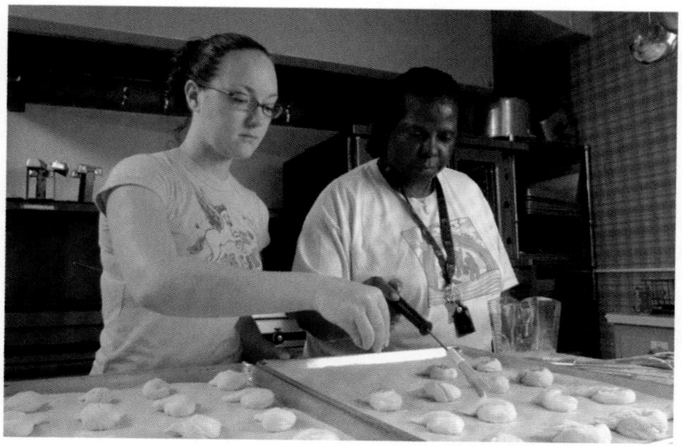

FIGURE 38.4 Jess and Janet at the Asbury Café. (Photo courtesy of C. Brown)

and need more extensive adaptations to the work environment. No formal assessments are completed; however, extensive skilled observation and task analysis are used to match employees with tasks and to make adaptations to the task and environment.

The second purpose of the Asbury Café is to reduce the stigma associated with serious mental illness by promoting positive social interactions between people with and without mental illness.

The Asbury Café demonstrates how occupational therapy can have an impact outside of a traditional service setting. The café is true to the values of the ecological models, which emphasize client-centered practice and full participation in community life. The program enhances occupational performance in the areas of work and social interaction by providing interventions targeting the person, environment, and occupation. The program itself is designed to change the stigmatizing social and cultural environment that is currently so pervasive for people with serious mental illness.

Target Area of Occupational Performance: Work

Ecological Model Components	Interventions
Person factors	
Individuals with serious mental illness often have cognitive impairments that slow information processing and interfere with learning of the job tasks.	Establish/restore: Provide simple instructions with demonstration, models, and regular feedback. Alter: Match worker with café task that best meets the person's interests and abilities. Adapt: Pair workers so that one with stronger skills can model, help focus, and provide feedback to the worker with developing skills.
Psychiatric symptoms such as anxiety and auditory hallucinations can make it more challenging to focus on work tasks.	Establish/restore: Teach the worker individual strategies to use when feeling anxious (e.g., deep breathing) or experiencing hallucinations (e.g., talk aloud to others). Adapt: Allow for frequent breaks, set up an environment of acceptance and support, use the environment to create distractions from hallucinations or worries.
Environmental factors	
Fewer job opportunities are available to the employees of the café in the neighborhoods where they live, and typical worksites do not offer the limited schedule needed and desired by current employees.	Adapt: The full Asbury Café program is an adapt strategy. Supervisors and volunteers have experience in mental health services. Employees at the café are individuals who need more extensive supports for successful work performance.
Employees at the café do not have cars, and no public transportation is available to the work location.	Adapt: Although this is not ideal, the mental health center provides transportation.
Occupation	
The major occupation is work in the area of meal preparation, serving, and cleanup. Each task has many subcomponents.	Adapt: The tasks are often adapted so that there are fewer steps or one task is done by two or three people so that the full task is not too difficult for an individual. Alter: Over time, the best matches become known; and individual workers assume responsibility for their tasks. They are able to perform these tasks without assistance or oversight.

(continued)

CASE STUDY 38.1 The Asbury Café (*Continued*)

Target Area of Occupational Performance: Social Interaction	
Ecological Model Components	**Interventions**
Person factors	
Many of the customers at the café have limited exposure to individuals with serious mental illness.	Alter: Employees with mental illness are assigned work tasks so that they have opportunities to interact directly with the café customers (taking money, serving meals). Employees with mental illness are also assigned work tasks that require regular contact with church staff. This provides an opportunity for real work relationships to develop.
Environmental factors	
Our culture tends to portray individuals with serious mental illness as dangerous, unpredictable, and in need of protection. Yet, the church is an environment that is open to accepting diverse individuals and welcomes the program.	Establish/restore: Educational opportunities are provided through the church in the form of lectures, articles in the newsletter, and presentations by consumers of the mental health center to provide accurate information to potential café customers about serious mental illness. Adapt: The program director and volunteers create an environment that models positive interactions with individuals with serious mental illness (e.g., avoiding distinguishing between those who do and do not have mental illness; in addition to working alongside one another, also socializing together during breaks).
Occupation	
Eating together socially.	Alter: The Asbury Café provides a naturally occurring opportunity for people to socialize in a natural setting. The café workers, supervisor, and volunteers eat during the time when the customers are eating so that there are more times for interaction.

Evidence Supporting the Ecological Models

The ecological models are large conceptual frameworks, making them difficult to study in their entirety. However, research indicating a relationship between environment and occupational performance and efficacy studies of environmental interventions provides support for the ecological models. This section provides examples of both types of research.

Research examining the relationship between the environment and occupational performance is increasing. For example, the following studies have implications for rehabilitation:

- Children with disabilities and their families identified physical, social, cultural, and institutional barriers as limiting transition to adulthood (Law et al., 1999).
- In a study of independence and employment for people with AIDS, environmental factors presented significant barriers to occupational performance (Paul-Ward, Kielhofner, Braveman, & Levin, 2005). One of the greatest barriers to independent living was the lack of low-income housing. Barriers to employment included procedures related to social security benefits and stigma by employers.
- A qualitative study of the home environment for people with physical disabilities found that social support was a major factor in overcoming impairments and inaccessibility in the home (Lund & Nygard, 2004). Time use was affected by the availability of support from others, and these individuals often spend much time waiting for others before they can engage in a desired occupation.
- Another study found that the physical environment of the home may present barriers for stroke survivors (Reid, 2004). For the most part, the stroke survivors were able to engage in desired occupations; however, getting through doorways and up and down stairs was difficult. Uneven ground outside the home was also a problem.
- A study examining environmental effects in healthy adults found better performance in familiar as compared to unfamiliar kitchens (Geusgen, van Heugten, Hagedoren, Jolles, & van den Heuvel, 2010).

There are several examples of research that support the efficacy of occupational therapy intervention with an ecological basis. Some of these interventions were intentionally designed with one of the ecological models in mind, whereas others are related in that they use the environment in the intervention approach. For example, Brown, Rempfer, and Hamera (2002) used the EHP model as a conceptual framework to develop a grocery shopping intervention for people with schizophrenia. In the intervention, participants were taught strategies to better use the naturally occurring environmental features of the grocery store (e.g., overhead signs, generic products). The intervention was effective in improving grocery shopping accuracy and efficiency.

The PEO model was used to develop a peer mentorship program for adolescents and young adults with physical disabilities (Stewart, 2003). The peer support of the mentorship program resulted in greater exploration of the self and the environment. This included an increased desire to try new things, socialize with others, and get out in the community.

The Environmental Skill-Building Program (ESP) (Corcoran et al., 2002), based on environmental press theory, incorporates environmental strategies to promote adaptive behavior in individuals with dementia. In ESP, the therapist works with a caregiver to adapt the home environment and teach interaction strategies. In a randomized controlled trial, caregivers who received the intervention were less upset with disruptive behaviors, had better affect, and had better overall well-being (Gitlin et al., 2003).

Another study considered the social environment as a factor in play skill development (Tanta, Deitz, White, & Billingsley, 2005). Using a single-subject design, preschool children with delayed play skills were paired with children who had a lower developmental play skills and a peer with a higher development play skills. The children with delayed play skills were more likely to initiate play and respond to the peer when paired with the child with higher play skills.

Intervention based on environmental assessment has become an integral component of practice for safety considerations with older adults. For example, a study of the CarFit assessment, which examines the match between an older driver and his or her vehicle, found that participants made changes to their car to increase safety while driving (Stav, 2010); and a study of environmental assessment with appropriate modifications of the home by occupational therapists found a reduction in falls (Pighills, Torgerson, Sheldon, Drummond, & Bland, 2011).

This growing body of research provides support for the impact of the environment on occupational performance and for the efficacy of environmental occupational therapy interventions. As the evidence continues to expand, occupational therapists will be better prepared to provide relevant and useful assessments and interventions using an ecological approach.

Conclusion

Occupational therapy practice is aimed at promoting occupational performance. Ecological models provide a framework for understanding the multiplicity of factors that must be taken into account in assessing and providing interventions to enhance occupational performance. These models require that the occupational therapist use a client-centered approach and always consider the importance of the environment in the occupational therapy process.

References

Bronfenbrenner, U. (1979). *The ecology of human development: Experiments by nature and design.* Cambridge, MA: Harvard University Press.

Brown, C., Rempfer, M., & Hamera, E. (2002). Teaching grocery shopping skills to people with schizophrenia. *Occupational Therapy Journal of Research, 22*(Suppl. 1), 90S–91S.

Brown, C., Rempfer, M., & Hamera, E. (2009). *Test of Grocery Shopping Skills Manual.* Bethesda, MD: AOTA Press.

Chamberlin, J. (1990). The ex-patients' movement: Where we've been and where we're going. *Journal of Mind and Behavior, 11*(3 & 4), 323–336.

Christiansen, C., & Baum C. (Eds.). (1997). *Occupational therapy: Enabling function and well-being* (2nd ed.). Thorofare, NJ: Slack.

Christiansen, C., Baum, C., & Bass-Haugen, J. (Eds.). (2005). *Occupational therapy: Performance, participation, and well-being* (3rd ed.). Thorofare, NJ: Slack.

Cooper, B., Letts, L., Rigby, P., Stewart, D., & Strong, S. (2001). Measuring environmental factors. In M. Law, C. Baum, & W. Dunn (Eds.), *Measuring occupational performance: Supporting best practice in occupational therapy* (pp. 229–256). Thorofare, NJ: Slack.

Corcoran, M. A., Gitlin, L. N., Levy, L., Eckhardt, S., Earland, T. V., Shaw, G., & Kearny, L. (2002). An occupational therapy home-based intervention to address dementia-related problems identified by family caregivers. *Alzheimer's Care Quarterly, 3*(1), 82–90.

Csikszentmihalyi, M. (1990). *Flow: The psychology of optimal experience.* New York, NY: Harper & Row.

Deegan, P. E. (1993). Recovering our self of value after being labeled. *Journal of Psychosocial Nursing, 31*(4), 7–11.

DeJong, G. (1979). Independent living: From social movement to analytic paradigm. *Archives of Physical Medicine and Rehabilitation, 60,* 435–446.

Dunn, W., Brown, C., & McGuigan, A. (1994). The ecology of human performance: A framework for considering the impact of context. *American Journal of Occupational Therapy, 48,* 595–607.

Dunn, W., McClain, L. H., Brown, C., & Youngstrom, M. J. (2003). The ecology of human performance. In E. B. Crepeau, E. S. Cohn, & B. A. B. Schell (Eds.), *Willard & Spackman's occupational therapy* (10th ed., pp. 223–226). Philadelphia, PA: Lippincott William & Wilkins.

Geusgen, C. A., van Heugten, C. M., Hagedoren, E., Jolles, J., & van den Heuvel, W. J. (2010). Brief report—Environmental effects in the performance of daily tasks in healthy adults. *American Journal of Occupational Therapy, 64,* 935–940.

Gibson, J. J. (1979). *The ecological approach to visual perception.* Boston, MA: Houghton Mifflin.

Gitlin, L. N., Winter, L., Corcoran, M., Dennis, M. P., Schinfeld, S., & Hauck, W. W. (2003). Effects of the home environmental skills building program on the caregiver-care recipient dyad: 6-month outcomes from the Philadelphia REACH initiative. *Gerontologist, 43,* 532–546.

Holm, M. B., & Rogers, J. C. (2008). The Performance Assessment of Self-Care Skills (PASS) (pp. 101–112). In B. Hemphill-Pearson (Ed.), *Assessment in occupational therapy in mental health: An integrative approach* (2nd ed.). Thorofare, NJ: Slack.

Kielhofner, G. (2004). *Conceptual foundations of occupational therapy* (3rd ed.). Philadelphia, PA: F. A. Davis.

Law, M., Cooper, B., Strong, S., Stewart, D., Rigby, P., & Letts, L. (1996). The person-environment-occupation model: A transactive approach to occupational performance. *Canadian Journal of Occupational Therapy*, *63*, 9–23.

Law, M., Haight, M., Milroy, B., Willms, D., Stewart, D., & Rosenbaum, P. (1999). Environmental factors affecting the occupations of children with physical disabilities. *Journal of Occupational Science*, *6*, 102–122.

Lawton, M. P. (1986). *Environment and aging* (2nd ed.). Albany, NY: Plenum Press.

Letts, L., Law, M., Rigby, P., Cooper, B., Stewart, D., & Strong, S. (1994). Person-environment assessments in occupational therapy. *American Journal of Occupational Therapy*, *48*, 608–618.

Letts, L., Rigby, P., & Stewart, D. (Eds.). (2003). *Using environments to enable occupational performance*. Thorofare, NJ: Slack.

Lund, M. L., & Nygard, L. (2004). Occupational life in the home environment: The experience of people with disabilities. *Canadian Journal of Occupational Therapy*, *71*, 243–252.

Nelson, D. L. (1988). Occupation: Form and performance. *American Journal of Occupational Therapy*, *42*, 633–641.

Paul-Ward, A., Kielhofner, G., Braveman, B., & Levin, M. (2005). Resident and staff perceptions of barriers to independence and employment in supportive living settings for persons with AIDS. *American Journal of Occupational Therapy*, *59*, 540–545.

Pighills, A., Torgerson, D., Sheldon, T., Drummond, A., & Bland, M. (2011). Environmental assessment and modification to prevent falls in older people. *Journal of the American Geriatrics Society*, *59*, 26–33.

Reid, D. (2004). Accessibility and usability of the physical housing environment of seniors with stroke. *International Journal of Rehabilitation Research*, *27*, 203–208.

Schkade, J. K., & Schultz, S. (1992). Occupational adaptation: Toward a holistic approach to contemporary practice, Part I. *American Journal of Occupational Therapy*, *46*, 829–837.

Shapiro, J. P. (1994). *No pity: People with disabilities forging a new civil rights movement*. New York, NY: Three Rivers Press.

Stark, S. L., Somerville, E. K., & Morris, J. C. (2010). In-Home Occupational Performance Evaluation (I-HOPE). *American Journal of Occupational Therapy*, *64*, 580–589.

Stav, W. (2010). CarFit: An evaluation of behavior change and impact. *British Journal of Occupational Therapy*, *73*, 589–597.

Stewart, D. (2003). Peer mentorship as an environmental support for adolescents and young adults with disabilities. In L. Letts, P. Rigby, & D. Stewart (Eds.), *Using environments to enable occupational performance* (pp. 197–206). Thorofare, NJ: Slack.

Tanta, K. J., Deitz, J. C., White, O., & Billingsley, F. (2005). The effects of peer-lay level on initiations and responses of preschool children with delayed play skills. *American Journal of Occupational Therapy*, *59*, 437–445.

For additional resources on the subjects discussed in this chapter, visit http://thePoint.lww.com/Willard-Spackman12e.

CHAPTER 39

The Model of Human Occupation

Kirsty Forsyth, Renée R. Taylor, Jessica M. Kramer, Susan Prior, Lynn Richie, Jaqueline Whitehead, Christine Owen, Jane Melton

LEARNING OBJECTIVES

After reading this chapter, you will be able to:

1. Describe the personal factors addressed by the Model of Human Occupation and articulate how each concept affects occupational life
2. Describe the environmental factors that are addressed by the Model of Human Occupation and articulate how each concept affects occupational life
3. Identify dimensions of doing that the Model of Human Occupation uses to describe and examine a person's engagement in occupations
4. Describe the steps of therapeutic reasoning in the Model of Human Occupation
5. Articulate how change occurs in occupational therapy and identify client actions and therapeutic strategies that lead to change
6. Describe how the Model of Human Occupation can be applied to clients with various diagnoses across the life course in different practice contexts

OUTLINE

Stephen is a man in his mid-30s who was diagnosed with schizophrenia in his final year of university. Due to fluctuating mental health, he became socially withdrawn and, throughout his adulthood, was unable to secure paid employment. Stephen's mental health improved recently, and he is keen to obtain an employment. He self-referred to occupational therapy (OT) vocational rehabilitation program with the goal of returning to paid employment.

John is a 7-year-old boy who wants to be a computer engineer like his dad when he grows up. He lives at home with his parents and his brother. His family describes him as a lovable, endearing boy. However, John's schoolteacher raised concerns about his awkward movement within classroom, distractibility, and laborious handwriting. The concern was raised that if these issues are not resolved, John will not be able to keep up with his class peers in terms of academic performance. As a result, it was decided that John would benefit from a specialist OT assessment.

Each of these clients' OT practitioners chose to use the Model of Human Occupation (MOHO) to guide their intervention. In the course of the chapter, these cases will be used to illustrate the theory and application of this model.

Introduction

The Model of Human Occupation (MOHO) (Kielhofner, 2008) is an occupation-focused (Pedretti & Early, 2001), theory-driven (Elenko, Hinojosa Blount, & Blount, 2000), client-centered (Law, 1998), evidence-based (Law et al., 1997) approach to OT practice. MOHO was introduced 30 years ago by three practitioners seeking to articulate an approach to occupation-based intervention. They described MOHO as a theory to guide thinking about clients and the therapy process (Kielhofner, 1980a, 1980b; Kielhofner & Burke, 1980; Kielhofner, Burke, & Heard, 1980). Evidence indicates that MOHO is now the most widely used occupation-based model in practice worldwide (Haglund, Ekbladh, Thorell, & Hallberg, 2000; Law & McColl, 1989; National Board for the Certification in Occupational Therapy, 2004; Wilkeby, Pierre, & Archenholtz, 2006). A national study of occupational therapists in the United States (Lee, Taylor, Kielhofner, & Fisher, 2008) indicated that 75.7% of therapists make use of MOHO in their practice. These therapists reported that MOHO allows them to have an occupation-focused practice and a clearer professional identity. They also reported that MOHO provides a holistic view of clients, supports client-centered practice, and provides a useful structure for intervention planning (Lee et al., 2008).

MOHO has been developed through the efforts of an international community of practitioners and scholars. It is supported by a substantial evidence base of well over 400 articles and chapters that present theoretical, applied, or research aspects of the model. A current bibliography of this literature is maintained on the Website, http://www.moho.uic.edu. The most comprehensive and authoritative discussion of MOHO is the book *A Model of Human Occupation: Theory and Application*, which is now in its fourth edition (Kielhofner, 2008). This chapter provides a brief overview of this model's focus, theory, and resources for application in practice.

Why the Model of Human Occupation Is Needed

MOHO emerged at a time when the field was just beginning to rediscover the importance of occupation as an outcome and means of intervention. In the 1970s, when MOHO was being formulated as an approach to practice, most OT theory and practice focused on understanding and reducing impairment. The impetus for developing MOHO was the recognition that many factors beyond motor, cognitive, and sensory impairments contribute to difficulties in everyday occupation. These include occupational barriers posed by the physical and social environment, difficulties in choosing and finding meaning in occupations, and the challenge of maintaining positive involvement in life roles and routines. MOHO was developed to address these factors.

Consequently, the MOHO concepts address (1) the motivation for occupation, (2) the routine patterning of occupations, (3) the nature of skilled performance, and (3) the influence of environment on occupation. These concepts serve as a framework for gathering data about a client's situation, enable therapists to identify the client's occupational strengths and limitations, and help therapists and clients plan and implement a course of OT. MOHO is appropriate for clients with a wide range of impairments (physical, mental, cognitive, and sensory) throughout the life course.

The Model of Human Occupation Concepts

MOHO explains how occupations are chosen, patterned, and performed (Kielhofner, 2008). MOHO is concerned with how people participate in daily occupations and achieve a sense of competence and identity (Figure 39.1). The model begins with the idea that a person's characteristics and his or her environment are linked together when someone is engaged in an occupation. Moreover, the model asserts that motives, patterns of performance, and skills are maintained and changed through engagement in occupations. MOHO understands OT as a process in which practitioners support client engagement in occupations in order to shape the clients' choices, their routine ways of doing things, and their skills.

Model of Human Occupation Concepts Related to the Person

To explain how occupations are chosen, patterned, and performed, MOHO conceptualizes people as composed of three interacting elements: volition, habituation, and performance capacity. The sections that follow will discuss these elements.

Volition

Volition refers to the process by which people are motivated toward and choose what activities they do. The concept of volition asserts that all humans have a desire to engage in occupations and that this desire is shaped

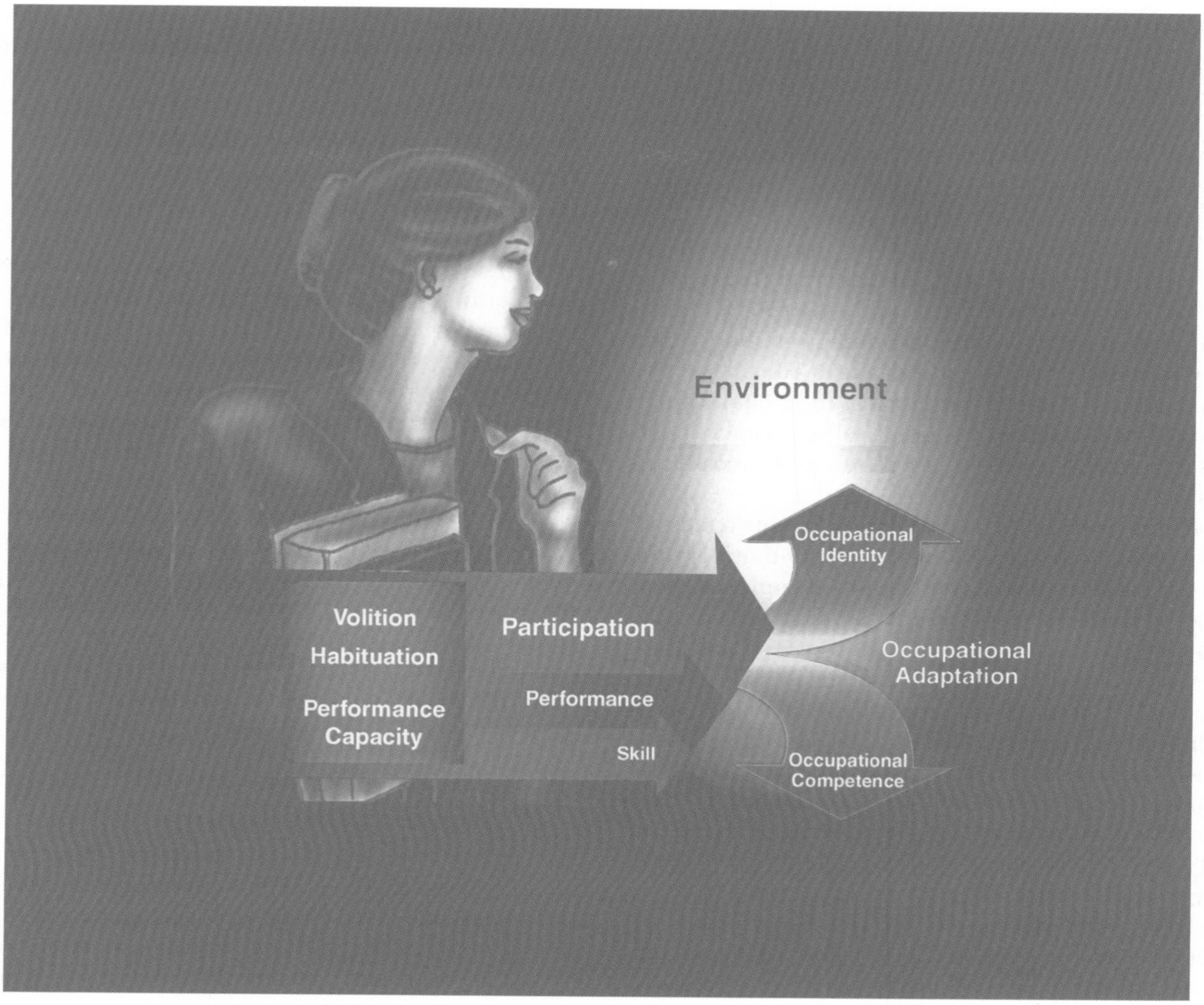

FIGURE 39.1 Model of Human Occupation concepts. (Reprinted with permission from Kielhofner, G. [2007]. *A model of human occupation: Theory and application* [4th ed.]. Baltimore, MD: Lippincott Williams & Wilkins.)

by previous experiences. Volition occurs in a cycle of anticipating possibilities for doing, choosing what to do, experiencing what one does, and subsequent interpretation of the experience. These thoughts and feelings are influenced by underlying personal factors, for example, how capable and effective one feels (called *personal causation*), what one holds as important (called *values*), and what one finds enjoyable and satisfying (called *interests*).

Personal causation refers to thoughts and feelings about one's abilities and effectiveness as he or she does everyday activities. These include, for example, recognizing one's strengths and weaknesses, feeling confident or anxious when faced with an occupation, and reflecting on how well one did after doing something.

Values are beliefs and commitments about what is good, right, and important to do. They include thoughts and feelings about activities that are worth doing, beliefs about the proper way to complete those activities, and the meanings that are ascribed to the things one does. Values specify what is worth doing, how to perform, and what goals or aspirations deserve commitment.

Interests develop through the experience of pleasure and satisfaction derived from occupational engagement (Matsutsuyu, 1969). Therefore, the development of interests depends on available opportunities to engage in occupations.

Volition has a pervasive influence on occupational life. Volition guides choices of what to do and determines the experience of doing. It shapes how people make sense of what they have done. Volition is also central to the OT process. All therapy requires that clients make choices to do things; therefore, it *must* engage clients' volition. Moreover, how clients experience what they do in therapy (a function of volition) to a large extent determines therapy outcomes.

Habituation

Habituation refers to a process whereby people organize their actions into patterns and routines. Through repeated action within specific contexts, people establish habituated patterns of doing. These patterns of action are governed by habits and roles, which shape how people go about the routine aspects of their lives.

Habits involve learned ways of doing things that unfold automatically. Habits operate in cooperation with context, using and incorporating the environment as a resource for doing familiar things. They influence how people perform routine activities, use time, and behave. For instance, habits shape how people intuitively go about self-care each morning, organize the weekly routine, and complete a familiar task.

Roles provide a cultural script for one's identity and provide a set of responsibilities and obligations that are associated with that identity. People see themselves as students, workers, and parents and recognize that they should behave in certain ways to fulfill these roles. Much of what people do is done as a spouse, parent, worker, or student. People learn how to acquire each of these roles successfully through the expectations that others have for a role and the social environment in which each role is located. Thus, through interaction with others, people internalize an identity and a way of behaving that is associated with each role they have internalized.

Habits and roles make up how people routinely interact with their physical and social environments. When habituation is challenged by impairments and/or environmental circumstances, people can lose a great deal of what has given life familiarity and consistency. One of the major tasks of therapy may be to reconstruct habits and roles so that the person can more routinely participate in life occupations within the everyday environment.

Performance Capacity

Performance capacity refers to a person's underlying mental and physical abilities and how those abilities are used and experienced in occupational performance. The capacity for performance is affected by the status of musculoskeletal, neurological, cardiopulmonary, and other bodily systems that are called on when a person does things. Biomechanical, motor control, cognitive, and sensory integration approaches to practice address these aspects of performance capacity that can be observed, measured, and modified (Ayres, 1979; Trombly & Radomski, 2001).

MOHO recognizes the importance of approaches that address physical and mental capacities for occupational performance, and it is typically used in conjunction with such models. MOHO stresses the importance of also paying attention to how people experience impairments. This includes paying attention to how people's bodies feel to them and how they perceive the world when they have impairments.

Model of Human Occupation Concepts Concerning the Environment

MOHO stresses that all occupation results from an interaction of the person (volition, habituation, and performance capacity) with the characteristics of the physical and social environment. The **environment** can be defined as the particular physical, social, cultural, economic, and political features within a person's context that influence the motivation, organization, and performance of occupation. There are several dimensions of the environment that may have an impact on an individual's occupational life. For example, people encounter different physical spaces, objects, and people as well as expectations and opportunities for doing things. At the same time, the larger culture, economic conditions, and political factors also exert an influence. Accordingly, the environment includes the following dimensions:

- The objects that people use when they do things
- The spaces within which people do things
- The tasks that are available, expected, and/or required of people in a given context and that provide a set of social norms and conventions for engaging in recognizable occupations (such as "studying," "cleaning the house," or "playing cards")
- The social groups (e.g., family, friends, coworkers, neighbors) that make up the context and the expectations those social groups hold
- The surrounding culture, political, and economic forces

Objects and spaces together comprise the **physical environment**. The **social environment** includes both tasks and social groups.

The things that people do and how they think and feel about these things reflect a complex interplay of motives, habits and roles, and abilities with the dimensions of the environment noted previously. Political and economic conditions determine what resources people have for doing things and what occupational roles are available to them. Culture shapes the formation of ideas about how one should perform and what is worth doing. The demands of a task can determine the extent to which a person feels confident or anxious. The match of objects and spaces to the capacity of the individual influences how the person performs. In these and a myriad of other ways, the environment has an impact on what people do and how they think and feel about their doing. In turn, people also choose and modify their environments. For instance, people select environments that match and allow them to realize their values and interests.

Dimensions of Doing

As Figure 39.1 shows, MOHO identifies three levels at which we can examine a person's engagement in occupations: occupational participation, occupational performance, and occupational skill.

Occupational participation refers to engaging in work, play, or activities of daily living (ADL) that are part of one's sociocultural context and that are desired and/or necessary to one's well-being. This is the highest "level" of conceptualizing engagement in occupations. Examples of occupational participation are volunteering for an organization, working in a full- or part-time job, regularly getting together with friends, doing self-care, maintaining one's living space, and attending school. Each area of occupational participation involves a cluster of related tasks that one does. For example, participating to maintain one's living space may include paying the rent, doing repairs, and cleaning. Doing a task related to participation in a major life area is referred to as **occupational performance**.

During occupational performance, we carry out discrete purposeful actions. For example, making tea is a culturally recognizable task in many cultures. To do so, one *gathers* together tea, kettle, and a cup; *handles* these materials and objects; and *sequences* the steps necessary to brew and pour the tea. These actions that make up occupational performance of a task are referred to as **skills**. Skills are goal-directed actions that a person uses while performing (Forsyth, Salamy, Simon, & Kielhofner, 1998). In contrast to *performance capacity*, which refers to underlying ability (e.g., range of motion and strength), skill refers to the actions *within* an occupational performance such as reaching or sequencing. There are three types of skills: motor skills, process skills, and communication and interaction skills. Detailed taxonomies of each of the three types of skills have been developed (Bernspang & Fisher, 1995; Doble, 1991; Fisher & Kielhofner, 1995; Forsyth, Lai, & Kielhofner, 1999; Forsyth et al., 1998).

Occupational Identity, Competence, and Adaptation

Over time, what people do creates their **occupational identity**. This identity, generated from experience, is the cumulative sense of who people are and who they wish to become as occupational beings. The degree to which people are able to sustain a pattern of doing that enacts their occupational identity is referred to as **occupational competence**. These two essential elements of **occupational adaptation** entail the creation of an occupational identity and the ability to enact this identity in various circumstances (Figure 39.1).

The Process of Change and Therapy

A basic premise of MOHO is that all change in OT is driven by clients' occupational engagement. The term **occupational engagement** refers to clients' doing, thinking, and feeling under certain environmental conditions in the midst of therapy or as a planned consequence of therapy.

When clients engage in tasks in therapy or as a result of therapy, volition, habituation, and performance capacity are all involved in some way. For example, a client may be (1) drawing on performance capacity to exercise skill in occupational performance, (2) evoking old habits that shape how the occupational performance is done, (3) enacting or working toward acquiring a role, (4) experiencing a level of satisfaction and enjoyment (or dissatisfaction) with occupational performance, (5) assigning meaning and significance to what is done (i.e., what this means for the client's life), or (6) feeling able (or unable) when doing an occupation.

Each of these aspects of what the client does, thinks, and feels shapes the change process. For this reason, practitioners using MOHO are mindful of their clients' volition, habituation, performance capacity, and environmental conditions in the midst of therapy and how these elements are interacting as the therapy unfolds. To help practitioners think about the process of occupational engagement, MOHO identifies the nine dimensions of occupational engagement shown in Table 39.1. These nine dimensions provide a basic structure for thinking about how clients achieve change and for planning how therapy goals will be achieved. This process is discussed in the next section.

Using Model of Human Occupation in Practice: Steps of Therapeutic Reasoning

Using MOHO in practice involves thinking with its concepts—a process referred to as *therapeutic reasoning*. Therapeutic reasoning refers specifically to the use of MOHO concepts in thinking about clients' needs throughout the OT process (American Occupational Therapy Association, 2002). The therapeutic reasoning process has six steps: (1) generating questions about the client, (2) gathering information on and with the client, (3) using the information gathered to create a theory-based explanation of the client's situation, (4) generating

TABLE 39.1 Dimensions of Client Occupational Engagement

Dimensions of Occupational Engagement	Definition
Choose/decide	Anticipate and select from alternatives for action.
Commit	Decide to undertake a course of action to accomplish a goal or personal project, fulfill a role, or establish a new habit.
Explore	Investigate new objects, spaces, social groups, and/or occupational forms/tasks; do things with altered performance capacity; try out new ways of doing things; and examine possibilities for occupational participation in one's context.
Identify	Locate novel information, alternatives for action, and new feelings that provide solutions for and/or give meaning to occupational performance and participation.
Negotiate	Engage in a give-and-take with others that creates mutually agreed-on perspectives and/or finds a middle ground between different expectations, plans, or desires.
Plan	Establish an action agenda for performance or participation.
Practice	Repeat a certain performance or consistently participate in an occupation with the intent of increasing skill, ease, and effectiveness of performance.
Reexamine	Critically appraise and consider alternatives to previously held beliefs, attitudes, feelings, habits, or roles.
Sustain	Persist in occupational performance or participation despite uncertainty or difficulty.

goals and strategies for therapy, (5) implementing and monitoring therapy, and (6) determining outcomes of therapy. Practitioners generally move back and forth between these steps over the course of therapy. Each step is briefly discussed subsequently.

Generating Questions

Practitioners must come to understand their clients in order to plan and implement therapy. This understanding begins with asking questions about their clients (Table 39.2). MOHO concepts allow a practitioner to generate these questions systematically. That is, the major concepts of the theory (environmental impact, volition, habituation, performance capacity, participation, performance, skills, occupational identity, and occupational competence) orient the practitioner to be concerned about certain things when learning about a client. For example, practitioners using MOHO would ask what their clients' thoughts and feelings are in relation to personal causation, values, and interests. Moreover, they would ask about their clients' roles and habits and how these affect the clients' routines. These questions would, of course, be tailored to the clients' circumstances.

Gathering Information

To answer the questions generated in the first step, practitioners must gather information on and with the client. Practitioners may take advantage of naturally occurring opportunities to gather information. For example, a practitioner might learn about a client's personal causation by observing the client's emotional reaction when attempting to learn a challenging new task. Practitioners may also use structured MOHO assessments. Some MOHO assessments will capture comprehensive information on several aspects of the person and the environment. Some MOHO assessments attempt to capture more in-depth information on one aspect of MOHO, such as assessments that focus on volition. A wide range of MOHO-based assessments has been developed; they are summarized in Table 39.3. Thus, practitioners using MOHO have a range of choices when they decide which assessment(s) to use. Some OT services have developed assessment protocols to indicate service response to assessment needs.

Creating a Theory-Based Understanding of the Client

The information that the practitioner gathers to answer questions about a client is used to create a theory-based understanding of that client. In this step, the practitioner uses MOHO theory as a framework for creating an explanation of that particular client's situation. As will be demonstrated in the cases of Stephen and John, the therapists use MOHO to create an explanation of each of these client's occupational circumstances to guide the next step of generating goals and strategies for therapy.

As part of creating an explanation of clients' circumstances, practitioners identify problems or challenges that need to be addressed in therapy as well as

TABLE 39.2 Model of Human Occupation (MOHO)–Based Therapeutic Reasoning Questions

MOHO Concept	Questions
Occupational identity	• What is the person's sense of who he or she has been, is, and wishes to become in relation to family life, school, friendships, hobbies, and interests? • What is the family's sense of who this person has been, is, and what do they wish him or her to become? How does this affect the person's occupational identity?
Occupational competence	• To what extent has this person sustained a pattern of satisfying occupational participation over time? • Does this person feel that he or she can do the things he or she needs to do in school, with friends, and in the community? • To what extent has this person's life sustained patterns of occupational participation over time that reflect their occupational identity?
Participation	• Does the person currently engage in work, play, and ADL that are part of his or her sociocultural context and that are desired and/or necessary for his or her well-being?
Performance	• Can this person do the occupations that are part of the work, play, and ADL that make up, or should make up, his or her life? • Can the person do the occupations that are expected of his or her roles?
Skill	• Does the person exhibit the necessary communication/interaction, motor, and process skills to perform what he or she needs and wants to do?
Environment	• Does the family support the person in developing the necessary volition, habituation and communication/interaction, motor, and process skills needed for participation? • What impact do the opportunities, resources, constraints, and demands (or lack of demands) of the environment have on how this person thinks, feels, and acts? • How do the opportunities, resources, constraints, or demands provided by spaces, objects, occupations/tasks, and social groups affect the person's skill, performance, and participation?
Volition	• What is this person's view of his or her personal capacity and effectiveness? • What does this person think is important? • What are this person's interests? What does this person enjoy doing?
Habituation	• What routines does this person participate in and how do routines influence what he or she does? • What are the roles with which this person identifies with and how do they influence what he or she routinely does?

ADL, activities of daily living.

strengths that can be drawn on in therapy. Problems and challenges may be a function of volition, habituation, performance capacity, or the environment.

Generating Measurable Goals and Strategies

This step involves creating therapy goals (i.e., identifying what will change as a result of therapy), deciding what kinds of occupational engagement will enable the client to change, and determining what kind of therapeutic strategies will be needed to support the client to change.

Goals (Table 39.4) indicate the kinds of changes that therapy will aim to achieve. Change is required when the client's characteristics and/or environment are contributing to occupational problems or challenges. For instance, if a client feels ineffective, therapy would seek to enable the client to feel more effective; or if a client has too few roles development of new roles would become the focus of therapy. In this way, identifying challenges or problems in the third step allows one to select the goals in the fourth step.

The next element in this step is to identify how the goals will be achieved. This involves indicating what occupational engagement on the part of the client will contribute to achieving these goals and how the practitioner will support the client. The previous section on change offered nine dimensions of occupational engagement and these serve as a framework for thinking in this step. MOHO also identifies key therapeutic strategies that practitioners will use; these are listed in Box 39.1.

The text *A Model of Human Occupation: Theory and Application* (Kielhofner, 2008) provides a comprehensive resource, the Therapeutic Reasoning Table, for this component of the therapeutic reasoning process. It identifies a wide range of problems and challenges that correspond to the concepts of MOHO along with types of changes that would be warranted. The table also indicates what types of occupational engagement could contribute to achieving those changes and what type of support from

TABLE 39.3 Model of Human Occupation (MOHO) Assessments Summary

MOHO Assessment	Method of Administration	Description
ACHIEVE assessment (Forsyth, Whitehead, Owen, & Gorska, 2012)	Questionnaire, interview or observation	The assessment can be administered by mail or over the telephone and is completed by the child's teacher with a separate rating scale for the parent or guardian. It affords an opportunity for teachers or parents to share their view of how the child is participating in everyday activities. It asks for information on the frequency of their child's engagement in home, community, and school activity and then asks MOHO orientated questions as to why this engagement is positive or negative.
Assessment of Communication and Interaction Skills (ACIS) (Forsyth et al., 1998)	Observation	Gathers information about the communication and interaction skills that a person displays while engaged in an occupation across the domains of physicality, information exchange, and relations. Used to generate goals for therapy related to communication/interaction skills and to assess outcomes/changes in skill.
Assessment of Motor and Process Skills (AMPS) (Fisher, 2003)	Observation	Gathers information about the motor and process skills that a person displays while engaged in an occupation. Used to generate goals for therapy related to motor and process skills and to assess outcomes/changes in skill.
Assessment of Occupational Functioning-Collaborative version (AOF-CV) (Watts, Hinson, Madigan, McGuigan, & Newman, 1999)	Interview and/or client self-report	Yields qualitative information and a quantitative profile of the impact of a client's personal causation, values, roles, habits, and skills on occupational participation. Used to inform intervention.
Child Occupational Self Assessment (COSA) (Keller, Kafkes, Basu, Federico, & Kielhofner, 2005)	Client self-report	Children and youths rate their occupational competence for engaging in 25 everyday activities in the home, school, and community and the importance of those activities. Used to generate goals and assess outcomes/change in competence and values.
Interest Checklist (Matsutsuyu, 1969)	Client self-report	Checklist that indicates strength of interest and past, present, and future engagement in 68 activities. Used to inform intervention.
Model of Human Occupational Screening Tool (MOHOST) (Parkinson, Forsyth, & Kielhofner, 2006)	Observation, interview(s), and/or chart review	Information gathered assesses impact of volition, habituation, skills, and environment on client's occupational participation. Used to generate goals and assess outcomes or changes in participation.
National Institutes of Health Activity Record (Frust, Gerber, Smith, Fisher, & Shulman, 1987; Gerber & Frust, 1992)	Client self-report	Self-report "log" records information in half-hour intervals throughout the day on perceptions of competence, value, enjoyment, difficulty, and pain experienced when engaging in various occupations in that time period. Used to inform intervention and assess outcomes or change in participation.
Occupational Circumstances Assessment-Interview and Rating Scale (OCAIRS) (Forsyth et al., 2005)	Interview	Interview yields information to assess values, goals, personal causation, interests, habits, roles, skills, readiness for change, and environmental impact on participation. Used to generate goals and assess outcomes or changes in participation.
Occupational Performance History Interview-II (OPHI-II) (Kielhofner et al., 2004)	Interview	Detailed life history interview that yields (1) scales measuring competence, identity, and environmental impact and (2) a narrative representation/analysis of the life history. Used as an in-depth, comprehensive assessment to generate goals, inform intervention, and build the therapeutic relationship.
Occupational Therapy Psychosocial Assessment of Learning (OT PAL) (Townsend et al., 1999)	Observation or interview	This assessment evaluates a student's volition (the ability to make choices), habituation (roles and routines), and environmental fit within the classroom setting. The manual includes reproducible assessment and data summary forms.

TABLE 39.3 Model of Human Occupation (MOHO) Assessments Summary (*Continued*)

MOHO Assessment	Method of Administration	Description
Occupational Questionnaire (OQ) (Smith, Kielhofner, & Watts, 1986)	Client self-report	Self-report "log" records information in half-hour intervals throughout the day on perceptions of competence, value, and enjoyment experienced when engaging in various occupations in that time period. Used to inform intervention and assess outcomes or change in participation.
Occupational Self Assessment (OSA) (Baron, Kielhofner, Iyenger, Goldhammer, & Wolenski, 2006)	Client self-report	Clients rate their occupational competence for engaging in 21 everyday activities and the importance of those activities. Allows clients to set priorities for change. Used to generate goals and assess outcomes or change in competence and values.
Pediatric Interest Profiles (PIP) (Henry, 2000)	Client self-report	Assessment includes three age-appropriate scales (some with line drawings) for children and adolescents to indicate participation, interest, and perceived competence in various play and leisure activities. Used to generate goals and assess outcomes or changes in participation.
Pediatric Volitional Questionnaire (PVQ) (Basu, Kafkes, Geist, & Kielhofner, 2002)	Observation	Guides a systematic observation of a child across multiple environments to assess volition and the impact of the environment on volition. Used as an in-depth assessment of volition to generate goals and assess outcomes or change in volition.
Residential Environment Impact Survey (REIS) (Fisher, Arriaga, Less, Lee, & Ashpole, 2008)	Observation or interview	Assesses how well the home environment is meeting the needs of the residents as a whole. Ratings in 24 areas provide a summary of the data and a structure for generating recommendations to enhance the qualities of the environment. The intent of this assessment tool is to not only assess the residential environment but also to determine the impact of the environment on the residents and to make recommendations to improve the quality of life for the residents and the work life of the staff.
Role Checklist (Oakley, Kielhofner, & Barris, 1985)	Client self-report	Checklist provides information on past, present, and future role participation and the perceived value of those roles. Used to inform intervention and assess outcomes or changes in role performance.
Short Child Occupational Profile (SCOPE) (Bowyer, Ross, Schwartz, Kielhofner, & Kramer, 2006)	Observation, interview(s), and/or chart review	Information gathered assesses impact of volition, habituation, skills, and environment on child's or adolescent's occupational participation. Used to generate goals and assess outcomes or changes in participation.
School Setting Interview (SSI) (Hemmingson, Egilson, Hoffman, & Kielhofner, 2005)	Interview	Interview works with students to gather information on student-environment fit and identify need for accommodations. Used to generate goals, inform intervention, and assess outcomes or changes in student-environment fit.
Volitional Questionnaire (VQ) (de las Heras, Lierena, & Kielhofner, 2003)	Observation	Guides a systematic observation of a client across multiple environments to assess volition and the impact of the environment on volition. Used as an in-depth assessment of volition to generate goals and assess outcomes or change in volition.
Worker Role Interview (WRI) (Braveman et al., 2005)	Interview	Interview yields information to rate the impact that volition, habitation, and perceptions of the environment have on psychosocial readiness for the worker role or return to work. Used to generate goals and assess outcomes or changes in psychosocial readiness for work.
Work Environment Impact Scale (WEIS) (Moore-Corner, Kielhofner, & Olson, 1998)	Interview	Interview works with client to assess environmental impact on participation in the worker role and to identify needed accommodations. Used to generate goals and inform intervention.

TABLE 39.4 Model of Human Occupation (MOHO)–Based Therapy Goals: Examples

MOHO Concept	Measurable Goal
Volition	Within [time frame], [client] will be *able to identify* (number of) occupations that are significant to his or her occupational life (or roles) and are consistent with his or her current skills and abilities [action] within [setting] independently [degree] Within [timeframe], [client] will *make the choice* to engage in (name occupation) having *identified* this as significant to his or her (successful performance of/or as a step in the progress towards) his or her performance as a (name role) [action] within [setting] with minimal support [degree]
Habituation	Within [time frame], [client] will be able to *identify* the responsibilities for roles that are valuable and meaningful to the person [action], this will be achieved with minimal support [degree] within [setting] Within [time frame], [client], will be able to *practice* and develop a habit pattern that will support achievement of a single occupation [action], this will be achieved with minimal support [degree] within [setting]
Skill	Within [time frame], [client] will be able to perform within (name the occupation) using (name skills) [action] within [setting], independently [degree] Within [time frame], [client] will be able to perform in (name the occupation) using adapted techniques to support lack of skill [action] within [setting], independently [degree]
Performance capacity	Within [time frame], [client] will be able to incorporate damaged or estranged parts of the body into completion of occupations [action], within [setting] independently [degree] Within [time frame], [client] will be able to manage symptoms while engaged in (name the occupations) [action] within [setting] independently [degree]
Environment	Within [time frame], [client] will be able to *perform* in (name the occupation) [action] within his or her physical and social home environment [setting], independently [degree] Within [time frame], [client] will be able to *perform* in the occupation using adapted objects or new objects [action] within [setting], independently [degree]

Adapted from Kielhofner, G. (2007). *A model of human occupation: Theory and application* (4th ed.). Baltimore, MD: Lippincott Williams & Wilkins.

the practitioner could facilitate change. Table 39.5 shows one small section from this Therapeutic Reasoning Table related to personal causation.

Implementing and Monitoring Therapy

To implement therapy means not only following the plan of action that was set out in the previous step but also monitoring how the therapy process unfolds. This monitoring process might confirm the practitioner's understanding of the client's situation or require the practitioner to reformulate the client's situation. The monitoring process also can confirm the usefulness of therapy and whether a change to the goals and/or plan is required. When things do not turn out as expected, the practitioner returns to earlier steps of generating questions, selecting methods to gather information, formulating the client's situation, setting goals, and establishing plans.

BOX 39.1 Therapeutic Strategies Identified by Model of Human Occupation

- **Validating:** Attending to and acknowledging the client's experience
- **Identifying:** Locating and sharing a range of personal, procedural, and/or environmental factors that can facilitate occupational performance
- **Giving feedback:** Sharing your understanding of the client's situation or ongoing action
- **Advising:** Recommending intervention goals/strategies
- **Negotiating:** Engaging in a give-and-take with the client
- **Structuring:** Establishing parameters for choice and performance by offering client alternatives, setting limits, establishing ground rules
- **Coaching:** Instructing, demonstrating, guiding, verbally and/or physically prompting
- **Encouraging:** Providing emotional support and reassurance in relation to engagement in an occupation
- **Physical support:** Using one's body to provide support for a client to complete an occupational form/task

TABLE 39.5 Excerpt from the Therapeutic Reasoning Table Showing a Problem/Challenge Related to Personal Causation and Corresponding Intervention Goals and Strategies

Problem/Challenge	Goal	Client Occupational Engagement	Therapeutic Strategies to Support the Client
• Feelings of lack of control over occupational performance leading to anxiety (fear of failure) within occupations.	• Reduce client's anxiety and fear of failure in occupational performance (e.g., "The client will complete a simple 3-step meal in 20 minutes without verbalizing anxiety or concern."). • Build up confidence to face occupational performance demands (e.g., "The client will identify and participate in 3 new leisure activities with minimal support in 1 week").	• *Reexamine* anxieties and fears in the light of new performance experiences. • *Choose* to do relevant and meaningful things that are within performance capacity. • *Sustain* performance in occupational forms tasks despite anxiety.	• *Validate* how difficult it can be to do things that provoke anxiety. • *Identify* client's strengths and weaknesses in occupational performance. • Give *feedback* to client about match/mismatch between choice of occupational forms/tasks and performance capacity. • Give *feedback* to support a positive reinterpretation of his or her experience of engaging in an occupation. • *Advise* client to do relevant and meaningful things that match performance capacity.

Collecting Information to Assess Outcomes

Determining therapy outcomes is an important final step in the therapy process. Typically, therapy outcomes are documented by examining the extent to which goals have been achieved and readministering structured assessments that were administered initially. Both of these approaches are valuable in documenting outcomes. Assessing outcomes by examining goal attainment is helpful in reflecting on the extent to which the therapeutic reasoning process resulted in good decisions for therapy. Using structured MOHO assessments also allows one to compare change across different clients or when different strategies are used. In this way, they can contribute to evidence-based therapy.

Case Studies

Collecting Information and Creating a Theory-Based Understanding of Stephen

Who Is Stephen?

Stephen is in his mid-30s and lives with his parents. He is very close to his supportive parents and younger brother who lives in the same city. He described himself as a helpful son, supportive brother, loyal friend, and devoted dog owner. He enjoys the outdoors and sports, and he is currently unemployed.

Background

Stephen did well academically at school but became unwell and was diagnosed with schizophrenia in his final year of university. He left without completing his degree. Throughout this period, Stephen worked part-time in various jobs: retail, hospitality, and caregiving. He also volunteered in local day center for the elderly. Throughout his 20s, Stephen's mental health was poor with regular long admissions to hospital. He became socially withdrawn, only spending time with family members and health professionals; he rarely participated in swimming and running, which had previously been daily occupations. During this period, Stephen's family helped him find several temporary jobs in retail and catering, all of which he left due to deterioration in his mental health.

Recently, Stephen's mental health has improved, which he attributes to an improved medication regime. He is engaging in sporting activities and is keen to return to employment. In the past, he attended an OT prevocational training project where he participated in office administration tasks. His goal was to return to employment. He gradually built confidence and on discharge from the project, went on to a college course. He attained a vocational qualification in office administration but had been unable to secure employment.

The OT service provides an evidence-based vocational MOHO rehabilitation program, based on supported employment, where service users are supported to find a job quickly and rehabilitation is focused on maintaining the job ("place then train") as opposed to prevocational training ("train then place"). More information about the service is contained in *The WORKS: Occupational Therapy and Evidence Based Vocational Rehabilitation* (Prior, Forsyth, & Ritchie, 2011). The service operates a self-referral system, and Stephen contacted the service with the goal of returning to paid employment.

Generating Questions

The occupational therapist was initially interested to explore Stephen's perceptions of his past, present, and future worker roles, including the following:

- What work activities does Stephen enjoy and value and how able does he feel doing these activities (volition)?
- How are his present roles and routines impacting on his engagement in work or impacting on work (habituation)?
- What level of support is offered in social and physical work environment?
- Stephen had not reported any specific challenges in motor, process, or communication and interaction skills and therefore early reflection on questions did not relate to these areas.

Gathering Information

The occupational therapist used the following assessment strategy to answer the previous questions:

Initial assessment

- Worker Role Interview (WRI) (Braveman et al., 2005)—The assessment was administered during the initial meeting between the occupational therapist and Stephen (**Figure 39.2**).
- Work Environment Impact Scale (Moore-Corner et al., 1998)—The assessment was selected by the occupational therapist to complement information gathered through the WRI to better understand the impact that previous work environments have had on Stephen's participation in his worker role (**Figure 39.3**).

Creating a Theory-Based Understanding of the Client

The following occupational formulation was created from the assessment findings.

- *What is Stephen's occupational identity?* Stephen is a son, brother, friend, and dog owner. He is a regular runner and swimmer. Stephen recognizes himself as an unemployed person who is seeking work.
- *What is Stephen's occupational competence?* Stephen enjoys and feels competent in all roles he is currently pursuing. He reported a tendency to underestimate his abilities; the standards he applies to his own work performance usually exceed those of his colleagues and managers. This has interfered with Stephen's personal causation in relation to work and has led him to doubt his competence in previous work roles. However, given improvements in mental health and his strong work ethic, he is confident that he will succeed in a worker role.
- *What are the occupational issues Stephen is having difficulty with?* Stephen reported frustration in his lack of success in applying for work. Previous worker roles had all been in entry-level jobs, and he had no aspirations for career development beyond attaining a paid job. Stephen described a lack of enjoyment of previous worker roles in hospitality and retail; in particular, he found the fluctuating demands of the role difficult to manage with high levels of noise and stress at busy times contrasting with lack of routine tasks in quiet periods. There was limited opportunity for Stephen to work with any autonomy in organizing his tasks. All the positions he had previously held were temporary, low paid entry-level jobs and had offered little reward. Stephen has previously had poor relationships with colleagues and managers and has felt stigmatized due to his mental health condition. Stephen's life at the time of assessment lacked structure and routines; his roles as family member, friend, and dog owner were important but demanded little time.
- *What are the positive occupational issues for Stephen?* Stephen has a strong commitment to being in paid employment. He has a clear understanding of the expectations of work roles he has held in the past. He has a strong supportive network of family and friends. They are very encouraging and had in the past used contacts to secure employment on his behalf.
- *Why is Stephen unable to work or having challenges engaging in work?* Previous worker roles Stephen has held were mainly in retail and hospitality and were a poor fit with his interest in office administration. His current methods for seeking employment have been unsuccessful, and he has been unable to adjust his strategies. His current routine lacks routine due to the absence of a worker role, and Stephen is concerned that he will find adjusting to the greater demands of a worker role challenging. Stephen has experienced difficulty in unsupportive relationships with coworkers and managers in past worker roles and is concerned this may occur in the future.

Generating Therapy Goals and Strategies

The following goals were jointly generated:

- Within 2 weeks, Stephen (with the support of the occupational therapist) will identify jobs that match his interests and preferred working style using online and paper-based career planning material at the therapy clinic.

Initial Assessment

Personal causation			Values		Interests		Roles		Habits			Environment			
Assesses Abilities & Limitations	Expectation of Success in Work	Takes Responsibility	Commitment to Work	Work Related Goals	Enjoys Work	Pursues Interests	Appraises Work Expectations	Influence of Others Roles	Work Habits	Daily Routines	Adapts Routine to Minimize Difficulties	Perception of Physical Work Setting	Perception of Family and Peers	Perception of Boss and/or Company	Perception of Co-workers
SS	**SS**	SS	**SS**	SS	**SS**	SS	**SS**	**SS**	SS	SS	SS	**SS**	**SS**	SS	SS
S	S	**S**	S	S	S	S	S	S	S	S	S	S	S	S	S
I	I	I	I	**I**	I	**I**	I	I	**I**	**I**	**I**	I	I	**I**	**I**
SI	SI	SI	SI	SI	SI	SI	SI	SI	SI	SI	SI	SI	SI	SI	SI
N/A	N/A	N/A	N/A	N/A	N/A	N/A	N/A	N/A	N/A	N/A	N/A	N/A	N/A	N/A	N/A

Outcome Assessment

Personal causation			Values		Interests		Roles		Habits			Environment			
Assesses Abilities & Limitations	Expectation of Success in Work	Takes Responsibility	Commitment to Work	Work Related Goals	Enjoys Work	Pursues Interests	Appraises Work Expectations	Influence of Others Roles	Work Habits	Daily Routines	Adapts Routine to Minimize Difficulties	Perception of Physical Work Setting	Perception of Family and Peers	Perception of Boss and/or Company	Perception of Co-workers
SS	**SS**	SS	**SS**	**SS**	**SS**	**SS**	**SS**	**SS**	SS	SS	SS	**SS**	**SS**	SS	SS
S	S	**S**	S	S	S	S	S	S	**S**	**S**	**S**	S	S	**S**	S
I	I	I	I	I	I	I	I	I	I	I	I	I	I	I	**I**
SI	SI	SI	SI	SI	SI	SI	SI	SI	SI	SI	SI	SI	SI	SI	SI
N/A	N/A	N/A	N/A	N/A	N/A	N/A	N/A	N/A	N/A	N/A	N/A	N/A	N/A	N/A	N/A

Rating Scale: SS Strongly Supports S Supports I Interferes SI Strongly Interferes N/A Not Applicable

WRI (Version 10.0), (Braveman et al., 2005)
Addresses psychosocial and environmental factors that impact return to work. Complimenting other work/physical capacity assessments to ensure a well rounded picture of the client and their needs that should be addressed to ensure return to work.

FIGURE 39.2 Stephen—Worker Role Interview (Version 10.0) ratings (From Braveman, B., Robson, M., Velozo, C., Kielhofner, G., Fisher, G., Forsyth, K., & Kerschbaum, J. [2005]. *The worker role interview* [WRI; Version 10.0]. Chicago, IL: Model of Human Occupation Clearinghouse.).

- Within 4 weeks, Stephen's (with the support of the occupational therapist) assistant will develop a résumé and begin applying for jobs in his local library.
- Within 6 weeks, Stephen will independently spend time daily identifying, researching, and applying for jobs at home, in the job center, and in the library.
- Within 6 weeks, Stephen and the occupational therapist will investigate potential opportunities for unpaid internship in positions relevant to preferred worker role.

The therapist used the format featured in Table 39.4 to create a clear goal structure for Stephen. For example, the first goal indicates the following:

- The time frame as "2 weeks"
- The degree (or amount of assistance) as "with the support of the occupational therapist"
- The action as "identify jobs which match his interests and preferred working style using online and paper-based career planning materials"
- The setting as "the therapy clinic"

Initial Assessment

Time demands	Task demands	Appeal of work tasks	Work schedule	Co-worker interaction	Work group membership	Supervisor interaction	Work role standards	Work role style	Interaction with others	Rewards	Sensory Qualities	Architecture / arrangement	Ambience / mood	Properties of objects	Physical amenities	Meaning of objects
4	**4**	4	4	4	4	4	**4**	4	4	4	4	**4**	4	**4**	**4**	**4**
3	3	3	**3**	3	3	3	3	3	**3**	3	3	3	3	3	3	3
2	2	**2**	2	**2**	**2**	2	2	**2**	2	**2**	**2**	2	**2**	2	2	2
1	1	1	1	1	1	**1**	1	1	1	1	1	1	1	1	1	1
N/A	N/A	N/A	N/A	N/A	N/A	N/A	N/A	N/A	N/A	N/A	N/A	N/A	N/A	N/A	N/A	N/A

Outcome Assessment

Time demands	Task demands	Appeal of work tasks	Work schedule	Co-worker interaction	Work group membership	Supervisor interaction	Work role standards	Work role style	Interaction with others	Rewards	Sensory Qualities	Architecture / arrangement	Ambience / mood	Properties of objects	Physical amenities	Meaning of objects
4	**4**	**4**	**4**	4	4	**4**	**4**	**4**	4	4	**4**	**4**	4	**4**	**4**	**4**
3	3	3	3	**3**	3	3	3	3	**3**	3	3	3	**3**	3	3	3
2	2	2	2	2	**2**	2	2	2	2	**2**	2	2	2	2	2	2
1	1	1	1	1	1	1	1	1	1	1	1	1	1	1	1	1
N/A	N/A	N/A	N/A	N/A	N/A	N/A	N/A	N/A	N/A	N/A	N/A	N/A	N/A	N/A	N/A	N/A

Rating Scale: 4 Strongly Supports 3 Supports 2 Interferes 1 Strongly Interferes N/A Not Applicable

WEIS (Version 2.0) (Moore-Corner et al., 1998)
Identifies environmental characteristics that facilitate successful employment experiences. Factors that inhibit worker performance and satisfaction and which may require accommodation are also addressed in order to maximize the "fit" of the worker and their skills to the job environment

FIGURE 39.3 Stephen—Work Environment Impact Scale (Version 2.0) ratings. (From Moore-Corner, R. A., Kielhofner, G., & Olson, L. [1998]. *A user's guide to work environment impact scale.* Chicago, IL: Model of Human Occupation Clearinghouse.).

The goals also include examples of occupational engagement that will help Stephen achieve the change necessary to obtain these goals. For example, the occupational engagement in the first goal is "identify."

Implementing and Monitoring Therapy

The intervention plan includes the therapeutic strategies (in italics) that will support Stephen's achievement of his goals.

- Stephen and the occupational therapist worked together, and exploring a range of employment options and *negotiating* which types of worker roles offered the best fit with his interests and working styles.
- The occupational therapist *coached* Stephen in how to use career-planning material and *encouraged* him to discuss his future worker roles with his natural social support network of family and friends.
- The OT assistant *coached* Stephen and assisted in *structuring* how to build a résumé and complete application forms.
- The therapist regularly met with Stephen to review his increasing work routine; during these sessions, the occupational therapist offered *advice* and *encouragement* and *gave feedback*.
- Initially, the occupational therapist *identified* opportunities and barriers for establishing a work routine for Stephen and offered support by *structuring* increasing participation. As he became more confident and independent, the occupational therapist offered *encouragement.*
- The occupational therapist with Stephen identified a relevant unpaid internship opportunity; they then met with the manager of the workplace to *negotiate* and *structure* a placement of gradually increasing demand.
- The occupational therapist and Stephen discussed the social environment of the work placement in advance of commencing the internship. Stephen was anxious about establishing new relationships with coworkers. The therapist listened to Stephen's

concerns based on previous negative experience and demonstrated respect by *validating* his perspective. The therapist *coached* Stephen in strategies for meeting and conversing with new people at work. Stephen chose not to disclose his mental health condition to coworkers and so role-playing allowed Stephen to practice tricky conversations.

- The therapist offered advice to Stephen and his manager about managing mental health and well-being in the workplace.
- The therapist regularly communicated with Stephen's wider mental health team to share information, feedback progress, and ensure compatibility of care plans and objectives.

Collecting Information to Assess Outcomes

After 3 months, Stephen was established in his internship—working 2.5 days per week, totaling 16 hours. He was also regularly applying for similar paid roles and had secured two interviews. The occupational therapist chose to assess outcomes to date (Figure 39.2 and Figure 39.3). The assessment strategy was

Goal attainment (i.e., review of initial goals)

- Stephen and the occupational therapist worked together, establishing that Stephen had gained the greatest levels of satisfaction in administrative roles; this had been his chosen course of study at college.
- Stephen has a résumé that he tailors and shares with local employers, and he regularly applies for relevant available jobs, recently securing two interviews.
- Stephen has established a work routine of activities related to applying for employment.
- The occupational therapist secured an unpaid internship at a local leisure center where Stephen gradually built up his routine from 3 half days per week to 2 full days and 1 half day. The manager of the leisure center is very positive about Stephen as a worker and has provided an excellent reference. The manager would be willing to appoint Stephen if a post was available.

Collecting Information and Creating a Theory-Based Understanding of John

Who Is John?

John is a 7-year-old boy who is a third grader in elementary school, a son, a grandson, a brother, a friend, a swimmer, and a bike rider. He wants to be a computer engineer like his dad when he grows up. He is described by his family as a lovable, endearing boy and by his schoolteacher as chaotic, disorganized, and worried.

Background

John lives at home with his two parents and his brother. John has been referred for a specialist assessment by his elementary schoolteacher who was concerned about his awkward movement within the classroom, distractibility, and laborious handwriting. These issues have been long standing; the strategies tried within the school have not been helpful and the challenges persist. The teachers within John's school had already tried some of the strategies from *Inclusive Learning and Collaborative Working: Teachers Ideas in Practice* (CIRCLE Collaboration, 2009b). This is a resource based on what teachers have found helpful when supporting children with additional support needs. They had identified supports and strategies from the motor skill section, namely, task breakdown, hand-over-hand support, modeling, and additional verbal instructions. There is a concern that if the issues are not resolved, John will not be able to keep up with his class peers in terms of academic performance. Following discussion between John's class teacher and the headmaster, it was decided that it would be appropriate to refer John for an OT assessment.

Generating Questions

The occupational therapist started with an intention to understand what was important to John, his teacher, and his family. The therapist wanted to use MOHO as a framework for understanding how the issues raised on the referral affected John's engagement and participation in everyday occupations. Therefore, the therapist asked the following questions:

- What is important to John (his values) and what motivates him to participate in occupations at school?
- How do John's distractibility and awkward movement impact his ability to fulfill his responsibilities, maintain his routines, interact with others, and organize activities?
- What is John's view of his abilities and his limitations?
- How does John's occupational performance vary in different environments (home and school)?

Gathering Information

When John was referred into a local therapy facility, the therapists chose an assessment pattern that would provide information for the previous questions.

Prior to Attendance at the Therapy Clinic

- Active in Children Health Integrating Evidence Valuing Experience (ACHIEVE) Assessment (Forsyth et al., 2012)—This assessment was administered by mail and was completed by John's mother and by John's teacher. It affords an opportunity for John's mother/teacher to share their view of how their child is participating in everyday activities (Figure 39.4).

SUMMARY SCORES - Baseline

Name: John..Date of Birth: ....

Age: 7..........Yrs...................................Months CHI Number: ....

Clinician(s) Scoring: ....

PARENT QUESTIONNAIRE

PARENTAL OBSERVATIONS OF ACTIVITY FREQUENCY - WHAT			None of the time	Some of the time	Most of the time	All of the time
	Home Activities	a. Able to dry after bath/shower	1	2	3	**4**
		b. Able to clean after toileting	1	2	3	**4**
		c. Able to get un/dressed	1	2	3	**4**
		d. Able to make a simple snack	1	2	**3**	4
		e. Able to use a knife and fork	1	2	**3**	4
		f. Able to get ready in the morning	1	2	3	**4**
	School Activities	a. Able to use learning materials	1	2	3	**4**
		b. Able to make effective shapes/letters/writing	1	2	3	**4**
		c. Able to engage in sports/leisure	1	2	3	**4**
		d. Able to engage in curriculum	1	2	3	**4**
		e. Able to clean after toilet at school	1	2	3	**4**
		f. Able to get dressed after P.E./gym	1	2	3	**4**
	Community Activities	a. Able to ride bike/rollerblade etc	1	2	3	**4**
		b. Able to play with friends in activities	1	2	3	**4**
		c. Able to take part in out of school clubs	1	2	3	**4**
		d. Able to take part in social events	1	2	3	**4**
		e. Able to take part with family in leisure activity	1	2	3	**4**
		f. Able to manage clothes before/after activities	1	2	3	**4**

PARENTAL OBSERVATIONS OF CHARACTERISTICS OF CHILD - WHY			None of the time	Some of the time	Most of the time	All of the time
	Routine	a. Understands sequence/structure of routine	1	2	3	**4**
		b. Organises routines	1	2	3	**4**
		c. Copes with changein routine	1	2	**3**	4
		d. Copes with change in how activity's done	1	2	3	**4**
		e. Copes with a variety of activities	1	2	3	**4**
	Responsibility	a. Understands their responsibilities	1	2	3	**4**
		b. Acceptstheir responsibilities	1	2	3	**4**
		c. Manages multiple responsibilities	1	2	3	**4**
		d. Understandsrules associated with activities	1	2	3	**4**
		e. Accepts leadership roles at home	1	2	3	**4**
	Confidence	a. Confident in their abilities	1	2	**3**	4
		b. Enjoys daily activities	1	2	3	**4**
		c. Satisfied with performance in activities	1	2	**3**	4
		d. Identifies what he/she wants to get better at	1	2	3	**4**
		e. Keeps trying despite challenges	1	2	**3**	4
	Social Skills	a. Plays well with others	1	2	3	**4**
		b. Chatty/sociable and talks with friends	1	2	3	**4**
		c. Speaks clearly when with others	1	2	3	**4**
		d. Understands other's feelings	1	2	**3**	4
		e. Can ask for the support he/she needs	1	2	3	**4**
	Organisational Skills	a. Organises and uses objects for activities	1	2	3	**4**
		b. Maintains concentration throughout activities	1	2	**3**	4
		c. Works out problems if stuck on a task	1	2	**3**	4
		d. Follows through instructions for activities	1	2	3	**4**
		e. Does the steps of an activity in the right order	1	2	3	**4**
	Environment	a. Can navigate around physical environment	1	2	3	**4**
		b. Community environment has opportunities	1	2	3	**4**
		c. Accessto the things to help them take part	1	2	3	**4**
		d. Family members are available for support	1	2	3	**4**
		e. School environment supports school activities	1	2	3	**4**
		f. Does activities in usual/accepted way	1	2	3	**4**

PARENTAL OBSERVATIONS OF MOTOR SKILLS (DCD Q) - WHY			Not at all	A bit like	Mod. like	Quite like	Extremely like
	Control During Movement	1. Throws ball	1	2	**3**	4	5
		2. Catches ball	1	2	**3**	4	5
		3. Hits ball/birdie	1	2	**3**	4	5
		4. Jumps over	1	2	3	**4**	5
		5. Runs	1	2	**3**	4	5
		6. Plans activity	1	2	3	**4**	5
		TOTAL					20/30
	Fine Motor/ Handwriting	1. Writing fast	1	**2**	3	4	5
		2. Writing legibly	1	2	**3**	4	5
		3. Effort and pressure	**1**	2	3	4	5
		4. Cuts	1	**2**	3	4	5
		TOTAL					8/20
	General Coordination	1. Likes sport	1	2	3	**4**	5
		2. Learning new skills	1	2	**3**	4	5
		3. Quick and competent	1	2	**3**	4	5
		4. "Bull in shop"	**1**	2	3	4	5
		5. Does not fatigue	1	2	3	4	**5**
		TOTAL					16/25
		OVERALL TOTAL					44/75

Children aged 5 years 0 months to 7 years 11 months (tick as appropriate)
15-46: Indication of DCD or suspect DCD ☑
47-75: Probably not DCD ☐

Children aged 8 years 0 months to 9 years 11 months (tick as appropriate)
15-55: Indication of DCD or suspect DCD ☐
56-75: Probably not DCD ☐

Children aged 10 years 0 months to 15 years (tick as appropriate)
15-57: Indication of DCD or suspect DCD ☐
58-75: Probably not DCD ☐

SCHOOL QUESTIONNAIRE

TEACHER OBSERVATIONS OF ACTIVITY FREQUENCY - WHAT			None of the time	Some of the time	Most of the time	All of the time
	Home Activities that relate to School	a. Able to clean after toileting	1	2	3	**4**
		b. Able to get dressed in morning	1	2	3	**4**
		c. Able to use a knife and fork	1	2	**3**	4
		d. Able to make a simple snack	1	2	**3**	4
		e. Able to prepare for school in the morning	1	2	3	**4**
		f. Able to prepare for school activities	1	2	3	**4**
	School Activities	a. Able to use learning materials	1	**2**	3	4
		b. Able to make effective shapes/letters/writing	1	**2**	3	4
		c. Able to engage in sports/leisure	1	2	**3**	4
		d. Able to engage in curriculum	1	2	**3**	4
		e. Able to organise themselves	1	2	**3**	4
		f. Able to get dressed after P.E./gym	1	2	3	**4**
	Community Activities	a. Able to ride bike/rollerblade etc	1	2	3	**4**
		b. Able to play withpeersin activities	1	2	**3**	4
		c. Able to take part inafter school clubs	1	2	3	**4**
		d. Able to take part in social events	1	2	3	**4**
		e. Able to take partwith family in leisure activity	1	2	3	**4**
		f. Able to manage clothes before/after activities	1	2	3	**4**

TEACHER OBSERVATIONS OF CHARACTERISTICS OF CHILD - WHY			None of the time	Some of the time	Most of the time	All of the time
	Routine	a. Understands sequence/structure of routine	1	2	3	**4**
		b. Organises routines	1	2	3	**4**
		c. Copes with change in routine	1	2	3	**4**
		d. Copes with change in how activity's done	1	2	3	**4**
		e. Copes with a variety of activities	1	2	3	**4**
	Responsibility	a. Understands their responsibilities	1	2	3	**4**
		b. Accepts their responsibilities	1	2	**3**	4
		c. Manages multiple responsibilities	1	2	**3**	4
		d. Understands rules associated with activities	1	2	**3**	4
		e. Accepts leadership roles at school	1	2	3	**4**
	Confidence	a. Confident in their abilities	1	**2**	3	4
		b. Enjoys school activities	1	**2**	3	4
		c. Satisfied with performance in activities	1	**2**	3	4
		d. Identifies what he/she wants to get better at	1	**2**	3	4
		e. Keeps trying despite challenges	1	**2**	3	4
	Social Skills	a. Plays well with others	1	**2**	3	4
		b. Chatty/sociable and talks with friends	1	2	3	**4**
		c. Speaks clearly when with others	1	2	**3**	4
		d. Understands other's feelings	1	2	**3**	4
		e. Can ask for the support he/she needs	1	2	**3**	4
	Organisational Skills	a. Organises and uses objects for activities	1	2	**3**	4
		b. Maintains concentration throughout activities	1	**2**	3	4
		c. Works out problems if stuck on a task	1	**2**	3	4
		d. Follows through instructions for activities	1	**2**	3	4
		e. Does the steps of an activity in the right order	1	2	**3**	4
	Environment	a. Can navigate around physical environment	1	**2**	3	4
		b. Community environment has opportunities	1	2	**3**	4
		c. Access to the things to help them take part	1	2	**3**	4
		d. School staff are available for support	1	2	**3**	4
		e. School environment supports school activities	1	2	3	**4**
		f. Does activities in usual/accepted way	1	2	3	**4**

TEACHEROBSERVATIONS OF MOTOR SKILLS (DCD Q) - WHY			Not at all	A bit like	Mod. like	Quite like	Extremely like
	Control During Movement	1. Throws ball	1	**2**	3	4	5
		2. Catches ball	1	2	**3**	4	5
		3. Hits ball/birdie	1	2	**3**	4	5
		4. Jumps over	1	2	**3**	4	5
		5. Runs	**1**	2	3	4	5
		6. Plans activity	1	2	**3**	4	5
		TOTAL					15/30
	Fine Motor/ Handwriting	1. Writing fast	**1**	2	3	4	5
		2. Writing legibly	1	**2**	3	4	5
		3. Effort and pressure	1	**2**	3	4	5
		4. Cuts	1	2	**3**	4	5
		TOTAL					8/20
	General Coordination	1. Likes sport	1	2	3	**4**	5
		2. Learning new skills	**1**	2	3	4	5
		3. Quick and competent	1	**2**	3	4	5
		4. "Bull in shop"	**1**	2	3	4	5
		5. Does not fatigue	**1**	2	3	4	5
		TOTAL					9/25
		OVERALL TOTAL					32/75

Children aged 5 years 0 months to 7 years 11 months (tick as appropriate)
15-46: Indication of DCD or suspect DCD ☑
47-75: Probably not DCD ☐

Children aged 8 years 0 months to 9 years 11 months (tick as appropriate)
15-55: Indication of DCD or suspect DCD ☐
56-75: Probably not DCD ☐

Children aged 10 years 0 months to 15 years (tick as appropriate)
15-57: Indication of DCD or suspect DCD ☐
58-75: Probably not DCD ☐

FIGURE 39.4 John—ACHIEVE Assessment scores: baseline and reassessment.

SUMMARY SCORES – Re-assessment

Name: ...John..Date of Birth: ....
Age: ..7.........Yrs...................................Months CHI Number: ....
Clinician(s) Scoring: ....

PARENT QUESTIONNAIRE

PARENTAL OBSERVATIONS OF ACTIVITY FREQUENCY - WHAT

		None of the time	Some of the time	Most of the time	All of the time
Home Activities	a. Able to dry after bath/shower	1	2	3	**4**
	b. Able to clean after toileting	1	2	3	**4**
	c. Able to get un/dressed	1	2	3	**4**
	d. Able to make a simple snack	1	2	**3**	4
	e. Able to use a knife and fork	1	2	**3**	4
	f. Able toget ready in the morning	1	2	3	**4**
School Activities	a. Able to use learning materials	1	2	3	**4**
	b. Able to make effective shapes/letters/writing	1	2	3	**4**
	c. Able to engage in sports/leisure	1	2	3	**4**
	d. Able to engage in curriculum	1	2	3	**4**
	e. Able to clean after toilet at school	1	2	3	**4**
	f. Able to get dressed after P.E./gym	1	2	3	**4**
Community Activities	a. Able to ride bike/rollerblade etc	1	2	3	**4**
	b. Able to play with friends in activities	1	2	3	**4**
	c. Able to take part in out of school clubs	1	2	3	**4**
	d. Able to take part in social events	1	2	3	**4**
	e. Able to take part with family in leisure activity	1	2	3	**4**
	f. Able to manage clothes before/after activities	1	2	3	**4**

PARENTAL OBSERVATIONS OF CHARACTERISTICS OF CHILD - WHY

		None of the time	Some of the time	Most of the time	All of the time
Routine	a. Understands sequence/structure of routine	1	2	3	**4**
	b. Organises routines	1	2	3	**4**
	c. Copes with change in routine	1	2	**3**	4
	d. Copeswith change in how activity's done	1	2	3	**4**
	e. Copes with a variety of activities	1	2	3	**4**
Responsibility	a. Understands their responsibilities	1	2	3	**4**
	b. Accepts their responsibilities	1	2	3	**4**
	c. Manages multiple responsibilities	1	2	3	**4**
	d. Understands rules associated with activities	1	2	3	**4**
	e. Accepts leadership roles at home	1	2	3	**4**
Confidence	a. Confident in their abilities	1	2	**3**	4
	b. Enjoys daily activities	1	2	3	**4**
	c. Satisfied with performance in activities	1	2	**3**	4
	d. Identifies what he/she wants to get better at	1	2	3	**4**
	e. Keeps trying despite challenges	1	2	**3**	4
Social Skills	a. Plays well with others	1	2	3	**4**
	b. Chatty/sociable and talks with friends	1	2	3	**4**
	c. Speaks clearly when with others	1	2	3	**4**
	d. Understands other's feelings	1	2	**3**	4
	e. Can ask for the support he/she needs	1	2	3	**4**
Organisational Skills	a. Organises and uses objects for activities	1	2	3	**4**
	b. Maintains concentration throughout activities	1	2	**3**	4
	c. Works out problems if stuck on a task	1	2	**3**	4
	d. Follows through instructions for activities	1	2	3	**4**
	e. Does the steps of an activity in the right order	1	2	3	**4**
Environment	a. Can navigate around physical environment	1	2	3	**4**
	b. Community environment has opportunities	1	2	3	**4**
	c. Access to the things to help them take part	1	2	3	**4**
	d. Family members are available for support	1	2	3	**4**
	e. School environment supports school activities	1	2	3	**4**
	f. Does activities in usual/accepted way	1	2	3	**4**

PARENTAL OBSERVATIONS OF MOTOR SKILLS (DCD Q) - WHY

		Not at all	A bit like	Mod. like	Quite like	Extremely like
Control During Movement	1. Throws ball	1	2	**3**	4	5
	2. Catches ball	1	2	**3**	4	5
	3. Hits ball/birdie	1	2	**3**	4	5
	4. Jumps over	1	2	3	**4**	5
	5. Runs	1	2	**3**	4	5
	6. Plans activity	1	2	3	**4**	5
	TOTAL					20/30
Fine Motor/ Handwriting	1. Writing fast	1	**2**	3	4	5
	2. Writing legibly	1	2	**3**	4	5
	3. Effort and pressure	**1**	2	3	4	5
	4. Cuts	1	**2**	3	4	5
	TOTAL					8/20
General Coordination	1. Likes sport	1	2	3	**4**	5
	2. Learning new skills	1	2	**3**	4	5
	3. Quick and competent	1	2	**3**	4	5
	4. "Bull in shop"	**1**	2	3	4	5
	5. Does not fatigue	1	2	3	4	**5**
	TOTAL					16/25
	OVERALL TOTAL					44/75

Children aged 5 years 0 months to 7 years 11 months (tick as appropriate)
15-46: Indication of DCD or suspect DCD ☑
47-75: Probably not DCD ☐

Children aged 8 years 0 months to 9 years 11 months (tick as appropriate)
15-55: Indication of DCD or suspect DCD ☐
56-75: Probably not DCD ☐

Children aged 10 years 0 months to 15 years (tick as appropriate)
15-57: Indication of DCD or suspect DCD ☐
58-75: Probably not DCD ☐

SCHOOL QUESTIONNAIRE

TEACHER OBSERVATIONS OF ACTIVITY FREQUENCY - WHAT

		None of the time	Some of the time	Most of the time	All of the time
Home Activities that relate to School	a. Able toclean after toileting	1	2	3	**4**
	b. Able to get dressed in morning	1	2	3	**4**
	c. Able to use a knife and fork	1	2	**3**	4
	d. Able to make a simple snack	1	2	**3**	4
	e. Able to prepare for school in the morning	1	2	3	**4**
	f. Able to prepare for school activities	1	2	3	**4**
School Activities	a. Able to use learning materials	1	2	3	**4**
	b. Able to make effective shapes/letters/writing	1	2	3	**4**
	c. Able to engage in sports/leisure	1	2	**3**	4
	d. Able to engage in curriculum	1	2	**3**	4
	e. Able to organise themselves	1	2	**3**	4
	f. Able to get dressed after P.E./gym	1	2	3	**4**
Community Activities	a. Able to ride bike/rollerblade etc	1	2	3	**4**
	b. Able to play with peers in activities	1	2	**3**	4
	c. Able to take part in after school clubs	1	2	3	**4**
	d. Able to take part in social events	1	2	3	**4**
	e. Able to take part with family in leisure activity	1	2	3	**4**
	f. Able to manage clothes before/after activities	1	2	3	**4**

TEACHER OBSERVATIONS OF CHARACTERISTICS OF CHILD - WHY

		None of the time	Some of the time	Most of the time	All of the time
Routine	a. Understands sequence/structure of routine	1	2	3	**4**
	b. Organises routines	1	2	3	**4**
	c. Copes with change in routine	1	2	3	**4**
	d. Copes with change in how activity's done	1	2	3	**4**
	e. Copes with a variety of activities	1	2	3	**4**
Responsibility	a. Understands their responsibilities	1	2	3	**4**
	b. Accepts their responsibilities	1	2	**3**	4
	c. Manages multiple responsibilities	1	2	**3**	4
		1	2	**3**	4
	e. Accepts leadership roles at school	1	2	3	**4**
Confidence	a. Confident in their abilities	1	2	3	**4**
	b. Enjoys school activities	1	2	3	**4**
	c. Satisfied with performance in activities	1	2	3	**4**
	d. Identifies what he/she wants to get better at	1	2	3	**4**
	e. Keeps trying despite challenges	1	2	3	**4**
Social Skills	a. Plays well with others	1	2	3	**4**
	b. Chatty/sociable and talks with friends	1	2	3	**4**
	c. Speaks clearly when with others	1	2	**3**	4
	d. Understands other's feelings	1	2	**3**	4
	e. Can ask for the support he/she needs	1	2	**3**	4
Organisational Skills	a. Organises and uses objects for activities	1	2	**3**	4
	b. Maintains concentration throughout activities	1	2	3	**4**
	c. Works out problems if stuck on a task	1	2	3	**4**
	d. Follows through instructions for activities	1	2	3	**4**
	e. Does the steps of an activity in the right order	1	2	**3**	4
Environment	a. Can navigate around physical environment	1	2	3	**4**
	b. Community environment has opportunities	1	2	**3**	4
	c. Access to the things to help them take part	1	2	**3**	4
	d. School staff are available for support	1	2	**3**	4
	e. School environment supports school activities	1	2	3	**4**
	f. Does activities in usual/accepted way	1	2	3	**4**

TEACHER OBSERVATIONS OF MOTOR SKILLS (DCD Q) - WHY

		Not at all	A bit like	Mod. like	Quite like	Extremely like
Control During Movement	1. Throws ball	1	**2**	3	4	5
	2. Catches ball	1	2	**3**	4	5
	3. Hits ball/birdie	1	2	**3**	4	5
	4. Jumps over	1	2	**3**	4	5
	5. Runs	**1**	2	3	4	5
	6. Plans activity	1	2	**3**	4	5
	TOTAL					15/30
Fine Motor/ Handwriting	1. Writing fast	**1**	2	3	4	5
	2. Writing legibly	1	**2**	3	4	5
	3. Effort and pressure	1	**2**	3	4	5
	4. Cuts	1	2	**3**	4	5
	TOTAL					8/20
General Coordination	1. Likes sport	1	2	3	**4**	5
	2. Learning new skills	**1**	2	3	4	5
	3. Quick and competent	1	**2**	3	4	5
	4. "Bull in shop"	**1**	2	3	4	5
	5. Does not fatigue	**1**	2	3	4	5
	TOTAL					9/25
	OVERALL TOTAL					32/75

Children aged 5 years 0 months to 7 years 11 months (tick as appropriate)
15-46: Indication of DCD or suspect DCD ☑
47-75: Probably not DCD ☐

Children aged 8 years 0 months to 9 years 11 months (tick as appropriate)
15-55: Indication of DCD or suspect DCD ☐
56-75: Probably not DCD ☐

Children aged 10 years 0 months to 15 years (tick as appropriate)
15-57: Indication of DCD or suspect DCD ☐
58-75: Probably not DCD ☐

FIGURE 39.4 *(Continued)*

TABLE 39.6 John—Movement Assessment Battery for Children-2 (ABC2) (Henderson & Sugden, 1992) Scores

Movement ABC2 Scores	Manual dexterity: 9th percentile, which is suggestive of being at risk of movement difficulties. Aiming and catching: 75th percentile, no movement difficulties detected Balance: 9th percentile, which is suggestive of being at risk of movement difficulties.
Overall Percentile	9th percentile, which is suggestive of being at risk of movement difficulties.

The Movement ABC2 assesses a child's fine motor ability, for example, pencils and scissors skills, performance with ball skills, and balance. The test scores provide information about how your child's motor performance compares to his or her peers and can provide an indication of the severity of the motor difficulties. Below 5th percentile: significant movement difficulties; 5th–15th percentile: suggestive of being at risk of movement difficulties; above 15th percentile: no movement difficulties detected.

- As the teacher indicated on the referral form that John's movement was awkward, the ACHIEVE Assessment also included a Developmental Coordination Disorder Questionnaire (DCDQ) (Wilson, Kaplan, Crawford, Campbell, & Dewey, 2000), which is a brief questionnaire designed to screen for coordination disorders in children aged 5 to 15 years.

During Therapy Clinic

- Review and verification of the findings of the ACHIEVE Assessment (Forsyth et al., 2012) with parent
- Movement Assessment Battery for Children (ABC) (Henderson & Sugden, 1992)—This assessment identifies, describes, and guides the treatment of motor impairment. It is used to assess children's motor skills disabilities and determine intervention strategies (Table 39.6).
- Standardized assessment of handwriting, *The Handwriting File* (Alston & Taylor, 1988), was completed to understand if John's writing skill was significantly slower that would be expected of a child his age (Table 39.7).

After the Therapy Clinic

- Short Child Occupational Profile (SCOPE) (Bowyer, et al., 2006)—This is an assessment that is completed by the therapist using information gathered in various ways.

TABLE 39.7 John—The Handwriting File (Alston & Taylor, 1988) Scores

Test	Handwriting file
Performance indicator	Letters per minute
Score	26 letters per minute (7-year-old normally able to manage 28 letters per minute)

- The therapist rated the SCOPE using information gathered from the other assessments as well as during an observation of John's participation within the classroom (Figure 39.5).
- This allowed for "triangulation" between the parents' view, the teacher's view, and the therapist's view on how different personal and environment factors impacted John's participation. This provides a range of views to build a comprehensive understanding of John.

Creating a Theory-Based Understanding of the Client

The following occupational formulation was created from the assessment findings.

- *What was important to John, his family, and his teacher?* John stated, "Writing is not my thing" and wanted to be able to keep up with his friends and not feel his cheeks getting hot and feeling panicky about being the last to complete writing tasks. John's mother wanted him to be able to write better and not find it so difficult to do this. John's teacher wants John to be less clumsy, less distractible, and for his writing to be less laborious.
- *What is John good at and what does he enjoy?* Comparing teacher and parent assessments, John performs more consistently in activities at home than at school. John has many areas of strength including home and community activities; for example, able to get dressed/undressed, able to ride a bike, able to take part in social events. John's teacher reports that John enjoys math and physical education.
- *Why does John have these strengths?* Despite concerns, John can achieve 26 letters per minute (normative performance is 28 letters per minute for a 7-year-old) *when focused.* John's mother, teacher, and therapists identified that John has structured routines at both home and school. His mother, teacher, and therapists agree that John mostly understands responsibilities, has appropriate social

Baseline

Volition				
Exploration	**1**	2	3	4
Expressions of enjoyment	**1**	2	3	4
Preferences & choices	**1**	2	3	4
Response to challenge	**1**	2	3	4

Habituation				
Daily activities	1	2	3	**4**
Response to transitions	1	2	3	**4**
Routine	1	2	3	**4**
Roles	1	2	3	**4**

Communication & Interaction skills				
Non verbal	1	2	**3**	4
Verbal expression	1	2	3	**4**
Conversation	1	2	**3**	4
Relationships	1	2	**3**	4

Process Skills				
Understands/uses objects	**1**	2	3	4
Orientation to environment	**1**	2	3	4
Plan/make decisions	**1**	2	3	4
Problem solving	**1**	2	3	4

Motor skills				
Posture/mobility	1	**2**	3	4
Coordination	1	**2**	3	4
Strength	1	2	3	**4**
Energy/Endurance	1	**2**	3	4

Environment				
Physical space	1	**2**	3	4
Physical resources	1	**2**	3	4
Social groups	1	2	**3**	4
Activity demands	1	**2**	3	4

Re-assessment

Volition				
Exploration	1	2	3	**4**
Expressions of enjoyment	1	2	3	**4**
Preferences & choices	1	2	3	**4**
Response to challenge	1	2	3	**4**

Habituation				
Daily activities	1	2	3	**4**
Response to transitions	1	2	3	**4**
Routine	1	2	3	**4**
Roles	1	2	3	**4**

Communication & Interaction skills				
Non verbal	1	2	**3**	4
Verbal expression	1	2	3	**4**
Conversation	1	2	**3**	4
Relationships	1	2	**3**	4

Process Skills				
Understands/uses objects	1	2	3	**4**
Orientation to environment	1	2	3	**4**
Plan/make decisions	1	2	3	**4**
Problem solving	1	2	3	**4**

Motor skills				
Posture/mobility	1	2	**3**	4
Coordination	1	2	**3**	4
Strength	1	2	3	**4**
Energy/Endurance	1	2	**3**	4

Environment				
Physical space	1	2	3	**4**
Physical resources	1	2	3	**4**
Social groups	1	2	**3**	4
Activity demands	1	2	3	**4**

Scale: 1 = Facilitates participation in occupation
2 = Allows participation in occupation
3 = Inhibits participation in occupation
4 = Restricts participation in occupation

FIGURE 39.5 John—Short Child Occupational Profile (SCOPE) scores: baseline and reassessment. (From Bowyer, P., Ross, M., Schwartz, O., Kielhofner, G., & Kramer, J. [2006]. *The short child occupational profile* [SCOPE; Version 2.1]. Chicago, IL: Model of Human Occupation Clearinghouse.)

skills, and has a supportive school and home environment matched to his abilities and skills.

- *What does John find challenging?* John doesn't have any areas of challenge at home. John was, however, observed in the classroom to have challenges using learning materials effectively (e.g., pens, pencils, crayons, rules, glue sticks, scissors) and being able to make effective shapes or letters and writing within a school context.
- *Why does John have these challenges?* Parents were concerned about John's motor skill development; however, from their point of view, there are no other health concerns. Indeed, John's teacher reported he has challenges navigating around his physical school environment. Although the DCDQ indicates challenges in fine motor or handwriting and general coordination within school and the Movement ABC was within the 9th percentile (which is suggestive of

being at risk of movement difficulties with manual dexterity and balance), it is likely that these scores have been significantly impacted by John's distractibility or lack of attention. John was observed to be *highly* distractible during both the therapy clinic and classroom. This is further supported by John's handwriting being normative for his age group when formally tested—when he was focused in a quiet environment. Moreover, John's teacher reports that John has significant challenges in the area of organizational ability in school (i.e., extremely poor concentration throughout written tasks, lack of effort in writing tasks, following through on instructions), which was consistent with the therapist's observation. The impact on John's confidence in school was noticeable in the classroom (i.e., having confidence in abilities, enjoyment or having satisfaction in school activities, and not trying despite challenges). This was consistent with John giving up easily within the therapy clinic, although he was competitive when performing against a timer.

Generating Therapy Goals and Strategies

Although the initial referral from the teacher was framed as challenges in movement and coordination, the assessment process identified that the main areas of occupational change to target in therapy was

- Improvement in use of learning materials through developing organizational skills and increase confidence for tasks completed within the classroom.

The joint measurable goal shared between therapy and education was therefore

- Within 4 weeks, John will be able to confidently use learning materials (such as books, writing utensils) through organizing objects and maintaining concentration within his classroom independently.

A meeting was arranged between the therapist, the parent, and the teacher to exchange strategies that worked for John at home and resulted in John performing better within the home environment (i.e., routine praise for completing activities regardless of outcome or speed), making eye contact with John before sharing instructions, and creating an environment with limited distractions when completing homework. The parent, teacher, and occupational therapists therefore identified strategies—from *Intervention Descriptions: Occupational Therapy* (CIRCLE Collaboration, 2009c)—of (1) modifying the school environment, (2) recreating volition, and (3) process skill building.

Implementing and Monitoring Therapy

The philosophy of the school therapist was to empower those around a child to provide therapeutic supports to allow for a more consistent approach to supporting a child's occupational participation. The understanding of John was shared with the teacher through the use of the *Collaborative Communication Chart* (CIRCLE Collaboration, 2009a) and *Therapy Manual: Occupational Therapy* (CIRCLE Collaboration, 2009d). This chart was created by therapists and teachers as a structured set of language to support consistent communication. This provided a common language for the therapist and teacher to discuss strategies that John could use to improve his organizational skills and concentration in the classroom.

The following was agreed as the intervention package:

- John was given a pencil grip.
- John's desk was moved to a front corner of the classroom from his current position in the center of the class to reduce distractions. He was also provided with a bigger desk that would have adequate space for work materials and support materials.
- John was provided with a range of objects that provide sensory feedback during writing (i.e., rubber grips, weighted pencils, weighted wrist bands).
- John's teacher provided praise on completion of activities and displayed work alongside others to show its equal value.
- John's teacher created writing tasks where John could write about strong interests.
- John's teacher made him more aware of when he was feeling enjoyment during writing tasks.
- Teacher facilitated positive feedback on his writing by his friends in the classroom.
- Teacher was positive about any perceived failure to support task perseverance despite challenges.
- Teacher was more aware of John disengaging from his writing task; and when she noticed disengagement, she supported John to use his concentration strategies to ensure continued focus.
- John's teacher made eye contact with John before providing instruction on writing task.
- Integrate into John's strong routines setting up and clearing away his work station space on daily basis.
- John was provided with a timer and taught how to use it to work in 10-minute increments.
- The therapist and John collaborated to make a checklist for materials and for checking task completion that John could then reference independently at the beginning and end of each class work period.

The teacher was encouraged to contact the therapist if there were any concerns or insurmountable challenges during the intervention period. Otherwise, the intervention was provided solely by the teacher.

Collecting Information to Assess Outcomes

The expected therapeutic change in John's occupational participation was within school. A reassessment after

4 weeks was arranged and the following review was completed.

- Goal attainment (i.e., review of joint therapy or educational goal)
- ACHIEVE Assessment (Forsyth et al., 2012) (Figure 39.4)
- SCOPE (Bowyer et al., 2006) (Figure 39.5)

John reached his 4-week goal of being able to perform within the classroom more confidently. This was supported by his teacher reporting (Figure 39.4) improved confidence and organizational skills. He was observed to use his self-monitored strategies. She also reflected that John was "calmer" and more "focused" within the classroom and less disruptive. Classroom observations using the SCOPE also revealed improved scores for confidence and organizational ability (Figure 39.5). Most importantly, John stated that he felt less panicked when writing tasks were assigned and his posture and demeanor were more relaxed. He proudly showed his workstation to the therapists as his space.

Conclusion

This chapter provided an overview of the concepts and practice resources of MOHO. Two cases were used to demonstrate how MOHO concepts are used to guide the process of therapeutic reasoning. As the cases illustrate, therapists can use MOHO to support a client-centered and occupationally focused practice. This chapter was able to demonstrate only a small fraction of the theoretical, empirical, and practical resources that are available under this model. Anyone who wishes to use MOHO is encouraged to take advantage of those resources.

References

Alston, J., & Taylor, J. (1988). *The handwriting file* (2nd ed.). Wisbech, United Kingdom: LDA.

American Occupational Therapy Association. (2002). Occupational therapy practice framework: Domain and process. *American Journal of Occupational Therapy, 56*, 609–639.

Ayres, A. J. (1979). *Sensory integration and the child.* Los Angeles, CA: Western Psychological Services.

Baron, K., Kielhofner, G., Iyenger, A., Goldhammer, V., & Wolenski, J. (2006). *The Occupational Self Assessment* (OSA; Version 2.2). Chicago, IL: Model of Human Occupation Clearinghouse.

Basu, S., Kafkes, A., Geist, R., & Kielhofner, G. (2002). *The Pediatric Volitional Questionnaire* (PVQ; Version 2.0). Chicago, IL: Model of Human Occupation Clearinghouse.

Bernspang, B., & Fisher, A. (1995). Differences between persons with a right or left cerebral vascular accident on the assessment of motor and process skills. *Archives of Physical Medicine and Rehabilitation, 75*, 1144–1151.

Bowyer, P., Ross, M., Schwartz, O., Kielhofner, G., & Kramer, J. (2006). *The short child occupational profile* (SCOPE; Version 2.1). Chicago, IL: Model of Human Occupation Clearinghouse.

Braveman, B., Robson, M., Velozo, C., Kielhofner, G., Fisher, G., Forsyth, K., & Kerschbaum, J. (2005). *The worker role interview* (WRI; Version 10.0). Chicago, IL: Model of Human Occupation Clearinghouse.

CIRCLE Collaboration. (2009a). *Collaborative communication chart.* Edinburgh, Scotland: City of Edinburgh Council, Queen Margaret University, and NHS Lothian.

CIRCLE Collaboration. (2009b). *Inclusive learning and collaborative working: Teachers' ideas in practice.* Edinburgh, Scotland: City of Edinburgh Council, Queen Margaret University, and NHS Lothian.

CIRCLE Collaboration. (2009c). *Intervention descriptions: Occupational therapy.* Edinburgh, Scotland: City of Edinburgh Council, Queen Margaret University, and NHS Lothian.

CIRCLE Collaboration. (2009d). *Therapy manual: Occupational therapy.* Edinburgh, Scotland: City of Edinburgh Council, Queen Margaret University, and NHS Lothian.

de las Heras, C. G., Lierena, V., & Kielhofner, G. (2003). *Remotivation process: Progressive intervention for individuals with severe volitional challenges* (Version 1.0). Chicago, IL: Department of Occupational Therapy, University of Illinois at Chicago.

Doble, S. (1991). Test-retest and interrater reliability of a process skills assessment. *Occupational Therapy Journal of Research, 11*, 8–23.

Elenko, B. K., Hinojosa, J., Blount, M.-L., & Blount, W. (2000). Perspectives. In J. Hinojosa & M.-L. Blount (Eds.), *The texture of life: Purposeful activities in occupational therapy* (pp. 16–35). Bethesda, MD: American Occupational Therapy Association.

Fisher, A. G. (2003). *Assessment of Motor and Process Skills* (5th ed.). Fort Collins, CO: Three Star.

Fisher, A., & Kielhofner, G. (1995). Skill in occupational performance. In G. Kielhofner (Ed.), *A model of human occupation: Theory and application* (2nd ed., pp. 113–137). Baltimore, MD: Lippincott Williams & Wilkins.

Fisher, G., Arriaga, P., Less, C., Lee, J., & Ashpole, E. (2008). *The residential environment impact survey* (REIS; Version 2.0). Chicago, IL: Model of Human Occupation Clearinghouse.

Forsyth, K., Deshpande, S., Kielhofner, G., Henriksson, C., Haglund, L., Olson, L., . . . Kulkarni, S. (2005). *The Occupational Circumstances Assessment Interview and Rating Scale* (OCAIRS; Version 4.0). Chicago, IL: Model of Human Occupation Clearinghouse.

Forsyth, K., Lai, J., & Kielhofner, G. (1999). The Assessment of Communication and Interaction Skills (ACIS): Measurement properties. *British Journal of Occupational Therapy, 62*(2), 69–74.

Forsyth, K., Salamy, M., Simon, S., & Kielhofner, G. (1998). *Assessment of Communication and Interaction Skills* (Version 4.0). Chicago, IL: Model of Human Occupation Clearinghouse.

Forsyth, K., Whitehead, J., Owen, C., & Gorska, S. (2012). *A users guide to the Active in Children Health Integrating Evidence Valuing Experience (ACHIEVE) Assessment.* Edinburgh: Queen Margaret University.

Frust, G., Gerber, L., Smith, C., Fisher, S., & Shulman, B. (1987). A program for improving energy conservation behaviors in adults with rheumatoid arthritis. *American Journal of Occupational Therapy, 41*, 102–111.

Gerber, L., & Frust, G. (1992). Scoring methods and application of the Activity Record (ACTRE) for patients with musculoskeletal disorders. *Arthritis Care and Research, 5*, 151–156.

Haglund, L., Ekbladh, E., Thorell, L., & Hallberg, I. R. (2000). Practice models in Swedish psychiatric occupational therapy. *Scandinavian Journal of Occupational Therapy, 7*(3), 107–113.

Hemmingson, H., Egilson, S., Hoffman, O., & Kielhofner, G. (2005). *School Setting Interview* (SSI; Version 3.0). Nacka, Sweden: Swedish Association of Occupational Therapists.

Henderson, E., & Sugden, D. (1992). *The Movement Assessment Battery for Children.* London, United Kingdom: Psychological Corporation.

Henry, A. D. (2000). *The pediatric interest profiles: Surveys of play for children and adolescents.* Unpublished manuscript, Model of Human Occupation Clearinghouse, Department of Occupational Therapy, University of Illinois, Chicago, Illinois.

Keller, J., Kafkes, A., Basu, S., Federico, J., & Kielhofner, G. (2005). *A user's guide to Child Occupational Self Assessment* (COSA; Version 2.1). Chicago, IL: University of Illinois, Chicago.

Kielhofner, G. (1980a). A model of human occupation: 2. Ontogenesis from the perspective of temporal adaptation. *American Journal of Occupational Therapy, 34*, 657–663.

Kielhofner, G. (1980b). A model of human occupation: 3. Benign and vicious cycles. *American Journal of Occupational Therapy, 34,* 731–737.

Kielhofner, G. (2008). *A model of human occupation: Theory and application* (4th ed.). Baltimore, MD: Lippincott Williams & Wilkins.

Kielhofner, G., & Burke, J. (1980). A model of human occupation: 1. Conceptual framework and content. *American Journal of Occupational Therapy, 34,* 572–581.

Kielhofner, G., Burke, J., & Heard, I. C. (1980). A model of human occupation: 4. Assessment and intervention. *American Journal of Occupational Therapy, 34,* 777–788.

Kielhofner, G., Mallison, T., Crawford, C., Nowak, M., Rigby, M., Henry, A., & Walens, D. (2004). *Occupational performance history interview-II* (OPHI-II; Version 2.1). Chicago, IL: Model of Human Occupation Clearinghouse.

Law, M. (1998). *Client-centered occupational therapy.* Thorofare, NJ: Slack.

Law, M., Cooper, B. A., Strong, S., Stewart, D., Rigby, P., & Letts, L. (1997). Theoretical contexts for the practice of occupational therapy. In C. Christiansen & C. Baum (Eds.), *Occupational therapy: Enabling function and well-being* (2nd ed., pp. 73–102). Thorofare, NJ: Slack.

Law, M., & McColl, M. A. (1989). Knowledge and use of theory among occupational therapists: A Canadian survey. *Canadian Journal of Occupational Therapy, 56,* 198–204.

Lee, S. W., Taylor, R., Kielhofner, G., & Fisher, G. (2008). Theory use in practice: A national survey of therapists who use the model of human occupation. *American Journal of Occupational Therapy, 62,* 106–117.

Matsutsuyu, J. (1969). The interest checklist. *American Journal of Occupational Therapy, 23,* 323–328.

Moore-Corner, R. A., Kielhofner, G., & Olson, L. (1998). *A user's guide to Work Environment Impact Scale.* Chicago, IL: Model of Human Occupation Clearinghouse.

National Board for the Certification in Occupational Therapy. (2004). A practice analysis study of entry-level occupational therapists registered and certifies occupational therapy assistant practice. *OTJR: Occupation, Participation and Health, 24*(Suppl. 1), s1–s31.

Oakley, F., Kielhofner, G., & Barris, R. (1985). An occupational therapy approach to assessing psychiatric patients' adaptive functioning. *American Journal of Occupational Therapy, 39,* 147–154.

Parkinson, S., Forsyth, K., & Kielhofner, G. (2006). *A user's manual for the model of human occupation screening tool* (MOHOST; Version 2.0). Chicago, IL: University of Illinois, Chicago.

Pedretti, L. W., & Early, M. B. (Eds.). (2001). Occupational performance and models of practice for physical dysfunction. In *Occupational therapy: Practice skills for physical dysfunction* (5th ed). St. Louis, MO: Mosby.

Prior, S., Forsyth, K., & Ritchie, L. (2011). *ActiVate Collaboration: Occupational therapy & evidence based vocational rehabilitation.* Edinburgh: Queen Margaret University, NHS Lothian.

Smith, N. R., Kielhofner, G., & Watts, J. (1986). The relationship between volition, activity pattern, and life satisfaction in the elderly. *American Journal of Occupational Therapy, 40,* 278–283.

Townsend, S., Carey, P. D., Hollins, N. L., Helfrich, C., Blondis, M., Hoffman, A., . . . Blackwell, A. (1999). *The Occupational Therapy Psychosocial Assessment of Learning* (OT PAL; Version 2.0). Chicago, IL: Model of Human Occupation Clearinghouse.

Trombly, C. A., & Radomski, M. V. (2001). *Occupational Therapy for Physical Dysfunction* (5th edition). Philadelphia, PA: Lippincott Williams & Wilkins.

Watts, J. H., Hinson, R., Madigan, M. J., McGuigan, P. M., & Newman, S. M. (1999). The assessment of occupational functioning—Collaborative version. In B. J. Hempill-Pearson (Ed.), *Assessments in Occupational Therapy in Mental Health.* Thorofare, NJ: Slack.

Wilkeby, M., Pierre, B. L., & Archenholtz, B. (2006). Occupational therapists' reflection on practice within psychiatric care: A Delphi study. *Scandinavian Journal of Occupational Therapy, 13,* 151–159.

Wilson, B. N., Kaplan, B. J., Crawford, S. G., Campbell, A., & Dewey, D. (2000). Reliability and validity of a parent questionnaire on childhood motor skills. *American Journal of Occupational Therapy, 54,* 484–493.

For additional resources on the subjects discussed in this chapter, visit http://thePoint.lww.com/Willard-Spackman12e.

CHAPTER 40

Theory of Occupational Adaptation

Sally W. Schultz

LEARNING OBJECTIVES

After reading this chapter, you will be able to:

1. State the features of occupational adaptation (OA) that most distinguish it from other occupation-based theories of practice
2. Describe the necessity of using the Guide to Therapeutic Reasoning for an OA-based treatment program
3. Describe key aspects of the OA Guide to Evaluation and Intervention
4. Explain why the therapeutic use of self is one of the most powerful therapeutic tools
5. Explain why it is necessary for therapists to use an articulated theory to develop an authentic occupation-based practice

OUTLINE

Alfonso is an 11-year-old boy attending public school in the fifth grade. He was referred to occupational therapy for help with attention deficit disorder, reading problems, and behavioral problems both in the classroom and at recess. His occupational therapist, Claudette, plans to include Alfonso in a therapy group with other boys who are having similar difficulties. This group is based on the theory of occupational adaptation. Some of Claudette's work with Alfonso is described in the case study later in the chapter.

Intellectual Heritage

In 1987, a group of Texas Woman's University occupational therapy faculty was charged by Dr. Grace Gilkeson (dean of the School of Occupational Therapy at the university) to develop a PhD program in occupational therapy. One of the group's challenges was to name and frame how the program would contribute to the discipline and practice of occupational therapy. After lengthy study and debate, the committee reached agreement that there were two concepts that were unquestionably fundamental to occupational therapy and should be emphasized throughout the doctoral program. These two concepts were occupation and adaptation. The committee saw occupation and adaptation as integral to the profession's beginnings, central to its philosophy, and essential for the integrity of its future. The research focus for the new doctoral program was thus identified as occupational adaptation (OA).

The design of the doctoral program progressed, and responsibilities were divided among the committee members. Sally Schultz and Janette Schkade were asked to develop the group's conceptualization of OA into the perspective that would be the core of the doctoral program. Drs. Anne Henderson, Lela Llorens, and Kathlyn Reed, noted occupational therapy scholars, provided ongoing consultation in the development of the PhD program and the research focus on OA. The program was established in 1994. By 2007, there were more than 30 graduates of the program. Schkade and Schultz expanded on the initial concept of **occupational adaptation**. They introduced OA as a frame of reference (Schkade & Schultz, 1992; Schultz & Schkade, 1992) and most recently (Schkade & Schultz, 2003) as an overarching theory for occupational therapy practice and research.

The theory of occupational adaptation describes the integration of two global concepts that have long been present in occupational therapy thinking: **occupation** and **adaptation**. Occupation has been presented as a paradigm for occupational therapy in numerous publications. The notion of adaptation as a paradigm for occupational therapy was alluded to by King (1978) and formally proposed by Schultz and Schkade (1997). The intellectual heritage of this theory dates back to the writings of William Dunton (1913) and Adolph Meyer (1922). Schkade and Schultz were also significantly influenced by the writings of several contemporary theorists both within and outside the field of occupational therapy (i.e., Gilfoyle, Grady, & Moore, 1990; King, 1978; Llorens, 1970; Selye, 1956). OA interventions for specific populations were first published in 1992 (Schkade & Schultz, 1992). A model outlining home health interventions appeared in 1994 (Schultz & Schkade, 1994). Numerous population-specific OA applications have appeared over the years (e.g., Ford, 1995; Garrett & Schkade, 1995; Jack & Estes, 2010; Johnson, 2006; Pasek & Schkade, 1996; Ross, 1994; Schkade, 1999; Schkade & McClung, 2001; Schkade & Schultz, 2003; Schultz, 1997, 2000, 2003; Schultz & Schkade, 1994; Stelter & Whisner, 2007; Werner, 2000).

Guiding Assumptions of Occupational Adaptation Theory

All theories are based on assumptions. Most occupational therapy is driven by the assumption that as clients become more functional, they will be more adaptive. The theory of occupational adaptation takes the opposite point of view. Practice based on OA is driven by the assumption that if clients become more adaptive, they will become more functional.

The founders of the theory of occupational adaptation (Schkade & Schultz, 1992) proposed six guiding assumptions about the relationship between occupational performance and human adaptation. The assumptions are presumed to be normative and applicable across the life course. These six assumptions are as follows:

1. Competence in occupation is a lifelong process of adaptation to internal and external demands to perform.
2. Demands to perform occur naturally as part of the person's occupational roles and the context (person–occupational environment interactions) in which they occur.
3. Dysfunction occurs because the person's ability to adapt has been challenged to the point at which the demands for performance are not met satisfactorily.
4. The person's **adaptive capacity** can be overwhelmed by impairment, physical or emotional disabilities, and stressful life events.
5. The greater the level of dysfunction, the greater is the demand for changes in the person's adaptive processes.
6. Success in occupational performance is a direct result of the person's ability to adapt with sufficient mastery to satisfy the self and others.

These six assumptions are not about occupational therapy. They are about the normative relationship between occupational performance and human adaptation. The assumptions are relevant to occupational therapy because they provide the practitioner with a way of viewing the client and the problems that are presented in therapy. The most common viewpoint the occupational therapy practitioner experiences is the medical model and its underlying assumptions. In medicine, patients are generally viewed in terms of their body systems. Treatment is focused on correcting the breakdown within the identified system(s). Medicine's underlying assumptions about illness and treatment shape the view and the interventions that are used. For example, a nurse reviews the chart's lab results, vital signs, and progress. The nurse visits the 68-year-old white male and asks, "How are you doing today?" The patient answers, "Pretty good, but I'm still having a lot of pain, and I get tired so easily." The nurse asks the physician to write an order for more pain medication and increased activity.

A practitioner whose practice is based on OA will view the client through the filter of the six assumptions that ground the theory. The OA constructs, models, and intervention methods are all based on these assumptions. They form the core of the theory of occupational adaptation. The OA-based practitioner visits the same 68-year-old client. The practitioner is aware that the man is a retired bus driver, that he is married to the mother of his four children, and that they have nine grandchildren. The practitioner wonders aloud to the client, "What would you be doing today if you hadn't broken your hip?" The client responds, "Oh, I don't know, the only thing that matters now is getting me back on my feet." The practitioner replies, "Yes, we'll focus on that. You had a pretty bad break, and you might need to do some things differently when you go home. I will help with that. Let's talk about what matters the most to you."

Introduction to the Theory of Occupational Adaptation

The first publication on the theory of occupational adaptation was presented in two parts (Schkade & Schultz, 1992; Schultz & Schkade, 1992). Part 1 presents the theory's assumptions about the relationship between human adaptation and the performance of everyday occupations. A normative model—the **occupational adaptation process**—was proposed to describe the interaction of the person, the environment, and the internal adaptive processes that occur when individuals engage in their occupations of daily living (Schkade & Schultz, 1992). The model is presented in a linear format. However, the author recognizes that the actual process of OA is characterized by complexity, randomness, and nonlinearity (e.g., Davies, 1988; Gleick, 1987; Prigogine & Stengers, 1984). Such human processes are inherently not describable in two-dimensional models. On the other hand, the benefit of a linear model is that it provides a rudimentary organization of highly interactive and complex phenomena. Such organization is necessary to engage in a systematic examination. In sum, the OA process is a highly interactive, complex, and self-organizing process that has the goal of achieving mastery over the environment.

The linear model provides a basis for scholarly dialogue. The objective in dynamic self-organizing processes is not to achieve a determined balance or equilibrium. The theory of occupational adaptation proposes that equilibrium or homeostasis can actually result in a state of dysadaptation. Personal adaptation is proposed in the theory as a human phenomenon that is in a continuous process of order and disorder and reorganization. Figure 40.1 presents a modified version of the original

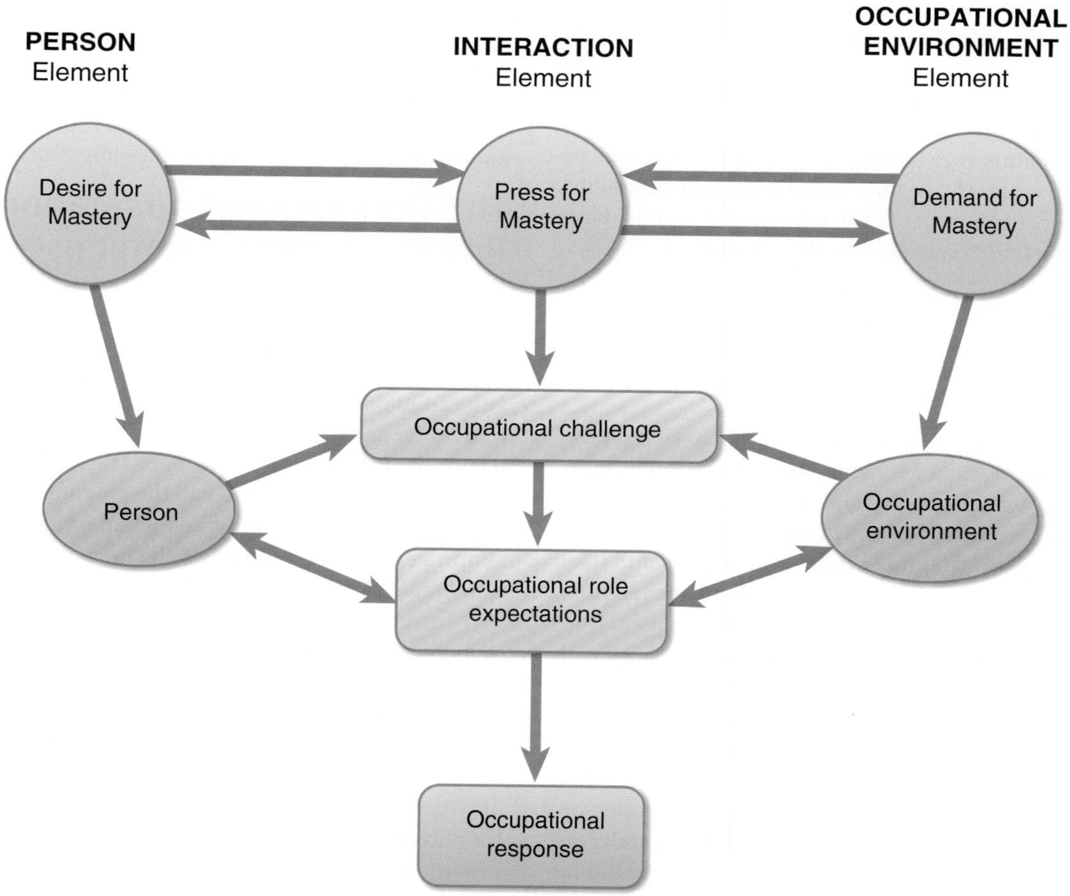

FIGURE 40.1 Model of the occupational adaptation process. (Adapted from Schkade, J. K., & Schultz, S. [1992]. Occupational adaptation: Toward a holistic approach to contemporary practice, Part 1. *American Journal of Occupational Therapy, 46*, 829–837. doi:10.5014/ajot.46.9.829)

1992 model. The revised model is somewhat simplified from the one that was presented in 1992. It is also a linear model that was created to serve as a vehicle for examining these very complex processes. Although dynamic models are often more inclusive of the multiple phenomena, an identifiable process is often elusive. The model of the OA process (Figure 40.1) is based on three overarching elements: the person, the **occupational environment**, and their interaction. Each is a dynamic, ever-changing state that influences the other. The following discussion elaborates on Figure 40.1. Terminology that is specific to the theory and/or model is initially presented in italics.

Person: Internal Factors of the Occupational Adaptation Process

The left side of the model is devoted to the internal factors: those that occur within the *person.* The process begins with a *desire for mastery.* The desire for mastery is proposed in the theory of occupational adaptation as a constant factor in the OA process; it is ever present. Even at the cellular level, there is constant demand for adaptation and mastery (Reilly, 1962). Seeking mastery over the environment is understood to be an innate human condition. The second factor, the person, is made up of the individual's unique sensorimotor, cognitive, and psychosocial systems. These person systems are unique to the individual, with specific attributes and deficits. They are also uniquely affected by the individual's genetic, biological, and phenomenological influences. The theory of occupational adaptation posits that all occupations are holistic. That is, all occupations involve the sensorimotor, cognitive, and psychosocial systems. The relative contribution of each system shifts on the basis of the circumstances surrounding the occupation.

Occupational Environment: External Factors of the Occupational Adaptation Process

The right side of the model is devoted to external factors that affect the *person* (see Figure 40.1). Correspondingly, the external process also begins with a constant factor: the *demand for mastery.* The theory of occupational adaptation proposes that any circumstance presents itself with at least a minimal degree of demand for mastery. The second external factor is the *occupational environment.* The term was coined by the founding authors with the intent to capture the dynamic meaning that they ascribed to the complexity of factors that are external to the person in the OA process. The occupational environment is highly significant in that it not only has an expectation of the person but also has a direct impact on the person. The occupational environment represents the overall context within which the person engages in the particular occupation and *occupational role.* There are three broad types of occupational environment: work, play/leisure, and self-care. Each type of occupational environment is affected by the physical, social, and cultural influences that are part of the individual's experiential context. The physical influence consists of the actual setting in which the occupation occurs. The social influence is made up of the individuals who are participants within the occupational environment. The cultural influence presents the habits, mores, and traditions and rituals that exist in the occupational environment. The occupational environment is also a continuously dynamic and experiential context.

The Occupational Adaptation Process: Interaction of Internal and External Factors

The internal and external factors are continuously interacting with each other through the modality of occupation. The ongoing interaction of the person's desire for mastery and the occupational environment's demand for mastery creates a third constant: the *press for mastery.* This constant forms the middle of the OA process model. The press for mastery yields the *occupational challenge.* The *occupational role expectations* of the person and of the occupational environment intersect in response to the unique occupational challenge that the individual experiences. A demand for adaptation occurs. The person makes an internal adaptive response to the situation and then produces an *occupational response.* The occupational response is the outcome—the observable by-product of the adaptive response. It is the action or behavior that the individual carries out in response to the occupational challenge. The OA process begins at the top of both the left and right sides of the model at the same time.

The Occupational Adaptation Process: Adaptive Response Subprocesses

Within the broad OA process, there are three subprocesses that are internal to the person. They are proposed to provide an explanation of the adaptive processes that the individual activates in response to an occupational challenge. The OA subprocesses enable the individual to plan the adaptive response, evaluate the outcome, and integrate the evaluation into the person as adaptation. The three subprocesses are identified as the generation subprocess, the evaluation subprocess, and the integration subprocess.

The *adaptive response generation subprocess* is the anticipatory portion of human adaptation (see Figure 40.2). The generation subprocess is activated by a mechanism that explains how an adaptive response is created. The *adaptive response mechanism* consists of *adaptation energy*, *adaptive response modes*, and *adaptive response behaviors.* The mechanism and the three components are interactive; they are neither linear nor hierarchical. These components provide the resources that the individual draws from to generate an adaptive response to an occupational challenge. The adaptive response mechanism is best understood as a dynamic system (e.g., Davies, 1988; Gleick, 1987; Prigogine & Stengers, 1984).

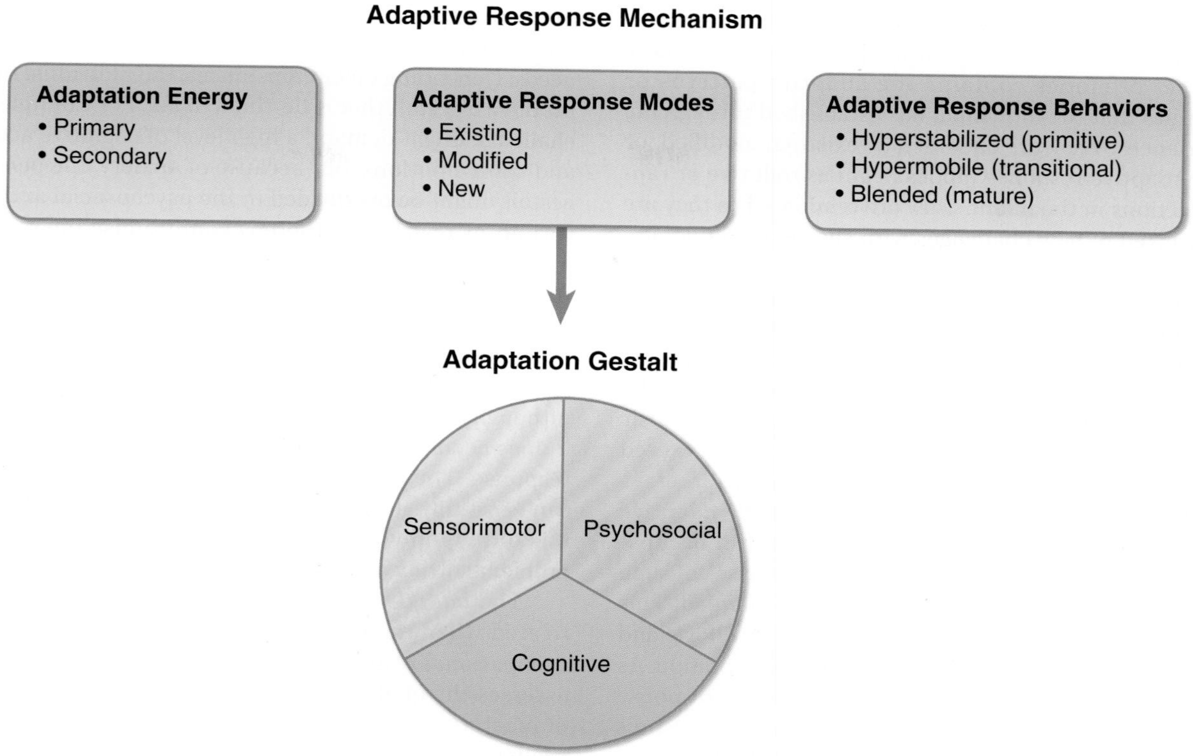

FIGURE 40.2 The adaptive response generation subprocesses are internal to the person.

The theory of occupational adaptation proposes that the individual uses adaptation energy at either a primary or a secondary level of cognitive awareness. If the individual is at a high level of cognitive awareness when attempting to generate an adaptive response, the *primary* level of adaptation energy is being used. If the individual is not highly engaged in creating an adaptive response, a *secondary* level of adaptation energy is being used. To illustrate, an individual may work and work on a problem (using primary energy). When a solution is not forthcoming, the individual might decide to mow the lawn or cook dinner (such routine activities allow secondary energy to continue to process and work on the problem). Often, when the individual returns to the original problem, a "light comes on," and the individual has a new idea—a solution that was elusive while the individual was focused on the problem. In some cases, the solution appears even sooner while the individual is still engaged in the routine activity. The common explanation for this occurrence is something like "I just had to get it off my mind." However, theory of occupational adaptation proposes that the problem was not off the individual's mind; rather, the problem was still being processed at another level, that is, with secondary energy. The following paragraph provides a more thorough discussion on this phenomenon.

The notion of adaptation energy is based on Selye's (1956) research on stress and its effect on adrenal glands in laboratory animals. Selye concluded that unremitting stress led to excessively high use of the adaptive capacity of the animals' endocrinological systems and led to premature death. He posited a general adaptation syndrome to describe this process and he extrapolated the presence of a similar process in humans. On the basis of Selye's work and that of Posner (1973), the theory of occupational adaptation posits that the previous example illustrates the use of adaptation energy, which occurs at both primary and secondary levels of cognitive attention. Posner's notion of information processing at simultaneous or parallel levels was a major influence on this assumption. A second influence was the literature on creative problem solving (Whetton & Cameron, 1984). Creative problem solving involves methods for seeking alternatives to existing approaches ("breaking set") when other attempts have failed to produce solutions.

In the first part of the previous scenario, the individual used adaptation energy at the primary level of cognitive awareness. When engaged in the routine activity, the individual had not "gotten it off his or her mind." As the individual changed to other activities, the problem was shunted to the secondary level of awareness. The secondary level is not inferior to the primary level. The secondary level of awareness continues to work on the problem (using adaptation energy) at a more efficient and sophisticated manner than that of the primary level. The idea of a secondary level of cognitive attention bears some conceptual similarities to Ayres' (1972) concept of subcortical processing. However, in the theory of occupational adaptation, the secondary level of cognitive processing is understood to remain within the cortical area of the brain.

The second component of the adaptive response mechanism is identified as the adaptive response modes. This set of modes contains the adaptive patterns or strategies that the individual has established through life experiences. They are classified as existing, modified, or new. Adaptive response modes begin as reflexive or random actions in the infant. They are reinforced as they are generalized to new challenges with successful outcomes. When first confronted with an occupational challenge, the individual usually selects an existing adaptive response mode and acts on it. If the outcome is unsuccessful, the individual may modify the mode and then achieve a successful outcome. The individual develops a new mode when the challenge is a significant departure from those previously experienced. However, the degree of challenge can exceed the individual's experiences and *adaptive capacity*.

The third component is identified as the adaptive response behaviors. According to the theory of occupational adaptation, there are three general classes of such behaviors: hyperstable, hypermobile, and blended. This classification system was drawn from that of Gilfoyle and colleagues' (1990) theory of spatiotemporal adaptation. As with the other two components of the adaptive response mechanism, these behaviors exist within the person's repertoire of experience. When faced with an occupational challenge, the individual selects one of the behaviors to use in response to the challenge. Hyperstable (primitive) behaviors are those in which the individual either continues to attempt the same solution or becomes "stuck" (e.g., the individual who sits and stares at the computer screen waiting for ideas to come). The individual who selects a hypermobile (transitional) behavior will move rapidly from one solution to another with a great deal of activity but no resulting product. Blended (mature) behavior is a blending of hyperstable and hypermobile that allows for greater opportunity for a positive outcome.

In summary, when an individual is faced with an occupational challenge, the adaptive response mechanism is activated. The individual will draw from prior experience that is available within the adaptive response mechanism. The individual selects a level of adaptation energy, an adaptive response mode, and an adaptive response behavior to use in adapting to the challenge. At this point, the plan of action has been created. This completes the first stage of generating an adaptive response.

The second stage is equally significant. The individual configures his or her person systems (sensorimotor, cognitive, and psychosocial) to carry out the plan. The configuration results in what is termed an **adaptation gestalt** of the individual's idiosyncratic sensorimotor, cognitive, and psychosocial functioning. Figure 40.2 presents the systems as equally balanced within the gestalt of the whole. However, in real-world situations, the relative balance of the person systems will adjust according to the occupational challenge and the individual's personal functioning. As with the adaptive response mechanism, the adaptation gestalt is also drawn from the individual's previous experience. Gestalts that the individual previously found effective might prove ineffective for future needs. Depending on circumstances, the individual might produce a gestalt that is destined to fail. For example, the challenge might demand a high level of cognitive activity and calm emotions; but because of anxiety, the person's gestalt might be overloaded in the psychosocial and sensorimotor realms and thereby compromise the remaining gestalt available for cognitive processing.

The adaptive response mechanism and the adaptation gestalt produce the internal adaptive response to the occupational challenge. The occupational response is the product of the individual's internal adaptive response. Although the adaptive response is not directly observable, it does become operationalized within the occupational response. The nature of the internal adaptive response can be readily gleaned from careful observation and analysis of the individual's approach to the task, his or her problem-solving methods, and the resulting outcome.

The *adaptive response evaluation subprocess* is activated when the individual assesses the quality of the occupational response (see Figure 40.3). The individual assesses the quality by evaluating his or her experience of mastery. Because this is a personal assessment, the evaluation is relative to the individual—hence the term *relative mastery* (Figure 40.4). There are four measures within **relative mastery**: efficiency (use of time, energy, resources), effectiveness (the extent to which the desired goal was achieved), satisfaction to self, and satisfaction to society. Relative mastery is inherently phenomenological. If the individual's assessment of the occupational response is positive overall, there is probably little need for further adaptation. If the result is negative, the *adaptive response integration subprocess* (see Figure 40.5) communicates this information to the person. The individual may then generate a modified or new adaptive response in order to better reach the desired level of mastery in any

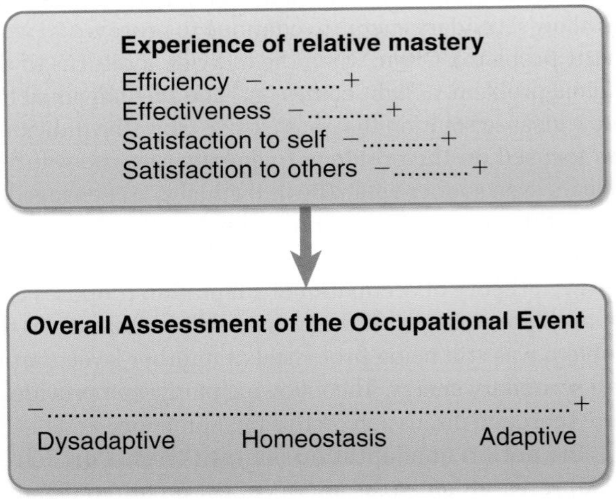

FIGURE 40.3 Adaptive response evaluation subprocess: The adaptive response subprocesses are internal to the person.

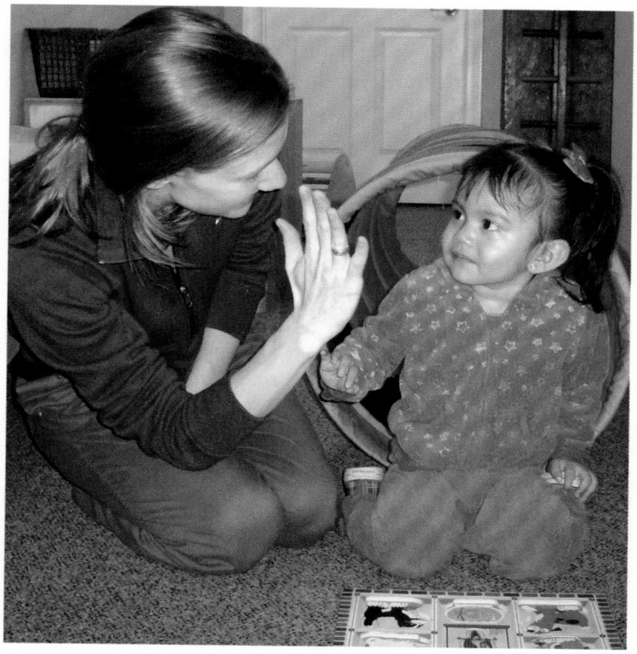

FIGURE 40.4 The therapist in the photo models one way to celebrate relative mastery to her young client.

one or all of the measures of relative mastery. The previous scenario describes the normative adaptive response generation, evaluation, and integration subprocess.

Introduction to Practice Based on the Theory of Occupational Adaptation

It is often difficult to distinguish between prominent theories of occupational therapy. Students and practitioners have often stated, "There's so much overlap, and it seems like there are only slight differences between the various theories." What is the uniqueness of occupational adaptation for practice? The following provides a reply to this question.

The theory of occupational adaptation directs practice to be focused on the therapeutic use of occupation to promote adaptation. Occupation is the tool. It is the medium that the practitioner uses to improve the client's **adaptiveness**. Therefore, the foremost intervention goal is to maximize the client's effectiveness in using his or her own ability to be adaptive. The theory of occupational adaptation is based on a unique core assumption that as the individual becomes more adaptive, he or she will become more able to be an active participant in daily life. This is a departure from other prominent occupation-based theories of practice, which emphasize increased function and/or occupational performance as the goal of therapy. All therapy is driven by core assumptions, whether or not these assumptions are in the consciousness of the practitioner. The theory of occupational adaptation focuses on developing the individual's adaptiveness. Occupation is the means to accomplish that goal. An OA-based practitioner selects interventions that are congruent with the theory's most basic assumption. The practitioner accomplishes the overarching therapy goal by presenting interventions that will activate and improve the individual's internal adaptation process. The practitioner guides the individual to select an occupational role on which he or she wants to focus. Individuals will readily identify activities that they want to be able to do. However, it is important for the practitioner to help clients tease out a life role in which they have a significant investment. OA theory posits that activities take on meaning only within the context of a role.

The theory asserts that it is the client's adaptiveness that determines occupational performance. Some individuals are characteristically very adaptive and will respond effectively whether they face a divorce, the birth of a child, a stroke, depression, or a major move to a new city. They take charge of their lives and adapt. They are adaptive people. Others are, by nature, more easily overwhelmed by life's challenges. Their adaptive capacity (ability to generate effective adaptive responses) is limited.

Each occupational therapy client presents with his or her own unique pattern of personal adaptation.

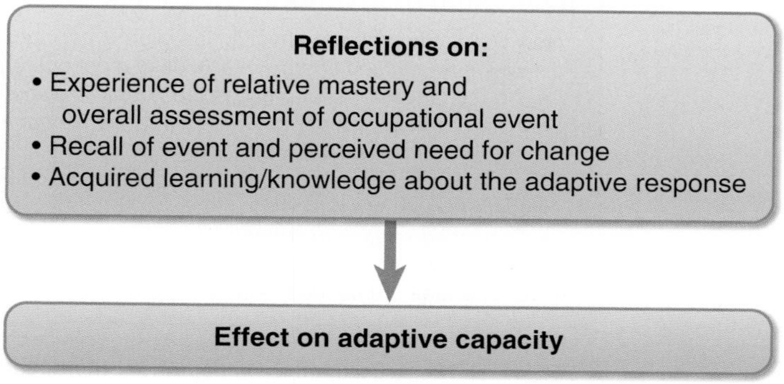
Reflections on:
• Experience of relative mastery and overall assessment of occupational event
• Recall of event and perceived need for change
• Acquired learning/knowledge about the adaptive response
Effect on adaptive capacity

FIGURE 40.5 Adaptive response integration subprocess: The adaptive response subprocesses are internal to the person.

Adaptiveness is relative to the individual. Each client also presents with various cognitive, sensorimotor, and psychosocial factors that may impair or facilitate the client's ability to be adaptive. With each added complication including internal and external role expectations, the demand on the individual to adapt becomes greater and greater.

In an OA-driven practice, the practitioner's focus must be on increasing the client's ability to adapt. The goal is not to help the client adapt. The goal is to help the client become adaptive. In the beginning stage of therapy, the practitioner might teach the client adaptive methods and might introduce assistive devices or teach specific skills (**occupational readiness**). However, the therapy must progress as quickly as possible to **occupational activities** that the client finds meaningful (Frankl, 1984). The OA Clinical and Professional Reasoning Process provides a systematic progression of questions that the practitioner uses to frame his or her overall thinking and therapeutic program (see Figure 40.6). Figure 40.7 presents the OA Guide to Assessment and Intervention.

Clients are most inclined to discover their own ability to adapt when they are challenged within occupational activities, that is, activities that are meaningful, have a beginning and an end, are process-oriented, and have an end product (Schkade & Schultz, 1992). It is human nature to be motivated to participate enthusiastically if the activity is personally meaningful. The individual's attraction to the activity fuels the desire to adapt. The client's *adaptive capacity* is triggered by meaning. Meaningful activity gives the practitioner a powerful tool to observe the client's internal adaptation process. Adaptation patterns that interfere with the client's ability to adapt can be readily observed. The practitioner intervenes when opportunities are presented during the client's engagement in the activity. Such opportunities are typically inherent in the activity and call for the client to make an adaptive response. The practitioner seizes this window of opportunity to facilitate the client's adaptiveness. The intervention may focus on the client's overall approach to the problem, difficulty generating an adaptive response or evaluating the effectiveness of responses, repetition of ineffective techniques, diminished adaptive capacity, depression, frustration, and so on. These are common roadblocks that interfere with the client's *adaptive response processes.* The practitioner intervenes through a progressive system of posing questions and making observations to the client. The framing of questions and observations is tailored to the client's cognitive and psychosocial functioning. The practitioner guides the client through questions and observations to assume the role of decision maker and problem solver. The practitioner provides no more direction than is absolutely essential. It is better to err

Data Gathering and Evaluation

What are the client's *occupational environments and occupational roles (OE/OR)?*
- Which role is of primary concern to client and family?
- What occupational performance is expected in the primary OE/OR?

What are the *physical, social, cultural* features of the primary OE/OR?
What is the client's *sensorimotor, cognitive, and psychosocial* status?
What is the client's level of *relative mastery* in the primary OE/OR?
What is facilitating or limiting *relative mastery* in the primary OE/OR?

Planning and Intervention

What combination of occupational readiness and occupational activity is needed to promote the client's *occupational adaptation process?*
What help will the client need to assess his or her *occupational responses* and use the results to increase his or her adaptiveness?
What is the best method to engage the client in the intervention process?

Evaluating Intervention Outcomes

How well is the program affecting the client's *occupational adaptation process?*
- Which *adaptation energy* level is used most often *(primary or secondary)?*
- What changes are occurring in the *adaptive response mode (existing, modified, or new)?*
- What is the most common *adaptive response behavior (hyper-stable, hyper-mobile, or blended)?*

What outcomes does the client show that reflect positive change in overall adaptiveness?
- Self-initiated adaptations?
- Enhanced *relative mastery?*
- Generalization to novel activities?

What changes are needed in the program to help the client maximize his or her adaptiveness?

FIGURE 40.6 Occupational adaptation: therapeutic reasoning process.

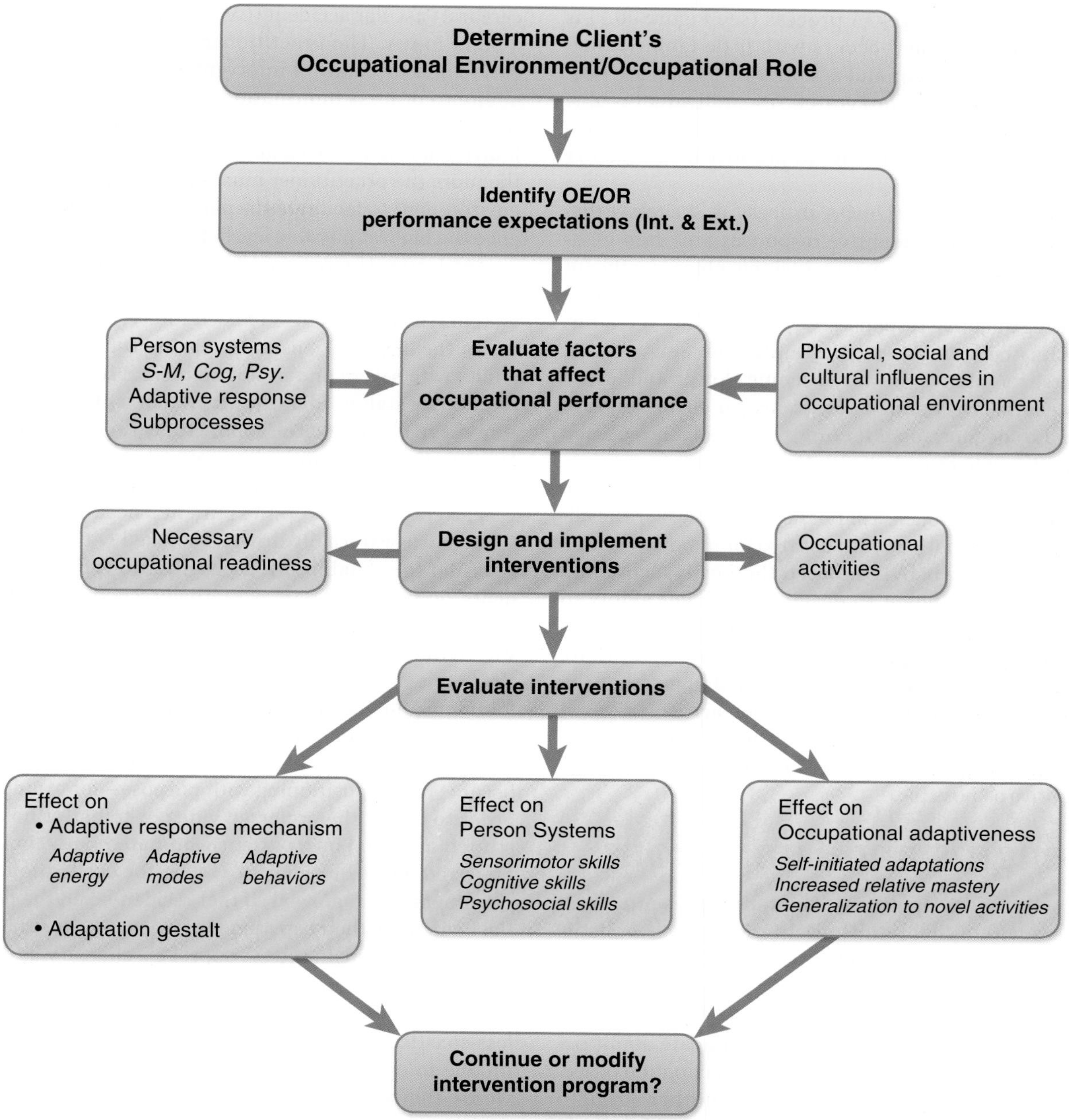

FIGURE 40.7 Occupational adaptation: guide to evaluation and intervention.

on the side of too little direction than too much. The more the practitioner directs, solves, and teaches, the less adaptive the client will become.

The therapeutic relationship is of critical significance in the theory of occupational adaptation. The relationship evolves into an artful dance between the client and practitioner. It is a partnership in which the client takes the lead. The practitioner becomes the facilitator. That is, the practitioner's function is to help the client discover his or her own ability to be adaptive. The practitioner is the agent of the occupational environment. The client is the agent of change (Schkade & Schultz, 1993).

Interruption in The Occupational Adaptation Process

Although the theory of occupational adaptation is not about mastery per se, it is the constant presence of the desire, demand, and press for mastery that provide the impetus for the individual to adapt. In other words, these constants are pervasive and ongoing influences. As long as the individual can reach a mutually satisfactory balance between the desire and demand for mastery, the normative OA process (see Figure 40.1) is working effectively and occurs with little fanfare. Day-to-day challenges occur and adaptive responses are generated, evaluated, and integrated. The individual is able to draw from the existing person systems and repertoire of adaptive responses in order to produce a satisfactory outcome.

When the normative OA process is seriously disrupted, the person's adaptive responses are often inadequate. Impairments in person systems place significant limits on the individual's ability to effectively use former or existing adaptive responses. Cognitive issues often further limit the ability to adapt. Depression emerges and the person's relative mastery becomes lower and lower. This scenario is a common occurrence for clients who are referred to occupational therapy. The challenges exceed the client's ability to adapt. See Case Study 40.1.

The case study depicts a school-based situation. However, the approach will be the same whether the client is a hospital patient with a stroke or a mother with a fragile premature baby. OA-based therapy is focused on working with the client to develop his or her ability to respond more adaptively to occupational challenges. At times, occupational readiness needs may supplant those for increased adaptiveness. This is a judgment that the practitioner makes. Many times, both can be addressed during therapy. The greater the severity of impairment or limitation, the greater is the need for the client to become as adaptive as possible.

Strengths and Limitations

The theory of occupational adaptation presents practitioners with a theoretical orientation that is holistic. Its assumptions adhere to the ideas of occupation and adaptation that are inherent in the profession's history and philosophy (Schultz & Schkade, 1997). It provides an organized way to think and communicate about occupational therapy intervention that is occupation based, process oriented, and client focused. Another strength is OA's compatibility with terminology from the World Health Organization (2004) and its concern with the ability of individuals and groups of individuals to participate fully in society. From an OA standpoint, occupation plays a significant role as a facilitator of social participation. Likewise, dysfunction in occupation becomes a significant factor in limiting social participation. The theory of occupational adaptation provides practitioners with one way to think about, describe, and plan occupation-based intervention.

Practitioners often question whether the theory of occupational adaptation is applicable to people with an impaired cognitive system. This is an unfortunate misunderstanding of the theory. The theory of occupational adaptation is as applicable to people with cognitive deficits as to those with sensorimotor or psychosocial deficits. The demand to adapt is as great for someone with a severe cerebral vascular accident (CVA) as it is for someone with a hand injury. The practitioner must adjust communication and methods of intervention to suit the person's ability to process information. The goal remains to help the person become as adaptive as possible. The more the individual is unable to manage his or her person systems, the more the practitioner must manage the occupational environment to facilitate the person's potential to experience the highest possible level of relative mastery.

At times, the primary avenue for communication with the person might be limited to the sensorimotor system. The effectiveness of such intervention was borne out in the author's consultation with a state hospital for adults with severe and profound mental retardation. The direct care staff used a reward system with the patients. When the clients were "good," that is, compliant with care routines and not yelling out, they were rewarded with the desired stuffed animal, music, or video. The staff was attempting to stop the patient's negative behavior. Change was externally driven. I worked with the staff to redesign the rehabilitation program to reflect the residents' occupational interests. A daily schedule of occupational activities was created for each person. Routine care was reframed from tasks that the staff must do for the patients to tasks that will help the patients to do what they found meaningful. The new objective was to increase the residents' experience of mastery over their environment. The necessity of turning the patient to prevent bedsores became one of positioning with purpose—for example, in order to watch the preferred video or to better hold the stuffed animal. For a patient who hated bath time, the preferred music helped her to relax. The occupational environment was managed so that residents had the potential to increase their experience of mastery over situations that they disliked. In the OA approach, change was driven by the patient's preferences. As a result of the patients' increased sense of relative mastery, they demonstrated less spasticity and fewer emotional outbursts. Although unable to communicate their relative mastery through words, they expressed it very clearly through their sensorimotor system.

Another limitation of this intervention approach lies within those practitioners who are willing to stay enmeshed in intervention practices and settings of the past 50 years. Such practitioners believe that intervention based on meaning is not practical in the everyday world of practice. These providers appear indifferent to the wide variety of modalities that a practitioner may use in practice. Outcomes are the issue at hand for practice. Research based on OA interventions supports the notion that clients whose therapy has been based on meaningful activity and the development of adaptiveness will outperform those whose therapy has concentrated on activities of daily living that might have little meaning for the clients (e.g., Buddenberg & Schkade, 1998; Dolecheck & Schkade, 1999; Ford, 1995; Jackson & Schkade, 2001; Johnson & Schkade, 2001).

CASE STUDY 40.1 Alfonso Learns a New Response to Frustration

Claudette greets Alfonso at the door as he enters the classroom. "Hello, Alfonso, my name is Ms. Murphy. Welcome to the group. Why don't you look around for a while . . . we can talk some later." As Alfonso begins to find his way into the occupational environment, there is a notable hum of activity—talking and doing. The group members (six altogether) notice Alfonso. Some greet him; others don't. He hesitantly observes a couple of the boys working on their individual projects. Claudette notices that Alfonso is waiting for her to take control. He is reluctant to touch any of the materials. He glances toward Claudette for direction. She slowly nods and turns her attention to another student. Claudette's manner of including the student in the group is integrally related to her intervention approach.

The group is grounded by the theory of occupational adaptation. This is reflected in the therapeutic tools that Claudette uses (see Box 40.1). One tool is her management, or agency, of the therapeutic occupational environment (OE). The second is Claudette's management of herself, that is, her ability to incorporate "therapeutic use of self" in the therapy sessions. This skill is intrinsically interwoven throughout the case study. The reader is referred to the early classical work of Gail Fidler and Jay Fidler (1963) for elaboration on specific methods and techniques. The third tool is Claudette's understanding of how occupation can be used to help an individual become more adaptive and respond more effectively to occupational challenges. The fourth and most powerful tool is her unwavering acceptance of the student as the agent of change.

Occupational activities (arts and crafts that are meaningful to the students) are the chosen intervention modality. The media are selected for their range of occupational challenge and attractiveness to the students. Some of the media are inherently structured; others are very open-ended. Claudette has very carefully created the nature and substance of the therapeutic OE; that is, she arranged the physical space, selected the media, and established the social climate and cultural standards for the therapy group.

Claudette follows the clinical and professional reasoning process identified in Figure 40.5. The practitioner must engage in the reasoning process to design appropriate OA-based interventions. The format in Figure 40.5 prompts the practitioner on what questions he or she must ask throughout the course of therapy. Figure 40.7 presents a model of intervention that puts into action the reasoning presented in Figure 40.6. Claudette's methods and interventions are consistent with both Figures 40.6 and 40.7.

In school-based therapy, the OE and related occupational role are predetermined. The overarching OE focuses on education-related work and play (each has its own physical, social, and cultural influences). The occupational role is, by definition, that of being a student. The OE has a specific demand for mastery and occupational role expectations (see Figure 40.1) of the student. These include a demand for a minimal level of performance in learning and behavior. Before meeting Alfonso, Claudette completed her assessment of the general OE in which Alfonso is a participant. She also assessed the OE's occupational role expectations for Alfonso. She found that school personnel expect Alfonso to cause trouble and to drop out of school when he is old enough. These are the actual occupational role expectations that Alfonso experiences, day in and day out.

As shown in the OA process model (Figure 40.1), an individual's occupational role expectations are affected by those of the OE. After the initial therapy sessions, Claudette deduces that Alfonso has been strongly affected by the school's expectations. In fact, he has integrated them as his own. His innate desire for mastery has become one of a power struggle with the OE. He and the school are enmeshed in a no-win situation.

Claudette has also reviewed the school's records on Alfonso's person system deficits. His attention deficit disorder, hyperactivity, and difficulty with reading are clearly documented. She could incorporate occupational readiness interventions with the goal of increasing his ability to stay on task and help him learn how to better regulate his hyperactivity. Claudette has also observed during the therapy groups that Alfonso has a severe developmental delay in his adaptive response subprocesses. See Figures 40.2, 40.3, and 40.5 for further clarification (these subprocesses are internal to the person). Claudette has observed that whenever Alfonso has difficulty with projects, he tends to generate the same adaptive response mode repeatedly: He experiences himself as a failure. He routinely acts out this mode by tearing up the project or work, making a joke out of his work, or causing trouble with another student in the group. Alfonso's teacher reports that this situation is also a frequent occurrence in the classroom.

As a result of his adaptive response mode, Alfonso's adaptation gestalt (Figure 40.2) is composed largely of angry emotion and sensorimotor agitation. Very little cognitive activity is present within the adaptation gestalt. As a result, the next step in his adaptive subprocesses, the evaluation of outcome, does not occur (see Figure 40.3). His adaptation gestalt doesn't allow room for very much cognitive reasoning. Claudette concludes that it is very unlikely that Alfonso will respond more effectively to occupational challenges unless he acquires new or modified adaptive response modes. His current sense of himself as a failure (the adaptive response mode) leads to an occupational response (behavior that is observed) that is not efficient, effective, or satisfying to himself or others. His relative mastery is very low.

Claudette completes her assessment of the factors that are affecting his occupational performance (see Figure 40.7) and concludes that her interventions should be focused on increasing Alfonso's ability to generate a more effective adaptive response mode. Because Claudette's practice is OA-based, she will not focus the therapy on changing Alfonso's behavior; this would be incongruent with the theory. Claudette's interventions will be designed to expand his adaptive response repertoire with a new mode such as "When I have trouble with a project, I can stop and figure out what the problem is." This will be an entirely new response mode for Alfonso. As he begins to acquire the new mode, it will affect his adaptation gestalt by decreasing the negative emotion and agitation that is present and freeing up space in the gestalt for cognitive processing. With his current adaptive response mode, Alfonso is at the mercy of his emotions. They are in control. As he experiences an adaptive response mode in which he has a greater sense of mastery, he will have the potential not only to control his emotions but also to control his behavior.

Claudette plans to work with Alfonso using occupational activities that he self-selects. Most occupational therapy is

(continued)

CASE STUDY 40.1 Alfonso Learns a New Response to Frustration (*Continued*)

driven by the assumption that if the client becomes more functional, he or she will be able to adapt. The theory of occupational adaptation takes the exact opposite point of view. Practice based on occupational adaptation is driven by the assumption that if the client becomes more adaptive, he or she will be able to function.

Through activities that Alfonso enjoys and finds meaningful, Claudette can more closely observe his adaptive processes and begin to intervene as appropriate. On the basis of the theory of occupational adaptation, Claudette believes that Alfonso must develop the wherewithal to respond to occupational challenges in new ways. Her method will be to facilitate this through the four core intervention tools listed in Box 40.1. Claudette's challenge is to seize the opportunities for intervention that Alfonso presents during occupational activities. Intervention in the adaptive response generation subprocess cannot occur after the occupational response (observed behavior). The intervention must occur at the same time that the client is beginning to generate an adaptive response. This is a brief "window" that tends to open and close very quickly. Catching the window is an artful skill that requires a great deal of practice. To accomplish the goal, Claudette realizes that she must use each of the four therapeutic tools. The following presents an example of how the four tools may actually play out in a practice situation.

As she continues to observe Alfonso's adaptive response patterns and resulting occupational responses, Claudette begins to recognize the cues for when the opportunity for intervention might present itself. She sits next to Alfonso, makes a general matter-of-fact comment, and begins to watch and wait. He has started a project, a soapbox derby–type wooden car. This is his second attempt. Claudette believes that his desire for mastery in the activity is beginning to emerge. The first car ended up in the trash after he tried to hammer the axle into the tire rather than sanding the axle. Soon, he faces the same challenge as he had with the first wooden car. He starts to pick up the hammer. The window for intervention has presented itself. Claudette believes that the most direct route to Alfonso's adaptive response mode will be through his adaptation gestalt. His adaptation gestalt is so overweighted with emotion and tension that the adaptive response mode is not readily available for therapeutic access. Claudette's therapy begins with a technique that she believes will have the desired positive effect on his gestalt. She will accomplish this through her role as agent of the OE. Claudette initiates the intervention by slowly stating to the student (as she reaches for the axle and wheel), "I wonder why this thing is so hard to get in here?" It is a rhetorical statement, not really a question to Alfonso. It is an observation that she is making aloud for the student to hear. It is as if she is giving a voice to the adaptive response mode ("I can stop and figure this out") that Alfonso lacks. She is not teaching it to him; she is showing it. As she quietly and slowly manipulates the objects, Claudette notices that Alfonso has sat back some in his chair; his adaptation gestalt appears to be changing. He relaxes somewhat; his affect softens. Claudette has used her agency of the OE to affect his adaptation gestalt. With calmness and curiosity, she has assumed physical control of the derby car. Her action reduces the sensorimotor demands that Alfonso was experiencing. The change in his OE allows him to distance himself from the emotions that he was experiencing as well. Through her management of the OE, Claudette has promoted a powerful shift in Alfonso's adaptation gestalt. Shortly, he exhales loudly, "Whew!" After a few moments, Claudette responds to his verbalized self-awareness. She comments, "It's frustrating when things don't work!" (The fewer the words, the more powerful is the impact.) Again, her comment is not being made directly to Alfonso. It is an observation that is presented for him to hear and perhaps use, allowing him to gain some control over his emotions by turning feelings into a cognitive thought.

As a result of the intervention, Alfonso experienced a new adaptation gestalt. Claudette now directs the intervention toward his first experience with the new adaptive response mode ("I can stop and figure things out") by presenting him with another observation. "Well," she says, "You tried hammering it in before, and that didn't work, so . . ." Claudette's observation is the first step in helping Alfonso to develop the new mode. She is prompting him to experience himself in the new mode—that is, to experience himself as a problem solver. The key to the interventions being described is that they are not artificial. They are not contrived or role-played; they occur in vivo. Alfonso interjects with excitement, "Maybe it's just a crummy kit. I'll get another one." Alfonso retrieves another car and soon discovers the same problem. His enthusiasm drains away. Claudette does not become enmeshed with his disappointment. She maintains her therapeutic focus and again initiates an intervention to affect his adaptation gestalt by managing the OE. She states aloud, "Hmm, I wonder if the directions say anything about how to put the axle in the wheel." She has again made a statement that prompts Alfonso to be in the problem solver role. Alfonso replies, "I don't know, I don't like directions." This is a pivotal point in the intervention. Because it is the first direct intervention with Alfonso, Claudette knows that she needs to provide enough support but no more than is absolutely necessary. Claudette also believes that Alfonso finds the project very meaningful and might be willing to risk trying to read the instructions. (The instructions are consistent with his reading potential.) As may be anticipated, he attempts to replay his typical battle with the OE by stating to Claudette, "Why don't you show me what to do? Isn't that your job?" Claudette matter-of-factly replies, "It's not my project . . . it's yours." She is careful to offer this statement with the same delivery as her others. It is presented merely as an observation. Through such a comment, she communicates her commitment to Alfonso that he is the agent of change. His comment was a test of her authenticity. Claudette will continue to work with Alfonso, following the principles of OA and using the four core therapeutic tools. Each intervention will be focused on helping him to acquire a new adaptive response mode ("I can stop and figure things out"). As he begins to assume the new mode, Claudette will shift her focus to the second subprocess: his ability to evaluate the outcome of his adaptive response. Figures 40.5 and 40.6 provide the reader with a more in-depth explanation of the complete process of evaluation and intervention. ■

BOX 40.1 Occupational Adaptation: Core Therapeutic Tools

1. Practitioner is the agent of the occupational environment.
2. Practitioner incorporates principles of therapeutic use of self.
3. Practitioner uses occupation to promote adaptiveness.
4. Client is the agent of change.

Another frequently mentioned limitation is the lack of an OA assessment tool. I have been reluctant to encourage development of such a tool for several reasons. From my point of view, the most significant deficit that the profession faces is that most practice is not theory driven. It appears that assessment tools are driving practice. Practitioners seem to prefer to use a static measure rather than a theory to guide their thinking process. This affects the nature of practice and the quality of research that can be carried out. A theory-driven practice is mandatory for occupational therapy to become clearly differentiated in health care. OA assessment is inherent in the Therapeutic Reasoning Process (see Figure 40.6). The OA Guide to Evaluation and Intervention (Figure 40.7) was developed to provide additional direction for the therapist. It appears that there are some dynamic systems process-oriented approaches to assessment that may be compatible with the theory of occupational adaptation and are worthy of exploration.

Research

Research on the effectiveness of OA intervention has included various methods. Most have been quasi-experimental with random assignment to treatment and control groups. There have been two main OA assumptions and related outcomes under study. The first assumption is that OA-based interventions will have a greater effect on functional independence than therapy based on traditional activities of daily living. The second OA assumption is that OA-based interventions will result in greater generalization of skills learned in therapy than traditional occupational therapy rehabilitation methods. The Functional Independence Measure (FIM) was used to test the first assumption. Performance on a patient-selected novel activity was used to test the second assumption.

In Gibson and Schkade (1997), the FIM scores of CVA inpatients were significantly higher on eight of the FIM scores than those of the control group. Jackson and Schkade (2001) conducted a similar study with hip fracture inpatients and found comparable FIM results. Buddenberg and Schkade (1998) researched generalization of skills learned in therapy to novel activities with hip fracture inpatients. The OA-based group performed significantly better on tasks on which they had not been previously trained than the control group. Dolecheck & Schkade (1999) studied the affects of an OA-based program with CVA inpatients. They served as their own control group over a period of 6 weeks. The patients were able to stand longer when engaged in personally meaningful occupation than when engaged in the facility's traditional occupational therapy.

Johnson & Schkade (2001) conducted a single-subject study with three CVA patients who had been discharged from home health because of insufficient progress in mobility. At the conclusion of the OA-based intervention, each of the patients made significant gains in mobility, self-care, and overall level of activity level. This description represents a portion of the research efforts to evaluate the effectiveness of OA-based interventions in practical applications.

Conclusion

The theory of occupational adaptation is presented as an overarching theory for practice. Traditional interventions such as neurodevelopmental approaches, sensory integration, and biomechanics are readily interfaced as part of the occupational readiness portion of intervention planning. Occupational readiness interventions are limited to addressing deficits in the person systems. The focus in such interventions is on improved performance. However, OA embraces a broader perspective. Intervention is focused on increasing the patient's adaptiveness.

Acknowledgments

This chapter on the theory of occupational adaptation is dedicated to those practitioners who embrace the importance of identifying the elements and parameters of scholarly practice. The work has been greatly advanced over the years by the wisdom and influence of students enrolled in the Texas Woman's University PhD program in occupational therapy. I continue to be inspired by and in awe of the drive that they have to pursue greater understanding of the practice of occupational therapy. OA was developed to provide a framework to name and frame what it is that actually goes on within the therapy session. That is, what does a therapist think about while engaged in the therapeutic process? On what does the therapist base a treatment program? How does the therapist go about establishing a meaningful collaboration with the client/patient? These questions aren't answered by assessment tools. They are answered by the therapist's use of a systematic framework to shape his or her clinical reasoning.

The theory of occupational adaptation is intended to be such a framework. It provides a systematic road map for the therapist to understand what actions need to occur, what needs to be assessed, and how to gauge treatment effectiveness. It emphasizes that the client/patient's perspective on treatment planning and outcomes are fundamental to the therapeutic process and achieving optimal results. In the last couple of years, students in the PhD program have begun to generate population-specific OA practice models. As these practice models continue to be refined, I anticipate that they will help to solidify a much more direct relationship between theory, practice, and treatment effectiveness.

References

Ayres, A. J. (1972). *Sensory integration and learning disorders.* Los Angeles, CA: Western Psychological Services.

Buddenberg, L. A., & Schkade, J. K. (1998). A comparison of occupational therapy intervention approaches for older patients after hip fracture. *Topics in Geriatric Rehabilitation, 13*(4), 52–68.

Davies, P. (1988). *The cosmic blueprint.* New York, NY: Simon & Schuster.

Dolecheck, J. R., & Schkade, J. K. (1999). Effects on dynamic standing endurance when persons with CVA perform personally meaningful activities rather than non-meaningful tasks. *Occupational Therapy Journal of Research, 19*(1), 40–53.

Dunton, W. (1913). Occupation as a therapeutic measure. *Medical Record, 3,* 388–389.

Fidler, G., & Fidler, J. (1963). *Occupational therapy: A communication process in psychiatry.* New York, NY: Macmillan Company.

Ford, K. (1995). Occupational adaptation in home health: A therapist's viewpoint. *Home Health and Community Special Interest Section Newsletter, 2*(1), 2–4.

Frankl, V. (1984). *Man's search for meaning* (3rd ed.). New York, NY: Simon & Schuster.

Garrett, S., & Schkade, J. K. (1995). The occupational adaptation model of professional development as applied to Level II fieldwork in occupational therapy. *American Journal of Occupational Therapy, 49,* 119–126. doi:10.5014/ajot.51.7.523

Gibson, J., & Schkade, J. K. (1997). Effects of occupational adaptation treatment with CVA. *American Journal of Occupational Therapy, 51,* 523–529. doi:10.5014/ajot.51.7.523

Gilfoyle, E., Grady, A., & Moore, J. (1990). *Children adapt.* Thorofare, NJ: Slack.

Gleick, J. (1987). *Chaos: Making a new science.* New York, NY: Penguin Books.

Jack, J., & Estes, R. (2010). Documenting progress: Hand therapy treatment shift from biomechanical to occupational adaptation. *American Journal of Occupational Therapy, 64*(1), 82–87. doi:10.5014/ajot.64.1.82

Jackson, J. P., & Schkade, J. K. (2001). Occupational adaptation model vs. biomechanical/rehabilitation models in the treatment of patients with hip fractures. *American Journal of Occupational Therapy, 55*(5), 531–537. doi:10.5014/ajot.55.5.531

Johnson, J., (2006). Describing the phenomenon of homelessness through the theory of occupational adaptation. *Occupational Therapy in Health Care, 20*(3/4), 63–80. doi:10.1300/J003v20n03_05

Johnson, J., & Schkade, J. K. (2001). Effects of occupation-based intervention on mobility problems following a cerebral vascular accident. *Journal of Applied Gerontology, 20*(1), 91–110. doi:10.1177/073346480102000106

King, L. (1978). Toward a science of adaptive responses. 1978 Eleanor Clarke Slagle Lecture. *American Journal of Occupational Therapy, 32*(7), 429–437.

Llorens, L. (1970). Facilitating growth and development: The promise of occupational therapy. *American Journal of Occupational Therapy, 24,* 93–101.

Meyer, A. (1922). The philosophy of occupational therapy. *Archives of Occupational Therapy, 1,* 1–10.

Pasek, P. B., & Schkade, J. K. (1996). Effects of a skiing experience on adolescents with limb deficiencies: An occupational adaptation perspective. *American Journal of Occupational Therapy, 50,* 24–31. doi:10.5014/ajot.50.1.24

Posner, M. I. (1973). *Cognition: An introduction.* Glenview, IL: Scott, Foresman.

Prigogine, I., & Stengers, I. (1984). *Order out of chaos: Man's new dialogue with nature.* New York, NY: Bantam Books.

Reilly, M. (1962). Occupational therapy can be one of the great ideas of 20th century medicine. Eleanor Clarke Slagle Lecture. *American Journal of Occupational Therapy, 16,* 1–9.

Ross, M. M. (1994, August 11). Applying theory to practice. *OT Week,* 16–17.

Schkade, J. K. (1999). Student to practitioner: The adaptive transition. *Innovations in Occupational Therapy Education, 1,* 147–156.

Schkade, J. K., & McClung, M. (2001). *Occupational adaptation in practice: Concepts and cases.* Thorofare, NJ: Slack.

Schkade, J. K., & Schultz, S. (1992). Occupational adaptation: Toward a holistic approach to contemporary practice, Part 1. *American Journal of Occupational Therapy, 46,* 829–837. doi:10.5014/ajot.46.9.829

Schkade, J. K., & Schultz, S. (1993). Occupational adaptation: An integrative frame of reference. In H. Hopkins & H. Smith, (Eds.), *Willard and Spackman's occupational therapy* (8th ed., pp. 87–91). Philadelphia, PA: Lippincott.

Schkade, J. K., & Schultz, S. (2003). Occupational adaptation. In P. Kramer, J. Hinojosa, & C. Royeen (Eds.), *Perspectives in human occupation* (pp. 181–221). Philadelphia, PA: Lippincott Williams & Wilkins.

Schultz, S. (1997, April). *Treating students with behavior disorder.* An institute presented at the American Occupational Therapy Association Convention, Orlando, FL.

Schultz, S. (2000). Occupational adaptation. In P. A. Crist, C. B. Royeen, & J. K. Schkade (Eds.), *Infusing occupation into practice* (2nd ed.). Bethesda, MD: American Occupational Therapist Association.

Schultz, S. (2003). Psychosocial interventions for students with behavior disorders: Identify challenges and clarify the role of occupational therapy in promoting adaptive functioning. *OT Practice, 8*(16), CE-1-CE-8.

Schultz, S., & Schkade, J. K. (1992). Occupational adaptation: Toward a holistic approach to contemporary practice, Part 2. *American Journal of Occupational Therapy, 46,* 917–926. doi:10.5014/ajot.46.10.917

Schultz, S., & Schkade, J. K. (1994). Home health care: A window of opportunity to synthesize practice. *Home & Community Health, Special Interest Section Newsletter, 1*(3), 1–4.

Schultz, S. & Schkade, J. (1997). Adaptation. In C. Christiansen & C. Baum (Eds.), *Occupational therapy: Enabling function and well being* (2nd ed., pp. 458–481). Thorofare, N.J.: Slack.

Selye, H. (1956). *The stress of life.* New York, NY: McGraw-Hill.

Stelter, L., & Whisner, S. (2007). Building responsibility for self through meaningful roles: occupational adaptation theory applied in forensic psychiatry. *Occupational Therapy in Health Care, 23*(1), 69–84. doi:10.1300/J004v23n01_05

Werner, E. (2000). *Families, children with autism and everyday occupations* (Unpublished doctoral dissertation). Nova Southeastern University, Fort Lauderdale, FL.

Whetton, D. A., & Cameron, K. S. (1984). *Developing management skills.* Glenview, IL: Scott, Foresman.

World Health Organization. (2004). *International classification of functioning, disability, and health (ICF).* Geneva, Switzerland: Author. Retrieved from http://www.who.int/classifications/en/

For additional resources on the subjects discussed in this chapter, visit http://thePoint.lww.com/Willard-Spackman12e.

CHAPTER 41

Occupational Justice

Ann A. Wilcock, Elizabeth A. Townsend

LEARNING OBJECTIVES

After reading this chapter, you will be able to:

1. Analyze occupational justice in relation to social, mental, and physical health
2. Appreciate, synthesize, and apply occupational justice within occupational therapy
3. Plan and evaluate approaches to advance occupational rights and reduce injustices

OUTLINE

Introduction

This chapter outlines the emergence and growth of occupational justice in conceptual terms and discusses how the physical, mental, and social health experiences of all people are potentially subject to injustices. The World Federation of Occupational Therapists (WFOT) supports occupationally just practice based on individual and population occupational "rights"; however, striving toward occupational justice is the major ethical dilemma facing occupational therapists in every corner of the world. Advancing the concept is complex. It demands a different mindset and focus and unfamiliar interventions within practice that are in line with the directives of the United Nations (UN) and World Health Organization (WHO). Occupational therapists are encouraged to consider the centrality of occupation to people's survival, health, and well-being as a human rights issue and to begin to incorporate action to address occupational injustices that lead to negative health outcomes experienced by individuals, communities, and populations.

Occupational Justice as an Idea and a Need

From the genesis of humankind, individuals and the communities in which they live have needed occupation to survive healthily or, indeed, to survive at all. They have had to find food, make shelter, and nurture their young as future occupational beings and their old as the custodians of accumulated occupational lore and wisdom. In those fundamental terms, an occupationally just situation is essential. An occupationally just society would be one in which each person and community could meet their own and others' survival, physical, mental, and social development needs through occupation that recognized and encouraged individual and communal strengths. An occupationally unjust situation would occur when only some individuals or groups could meet occupational needs because of imposed external factors that advantaged a favored few. A central ethical dilemma for occupational therapists is a lapsed duty or responsibility when work focuses only on bodily issues such as cognition or the physical performance of daily living skills. Frequently encountered occupational injustices in occupational therapy practices around the world are structures that perpetuate injustice and undermine health. Common examples that are well known by occupational therapists are absent or insufficient housing, lack of employment or employment accommodations, and inadequate financial support for youth, adults, and seniors who lack the resources to live and sustain their mental, physical, and spiritual health.

Despite an apparent need for "occupational justice" throughout human time, it was not named as such until the mid-1990s. That arose from two directions of study in different parts of the globe. One direction of study, concerned with understanding the relationship between occupation and health, discovered that beneficial or negative health outcomes of the relationship were dependent on sociopolitical and cultural determinants, which could be framed in social justice terms (Wilcock, 1993, 1995, 1998, 2006). The other direction of study discovered that many societal and practice determinants "overruled" occupational therapists' "good intentions" of enabling social justice with clients who could be populations, organizations, communities, groups, families, or individuals (Townsend, 1993, 1996, 1998, 2003a, 2003b, 2007). Both research directions generated reflections on whether or not social justice sufficiently addresses the rights of people, individually or collectively, to participate in what they define as meaningful occupations. With this common focus, Townsend and Wilcock (2004) have explored together what they describe as occupational justice.

Cultural, linguistic, and social differences make it difficult to describe the concept. The following outline the meanings that the authors ascribe to occupation, social justice, and occupational justice.

Occupation

Occupation is used to mean all the things that people want, need, or have to do whether of a physical, mental, social, sexual, political, or spiritual nature and is inclusive of sleep and rest. It refers to all aspects of actual human doing, being, becoming, and belonging. The practical, everyday medium of self-expression or of making or experiencing meaning, occupation is the activist element of human existence whether occupations are contemplative, reflective, and meditative or action based. Occupation enables populations and communities to participate actively in creating their own destiny and sustainability (Thibeault, 2002) and is a unit of economy shaped by time, place, and social conditions. It is a fundamental means of achieving implicit or explicit goals, so power relations are central to possibilities and limitations: the power to participate in occupations may be controlled through physical force or invisibly through regulation, the media, and sociocultural expectations. Those can provide the means to suppress or express the self, being, belief, spirit, autonomy, and individual or group identity and can therefore be health threatening, as well as health enhancing.

Social Justice

Social justice is applied to the ethical distribution and sharing of resources, rights, and responsibilities between people recognizing their equal worth, "their equal right to be able to meet basic needs, the need to spread opportunities and life chances as widely as possible, and finally, the requirement that we reduce and where possible eliminate unjustified inequalities" (Commission on Social Justice, 1994, p. 1). An accepted value in many ancient and a growing number of postmodern societies, social justice centers on just social relations and conditions regardless of differences related, for example, to race, class, gender, income, ability or disability. In ideological terms, social justice grew, in part, as a central theme of the Arts and Crafts socialist movement founded in England in the late 19th century. The Movement's ideology quickly became popular in the United States where it was reinterpreted from a communal to an individual concern (MacCarthy, 1994). "A new kind of reform" was pioneered aimed at "manipulating psychic well-being" to try to fit individuals into emerging hierarchies (Jackson Lears, 1981, p. 79). Along with other progressives, social reformer, and Arts and Crafts devotee, Jane Addams at Hull House in Chicago—where the first school of occupational therapy was located—sought to revitalize people's lives toward personal fulfillment within the emerging economy. Individualism was seen as "the route to perfection—a spontaneous social order of self-determined, self-reliant, and fully developed humans" (Emerson's lecture on New England reformers as cited in Lukes, 1973). So, in both "Old" and "New" Worlds, the unhealthy nature of the industrially developing world was challenged in social justice terms from both individual and communal perspectives.

Occupational Justice

Occupational justice and **occupational rights**, like social justice and human rights in general, are concerned with ethical, moral, and civic issues such as equity and fairness for both individuals and collectives but specific to engagement in diverse and meaningful occupation. Conditions of occupational injustice undermine the occupational rights of both communities and individuals across the globe to meet basic occupational needs and have equal opportunities and life chances to reach toward their potential. Although those who live in poverty are the most likely to suffer the direct effects of injustices of an occupational nature, the affluent, too, are conditioned to particular occupations and ways of life that may not meet their needs.

In their exploratory theory of occupational justice (see Figure 41.1), Townsend and Wilcock (2004) proposed that occupation highlights the reality of justice in daily life. It exposes the everyday individual, group, and population experiences within broad social conditions and structures that shape options for and against justice in different cultures around the world. Their theory accepts that people are occupational beings and participate in occupations as autonomous beings and as members of particular communities, that participation is interdependent and contextual, and that it is a determinant of health and well-being. The theory proposes the principles of ***empowerment*** through occupations; the need for a more inclusive classification of occupations to recognize the economic and social value of occupations not currently defined as work; individual and collective enablement of occupational potential; and diversity, inclusion, and shared advantage for everyone in their occupational participation. However, for justice to prevail, there must be an ethical distribution and sharing of resources, rights, and responsibilities with regard to what both individuals and population groups want, need, or are obliged to do within their social milieu.

The naming of occupational justice may be new; but respected scholars, over millennia, have considered the notion that what people do, and their actions toward being, becoming, and belonging are not necessarily a matter of individual choice. Some have deplored the occupational injustices caused by biased expectations, assumptions, rules, protocols, and political expediencies. Ruskin (1865/1892), for example, asked, "Which of us . . . is to do the hard and dirty work for the rest, and for what pay? Who is to do the pleasant and clean work, and for what pay?" (p. 107).

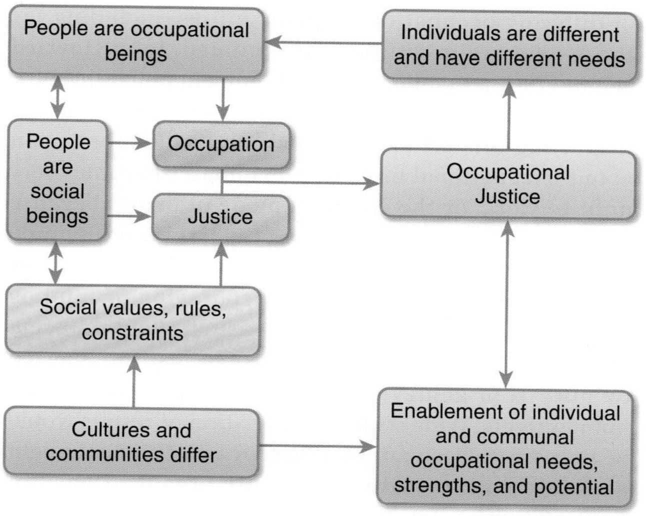

FIGURE 41.1 An exploratory theory of occupational justice: intersecting ideas. (Reproduced with permission from Prentice Hall.)

Within postindustrial nations, the division between desirable and undesirable occupations is less obvious than it was in earlier centuries. However, even though people may appear empowered to direct their lives, for a variety of sociopolitical reasons many flounder, unable to realize their talents or achieve their aspirations. It is easy to ignore that many people are channeled into occupations by social and family expectation, class systems, and financial circumstances. Commonly, children and adolescents, for example, are pressured to put aside particular interests and talents to excel within a limited range of occupations in order to be financially successful as adults. That may be a contributing factor to the probability that young people are experiencing increased unhappiness in life as evidenced by the growing numbers of suicides. In the United States, for example, suicide rates are the third leading cause of death among those aged 15 to 24 years, having tripled in the past half century. Equally common is the pressure put on older people to change their interests and levels of activity at a given chronological age whatever they feel about it themselves or whatever their health status (Nilsson & Townsend, 2010). A significant 13-year study of 2,761 older Americans found that doing social and productive occupations carried as much weight in terms of lowering the risk of all causes of death as doing exercise (Glass, de Leon, Marottoli, & Berkman, 1999, pp. 478–483).

Concerns about occupational justice can be linked without much effort to the politics of economic growth and the growing disparity of wealth and power (Werner, 1998). The disparity is pronounced between agrarian, industrializing, industrialized, and postindustrial countries; but in the first two of these, many people are unable to provide the necessities of life that are prerequisite to health; and in all of them, some people are unable to achieve positive well-being through what they do. The primary purpose for developing a theory of occupational justice was to draw attention to the fact that, throughout the world, many individuals and population groups are constrained, deprived, and alienated from engaging in occupations that provide personal, family, and/or community necessities, satisfaction, meaning, and balance (Wilcock, 1998, 2006).

Occupational justice draws together three powerful biological needs: to survive, to do, and to be part of a social group. These are innate mechanisms, as archaeological and anthropological research demonstrates (Wilcock, 2006). Occupational justice also draws on two powerful

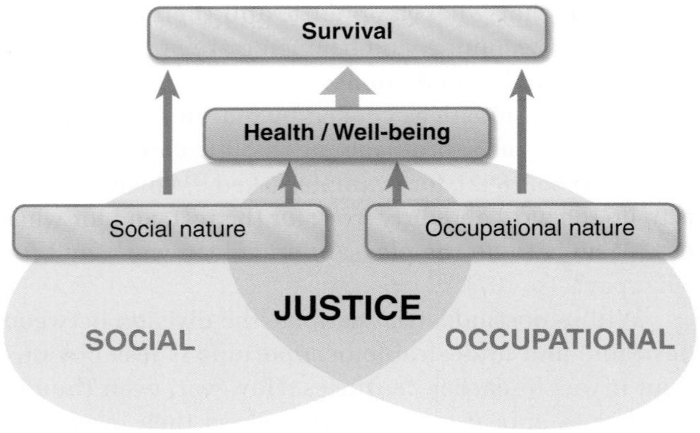

FIGURE 41.2 Occupational justice and social justice enabling survival through the meeting of biological needs and providing the means to health.

social needs: to create families, groups, and communities as structures in which people define who they will be and become and how they belong or not in particular social contexts; and to organize economic and human resources so that everyone is enabled to participate, experience well-being, and thrive (Stadnyk, Townsend, & Wilcock, 2010; Whiteford & Townsend, 2011). Health and well-being are dependent upon meeting primary survival requirements, the biological needs to do and to belong, and the structure of social groups (Argyle, 1987; Blaxter, 1990; Cohen et al., 1982; Isaksson, 1990; Warr, 1990; Wilcock et al., 1998; WHO, Health and Welfare Canada, Canadian Public Health Association, 1986). Figure 41.2 depicts the relationships between occupational justice, social justice, and health.

Occupational Justice and Health

Because the WHO is, arguably, the ultimate global authority on health issues, it is appropriate that its relevant directives are woven through this section about occupational justice and health. From its inception in 1946, the WHO recognized that health encompasses social, mental, and physical well-being as well as the absence of illness. Because health encompasses social well-being, the responsibilty of health professionals, including occupational therapists, must extend to the population at large as well as to people with medically defined conditions or disabilities. In 1986, the WHO built on that initial concept with the definitive call for action found within the Ottawa Charter for Health Promotion, a call for "reducing differences in current health status and ensuring equal opportunities and resources to enable all people to achieve their fullest health potential" (WHO, 1998, p. 1). WHO called not only for people being able to satisfy needs and cope with the environment but also to realize aspirations if positive health and well-being are to be reached. The Charter remains current, having been reaffirmed many times over the ensuing years in subsequent worldwide health promotion conferences.

Occupational Justice, Social Health, and Well-Being

The Universal Declaration of Human Rights (UN, 1998) advocates for all people having a standard of living adequate for health and well-being, with equal rights to work; to free choice of employment; and to rest, leisure, and holidays. This landmark UN declaration advocates for all to participate in the cultural life of a community, in the arts and scientific advancement, in national governments, and in education directed to the full development of the human personality. These fundamental rights of all people clearly provide topics for debate about **social health** in relation to empowerment, choice, and opportunity centering around the realities of occupation, on the tension between individual and communal rights, and between justice for individuals and the common good. This tension between individual and community interests is central to debates about the scope, nature, and responsibilities that go with asserting occupational rights. For example, the occupational right of seniors to participate in meaningful occupations requires a community that encourages and values their opinions and expertise. Societies need to ensure that buildings, housing, transportation, and everyday technology are fully accessible and also that facilities are designed for active living, not only for caregiving (Nilsson & Townsend, 2010; Townsend, 2007; Townsend & Wilcock, 2004). Indeed, occupational therapists should seek opportunities to be involved in developing occupationally just solutions for older people in emerging policies toward "aging in place" rather than accepting that life ends by aging in institutions (Trentham & Cockburn, 2011).

Occupational injustices are not recent phenomena. Over the centuries, many have questioned the fairness of differing occupational opportunities, including for those who are institutionally confined. John Howard (1726–1790), a well-known Enlightenment philanthropist, is a case in point. He travelled widely throughout Europe inspecting prisons and hospitals and called for action about occupational injustices as inmates became "very unfit to work, or the common mode of living" because of a lack of provision for them to maintain or upgrade skills (Howard, 1789, pp. 140–142). Occupational therapy organizations might consider encouraging or funding similar broad scale investigative research about the occupational injustices that prevent people, institutionalized or not, from achieving the UN occupation-focused human rights. Wide scale dissemination of results would be necessary. Occupational therapy practitioners might consider working with community organizations, for example with "street kids." In Nova Scotia, Canada's Mobile Outreach Street Health (MOSH) program, the occupational therapist is "mobile." Practice is not office based; instead, it includes texting and phoning team members and community organizations, always engaging youth where possible, to identify and develop housing, employment, coffee house, health promotion, and other opportunities for street youth. Guided by the Canadian Model of Occupational Performance and Engagement (CMOP-E) (Townsend & Polatajko, 2007), youth explore their present lifestyle and future options and develop their life skills and negotiation strategies from completing funding or housing and job applications to cooking, communication, and advocacy. Similarly, Kielhofner, de las Heras, and Suarez-Balcazar (2011) report using the Model of Human Occupation (MOHO) as a framework to address social injustice, one example being to engage street youth in sports occupations while also advocating for changes in the local school system.

In recent times, health has become so associated with medical care alone that key understanding about the many negative or positive health consequences of occupation is frequently overlooked. As well, the notion of social health is hardly paid lip service. This is despite current recognition that the fundamental conditions and resources for health are peace, shelter, education, food, income, a stable ecosystem, sustainable resources, social justice, and equity (WHO, Health and Welfare Canada, Canadian Public Health Association, 1986). Those conditions and resources relate directly or indirectly to what people do, but millions around the world are unable to meet those primary occupational needs. In addition, the WHO recognizes that "changing patterns of life, work, and leisure have a significant impact on health"; indeed, should be a "source of health for people," and that communities as well as individuals "must be able to identify and realize aspirations, to satisfy needs and to change or cope with the environment" (p. 3).

That authoritative recognition stimulated contentious argument during the 1990s about the need to put aside "power plays" in order to meet the fundamental conditions required for health for all people. The argument called for intervention beyond the provision of conventional medical and health services because "the struggle for health is essentially a struggle for equity and compassion" in "all sectors and aspects of life" (Werner, 1998, p. 2). The development of "active societies" and "enabling states" began to be addressed within international organizations (Gilbert, 1995; Kalisch, 1991, pp. 3–9; Organization for Economic Cooperation and Development [OECD], 1989). The Clinton administration, for example, encouraged a "blueprint for a new America" in which

> . . . the enabling state be organized around the goals of work and individual empowerment . . . Above all, it should help poor Americans develop the capacities they need to liberate themselves from poverty and dependence. . . . An enabling strategy should see the poor as the prime agents of their own development, rather than as passive clients of the welfare system. (Marshall & Schram, 1993)

The rhetoric is impressive but cannot be achieved without major economic and political change as well as acceptance within conventional health care, that marked disparities in health and illness experiences are rooted in social and economic inequalities. "If health is ever to be construed as a human right" . . . "disparities of outcome in and between countries" are major challenges (Farmer, Furin, & Katz, 2004, p. 1832). To right such wrongs, action is required at all levels to advance occupational justice as an inseparable part of social health care. Three major ethical dilemmas facing occupational therapists in this regard are accepting social health as a legitimate field of work, accepting the professional responsibility of raising awareness of occupational injustices within communities, and accepting the professional responsibility to develop programs that address occupational injustices, such as occupational deprivation, imbalance, and alienation (Trentham & Cockburn, 2011; Wilcock 1993, 2006).

Occupational Justice, Mental Health, and Well-Being

The WHO's (1998) *Health for All in the Twenty-first Century* validates personal uniqueness and the "need to respond to each individual's spiritual quest for meaning, purpose and belonging." A 2005 WHO report claims that mental as well as social and physical health is a state in which people realize their own abilities, cope with the normal stresses of life, and work productively and fruitfully. In a healthy state, people seek response to their spiritual quest for meaning, purpose, and belonging and are able to make a contribution to their community. The report recognizes that mental health can be enhanced by interventions that "respect and protect basic civil, political, economic, social, and cultural rights" (Herrman, Shekhars, & Moodie, 2005, p. XIX). Programs that followed these socially and occupationally just recommendations would provide all people with a better chance of experiencing mental health and well-being.

Currently, with mental health or illness, rich or poor people alike may be unable to meet those needs, albeit for differing occupational reasons such as the restrictions imposed by requirements or expectations of their social world. Within particular societies and communities, occupations are often biased, with good health, choice, and opportunity skewed in favor of a controlling minority. Such bias is a matter of occupational injustice and can lead to an increasing number of people experiencing mental illness, thus adding barriers to achieving WHO goals.

Despite a long and varied history, the treatment of mental illness is now medicalized. There were times when therapeutic milieus included religion, peace or tranquility, and others when ridicule, neglect, mental, and physical abuse were the order of the day. As a counter to the latter regime, 19th century Scottish psychiatrist, W. A. F. Browne (1837), based his revolutionary treatment on "justice, benevolence and occupation" in which without compulsion, gradually increasing occupation was planned to meet individual needs. Ladies, for example, could read; play the harp; flower muslin; or be out walking, riding, or driving to church, market, or the country. Gentlemen might follow intellectual pursuits, billiards, or outside work structured and apportioned to suit the "tastes and powers of each." Browne (1837) saw the outcome of such occupationally just regimes as self-applause, the approbation of others, a lessening of pain and disagreeable thoughts, and sound sleep at night (pp. 229–230). Occupation-focused programs for people with mental illness have decreased with economic rationalism despite an increase of modern-day disorders of mental health such as child, gender, and substance abuse; violence; depression; and anxiety. These are more problematic where there is low income, high unemployment, stressful work conditions, limited education, gender discrimination, human rights violations, and unhealthy lifestyles (Herrman et al., 2005). Advocacy by occupational therapists is called for to address the current lack of occupation-based programs for such problems. These should be founded on well-developed but flexible program ideas that could be implemented within communities without a great deal of expense or preferably be self-supporting.

An ethical dilemma facing occupational therapists is inadequate understanding of occupational injustices that compound mental health problems. Increasing understanding and raising community awareness is a primary requirement to address this dilemma. Only with greater awareness of occupational injustices can occupational therapy initiatives be developed to enable all people to access a range of occupations that individuals and communities define as meaningful, that promote optimal well-being, and that rehabilitate those affected by mental illness. In line with WHO directives, initiatives must enable the development of programs that assist people to cope with the normal stresses of life, contribute to their community, strive toward their occupational potential, and forward their needs for meaning, purpose and belonging. Such intiatives must respect, protect, and further basic civil, political, economic, sociocultural, and, most importantly in this case, occupational rights.

Occupational Justice, Physical Health, and Well-Being

Occupational justice is an essential aspect of physical health and well-being. Too much, too little, or ill-chosen occupation can lead directly to illness or death. Bernardino Ramazzini (1705), a pioneer figure of occupational health, raised very practical concerns about the early death and disorders suffered by workers in many types of basic and necessary employment in the 18th century. His extensive research is a testament to the occupational injustices of that time and resonates with what still happens in many poor communities around the world in agrarian, industrializing, and industrialized countries. Currently, opportunities to inform and assist people to prevent physical illness or to assist in recovery from it through occupation are haphazard. Such a notable bias within the provision of health care is a global injustice, given that physical inactivity has now been identified as the fourth leading risk factor in global mortality. It is one of only a few largely preventable risk factors that accounts for most illness throughout the world (WHO, 2004).

The WHO (2011a, 2011b) argues that increasing industrialization, urbanization, economic development, and food market globalization have led to significant changes in physical activity and that regular moderate physical occupations can reduce the risk of a range of common disorders such as cardiovascular diseases, diabetes, hip and vertebral fractures, disorders of weight, some cancers, and depression. Eighty percent of deaths caused by such diseases occur in low- and middle-income countries where poverty hinders economic development. Occupational therapists should be at the forefront of developing programs addressing changed physical activity levels, enabling individuals and communities to recognize that physical activity is not restricted to exercises to keep fit, and can meet personal and group occupational needs and interests while improving health. This may mean being entrepreneurial away from the comfort zone of medically based organizations.

In all parts of the world, a reduction in physical occupations can be the result of unintentional occupational injustices. For example, multinational corporations that make money out of encouraging people to engage in addictive, low-level physical occupations are as guilty of occupational injustice as are those who encourage drinking or smoking for recreation. The WHO (2011a) recommendations to increase physical activity levels across the globe require population-based and culturally relevant policies that are multidisciplinary and multisectorial.

At the other extreme, well-chosen occupations can be a source of health, for both individuals and communities and aid in the repair of illness. Widely recognized at the start of the 20th century, this led to the advent of occupational therapy as a formal discipline. However, occupation-focused remedial programs have decreased in regular health care facilities for people experiencing physical illness, except perhaps for those aimed at improving independence in personal care. The decrease can be blamed on increased medical costs and priorities, shortened stays within health facilities, and a general change in appreciation that what people do in their lives affects physical health and well-being. Reliance on medication and surgery has become paramount. When this is to the exclusion or reduction of appropriate activity levels, this, too, is occupationally unjust. Ethical dilemmas for occupational therapists include how to increase community understanding of the physical health benefits of meeting wide ranging occupational needs, how to continue occupation-based rehabilitation programs beyond shortened institutional stays, and how to assist compensatory cases to improve their fitness while under the restrictive jurisdiction of insurers.

Occupational Justice within Occupational Therapy

Occupational injustice is an ethical dilemma for occupational therapists and for every society on earth if the move toward an occupationally just and healthy world is to be achieved. It is timely that the concept of occupational justice is influencing the governance, planning, and policies of occupational therapy's professional organizations. In 2006, the WFOT endorsed fully the UN Universal Declaration of Human Rights when it published a position statement that includes its stand on occupational justice. This accepts that the "right to occupation is subject to cultural beliefs and customs, local circumstances and institutional power and practices" and condemns the global conditions that threaten the right, including "poverty, disease, social discrimination, displacement, natural and man-made disasters, and armed conflict." It calls for occupational therapists to identify and support individuals, groups, communities, and societies experiencing occupational injustices and to work with them to enhance participation in occupation.

The position paper was prompted by interest in occupational justice evinced in various corners of the world, not least *Australasia* (a term that encompasses Australia, New Zealand, and the Asian continent) and Canada where the idea evolved. The European Network of Occupational Therapists in Higher Education (ENOTHE) embraced occupational justice as the theme of its 2003 annual conference. At that meeting, Townsend (2003a) asked, "Why would occupational therapists be concerned with occupational justice?" Responses related to the injustices experienced when people are barred, trapped, confined, segregated, restricted, prohibited, unable to develop, disrupted, alienated, imbalanced, deprived, or marginalized in ways that exclude them from participating optimally in the occupations they need and want to do to sustain health throughout the life course.

In 2005, the British College of Occupational Therapists (COT) proposed that "occupational justice provides a framework for asking questions about inequities of opportunity for occupational development, or inequities related to lack of appropriate enablement for those living with a disability" (pp. 2–3).

In the same year, Wood, Hooper, and Womack (2005) discussed the place of occupational justice within occupational therapy education; and textbooks began to appear in which occupational therapists were encouraged to work in underresourced countries to help overcome occupational injustice. However, to do so, it was recognized that they themselves might need support because of potential professional isolation (Newton & Fuller, 2005). When Kronenberg, Algado, and Pollard (2005) challenged occupational therapists to work in places and situations where people are occupationally marginalized and exploited, they argued that occupational justice is a professional responsibility. They explained it as an ethical issue of global citizenship, introducing the notion of occupational apartheid to raise critical awareness and understanding about the political nature of occupation. Following up on that work, Pollard, Sakellariou, and Kronenberg (2009) advanced ideas to assist occupational therapists to improve political awareness in order to achieve occupationally just goals in community development.

Although the first initiatives recognizing occupational justice came from the West, occupational therapists throughout the world are now exploring the idea with attention to cultural variations. Exploration is a regular feature in textbooks, on the Web, and at formal venues with discussions covering diverse practice, community, and population health initiatives (Sakellariou & Simó Algado, 2006; Smith & Hilton, 2008; Trentham & Cockburn, 2011; Wilcock, 2006; Windley, 2011). Some see occupational justice and occupational rights as the profession's core purpose guiding practice according to "a whole new way of viewing the world" (Hammell, 2008; Molineux & Baptiste, 2011, p. 3; White, 2009). Future practice of occupational therapy may rest on the profession's success in putting occupational justice explicitly on the public agenda and showing what an occupation-focused, justice-driven profession can accomplish.

Reducing Occupational Injustices and Advancing Occupational Rights

Because occupational therapy is founded on the belief that participation in occupation is central to health, a lack of understanding about occupational justice is the major ethical dilemma that all occupational therapists need to address. It is their responsibility to advance understanding of occupational injustices, to educate others, and to effect change. The task of reducing occupational injustices and advancing occupational rights demands a committed effort; the task is actually about changing the world. This may sound both grandiose and overwhelming, yet Margaret Mead (1901–1978) reminded us to "never doubt that a small group of thoughtful, committed citizens can change the world. Indeed, it is the only thing that ever has" (para. 1).

Advancing occupational justice and rights while also reducing occupational injustices requires a group of thoughtful committed occupational therapists, occupational scientists, and others who recognize the centrality of occupation in human existence and health. To that end, a questionnaire is proposed as a checklist and guideline to prompt attention to occupational injustice in a busy practice day. The questionnaire shown in Table 41.1, based on UN, WHO, and WFOT directives,

TABLE 41.1 Occupational Justice and Health Questionnaire (OJHQ)

Instructions: Tick column 2 if client or community is able to meet the right listed in column 1.
Tick one or more of columns 3–6 if client or community is unable according to the reason(s) stated.

Client: Individual, Community or Population: ____________ **Date:** ____________

DETERMINANTS	ABLE	UNABLE Health	UNABLE Political	UNABLE Social	UNABLE Economic	COMMENT
Basic Needs (WHO)						
Peace						
Shelter						
Education						
Food						
Income						
Sustainable resources						
Social equity						
Social, Physical, and Mental Well-being (WHO)						
Life pattern = well-being						
Work = well-being						
Leisure = well-being						
Can realize aspirations						
Can satisfy specific needs						
Has regular physical activity						
Change/Cope with environment						
Validate personal uniqueness						
United Nations Rights—Living Standard Adequate for Health and Well-being. Free Choice to:						
Employment						
Rest						
Leisure						
Holidays						
Community cultural life						
The arts						
Scientific advancement						
Participate in government						
Education toward full development of personality						
World Federation of Occupational Therapists (WFOT) Rights 5 As above plus free choice to participate in:						
Cultural beliefs and customs						
Local events						

TABLE 41.1 Occupational Justice and Health Questionnaire (OJHQ) (*Continued*)

SUMMARY: Instructions: Tick one or more if occupational injustice results from the community issues listed below.	
WHO and WFOT—The right to health and well-being through occupation is decreased because of:	
Poverty	Low incomes
High unemployment	Stressful work conditions
Gender discrimination	Social discrimination
Limited education	Occupational discrimination
Unhealthy lifestyles	Displacement
Lack of health facilities	Political unrest
Lack of recreational opportunities	Human rights violations
Natural/Man-made disasters	Armed conflict
RECOMMENDATIONS/ACTION	

provides a starting point to document injustices and encourage action. Some readers may wish to begin testing and validating the questionnaire if their interests are in quantifying the issues named.

Occupational therapists can start their commitment where they work, linking their individual, local actions to a global vision of an occupationally just world. Some occupational therapists may find like-minded colleagues to form a local group or to network nationally and internationally. For occupational therapists with a passion to influence global change, there are collective options to work through the WFOT, through nongovernmental organizations (NGOs), through media consumer-based programs, through local political networks, or through individual efforts to generate collective action.

Because occupational justice requires proactive initiatives that explore, inform, and inspire changes to basic community structures and organizational health strategies, the cases provided subsequently suggest what therapists could do in various spheres of work instead of case examples of individual therapists working with individual clients. Figure 41.3 illustrates three "cases" of occupational therapy practice to address occupational injustices as a visual tool to stimulate ideas beyond the suggested examples. The figure shows how local, group, and collective actions are linked. The opening questions in this figure emphasize the importance of partnerships, media attention, documentation, and daily life occupation as important media for change. The arrows suggest actions that are targeted for individual, group, or collective action but are interrelated. An individual may start actions that attract others to engage in collective action; conversely, collective action, such as joining a justice-based NGO, could stimulate ideas for individual or group action in particular directions or situations. Evaluation of individual, group, and collective action can be facilitated by setting objectives that can be measured, narrated, or otherwise documented for review in a stated time frame and place for funders, managers, the public, insurers, or other interested audiences.

The three cases suggest individual, group, and collective action on occupational injustice, with questions to stimulate dialogue, take action, and evaluate progress toward occupational justice and occupational rights.

The first case relates to rehabilitation practices in health facilities where occupational therapists work with individuals who have physical, mental, cognitive, and other challenges related to long-term discrimination on the basis of disability or old age. The question is often raised whether occupational therapists in these traditional places of work should focus on enabling occupational justice when work to change the environment or address client rights is not funded or recognized as necessary by those in charge. Not to do so demonstrates a failure to further the profession's philosophical foundations and failure to benefit similar client needs in the future. Each therapist is an agent with the power to shape future health care, other sectors in society from housing to education and transportation, and the profession—that is, if the evaluation of actions is documented in reports that can be distributed to health and other hierarchies, the media, or interested parties. An action by therapists could be to develop occupational injustice checklists suited to particular situations, such as the Occupational Justice and Health Questionnaire (OJHQ) (Table 41.1) and the Occupational Injustice and Seniors Checklist (Box 41.1).

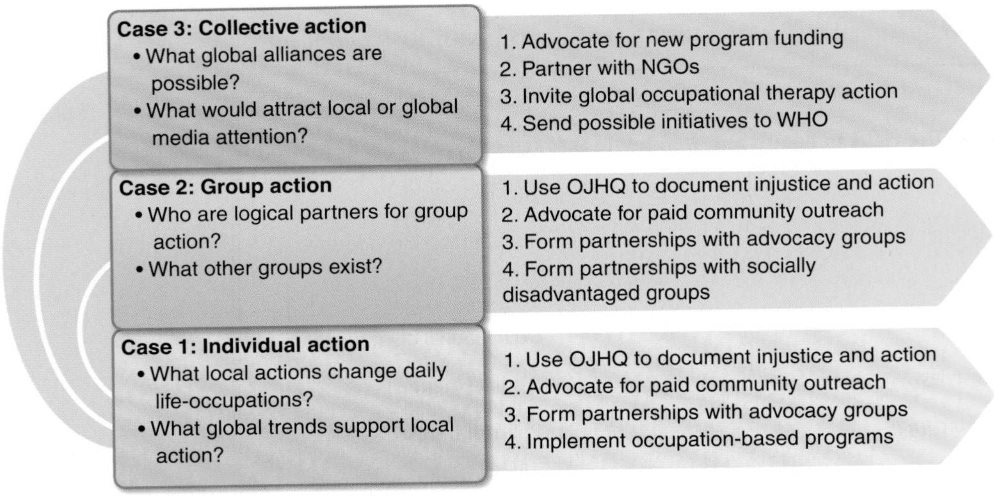

FIGURE 41.3 Linking individual, group, and collective action for local and global change. *OJHQ*, Occupational Justice and Health Questionnaire; *NGOs*, nongovernmental organizations; *WHO*, World Health Organization.

The second case in Figure 41.3 addresses occupational injustice relating to the promotion of mental health. It suggests action with a group of interested colleagues. There are advantages in the strength and support of numbers and in brainstorming opportunities to discover innovative, feasible group action about occupational injustice in communities and health services. Whether face to face, e-mail, teleconference, or other means, occupational therapists can access colleagues working in the geographical area or belonging to the same interest groups. The challenge to a group is to be daring and innovative in using occupational therapy knowledge, occupational injustice checklists, and questionnaires. With such tools and using data from multiple occupational therapists to record occupational justice issues, group action could start by raising awareness of "real" injustices and progress to enlisting community action toward changing them.

The third case suggests collective action through raising questions capable of generating debate and innovation to change an occupationally unjust world. Action could take many forms such as innovative programming; media arousal, perhaps through presenting at rallies and meetings; publicizing stories about occupationally unjust situations and actions; presenting statistics of concern and using population data to monitor change; creating and critiquing visual images of occupational injustices and actions; and consultation, cooperation, and contributions to national and international organizations such as the WHO. The use of occupational justice language to pinpoint the issues is the most powerful aspect of this case.

Initiatives of this kind continue the tradition of the collective action that was central to the emergence of occupational therapy in the early 20th century and to the

BOX 41.1 Occupational Injustice and Seniors Checklist

Check all that apply.

- ❑ Not attended to when they talk about what they have done in their lives
- ❑ Not asked for advice or listened to if they give it
- ❑ Given no chance to help others
- ❑ Taken for outings in which they have no interest
- ❑ Are told they can't do something they would enjoy "for their own good"
- ❑ Insufficient advice, practical assistance, equipment, or support to remain in their own environment if they wish to do so
- ❑ Prevented from doing what they want in the name of risk management
- ❑ Placement in sheltered accommodation away from their own people, pets, interests, and environment
- ❑ Sitting alone in nursing homes or other confined settings with nothing to do except watch others in the same situation or a television that shows program after program they did not choose
- ❑ Lack of resources, helpers, services, or support to enable satisfying occupations to match their interests
- ❑ Social contact restricted to paid service providers who bring food, help with personal care, and change beds
- ❑ Restricted, deprived, or alienated by the policies of people in authority or by legislation

profession's growth around the world. Early occupational therapists, despite minuscule numbers, stimulated the profession's rapid growth because of their belief in the effectiveness of occupation as therapy and their commitment to it demonstrated through collective action. Since then, the profession's leaders have negotiated positions based on client need, workplace agreements, professional regulation, and other structures to meet people's occupational needs, contribute to society, and develop the profession.

Conclusion

Proactivity toward an occupationally just world is the next challenge in the occupation for health journey. It is a major ethical dilemma facing occupational therapists in all corners of the world. Advancing the concept is complex. It demands a different mindset and focus and requires the development of unfamiliar proactive interventions within personal, community, national, and world stages and the development of occupational therapy practice clearly in line with the directives of the UN, WHO, and occupational justice principles.

References

Argyle, M. (1987). *The psychology of happiness*. New York, NY: Methuen.

Blaxter, M. (1990). *Health and lifestyles*. London, United Kingdom: Tavistock/Routledge.

British College of Occupational Therapists. (2005). *Making the connections: Delivering better services for Wales. Clause 3.1.4*. London, United Kingdom: Author.

Browne, W. A. F. (1837). *What asylums were, are, and ought to be*. Edinburgh, Scotland: Adam & Charles Black.

Cohen, P., Struening, E. L., Genevie, L. E., Kaplan, S. R., Muhlin, G. L., & Peck, H. B. (1982). Community stressors, mediating conditions and wellbeing in urban neighborhoods. *Journal of Community Psychology, 10*, 377–390.

Commission on Social Justice. (1994). *Social justice: Strategies for national renewal. The report of the Commission on Social Justice*. London, United Kingdom: Vintage.

Farmer, P. E., Furin, J. J., & Katz, J. T. (2004). Global health equity. *The Lancet, 363*, 1832.

Gilbert, N. (1995). *Welfare justice: Restoring social equity*. London, United Kingdom: Yale University Press.

Glass, T. A., de Leon, C. M., Marottoli, R. A., & Berkman, L. F. (1999). Population based study of social and productive activities as predictors of survival among elderly Americans. *British Medical Journal, 319*, 478–483.

Hammell, K. W. (2008). Reflections on well-being and occupational rights. *Canadian Journal of Occupational Therapy, 75*, 61–64.

Herrman, H., Shekhars, S., & Moodie, R. (Eds.). (2005). *Promoting mental health. Concepts, emerging evidence, practice: A report of the World Health Organization*. Geneva, Switzerland: World Health Organization. Retrieved from http://whqlibdoc.who.int/publications/2005/9241562943_eng.pdf

Howard, J. (1789). *An account of the Principal Lazarettos in Europe*. Warrington, United Kingdom: William Eyres.

Isaksson, K. (1990). A longitudinal study of the relationship between frequent job change and psychological well-being. *Journal of Occupational Psychology, 63*, 297–308.

Jackson Lears, T. J. (1981). *No place of grace: Antimodernism and the transformation of American culture 1880–1920*. New York, NY: Pantheon Books.

Kalisch, D. (1991). The active society. *Social Security Journal*, August, 3–9.

Kielhofner, G., de las Heras, C. G., & Suarez-Balcazar, Y. (2011). Human occupation as a tool for understanding and promoting social justice. In F. Kronenberg, N. Pollard, & D. Sakellariou (Eds.), *Occupational therapy without borders. Vol. 2. Towards an ecology of occupation-based practices* (pp. 269–277). Edinburgh, Scotland: Elsevier/Churchill Livingstone.

Kronenberg, F., Algado, S. S., & Pollard, N., (Eds.). (2005). *Spirit of survivors: Occupational therapy without borders*. Edinburgh, United Kingdom: Elsevier/Churchill Livingstone.

Lukes, S. (1973). *Individualism*. Oxford, United Kingdom: Basil Blackwell.

MacCarthy, F. (1994). *William Morris: A life for our time*. London, United Kingdom: Faber and Faber.

Marshall, W., & Schram, M., (Eds.). (1993). *Mandate for change*. New York, NY: Berkley.

Mead, M. (1901–1978). *Laura Moncur's motivational quotations*. Retrieved from http://www.quotationspage.com/quote/33522.html

Molineux, M., & Baptiste, S. (2011) Emerging occupational therapy practice: Building on the foundations and seizing the opportunities. In M. Thew, M. Edwards, S. Baptiste, & M. Molineux (Eds.), *Role emerging occupational therapy: Maximising occupation-focused practice*. West Sussex, United Kingdom: John Wiley & Sons.

Newton, E. & Fuller, B. (2005). The Occupational Therapy International Outreach Network: Supporting occupational therapists without borders. In F. Kronenberg, S. S. Algado, & N. Pollard (Eds.), *Occupational therapy without borders: Learning from the spirit of survivors* (pp. 361–373). Edinburgh, Scotland: Elsevier/Churchill Livingstone.

Nilsson, I., & Townsend, E. A. (2010). Occupational justice—Bridging theory and practice. *Scandinavian Journal of Occupational Therapy, 17*, 57–63.

Organization for Economic Cooperation and Development. (1989, July). Editorial: The path to full employment: Structural adjustment for an active society [Editorial]. *Employment Outlook*. Retrieved from http://www.oecd.org/dataoecd/48/28/3247295.pdf

Pollard, N., Sakellariou, D., & Kronenberg, F. (Eds.). (2009). *A political practice of occupational therapy*. Edinburgh, Scotland: Elsevier/Churchill Livingstone.

Ramazzini, B. (1705). *A treatise of the diseases of tradesmen: Shewing the various influence of particular trades upon the state of health*. London, United Kingdom: Andrew Bell.

Ruskin, J. (1982). *Sesame and Lilies* (13th ed.). Orpington, United Kingdom: George Allen. (Original work published 1865)

Sakellariou, D., & Simó Algado, S. (2006). Sexuality and disability: A case of occupational injustice. *British Journal of Occupational Therapy, 69*(2), 69–76.

Smith, D. L., & Hilton, C. L. (2008). An occupational justice perspective of domestic violence against women with disabilities. *Journal of Occupational Science, 15*, 166–172.

Stadnyk, R., Townsend, E. A., & Wilcock, A. (2010). Occupational justice. In C. Christiansen & E. A. Townsend (Eds.), *Introduction to occupation: The art and science of living* (2nd ed., pp. 329–358). Thorofare, NJ: Prentice Hall.

Thibeault, R. (2002). Occupation and the rebuilding of civic society: Notes from the war zone. *Journal of Occupational Science, 9*(1), 38–47.

Townsend, E. (1993). Muriel Driver Memorial Lecture: Occupational therapy's social vision. *Canadian Journal of Occupational Therapy, 60*, 174–184.

Townsend, E. (1996). Enabling empowerment: Using simulations versus real occupations. *Canadian Journal of Occupational Therapy, 63*, 113–128.

Townsend, E. (1998). *Good intentions overruled: A critique of empowerment in the routine organization of mental health services*. Toronto, Canada: University of Toronto Press.

Townsend, E. A. (2003a). *Occupational justice: Ethical, moral and civic principles for an inclusive world. European Network of Occupational Therapy Educators. Prague, Czech Republic*. Retrieved from www.enothe.hva.nl/meet/ac03/acc03-text03.doc

Townsend, E. A. (2003b). Power and justice in enabling occupation *Canadian Journal of Occupational Therapy, 70*, 74–87.

Townsend, E. A. (2007). Justice and habits: A synthesis of habits III. *OTJR: Occupation, Participation and Health, 27*, 69S–78S.

Townsend, E. A., & Polatajko, H. J. (2007). *Enabling occupation II: Advancing an occupational therapy vision of health, well-being and justice through occupation*. Ottawa, Canada: Canadian Association of Occupational Therapists.

Townsend, E. A., & Wilcock, A. A. (2004). Occupational justice and client-centered practice: A dialogue in progress. *Canadian Journal of Occupational Therapy, 71*, 75–87.

Trentham, B., & Cockburn, L. (2011). Promoting occupational therapy in a community health centre. In M. Thew, M. Edwards, S. Baptiste, M. Molineux (Eds.), *Role emerging occupational therapy: Maximising occupation-focused practice* (pp. 97–110). West Sussex, United Kingdom: John Wiley & Sons.

United Nations. (1998). *Universal declaration of human rights*. Geneva, Switzerland: UN General Assembly.

Warr, P. (1990). The measurement of well-being and other aspects of mental health. *Journal of Occupational Psychology, 63*(4), 193–210.

Werner, D. (1998, November). *Health and equity: Need for a people's perspective in the quest for world health*. Paper presented at the "PHC21—Everybody's Business" Conference, Almaty, Kazakhstan.

White, J. A. (2009). Questions for occupational therapy. In E. B. Crepeau, E. S. Cohn, & B. B. Schell (Eds.), *Willard and Spackman's occupational therapy* (11th ed.). Philadelphia, PA: Lippincott Williams & Wilkins.

Whiteford, G., & Townsend, E. A. (2011). A participatory occupational justice framework: Enabling occupational participation and inclusion. In F. Kronenberg, N. Pollard, & D. Sakellariou (Eds.), *Occupational therapy without borders: Learning from the spirit of survivors* (2nd ed., pp. 65–84). Elsevier.

Wilcock, A. (1993). A theory of the human need for occupation. *Journal of Occupational Science: Australia, 1*(1), 17–24.

Wilcock, A. (1995). The occupational brain: A theory of human nature. *Journal of Occupational Science: Australia, 2*(1), 68–73.

Wilcock, A. (1998). *An occupational perspective of health*. Thorofare, NJ: Slack.

Wilcock, A. (2006). *An occupational perspective of health* (2nd ed.). Thorofare, NJ: Slack.

Wilcock, A., van der Aren, H., Darling, K., Scholz, J., Sidall, R., Snigg, C., & Stephens, J. (1998). An exploratory study of people's perception and experiences of wellbeing. *British Journal of Occupational Therapy, 61*(2), 75–82.

Windley, D. (2011). Community development. In M. Thew, M. Edwards, S. Baptiste, M. Molineux, (Eds.), *Role emerging occupational therapy: Maximising occupation-focused practice* (pp. 97–110). West Sussex, United Kingdom: John Wiley & Sons.

Wood, W., Hooper, B., & Womack, J. (2005). Reflections on occupational justice as a subtext of occupation-centred education. In F. Kronenberg, S. S. Algado, & N. Pollard (Eds.), *Occupational therapy without borders: Learning from the spirit of survivors* (pp. 378–389). Edinburgh, Scotland: Elsevier/Churchill Livingstone.

World Federation of Occupational Therapists. (2006). *Position statement on human rights*. Retrieved from http://www.wfot.org/office_files/Human%20Rights%20Position%20Statement%20Final%20NLH%281%29.pdf

World Health Organization. (1946). *Constitution of the World Health Organization*. Geneva, Switzerland: Author.

World Health Organization. (1998). *Health for all in the twenty-first century. Document A51/5*. Geneva, Switzerland: Author.

World Health Organization. (2004). *Global strategy on diet, physical activity and health*. Geneva, Switzerland: Author.

World Health Organization. (2011a). *Global strategy on diet, physical activity and health*. Geneva, Switzerland: Author.

World Health Organization. (2011b). *Physical activity*. Geneva, Switzerland: Author.

World Health Organization, Health and Welfare Canada, Canadian Public Health Association. (1986). *Ottawa charter for health promotion*. Ottawa, Canada: Author.

For additional resources on the subjects discussed in this chapter, visit http://thePoint.lww.com/Willard-Spackman12e.

CHAPTER 42

Emerging Theories

Debra Tupe

LEARNING OBJECTIVES

After reading this chapter, you will be able to:

1. Identify key occupational therapy trends, issues, and concepts that contribute to emerging theory
2. Describe the contributions of systems theories, cultural approaches, and transdisciplinary frameworks in understandings of occupational performance, social participation, and civic engagement
3. Describe the role and application of social entrepreneurship and service learning in novel and community-based occupational therapy contexts

OUTLINE

Introduction

An emerging issue should be "disturbing, provocative, forcing one to change how one thinks" (Dator, as cited in Inayatullah, 2007, p. 49). Emerging ideas can evolve as trends or have a long-lasting or dramatic impact on society, the ways we think, and everyday experiences. Emerging theory communicates the need for a profession to rethink conceptual constructs or assess practice. It is our professional responsibility to create knowledge and develop theoretical models that align with our core values (Royeen, 2003). Occupational therapy is a reflexive profession. We are required to reflect, question, and identify which events, trends, or phenomena will give rise to new conceptual models and determine if existing theories adequately address issues in contemporary practice. This chapter imparts new ways occupational therapists are thinking about the profession's conceptual constructs, practice beyond traditional borders, and professional roles as change agents in the global community. How, then, can practice provoke revisions of outdated perspectives, reconfigure conceptual constructs, or produce new and emerging approaches?

The Impact of Globalization on Practice and Theory

Globalization is the defining issue of our time. Over the past two decades, revolutionary advances in technology and commerce have reconstructed the notion of the *global community*. With the push of a button or click of a mouse, we can share ideas, communicate with friends in distant lands, purchase products from virtual stores, download publications, and access the latest news or social commentary with a tweet. Our world of villages, communities, and cities is now interconnected, complex, dynamic, and reachable through cyberspace. Globalization has impacted how we live our day, acquire knowledge, enact occupations, make sense of the world, and how we conceive and deliver occupational therapy services.

The complexity of the global world requires new methodologies and conceptual approaches that inform, describe, evaluate, and advance understandings of occupation. In addition, efforts are required to address how cultural, political, social, and economic environments impact occupational choices, support access to occupation, and facilitate or restrict full social participation. As occupational therapy interfaces with the dynamic and rapidly changing global community, existing theories may not adequately address deficiencies and advances in our practice. Current occupational therapy literature, however, provides a path in which to navigate key issues that are relevant to the postmodernist global context and development of contemporary theoretical approaches. The literature calls for (1) expansion of theoretical frameworks beyond the clinic and community to complex societal contexts (Galheigo, 2011a); (2) adoption of a multilevel perspective that evaluates structural, institutional, and individual contributions to occupation, health, and well-being (Aldrich, 2008; Dickie, Cutchin, & Humphry, 2006; Fogelberg & Frauwirth, 2010); (3) movement away from a reductionist framework to a contextual and population-based approach that incorporates transdisciplinary worldviews and principles of occupational justice (Sinclair, 2009; Whiteford & Townsend, 2011); and (4) expand research evidence to include judgment-based practice, client narratives, and phenomenological approaches (Galheigo, 2011a; Law, 2010; Polkinghorne, 2004; Tomlin & Borgetto, 2011).

Occupational therapy has consistently responded to changes and trends in health care, education, and political agendas and is now called to address globalization's potential to influence our practice and challenge our theoretical models. In her Slagle lecture, Elnora M. Gilfoyle (1984) acknowledged a paradigmatic shift in occupational therapy thinking and practice stating, "Regardless of the future, legal, political, economic, professional, and organizational issues will influence our transformation. By recognizing both internal and external issues and identifying strategies, we can influence our own future" (p. 363). Gilfoyle's visionary view led to recommendations for our profession's ongoing development. Suggestions included diminish allegiance to the biomedical model, new understandings of occupation, transdisciplinary collaborations, attention to relationships of power and gender, and further development of theories that represent the breadth and scope of our practice. This proposal continues to be relevant to contemporary occupational therapy practice in today's global world.

The Need for New Theoretical Perspectives

The World Federation of Occupational Therapists has responded to the influence of the global environment on occupational therapy practice and has taken into account emerging issues such as global labor markets, new medical technologies, and extension of occupational therapy practice to groups affected by migration, disaster, or human conflict (Sinclair, 2009). As our profession moves forward in developing practice in emerging areas, new theories, frameworks, and models are required to communicate and demonstrate the range of our skill set and how occupational therapists think differently about illness, disability, and social exclusion (Thew, Edwards, Baptiste, & Molineux, 2011). Armed with a central and evolving occupational perspective, our profession has the opportunity to influence the health of collective groups and societies while enhancing understandings of the impact of structural systems on occupational engagement (Thew et al., 2011). These new ways of thinking about current issues and opportunities have prompted a movement in occupational therapy theory and practice that embraces the social field and recognizes occupational therapy's role as agents of social change (Galheigo, 2011a; Sinclair, 2009). This shift expands our view beyond the clinic to larger contextual aspects in the global community.

The power of an occupational perspective to address social issues facing the global community is now acknowledged within occupational therapy (Thew et al., 2011). Galheigo (2011b) proposes that a theory grounded in *complexity* and embedded in *cultural* and *political analysis* may lead occupational therapy to new insights on occupation, agency, culture, and human rights. The possibility of thoughtful discussions across borders and disciplines underscores the importance of ongoing and vigilant rethinking and reconstructing of our practice. Galheigo (2011b) asks a simple yet profound question, "What needs to be done?" (p. 60).

The global context has necessitated occupational therapy's rapid and keen anticipation of and attention to evolving social, cultural, economic, and political trends and processes and procedures that influence our practice, educational models, and theoretical underpinnings. Occupational therapy theoretical models based on systems approaches are presented to enhance understandings of the influence and interactions of structural systems on occupation at individual, group, and population levels. Sociocultural approaches are included to further advance notions of cultural relevance, situated meaning, and contextual experiences. The final section brings in contributions from other disciplines that inform our perspectives around current professional issues such as power relations, professional identities, and knowledge creation.

Complexity and Systems Theories

Occupational therapy's exploration of complexity theory can, in part, be attributed to limitations of the biomedical model, particularly its displacement of occupation. As occupational therapy began to challenge the dominant paradigm of biomedicine, occupation was viewed as a broader, more complex phenomenon that required a conceptual approach beyond reductionistic models (Whiteford & Townsend, 2011). Movement away from the Western perspective of linear relationships afforded opportunities to adapt and create concepts and constructs that perhaps are more appropriate to how occupational therapy practitioners think about occupation. Since our world and our profession continues to acquire new knowledge, embrace innovative practice models, and advance science and technology, old and new theory can not only work together, they can strengthen and inform practice, research, and education. Foundational and existing conceptual models, such as the Model of Human Occupation, Person-Environment-Occupation, and Occupational Adaptation, have firmly situated occupation as the central element of our profession and the core unit of analysis. These theoretical approaches clearly continue to have a relevant and essential role in how we conceptualize, describe, and enact occupation-based evaluations, planning, and intervention procedures. At the same time, in this swift and revolutionary global environment, new ways of thinking about occupation and practice call for emerging and more expansive approaches that consider the interrelatedness and interdependences of physical, biological, psychological, social, and cultural phenomenon (Aldrich, 2008; Fogelberg & Frauwirth, 2010; Gilfoyle, 1984). Furthermore, integration of a systematic framework, such as a complexity theory that examines occupational phenomenon from micro to macro levels, is vital to understandings of larger health and social problems.

Complexity Theory

Complexity theory is grounded in the principles of systems theory. Systems thinkers focus on broader social or institutional dimensions of a given problem in order to understand the relationship of individuals and disciplines. The Model of Human Occupation is an example of a foundational theoretical approach anchored in systems theory. This model understands occupation as a complex and interactive system in which bidirectional change occurs between the individual and the context (Reed & Sanderson, 1999). Yet, according to Fogelberg and Frauwirth (2010), although systems theory is useful in describing, understanding, and modeling occupation, it is limited in analyzing occupation beyond the individual level. Complexity theory expands aspects of systems theory to include the interactional components within the environment or context. Whiteford, Klomp, and Wright-St. Clair (2004) describe complexity within this theory as "the richness and variety of structure and behavior that arises from interactions between components of the system and sources outside of the phenomenon" (p. 5). Sources outside of the phenomenon may be politics, historical context, or means of production. This theoretical approach holds that no action occurs in isolation. Individuals and processes interact to form complex systems. Given its focus on complexity, attention to multilayered contexts and recognition of the diversity of individual behaviors is a part of this framework. Complex systems are inherently unpredictable, thus, they are in a constant state of disequilibrium.

Complexity theory provides occupational therapy with a conceptual model in which to understand phenomena, as well as interconnectedness of individuals and context, social processes, and structural arrangements. Viewed from the lens of occupational therapy, this framework can be employed to examine how human influences and structural arrangements relate to occupational choices, occupational production, and individual interactions within the given system. Similar to the Person-Environment-Occupation Model of Occupational Performance, complexity theory views occupation as a socially mediated and complex phenomenon grounded in and influenced by cultural, social, economic, historic, and political forces. Royeen (2003) employs the term *occupational complexity* to describe the many processes and variables that influence or co-affect one another within the context occupation occurs. Occupational processes are interrelated and evolve over time. Complex systems display constant novelty; and as such, the occupational phenomenon is always unfolding and in transition (Fogelberg & Frauwirth, 2010).

Complexity theory contributes to occupational therapy knowledge and practice by elucidating relationships, influences, and interactions within a system. Moreover, complexity approaches are useful in refining understandings of the impact of social structures and cultural institutions on occupational participation. Aldrich (2008), however, acknowledges the value of complexity theory's challenge to linear models of behavior, although she questions the usefulness of complexity theory in explaining occupational phenomena and understanding notions of occupational behavior. Critiques of this model raise issues concerning occupational therapy's fidelity to complexity theory concepts, its application to non-Western and international environments, and separation of the individual and context within the system. In response to these concerns, Aldrich presents an alternative to complex systems model approaches offering transactionalism as a more comprehensive framework in which to understand occupational behavior.

Transactionalism

Dickie et al. (2006) introduced the notion of transactionalism as an alternative perspective of understanding occupation as well as challenging customary understandings of occupation as an individual experience. Finding that occupation is seldom individual in nature, the authors call for exploration of occupation in a larger context that extends beyond the singular person and views the individual and context as an integrated whole. Based on Dewey's concept of transaction, this approach addresses the nature of phenomena whether it is individuals, occupation, or context on the basis of their relationship with other phenomena. Within this model, phenomena not only interact with other forms or systems, "they move through one another and transact as co-constituted entities" (Aldrich, 2008, p. 151). As ideas surrounding shared and collective occupations further develop, transactional and relational aspects of context and occupation become more essential to theoretical conceptions. Whereas complexity theory separates the study of nature and behavior, transactionalism views context and behavior as symbiotic components (Cutchin as cited in Aldrich, 2008).

Transactionalism, like complexity theory, moves away from linear models of understanding occupation; however, the approaches differ in the location of occupation within the model and relationships between occupation and the actor. An association between transactionalism and the model of Occupational Adaptation can be seen in this existing theory's interaction element of occupational challenge as a situational event that promotes mastery of the desired task or skill (Reed & Sanderson, 1999). The transactional aspect of Sensory Processing theory is noted in the role of sensory modulation in organizing sensory information and in turn contributing to individual–occupation goodness of fit in an adaptive manner (Tomchek & Dunn, 2007). Transactionalism conceptualizes occupation as shaped by the situation in which the actor occupies, shifting the location of occupation from the level of the individual to the level of the situation of which the individual is a constituent part (Dickie et al., 2006). Thus, occupational participation is anchored in the holistic aspects of person–environment interdependence and immersed in contextual factors of the physical, social, cultural, and political local and global community. It is through occupation that the individual and situation experience ongoing change (Dickie et al., 2006).

Occupational Systems Approach

Although occupational therapy's adoption of complexity theory is useful in understanding the relationships between systems and individuals, Fogelberg and Frauwirth (2010) present a broader perspective on occupation and multilevel analysis within the theory. Applying a complexity science approach, the authors focus on occupations within the context of social collectives—groups, communities, and populations. Fogelberg and Frauwirth introduce a framework that has *occupational systems* as its foundation. This perspective is also based on systems theory and contends, "Occupation is central to organization of many social systems and furthermore the production of occupation is distributed among multiple elements of such systems" (p. 134). An occupational system considers not only the influence of the individual on occupation but also addresses external factors on the production of occupation. In concert with systems theory, occupational systems view the occupational actor and the context as integrated in the whole system.

This model aims to advance theory beyond the level of the individual and therefore focuses on collective occupations that are produced, shared, and enacted among multiple individuals at group, community, and population levels. The term **distributive occupations** describe elements that produce occupation distributed among multiple individuals working within a particular system.

Sociocultural Approaches

New definitions and reconceptualization of culture hold critical implications for how we create knowledge, how we understand our clients, and the meaningfulness of our interventions. Iwama (2003) asserts that occupational therapy core values are embedded in Western cultural assumptions that undermine cross-cultural constructs and meanings of occupation. Thus, a more meaningful occupational therapy that is relevant and appropriate to the client's cultural world and local reality is essential.

The work of Bonder, Martin, and Miracle (2004) builds on Iwama's (2003) perspective and emphasizes the importance of the therapist as an interpretive participant in the treatment encounter. Bonder et al. contend that individuals collectively negotiate cultural events, including treatment encounters, through interactions within culturally supported boundaries. Culture is reconfigured as an emergent phenomenon growing out of interactional moments within the therapeutic session. In other words, this approach holds that culture, as it relates to theory and practice of occupational therapy, needs to be understood from the perspectives of those we serve within their contextualized reality. In response, Iwama (2006) developed *The Kawa Model: Culturally Relevant Occupational Therapy.*

Kawa Model

The Kawa Model challenges our profession's ability to evaluate contemporary theory beyond Western-based cultural contexts and assumptions. The Kawa Model defines *culture* as "'shared experiences and common spheres of meaning' and the collective social processes by which distinctions, meanings, categorizations of objects, and phenomenon are created and maintained" (Iwama, 2006, p. 8). This theoretical approach views culture as a particular concept as well as a dynamic process. Cultural meanings vary according to individual's shared understanding and are bound by time and place. Occupation is considered in context with social interactions shaping context. The Kawa Model calls into question occupational therapy's privileging of Western notions of individualism, independence, and ableism. The notions of *cultural relevance and safety* are distinctive attributes of this model. The intention of this model is to develop understandings of client's occupational needs in a complex, holistic, and integrated way and to affirm the inseparability of the individual from context (Iwama, Thomson, Macdonald, 2011).

The image of a river serves as a metaphor for the representation of life in the Kawa Model (Figure 42.1). The river is employed to transmit the complexity surrounding the relationship and integration of self and context. Aspects of self, society, and circumstances are seen as one element, an inseparable whole with all components interrelated and connected. Nature, or context, is viewed to set certain conditions in which particular action or occupation occurs. The surrounding social and physical environment influences the meaning and value ascribed to phenomena or an action. This model focuses on the value of belongingness and interdependence, not unilateral agency and self-determinism. In this worldview, consequences and the impact of particular disability emanate to wider social sphere with the surrounding context enabling or disabling people. Well-being is attributed to the state in which all elements coexist in harmony within the context. The conceptual structure of the Kawa Model is illustrated by the flow of a river. Table 42.1 identifies and describes the components and functions of the model, whereas Figure 42.2 depicts the relationships among the components.

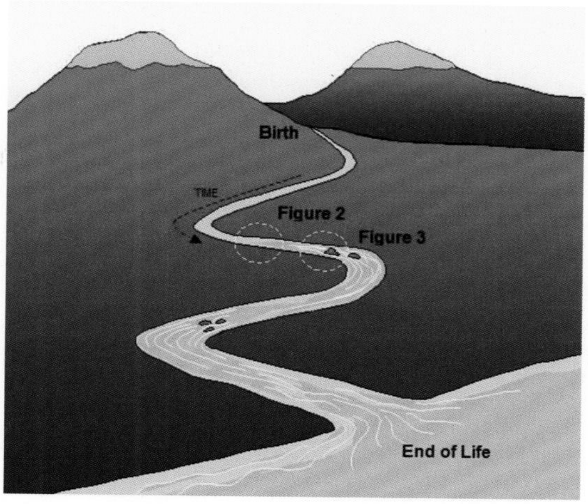

FIGURE 42.1 Life is like a river, flowing from birth to end of life. (From Iwama, M. K. The Kawa Model: Culturally Relevant Occupational Therapy. Oxford, UK: Elsevier Limited, 2006. Used with permission.)

Healthy life flow can be impeded by obstructions (rocks and driftwood) and environmental constrictions (thickening of the river side walls and bottom) as depicted by Figure 42.3. The aim of occupational therapy intervention in this framework is to facilitate and enhance life flow at individual and community levels. The client is viewed as a partner in the intervention process and, in turn, the process values the client's experiences and concerns. Intervention is based on discussions between the therapist, partner, and community. The Kawa Model requires occupational therapy to view and treat occupational issues within a holistic framework that identifies issues as inseparable from their contexts.

Social Field Approaches

As occupational therapy practitioners look toward expanding our roles around collective occupations, inadequacies of the medical model can promote opportunities to gain insights from the social context (Kronenberg, Pollard, &

TABLE 42.1 Kawa Model Components and Functions

Components		**Function/Roles**
Mizu	Water	Represents client's life flow
Kawa no soku and Kawa no zoko	River side wall and river bottom	Structures and concepts in client's environment
Iwa	Rocks	Circumstances that impede client's life flow
Ryuboku	Driftwood	Client's personal attributes and liabilities; values, character, and material assets
Sukima	Space between obstructions	Allows potential channels to determine points of intervention

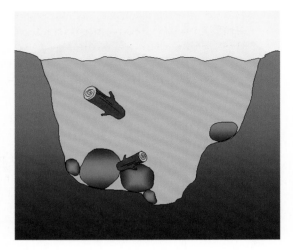

FIGURE 42.2 Cross-section view of the early Kawa Model showing the basic concepts. (From Iwama, M. K. The Kawa Model: Culturally Relevant Occupational Therapy. Oxford, UK: Elsevier Limited, 2006. Used with permission.)

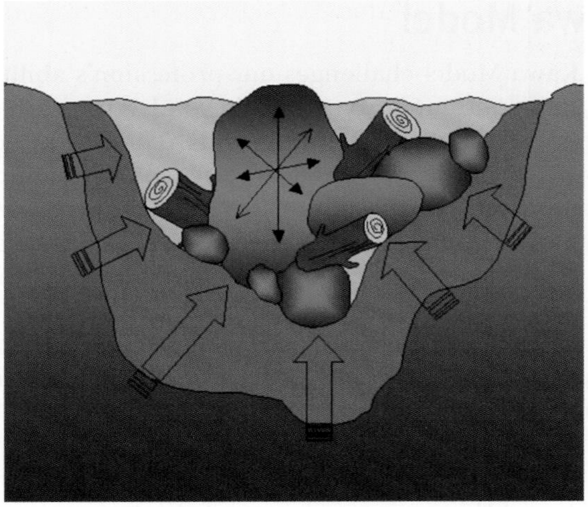

FIGURE 42.3 Cross-section view of a client's Kawa showing the effect of river components on flow. (From Iwama, M. K. The Kawa Model: Culturally Relevant Occupational Therapy. Oxford, UK: Elsevier Limited, 2006. Used with permission.)

Sakellariou, 2011). Galheigo (2011b) maintains that when our profession addresses the needs of individuals or groups who are marginalized, socially excluded, or vulnerable, occupational therapy enters an area of practice that differs from physical rehabilitation and healthcare. As such, theoretical models and practice in the social field may hold alternative views that differ from conventional occupational therapy perspectives. In identifying theoretical limitations of our practice in the social field, Galheigo brings in the work of Pierre Bourdieu to assist in understandings of social life.

Bourdieu's notion of *habitus* views social space as embedded in conflict and social stratification. The social field is dynamic, structured, and organized in networks with members taking on different roles. The dispositions of individuals within the field are acquired through the process of socialization and life experiences. The social space produces and disputes issues and assigns capital and power. Within this view, capital is conceptualized as being social, cultural, political, and symbolic. Access to resources varies depending on individual or group capability to accumulate and make use of capital. Within the social field, the execution of power, or social control, can legitimize the status quo of social stratification or reduce social inequality and promote human rights (Galheigo, 2011a).

Bourdieu's contributions remind occupational therapy of the relationship between the individual and context, drawing our attention to the influence of structural arrangements on social participation. Structural consequences of social stratification and distributive inequality direct our occupational therapy lens to new paradigms with innovative approaches (Pattison, 2011). As occupational therapy practice reaches further into the social context, concepts of service learning and social entrepreneurship can anchor our work with communities, foster alternative practice models, and expand our skill set in community and international development.

Social Entrepreneurship

Growing interest in social entrepreneurship has developed over the past decade. Occupational therapy has applied social entrepreneurship concepts to practice in community-based rehabilitation, disaster preparedness, and response situations (Pattison, 2011). *Social entrepreneurship* is described as variation of business entrepreneurship with the focus on a social mission rather than generating wealth (Katzenstein & Chrispin, 2011). Social entrepreneurs function as change agents for society and focus on the process as well as the outcomes (Katzenstein & Chrispin, 2011; Kronenberg et al., 2011). Efforts are directed toward larger social issues in the local context. Reduction of poverty, access to health care, and services for individuals with disabilities are the types of conditions addressed by social entrepreneurs.

The social entrepreneur is responsible for establishing and sustaining relationships that support the needs of the target population and the success of the program. Aspects of systems and complexity theories ground social entrepreneurship by informing how relationship patterns evolve and sustain themselves. Complexity theory provides the view that organizations evolve as they adapt and interact with other systems. As all things in the organization are interconnected, organizational change emerges from the evolution of the individual and small groups. Hence, an essential role of the social entrepreneur is to identify individuals who will facilitate relationships needed to sustain new patterns of interaction and contribute to the success of the project. In this model, systems theory concepts of interdependent and independent networks allow the organization to center on activities it does best and to partner with other sources where the organization is deficient.

Comparable to Galheigo's (2011b) view of occupational therapy's technical approach to social issues,

Katzenstien and Chrispin (2011) contend that conventional models of development in international contexts do not work "because they stress technical solutions to problems that have their roots in the cultural environment" (p. 10). The literature suggests that *service learning*, a theoretical and educational approach that is grounded in experiential learning, may bridge the gap between technical solutions and cultural understandings.

The Impact of Emerging Theory on Occupational Therapy Practice, Research, and Education

New ways of thinking have the potential to advance and transform the profession of occupational therapy. As occupational therapy practice, research, and education reaches beyond traditional settings, responds to global trends, and broadens our scope of inquiry, emerging theoretical models are needed. These models draw attention to the delivery of culturally relevant occupation-based procedures and the impact of structural and institutional arrangements on occupational choices and service delivery, as well as an enhanced focus on collective occupation. Marilyn Pattison (2011) suggests that new areas of occupational therapy practice and innovative ways of thinking can be viewed as a form of social entrepreneurism that values and addresses social determinants of health and occupational therapy's role in building healthy communities. The following is an illustration of how new formulations of existing and emerging theory can inform practice models and be applied in clinical and community contexts. The Modified Instrumentalism in Occupational Therapy (MIOT) is one example of the transactional relationship between theory and practice.

The Modified Instrumentalism in Occupational Therapy

The MIOT was developed to empower individuals and communities in addressing social challenges through occupational performance (Ikiugu, 2011). The first version of this model, Instrumentalism in Occupational Therapy (IOT), was based on Dewey's pragmatic construct of instrumentalism. This model views the mind as an instrument for adaptation to the environment through occupational performance. The IOT's foundational concept was then revised to achieve better understanding of complex occupational performance and brought in aspects of dynamic systems theory to better address the needs of individuals and the community to identify and alter maladaptive occupational choices. This model guides the process of empowering and sensitizing individuals and communities to enable them to positively influence individual and global events. The MIOT considers the influences of the individual, community, and structure on occupational performance. The MIOT can be applied to a range of social challenges such as poverty or disease. This theoretical approach underscores the complexity in our practice and draws attention to social and cultural aspects of community practice.

Addressing Complexity in Research

The complex nature of occupation and occupational therapy practice has also led to an acknowledgement of the limitations of quantitative research studies. Tomlin and Borgetto (2011) advocate for broader conceptual approaches that relate not only to theory development but to research procedures as well. The researchers propose an alternative hierarchical model, the Research Pyramid. The intent of this model is to foster a more comprehensive integrated approach that values contributions of qualitative procedures in informing judgment-based decision making. The researchers contend that the addition of family narratives, observational participation, and interviews as legitimate data sources can address research complexities such as client perceptions and cultural relevance and enhance understandings of the experiences of our clients. In support of Tomlin and Borgetto's perspective, Law (2010) asserts occupational knowledge is derived from multiple sources including clients' needs and practitioner's wisdom as valuing knowledge from all participants as evidence for practice.

Service Learning

Based on John Dewey's ideas of democratic and public education, service learning is a form of experiential learning. Kolb and Schon further developed Dewey's notion of experiential learning by linking the role of everyday experiences to knowledge creation and reflection to understanding of the experience (Flecky, 2011). Therefore, it is in understanding and transforming the experience that new knowledge is produced (Law, 2010). In alignment with occupational therapy practice, students who engage in service activities learn by doing (Gitlow & Flecky, 2005). Crist (2011) describes service learning as "a structured, community activity where students apply their professional and academic learning to real-world problems or challenges that have been negotiated with a community partner as potentially beneficial or meaningful" (p. 281). A key component of service learning is putting the needs of the community first. Akin to conceptions of occupation, service learning is complex and incorporates diverse theoretical perspectives including critical theory and feminist pedagogy. Albeit, the adoption of multiple theoretical approaches has raised concerns regarding clarity and substance of service learning theoretical foundations (Flecky, 2011).

Service learning allows students to apply classroom theory to community social issues. Partnership within the community affords participants opportunities to engage in social problem solving, understand disability as a multilevel construct, locate professional roles in the larger social context, take on advocacy roles and further advance understandings of cultural interactions (Crist, 2011; Doll, 2011; Flecky & Gitlow, 2011; Gitlow & Flecky, 2005). Service learning is shown to be a valuable approach in teaching health professional concepts of cultural competence (Doll, 2011). Moreover, through service-learning occupational therapy, students can develop knowledge relating to occupation, social justice, and cultural diversity (Law, 2010).

Kronenberg et al. (2011) view service learning as a form of *social responsiveness initiatives.* Social responsiveness is explained as the role of academia in supporting or promoting the public good through active engagement with local communities and constituents. The intent of social responsiveness initiatives is to create and distribute knowledge and demonstrate the application of scholarly activities in addressing social problems. As offered by Mary Law, (2010) occupational therapy has a social responsibility to create and use knowledge consistent with our values. Law also recognizes the benefits of knowledge created within other disciplines in informing occupational therapy theory and practice. In turn, Iwama (2006) questions our profession's ambition to engage in transdisciplinary and global discourse stating "as post-modernism discourse of social constructionism and cultural relativism take greater hold in the social sciences and find their way to occupational therapy . . . it might be simply a matter of time before the profession realizes and embraces a more diverse and socially just regard for its theory" (p. 229).

Occupational Therapy Case Studies

Case studies 42.1 and 42.2 are presented to provoke new ways of thinking about relationships between emerging theory, context, and practice. For each case study, please respond to the following questions.

1. What are the contextual factors that restrain, support, or influence the client's occupational participation?
2. Identify emerging theories or approaches that are useful in understanding the client's occupational performance and social participation in the particular context?
3. How may the selected theoretical approach influence intervention priorities and goals?

CASE STUDY 42.1 Ben—Cultural Safety and Occupational Deprivation

Ben is a 40-year-old man of Asian descent living in a large urban shelter in northeast United States. Ben has lived in the shelter for 5 years, even though the local government has imposed a 9-month limit on shelter stays. Due to his loss of immigration documents, he is the longest dwelling resident at the shelter. Ben came to the United States when he was 17 years of age. His family sent him to the United States when he began to display paranoid behaviors. He has the diagnosis of paranoid schizophrenia. Ben is fluent in English, and he obtained a bachelor's degree in business management. He has worked in restaurant services, office jobs, and data management for short intervals. Ben has little insight into his condition and difficulty with self-care. He requires reminders to groom and change his clothes. Ben wakes early to take his shower privately. He believes his difficulties with socialization and time management are related to not having a job. Ben spends a lot of time alone walking around the building or engaged in passive solitary activities. He says that he just sits on his bed and does nothing before he goes to bed. Ben performs tasks at a slow pace and often takes naps in the afternoon. He exhibits good use of knowledge but does not always inquire for additional information when needed. He is hesitant to initiate conversations.

CASE STUDY 42.2 Belkis—Accessing Resources for Child: Agency and Context

Belkis lives with her family in the countryside of Cuba. Her family includes her husband, 3-year-old daughter, and 11-year-old son. Belkis is 33 years old and has completed a preuniversity program. She describes her 3-year-old daughter with spastic diplegia cerebral palsy as spontaneous, smart, and difficult at times. Belkis learned about her daughter's condition when the child was 9 months old. Belkis explains her daughter's condition as "a brain lesion that will not get better or worse." Belkis envisions her child doing things for herself and walking. To attain this vision, Belkis puts all her faith in the expert therapists, does the assigned exercises daily, and gives her child everything. She lacks access to resources and does not value the way resources can be attained through institutional arrangements. Belkis wants to have parallel bars in her home. Her family in the United States has sent a therapy ball and a stroller for her daughter. A community friend referred Belkis to a wheelchair organization though she was not eligible to receive the equipment. When asked if she could make a difference in daughter's progress, Belkis just shrugged.

Conclusion

As occupational therapy ventures into novel and complex contexts, broader theories that are multilevel, culturally relevant, and counter the dominant discourse are required to promote diversity of thought, innovation in practice, and retain the relevance of occupational therapy in health, educational, and social sectors. The development of political competence skills is essential to our profession's capability to remain relevant in health and social discourses and to work with problems generated by social, political, economic, and environmental contexts. Pollard, Sakellariou, and Kronenberg (2009) describes political competence as a mixture of experience and use of analytical tools to assess information within a multiperspective environment.

New theories and practice approaches are needed that expand occupational therapy roles in local, global, and political landscapes. As occupational therapy theories and practice are reconceptualized, a wider appreciation of global and social responsibility and principles of occupational justice is needed to meet the challenges of poverty and inequality relating to class, race, and gender.

Issues that remain unresolved are occupational therapy philosophy as unified and universal or local and contextualized, professional identity as the generic practitioner or the highly specialized clinician, allegiance to the dominant medical model or professional autonomy, and valuing clinical wisdom and client narratives or the insistence on empirical evidence in the production of occupational therapy knowledge. As occupational therapy practitioners debate the direction of the profession, hopefully, we will choose to adopt an attitude of forward thinking, value diverse perspectives, and support professional autonomy as our practice, student training, and theoretical approaches develop and evolve in the ever-changing global community.

References

Aldrich, R. M. (2008). From complexity theory to transactionalism: Moving occupational science forward in theorizing the complexities of behavior. *Journal of Occupational Science, 13*, 147–156.

Bonder, B. R., Martin, L., & Miracle, A. W. (2004). Culture emergent in occupation. *American Journal of Occupational Therapy, 58*, 159–168.

Crist, P. (2011). Involve me and I understand: Differentiating service-learning and fieldwork. In K. Flecky & L. Gitlow (Eds.), *Service-learning in occupational therapy education: Philosophy and practice* (pp. 275–288). Boston, MA: Jones and Bartlett.

Dickie, V., Cutchin, M. P., & Humphry, R. (2006). Occupation as transactional experience: A critique of individualism in occupational science. *Journal of Occupational Science, 13*, 83–93.

Doll, J. D. (2011). Cross-cultural service-learning: An introduction and best practices. In K. Flecky & L. Gitlow (Eds.), *Service-learning in occupational therapy education: philosophy and practice* (pp. 59–86). Boston, MA: Jones and Bartlett.

Flecky, K. (2011). Foundations of service learning. In K. Flecky & L. Gitlow (Eds.), *Service-learning in occupational therapy education: philosophy and practice* (pp. 1–18). Boston, MA: Jones and Bartlett.

Flecky, K., & Gitlow, L. (Eds.). (2011). *Service-learning in occupational therapy education: philosophy and practice.* Boston, MA: Jones and Bartlett.

Fogelberg, D., & Frauwirth, S. (2010). Complexity science approach to occupation: Moving beyond the individual. *Journal of Occupational Science, 17*, 131–139.

Galheigo, S. M. (2011a). Occupational therapy in the social field: Concepts and critical considerations. In F. Kronenberg, N. Pollard, & D. Sakellariou (Eds.), *Occupational therapies without borders: Vol. 2. Towards an ecology of occupation-based practice* (pp. 47–56). London, United Kingdom: Churchill Livingstone Elsevier.

Galheigo, S. M. (2011b). What needs to be done? Occupational therapy responsibilities and challenges regarding human rights. *Australian Occupational Therapy Journal*, 58, 60–66.

Gilfoyle, E. (1984). Transformation of a profession. *American Journal of Occupational Therapy, 38*, 575–584.

Gitlow, L., & Flecky, K. (2005). Integrating disability concepts into occupational therapy education using service learning. *American Journal of Occupational Therapy*, 58, 546–553.

Ikiugu, M. N. (2011). Influencing social challenges through occupational performance. In F. Kronenberg, N. Pollard, & D. Sakellariou (Eds.), *Occupational therapies without borders: Vol. 2. Towards an ecology of occupation-based practice* (pp 113–122). London, United Kingdom: Churchill Livingstone Elsevier.

Inayatullah, S. (2007). Alternative futures of occupational therapy and therapists. *Journal of Future Studies, 11*, 41–58.

Iwama, M. K. (2003). Toward culturally relevant epistemologies in occupational therapy. *American Journal of Occupational Therapy, 57*, 582–588.

Iwama, M. K. (2006). *The Kawa model: Culturally relevant occupational therapy.* Toronto, Canada: Churchill Livingstone Elsevier.

Iwama, M. K., Thomson, N. A., & Macdonald, R. M. (2011). Situated meaning: A matter of cultural safety, inclusion and occupational therapy. In F. Kronenberg, N. Pollard, & D. Sakellariou (Eds.), *Occupational therapies without borders: Vol. 2. Towards an ecology of occupation-based practice* (pp. 85–92). London, United Kingdom: Churchill Livingstone Elsevier.

Katzenstein, J., & Chrispin, B. (2011). Social entrepreneurship and a new model for international development in the 21st century. *Journal of Developmental Entrepreneurship*, 16, 87–102. Retrieved from http://econpapers.repec.org/article/w8ijd

Kronenberg, F., Pollard, N., & Sakellariou, D. (Eds.). (2011). *Occupational therapies without borders: Vol. 2. Towards an ecology of occupation-based practice.* London, United Kingdom: Churchill Livingstone Elsevier.

Law, M. (2010). Learning by doing: Creating knowledge for occupational therapy. *WFOT Bulletin, 62*, 12–18.

Pattison, M. (2011). Foreword. In F. Kronenberg, N. Pollard, & D. Sakellariou (Eds.), *Occupational therapies without borders: Vol. 2. Towards an ecology of occupation-based practice* (pp. 133–142). London, United Kingdom: Churchill Livingstone Elsevier.

Polkinghorne, D. (2004). *Practice and the human sciences: The case for a judgment base practice of care.* In L. Fazio (Ed.), *Developing occupation-centered programs for the community.* Upper Saddle River, NJ: Pearson Prentice Hall.

Pollard, N., Sakellariou, D., & Kronenberg, F. (Eds.). (2009). Political competence in occupational therapy. In *A political practice of occupational therapy* (pp. 21–38). London, United Kingdom: Churchill Livingstone Elsevier.

Reed, K. L., & Sanderson, S. N. (1999). *Concepts of occupational therapy* (4th ed.). Philadelphia, PA: Lippincott Williams & Wilkins

Royeen, C. B. (2003). Chaotic occupational therapy: Collective wisdom for a complex profession, 2003 Eleanor Clarke Slagle lecture. *American Journal of Occupational Therapy, 57*, 609–624.

Sinclair, K. (2009). Working for the future of occupational therapy: Strategic activities of the World Federation of Occupational Therapists. *TOG, 6*, 1–11. Retrieved from http://www.revistatog.com

Thew, M., Edwards, M., Baptiste, S., & Molineux, M. (2011). *Role emerging occupational therapy: Maximising occupation-focused practice*. West Sussex, United Kingdom: Wiley-Blackwell.

Tomchek, S. D., & Dunn, W. (2007). Sensory processing in children with and without autism: A comparative study using the Short Sensory Profile. *American Journal of Occupational Therapy, 61*, 190–200.

Tomlin, G., & Borgetto, B. (2011). Research pyramid: A new evidence based-practice model for occupational therapy. *American Journal of Occupational Therapy, 65*, 189–196.

Whiteford, G., Klomp, N., & Wright-St. Clair, V. (2004). Complexity theory: Understanding occupation, practice and context. In G. Whiteford & V. Wright-St. Clair (Eds.), *Occupation and practice in context* (pp. 3–15). Sydney, Australia: Elsevier.

Whiteford, G., & Townsend, E. (2011). Participatory occupational justice framework (POJF 2010): Enabling occupational participation and inclusion. In F. Kronenberg, N. Pollard, & D. Sakellariou (Eds.), *Occupational therapies without borders: Vol. 2. Towards an ecology of occupation-based practice* (pp. 65–84). London, United Kingdom: Churchill Livingstone Elsevier.

For additional resources on the subjects discussed in this chapter, visit http://thePoint.lww.com/Willard-Spackman12e.

Broad Theories Informing Practice

UNIT X

"Whether you can observe a thing or not depends on the theory which you use.

It is the theory which decides what can be observed.

—Albert Einstein

CHAPTER 43

Recovery Model

Terry Krupa

OUTLINE

LEARNING OBJECTIVES

After reading this chapter, you will be able to:

1. Describe contemporary perspectives on recovery in the mental health field
2. Identify elements or components of the recovery process
3. Integrate various frameworks or models of the recovery process
4. Apply recovery-oriented principles in occupational therapy practice

Introduction

> The concept of recovery is rooted in the simple and yet profound realization that people who have been diagnosed with mental illness are human beings . . . The goal is to become the unique, awesome, never to be repeated human being that we are called to be. Those of us who have been labeled with mental illness are not de facto excused from this fundamental task of becoming human. In fact, because many of us have experienced our lives and dreams shattered in the wake of mental illness, one of the most essential challenges that face us is to ask who can I become and why should I say yes to life. (Deegan, 1996, p. 92)

This opening quote is by Patricia Deegan, who is widely credited with coining the term "recovery" to describe the phenomena whereby people come to live rich and meaningful lives despite experiencing mental illness. As a person with lived experience of mental illness, Deegan provides a powerful real-life example of how recovery can unfold within a life situation characterized by despair, isolation, and deprivation. Deegan has poignantly described how mental health service providers have the power to be either insensitive and hardened or enabling and supportive of the struggles that people with mental illness experience in determining "who to become" and in "saying yes to life." Indeed, becoming familiar with the range of Deegan's writings and speeches might be considered foundational

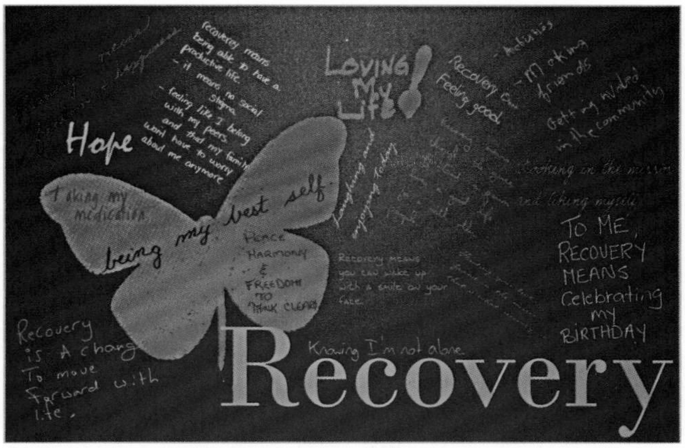
Hope
LOVING MY LIFE!
being my best self
TO ME, RECOVERY MEANS Celebrating my BIRTHDAY
Knowing I'm not alone
Recovery

FIGURE 43.1 Recovery-oriented services create a vision of recovery that includes the voices of people served.

knowledge for occupational therapists learning about recovery (see for example, Deegan, 1988, 1990, 1996, 2001).

In this chapter, the reader is introduced to recovery as it is evolving in the mental health field. Multiple perspectives on recovery are presented, but particular emphasis is placed on the perspectives of people with lived experience of mental illness (Figure 43.1). The recovery construct is not free of debate in the mental health field. Understanding the controversy surrounding recovery can position occupational therapists to better evaluate their own practice and to contribute to the ongoing evolution of the recovery vision. This chapter begins with the definitions of recovery. Conceptual frameworks and models of recovery are then presented. These are followed by a discussion of recovery in practice that reviews recovery intervention programs and issues related to evaluation. In the final section of this chapter, the relationship between recovery and occupational therapy are discussed.

Defining Recovery

Recovery as a Personal Life Journey

In this chapter, **recovery** is defined as a process experienced by people with mental illness whereby they come to a life that is defined less by illness and pathology and defined more by a personal sense of purpose, agency and control, and active participation in valued and meaningful activities (Noordsy et al., 2002). The understanding of recovery as a *process* is important; it denotes an ongoing personal life journey, rather than an endpoint, or some final outcome. As with everyone's life journey, it suggests that there will be ups and downs, high points and low points, and successes and failures. Yet the overarching expectation is that the journey of recovery will provide opportunities for greater well-being, positive growth, and community participation.

This definition of recovery also highlights that the process of recovery belongs to, and is the personal responsibility of, people with mental illness themselves. It is consistent with what Slade (2009) has referred to as "personal recovery." Deegan stresses that service providers are not responsible for making people recover, but they can play an important role by creating conditions that will invite people to engage in the recovery journey and to negotiate the struggles that will inevitably present (Deegan, 1988, 1996).

Conflicting Perspectives on Recovery

Recovery has gained international prominence as a guiding vision for the development of mental health services and systems. Yet, despite its influence, confusion persists; and there is no guarantee that discussions about recovery in mental health will start from a shared agreement about its meaning. The Practice Dilemma illustrates

Practice Dilemma

Shandra, an occupational therapist, works for a community mental health program that is focused on helping people with serious mental illness to live successfully in the community. At their annual retreat, the agency set aside time to discuss practices related to employment and other vocational or productive activities. Shandra examined the employment and productivity participation of the people receiving services and informed the team that fewer than 15% of the 90 people served identified any regular involvement in productivity activities such as work, school, or volunteering. During the ensuing discussion, team members made comments such as "the people we serve are too sick to work," "we don't have the time or resources to focus on work—that isn't our job," "no one I work with has said they want to work" and "work will make their symptoms flare up." The team encouraged Shandra to follow up on her interest in employment and productivity but left the discussions without any firm plans for follow-up.

Questions

1. Evaluate the service response to the issue of employment and productivity with respect to contemporary perspectives on recovery.
2. Shandra decides to give some thought to how she might respond to this discussion, so that she can facilitate a shift to more recovery-oriented services. What might she say to challenge the idea that addressing employment and productivity is not within the scope of the service?
3. The practice dilemma does not reflect the voices of people with mental illness. How might Shandra engage their involvement in this discussion about employment and productivity?

divergent views on the meaning of recovery and expectations regarding participation in occupations for persons with mental illness.

Clinical versus Personal Perspectives on Recovery

Definitions of recovery that have emerged from mental health professionals have tended to focus on the amelioration of the mental illness, evidenced by symptom remission and the reduction in the need for intensive treatment services. Slade (2009) refers to this as a definition of "recovery as cure" and distinguishes it as a clinical perspective on recovery rather than the personal perspective of recovery that emerges from people with lived experience. Davidson and Roe (2007) suggest that *clinical interpretations* are perhaps best described as "recovery from mental illness," whereas *personal interpretations* are best described as "being in recovery." The ongoing confusion between personal and clinical definitions of recovery has historical roots. It is occurring within a mental health system that has long been dominated by biomedical perspectives on illness.

The assumption underlying the clinical perspective is that illness management is central to recovery and occurs in the context of treatments—treatments that are largely developed and offered by mental health professionals who have expertise. The assumptions underlying personal recovery—that people with mental illness can be largely in control of managing their illnesses, that effective illness management strategies exist outside the realm of the authority of mental health professionals, and that people with mental illness can enjoy a life of inclusion in their communities—has been largely overlooked and, at worst, depreciated. Davidson, Rakfeldt, and Strauss (2010), in their study of the historical roots of the recovery movement, point out that although other branches of health care have largely accepted that people who experience chronic forms of disease or significant disability should not "put their lives on hold until the illness resolves" (p. 4), this notion has not received the same broad acceptance in the mental health service arena.

Recovery as a Citizenship Movement

Another perspective on recovery, although perhaps less prevalent, is the argument that definitions of recovery have been highly individualistic and ultimately unable to integrate the influence of exceptional levels of disadvantage and marginalization that characterize the social position of people with mental illness. From this perspective, it is argued that people with mental illness in their recovery process encounter injustices embedded within social structures, such as discrimination, oppressive public policies, and social segregation. Social perspectives on recovery highlight the extent to which the daily lives of people with serious mental illness are characterized by conditions of social and economic poverty, marginalization, and stigma. There is evidence to support that these social and financial strains will have a negative impact on the recovery process (Mattson, Topor, Cullberg, & Forsell, 2008). From this social perspective, recovery is conceptualized as a civil rights movement focused on securing full citizenship rights and responsibilities for people with mental illness.

The Definition Matters

More than a play of words, the definition of recovery does matter—a great deal. With recovery being adapted as a guiding vision for mental health services in many jurisdictions, the definition selected will ultimately influence how human and material resources are distributed, how success in the system will be evaluated, and what kinds of service activities and supports will be expected.

The perspective of personal recovery offers an important opportunity for a fundamental transformation in the mental health service arena toward a integrated system that is able to address illness, health, well-being, and citizenship in a synergistic fashion. In response to this challenge, efforts have been directed to describing how the concepts and ideals of personal recovery can be translated to reform service delivery and service systems, avoiding the very real risk that conflicting perspectives on recovery will lead to the conclusion that only small tweaks are required or worse, that recovery-oriented practices are already in place. For example, Tondora and Davidson (2006) and Davidson et al., (2007) have advanced practice guidelines to direct the development of recovery-oriented services and to identify what people in recovery should expect from the mental health service system.

Recovery Frameworks or Models

To date, no single theory or conceptual model of recovery has been developed and accepted, but the mental health field is replete with systematic efforts to capture critical elements of an overarching framework for recovery. Empirically constructed conceptualizations of the personal recovery process incorporate a common understanding of the components or elements of the recovery process and the phases and tasks central to the process.

Elements of the Recovery Process

Based on an analysis of published qualitative accounts of recovery, Davidson (2005) identified and described elements that appear common to the experience of the recovery process, including

- Renewing hope and commitment,
- Redefining self,
- Incorporating illness,
- Being involved in meaningful activities,
- Overcoming stigma,

- Assuming control,
- Becoming empowered,
- Exercising citizenship,
- Managing symptoms, and
- Being supported by others.

The elements provide an understanding of the nature of the personal transformations that are experienced in the recovery process. The renewal of hope provides the individual with a growing sense that the future holds possibilities. The individual develops a growing sense that the illness need not be the defining feature of one's identity; there are other stories about the self that are waiting to be explored and developed. A transition from passive acceptance of circumstances to a growing sense of control and personal agency occurs. The illness experience is not ignored but becomes integrated into this broader view of the self and the self in the world. The sense of personal agency, or self-determination, is extended to developing a personal understanding of the illness that supports these processes of growth and change and the development of strategies to manage the illness experience. The critical elements include actions that connect the individual to living a full life in the broader community.

The 10 components of recovery identified in the *National Consensus Statement on Mental Health Recovery* by the U.S. Substance Abuse and Mental Health Services Administration (SAMHSA; 2006) have similarities to those proposed by Davidson (2005) but are written more from a perspective that guides mental health service delivery and the design of service systems (see Box 43.1). The components highlight important elements of the mental health service system, such as peer support. At its core,

BOX 43.1 National Consensus Statement on Mental Health Recovery: The 10 Fundamental Components of Recovery

Self-direction: Consumers lead, control, exercise choice over, and determine their own path of recovery by optimizing autonomy, independence, and control of resources to achieve a self-determined life. By definition, the recovery process must be self-directed by the individual, who defines his or her own life goals and designs a unique path toward those goals.

Individualized and person centered: There are multiple pathways to recovery based on an individual's unique strengths and resiliencies as well as his or her needs, preferences, experiences (including past trauma), and cultural background in all of its diverse representations. Individuals also identify recovery as being an ongoing journey and an end result as well as an overall paradigm for achieving wellness and optimal mental health.

Empowerment: Consumers have the authority to choose from a range of options and to participate in all decisions—including the allocation of resources—that will affect their lives, and are educated and supported in so doing. They have the ability to join with other consumers to collectively and effectively speak for themselves about their needs, wants, desires, and aspirations. Through empowerment, an individual gains control of his or her own destiny and influences the organizational and societal structures in his or her life.

Holistic: Recovery encompasses an individual's whole life, including mind, body, spirit, and community. Recovery embraces all aspects of life, including housing, employment, education, mental health and health care treatment and services, complementary and alternative health services, addictions treatment, spirituality, creativity, social networks, community participation, and family supports as determined by the person. Families, providers, organizations, systems, communities, and society play crucial roles in creating and maintaining meaningful opportunities for consumer access to these supports.

Nonlinear: Recovery is not a step-by-step process but one based on continual growth, occasional setbacks, and learning from experience. Recovery begins with an initial stage of awareness in which a person recognizes that positive change is possible. This awareness enables the consumer to move on to fully engage in the work of recovery.

Strengths-based: Recovery focuses on valuing and building on the multiple capacities, resiliencies, talents, coping abilities, and inherent worth of individuals. By building on these strengths, consumers leave stymied life roles behind and engage in new life roles (e.g., partner, caregiver, friend, student, employee). The process of recovery moves forward through interaction with others in supportive, trust-based relationships.

Peer support: Mutual support—including the sharing of experiential knowledge and skills and social learning—plays an invaluable role in recovery. Consumers encourage and engage other consumers in recovery and provide each other with a sense of belonging, supportive relationships, valued roles, and community.

Respect: Community, systems, and societal acceptance and appreciation of consumers—including protecting their rights and eliminating discrimination and stigma—are crucial in achieving recovery. Self-acceptance and regaining belief in one's self are particularly vital. Respect ensures the inclusion and full participation of consumers in all aspects of their lives.

Responsibility: Consumers have a personal responsibility for their own self-care and journeys of recovery. Taking steps toward their goals may require great courage. Consumers must strive to understand and give meaning to their experiences and identify coping strategies and healing processes to promote their own wellness.

Hope: Recovery provides the essential and motivating message of a better future—that people can and do overcome the barriers and obstacles that confront them. Hope is internalized but can be fostered by peers, families, friends, providers, and others. Hope is the catalyst of the recovery process. Mental health recovery not only benefits individuals with mental health disabilities by focusing on their abilities to live, work, learn, and fully participate in our society but also enriches the texture of American community life. America reaps the benefits of the contributions individuals with mental disabilities can make, ultimately becoming a stronger and healthier nation.

Adapted from Substance Abuse and Mental Health Services Administration. (2006). *National consensus statement on mental health recovery*. Rockville, MD: U.S. Department of Health and Human Services. Retrieved from http://store.samhsa.gov/shin/content//SMA05-4129/SMA05-4129.pdf

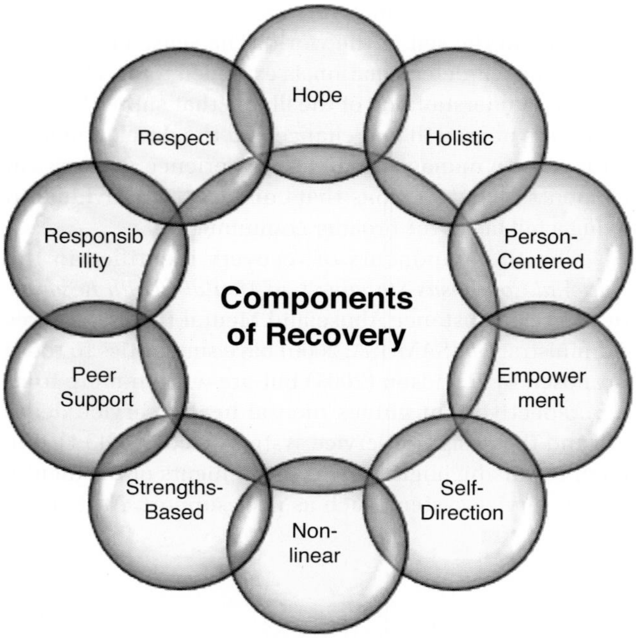

FIGURE 43.2 A synergistic model of recovery.

the recovery process reflects a release of strengths and a growth of abilities, capacities, and possibilities that should be valued and nurtured by others. All of the components are interdependent and act synergistically toward the goal of recovery (see Figure 43.2). The consensus statement concludes with a very powerful statement that recovery benefits not only the individual in recovery but also society.

Stage and Task Models of Recovery

There have been several efforts to understand how the recovery process unfolds and how the various defined elements of the process are related to each other over time. These have led to the development of several stage models of the process, largely developed empirically from persons in recovery (see Andresen, Oades, & Caputi, 2003 for an integrated review of several stage models).

One such model was developed by people with lived experience of mental illness who are considered leaders across the United States in their roles as members of a Recovery Advisory Group (Ralph, 2005). They described a six-stage model of the recovery process: (1) anguish, described as an experience of despair related to the accepted label of "mentally ill"; (2) awakening, reflecting the beginning sense that things can change; (3) insight, or the growing understanding and personalization of possibilities of change; (4) action planning, reflecting the increase in doing toward well-being and meaning; (5) determined commitment to become well, describing the growing resolution for action and self-determination; and (6) well-being and empowerment, an experience of belief in the self to help the self and others. A particularly helpful feature of the model is the inclusion of specific domains of change—four internal (occurring within the self) and four external (responses or actions)—and descriptions of changes that occur in these domains across the six stages.

Although stage models advance our understanding and provide empirical support for the recovery process, they are inherently problematic. If we are to conceptualize recovery as an individual and nonlinear process, then how can defining moments of the recovery process be ordered in any sort of generalizable way? The field will need to evaluate how stage models capture the range of expressions of recovery.

In contrast to stage models, Slade (2009) proposed a model of recovery based on the tasks that people are engaged in over the course of the recovery process. The tasks are highly consistent with empirically derived elements of recovery; account for recovery as both an internal process and a process that is positioned within a larger social environment; and are only loosely ordered, acknowledging considerable individual variability. The four tasks include (1) developing a positive identity—developing a multifaceted view of a valued sense of self, (2) framing the mental illness—making sense of the illness experience as an important challenge to be negotiated within the context of important broader life experiences, (3) self-managing the illness—developing expertise in controlling the experience of mental illness, and (4) developing valued social roles—connecting to others and the broader world through personally and socially valued activities.

Recovery in Practice

Evaluating Recovery

The complexity of the recovery process extends to design and methodological issues related to research and evaluation. If, for example, recovery is an ongoing process, how can any meaningful outcome associated with recovery be conceptualized and evaluated? How can we reconcile the notion of recovery as a process experienced and owned by people with mental illness within a health care system (and research funding system) that highly values controlled trials, researcher objectivity, and quantified results?

People with mental illness have long been concerned that innovations in practice and advances in research have largely occurred without their input and voice. The popular slogan "Nothing about us without us" became a sort of rallying call against a mental health system that did not, in any meaningful way, include the voices of the people it served. The understanding of recovery as a personal journey experienced and owned by people with mental illness has advanced this movement because it has relied on first-person narratives of the lived experience. This has led to a greater understanding of the value of the experiential knowledge of people who live with mental illness and has subsequently contributed to the growth of valued, formal peer support services in the mental health system and the development of research relationships with people in recovery that engage them to a varying extent—from seeking their perspectives to involving them as coresearchers (Figure 43.3).

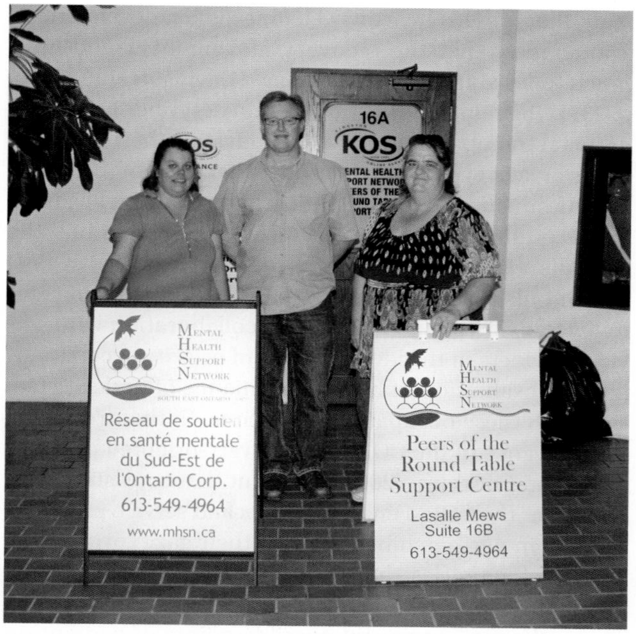

FIGURE 43.3 Peer involvement including formal peer support services are a critical element of a recovery oriented service system.

Advances in the conceptual development of recovery are providing a good foundation for advancing evaluation. A wide array of measures to evaluate individual recovery have now been developed and been subject to psychometric testing. Most measures are self-report measures, such as the Recovery Process Inventory (Jerrell, Cousins, & Roberts, 2006) which asks people with mental illness to rate themselves on six dimensions (anguish, connection to others, confidence or purpose, others care or help, living situation, and hopeful). Many of these measurement tools are available electronically on the web and are not subject to restrictive copyright rules (see for example, Campbell-Orde, Chamberlin, Carpenter, & Leff, 2005).

In addition to generic measures of recovery, evaluation can be designed to focus on particular elements of the recovery process. For example, it is widely accepted that a fundamental shift in agency occurs in the recovery process whereby individuals with mental illness move from attitudes and behaviors that reflect passivity, internalized stigma, the absence of expectations, and helplessness to positions of control and a growing sense of expectations for the self in the larger world. With this in mind, evaluators may choose to focus on the changing sense of empowerment within the recovery process and use established measures such as the Empowerment Scale (Rogers, Chamberlin, Ellison, & Crean, 1997)—a self-report scale developed by individuals with mental illness, which operationalizes the many dimensions of empowerment in 28 items reflecting five factors of self-efficacy and self-esteem, power and powerlessness, community activism, righteous anger, and optimism toward the future.

Remembering that the personal journey of recovery occurs within a larger mental health care context, recovery-related evaluation has also been directed to operationalizing and measuring the shifts expected within this context. Clear descriptions of how programs and services are structured and administered within a recovery-oriented system have contributed to the ability to evaluate system change. For example, the Recovery Self-Assessment (RSA) tool has been used to engage services in adopting a recovery orientation (O'Connell, Tondora, Evans, Croog, & Davidson, 2005). Similarly, shifts in service provider knowledge and practice are expected, and this has included the clear articulation of recovery competencies or the attitudes, knowledge, and behaviors expected from providers in a recovery-oriented system. In New Zealand, for example, a set of recovery competencies was developed for all mental health service providers to inform the development of standards in care (Mental Health Commission, 2001). With the development of evaluation tools such as the Recovery Knowledge Inventory (RKI) (Bedregal, O'Connell, & Davidson, 2006), changes in provider attitudes and knowledge about recovery can be evaluated over time.

Recovery Approaches and Strategies

Various intervention approaches and strategies have been developed in response to the growing understanding of the recovery process. Evidence demonstrating the effectiveness of these strategies is emerging. Generally, these intervention approaches attempt to operationalize key elements of recovery-oriented practice. The *Recovery Workbook* (Spaniol, Koehler, & Hutchinson, 1994) takes individuals with mental illness through a series of activities meant to increase their awareness of recovery, increase their knowledge about and control of psychiatric conditions, understand the importance of stress, build a meaningful and enjoyable life and personal supports, and begin to develop sustained plans of action. A pilot research study, using a randomized controlled trial design, evaluated the effectiveness of a modified version of the workbook that shortened the 30 weekly sessions to 12 sessions. Findings suggested that participants experienced positive changes in perceived levels of hope, empowerment, and general measures of recovery (Barbic, Krupa, & Armstrong, 2009). The well-known *Wellness Recovery Action Plan* (Copeland, 1997) engages people with mental illness in activities designed to identify and implement personalized wellness strategies and raise awareness of benefits of peer support. A large-scale study using randomized controlled trials demonstrated positive changes in experiences of psychiatric symptoms, increased levels of hopefulness, and enhanced quality of life (Cook et al., 2012). Finally, the Illness Management and Recovery intervention program uses a series of activities based on five practices for teaching illness self-management, including psychoeducation, behavioral training focused on integrating medications into daily routines, relapse prevention planning, coping skills training, and social skills training to enhance social support (Gingerich & Mueser, 2005). A randomized controlled trial of the intervention program suggested that participants experienced improvements in illness self-management, as evaluated by both self and clinician ratings (Levitt et al., 2009).

Recovery and Occupational Therapy

Recovery-oriented practice is not considered the domain of any one discipline or professional group. Rather, efforts to instill a recovery-oriented vision in our mental health systems have depended on all providers to consider their own practice with respect to the evolving understanding of recovery processes. The relationship between recovery and occupational therapy is reciprocal. Occupational therapy can contribute to the growing knowledge and evidence base of recovery, and recovery concepts can inform occupational therapy practice.

Many occupational therapists have actively contributed to efforts to realize the vision of recovery in the mental health services sector. They have served as study investigators on research advancing our understanding of recovery. Occupational therapists have been hired to serve as recovery facilitators to assist mental health organizations in achieving the difficult transformation to recovery-oriented care. Occupational therapists have worked in close collaboration with groups of individuals with lived experience to advocate for and implement structures that ensure their meaningful involvement in creating recovery-oriented practices, services, and systems.

Of particular interest in this chapter, however, is the consideration of how the distinct knowledge and practice base of the occupational therapy profession might contribute to the ongoing evolution of recovery. From this perspective, the question engages occupational therapists in considering how their particular focus on their domain of concern—occupation—can advance recovery knowledge and practice. The connection between occupation and recovery is fairly explicit, given that participation in personally and socially meaningful activities and roles has been considered a critical element of the recovery process. Davidson and colleagues (2010) in their history of the roots of the recovery movement, express that participation in the everyday but meaningful activities of daily life is not the outcome of recovery but rather the foundation of recovery. Consistent with occupational therapy theory and practice, the authors contend that the recovery process can be positively influenced by the actual doing of activities, particularly when supported by others in their engagement in occupations. Lamenting the loss of attention to activity-based approaches within the mental health service system with the closure of psychiatric hospitals, they suggest, "There currently are glimmers of hope that the recovery movement may bring about a bit of renaissance of occupational therapy and science within psychiatry" and state they would "heartily welcome such a development, and suggest that the recovery movement would have much to learn from this discipline" (Davidson et al., 2010, p. 237). The remainder of this section describes how occupational therapists have or could advance their expertise in the area of occupation to further the vision of recovery.

Although goal identification and planning has been an integral element of several recovery interventions, the Canadian Occupational Performance Measure (COPM) (Law et al, 1990) is a client-centered tool that engages individuals with mental illness in collaboration with service providers in the identification of priority occupations and the evaluation of both performance of and satisfaction with these occupations over time. In their review of the relevance of the COPM to recovery-oriented practice, Kirsh and Cockburn (2009) point out that consistent with recovery, "the COPM enables clients and service providers to work in partnership and direct their gaze towards the roles and activities that compromise people's identity, enhancing opportunities for self-actualization" (p. 174). The authors raise several possible points of contention surrounding the COPM, including concerns about its sensitivity to diversity and culturally specific occupations, as well as the susceptibility of clients to the perspectives of clinicians even in the context of interactions that are meant to be collaborative. These are not concerns exclusive to the COPM but rather reflect healthy critical discourse that should underlie all recovery practice.

A recent systematic review of occupation- or activity-based interventions examines the extent to which these interventions lead to positive changes in areas of community integration and normative life roles for adults with serious mental illness (Gibson, D'Amico, Jaffe, & Arbesman, 2011). The study considered a range of interventions from training in social skills to instrumental activities of daily living (IADL) and life skills training and role development. Not all interventions were developed specifically by occupational therapists (e.g., supported employment and education and neurocognitive training), but all interventions were considered within the occupational therapy scope of practice. The review suggested that the evidence for social skills training was strong, whereas the evidence supporting the effectiveness of neurocognitive training paired with skills training across domains of occupational performance and training in life skills and IADL was only moderate. The review provides a valuable summary of evidence-based, occupation-focused interventions and perhaps offers a prototype for how a range of seemingly disparate interventions might be organized conceptually within the framework of recovery.

People with mental illness frequently experience profound disruptions in both their performance of important occupations and in their experience of these occupations. Descriptions of the nature of these disruptions are being advanced by the profession with a view to connecting the experience of occupations closely with intervention and support approaches. For example, an individual whose occupational patterns are characterized by an exceptional lack of involvement might best be characterized as disengagement or difficulties associated with emotional detachment, or it might be more characterized by deprivation or exceptional levels of disadvantage with respect to opportunities (Krupa, Fossey, Anthony, Brown, & Pitts, 2009). In the former case, the individual in recovery and the therapist might work together to identify and build sources of meaning in occupation, whereas in the latter, they might assertively organize opportunities and resources of occupation. Developing ways to talk directly about occupation is important for the evolution of recovery as a guiding vision for mental health service delivery. It can, for example, provide a way to talk about people who experience mental illness as social and community beings rather than focusing on illness and pathology. Rebeiro Gruhl (2008) suggests that the occupational issues facing people with serious mental illness needs to be conceptualized as an issue of occupational injustice, highlighting that social and structural issues constrain and restrict their occupational lives and that this needs to be reconciled if the recovery vision in mental health is to be realized. These highlight the importance of advocacy as a fundamental element of occupational therapy practice within a recovery framework.

Consistent with recovery, occupational therapists have advanced the development of a range of approaches to collaboratively develop occupational lives that are characterized by health and well-being. Assessment tools, such as the Occupational Performance History Interview, have been developed to engage individuals in telling their occupational stories in a way that can build on the individual's lived experiences and reveal strengths and potential opportunities (Ennals & Fossey, 2009). Similarly, assessment tools that measure time use help to capture the actual occupational patterns of people with mental illness to facilitate collaborative planning (Eklund, Leufstadius, & Bejerholm, 2009). Other tools such as the Profile of Occupational Engagement (Bejerholm, Hansson, & Eklund, 2006) can help with the interpretation of occupational patterns by considering how elements of well-being and health are being experienced through occupation For example, occupational patterns might be explored with respect to the extent to which they provide the individual with structure and routine, provide a good level of satisfaction, and provide opportunities for social interactions and access to a range of community environments. Occupational therapists have used the evidence-based practice of psychoeducation to explicitly inform people with mental illness and their support networks about the link between activity, occupation, and recovery. Figure 43.4 provides an example of

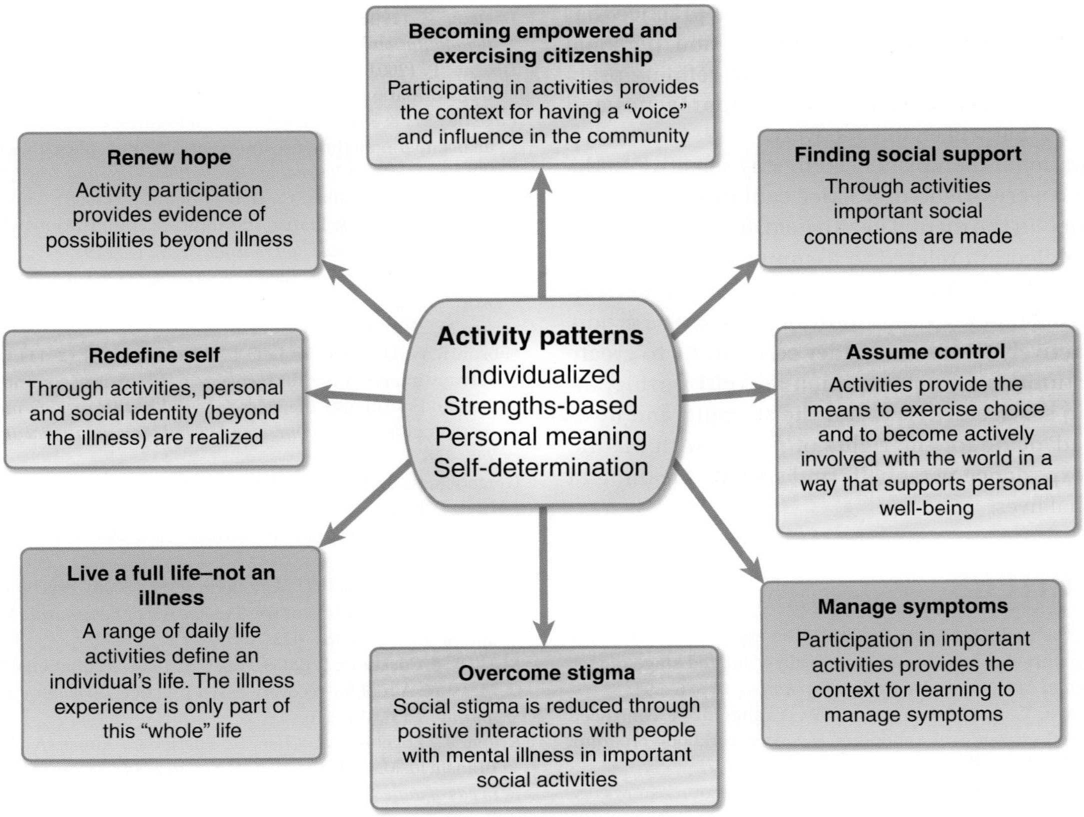

FIGURE 43.4 The recovery benefits of activity participation. (Adapted from Krupa, T., Edgelow, M., Chen, S., Mieras, C., Almas, A., Perry, A., . . . Bransfield, M. [2010]. *Action over Inertia: Addressing the activity health needs of people with serious mental illness.* Ottawa, Canada: CAOT Publications ACE. Reprinted with permission.)

a handout used in one such initiative, *Action over Inertia*, which addresses the activity health needs of people with serious mental illness. Initial testing of *Action over Inertia* has suggested that it may be effective in enabling people to make meaningful changes in their occupational patterns (Edgelow & Krupa, 2011; Krupa et al., 2010).

Conclusion

The core values, assumptions, and philosophy of occupational therapy are remarkably consistent with those espoused within contemporary perspectives on personal recovery. It is important to remember, however, that occupational therapists have and do practice within a health service delivery system where there have been major challenges and obstacles to implementing a recovery-oriented vision. It would be unreasonable to think that occupational therapists have somehow not been influenced by these obstacles and that their practice has always been recovery oriented within a larger system that has had such difficulty with this transformation. For example, Davidson, O'Connell, Tondora, Styron, and Kangas (2006) identified several concerns about recovery that emerged during efforts to transform a state mental health system. These concerns include such difficulties as practicing from the assumption that recovery is possible for only a selection of people with mental illness; difficulties with orienting professional expertise to practice that is assertively supportive of self-determination, personal agency, and control; and difficulties with refining practice to actively develop evidence-based approaches and interventions that will enable recovery.

Occupational therapists need to stay sensitive to the fact that recovery-oriented practice cannot reflect "business as usual" in the mental health field. It will necessitate continual reflection related to assumptions underlying practice, the development of new forms of partnership with the people they serve as individuals and as a group, engaging actively with the broader community to create real opportunities for participation and citizenship, innovation in service delivery, and the strength and leadership to advocate for the rights of people with mental illness to experience personally and socially meaningful occupational lives.

References

Andresen, R., Oades, L., & Caputi, P. (2003). The experience of recovery from schizophrenia: Towards an empirically-validated stage model. *Australian and New Zealand Journal of Psychiatry, 37*, 586–594.

Barbic, S., Krupa, T., & Armstrong, I. (2009). A randomized controlled trial of the effectiveness of a modified recovery workbook program: Preliminary findings. *Psychiatric Services, 60*, 491–497.

Bedregal, L. E., O'Connell, M., & Davidson, L. (2006). The Recovery Knowledge Inventory: Assessment of mental health staff knowledge and attitudes about recovery. *Psychiatric Rehabilitation Journal, 30*(2), 96–103.

Bejerholm, U., Hansson, L., & Eklund, M. (2006). Profiles of occupational engagement in people with schizophrenia (POES): The development of a new instrument based on time-use diaries. *British Journal of Occupational Therapy, 69*(2), 58–69.

Campbell-Orde, T., Chamberlin, J., Carpenter, J., & Leff, H. S. (2005). *Measuring the promise: A Compendium of Recovery Measures* (Vol. 2). Retrieved from http://www.power2u.org/downloads/pn-55.pdf

Cook, J. A., Copeland, M. E., Jonikas, J. A., Hamilton, M. M., Razzano, L. A., Grey, D. D., . . . Boyd, S. (2012). Results of a randomized controlled trial of mental illness self-management using wellness recovery action planning. *Schizophrenia Bulletin, 38*(4), 881–891.

Copeland, M. E. (1997). *Wellness recovery action plan*. Brattleboro, VT: Peach Press.

Davidson, L. (2005). Recovery in serious mental illness: Paradigm shift or shibboleth. In L. Davidson, C. Harding, & L. Spaniol (Eds.), *Recovery from severe mental illnesses: Research evidence and implications for practice* (pp. 5–26). Boston, MA: Centre for Psychiatric Rehabilitation, Boston University.

Davidson, L., O'Connell, M., Tondora, J., Styron, T., & Kangas, K. (2006). The top ten concerns about recovery encountered in mental health system transformation. *Psychiatric Services, 57*, 640–645.

Davidson, L., Rakfeldt, J., & Strauss, J. (2010). *The roots of the recovery movement in psychiatry*. West Sussex, United Kingdom: Wiley-Blackwell.

Davidson, L., & Roe, D. (2007). Recovery from versus recovery in serious mental illness: One strategy for lessening confusion plaguing recovery. *Journal of Mental Health, 16*(4), 459–470.

Davidson, L., Tondora, J., O'Connell, M., Kirk, T., Rockholz, P., & Evans, A. (2007). Creating a recovery-oriented system of behavioural health care: Moving from concept to reality. *Psychiatric Rehabilitation Journal, 31*, 23–31.

Deegan, P. (1988). Recovery: The lived experience of rehabilitation. *Psychosocial Rehabilitation Journal, 11*(4), 11–19.

Deegan, P. (1990). Spirit breaking: When the helping professions hurt. *The Humanistic Psychologist, 18*(3), 301–313.

Deegan, P. (1996). Recovery as a journey of the heart. *Psychiatric Rehabilitation Journal, 19*(3), 91–97.

Deegan, P. (2001). Recovery as a self-directed process of healing and transformation. *Occupational Therapy in Mental Health, 17*, 5–21.

Edgelow, M., & Krupa, T. (2011). Randomized controlled pilot study of an occupational time-use intervention for people with serious mental illness. *American Journal of Occupational Therapy, 65*(3), 267–276.

Eklund, M., Leufstadius, C., & Bejerholm, U. (2009). Time use among people with psychiatric disabilities: Implications for practice. *Psychiatric Rehabilitation Journal, 32*(3), 177–191.

Ennals, P., & Fossey, E. (2009). Using the OPHI-II to support people with mental illness in their recovery. *Occupational Therapy in Mental Health, 25*(2), 138–150.

Gibson, R. W., D'Amico, M., Jaffe, L., & Arbesman, M. (2011). Occupational therapy interventions for recovery in the areas of community integration and normative life roles for adults with serious mental illness: A systematic review. *American Journal of Occupational Therapy, 65*(3), 247–256.

Gingerich, S., & Mueser, K. T. (2005). Illness management and recovery. In R. E. Drake, M. R. Merrens, & D. W. Lynde (Eds.), *Evidence-based mental health practice: A textbook* (pp. 395–424). New York, NY: Norton.

Jerrell, J. M., Cousins, V. C., & Roberts, K. M. (2006). Psychometrics of the Recovery Process Inventory. *The Journal of Behavioral Health Services and Research, 33*, 464–473.

Kirsh, B., & Cockburn, L. (2009). The Canadian Occupational Performance Measure: A tool for recovery-based practice. *Psychiatric Rehabilitation Journal, 32*(3), 171–176.

Krupa, T., Edgelow, M., Chen, S., Mieras, C., Almas, A., Perry, A., . . . Bransfield, M. (2010). *Action over inertia: Addressing the activity-health needs of individuals with serious mental illness*. Ottawa, Canada: CAOT Publications ACE.

Krupa, T., Fossey, E., Anthony, W. A., Brown, C., & Pitts, D. (2009). Doing daily life: How occupational therapy can inform psychiatric rehabilitation practice. *Psychiatric Rehabilitation Journal, 32*(3), 155–161.

Law, M., Baptiste, S., McColl, M. A., Opzoomer, A., Polatajko, H., & Pollock, N. (1990). The Canadian Occupational Performance Measure: An outcome measure for occupational therapy. *Canadian Journal of Occupational Therapy, 57*, 82–87.

Levitt, A. J., Mueser, K. T., DeGenova, J., Lorenzo, J., Bradford-Watt, D., Barbosa, A., . . . Chernick, M. (2009). Randomized controlled trial of illness management and recovery in multiple-unit supportive housing. *Psychiatric Services, 60*, 1629–1636.

Mattson, M., Topor, A., Cullberg, J., & Forsell, Y. (2008). Association between financial strain, social network, and five year recovery from first episode psychosis. *Social Psychiatry and Psychiatric Epidemiology, 43*, 947–952.

Mental Health Commission. (2001). *Recovery competencies for New Zealand mental health workers*. Wellington, New Zealand: Mental Health Commission. Retrieved from http://www.mhc.govt.nz

Noordsy, D., Torrey, W., Mueser, K., Mead, S., O'Keefe, C., & Fox, L. (2002). Recovery from severe mental illness: An intrapersonal and functional outcome definition. *International Review of Psychiatry, 14*(4), 318–326.

O'Connell, M. J., Tondora, J., Evans, A. C., Croog, G., & Davidson, L. (2005). From rhetoric to routine: Assessing recovery-oriented practices in a state mental health and addiction system. *Psychiatric Rehabilitation Journal, 28*(4), 378–386.

Ralph, R. (2005). Verbal definitions and visual models of recovery: Focus on the recovery model. In R. O. Ralph & P. W. Corrigan (Eds.), *Recovery in mental illness: Broadening our understanding of wellness* (pp. 131–145). Washington, DC: American Psychological Association.

Rebeiro Gruhl, K. (2008). Strengths and challenges to practice: Reconciling occupational justice issues as a prerequisite to mental health recovery. In E. A. McKay, C. Craik, K. H. Lim, & G. Richards (Eds.), *Advancing occupational therapy in mental health practice* (pp.103–117). Malden, MA: Blackwell.

Rogers, E. S., Chamberlin, J., Ellison, M. L., & Crean, T. (1997). A consumer-constructed scale to measure empowerment among users of mental health services. *Psychiatric Services, 48*(8), 1042–1047.

Slade, M. (2009). *Personal recovery and mental illness: A guide for mental health professionals*. Cambridge, United Kingdom: Cambridge University Press.

Spaniol, L., Koehler, M., & Hutchinson, D. (1994). *Recovery workbook: Practical coping and empowerment strategies for people with psychiatric disability*. Boston, MA: Centre for Psychiatric Rehabilitation, Boston University.

Substance Abuse and Mental Health Services Administration. (2006). *National consensus statement on mental health recovery*. Rockville, MD: U.S. Department of Health and Human Services. Retrieved from http://store.samhsa.gov/shin/content//SMA05-4129/SMA05-4129.pdf

Tondora, J., & Davidson, L. (2006). *Practice guidelines for recovery-oriented behavioural health care*. Hartford, CT: Connecticut Department of Mental Health and Addiction Services.

For additional resources on the subjects discussed in this chapter, visit http://thePoint.lww.com/Willard-Spackman12e.

CHAPTER 44

Health Promotion Theories

S. Maggie Reitz

OUTLINE

LEARNING OBJECTIVES

After reading this chapter, you will be able to:

1. Describe theories of health behavior and health promotion that can be used to inform occupational therapy practice
2. Discuss considerations in combining occupational therapy theories with health behavior theories
3. Apply theory to the development of occupation-based occupational therapy health promotion interventions in interdisciplinary health promotion practice
4. Examine the evidence available related to occupational therapy health promotion and health behavior health promotion interventions

Introduction

Health promotion activities have long been engaged in by a small portion of occupational therapy practitioners (American Occupational Therapy Association [AOTA], 2010a; Reitz, 1992) and seen as an appropriate role for the profession (Brunyate, 1967; Finn, 1972; Jaffe, 1986; Johnson, 1986; Kaplan & Burch-Minakan, 1986; West, 1967, 1969; Wiemer, 1972). More recently, health and wellness was identified as one of the major practice areas in the AOTA's Centennial Vision (Baum, 2006). In addition, health promotion is an important part of the remaining five identified practice areas, which include children and youth; productive aging; mental health; rehabilitation, disability, and participation; and work and industry (Baum, 2006). Health and wellness also has been identified as one of the possible outcomes of occupational therapy intervention in the AOTA (2008b) "Occupational Therapy Practice Framework."

Within this chapter, occupational therapy's potential to enhance the health of clients through the use of health promotion interventions will be detailed in the hope of encouraging greater involvement in this important area of practice. Clients can be individuals, families, communities, or populations (AOTA, 2008b). This information will be provided through a lens of theory-driven practice, based on the assumption that ethical occupational therapy practice is theory based, occupation based, and evidence driven (AOTA, 2008b, 2010b, 2010c). The objective is to demonstrate how theory can be used to support and strengthen the profession's role in health promotion thereby maximizing the health and well-being of the society we serve.

Definitions of Health, Health Promotion, and Wellness

Definitions of health promotion and the focus of health promotion interventions vary across the many disciplines that engage in this type of practice; however, the definition of health is generally agreed on. The following definition of health from the World Health Organization (WHO) is probably the most frequently cited. **Health** is "the complete state of physical, mental and social well-being and not just the absence of disease or infirmity" (WHO, 1947, p. 29). **Health promotion** is the use of discipline-specific techniques to assist people in achieving their health-related goals. ***Occupational therapy–directed health promotion*** is the client-centered use of occupations, adaptations to context, or alteration of context to maximize individuals', families', communities', and groups' pursuit of health and quality of life. Health promotion is a process of maximizing health through structured interventions, whereas **wellness** is the outcome of health promotion and ultimately is the responsibility of the individual, family, community, or society (Reitz & Scaffa, 2010).

Determinants of Health

Before an appropriate theory can be selected for a health promotion initiative, a clear understanding of the health and occupation needs and desires of the population being served is required. Health is determined by many factors. In a U.S. national government report entitled *Healthy People 2020*, determinants of health are described within five broad categories: biology and genetics, individual behavior, social environment, physical environment, and health services (U.S. Department of Health and Human Services [USDHHS], 2010). These five determinants are shown in Figure 44.1 together with the mission of *Healthy People 2020* and the overarching goals for the next decade for improving health of the nation. *Healthy People 2020* is a framework available for usage by federal, state, and local governments; nonprofits; and businesses to address and assess outcomes of programs and policies that aim to improve the health and quality of life of populations living in the United States (USDHHS, 2010). If a community or population has not already identified a health need, then a review of the objectives identified in this report may be of assistance to start the conversation.

WHO, through a document entitled *Ottawa Charter for Health Promotion* published in 1986, identified eight prerequisites for health. These prerequisites (WHO, 1986, p. 1) include the following:

- Education
- Food
- Income
- Peace
- Shelter
- Social justice and equity
- Stable ecosystem
- Sustainable resources

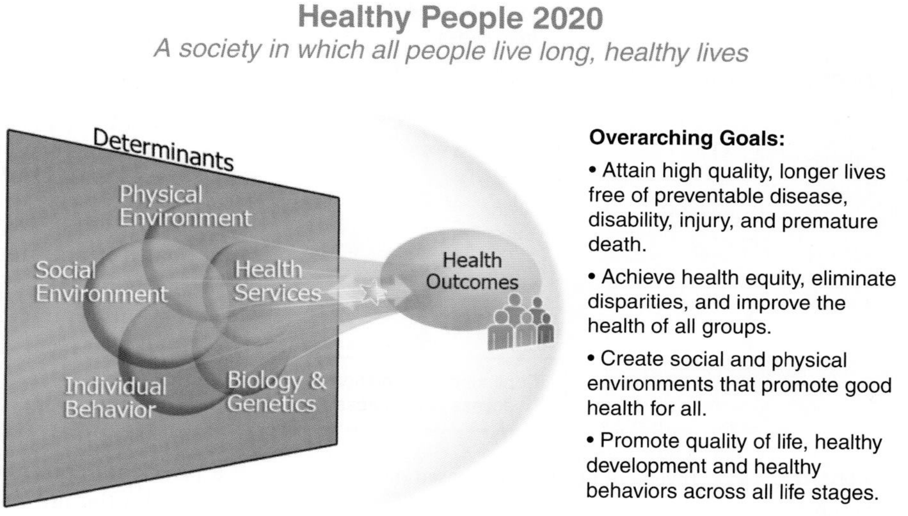

Healthy People 2020
A society in which all people live long, healthy lives
Determinants
Physical Environment
Social Environment
Health Services
Individual Behavior
Biology & Genetics
Health Outcomes
Overarching Goals:
• Attain high quality, longer lives free of preventable disease, disability, injury, and premature death.
• Achieve health equity, eliminate disparities, and improve the health of all groups.
• Create social and physical environments that promote good health for all.
• Promote quality of life, healthy development and healthy behaviors across all life stages.

FIGURE 44.1 Graphic model of Healthy People 2020. (U.S. Department of Health and Human Services, n.d., p. 3).

TABLE 44.1 Occupational Deprivation and Health Impacts

Occupational Deprivation	Relationship to Health Determinants
Children with congenital sensory and motor challenges who do not have opportunities to play with peers on adaptive playgrounds	• Biology and genetics • Social environment • Physical environment
Rural teenagers with limited opportunities to access various positive group occupations with peers turn to unhealthy habits to cope with boredom and isolation	• Individual behavior • Social environment • Physical environment
Working parents' limited access to health care and/or educational services due to lack of proof of citizenship	• Health services • Social environment
Older adults who cannot negotiate exit from house become imprisoned in own home	• Social environment • Physical environment

A comparison of the determinants of health identified by the USDHHS to the prerequisites for health developed by WHO shows the WHO places less emphasis on the individual and health services and a greater emphasis on access to basic human needs that are required to live a healthy life. Successful health promotion programs should address both those prerequisites and determinants of health that are applicable to the population, based on the population's self-determination, which will be influenced by geopolitics, geographical location, and other contextual features.

Access to occupations, or occupational enrichment (Molineux & Whiteford as cited in Polatajko et al., 2007, p. 26), is an important contributor to health mediated through health determinants and prerequisites for health. Lack of access to occupation can result in occupational deprivation, which in turn can have a significant negative impact on the health of individuals, families, and communities. **Occupational deprivation**, which is the lack of access to engagement in an array of self-selected occupations that have meaning to the individual, family, or community, can result in ill health (Wilcock, 2006) and cascading occupational injustice. The divergent paths for those who experience occupational enrichment, and thus the prerequisites for health, from those who experience occupational deprivation are displayed in Figure 44.2. The potential relationships between occupational deprivation and health determinants are depicted in Table 44.1.

Each of the examples in Table 44.1 can be the beginning of a negatively reinforcing relationship leading to additional threats to health as occupational deprivation increases. For example, the rural teenager with limited access to age-appropriate, group occupations can move from using tobacco and abusing alcohol alone near home to driving long distances after drinking. This in turn could lead to a driving under the influence (DUI) conviction, a manslaughter charge, or the use of illegal drugs, any of which could result in a period of incarceration, which then can result in decreased access to various self-chosen occupations and an acceleration of health problems. An adaption of a well-known Ben Franklin quote summarizes the potential benefit of occupation-based interventions on health determinants—an ounce of occupation can prevent the need for pounds and dollars of cure.

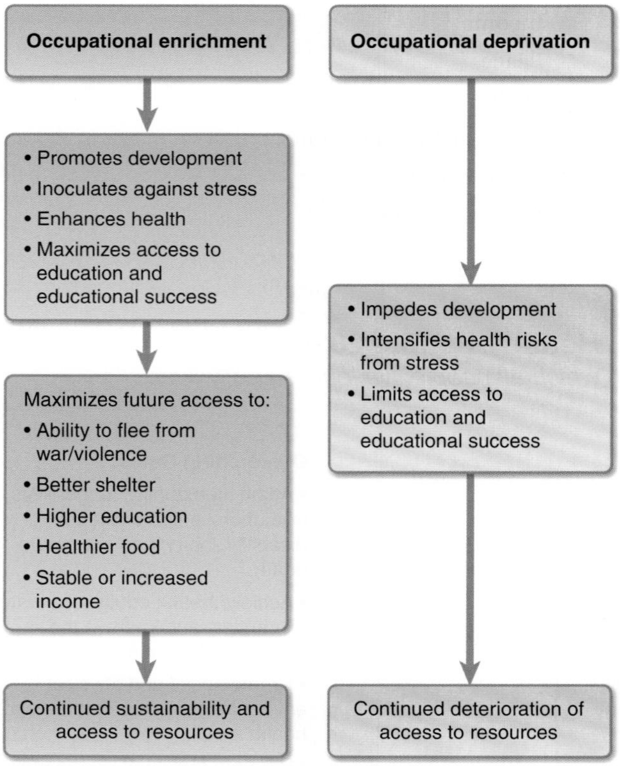

FIGURE 44.2 Divergent health paths based on access to occupation.

Health Promotion and Occupational Therapy

The question of why the profession should be involved in health promotion can be answered by reflecting on the early history of the profession as well as more recent events. Founders and early leaders in the profession studied and used the health promoting as well as the healing properties of occupation (Reitz, 2010). Besides these well-known leaders, others articulated the value of occupation to health. For example, as early as the 1930s, a physician commented that occupational therapy had the potential not only to do more than quicken the rate of recovery from injury or disease but to also "be an agent for positive health" (Losada, 1936, p. 285).

Historically, there has been limited engagement in health promotion among occupational therapy practitioners (Reitz, 1992). Although many occupational therapy practitioners engage in limited health promotion activities through instructing clients in basic preventive strategies such as energy conservation or the use of ergonomic principles, fewer engage in community- or population-based health promotion activities. Data from AOTA membership surveys indicate that from 1970 to 2010, few occupational therapy practitioners taking part in the surveys practiced primarily with the well population, in health promotion, or at the population level (AOTA, 1982, 1987, 1991, 2001, 2006a, 2010a; Jantzen, 1979).

There are many barriers that have limited occupational therapy practitioners' engagement in community- or population-based health promotion practice. Besides difficulty in seeking and receiving reimbursement, minimal education and exposure to health promotion, a shortage of mentors and evidence, and confusion about role delineation also can be contributing factors.

In more recent times, the development of noteworthy documents has helped to support and communicate the profession's contribution to health promotion. A sample of these documents is listed in Box 44.1. AOTA, through the statement "Occupational Therapy in the Promotion of Health and the Prevention of Disease or Disability" (AOTA, 2008a), describes the role of occupational therapy in health promotion for not only individuals but also for families, communities, and populations. The philosophical link and match of occupational values to national and international policies on health promotion are reviewed to provide the context for a series of examples of potential assessments, interventions, and strategies. Examples are provided for each of the three levels of prevention (i.e., primary, secondary, and tertiary) and with various clients (i.e., individuals, communities, populations) and are an excellent source of ideas for potential interventions at the person and policy levels.

The AOTA, World Federation of Occupational Therapists (WFOT), and other national occupational therapy associations, through publication of documents, also advocate for access to prerequisites for health, including access to meaningful occupations in the community. For example, the document entitled "AOTA's Societal Statement on Livable Communities" (AOTA, 2009), informs the public, students, and new practitioners about the profession's support for access to services, establishment of policies, and implementation of design features that will allow both older adults to age in place and individuals with disabilities to fully engage in the community and reach their full occupational potential. The WFOT 2004, through the *Position Paper on Community Based Rehabilitation*, also advocates for equal access to the right of occupational engagement of individuals with disabilities and their families. Lack of such access or occupational deprivation leads to cascading health problems and further injustices as was depicted earlier in Figure 44.2. Understanding the role of occupational therapy and the potential to assist in making meaningful change is the first step. The next steps include identifying the clients' needs and wants and selecting an appropriate theory that can guide the development of an intervention.

Health Promotion Theories

Health promotion interventions beyond those typically offered to individual clients or families are most often conducted by interdisciplinary teams or in close consultation with other disciplines. Thus, an understanding of theories commonly used in health promotion is important in enhancing communication and understanding. Three health behavior theories will be briefly introduced—the Health Belief Model (HBM), the Stages of Change Model, and Social Cognitive Theory (SCT). In addition, one planning framework will be described. These theories and framework were selected from many possibilities due to either past experience combining them with occupational therapy theories or easily seen commonalities for future blending. An additional potential model is the Social Ecological Model, which is described elsewhere (Reitz, Scaffa, Campbell, & Rhynders, 2010). Prior to using any of these theories or framework, additional knowledge should be sought through reading,

BOX 44.1 Sampling of Occupational Therapy Documents Related to Health Promotion

- "American Occupational Therapy Association's (AOTA) Societal Statement on Health Disparities" (AOTA, 2006b)
- "AOTA's Societal Statement on Health Literacy" (AOTA, 2011a)
- "Health Promotion in Occupational Therapy" (British Association of Occupational Therapists and College of Occupational Therapists, 2008)
- "AOTA's Societal Statement on Livable Communities" (AOTA, 2009)
- "Role of Occupational Therapy in Disaster Preparedness, Response, and Recovery: A Concept Paper" (AOTA, 2011b)
- "Occupational Therapy in the Promotion of Health and the Prevention of Disease or Disability" (AOTA, 2008a)
- "World Federation of Occupational Therapists' (WFOT) Position Paper on Community Based Rehabilitation" (WFOT, 2004)

mentoring, continuing education, or working toward a specialized doctoral degree.

Health Belief Model

The HBM is one of the first and most widely used models to explore and facilitate health behavior change. It was originated by public health social psychologists in the 1950s (National Cancer Institute [NCI], 2005). Occupational therapy practitioners frequently recommend that their clients change occupational behaviors. This model explores the way people examine and balance competing factors when deciding to adopt or not adopt health recommendations. The constructs of the model are described together with strategies to promote behavior change related to each specific construct in Table 44.2. Various health promotion programs can be designed using these constructs.

The basis of this model is the balancing of threats (i.e., perceived susceptibility and perceived seriousness) with barriers (e.g., time, financial cost) of taking the recommended action (e.g., time, financial cost) and the potential benefits. When the individual, family, or community believes the threat outweighs the cost of action, then change will occur (NCI, 2005). Other components of the model include **self-efficacy** and cues to action. A cue to action can be an artifact such as the "save the ta-tas" bumper stickers that can serve as a reminder to perform breast self-examinations. The bumper sticker cue to action will be more likely to result in a woman performing a breast self-exam if the woman feels competent to perform the exam (e.g., self-efficacy).

The impact and relationship of these constructs can be shown through a description of the potential roles of a health educator and an occupational therapy practitioner on an interdisciplinary smoking cessation program development team. Health educators have the background knowledge and expertise to ensure the perceived seriousness (e.g., ill health, death, decreased life span) and susceptibility are appropriately represented in the program without causing undue fear. Although both health educators and occupational therapists can be familiar with barriers to behavior change, occupational therapists can add a perspective in terms of establishing new habits to support health decisions while unhealthy habits are extinguished through an occupation lens. For example, an occupational therapy practitioner may suggest to highlight additional negative aspects of smoking related to social consequences that health educators may not as readily identify but could increase the level of perceived seriousness (e.g., social ostracization due to tobacco odor, marginalization of smokers due to smoking bans).

In order to strengthen the likelihood of a person taking a positive health action and decreasing the negative consequences of smoking, an occupational therapist may suggest implementing a peer buddy occupation-based strategy. In order to successfully stop smoking, a change in social occupations and friends often is needed to prevent relapse. When first stopping smoking, for example, it is best to avoid social and physical contexts that reinforce smoking such as happy hours at an outside bar that permits smoking (e.g., barrier). The buddy strategy pairs successful ex-smokers (e.g., a cue to action) with individuals desiring to stop smoking. Through the use of an

TABLE 44.2 Health Belief Model

Concept	Definition	Potential Change Strategies
Perceived susceptibility	Beliefs about the chances of getting a condition	• Define what populations(s) are at risk and their levels of risk • Tailor risk information based on an individual's characteristics or behaviors • Help the individual develop an accurate perception of his or her own risk
Perceived severity	Beliefs about the seriousness of a condition and its consequences	• Specify the consequences of a condition and recommended action
Perceived benefits	Beliefs about the effectiveness of taking action to reduce risk or seriousness	• Explain how, where, and when to take action and what the potential positive results will be
Perceived barriers	Beliefs about the material and psychological costs of taking action	• Offer reassurance, incentives, and assistance; correct misinformation
Cues to action	Factors that activate "readiness to change"	• Provide "how to" information, promote awareness, and employ reminder systems
Self-efficacy	Confidence in one's ability to take action	• Provide training and guidance in performing action • Use progressive goal setting • Give verbal reinforcement • Demonstrate desired behaviors

Reprinted from National Cancer Institute. (2005). *Theory at a glance* (2nd ed.). Bethesda, MD: National Institutes of Health. p. 14. Retrieved from http://www.cancer.gov/theory.pdf

instrument such as the activity checklist, alternate activities and identification of a new peer group of nonsmokers could be identified. Engagement in one of more of these occupations with the buddy can increase the likelihood of success while broadening a person's occupational repertoire and social supports. Thus, instead of losing an identity and pleasurable occupation, they gain a friend, a new identity as an ex-smoker, and one or more new pleasurable occupations.

Although the HBM's use by occupational therapy has not been widely reported in the literature, other researchers have used it to explore occupation-based health behaviors such as eating habits (Deshpande, Basil, & Basil, 2009), physical activity engagement (Juniper, Oman, Hamm, & Kerby, 2004), and weight management (James, Pobee, Oxidine, Brown, & Joshi, 2012).

Transtheoretical Model of Change/Stages of Change Model

The originators of this model first investigated why some people were better able to quit smoking than others (Prochaska & DiClemente, 1982, 1983). Their work led to the development of a model that can be used to study people's readiness for change—ceasing a poor health habit such as smoking or starting a good health habit such as exercise. Literature regarding the model refers to it as either the *transtheoretical model of change* or the *stages of change model.* According to the proponents of the model, there are potentially five stages that an individual goes through as he or she change a health-related behavior. These stages include precontemplation, contemplation, decision, action, and maintenance (NCI, 2005). The components of this model are presented in Table 44.3 and discussed in greater detail in other sources (NCI, 2005; Reitz et al., 2010) and in a table later in this chapter.

There are two aspects of the model that are particularly helpful to occupational therapy health promotion practice. One is the belief that relapse can be part of the normal cycle of behavior change. Therefore, neither the occupational therapy practitioner nor the client should give up hope. The second is the belief that specific strategies can be matched to each of the stages. For example, *consciousness-raising* is a process that is well matched for moving someone from the precontemplation to the contemplation stage. Occupational therapy practitioners can be helpful in moving someone closer to smoking cessation through consciousness-raising. For example, if a smoker reports concerns about walking to the corner store for milk, the occupational therapy practitioner, besides offering energy conservation strategies, also can suggest that they may be less out of breath walking if they stopped or decreased the number of cigars smoked.

Contingency management can help people be successful once they take action and to then maintain their new behavior. Following the earlier smoking cessation example, if a new ex-smoker was invited to a work event where people may be smoking, he or she may want to have a contingency plan such as inviting their antismoke buddy for support and suggestions on how to negotiate the experience. This model has contributed to the design and success of various health behaviors at the individual and group levels. One such example is a faith-based community weight loss program (Kim et al., 2008) named WORD (wholeness, oneness, righteousness, deliverance).

Social Cognitive Theory

SCT is a model that is a good fit for occupational therapy health promotion program development and evaluation due to its emphasis on "how" to change behavior, the importance placed on self-efficacy, and mastery gained through doing (Cook, 2004). According to Bandura (2004), the developer of SCT, this type of approach promotes "effective self-management of health habits that keep people healthy through their lifespan" (p. 144). The primary construct of the model is self-efficacy. Additional constructs include knowledge, a prerequisite for behavior change; outcome expectations, including physical, social, and self-evaluative; health goals; and sociostructural

TABLE 44.3 Stages of Change Model

Stage	Definition	Potential Change Strategies
Precontemplation	Has no intention of taking action within the next six months	Increase awareness of need for change; personalize information about risks and benefits
Contemplation	Intends to take action within the next six months	Motivate; encourage making specific plans
Preparation	Intends to take action within the next thirty days and has taken some behavioral steps in this direction	Assist with developing and implementing concrete action plans; help set gradual goals
Action	Has changed behavior for less than six months	Assist with feedback, problem solving, social support, and reinforcement
Maintenance	Has changed behavior for more than six months	Assist with coping, reminders, finding alternatives, avoiding slips/relapses (as applicable)

Reprinted from National Cancer Institute. (2005). *Theory at a glance* (2nd ed.). Bethesda, MD: National Institutes of Health. p. 15. Retrieved from http://www.cancer.gov/theory.pdf

TABLE 44.4 Social Cognitive Theory

Concept	Definition	Potential Change Strategies
Knowledge	Information related to health practices and their benefits and risks	• Provide tailored information connected to people's values, cultural, contextual, and educational level
Self-efficacy	Confidence in the ability to implement a health behavior change(s)	• Provide authentic positive feedback from a respected source at each stage of health behavior change • Build on effective behavior change strategies previously used
Outcome expectations	Determination whether the effort of the person or group to overcome the perceived barriers is worth the potential benefits of taking action	• Assist client or group in weighing of potential cost and benefits through a listing or section activity
Goals	Concrete, measurable goals and action steps to achieving goals	• Facilitate development of a system such as a blog, diary, or computerized reminder system to review progress toward steps and goal(s) on a predetermined schedule
Perceived facilitators	Social and physical supports for change	• Develop an artifact that symbolically represents assets for change
Perceived impediments	Social and physical barriers to change	• Develop an artifact that symbolically represents barriers to change, which can be either physically removed or erased and crossed out when barrier is no longer a threat

Adapted from National Cancer Institute. (2005). *Theory at a glance* (2nd ed.). Bethesda, MD: National Institutes of Health. p. 20, Table 5. Retrieved from http://www.cancer.gov/theory.pdf

factors, including facilitators and impediments. The constructs of the model are described in Table 44.4 together with strategies to promote behavior change (Bandura, 2004; Cook, 2004) specific to each construct.

Returning to the earlier smoking cessation example, the SCT could be used to support both health educator and occupational therapy contributions to the smoking cessation program. Prior to instituting the antismoking buddy intervention, the health educators would again be responsible for ensuring the participants had sufficient knowledge regarding the relationship of smoking to ill health. In this example, the buddy intervention is supported by the SCT because it serves to maximize self-efficacy through the use of social supports to achieve client-selected goals. A good resource for using this model in occupational therapy is Cook (2004) who used the SCT to develop an occupational therapy health promotion program for older adults.

PRECEDE-PROCEED: A Framework for Planning Health Promotion Programs

The Predisposing, Reinforcing, and Enabling Constructs in Educational/Environmental Diagnosis and Evaluation (PRECEDE)-Policy, Regulatory, and Organizational Constructs in Educational and Environmental Development (PROCEED) model is not a theory; it is a planning framework comprising eight phases. These phases are helpful to guide ethical health promotion interventions at the community or population level (Green & Kreuter, 2005; NCI, 2005). The originators clearly share occupational therapy's value of client-centered care by communicating the importance of the community or population as decision makers. Community engagement starts immediately in the PRECEDE portion of the framework in which the community guides the health promotion experts in the selection of the priority health concern that is to be addressed. In the next group of steps called the PROCEED section, models such as the ones describe earlier are used to guide the specific details of the chosen intervention. The PROCEED portion of the framework also details the evaluation process of the intervention. The phases of the PRECEDE-PROCEED framework (Green & Kreuter, 2005; NCI, 2005) and potential actions for each phase are described in Table 44.5. This is an introductory table; additional reading on the framework would be required before using it to plan or evaluate a health promotion program.

The PRECEDE-PROCEED framework has the potential to work well with the occupational therapy framework (AOTA, 2008b) and other theories to develop occupation-based health promotion programs such as a dating etiquette program to decrease dating and partner violence among adolescents and young adults. There is a need for such programs because 12 million individuals each year are impacted by intimate partner violence (IPV), and data indicate that the first rape or IPV experience most often happens before the age of 24 years (Centers for Disease Control and Prevention [CDC], National Center for Injury Prevention and Control, 2010).

TABLE 44.5 PRECEDE-PROCEED Planning Framework

Section	Phase	Description	Potential Change Strategies
PRECEDE	1. Social assessment and situational analysis	Engaging the community in identifying current social problems and their vision of an improved quality of life	• Review available data on the status of the prerequisites of health in the community • Share data at meetings with community stakeholders; focus groups with community members to elicit their decision as to priorities for interventions and assets and community capacities that can be tapped • Formalize relations with a community-identified group or institute a community board
	2. Epidemiological assessment	Reviewing health and health-related data that is linked to the social health concerns identified in Phase 1	• Review summary of data and data sources with community board • Identify need for additional data or sources for data
	3. Educational and ecological assessment	Identifying the predisposing factors, enabling factors, and reinforcing factors linked to the identified social problem	• Review summary of data and data sources with community board and government leaders if none are on the board • Identify need for additional data or sources for data
	4. Administrative and policy assessment and intervention alignment	Identifying potential policy and resource barriers to initiate and maintain program; developing and securing needed policy changes and additional resources	• Review findings with community board and local government leaders
PROCEED	5. Implementation	Launching and conducting the program	• Facilitate a culturally relevant kickoff for the program with the community board
	6. Process evaluation	Evaluating success of continued community involvement and utilization of community resources	• Review program implementation as it is occurring and solicit feedback from community board, stakeholders, and participants
	7. Impact evaluation	Evaluating short-term progress toward goals of program such as access to resources and gaining of skills and knowledge	• Collect data from participants through previously planned strategy (e.g., post portion of a pretest posttest plan, focus group)
	8. Outcome evaluation	Evaluating long-term achievement of goals of program related to quality of life and health indicators	• Continue to collect data from participants through previously planned strategy (e.g., post portion of a pretest posttest plan, focus group) • Review and share with community board the current social and epidemiological data to determine if there were changes in desired quality of life and health indicators

Adapted from National Cancer Institute. (2005). *Theory at a glance* (2nd ed.). Bethesda, MD: National Institutes of Health. p. 42, Table 10. Retrieved from http://www.cancer.gov/theory.pdf

A potential example of the use of the PRECEDE-PROCEED framework to combat IPV will be described next. An occupational therapy student and a health education student approached the Student Government Association (SGA) with a request for funds to develop a program to increase awareness of IPV. They shared that fellow students were concerned about campus safety and had approached their respective student organizations to take the lead in developing a solution (Phase 1). The two were identified by the groups to represent them and their plan to take action. The pair also shared with the SGA data that showed the incidence of IPV both on their campus and other campuses as well as reports from the literature of health impacts of such violence that had been gathered and vetted by the leadership of both student groups (Phases 2 and 3). Meeting with the SGA, requesting funds, and meetings with the vice president of student affairs, which preceded the request for funds, were parts of Phase 4. An evaluation plan for the program was shared with the SGA, which included process, impact, and outcome evaluation (Phases 6, 7, 8).

Health Promotion Theories and Occupational Therapy

Health promotion is a process that can vary in length, intensity, and audience. For example, it can include providing a specific short-term standardized intervention such as a fall prevention program or a more complex, community-wide initiative such as developing a community garden in an urban food desert. A *food desert* is a geographic area where inhabitants "lack access to affordable fruits, vegetables, whole grains, low-fat milk, and other foods that make up the full range of a healthy diet" (CDC, 2010, para. 2). The client can be an individual, group, family, school, business, local community, or government.

The occupational profile can easily be used to determine and guide a single client's desire to address his or her health through occupation; it also can be adapted to conduct an initial needs assessment for a group or small community (AOTA, 2008b). For example, at the individual level, it can be used to discover that a client wishes to quit smoking so that he or she has sufficient energy to play with his or her grandchildren. Using the occupational profile helps the occupational therapist gain an initial broad perspective of the client's "occupational history and experiences, patterns of daily living, interests, values, and needs" (AOTA, 2008b, p. 649). The occupational therapist could then blend the transtheoretical model described earlier and the Model of Human Occupation (Dumont & Kielhofner, 2007; Yamada, Kawamata, Kobayashi, Kielhofner, & Taylor, 2010) to develop strategies to quit smoking and adopt new healthy habits. Whether working with an individual, family, or a community, when this process is effectively used, it helps to ensure a client-centered or community-centered approach.

Selecting and Blending Theories

Weighing possible theories for the best fit should take place throughout the health promotion process but at a minimum should be a part of decision making when determining the occupation and health need to be addressed and how. There are a variety of factors to consider in the selection of a health promotion theory; first and foremost must be the ease with which the theory and its constructs can be translated into lay language or the language of the cultural group requesting the intervention or assistance. Second is whether there is evidence that this theory has been useful in developing programs or evaluating health promotion interventions.

There are various health behavior theories as well as occupational therapy theories available to guide health promotion interventions as well as research that can inform interdisciplinary health promotion efforts. Health behavior theories generally lack an essential occupation perspective, whereas occupational therapy theories often can be strengthened through the application of constructs from one or more health behavior theories. A selection of the available theories to use in health promotion intervention and research that were introduced earlier is described in Table 44.6 together with a selection of occupational therapy theories. This was done in order to identify potential natural pairings between complementary occupational therapy theories and health behavior theories (see Box 44.2). Table 44.7 provides an example of the use of a blended theory approach to developing a healthy weight program for high school girl students. This is discussed further in the Practice Dilemma that appears later in this chapter. Although pragmatic blending of theories can strengthen health programs, this work should be extended beyond simple evaluation of program outcomes in order to facilitate the creation of new, more powerful theories from the initial constituent theories, thus leading to broader benefit.

In addition to incorporating theory, occupational therapy health promotion interventions should be based on evidence. An example of evidence is provided in the "Commentary on the Evidence" box. Several systematic reviews also are available in a special issue of the *American Journal of Occupational Therapy* that directly relate to the impact of health promotion on the health and well-being of older adults (AOTA, 2012). Although randomized trials are seen by many as the most important level of evidence, by their nature, they require tight control over all aspects of the program development and evaluation. A participatory action research approach supports more of the desired community involvement.

Examples of Occupational Therapy Health Promotion in Action

Although there are many examples of occupational therapy health promotion activities, the link of the program to theory is not always explicit. A small sampling of initiatives is provided here to show the potential for occupational therapy's role in the promotion of health via research, program development, and program evaluation. These examples primarily fall into two categories: school-aged children and older adults. Each initiative will be linked to a potentially supporting health promotion theory, either identified by the developer of the program or suggested by this author.

One initiative for children and youth is the AOTA National School Backpack Awareness Day (Jacobs, Wuest, Markowitz, & Hellman, 2011). The AOTA National School Backpack Awareness Day happens annually in September with the express goal of having students wear their backpack over both shoulders and to monitor the weight they carry. The programs can use a combination of fun activities to ensure that the students understand their potential susceptibility for an injury and the potential seriousness of an injury (two constructs from the HBM) as well as the proper techniques. Self-efficacy also can be promoted by students performing the correct techniques, which provide feedback about their ability to perform the task (SCT and HBM constructs) as well as to feel firsthand the benefits (HBM construct).

Barnard and colleagues (2004) describe an initiative that was developed by occupational therapy faculty and students in partnership with older adults in a small North Carolina town. They developed a 5-week wellness

TABLE 44.6 Comparison of Theories to Support Health Promotion

Theory	Focus	Key Constructs
Ecology of Human Performance (Dunn, Brown, & McGuigan, 1994)	How performance range can be maximized through skill, habit, or role development and/or modification of the environment	Establish or restore Adapt Alter Prevent Create
Health Belief Model (National Cancer Institute [NCI], 2005)	How individuals or communities balance the threat posed by a health problem with the benefits of avoiding the threat, the cost to avoid the threat, and other factors that influence the decision to act	Perceived susceptibility Perceived severity Perceived benefits Perceived barriers Cues to action Self-efficacy
Occupational Adaptation (Schultz, 2009)	How the ability to use adaptive capacities to solve problems, experience relative mastery, and enhance occupational performance can be enhanced	Adaptive capacity Adaptation energy Adaptive response Relative mastery
Model of Human Occupation (Kielhofner, 2009)	How individuals and communities develop performance capacity to perform habitual occupations to support participation and occupational adaption	Volition Habituation Performance capacity Occupational adaptation Occupational competency Occupational identity
Stages of Change Model (Prochaska & DiClemente, 1982, 1983)	Identification of when individuals or communities are ready to change a problem behavior, their current stage of change, and the optimal matching of intervention to current stage of change	Precontemplation Contemplation Decision Action Maintenance Relapse

Adapted from National Cancer Institute. (2005). *Theory at a glance* (2nd ed.). Bethesda, MD: National Institutes of Health. p. 45, Table 11. Retrieved from http://www.cancer.gov/theory.pdf

program, based on "community-built approach" (p. 152), that focused on physical activity, using spirituality as a means of expression, increasing awareness of nutrition and cooking, and increasing cognitive functions. Miller and colleagues (2001) describe the Microwave Project, in which occupational therapy students worked with an interdisciplinary team and older adults who received Meals on Wheels to address a challenge that some recipients were having in reheating their meals adequately and safely. Two theories were used to support the development of the program: occupational adaptation (Schultz, 2009) and the transtheoretical model of change (Prochaska & DiClemente, 1982). Older adults who were at risk of health problems because of difficulty with food preparation were involved in a luncheon program (if they were able to leave their homes to attend) or the homebound program so that they could gain skills in food preparation and reheating using a microwave oven.

BOX 44.2 Potential Theory Pairings

Health Belief Model and Ecology of Human Performance
Health Belief Model and Model of Human Occupation
Stages of Change and Occupational Adaptation
Stages of Change and Model of Human Occupation
Stages of Change and Person-Environment-Occupation

TABLE 44.7 Use of Multiple Frameworks and Theories in a Health Promotion Intervention to Reduce Obesity

Step	Models to Partially Apply	Objective	Healthy Weight Example
1	PRECEDE portion of PRECEDE-PROCEED	Apply structure to work with community to identify occupation and health needs	Parents and school officials raise concerns regarding an increase in obesity rates among high school students
2	Health Belief Model	Determine level of threat (i.e., perceived seriousness and susceptibility weighed against benefits), relevant cues to action, and self-efficacy	Conduct separate groups prior to program development with parents, school employees, students, and local pediatricians to discuss culturally relevant cues to actions and approaches
	Stages of Change	Determine readiness for change	Develop mechanisms to identify and recruit students in the precontemplation, contemplation, and preparation stages
	Ecology of Human Performance	Determine which skills need to be established or restored through appropriate occupation-based intervention, which context or tasks be adapted or context altered to prevent harm; determine what programs or initiatives warrant being created	Assess environmental supports by identifying what foods are available for meals and snacks; observe meal and snack time behaviors of students; conduct formative or process evaluations with student participants to modify program as needed to ensure needed skills and knowledge are being obtained
3	PROCEED portion of PRECEDE-PROCEED	Plan and implement program evaluation to include process, impact, and outcomes evaluations	Involve student leaders, parents, and school officials in program evaluation planning

Community outreach was undertaken to give older adults with low incomes access to microwave ovens.

Stav (2010) has linked CarFit, a program developed jointly by AOTA, AARP (formerly the American Association of Retired Persons), and the American Automobile Association (AAA) to assess the fit between older drivers and their vehicles to theoretical constructs from the HBM and the Person-Environment-Occupation (PEO) model (Law et al., 1996). CarFit sessions are offered in the community often in between rush hours when older adults are more typically running errands. The evaluations are scheduled in 30-minute increments to ensure that the 12-step checklist can be completed in a nonrushed manner.

The primary purpose of the program is for older adults to gain information about the fit between their body and their car while sitting in their car (PEO constructs). Needed mirror, steering wheel, and seat adjustments can be made immediately and other recommendations for additional adaptations when

Commentary on the Evidence

The Well Elderly Study (Clark et al., 2001; Clark et al., 1997) and falls prevention initiatives (e.g., Clemson et al., 2004) are examples of interventions that have been evaluated through randomized controlled trials. The Well Elderly Study in California demonstrated through a randomized clinical trial design that a preventive occupational therapy intervention (i.e., Lifestyle Redesign) resulted in measurable benefits in health, function, and quality of life (Clark et al., 1997), and these results were sustained after a 6-month follow up (Clark et al., 2001). The 9-month occupational therapy intervention in the Well Elderly study focused on helping older adults to build positive changes into their lifestyles, covering areas such as transportation, safety, finances, and social relationships (Carlson, Clark, & Young, 1998).

The Well Elderly Trial 2 was conducted over a 5-year period for the purpose of replicating and assessing the effectiveness and cost-effectiveness of Lifestyle Redesign among a more ethnically and economically diverse group of elders from a great number of sites around Los Angeles than in the first well-elderly trial. "The primary goal of the intervention was to enable the elders to develop a sustainable and customized healthy lifestyle in their daily context" (Clark & Jackson, 2010, para. 2). Results indicated that the intervention had a greater impact on measures of mental well-being (e.g., vitality, social function, life satisfaction) at statistically significant levels than on physical, health, and well-being measures (Clark et al., 2011). Lifestyle Redesign was found to be a cost-effective intervention for use in ethnically diverse urban communities (Clark et al., 2011; Clark & Jackson, 2010).

Practice Dilemma

At the request of a high school, you, together with a health educator, have successfully developed a weight management program for female high school students based on the theories shown in Table 44.7. The program includes occupation-based activities such as complicated line or group dances; healthy cooking classes, which emphasize portion control; a dress for success for all body types lecture series; and a culminating fashion show. Each of these activities focused on establishing skills (Ecology of Human Performance [EHP] construct) and self-efficacy (HBM and SCT construct) as well as social support to live a healthy life. A series of outings also were taken to local healthy fast food restaurants to sample healthier alternatives to fried food and red meat with the goal of permanently altering locations (EHP construct) of after-school meals to foster continued healthy food choices. The use of nondieting strategies were incorporated into the education portion of the program based on the work of Cole and Horacek (2009) who used the PRECEDE-PROCEED framework to develop an intuitive eating approach to weight management.

Based on your success, you have been asked to replicate your program with middle school boys and girls. The health educator you developed the program with has retired and is no longer available to assist you.

1. Given the retirement of the health educator, do you have the knowledge and skills to deliver an effective adaption of the current program to the new population? Explain your answer.
2. What are the implications to the use of the currently chosen theories with the new population?
3. Is there a place for developmental theory or other theory to guide you in adaptations to the programs for the new populations?

indicated are provided. Participants are educated to the finding that proper seating and alignment of mirrors decreases risk for a crash (HBM construct) due to increased visibility. At the end, participants walk around the car and reenter and can reassess the increased visibility leading to self-efficacy (HBM and SCT construct). The social atmosphere and encouragement in a group of peers acts as a sociostructural facilitator (SCT construct).

Conclusion

Occupation can be prescribed to promote health and well-being of individuals, families, and communities. However, this prescription must be unique and designed to be culturally relevant, client centered, and based on theory and the most current evidence available. Using a blend of theories drawn from health behavior and occupational therapy has the potential to strengthen occupational therapy health promotion program design and success. The prescription or intervention then must be evaluated to determine if outcomes are achieved, whether the prescription or program needs to be modified, and whether the theoretical foundation needs to evolve.

Although the potential contributions of health promotion to social participation and the health of society have been and are currently a focus of the profession's leadership, they also are a current focus of governmental efforts to enhance the nation's health while controlling costs (USDDHS, 2010). Occupational therapy practitioners can contribute to efforts to reduce costs while improving quality of life and overall well-being through health promotion initiatives crafted with clients and built on evidence and theory.

Acknowledgment

Melissa Kellner assisted in the production of this chapter while she was a graduate assistant in the Department of Occupational Therapy and Occupational Science, Towson University.

References

American Occupational Therapy Association. (1982). *1982 Member data survey*. Rockville, MD: Author.

American Occupational Therapy Association. (1987). *1986 Member data survey: Interim report #1*. Rockville, MD: Author.

American Occupational Therapy Association. (1991). *1990 Member data survey: Summary report*. Rockville, MD: Author.

American Occupational Therapy Association. (2001). *AOTA 2000 Member compensation survey*. Rockville, MD: Author.

American Occupational Therapy Association. (2006a). *AOTA 2006 Workforce and compensation report*. Rockville, MD: Author.

American Occupational Therapy Association. (2006b). AOTA's societal statement on health disparities. *American Journal of Occupational Therapy, 60*(6), 679.

American Occupational Therapy Association. (2008a). Occupational therapy in the promotion of health and the prevention of disease or disability. *American Journal of Occupational Therapy, 62*(6), 694–703.

American Occupational Therapy Association. (2008b). Occupational therapy practice framework: Domain and process, 2nd edition. *American Journal of Occupational Therapy, 62*(6), 625–683.

American Occupational Therapy Association. (2009). AOTA's societal statement on livable communities. *American Journal of Occupational Therapy, 63*(6), 847–848.

American Occupational Therapy Association. (2010a). *2010 Occupational therapy compensation and workforce study*. Bethesda, MD: Author.

American Occupational Therapy Association. (2010b). Occupational therapy code of ethics and ethics standards (2010). *American Journal of Occupational Therapy, 64*(Suppl.), S17–S26. doi:10:5014/ajot2010.62S17-64S26

American Occupational Therapy Association. (2010c). Standards of practice for occupational therapy. *American Journal of Occupational Therapy, 64*(Suppl.), S10–S11. doi:10.5014/ajot.2010.64 S106–64S111

American Occupational Therapy Association. (2011a). AOTA's societal statement on health literacy. *American Journal of Occupational Therapy*, *65*(Suppl.), S78–S79.

American Occupational Therapy Association. (2011b). Role of occupational therapy in disaster preparedness, response, and recovery: A concept paper. *American Journal of Occupational Therapy*, *65*(6, Suppl.), S11–S25. doi:10.5014/ajot.2011.65S8

American Occupational Therapy Association. (2012). Special issue on productive aging: Evidence and opportunities for occupational therapy practitioners. *American Journal of Occupational Therapy*, *66*(3), 263–265.

Bandura, A. (2004). Health promotion by social cognitive means. *Health Education & Behavior*, *31*(2), 143–164.

Barnard, S., Dunn, S., Reddic, E., Rhodes, K., Russell, J., Tuitt, T. S., . . . White, K. (2004). Wellness in Tillery: A community-built program. *Family and Community Health*, *27*(2), 151–157.

Baum, M. C. (2006). Presidential address, 2006: Centennial challenges, millennium opportunities. *American Journal of Occupational Therapy*, *60*(6), 609–616.

British Association of Occupational Therapists and College of Occupational Therapists. (2008). *Health promotion in occupational therapy*. London, England: College of Occupational Therapists.

Brunyate, R. W. (1967). From the President: After fifty years, what stature do we hold? *American Journal of Occupational Therapy*, *21*(5), 262–267.

Carlson, M., Clark, F., & Young, B. (1998). Practical contributions of occupational science to the art of successful ageing: How to sculpt a meaningful life in older adulthood. *Journal of Occupational Science*, *5*, 107–118.

Centers for Disease Control and Prevention. (2010). *Food deserts*. Retrieved from http://www.cdc.gov/Features/FoodDeserts/

Centers for Disease Control and Prevention, National Center for Injury Prevention and Control. (2010). *National intimate partner and sexual violence survey*. Retrieved from http://www.cdc.gov/ViolencePrevention/pdf/NISVS_FactSheet-a.pdf

Clark, F., Azen, S. P., Carlson, M., Mandel, D., LaBree, L. Hay, J., . . . Lipson, L. (2001). Embedding health-promoting changes into the daily lives of independent-living older adults: Long-term follow-up of occupational therapy intervention. *Journal of Gerontology: Psychological Sciences*, *56B*, P60–P63.

Clark, F., Azen, S. P., Zemke, R., Jackson, J., Carlson, M., Mandel, D., . . . Lipson, L. (1997). Occupational therapy for independent-living older adults: A randomized controlled trial. *Journal of the American Medical Association*, *278*, 1321–1326.

Clark, F., & Jackson, J. (2010). *Well Elderly II clinical trial results: Effectiveness and cost-effectiveness of the Lifestyle Redesign intervention in community settings*. Retrieved from http://www.wfot.org/wfot2010/program/pdf/1457.pdf

Clark, F., Jackson, J., Carlson, M., Chou, C., Cherry, B. J., Jordan-Marsh, M., . . . Azen, S. P. (2011). Effectiveness of a lifestyle intervention in promoting the well-being of independently living older people: Results of the well elderly 2 randomised controlled trial. *Journal of Epidemiology and Community Health*, 1–9. Advance online publication. doi:10.1136/jech.2009.099754

Clemson, L., Cumming, R. G., Kendig, H., Swann, M., Heard, R., & Taylor, K. (2004). The effectiveness of a community-based program for reducing the incidence of falls in the elderly: A randomized trial. *Journal of the American Geriatrics Society*, *52*, 1487–1494.

Cole, R. E., & Horacek, T. (2009). Applying PRECEDE-PROCEED to develop an intuitive eating nondieting approach to weight management pilot program. *Journal of Nutrition Education and Behavior*, *41*, 120–126.

Cook, A. (2004). Health education programming for older adults based on social cognitive theory. *American Occupational Therapy Association Gerontology Special Interest Section Quarterly*, *27*(1), 1–4.

Deshpande, S., Basil, M. D., & Basil, D. Z. (2009). Factors influencing healthy eating habits among college students: An application of the health belief model. *Health Marketing Quarterly*, *26*(2), 145–164.

Dumont, C., & Kielhofner, G. (2007). *Positive approaches to health*. New York, NY: Nova Science.

Dunn, W., Brown, C., & McGuigan, A. (1994). The ecology of human performance: A framework for considering the effect of context. *American Journal of Occupational Therapy*, *48*, 595–607.

Finn, G. (1972). The occupational therapist in prevention programs. *American Journal of Occupational Therapy*, *26*(2), 59–66.

Green, L. W., & Kreuter, M. W. (2005). *Health promotion planning: An educational and ecological approach* (4th ed.). New York, NY: McGraw Hill.

Jacobs, K., Wuest, E., Markowitz, J., & Hellman, M. (2011). Get packing: Planning your own National School Backpack Awareness Day event. *OT Practice*, *16*(13), 11–14.

Jaffe, E. (1986). Nationally speaking—The role of occupational therapy in the disease prevention and health promotion. *American Journal of Occupational Therapy*, *40*(11), 749–752.

James, D. C. S., Pobee, J. W., Oxidine, D., Brown, L., & Joshi, G. (2012). Using the health belief model to develop culturally appropriate weight-management materials for African-American women. *Journal of the Academy of Nutrition and Diuretics*, *112*(5), 664–670.

Jantzen, A. (1979). The current profile of occupational therapy and the future—Professional or vocational. In American Occupational Therapy Association (Ed.), *Occupational therapy: 2001* (pp. 71–75). Rockville, MD: American Occupational Therapy Association.

Johnson, J. A. (1986). *Wellness: A context for living*. Thorofare, NJ: Slack.

Juniper, K. C., Oman, R. F., Hamm, R. M., & Kerby, D. S. (2004). The relationships among construct in the health belief model and the transtheoretical model among African-American college women for physical activity. *American Journal of Health Promotion*, *18*(5), 354–357.

Kaplan, L. H., & Burch-Minakan, L. (1986). Reach out for health: A corporation's approach to health promotion. *American Journal of Occupational Therapy*, *40*, 777–780.

Kielhofner, G. (2009). *Conceptual foundations of occupational therapy* (4th ed.). Philadelphia, PA: F. A. Davis.

Kim, K. H., Linnan, L., Campbell, M. K., Brooks, C., Koenig, H. G., & Wiesen, C. (2008). The WORD (wholeness, oneness, righteousness, deliverance): A faith-based weight-loss program utilizing a community-based participatory action research approach. *Health Education & Behavior*, *35*(5), 634–650.

Law, M., Cooper, B., Strong, S., Stewart, D., Rigby, P., & Letts, L. (1996). The person-environment-occupation model: A transactive approach to occupational performance. *Canadian Journal of Occupational Therapy*, *63*(1), 9–23.

Losada, C. A. (1936). Some values in occupational therapy. *Occupational Therapy and Rehabilitation*, *15*(5), 285–289.

Miller, P. A., Hedden, J. L., Argento, L., Vaccaro, M., Murad, V., & Dionne, W. (2001). A team approach to health promotion of community elders: The microwave project. *Occupational Therapy in Health Care*, *14*(3/4), 17–34.

National Cancer Institute. (2005). *Theory at a glance* (2nd ed.). Bethesda, MD: National Institutes of Health. Retrieved from http://www.cancer.gov/theory.pdf

Polatajko, H. J., Davis, J., Stewart, D., Cantin, N., Amoroso, B., Purdie, L., & Zimmerman, D. (2007). Specifying the domain of concern: Occupation as core. In E. A. Townsend & H. J. Polatajko (Eds.), *Enabling occupation II: Advancing an occupational therapy vision for health, well-being, & justice through occupation*. Ottawa, Canada: Canadian Association of Occupational Therapists Publications ACE.

Prochaska, J. O., & DiClemente, C. C. (1982). Transtheoretical therapy: Toward a more integrative model of change. *Psychotherapy: Theory, Research and Practice*, *19*(3), 276–288.

Prochaska, J. O., & DiClemente, C. C. (1983). Stages and processes of self-change of smoking: Toward an integrative model of change. *Journal of Counseling and Clinical Psychology*, *51*(3), 390–395.

Reitz, S. M. (1992). A historical review of occupational therapy's role in preventive health and wellness. *American Journal of Occupational Therapy*, *46*, 50–55.

Reitz, S. M. (2010). Historical and philosophical perspectives of occupational therapy's role in health promotion. In M. E. Scaffa, S. M. Reitz, & M. A. Pizzi (Eds.), *Occupational therapy in the promotion of health and wellness* (pp. 1–21). Philadelphia, PA: F. A. Davis.

Reitz, S. M., & Scaffa, M. E. (2010). Public health principles, approaches, and initiatives. In M. E. Scaffa, S. M. Reitz, & M. A. Pizzi (Eds.), *Occupational therapy in the promotion of health and wellness* (pp. 70–95). Philadelphia, PA: F. A. Davis.

Reitz, S. M., Scaffa, M. E., Campbell, R. M., & Rhynders, P. A. (2010). Health behavior frameworks for health promotion practice. In M. E. Scaffa, S. M. Reitz, & M. A. Pizzi (Eds.), *Occupational therapy in the promotion of health and wellness* (pp. 46–69). Philadelphia, PA: F. A. Davis.

Schultz, S. (2009). Occupational adaptation. In E. B. Crepeau, E. S. Cohn, & B. A. B. Schell (Eds.), *Willard & Spackman's occupational therapy* (11th ed., pp. 462–475). Philadelphia, PA: Lippincott Williams & Wilkins.

Stav, W. (2010). CarFit: An evaluation of behavior change and impact. *British Journal of Occupational Therapy, 73*(12), 589–597.

U.S. Department of Health and Human Services. (2010). *Healthy people 2020* [Brochure]. Retrieved from http://www.healthypeople.gov/2020/TopicsObjectives2020/pdfs/HP2020_brochure.pdf

U.S. Department of Health and Human Services. (n.d.). *Healthy people 2020: Framework*. Retrieved from http://healthypeople.gov/2020/consortium/HP2020Framework.pdf

West, W. (1967). The occupational therapist's changing responsibility to the community. *American Journal of Occupational Therapy, 21*(5), 312–316.

West, W. (1969). The growing importance of prevention. *American Journal of Occupational Therapy, 23*(3), 226–231.

Wiemer, R. (1972). Some concepts of prevention as an aspect of community health. *American Journal of Occupational Therapy, 26*(1), 1–9.

Wilcock, A. A. (2006). *An occupational perspective of health* (2nd ed.). Thorofare, NJ: Slack.

World Federation of Occupational Therapists. (2004). *WFOT position paper on community based rehabilitation*. Retrieved from World Federation of Occupational Therapists Document Centre website: http://www.wfot.org/ResourceCentre.aspx

World Health Organization. (1947). Constitution of the World Health Organization. *Chronicle of the World Health Organization, 1*(1), 29–40.

World Health Organization. (1986). *Ottawa charter for health promotion*. Retrieved from http://www.who.int/hpr/NPH/docs/ottawa_charter_hp.pdf

Yamada, T., Kawamata, H., Kobayashi, N., Kielhofner, G., & Taylor, R. (2010). A randomized clinical trial of a wellness programme for healthy older people. *British Journal of Occupational Therapy, 73*(11), 540–548.

For additional resources on the subjects discussed in this chapter, visit http://thePoint.lww.com/Willard-Spackman12e.

CHAPTER 45

Principles of Learning and Behavior Change

Christine A. Helfrich

OUTLINE

LEARNING OBJECTIVES

After reading this chapter, you will be able to:

1. Identify and describe five theories of learning: behaviorist, social cognitive, constructivist, self-efficacy, and motivational
2. Compare the essential elements and assumptions of each theory of learning
3. Explain how different theories of learning contribute to occupational therapy intervention
4. Analyze a learning need and synthesize information to select the most appropriate strategy

Introduction

Think of the many things you may have taught different people. Perhaps you taught a younger sibling how to share toys, a friend how to navigate a bus or subway system, grandparents how to keep track of their medicines, a classmate how to organize information and prepare for an important test, a son or daughter how to overcome a fear or anxiety, and yourself a new leisure activity or how to use a new cell phone. How did you decide *how* to teach the person? Why did you teach the skill or behavior *in a particular way*? What *strategies* did you use? *What beliefs about how people learn guided you in your selection of strategies?* In your efforts to teach others, you have likely developed a beginning set of beliefs about how people learn best. Hopefully, you have also begun to notice that different strategies work best for different people and/or different situations.

This chapter presents an overview of selected *theories of learning*. In general, "learning theories" explain a perspective on what is "knowing" and how a person "comes to know" (Fosnot, 1996, p. ix). Learning theories have provided the foundation for many occupational therapy theories and frames of reference such as Cognitive Disabilities and the Model of Human Occupation. It is important to understand the basic concepts of learning when using theoretical approaches considered unique to occupational therapy. Five different overall ways of thinking about and conceptualizing theories of learning are reviewed in this chapter: behaviorist, social cognitive, constructivist, self-efficacy, and motivational.

Why Should Occupational Therapists Study Theories of Learning?

Suinicki (2004) identified several reasons to study theories of learning. Many of these are relevant to occupational therapists. Box 45.1 summarizes six important reasons for occupational therapy practitioners to study theories of learning as well as theory in general.

- Theory provides an overall *foundation for assessment and treatment* in all areas of practice. People often come to occupational therapy because they want to learn new ways of doing what is important to them, and occupational therapy practitioners help people to change behaviors so that they can engage in meaningful occupations. Theory provides the basis for designing specific interventions to address client issues.
- Theory *guides* and *informs* practice. Theory provides us with a conceptual framework related to observations of human behavior. Theories offer guidance about what to observe and answer questions about how best to facilitate behavior change.
- Theory presents an organizing framework of ideas about how people learn that leads to questions that can be tested in practice—in other words, *research*. Asking and answering questions about occupational therapy practice through research is a core responsibility for all occupational therapy practitioners.
- The primary goal of occupational therapy is to help people function in their daily occupations. Interventions may be designed, suggested, and implemented in many different ways. Practitioners who understand different perspectives on how people learn are likely to be more *effective* at presenting a range of interventions that match their clients' learning needs and learning styles. And when problems do arise, it is important to be able to analyze why the intervention may not be working. Understanding theories of learning will help you to *solve problems* that emerge during intervention and generate new approaches with your client when an intervention strategy is not effective.
- Each client with whom you work will have different values, interests, needs, abilities, and preferred ways of learning. Understanding theories of learning will help you to design *individualized* and *creative* interventions that respond to each client's unique strengths and limitations.
- Occupational therapy practice should always be moving forward; it is not static. Neither is theory. Ongoing exploration of theory and theory development is a *professional responsibility* of all occupational therapy practitioners.

In addition to the reasons to study theories of learning listed in Box 45.1, theories of learning serve several other purposes as well. At perhaps the most basic level, they provide us with a way to organize vast amounts of knowledge that are used in practice. Theory helps us to put our knowledge together, to organize otherwise random knowledge into a cohesive set of ideas that explains some phenomenon—in this case, learning. Theories of learning enable us to see how interesting and complex even the most seemingly simple things can be. This does not mean that theory makes things more *complicated.* Rather, theory helps you to see that there is usually more to any teaching-learning situation than meets the eye. Theories of learning reflect beliefs about how people think and how they store and use information (Suinicki, 2004). According to Hergenhahn (1976),

> since most human behavior is learned, investigating the principles of learning will help us understand why we behave as we do. An awareness of the learning process will not only allow greater understanding of normal and adaptive behavior, but will also allow greater understanding of the circumstances that produce maladaptive and abnormal behavior. (p. 12)

Therefore, in any intervention situation, practitioners need to understand the reason or reasons that contribute to problematic behavior.

BOX 45.1 Reasons to Study Theories of Learning

1. Provides a foundation for practice
2. Guides and informs practice
3. Leads to researchable questions
4. Enhances practitioners' effectiveness and ability to solve problems
5. Promotes individualized and creative interventions
6. Core professional responsibility

Where to Begin?

What is learning? How do we know when someone is learning? Under what conditions does learning occur? Why does learning occur? What does the learner do to cause the learning? What are the outcomes of learning? The answer to all of these questions is "it depends." It depends because different learning theories attribute different causes, reasons, actions, and circumstances to learning. And, because the therapist is treating an individual, who is unique, the challenge may be to determine the most appropriate theory to treat that person.

Behaviorist Theory

Behaviorist theory focuses on how observable, tangible behaviors are learned in response to some environmental stimulation (Martin & Pear, 2011). Behaviorist theorists focus on observable events rather than mental processes. For example, how does a child learn to take turns while playing a game with friends, how might a person with a developmental disability learn to respond appropriately in a conversation, and how would a person learn to propel and navigate a wheelchair in an urban community? In these examples, the observable events are the child waiting for and taking his or her turn during a game of kickball, a person waiting for a conversation partner to finish speaking before providing new information, and a person successfully navigating curbs and crowds in a wheelchair. The overall emphasis in behavioral theories of learning is on the relationship between an environmental stimulus and a behavioral response and on how learning is indicated by an observed change in behavior.

What Are the Essential Elements and Assumptions of Behaviorist Learning Theory?

Behaviorists use the term *conditioning* to explain changes in behavior rather than learning because behaviorist theory asserts that a person's behavior is conditioned by events in the environment. A behavior is gradually shaped, changed, and molded as it reflects the environment's response to the behavior. There are several key terms that you will notice in most types of behavioral theory: **conditioning** (a behavior modification process that increases or decreases the likelihood of a behavior being performed), **stimulus** (verbal, sensory, or environmental input that prompts a behavior), **response** (the reaction to the stimulus), **fading** and **shaping** (strategies to develop closer and closer approximations of a behavior), **chaining** (a stepwise process for teaching a multistep task), **reinforcement** (a stimulus that causes a behavior to be strengthened and performed again [positive or negative reinforcement]), **punishment** (an aversive stimulus that causes a behavior to decrease in frequency), and **extinction** (the process of reducing the frequency of a behavior by withholding reinforcement). Each of these terms will be further defined and discussed in more detail.

Behavioral Theorists

Many well-known theorists have contributed to the development of the behavioral perspective, such as Ivan Pavlov (1849–1936), Edward Thorndike (1874–1949), John Watson (1878–1958), and Burrhus Frederic (B. F.) Skinner (1904–1990). Although their theories are slightly different from each other, they do share common assumptions about the nature of learning—chiefly the need to focus on external, observable events as evidence of learning (Ormrod, 1990).

Ivan Pavlov developed the theory of *classical conditioning*, which resulted from his initial studies of a dog's salivation response to a neutral stimulus paired with an *unconditioned stimulus* (*food*), which caused an *unconditioned response* (*salivation*). After many pairings, the *neutral stimulus* (*bell*) became a *conditioned stimulus*, which then caused a *conditioned response* (*salivation*). As a result of his experiments and observations, Pavlov concluded that changes in behavior (learning) are due to *experience*.

Edward Thorndike's perspective is known as *connectionism*, whereby learning is seen as a process of making connections between things, understanding the relationship of a stimulus to a response. This concept may also be referred to as the *Law of Effect* (Driscoll, 2005). Thorndike studied how people established those connections and therefore how people developed and maintained behaviors. He emphasized the role of practice and experience in strengthening or weakening the connections between a stimulus and a response. Through a series of experiments, Thorndike concluded that behavior is learned via the consequences of the behavior. So responses to a behavior that were followed by a satisfying experience would be rewarded, thus strengthening the connection, the neural bond between the stimulus and the response, and increasing the likelihood that the behavior would be produced again.

John Watson introduced the term *behaviorism*. He emphasized the importance of focusing on observable behaviors. Watson was greatly influenced by the work of Pavlov. As he expanded on Pavlov's work, Watson proposed two "laws" that explained the relationship between stimulus and response and ultimately how behavior is learned. The *Law of Frequency* proposes that "the more frequently a stimulus and response occur in association with each other, the stronger that Stimulus-Response habit will become" (Ormrod, 1990, p. 20). The *Law of Recency* proposes that "the response that has most recently occurred after a particular stimulus is the response most likely to be associated with that stimulus" (Ormrod, 1990, p. 20).

B. F. Skinner was influenced by both Pavlov and Watson. He coined the term **operant conditioning**. Skinner's basic principle was that a response followed by some reinforcement is likely to be strengthened. And because a response is a change in behavior, then from a behaviorist perspective, this indicates learning. Any behavior, positive or negative, can be reinforced. Skinner used the term *reinforcement* rather than *reward* for two reasons. First, he believed that the term *reward* implies something pleasant or desirable, but sometimes people intentionally do things to produce an unpleasant consequence (e.g., Sally might wear her sister's clothes just to annoy her because Sally enjoys watching her sister get angry). Second, the terms *reward*, *pleasant*, and *desirable* are highly subjective terms.

There are three important factors in operant conditioning. First, the reinforcement must follow, not precede the response. Second, the reinforcement should immediately follow the behavior in order to have the greatest effect. Third, the reinforcement must be contingent on the response; it should not be given for an unintended or unrelated response.

How is operant conditioning different from classical conditioning? In classical conditioning, there is an unconditioned stimulus and a conditioned stimulus. The conditioned stimulus brings about the conditioned response. The response is *automatic and involuntary*. In operant conditioning, a response is *followed by* a reinforcing stimulus. The response is *voluntary*. The organism has control over whether it emits the response. For example, consider John, a 77-year-old man attending a community independent living center. An example of *classical conditioning* would be if the living center was playing old songs (stimulus) that reminded John of past experiences with friends. This could make John feel comfortable and pleasant (response) and cause John to want to attend the center more often. *Operant conditioning* would occur if after John went to the community independent living center (response), he received praise and enthusiasm (reinforcing stimulus) and then attended the center more regularly as a result.

Behavioral Intervention Approaches: Positive Reinforcement, Negative Reinforcement, Punishment, and Extinction

There are several different types of interventions that are designed to strengthen or increase behavior, whereas others decrease or eliminate behavior.

- **Positive reinforcement** is the presentation of a reinforcer (stimulus) immediately following a behavior that causes the behavior to be more likely to reoccur. Different types of reinforcement may include consumable (i.e., food), manipulative (i.e., toy to play with), social (i.e., positive feedback or attention), activity (i.e., swinging or bouncing on lap or watching television), and possession (i.e., money or tokens). The reinforcer must be appealing to the individual for it to be effective.
- **Negative reinforcement** occurs when the removal of a stimulus immediately after a response causes the response to be strengthened or to increase in frequency (Martin & Pear, 2011). For example, if Anna gets in her car and begins pulling out of her driveway, a seatbelt alarm will sound until Anna fastens her seatbelt. In this case, removal of the aversive stimulus of the alarm causes the seatbelt wearing response to be strengthened.
- **Punishment** is the presentation of an aversive stimulus contingent upon a response that reduces the rate of that response.
- **Extinction** is the process of reducing the frequency of a behavior by withholding reinforcement. Extinction can be challenging to enact because it may be difficult to know which reinforcer is the one actually reinforcing the undesirable behavior. For example, a child who hits other children and is given a time-out for that behavior may actually be receiving positive reinforcement (in the form of social contact) for that behavior from the adult giving the time-out. When trying to extinguish a behavior, you may also see an **extinction burst** or **spontaneous recovery**. An *extinction burst* occurs when the behavior being extinguished gets worse before it gets better. For example, an individual who is diagnosed with diabetes and told she must eliminate all sweets from her diet goes out to a dessert buffet every night for a week before starting her new diet. **Spontaneous recovery** occurs when the behavior being extinguished reappears after a delay, even though typically it is not as severe. An example of this is a child who has stopped taking other's toys and then begins to do so again, seemingly for no reason. Often, spontaneous recovery can be linked to a stressful or anxiety-producing event for the individual. Reimplementing the behavioral strategies that extinguished the behavior initially can usually be done quite quickly and successfully.

Reinforcement Schedule, Differential Reinforcement, Stimulus Discrimination, and Generalization

Each type of reinforcement used to change a behavior is delivered on a schedule. A **reinforcement schedule** indicates which instances of behavior, if any, will be reinforced. There are two main types of reinforcement schedules. **Continuous reinforcement** reinforces every instance of the behavior and is most often used at the beginning of treatment. **Intermittent reinforcement** only reinforces certain demonstrations of the behavior and is more effective at maintaining the desired response. Intermittent reinforcement can be delivered using one of the following four types of reinforcement schedules: (1) *ratio schedules*: reinforcement is based on the number of behaviors required; (2) *interval schedules*: reinforcement is based on the passage of time between behaviors occurring; (3) *fixed schedules*: the requirements for reinforcement are always the same; and (4) *variable schedules*: the requirements for reinforcement change randomly. It is easiest for someone to change his or her behavior initially when he or she knows when he or she will receive his or her next reinforcement; however, variable reinforcement is more effective at maintaining behavior change. For example, if the goal is for Bobby to get to school on time every day, you would begin by giving him positive reinforcement *each* day he arrived on time (*continuous*). Once he was arriving on time consistently, you might only reward him each time he arrived 3 days in a row (*ratio*) or every fourth day (*interval*) he arrived on time. Once either or both of these patterns were achieved, you would provide random reinforcement (*variable schedule*) for his on-time arrival to school.

Differential reinforcement teaches individuals to discriminate between *desired* and *undesired* behavior and can be used to *increase* or *decrease* behavior. There are four types of differential reinforcement. *Differential reinforcement at low rates* (DRL) and *differential reinforcement of zero responding* (DRO) involves the simple decrease or absence of behavior (i.e., decreases or stops talking out in class) (DRL or DRO). *Differential reinforcement of incompatible responding* (DRI) and *differential reinforcement of alternative behavior* (DRA) involve adding an incompatible or alternative behavior to replace the original behavior (i.e., eating a lollipop instead of sucking one's thumb [DRI], rolling cigarettes instead of spending food money on expensive cigarettes [DRA]). Note: Harm reduction programs use forms of differential reinforcement by reinforcing less harmful behaviors that replace more harmful behaviors (e.g., going to a needle exchange program instead of sharing needles to use heroin [DRA], taking Antabuse to decrease alcohol use [DRI]).

Stimulus discrimination learning is the procedure by which an individual can learn to emit a behavior under certain conditions instead of others. For example, children learn to raise their hands to be called on in the classroom if they wish to speak, whereas at the family dinner table, they wait for a pause in the conversation to speak (without raising their hands). In contrast, **stimulus generalization** occurs when a behavior becomes more probable in the presence of one stimulus as a result of being reinforced in the presence of another similar stimulus. For example, a child who has been abused by his father may *generalize his response* to being fearful of all men and demonstrate this fear by avoiding males, in general.

Behavioral Techniques: Fading, Shaping, and Chaining

Whereas different types of reinforcement are used to *increase* or *decrease* specific behaviors, *fading, shaping*, and *chaining* are behavioral methods used to teach skills that involve *more than one step*.

- **Fading** occurs when prompts or cues that guide the performance of a complex behavior are gradually withdrawn. A *prompt* is a stimulus (physical, verbal, or visual) introduced to control the desired behavior during the early part of a learning program. For example, when Tom is learning how to swing a golf club, the instructor will first provide hand-over-hand guidance to show Tom how to hold and swing the club, then will move to using only verbal cues, and next will use fewer and fewer verbal cues until eventually Tom is swinging the club on his own.
- **Shaping** occurs by reinforcing successively closer approximations to the target behavior while extinguishing preceding approximations of the behavior. For example, when baby Jennifer is learning how to talk and says "Je" when first attempting to say her own name, her parents reinforce her behavior with smiles and verbal praise. With practice, Jennifer next refers to herself as "Jen," then "Jen-fer," and finally as "Jennifer." As Jennifer's pronunciation improves, her parents provide smiles and verbal praise for each improved pronunciation while no longer reinforcing previous versions. For example, once Jennifer learns to say "Jen-fer", she is no longer praised for referring to herself as "Je."

Both fading and shaping involve a gradual change. Fading involves a gradual change in stimulus while the response stays the same. Shaping uses the same stimulus to establish a gradual change in the response.

- **Chaining** is used to teach a complex behavior by reinforcing the performance of each part of the behavior separately, but in order, until the individual can complete the entire sequence.

There are three types of chaining: (1) *Forward chaining* begins with reinforcing the first step and then adding sequential steps while fading the prompts/reinforcers for previous steps as they are learned. Forward chaining is the natural way that you would teach yourself a task that you had to read directions for, such as setting up a new computer system. (2) *Backwards chaining* begins with reinforcing the final step of the complex behavior and then the second-to-last step, and so on, until the behavior is learned. For example, Betty recently had a cerebrovascular accident (CVA) and needs to learn to feed herself again. You would prepare her food, cut it into pieces and place her fork correctly in her hand, and then she would complete the last step: placing the food in her mouth—a natural reinforcement. The advantage of backwards chaining is that it is a natural reinforcer because the task is already completed and sometimes there is less frustration (see Figure 45.1). (3) *Total task training* occurs when the individual is asked to attempt to do all the steps from the beginning to the end. Prompting may be provided along the way, and reinforcement is provided following the last step. This method often instills confidence when an individual is relearning a previously learned skill or learning a skill he or she may consider insulting to be taught yet may be necessary for safety or independence evaluations (i.e., dressing, cooking).

Behavior Modification: Assessment and Treatment

There are four phases of a successful behavioral modification program: (1) screening, (2) baseline, (3) treatment, (4) follow-up. Behavioral assessment can be carried out throughout the whole behavioral modification program or during each phase of the program.

Three sources of getting information for the baseline assessment include indirect assessment, direct assessment, and functional assessment. **Indirect assessment** includes interviews, questionnaires, role-playing, consulting with other professionals, and client self-monitoring.

Direct assessment records the *characteristics* of behaviors that are observed, including (1) *topography*: form of a particular response, (2) *amount*: frequency and duration of the behavior, (3) *intensity* (*force* or *magnitude*), (4) *stimulus control*: a certain behavior occurs in the presence of certain stimuli, (5) *latency*: the time between the occurrence of a stimulus and the beginning of a response, and (6) *quality of behavior*.

Functional assessment is used to identify the *cause* of a problem behavior. There are several approaches to completing a functional assessment including (1) *questionnaires*, (2) *observations*: observes and describes the antecedents and immediate consequences of the behavior in natural settings, and (3) *functional analysis*: directly assesses the effects of controlling variables on the problem behavior. In functional analysis, environmental events are systematically manipulated to test their roles as antecedents or as consequences in controlling and maintaining specific behaviors.

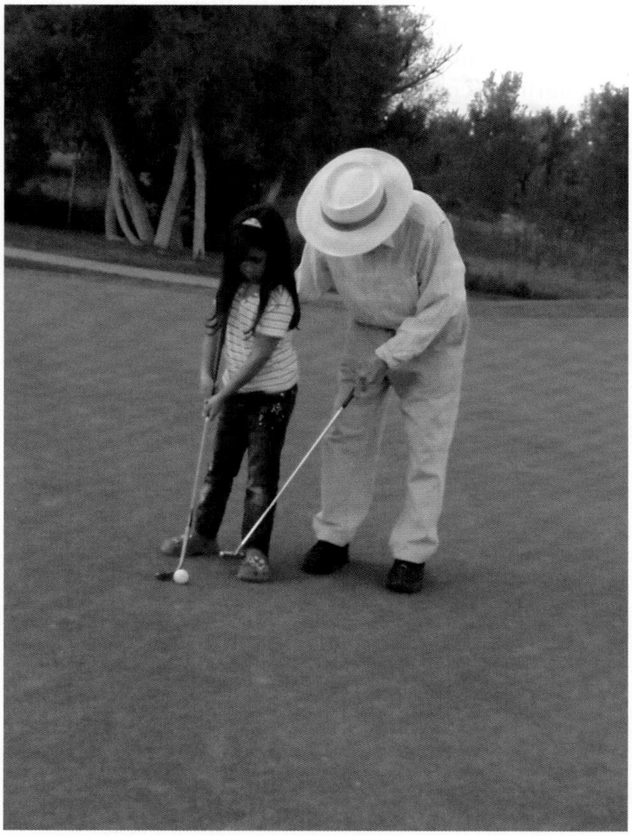

FIGURE 45.1 A great uncle uses backwards chaining to teach his young niece to golf by first reinforcing the final step of putting the golf ball into the hole.

Occupational Therapy and Behaviorist Theory

Occupational therapy practitioners using behaviorist theory to understand human learning and guide their intervention would analyze a complex behavior that needs to be learned (e.g., a child's need to take turns when she plays) and sequence that behavior from simple to complex. Sometimes the process of *learning* a new behavior also involves *extinguishing* a problem behavior. Intervention would consist of opportunities for the person to participate in increasingly complex behaviors, using behaviorist principles such as reinforcement, shaping, and chaining. Progress would be measured by clients' observed occupational performance and their ability to complete increasingly complex behaviors necessary for occupational performance.

Occupational therapy practitioners have used the behavioral theory of learning in several ways to guide their interventions with clients. For example, Giles and Wilson (1988) and Giles, Ridley, Dill, and Frye (1997) described programs to help retrain people who had sustained severe brain injuries. The clients had severe physical and cognitive impairments and needed help with washing and dressing: basic self-care behaviors. The practitioners designed and implemented a program that consisted of individualized plans to break down each larger activity (getting dressed) into its smaller elements. Practitioners used a specific set of instructions to gradually add skills to each person's repertoire (*shaping*) and eventually teach the entire behavior.

Katzmann and Mix (1994) presented a case report of a 34-year-old woman with viral encephalitis. The woman had difficulty processing written and verbal information and had great difficulty with various complex self-care tasks. The practitioners' intervention was influenced by behavioral theories, using such techniques as prompting with step-by-step instructions, shaping, and verbal or physical cues. The practitioners identified and sequenced all of the steps required for the woman to complete her washing, dressing, and grooming routine, which began with getting out of bed and ended with going to breakfast in the rehabilitation facility. A series of step-by-step instructions, gradual and consistent shaping of behavior, verbal cues, and physical assistance helped the woman to improve her overall activities of daily living (ADL) functioning. The practitioners used forward chaining by cueing the woman with directions or providing physical assistance for a step that needed to be completed and gradually removed the cues as she initiated and completed the task independently.

Behaviorist theories emphasize observable behavior, rewarding and reinforcing desirable behavior and reducing problematic behaviors. Clients who might benefit from intervention approaches that are grounded in behaviorist theories of learning include people who have difficulty planning and organizing activities, those who have problems with memory and/or attention, those who have deficits in sequencing activities, and those who demonstrate inappropriate social behaviors. Some strategies that could help a child to develop sharing and turn-taking skill include praising appropriate behavior (to provide positive reinforcement for sharing), not giving attention every time she takes toys from others (to decrease the negative reinforcement for the undesired behavior), using a sticker chart to document sharing (to gradually shape appropriate behavior), and providing rewards for good sharing, such as letting her stand first in line to go to the playground.

Social Learning and Social Cognitive Theory

The social learning and social cognitive theory of learning are an outgrowth of behaviorist theories. Theorists such as Piaget (1970) and Bandura (1977b) were dissatisfied with the limits of behaviorist theory because they believed that there was more to learning than just the interaction of a person with the environment. They developed theories of learning that integrated *social* and *cognitive* processes with behavioral processes. Although there are individual variations and areas of focus, in general, social cognitive theory explains learning as occurring in a social context, that is, the "where, what, when, with whom, how often, and under what circumstances" aspects of our lives. Humans learn by observing others, cognitively processing observations, storing those observations and thoughts, and then using them, sometimes at a much later time. This is an important contrast with behavioral theorists, who view learning as an observable change in behavior at a specific point in time. Social learning/social cognitive theorists disagree and say that *learning can occur even in the absence of an observable change in behavior* (Ormrod, 2006). Social and cognitive processes such as observation, storing observations in memory, self-assessment, and self-appraisal promote learning. The *interactions* between a person, behavior, and the environment are emphasized.

Five major assumptions are inherent to social learning/social cognitive theory (Ormrod, 2006).

1. *People can learn by observing others.* For example, a college freshman, new to living and eating in a dormitory, may be unfamiliar with a waffle maker available to her in the breakfast line. She might casually watch others make waffles until she feels confident that she knows the process well enough to try it herself.
2. *Learning is an internal process* that may or may not lead to an observable change in behavior. For example, people might observe various social skills, such as how to introduce themselves to someone they meet, how to end a conversation politely, and how to maintain an appropriate social distance during a conversation. These skills might be stored in memory for future use and not be immediately demonstrated.
3. *People are generally motivated to achieve goals for themselves*, and their behavior is typically directed toward those goals.
4. *Learning occurs as people regulate and adjust their own behavior*, instead of learning being a direct response to and dependent on environmental stimuli. This means that people would observe others, determine their own individual standards, and then work to behave according to those standards.
5. *Feedback via reinforcement and punishment affect learning and behavior indirectly* (not directly, as behaviorists believe). This means that people can adjust their behavior on the basis of *anticipated* (positive or negative) consequences. Or, people might observe the outcomes of a behavior demonstrated by others and adjust their behaviors on the basis of that observation (Ormrod, 2006). Box 45.2 summarizes these major assumptions.

It is important for a person to observe skills and behaviors via models and to note the reinforcement that models receive for behaviors. Models can be *live* (a person with whom the learner has actual contact) or *symbolic* (a pictorial or abstract representation of behavior, such as through television or other media). Whatever the

BOX 45.2 Major Assumptions of Social Cognitive Theory of Learning

- People can learn by observing others.
- Learning is an internal process.
- People are motivated to achieve goals.
- People regulate and adjust their own behavior.
- Reinforcement and punishment may have an indirect effect on behavior.

source, the modeled behavior serves as information for the observer/learner. A person can also learn *vicariously*, increasing or decreasing a given behavior on the basis of the reinforcement that the person observes someone else is receiving (also an indirect form of modeling because the reinforcement is being modeled). For example, if a model's behavior is positively reinforced, the observer might increase that behavior. Other determining factors include how much attention gets paid to the model, how credible or prestigious the model is, and how the model is rewarded (Ormrod, 2006).

Because people can learn by observing others, *attention* to the behavior is a very important factor. A learner is more likely to remember information when the learner consciously attends to the behavior, rehearses it in his or her own mind, and develops personal verbal or visual ways to represent the information (Ormrod, 1990). A person should be able to describe the behavior or have a picture of that behavior in his or her mind, stored for future use.

People develop expectations about what they think will happen as a result of different behaviors. Thus, *incentive* is an important consideration. Incentive is the anticipation that something will happen (reinforcement) if a particular behavior is performed or not performed. This is another difference from behaviorist theory. According to operant conditioning theory, the reinforcement must come after the behavior has been performed. According to social cognitive theory, an anticipated outcome might precede the behavior being performed (or not performed).

Occupational Therapy and Social Learning/Social Cognitive Theory

An occupational therapy practitioner working with Jake, a 14-year-old who is having difficulty at school, might have Jake *identify* specific problem situations (e.g., being distracted in class, using minimal effort to complete projects, or becoming bored in class) and then identify specific strategies to address these difficulties (e.g., sitting at the front of the classroom, setting "effort goals" for himself, identifying at least one interesting aspect of any project), *set* manageable and measurable goals, and then *develop* a mechanism to determine how well he has achieved his goals. The occupational therapy practitioner might also encourage Jake's teacher to pair him with classmates who demonstrate good study habits and who are highly motivated for learning. Or, the practitioner might role-play conversations that Jake is likely to have with his parents or teachers about his feelings and attitudes toward schoolwork. The role-play conversations could help Jake to articulate his concerns and then work to support his learning.

A variety of occupational therapy intervention programs have incorporated aspects of social learning theories. Jao and Lu (1999) studied the effects of a problem-solving intervention on the interpersonal skills of people with chronic schizophrenia. They found that helping people with schizophrenia to recognize and define problems, think of alternative solutions, and determine the best course of action facilitated the development of interpersonal problem-solving skills.

Helfrich, Chan, and Sabol (2011) described a life skills intervention in the community for individuals who were homeless using *Situated Learning*. Situated learning theory, which is derived from social learning theory (Lave & Wenger, 1991), posits that behavior results from interaction between the person and the situation. The learner is placed in contexts that allow for simulated and actual application to everyday situations, whereas peers enhance the learning experience with feedback. In social situations, individuals gain motivational support from others and access both expertise and collaborative thinking, increasing opportunities to acquire and apply new knowledge. This approach allowed group participants functioning at a variety of levels to benefit from others' experiences with the life skills being taught.

Most of these programs emphasize the importance of learning in a social context, providing numerous opportunities for clients to develop or relearn essential skills for living, and employ activities such as role-play, observation, problem solving, and practice in real-life situations.

Constructivist Theory

Suppose you are an occupational therapy practitioner working in a community independent living center. Your clients are typically recovering from substance abuse or might have chronic mental illness. Part of your intervention includes a series of life skills sessions that are designed to help people learn or relearn different instrumental ADLs. A new session will begin next week with

BOX 45.3 Major Assumptions of Constructivist Theory of Learning

- Learners must be active participants in their learning.
- Learners are capable of discovering and creating their own knowledge.
- Active participation in the learning environment enhances critical thinking and problem-solving abilities.
- In learning, people gather information and develop problem-solving strategies simultaneously.
- Active participation in the learning environment enhances the meaning and relevance of the learning experience and motivation for learning.

five new clients. One segment of your program focuses on time use and leisure planning. Will all five clients come to the course with the same life experiences? Will all five people have the same outlook on life? How might you understand the teaching-learning process, given these individual differences and experiences?

A constructivist would assert that individual differences are to be expected, that "everyone's construction of the world is unique even though we share a great many concepts" (Suinicki, 2004, p. 14). Although there are several "traditional" methods of providing information, such as through imparting information or finding information in books or on the Internet, this does not necessarily indicate or result in learning, according to constructivism. For constructivists, the learner must *access* information, use this information to *alter* or modify existing knowledge and understanding, and *integrate* the new information with previous information to *create* a new understanding that is relevant to himself or herself (Marlowe & Page, 1998). For the life skills challenge posed earlier, a constructivist would embrace the members' different perspectives and perceive them as essential to individual learning. Although this approach may sound very similar to situated learning as described previously, *constructivism* speaks more to the role of the client as an individual-learner, responsible for his or her own learning. Situated learning places the role of learning more in the context of an apprenticeship or mentoring model.

There are some basic assumptions about the teaching-learning process that are common to constructivism. First, learners must be *active participants* in their learning. Second, the learner is capable of *creating* his or her own *knowledge* through interaction with the human and nonhuman environment. Third, when learners participate in this type of learning environment, they develop the *ability to think critically* to solve problems. Fourth, when actively engaged in constructing their own knowledge, people *gather information and develop strategies* at the same time (Marlowe & Page, 1998).

Bruner (1961) has had a major influence in the development of constructivism or "discovery" learning. According to Bruner, a constructivist approach fosters *intellectual potency*, meaning that when people seek and find information for themselves, that information is more meaningful, relevant, and powerful for them. Furthermore, people organize information they find for themselves so that it is more efficiently and effectively retrieved for future use. Constructivists call this a *conservation of memory*. Second, because the learners "own" the information, this approach fosters *intrinsic motivation*. Rather than settling into a pattern in which learners conform to what the instructor wants them to learn, learners *discover* for themselves. This promotes motivation to learn. Third, the only way to improve one's ability to think, question, and discover is to do it actively and repeatedly; to engage in the process. Constructivism fosters people's learning the *process of discovery*. Box 45.3 summarizes the major assumptions of constructivism.

A practitioner who uses a constructivist approach in the teaching-learning process emphasizes skills and activities such as asking questions, independent exploration, identifying problems, brainstorming, and generating individual solutions to problems. The practitioner emphasizes the *client's essential role in the process* and sees his or her own role as facilitating client's progress. The practitioner views the therapy process as recognizing, embracing, respecting, and encouraging people to develop individual meanings, to promote and enhance the client's knowledge and skill.

In this perspective, clients are expected to actively direct what needs to be learned and how the learning will occur. Clients help to determine the resources that will enhance their learning. Independent thinking, collaborative problem solving, and using past experience to reframe and revise new learning are all important. The practitioner's knowledge and expertise are still very essential; however, in this perspective, the practitioner uses his or her knowledge and expertise as a point of reference. In many ways, the practitioner takes a "back seat" as the client pursues learning; the practitioner's role is to address problems that arise. The practitioner facilitates the process, using himself or herself to promote the client's ability to identify, address, and solve problems. The occupational therapy practitioner does not provide "the intervention" but instead works to facilitate the person's developing his or her own strategies to deal with his or her own issues. The practitioner is alert to major issues but is neither prescriptive nor directive (Lederer, 2000) (see Figure 45.2).

Practice Dilemma

Constructivist Perspective on Learning

If each person constructs his or her own learning and therefore there is no "objective reality," what challenges does that present to an occupational therapy practitioner who advocates a constructivist perspective on learning? What opportunities does it provide to the practitioner and/or to the person with whom the practitioner is working? What are some strategies that you could implement to address clients' time use and leisure skill development in the life skills program described earlier? How would you address this individual's goals in a group setting?

Self-Efficacy Theory

The self-efficacy theory of learning focuses on a person's individual beliefs about how effective he or she is or will be at learning or completing a new skill or behavior. Albert Bandura (1977a) first articulated a theory of self-efficacy. His perspective on how behaviors are learned and changed involved behavioral *and* cognitive processes. His central thesis is that a person's **efficacy expectations**, the person's beliefs about how successful or unsuccessful he or she will be at performing a skill or occupation, will greatly influence his or her execution of that skill or occupation. The emphasis here is on the *person's beliefs* and *how those beliefs influence his or her performance.* For example, a person might believe that a particular action performed or executed by a person *in general* will produce a certain outcome. However, this is different from the person's belief that he or she has the ability to perform the action and that it will result in a successful outcome. A person's efficacy expectations also influence the person's *persistence* with different occupations. "Efficacy expectations determine how much effort people will expend and how long they will persist in the face of obstacles and aversive experiences. The stronger the perceived self-efficacy, the more active the efforts" (Bandura, 1977a, p. 194).

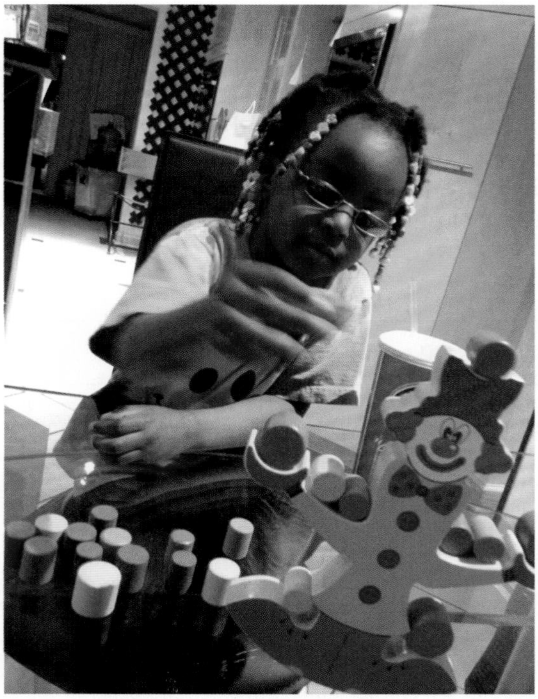

FIGURE 45.2 A young girl actively participates in her own learning by exploring principles of balance through play with blocks of different sizes and weights.

Efficacy expectations have three important dimensions: magnitude, generality, and strength (Bandura, 1977a). *Magnitude* involves the level of difficulty for a task—for example, making a sandwich versus making an elaborate dinner. *Generality* involves the degree to which a person's perceived self-efficacy for one task transfers to another—for example, maneuvering a wheelchair around the occupational therapy clinic versus maneuvering a wheelchair in a busy urban community. *Strength* refers to the degree to which people believe they can be successful—for example, being very confident about one's success versus being only slightly confident.

Typically, a person's self-efficacy is developed over time and through four sources of information: outcomes that were generated by the person's own *personal accomplishments*; through *vicarious experience*, that is, seeing others perform a skill and through that vicarious experience believing that "if the other person can accomplish the skill, so can I"; by being *persuaded* by others that the person can be successful; and by *feeling calm and relaxed* when performing a skill (Bandura, 1977a). Given these information sources, the person's *own cognitive appraisal* of how successful or unsuccessful he or she will be has the greatest impact on the person's efficacy expectation.

Although perceived self-efficacy and self-esteem are related, the two concepts are not the same. Perceived self-efficacy is what you believe you can do with your skill. *Self-esteem* refers to a person's negative or positive sense of self. So a person might feel that he or she is competent and successful in completing a variety of occupations but might have an overall negative feeling about himself or herself. Certainly, perceived self-efficacy might contribute to a person's self-esteem; but they are two separate concepts (Gage & Polatajko; 1994).

According to Bandura (1977b), self-efficacy relates to behavior change very directly. If a person has only weak expectations for his or her success, it is likely that unsuccessful experiences will quickly result in the person's not performing the skill or behavior. If the person's beliefs about his or her success are strong, then it is likely that the person will persist, even through negative or unsuccessful experiences.

Motivational Theory

Motivational theories view change as coming from within the person and his or her motivation to make a change. The most common and well-developed theory is the Transtheoretical Model (TTM) of intentional change, which assesses individuals' readiness to change and measures progress toward goals over the course of an intervention (Brady et al., 1996; Finnell, 2003; J. O. Prochaska, Redding, & Evers, 1997). The theory, developed from the disciplines of psychology and psychotherapy, proposes that a person may progress through five stages of behavior change: precontemplation, contemplation, preparation, action, and maintenance (J. O. Prochaska, 2001; J. O. Prochaska & DiClemente, 1983). The TTM proposes that effective interventions address an individual's present stage of change and cautions that without intervention, individuals may not progress (Finnell, 2003; Haggerty & Goodman, 2006). The transtheoretical stages of change model has been applied to a variety of health behaviors and systems issues, such as smoking cessation (J. O. Prochaska & DiClemente, 1983), addressing health risk behaviors (Nigg et al., 1999), arthritis self-management (Keefe et al., 2000), organizational change (J. M. Prochaska, Prochaska, & Levesque, 2001), and weight control (Plotnikoff et al., 2009; Sarkin, Johnson, Prochaska, & Prochaska, 2001). This model has two essential elements: the five integrated *stages* of change and the various *processes* that can facilitate a person's moving from one stage to the next.

The stages of change begin with *precontemplation*. Here, a person demonstrates a behavior that is perceived by others as needing to be changed. These behaviors are often harmful or destructive (e.g., a substance use or addiction, poorly controlled anger or stress, or general health and wellness issues). The person might be unaware or minimally aware of his or her problem, or the person might be aware of the problem but resistant to fully acknowledging or addressing it. In the second stage, *contemplation*, the person is likely to be aware of his or her problem and is thinking about overcoming it but is not quite ready to take action. In the third stage, *preparation*, the person begins to make some small changes in his or her behavior. In the fourth stage, *action*, the person is committed to making the change and is involved in change behaviors on a regular basis. The person is putting forth great energy to modify behaviors, the environment, or his or her experiences to effect serious change. In the fifth stage, *maintenance*, the person struggles to maintain the change, working to sustain accomplishments and prevent relapse (J. O. Prochaska, Norcross, & DiClemente, 1992).

These stages might appear to be linear, occurring in a step-by-step progression from one stage to the next. However, J. O. Prochaska et al. (1992) explain change as occurring in a spiral fashion, because most people experience relapses or other setbacks as they work to change behaviors. In fact, relapse is expected! Relapse can occur back to *any* stage; however, the subsequent progress usually is easier for the individual. Think about a time that you or a friend set out to change a certain behavior and achieved stage three (preparation) or stage four (action) only to experience some setback and spiral back down to an earlier stage? According to the TTM, this is common and to be expected.

The *processes* of change explain *how* to promote the shifts. Because individuals may lack self-efficacy regarding their ability to change, it may be critical to increase the skills needed for change and to allow opportunities to practice change behaviors. According to J. O. Prochaska et al. (1992), people who have reached the contemplation stage are ready to understand the processes that

BOX 45.4 Principles of Motivational Interviewing

1. *Express empathy about the change being considered* is showing your acceptance of an individual no matter what the individual says or does. Expressing empathy and reflective listening are fundamental for the interviewee to feel that you are invested in the conversation.
2. *Develop discrepancy between present behavior and important personal goals or values* occurs when the therapist gently points out how the client's present goal does not match his or her current behavior. For example, Laura wants to be a good mother and maintain custody of her children, but she goes out every Friday night to the bar and spends her paycheck on alcohol while her young children are left alone at home. Once the client can see the discrepancy between her present behavior and the goal behaviors that are important to her, the discrepancy can help to motivate change.
3. *Roll with resistance by avoiding arguing for change and inviting new perspectives.* Being client centered is essential here. In a life skills study involving a money management group, Bill indicated he would not participate if the therapist was going to "make" him spend less money on cigarettes by *quitting* or *cutting down*. Instead, they worked together to find ways to smoke less expensively with roll-your-own cigarettes and smokeless tobacco. Both strategies ultimately helped move Bill toward decreasing his smoking.
4. *Support self-efficacy through the person's belief in the possibility of change.* This principle involves conveying your belief and hope in the possibility of change while supporting the client to develop a sense of self-efficacy and choose his or her own personal goals.

BOX 45.5 Six Themes of Change Talk

1. ***Desire*:** Verbs include *want, like,* and *wish*. These tell you something that the person wants. (i.e., I *wish* I could lose some weight.)
2. ***Ability*:** The prototypical verb is *can* (*could*). These show you what the person perceives as within his or her ability. (i.e., I *could* probably cut down a bit.)
3. ***Reasons*:** There are no particular verbs here, but words used always express specific reason for a certain change. (i.e., This pain keeps me from playing the guitar!)
4. ***Need*:** Marker verbs include *need, have to, got to, should, ought,* and *must*. These tell you some necessity. (i.e., I *must* quit smoking.)
5. ***Commitment*:** Most used verbs are *will, intend to,* and *going to*. These can be presented with strong or lower level of commitment. (i.e., I *will* go to Alcoholics Anonymous [AA] group once a month.)
6. ***Taking steps*:** Reporting recent specific action (step) towards change. (i.e., I quit drinking for a couple of weeks but then started again.)

can contribute to behavioral change. Their research indicates that people who are in the precontemplation stage lack the awareness to engage in or benefit from the processes of change. Others (Helfrich, Chan, Simpson, & Sabol, 2011) have disputed this assumption. Their research has demonstrated that people in the precontemplation stage of change may move to the contemplation stage, or yet a higher stage, through the process of being exposed to treatment interventions. The process of introducing the possibility of change may allow an individual to risk changing. People who have progressed to the contemplation stage may benefit from *consciousness-raising* strategies that help them to get information about their problem and themselves, by being encouraged to express their feelings about their problems through various *dramatic relief* strategies such as role-playing, and by *environmental reevaluation* to assess how their behavior affects their physical and social surroundings (e.g., perhaps a person's smoking deters family or friends from visiting or there are stains and cigarette burns on the person's furnishings). Strategies such as values clarification exercises to enhance *self-reevaluation*, or how one thinks and feels about himself or herself, can be helpful as one moves to the preparation stage. Making a real commitment to change, believing in one's ability to change, and using techniques such as personal goal setting to enhance *self-liberation* or will power can be helpful during the action stage. Several processes are important in the maintenance stage, such as fostering *helping relationships* and social supports that encourage the person to be open and honest about his or her problems; avoiding things that elicit the problem behavior and substituting alternatives (*stimulus control* and *counterconditioning*); and *reinforcement management*, rewarding oneself for making changes. *Social liberation* helps to promote change across various stages through advocacy, empowerment, and social change mechanisms (J. O. Prochaska et al., 1992).

Motivational interviewing is another clinical process (technique) that encourages people to consider and implement change. The principles of motivational interviewing include (1) express empathy about the change being considered, (2) develop discrepancy between present behavior and important personal goals or values, (3) roll with resistance by avoiding arguing for change and inviting new perspectives, and (4) support self-efficacy through the person's belief in the possibility of change (Miller & Rollnick, 1991). Box 45.4 summarizes the principles of motivational interviewing.

There are four primary skills that are suggested to implement these principles of motivational interviewing: (1) asking open questions, (2) reflective listening, (3) affirming, and (4) summarizing. In addition, the therapist should always be listening for *change talk* and to elicit the possibility of change talk during conversation with the client. Box 45.5 describes the six themes of change talk.

The key to success for this model is the careful, systematic, and close fit between the person, the stage, and the process. According to J. O. Prochaska et al. (1992), "efficient self-change depends on doing the right things (processes) at the right time (stages)" (p. 1110). Table 45.1 summarizes J. O. Prochaska et al. (1992) stages and processes of change.

TABLE 45.1 Stages and Processes of Change

Stage	Process (How to Promote Change)
Precontemplation	Strategies are not effective because the person lacks awareness to engage in or benefit from change
Contemplation	Consciousness-raising strategies to learn about problem, role-play strategies to express feelings, assessment of how behavior affects physical and social environment
Preparation	Values clarification exercises to promote reevaluation of feelings or self-perception
Action	Goal-setting strategies and techniques
Maintenance	Development of social supports, substitution of alternatives to problem behavior, avoidance of experiences that elicit the problem behavior, rewarding oneself for making changes

Occupational Therapy, Self-Efficacy Theory, and Motivational Theory

Both self-efficacy theories and motivational theories have great relevance for occupational therapy. Often, a person's self-perceptions and beliefs about his or her ability to be successful with an occupation influence the person's decision about whether to participate in that occupation. For example, a person who believes that he or she has good interview skills will be more likely to respond to a job advertisement even though he or she might not have direct experience with the type of work that needs to be done. A person who did not have that sense of effectiveness might be less likely to pursue the job. Intervention strategies to promote a person's perceived self-efficacy in the job interview situation described here would include determining with the person that he or she had all the requisite skills to be successful, using peer role models so that the person could practice or "try on" the essential skills and behaviors, having the person practice interview skills, providing feedback on specific successes, and encouraging the person to evaluate his or her skills in a personal way rather than comparing these skills to someone else's. These theories all emphasize the importance of an individual's participation in *meaningful* occupations as both the foundation and result of motivation and self-efficacy (see Figure 45.3).

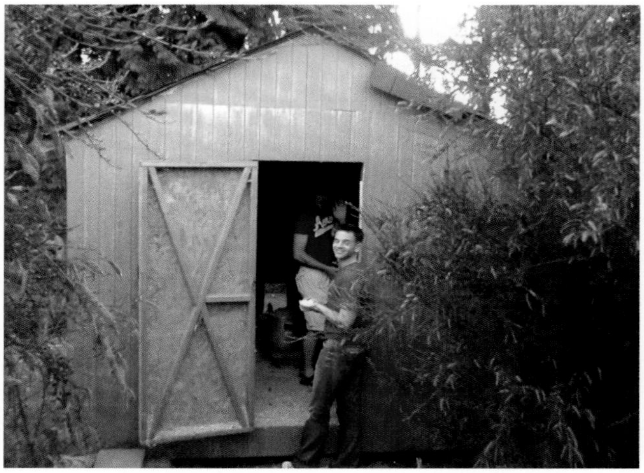

FIGURE 45.3 Two men who work in finance and value sustainability successfully build their own chicken coop to raise chickens and sell eggs, demonstrating self-efficacy and Prochaska's "action" stage of change.

Practice Dilemma

Promoting Self-Efficacy

If you are asked to evaluate an individual who presents with severe problems with activities of daily living, and he self-rates himself as not having a problem (not needing to change his behavior), what do you do? How would you discuss the problem behavior with the individual? Which theories of learning would be most helpful in working with this individual? Would you start with one theory and then shift to another theory at a different point in treatment? How might your approach be different for different diagnoses?

CASE STUDY 45.1 Olivia: Behavior Change

Olivia, a 55-year-old woman, has always been severely overweight. Over the years, she has tried many different diets and has joined (and quit) numerous exercise programs and groups. After a recent episode of chest pain, Olivia's health care provider strongly recommended that she participate in organized nutrition, exercise, and overall health-promotion activities.

- How might you help Olivia to understand and reflect on her challenges with health and wellness issues over the years through the transtheoretical perspective?
- What stage might she be at currently?
- How might you help her move from one stage to the next?
- How might you work to minimize any setbacks to the process and remedy those setbacks when they occur?
- How would each theory of learning presented in this chapter be helpful with this case?

Strategies might include the following:

- The occupational therapy practitioner would first work with Olivia to help her understand the processes of change. Their work together would include helping Olivia to understand how change occurs, the spiraling nature of change, and the natural, to-be-expected gains and setbacks that occur. The occupational therapy practitioner would use counseling and discussion to encourage Olivia's conscious reflection on her behavior and recognition of the different stages of change. Olivia's current stage could be seen as preparation.

CASE STUDY 45.1 Olivia: Behavior Change (*Continued*)

- Olivia would be presented with the behaviors she has demonstrated that have contributed to her weight gain and interfered with her weight loss. She would also be presented with the health consequences of those behaviors. With support, as needed, from the therapist, Olivia would go to the health library and identify the long-term results of not addressing these concerns.
- A variety of intervention strategies, such as personal goal setting, developing social supports, creating a self-reward system for positive change or progress, and evaluation and reevaluation of progress, could be introduced using motivational interviewing techniques. As Olivia applied and practiced these strategies in her life, she could come back to the occupational therapist to problem-solve and revise those that did not work as well as update her self-reward system for those that were successful.
- The occupational therapy practitioner would recommend that Olivia participate in a group based on social learning principles so that she could benefit from hearing others' strategies. This type of group would also help to build her self-esteem as she shared her own accomplishments and strategies with others as well. After the group sessions, Olivia would meet individually with the occupational therapy practitioner to identify one or two new strategies that she heard to try each week. Olivia would develop a plan, with coaching, as needed from the occupational therapist, to go out and try the new strategy.
- Olivia would also be encouraged to view earlier obstacles or setbacks to change as typical and predictable. When setbacks do occur, the occupational therapy practitioner would reinforce the importance of conscious understanding of the spiraling nature of progress, the success of identifying setbacks when they occur, the opportunity to prevent any setback from spiraling too far down, and a return to strategies that were successful in the past or continuing to develop new strategies. The occupational therapy practitioner would reinforce the ongoing nature of change and progress. ■

Conclusion

Behaviorist, social cognitive, constructivist, self-efficacy, and motivational theories of learning have great relevance and use for occupational therapy practitioners. Table 45.2 summarizes the five different theories of learning that were presented in this chapter and highlights their relevance to occupational therapy practice. The information presented in this chapter can be used to influence how you think about the learning needs of patients and clients, to reinforce the importance of designing optimal learning environments, to contribute to your ongoing professional development, and to promote your clients' abilities to achieve their goals.

Acknowledgment

We would like to acknowledge Perri Stern for her contributions to the previous edition of this chapter.

TABLE 45.2 Summary Table

Theory	Major Emphases	Application to Occupational Therapy Practice
Behaviorist	• Learned behavior as an observable event (not a mental process) • Behavior is conditioned by the environment • Environmental response alters subsequent behaviors	• Analyze and sequence behaviors from simple to complex • Measure progress as the person completes increasingly complex behaviors • Use strategies including reinforcement, shaping, and rewards
Social learning/social cognitive	• Integrates behavior, social, and cognitive processes • Learning occurs in a social context • Learning may occur without observable behavior change • Person regulates and adjusts his or her own behavior	• Emphasize client learning essential skills for living • Use role-play, peer observation, role modeling, problem solving, and real-life practice activities to promote learning • Encourage the client to identify the problem, set goals, develop a plan, evaluate outcomes
Constructivist	• Learner is an active participant in his or her own learning • Learner creates/constructs knowledge through past experience and interaction with the environment • Self-constructed knowledge has great meaning and relevance for the learner • Self-constructed knowledge promotes the learner's motivation for learning	• Client actively directs what is to be learned and how learning will occur • Use strategies including brainstorming, individual problem solving, independent exploration, asking questions. • Occupational therapist facilitates but does not direct the learning process

(continued)

TABLE 45.2 Summary Table (*Continued*)

Theory	Major Emphases	Application to Occupational Therapy Practice
Self-efficacy	• Emphasize a person's beliefs about how effective he or she is or will be • Efficacy expectations influence a person's persistence with an activity • Efficacy expectations are influenced by the difficulty of the task, how well completing a task transfers to other situations, and the degree to which a person believes that he or she will be successful • Self-efficacy is developed over time and through experience	• Personal accomplishment has the greatest effect • Self-evaluation, and personal appraisal are important • Tasks should be challenging but not overwhelming, should be transferable to other situations • Vicarious, observation experiences and/or persuasion to enhance the person's beliefs that he or she can be successful are less effective
Motivational	• Learning and change occurs in a spiral fashion. It is not linear. • A person's readiness for change will influence the outcomes • Relapses are common and to be expected	• Intervention processes must match behavior stage • Intervention processes become increasingly active, self-directed, and self-monitored

References

Bandura, A. (1977a). Self-efficacy: Toward a unifying theory of behavioral change. *Psychological Review, 84*(2), 191–215.

Bandura, A. (1977b). *Social learning theory*. Upper Saddle River, NJ: Prentice Hall.

Brady, S., Hiam, C. M., Saemann, R., Humbert, R., Fleming, M. Z., & Dawkins-Brickhouse, K. (1996). Dual diagnosis: A treatment model for substance abuse and major mental illness. *Community Mental Health Journal, 32*, 573–578.

Bruner, J. S. (1961). The act of discovery. *Harvard Educational Review, 31*(1), 21–32.

Driscoll, M. P. (Ed.). (2005). *Psychology of learning for instruction* (3rd ed.). Boston, MA: Allyn & Bacon.

Finnell, D. S. (2003). Addiction services: Use of the transtheoretical model for individuals with co-occurring disorders. *Community Mental Health Journal, 39*, 3–15.

Fosnot, C. T. (Ed.). (1996) *Constructivism: Theory, perspectives and practice*. New York, NY: Teachers College Press.

Gage, M., & Polatajko, H. J. (1994). Enhancing occupational performance through an understanding of perceived self efficacy. *American Journal of Occupational Therapy, 48*, 452–461.

Giles, G. M., Ridley, J. E., Dill, A., & Frye, S. C. (1997). A consecutive series of adults with brain injury treated with a washing and dressing retraining program. *American Journal of Occupational Therapy, 51*, 256–266.

Giles, G. M., & Wilson, J. C. (1988). The use of behavioral techniques in functional skills training after severe brain injury. *American Journal of Occupational Therapy, 42*, 658–665.

Haggerty, L. A., & Goodman, L. A. (2006). Stages of change-based nursing interventions for victims of interpersonal violence. *Journal of Obstetric, Gynecologic, and Neonatal Nursing, 32*(1), 68–75.

Helfrich, C. A., Chan, D. V., & Sabol, P. (2011). Cognitive predictors of life skill interventions: Outcomes for adults with mental illness at risk for homelessness. *American Journal of Occupational Therapy, 65*, 277–286. doi:10.5014/ajot.2011.001321

Helfrich, C. A., Chan, D. V., Simpson, E., & Sabol, P. (2011). Readiness-to-change cluster profiles among adults with mental illness who were homeless participating in a life skills intervention. *Community Mental Health Journal*. Advance online publication. doi: 10.1007/s10597-011-9383-z

Hergenhahn, B. R. (1976). *An introduction to theories of learning*. Englewood Cliffs, NJ: Prentice Hall.

Jao, H. P. I., & Lu, S. J. (1999). The acquisition of problem-solving skills through instruction in Siegel and Spivack's problem solving therapy for the chronic schizophrenic. *Occupational Therapy in Mental Health, 14*(4), 47–63.

Katzmann, S., & Mix, S. (1994). Improving functional independence in a patient with encephalitis through behavior modification shaping techniques. *American Journal of Occupational Therapy, 48*, 259–262.

Keefe, F. J., Lefebvre, J. C., Kerns, R. D., Rosenberg, R., Beaupre, P., Prochaska, J., . . . Caldwell, D. S. (2000). Understanding the adoption of arthritis self-management: Stages of change profiles among arthritis patients. *Pain, 87*, 303–313.

Lave, J., & Wenger, E. (1991). *Situated learning*. New York, NY: Cambridge Press.

Lederer, J. M. (2000). The application of constructivism to concepts of occupation using a group process approach. *Occupational Therapy in Health Care, 13*(1), 81–93.

Marlowe, B. A., & Page, M. L. (1998). *Creating and sustaining the constructivist classroom*. Thousand Oaks, CA: Corwin Press/Sage.

Martin, G., & Pear, J. (2011). Behavior modification: What it is and how to do it (9th ed.). Upper Saddle River, NJ: Prentice Hall.

Miller, W. R., & Rollnick, S. (Eds.). (1991). *Motivational interviewing: Preparing people for change*. New York, NY: Guilford Press.

Nigg, C. R., Burbank, P. M., Padula, C., Dufresne, R., Rossi, J. S., Velicer, W. F., . . . Prochaska, J. O. (1999). Stages of change across ten health risk behaviors for older adults. *Gerontologist, 39*, 473–482.

Ormrod, J. E. (1990). *Human learning: Principles, theories and educational applications* (2nd ed.). New York, NY: Macmillan.

Ormrod, J. E. (2006). *Educational psychology: Developing learners* (5th ed.). Upper Saddle River, NJ: Prentice Hall.

Piaget, J. (1970). Piaget's theory. In P. H. Mussen (Ed.), *Carmichael's manual of psychology*. New York, NY: Wiley.

Plotnikoff, R. C., Hotz, S. B., Johnson, S. T., Hansen, J. S., Birkett, N. J., Leonard, L. E., & Flaman, L. M. (2009). Readiness to shop for low-fat foods: A population study. *Journal of the American Dietetic Association, 109*, 1392–1397.

Prochaska, J. M., Prochaska, J. O., & Levesque, D. A. (2001). A transtheoretical approach to changing organizations. *Administration & Policy in Mental Health, 28*, 247–261.

Prochaska, J. O. (2001). Treating entire populations for behavior risks for cancer. *The Cancer Journal, 7*, 360–368.

Prochaska, J. O., & DiClemente, C. C. (1983). Stages and processes of self change of smoking: Toward an integrative model of change. *Journal of Consulting and Clinical Psychology, 51*, 390–395.

Prochaska, J. O., Norcross, J. C., & DiClemente, C. C. (1992). In search of how people change: Applications to addictive behaviors. *American Psychologist, 47*, 1102–1113.

Prochaska, J. O., Redding, C. A., & Evers, K. E. (1997). The transtheoretical model and stages of change. In K. Glanz, F. M. Lewis, & B. K. Rimer (Eds.), *Health behavior and health education: Theory, research, and practice* (2nd ed., pp. 60–80). San Francisco, CA: Jossey-Bass.

Sarkin, J. A., Johnson, S. S., Prochaska, J. O., & Prochaska, J. M. (2001). Applying the transtheoretical model to regulate moderate exercise in an overweight population: Validation of a stages of change measure. *Preventive Medicine, 33*, 462–469.

Suinicki, M. D. (2004). *Learning and motivation in the postsecondary classroom.* Bolton, MA: Anker.

For additional resources on the subjects discussed in this chapter, visit http://thePoint.lww.com/Willard-Spackman12e.

UNIT XI

Evaluation, Intervention, and Outcomes for Occupations

"... the small experiences of everyday life and everyday occupation have complexity; beauty, meaningfulness, and relevance to health and well-being that belie their aura of ordinariness and routine."

—Betty Risteen Hasselkus

CHAPTER 46

Introduction to Evaluation, Intervention, and Outcomes for Occupations

Glen Gillen, Barbara A. Boyt Schell

OUTLINE

LEARNING OBJECTIVES

After reading this chapter, you will be able to:

1. Understand classification systems used to discuss areas of occupation
2. Appreciate the complexity of occupation and the potential difficulties in applying these classification systems

Categories of Occupation

As occupational therapists, we consider the many types of occupations in which clients engage across the course of the day. These occupations fall under the category of **activities** and **participation** in the World Health Organization's (WHO, 2001) *International Classification of Functioning, Disability, and Health* (ICF). The WHO (2001) defines activity as "the execution of a task or action by an individual" and participation as "involvement in a life situation" (p. 123). Further, they define the term **activity limitations** as "difficulties an individual may have in executing activities" and ***participation restrictions*** as "problems an individual may experience in involvement in life situations" (WHO, 2001, p. 123). Within the ICF, the domains for the Activities and Participation component are presented as a single list that covers the full range of life areas. Examples of included areas are mobility, self-care, domestic life, interpersonal interactions, major life areas (e.g., education, work, economic life), communication, etc.

Occupational therapy classification systems typically sort the broad ranges of activities or occupations into categories called **areas of occupation**. There is no standardized classification system, and these areas of occupation have been categorized and classified in a variety of ways. For example, the Canadian Occupational Performance Measure (Law et al., 2005), which is a standardized measure of occupational performance, uses a three-category system of self-care, productivity, and leisure. On the other hand, the American Occupational Therapy Association (AOTA, 2008) categorizes these areas of occupation as eight kinds of life activities in which people, populations, or organizations engage. Because the AOTA categories for the areas of occupation are used as the basis for the major chapters in this unit, they are briefly described here, using the AOTA Practice Framework (AOTA, 2008) as the primary source. Readers are referred to the chapters themselves for more in-depth definitions and discussions about each category of occupations.

Activities of Daily Living

Activities of daily living (ADL) are activities that focus on caring for one's body and which are directed toward basic survival. Examples include bathing, grooming, dressing, feeding, functional mobility, sexual activity, personal device care, etc.

Instrumental Activities of Daily Living

Instrumental activities of daily living (IADL) are grouping of activities that also are necessary for daily life but which go beyond basic bodily care and survival. They typically involve a broader context, including family and community. A variety of activities are categorized as IADL including child rearing, pet care, financial management, meal preparation, shopping, and home management.

Education

Educational occupations are focused on formal and informal learning. Examples include formal educational participation (academic, nonacademic, extracurricular, and vocational participation), informal personal educational needs or interests exploration, and informal personal education participation.

Work

The category of work includes productive activities such as work and volunteer activities. It includes employment interests and pursuits, employment seeking and acquisition, job performance, retirement preparation and adjustment, volunteer exploration, and volunteer participation.

Play and Leisure

Play and leisure are activities that are characterized by enjoyment or diversion, and which typically arise out of interests and motivation of the person, as opposed to social obligation or survival requirements. This grouping encompasses play exploration and play participation and includes both leisure exploration and participation.

Rest and Sleep

The activities associated with rest and sleep are more recently included in the AOTA Practice Framework, in recognition of the role they play in supporting all other occupational functioning. Beyond rest and sleep, this area of occupation also includes sleep preparation and sleep participation. Examples include bedtime routines, ability to manage cues for waking such as the use of wake-up signals, as well as the management of the physical environment for comfort and safety. Occupations in this category may include negotiating the needs and requirements of others within the social environment such as sleep partners and children.

Social Participation

Social participation refers to the interweaving of occupations to support desired engagement in community and family activities as well as those involving peers and friends.

Cautions about Categorization

Personal Perspectives

An important consideration when using any classification system to guide evaluation and intervention is to fully understand the way that the person engaging in the occupation perceives the particular activity. For instance, making a meal may be considered work to a busy parent who sees it as part of his or her "job" as a parent to feed the family. Individuals who live by themselves or who take responsibility for this occupation as a part of family chores may consider meal preparation an IADL. Others may classify meal preparation as a leisure activity because it may help them to relax or decrease their stress levels. A chef in a restaurant is most likely to classify meal preparation as work. Finally, meal preparation may be considered under the heading of social participation. Examples include participating in a weekly neighborhood soup kitchen to serve meals to the homeless or being part of a group of friends or family engaged in making a holiday feast. Care of pets is just one of many other examples that can be considered. Depending on one's perspective, this may be considered as an IADL, as part of leisure/play, or as work for someone employed as a part-time dog walker (see Figure 46.1).

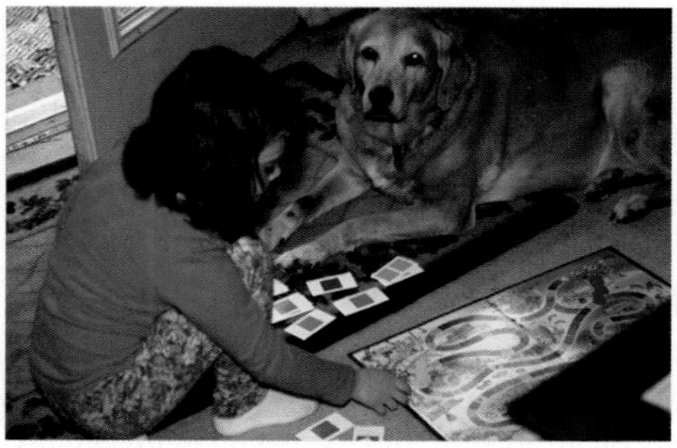

FIGURE 46.1 In this picture, the child is hard at work playing . . . but is the dog resting or playing? Or both? Or perhaps engaged in child care?

Occupational Blends versus Categories

Some occupational scientists suggest that rather than trying to classify occupations into discrete categories, it might be more helpful to consider the relative mix within a particular activity. For example, someone who loves his or her job may have parts of the job that really feel like work, parts that are fun and feel like play, and parts that feel like IADL, such as using a calendar to coordinate work and home life. Indeed, in her paper "Work and Leisure: Transcending the Dichotomy," Primeau (1996a) cites the work of Csikszentmihalyi (1975) who was an early challenger of the work versus leisure dichotomy. "One way to reconcile this split is to realize that work is not necessarily more important than play and play is not necessarily more enjoyable than work" (p. 202). Thus, client-centered care relies in part on the practitioner seeking to understand the client's particular perspective on their daily occupations in order to avoid incorrect assumptions. This knowledge of the personal meaning of various occupations is essential to understand the significance of the occupation to an individual (Primeau, 1996b).

Attention to Scope and Detail

In her discussion of using broad categories to classify occupations, Hasselkus (2006) expressed concern that we as occupational therapy practitioners ". . . risk losing sight of the unique contexts and individual small behaviors of everyday life and everyday occupation that make up those sweeping categories" (p. 629). However, a positive aspect of having a variety of classification systems is that it serves as a reminder to occupational therapy practitioners to inquire and evaluate a person's occupational engagement as a whole. Too often, occupational therapy may be overfocused on an occupation of particular interest in that setting. For instance, in medical rehabilitation, there is a strong focus on self-care retraining. We need to always reflect that our scope is much greater and holistic. As far back as 1995, Radomski reminded us that "there is more to life than putting on your pants" (p. 487). Likewise, in school-based practice, the need in the United States to justify services to be educationally related does not preclude the importance of appreciating that a child engages in a range of occupations during a school day and goes home to even more with his or her family.

Client Values and Choice

It is of critical importance to understand the value that our clients place on chosen occupations. Although self-care may be important and valued by many clients, exclusive focus on this area of occupation may not serve our clients well in terms of giving them the ability to engage in occupations that are considered quality-of-life changers. For one client, this may be focused on regaining the ability to drive, for another to be able to interact with grandchildren, for another to access e-mail via the Internet, and for another to feed himself or herself independently. The occupational therapy profession has discussed the importance of client-centered care and client-centered assessment for more than two decades. A continued emphasis on this aspect of care will assure that we are truly collaborating with our clients and placing our therapy focus on meaningful client-chosen occupations regardless of how they might be classified.

Orchestrating Life

Finally, practitioners must not only consider specific occupations and engagement in occupations but also understand how clients orchestrate their engagement over time and within various environments (Larson, 2000; Molineux, 2007). Many of our clients are required to engage in multiple occupations at the same time, alternate back and forth between occupations based on changing priorities. They must organize and sequence occupations into a routine, which is satisfactory to themselves and those important to them. This may require that they balance participation in an array of occupations in a variety of familiar and unfamiliar contexts.

No Simple Hierarchies

The chapters that follow in this unit place specific focus on evaluating and intervening to maximize participation in specific categories of areas of occupation. Readers are cautioned that the order of presentation of these topics does not represent a hierarchy. New practitioners may wrongly assume that basic ADL are foundational skills, and that clients must gain competence in these before tackling other areas. However, both clinical experience and current research suggests that other activities such as making a hot beverage or hand washing dishes may be much easier as compared to upper body grooming and total body dressing, depending on the patterns of performance skill deficits that a client presents with (Fisher & Jones, 2011).

Conclusion

In summary, the domain of occupational therapy is best described as "supporting health and participation in life through engagement in occupation" (AOTA, 2008, p. 626). Knowledge gained from this unit should give the readers a range of therapy options to help our clients engage in their chosen occupations, maximize our clients' ability to participate fully, and assure satisfaction with the care we provide.

References

American Occupational Therapy Association. (2008). Occupational therapy practice framework: Domain and process, 2nd edition. *American Journal of Occupational Therapy, 62*, 625–683.

Csikszentmihalyi, M. (1975). *Beyond boredom and anxiety: Experiencing flow in work and play*. San Francisco, CA: Jossey-Bass.

Fisher, A. G., & Jones, K. B. (2011). *Assessment of Motor and Process Skills: Development, standardization, and administration manual* (7th ed.). Fort Collins, CO: Three Star Press.

Hasselkus, B. R. (2006). 2006 Eleanor Clarke Slagle Lecture—The world of everyday occupation: Real people, real lives. *American Journal of Occupational Therapy, 60*, 627–640.

Larson, E. A. (2000). The orchestration of occupation: The dance of mothers. *American Journal of Occupational Therapy, 54*, 269–280.

Law, M., Baptiste, S., McColl, M. A., Polatajko, H., Carswell, A., & Pollock, N. (2005). *Canadian Occupational Performance Measure* (4th ed.). Ottawa, Canada: Canadian Association of Occupational Therapists.

Molineux, M. (2007). The occupational careers of men living with HIV infection in the United Kingdom: Insights into engaging in and orchestrating occupations. *Australian Occupational Therapy Journal, 54*, 85.

Primeau, L. A. (1996a). Work and leisure: Transcending the dichotomy. *American Journal of Occupational Therapy, 50*, 569–577.

Primeau, L. A. (1996b). Work versus nonwork: The case of household work. In R. Zemke & F. Clark (Eds.), *Occupational science: The evolving discipline* (pp. 57–70). Philadelphia, PA: F. A. Davis.

Radomski, M. V. (1995). There is more to life than putting on your pants. *American Journal of Occupational Therapy, 49*, 487–490.

World Health Organization. (2001). *International classification of functioning, disability, and health*. Geneva, Switzerland: Author.

For additional resources on the subjects discussed in this chapter, visit http://thePoint.lww.com/Willard-Spackman12e.

CHAPTER 47

Activities of Daily Living and Instrumental Activities of Daily Living

Anne Birge James

OUTLINE

LEARNING OBJECTIVES

After reading this chapter, you will be able to:

1. Describe the purposes of an occupational therapy activities of daily living (ADL) and instrumental activities of daily living (IADL) evaluation
2. Given a client case, identify client and contextual factors that would influence the evaluation plan
3. Develop individualized client goals that will drive the intervention process
4. Describe contextual considerations that influence goal development
5. Explain the most common approaches to ADL and IADL intervention
6. Describe the role of client and caregiver education in treatment of ADL and IADL deficits
7. Grade treatment activities to progress clients toward increased participation in ADL and IADL

This chapter focuses on the evaluation and treatment of areas of occupation that are classified as **activities of daily living** (ADL) and **instrumental activities of daily living** (IADL) in the "Occupational Therapy Practice Framework" (OTPF) (American Occupational Therapy Association [AOTA], 2008). Dysfunctions in ADL and IADL are termed *activity limitations* in the *International Classification of Functioning, Disability, and Health* (ICF) (World Health Organization, 2002) framework. Evaluation and treatment of ADL and IADL dysfunction are central to individuals' participation in meaningful occupation. Individuals may value ADL and IADL as meaningful in and of themselves and as prerequisite tasks to meaningful engagement in education, work, play, leisure, and social participation.

Definition of Activities of Daily Living and Instrumental Activities of Daily Living

Conceptually, the term *activities of daily living* could apply to all activities that individuals perform routinely. In the OTPF, however, ADL are defined more narrowly as "activities that are oriented toward taking care of one's own body" (AOTA, 2008, p. 631), which include 10 activity categories: bathing/showering, bowel and bladder management, dressing, eating, feeding, functional mobility, personal device care, personal hygiene and grooming, sexual activity, and toilet hygiene. IADL are defined as "activities to support daily life within the home and community that often require more complex interactions than self-care used in ADL" (AOTA, 2008, p. 631). IADL include 12 activity categories: care of others, care of pets, child rearing, communication management, community mobility, financial management, health management and maintenance, home establishment and management, meal preparation and cleanup, religious observance, safety and emergency maintenance, and shopping. Although both ADL and IADL include essential occupational performance tasks, IADL may be easier to delegate to another person.

The OTPF (AOTA, 2008) provides a nomenclature for the domains of occupational therapy practices and description of the process for occupational therapy practitioners in the United States. The OTPF's definitions of ADL and IADL are consistent with those of the National Center for Health Statistics (2009); however, other health care and social services practitioners or occupational therapists outside the United States might use other terms to refer to these same ADL and IADL concepts or use the same terms but define them differently. The term *activities of daily living* is typically restricted to activities involving functional mobility (ambulation, wheelchair mobility, bed mobility, and transfers) and personal care (feeding, hygiene, toileting, bathing, and dressing) consistent with the OTPF, although some define ADL more broadly, referring to activities performed in daily life (e.g., Archenholtz & Dellhag, 2008; Hsueh, Wang, Sheu, & Hsieh, 2004). Other terms that are used to refer specifically to functional mobility and personal care are *basic ADL* and *personal ADL* (AOTA, 2008). The term *instrumental activities of daily living* appears outside the occupational therapy literature in a less consistent way. Measures of IADL vary considerably according to the activities that are included in the scales (Chong, 1995); for example, the Nottingham Extended ADL Scale includes leisure activities and feeding (Nouri & Lincoln, 1987), tasks that fall outside the OTPF definition of IADL. Synonyms for IADL are *independent living skills* and *extended ADL* (Nouri & Lincoln, 1987). *Advanced ADL* is a construct that includes IADL but focuses on more physically demanding activities, such as running errands and driving more than 5 miles (Pincus, Swearingen, & Wolfe, 1999), and may include activities such as hobbies, recreation, and volunteer work (Moore, Endo, & Carter, 2003), which are more in line with the OTPF concept of play or leisure rather than IADL. The crucial point is to understand that terms that refer to daily activities are used in variable ways; so it is important, in referring to written work, to look for operational definitions of terms used by authors and, in a clinical setting, to find out the conventional language used by practitioners. Occupational therapy practitioners need to be aware of the differences in terminology and use commonly accepted terms for the context when communicating with other professionals and when selecting assessment instruments.

This chapter focuses on the evaluation and treatment of occupational performance limitations specifically related to ADL and IADL as defined by the OTPF. It is essential to have a fundamental understanding of the occupational therapy process before reading this chapter; the process is described in Chapter 23. The reader should be aware that ADL and IADL, although often a primary focus of occupational therapy practice, do not typically represent the full complement of occupational performance tasks needed for satisfying and meaningful participation in individual and societal roles. Evaluation and treatment should always begin with a comprehensive occupational profile (AOTA, 2008). Treatment should address all of the client's priorities, which will typically extend beyond ADL and IADL, although the rest of this chapter will focus exclusively on ADL and IADL.

Evaluation of Activities of Daily Living and Instrumental Activities of Daily Living

Evaluation refers to the overall process of gathering and interpreting data needed to plan intervention, including developing an evaluation plan, implementing the data collection, interpreting the data, and documenting the evaluation results (AOTA, 2010). **Assessment** refers to the specific method or tools that are used to collect data, which is one component of the evaluation process (AOTA, 2010). Standardized assessment methods are referred to as *assessment tools* or *instruments*. The evaluation is carried out by an occupational therapist. An occupational therapy assistant may participate in selected assessments under the supervision of an occupational therapist who is responsible for interpreting assessment data for use in intervention planning.

The ADL/IADL evaluation is discussed in two stages in this chapter: (1) planning the evaluation, which includes selecting specific assessment methods; and (2) implementing the evaluation, which includes gathering assessment data, making critical observations, generating hypotheses, and performing ongoing revision of the evaluation plan until adequate data have been collected. Keep in mind that ADL and IADL evaluation is only one part of a more comprehensive occupational therapy evaluation.

Evaluation Planning: Selecting the Appropriate Activities of Daily Living and Instrumental Activities of Daily Living Assessments

Occupational therapists can choose from various ADL and IADL assessments designed to meet the varied needs of clients and treatment settings. Selecting an appropriate assessment will facilitate optimal treatment planning and can be initiated by following these steps:

1. Identify the overall purpose(s) of the evaluation.
2. Have clients identify their needs, interests, and perceived difficulties with ADL and/or IADL as part of the occupational profile.
3. Further explore the client's relevant activities so that the activities are operationally defined.
4. Estimate the client factors that affect occupational performance and/or the assessment process.
5. Identify contextual features that affect assessment.
6. Consider features of assessment tools.
7. Integrate the information from steps 1 to 6 to select the optimal ADL and IADL assessment tools.

In practice, the experienced occupational therapist completes this process quickly so that much of the ADL and IADL evaluation is completed in the first occupational therapy session. Also, although these steps appear to follow a linear progression, in practice, the steps become integrated because the occupational therapist continually blends knowledge and experience with information from and about the client. For the developing therapist, however, it is helpful to explore each step independently to examine critical factors that contribute to the complex clinical reasoning process that is employed in planning an evaluation.

Step 1: Identify the Purpose of the Activities of Daily Living/Instrumental Activities of Daily Living Evaluation

ADL and IADL may be evaluated for different purposes. At the level of individual client care, evaluation may be done to assess activity limitations to plan occupational therapy intervention or to facilitate decision-making concerning discharge environment, competency, conservatorship, and/or involuntary commitment. At the programmatic level, evaluation may be done to document the need for program development and to appraise outcomes. Before starting an evaluation, the occupational therapist must determine how the information will be used so that appropriate and sufficient data are obtained. The extent of data gathering depends on the specific purpose for which the evaluation is being conducted.

Evaluation to Plan and Monitor Occupational Therapy Interventions. Before practitioners intervene to improve performance of ADL or IADL, they must evaluate clients' baseline performance. When an evaluation is conducted to plan occupational therapy intervention, certain types of data are needed (Dunn, 2005). First, activities in which performance is deficient need to be identified so that intervention can focus on components that are dysfunctional while simultaneously maintaining and enhancing those that are functional. Second, data are needed about the cause or causes of the activity limitation. For example, a limitation in cooking might be caused by low vision, a kitchen that is not wheelchair accessible, or poor motivation to cook. Occupational therapy intervention for a limitation in cooking is different for each of these causes. To understand the etiology of an activity limitation in ADL or IADL, data about occupational performance needs to be supplemented with data about the client's performance patterns and skills, client factors, activity demands, and contexts (Dunn, 2005). Third, the occupational therapy evaluation should provide data about the possibilities for modifying the client's activity performance. Information about the activity demands and context should include consideration of which aspects might be modifiable to support performance and which features cannot be changed. The potential to change performance patterns and skills or client factors must also be assessed. Interventions that involve skill acquisition are feasible for some clients, depending on the factors that are interfering with task performance. For example, a child with balance deficits secondary to cerebral palsy might have the potential to increase balance skills to support participation across several ADL and IADL, whereas a person with similar deficits from Parkinson's disease might not because the disorder is progressive. All three types of data (performance deficit, underlying causes, and potential for change) are needed to devise adequate intervention plans.

Evaluation to Facilitate Decision Making about Eligibility or Discharge Environment. Clients may also be referred for evaluation of ADL and IADL to facilitate decision making about eligibility or discharge environment. The ability to care for oneself and one's home can make the difference between independent and supported or assisted living. Supported living represents a continuum of options that includes in-home services (e.g., chore services), personal care assistants, assisted living centers, foster homes, group homes, independent living centers, supervised apartments, transitional apartments, and long-term care facilities. Varied levels of support are offered within these settings to maintain or enhance daily living skills. When ADL and IADL are evaluated to serve eligibility or discharge decisions, the evaluation may be less comprehensive and detailed than when it is done to plan individual interventions. The primary question to be answered through the evaluation is: "Does the client meet the functional criteria?" This question can generally be answered by identifying activities in which limitations are present.

A somewhat similar evaluation objective occurs when occupational therapy practitioners are asked to make recommendations regarding legal competence for independent living. This usually involves competence in caring for oneself or competence in managing one's property. **Guardianship** is a legal association in which a protected individual's personal affairs are managed by one or more people or an agency. **Conservatorship** is a legal relationship, like guardianship, but is limited to managing the protected individual's financial affairs and property (Moye, 2005). Evaluation may also be requested in conjunction with involuntary commitments to psychiatric facilities to appraise the influence of psychiatric status on daily living. When competence is used in the legal sense, the capacity to make judicious or responsible decisions usually takes precedence over the capacity to perform activities. Individuals who have the ability to procure services and supervise caregivers in managing their personal care and living situation are viewed as competent, even though they might not be able to perform these activities themselves. Thus, occupational therapy evaluations that are conducted with guardianship, conservatorship, or involuntary commitment in mind must take into account the decisional capacities and supervisory skills needed by clients.

Evaluation for Programmatic Uses. Although this chapter emphasizes evaluation for individual client care, it is important to recognize that data gathered about clients may be aggregated for programmatic purposes (Law, King, & Russell, 2005). For example, data about the ADL and IADL characteristics of clients who are served in an occupational therapy clinic can be used to document the extent of particular activity limitations and to support the development of new or expanded programs to manage them. In the current health care climate of cost-effectiveness and cost containment, group data are increasingly being used to evaluate the outcomes of occupational therapy programs and occupational therapy interventions (Robertson & Colburn, 2000). Occupational therapy practitioners are often expected to measure and document ADL and IADL data consistently across clients so that they can be used effectively for program evaluation, such as the Uniform Data System for Medical Rehabilitation (2005).

Step 2: Have Clients Identify Their Needs, Interests, and Perceived Difficulties with Activities of Daily Living and/or Instrumental Activities of Daily Living

Once the purpose of the ADL/IADL evaluation has been determined, the occupational therapist must identify the specific activities to be evaluated. This is *one* component of the occupational profile, which will also encompass other aspects of occupational performance, including education, play, leisure, work, and social participation (AOTA, 2008). Developing the client's occupational profile is a crucial step in a client-centered evaluation, which enhances both the process and outcomes of occupational therapy (Law & Baum, 2005). A client-centered approach to ADL and IADL evaluation requires practitioners to begin by discovering the ADL and IADL problems of concern to the *client* (Law & Baum, 2005). Practitioners can expect the activities of concern to vary significantly for a 10-year-old elementary school student, a 29-year-old homemaker caring for three young children, and a 49-year-old business executive; the evaluations of these clients need to be tailored to take clients' lifestyle differences into account. It is easy to make assumptions about a client's priorities based on both clinical and personal experience and values; however, it is important to remember that unique circumstances may affect clients' selection of the ADL or IADL that they wish to address in treatment. Clients' perception of their ADL and IADL problems, needs, and goals can be gathered through a semistructured interview process or through a more formal assessment, such as the Canadian Occupational Performance Measure (COPM) (Law, Baptiste et al., 2005) or Occupational Performance History Interview II (Kielhofner et al., 2004). More informally, practitioners may have clients rate activities on a Likert scale, for example where 1 = "not at all important to perform effectively" and 10 = "crucial to perform," in order to quantify the relative value of activities. Alternatively, clients can be asked to rank a list of ADL and IADL in order of importance to identify priorities.

Step 3: Further Explore Clients' Relevant Activities So That the Activities are Operationally Defined

The nature of the tasks that make up selected ADL and IADL can vary among individuals. Before activities can be evaluated, they must have an operational definition; that is, the occupational therapy practitioner and client must be clear on the precise meaning of each term. For example, meal preparation for a middle school student might consist of making cereal for breakfast and packing a lunch, whereas meal preparation for a homemaker feeding a family of five involves a much wider range of food preparation tasks and a very different set of skills. Because different assessment tools define activities differently, it is important to select an instrument that is congruent with the activities as defined by the client. For example, in using the Barthel Index to assess feeding, clients are rated "independent" if they can feed themselves, which includes cutting up food and spreading butter on bread (Mahoney & Barthel, 1965). Clients are rated as "needing assistance" if they can get food from the plate to the mouth but need help cutting food into bite-sized pieces. The Katz Index of ADL, however, does not include preparation of food on the plate (e.g., cutting and spreading butter on bread) in the operational definition of feeding, so clients are rated independent if they can get food from the plate to the mouth, even if they cannot cut food or butter bread (Katz, Ford, Moskowitz, Jackson, & Jaffe, 1963). Many adolescents and adults would be dissatisfied with their feeding performance if their food had to be cut or their bread buttered by another person, so the Katz Index of ADL would not be an appropriate measure for individuals who consider cutting and buttering to be essential components of feeding.

The operational definitions of IADL are more varied than those for ADL because of their greater complexity. Consider the task of meal preparation. On the IADL Scale, which is generally considered to be the prototype assessment instrument for IADL, the highest level of competence is described as "plans, prepares, and serves adequate meals independently" (Lawton, 1972, p. 133). Comparable items on the Nottingham Extended ADL Scale examine the ability to make a hot drink and hot snack alone and easily (Nouri & Lincoln, 1987). Thus, a rating of independence in cooking achieved on the Nottingham Extended ADL Scale implies a lower level of competence than does a rating of independence on the IADL Scale.

Occupational therapy practitioners also need to consider relevant performance parameters when planning an evaluation. Performance parameters include independence, safety, and adequacy. Operational definitions of acceptable ADL and IADL performance should include attention to all relevant parameters in order to establish appropriate baseline data and intervention outcomes.

Level of Independence. Although clients often wish to be independent in ADL and IADL, practitioners should not make this assumption; because some level of assistance, either verbal or physical, might be acceptable. For example, many clients who undergo total hip replacements must follow movement precautions for 2 months that make it impossible to don shoes and socks independently without adaptive equipment. Some clients who live with others might prefer to have assistance with this task rather than purchasing and using the required adaptive equipment. As long as the context supports this, that is, as long as they have someone who is willing and able to assist, a goal for assisted lower extremity dressing is perfectly appropriate; and treatment may focus on making sure that the patient and caregiver can complete the task together while adhering to total hip precautions. Independence is the performance parameter that is the focus of most assessment tools, so occupational therapists can select from various assessment tools that measure independence. Several other considerations, discussed later in this chapter, can help the occupational therapist to identify which of the many assessment tools is best for the situation.

Safety. Many assessment tools address safety indirectly by specifying that performance be completed in a safe manner in order to be rated as independent (e.g., the Functional Independence Measure [FIM™]). Some tools do not address safety directly (e.g., the Katz Index of ADL; Katz et al., 1963), and a few rate safety separately from independence (e.g., the Performance Assessment of Self-Care Skills; Holm & Rogers, 2008; Rogers & Holm, 1994). When safety is a particular concern, for example, with clients who have cognitive deficits that impair judgment, a separate measure of safety can be more effective for documenting progress toward treatment goals. A separate safety measure also makes it clear in the occupational therapy documentation that safety has been addressed.

Adequacy. Clients may have criteria regarding the efficiency of task performance and the acceptability of the outcome of the performance, and these should be considered in selecting assessment tools. For example, a client might be safe and independent in lower body dressing but deem her performance inefficient because it takes her over an hour to complete the task and she is too physically exhausted after dressing to attend to work duties; or a client might be independent and safe in feeding himself but find his performance outcome unacceptable if he drops food onto his clothing during each meal. If an assessment tool measured only independence and safety, it would be hard to justify intervention in either of the aforementioned examples because both clients were safe and independent. There are, however, occupational performance problems in both cases that might be addressed effectively through treatment; that is, reducing the time needed to complete lower body dressing or reducing the amount of food spilled on clothing during eating. Adequacy parameters that warrant consideration in the context of ADL and IADL performance include perceived difficulty, pain, fatigue, dyspnea (shortness of breath), societal standards, satisfaction, aberrant behaviors, and past experience with the activity. Practitioners must keep in mind that independence might not be the only important performance parameter to assess in the occupational therapy evaluation.

Step 4: Estimate the Client Factors That Affect Activities of Daily Living/Instrumental Activities of Daily Living and the Assessment Process

One purpose of the ADL/IADL evaluation is to provide insight into the problems underlying occupational performance deficits. However, some estimate of these deficits prior to the assessment can help the occupational therapist to select the assessment tools that will be most effective in identifying and documenting occupational performance problems and the underlying deficits. Occupational therapists use their knowledge of pathology and how it affects occupational performance when selecting assessment tools. For example, some instruments rely on self-report, which is a very efficient way to gather information about a wide range of activities. However, self-reported measures could be inaccurate if the client has significant cognitive deficits (e.g., a person with Alzheimer's disease), distorted thought functions (e.g., a person with schizophrenia), or little experience with the disorder (e.g., a teenager who sustained a spinal cord injury with quadriplegia just 5 days earlier). For many types of deficits, insight into clients' underlying problems will be enhanced by actually seeing the client attempt to perform tasks rather than relying on a description of the problem. For example, a client who has had a stroke might report that he or she is unable to reach items stored above chest height with his or her affected hand, but the occupational therapy practitioner can gain additional information needed for treatment by observing the client while he or she is reaching by looking for clues whether the movement problem is due to limitations in movement of the scapula, glenohumeral joint, or elbow or some combination of the three.

See **Appendix I, Common Conditions, Resources, and Evidence**, for more information about stroke.

Knowledge of underlying pathology and anticipated impairments also enables occupational therapists to select appropriate assessment tools that are designed for specific diagnostic groups, focusing on activities that are more commonly problematic for that population. For example, the Arthritis Impact Measurement Scale was developed for adults with rheumatic diseases and includes not only measures of ADL and IADL performance but also symptoms that are commonly experienced by people with arthritis during or following activities, such as pain and fatigue (Meenan, Mason, Anderson, Guccione, & Kazis, 1992).

Step 5: Identify Contextual Features That Affect Assessment

In this step, the occupational therapist considers the intervention context and its impact on the evaluation of ADL and IADL. These include physical context, social context, safety, the client's experience, time constraints, the practitioner's training and experience, availability of resources, and mandates from facilities or **third-party payers**.

Physical Context. Practitioners may observe activity performance under natural or clinical conditions. Under natural conditions, performance is observed within the context in which it usually takes place or is expected to take place, including the location (e.g., home), the objects that are usually used for activities (e.g., bathtub, soap), and the routine time when activities take place, when possible. These conditions, which can often be met in long-term care settings and home-based care, provide the most accurate assessment of clients' performance (Rogers et al., 2003). When clients are seen in the hospital or outpatient clinics, observation of activity performance takes places under clinical conditions. Regardless of where an assessment takes place, the influence of the physical context on activity performance must be taken into account so that valid conclusions about performance can be drawn. Occupational therapy clinics are designed to promote function and have numerous adaptive features to compensate for impairments. These features can make it easier for clients to perform activities in the clinic than in their own homes. Conversely, performance might be more difficult for some tasks because clients are unfamiliar with the clinic setting. When an evaluation is done in the home, clients have the advantage of using their own activity objects in the confines of familiar architecture. Research in this area is limited but demonstrates the variable impact of context on performance. For example, Brown, Moore, Hemman, and Yunek (1996) found that clients with mental illness performed similarly on a simulated purchasing task in the clinic and an actual purchasing task in a store, whereas Park, Fisher, and Velozo (1994) found that older adults' process skills during IADL were higher in their homes than in clinic settings. Provencher, Demers, and Gélinas (2009) completed a systematic review to examine the impact of setting (home versus clinic) on IADL performance in adults and found varied results for studies of mixed-aged populations and some evidence that performance in home settings was better for older adults. The home advantage seemed to be more evident in activities that require interaction with the environment and not just task objects (e.g., cooking versus managing finances). More research is needed to identify the relationships among different types of client impairments and varied evaluation contexts.

Social Context. The occupational therapy evaluation also occurs in a social context. Practitioners must oversee activity performance during assessment, and their very presence can affect the manner and adequacy of the activities performed. The practitioner's presence especially affects the client's ability to initiate participation in ADL or IADL because the structure of the assessment process itself prompts clients to engage in the tasks. If initiation of task performance is impaired, the practitioner must supplement performance measures from a structured therapy session. For example, the Independent Living Scale includes a subscale for initiation (Ashley, Persel, & Clark, 2001). Alternatively, family members might be asked to keep track of the number of days the client completed pet care responsibilities without being asked, for example. Clients' occupational performance might be also be impaired or enhanced in the natural environment compared to the clinic, depending on their needs and the differences in social context between clinic and natural environments. For example, a client with a spinal cord injury who must be skilled in directing a personal care attendant during ADL might give directions effectively to a rehabilitation aide who is familiar with caring for people with similar needs but might not give detailed enough instructions for an employee in the home who has less experience. Conversely, a client who requires setup to feed himself or herself will be more independent at home than in the clinic if he or she lives in a family where meals are routinely set up for the entire family by a parent who does all the cooking.

Safety. Occupational therapists must assess risks associated with ADL or IADL that have been identified as priorities by clients and might need to defer assessment of a task that they believe could be unsafe. Identifying the potential risk of a given assessment is based on occupational therapists' expertise in determining activity demands combined with their estimate of client problems, outlined in step 4 earlier. Occupational therapists may opt to defer or modify an assessment that they deem is unsafe. For example, a client who experienced a recent stroke resulting in very poor sitting balance might identify showering as an important goal; however, getting the client onto a shower chair in a wet and slippery environment for an assessment might be unsafe, given the level of assistance she needs for maintaining balance so soon after the stroke. Instead, the occupational therapist might suggest beginning with an assessment of bathing skills that can be completed at bedside and defer a shower assessment until sitting balance is improved and the shower can be completed safely. Simulating an occupational performance task may also be a way to minimize risk during an evaluation. For example, driving is an IADL with a critical safety component and although on-road assessments are considered to be the most accurate, driving simulators offer therapists a safe alternative for gathering data to determine whether or not the client is appropriate to assess on city streets (Bédard, Parkkari, Weaver, Riendeau, & Dahlquist, 2010).

The Client's Experience. Clients will come with varied experience with ADL and IADL based on personal context. Typically, ADL practice begins in childhood, and the societal expectation is that adolescents and adults have a wide range of experience with these activities and can perform them adequately. However, a similar expectation does not hold for IADL, for which people have more options. Therefore, clients might not have developed proficiency in all IADL activities. Some might have no experience in planning and preparing meals, doing the laundry, or managing finances. Children with developmental disabilities often experience delays in the acquisition of ADL and IADL skills and might lack experience that a typically developing child would have at a given age. Clients' activity performance history is essential for understanding their current performance level. An activity limitation is interpreted differently for a client who has had no or little prior experience performing the activity than for one who had been doing it immediately premorbidly.

Time Constraints. The time that is available for occupational therapy assessment and intervention is often limited by several factors, including reimbursement policies, so the evaluation process must be done efficiently. For clients with a long list of ADL and IADL goals, selecting key activities will be necessary so that the intervention designed to enhance occupational performance can be initiated in a timely manner. As goals are met, additional assessments may be initiated to document baseline performance of other ADL or IADL and to justify additional occupational therapy goals and treatment.

The Occupational Therapy Practitioner's Training and Experience. An occupational therapy practitioner's experience can also affect the selection of assessment tools. Familiarity with an instrument can increase efficiency of use and effectiveness of interpreting assessment results. Some assessment tools require specialized training, so they are not options for therapists who lack the training. For example, the Assessment of Motor and Process Skills (AMPS) (Fisher & Jones, 2011a, 2011b) relies on software that can be accessed only by practitioners who have completed the training course and calibration process (Gitlin, 2005).

Availability of Resources. The materials that are required for ADL and IADL assessments vary, and the occupational therapist must make sure that the necessary materials are readily available. Completing a cooking assessment using a client's favorite cookie recipe might be an excellent choice for examining the client's performance, but the logistics and cost of procuring the ingredients for this activity make it impractical for an occupational therapy practitioner in a hospital setting. However, a client who is being seen in home-based therapy might have the required resources for making cookies readily available in the home. Some assessments require special test kits, which can be costly, and facilities might have only a few such tools available for use.

Mandates from Facilities or Third-Party Payers. Many facilities or third-party payers have assessment forms or procedures that must be completed for all clients. For example, rehabilitation facilities must use the Inpatient Rehabilitation Facility–Patient Assessment Instrument (IRF-PAI), which includes the FIM™ for measuring ADL (Department of Health and Human Services Centers for Medicare & Medicaid Services, 2006). If a client's description of a selected ADL differs from that of the FIM™ or if the client would like to address adequacy parameters in addition to independence and safety, then the occupational therapist must use a supplemental assessment, because documentation of the FIM™ scores is required.

Step 6: Consider Features of Assessment Tools

The occupational therapist must be familiar with available assessments and consider what tasks are included in the assessment, how tasks are defined, the psychometric properties, the type of data to be collected, and the method of data collection.

Tasks Assessed. Tasks that are included in an ADL or IADL assessment should be consistent with clients' priorities, and the operational definition of effective performance should fit clients' needs and address all parameters of importance. For example, many assessment instruments measure independence; but if clients would also like to complete tasks independently without experiencing shortness of breath or pain, occupational therapists might want to use a dyspnea or pain scale in conjunction with the independence measure.

Standardized versus Nonstandardized Assessments. Some assessments are not **standardized assessments**; that is, the individual therapist designs the assessment and decides the type of information to gather or practitioners in a clinic might develop their own instrument for assessment. Nonstandardized assessments lack testing of psychometric properties, such as reliability, validity, or sensitivity to change in a client's status (Lorch & Herge, 2007). Standardized assessments rely on a well-described, uniform approach. There is a lot of variability in the extent to which the psychometric properties of standardized assessments have been established. Some assessments have been extensively studied and include a wide range of psychometric statistics to support the reliability and validity of the tool. The psychometric properties of test instruments may be published in the test manual or through peer-reviewed publications, such as the *American Journal of Occupational Therapy* (AJOT). When possible, it is best to use an assessment with established psychometric properties (Lorch & Herge, 2007).

There are different types of standardized assessments, including **norm-referenced tests** and **criterion-referenced tests**. Types of evaluations are described in more detail in Chapter 25. The purpose of norm-referenced testing is to compare a client's performance on a test to that of other people on the same test (Kielhofner, 2006). ADL and IADL assessments are not usually norm-referenced tests, which tend to be used to assess developmental levels, performance skills, or client factors such as visual perception, grip strength, or coordination. ADL and IADL assessments are typically criterion based, that is, tests that compare a client's performance to a performance standard (Portney & Watkins, 2009). Criterion-referenced tests stress activity mastery and address questions such as: "Can clients perform all activities, or procure the services, needed to live in the community on their own?" Criterion-referenced tests often incorporate activity analyses, and the degree of structure that is imposed on testing is usually more flexible than those for norm-referenced testing, allowing therapists to tailor tests appropriately. For example, a dressing assessment is typically done with clothes that the client needs to and wants to wear, which can have an impact on performance. If a patient needs to be able to manage buttoning, that should be incorporated into the assessment even if it is difficult for the patient; however, if the patient has not worn garments with buttons for many years, there is no reason to assess buttoning ability.

Descriptive versus Quantitative Data. Some nonstandardized assessments use a descriptive approach; that is, the salient characteristics of clients' activity performance are observed or obtained through client or caregiver descriptions. Clients' status is documented by simply describing their performance. Quantitative ADL and IADL measures use a scale that converts observed or reported behavior into a number. Standardized quantitative measures include instructions for the person who is completing the assessment, which makes the assessment more reliable when the tool is used for reassessment or when there are multiple therapists in a facility. For example, the term *moderate assistance* could be interpreted in several ways, but if it is specifically described as "The patient requires more help than touching, or expends between 50% and 74% of the effort" (Uniform Data System for Medical Rehabilitation, 2005), there is likely to be better agreement among therapists using the instrument. Reducing observed behavior to a number also makes it efficient for reporting data in documentation. However, loss of descriptive data can make it difficult for the reader to get a clear understanding of the client's limitations. Often, documentation includes quantitative assessment data that are accompanied by some descriptive data to provide a more comprehensive picture of client performance. A brief case, presented in Table 47.1, compares descriptive and quantitative data from two cases.

It is possible to use descriptive data to document a client's baseline status, which is needed to determine

TABLE 47.1 Comparison of Descriptive and Quantitative Data from a Dressing Assessment of Two Children

Aiden	Brody
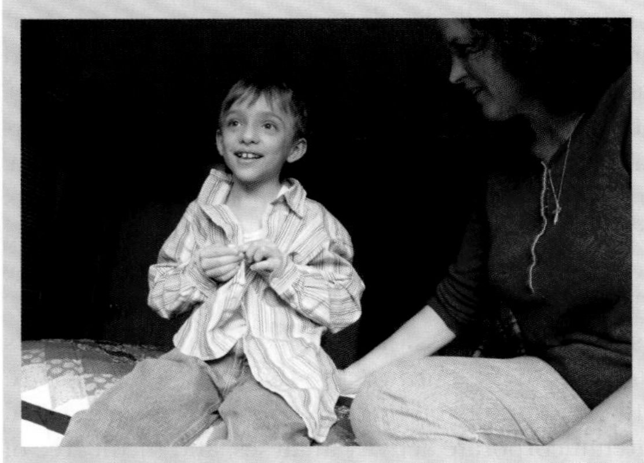	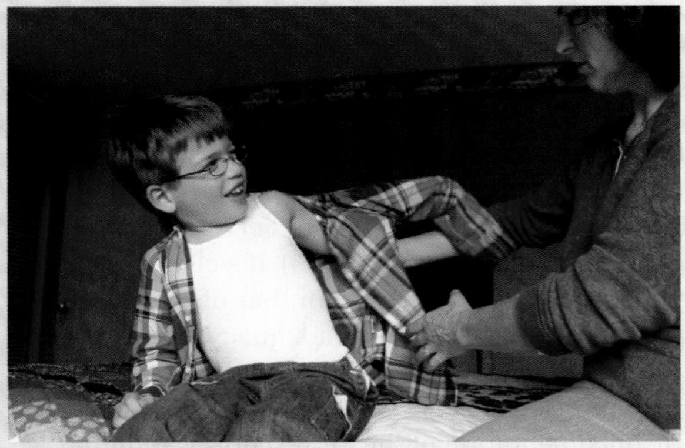
Client Description	
Aiden is a 7-year-old child who sustained a traumatic brain injury. Before his injury, he was a typically developing child who dressed himself independently.	Brody is a 7-year-old child with cerebral palsy affecting the right side of his body. His mother has been helping him dress prior to this assessment.
Descriptive Data From Observing Dressing	
• Well-coordinated and smooth movements of both upper extremities (UEs) when manipulating clothing. • Maintenance of appropriate posture, sitting unsupported on the bed. • Reached all areas of his body (behind, overhead, feet) without loss of balance or postural instability. • Frequently stopped midtask to verbally express thoughts, which were disjointed and difficult to follow. • Made repeated (total of five) attempts to get his left arm in a sleeve turned inside out. Did not attempt to self-correct or respond to verbal directions to turn the sleeve right side out. The practitioner turned the sleeve right side out after giving three verbal cues and gesturing toward the sleeve. • Aiden left the dressing task to look out the window when he heard a plane passing overhead and continued to talk about the plane when asked to return to the dressing task. • Aiden returned to the task when the practitioner physically guided him to the bed and placed one of his arms in the sleeve. Aiden then completed putting the shirt on his other arm without physical assistance or cues. • When asked to button his shirt, he completed 2 of 6 buttons, which were misaligned. When asked how well his shirt was buttoned, he looked down at himself and said, "It's perfect," then skipped out of the room saying that he wanted to go to the TV room.	• Started to put left (stronger) arm in his shirtsleeve first. Responded immediately to verbal cue to dress the right side of the body first. • Wavering of trunk when using both UEs to position the shirt. Practitioner steadied Brody's trunk to prevent him from falling forward when he pulled the shirt across his back. He could not get the shirt far enough around to reach the sleeve. The practitioner moved the shirt so he could reach it with the left arm. • Left UE movements were smooth and well coordinated. • Right UE movement was minimal, and he could not use his hand for fine tasks, such as buttoning. Several attempts were required to complete the bottom three buttons with the left hand, and the practitioner had to complete the top three. • Putting on his shirt took 15 minutes. Brody reported he felt "pretty tired" at the end. Brody was focused during the task, even when his little brother ran into and out of the room. • Brody followed instructions consistently and made five attempts to help solve problems encountered along the way, for example, suggesting he wear pullover shirts that do not have buttons. • When asked which arm he will dress first when he tries the task tomorrow, Brody responded, "My right arm."
Quantitative Data Based on the Wee FIM™	
Upper Body Dressing = 4	Upper Body Dressing = 4

whether or not progress is made in treatment; however, this can be difficult and time consuming. For example, if Aiden's and Brody's occupational therapists had to document the status of *all* ADL and IADL as in Table 47.1, the evaluation report would take a great deal of time to write and to read. Additionally, the occupational therapy practitioner who is documenting descriptive data should be very careful to distinguish between *observations* and *clinical judgments* (subjective interpretations about the observations). The statements listed in Table 47.1 are observations. A statement of clinical judgment is interpretive, and several plausible interpretations could be made from the more objective observations. For example, the occupational therapy practitioner could conclude that Brody has weak trunk muscles that interfere with balance. This conclusion should be presented as a hypothesis, not as an observation; because Brody's inability to maintain balance while dressing could be due to other factors, such as impaired vestibular and proprioceptive input that interferes with his ability to detect when he is starting to fall to one side.

Quantitative methods provide a more efficient way to document progress, although it might not provide the reader with adequate information. For example, although Aiden and Brody have the same quantitative score on the WeeFIM™, the descriptive information enables readers to see that there are very different underlying problems. Occupational therapists can document some key descriptive data to support their evaluation and treatment plan, but most descriptive observations are simply used by therapists for planning treatment, whereas quantitative data are recorded in documentation (Gateley & Borcherding, 2011). Many quantitative ADL scales are available; however, it can be difficult for occupational therapy practitioners to find standardized assessments for some IADL, so a descriptive approach also provides a reasonable option for the assessment of selected tasks for which no quantitative measure exists.

Reported versus Observed Performance. Data about ADL and IADL performance can be gathered by report or through direct observation. Reported data about the client's abilities and limitations in performance can be gathered from the client, the caregiver, and/or another health professional. The occupational therapy practitioner poses questions about ADL and IADL performance. The questioning method may be implemented in an oral or a written format, using interviews or questionnaires, respectively. Although the questioning is frequently done face to face, either format can be done without physical interaction. Interviews may be conducted over the telephone. Questionnaires may be completed while the client is waiting for an appointment or can be mailed out in advance of a session. Gathering data via report can be done informally; that is, the practitioner develops the questions to be asked and the actual data that are gathered or through the use of a standardized instrument such as the COPM (Law, Baptiste et al., 2005), the Occupational Self Assessment (Baron, Kielhofner, Iyenger, Goldhammer, & Wolenski, 2006), or the Child Occupational Self Assessment (Keller, Kafkes, Basu, Federico, & Kielhofner, 2005). Although self-report is an efficient way to measure ADL and IADL, it is not always consistent with actual performance (Brown et al., 1996; Goverover, Chiaravalloti, Gaudino-Goering, Moore, & DeLuca, 2009; Hilton, Fricke, & Unsworth, 2001; Rogers et al., 2003); and the occupational therapist should do selected performance-based assessments when the client's accuracy is in question. Additionally, gathering data about selected ADL or IADL through both self-report and performance-based measures can provide the occupational therapist with valuable insight into the accuracy of the client's self-awareness regarding the impact of his or her disability.

In some situations, clients might be unable to respond on their own behalf. For example, they might be too physically ill or depressed to participate in questioning or they might lack insight into their problems because of cognitive deficits. In these situations, caregivers or other proxies can be asked to respond on behalf of clients. The usefulness of the information that is obtained from caregivers or proxies depends on their familiarity with the client's ADL and IADL. For example, if the caregiver or proxy has not actually observed a client bathing recently, the information that this person gives about bathing might be based more on opinion than on concrete knowledge of performance. In addition, there are known biases in the reporting tendencies of caregivers and proxies. Cohen-Mansfield and Jensen (2007) examined accuracy of spouses' perceptions of each other's self-care practices and found spouses agreed "exactly" 58% of the time and had "close/partial agreement" 75% of the time. Family proxies of people post stroke reported their family members as being more disabled compared to self-report, although the size of the difference was small (Carod-Artal, Coral, Trizotto, & Moreira, 2009). Caregivers and proxies can readily observe evaluation parameters such as independence, safety, and aberrant activity behaviors. For some evaluation parameters, however, clients are the only appropriate respondents. For example, values, satisfaction with performance, and activity-related pain are subjective; and indices of these parameters are difficult for others to observe.

Assessments that rely on self-report or caregiver's report are particularly useful for screening for activity limitations because a large number of activities can be queried in a short amount of time. Questioning is also the data-gathering method of choice when information is needed about daily living *habits*—that is, about what clients usually do on a daily basis—or to learn about clients' ADL and IADL experience. However, reporting is less useful in evaluating limitations for the purposes of intervention because clients might not be able to describe their limitations in sufficient detail to target the components of activities that are problematic.

Assessment data can also be gathered through direct observation of ADL and IADL, which gives the practitioner more information about how the client performs a task. Observation of performance, however, requires more time and material resources and is therefore more costly. Direct observation of performance can also be done in a nonstandardized way or through use of a standardized assessment. The constraints of practice settings, often imposed by third-party payers or limited funding, can place restrictions on the time an occupational therapist has available for evaluation. Occupational therapists must be strategic in selecting ADL and IADL assessments that will provide information relevant to the client and can be generalized to other tasks so that the practitioner does not have to observe all meaningful ADL and IADL that may be addressed in treatment. For example, if a client requires assistance with cooking because of an inability to transport food and cooking equipment safely while using a walker, the occupational therapist can reasonably project, without having to observe performance, that the same client will require assistance in doing laundry because laundry also requires the transportation of task objects.

Selected standardized ADL and IADL assessments are listed in Tables 47.2 and 47.3. The ADL assessments that are included in Table 47.2 are readily available and either are commonly used in practice (e.g., the FIM™) or research (e.g., the Barthel Index) or provide a unique approach to assessment. For example, the Independent Living Scale measures task initiation (Ashley et al., 2001). Information for learning to use each assessment is also provided. The IADL instruments that were selected include a range of activities. More ADL and IADL assessments can be found in the resources listed in Box 47.1, and a more comprehensive list of assessments can be found in Appendix II.

Step 7: Integrate the Information from Steps 1 to 6 to Select the Optimal Activities of Daily Living and Instrumental Activities of Daily Living Assessment Tools

After establishing the purpose of the evaluation and the client's priorities and gathering some preliminary information about the client and relevant contextual features, assessment instruments can be selected that are client centered, yield appropriate data, are reliable and valid, and are feasible to administer. Occupational therapists should engage in best practice by considering the evidence regarding the selection and use of assessments, for example, the reliability of instruments and the validity for a given clinical situation. Additional considerations for evidence-based evaluation are discussed in the "Commentary on the Evidence" box on putting evidence into practice through the use of standardized assessments. Perhaps the best data-gathering strategy is to use a combination of methods and sources, relying on the convergence of data for the best profile of clients' activity abilities and limitations.

It is often most effective to begin the evaluation with a questioning approach to provide an overall profile of the client's abilities and limitations, to understand clients' priorities, and to target activities that require in-depth evaluation. Questioning is then followed by observational assessments. If observational assessments raise additional questions about the client's activity performance abilities, the evaluation plan can be modified to gather more or different data.

Planning an effective ADL and IADL evaluation is best illustrated by an example case study that follows the steps described earlier.

Implementing the Evaluation: Gathering Data, Critical Observation, and Hypothesis Generation

Gathering Data and Critical Observation

Once occupational therapists develop an evaluation plan, they must carry it out. The thoughtful and deliberate selection of appropriate assessments described previously is key in making the data gathering run smoothly. A few additional considerations about the actual implementation of the evaluation warrant discussion. The occupational therapy practitioner who is doing an assessment should do the following:

- *Collect all equipment and supplies* needed for carrying out the evaluation plans, making sure test kits are complete and organized and that necessary equipment and supplies are available, including clients' personal items (e.g., clothing from home). Novice practitioners might find it helpful to create a list of needed items to make sure that everything is available and in working order.
- *Schedule assessment sessions in the best environment available and the most appropriate time of day.* For example, a client in an inpatient rehabilitation center would find it more comfortable to dress in his or her room than in a curtained-off area in a busy clinic and may find it more meaningful and motivating to dress early in the day.
- *Be sensitive to individual needs for modesty*, which can vary greatly among clients. Many ADL are personal tasks that are typically done alone, including dressing, bathing, and toileting. Assessment for potential impairment in sexual activity should be included in ADL assessments but must be handled with sensitivity.
- *Structure the optimal social context.* For example, the practitioner might wish to have family members present during an interview to gain their perspectives about a client's abilities or needs, whereas having several family members observing a performance-based assessment of cooking might be distracting to the client and interfere with the evaluation process.
- *Bring appropriate tools to record data.* A well-planned evaluation session will reveal a lot of information about a client. Standardized tests often come with forms for recording data. Facilities may also have forms for recording data using assessments typically performed in that setting. The practitioner might also want to jot down relevant observations, for example, noting that a client complained of shoulder pain when putting a shirt on overhead or that a client's grocery list included

CASE STUDY 47.1 Evaluation of a Client with Morbid Obesity and Respiratory Failure

Mrs. Howard is a 59-year-old woman with a history of morbid obesity (she is 5 ft 1 in tall and weighs 376 lb). She was admitted to a hospital with difficulty breathing secondary to an allergic reaction to an over-the-counter medication. She subsequently went into respiratory arrest and required a tracheostomy and mechanical ventilation. She was weaned from the ventilator 6 weeks later and placed on supplemental oxygen. She developed a right foot drop, secondary to peroneal nerve compression that occurred during her prolonged bedrest. After 2 months in acute care, Mrs. Howard was transferred to a rehabilitation hospital where she participated in occupational therapy (OT) for activities of daily living (ADL) and instrumental activities of daily living (IADL) training and physical therapy (PT) for mobility training. She was dependent in all areas of ADL and IADL on admission and made considerable gains in function before her discharge home 6 months after her initial hospitalization. At discharge, she was ambulating short distances (up to 50 ft) independently with a rolling walker and a brace on the right foot. She had an extra wide wheelchair for limited community outings (e.g., doctor's appointments), but the chair did not fit in her home. She continued to require supplemental oxygen and was independent in tracheostomy care and suctioning. Mrs. Howard was referred for home-based services, including skilled nursing, nutritional counseling, home health aide (3 days a week, 2 hours each day), PT, and OT.

Occupational Profile

Mrs. Howard has lived with her husband of 30 years. He worked full time but was physically able and willing to assist his wife when he was home. Mr. and Mrs. Howard had two grown children and two school-aged grandchildren who lived in the area. Before hospitalization, Mrs. Howard was independent in ADL and IADL. She had primary responsibility for cooking, light housekeeping, and laundry. She worked 20 hours a week at the public library. Mrs. Howard had several close friends she enjoyed meeting for lunch or shopping, especially bargain hunting at flea markets. She and her husband also frequently attended their grandchildren's sports events in a nearby town. The following considerations were used to select appropriate ADL and IADL assessments for Mrs. Howard:

1. **Identify the overall purpose(s) of the evaluation.** The primary purpose was to plan and monitor OT intervention, so baseline data must be effective for determining progress toward goals.
2. **Have clients identify their needs, interests, and perceived difficulties with ADL and/or IADL.** Mrs. Howard's primary goal was to regain her independence in ADL, IADL, and leisure. She identified ADL and IADL, including driving, as priorities because she was concerned about being a burden on her husband. She reported that her biggest difficulties were with lower body ADL (unable to reach) and with all IADL (fatigue, shortness of breath, limited reach, and mobility). She had frequent medical appointments and lived in a rural area, and she hated relying on others for getting to and from appointments.
3. **Further explore the client's relevant activities so that the activities are operationally defined.** The "problem activities" that Mrs. Howard identified were briefly discussed for more detail. ADL were completed in the typical fashion, except for the brace that she wore on the right foot. She reported that sexual activity was not currently a priority but that she would like to address it later, once she had sufficient energy for and independence in other ADL. IADL priorities for Mrs. Howard included the following:
   - Transporting laundry from the bedroom to the kitchen (top-loading washer) and out to the clothesline to dry (no dryer).
   - Cooking complete dinners, including accessing the refrigerator, oven, stovetop, cooking utensils, dishwasher, and sink. A sample dinner would include fish, baked potatoes, steamed green beans, and a salad.
   - Driving and riding in her minivan.
   - Accessing all areas of her one-story home except the basement, including home office for doing finances and using the computer, linen closets, and so forth.

   Additionally, Mrs. Howard reported adequacy parameters, including the ability to complete ADL and IADL in a timely manner and regain the ability to sustain activity without fatigue or shortness of breath.
4. **Estimate the client factors that affect occupational performance and/or the assessment process.** Mrs. Howard's primary problems limiting function were caused by her obesity, which limited her reach and ability to move and caused fatigue and dyspnea. Cognition and perception did not appear to be factors that interfered with function on review of her rehabilitation records and the initial interview.
5. **Identify contextual features that affect assessment.** Contextual features that supported the evaluation process included the following:
   - The assessment occurred in Mrs. Howard's home, providing the advantage of a natural environment.
   - There was a ramp into the home, providing access to the yard and driveway.
   - Mrs. Howard had years of experience with all of the tasks she wished to return to, which would support performance of tasks.

   Contextual features that were barriers to the evaluation process included the following:
   - Clutter in the home that presented a potential safety issue and restricted mobility and access.
   - Mrs. Howard was on oxygen, with the unit in the bedroom and a very long tube connected to her nasal cannula, so she had to manage the tubing as she moved around the house.
   - The evaluation occurred during the week, and the therapist was alone with a client whose weight presented a potential safety problem to the therapist who had no

(continued)

CASE STUDY 47.1 Evaluation of a Client with Morbid Obesity and Respiratory Failure (*Continued*)

assistance for guarding Mrs. Howard when trying a new task.

- Mrs. Howard had private insurance, which required that the OT evaluation be completed in one visit.

6. **Consider features of assessment tools.** This step is included in the discussion of step 7.
7. **Integrate the information from steps 1 to 6 to select the optimal ADL and IADL assessment tools.** The time limit of one visit (approximately 60–75 minutes) had a significant impact on which assessments were selected. The occupational therapist decided to start with the COPM based on the following considerations:
   - The COPM had well-established psychometric properties and assessed both ADL and IADL and leisure (Law, Baptiste et al., 2005).
   - The COPM relied on self-report; however, Mrs. Howard was cognitively intact and had been learning to live with her disability for the past 4 months. One advantage of the self-report format is that it did not pose any safety hazards. For example, the occupational therapist got a baseline performance and satisfaction rating on driving her car (including getting in and out) without having to attempt the task alone with Mrs. Howard.
   - Mrs. Howard indicated that she felt stress about burdening her husband. The COPM would help Mrs. Howard and the occupational therapist to prioritize the ADL and IADL that would reduce caregiver burden.
   - The COPM included a satisfaction measure, which reflected some of the adequacy parameters that Mrs. Howard identified (e.g., if she could dress independently but it took her 45 minutes, she would give that a low satisfaction score).
   - The COPM could be completed in about 20 minutes.

After the COPM, the occupational therapist selected the FIM™ subtests of transfers, lower body dressing, and grooming. Other subtests were not observed because they were activities that Mrs. Howard reported no difficulty with (including feeding, toileting, and upper body dressing) or because of time constraints (e.g., bathing). The FIM™ was identified as an appropriate measure for the following reasons:

- Mrs. Howard reported that she required physical assistance for lower body dressing and getting out of bed (on the FIM™, transfers start from supine and end in standing for people who do not use a wheelchair), and the scale was believed to have adequate sensitivity in levels of physical assistance to document progress.
- The FIM™ included client appliances in the lower body dressing measure, and Mrs. Howard reported that her brace was one thing she was not able to master while in the rehabilitation center.
- The occupational therapist had discharge FIM™ scores from the rehabilitation center, so performance in the clinic could be compared to performance in the home with the same tool to examine the impact of the home context on performance and aid in problem solving for intervention.
- These tasks could all be completed in 25 minutes.

Two additional parameter measures were used to supplement the FIM™. Lower body dressing and grooming were timed, which required no additional assessment time. Dyspnea was measured after each of the three subtasks, using a 100-mm visual analogue scale where 0 = "no shortness of breath," 50 mm = "moderate shortness of breath," and 100 mm = "severe shortness of breath" (Lansing, Moosavi, & Banzett, 2003). Mrs. Howard was asked to place a mark on the line that best represented her dyspnea. Completion of the dyspnea scales required little additional time, fitting into the 25 minutes allowed for the FIM™.

At this point, Mrs. Howard needed a rest, although the occupational therapist wanted to include some observation of IADL in the evaluation. While Mrs. Howard took a rest, the therapist used the walker to do an informal accessibility assessment for several key areas in the home, including Mrs. Howard's dresser, closet, personal computer, kitchen appliances, and cabinets. Although standardized assessments are available, the occupational therapist used a nonstandardized approach because Mrs. Howard's walker required additional room for accessibility and the therapist needed to focus on a few key areas because time was limited. The occupational therapist also began some intervention by making a list of suggestions that would make Mrs. Howard's environment more accessible. The therapist reviewed the recommendations with Mrs. Howard so that she could enlist a friend or family member in modifying the context, making treatment sessions more effective. The informal assessment of context and review with Mrs. Howard could be completed in 15 minutes.

At this point, Mrs. Howard and her occupational therapist were about 1 hour into the initial evaluation. The therapist would have liked to observe Mrs. Howard complete a simple cooking task and also assess her potential to return to driving by having her get in and out of her car, including folding and storing the walker. However, Mrs. Howard was fatigued and 15 minutes was not enough time for both. The therapist's quick analysis of the varied demands of the two tasks lead her to conclude the session with a nonstandardized assessment of a kitchen task. Mrs. Howard had a minivan that would require a significant step up. Given her level of fatigue with lighter activities and concerns about safely guarding someone of her size, the occupational therapist opted to have Mrs. Howard make a cup of tea, deferring the car assessment to another session. The kettle was placed in a low cabinet to assess her ability to retrieve it. The tea was in an over-counter cabinet. The therapist gathered descriptive data and also timed the task and used the visual analogue scale to measure dyspnea on completion. The task took less than 10 minutes. After the assessment, Mrs. Howard settled into her favorite chair to enjoy her cup of tea.

TABLE 47.2 Summary of Selected ADL and IADL Instruments

Title	Areas Addressed	Population	Method/Rating	Learning to Use the Assessment
ADL-Focused Occupation-Based Neurobehavioral Evaluation (A-ONE; formerly, Árnadóttir OT-ADL Neurobehavioral Evaluation)	Feeding, dressing, grooming and hygiene, transfers and mobility, and communication	Those 16 years and older with central nervous system dysfunction	Observation of ADL; uses an ordinal scale.	Training required to rate reliably (Árnadóttir, 1990, 2011).
Assessment of Living Skills and Resources (ALSAR)	11 IADL skills	Adults	Interview with guiding questions; uses a three-point ordinal scale.	Self-study using published references, including Williams et al. (1991); Hilton et al., (2001); Kuo et al. (2007); and Clemson, Bundy, Unsworth, and Singh (2009).
Assessment of Motor and Process Skills (AMPS)	Over 100 calibrated ADL and IADL activities; client and therapist select 2 or 3 for assessment	Children (> age 2 years) and adults	Interview to identify 2 to 3 tasks for performance testing; activities rated on 16 motor skills (e.g., reaches, lifts) and 20 process skills (e.g., initiates, searches); uses a 4-point ordinal scale.	Training required. Software for scoring and required rater calibration available only through course. Course information and extensive reference list are available from the AMPS Project International Website: http://www.ampsintl.com
Barthel Index	10 ADL skills	Adults	Each item is rated on a 10- or 15-point scale; total ADL performance ranges from 0 to 100.	Test items and guidelines for administering can be found at http://strokecenter.org/trials/scales/barthel.html
Canadian Occupational Performance Measure (COPM)	Activities classified into three areas: self-care (ADL and some IADL), productive (some IADL and work), and leisure	Children and adults	Self-report using a semistructured interview; problems identified by client are rated for importance (scale of 1–10); the five most important problems are rated for both performance and satisfaction (also scales of 1–10).	Self-guided training available through the manual (Law et al., 2005) and on DVD/video from the Canadian Occupational Therapy Association: www.caot.org
Functional Independence Measure (FIM™)	18 activities, 13 ADL tasks, and 5 involving communication and social cognition (no IADL tasks)	Adolescents and adults	Observation by a trained observer; uses a 7-point ordinal scale, grading amount of assistance needed by clients to complete activity.	Training is recommended for interrater reliability. Training often provided by employer. Also available from the Uniform Data System for Medical Rehabilitation: http://www.udsmr.org
Independent Living Scale (ILS)	6 ADL tasks and 10 IADL tasks; also rates behaviors in the context of tasks, including initiation and aberrant task behaviors	Adolescents and adults with traumatic brain injury	Observation over the course of a week (needed for measuring initiation and aberrant task behaviors); data may be supplemented by other team members.	Instructions for the test are available in Ashley et al. (2001). The ILS form and general information can be purchased for a nominal fee at http://www.neuroskills.com/cgi-bin/store/CNSstore.cgi?user_action=detail&catalogno=cns00065

(continued)

TABLE 47.2 Summary of Selected ADL and IADL Instruments (*Continued*)

Title	Areas Addressed	Population	Method/Rating	Learning to Use the Assessment
Instrumental Activities of Daily Living (IADL) Scale	8 IADL tasks	Adults	Scoring is based on what clients can do rather than what they actually do; scale ranges from 0 to 17.	The instrument is available at http://strokecenter.org/trials/scales/lawton.html
Kohlman Evaluation of Living Skills (KELS)	17 activities grouped into categories: ADL, safety and health, selected IADL, work, and leisure; tends to emphasize knowledge component of activities	Adults with cognitive impairments	Combination of interview and performance; uses a 3-point ordinal scale.	Manual included in test kit describes testing procedures. The KELS can be purchased from the AOTA: http://www.aota.org
Melville-Nelson Self-Care Assessment	7 ADL that are consistent with the Minimum Data Set	Adults in skilled nursing facilities	Performance-based; tasks are rated on 2 scales: how much the client does and how much/what type of assistance is given. Client performance ratings are made for subtasks and sub-subtasks to help with planning intervention	Protocol describes standardized administration procedures. The form and protocol are available at http://www.utoledo.edu/hshs/ot/melville.html
Minimum Data Set (MDS) 3.0 —Section G: Functional Status Scale	10 ADL tasks activities	Residents in long-term care	Performance, ascertained from multiple health care professionals, overall shifts during past 7 days; activities rated for self-performance and support provided.	The Centers for Medicare and Medicaid has training resources at http://www.cms.gov/NursingHomeQualityInits/25_NHQIMDS30.asp#TopOfPage
Outcome and Assessment Information Set (OASIS)	Eight ADL and six IADL tasks	Clients in home care	Data may be obtained through various methods (observation, client, or proxy report); ratings differentiated by task characteristics; scale varies from item to item.	The Centers for Medicare and Medicaid has training resources at https://www.cms.gov/OASIS/01_Overview.asp#TopOfPage
Pediatric Evaluation of Disability Inventory (PEDI)	ADL, including mobility, social function; has broad IADL tasks (household chores and community function)	Children 6 months to 7½ years (or older if development is delayed)	Report of clinicians or educators familiar with the child or through parental interview; the PEDI is a normed test.	Manual includes detailed instructions and cases to practice scoring the PEDI. Available for purchase at Pearson Assessments: http://www.pearsonassessments.com

TABLE 47.2 Summary of Selected ADL and IADL Instruments (*Continued*)

Title	Areas Addressed	Population	Method/Rating	Learning to Use the Assessment
Performance Assessment of Self-Care Skills (PASS)	26 tasks, including ADL and home management IADL tasks; there are different protocols for use in the client's home and an occupational therapy clinic.	Adults	Performance-based observational tool; yields summary scores of activity independence, safety, and adequacy; uses a 4-point ordinal scale.	Validity, reliability, and standardized procedures are described in the manual. The PASS is available from Dr. Margo Holm at the University of Pittsburgh, Pittsburgh, PA (mbholm@pitt.edu). Manual includes detailed instructions and clinicians and researchers can arrange to go to the University of Pittsburgh to establish interrater reliability with experienced PASS users if desired.
WeeFIM™ II	Measure disability severity related to physical impairment, across health, development, educational, and community settings. 0 to 3 module measures precursors to function.	Children from 6 months to 7 years	Observation, interview or both; uses same rating system as FIM™; scores range from 18 (total dependence) to 126 (complete independence).	Training information at http://www.udsmr.org/WebModules/WeeFIM/Wee_About.aspx

primarily nonnutritious foods. If possible, practitioners should record directly on facility-based documentation forms or electronic forms to reduce the time needed for completing the evaluation report later on.

During the evaluation, the practitioner should engage in critical observation, which can be framed by questions the practitioners ask themselves throughout the process, such as the following:

- *What are some of the possible underlying causes of the occupational performance deficits that are being observed or reported?* For example, various different factors may limit a client's ability to reach the clothes in his or her closet, including upper extremity weakness, impaired range of motion (ROM), poor coordination, diminished standing balance, or a clothes rod that is out of reach for the client's height. Observations that are made as the client tries to get clothes from the closet can provide clues to the underlying causes that will aid the occupational therapist in making sound treatment decisions, as shown in Figure 47.1.
- *What changes might need to be made in the initial evaluation plan based on the data from the first assessments?* For example, a cooking assessment might reveal mild cognitive deficits that were not apparent during initial interactions with a client, so the occupational therapist would add a cognitive assessment to the evaluation plan.
- *Are there discrepancies in the evaluation data that were collected?* Discrepancies need to be clarified and reconciled and can provide valuable insight into the nature of the client's ADL and IADL limitations. For example, a practitioner might ascertain through performance testing that a client can execute bed-to-wheelchair transfers, yet the client might insist that he cannot. The inconsistency might arise because although the client performs the transfer independently with the practitioner present, he feels insecure about his abilities and will not transfer on his own. In this example, the use of different data sources identified a performance discrepancy between skill and habit that would not have been apparent from the use of one source alone.

Hypothesis Generation

The evaluation data that are obtained through questioning, observing, and testing methods must be analyzed, synthesized, and integrated into a cohesive problem statement (Gateley & Borcherding, 2011). This integration of data is accomplished through diagnostic reasoning, which is a component of clinical reasoning (Schell & Schell, 2008). The clinical reasoning of practitioners occurs as a kind of internal dialogue about the interpretation of the data. Evidence supporting one interpretation is weighed against evidence rejecting that interpretation, and the interpretation that has the most supporting or compelling evidence is selected. If the evidence fails to sufficiently support one interpretation over another, more evaluative

TABLE 47.3 Classification of Selected ADL and IADL Instruments

	Areas of Occupation			Client Factors					
	Activity	**Participation**	**Quality of Life**	**Body Structures and Functions**	**Values, Beliefs, Spirituality**	**Performance Skills**	**Performance Patterns**	**Activity Demands**	**Environmental Factors/Context and Environment**
Assessment									
Arthritis Impact Scale	X			X					
Assessment of Motor and Process Skills	X	X				X			
ADL-Focused Occupation-Based Neurobehavioral Evaluation (A-ONE; formerly Árnadóttir OT-ADL Neurobehavioral Evaluation)	X			X					
Barthel Index	X								
Canadian Occupational Performance Measure	X	X							
Child Occupational Self-Assessment	X	X							
Functional Independence Measure (FIM™)	X								
Independent Living Scale	X						X		
Instrumental Activities of Daily Living Scale	X								
Katz	X								
Nottingham Extended Activities of Daily Living Scale	X	X							
Occupational Performance History Interview	X	X							X
Occupational Self-Assessment	X	X							
Performance Assessment of Self-Care Skills	X								
WeeFIM™	X								

BOX 47.1 Resources for ADL and IADL Assessments

Asher, I. A. (2007). *Occupational therapy assessment tools: An annotated index* (3rd ed.). Bethesda, MD: American Occupational Therapy Association.

Bolton, B. F., & Parker, R. M. (2008). *Handbook of measurement and evaluation in rehabilitation* (4th ed.). Austin, TX: Pro-Ed.

Gallo, J., Bogner, H. R., Fulmer, T., & Paveza, G. J. (2007). *Handbook of geriatric assessment* (4th ed.). Boston, MA: Jones & Bartlett.

Hemphill-Pearson, B. J. (Ed.). (2008). *Assessments in occupational therapy mental health: An integrative approach* (2nd ed.). Thorofare, NJ: Slack.

Law, M., Baum, C., & Dunn, W. (Eds.). (2005). *Measuring occupational performance: Supporting best practice in occupational therapy* (2nd ed.). Thorofare, NJ: Slack.

McColl, M. A., Carswell, A., Law, M., Pollock, N., Baptiste, S., & Polatajko, H. (2006). *Research on the Canadian Occupational Performance Measure (COPM): An annotated resource.* Toronto, Canada: Canadian Association of Occupational Therapists.

McDowell, I., & Newell, C. (2006). *Measuring health: A guide to rating scales and questionnaires* (3rd ed.). New York, NY: Oxford University Press.

Osterweil, D., Brummel-Smith, K., & Beck, J. C. (2000). *Comprehensive geriatric assessment.* New York, NY: McGraw-Hill.

Commentary on the Evidence: Standardized Assessments

Putting Evidence into Practice through the Use of Standardized Assessments

Best practice in occupational therapy indicates that standardized activities of daily living (ADL) and instrumental activities of daily living (IADL) assessments should be used because they provide objective measures that are both reliable and valid (Dunn, 2005; Fasoli, 2008; Lorch & Herge, 2007). Reliable assessments enable practitioners to trust that differences in scores measured at different times represent true changes in ADL or IADL status and that reassessments done by another clinician can be reliably compared to a client's prior scores (Fasoli, 2008; Richardson, 2010). Third-party payers also prefer documentation that describes clients' status and progress toward goals with standardized assessments. In spite of this, many clinicians continue to rely on nonstandardized assessments in clinical practice, often citing barriers, including beliefs that standardized outcome measures are not clinically relevant (Colquhoun, Letts, Law, MacDermid, & Edwards, 2010) and are too time consuming to be practical (Lorch & Herge, 2007). Clinicians also report they lack the necessary knowledge and skills to select and administer assessments (Colquhoun et al., 2010).

Many of these barriers may be relatively easy to overcome. Some standardized ADL and IADL assessments do not require much, if any, additional time or effort to conduct once practitioners are familiar with assessment protocols and scoring. For example, clinicians frequently begin their assessment with an interview to establish an occupational profile and clients' priorities (Radomski, 2008; Stewart, 2010). The Canadian Occupational Performance Measure (COPM) gathers descriptive data, as an informal interview does, but also includes reliable and valid quantitative measures of clients' self-reported performance ability and satisfaction on client-selected occupational performance tasks (Law, Baptiste et al., 2005). Clients' initial COPM scores serve as an objective baseline measure, and reassessment of clients' perceived progress can be quickly done by asking clients to rerate their performance and satisfaction on previously rated tasks. Practitioners who volunteered to begin using the COPM as part of a research study did not find that it required additional evaluation time and reported that the information gained enhanced their ability to plan and carry out treatment (Colquhoun et al., 2010).

Standardized tests that do not require extensive additional time can also be selected when practitioners need to observe clients' actual performance. For example, the Performance of Self-Care Skills (PASS) uses a standardized approach in assessing several ADL and IADL, often by structuring observations of key elements of a task, such as sweeping up cereal placed on the floor by the therapist rather than having to observe the client sweep the entire kitchen (Holm & Rogers, 2008; Rogers & Holm, 1994). The assessment yields measures of three different parameters: independence, safety, and adequacy. Any or all of these performance parameters can be tracked and reported to document clients' progress toward goals. At first glance, the PASS administration and scoring procedures may seem complicated, but the assessment is very user friendly once practitioners become familiarized with the instrument.

Many standardized assessments are available for measuring ADL performance (Letts & Bosch, 2005), but many practitioners continue to use informal ADL assessments in clinical practice. Klein, Barlow, and Hollis (2008) conducted an action research design to identify ADL measures that were most reflective of the principles of occupational therapy practice and identified six instruments, including the ADL Profile, Assessment of Motor and Process Skills (AMPS), Functional Performance Measure, Rivermead ADL Assessment, Edmans ADL Index, and the Melville-Nelson Self-Care Assessment.

Appropriate assessment tools for IADL are more difficult to find. Standardized assessment of IADL is more challenging because of the variability and complexity of IADL tasks. One potential limitation in using standardized assessments for IADL is that many IADL assessments that examine a range of IADL tasks (rather than a single skill, such as cooking) rely on self-report or proxy report; examples are the Extended ADL (Nouri & Lincoln, 1987), COPM (Law, Baptiste et al., 2005), Assessment of Living Skills and Resources (Williams et al., 1991), and some parts of the *Kohlman Evaluation of Living Skills* (Kohlman Thomason, 1992). The limitations of using reported performance were addressed earlier in this chapter. The development of reliable and valid IADL assessments that enable occupational therapy practitioners to objectively measure observed performance across many IADL tasks would increase their ability to engage in evidence-based evaluation.

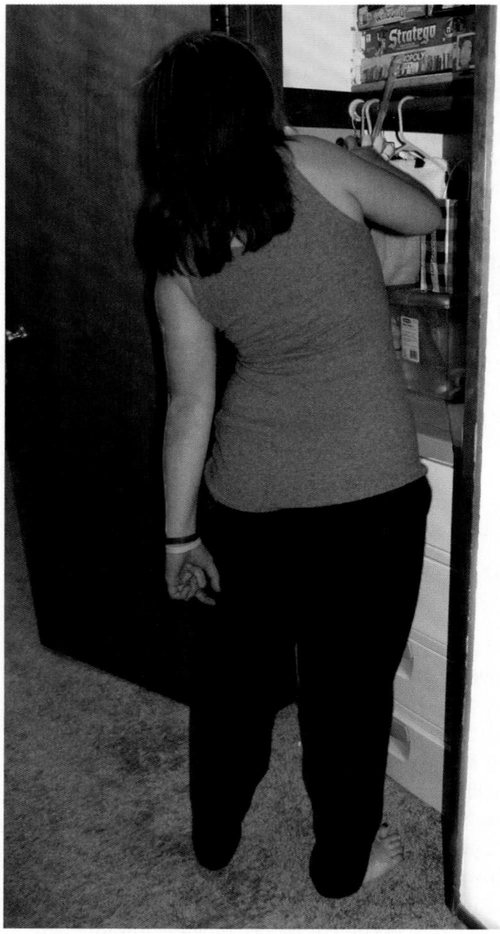

FIGURE 47.1 Observations made during reach: Lateral flexion of the trunk suggests that the client is compensating for an inability to raise the arm, which could be from limited passive range of motion or decreased strength. The height of the closet rod relative to the client's size should require only about 50% of typical shoulder flexion. Balance does not appear to be an issue because the client appears stable even while shifting her center of gravity toward the left as she reaches.

data are collected to supplement the reasoning process. This process is best illustrated through an example, based on the cases presented in Table 47.1. Aiden and Brody had the same dressing scores on the FIM™, a quantitative ADL assessment, but the occupational therapist's clinical interpretation of the descriptive data will lead to very different assumptions about the problems that are causing dressing impairments for the two children. Before reading on, take a minute to reflect on the different observations reported in Table 47.1, and consider the following:

- What are the underlying factors that interfere with Aiden's ability to dress independently? What are Aidens's strengths, that is, what skills support his dressing performance? What observed behaviors led to your conclusions about Aiden's strengths and limitations?
- What are the underlying factors that interfere with Brody's ability to dress independently? What are Brody's strengths, that is, what skills support his dressing performance? What observed behaviors led to your conclusions about Brody's strengths and limitations?

For Aiden, limited attention, impaired awareness of occupational performance deficits, and inconsistent response to feedback seemed to be underlying problems that limited his ability to dress independently. This is a hypothesis or clinical judgment rather than an objective observation, because constructs such as attention and awareness of deficits cannot be directly observed and must be inferred from specific behaviors. At the same time, Aiden's physical capabilities seemed to be an asset and supported performance in many ways. Compare the observations and clinical judgments made by the occupational therapist about Aiden to those made about Brody. In both cases, the children required verbal cueing and occasional physical assistance; however, descriptive data led the occupational therapist to a very different hypothesis about Brody's dressing limitations. The underlying problems for Brody were physical impairments, for example, diminished sitting balance, incoordination of the right upper extremity, and decreased endurance. Behaviors that supported performance included attention to task, follow-through with feedback, the ability to recall adaptive strategies, and engagement in active problem solving. Generating hypotheses about the nature of the occupational performance deficit is crucial for selecting effective intervention, which must address the underlying problem. For example, adaptive equipment could be provided to help Brody reach his feet independently or to compensate for limited right hand function during buttoning; however, this equipment would be of no help to Aiden and would likely impede performance by distracting him from the task.

Through this process, the occupational therapist arrives at a cohesive understanding of the ADL and IADL performance of the client, factors that are interfering with performance, and appropriate therapeutic actions given the nature of the client's deficits. This understanding is presented to clients or their proxies for verification and collaborative decision making concerning the therapeutic action to be implemented.

Establishing Clients' Goals: The Bridge between Evaluation and Intervention

The OTPF includes the establishment of clients' goals as the final step in the evaluation process and as the first component of the intervention plan (AOTA, 2008), so this important step really serves as a transition from evaluation to intervention. Synthesizing evaluation that results into a meaningful, individualized intervention plan is a complex cognitive task and can be overwhelming for the student or new occupational therapy practitioner. The process of planning and implementing interventions is much easier for practitioners who have reasonable, attainable, and measurable goals or outcomes. The following section is focused on the multiple factors that influence outcomes to help guide novice practitioners in the clinical reasoning for establishing effective client goals and to structure the problem-solving process for more experienced practitioners, especially when they are managing particularly complex or challenging clients.

Establishing goals requires analysis of the evaluation results in conjunction with additional factors that influence outcomes, namely, the client's self-awareness and ability to learn, the client's prognosis, the time allocated for intervention, the client's discharge disposition, and the client's ability to follow through with new routines or techniques. The next section focuses on using performance parameters to establish meaningful goals for clients that have a clearly identified behavior; that is, what the client is expected to *do*. The behavior must be observable and include an appropriate *degree of performance*; that is, a characteristic of the behavior that is measurable (e.g., "independently" or "without pain"; Sames, 2010). Goal behaviors may be aimed at underlying skills, for example, increasing strength or ROM to support participation in ADL. However, examples in this chapter will focus on establishing goals with occupational performance behaviors, such as bathing or doing laundry.

Identifying Appropriate Goal Behaviors

A comprehensive evaluation examines ADL and IADL performance across relevant performance parameters. Four of these performance parameters—value, level of difficulty, safety, and fatigue and dyspnea—are particularly relevant to consider in order to identify goals for intervention that target realistic and appropriate client behaviors.

Value

Occupational therapists should select goal behaviors (i.e., ADL and IADL tasks) that reflect the values defined by the client during the evaluation. The value that clients place on given activities influences their motivation for participation in any intervention aimed at improving performance for that activity (Doig, Fleming, Cornwell, & Kuipers, 2009: Jack & Estes, 2010). Because many occupational therapy interventions require the acquisition of new skills through practice, motivation can greatly influence the ultimate functional outcome. Clients who put little value on the activity that is being addressed during an intervention might appear to be uncooperative in treatment and are unlikely to follow through with programs outside of direct treatment that are necessary for improving skill in that activity.

Clients' self-awareness of ADL and IADL performance deficits can have an impact on identifying goals and their relative value. Clients with cognitive deficits and poor self-awareness may not value selected ADL or IADL goals if they perceive they are already independent, efficient, and effective in their performance of those tasks. Doig et al. (2009) found that the process of collaborative goal setting with clients with traumatic brain injury and their significant others actually facilitated clients' self-awareness and increased their participation in occupational therapy. Occupational therapy practitioners who work with children may also face challenges in collaborative goal setting, although young school-age children with neurodevelopmental disabilities were able to engage effectively in setting goals with support of an assessment instrument that measured their perceived competence in various physical tasks (Missiuna, Pollock, Law, Walter, & Cavey, 2006). Clients who have good insight into their occupational performance challenges may be more easily engaged in a collaborative goal-setting process, but occupational therapy practitioners must carefully attend to the complex issues that can impact clients' priorities.

ADL and IADL are often highly valued by both children and adults because of the dependency on others that accompanies role dysfunction (Robinson-Smith, Johnston, & Allen, 2000). However, occupational therapy practitioners should be careful not to assume that ADL and IADL are immediate priorities. Some people, especially those with severe activity limitations, might need or want to accept assistance from others in ADL so that they can focus on improving other areas of occupational performance. This was the case with Mr. Fritz, a 32-year-old with a recently sustained spinal cord injury resulting in C6 quadriplegia. He was married, had three small children, and was self-employed as a tax accountant. His wife worked part time as a nurse and took care of their children before and after school. The family depended on Mr. Fritz's income and he had no disability insurance coverage. Although outcomes in ADL were initially established for Mr. Fritz, it soon became apparent that attempts at self-care retraining were being met with resistance and frustration. Further discussion of the targeted intervention outcomes revealed that Mr. Fritz was anxious to return to work and that he could do this if he could use the computer in his home office. Although he expressed an interest in becoming independent in self-care, he felt that the best option for him was to return to work as quickly as possible to minimize the financial burden on his family from his current inability to work. His wife was able and willing to help him with self-care tasks at home. The couple felt that self-care retraining could be delayed until the family business was again operational. With intervention outcomes refocused on activities most valued by Mr. Fritz—namely, computer access and home mobility—he became highly motivated to participate in therapy.

Clients' values should drive long-term goals, but occupational therapy practitioners may need to help clients focus on ADL initially when they have identified priorities for more complex occupational performance areas (e.g., IADL, work, or leisure) that may be difficult to treat efficiently and effectively early in the intervention process (Cipriani et al., 2000). Self-care training often helps clients to develop capacities and problem-solving skills that can later be applied to activities that are more complex than self-care, particularly when dealing with severe disorders of sudden onset (e.g., stroke and traumatic injuries). For example, suppose Mr. Fritz could not work from a home office and wanted to focus on driving in order to get to work, which is a realistic long-term goal for someone with C6 quadriplegia. Initiating occupational therapy intervention with driver training, however, would be impractical because Mr. Fritz lacked the prerequisite functional mobility skills early in his rehabilitation. ADL training—involving bathing, dressing, transferring, and wheelchair mobility—can facilitate the development of functional mobility skills. Such training, therefore, would logically precede driver training. If Mr. Fritz had been in this situation, his needs may have been met through a referral to social services for assistance with financial planning to help the family manage until he could return to work. The occupational therapy practitioner would have also needed to educate Mr. Fritz about the commonalities among skills needed for both self-care and driving. This plan would simultaneously recognize Mr. Fritz's valued roles and progress him to the desired outcome in the most efficient way possible.

When the most valued activities and roles are beyond the client's potential skill level, the occupational therapy practitioner helps the client to refocus priorities so that goals are realistic and achievable. If Mr. Fritz were the owner and cook of a small restaurant, for example, it is unlikely that he would meet the essential job requirements of a short-order cook even if the kitchen were adapted for wheelchair accessibility because the activities require bilateral hand function and must be done quickly. It is possible, however, that he could perform the activities of restaurant owner. For example, he could manage personnel, handle the finances, operate the cash register, and seat customers. In this and similar situations, occupational therapy practitioners use their expertise in activity analysis and functional adaptation to assist clients in creating a realistic yet meaningful life for themselves and help them establish achievable goals to progress them to that vision (Doig et al., 2009; Liddle & McKenna, 2000).

Difficulty

The perceived ease with which a client completes an activity and the projected difficulty that will remain after intervention are important considerations in selecting goal behaviors (Thornsson & Grimby, 2001). The occupational therapy practitioner, who is skilled in activity analysis and has knowledge of pathology and impairment, must determine the prognosis for functional difficulty. This prognosis must then be communicated to clients so that decisions about acceptable levels of difficulty can be made collaboratively. Clients set intervention priorities, in part, by weighing the projected level of difficulty within the context of value—that is, how much difficulty they are willing to tolerate to be independent in an activity. The frequency with which an activity is performed should also be considered in establishing goals for ADL and IADL that are likely to remain difficult for a client to perform. In general, a higher level of proficiency or ease of performance is needed for activities that need to be done routinely, whereas a lower level of proficiency or ease of performance may be acceptable for activities that are done only occasionally.

For example, James is a 7-year-old boy with spina bifida, which damaged his spinal cord at T6 resulting in paralysis from the waist down. He has a neurogenic bladder and requires routine intermittent catheterization. He identified self-catheterization as a critical task for fulfilling his roles as self-carer and student, because he would prefer not to have help with this personal task from family or school personnel. James will need to be able to self-catheterize independently and efficiently for this task to fit into his school day. The occupational therapist believes that James will be capable of achieving independence with little difficulty after a period of practice. The goal is agreed upon, and treatment begins. Another client, Amy, also has spina bifida, which resulted in incomplete spinal cord damage at C7, which affects her upper extremities as well as her trunk and lower extremities. Because the spinal cord damage is incomplete, she can typically get adequate emptying of her bladder without self-catheterization. On rare occasions, however, she has episodes of urinary retention, requiring catheterization within about 1 hour of experiencing symptoms. Amy would also like to be independent so that when she must be catheterized at school, she does not need help. The occupational therapist thinks that independent self-catheterization using safe and clean technique is a reasonable goal for Amy, but it will always be difficult because she has impaired hand function and positioning herself so that she can see and reach to insert the catheter is challenging. Amy will need to go to the nurse's office to transfer to a bed. Despite the difficulty, Amy opts to work on this goal. Because she has to catheterize herself so infrequently, she believes that her skill level will be adequate for meeting her needs.

Safety

The degree of risk inherent in the person-task-environment transaction must also be considered when establishing client goals. IADL tasks tend to pose more safety risks, for example, working with sharp or hot objects while cooking, driving, or operating snow blowers or lawn mowers for home maintenance. However, some ADL can also pose safety risks for people, such as bathing, managing medications, or using safe-sex practices during sexual activity. Oftentimes, treatment is effective in reducing safety risks to an acceptable level; however, if the occupational therapist believes a person-task-environment transaction that leads to unsafe performance cannot be effectively modified to meet safety standards, then those tasks may not be appropriate goals.

Safe driving has received increasing attention in the health care literature as the number of older drivers, many with health-related impairments, continues to increase. Occupational therapists are often the health professionals who evaluate and treat this important IADL (Korner-Bitensky, Menon, von Zweck, & Van Benthem, 2010). Because of the potentially grave consequences of unsafe driving, occupational therapists must develop the skills to identify when it is appropriate to pursue driving goals and when safety precludes a return to driving and treatment should focus on driving cessation and goals that address alternative transportation methods, such as using public transportation (Kartje, 2006).

Understanding and implementing "safe-sex" practices to prevent sexually transmitted diseases may be an important safety-related goal for clients that is frequently unaddressed by occupational therapy practitioners. Clients with cognitive deficits that may impair decision making (e.g., developmental disability, traumatic brain injury, or mental health disorders such as bipolar disorder or schizophrenia) may benefit from education about the potential health threats associated with unprotected sex. Clients with physical disabilities may require adaptations for safe-sex tasks, such as applying condoms.

Fatigue and Dyspnea

Fatigue, the sensation of tiredness that is experienced during or following an activity, and dyspnea, difficult or labored breathing, can interfere with activity performance (Seo, Roberts, LaFramboise, Yates, & Yurkovich, 2011; Vanage, Gilbertson, & Mathiowetz, 2003). Both fatigue and dyspnea are likely to be exacerbated by activity performance. The occupational therapist uses activity analysis to take into account the effort that is required to perform a task and its typical duration. In addition, the client's entire daily routine must be examined so that the energy demands of one activity can be weighed in relation to the client's other activities (Mathiowetz, Matuska, & Murphy, 2001). Assisting clients to examine the physical demands of their preferred activities can help them to prioritize activities so that appropriate goals can be established. Similar to budgeting money, clients must be encouraged to look at their "energy dollars" and decide how they wish to spend them. The occupational therapy practitioner contributes to this decision-making process by bringing valuable information about options for activity adaptation that can reduce the energy demands of activities, thereby saving clients' energy for other tasks.

For example, Mrs. Hernandez lived alone in an apartment in a retirement community. Her sister and brother-in-law also resided in the community, and she had many close friends there. She has had multiple sclerosis for many years, with some weakness and spasticity; but she remained independent in her ADL until a recent exacerbation, which required hospitalization.

See **Appendix I, Common Conditions, Resources, and Evidence**, for more information about multiple sclerosis.

An increase in fatigue and decrease in strength resulted in the need for physical assistance with dressing and bathing and the use of a wheelchair for mobility. The retirement community required residents to manage their own ADL and prepare breakfast and a light evening snack. A hot meal was provided at midday. Mrs. Hernandez reported that she could not afford to hire an aide to help her daily with these tasks. The occupational therapy practitioner explained to Mrs. Hernandez that although independence in ADL and simple meal preparation were reasonable goals, completing her ADL would likely be time consuming and fatiguing, leaving her limited energy for other activities. Mrs. Hernandez was enthusiastic about beginning therapy, indicating that she was willing to engage in fewer IADL and leisure activities in order to be independent in ADL and simple meal preparation because it would enable her to remain in the retirement community with family and friends.

A different scenario played out with Mrs. McKay, who also had multiple sclerosis. Like Mrs. Hernandez, she had a recent exacerbation that caused a functional decline, and achieving independence in ADL was likely to expend much of her daily energy. Mrs. McKay had been working full time as a programmer for a local radio station and was the mother of two young children. She perceived her role as a self-carer to be important, along with those of worker and mother. However, when it became apparent that independence in ADL would leave her with little energy for performing work and parenting roles, she decided not to establish goals for independence in ADL, opting instead to hire a personal care attendant for assistance so she could focus on work and parenting goals.

Identifying an Appropriate Degree of Performance

Treatment goals must include a measurable outcome that indicates how well or at what level the identified behavior will be done, sometimes referred to as the *degree of performance* (Kettenbach, 2009). Independence is the most common degree of performance; however, several performance parameters can also provide effective goals, especially when the client is independent but occupational performance deficits remain that warrant treatment. For example, this would be the case when a client can open jars independently, but it is painful and results in deforming forces to the hand joints.

Independence

The performance parameter that is most commonly focused on in occupational therapy interventions is independence in activity performance, which becomes the degree or measurable part of the goal (Sames, 2010). Across all ages and disabilities, the goal is generally to increase the level of independence (Eyres & Unsworth, 2005; Gavacs, 2009; Healy & Rigby, 1999; Johansson, Lilja, Petersson, & Borell, 2007; Legg, Drummond, & Langhorne, 2006; Pillastrini et al., 2008). Independence in activity performance may be divided into three phases: initiation of a task, continuation of a task, and completion of a task. The most common occupational therapy goals focus on the completion of the task, which implies that initiation and continuation of the task occurred; for example, a goal might be: "Client will be independent in feeding her cats 3/3 meals a day by December 12, 2012" or "Client will require moderate assistance for bed to/from wheelchair transfers in 1 week." Occupational therapy practitioners might also want to focus an independence goal on initiation of task performance when that is particularly difficult for a client.

Initiation is an aspect of activity performance that is frequently overlooked when goals are established, in part because it is difficult to evaluate and treat. The very presence of the occupational therapy practitioner may be a cue to initiate a task; and certainly a greeting, such as "Good morning, Mrs. Smith, today we will work on dressing," serves as a prompt for action. Adults are typically expected to initiate ADL and IADL independently. Expectations for children also exist, depending on the children's ages and skills and the division of task responsibilities among family members. Impairments in activity initiation may occur as a result of many diseases and disorders, such as attention deficit disorder, dementia, depression, schizophrenia, brain injury from trauma or stroke, multiple sclerosis, and Parkinson's disease. Family members generally find it frustrating to have to cue ("constantly nag") a client with impaired initiation for each aspect of a daily routine. The occupational therapist may write an independence goal that includes initiation, such as, "Client will initiate and complete bathing independently three to seven times a week by November 30, 2012." In this example, measuring progress toward the goal would require the client or a proxy to record the number of times in a week that the client initiated bathing without cueing or assistance from another person.

Safety

Although some goals may not be feasible at all because of safety concerns, other times, it is possible to improve a person's safe performance of ADL/IADL, so safety becomes a part of the goal. Because safety is a quality of the person-task-environment transaction, it cannot be observed or treated in isolation from independence (Chui & Oliver, 2006; Russell, Fitzgerald, Williamson, Manor, & Whybrow, 2002). Goals related to safety are typically linked to independence outcomes; that is, independent performance is assumed to be safe because an occupational therapist could not ethically create a goal for independent performance that was not deemed to be safe. Although occupational therapy practitioners agree that safety is an intervention priority, there is less consensus about specific activity behaviors that are safe or unsafe. Many behaviors fall into a questionable zone, where some would rate them as safe, whereas others perceive them as unsafe. In determining acceptable risk for setting independence goals, it is useful to consider clients' comfort level with risk; their ability to analyze the risks associated with a particular activity and devise a plan for managing them; and, most important, their ability to implement the plan expeditiously despite impairments. At times, the goal for level of independence in activity performance might need to be sacrificed for safety. A comparison of two clients with bilateral lower extremity fractures sustained in car accidents who are learning independent transfers illustrates this point.

Ted and Ryan were both recently injured, are non–weight bearing on both lower extremities, and are learning sliding board transfers. Ted demonstrates good judgment and a realistic perception of his skills. The occupational therapist has determined that the following goal is realistic: "Client will be independent in sliding board transfers from wheelchair to/from bed within three therapy sessions." Through training, Ted learns to transfer safely with a sliding board by following specific guidelines (e.g., position wheelchair at a 45-degree angle to the bed, secure brakes on wheelchair, ascertain that bed height is level with the wheelchair). After a couple of sessions, he is able to follow these guidelines consistently; therefore, his goal of independence in transferring from wheelchair to bed and back is met. Ryan's injuries are similar to Ted's, but he also incurred a mild brain injury. Although Ryan's motor skills are comparable to Ted's, Ryan has difficulty recalling the guidelines for transfers and is at risk for bearing weight on his lower extremities during transfers, which could interfere with fracture healing. Therefore, the occupational therapist believes that independent transfers could be unsafe because Ryan's memory deficits place him at risk for violating weight-bearing precautions. The occupational therapist incorporates safety considerations by setting a goal for Ryan that is aimed at a lower level of independence, for example, "Client will require supervision and occasional verbal cues for sliding board transfers from wheelchair to/from bed while adhering to weight-bearing precautions within six therapy sessions." The degree of independence in Ryan's goal was adjusted to realistically reflect his capacity for safe transfer performance.

In some situations, it may be better to establish client goals in which the goal behavior is directly related to safety rather than being assumed in the degree of independence indicated. Goals can be aimed at the occupational performance level, that is, the IADL "safety and emergency maintenance" (AOTA, 2008); for example, the goal might be, "Client will verbally describe correct responses to a minimum of 10 potential home emergencies with 100% accuracy within 3 weeks." Safety goals may also be aimed at developing safe habits; for example, "Client will pause when entering a room and scan for obstacles on the floor 100% of the time to reduce fall risk during functional mobility by December 1, 2012," or "Client will report 100% compliance with condom use to reduce the risk of sexually transmitted diseases within 3 weeks."

Adequacy

Several aspects of activity performance contribute to the adequacy or quality of the behavior stated in the goal, which can also be reflected in the goal as the degree to which the behavior is expected to be done. In addition to independence, these performance parameters may be crucial components of meaningful goals, especially for clients who are independent and safe with their performance but who feel dissatisfied with the process or some other aspect of the outcome. Goals with measurable adequacy parameters can be used to justify treatment even if clients are independent in tasks. Six adequacy parameters can be used as measurable outcomes: pain, fatigue and dyspnea, duration, societal standards, satisfaction, and aberrant task behaviors. Some of these parameters may be interdependent within a single client. For instance, pain might lead to changes in duration of activity performance (e.g., the activity takes longer) as well as the ability to meet normative standards and personal satisfaction. A goal should include only one measurable parameter so that it is clear what has changed in documenting progress toward goals.

Pain. Pain, either during or following an activity, can negatively influence engagement in ADL or IADL even if the activity is completed independently (Covinsky, Lindquist, Dunlop, & Yelin, 2009; Dudgeon, Tyler, Rhodes, & Jensen, 2006; Liedberg & Vrethem, 2009; Mullersdorf, 2000). The source of pain and the prognosis for it must be carefully considered in establishing goals and selecting an intervention approach. Both the evaluation and the goals must include an index of pain so that intervention remains focused on achieving the projected level of independence while simultaneously reducing the presence of pain. Often, the pain assessment can be incorporated into the goal as an indicator of the degree of pain; for example, the goal might be, "Client will prepare a simple meal (soup, sandwich, and beverage) independently with a maximum pain level of 2 cm on a 10-cm visual analogue scale 4/5 times within 2 weeks."

Fatigue and Dyspnea. Fatigue and dyspnea can influence the actual task behaviors that are selected for client goals, as was described earlier in this section; but when fatigue or dyspnea can be reduced through task adaptation or conditioning, goals can be established that use these performance parameters as performance criteria outcomes. The initial evaluation should include baseline data for comparison. For example, a goal might be, "Client will complete morning care routine (shower, grooming, dressing) with a maximum score of 6 on the Borg Reported Perceived Exertion Scale 75% of the time by November 28, 2012." As long as the Borg Scale (Borg, 1998) was used during the initial evaluation, a lower number (meaning less exertion) can be used in a goal to indicate progress toward becoming less fatigued during ADL or IADL tasks. Dyspnea can be monitored in a similar way, using a visual analogue scale or numerical rating scale (Gift & Narsavage, 1998). Diagnosis is important to consider when goals are formulated relative to fatigue and dyspnea. Overexertion can exacerbate symptoms or even the disease process itself for conditions such as cardiac disease and multiple sclerosis. Prognosis is another important diagnostic consideration in setting goals that measure fatigue or dyspnea. Clients with chronic obstructive pulmonary disease are likely to become worse; therefore, goals must be reasonable to achieve through activity adaptations and might need to accommodate a decline in function. A client with paraplegia secondary to spinal cord injury, by contrast, experiences fatigue from having to use the smaller muscles of the upper extremity for wheelchair mobility to compensate for the larger lower extremity muscles previously used for walking.

Endurance is likely to improve significantly as upper extremity strength increases with use, and more ambitious goals for reducing fatigue could be appropriate.

See **Appendix I, Common Conditions, Resources, and Evidence**, for more information about chronic obstructive pulmonary disease and spinal cord injury.

Duration. The length of time that is required to complete activities is typically thought of as a reflection of efficiency, which may be affected by many types of impairments, including poor endurance, impaired coordination, and cognitive deficits such as reduced attention for tasks, which is common in people with various mental health disorders. Although measuring performance time may be relatively simple, interpreting time data in a meaningful way is often difficult. The duration of ADL/IADL depends highly on the nature of the activity and the task objects that people choose to use in performing the activity. It takes longer to prepare dinner than it does to fix a light snack. Most of us spend more time dressing when we are going out to dine in an elegant restaurant than we do we when are going to a fast-food establishment. Therefore, it is difficult to establish meaningful time norms for ADL and IADL, but duration is often a parameter that clients wish to incorporate into their occupational therapy goals when they are frustrated by slow performance.

Establishing acceptable time frames for ADL goals must be done collaboratively with clients and their significant others. Occupational therapists also should consider safety and independence parameters when establishing goals with time frames. Clients may be at increased risk when they rush through activities or even when they attempt them at a typical pace. For example, clients with swallowing deficits might need to eat more slowly than people without such deficits to avoid choking. People with poor fine motor coordination or sensory deficits might need to slow down when using sharp knives to improve control of the knives and prevent injury. In these examples, setting goals to decrease the duration of performance would be inappropriate because it could result in unsafe performance.

Societal and cultural standards also need to be taken into consideration in establishing outcomes for activity duration. In the United States, timeliness is highly valued, and efficient performance in community skills is expected. Shoppers might become irritated when they are standing in a checkout line behind a customer who takes 5 minutes to identify and count currency, even though in other cultures, this delay might go unnoticed. An American with cognitive or visual impairments that interfere with the ability to count currency might wish to decrease the time required for this activity to reduce embarrassment when shopping. The goal, then, needs to include an efficiency measure to reflect this performance parameter, for example, "Client will independently complete a simple cash transaction (select appropriate currency and count change) in less than 1 minute within 3 weeks to support participation in shopping."

Societal Standards. Performance standards, determined by the society and culture in which the client lives, are likely to exist in terms of both the end result and the process through which it is achieved. The line between acceptable and unacceptable performance is likely to be thick rather than narrow and may vary considerably, depending on characteristics such as age, gender, and cohort (generation) membership.

Societal standards exist for neatness, for example. A client might dress safely and independently, but if clients select clothing with clashing colors or their appearance is disheveled (the end product), then dressing might not meet societal standards. If the client is a teenager, such an appearance might be considered acceptable. However, if the client is a public relations manager going to work, it is likely to be labeled unacceptable and could well put the client's job in jeopardy. Occupational therapists and clients may identify relevant societal standards for inclusion in goals. Identifying societal standards might seem subjective and difficult, but the use of measurable indicators of societal standards is critical for effective goals and can justify intervention. A goal for a client who eats rapidly, putting food in his mouth when it is still full, might include a measure of societal standard, such as: "When eating during a social event, the client will demonstrate appropriate pacing as evidenced by completing a meal in no less than 15 minutes, swallowing each bite before putting additional food in his mouth, and conversing between bites of food by December 10, 2012."

Satisfaction. In addition to societal standards, clients have their own standards of acceptable performance, which also need to be incorporated into goals (Eklund & Gunnarsson, 2008). Setting goals with satisfaction measures requires collaboration with clients because personal standards will vary greatly from person to person. Mr. Balouris, for example, is always losing things. He never seems to know where his wallet and keys are, and he is always searching for something. Nonetheless, items seem to turn up, and he sees no reason to go to the trouble of organizing his apartment better to help him keep track of his belongings. Mr. Johnson, however, has always been meticulously neat and could put his hands on items the minute he wanted them. Recently, he sought medical attention for memory problems. He complained that he needed to search for items because he failed to put them in their usual places. He was particularly concerned about his memory problem because of a family history of Alzheimer's disease.

See **Appendix I, Common Conditions, Resources, and Evidence**, for more information about Alzheimer's disease.

He was referred to occupational therapy to learn strategies to help him remember where items are placed. Objectively, Mr. Johnson's performance is similar to Mr. Balouris; however, Mr. Johnson is dissatisfied with his performance, which he views as impaired.

Clients must rate their own level of satisfaction with a task because it is a subjective experience. Client satisfaction can be measured quickly and easily with a visual analog scale or numerical scale, such as the 10-point scale that is used in the COPM (Law, Baptiste et al., 2005). Satisfaction measures are easily incorporated into goals to reflect the degree of performance, for example, "Client will be independent in locating items needed for ADL and IADL in the home with a satisfaction rating of at least 8/10 within 3 weeks to support participation in ADL and IADL."

Aberrant Task Behaviors. Goals and interventions may also address any aberrant task behaviors that interfere with activity performance (Ashley et al., 2001; Rogers et al., 2000). Aberrant task behaviors vary widely and include unwanted motor behavior such as athetoid or ballistic movements and behavioral problems such as self-stimulation or hitting caregivers. Exploration of the underlying cause of the aberrant task behavior facilitates the establishment of realistic goals and the selection of effective intervention strategies. Goals are aimed at eliminating or diminishing aberrant task behavior in the context of ADL and IADL tasks, for example, "Client will decrease tongue-thrusting behaviors during feeding to a maximum of 3 episodes a meal within 2 months to support oral feeding that meets the client's nutritional needs."

Additional Considerations for Setting Realistic Client Goals

The occupational therapist uses performance parameters to identify goal behaviors and degrees of performance, but several additional factors that can affect goal achievement must also be considered. The process of setting goals is complex and must be based not only on clients' hopes but also what changes are realistic (Wade, 2009). Several contextual factors must be considered, such as physical and social environment, financial resources, time available for intervention, and the client's past experience and learning ability. The prognosis for impairments, given the client's disability, can also affect goal achievement.

Prognosis for Impairments

The client's potential for improvement of performance skills and patterns and client factors must be examined within the context of any existing disease or disorder and resulting impairments (Radomski, 2008; Sames, 2010). First, the practitioner must consider any precautions or contraindications pursuant to the diagnosis that could preclude the use of certain intervention strategies. For example, compare two clients whose endurance significantly limits their performance. Mrs. Tanaka has chronic fatigue syndrome, a disorder that may worsen if she becomes overfatigued.

See **Appendix I, Common Conditions, Resources, and Evidence**, for more information about chronic fatigue syndrome.

An aggressive program to increase endurance is contraindicated for her, so alternative intervention strategies should be explored, and goals for increasing endurance for ADL must be reasonable, given Mrs. Tanaka's potential for exacerbation of her disease. Conversely, Mr. Krull is very deconditioned from inactivity resulting from major depressive illness and would like to increase his endurance to support participation in heavy home maintenance tasks, such as mowing the lawn and finishing an addition on his house. A rigorous activity program to increase endurance is not contraindicated and would help to increase Mr. Krull's participation in IADL.

Second, the prognosis for improvement of impairments, given the client's diagnosis (i.e., disease, disorder, or condition), must be considered. Increasing impairment is expected in progressive disorders, such as muscular dystrophy, Alzheimer's disease, and rheumatoid arthritis. Goals must be established with these potential declines in mind so that the goals are realistic. Occupational therapy practitioners must evaluate impairments separately, however, because progressive diseases might not affect all bodily structures and functions directly. Jorge, a teenager who has muscular dystrophy, illustrates this point. He has significant muscle weakness in the trunk and all four extremities and has developed some limitations in pelvic and ankle passive range of motion (PROM) that preclude maintaining an optimal position for functioning from his wheelchair. His muscle strength is expected to decline, even with intervention. His PROM restrictions, however, are secondary to the muscle weakness, not a direct result of the muscular dystrophy. Intervention gains can be expected in PROM with treatment, despite the overall prognosis. In turn, increased PROM can enhance function by increasing the options available for positioning Jorge in his wheelchair.

Stable or diminishing impairments may be anticipated in many disorders and after injury. Pharmacological intervention, for example, may improve the impairments associated with depression so that occupational therapy intervention can be focused on transferring gains made in mental and psychological capacities into ADL and IADL performance.

See **Appendix I, Common Conditions, Resources, and Evidence**, for more information about mood disorders and depression.

Typically, clients of all ages who have had brain injuries from trauma or strokes can expect some spontaneous return of motor function in the early stages of recovery. Projected intervention goals should take into account the typical improvements for this diagnosis. Accuracy in predicting "typical improvements" takes time and experience to develop, and the novice practitioner might find it helpful to consult with more experienced clinicians to facilitate the ability to set realistic goals.

Experience

Information gathered in the evaluation about a client's past and recent experience with an activity is important to consider so that relevant and attainable goals can be established. Recent experience may facilitate progress in reestablishing independence in an activity because the client is learning a new way to do the activity rather than developing a new skill. For example, Mrs. McCarthy needs to relearn cooking skills following a stroke. She uses a wheelchair for mobility and has minimal use of her right (dominant) hand. Her cognitive skills are intact, and she can easily follow a recipe. Furthermore, she demonstrates good problem-solving skills in adapting cooking activities to improve her performance. Miranda, a 19-year-old with spastic hemiplegia secondary to cerebral palsy, like Mrs. McCarthy, has limited use of one hand and uses a wheelchair for mobility.

See **Appendix I, Common Conditions, Resources, and Evidence**, for more information about cerebral palsy.

Miranda wants to cook simple meals and bake cookies. Her intervention is likely to require more time and guidance than Mrs. McCarthy's intervention, because Miranda has to learn basic cooking skills along with the activity adaptations that are required to compensate for her impairments.

At times, adults are also confronted with needing to learn new activities. Some of these activities relate to skills that are needed to manage new impairments, such as performing self-catheterization, donning pressure garments, or learning to operate electronic aids to independence. New learning may also be needed when new roles are assumed, for example, when a spouse becomes disabled or dies and the partner has to take on new responsibilities. Whenever a skill is unfamiliar to a client, additional intervention time and education from the occupational therapy practitioner might be needed for basic skill acquisition and should be incorporated into the goal and the intervention plan.

Client's Capacity for Learning and Openness to Alternative Methods

The client's capacity for learning and openness to using alternative methods for task completion must be evaluated because intervention often requires learning new methods of completing activities (Flinn & Radomski, 2008). Clients with limited learning capacity due to cognitive or affective impairments can still learn new skills if appropriate teaching approaches are used and the duration of the intervention is adequate (Davis, 2005). Some clients might resist treatment that incorporates adaptive equipment if they do not want to use a special device to do a task that most people do without a device (Lund & Nygård, 2003). Clients with a good capacity for learning and openness to alternative methods may be able to address more task deficits because of increased intervention options and the reduced time required for learning. It is important to view capacity for learning on a continuum; clients can fall between the extremes, and capacity might be better for some tasks than for others. A client might be capable of learning the relatively simple task adaptation of using a joystick to drive a wheelchair but be unable to master a more complex electronic aid to daily living, even one that relies on the same movements that are used to control the joystick.

Clients' capacity for learning may also change as they progress through the rehabilitation process, particularly for clients with a new disability. The focus of learning should progress from more directive, therapist-initiated learning for specific tasks to client-initiated learning, where the client is more autonomous in identifying goals and directing his or her own learning (Greber, Ziviani, & Rodger, 2007; Jack & Estes, 2010). Autonomous learning strategies enable clients to solve problems long after therapy has ended and enables them to develop their own adaptive strategies. The ability to be an independent problem solver can be learned, and occupational therapists should consider clients' potential for becoming autonomous learners and structure treatment activities that promote self-directed learning (Greber et al., 2007).

Projected Follow-Through with Program Outside of Treatment

Efforts to contain health care costs have led to increasingly shorter lengths of stay in hospitals and rehabilitation centers and a reduction in outpatient and home health visits. Clients are expected to take a more active role in their therapy programs and to supplement formal interventions with home programs (Novak, Cusick, & Lannin, 2009). Goals therefore need to be established with some estimate of the client's capacity to follow through with a self-directed program because this may influence the success of an intervention (Jan et al., 2004).

Several of the performance parameters that were previously described can give the occupational therapy practitioner guidance in this area. Clients have more motivation for programs aimed at activities that they highly value than at those that they do not value, making a client-centered approach critical for success (Doig et al., 2009). In addition, performance parameters such as difficulty, fatigue, pain, and satisfaction must be graded so that self-directed programs are manageable within the context of the client's daily routines. The meaning of *manageable* must be established by clients in consultation with the occupational therapy practitioner and should take into consideration clients' daily activities and responsibilities, tolerance for frustration, and perseverance.

Many clients require some assistance to practice activities, and the occupational therapy practitioner must be sure that these resources are available. This assistance may include setting up an activity, providing assistance for specific activity steps, and allowing ample time (as prescribed) for effective practice. It is important to remember that impairments can affect the client's ability to initiate or persevere with everyday activities. For these clients, assistance is needed for initiation and follow-through in the home program. This responsibility often falls on family members, and occupational therapy practitioners need to interact with and educate family members about their critical role.

Time for Intervention

The projected timeline for occupational therapy may be influenced by multiple factors, including the functional prognosis, the client's motivation for improvement, and the client's finances. Third-party payers vary in their reimbursement allowances for therapy visits, which can impact access to services and treatment outcomes

(Nof, Rone-Adams, & Hart, 2007). Ongoing changes in Medicare impact services across settings, such as home health (FitzGerald et al., 2006). Occupational therapy goals must be tailored to meet a client's needs as much as possible within the time allotted. Nonetheless, it must also be recognized that best practice takes into account *all* the client's needs. Often, with clear and complete documentation of adequate progress toward established goals, third-party payers will approve additional occupational therapy visits. Occupational therapy practitioners need to be aware of their professional responsibility to clients to request intervention extensions and to support these requests through detailed documentation and to appeal payment denials for needed services (Sames, 2010). They must also ensure that intervention timelines are established to meet the needs of the client, rather than the needs of the facility, which may benefit from providing services that extend beyond the client's needs or tolerance level, as described in the "Ethical Dilemma" box.

Ethical Dilemma

Can Client-Centered Care Conflict with the Needs of an Organization?

Jessica is an occupational therapist working in a subacute rehabilitation unit in a skilled nursing facility. She completed an evaluation on Mrs. Cabrini, an 82-year-old woman with multiple medical problems, including a recent total hip replacement secondary to a fracture, cardiovascular disease, and rheumatoid arthritis.

See **Appendix I, Common Conditions, Resources, and Evidence**, for more information about joint replacements, cardiopulmonary conditions, and rheumatoid arthritis.

Mrs. Cabrini would like to be independent in transfers, indoor mobility, and toileting, which would enable her to return to her home in an assisted living facility. She reported that she could get daily help with dressing and bathing and would prefer to do that because she fatigues quickly and wants to save her energy for the daily morning craft group. During the evaluation, Mrs. Cabrini tolerated about 30 minutes of therapy in the morning and 30 minutes in the afternoon, divided between occupational therapy and physical therapy. Jessica established client-centered goals collaboratively with Mrs. Cabrini. The physical therapist agreed that the client could work productively for only two 30-minute treatments a day, and they opted to split the time, so Jessica documented that the intensity of occupational therapy would be 30 minutes daily, 7 days a week.

Jessica's supervisor approached Jessica and asked her to increase Mrs. Cabrini to 45 minutes a day so that Mrs. Cabrini would qualify for a higher Resource Utilization Group (RUG) under the Medicare prospective payment system. The supervisor told Jessica that if the facility cannot increase reimbursement rates by having more clients in higher RUGs, they might need to lay off staff, which would have a negative impact on client care. Jessica's supervisor also suggested that it would be easy to justify the increased treatment if Jessica added more ADL goals, such as independence in dressing and bathing, to Mrs. Cabrini's care plan.

1. What should Jessica do in this situation?
2. How might client-centered care influence Jessica's actions?
3. How can Jessica balance the needs and wishes of her client with the needs of the facility?

Expected Discharge Context and Resources

Clients' expected discharge environments must be considered in establishing goals and selecting interventions that will be relevant to the environment in which clients will ultimately perform tasks (Dunn, Brown, & McGuigan, 1994; Law & Dunbar, 2007; Nakanishi, Sawamura, Sato, Setoya, & Anzai, 2010). The social context is critical for clients who require assistance from others after discharge; that is, it is important to determine whether there are people who are willing and able to provide needed assistance. Clients' needs vary broadly in terms of the type and duration of assistance required. Some clients need only supportive services, such as help with shopping or housecleaning. Those with significant activity limitations and intact cognition might require considerable physical assistance but can be left alone once ADL have been completed, they have eaten, and they are mobile in their wheelchairs. Clients with cognitive impairments do not always need physical assistance but might need verbal cueing to initiate or sustain activities or to perform them in a safe manner. This assistance might be specific to certain tasks (e.g., when cooking or interacting with small children) or it may need to be constant. Inadequate support in the client's expected environment may necessitate a change in the discharge plan. Some families or friends might be able to provide the level and type of assistance needed, whereas other families might be unable or unwilling to do this.

The physical environment must also be considered in setting realistic goals (Gitlin, Corcoran, Winter, Boyce, & Hauck, 2001). For example, Mr. Feng has reached his goal of independence in bathing during his hospital-based rehabilitation. He requires a transfer tub seat, a handheld shower hose, and a grab bar to bathe safely without help (see Figure 47.2). The occupational therapy practitioner wants to order this equipment for him. However, Mr. Feng reports that he must shower in a 4 × 4 foot shower stall because the only bathtub is on the second floor and he cannot manage stairs. His shower will not accommodate the transfer tub bench that he requires for safe transfers and balance during showering. An alternative bathing goal should have been established at the beginning of intervention so that Mr. Feng's program focused on developing skills he could use at home, such as sponge bathing at the sink.

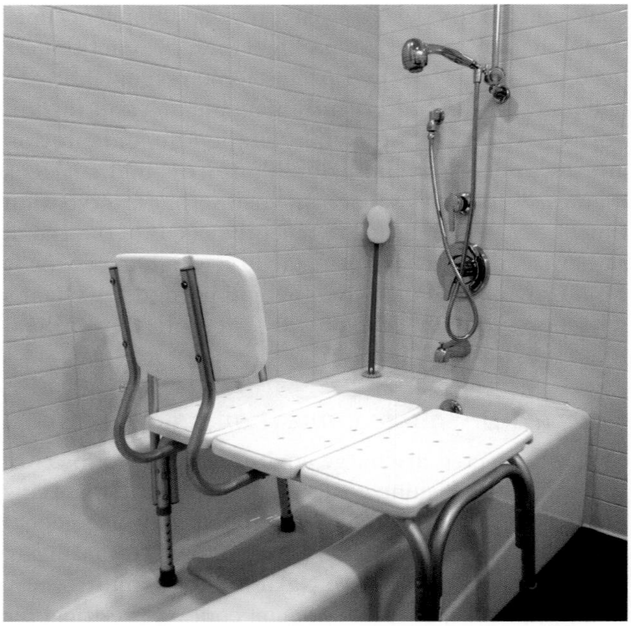

FIGURE 47.2 A transfer tub seat requires more space than Mr. Feng's small bathroom and shower can accommodate. Knowing the client's discharge environment can help practitioners determine interventions that will be successful after discharge.

The adaptability of the discharge environment must also be explored before setting goals. A house that is high above the street on a small lot with 21 steps to the front door makes the installation of a properly graded ramp impossible. Wall grab bars cannot be installed on some fiberglass tub surrounds, making a safety rail placed on the side of the bathtub the only feasible option regardless of where the client really needs the most support.

Established functional goals must also be achievable within the client's available resources, including property and financial resources. For example, clients living in rental units might be unable to make structural alterations as desired because they do not own the unit. Some individuals may benefit from equipment or devices that they cannot afford and are not covered by their third-party payer. This situation can result in a practice dilemma for the occupational therapist, as described in the Practice Dilemma box.

Last, all of the various places in which a client expects to function after discharge must be explored if activities are likely to be performed in more than one place. Clients in a hospital-based setting may be focused primarily on returning home, but most people do not confine themselves to a single environment. Adaptations for toilets, such as raised toilet seats and toilet armrests, are commonly used for people with limited mobility. Home adaptations are easily made, but clients are often in environments that have not been adapted, such as public buildings, friends' homes, airplanes, hotels, and portable toilets at the local fair. If clients are likely to be in these environments, their goals should address their ability to perform tasks in varied settings.

Interventions for Activities of Daily Living and Instrumental Activities of Daily Living Deficits

Interventions for ADL and IADL deficits are based on clients' goals and involve selecting treatment approaches and activities, carrying out the treatment, and reviewing the intervention to ensure that it is effective in progressing clients toward their goals.

Practice Dilemma

How Does One Provide Optimal Care with Limited Resources?

Jon is an occupational therapist in a large rehabilitation hospital in a major city. The occupational therapy department recently installed the latest **electronic aids to independent living (EADL)** in an on-site apartment that they use for treatment. Henry is a 16-year-old who has muscular dystrophy. He has a reclining power wheelchair that he can drive independently with a head switch. He has very limited use of his upper extremities. Henry lives alone with his mother who works in a low-wage job. He receives Medicaid.

Henry's disease has progressed such that he is no longer able to get into and out of his home without assistance or operate common electronic devices, including the television, telephone, and lights. Because his mother works during the day, Henry must attend an after-school program, which is primarily for small children. Henry has told his occupational therapist that his most important goal is to be able to go home from school and access his home. The occupational therapist is sure that this could be an achievable goal for Henry with an EADL system that would enable him to be independent in unlocking and opening the door, turning lights and electronic devices on and off, and using the telephone and computer. The therapist is also aware, however, that Medicaid will not pay for an EADL in his state.

1. How should Jon proceed? Should he train Henry in the use of the EADL, even if it will not be possible for him to purchase it?
2. What team members might the occupational therapist consult with to help him progress Henry toward his goal?
3. Does the diagnosis of muscular dystrophy, a progressive disorder, affect the approach that Jon would take to solve this problem?
4. How can Jon help Henry to achieve his goal?

Planning and Implementing Intervention

Five intervention approaches are described in the OTPF: create/promote, establish/restore, maintain, modify, and prevent (AOTA, 2008). Although all of these approaches can be used to support or enhance ADL and IADL performance, modify and establish/restore are the most commonly used in practice for addressing ADL and IADL and will be the focus of intervention discussed in this chapter. Both modify and establish/restore approaches need to be combined with client and/or caregiver education to ensure carryover of the program to function in everyday life (Flinn & Radomski, 2008). Often, the client/caregiver education shifts into a maintain approach, because the focus is on modifications and/or restorative programs that enable clients to preserve gains in ADL and IADL after therapy is discontinued. Occupational therapy practitioners select specific treatment activities for clients that are guided by a range of theory-based intervention approaches, often referred to as *frames of reference*. Specific occupational therapy treatment theories are beyond the scope of this chapter, but examples can be found in Unit XII. The following subsection focuses on broader intervention approaches and their related strategies. It also includes a discussion of client and caregiver education and strategies for grading activities to progress clients to the established goals.

Selecting an Intervention Approach

The occupational therapy practitioner considers several variables when deciding whether it is more appropriate to focus on compensating for a client's deficits through adaptation or restoring underlying skills needed to reach goals or a combination of both. These considerations are addressed in the sections that follow.

Modify. Activity performance can be enhanced through modifications that compensate for activity limitations rather than restore previous capacities. This is often necessary when restoration is not an option. For example, at this time, a client with a complete C5 quadriplegia will not regain previous hand function regardless of the restorative approach used. Compensation for impairments is needed for successful participation in ADL and IADL. Even for clients for whom restoration is possible, a modify approach might be more appropriate if time limitations or client motivation would lead to less than optimal outcomes. Compensatory strategies may also be warranted when some, but not full, restoration of function is achieved. Generally, compensatory strategies require less intervention time for achieving functional outcomes compared with restorative strategies.

Three general intervention strategies may be employed under the compensatory approach. The activity or task method may be altered, the task objects may be adapted, or the environment may be modified. Combinations of these methods may be used to maximize client performance. Examples of these three intervention strategies for selected ADL and IADL are included in Table 47.4.

- **Alter the Task Method.** When the task method is altered, the task objects and contexts are unchanged; but the method of performing the task is altered to make the task feasible given the client's impairments. Many one-handed techniques for tasks that are normally done with two hands use this strategy, including one-handed dressing, one-handed shoe-tying (Figure 47.3), and one-handed typing techniques.

Clients with low back injuries or movement limitations secondary to total hip replacements may find they need to modify positions used during sexual activities in order to avoid movements or positions that could damage joints. Individuals with tremors or **ataxia** may improve performance in a range of ADL by stabilizing their forearms on tabletops, armrests, or walls to improve coordination of the hands (Gillen, 2000). To master an altered task method successfully, clients require the capacity to learn. The necessary level of learning capacity depends on the complexity of the method that is to be learned (Flinn & Radomski, 2008). Occupational therapy practitioners should also attend to the level of automaticity clients may wish to achieve for specific ADL and IADL. People often rely on automatic processing for well-learned tasks, which means they require little direct attention. Automatic processing of routine tasks frees the individual for other things, such as planning one's workday while getting ready in the morning or chatting with a child while grocery shopping. Practice is a necessary component of all learning and is especially crucial for clients who wish to develop or return to automatic performance of ADL or IADL because brain activity patterns shift from relying on conscious attention mediated primarily by prefrontal cortex activity to more automatic movements mediated predominantly by subcortical structures (Floyer-Lea & Matthews, 2004). Clients benefit from follow-through with a training program that includes the practice and repetition needed to meet adequacy parameters, such as reducing difficulty and duration of performance and increasing satisfaction.

- **Adapt the Task Objects or Prescribe Assistive Devices.** The objects that are used for the task may be altered to facilitate performance. For example, handles can be built up on utensils for clients with decreased active finger range of motion or training in the use of memory aids (e.g., memory notebooks, checklists, cue cards, and electronic cueing devices) may help clients who have difficulty initiating tasks (Gillen, 2009; specifically Chapter 9). For some task adaptations, the task objects do not significantly alter the task method, so the need for learning is less than it is when the method is altered. When this is the case, the need for practice is also reduced, and performance can improve quickly. Examples of simple adaptations include utensils with enlarged or extended handles, a

TABLE 47.4 Examples of the Three Approaches to Modifying Tasks to Compensate for Impairments

Task	Alter the Method	Alter the Task Objects	Modify the Task Environment
Bathing	Substitute washing at the sink for someone who is unable to get into and out of the tub safely even with adaptive equipment.	Use a bath mitt and soap on a rope so that a person who cannot retrieve objects does not drop them.	Install grab bars and a transfer tub seat to enable a client to remain seated during bathing.
Grooming	Client learns to stabilize small containers with the ulnar digits while unscrewing lids with the radial digits of the same hand to compensate for loss of the use of one hand.	An extended handle is added to a razor so that a woman can shave her legs without bending forward.	A daily schedule is posted in the bathroom for a client with impaired attention or initiation to improve adherence to a daily grooming routine.
Toileting	Use an alarm watch to encourage regular emptying of the bladder.	Use a toilet aid to extend the range of reach for toilet hygiene.	Install a bidet on the toilet to eliminate the need for manipulating toilet paper for hygiene.
Dressing	Learn to dress the affected side first to compensate for loss of use of one side of the body.	Use a sock aid to put socks on without having to reach the feet.	Lower clothing racks or replace a high dresser with a low one to increase access to clothes.
Feeding	Serve different food items (e.g., meat, starch, vegetable) in consistent places on the plate for someone who is blind.	Use a built-up handled utensil to compensate for diminished prehension in the hand.	Have a second-grader with an attention disorder eat with a few friends in a small room rather than the loud and busy cafeteria.
Sexual activity	Identify alternate erogenous zones for a person who has lost sensation in the genital area.	Use a vibrator for satisfying a female partner for a male partner with erectile dysfunction.	Provide bed rails or overhead trapeze to facilitate repositioning during sexual activity in bed.
Transfers	Sit first in the car seat before swinging the legs in rather than entering the car by leading with the leg.	Use a sliding board to eliminate the need for the lower extremities to support body weight.	Rearrange furniture to allow the wheelchair to be positioned near to the bed or a favorite chair.
Child care	Use safe lifting techniques when lifting a child out of a crib or onto a changing table.	Add a handle to a baby bottle to reduce the amount of finger grip needed to securely hold and position the bottle.	Install a wall-mounted changing table that allows for easy wheelchair access.
Caregiving for an adult	Change from showers to sponge baths to reduce the need for multiple transfers during the morning care routine.	Use of a slip sheet to reduce friction when repositioning a person in bed.	Add high contrast stickers to the bottom of the tub to make the bottom visible and reduce fear of bathing for an adult with dementia.
Cooking	Sit at the kitchen table to chop vegetables to conserve energy.	Use a cutting board with aluminum nails to hold vegetables for cutting or peeling.	Install a mirror above the stove to enable a wheelchair user to see items cooking.
Paying bills	Round check entries to the nearest dollar to simplify the math for a client with cognitive impairment.	Use large checks, a dark pen, and a writing guide to compensate for low vision.	Install four plastic wall pockets to sort bills due each week of the month for a client with poor attention or memory.
Driving	Enter the vehicle by sitting first then swinging the legs in.	Provide hand controls to compensate for lower extremity paralysis	Restrict driving to daylight or low-volume hours.
Shopping	Shift to online and catalogue shopping to reduce the need for community mobility.	Purchase a walker basket for carrying items.	Request assistance from a grocery store employee to help reach items.

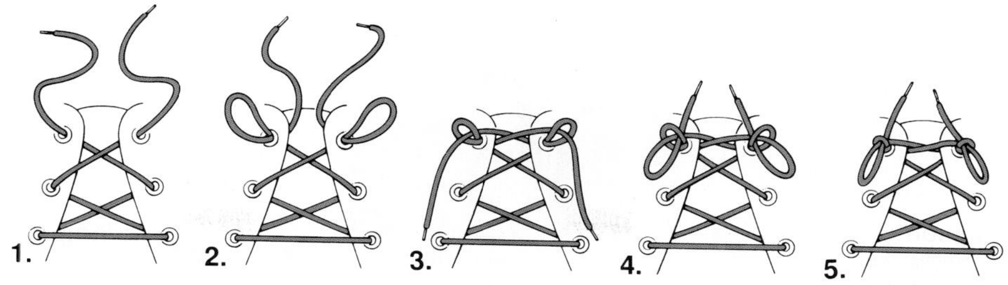

1. Lace laces in usual way.
2. Put both lace ends back through the holes they exited until the loops formed are small.
3. Put the lace ends through the opposite loops and pull to tighten loops, allowing just enough room to put the lace end back through the loop.
4. Put lace ends back through the loops, forming another loop.
5. Pull on these loops alternately to tighten.

FIGURE 47.3 One-handed shoe-tying method.

cutting board with nails to stabilize food while cutting, and elastic shoelaces. Some adaptations, however, require more extensive training, for example, learning to drive with hand controls.

The prescription of assistive devices must take into account the client's capabilities and willingness to use the device as well as the features of the device—a process that is frequently oversimplified. For example, a sock aid can help a client with poor sitting balance to reach her feet without leaning forward, which could throw her off balance. However, if the client's balance deficit is secondary to hemiplegia and she also has poor use of one hand, it will be very difficult or impossible for her to get the sock onto the sock aid, which typically requires both hands (Figure 47.4). Figure 47.5 depicts the number

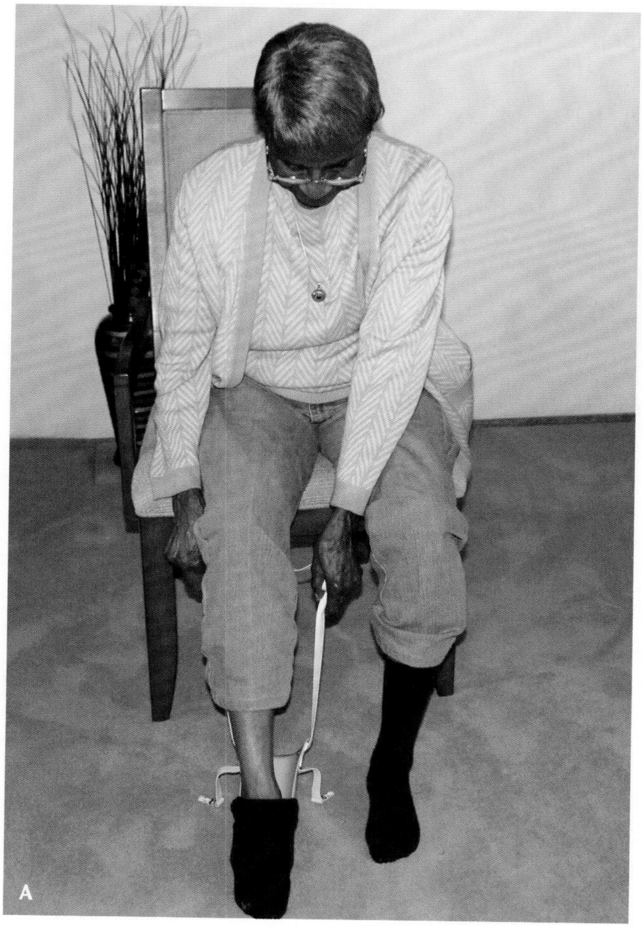

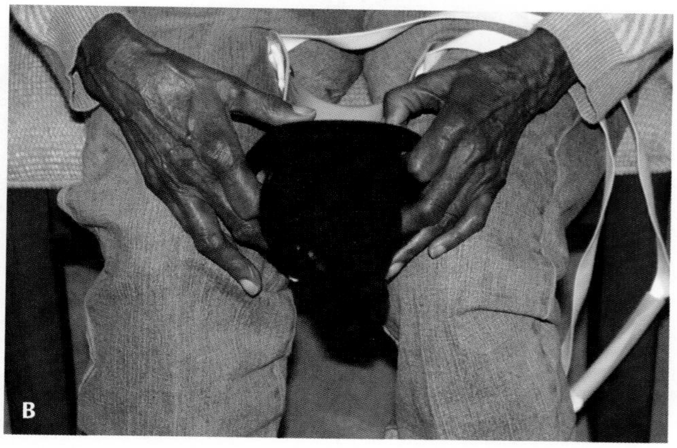

FIGURE 47.4 **A.** A sock-aid is useful for people with limited reach, for example, from limited balance or range of motion. **B.** However, the client needs to have the use of both hands to get the sock onto the device, which could make it impractical for some clients.

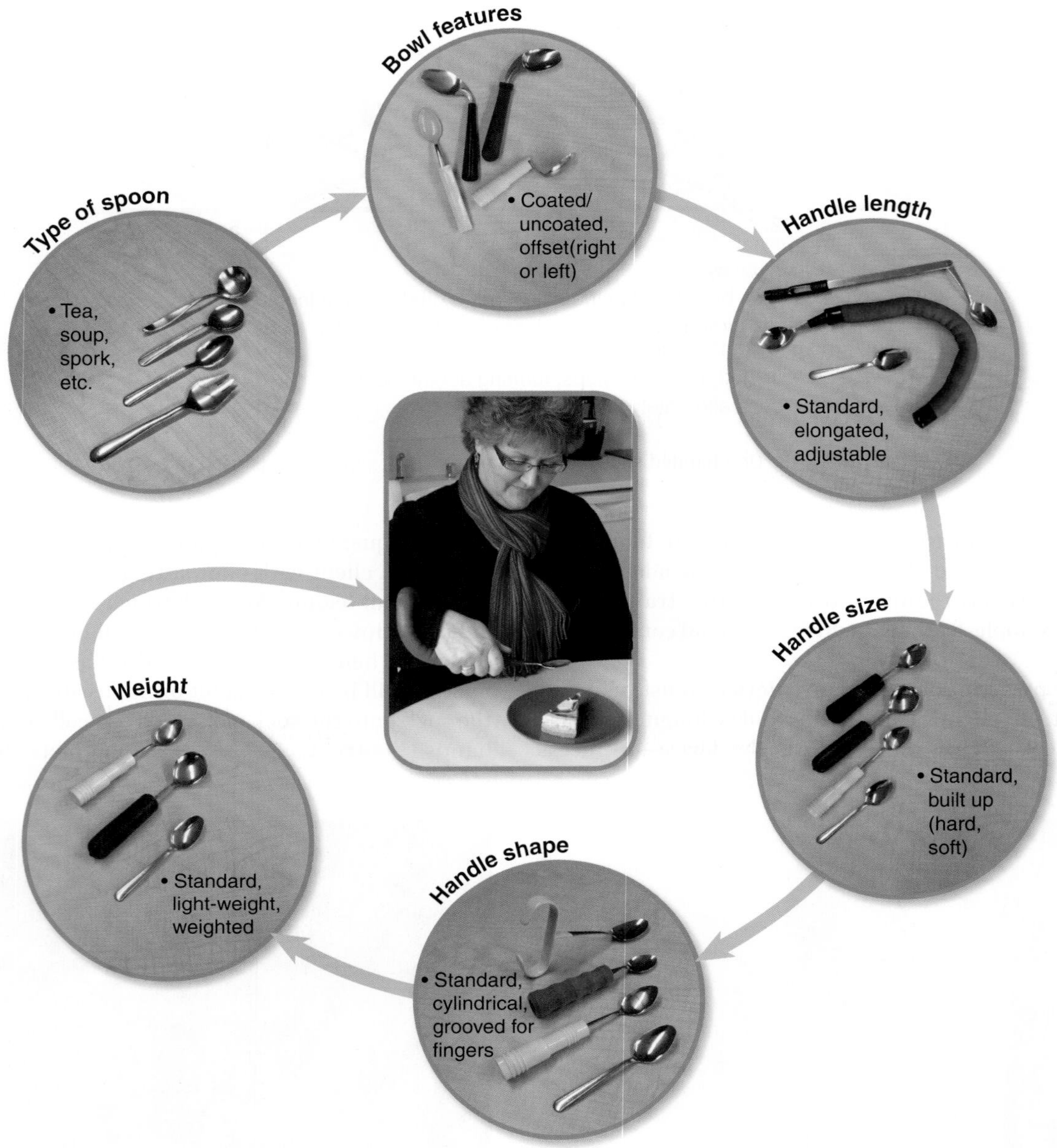

FIGURE 47.5 Potential decisions for prescribing an adapted spoon, a simple assistive device.

of decisions that an occupational therapy practitioner makes when selecting an adapted spoon, a very simple type of adaptive equipment. Although many assistive devices that occupational therapy practitioners prescribe are quite simple mechanically, some are sophisticated and include complex electronics, circuits, and microprocessors, such as augmentative communication devices.

One disadvantage of adapting task objects is that the adapted or assistive device must be available to clients whenever and wherever they engage in the task. This might or might not pose a problem, depending on the task and the adaptation. Clients who use memory books at work to compensate for cognitive impairments can incorporate the structure and cues needed into a daily planner or a handheld personal data assistant, a tool that was used habitually before the impairment. If a client requires built-up utensils for eating, however, and wishes to eat at a restaurant, the utensils must be taken along. This is cumbersome, and some clients find it embarrassing.

Finally, some clients find that the use of adaptive equipment reduces satisfaction with task performance. To enhance personal satisfaction with task performance, they might be willing to cope with the increased difficulty of doing a task without adapted tools. For example, Ms. Lindstrom, a woman with multiple sclerosis, found that her mobility was safer and easier in a wheelchair, but she preferred to walk when out in the community.

Her dissatisfaction with the wheelchair overrode other considerations.

- **Modify the Task Environment.** Modification of the environment itself may be used to facilitate task performance (Chard, Liu, & Mulholland, 2009; Østensjø, Carlberg, & Vøllestad, 2005). Typically, when the environment is modified, the demand for learning and practice is less than that required for learning an alternative method or using adapted task objects. Environmental modifications are often fixed in place so that clients do not need to remember to bring along the necessary adaptations and the adaptations cannot be easily displaced (e.g., they cannot be dropped out of reach). The task method is often unchanged, or only minimally changed, so that clients can rely on previous experience. Examples include installing a wheelchair ramp, recessing plumbing under the sink to accommodate a wheelchair user, increasing available light, labeling cupboard doors to compensate for cognitive deficits, and installing a toilet seat frame (Figure 47.6). Electronic aids to daily living are also environmental modifications that enable people with severe physical impairments to operate home electronics (e.g., computer, phone, lights, stereo, television) and even open doors by using an accessible switch, user display, and a processor (Ripat, 2006).

The biggest drawback of environmental modifications is that clients might become limited in terms of performance context. They must do the task in the modified environment or in one that has been similarly modified because the modifications are not easily transportable and might be custom designed for a specific setting.

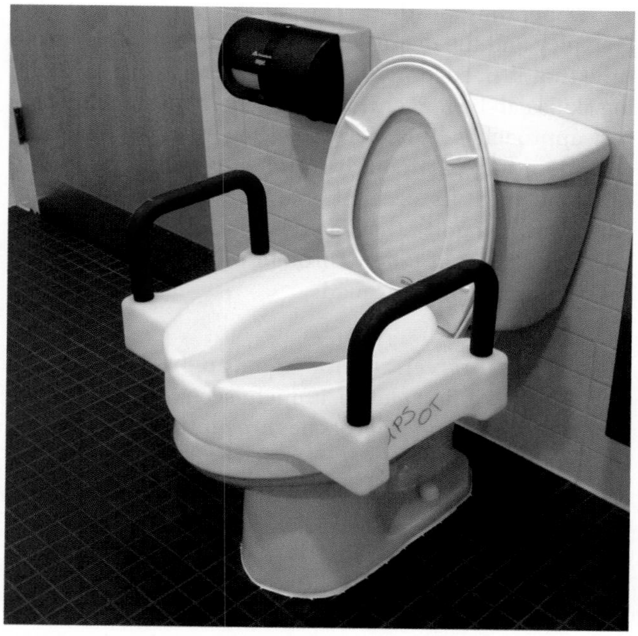

FIGURE 47.6 A toilet frame used to help the individual move between sitting and standing and to increase stability during transfers.

Establish/Restore. A restorative approach typically focuses intervention at the impairment level with the aim of restoring or establishing the capacities that are needed for functional tasks (AOTA, 2008). Intervention may be used to restore capacities such as strength, endurance, range of motion, short-term memory, visual scanning, and interests. More information about specific techniques can be found in the chapters in Unit XII. Regardless of the underlying theories or techniques used, however, one must always establish the link between the impairment and the resulting activity limitations. Careful documentation of the evaluation assists other health professionals and third-party payers to understand the connection between the intervention and the established occupation-based outcomes. Clients must also be educated about the relationship between their inherent capacities and the everyday tasks that they pursue so that they understand how the intervention will ultimately lead to improved task performance.

All intervention programs that are designed to restore or establish inherent capacities must provide clients with a structured opportunity to transfer the gains made in these capacities to relevant functional tasks (Latham, 2008a). This ensures that the intervention outcome is occupation based. Using new or regained capacities in a functional context also helps clients to maintain or enhance gains by using them within the daily routine, increasing opportunities for practice. For example, stretching exercises that result in increased right shoulder flexion passive and active ROM should be accompanied by functional tasks that require movement into the newly acquired range, such as using the right upper extremity to reach up to pin pictures on a bulletin board or dusting bookshelves (Figure 47.7). Other examples can be found in Table 47.5.

Intervention that is aimed at establishing or restoring capacities is often most efficient for clients for whom a few impairments affect many tasks and for whom diminished capacities can be expected to improve. For example, Mr. Stapinski had circumferential second-degree burns to both upper extremities.

See **Appendix I, Common Conditions, Resources, and Evidence** for more information about burns.

The resulting bilateral restrictions in elbow flexion prevented him from completing most ADL owing to an inability to reach his face, head, or trunk. Tasks could be easily adapted by using long-handled devices, but extended tools would have been needed for many ADL tasks (e.g., eating utensils, toothbrush, comb, brush, bath sponge). Because clients with burns can be expected to increase ROM with passive stretching, scar management,

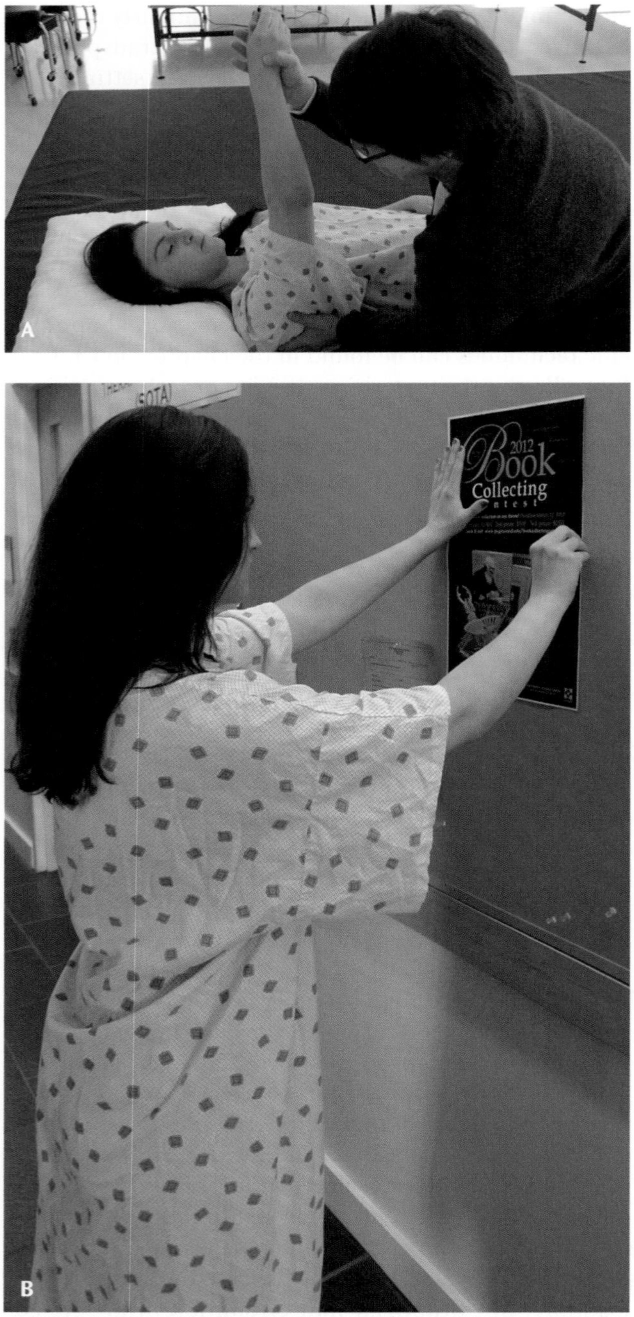

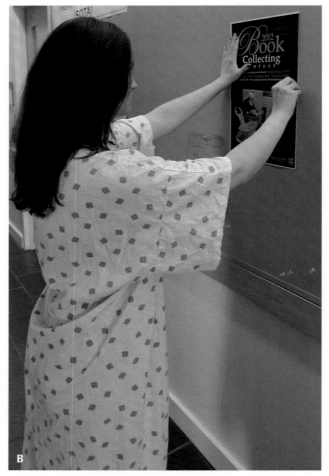

FIGURE 47.7 Stretching to restore passive range of motion (PROM) may be an effective treatment for improving reach (**A**), but practitioners should be sure to incorporate PROM gains into occupation-based activities (**B**).

and exercise, intervention was most efficient when it was aimed at increasing Mr. Stapinski's elbow flexion. Adapting selected task objects improved his ADL performance in the short term; however, the long-term goal of restoring Mr. Stapinski's capacity to flex his elbows enhanced function across many different tasks.

A restorative approach may be appropriate for some clients with progressive disorders even though their capacities are expected to deteriorate, given the typical course of the condition. The focus, however, becomes slowing the decline of specific capacities and skills. For example, clients with Parkinson's disease may have reduced bradykinesia with the use of a movement exercise program (Dibble, Hale, Marcus, Gerber, & LaStayo, 2009).

See **Appendix I, Common Conditions, Resources, and Evidence** for more information about Parkinson's disease.

For clients with some types of impairments, carefully structured everyday activities can restore or establish capacities while simultaneously permitting the practice of the activities. Clients who are severely deconditioned might find their activity level limited by poor endurance. Intervention could rely on aerobic exercise to increase cardiopulmonary endurance, with the goal of participating in functional activities when an adequate increase in cardiopulmonary capacity is achieved. Instead, an intervention that graded the intensity and duration of daily activities could be as effective in increasing cardiovascular fitness while enabling the client to participate in desired tasks. In addition, gains that are made in endurance are immediately transferred into functional activities. Children and adults may engage more effectively in play or leisure activities that incorporate the necessary repetitive movements compared to a rote exercise (Melchert-McKearnan, Deitz, Engel, & White, 2000). Practice and participation in ADL and IADL programs also give clients with a new disability an opportunity to become familiar with their new bodies (Guidetti, Asaba, & Tham, 2007).

Depending on the nature of the performance discrepancy and the degree of impairment, the intervention time that is needed in establishing or restoring underlying skills can be longer than that required for compensatory approaches. This increased time must be taken into consideration, particularly for clients who have limited reimbursement for occupational therapy. In addition, clients must recognize that the rehabilitation period might be longer and that follow-through with a home program is vital if gains are to be made.

Integrating Intervention for Impairments and Activity Limitations. At first glance, it might seem that the *modify* and *establish/restore* approaches are mutually exclusive—that is, that the outcome is either to establish/restore the impaired capacity or to compensate for it. Using both approaches simultaneously might seem a bit like using a belt and suspenders. However, a carefully crafted program enables clients to be more functional through the use of compensatory strategies while at the same time working to restore functional capacities. It is critical that the occupational therapy practitioner reduce the use of compensatory strategies as clients make gains in skill performance when using the two approaches.

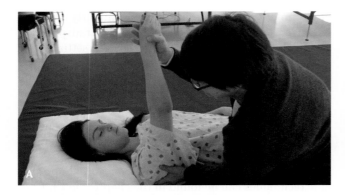

TABLE 47.5 Integrating Treatment Gains from an Establish or Restore Approach into Functional Tasks

Impairment	Preparatory Activity to Reduce Impairment	Task to Integrate Gains Made into ADL/IADL	Functional Outcomes
Impaired grip strength	Hand putty exercises	Cooking task that begins with light resistance (e.g. stirring Jello) and progresses to more resistive tasks (e.g., brownies then cookies)	Increased ability to grasp task objects firmly (e.g. opening containers, doors, pulling up pants)
Decreased upper extremity muscle endurance	Using an arm ergometer	Wheelchair mobility, increasing time and difficulty (e.g., progress from flat surfaces to ramps)	Increased ability to engage in sustained upper extremity work (e.g., propelling a wheelchair, shampooing hair, washing windows)
Hyperresponsiveness to tactile stimuli	Brushing skin	Progress from bathing in a tub to a shower, which provides a stronger stimulus	Ability to tolerate tactile stimuli in everyday tasks, including dressing, brushing teeth, and interacting with others
Poor visual scanning	Paper-and-pencil cancellation tasks (e.g., cross out all the *M*'s on a sheet of letters) using a left to right, right to left, top to bottom scanning pattern	Find items in a kitchen cupboard or grocery store shelf	Ability to use a more organized scanning process for locating objects (e.g., finding a blouse in the closet, a brush on a cluttered dresser, the milk in the refrigerator)
Anxiety in new situations	Practice progressive relaxation in a quiet place to reduce anxiety	Use progressive relaxation in community outings with the therapist	Ability to function effectively in new situations without experiencing excessive anxiety (e.g., job interview, cultural events, travel).

For example, Mr. Stapinski, whose burns resulted in bilateral limitations in elbow flexion, might benefit from using utensils with extended handles. With the extended handles on the utensils, he can feed himself independently during the 2 to 3 weeks that it takes to increase his elbow flexion sufficiently for him to feed himself without these utensils. The extended handles should be fabricated to require him to flex fully within his available range and should be shortened as gains in PROM are made so that the new range is incorporated into the feeding task.

Whenever occupational therapy practitioners anticipate that task or environmental adaptations will be temporary, they must consider the cost in relationship to the anticipated time the devices or adaptations will be needed and the potential benefit to clients. Thermoplastic or wood extensions can be added temporarily to the handles of regular utensils rather than prescribing the more costly commercially available utensils with elongated handles. For some tasks, safety concerns supersede cost considerations. Using a collapsible lawn chair in the shower would be an inexpensive alternative to a shower chair, but it would not provide adequate stability for most clients.

Education of the Client or Caregiver

Caregiver training may be implemented to maximize a client's functional outcome (Chard et al., 2009) while minimizing the efforts of the caregiver (Dooley & Hinojosa, 2004). For example, Mr. Ford sustained a left cerebrovascular accident and required minimal physical assistance with verbal cueing from the occupational therapy practitioner for wheelchair transfers. Mrs. Ford was physically able to help her husband but had no prior experience in transferring a person with hemiparesis. One day, she decided to help her husband move from his hospital bed to the chair. Because she did not block his right knee or tell him to wait for her cue before standing, they both fell onto the bed while attempting to execute the transfer. Fortunately, no one was hurt. As a consequence of this experience, Mrs. Ford was convinced that she could not care for her husband at home. At the same time, she was distressed by the thought of having to admit him to a long-term care facility. She was receptive to receiving transfer training from the occupational therapy practitioner and was delighted to find that by using the proper physical and verbal techniques, she could easily and safely assist her husband. In this example, caregiver training increased the client's level of independence and the probability that he could go home at discharge.

Instructional Methods. Various instructional methods are available for client and caregiver education (Greber et al., 2007), and methods should be selected that best meet the person's needs. When a facility has a homogeneous client population, group instruction can be an efficient and effective method for providing basic education. Many arthritis centers provide group instruction in joint protection techniques. Teaching a group is cost-effective and, when well structured, can facilitate learning through peer interaction. For caregiver groups, the contact with others who are experiencing similar problems in their caregiving roles can provide valuable emotional support and an opportunity for constructive group problem solving.

Some type of individualized instruction is typically needed to complement group instruction so that information can be tailored to meet the specific and unique needs of each person. If group instruction has preceded the individualized instruction, the client-specific sessions can be relatively short and focused on application of the information learned in the group to the client's particular circumstances. For example, clients would be taught how to apply proper lifting techniques to the weights and dimensions of objects in their own homes.

Individualized instruction is more appropriate for many clients and caregivers because the personal nature of the tasks that need to be learned does not lend itself to group instruction (e.g., bathing). Furthermore, in intervention settings that serve a diverse case mix, the opportunity for group instruction may not occur. One-to-one client or caregiver education and training enables the occupational therapy practitioner to obtain immediate feedback from the person as the session progresses and to alter the amount and focus of learning accordingly.

A vast array of media are available to occupational therapy practitioners to facilitate the client's or caregiver's learning process. Written materials may be developed specifically for a client or caregiver or published materials can be used if appropriate ones are available. Videocassette or digital recorders are widely available, even in clients' homes, and custom or commercially made videotapes or DVDs can be effective teaching tools. Audiotapes can also be useful, particularly when visual input would be distracting. For example, an audiotape may be used to facilitate visual imagery for relaxation or stress reduction. The Internet contains a wealth of information about various disorders that is specifically geared toward clients and caregivers, or practitioners can develop and upload customized educational content to accessible sites, such as YouTube, as long as careful attention is paid to client confidentiality. Clients can also find peer support groups through chat rooms, Web forums, or e-mail lists. Health care professionals, including occupational therapists, are using teleconferencing for educational purposes, for example, to teach energy conservation strategies to people with multiple sclerosis living in the community (Finlayson & Holberg, 2007).

It is important that occupational therapy practitioners take care to assess the match between client and caregiver skills and the educational media used. In addition, type of media and the content included must be accessible and presented at the appropriate level. For example, adults living in developed countries have mean reading skills that range from fifth to eighth grade, so written materials should be designed with these literacy levels in mind in order to improve clients' learning (McKenna & Scott, 2007). More information on client education can be found in the "Commentary on the Evidence" box.

Commentary on the Evidence

Client Learning

Finding the Best Educational Strategies for Client Learning

As individual treatment time has been reduced by third-party reimbursement plans, client and caregiver education has played a more important role in treatment. Many studies have demonstrated the effectiveness of different and varied educational programs. For example, patient education programs have been effective in improving self-management and reducing pain and disability for people with rheumatoid arthritis (Hammond, 2004), reducing the impact of fatigue on occupational performance in people with multiple sclerosis (Vanage et al., 2003), and increasing confidence and activity participation in older adults who have a fear of falling (Cheal & Clemson, 2001). Eklund, Sonn, and Dahlin-Ivanoff (2004) compared a health education program for people who have visual impairment with traditional individualized intervention and reported that participants in the health education program had higher perceived security for several ADL and IADL. Researchers typically describe the educational programs that were used in their studies, and the educational methods reported vary significantly. Although there is ample research to support the efficacy of patient education programs on client outcomes, few studies were found that compared varied educational approaches for clients to identify best practice in this area. For example, research on group intervention that includes active participation, collaborative problem solving, and learning tasks that relate to a current, relevant problem seem to be more effective in equipping clients with tools needed to meet challenges in the future (Eklund & Dahlin-Ivanoff, 2006). Learning is a complex process, and factors such as motivation and self-efficacy should be addressed in planning learning experiences (Edelstein, 2005). Clients must be ready to learn, so the timing of education can also affect its effectiveness (Hammond, 2004; Kendall et al., 2007) and should be further explored. Many educational programs are aimed at changing clients' habits, such as engaging in home exercise programs or incorporating energy conservation techniques into daily activities, which require behavioral approaches for supporting the development of new habits and follow-up studies to examine program effectiveness (Mathiowetz, Matuska, Finlayson, Luo, & Chen, 2007). Future research should also examine the impact of varied impairments on the effectiveness of education, for example, problems with initiation, attention, or executive function. Gathering additional evidence will enable practitioners to become even more effective in helping clients to reach their goals. See Chapters 28 and 44.

Caregiver Training. In addition to evaluating clients' learning capacity, the learning capacity of their caregivers needs to be appraised. Like clients, caregivers have varied learning styles, capacities, and experience. In many situations, the caregiver is a family member who is still coping with the emotional impact of having a family member with a disability, whether a new parent with a child with cerebral palsy or the spouse of someone who has had a stroke. Caregivers experiencing emotional stress have impaired learning and memory (Mackenzie, Wiprzycka, Hasher, & Goldstein, 2009) and often need more time and repetition to process information accurately. In other cases, caregivers have been providing care for years and bring a wealth of caring expertise to the treatment session. The occupational therapy practitioner should work collaboratively with all caregivers but may move into a more consultative role with experienced caregivers who can articulate problems and engage actively in problem solving based on prior learning (Toth-Cohen, 2000). When caregivers are expected to assist clients physically, their physical capacity for providing this assistance also warrants evaluation, and training must be designed that matches their physical capacity.

Caregivers have varied learning styles, and instruction that caters to their preferred style is likely to be the most efficient and effective (Banford et al., 2001). Some people, for example, are kinesthetic learners. They learn most quickly through doing. Visual learners might prefer to watch a demonstration of the activity several times before attempting it themselves. Others might prefer written instructions. All learners benefit from the opportunity to ask questions to clarify instructions. Media that support teaching by a practitioner can be a great asset. Videotapes or DVDs, for example, provide caregivers with an excellent visual image of how an exercise or activity is to be done. Often, home- or clinic-made videotapes can be made of a client's activity performance. These productions add little time to the intervention session because they are recorded as activities are practiced during regular therapy. They have the advantage of providing richer and more detailed information than is feasible in oral or written instructions.

When caregivers are helping to carry out an intervention program, the goals and general intervention strategies should be made clear to them (McKenna & Scott, 2007). For programs using an establish/restore approach, clients might need assistance with implementing specific exercises or grading of activities in a way that will help to enhance skills. Caregivers need to learn specific cueing strategies so that home programs are carried out accurately, whether in clients' homes, group homes, or long-term care settings. Caregivers are often pivotal in motivating clients. Spurring clients on who have disorders that impact motivation, such as depression, can be particularly challenging. Helping caregivers to understand that disinterest and lack of motivation are a part of the disorder, and providing concrete strategies for managing the "getting going" phase of the home program will foster its success (Resnick, 1998). For clients with behavior problems, such as the reactions that may accompany autism or Alzheimer's disease, teaching caregivers behavior management strategies that defuse potentially volatile situations can be invaluable to their success as caregivers.

Caregiver training for assisting clients with ADL and IADL should focus first on safety for clients and caregivers. The occupational therapy practitioner should emphasize components of the activity that promote safety, such as locking the wheelchair brakes or blocking the client's knee to prevent buckling when transferring to and from the wheelchair. As intervention progresses, the occupational therapy practitioner should inform caregivers of the activities that are safe and unsafe to perform outside of the therapy situation. For example, although a client might be working on bathtub transfers during therapy, skilled facilitation to get into and out of the tub safely might be required, making it premature for the client to practice these transfers at home.

When caregivers need to provide physical assistance, they should be trained in using proper body mechanics, especially during transfers or bed mobility and for wheelchair positioning. Assisting a client in a wheelchair with ADL, such as brushing teeth or feeding, while the caregiver is standing can fatigue the caregiver's lower back muscles; and tasks that requiring lifting or positioning increase the risk of back injuries. Hinojosa and Rittman (2009) found that caregivers with greater educational needs were more likely to have sustained a physical injury, suggesting that caregiver education may reduce the risk of injury. Taking care of the caregiver is frequently overlooked in occupational therapy interventions, but it is an essential component of the person-task-environment transaction, particularly when it is anticipated that the client will require assistance over a long period of time.

Grading the Intervention Program

Intervention programs should never be static. It is important to progress the client continually toward the established intervention goals and to set new goals as initial goals are met. The specific means of grading intervention when a restoration approach is being implemented depends on the impairments and the intervention strategies that are being used (Latham, 2008b). If the intervention plan blends establish/restore and modify/adapt approaches, the program can be graded by reducing the amount of task and environmental adaptations as clients' capacities are restored. Intervention for activity limitations can be graded by modifying many of the performance parameters that were described earlier in the chapter. Clients may increase their level of independence in task performance, take more responsibility for safety, feel more personal satisfaction from a task, reduce the level of difficulty or required exertion, or decrease the task duration or the occurrence of aberrant task behaviors.

Grading Task Progression from Easier to Harder. One means of grading an intervention program is to begin with easier ADL or IADL tasks and progress to more difficult ones. Task difficulty will be relative to a client's activity limitations and underlying impairments. For example, paying bills might be relatively easy for a client with quadriplegia to perform once the use of a writing tool is mastered, whereas lower extremity dressing is much more difficult. Conversely, a client with an acquired brain injury who has significant cognitive impairment but relatively preserved motor skills is likely to find lower extremity dressing to be relatively easy but money management extremely difficult.

Increasing Complexity within the Task. Rather than progressing only from easier to harder activities, intervention may also be graded by increasing the complexity within an activity or by progressing from simple to more complex ways of doing it. Cooking skills might extend from simple preparations such as cold sandwiches to more complex, multiple-course dinners. Even seemingly simple tasks can often be graded. A sock-donning intervention, for example, might be scaled from using looser ankle socks to tighter knee socks and finally to tight anti-embolus hose.

Same Task in Varied Performance Environments. A critical part of a graded intervention program involves progression from the intervention environment to the real-life environment in which the activity will actually be performed. This can involve transfer from a clinic to a home setting or the more subtle dynamics associated with the transfer of help from the occupational therapy practitioner to the natural caregiver. The client who is independent in donning a jacket while sitting on a mat table in the clinic might be unable to do so when sitting on a chair with a back or when standing (the way a jacket is typically donned by people who are able to walk). Providing practice in increasingly demanding performance environments can facilitate the generalization of skills, thereby enhancing the client's functional flexibility.

Therapist-Facilitated to Client-Facilitated Problem Solving. Clients with permanent disabilities or chronic diseases must develop problem-solving skills in order to meet new challenges in their lives after discharge from occupational therapy services. Initially, when facing a new task or becoming familiar with a changed body or mind, therapists may use explicit instruction or demonstration to help clients learn new approaches to ADL and IADL. Treatment can be graded by engaging the client in problem solving, for example, by asking a client who is a new wheelchair user to come up with strategies for traveling after completing more direct training in community mobility in a familiar setting.

Intervention Review: Reevaluation to Monitor Effectiveness

ADL and IADL are evaluated on entry to occupational therapy to provide a measure of the client's baseline performance status. Regardless of the extent and length of the intervention, reevaluation of ADL and IADL performance is needed to ascertain whether the intervention is resulting in improvement, whether the intervention should be continued or changed, or whether maximal benefit from occupational therapy has been achieved and activity performance has reached a plateau (AOTA, 2008). Occupational therapy practitioners routinely engage in informal review of interventions by observing clients' performance during treatment and considering the actual or potential impact of their performance on established goals.

Periodically, a more formal intervention review or reevaluation is needed to objectively measure clients' progress toward goals and to document their progress in clinical records. The best strategy for reevaluation is to readminister the assessments done during the initial evaluation. Using the same ADL and IADL content, the same measurement parameters, and the same data-gathering methods enhances the possibility of detecting change in the client's performance that is attributable to intervention. If the reevaluation varies from a prior evaluation, the potential for detecting change is reduced. For example, if ADL performance is assessed initially with a self-report measure regarding the amount of assistance needed but then is reassessed with a performance-based measure, differences in level of assistance may reflect an actual change in performance or simply varied perceptions of the client and the therapist. The realities of practice, however, may make it difficult to repeat all initial measures, so occupational therapists must consider variations in reassessment when drawing conclusions about the effectiveness of the intervention.

Conclusion

This chapter described the complex practice of evaluating and treating clients with ADL and IADL deficits. Performance parameters of value, independence, safety, and adequacy were reviewed; and their relevance to the selection of specific assessment tools was described. Occupational therapists should establish objective baseline measures through the use of standardized ADL and IADL assessments whenever possible; however, the realities of the treatment setting may also require the use of nonstandardized assessments. Developing objective goals that address all relevant performance parameters is a crucial first step in implementing treatment by providing a "road map" for guiding client care. General treatment approaches that occupational therapists use to increase participation in ADL and IADL include modifying the task or environment, establishing or restoring underlying impairments, and providing client and caregiver education. Grading activities effectively will maximize clients' progress toward goals. Specific treatment activities vary significantly according to the clients' ages and disabilities and are beyond the scope of this chapter. Readers should use this chapter to guide them in the overall process of ADL and IADL intervention and refer to sources that focus on specific client populations and service delivery models when selecting specific treatment activities.

Acknowledgments

I would like to thank Dr. Margo B. Holm and Dr. Joan Rogers for inviting me to coauthor earlier editions of the ADL/IADL treatment chapters for *Willard & Spackman's Occupational Therapy*, which led to the opportunity to author this chapter. Dr. Holm and Dr. Rogers conceptualize occupational therapy practice in ways both scholarly and practical. Their contributions from prior editions continue to shine brightly through in this chapter. I also wish to thank clients, students, and colleagues who posed for photographs and especially Lucretia and Michael Berg for their generous assistance taking and editing photos.

References

American Occupational Therapy Association. (2008). Occupational therapy practice framework: Domain and process, (2nd ed.) *American Journal of Occupational Therapy, 62*, 625–683.

American Occupational Therapy Association. (2010). Standards of practice for occupational therapy. *American Journal of Occupational Therapy, 64*(Suppl.), S10–S11.

Archenholtz, B., & Dellhag, B. (2008). Validity and reliability of the instrument Performance and Satisfaction in Activities of Daily Living (PS-ADL) and its clinical applicability to adults with rheumatoid arthritis. *Scandinavian Journal of Occupational Therapy, 15*, 13–22. doi:10.1080/11038120701223165

Árnadóttir, G. (1990). *The brain and behavior: Assessing cortical dysfunction through activities of daily living*. St. Louis, MO: Mosby Elsevier.

Árnadóttir, G. (2011). Impact of neurobehavioral deficits on activities of daily living. In G. Gillen (Ed.), *Stroke rehabilitation: A function-based approach* (3rd ed., pp. 456–500). St. Louis, MO: Mosby Elsevier.

Ashley, M. J., Persel, C. S., & Clark, M. C. (2001). Validation of an Independent Living Scale for post-acute rehabilitation applications. *Brain Injury, 15*, 435–442.

Banford, M., Kratz, M., Brown, R., Emick, K., Ranck, J., Wilkins, R., & Holm, M. (2001). Stroke survivor caregiver education: Methods and effectiveness. *Physical and Occupational Therapy in Geriatrics, 19*, 37–51.

Baron, K., Kielhofner, G., Iyenger, A., Goldhammer, V., & Wolenski, J. (2006). *The Occupational Self-Assessment* (Version 2.2). Chicago, IL: University of Illinois at Chicago, College of Applied Health Sciences, Department of Occupational Therapy, Model of Human Occupation Clearinghouse.

Bédard, M., Parkkari, M., Weaver, B., Riendeau, J., & Dahlquist, M. (2010). Brief report—Assessment of Driving Performance using a Simulator Protocol: Validity and reproducibility. *American Journal of Occupational Therapy, 64*, 336–340.

Borg, G. (1998). *Borg's Perceived Exertion and Pain Scales*. Champagne, IL: Human Kinetics.

Brown, C., Moore, W. P., Hemman, D., & Yunek, A. (1996). Influence of instrumental activities of daily living assessment method on judgments of independence. *American Journal of Occupational Therapy, 50*, 202–206.

Carod-Artal, F. J., Coral, L. F., Trizotto, D. S., & Moreira, C. M. (2009). Self- and proxy-report agreement on the Stroke Impact Scale. *Stroke, 40*, 3308–3314. doi:10.1161/STROKEAHA.109.558031

Chard, G., Liu, L., & Mulholland, S. (2009). Verbal cueing and environmental modifications: Strategies to improve engagement in occupations in persons with Alzheimer's disease. *Physical & Occupational Therapy in Geriatrics, 27*, 197–211. doi:10.1080/02703180802206280

Cheal, B., & Clemson, L. (2001). Older people enhancing self-efficacy in fall-risk situations. *Australian Occupational Therapy Journal, 48*, 80–91.

Chong, D. K. (1995). Measurement of instrumental activities of daily living in stroke. *Stroke, 26*, 1119–1122. Retrieved from http://stroke.ahajournals.org/cgi/content/full/26/6/1119

Chui, T., & Oliver, R. (2006). Factor analysis and construct validity of the SAFER-HOME. *OTJR: Occupation, Participation, & Health, 26*, 132–142.

Cipriani, J., Hess, S., Higgins, H., Resavy, D., Sheon, S., Szychowski, M., & Holm, M. (2000). Collaboration in the therapeutic process: Older adults' perspectives. *Physical and Occupational Therapy in Geriatrics, 17*(1), 43–54.

Clemson, L., Bundy, A., Unsworth, C., & Singh, M. (2009). Validation of the Modified Assessment of Living Skills and Resources, an IADL measure for older people. *Disability & Rehabilitation, 31*, 359–369. doi:10.1080/09638280802105881

Cohen-Mansfield, J., & Jensen, B. (2007). Adequacy of spouses as informants regarding older persons' self-care practices and their perceived importance. *Families, Systems, & Health, 25*, 53–67. doi:10.1037/1091-7527.25.1.53

Colquhoun, H., Letts, L., Law, M., MacDermid, J., & Edwards, M. (2010). Feasibility of the Canadian Occupational Performance Measure for routine use. *British Journal of Occupational Therapy, 73*, 48–54. doi:10.4276/030802210X12658062793726

Covinsky, K. E., Lindquist, K., Dunlop, D. D., & Yelin, E. (2009). Pain, functional limits, and aging. *Journal of the American Geriatric Society, 57*, 1556–1561. doi:10.1111/j.1532-5415.2009.02388.x

Davis, L. A. (2005). Educating individuals with dementia: Perspectives for rehabilitation professionals. *Topics in Geriatric Rehabilitation, 21*, 304–314.

Department of Health and Human Services Centers for Medicare & Medicaid Services. (2006). *Inpatient Rehabilitation Facility–Patient Assessment Instrument*. Retrieved from http://www.cms.gov/InpatientRehabFacPPS/04_IRFPAI.asp#TopOfPage

Dibble, L., Hale, T., Marcus, R., Gerber, J., & LaStayo, P. (2009). High intensity eccentric resistance training decreases bradykinesia and improves quality of life in persons with Parkinson's disease: a preliminary study. *Parkinsonism & Related Disorders, 15*, 752–757.

Doig, E., Fleming, J., Cornwell, P. L., & Kuipers, P. (2009). Qualitative exploration of a client-centered, goal-directed approach to community-based occupational therapy for adults with traumatic brain injury. *American Journal of Occupational Therapy, 64*, 559–568.

Dooley, N. R., & Hinojosa, J. (2004). Improving quality of life for persons with Alzheimer's disease and their family caregivers: Brief occupational therapy intervention. *American Journal of Occupational Therapy, 58*, 561–569.

Dudgeon, B. J., Tyler, E. J., Rhodes, L. A., & Jensen, M. P. (2006). Managing usual and unexpected pain with physical disability: A qualitative analysis. *American Journal of Occupational Therapy, 60*, 92–103.

Dunn, W. (2005). Measurement issues and practices. In M. Law, C. Baum, & W. Dunn (Eds.), *Measuring occupational performance: Supporting best practice in occupational therapy* (2nd ed., pp. 21–32). Thorofare, NJ: Slack.

Dunn, W., Brown, C., & McGuigan, A. (1994). The ecology of human performance: A framework for considering the effect of context. *American Journal of Occupational Therapy, 48*, 595–607.

Edelstein, J. E. (2005). Motivating elderly patients with recent amputations. *Topics in Geriatric Rehabilitation, 21*, 116–122.

Eklund, K., & Dahlin-Ivanoff, S. (2006). Health education for people with macular degeneration: Learning experiences and the effect on daily occupation. *Canadian Journal of Occupational Therapy, 73*, 272–280. doi:10.2182/cjot.06.004

Eklund, K., Sonn, U., & Dahlin-Ivanoff, S. (2004). Long-term evaluation of a health education programme for elderly persons with visual impairment. A randomized study. *Disability and Rehabilitation, 26*, 401–409.

Eklund, M., & Gunnarsson, A. B. (2008). Content validity, clinical utility, sensitivity to change and discriminant ability of the Swedish Satisfaction with Daily Occupations (SDO) instrument: A screening tool for people with mental disorders. *British Journal of Occupational Therapy, 71*, 487–495.

Eyres, L., & Unsworth, C. A. (2005). Occupational therapy in acute hospitals: The effectiveness of a pilot program to maintain occupational performance in older clients. *Australian Occupational Therapy Journal, 52*, 218–224. doi:10.1111/j.1440-1630.2005.00498.x

Fasoli, S. E. (2008). Assessing roles and competence. In M. V. Radomski & C. A. T. Latham (Eds.), *Occupational therapy for physical dysfunction* (6th ed., pp. 65–90). Philadelphia, PA: Lippincott Williams & Wilkins.

Finlayson, M., & Holberg, C. (2007). Evaluation of a teleconference-delivered energy conservation education program for people with multiple sclerosis. *Canadian Journal of Occupational Therapy, 74*, 337–347.

Fisher, A. G., & Jones, K. B. (2011a). *Assessment of Motor and Process Skills: Development, standardization, and administration manual* (7th ed. revised). Ft. Collins, CO: Three Star Press.

Fisher, A. G., & Jones, K. B. (2011b). *Assessment of Motor and Process Skills: User manual* (7th ed. revised). Ft. Collins, CO: Three Star Press.

FitzGerald, J., Mangione, C., Boscardin, J., Kominski, G., Hahn, B., & Ettner, S. (2006). Impact of changes in Medicare home health care reimbursement on month-to-month home health utilization between 1996 and 2001 for a national sample of patients undergoing orthopedic procedures. *Medical Care, 44*(9), 870–878.

Flinn, N. A., & Radomski, M. V. (2008). Learning. In M. V. Radomski & C. A. T. Latham (Eds.), *Occupational therapy for physical dysfunction* (6th ed., pp. 382–401). Philadelphia, PA: Lippincott Williams & Wilkins.

Floyer-Lea, A., & Matthews, P. (2004). Changing brain networks for visuomotor control with increased movement automaticity. *Journal of Neurophysiology, 92*(4), 2405–2412.

Gateley & Borcherding, 2011. *Documentation manual for writing SOAP notes in occupational therapy* (2nd ed.). Thorofare, NJ: Slack.

Gateley, C., & Borcherding, S. (2011). *Documentation manual for writing SOAP notes in occupational therapy* (3rd ed.). Thorofare, NJ: Slack.

Gavacs, M. (2009, June). The dance of independence. *OT Practice, 14*(10), 32.

Gift, A. G., & Narsavage, G. (1998). Validity of the numeric rating scale as a measure of dyspnea. *American Journal of Critical Care, 7*, 200–204.

Gillen, G. (2000). Improving activities of daily living performance in an adult with ataxia. *American Journal of Occupational Therapy, 54*, 89–96.

Gillen, G. (2009). *Cognitive and perceptual rehabilitation: Optimizing function*. St. Louis, MO: Mosby Elsevier.

Gitlin, L. N. (2005). Measuring performance in instrumental activities of daily living. In M. Law, C. Baum, & W. Dunn (Eds.), *Measuring occupational performance: Supporting best practice in occupational therapy* (2nd ed., pp. 227–247). Thorofare, NJ: Slack.

Gitlin, L. N., Corcoran, M., Winter, L., Boyce, A., & Hauck, W. W. (2001). A randomized, controlled trial of a home environmental intervention: Effect on efficacy and upset in caregivers and on daily function of persons with dementia. *Gerontologist, 41*, 4–14.

Goverover, Y., Chiaravalloti, N., Gaudino-Goering, E., Moore, N., & DeLuca, J. (2009). The relationship among performance of instrumental activities of daily living, self-report of quality of life, and self-awareness of functional status in individuals with multiple sclerosis. *Rehabilitation Psychology, 54*, 60–68. doi:10.1037/a0014556

Greber, C., Ziviani, J., & Rodger, S. (2007). The four-quadrant model of facilitated learning (Part 2): Strategies and applications. *Australian Occupational Therapy Journal, 54*, S40–S48. doi:10.1111/j.1440-1630.2007.00663.x

Guidetti, S., Asaba, E., & Tham, K. (2007). The lived experience of recapturing self-care. *American Journal of Occupational Therapy, 61*, 303–310.

Hammond, A. (2004). Rehabilitation in rheumatoid arthritis: A critical review. *Musculoskeletal Care, 2*, 135–151.

Healy, H., & Rigby, P. (1999). Promoting independence for teens and young adults with physical disabilities. *Canadian Journal of Occupational Therapy, 66*, 240–249.

Hilton, K., Fricke, J., & Unsworth, C. (2001). A comparison of self-report versus observation of performance using the Assessment of Living Skills and Resources (ALSAR) with an older population. *British Journal of Occupational Therapy, 64*, 135–143.

Hinojosa, M. S., & Rittman, M. (2009). Association between health education needs and stroke caregiver injury. *Journal of Aging and Health, 21*, 1040–1058. doi:10.1177/0898264309344321

Holm, M. B., & Rogers, J. C. (2008). Performance Assessment of Self-Care Skills. In B. J. Hemphill-Pearson (Ed.), *Assessments in occupational therapy mental health: An integrative approach* (2nd ed., pp. 101–110). Thorofare, NJ: Slack.

Hsueh, I. P., Wang, W. C., Sheu, C. F., & Hsieh, C. L. (2004). Rasch analysis of combining two indices to assess comprehensive ADL function in stroke patients. *Stroke, 35*, 721–726. doi:10.1161/01.STR.0000117569.34232.76

Jack, J., & Estes, R. I. (2010). Documenting progress: Hand therapy treatment shift from biomechanical to occupational adaptation. *American Journal of Occupational Therapy, 64*, 82–87.

Jan, M. H., Hung, J. Y., Lin, J. C., Wang, S. F., Liu, T. K., & Tang, P. F. (2004). Effects of a home program on strength, walking speed, and function after total hip replacement. *Archives of Physical Medicine and Rehabilitation, 85*, 1943–1951. doi:10.1016/j.apmr.2004.02.011

Johansson, K., Lilja, M., Petersson, I., & Borell, L. (2007). Performance of activities of daily living in a sample of applicants for home modification services. *Scandinavian Journal of Occupational Therapy, 14*, 44–53. doi:10.1080/11038120601094997

Kartje, P. (2006, October). Approaching, evaluating, and counseling the older driver for successful community mobility. *OT Practice, 11*(19), 11–15.

Katz, S., Ford, A. B., Moskowitz, R. W., Jackson, B. A., & Jaffe, M. A. (1963). Studies of illness in the aged. The Index of ADL: A standardized measure of biological and psychosocial function. *Journal of the American Medical Association, 185*, 914–919.

Keller, J., Kafkes, A., Basu, S., Federico, J., & Kielhofner, G. (2005). *The Child Occupational Self Assessment* (Version 2.1). Chicago, IL: University of Illinois at Chicago, College of Applied Health Sciences, Department of Occupational Therapy, Model of Human Occupation Clearinghouse.

Kendall, E., Catalano, T., Kuipers, P., Posner, N., Buys, N., & Charker, J. (2007). Recovery following stroke: The role of self-management education. *Social Science & Medicine, 64*, 735–746. doi:10.1016/j.socscimed.2006.09.012

Kettenbach, G. (2009). *Writing patient/client notes: Ensuring accuracy in documentation* (4th ed.). Philadelphia, PA: F. A. Davis.

Kielhofner, G. (2006). Developing and evaluating quantitative data collection instruments. In G. Kielhofner (Ed.), *Research in occupational therapy: Methods of inquiry for enhancing practice* (pp. 155–176). Philadelphia, PA: F. A. Davis.

Kielhofner, G., Mallinson, T., Crawford, C., Nowak, M., Rigby, M., Henry, A., & Walens, D. (2004). *Occupational Performance History Interview II (OPHI-II)* (Version 2.1). Chicago, IL: University of Illinois at Chicago, College of Applied Health Sciences, Department of Occupational Therapy, Model of Human Occupation Clearinghouse.

Klein, S., Barlow, I., & Hollis, V. (2008). Evaluating ADL measure from an occupational therapy perspective. *Canadian Journal of Occupational Therapy, 75*, 69–81.

Kohlman Thomason, L. (1992). *Kohlman Evaluation of Living Skills* (3rd ed.). Bethesda, MD: American Occupational Therapy Association.

Korner-Bitensky, N., Menon, A., von Zweck, C., & Van Benthem, K. (2010). Occupational therapists' capacity-building needs related to older driver screening, assessment, and intervention: A Canadawide survey. *American Journal of Occupational Therapy, 64,* 316–324.

Kuo, J., Fleming, J., Dermer, B., Cullen, C., Jack, C., Bacon, E., & O'Shea, K. (2007). Reliability of the original and revised versions of the Assessment of Living Skills and Resources. *Australian Occupational Therapy Journal, 54,* 194–202. doi:10.1111/j.1440-1630.2006.00625.x

Lansing, R. W., Moosavi, S. H., & Banzett, R. B. (2003). Measurement of dyspnea: Word labeled visual analog scale vs. verbal ordinal scale. *Respiratory Physiology & Neurobiology, 3,* 77–83.

Latham, C. A. T. (2008a). Conceptual foundations for practice. In M. V. Radomski & C. A. T. Latham (Eds.), *Occupational therapy for physical dysfunction* (6th ed., pp. 1–20). Philadelphia, PA: Lippincott Williams & Wilkins.

Latham, C. A. T. (2008b). Occupation as therapy: Selection, gradation, analysis, and adaptation. In M. V. Radomski & C. A. T. Latham (Eds.), *Occupational therapy for physical dysfunction* (6th ed., pp. 358–381). Philadelphia, PA: Lippincott Williams & Wilkins.

Law, M., Baptiste, S., Carswell, A., McColl, M. A., Polatajko, H., & Pollock, N. (2005). *The Canadian Occupational Performance Measure* (4th ed.). Toronto, ON: Canadian Association of Occupational Therapists.

Law, M., & Baum, C. (2005). Measurement in occupational therapy. In M. Law, C. Baum, & W. Dunn (Eds.), *Measuring occupational performance: Supporting best practice in occupational therapy* (2nd ed., pp. 3–20). Thorofare, NJ: Slack.

Law, M., & Dunbar, S. B. (2007). Person-environment-occupation model. In S. B. Dunbar (Ed.), *Occupational therapy models for intervention with children and families* (pp. 27–49). Thorofare, NJ: Slack.

Law, M., King, G., & Russell, D. (2005). Guiding therapist decisions about measuring outcomes in occupational therapy. In M. Law, C. Baum, & W. Dunn (Eds.), *Measuring occupational performance: Supporting best practice in occupational therapy* (2nd ed., pp. 33–47). Thorofare, NJ: Slack.

Lawton, M. P. (1972). Assessing the competence of older people. In D. P. Kent, R. Kastenbaum, & S. Sherwood (Eds.), *Research planning and action for the elderly: The power and potential of social science* (pp. 122–143). New York, NY: Behavioral Publications.

Legg, L., Drummond, A., & Langhorne, P. (2006). Occupational therapy for patients with problems in activities of daily living after stroke. *Cochrane Database of Systematic Reviews,* (4), 1–47. doi:10.1002/14651858.CD003585.pub2

Letts, L., & Bosch, J. (2005). Measuring occupational performance in basic activities of daily living. In M. Law, C. Baum, & W. Dunn (Eds.), *Measuring occupational performance: Supporting best practice in occupational therapy* (2nd ed., pp. 179–225). Thorofare, NJ: Slack.

Liddle, J., & McKenna, K. (2000). Quality of life: An overview of issues for use in occupational therapy outcome measurement. *Australian Occupational Therapy Journal, 47,* 77–85.

Liedberg, G. M., & Vrethem, M. (2009). Polyneuropathy, with and without neurogenic pain, and its impact on daily life activities—A descriptive study. *Disability and Rehabilitation, 31,* 1402–1408. doi:10.1080/09638280802621382

Lorch, A., & Herge, E. A. (2007). Using standardized assessments in practice. *OT Practice,* 17–22.

Lund, M. L., & Nygård, L. (2003). Incorporating or resisting assistive devices: Different approaches to achieving a desired occupational self-image. *OTJR: Occupation, Participation, and Health, 23,* 67–75.

Mackenzie, C., Wiprzycka, U., Hasher, L., & Goldstein, D. (2009). Associations between psychological distress, learning, and memory in spouse caregivers of older adults. *Journals of Gerontology Series B: Psychological Sciences & Social Sciences, 64B,* 742–746. doi:10.1093/geronb/gbp076

Mahoney, F. I., & Barthel, D. W. (1965). Functional evaluation: The Barthel Index. *Maryland State Medical Journal, 14,* 61–65.

Mathiowetz, V., Matuska, K. M., & Murphy, M. E. (2001). Efficacy of an energy conservation course for persons with multiple sclerosis. *Archives of Physical Medicine and Rehabilitation, 82,* 449–456.

Mathiowetz, V. G., Matuska, K. M., Finlayson, M. L., Luo, P., & Chen, H. Y. (2007). One-year follow-up to a randomized controlled trial of an energy conservation course for persons with multiple sclerosis. *International Journal of Rehabilitation Research, 30,* 305–313.

McKenna, K., & Scott, J. (2007). Do written education materials that use content and design principles improve older people's knowledge? *Australian Occupational Therapy Journal, 54,* 103–112. doi:10.1111/j.1440-1630.2006.00583.x

Meenan, R. F., Mason, J. H., Anderson, J. J., Guccione, A. A., & Kazis, L. E. (1992). AIMS2: The content and properties of a revised and expanded Arthritis Impact Measurement Scales Health Status Questionnaire. *Arthritis and Rheumatism, 35,* 1–10.

Melchert-McKearnan, K., Deitz, J., Engel, J. M., & White, O. (2000). Children with burn injuries: Purposeful versus rote exercise. *American Journal of Occupational Therapy, 54,* 381–390.

Missiuna, C., Pollock, N., Law, M., Walter, S., & Cavey, N. (2006). Examination of the Perceived Efficacy and Goal Setting System (PEGS) with children with disabilities, their parents, and teachers. *American Journal of Occupational Therapy, 60,* 204–214.

Moore, A. A., Endo, J. O., & Carter, M. K. (2003). Is there a relationship between excessive drinking and functional impairment in older persons? *Journal of the American Geriatric Society, 51,* 44–49.

Moye, J. (2005). Guardianship and conservatorship. In T. Grisso (Ed.), *Evaluating competencies: Forensic assessments and instruments* (2nd ed., pp. 309–390). doi:10.1007/b106006

Mullersdorf, M. (2000). Factors indicating need of rehabilitation: Occupational therapy needs among persons with long-term and/or recurrent pain. *International Journal of Rehabilitation Research, 23,* 281–294.

Nakanishi, M., Sawamura, K., Sato, S., Setoya, Y., & Anzai, N. (2010). Development of a clinical pathway for long-term inpatients with schizophrenia. *Psychiatry and Clinical Neurosciences, 64,* 99–103. doi:10.1111/j.1440-1819.2009.02040.x

National Center for Health Statistics. (2009). *Limitations in activities of daily living and instrumental activities of daily living, 2003-2007.* Retrieved from http://www.cdc.gov/nchs/health_policy/ADL_tables.htm

Nof, L., Rone-Adams, S., & Hart, D. L. (2007). Relation between payer source and functional outcomes, visits and treatment duration in US patients with lumbar dysfunction. *Internet Journal of Allied Health Sciences and Practice, 5*(2). Retrieved from http://ijahsp.nova.edu/articles/vol5num2/nof.htm

Nouri, F. M., & Lincoln, N. B. (1987). An Extended Activities of Daily Living Scale for stroke patients. *Clinical Rehabilitation, 1,* 301–305.

Novak, I., Cusick, A., & Lannin, N. (2009). Occupational therapy home programs for cerebral palsy: Double-blind, randomized, controlled trial. *Pediatrics, 124,* e606–e614. doi:10.1542/peds.2009-0288

Østensjø, S., Carlberg, E., & Vøllestad, N. (2005). The use and impact of assistive devices and other environmental modifications on everyday activities and care in young children with cerebral palsy. *Disability & Rehabilitation, 27,* 849–861. doi:10.1080/09638280400018619

Park, S., Fisher, A. G., & Velozo, C. A. (1994). Using the Assessment of Motor and Process Skills to compare occupational performance between clinic and home settings. *American Journal of Occupational Therapy, 48,* 697–709.

Pillastrini, P., Mugnai, R., Bonfiglioli, R., Curti, S., Mattioli, S., Maioli, M. G., . . . Violante, F. S. (2008). Evaluation of an occupational therapy program for patients with spinal cord injury. *Spinal Cord, 46,* 78–81.

Pincus, T., Swearingen, C., & Wolfe, F. (1999). Toward a Multidimensional Health Assessment Questionnaire (MDHAQ). *Arthritis & Rheumatism, 42,* 2220–2230.

Portney, L. G., & Watkins, M. P. (2009). *Foundations of clinical research: Applications to practice* (3rd ed.). Upper Saddle River, NJ: Pearson.

Provencher, V., Demers, L., & Gélinas, I. (2009). Home and clinical assessments of instrumental activities of daily living: What could explain the difference between settings in frail older adults, if any? *British Journal of Occupational Therapy, 72,* 339–348.

Radomski, M. V. (2008). Planning, guiding, and documenting practice. In M. V. Radomski & C. A. T. Latham (Eds.), *Occupational therapy for physical dysfunction* (6th ed., pp. 40–64). Philadelphia, PA: Lippincott Williams & Wilkins.

Resnick, B. (1998). Motivating older adults to perform functional activities. *Journal of Gerontological Nursing, 24*(11), 23–30.

Richardson, P. K. (2010). Use of standardized tests in pediatric practice. In J. Case-Smith & J. C. O'Brien (Eds.), *Occupational therapy for children* (6th ed., p. 243). Maryland Heights, MO: Mosby Elsevier.

Ripat, J. (2006). Function and impact of electronic aids to daily living for experienced users. *Technology & Disability, 18*, 79–87.

Robertson, S. C., & Colburn, A. P. (2000). Can we improve outcomes research by expanding research methods? *American Journal of Occupational Therapy, 54*, 541–543.

Robinson-Smith, G., Johnston, M. V., & Allen, J. (2000). Self-care, self-efficacy, quality of life, and depression after stroke. *Archives of Physical Medicine and Rehabilitation, 81*, 460–464.

Rogers, J. C., & Holm, M. B. (1994). *Performance Assessment of Self-Care Skills (PASS)* (Version 3.1). Unpublished manuscript, University of Pittsburgh, Pennsylvania.

Rogers, J. C., Holm, M. B., Beach, S., Schulz, R., Cipriani, J., Fox, A., & Starz, T. W. (2003). Concordance of four methods of disability assessment using performance in the home as the criterion method. *Arthritis Care & Research, 49*, 640–647.

Rogers, J. C., Holm, M. B., Burgio, L. D., Hsu, C., Hardin, J. M., & McDowell, B. (2000). Excess disability during morning care in nursing home residents with dementia. *International Psychogeriatrics, 12*, 267–282.

Russell, C., Fitzgerald, M. H., Williamson, P., Manor, D., & Whybrow, S. (2002). Independence as a practice issue in occupational therapy: The safety clause. *American Journal of Occupational Therapy, 56*, 369–379.

Sames, K. M. (2010). *Documenting occupational therapy practice* (2nd ed.). Upper Saddle River, NJ: Pearson.

Schell, B. A. B., & Schell, J. W. (Eds.). (2008). Professional reasoning as the basis of practice. In *Clinical and professional reasoning in occupational therapy* (pp. 3–35). Philadelphia, PA: Lippincott Williams & Wilkins.

Seo, Y., Roberts, B. L., LaFramboise, L., Yates, B. C., & Yurkovich, J. M. (2011). Predictors of modifications in instrumental activities of daily living in persons with heart failure. *Journal of Cardiovascular Nursing, 26*, 89–98.

Stewart, K. B. (2010). Purposes, processes, and methods of evaluation. In J. Case-Smith & J. C. O'Brien (Eds.), *Occupational therapy for children* (6th ed., pp. 193–211). Maryland Heights, MO: Mosby Elsevier.

Thornsson, A., & Grimby, G. (2001). Ability and perceived difficulty in daily activities in people with poliomyelitis sequelae. *Journal of Rehabilitation Medicine, 33*, 4–11.

Toth-Cohen, S. (2000). Role perceptions of occupational therapists providing support and education for caregivers of persons with dementia. *American Journal of Occupational Therapy, 54*, 509–515.

Uniform Data System for Medical Rehabilitation. (2005). *IRF PAI rating tutorial* [DVD]. Retrieved from http://www.udsmr.org/WebModules/Brochures.aspx

Vanage, S. M., Gilbertson, K. K., & Mathiowetz, V. (2003). Effects of an energy conservation course on fatigue impact for persons with progressive multiple sclerosis. *American Journal of Occupational Therapy, 57*, 315–323.

Wade, D. T. (2009). Goal setting in rehabilitation: An overview of what, why, and how. *Clinical Rehabilitation, 23*, 291–295.

Williams, J. H., Drinka, T. J. K., Greenberg, J. R., Farrel-Holtan, J., Euhardy, R., & Schram, M. (1991). Development and testing of the Assessment of Living Skills and Resources (ALSAR) in elderly community-dwelling veterans. *Gerontologist, 31*, 84–91.

World Health Organization. (2002). *Towards a common language for functioning, disability, and health: ICF*. Retrieved from http://www.who.int/classifications/icf/training/icfbeginnersguide.pdf

For additional resources on the subjects discussed in this chapter, visit http://thePoint.lww.com/Willard-Spackman12e.

CHAPTER 48

Education

Yvonne L. Swinth

LEARNING OBJECTIVES

After reading this chapter, you will be able to:

1. Identify different educational settings in which an occupational therapist may provide services
2. Describe the occupational therapy process within an educational setting
3. Recognize key requirements of occupational therapy services under the Individuals with Disabilities Education Improvement Act
4. Describe the difference between an Individualized Family Service Plan (IFSP), Individualized Education Program (IEP), and Individualized Transition Plan (ITP)
5. Describe how a disability may affect the occupation of student

OUTLINE

Occupational Therapy in Educational Settings

Occupational therapy practitioners work in a variety of educational settings. These may include public schools, charter schools, private schools, alternative schools, vocational schools, and university settings. Across these settings, practitioners work with children and adolescents, generally from birth to 21 years old in a variety of contexts. For example, an occupational therapy practitioner might work with infants and families in a 0 to 3 center, young children in a preschool on the playground, elementary school age children in the classroom, or adolescents in an alternative high school at a worksite. Occupational therapists might also work with an older adult client who is returning to school to learn a new skill after an injury (e.g., work hardening, job retraining) or for personal enhancement (i.e., leisure activity). Public schools and early intervention are the most common work setting for occupational therapy practitioners; more than 24% of all practitioners who are members of the American Occupational

Therapy Association (AOTA) identify public school/early intervention as their primary work setting (AOTA, 2009a). According to the Bureau of Labor Statistics, U.S. Department of Labor (2012), continued growth is expected for the profession of occupational therapy, including working in educational settings, early intervention, and transition to work environments. It is also anticipated that the niche for occupational therapists working in other educational settings (e.g., colleges, universities, community colleges, and continuing education venues) will grow as these children become young adults and desire to continue their education.

The primary focus of this chapter is on occupational performance within early intervention and public schools because this is the most common educational setting that employs occupational therapy practitioners. However, the reader is encouraged to consider the wide variety of educational settings that may benefit from the skills and expertise of an occupational therapist. These types of occupational therapy services may be innovative and preventive and may increase the occupational performance of individuals in ways that historically have not been explored or considered. For example, occupational therapy practitioners might develop a health promotion program for an entire school system to increase students' engagement in physical activity or work in collaboration with the school counselor to develop a social skills program that recognizes and addresses the complexity of needs in today's schools. Colleges or universities may benefit from an occupational therapist's expertise in addressing universal design, access to curricular materials for students with disabilities, or ergonomic needs of staff and students. For example, an occupational therapist may work with a disability counselor at a university to help with the decision making, procurement, and implementation of assistive technology to support written communication for a student with physical disabilities. Many of the principles that are discussed in this chapter can be generalized to any educational setting.

Legislation Guiding Practice

A variety of legislative and funding sources support occupational therapy services in different educational settings. Although the Individuals with Disabilities Education Improvement Act (2004) specifically addresses services in early intervention and schools that receive public funds, every educational setting must meet the requirements of Section 504 of the Rehabilitation Act (1973) as well as the Americans with Disabilities Act of 1990 (ADA) (P.L. 101-336). Thus, occupational therapy services in settings such as private schools, universities, and continuing education venues can be provided under Section 504 and the ADA. Section 504 supports reasonable accommodations for individuals with a disability, a history of a disability, or a perceived disability if accommodations are needed to allow the individual to participate in educational settings. The ADA is a civil rights act and provides protection to individuals with disabilities similar to those provided to individuals on the basis of race, color, sex, national origin, age, and religion. Further, the ADA supports the right of individuals with disabilities to have equal opportunities to live, work, and play within society (including educational settings). Table 48.1 provides an overview of legislation and funding that support occupational therapy services in educational settings.

Practice within the public schools is guided by federal legislation, with a focus on the occupation of education and the role of the student. Occupational therapists began working in the schools after 1935 when federal grants to the states created Crippled Children's Services under a special section of the Social Securities Act. Initially, these services were provided in segregated settings or special schools and primarily to children with orthopedic and neurological impairments. In 1975, the Education for All Handicapped Children Act (EHA) (P.L. 94-142) was enacted. This act required states to provide special education and **related services**, including occupational therapy, to all eligible children ages 6 through 21 years. Amendments to the EHA in 1986, P.L. 99-457, added services for preschoolers (ages 3 to 5 years) and provided incentives for states to develop statewide systems for providing early intervention services to infants, toddlers, and their families. In 1990, the EHA was renamed the Individuals with Disabilities Education Act, or IDEA (P.L. 101-476), and additional services were added. These included assistive technology devices and services, services for children from birth to 3 years old, transition services (to prepare them for life after school), and increased focus, funds, and programs for children with emotional disturbances. Further amendments were made to the IDEA in 1997 (P.L. 105-117), which mostly fine-tuned the original intent of the law (AOTA, 2007). Increasingly, there has been a greater emphasis on access to and participation in the general education curriculum for students with disabilities (see Box 48.1).

The latest amendments were completed in December 2004, and the name was changed to the Individuals with Disabilities Education Improvement Act—IDEA 2004 (P.L. 108-446). These amendments continued the trend toward increased access to and participation and performance in the general education curriculum. This latest reauthorization also increased the emphasis on prereferral intervention or **early intervening services** (commonly referred to as *response to intervention* or RtI) by bringing more of the IDEA 2004 in line with the No Child Left Behind Act of 2001. The amendments also place an emphasis on the use of scientifically based (research-based, evidence-based) practices, high-quality preservice training and professional education, dispute resolution without going to court, increased representation of minorities in fields such as teaching and occupational therapy, and the use and development of appropriate technology

TABLE 48.1 Occupational Therapy Services in Educational Settings

Legislation/Sources of Funding	Population Served	Role of Occupational Therapist
Individuals with Disabilities Education Improvement Act (IDEA) of 2004	Students who are eligible for special education and require the related service of occupational therapy in order to receive free appropriate public education (FAPE) in the least restrictive environment (LRE). (IDEA 2004 is applicable only for students [age 0 to 21 years] who receive special education services through their public school setting.)	To collaborate with the Individualized Education Program (IEP) team to determine the student's needs and then to provide services as outlined in the IEP in order to support student performance relevant to the educational environment.
Section 504 of the Rehabilitation Act	Students who have a disability, a history of a disability, or a perceived disability that affects their performance in school. (In the public schools, these are generally students who are not eligible for special education.) Students who meet the definition of "individual with a disability" are defined as those individuals who have a physical or mental impairment that substantially limits one or more major life activities.	To collaborate with the 504 team to provide the accommodations and adaptations that the student needs to access the school environment and services.
Americans with Disabilities Act (ADA)	The ADA ensures equal opportunity for individuals with disabilities in employment, state and local government services, public accommodations, commercial facilities, and transportation. Thus, it is a civil rights legislation that supports participation in the educational setting by students who have a disability.	To provide support through consultation and monitoring to ensure that students with disabilities have access to and can participate in the educational setting. It often involves working with environmental adaptations, accommodations, and the use of assistive devices.
Other funding sources • General education funds (for public schools) • Private insurance • Private agencies (e.g., United Cerebral Palsy) • State agencies (e.g., Division of Vocational Rehabilitation)	Any student who needs the support of an occupational therapy practitioner.	To support student performance in occupations relevant to the educational environment.

Adapted from Swinth, Y., Chandler, B., Hanft, B., Jackson, L., & Shepherd, J. (2003). *Personnel issues in school-based occupational therapy: Supply and demand, preparation, and certification and licensure.* Gainesville, FL: Center on Personnel Studies in Special Education. Retrieved from http://www.coe.ufl.edu/copsse

BOX 48.1 Key Changes in the Individuals with Disabilities Education Act of 1997

1. Participation of children and youths with disabilities in state and districtwide assessment programs
2. Expanded parent participation in any decisions made about their child
3. Addition of transition planning starting at age 14 years and younger if needed
4. Supporting professional development to ensure that all school personnel have the needed knowledge and skills to educate children with disabilities

Adapted from National Information Center for Children and Youth with Disabilities. (1998). The IDEA amendments of 1997. *NICHY News Digest, 26* (Rev. ed.). Retrieved from http://nichcy.org/wp-content/uploads/docs/nd26pdf.pdf

BOX 48.2 Key Assumptions of the Individuals with Disabilities Education Act

1. Equality of opportunity for all individuals
2. Full participation (empowerment)
3. Independent living
4. Economic self-sufficiency

Adapted from Silverstein, R. (2000). An overview of the emerging disability policy framework: A guidepost for analyzing public policy. *Iowa Law Review, 85*, 1757–1802.

(including assistive technology). It should be noted that this emphasis on the use of research to inform practice is applicable across all educational settings, not just the public schools, owing to both policy priorities and the priorities of the AOTA.

Since 1975, the key goals of the IDEA 2004 (originally the EHA) have remained the same (see Box 48.2), with an increasing shift from the old paradigm of "if we cannot fix them, we exclude them" to a new paradigm of "disability as a natural and normal part of the human experience" (Silverstein, 2000, p. 1761). Thus, the role of occupational therapy under the IDEA 2004 has shifted to include a focus on contextual factors such as access to the environment so that individuals with disabilities can participate in their environments rather than on "fixing" the disability of the child or adolescent.

The IDEA 2004 has four parts, A through D; however, this chapter will primarily address Parts B and C. (Part A addresses the general provisions of the IDEA, and Part D addresses research and training.) A positive addition to the 2004 amendments is the inclusion of related service providers, including occupational therapists, as a priority for monies and support, under Part D, related to research and training. Under Part C of the IDEA 2004, occupational therapy can be a primary service for infants and toddlers from birth to 2 years of age who are eligible for early intervention services (AOTA, 2007). Part B of the IDEA 2004 identifies occupational therapy, as a related service, for children ages 3 through 21 years for whom the team determines the service is *necessary* in order for students to benefit from their special education program. Two key concepts of Part B of the IDEA 2004 are a **free appropriate public education** (**FAPE**) in the **least restrictive environment** (**LRE**) (see Box 48.3 for definition of key terms found within the IDEA 2004). The IDEA 2004 allows each state and local education agency some latitude in how the federal legislation will be implemented as long as the FAPE and LRE provisions

BOX 48.3 Common Terms in the Individuals with Disabilities Education Act 2004

Early intervening services: Academic and behavior support to succeed in general education but is not part of special education.

Free appropriate public education (FAPE): Special education and related services provided at public expense that meets the standards of the state education agency (SEA).

General education: The environment, curriculum, and activities that are available to all students.

General education curriculum: The same curriculum as for nondisabled children.

Individualized Education Program (IEP): A commitment of services that ensures that an appropriate program is developed that meets the unique educational needs of children ages 3 to 21 years.

Individualized Family Services Plan (IFSP): A commitment of services that ensures that an appropriate program is developed that meets the unique developmental and preeducational needs of children 0 to 3 years old and their families.

Least restrictive environment (LRE): The environment that provides maximum interaction with nondisabled peers and is consistent with the needs of the child/student.

No Child Left Behind: P.L. 107-110, aimed at improving the educational performance of all students by increasing accountability for student achievement. It emphasizes standards-based education reform with the belief that high expectations will result in success for all students.

Related services: Transportation and such developmental, corrective, and other supportive services (including speech-language, audiology, psychological, and physical and occupational therapy services) needed to help the child benefit from special education.

Response to intervention (RtI): An integrated approach to service delivery that includes both general and special education and includes high-quality instruction, interventions matched to student need, frequent progress monitoring, and data-based decision making.

Special education: Specially designed instruction at no cost to parents to meet the unique needs of a child with a disability.

Adapted from National Council on Disabilities. (2000). *Back to school on civil rights: Advancing the federal commitment to leave no child behind.* Washington, DC: Author.

are not compromised. Thus, there are differences across states and local programs regarding the specifics of how services are provided.

The purpose of the IDEA 2004 is "to ensure that all children with disabilities have available to them a free appropriate public education that emphasizes special education and related services designed to meet their unique needs and prepare them for further education, employment and independent living" (Section 300.1). Occupational therapy practitioners in the public school setting provide services within this structure and are generally a related (supportive) service to the educational program (specially designed instruction). Students come to school to get an education; and in the schools, occupational therapy serves this priority.

Occupational Therapy Process in Educational Settings

A variety of factors affect the occupational therapy process in educational environments. Services that are provided under the structure of the IDEA 2004 often are influenced by the educational team. Collaboration across stakeholders through effective teaming often results in positive outcomes for children and adolescents (Hanft & Shepherd, 2008). Regardless of the educational setting in which the practitioner works, a team of professionals typically influence the occupational therapy process.

Decision Making

Effective and efficient delivery of services in the school environment requires a systematic process for team decision making and problem solving. There is a tendency by professionals to identify a need and immediately start proposing and implementing solutions without first identifying the necessary outcomes needed for the student to participate in the educational environment. Educational teams have access to a variety of tools that support a systematic process of decision making and team problem solving (e.g., McGill Action Planning System [MAPS], Choosing Outcomes and Accommodations for Children). Through working with educational teams, practitioners are better able to identify and address priority educational needs.

Educational Teams

The concept of teaming, or collaborating as a team, to make decisions about the program and services to be provided has been a guiding principle of occupational therapy services in public schools since the inception of federal law (Hanft & Shepherd, 2008). With the reauthorization in 1997, the IDEA became more explicit regarding the emphasis on teaming and collaboration among professionals and families to make effective decisions about student need(s). The IDEA 1997 clearly specified that whenever decisions are made about a student, the parents or caregivers must be involved. Two types of teams are involved in a student's program: the evaluation team and the Individualized Education Program (IEP) team (Individualized Family Service Plan [IFSP] for children 0 to 3 years and Individualized Transition Plan [ITP] for adolescents 16 years and older). Both teams must include qualified professionals who are knowledgeable about the student and his or her need(s). If a decision is being made about occupational therapy involvement in a student's program, then an occupational therapist must be involved in the teaming process. In the public schools, the specific composition of each team is driven by the student's needs and may include general and special education teachers, therapists (physical, occupational, and speech), psychologists, counselors, parents, the student, and different community members. The focus of the team decision-making process must be on student outcomes and performance with an emphasis on participation in the general education environment as appropriate.

In the public schools, a team of qualified individuals, which may include an occupational therapist, school psychologist, special education and general education teachers, physical therapist, speech-language pathologist, and others, is responsible for conducting the evaluation. The purpose of the evaluation process is not only to determine the student's needs in order to have access to and participate in the educational environment to the maximum extent appropriate but also to determine the student's needs in order to perform within the school setting. Additionally, the IDEA 2004 requires that the evaluation help to determine services that will support a student's ability to demonstrate outcomes with a focus on the general education curriculum. Therefore, the evaluation process is driven by contextual factors (the school environment) and student (client) needs (Bazyk & Case-Smith, 2010; Chapparo & Lowe, 2012; Dunn, Brown, & McGuigan, 1994). In other educational settings, although the IDEA 2004 requirement to have a "team of qualified professionals" is not mandated, it is consistent with best practice. In most other settings, the team will be smaller but seldom does an occupational therapy practitioner make decisions in isolation. Regardless of the setting, the emphasis of the evaluation is on the occupational performance area of *education*. However, other areas of occupation such as social participation might need to be addressed if participation in these areas is affecting educational performance.

Evaluation Requirements in the Schools

One primary role of the occupational therapy practitioner, as part of the team, under IDEA 2004, is to contribute to the evaluation process. Ideally, this is a collaborative process across team members (Hanft & Shepherd, 2008). The practitioner's contribution might help the educational team determine eligibility for special education and/or related services as well as identify needed supports, accommodations, adaptations and/or modifications. Several key requirements underlie the evaluation process in schools under the IDEA 2004 that occupational therapy practitioners may not have to address in other settings. These requirements are briefly discussed.

Referral

Generally, the process of referral within the school setting is different from that in a clinical setting. As with any procedures within special education, specific steps can vary from state to state or from setting to setting. However, in most public school situations, if there is a concern about student performance, a team of professionals will discuss and implement different strategies within the general education classroom before referring the student for special education. If these strategies are not successful, then the student is referred for a special education evaluation to determine eligibility for services. Occupational therapy may or may not be involved in this step of the process. If the occupational therapist is not involved in the initial evaluation process, then the team may request an occupational therapy evaluation at any time after determining that the student is eligible for special education. If the occupational therapist is working in a state where the occupational therapy practice act requires a physician referral for services, then such a referral may be necessary before the implementation of services. If a physician refers a student for an occupational therapy evaluation, this referral does not guarantee services in a school setting. Generally, the occupational therapist in the public school must first ensure that the student is eligible for special education and then determine whether services are necessary for the student to benefit from his or her education program.

In other educational settings, the referral process may be less formal. For example, in some university settings, a referral might come through the center for disability access (e.g., a student access concern) or human resources (e.g., a staff ergonomic concern). Therapists who provide services in these types of settings might need to develop a referral system to ensure that the process meets the needs of the client(s). If a physician referral is required by a state practice act, then the occupational therapist must comply with this requirement regardless of the setting.

As with other occupational therapy practice areas, the **evaluation** process in the schools is dynamic and ongoing and often continues during intervention (Stewart, 2010). According to the IDEA 2004, the evaluation determines whether a child has a disability and the nature and extent of the special education and related services that the child needs (Section 300.15). The IDEA 2004 does not require use of a specific type of **assessment** method or tool. Rather, it requires that a variety of tools and strategies be used to gather relevant "functional and developmental information" related to enabling the child to "be involved in and progress in the general education curriculum" (Section 300.304[1]). In addition, the evaluation should help to determine the child's educational needs and how the disability affects the child's participation in school activities.

A child does not "qualify" for occupational therapy on the basis of testing under the IDEA 2004. Instead, occupational therapy services should be recommended by the occupational therapist, based on the evaluation results, and provided for a child if necessary for the child to "benefit from their special education program." Even though the evaluation process in the schools is guided by federal law, occupation remains the core of the occupational therapy practitioner's theoretical perspective. Within the educational setting, therapy practitioners draw on the appropriate frames of reference to guide the evaluation process (Frolek-Clark, Polichino, & Jackson, 2004).

The evaluation process should be individualized (student centered) and should use a top-down approach (Chapparo & Lowe, 2012; Coster, 1998). This means that the occupational therapy evaluation should start by looking at student performance within context versus evaluating specific client factors out of context. As with any occupational therapy evaluation, a broad view of the student (client) must be considered. Thus, the emphasis is on the educational context, including physical, temporal, social, and cultural considerations. Within the educational setting, the focus of special education and related services is on student outcomes. If the educational staff and/or parents require services (e.g., specialized training) for the student to reach his or her outcomes, then the practitioner is responsible for addressing these needs (Kramer & Hinojosa, 2009) as well as broader systems issues (e.g., curriculum, environmental adaptations) that might require occupational therapy input and support (Bazyk & Case-Smith, 2010; Chapparo & Lowe, 2012; Muhlenhaupt, 2003; Ziviani, Kopeshke, & Wadley, 2006). Under the IDEA 2004, occupational therapy services are supportive in nature in order to help the child be successful in school as well as in after-school activities (Giangreco, 2001). Additionally, services can be provided "on behalf of" the child and "to the parents, teachers, and other staff" so that these individuals can better support the child's learning (see Table 48.2).

The occupational therapist in the school setting focuses his or her evaluation on what is needed for the student to engage and participate in meaningful and purposeful school occupations. The occupational therapy evaluation addresses the student's areas of strengths and concerns in areas of occupation, including activities of daily living (ADL), education/work, play/leisure, and social participation. In each of these areas, the

TABLE 48.2 Clients to Consider during the Occupational Therapy Evaluation Process

Client	Evaluation Consideration(s)
Student	Gather data regarding the occupational profile and occupational performance
Parents/educational staff	On the basis of the student's occupational profile and occupational performance, determine whether there is any need for specific training, support, and/or dissemination of information.
System	On the basis of the student's occupational profile and occupational performance, determine whether any system supports (e.g., environmental modifications, curriculum development) are needed.

occupational therapist addresses the performance skills and the student's physical, sensory, neurological, and cognitive/mental function. First, an occupational profile is developed in collaboration with the team, including the family and student, as appropriate. This profile is followed by an analysis of the student's occupational performance within the educational setting.

Following is a brief description of the occupational therapy evaluation process. The specific role of the occupational therapist during the evaluation process for any given student will depend on the expertise and skills of all the team members as well as the referral concerns. There may be overlap across professional disciplines regarding specific skills assessed (e.g., gross motor skills with physical therapy, feeding with speech therapy, or psychosocial issues with psychology), but the input of an occupational therapist is needed because of the unique emphasis of occupational therapy on occupation and context/environmental factors that affect occupational performance.

As in all other settings in which occupational therapy practitioners work, the occupational therapist is responsible for the administration of the evaluation methods and measures, the interpretation and documentation of results, and the communication of evaluation results with other team members. However, if an occupational therapy assistant is part of the team, he or she may contribute to any part of the process under the direct supervision of the occupational therapist.

When occupational therapy is involved in the evaluation process, the occupational therapist can use the "Occupational Therapy Practice Framework" (AOTA, 2008a) as a guide to the process. As described in the following section, the special education process closely parallels the occupational therapy process described in the framework.

Occupational Profile

The occupational profile is developed by gathering data from the student, family, and educational staff (AOTA, 2008a). The occupational therapy assistant, community providers, and others who know the student also may contribute to this process. Often, the development of the occupational profile occurs over time. Several assessments and procedures that have been designed for use in the educational setting may be used to develop the occupational profile. Table 48.3 and Appendix II lists some of the assessments and procedures that are used in educational settings.

Most of these assessments are process oriented and must be completed with input from all team members, including the student and family. Ideally, the assessments should have a problem-solving focus that addresses the student's strengths and concerns as well as contextual factors that may affect student performance and outcomes. The assessments also will help the occupational therapy practitioner to identify strengths and challenges specific to the student's performance patterns and activity demands. By completing one or more of these process-oriented assessments, the occupational therapy practitioner will have addressed most of the occupational profile questions that are outlined within the "Occupational Therapy Practice Framework" (see Box 48.4).

For example, the MAPS consists of seven specific questions that support the planning process and identification of team-generated outcomes for students with disabilities (O'Brien, Forest, Snow, Pearpoint, & Hasbury, 1989). The questions include the following:

1. What is the student's history?
2. What are your dreams for the student?
3. What are your fears for the student?
4. Who is the student? (one-word statements that describe the student)
5. What are the student's strengths, gifts, and abilities?
6. What are the student's needs?
7. What would the student's ideal day at school look like and what must be done to make it happen?

A typical MAPS planning session can take up to 2 hours. The entire team (parents, students, therapists, and teachers) as well as other invited members (siblings, other family members, or community members) provide input in answer to each question. The questions are not quick or easy to answer, but the result of a good planning session is a strong foundation from which to develop the student's program, including any occupational therapy services. The process focuses on the value of integrating the student in neighborhood schools and in general education classes in order to develop friendships and to ensure a high-quality education for the child.

TABLE 48.3 Common Evaluation Methods and Tools Used in Educational Settings

Assessment	Participation		Areas of Occupation					Client Factors	
	Characteristics	*Contextual Factors*	*Activity*			*Experience*		*Performance Skills*	*Abilities*
			Activity Interests	*Activity Choices*	*Subjective Experience*	*Personal Meaning*	*Satisfaction*		
Part I: Process-Oriented Assessment Tools: support gathering data for the occupational profile and analysis of occupational performance									
Assessment of Motor and Process Skills (School Version [AMPS])	♦	♦	♦	♦	♦	♦	♦	♦	♦
Children's Assessment of Participation and Enjoyment (CAPE)/Preferences from Activities of Children (PAC)	♦	♦	♦	♦	♦	♦	♦	♦	♦
Choosing Outcomes and Accommodations for Children (COACH)	♦	♦	♦	♦	♦	♦	♦	♦	♦
Canadian Occupational Performance Measure (COPM)	♦	♦	♦	♦	♦	♦	♦	♦	♦
Making Action Plans (MAPs)	♦	♦	♦	♦	♦	♦	♦	♦	♦
Miller Fun Scales			♦	♦		♦	♦	♦	♦
Planning Alternative Tomorrows with Hope (PATH)	♦	♦	♦	♦	♦	♦	♦	♦	♦
Perceived Efficacy and Goal Setting Scale (PEGS)	♦	♦	♦	♦	♦	♦	♦	♦	♦
Interview with the student, educational staff, parents, and others	♦	♦	♦	♦	♦	♦	♦	♦	♦
School Function Assessment (SFA)	♦	♦		♦				♦	♦
Skilled observation	♦	♦	♦	♦	♦	♦	♦	♦	♦
Vermont Interdependent Services Team Approach (VISTA)	♦	♦	♦	♦	♦	♦	♦	♦	♦
Part II: Assessments of Client Factors: supports analysis of occupational performance with specific performance skills, patterns, and tasks									
Beery Developmental Test of Visual Motor Skills (Beery VMI)								♦	♦
Bruininks-Oseretsky Test of Motor Proficiency-2 (BOT-2)								♦	♦
Children's Handwriting Evaluation Scale (CHES)								♦	♦
DeGangi-Berk Test of Sensory Integration								♦	♦
Development Test of Visual Perception (DVPT)								♦	♦
Evaluation Tool of Children's Handwriting (ETCH)								♦	♦
Gross Motor Function Measure (GMFM)	♦						♦	♦	
Knox Preschool Play Scale				♦				♦	
Interest Checklist			♦						
Leisure Diagnostic Battery	♦	♦		♦	♦				
Minnesota Handwriting Assessment								♦	♦
Motor Free Visual Perception Test (MVPT)								♦	♦
Peabody Developmental Motor Scales -2 (PDMs-2)								♦	♦
Pediatric Evaluation of Disability Inventory (PEDI)	♦	♦						♦	♦
Sensory Integration and Praxis Test (SIPT)	♦	♦						♦	♦
Sensory Profile (Infant/Toddler)	♦							♦	♦
Sensory Profile (Adolescent/Adult)									
Social Skills Rating System	♦					♦	♦	♦	
Test of Handwriting Skills								♦	♦
Test of Visual Perceptual Skills (TVPS)								♦	♦
Test of Visual Motor Skills (TVMS)								♦	♦

BOX 48.4 Occupational Profile Questions from the Occupational Therapy Practice Framework (Adapted for the Educational Setting)

1. Who is the student?
2. Why was the student referred to special education and/or for an occupational therapy evaluation in the schools?
3. In what areas of educational occupations (activities of daily living, education, work, play/leisure, and/or social participation) are the student successful, and what areas are causing problems or risks?
4. What contexts support engagement in desired educational occupations, and what contexts are inhibiting engagement?
5. What is the student's occupational history?
6. What are the student's, family's, and educational staff's priorities and desired target outcomes?

Adapted from American Occupational Therapy Association (2008a). Occupational therapy practice framework: Domain and process, 2nd edition. *American Journal of Occupational Therapy, 62,* 625–683.

By the time the team members are addressing question 6 ("What are the student's needs?"), they have the background to be able to establish both short- and long-term outcomes. These outcome goals are then used to guide a discussion regarding the student's ideal day and how to get there.

Analysis of Occupational Performance

Often concurrent with the development of the occupational profile, the occupational therapist works with the team to determine whether more specific assessments are needed to help further determine a student's needs. Within the educational setting, the occupational therapist addresses performance in all areas of occupation as it relates to the child's educational needs (see Table 48.4). Often, the process-oriented tools not only help with the development of the occupational profile but also help the occupational therapist better understand contextual factors, potential "whole-school approaches," and curricular and extracurricular issues. These tools help the occupational therapist to communicate observations of the person-activity-environment fit as it relates to the student's occupational performance in school.

If it is determined that additional information about occupational performance related to physical, sensory, neurological, and/or mental functions of the student is needed, the occupational therapist may use standardized or nonstandardized assessments that focus on client factors (see Chapter 19). These

TABLE 48.4 Occupational Performance Areas Addressed from the Occupational Therapy Practice Framework (Adapted for the Educational Setting)

Occupational Performance Area	How Addressed in the Educational Setting
Activities of daily living (basic and instrumental)	Cares for basic self needs in school (e.g., eating, toileting, managing shoes and coats, dressing up and down for physical education [PE]); uses transportation system and uses communication devices to interact with others
Education	Participates and performs in the educational environment including academic (e.g., math, reading, writing), nonacademic (e.g., lunch, recess, after-school activities), prevocational, and vocational activities
Work	Develops interests, aptitudes, and skills necessary for engaging in work or volunteer activities for transition to community life on graduation from school
Play/leisure	Identifies and engages in age-appropriate toys, games, and leisure experiences; participates in art, music, sports, and after-school activities
Social participation	Interacts with peers, teachers, and other educational personnel during academic and nonacademic educational activities including extracurricular and preparation for work activities

Adapted from Swinth, Y., Chandler, B., Hanft, B., Jackson, L., & Shepherd, J. (2003). *Personnel issues in school-based occupational therapy: Supply and demand, preparation, and certification and licensure.* Gainesville, FL: Center on Personnel Studies in Special Education. Retrieved from http://www.coe.ufl.edu/copsse

assessments can help to determine specific information about occupational performance but should not be used without one or more of the process-oriented assessments. Additionally, the occupational therapist may use observation, parent or teacher interviews, and file review to support the analysis of a student's performance. Case Study 48.1 describes the process of developing an occupational profile for Kristi, a junior high school student with cerebral palsy, as well as other steps of the occupational therapy process.

These findings and recommendations were included in the special education evaluation report, and the team used them to develop Kristi's special education program. Once her program was developed, the team discussed Kristi's need for occupational therapy support to meet her educational goals and objectives.

CASE STUDY 48.1 Process for Developing an Occupational Profile for Kristi, a 13-Year-Old Student with Cerebral Palsy

Background

Kristi is a 13-year-old student with tetraplegia cerebral palsy. See Appendix I for more details about cerebral palsy. She has received occupational therapy in the past in both clinical and school-based settings. Kristi and her family had recently moved, and the education team in her new school district decided to complete an evaluation to determine her educational needs.

Occupational Profile

The occupational therapist started gathering data for the occupational profile by talking to Kristi and her family and reviewing Kristi's past records. Through this process, the occupational therapist began to develop a summary of Kristi's occupational history and her strengths and concerns in the areas of occupation related to Kristi's educational program. The therapist then observed Kristi in her academic courses, physical education (PE) class, lunch, and transitional periods (e.g., on and off the bus, between classes). The team also met with Kristi and her parents to complete a McGill Action Planning System.

Analysis of Occupational Performance

On the basis of the data that had been gathered, the occupational therapist summarized Kristi's occupational performance (strengths and concerns) related to most of Kristi's physical, sensory, neurological, and/or mental functions. Because Kristi had some difficulty with handwriting, the therapist also completed a Test of Visual Perceptual Skills and a Test of Visual Motor Skills to assess potential underlying client factors affecting Kristi's handwriting performance. The therapist also completed a manual muscle test to determine Kristi's strength and range of motion.

Summary

The occupational therapist summarized the following findings and recommendations to the educational team:

Occupational Performance Area	Strengths and Concerns
Activities of daily living (basic and instrumental)	Kristi is able to take care of her basic self-care needs within her school environment at this time. However, she has difficulty with some dressing activities that could affect her ability to participate in PE activities when she moves to the junior high and high school settings. Kristi and her mother also want Kristi to take a cooking class as soon as possible to determine Kristi's need for adaptive equipment for cooking. Kristi uses a school bus with a lift to get to and from school. She is able to communicate with her peers and teachers without any difficulty.
Education	Kristi is able to participate and complete assignments in her general education classes with accommodations and adaptations. She requires additional time to complete written assignments and uses a computer for longer papers. She needs to develop the self-determination skills necessary to independently problem-solve and implement accommodations/adaptations.
Work	Kristi states that she would like to be a lawyer or special education teacher. At age 14 years, the team will collaborate with Kristi and her parents to begin to develop her transition plan. This plan will support the assessment and address her needs for future environments.
Play/leisure	Kristi rides horses, swims at the YMCA, and enjoys playing computer games and watching television
Social participation	Kristi tends to keep to herself at school. Her mother states that Kristi is very social when at home with her family but that she has minimal interaction with other students her age. Kristi reports that she enjoys sports and that even though she cannot play, she would like to be involved by keeping scores or helping in some other way.

Intervention

Occupational therapy services address a student's performance based on the evaluation results in order to support the student's participation in the curriculum, access to the school environment, and participation in extracurricular activities (see Figures 48.1 and 48.2). Within educational settings, occupational therapy practitioners need to be familiar with and understand the educational environment in which they work as well the legislation and/or funding source(s) that support their involvement in the particular education setting.

Factors That Influence Occupational Therapy Interventions in Educational Environments

In addition to the setting and legislation, a variety of factors affect the planning and implementation of intervention by occupational therapy practitioners within educational environments. These include the unique characteristics of the system, the range of services provided, and the research evidence supporting intervention.

Unique Characteristics of the System

Each educational setting has unique characteristics that must be considered in planning and implementing intervention. Even within the same school district, different schools have unique strengths and barriers. Many occupational therapists working in educational settings are itinerant and work among three or more schools. Variability can make it challenging for therapists to keep track of the uniqueness of different settings. Additionally, the different legislation (e.g., Section 504 of the Rehabilitation Act, 1973; ADA, 1990) and different emphasis (e.g., public schools, universities, continuing education, virtual classroom) also affect the uniqueness of the system. Therapists in educational settings need to attend to systemic issues, changes, and challenges in order to provide the most effective services.

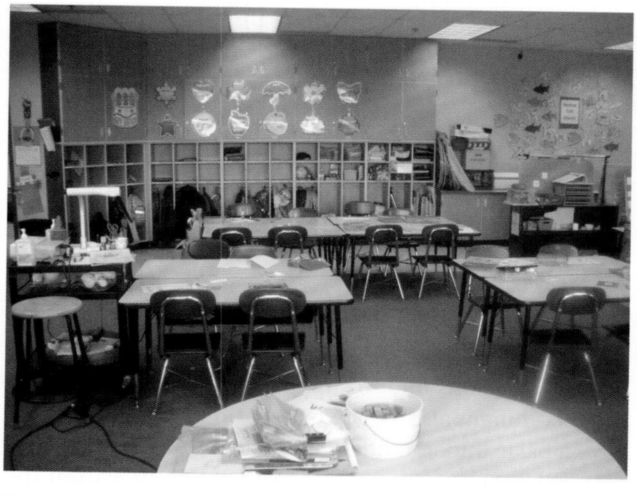

FIGURE 48.1 Occupational therapists may work with teachers to help engineer a classroom to support student participation.

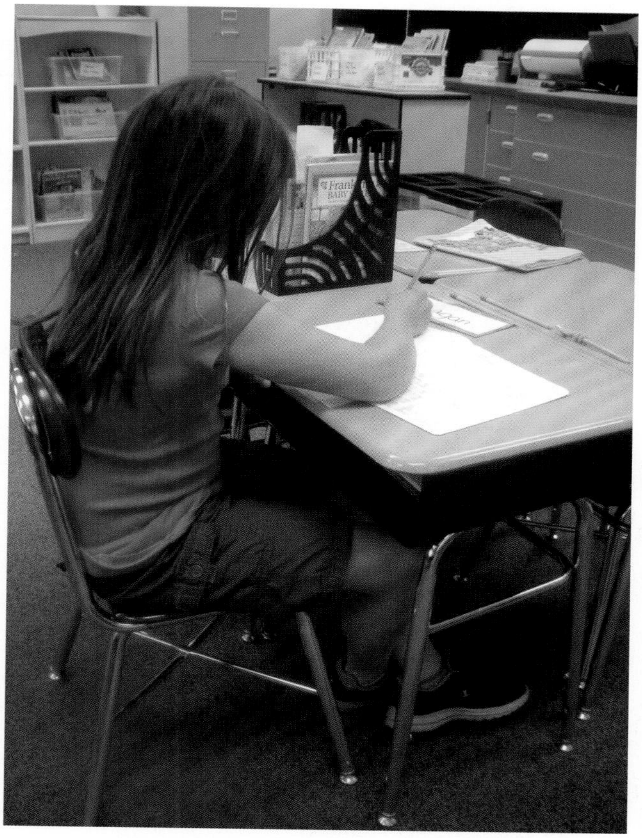

FIGURE 48.2 Occupational therapy works with classroom staff to support proper positioning in the classroom.

Range of Services

Occupational therapy practitioners provide a range of services in educational settings. Intervention may include hands-on services (such as one-on-one or group activities) or team supports to identify and implement environmental adaptations and modifications to the physical layout of the school campus or the classroom. Finally, services may include system supports, which are activities such as working with the curriculum committee of a district to establish a handwriting curriculum or working with an elementary school principal to help design an accessible play area to be used during recess (AOTA, 2012a; Hanft & Shepherd, 2008) (see Table 48.5 for examples of the range of services in the schools). Regardless of how services are provided, practitioners working in public schools must be aware of curricular issues such as education reform, standards-based assessment, and the requirements of general education. The IDEA 2004 requires

TABLE 48.5 Occupational Therapy Interventions in School Settings[a]

Performance Skill	Student Interventions	Educational Staff Interventions	Systems Intervention
Process skills			
• Energy • Knowledge • Temporal orientation • Organizing space and objects • Adaptation	• Learning about self-regulation/ levels of arousal and attention • Use of sensory media during intervention • Sensory integrative techniques • Initiates activities and sustains attention to complete them • Organization of desk and other work areas • Accommodates/adapts to changes in the routine • Work on visual perceptual skills • Orientation to time and place • Problem-solving • Self-determination • Behavior management	• Teach staff how to use sensory processing techniques in the classroom • Provide in-services on programs such as the Alert Program (Williams & Shellenberger, 1994) to help students learn to recognize how alert they are feeling and to identify sensorimotor experiences that can be used to change the level of alertness • Training and collaborative program development	• Participate on curriculum committees • Educate the system about specific environmental factors that support self-regulation and arousal in the school • Environmental modifications
Motor skills			
• Posture • Mobility • Coordination • Strength and effort • Energy	• Participation in physical education and recess activities • Participation in classroom activities such as written work • Posture/body alignment during school activities • Mobility within the school environment • Accessing assistive technology • Teach energy conservation techniques	• Training on use of adaptive equipment and accommodations and modifications • Training on positioning, lifting, and transferring	• Work with the school system to adopt a handwriting curriculum • Application of universal design to physical environment and the curriculum • Ordering appropriate adaptive equipment (e.g. lifts) for staff safety • Campaign for proper use of backpacks • Adapted equipment (e.g., weight training machines)
Communication/interaction skills			
• Physicality • Information exchange • Relations	• Social skill development • Psychosocial skill development • Peer interactions • Development of self-determination skills	• Training and collaborative program development	• Staff development activities • Participation on curriculum committees

[a]This is not an inclusive list of interventions; rather, it is an outline of some possibilities. Specific needs of the student, staff, and system would help to define the specific interventions to be used.

that students with disabilities be considered for and have access to the general education curriculum whenever possible and be included in education reform and statewide assessments. Therefore, occupational therapy services should consider and address the requirements of general education as well. For example, in some states, occupational therapists are being asked to address alternative assessments for students who have severe disabilities, or occupational therapists are involved in making decisions about reasonable testing accommodations for students with learning disabilities. To fully participate in these discussions and to support the implementation of the recommendations, the occupational therapist must have a basic understanding of the identified general educational outcomes and testing requirements within the education system.

Additionally, occupational therapists need to understand the difference between accommodations

TABLE 48.6 Examples of Accommodations and Modifications

Accommodations	Modifications
Alternative acquisition modes • Sign-language interpreters • Voice-output computers • Tape-recorded books	Teaching less content • Discriminating between animals and plants versus telling the distinguishing characteristics of animal and plant cells
Content enhancements • Advance organizers • Visual displays • Study guides • Peer-mediated instruction	Teaching different content • Identifying different animals versus learning the human anatomy
Alternative response modes • Scribe • Untimed response situations	

and modifications and how these affect learning outcomes. Often, these terms are used interchangeably; but in educational settings, the same strategies may be used in both categories, yet they have very different outcomes. *Accommodations* are adaptations or strategies that support student learning but require the same learning outcome as other students. *Modifications* are adaptations or strategies that change the learning outcome by requiring the student to learn something different or to learn less (Nolet & McLaughlin, 2000). Table 48.6 provides some examples of accommodations and modifications to illustrate these differences.

In educational systems such as universities or continuing education settings, a range of occupational therapy services may be provided as well. However, at this time, most occupational therapy services in these settings tend to be more collaborative/consultative or focus on accommodations rather than direct hands-on therapy services. For example, an occupational therapist might consult to a university computing center to recommend appropriate ergonomic arrangements or provide resources related to healthy computing.

Development of the Individualized Family Service Plan, Individualized Education Program, or Individualized Transition Plan

Once the evaluation has been completed, the IFSP, IEP, or ITP team collaborates to design the child or student's program (Giangreco, 2001). *IFSPs* are plans that include the child and family needs and are used in early intervention (age 0 to 3 years services) programs. *IEPs* are programs that address the needs of students in preschool through high school. *ITPs* are developed by the time a student turns 16 years and reflect the student's skills and aptitudes and guides teams to discuss and prepare the student for postschool programs (i.e., work, higher education, adult day health) (Figure 48.3). When developing the IFSP, IEP, or ITP, the team, which includes the parents and student (whenever appropriate), first reviews the evaluation results and writes a summary of the student's educational performance, called *present levels of academic achievement and functional performance*. The present levels describe the student's strengths and areas of concern in relation to the expectations of the general education curriculum. The team then develops the student's *goals and objectives* on the basis of the data summarized in the present levels and the agreed-upon outcomes that the team has identified.

Different settings have different requirements for how goals and objectives are written. Under the IDEA 2004, the ideal is that goals and objectives are developed as a team. Thus, there might not be an "occupational therapy goal page." This is particularly common in some early intervention settings and is becoming increasingly common across all settings. Generally, it is expected that goals and objectives will identify a functional outcome, will state what the student will do and under what conditions the skill or behavior will be performed, and will

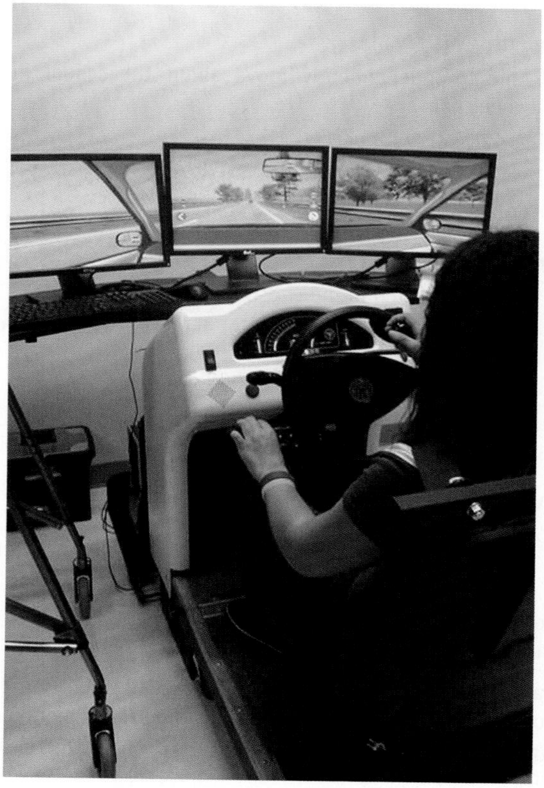

FIGURE 48.3 School-based therapists can support transition planning through activities such as adaptive driving.

include a timeline for completion (Borcherding, 2012; Mulligan, 2003; Park, 2012).

As discussed previously, collaborating with the team is an important aspect of occupational therapy service delivery in the schools. This collaboration sets the stage for focusing intervention strategies on specific student outcomes. Because parents (and older students) are involved in the team planning and decision-making process, their perspectives are well represented in the occupational profile that the occupational therapist develops. Throughout the collaborative process, the occupational therapist identifies where he or she may be able to support the student's occupational performance in the educational environment. The following case study provides an example of the goal-setting documentation for Shanna, a sixth grade middle school student with spina bifida.

After the goals and objectives have been developed, the team discusses which professional(s) should address particular goals (e.g., teacher and occupational therapist or maybe occupational therapist and speech-language pathologist), when they will be addressed (e.g., during physical education, during art, when walking in the hall), and where they will be addressed (e.g., in the general education classroom, in the cafeteria, on the playground). Each of these decisions is made on the basis of the student's need, not the personal preferences of professionals. Thus, if needed, the occupational therapist designs the occupational therapy intervention plan on the

CASE STUDY 48.2 Goal-Setting Documentation for Shanna

Shanna is in the sixth grade at the Norwood Middle School. She has spina bifida and some cognitive delays. The school psychologist, Shanna's teacher, the occupational therapist, the physical therapist, and the speech therapist each completed an individualized evaluation. The occupational therapy evaluation included an occupational profile and an analysis of Shanna's occupational performance in her educational setting. As a result of the individual assessments, an evaluation report was written, and the following are some of the strengths and concerns identified:

Strengths

- Able to independently move about the school in her wheelchair
- Social skills with peers
- Verbal expressive language
- Creativity

Concerns

- Easily distracted in the classroom
- Cannot transfer in and out of her wheelchair independently
- Receptive language
- Written language
- Fine and gross motor skills

(This is not an inclusive list of strengths and concerns.)

Excerpts from Shanna's Present Levels of Academic Achievement and Functional Performance

(Note: These excerpts and goal examples were developed and written as a team, not solely by the occupational therapist.)

Shanna currently participates in her general education classroom throughout her day. Her assignments are modified so that she can complete them in the same amount of time as her peers. Noise and visual stimuli can easily distract Shanna within her classroom environment. She goes to the resource room for assistance with math and written language when she cannot complete the assignment independently in her general education classroom.

Shanna can move about her school environment without assistance using her manual wheelchair. In the classroom, she requires physical assistance to transfer from her wheelchair to desk chair and back. She has difficulty with fine motor skills. She is unable to control a writing utensil for a sustained period (more than 5 minutes). Her difficulty with writing affects her ability to complete written assignments and art projects with her peers. Her delays in gross motor skills affect her ability to participate in physical education and recess activities.

Shanna demonstrates good adaptive skills during social interactions with her peers. However, she is becoming increasingly aware of her disability and limitations. This awareness has caused some episodes of depression and has resulted in extended absences from school. Shanna demonstrates emerging self-determination skills in other areas as well. She can describe potential accommodations and adaptations that she would like to her parents and other familiar adults, but she does not advocate for herself during school.

Goal Examples

To address psychosocial skills: Shanna will demonstrate improved self-determination and self-advocacy by collaborating with her therapists and teachers to identify and implement any needed modifications and adaptations into her educational program from less than 50% of the time to 90% of the time as measured by therapist and teacher data by June.

To address written language: Shanna will use identified accommodations/adaptations and/or assistive technology (e.g., word processor, spell-checker, adapted writing utensil) in order to complete her classroom assignments within the general education setting within the same amount of time as her peers from 75% of the time to 100% of the time as measured by therapist and teacher data by June.

basis of the outcomes that the entire educational team has identified.

The Occupational Therapy Intervention Plan

Once the team has developed the program and determines that a student would benefit from receiving occupational therapy services, in order to reach anticipated outcomes, the occupational therapy practitioner develops a specific occupational therapy intervention plan. The intervention plan addresses the occupational performance areas as well as the performance skill or student factor(s) that are affecting the student's ability to fully participate in the educational environment.

As in other settings, the occupational therapy practitioner considers student factors such as motor skills, process skills, and communication/interaction skills when determining student needs. Additionally, the practitioner considers performance patterns, such as habits and routines, the activity demands in the school setting, and the entire school context when determining student needs. With occupational performance as the core, a variety of conceptual frameworks for practice and frames of references guide occupational therapy interventions in educational settings. The primary perspectives may include occupational behavior, developmental, neurodevelopmental, learning, biomechanical, sensory integration, and coping perspectives (Kramer & Hinojosa, 2009). However, there are limited randomized controlled trials supporting or refuting specific occupational therapy interventions strategies in the schools. Therefore, as much as possible, intervention needs to relate to the student's response to the intervention based on the occupational therapy and teacher data. Throughout occupational therapy intervention, the occupational therapy practitioner uses systematic data collection to inform intervention decisions, ensure the effectiveness of the intervention for the specific student, and help to support the best outcomes for the student (see the following section for information about Shanna's intervention plan).

Service Delivery

Planning Intervention

When planning the intervention implementation, occupational therapists must consider the least restrictive environment requirement of the IDEA 2004: "to the maximum extent appropriate, children with disabilities are to be educated with children who are not disabled . . . removal of these children from the general educational environment occurs only when the nature or severity of the disability is such that education in regular classes with the use of supplementary aids and services cannot be achieved satisfactorily (Least Restrictive Environment)" (Section 300.114[a][2][i]). Thus, occupational therapy is provided in the student's typical environment to the extent possible. Such environments may include the classroom, lunchroom, bathroom, or playground.

Historical Background

With the start of P.L. 94-142 and through each reauthorization, service delivery by occupational therapy practitioners, in the schools, has been refined. Historically, the three most commonly described models in the occupational therapy literature are direct services, consultation, and monitoring (Bazyk & Case-Smith, 2010; Dunn, 1988). However, recently, there has been an increased recognition of the need for practitioners to work more deliberately within the general education environment and the system as a whole. Newer publications (Hanft & Shepherd, 2008) are using terms such as *hands-on* (includes one-on-one, small group services, and the like in pullout or natural contexts), *team supports*, and *system supports* to describe services in the schools. Although terms to describe services in the schools continue to be refined, a variety of different terms, including *direct*, *consult*, and *monitoring* continue to be used to describe occupational therapy services depending on the setting, state, or system in which the therapist works.

CASE STUDY 48.2 Outline of Shanna's Occupational Therapy Intervention Plan (*Continued*)

Using the team-identified goals and objectives as a guide, Shanna's occupational therapist developed an intervention plan. This plan included some direct therapy to identify and to teach Shanna how to implement any needed accommodations or adaptations and how to use any assistive technology. The occupational therapist also worked with Shanna to teach other school district personnel about her accommodations and adaptations and assistive technology. Ongoing consultation and monitoring were included to ensure that Shanna was able to participate within her educational environment. Finally, because Shanna also received therapy from a community-based occupational therapist, the school therapist contacted the community therapist at least every 6 months to discuss Shanna's program. The therapist did not directly address written language or work on improving handwriting. This was part of the teacher's lesson plan. The occupational therapist collaborated with the teacher to address the underlying concerns affecting handwriting performance, including the implementation of accommodations and adaptations.

Service Delivery Models

Many different service delivery models are used within the educational setting. The IDEA 2004 defines four different categories for service delivery:

- Specially designed instruction
- Related services
- Supplemental aids and services
- Services on behalf of the child

In most educational settings, occupational therapists provide related services, supplemental aids and services, and services on behalf of the child. Depending on the rules and regulations in a particular state, an occupational therapist might provide the specially designed instruction. Generally, it would be rare that an occupational therapist would be the only professional providing special education services to a student with a disability. However, a student with normal cognition but significant motor delays (e.g., muscular dystrophy, spina bifida, cerebral palsy) might require more support than just accommodations or adaptations in order to participate within his or her educational setting.

The rest of this section will use a model (Hollenbeck, 2012b) to contextualize services (see Figure 48.4) that recognize the unique skills and expertise of occupational therapy practitioners and represents current research and best practice trends in schools. Student need is the driving factor in deciding how services should be provided. As discussed previously, the need of a student represents the interaction among the client factors, performance skills and patterns, and program and placement (Giangreco, 2001). IDEA 2004 mandates that services be provided in the least restrictive environment as much as possible. Thus, practitioners in the schools may provide systems supports (AOTA, 2012a). At times, services provided at a systems level, such as playground redesigned to address universal access, has a greater impact on a larger number of children rather than working one on one with a student to learn to navigate a traditional climbing structure (Figure 48.5). Information sharing can be a powerful service delivery option in the schools. Occupational therapy practitioners in the schools can help other partners in the schools better understand the unique needs of students in the schools. Key areas of information sharing can include AOTA initiatives such as backpack awareness (Figure 48.6), obesity prevention, and social skills. If the information sharing and training would result in the child receiving FAPE in the LRE, then a greater intensity of services (e.g., hands-on services in context) may not be needed. Accommodations are defined previously. The occupational therapy practitioners' skills in activity analysis enable them to be able to support the team in determining the best fit related to the accommodation.

The need for increased collaboration in the schools, by all partners, has been receiving increased

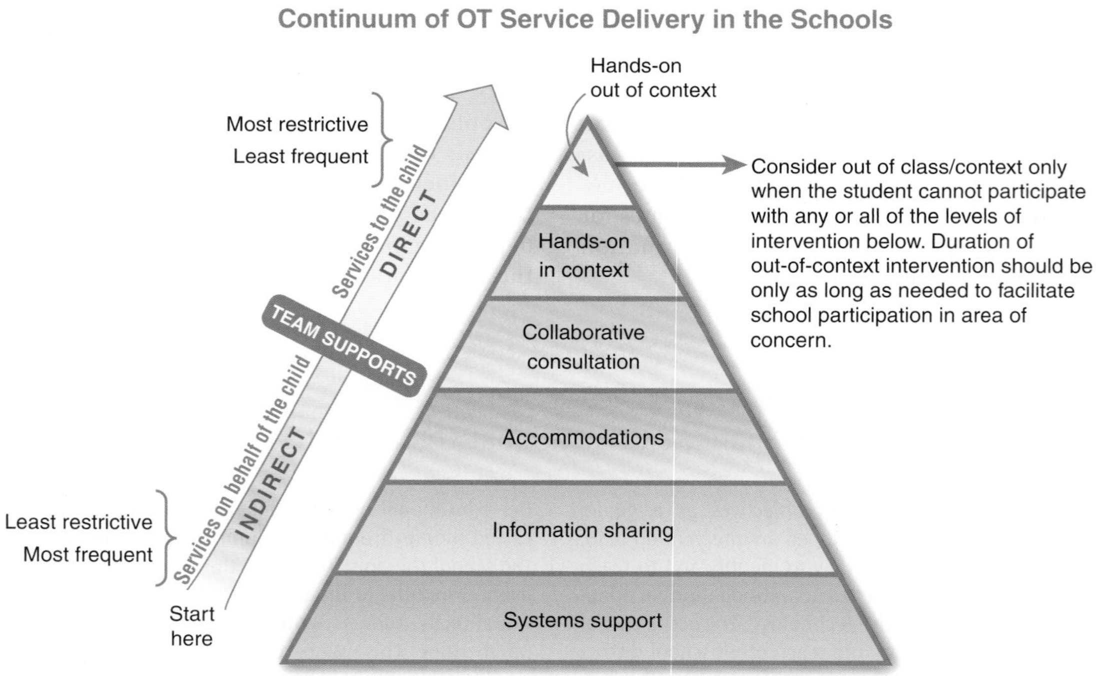

FIGURE 48.4 Occupational therapy service delivery in the schools. (Adapted with permission from Hollenbeck, J. (2012b). *Supporting students with SPD in school*. Retrieved from http://publicschoolot.com/currenttopics/sensory-integration/how-to-guides/115-supporting-students-with-spd-in-school.)

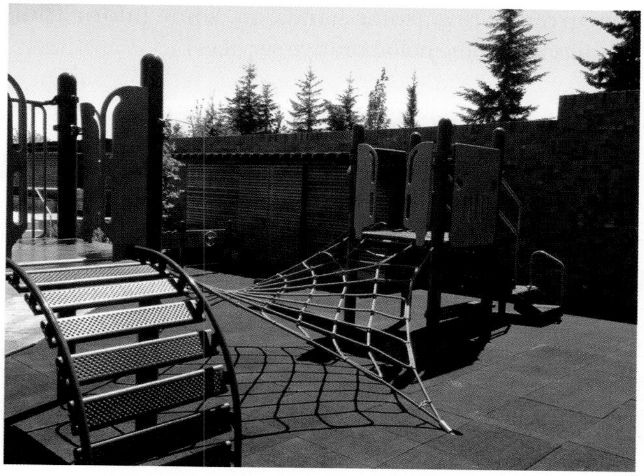

FIGURE 48.5 Occupational therapists support student participation on the playground and may be involved in playground design.

attention (Glennon, 2011; Hanft & Shepherd, 2008; Hanft & Swinth, 2011; Sayers, 2008) with positive results for students, families, and school staff (Henry & McClary, 2011; Moser, 2011; Shasby & Schneck, 2011). Collaboration reflects the interactive communication among team members (Friend & Cook, 2009; Snell & Janney, 2005; Thousand & Villa, 2000; Villa, Thousand, Nevin, & Malgeri, 1996; Walther-Thomas, Korinek, McLaughlin, & Williams, 2002). Collaborative consultation involves working closely with other team members to support student outcomes. For example, the practitioner may collaborate with the school counselor to integrate sensory processing strategies into a social skills curriculum used by the counselor or the practitioner may work with the classroom teacher on classroom redesign and dynamic seating options to help increase attention and engagement (Bill, 2008; Eingle et al., 2008; Pfeiffer, Henry, Miller, & Witherell, 2008; Schilling & Schwartz, 2004).

The previous examples of service delivery reflect *indirect services* or services where the occupational therapist is not working hands-on with the child. In IDEA terms, these can be included as a related service; but some districts document these services as supplemental aid and services (especially if provided in the general education setting) or services on behalf of the child when they are provided around a specific need of a specific student. Some systems supports, information sharing, and accommodations may be provided not only as part of special education but also as part of programs such as RtI or may not be specific to any student but benefit all students.

For some students, a greater intensity of services may be needed. These services are often referred to as *direct services* and may include hands-on services either in context or out of context. The goal is to provide services *in context* (e.g., in the classroom, lunchroom, during recess) whenever possible. Removing a student from the educational setting to go to a therapy room (or any other specialize space) should only be done if the skill cannot be addressed in context because this is a more restrictive environment. As soon as possible, an LRE option of service delivery should be implemented. Often, services are provided *out of context* for brief periods of time to help a child learn a

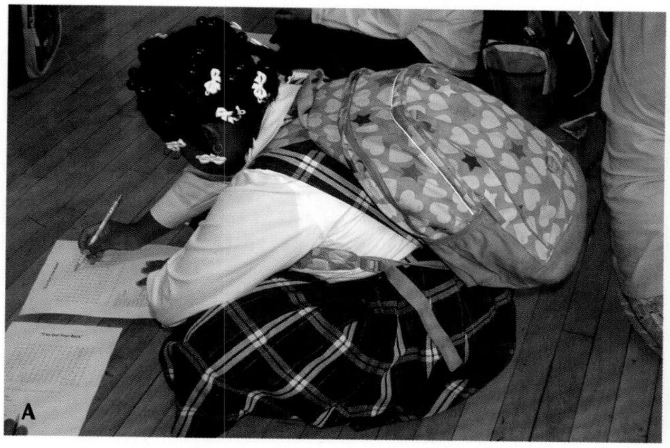

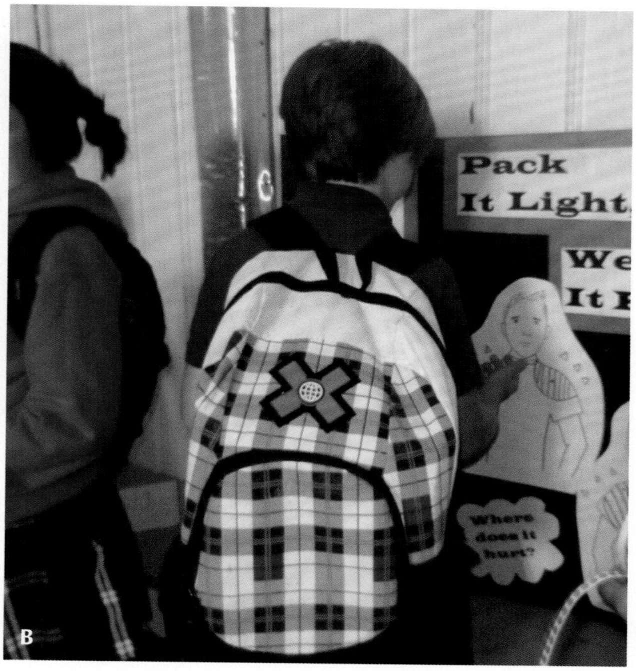

FIGURE 48.6A&B Participating in the American Occupational Therapy Association's (AOTA's) backpack campaign in the schools may prevent future injury for some students. (Photo courtesy of Karen Jacobs, EdD, OTR/L, CPE, FAOTA.)

new skill (e.g., a dressing technique). But once the skill is learned in a 1:1 setting, the student should practice and refine the skill as part of the natural school routine. Regardless of the type of service delivery provided by the practitioner, *team supports* should be considered (AOTA, 2007; Hanft & Shepherd, 2008). Table 48.7 provides a definition and additional examples of the different service delivery options.

Each type of service delivery is important and valuable and should be viewed as integrated features of an entire service delivery approach. In many cases, to meet a student's identified need(s), therapy practitioners working in the schools may use a variety of approaches concurrently (e.g., some hands-on, some information sharing, and some collaborative services).

Interagency Collaboration

Another important aspect of occupational therapy service delivery in educational settings includes collaboration between school personnel and staff from any clinic a child might be attending as well as collaboration with other agencies. Interagency collaboration is particularly necessary if the occupational therapy practitioner is providing services for students who use assistive technology or during transition planning for older students.

TABLE 48.7 Service Delivery Examples[a]

Type of Service	Definition	Example
Systems support	Working at a systems level (e.g., school, district) to meet the needs of all students, not just students with disabilities	Playground redesign Schoolwide approaches to address sensory needs Implementation of a handwriting curriculum Support policies related to evacuation Positive behavioral supports Address child mental health needs or psychosocial needs
Information sharing	Reframing, educating, teaching, supporting, and other ways to share information regarding a student, disability, program, or need	Provide in-services Information sheets for teacher Reframe a student behavior based on the disability Occupational therapy corner in school newsletter Participate in teacher meetings Participate on curriculum committees
Accommodations (see Table 48.6 for additional information)[a]	Support is provided without changing the content or outcome expectations	Dynamic seating Sensory tools Assistive technology supports
Collaborative Consultation	An interactive process that focuses teams and agencies on enhancing the functional performance, educational achievement, and participation of children and youth with disabilities in school, community, and home environments (Hanft & Shepherd, 2008)	Team meetings Evaluate/observe collaboratively Collaborative e-mails Feedback regarding collaborative goals
Hands-on in context	Contextual hands-on interventions designed to support student across settings, routines, and skills	Addressing needs: In the classroom On the playground During extracurricular activities On field trips In the bathroom During physical education In the lunchroom On the bus In the community Small social skills groups
Hands-on out of context	Hands-on interventions in settings that are not part of the naturally occurring school/classroom routines	Working in the therapy room Working 1:1 in the gym

[a]This is not an inclusive list; rather, it represents examples of possibilities.

Adapted with permission from Hollenbeck, J. (2012a). *Service delivery*. Retrieved from http://publicschoolot.com/sped-process/service-delivery.

Interagency collaboration is important for any educational setting. For example, if a student with a disability who is attending university needs specialized adaptive equipment in order to fully participate in the setting, the Department of Vocational Rehabilitation might help with the procurement of such device. Or if an occupational therapist is providing a continuing education course and one of the attendees is deaf, a sign-language interpreter might be needed.

Periodic Review

Inherent in service delivery in any setting is the documentation of services. Documentation serves as a communication tool to the students and families regarding the individualized program. Additionally, all decision making about occupational therapy intervention in the schools should be based on data, including research to the maximum extent possible. IDEA 2004 requires that the IFSP or IEP be reviewed at least annually, with regular updates to the family regarding the student's progress. (The IDEA 2004 requires that updates regarding student progress on IEPs be at least at the same intervals as general education report cards.) However, the occupational therapist should consistently (more often than quarterly) reevaluate the intervention plan to ensure that the student is moving toward achieving targeted outcomes. If necessary, the occupational therapy intervention plan or even the IFSP or IEP might need to be modified before the annual review.

Emerging Practice Considerations

Services in the schools continue to evolve to meet the unique needs of the students and system. Occupational therapy practitioners with their unique skills in activity analysis and their awareness of the interaction among the client, occupation and environment are well equipped to collaborate and partner with many other professionals in the schools in order to support participation and performance. Some emerging practice considerations include early intervening services, child mental health, social skills, and obesity. These areas are addressed as part of the AOTA Centennial Vision, the AOTA evidence review project, and AOTA workgroups.

Early Intervening Services

Within the IDEA 2004, *RtI* is defined as services that are provided for students, not in special education, who need "additional academic and behavioral support to succeed in a general education environment" (Section 300.226). Increasingly, research is suggesting that students need effective support when they first start having difficulty in school. Thus, IDEA 2004 has included early intervening services within the statutes. These services are for students "kindergarten through 12th grade (with particular emphasis on kindergarten through grade 3) who are not currently identified as needing special education or related services, but who need additional academic and behavioral support to succeed in a general education environment" (CFR, Section 300.226[a]). These supports are often referred to as *early intervening services*, *prereferral interventions* or *whole-school approaches*. Many districts are now implementing the RtI model to address this need (National Association of State Directors of Special Education [NASDSE], 2005).

RtI, which is based on research evidence and student outcome data, is an integrated approach to service delivery that includes both general and special education and includes high-quality instruction, interventions matched to student need, frequent progress monitoring, and data-based decision making (NASDSE, 2005). It is a whole-school approach to services that are specifically directed at student need. RtI is based on a problem-solving model in which the team defines the problem, analyzes what is happening, develops a plan, and evaluates the effectiveness of the plan. This model generally uses a three-tiered approach to support (see Figure 48.7). The first tier involves screening and group intervention; this approach will generally address about 80% of the problems. The second tier is targeted, short-term interventions,

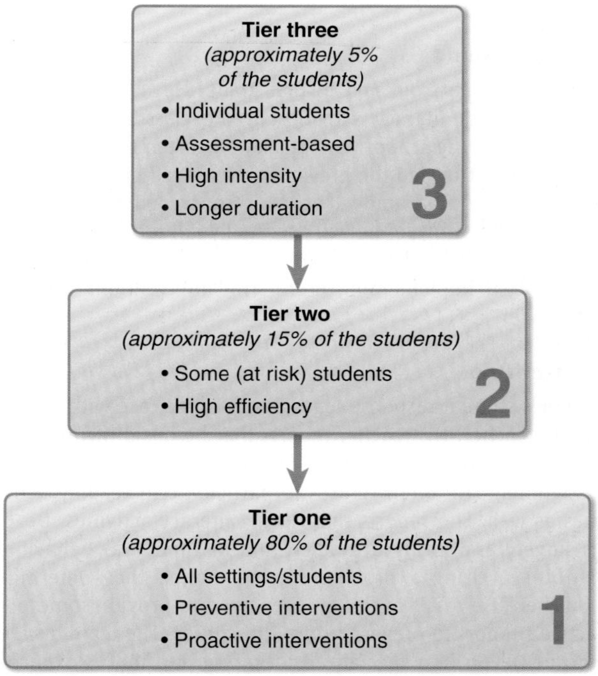

FIGURE 48.7 Response to intervention (RtI) three-tiered model. (Adapted from National Association of State Directors of Special Education. [2005]. *Response to intervention: Policy considerations and implementation*. Alexandria, VA: Author.)

addressing another 15% of the student needs. The final tier is intensive instruction, which is required by about 5% of the students. The role of occupational therapy at each tier varies across school districts. Some districts feel that the first tier should be addressed by the immediate team, whereas others include the occupational therapist early in the process. If the underlying concern is within the domain of occupational therapy, a therapist may be involved in the second or third tier of interventions. The following case study provides an illustration of how occupational therapy may be involved in early intervening services. At this time RtI, although a promising practice, is not mandated in the IDEA 2004 and thus not all occupational therapists or schools are involved in early intervening services.

If the early intervening services are not effective, the student is then referred to a special education evaluation team. The evaluation team determines whether the special education process, as outlined in the IDEA 2004, should be initiated or whether the student should be referred for some other type of support. Such support is provided under Section 504 of the Rehabilitation Act. For example, if a student requires additional accommodations or adaptations but does not require specially designed instruction to meet educational outcomes, then the evaluation team might not recommend a full special education evaluation. They would then refer the student to the school's 504 team. If the evaluation team feels that the student might need specially designed instruction (special education) in order to receive FAPE in the LRE, then the special education evaluation process would be initiated. Ideally, the occupational therapist should be involved throughout the decision-making process if the evaluation team feels that the student might require the services of an occupational therapy practitioner or that the student has needs that might require the expertise of an occupational therapist.

In the public schools, when a classroom teacher is concerned about a student, initial interventions can be developed and implemented through a collaborative team process before the student is referred to special education. Increasingly, occupational therapy practitioners are involved with the planning and implementation of such prereferral or early intervening services (AOTA, 2008b). In some cases, effective prereferral interventions, such as the use of a move-and-sit cushion for a fidgety student or the development and implementation of a handwriting curriculum, may successfully support the student within the educational environment; and further intervention might not be needed (see Case Study 48.3).

CASE STUDY 48.3 Early Intervening Services to Support Devon's Educational Program

Background

Devon is 7 years old and in first grade. He has been having difficulty with literacy activities in the classroom since the beginning of the school year. His kindergarten teacher reports that Devon struggled the previous year as well but always "just made it." His first grade teacher is concerned that if Devon continues to struggle, he will eventually fall too far behind his peers to catch up. The elementary school that he attends has just started implementing prereferral interventions using an RtI model.

Tier One

Devon's student response team discusses his case with his first grade teacher. His teacher reports that he has difficulty copying and writing more than one or two words during any writing assignment. He often refuses to participate in reading activities as well. She reports that during literacy activities, Devon is fidgety and easily distracted and at times has behavioral outbursts. Using a problem-solving model, they determine that because it is November, they need to provide some proactive support to prevent future difficulties. The team decides to put Devon in a specialized literacy group that is explicitly designed to target first grade literacy outcomes. Occupational therapy was not involved during this first meeting because the team did not feel that there were concerns about Devon's performance that required the skills and expertise of an occupational therapist.

Tier Two

For 3 months, Devon participated in the specialized literacy group, and data were systematically recorded to track the interventions that were used and Devon's progress. Devon's reading and writing skills improved, but he continued to be fidgety and easily distracted and to exhibit behavior problems during literacy activities. The team invites an occupational therapist to the second team meeting, wondering whether sensory processing might be affecting Devon's performance. The occupational therapist recommends strategies to the classroom teacher that can support Devon's sensory processing (e.g., use of a move-and-sit cushion, allowing Devon to hold small objects in his hand to fidget, use of a water bottle) during literacy activities. Devon's parents also agree to try these strategies at home. The teacher introduced the strategies to the entire group and allowed anyone to use them. Data were recorded to help Devon and the team determine the best strategies for him. The combination of the targeted instruction by the teacher and sensory strategies recommended by the occupational therapist resulted in improved performance, and Devon did not need to receive Tier Three intervention. One year later, he was still doing well. ■

Child Mental Health

Occupational therapy has strong roots in mental health and addressing psychosocial needs of children and youth. There has been an increase emphasis on mental health and the link to learning and school participation in the educational community (AOTA, 2009b, 2010a). Some of this increased awareness is being driven by the increasing numbers of students on the spectrum. Occupational therapists are well positioned to be able to support this need and help school teams address mental health and psychosocial needs. Therapy practitioners in the schools may collaborate with school counselors or school psychologists to run social groups. They may be part of preventative teams to address bullying or other such initiatives. Bazyk (2011) lays a foundation in her book, *Mental Health Promotion, Prevention, and Intervention with Children and Youth,* that can be used by occupational therapy practitioners to talk to other professionals about occupational therapy's contribution to this need.

Social Skills

With the emphasis on social participation in the "Occupational Therapy Practice Framework" (AOTA, 2008a) and the necessity of appropriate social skills to be successful in postschool outcomes (AOTA, 2010b), occupational therapy practitioners may work as part of the team to support student engagement in this area of occupation There is increasing awareness of the need to explicitly teach social skills and social thinking (Winner, 2007). Additionally, for some children, particularly those on the spectrum, sensory processing needs may impact social participation; and so the two issues may need to be addressed simultaneously (Baltazar-Mori & Piantanida, 2007; Kuypers, 2011). Again, the unique skills and expertise of the school-based practitioner is well served to work with the team to help address this area of need (see Chapter 58 for more details).

Obesity

Occupational therapy practitioners can play important roles in addressing childhood obesity in a variety of settings, including in schools and communities and at home. In each setting, intervention may focus on a number of areas, including culturally appropriate healthy food preparation and meals, enjoyable physical and social activities, and strategies for decreasing weight bias/stigma and bullying. Messages should focus on "health and a healthy lifestyle" rather than weight loss. Services can help children identify personal character strengths (e.g., creativity, humor, thoughtfulness) and build on them. Occupational therapy practitioners can play a critical role in working with school teachers, nutritionists, and other professionals to enhance healthy lifestyles in all children and youth. (AOTA, 2011, p. 2). See Appendix I for more details on obesity.

With the Centennial Vision emphasis on Health and Wellness and the statistics regarding the increase in childhood obesity, there are many things school-based practitioners can consider as part of their intervention for students with special needs as well as within the school system as a whole. This area of intervention is one that is recently getting increased attention both within the field of occupational therapy and the American population as a whole.

Outcomes

Whether addressing traditional practice arenas or emerging practice trends in educational settings, outcomes are determined by increased ability of the client (child, student, other professional[s], family, etc.) to participate (or support participation) in the occupation of being a student (see Figure 48.8). With the emphasis in today's educational settings on evidence-based practices, it is important that occupational therapists working in these settings use strategies and techniques that are supported by research or effective or promising practices (Swinth, Spencer, & Jackson, 2007). The challenge for most therapists in these settings is that there is limited research and the research that exists tends to be descriptive. However, in the public schools, the federal government has recognized this dearth in research and therefore supports promising practices. Occupational therapy practitioners working in educational settings can respond to this challenge by systematically collecting data when working with their clients and then using these data to support or change intervention. It is important that occupational therapists use research-based reasoning to inform their practice but that they not allow the lack of more experimental research to limit the scope of their practice in education settings. See the "Commentary on the Evidence" box for an example.

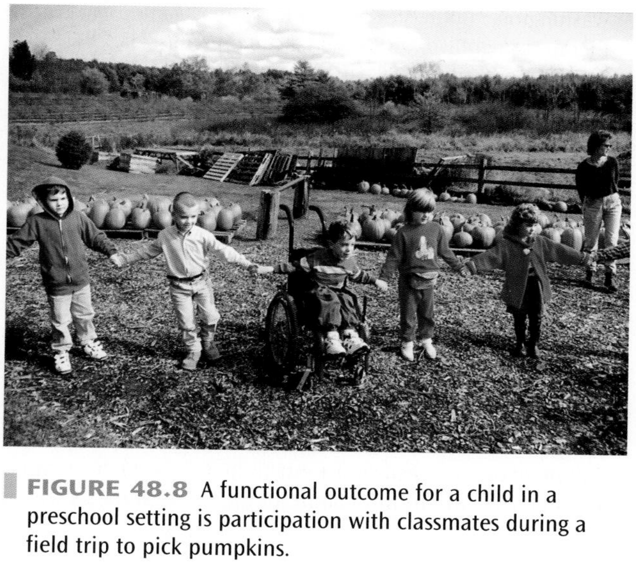

FIGURE 48.8 A functional outcome for a child in a preschool setting is participation with classmates during a field trip to pick pumpkins.

Commentary on the Evidence

School-Based Practice

The Individuals with Disabilities Education Act (IDEA) 2004 requires that therapists use "scientifically based instructional practices, to the maximum extent possible" (Section 601[c][5][E]). This requirement is congruent with occupational therapy in any setting and is applicable to all professionals who provide services in public schools. Occupational therapy practitioners can use research evidence to examine the assumptions that guide their practice. For example, the value of consultation and education approaches and providing intervention within natural performance contexts is well documented in the research literature and serves as a guideline for best practice (Spencer, Turkett, Vaughan, & Koenig, 2006).

Although some research evidence is available, rigorous studies supporting effective practice in schools are still emerging. Swinth et al. (2007), in a paper developed for the Center on Personnel Studies in Special Education (COPSSE), summarized the current state of research supporting effective practices in the schools. (The reader is referred to the full report for specifics and in-depth information.) Because the mandate of IDEA is for services to be provided within the natural context as much as possible, Swinth and colleagues recommend that "occupational therapists working within the schools must consider outcomes within the context of the environment as well as the expectations in which their services are provided" (p. 8). Considering outcomes within the educational setting creates a challenge for therapy practitioners because some intervention strategies that have a strong research base in a clinical setting might not be as appropriate or as effective in educational settings. For example, rather than working on sensory processing in a one-on-one setting down the hall from the classroom in an environment that simulates a clinical setting, therapists in the schools might work with the teacher and student to implement sensory processing strategies in the classroom. The school-based therapist might work with the teacher to integrate tools such as move-and-sit cushions, a ball chair, and fidgets into the classroom routine (Bill, 2008; Eingle et al., 2008; Pfeiffer et al., 2008; Schilling & Schwartz, 2004; Schilling, Washington, Billingsley, & Deitz, 2003). Additionally, the therapist might work with the teacher to adjust the classroom environment, such as playing low music, decreasing the lights or using natural lighting, or developing a "quiet corner" where students can go to decrease the amount of sensory input they are receiving.

The COPSSE review of the evidence specific to school-based practice revealed a lack of high-level research-based evidence due to the few randomized controlled trials or meta-analyses of such trials related to school-based occupational therapy services. Despite this finding, a growing body of descriptive research does exist. "Thus, currently occupational therapists must rely more on effective or promising practices, clinical expertise and client values as well as systematically collected data when delivering effective practices" (Swinth et al., 2007, p. 34). To increase the breadth and depth of the evidence, a culture of inquiry needs to be established among school-based practitioners. Within this culture of inquiry, a strong research agenda should be established to help inform and shape school-based practice. This research agenda should study current practice strategies (e.g., the use of sensory principles in the classroom, the best use of the skills and expertise of an occupational therapist to address handwriting) as well as the current assumptions of school-based occupational therapy service delivery (e.g., therapy in a therapy room versus in the classroom, the effectiveness of collaborative service delivery). It should be noted that several studies support the idea that intervention in natural contexts is effective (Dunn, 1991; Friend & Cook, 2009; Snell & Janney, 2005; Thousand & Villa, 2000; Walther-Thomas et al., 2002) However, many systems and school-based therapists continue to struggle with how and when to effectively move services out of a direct approach in a pullout environment. Research is needed to help inform occupational therapy practitioners and others about how direct services can be provided effectively within natural contexts as well as how other approaches to service delivery (such as team supports or system supports) can be provided efficiently and effectively to improve student outcomes. Finally, high-level experimental and quasi-experimental studies that address the effectiveness of specific occupational therapy practices on students' educational access, participation, and performance (outcome measures) are needed.

Evidence reviews related to school-based practice are available from AOTA (AOTA, 2012b; Jackson & Arbesman, 2005). Although these reviews are not specific to occupational therapy services under the IDEA 2004, some of the summaries and data that are contained in the reviews can help to inform occupational therapy services in the schools. Additionally, there are individual critical appraisals of papers (CAPS) available on AOTA's Web page that are specific to interventions in the schools, such as handwriting that can help inform practitioner decision making.

School-based occupational therapy practitioners must balance the current state of the research with the need to make the best decisions possible to support student outcomes. Ilott (2004) has noted that occupational therapy is a "research emergent" profession. At times, the profession, including practitioners working in the schools, lacks a sufficient evidence base to fully determine which practices and interventions are most effective.

> As a result, the competent school-based occupational therapist must think about "effective practice" and engage in systematic data collection related to desired student outcomes. At all times, the therapist must utilize student/client evaluation and intervention activities to collect and document student performance (outcomes) which justify on-going decisions [related to] occupational therapy service continuation, modification, or discontinuation. (Swinth et al., 2007, p. 35)

The following table provides an example of how school-based therapists can use research evidence to support their reasoning about intervention.

Commentary on the Evidence (*Continued*)

Intervention Question	Evidence Reviewed	Implications for Intervention Outcomes
Should school-based occupational therapists provide hands-on direct services in a one-on-one setting to address the handwriting needs of students?	• Case-Smith (2000) • Case-Smith (2002) • Denton, Cope, & Moser (2006) • Cooley (2004) • Mackay, McCluskey, & Mayes (2010) • Ratzon, Efraim, & Bart (2007)	Occupational therapy practitioners should consider the following when determining the type(s) of intervention provided to support a student's handwriting performance: • Although the research supports direct intervention to improve handwriting, it might not be the best use of the skills and expertise of an occupational therapist to address this need • Use of a specific handwriting curriculum may support better outcomes • The implementation of a sensorimotor aspect to handwriting instruction may not be as effective as therapeutic practice • Use of play with younger children may support improved fine motor skills • Occupational therapy may help to improve letter legibility but might not affect speed or numerical legibility • The dynamic tripod grasp is not the only functional pencil grip used in handwriting activities • Short periods of intervention in small groups may be an effective intervention strategy

Conclusion: On the basis of the evidence review, the occupational therapist determined that a greater emphasis on team and system support might better support the handwriting needs of the students in his district. The therapist felt that intervention for each student who is referred to occupational therapy could be best served through collaboration with teachers to develop handwriting clubs, implement adaptations in the classroom (e.g., pencil grasps, writing templates, assistive technology), promote fine motor practice and activities within the natural context of the classroom, and implement a comprehensive handwriting curriculum across the district. Direct occupational therapy services through one-on-one or group intervention would be provided only if it was determined through an occupational therapy evaluation that a student had underlying client factors (e.g., biomechanical, visual-motor, fine motor) affecting handwriting performance that could be improved through such direct intervention and then for short periods of time. The therapist hypothesized that by providing services through a team or system support approach, more children would benefit from occupational therapy, albeit indirectly, and that the number of referrals to occupational therapy would decrease so that the therapist would be evaluating only those children with handwriting concerns that had underlying client factors.

Summary

Occupational therapy intervention in the schools is guided by the IDEA 2004. Practitioners working in the schools collaborate with the IEP team to determine student needs and targeted outcomes. Once these needs and outcomes have been defined in the IEP and the team determines that occupational therapy services are needed, then the occupational therapist designs the specific occupational therapy intervention plan. Occupational therapy intervention in the schools focuses on the occupational performance of the student within the educational environment. Practitioners may also provide services that are directed to the needs of the educational staff, parents, or system. Specific intervention strategies and approaches should be based on research to the maximum extent possible. When research is not available but preliminary data indicate that a particular intervention or service delivery could be effective (promising), then the occupational therapy practitioner should use systematic data-based decision making to inform decisions about intervention for individual students.

References

American Occupational Therapy Association. (2007). *Occupational therapy services for children and youth under the Individuals with Disabilities Education Act* (3rd ed.). Bethesda, MD: AOTA.

American Occupational Therapy Association. (2008a). Occupational therapy practice framework: Domain and process, 2nd edition. *American Journal of Occupational Therapy, 62*, 625–683.

American Occupational Therapy Association. (2008b). *FAQ on response to intervention for school-based occupational therapists and occupational therapy assistants.* Bethesda, MD: Author.

American Occupational Therapy Association. (2009a). *AOTA member participation survey overview report.* Bethesda, MD: Author.

American Occupational Therapy Association. (2009b). *Occupational therapy and school mental health.* Bethesda, MD: Author.

American Occupational Therapy Association. (2010a). *Occupational therapy in school settings.* Bethesda, MD: Author.

American Occupational Therapy Association. (2010b). Occupational therapy services in the promotion of psychological and social aspects of mental health. *American Journal of Occupational Therapy, 64,* 578–591.

American Occupational Therapy Association. (2011). *Occupational therapy's role in mental health promotion, prevention, & intervention for children and youth: Childhood obesity.* Bethesda, MD: Author.

American Occupational Therapy Association. (2012a). *Occupational therapy's role in mental health promotion, prevention, & intervention for children and youth: Recess promotion,* Bethesda, MD: Author.

American Occupational Therapy Association (2012b). *School based interventions. Evidence brief series.* Retrieved from http://www.aota.org/Educate/Research/EB/School.aspx

Americans with Disabilities Act of 1990, 42 U.S.C.A. § 12134 (1990).

Baltazar-Mori, A., & Piantanida, D. B. (2007). *Every child wants to play: Simple and effective strategies for teaching social skills.* Torrance, CA: Pediatric Therapy Network.

Bazyk, S. (2011). *Mental health promotion, prevention, and intervention with children and youth: A guiding framework for occupational therapy.* Bethesda, MD: AOTA.

Bazyk, S., & Case-Smith, J. (2010). School-based occupational therapy. In J. Case-Smith & J. O'Brien (Eds.), *Occupational therapy for children* (6th ed., pp. 713–743). Philadelphia, PA: Mosby.

Bill, V. N. (2008). *Effects of stability balls on behavior and achievement in the special education classroom* (Unpublished master's thesis). Southwest Minnesota State University, Marshall, MN.

Borcherding, S. (2012). *Documentation manual for writing SOAP notes in occupational therapy* (3rd ed.). Thorofare, NJ: Slack.

Bureau of Labor Statistics, U.S. Department of Labor. (2012). *Occupational outlook handbook, 2012–2013 Edition. Occupational therapists.* Retrieved from http://www.bls.gov/ooh/healthcare/occupational-therapists.htm

Case-Smith, J. (2000). Effects of occupational therapy services on fine motor and functional performance in preschool children. *American Journal of Occupational Therapy, 54,* 372–380.

Case-Smith, J. (2002). Effectiveness of school-based occupational therapy intervention on handwriting. *American Journal of Occupational Therapy, 56,* 17–25.

Chapparo, C., & Lowe, S. (2012). School: Participating in more than just the classroom? In S. Lane & A. Bundy (Eds.), *Kids can be kids: A childhood occupations approach* (pp. 83–101). Philadelphia, PA: F. A. Davis.

Cooley, C. (2004). *Is the dynamic tripod grasp the most functional grip for handwriting?* UPS Evidence-Based Practice Symposium. Retrieved from http://www.region10.org/ssvi/EBPXEvidenceResearch/documents/Tripod_Grasp.pdf

Coster, W. (1998). Occupation-centered assessment of children. *American Journal of Occupational Therapy, 52,* 337–344.

Denton, P. L., Cope, S., & Moser, C. (2006). The effects of sensorimotor-based intervention versus therapeutic practice on improving handwriting performance in 6- to 11-year-old children. *American Journal of Occupational Therapy, 60,* 16–27.

Dunn, W. (1988). Models of occupational therapy service provision in the school system. *American Journal of Occupational Therapy, 42,* 718–723.

Dunn, W. (1991). A comparison of service provision models in school-based occupational therapy services: A pilot study. *Occupational Therapy Journal of Research, 10,* 300–320.

Dunn, W., Brown, C., & McGuigan, M. (1994). The ecology of human performance: A framework for considering the effect of context. *American Journal of Occupational Therapy, 48,* 595–607.

Education for All Handicapped Children Act of 1975, Pub. L. No. 94-142, 20 U.S.C., §1401, Part H, § 677 (1975).

Education of the Handicapped Act Amendments of 1986, Pub. L. No. 99-457, 20 U.S.C. §1400 (1986).

Eingle, K. L., Hamilton, C. B., McLane, M. C., Mun-Bryce, S., Frank, J., & Scheerer, C. (2008). *Seating that makes "sense": A sensory-based classroom technique* (Unpublished master's thesis). Xavier University, Cincinnati, OH.

Friend, M., & Cook, L. (2009). *Interactions: Collaboration skills for school professionals* (6th ed.). Boston, MA: Allyn & Bacon.

Frolek-Clark, G., Polichino, J., & Jackson, L. (2004). Occupational therapy services in early intervention and school-based programs. *American Journal of Occupational Therapy, 58,* 681–685.

Giangreco, M. (2001). Interactions among program, placement, and services in educational planning for students with disabilities. *Mental Retardation, 39,* 341–350.

Glennon, T. J. (2011). Human factors: Just as important as knowledge factors in collaborative experiences. *Journal of Occupational Therapy, Schools, & Early Intervention, 4,* 13–21.

Hanft, B., & Shepherd, J. (2008). *Collaboration and teamwork: Essential to school-based occupational therapy.* Bethesda, MD: AOTA.

Hanft, B., & Swinth, Y. (2011). Commentary on collaboration. *Journal of Occupational Therapy, Schools, & Early Intervention, 4,* 2–7.

Henry, D. A., & McClary, M. (2011). The Sensory Processing Measure-Preschool (SPM-P)—Part two: Test-retest and collective collaborative empowerment, including a father's perspective. *Journal of Occupational Therapy, Schools, & Early Intervention, 4,* 53–70.

Hollenbeck, J. (2012a). *Service delivery.* Retrieved from http://publicschoolot.com/sped-process/service-delivery

Hollenbeck, J. (2012b). *Supporting students with SPD in school.* Retrieved from http://publicschoolot.com/currenttopics/sensory-integration/how-to-guides/115-supporting-students-with-spd-in-school

Ilott, I. (2004). Evidence-based practice forum: Challenges and strategic solutions for a research emergent profession. *American Journal of Occupational Therapy, 58,* 347–352.

Individuals with Disabilities Education Act Amendments of 1990, Pub. L. No. 101-476, 20 U.S.C. §1400–1485.

Individuals with Disabilities Education Act Amendments of 1997, Pub. L. No. 105-117, 111 Stat. 37 (1997).

Individuals with Disabilities Education Improvement Act of 2004, Pub. L. No. 108-446, 20 U.S.C. §1400 *et seq* (2004).

Jackson, L., & Arbesman, M. (2005). *Children with behavioral and psychosocial needs: Occupational therapy practice guidelines.* Bethesda, MD: American Occupational Therapy Association.

Kramer, P., & Hinojosa, J. (2009). *Frames of reference for pediatric occupational therapy* (3rd ed.). Philadelphia, PA: Lippincott Williams & Wilkins.

Kuypers, L. (2011). *The zones of regulation.* San Jose, CA: Think Social.

Mackay, N., McCluskey, A., & Mayes, R. (2010) The log handwriting program improved children's writing legibility: A pretest–posttest study. *American Journal of Occupational Therapy, 64,* 30–36.

Moser, C. S. (2011). Reviews, tools, and resources. *Journal of Occupational Therapy, Schools, & Early Intervention, 4,* 8–12.

Muhlenhaupt, M. (2003). Enabling student participation through occupational therapy services in the schools. In L. Letts & D. Stewart (Eds.), *Using environments to enable occupational performance* (pp. 177–196). Thorofare, NJ: Slack.

Mulligan, S. (2003). *Occupational therapy evaluation for children: A pocket guide.* Philadelphia, PA: Lippincott Williams & Wilkins.

National Association of State Directors of Special Education. (2005). *Response to intervention: Policy considerations and implementation.* Alexandria, VA: Author.

National Council on Disabilities. (2000). *Back to school on civil rights: Advancing the federal commitment to leave no child behind.* Washington, DC: Author.

National Information Center for Children and Youth with Disabilities. (1998). The IDEA amendments of 1997. *NICHY News Digest, 26* (Rev. ed.). Retrieved from http://nichcy.org/wp-content/uploads/docs/nd26pdf.pdf

No Child Left Behind Act of 2001, Pub. L. No. 107-110, 115 Stat. 1425 (2002).

Nolet, V., & McLaughlin, M. J. (2000). *Accessing the general curriculum: Including students with disabilities in standards-based reform.* Thousand Oaks, CA: Corwin Press.

O'Brien, J., Forest, M., Snow, J., Pearpoint, J., & Hasbury, D. (1989). *Action for inclusion: How to improve schools by welcoming children with special needs into regular classrooms.* Toronto, Canada: Inclusion Press.

Park, S. (2012). Setting goals that express the possibilities: If we don't know where we are going, how will we know when we get there?

In S. Lane & A. Bundy (Eds.), *Kids can be kids: A childhood occupations approach* (pp. 349–367). Philadelphia, PA: F. A. Davis.

Pfeiffer, B., Henry, A., Miller, S., & Witherell, S. (2008). The effectiveness of Disc 'O' Sit cushions on attention to task in second-grade students with attention difficulties. *American Journal of Occupational Therapy, 62*, 274–281.

Ratzon, N. Z., Efraim, D., & Bart, O. (2007). A short-term graphomotor program for improving writing readiness skills of first-grade students. *American Journal of Occupational Therapy, 61*, 399–405.

Rehabilitation Act of 1973, 29 U.S.C., § 504 (1973).

Sayers, B. (2008). Collaboration in school settings: A critical appraisal of the topic. *Journal of Occupational Therapy, Schools, & Early Intervention, 1*, 170–179.

Schilling, D. L., & Schwartz, I. S. (2004). Alternative seating for young children with autism spectrum disorder: Effects on classroom behavior. *Journal of Autism and Developmental Disorders, 34*, 423–432.

Schilling, D. L., Washington, K., Billingsley, F. F., & Deitz, J. (2003). Classroom seating for children with attention deficit hyperactivity disorder. *American Journal of Occupational Therapy, 57*, 534–541.

Shasby, S., & Schneck, C. (2011). Commentary on collaboration in school-based practice: Positives and pitfalls. *Journal of Occupational Therapy, Schools, & Early Intervention, 4*, 22–33.

Silverstein, R. (2000). An overview of the emerging disability policy framework: A guidepost for analyzing public policy. *Iowa Law Review, 85*, 1757–1802.

Snell, M., & Janney, R. (2005). *Collaborative teaming* (2nd ed.). Baltimore, MD: Paul H. Brookes.

Spencer, K. C., Turkett, A., Vaughan, R., & Koenig, S. (2006). School-based practice patterns: A survey of occupational therapists in Colorado. *American Journal of Occupational Therapy, 60*, 81–91.

Stewart, K. (2010). Purposes, processes, and methods of evaluation. In J. Case-Smith & J. O'Brien (Eds.), *Occupational therapy for children* (6th ed., pp. 218–245). St. Louis, MO: Elsevier.

Swinth, Y., Chandler, B., Hanft, B., Jackson, L., & Shepherd, J. (2003). *Personnel issues in school-based occupational therapy: Supply and demand, preparation, and certification and licensure.* Gainesville, FL: Center on Personnel Studies in Special Education. Retrieved from http://www.coe.ufl.edu/copsse

Swinth, Y. L., Spencer, K. C., & Jackson, L. (2007). *Occupational therapy: A report on effective school-based practices within a policy context.* Gainesville, FL: Center on Personnel Studies in Special Education.

Thousand, J., & Villa, R. (2000). Collaborative teaming: A powerful tool in school restructuring. In R. Villa & J. Thousand (Eds.), *Restructuring for caring and effective education* (pp. 254–291). Baltimore, MD: Paul H. Brookes.

Villa, R., Thousand, J., Nevin, A., & Malgeri, C. (1996). Instilling collaboration for inclusive schooling as a way of doing business in public education. *Remedial and Special Education, 1793*, 169–181.

Walther-Thomas, C., Korinek, L., McLaughlin, V., & Williams, B. (2002). *Collaboration for inclusive education: Developing successful programs.* Boston, MA: Allyn & Bacon.

Williams, M. S., & Shellenberger, S. (1994). *How does your engine run? A leader's guide to the alert program for self-regulation.* Albuquerque, NM: TherapyWorks.

Winner, M. G. (2007). *Thinking about YOU thinking about ME* (2nd ed.). San Jose, CA: Think Social.

Ziviani, I., Kopeshke, R., & Wadley, D. (2006). Children walking to school: Parent perceptions of environmental and psychosocial influences. *Australian Occupational Therapy Journal, 53*, 27–34.

For additional resources on the subjects discussed in this chapter, visit http://thePoint.lww.com/Willard-Spackman12e.

CHAPTER 49

Work

Phyllis M. King, Darcie L. Olson

OUTLINE

LEARNING OBJECTIVES

After reading this chapter, you will be able to:

1. Differentiate between the definition and meaning of work and occupation in occupational therapy practice
2. Describe work practice in occupational therapy as it applies to populations described across the life span and by physical, mental, and social conditions
3. Identify services offered by occupational therapy in work practice
4. Identify the various types of practice settings in which occupational therapy provides work evaluation and interventions

Introduction

Occupational therapists and occupational therapy assistants strive to promote optimal levels of work performance for all individuals to promote a sense of well-being. The profession of occupational therapy supports the use of **work** as an evaluation and treatment medium, essential to providing a sense of meaning and productivity that is vital to health.

Work and work-related treatments have always been at the core of occupational therapy. *Merriam-Webster's Collegiate Dictionary* (2003) defines work as "exertion or effort directed to produce or accomplish something" (p. 906). In occupational therapy, the focus is directed more to the intrinsic value of work as "meaningful occupation." **Occupation** can be defined as a meaningful, purposeful activity (Primeau, 1996). In other words, occupational therapy considers work an occupation. Work is "any activity that contributes to the goods and services of society, whether paid or unpaid" (Primeau, 1996, p. 57). It is one of the major human performance areas that encompasses life roles such as wage earner, homemaker, volunteer, and student.

Role of Work

Work plays an important role in an individual's life, contributing to the development of self-esteem, volition, sense of belonging, and competence (Westmorland, Williams, Strong, & Arnold, 2002). "Work can offer a sense of mastery over the environment, as well as a sense of accomplishment and competence leading to an improved quality of life" (Siporin, 1999, p. 23). It provides structure to a person's life; fulfills the work ethic; and improves an individual's morale, discipline, self-worth, and dignity (Harvey-Krefting, 1985). One's culture and social environment may further provide meaning to work and define what is acceptable, providing incentives and/or constraints in relation to choice. Engagement in meaningful occupations, including work, is known to promote health and occupational balance (Wilcox, 1998). For many, an interruption in work can disrupt that balance and have a significant impact on health.

Role of Occupational Therapy

Work performance can be influenced by physical, cognitive, perceptual, psychological, social, and/or developmental factors. Occupational therapists have knowledge of disease, disability, and the process of occupational analysis and engagement to develop appropriate evaluation, treatment, and prevention programs. See Appendix I and Chapter 21. Evaluation includes client factors such as body functions (e.g., neuromuscular, sensory, visual, perceptual cognitive) and body structures (e.g., cardiovascular); habits; routines; roles and behavior patterns; cultural, physical, environmental, social, and spiritual contexts; and activity demands that affect performance and performance skills, including motor, process, and communication/interaction skills (American Occupational Therapy Association [AOTA], 2008). See Units IV, V, and VI.

The occupational therapist or the occupational therapy assistant (under the supervision of the occupational therapist) collaborates with the individual, other team members (e.g., employers, case managers), or agencies (e.g., educational, local/state mental health, vocational rehabilitation) to develop intervention strategies. These strategies are based on the individual's interests, abilities, and needs and are designed to explore and expand work options, to enhance or develop work-related capabilities, and to obtain or retain employment (AOTA Commission on Practice, 2010).

Interventions include development, remediation, or compensation of physical, cognitive, neuromuscular, sensory functions, and behavioral skills. Education and training of individuals, care coordination, case management, transition services, and consultative services can be additional contributions by occupational therapists. To enhance the client's performance skills, occupational therapists may modify environments and create adaptive processes and devices to enhance functional mobility, and to enhance sensory, perceptual, and cognitive processing (AOTA, 2008).

Historical Context

The precursors of occupational therapy and work programs date back to the 1800s where "work programs" were formed to promote sanity and morale in people with mental illness (Paterson, 1997). Soon after, work-related therapy was also used with people with physical disabilities to promote health. Adolph Meyer (1977),

CASE STUDY 49.1 The Definition of Work: The Perspectives of Amy and George

Amy, a young woman in her early-20s, defines work as clearing tables and washing dishes in two restaurants. The two jobs provide health insurance and enough income to pay for a small apartment and a car, big accomplishments for a young woman who struggled to complete high school.

When Amy fractured her fingers by pinching them in a folding banquet table, she did not envision the complex road to recovery. The stitches and damaged fingernails prevented Amy from working at either job for several months. The reduced income and the complicated paperwork associated with work restrictions caused financial and emotional problems. The independent lifestyle she had worked so hard to achieve was unraveled because she had to rely on family members for daily assistance.

George, a retired butcher in his early 70s, defines work as driving the courtesy van for the local medical center 2 days per week. The early morning transport of community members to medical appointments provides conversation and purpose.

George was injured when he fell off of a ladder while washing windows. The resulting shoulder injury halted his driving, and therefore his work. His wife became the primary driver, transporting George to his medical appointments. She disliked the responsibility of driving and George disliked being the patient. Both George and his wife expressed frustration at the changes in their daily routines.

Both Amy and George provide examples of how lives are affected when work is interrupted. Their stories highlight the intrinsic meaning of work. ■

one of the founders of occupational therapy, provided the first philosophy of the profession when he wrote that healthy living involved a "blending of work and pleasure" (p. 640). During World War I, occupational therapists used productive occupation to physically restore injured soldiers to work roles. The use of occupation soon gained a reputation as being therapeutic. In the early 1900s, the "work cure" was incorporated into workshops where clients actually received profits from producing marketable goods. Therapeutic occupations, habit training, handiwork occupations, and preindustrial shops as curative work became more common (Jacobs & Baker, 2000).

Today, occupational therapy continues to be committed to work and work-related activities, with a greater focus and expansion on injury prevention services (e.g., ergonomics, preplacement screenings, joint protection education, and postural awareness) and engagement in partnerships to serve industry. Therapists increasingly practice outside of the medically based facilities and more in the workplace engaging with employees and employers.

Occupational Therapy Theory and Frame of Reference

Occupational therapy theory, practice, and research have always approached performance from a holistic perspective. One model, the Person-Environment-Occupation Model (see Chapter 38), emphasizes the complex, dynamic relationships between the person, environment, and occupation. It describes occupational performance as the outcome of a dynamic, interwoven relationship that exists among persons; their roles and occupations; and the environments in which they live, work, and interact. According to this model, occupational therapy intervention seeks to enable optimal performance in occupations defined as important by the client (Kornblau, Lou, Weeder, & Werner, 2002). For example, Lori, an occupational therapist, assisting Jim, a 42-year-old husband and father of two children who seeks to return to his job as an office manager following a T12–L1 spinal cord injury, must consider his personal strengths and limitations in the performance of self-care, his psychological and social adjustment to his disability, and mobility skills in preparation for return to work. Variables in the home and office environment must be assessed and modified to optimize independence in functioning. Doorways may need to be widened and a ramp installed for entry and exit to both environments. Transportation issues will need to be addressed with Jim's motor vehicle adapted for incorporation of hand controls. An analysis of his office job will need to be conducted to identify work accommodations that would enable him to perform his job independently. Such accommodations may include a larger office space, a desk that accommodates a wheelchair, and relocating office equipment for ease in reach.

Occupational adaptation suggests competence in a person's occupational response (see Chapter 40). In order to obtain competence, the person must interact with the occupational challenges within the environmental context. A person's performance is largely dependent upon the level of desire for mastery, the environment's demand for mastery, and the resulting press for mastery (Schkade & Schultz, 1992). How a person responds adaptively determines whether the person will experience relative mastery in his or her occupations. The strength of this desire largely influences the achievement of mastery.

The occupational environment presents challenges to an individual's performance. Physical, social, and cultural aspects of the environment can either facilitate or impede performance based upon the aptitudes and adaptive capacity of the individual. Occupational therapists can act as facilitators of the environment. They can address both the person-system deficits and the environmental demands to facilitate a person's mastery in his or her preferred work occupation (Kornblau et al., 2002).

According to the occupational adaptation frame of reference, Lori will need to consider Jim's level of motivation to return to work and the job tasks required. He may need to return to his job to financially support his family. In this case, Jim's desire for mastery is high. The office setting may present physical challenges for him with limitations in space in the office and bathroom to accommodate a wheelchair. Adaptation and relocation of office equipment such as a computer, telephone, desk, and file cabinets will need to be considered to optimize his ability to perform his job.

Populations

"Occupational therapists and occupational therapy assistants provide services to individuals or populations with deficits or problems in the area of work performance" (AOTA, 2005, p. 676). Work-related services can be provided to individuals of all ages. Throughout the life span, participation in work provides social, developmental, and economic benefits.

Children and School Programs

E. A. Larson (2004) suggested that children benefit from culturally acceptable work roles such as cleaning up after oneself or participating in household chores. Early exposure to self-care and chores may impact the child's relationships with family members and provide the foundation for other work skills in the future (see Figure 49.1).

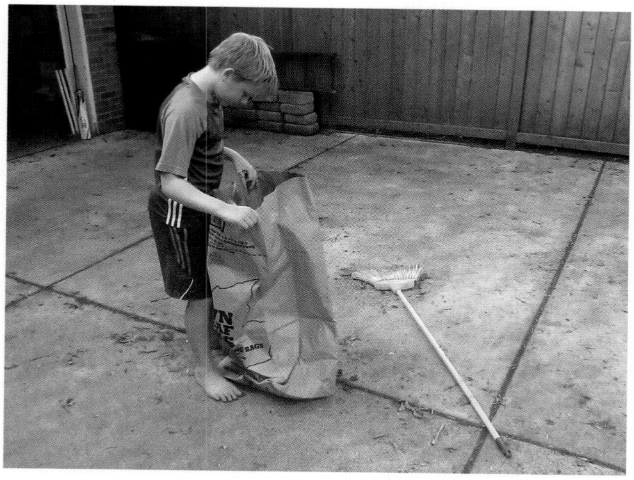

FIGURE 49.1 Exposure to chores sets the foundation for other work skills.

In 1997, the Individuals with Disabilities Education Act (1997) mandated that along with the Individualized Education Plan (IEP), each adolescent in special education would have an Individualized Transition Plan before reaching age of 14 years. See Chapter 48. **Transition** is the process where the education and rehabilitation team prepare the student to leave the school setting and enter into employment and community living (Kardos & White, 2005). Transition planning includes four primary areas: postsecondary education, community participation, postsecondary employment needs, and residential outcomes (K. C. Spencer, 2000).

Occupational therapists offer a unique role in the transition process by promoting movement from school to post-school activities through occupation-based evaluation and interventions (J. E. Spencer, Emery, & Schneck, 2003). Career interest inventories and job exploration may be conducted. Interventions such as use of adaptive equipment or assistive technologies may be considered to maximize function in chosen post-school activities. Occupational therapists incorporate daily living skills, work readiness, and community involvement into the students' therapy programs to prepare for eventual employment and community living.

Occupational therapists participate in achieving transition outcomes for each student by addressing their specific needs. Working with the student ensures that his or her preferences and interests provide the foundation for transition planning. Along with the students, their families, and the transition team, the occupational therapist may develop and provide prevocational programs, facilitate functional living skills development, modify environments, facilitate inclusion in community experiences, and provide education to parents and other staff. Occupational therapy in transition planning uses functional, real-life tasks and task analysis to help students develop functional living skills.

Adults

Studies of adults with disabilities have shown that quality of life is improved through participation in competitive employment and meaningful occupations (Bond, 2004; Dickie, 2003). Whether an adult has a disability or not, the therapist must recognize the fact that occupational repertoires in adults differ between different stages of life (Singleton & Harvey, 1995). Occupations provide challenges that contribute to personal and professional growth and development. Major occupations in an individual's everyday life will therefore change with age. For example, an adult in his or her early 20s is more inclined to seek an occupation that will build a career, whereas adults entering retirement may be more interested in maintenance occupations and those that provide personal value.

Older Adults: Work as a Focus with the Aging Population

Working with older adults to promote participation in work is an emerging practice area for occupational therapists. As the proportion of older adults in the population grows, the role of the occupational therapist will be expanded to accommodate the needs of the older worker. Occupational therapy services are not limited to individuals with physical and developmental disabilities. Work participation is a part of occupational therapy programs for all individuals, including those with mental and behavioral disabilities.

Having a work identity is central to being an adult in America. "In contemporary American society, a sense of being something (at minimum, being a productive person) seems critical to perceptions of belonging and status as well as one's sense of personal worth" (Dickie, 2003, p. 251). According to Mosisa and Hipple (2006), the median age of the American workforce is rising sharply and expected to continue to rise through 2015 as the baby boomers (individuals born between 1946 and 1964) approach retirement age. The average American worker is projected to be over 40 years old in 2012, constituting more than 40% of the labor force. The increased age of the American worker is affected by both the aging of the baby boomers and the projected increased participation rates of workers over age 55. As the workforce continues to age, significant challenges face employers and rehabilitation providers. Neurological, cognitive, physical, and psychological age-related changes need to be considered when working with older adults (Gupta & Stoffel, 2001). Older workers have been found to require more days off of work to recover from injuries than their younger counterparts

(Bureau of Labor Statistics, 2005). This is suggested to be due to slower recovery and comorbid conditions.

Kornblau (2000) viewed the changing workforce as a trend to be embraced by occupational therapists. "Occupational therapists can play a big role in designing and adapting the workplace for the changing workforce" (p. 1). Occupational therapists provide services to facilitate successful aging in the workplace. They assist older workers and employers to understand occupational performance issues and strategies specific to older employees (Gupta & Stoffel, 2001). Occupational therapists assist older workers and their employers to optimize the fit between a person's abilities and the contextual demands imposed by the occupation and the environment (Sterns & Miklos 1995).

Conditions

Problems in work performance can arise from aging, physical or mental illness or injury, and/or developmental or behavioral impairments. Occupational therapists provide services to individuals with a wide variety of conditions with a particular goal of enhancing participation in work. The practice settings often, but not always, define the age and conditions of the population served. School systems serve youth with learning and developmental disabilities as they transition to adult life and employment opportunities. Individuals with mental or behavioral illness are served in a variety of settings, including hospitals, community clinics, and homeless shelters. Work-focused interventions for individuals with these conditions include assessment, education, and training in key areas to enhance successful integration into competitive employment.

Occupational therapists working in hospitals, clinics, and on-site in industry provide services for adults with a wide array of medical conditions. Physical injuries and illnesses related to employment, such as musculoskeletal disorders and traumatic workplace injuries, benefit from integrated services that involve the worker, employer, health care providers, and others involved in safe return-to-work planning. Non-work-related medical conditions, such as traumatic injuries or illnesses, also require integrated planning to enhance the opportunities for participation in work. Individuals with disabilities benefit from the education provided by occupational therapists regarding services and programs that promote safe employment.

Legislation, federal, and community agencies provide incentives to work, although many individuals lack awareness of the programs or are fearful that working will impact their benefits from Medicare, welfare, disability, insurance, or workers' compensation (Fiedler, Indermuehle, Drobac, & Laud, 2002). Work-focused assessments, education, interventions, and the integration of services are apparent in all practice areas of occupational therapy for individuals of all ages and conditions.

Services

Wellness, Health Promotion, and Injury Prevention

Wellness integrates fitness, nutrition, healthy relationships, a positive self-image, and the ability to take personal responsibility for self-care. It is the *process* of taking responsibility for realizing one's maximum health potential (Rothman, 1998). **Health promotion** is the movement toward optimal health and high-level wellness. These concepts are the basic tenets of occupational therapy. Rehabilitation programs commonly include strategies for empowering the client to gain or regain responsibility for optimal health and function. Community education programs including topics such as energy conservation and work simplification have long been part of occupational therapy's health promotion campaign. On-site educational programs in industries encourage personal responsibility for wellness through prevention programs. These prevention programs include stretching, fitness, safe work practices and early recognition, reporting, and management of physical problems associated with work (Olson, 1999). Prevention, an important dimension of wellness, is defined as taking steps to avert the development of disease or illness (Rothman, 1998).

Wellness and prevention programs positively influence health and prevent injury (Massy-Westropp & Rose, 2004; Yassi, Gilbert, & Cvitkovich, 2005). Two major factors motivating companies to initiate wellness programs are the reduction of work-related injuries and the associated costs savings of a healthier workforce (Melnik, 2000; Naso, 2003; Rothman, 1998). Occupational therapists can incorporate wellness and health promotion into any practice setting. Siporin (1999) emphasized the importance of training programs for individuals with mental or behavioral disabilities in areas such as social skills, proper hygiene, and dressing for work. In this context, health promotion involves training in areas that prepare for more successful integration into community environments. Health promotion programs can include the assessment of health risk factors, such as problem assessments, workforce symptom surveys or hazard checklists, education and training in lifestyle improvements, safety precautions, safe working techniques, and fitness programs (Olson, 1999; Rothman, 1998). In industry, on-site wellness programs result in decreased absenteeism, reduced health care costs, protection from lower back problems and musculoskeletal injuries, and can improve productivity (Carrivick, Lee, Yau, & Stevenson, 2005; Melnick, 2000; Naso, 2003; Rothman, 1998).

Ergonomics

Ergonomics is a relatively new profession that focuses on the use of a **systems approach** for improving safety and productivity through the design of work systems and environments. The *practice* of ergonomics has been evident through documents dating back to the 1800s; however, the term "ergonomics" was not coined until 1949 (Dahl, 2000; Vitalis, Walker, & Legg, 2001). The most recent definition of the term "**ergonomics**" was established in 2000 by the International Ergonomics Association (IEA; 2005) as "the scientific discipline concerned with the understanding of interactions among humans and other elements of a system, and the profession that applies theory, principles, data and methods to design in order to optimize human well-being and overall system performance" (Marshall, 2000, p. 1). In short, ergonomics has been defined as considering the whole system in the process of "fitting the job to the man" (Vitalis et al. p. 1295).

A systems approach views the properties of the "whole," or system, as arising from interactions and relationships among the parts. In this framework, the practitioner integrates the biological, psychological, and social factors of human performance within the environmental context (Dahl, 2000). Occupational therapists provide ergonomic services for individuals and populations in a variety of systems and settings. They use the principles of ergonomics to design safe and efficient living environments, workplaces, and products. The role of the occupational therapist in ergonomics is informed by knowledge of human performance and potential and the legislation mandating safe, accessible workplaces.

Workplace environments or systems include the organizational structure, environmental factors, tools and equipment, job tasks, and the workers (Dahl, 2000). All aspects of the system are considered in ergonomics. The occupational therapist assesses and analyzes the system to identify the presence of ergonomic risk factors. Workplace surveys, hazard assessments, and job task analyses are tools available to the practitioner. Collaboration with others within the system is necessary for an accurate and thorough assessment and intervention. The other members of the system include the workers, supervisors, engineers, and administration. The occupational therapist benefits from skillful communication skills as well as comprehensive knowledge in the field of ergonomics (see Figure 49.2).

Ergonomic interventions generally fit within three primary categories: administrative, engineering and individual. **Administrative controls** or interventions include changes in the nature of work such as scheduling, worker rotation, or the assignment of work tasks. **Engineering controls** include equipment and workplace designs or changes that reduce the human efforts needed. **Individual controls** include the physical, cognitive and social skills, and performance of the workers. Safe, efficient job design is dependent upon coordination of all aspects of the system.

Matoushek (2005) used the term "**work integration programs**" to refer to the coordination of the clinical features of the injured worker into the organizational and ergonomic aspects of the system. Occupational therapists address both the accessibility of the workplace for all workers as well as the reasonable placement of individuals who have physical, psychological, or behavioral issues. Awareness of ergonomic principles provides a foundation for safely integrating workers into work.

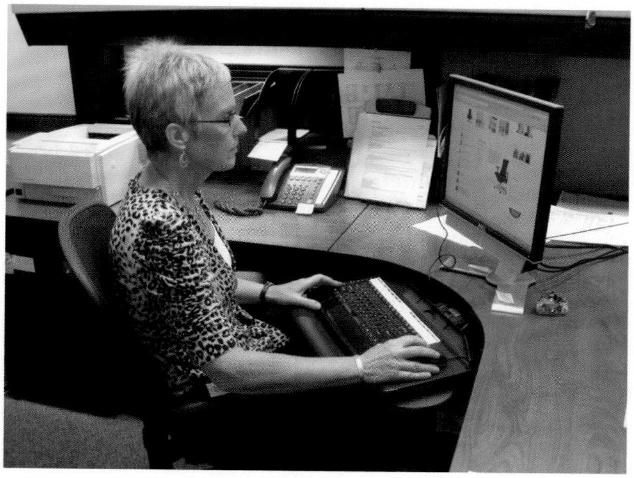

FIGURE 49.2 Those who spend many hours keyboarding may benefit from ergonomic services.

Job Analysis

"Work performance supports participation and productivity, which are essential to the health and well-being of each individual" (AOTA, 2005, p. 676). The role of the occupational therapist in enhancing participation in occupation may include an analysis of work settings. A job analysis provides an objective basis for hiring, evaluating, training, accommodating, and supervising persons with disabilities (United States Department of Labor Office of Disability Employment Policy, 1994).

Regardless of the practice setting, the principles of job analysis are beneficial tools for the occupational therapist. Occupational therapists use these tools when planning the school-to-work transition for school-aged students and participation in supported employment or sheltered workshops by individuals with physical and/or mental disabilities. A job analysis also benefits the clients who are preparing for their first experience with competitive employment or who are returning to employment after illness or injury. In addition, therapists employed in industrial programs may be called upon to assist employers in describing jobs and/or determining the safety of the workplace.

The occupational therapist may be engaged in assessing the job site with a thorough investigation of all aspects of the work environment or perhaps simply to explore discrete components of the job. "Approaches and techniques are intended to provide a foundation for analysis that can be applied to reducing the likelihood of injury, interrupting or minimizing the progression of an illness, or reducing the resultant disability of an injured worker" (Bohr, 1998, p. 229). Job analysis is a dynamic process appropriate to all practice settings that considers the worker, work environment, and work demands. Box 49.1 and Table 49.1 lists references and resources for conducting a job analysis.

Job Description

A **job description** defines the essential functions of the job and how the job relates to other jobs and to the workplace (Bohr, 1998; Ellexson, 2000). An accurate and functional job description must define the essential work tasks, the physical and mental requirements of the worker, the necessary tools and equipment, and a description of the work space and environmental conditions of the job.

Essential tasks are the basic job duties that all employees must be able to perform with or without reasonable accommodation (Ellexson, 2000). The Americans with Disabilities Act (ADA, 1990) mandated that job descriptions include the essential job functions. The essential duties are the reason that the position exists and the degree of expertise or skill that is necessary to perform the task. The job description also includes the **marginal functions** of a job. These are tasks that are not essential to the specific job, or tasks that could, if necessary be completed by another worker. Identification of marginal tasks assists the therapist in determining job placement and provides guidelines for training the worker for work.

Task Analysis

Job analysis and job task analysis refer to a thorough assessment of the physical, cognitive, and psychological demands of the job. **Job analysis** includes a formal methodology that details the interaction between the worker and the equipment of a system. It defines the performance requirements of the worker by a detailed description of the human task requirements. Job task analysis is the specific assessment of a particular task or procedure. A thorough job analysis includes employer and worker interviews, observation of multiple workers performing the task (if possible), measurement of the forces, frequencies and durations of work tasks, the postural requirements such as reaching and leaning, and the environmental and psychosocial conditions present in the workplace.

Methods

Prior to conducting a job analysis, it is imperative to discuss with management or the supervisor several issues regarding the assessment process. The employer will be able to provide information on the least disruptive methods for conducting the evaluation and the necessary safety precautions for the evaluator. Personal protective equipment, such as safety glasses, steel-toed shoes, hearing protection, or special clothing may be required

BOX 49.1 Job Analysis Tools

- General Assessments
  http://www.osha.gov/SLTC/ergonomics/analysis_tools.html
- Rapid Entire Body Assessment (REBA)
  http://www.osha.gov/SLTC/ergonomics/analysis_tools.html
  http://personal.health.usf.edu/tbernard/HollowHills/REBA.pdf
  Hignett, S., & McAtamney, L. (2000). Rapid Entire Body Assessment (REBA). *Applied Ergonomics, 31*, 201–205.
- Rapid Upper Limb Assessment RULA
  http://ergo.human.cornell.edu/ahRULA.html
  McAtamney, L., & Corlett, E. N. (1993). RULA: a survey method for the investigation of work-related upper limb disorders. *Applied Ergonomics, 24*, 91–99.
- Lifting Assessments
  1) http://www.cdc.gov/niosh/docs/94–110/pdfs/94–110.pdf
  Waters, T. R., Putz-Anderson, V., Garg, A., & Fine, L. (1993). Revised NIOSH equation for the design and evaluation of manual lifting tasks. *Ergonomics*, 36, 749–776.
  2) http://www.lni.wa.gov/Safety/Topics/Ergonomics/Services Resources/Tools/default.asp
- Threshold Limit Values for Lifting adapted from American Conference of Governmental Industrial Hygienist® (ACGIH®)
  http://personal.health.usf.edu/tbernard/HollowHills/Lifting TLV11.pdf
- Force Measurement
  Chatillion Force Pressure Gauge
  http://www.chatillon.com
- Vibration
  1) http://wisha-training.lni.wa.gov/training/presentations/HandArmVibrPrimer.ppt
  2) Washington Industrial Safety and Health Act (WISHA) Hand-Arm Vibration Analysis http://personal.health.usf.edu/tbernard/HollowHills/WISHA_HAV.pdf
- Illumination
  Recommended lighting levels by the Illuminating Engineering Society of North America
- Noise
  Occupational Safety and Health Administration (OSHA) Noise standard, 29, DFR 1910.95 (a) and (b)
- Repetition
  http://www.lni.wa.gov/WISHA/Rules/GeneralOccupational Health/PDFs/ErgoRulewithAppendices.pdf
- Posture
  Appendix I: Illustrations of physical risk factors (WAC 296-62-05172).
  http://www.lni.wa.gov/WISHA/Rules/GeneralOccupational Health/PDFs/ErgoRulewithAppendices.pdf
- Monitor Display
  Washington State Department of Labor and Industries. (2002). *Office ergonomics: Practical solutions for a safer workplace*. Retrieved from http://www.lni.wa.gov/IPUB/417-133-000.pdf

TABLE 49.1 Assessments for Conducting a Job Analysis

	Areas of Occupation			Client Factors					
ASSESSMENT	Activity	Participation	Quality of Life	Body Structures and Functions	Values, Beliefs, Spirituality	Performance Skills	Performance Patterns	Activity Demands	Environmental Factors/Context and Environment
Rapid Entire Body Assessment (REBA)				X					
Rapid Upper Limb Assessment (RULA)				X					
National Institute for Occupational Safety and Health (NIOSH) Lifting Equation						X	X	X	X
Threshold Limit Values for Lifting (adapted from ACGIH)						X	X	X	X
Force Pressure Gauge								X	
WISHA Hand-Arm Vibration Analysis									X
Illumination: Recommended lighting levels by the Illuminating Engineering Society of North America									X
Occupational Safety and Health Administration Noise standard, 29, DFR 1910.95 (a) and (b)									X
Repetition								X	
Monitor Display									X

while on the job site. There may be restrictions to interviewing workers while in the performance of their work. Interviews may need to occur during the worker's lunch or break periods. In addition, the therapist should discuss and receive permission in advance for use of any audio, photographic, or video equipment.

Detailed, organized documentation of the information gained during the job analysis will be the most useful. Many checklists or forms are available to use as a starting point allowing the therapist to highlight specific areas to target for more thorough analysis (Occupational Safety and Health Administration [OSHA], 2002; Washington State Department of Labor and Industries, 2005). It is also helpful to use audiotape, photographic, or video equipment to record the worker or workers performing the job, allowing a more thorough analysis at a later time. Other common supplies helpful in job analysis are a tape measure, force pressure gauge, stop watch, and goniometer. In addition, specific tools can be investigated for measuring noise, heat, and vibration.

Supervisor and worker interviews provide valuable insight into all aspects of the job. According to OSHA (2002), "involving employees will help minimize oversights and ensure a quality analysis" (p. 9). The interviews can be a method of learning about routine and infrequent tasks, flow patterns and sequences, and to obtain worker perspectives of physical and mental work stresses (Bohr, 1998; OSHA, 2002).

Formal Measurements

The job analysis involves measurements of many of the aspects of the job (Ellexson, 2000). This includes the dimensions of the workspace and the materials handled. Measuring the workspace includes measuring the dimensions of reach required for the various tasks, the distances required to transport items, and the heights of work surfaces. The weight of objects that are lifted or lowered is documented as well as the frequency, duration, distance, and quality of the task, such as the handholds or the stability of the load. Other forces encountered by the worker are also measured, such as pushing and pulling and use of tools, gloves, and other personal protective equipment.

The body positions of the worker, such as leaning, reaching, or other postures, should be measured or estimated; and the duration and frequency should be recorded. It may only be possible to record the initial and terminal postures for dynamic motions. Video or photographic equipment aid in the assessment of body postures by allowing the evaluator to assess angles, frequency, duration, or other variables later (Bohr, 1998).

Finally, the conditions of the workspace and the environmental considerations such as the ambient temperature, the surface temperatures, the humidity, noise level, illumination, vibration, and so forth are also documented and measured. To assist the therapist in identifying the safe working levels, databases of acceptable working conditions are available. These are based on **epidemiological**, **biomechanical**, psychophysical, and **physiological** approaches (Eastman Kodak, 1983; Snook & Cirello, 1991; Washington State Department of Labor and Industries, 2005; Waters, Putz-Anderson, Garg, & Fine, 1993).

The job analysis is completed by preparing a summary that is specifically developed for the customer. Generally the report will include an overview of the data collected, the problems identified, and recommendations for addressing the problems. "It is often a good idea to offer staged solutions for addressing the problems" (Bohr, 1998, p. 244). The therapist should prioritize solutions that will be the most effective in the short term to assist the employer in analyzing the cost benefit ratio. The emphasis of the report will vary depending on the customer. When the customers are concerned about job placement for a client, the focus of the report will be on the individual. The report will highlight the necessary physical demands and rehabilitation needs such as strengthening, endurance, and/or flexibility. When the focus is on workplace safety, the report will highlight hazardous conditions with recommendations for safety, efficiency, and productivity. Regardless of the purpose of the assessment, the job analysis will identify factors that will either enhance or restrict participation in the occupation of work with recommendations for the client, the rehabilitation team, and/or the employer. "Through observation, demonstration, participation, documentation and analysis, the skilled occupational therapist can develop a clear and concise picture of a specific job" (Ellexson, 2000, p. 6).

Functional Capacity Evaluation

The **functional capacity evaluation** (FCE) is an integral assessment tool used for work injury prevention and rehabilitation. FCEs define an individual's functional abilities and/or limitations in the context of safe, productive work tasks. An FCE itself involves a process of systematically gathering and testing information and making and testing hypotheses about performance, often in relation to an occupation in context. The therapist begins by reviewing referral information related to a client's medical and work history. A series of test activities are then administered to measure whether the person has the abilities to meet the required job demands, determine a level of disability, or demonstrate the need for, and progress in, rehabilitation (Harwood, 2004). Physicians, employers, insurers, and benefits adjudicators often rely upon FCEs to provide definitive answers in a variety of situations involving work. Results of these evaluations have significant implications for further rehabilitation efforts, employment, compensability determinations, and cash benefits.

FCEs include a wide range of evaluation activities. The simplest evaluations involve a series of standardized tasks with measured weights and distances, and a trained observer; these are available for upper extremity as well as back/lower extremity activities. Other approaches use machines to measure average and peak forces, velocity, and range of motion in several different planes. In these situations, workers are generally asked to exert a maximal effort. Job simulation, using tasks and equipment specific to a particular job, has recently become more popular, in part due to the ADA requirement that valid testing should be job-specific and focus on a comparison of capacity to actual job demands (Lechner, 1998).

The concept of matching job/workplace demands to the capabilities and limitations of a worker is a fundamental assumption underlying FCE application. One of the most important aspects of an FCE is that the measurement of capacity is specific to the demands posed by the job. The estimates of job demands are inexact generalizations that have not been scientifically validated. A formal job analysis is desirable for those FCEs intended to measure ability to work at a specific job. Discussions with employees and written company job descriptions are helpful also in obtaining accurate assessments of job demands.

FCEs are usually performed in the clinic and may range from 2 to 4 hours in duration over the course of a 2-day period. Protocols often extrapolate from tasks that are stereotypical, or performed at near-maximal levels for a short period of time, to predict ability to sustain job activities for a full workday and workweek. Performance on FCE tasks are often compared with population or coworker norms because actual job force requirements are not often estimated during this process. It is important for therapists to use good observational skills throughout the assessment to ensure a client's safe performance (King, 2005).

FCEs are generally classified into two broad categories: comprehensive and job-specific (Frings-Dresen & Sluiter, 2003; King, Tuckwell, & Barrett, 1998). When administering the comprehensive FCE, most evaluators use a complete battery of tasks that cover all 20 physical demands listed in the Dictionary of Occupational Titles (United States Department of Labor Employment and Training Administration, 1977).

In job-specific testing, the evaluator tests only those tasks directly related to the job. The job specific testing is more cost-effective and often used for disability determination. However, if the client cannot return to the former job, then additional testing may be required.

FCE reporting formats vary in length from 1 page to 35 pages or more. The primary objective is to describe the client's safe level of overall exertion, ranging from sedentary to very heavy. A summary cover page is usually attached to the FCE data collection forms when submitting FCE information to referral sources.

In these times of unprecedented workers' compensation costs and disability costs, there is a pressing need to return workers to gainful employment if possible and to make appropriate disability decisions for those who are unable to work. A well-designed FCE can provide objective information on a wide range of functional activities for clinical decision making (Isernhagen, 1988; Lechner, Jackson, Roth & Straaton, 1994; Lechner, Roth, & Straaton, 1991)

Preplacement Assessment

Preplacement assessments (PPAs) are used by employers to determine if an individual is capable of performing the job. The results of these assessments help employers make appropriate decisions related to the placement of individuals in jobs without hazards to the safety of themselves or others. Proper PPAs may reduce the number and costs of employee injuries as well as absenteeism attributed to ill health (Nachreiner et al., 1999).

Prior to the passage of the ADA of 1990, pre-work screening was performed for the purpose of excluding individuals from employment if they presented an increased risk of any type of illness or injury (Andstadt, 1989). These screenings are no longer legal. PPAs have taken the place of these screenings. Applicants must now be given a conditional offer of hire based on successful completion of the PPA. The preplacement screen is viewed as an injury prevention strategy and not as a means to screen out applicants. The employer's decision to withdraw a job offer must be based on the applicant's inability to perform the essential functions of the job with or without accommodations. A prospective employee can be denied the job only if he or she is at definite risk of specific injury or illness while performing the essential functions of the job. Employers are required to provide reasonable accommodation to mitigate these risks as much as possible (Nachreiner et al., 1999).

Occupational therapists design and administer preplacement screenings. The screening occurs after a conditional offer of hire, and it must apply to all applicants for a specific job position. First, a job description is requested by the therapist to ascertain the essential functions of the job. If a job description is not available, the therapist must perform a job analysis to determine the physical demands of the job. This entails observing job tasks, videotaping employees performing the job, and collecting workstation measurements to obtain accurate information to design an appropriate preplacement screen. Once the job description is developed, the therapist develops a standardized test of the physical demands of the job. To verify that the preplacement screen tests what it is intended to test, a sample of current employees performing the particular job is selected to validate the job description and pilot the test. The therapist rates the performance of the individual according to the validated physical demands of the job. The applicant receives the scoring information. The evaluator does not make hiring interpretations. The ultimate decision to hire is in the hands of the employer.

Work Hardening and Work Conditioning Programs

The term *work hardening* came into being in the late 1970s as professionals used work as a treatment or evaluation modality. Other terms used synonymously are *work conditioning, work readiness, and work capabilities* (Isernhagen, 1988). In 1989, the Commission on Accreditation of Rehabilitation Facilities (CARF, 1988) officially defined **work hardening** as "a highly structured, goal-oriented, individualized treatment program designed to maximize the individual's ability to return to work" (p. 69). The guidelines recommended that work hardening programs be interdisciplinary in nature and capable of addressing the functional, physical, behavioral, and vocational needs of the person served. CARF suggested the use of real or simulated work activities in conjunction with conditioning activities to improve biomechanical, neuromuscular, cardiovascular/metabolic, behavioral, and vocational functioning (King, 1998). Work hardening programs usually employ exercise equipment, a work-simulation area, and quiet, private areas for testing and evaluation.

Work conditioning programs emphasize physical conditioning, which addresses issues of strength, endurance, flexibility, motor control, and cardiopulmonary function (Helm-Williams, 1993). They are shorter in duration than work hardening programs, use exercise, aerobic conditioning, education and limited work task simulation, and require less physical space than work hardening programs. Work conditioning programs usually involve only one or two disciplines and are usually half-day programs. Work hardening and work conditioning programs are increasingly being located in nonmedical settings such as industrial parks, strip shopping malls, office complexes, and at the work site. Programs implemented at the work site provide a more realistic environment and place the employee back at work and in close communication with the employer.

The work hardening and work conditioning evaluation and treatment process consists of entrance criteria whereby clients are unable to return to work due to pain or dysfunction following injury and the clients agree to participate in the program. The clients must also have a reasonably good prognosis for improvement of employment capacity and a job-oriented goal (King, 1998). The occupational therapist initially interviews the client to gather valuable information related to his or her medical and work history. Insight into what procedures have worked or failed in the past, as well as the client's beliefs or misperceptions about his or her condition, can be ascertained. Job history, preinjury and postinjury, and how long the client has been off work or on light duty is important information in designing a work rehabilitation program. An evaluation of a client's functional capabilities is performed prior to performance of any conditioning and/or work-related activities. The purpose of this evaluation is to become familiar with the client's current functional status, behaviors associated with work activity, potential latent symptom responses after activity, and body mechanics techniques. This information is compared with the client's job demands and goals for progress.

The client's length of time in work hardening and work conditioning programs depends on his or her individualized treatment needs and the treatment protocols established by the program. Typically, clients are started in programs for 2 hours per day, eventually progressing to 4 hours as tolerated. This requires highly focused and well managed treatment plans. Most programs start with warm-up exercises, followed by strengthening and job simulation activities. Education on risk factors to injury and prevention of injuries with use of proper body mechanics and work methods is woven into the program. Clients are discharged when (1) they meet their goals, (2) progress has stopped or slowed to an imperceptible level, (3) the client has medical complications, or (4) the client is noncompliant with the program.

Work rehabilitation is the term most recently coined to reflect programs that combine aspects of work hardening and work conditioning programs. Work rehabilitation is a structured program of graded physical conditioning/strengthening exercises and functional tasks in conjunction with real or simulated job activities. Treatment is designed to improve the individual's cardiopulmonary, neuromusculoskeletal (strength, endurance, movement, flexibility, stability, and motor control) functions, biomechanical/human performance levels, and **psychosocial** aspects as they relate to the demands of work. Work rehabilitation provides a transition between acute care and return to work while addressing issues of safety, physical tolerances, work behaviors, and functional abilities (Ellexson, 2000).

Case Management

An increasing number of occupational therapists are assuming case management roles. Interestingly enough, case management is not a profession. It is an area of practice within a profession. Therapists, nurses, social workers, and rehabilitation counselors may all serve as case managers. Their goal is to achieve a successful, cost-effective method to return clients to work.

The non-profit organization Case Management Society of America (CMSA, 1995) was established in 1989. Their *Standards of Practice for Case Management* document defines **case management** as "a collaborative process which assesses, plans, implements, coordinates, monitors, and evaluates options and services to meet an individual's health needs through communication and available resources to promote quality cost effective outcomes" (p. 8). A certification process was established to monitor professional conduct and provide standards of practice to those who perform case management functions. Certified or not, a successful case manager must be skilled in communication, diplomacy, and relationship building. He or she must demonstrate skill in identifying cost-effective resources and make appropriate referrals to promote case closure.

In a work injury case, where workers' compensation is involved, the case manager may interact with several players: the injured employee, the employer, the insurance carrier, and the physician. Each player has a different perspective on the injury. Case management services are not restricted to workers' compensation cases, however. Case management services are just as important in other areas of work rehabilitation such as those that involve individuals with mental illness and developmental disabilities. The primary difference between case management practice with different populations is the team of players and the resources investigated to facilitate a successful outcome. Regardless of the population served, case management requires the ability to coordinate a complex mix of resources and services. These skills are dependent, at least in part, on clinical experience.

Settings

Work programs in occupational therapy are evident in a variety of different settings. Traditional settings include hospitals, clinics, and schools. Non-traditional occupational therapy settings include on-site programs in industry, fitness centers, and community rehabilitation programs. Regardless of the setting, the focus on the therapeutic value of work is a key aspect of occupational therapy. Occupational therapy services in these various settings continue to receive attention regarding how effective they are. See Table 49.2 for examples of evidence that support interventions in these settings.

On-site Rehabilitation and Injury Management

The industrial rehabilitation movement in the 1980s provided the impetus for the development of on-site rehabilitation programs in industry. Although therapists working on-site in industry represent only a fraction of those involved in occupational rehabilitation, the many benefits of these programs foster their continued growth (Jundt & King, 1999; Tramposh, 1998). Occupational therapists working on-site or consulting with industry have many roles that include prevention, assessment, and rehabilitation programming. The benefits of on-site programming are decreased overall costs and improved quality care (B. A. Larson, 2000; Melnik, 2000). Therapists working on-site in industry enjoy improved communication with the employer, increased autonomy, and the ability to assess and intervene from an informed perspective, consistent with the holistic philosophy of occupational therapy.

The clients benefit from on-site programs in several ways. On-site programs may reduce the waiting time for appointments, enhancing recovery through immediate care. The integration of the on-site therapist into the culture of the industrial setting may improve reasonable restricted duty placement and progression toward full duty work. Awareness of the job demands and the worker's

TABLE 49.2 Work: Samples of Evidence-Based Interventions

Authors	Objective or Research Question	Findings
Amini, 2011	What occupational therapy interventions are effective in the rehabilitation of individuals with work-related injuries or conditions of the forearm, wrist, and hand?	The use of occupation-based activities has reasonable yet limited evidence to support its effectiveness. This review supports the premise that many client factors can be positively affected through the use of several commonly used occupational therapy–related modalities and methods.
Bond, Drake, & Becker, 2008	What evidence supports the Individual Placement and Support (IPS) model of supported employment for clients with severe mental illness?	The number, consistency, and effect sizes of studies of evidence-based supported employment establish it as one of the most robust interventions available for persons with severe mental illness.
de Boer et al., 2011	To evaluate the effectiveness of interventions aimed at enhancing return-to-work in cancer patients.	Moderate quality evidence showed that employed patients with cancer experience return-to-work benefits from multidisciplinary interventions compared to care as usual.
Schaafsma et al., 2010	To compare the effectiveness of physical conditioning programs in reducing time lost from work for workers with back pain.	The effectiveness of physical conditioning programs in reducing sick leave when compared to usual care or other exercises in workers with back pain remains uncertain. In workers with acute back pain, these programs probably have no effect on sick leave; but there may be a positive effect on sick leave for workers with subacute and chronic back pain. Workplace involvement might improve the outcome. Better understanding of the mechanism behind physical conditioning programs and return-to-work is needed to be able to develop more effective interventions.
Cheng & Hung, 2007	What is the effect of workplace-based rehabilitation program on the return to work outcome of work-related rotator cuff disorder, which is based on the therapeutic use of actual work facilities and work environment?	The workplace-based work hardening program appeared to be more effective in facilitating the return-to-work process of the injured worker as assessed immediately following intervention as compared to the clinic-based work hardening program.
Snodgrass, 2011	What occupational therapy interventions are effective in the rehabilitation of individuals with work-related low back injuries and illnesses?	For interventions to be effective, occupational therapy practitioners should use a holistic, client-centered approach. The research supports the need for occupational therapy practitioners to consider multiple strategies for addressing clients' needs. Specifically, interventions for individuals with low back injuries and illnesses should incorporate a biopsychosocial, client-centered approach that includes actively involving the client in the rehabilitation process at the beginning of the intervention process and addressing the client's psychosocial needs in addition to his or her physical impairments.
van Geen, Edelaar, Janssen, & van Eijk, 2007	To determine the long-term effect of multidisciplinary back training on the work participation of patients with nonspecific chronic low back pain.	In the long term, multidisciplinary back training has a positive effect on work participation in patients with nonspecific chronic low back pain.
Webb et al., 2009	One of the aims of this study was to determine which interventions most effectively reduce workplace-related alcohol problems.	It appears from the evidence that brief interventions, interventions contained within health and lifestyle checks, psychosocial skills training, and peer referral have potential to produce beneficial results.

physical capacity may prevent reinjury while allowing the worker to safely continue in productive employment.

The employer also benefits from on-site programming. Successful programs allow the employer to oversee an employee's path through rehabilitation. Communication is improved through on-site interactions between the employee, the supervisor, and the practitioner. Improved communication speeds the rehabilitation process, reducing overall workers' compensation costs (Tramposh, 1998). The costs associated with travel to and from off-site clinics are also reduced by keeping the workers on-site for their therapy visits.

On-site therapists enjoy immersion in the culture of the industry, enhancing their realistic programming for the client, and adding the benefits of early rehabilitation. Therapists who work on-site often work autonomously and require a thorough understanding of work injury assessment, rehabilitation, prevention, and the psychosocial aspects of disability (B. A. Larson, 2000; Tramposh, 1998). In addition, knowledge of the rehabilitation system, the ability to analyze tasks, and the ability to creatively adapt the physical environment are all important skills. The setting requires skills in decision making and in dealing with persons from various socioeconomic and cultural backgrounds. The therapist's role is often an intermediary between the injured worker, the employer, and the workers' compensation carrier, each bringing forth their own perspectives and issues.

On-site prevention programs include educational offerings such as back schools, stretching programs, fitness programs, and other health promotion or wellness activities (Melnik, 2000). Prevention can also include worker symptom surveys, hazard assessments, ergonomic assessments, writing job descriptions, and participation in safety teams and committees (Rothman, 1998). Prevention programs must be continually adapted to the constantly changing industrial environment. Successful programs require management support, supervisor buy-in, employee participation, and ongoing support and reinforcement (Melnick, 2000). See Figure 49.3

Assessment and rehabilitation of injured workers in on-site clinics include a vast array of services. Early intervention assessments may involve screening, education, and prevention activities for workers who have experienced mild symptoms or discomfort (Olson, 1999). Comprehensive assessments include worker evaluations for specific injuries as well as functional capacity evaluations. Rehabilitation programming can include the management of a specific injury, such as carpal tunnel, or more intensive work hardening and work conditioning programs. On-site therapists have the advantage of integrating services within the context of the worker's physical job demands. On-site therapists may also be involved in job analysis, ergonomic analysis, job placement, and the design of restricted duty programs. The occupational therapist's role on-site in industry is to provide prevention, assessment, and intervention services to enhance a safe, efficient, and productive work environment for the worker and the employer.

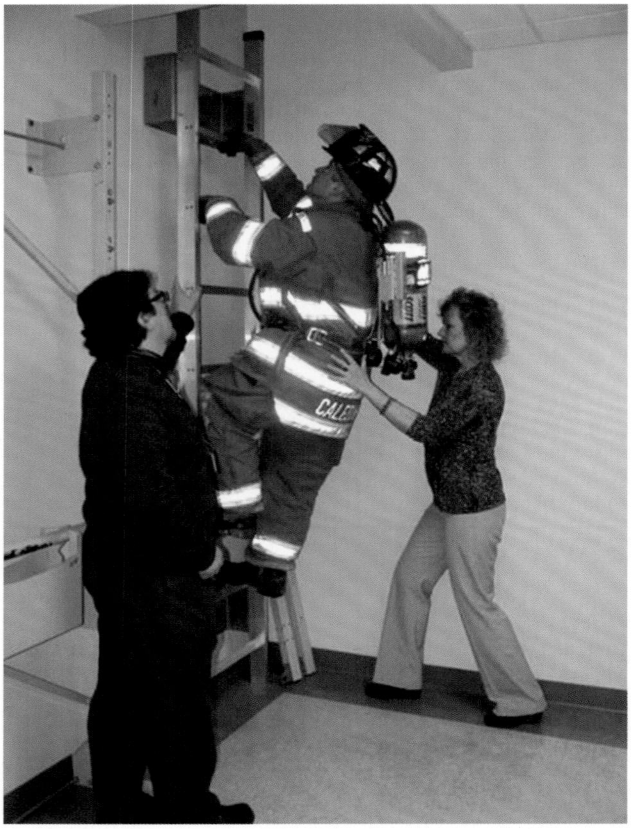

FIGURE 49.3 A therapist conducting a work site job analysis.

Work Clinics

Throughout the history of occupational therapy, participation in valued occupations, including work, has provided the foundation of rehabilitation (Lysaght & Wright, 2005). In the late 1970s and 1980s, many industrial rehabilitation clinics emerged providing services that focused on return-to-work as the outcome of intensive rehabilitation programs (Jacobs & Baker, 2000; Tramposh, 1998). The individualized therapy programs included functional capacity evaluations and progressive strengthening based on simulating the critical aspects of the client's work. Rehabilitation included creating workstations that represented the client's actual work tasks. The integrated services were designed to safely identify a client's tolerance for work tasks and to progress toward returning the client to productive employment. Although the primary focus of work has been obvious in these "end of rehabilitation programs," it has been no less evident in other rehabilitation settings. Safe, productive return to work has been included to some extent in all contexts of occupational therapy.

Hospital-Based and Freestanding Clinics

Traditional occupational therapy programs exist in hospitals and clinics providing inpatient and outpatient services to individuals with illnesses or injuries. Work, as a focus of rehabilitation, can be enhanced by the occupational therapy practitioner who analyzes the multidimensional issues faced by these individuals. Standardized rehabilitation assessment tools are available and can be customized to assess the physical, cognitive, and behavioral abilities of the individual in relation to the demands of the workplace. These skills are measured within the framework of productivity, interpersonal skills, and safety (Chappell, Higham, & McLean, 2003; Jackson, Harkess, & Ellis, 2004). Treatment programs address the identified deficit areas in performance and simulate the unpredictable nature of actual workplace demands. Studies have shown that use of a formal tool for addressing work abilities improved the decisiveness and clear recommendations by the therapist and provided a clear standard for formatting reports, and the clients expressed satisfaction that alternatives were suggested, which included alternative work, further education, and voluntary work options (Jackson et al., 2004). Also, use of a standardized assessment resulted in increased participation of the clients in hobbies and leisure pursuits.

Occupational therapists must consider the barriers to employment when designing rehabilitation programs. Awareness of problem areas can guide assessment, training, and intervention. Lack of transportation, concerns about loss of financial benefits, and lack of awareness of social and federal programs have been cited as barriers to employment among the disabled (Fiedler et al., 2002). Occupational therapy interventions focus on overcoming barriers through specifically designed rehabilitation programs and education that is presented in a timely fashion. In a study of individuals with spinal cord injuries who were discharged from an inpatient rehabilitation unit, Fiedler and colleagues found that information on vocational services was presented too early in the rehabilitation process, limiting retention and usefulness. Although provision of the vocational information was a standard aspect of care, the majority of the study participants were unaware of federal vocational programs that were available to them.

The rehabilitation phase provides multiple opportunities for occupational therapists to explore issues and barriers to participation in work activities. The comprehensive occupational therapy program for individuals receiving services in hospital or clinic settings should include a work-focused standardized assessment, individualized intervention guided by the assessment, and education and training in areas informed by awareness of the barriers to employment.

Community Work Programs

Occupational therapy practitioners play major roles in using and developing the social context for vocational exploration and placement of persons with mental illness and developmental delays. Therapists are instrumental in developing community programs that are built on strong support networks and relationships with employers and other community job service agencies and health personnel. To influence the social context, practitioners use various management skills: needs evaluation, program development, work site development, evaluation and monitoring of placements, and advocacy at the community level (Ramsey, Starnes, & Robertson, 2000).

Occupational therapy practitioners involved in vocational programming must be knowledgeable about work incentive issues that help persons make the transition to work. Supplemental Security Income (SSI), Social Security Disability Insurance (SSDI), Welfare-to-Work incentives, and other public assistance programs must be well understood in order to adhere to the policies that qualify recipients to continue receipt of benefits while transitioning to gainful employment.

Many different program models exist to address vocational needs of persons with serious mental illness and developmental delays. Overall, program models fall into two categories: programs that train and programs that both train and place.

Training Programs

Both simulated and actual work settings are used in training programs that are designed to train the client for general work habits and specific work skills. These programs encourage clients to obtain employment paying at least minimum wage. Integrated environments provide

CASE STUDY 49.2 Mr. Todd: An Injured Sheet Metal Worker

Mr. Todd is 42 years old and employed as a sheet metal worker. He is the primary source of income for his family of four: two sons and a wife. Two months ago, a machine malfunctioned and a stamping machine crushed his right hand. He has had multiple surgeries to structurally restore the right hand. Impairments in sensation, muscle strength, and coordination exist in his hand. Workers' compensation is providing him financial assistance in the form of income and medical expense coverage, but he is concerned about his job and when and whether he will be able to return to work. His physician has referred him to a work rehabilitation program.

Questions

What is the occupational therapy process for Mr. Todd's rehabilitation?
How does the therapist determine Mr. Todd's functional abilities to return to work?

Discussion

The therapist should review Mr. Todd's work, social, and medical history. Intake interview information will likely reveal Mr. Todd's desire to return to his previous job. A job description from the employer and/or reported by Mr. Todd should be obtained. An initial musculoskeletal assessment should be conducted to determine the extent of Mr. Todd's impairments. A work rehabilitation program is then established to address these impairments. This program should include job simulation tasks to facilitate functional capabilities to perform his previous job. Communication with the employer and/or case manager is crucial to promote an early return to work plan. The employer may be willing to accept Mr. Todd back sooner if the employer understands Mr. Todd's abilities and the therapist articulates job accommodation measures.

for additional learning opportunities with individuals without mental illnesses or developmental disabilities.

Place and Train Programs

Place and train programs put clients into actual work environments that require them to learn to solve problems and adapt to work styles in a real work environment. Initially, the occupational therapist will evaluate the client's vocational potential by assessing medical and work history, work skills, social skills, specific job stresses, transportation needs, and so forth to determine an appropriate job placement. No best way exists for designing work programs that meet all clients' needs. Instead, occupational therapy programs that offer a range of services best respond to client and employer needs.

Vocational programs require a continuum of services. The developer of these programs must help clients build work habits and skills at one end of the continuum and locate independent part-time or full-time paid employment at the other end of the continuum.

Sheltered Workshops

Sheltered workshops are noncompetitive employment settings intended to provide many of the positive benefits of a work atmosphere for individuals with disabilities. A longstanding model of vocational rehabilitation, sheltered workshops strive to provide a protected work environment while developing vocational competency and providing behavioral interventions if needed (Siporin, 1999). Some individuals with physical or mental disabilities struggle with many issues in competitive employment settings such as social skills, personal hygiene, and appearance. Difficulties in these areas can further isolate individuals rather than foster inclusion (Krupa, Lagarde, & Carmichael, 2003).

Siporin (1999) suggested that the occupational therapist is ideally suited to work in the sheltered workshop setting by assisting clients to build on existing skills or train for new skills aimed at successful employment. The occupational therapists' role in sheltered workshop settings includes assessment and training in activities of daily living, sensorimotor skills, cognitive abilities, and social skills. Whereas the protected environment of the sheltered workshop remains a successful option for some individuals with disabilities, studies have indicated that supported employment has proved to be a better option for many to enhance quality of life while allowing clients to earn competitive wages in the community (Bond, 2004; Siporin & Lysack, 2004).

Supported Employment

Supported employment refers to competitive work in an integrated work environment consistent with the strengths, resources, priorities, concerns, abilities, capabilities, interests, and informed choice of the individuals (Rehabilitation Act Amendments, 1998). The Rehabilitation Act Amendments of 1986 provided the initial springboard for the transition from sheltered workshops into supported employment programs. It was intended to foster inclusion and integration of persons with disabilities into the economic, political, social, cultural, and educational mainstream of American society. It was based on the premise that work is a valued activity for everyone, including persons with disabilities. It stated that work fulfilled the need of an individual to be productive, promoted independence, enhanced self-esteem, and allowed for participation in the mainstream of life in the United States, which included earning competitive wages.

The three essential characteristics of supported employment are paid work, employment in an integrated work setting, and ongoing support services available to meet continuous or periodic training needs. The ongoing services may include a job coach, job trainer, work-study coordinator, and/or an employment counselor. Studies have shown that participation in supported employment improved the quality of life for persons with disabilities (Bond, 2004; Siporin & Lysack 2004). Greater benefits were realized by consumers who held their competitive jobs for sustained periods of time, worked in jobs that reflected their choices, and when clients were placed directly into the work environment rather than undergoing training prior to placement.

Strong evidence supports the integration of rehabilitation and vocational services (Bond, 2004). The occupational therapist in many different practice settings can play an integral role in preparing a client for supported employment. School systems, mental health settings, and rehabilitation units all promote work as a valued outcome of occupational therapy intervention. The occupational therapist is ideally positioned to include motor skills function, cognitive function, social skills, activities of daily living, and adaptive equipment as part of the comprehensive treatment program. "Occupational therapists can contribute to closing the gap between the impairments of individuals with developmental disabilities and the complex demands of supported employment and even the competitive workplace" (Siporin & Lysack, 2004, p. 463).

Funding and Legal Issues

There are specific laws that govern and influence practice in work programs. Therapists should become familiar with this legislation and how it impacts practice and the various populations they serve.

Workers' Compensation

The workers' compensation law is actually a system of individual state workers' compensation laws. These laws were designed to (1) cover the medical expenses and wage loss of workers who are injured or develop illnesses on the job, and (2) shield employers from costly negligence lawsuits. Box 49.2 outlines the features of a typical workers' compensation system. Most states require

Practice Dilemma

Issues in Work Practice

Imagine that you are an occupational therapist in the following practice settings, and describe the assessments and interventions that you would pursue for your clients.

- You are a school-based therapist working with a 16-year-old boy who has spasticity of the upper extremities due to cerebral palsy.
- The factory where you provide on-site services employs many workers over the age of 50 years.
- You are working in a homeless shelter with a 27-year-old single mother who has two small children and an eighth-grade education.
- The inpatient rehabilitation unit is well known for treatment of individuals with spinal cord injuries. Your caseload includes individuals between 16 and 35 years of age.

employers to carry workers' compensation insurance. The states differ in respect to employers' insurance arrangements and their benefits offered to employees. However, most states cover medical expenses (including rehabilitation), disabilities (partial, total, temporary, permanent), and survivors' benefits (Business and Legal Reports, 1997; Fishback, 2010).

Americans with Disabilities Act

The ADA was passed in 1992 to prohibit discrimination against qualified individuals with physical or mental disabilities in all employment settings. The ADA is divided into five titles. Table 49.3 provides an outline of the areas of coverage. In 2008, the ADA Amendments Act was signed into law. The amendments focus on the discrimination at issue instead of the individual's disability. Among the significant changes to the law were the definition of "disability" and the definition of "major life activities" (U.S. Equal Employment Opportunity Commission, 2008).

Rehabilitation Act of 1973

Many of the concepts contained in the ADA have as their origin the Rehabilitation Act of 1973. By its terms, the Rehabilitation Act of 1973 was limited in scope. It prohibited discrimination only by federal agencies, entities that have contracts with the federal government, and recipients of federal financial assistance. Three major classes of recipients of federal funds are (1) public school systems; (2) colleges and other institutions of higher learning; and (3) health, welfare, and social service providers (Domer, 1998).

In 1992, the Rehabilitation Act of 1973 was amended so that its terms would conform to those set forth in the ADA. State plans were developed that allowed each state to

BOX 49.2 Features of Workers' Compensation Systems

- Coverage of workers' compensation is limited to employees who are injured on the job.
- Workers' compensation is automatic.
- Employee injuries and illnesses that arise out of the course of employment are usually considered compensable.
- Most workers' compensation systems include wage-loss benefits, which are usually between one-half and three-fourths of the employee's average weekly wage.
- Most workers' compensation systems require payment of all medical expenses, including such expenses as hospital expenses, rehabilitation, and prosthesis expenses.
- Administration of workers' compensation is usually assigned to a commission or board within each state.
- In accepting workers' compensation, injured employees waive any common law action to sue the employer.
- When an injury is of a permanent nature, a dollar value for the percentage of loss to the injured employee is assigned and known as permanent partial disability or permanent total disability.
- In most states, employers with one or more employees are normally required to possess workers' compensation.
- Workers' compensation benefits are generally separate from the employment status of the injured employee.
- The workers' compensation commission/board in each state normally develops administrative rules and regulations for the administration and hearing procedures (Schneid & Schumann, 1997).
- Virtually all workers' compensations systems are fundamentally a no-fault mechanism through which employees who incur work-related injuries and illnesses are compensated with monetary and medical benefits. Either party's potential negligence is usually not an issue as long as there is an employer/employee relationship. Employees are guaranteed a percentage of wages (usually two-thirds) and full payment for their medical costs when injured on the job. Employers are guaranteed a reduced monetary cost for these injuries or illnesses and are provided a protection from additional or future legal action by the employee for the injury.

TABLE 49.3 Five Titles of the Americans with Disabilities Act

Title	Area	Description
I	Employee Provisions	Protects employees with disabilities from discrimination with regard to job applications, hiring, advancement, discharge, compensation, training and other terms, and conditions and privileges of employment.
II	Public Services	Prohibits discrimination against persons with disabilities by public entities. This covers all governmental programs, services, activities and employment, but not the private sector. Requires that public transportation entities make a good faith effort to obtain or make vehicles accessible to persons with disabilities.
III	Public Accommodations	Extends the requirements in Title II to the private sector public facilities. Requires that all goods, services, privileges, advantages or facilities of any public place be offered to those with disabilities.
IV	Telecommunications	Requires telecommunication services provide individuals with speech-related disabilities the ability to communicate with hearing individuals through the use of telecommunication devices for the deaf.
V	Miscellaneous Provisions	Addresses insurance-related issues such as allowing insurance providers to continue to use the pre-existing condition clause but prohibits denial of health insurance coverage to individuals based on their disability. Does not limit or invalidate other federal or state laws that provide equal or greater protection to persons with disabilities.

submit to the commissioner of the Rehabilitation Services Administration a plan for **vocational rehabilitation** and assigned a state agency to administer or supervise the plan. The 1992 amendments to the act emphasized individual written rehabilitation programs, which were designed to achieve an employment objective consistent with the individual's unique strengths, resources, priorities, concerns, abilities, and capabilities and include a statement of the long-term rehabilitation goals. The term *disability* was substituted for *handicap* in the statute.

The act provided for training and community rehabilitation programs. It authorizes grants and contracts to ensure that skilled personnel are available to provide rehabilitation services to individuals with disabilities through vocational, medical, social, and psychological rehabilitation programs, and through supported employment programs, independent living services programs, and client assistant programs (Domer, 1998). The grants and contracts exist to provide training and information to individuals with disabilities and to their parents, families, guardians, advocates, and authorized representatives.

Social Security Disability

In the mid-1950s, the Social Security Act (SSA) established a social insurance program designed to provide guaranteed income to individuals with disabilities when they are found to be generally incapable of gainful employment. Its purpose is to provide a basic level of financial support for people who cannot support themselves because of disability. The SSA provides for disability benefit programs administered by the SSA, including SSDI and SSI programs. The SSDI program provides benefits to disabled workers, dependents, and widows/widowers if the worker is insured under the provisions of the program. The SSI program provides benefits to disabled individuals whose incomes and assets fall below a specified level (Domer, 1998).

Conclusion

Occupational therapists address work issues for clients as young as 14 years old in school-based transition programs and across the life span to older adults who continue to benefit from work activities. The practice settings are varied including both traditional and non-traditional environments. Work-related assessments and interventions require the occupational therapist to integrate medical, psychological, behavioral, and philosophical dimensions to address the specific needs of the client, the population, the setting, and the system. Communication and collaboration with the clients, their families, and the team members enhance the success of work programs in all settings. The basic premise of work as a meaningful occupation provides the foundation for occupational therapy in work programs.

Reference

American Occupational Therapy Association. (2005). Occupational therapy services in facilitating work performance. *American Journal of Occupational Therapy, 59*, 676–679.

American Occupational Therapy Association. (2008). Occupational therapy practice framework: Domain and process, 2nd edition. *American Journal of Occupational Therapy, 62*, 625–683.

American Occupational Therapy Association Commission on Practice. (2010). Standards of practice for occupational therapy. *American Journal of Occupational Therapy, 64*, S106–S111.

Americans with Disabilities Act of 1990, Pub. L. No. 101-336, 42 U.S.C.A. § 12101 *et seq.*

Amini, D. (2011). Occupational therapy interventions for work-related injuries and conditions of the forearm, wrist, and hand: A systematic review. *American Journal of Occupational Therapy, 65*, 29–36.

Andstadt, G. W. (1989). Occupational medicine forum: Preplacement/pre-employment physical examinations. *Journal of Occupational Medicine, 32*, 295–299.

Bohr, P. C. (1998). Work analysis. In P. M. King (Ed.), *Sourcebook of occupational rehabilitation* (pp. 229–245) New York, NY: Plenum Press.

Bond, G. R. (2004). Supported employment: Evidence for an evidence-based practice. *Psychiatric Rehabilitation Journal, 27*, 345–360.

Bond, G. R., Drake, R. E., & Becker, D. R. (2008). An update on randomized controlled trials of evidence-based supported employment. *Psychiatric Rehabilitation Journal*, 31,280–290.

Bureau of Labor Statistics. (2005). *Older workers and severity of occupational injuries and illnesses involving days away from work.* Retrieved from http://www.bls.gov/opub/cwc/sh20050713ch01.htm

Business and Legal Reports. (1997). *Encyclopedia of workers' compensation.* Madison, CT: Business & Legal Reports Inc.

Carrivick, P. J. W., Lee, A. H., Yau, K. K. W., & Stevenson, M. R. (2005). Evaluating the effectiveness of a participatory ergonomics approach in reducing the risk and severity of injuries from manual handling. *Ergonomics, 48*, 907–914.

Case Management Society of America. (1995). *CMSA standards of practice for case management guidebook.* Little Rock, AR: Author.

Chappell, I., Higham, J., & McLean, A. M. (2003). An occupational therapy work skills assessment for individuals with head injury. *The Canadian Journal of Occupational Therapy, 70*, 163–169.

Cheng, A. S., & Hung, L. K. (2007). Randomized controlled trial of workplace-based rehabilitation for work-related rotator cuff disorder. *Journal of Occupational Rehabilitation, 17*, 487–503.

Commission on Accreditation of Rehabilitation Facilities. (1988). *1988 standards manual for organizations serving people with disabilities.* Tucson, AZ: Author.

Dahl, R. (2000). Ergonomics. In B. L. Kornblau & K. Jacobs (Eds.), *Work: Principles and practice—A self-paced course from AOTA, Lesson 12*, Bethesda, MD: American Occupational Therapy Association.

de Boer, A. G., Taskila, T., Tamminga, S. J., Frings-Dresen, M. H., Feuerstein, M., & Verbeek, J. H. (2011). Interventions to enhance return-to-work for cancer patients. *Cochrane Database of Systematic Reviews*, (2), CD007569.

Dickie, V. A. (2003). Establishing worker identity: A study of people in craft work. *American Journal of Occupational Therapy, 57*, 250–261.

Domer, T. (1998). Regulatory agencies and legislation. In P. M. King (Ed.), *Sourcebook of occupational rehabilitation* (pp. 43–68). New York, NY: Plenum.

Eastman Kodak Company. (1983). *Ergonomic design for people at work: a sourcebook for human factors practitioners in industry including safety, design, and industrial engineers, medical, industrial hygiene, and industrial relations personnel, and management.* Belmont, CA: Lifetime Learning.

Ellexson, M. T. (2000). Job analysis. In B. L. Kornblau & K. Jacobs (Eds.), *Work: Principles and practice—A self-paced course from AOTA, Lesson 5* (pp. 1–14). Bethesda, MD: American Occupational Therapy Association.

Fiedler, I. G., Indermuehle, D. L., Drobac, W., & Laud, P. (2002). Perceived barriers to employment in individuals with spinal cord injury. *Topics in Spinal Cord Injury Rehabilitation, 7*, 73–82.

Fishback, P. V. (2010). *Worker's compensation.* Retrieved from http://eh.net/encyclopedia/article/fishback.workers.compensation

Frings-Dresen, M. H., & Sluiter, J. K. (2003). Development of a job-specific FCE protocol: The work demands of hospital nurses as an example. *Journal of Occupational Medicine, 13*, 233–248.

Gupta, J., & Stoffel, S. (2001). Take action: Occupational therapy and older workers. *Gerontology, Special Interest Section Quarterly, 24*(1), 1–2.

Harvey-Krefting, L. (1985). The concept of work in occupational therapy: A historical review. *American Journal of Occupational Therapy, 39*, 301–317.

Harwood, K. J. (2004). A review of clinical practice guidelines for functional capacity evaluations. *Journal of Forensic Vocational Analysis, 7*, 67–74.

Helm-Williams, P. (1993, March). Industrial rehabilitation (Developing guidelines). *Magazine of PT*, 65–68.

Individuals with Disabilities Education Act Amendments of 1997, Pub. L. 105-17, § 602. (2002). Retrieved from http://www2.ed.gov/offices/OSERS/Policy/IDEA/index.html

International Ergonomics Association. (2010). What is ergonomics? Retrieved from http://www.iea.cc/01_what/What%20is%20Ergonomics.html.

Isernhagen, S. J. (1988). *Work injury: Management and prevention.* Gaithersburg, MD: Aspen Publishers.

Jackson, M., Harkess, J., & Ellis, J. (2004). Reporting patients' work abilities: How the use of standardized work assessments improved clinical practice in Fife. *British Journal of Occupational Therapy, 67*, 129–132.

Jacobs, K., & Baker, N. A. (2000). The history of work-related therapy in occupational therapy. In B. L. Kornblau & K. Jacobs (Eds.), *Work: Principles and practice-A self-paced course from AOTA, Lesson 1.* Bethesda, MD: American Occupational Therapy Association.

Jundt, J., & King, P. M. (1999). Work rehabilitation programs: A 1997 survey. *Work: A Journal of Prevention, Assessment, & Rehabilitation, 12*, 139–144.

Kardos, M., & White, B. P. (2005). The role of the school-based occupational therapist in secondary education transition planning: A pilot survey study. *American Journal of Occupational Therapy, 59*, 173–180.

King, P. M. (1998). *Sourcebook of occupational rehabilitation.* New York, NY: Plenum.

King, P. M. (2005). Analysis of the reliability and validity supporting functional capacity evaluations. *Journal of Forensic Vocational Analysis, 7*, 75–83.

King, P. M., Tuckwell, N., & Barrett, T. E. (1998). A critical review of functional capacity evaluations. *Physical Therapy, 78*, 852–866.

Kornblau, B. L. (2000). The future of OT work practice. *Work programs: Special Interest Section Quarterly, 14*(4), 1–2.

Kornblau, B. L., Lou, J. Q., Weeder, T. C., & Werner, B. (2002). Occupational therapy and theories of career choice and vocational development. In B. L. Kornblau & K. Jacobs (Eds.), *Work: Principles and practice—A self-paced course from AOTA, Lesson 2* (pp. 1–23). Bethesda, MD: American Occupational Therapy Association.

Krupa, T., Lagarde, M., & Carmichael, K. (2003). Transforming sheltered workshops into affirmative businesses: An outcome evaluation. *Psychiatric Rehabilitation Journal, 26*, 359–367.

Larson, B. A. (2000). On-site work programs. In B. L. Kornblau & K. Jacobs (Eds.), *Work: Principles and practice—A self-paced course from AOTA, Lesson 8* (pp. 1–12). Bethesda, MD: American Occupational Therapy Association.

Larson, E. A. (2004). Children's work: The less-considered childhood occupation. *American Journal of Occupational Therapy, 58*, 369–379.

Lechner, D. E. (1998). Functional capacity evaluation. In P. King (Ed.), *Sourcebook of occupational rehabilitation* (pp. 209–227). New York, NY: Plenum.

Lechner, D. E., Jackson, J. R., Roth, D. L., & Straaton, K. V. (1994). Reliability and validity of a newly developed test of physical work performance. *Journal of Occupational Medicine, 36*, 997–1004.

Lechner, D., Roth, D., & Straaton, K. (1991). Functional capacity evaluation in work disability. *Work, 1*, 37–47.

Lysaght, R., & Wright, J. (2005). Professional strategies in work-related practice: An exploration of occupational and physical therapy roles and approaches. *American Journal of Occupational Therapy, 59*, 209–217.

Marshall, A. (2000). IEA Executive council defines ergonomics. *Congress Current*, August 1, 1.

Massy-Westropp, M., & Rose, D. (2004). The impact of manual handling training on work place injuries: A 14 year audit. *Australian Health Review, 27*, 80–87.

Matoushek, N. (2005). Work integration programs: Improving return to work. *Advance for Occupational Therapy Practitioners, 21*(23), 15–16.

Melnik, M. S. (2000). Injury prevention. In B. L. Kornblau & K. Jacobs (Eds.), *Work: Principles and practice-A self-paced course from AOTA, Lesson 11* (pp. 1–14), Bethesda, MD: American Occupational Therapy Association.

Meyer, A. (1977). The philosophy of occupational therapy. *American Journal of Occupational Therapy, 31*, 639–642.

Mosisa, A., & Hipple, S. (2006). Trends in labor force participation in the United States. *Monthly Labor Review Online*. Retrieved from http://www.bls.gov/opub/mlr/2006/art3exc.htm

Nachreiner, N., McGovern, P., Kochevar, L. K., Lohman, W. H., Cato, C., & Ayers, E. (1999). Preplacement assessments. Impact on injury outcomes. *AAOHN Journal: Official Journal of the American Association of Occupational Health Nurses, 47*, 245–253.

Naso, M. (2003). Stretching the limits. *Safety and Health*, 48–50.

Occupational Safety and Health Administration. (2002). Job hazard analysis (Publication No. OSHA 3071). Retrieved from http://www.osha.gov/Publications/osha3071.pdf#search='job%20analysis

Olson, D. L. (1999). An on-site ergonomic program: A model for industry. *Work: A Journal of Prevention, Assessment & Rehabilitation, 13*, 229–238.

Paterson, C. (1997). An historical perspective of work practice services. In J. Pratt & K. Jacobs (Eds.), *Work practice: International perspectives* (pp. 25–38). Boston, MA: Butterworth-Heinemann.

Primeau, L. A. (1996). Work versus non-work the case of housework. In R. C. Zemke & F. Clark (Eds.), *Occupational Science: The evolving discipline* (pp. 57–69). Philadelphia, PA: F. A. Davis.

Ramsey, D. L., Starnes, W., & Robertson, S. C. (2000). Work programs for persons with serious and chronic mental illnesses. In B. L. Kornblau & K. Jacobs (Eds.), *Work: Principles and practice-A self-paced course from AOTA, Lesson 9* (pp. 1–22). Bethesda, MD: American Occupational Therapy Association.

Rothman, J. (1998). Wellness and fitness programs. In P. M. King (Ed.), *Sourcebook of occupational rehabilitation* (pp. 127–144). New York, NY: Plenum Press.

Rehabilitation Act Amendments of 1986, 4 Pub. L. No. 99-506, 39 (1986).

Rehabilitation Act Amendments of 1998, 4 Pub. L. No. 105-220, 112 Stat. 936 (1998). Retrieved from http://www.access-board.gov/sec508/guide/act.htm

Schaafsma, F., Schonstein, E., Whelan, K. M., Ulvestad, E., Kenny, D. T., & Verbeek, J. H. (2010). Physical conditioning programs for improving work outcomes in workers with back pain. *Cochrane Database of Systematic Reviews*, (1), CD001822.

Schneid, T. D., & Schumann, M. S. (1997). *Legal liability: A guide for safety and loss prevention professionals*. Sudbury, MA: Jones and Bartlett.

Schkade, J. K., & Schultz, S. (1992). Occupational adaptation: Toward a holistic approach for contemporary practice, Part 1. *American Journal of Occupational Therapy, 46*, 829–837.

Singleton, J. F., Harvey, A. (1995). Stage of lifecycle and time spent in activities. *Journal of Occupational Science, 2*, 3–12.

Siporin, S. (1999). Help wanted: Supporting workers with developmental disabilities. *Occupational Therapy Practice*, 19–24.

Siporin, S., & Lysack, C. (2004). Quality of life and supported employment: A case study of three women with developmental disabilities. *American Journal of Occupational Therapy, 58*, 455–465.

Snodgrass, J. (2011). Effective occupational therapy interventions in the rehabilitation of individuals with work-related low back injuries and illnesses: A systematic review. *American Journal of Occupational Therapy, 65*, 37–43.

Spencer, J. E., Emery, L. J., & Schneck, C. M. (2003). Occupational therapy in transitioning adolescents to post-secondary activities. *American Journal of Occupational Therapy 57*, 435–441.

Spencer, K. C., (2000), Transition from school to adult life. In B. L. Kornblau & K. Jacobs (Eds.), *Work: Principles and practice-A self-paced course from AOTA, Lesson 3* (pp. 1–24). Bethesda, MD: American Occupational Therapy Association.

Snook, S. H., & Cirello, V. M. (1991). The design of manual handling tasks: Revised tables of maximum acceptable weights and forces. *Ergonomics, 34*, 1197–1213.

Sterns, H. L., & Miklos, S. M. (1995). The aging worker in a changing environment: Organizational and individual issues. *Journal of Vocational Behavior, 47*, 248–268.

Tramposh, A. K. (1998). On-site therapy programs. In: P. M. King (Ed.), *Sourcebook of occupational rehabilitation* (pp. 275–286). New York, NY: Plenum.

United States Department of Labor Employment and Training Administration. (1977). *Dictionary of occupational titles* (4th Ed.). Washington, DC: U.S. Government Printing Office.

United States Department of Labor Office of Disability Employment Policy. (1994). *Job analysis: An important employment tool*. Retrieved from http://www.dol.gov/odep/pubs/fact/analysis.htm

U.S. Equal Employment Opportunity Commission. (2008). *Notice Concerning Americans With Disabilities Act (ADA) Amendments Act of 2008*. Retrieved from http://www.eeoc.gov/ada/amendments_notice.html

van Geen, J.-W., Edelaar, M. J. A., Janssen, M., & van Eijk, J. (2007). The long-term effect of multidisciplinary back training: A systematic review. *Spine, 32*, 249–255.

Vitalis, A., Walker, R., & Legg, S. (2001). Unfocused ergonomics? *Ergonomics, 44*, 1290–1301.

Washington State Department of Labor and Industries. (2005). *Evaluation tools*. Retrieved from http://www.lni.wa.gov/Safety/Topics/Ergonomics/ServicesResources/Tools/default.asp

Waters, T. R., Putz-Anderson, V., Garg, A., & Fine, L. J. (1993). Revised NIOSH equation for the design and evaluation of manual lifting tasks. *Ergonomics, 36*, 749–776.

Westmorland, M. G., Williams, R., Strong, S., & Arnold, E. (2002). Perspectives on work (re)entry for persons with disabilities: Implications for clinicians. *Work: A Journal of Prevention Assessment & Rehabilitation, 18*, 29–40.

Webb, G., Shakeshaft, A., Sanson-Fisher, R., & Havard, A. (2009). A systematic review of work-place interventions for alcohol-related problems. *Addiction, 104*, 365–377.

Wilcox, A. A. (1998). *An occupational perspective of health*. Thorofare, NJ: SLACK Incorporated.

Work. (2003). *Merriam-Webster's collegiate dictionary* (11th ed.). Springfield, MA: Merriam-Webster, Inc.

Yassi, A., Gilbert, M., & Cvitkovich, Y. (2005). Trends in injuries, illnesses, and policies in Canadian healthcare workplaces. *Canadian Journal of Public Health, 96*, 333–339.

For additional resources on the subjects discussed in this chapter, visit http://thePoint.lww.com/Willard-Spackman12e.

CHAPTER 50

Play and Leisure

Loree A. Primeau

LEARNING OBJECTIVES

After reading this chapter, you will be able to:

1. Describe four definitions of play and leisure
2. Describe guidelines and parameters for evaluation of play and leisure
3. Identify selected assessments that can be used to develop an occupational profile and to evaluate play and leisure
4. Describe three purposes of play and leisure in intervention
5. Define play and leisure as lures or rewards, as means, and as ends
6. Explain how play and leisure as means can be used for intervention
7. Describe four types of occupational therapy intervention to facilitate play and leisure as ends

OUTLINE

What Are Play and Leisure?

Occupational therapy practitioners have a long tradition of considering play and leisure in the lives of people with whom they work (Parham, 2008). In the founding years of the profession, the "play spirit" was seen as essential for living a worthwhile life (Saunders, 1922; Slagle, 1922; Ziegler, 1924). Over time, as occupational therapy practitioners became increasingly concerned with scientific and technical aspects of intervention, play and leisure were thought to be unscientific and inappropriate for use in practice. Late in the 20th century, scholars in occupational therapy and occupational science reclaimed play and leisure (Bundy, 1993; Canadian Association of Occupational Therapists [CAOT], 1996; Parham, 1996; Primeau, 1996; Reilly, 1974; Suto, 1998).

The "Occupational Therapy Practice Framework: Domain and Process, 2nd Edition" (American Occupational Therapy [AOTA], 2008) provides definitions of play and leisure to guide occupational therapy practice. Play is defined as "any spontaneous or organized activity that provides enjoyment, entertainment, amusement, or diversion" (p. 632). Leisure is defined as "a non-obligatory activity that is intrinsically motivated and engaged in during discretionary time, that is, time not committed to obligatory occupations such as work, self-care, or sleep" (p.632). As defined here as well as elsewhere in the occupational therapy literature and the literature in general, play and leisure are separate and distinct concepts. This distinction between the concepts of play and leisure is vital for theory development and research needed to further our understanding of these concepts. Readers are referred to the following sources to expand their understanding of the differences between play and leisure (Edginton, DeGraaf, Dieser, & Edginton, 2006; Fenech, 2008; McMahon, Lytle, & Sutton-Smith, 2005; Parham & Fazio, 2008; Rojek, Shaw, & Veal, 2007; Scarlett, Naudeau, Salonius-Pasternak, & Ponte, 2005). Nevertheless, as used in occupational therapy practice, specifically for evaluation and intervention purposes, these concepts are more similar than dissimilar. Therefore, for these purposes, play and leisure will be used here as synonymous terms.

Multiple definitions of *play* and *leisure* have been proposed in the literature, including those provided by the AOTA (AOTA, 2008); however, consensus has not been reached on how to define these terms (Hurd & Anderson, 2011; Parham, 2008). Lack of definitional clarity for these terms should not prevent occupational therapy practitioners' consideration of their clients' performance in these areas of occupation. From a pragmatic point of view, play and leisure are powerful tools for practice; but single, precise, and all-purpose definitions that are responsive to the needs of an entire profession might not be required or desired, even if they were possible (Hurd & Anderson, 2011; Parham, 2008). Nevertheless, definitions of play and leisure in the literature tend to converge into four major categories: (1) play and leisure as discretionary time, (2) play and leisure as context, (3) play and leisure as observable behavior or activity, and (4) play and leisure as disposition or experience (Hurd & Anderson, 2011; Rubin, Fein, & Vandenberg, 1983).

Play and Leisure as Time

The category of play and leisure as discretionary time views them as free time away from obligatory activities, such as paid or unpaid work and self-maintenance tasks, or as leftover time after obligatory activities have been completed (Hurd & Anderson, 2011; Stebbins, 2008). Play and leisure are defined by what they are not: They are not work or school activities; they are not activities of daily living (ADL) or instrumental ADL. By definition, play and leisure are quantified as the time that is spent by the individual who is engaged in them. This view of play and leisure lends itself easily to measurement and is often the focus of evaluation in occupational therapy through the use of activity configurations as an assessment tool (Suto, 1998). Although practitioners need to know about their clients' use of time and its relationship to their health and well-being, equally important for evaluation of play and leisure are the contexts in which they occur, the clients' activities, and their experience of those activities.

Play and Leisure as Context

The category of play and leisure as context identifies and describes them in terms of the conditions under which they occur. Contexts that are friendly, safe, and comfortable with a variety of materials, objects, people, and activities and that also denote cultural sanctions for play and leisure are more likely to elicit them (Figure 50.1). Freedom of choice to engage or not to engage in play and leisure and freedom from hunger, fatigue, illness, or other stressors are also identified as conditions that are conducive to play and leisure (Rubin et al., 1983). Beliefs held by people in a specific culture will determine what is and is not considered to be play and leisure and the conditions under which they will occur. Practitioners often draw from this category when they evaluate supports and barriers in their clients' contexts and environments that facilitate or hinder their engagement in play and leisure. One problem with the view of play and leisure as context is that although the conditions described above are necessary for play and leisure, they are not sufficient, meaning that producing such a context does not ensure that play and leisure will emerge in it (Rubin et al., 1983). Because play and leisure are transactions between clients and their contexts/environments (Bundy, 2001), clients' play and leisure activities and their experience of them must also be considered.

Play and Leisure as Activity

The category of play and leisure as activity views them as behaviors or activities that can be observed and named.

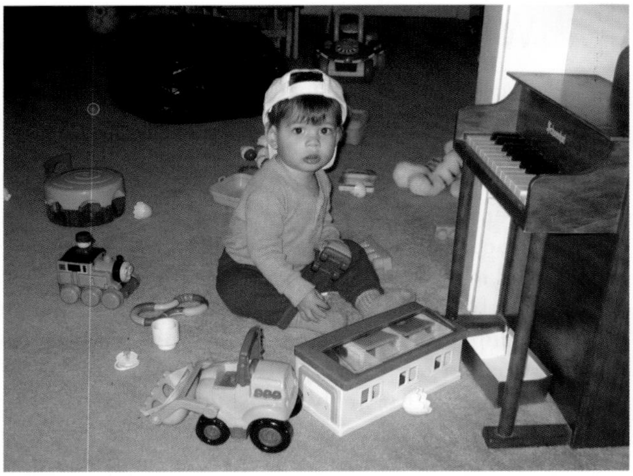

FIGURE 50.1 The definition of play as context can be seen in this boy's enjoyment of conditions that support his engagement in play.

Taxonomies are used to identify and describe types of play and leisure activities. Such taxonomies are useful because they provide descriptive criteria for observation and evaluation of clients' play and leisure behaviors (Rubin et al., 1983), including their interests (Primeau, 1996). This view of play and leisure as activity is also easily quantified and measurable. It is familiar to practitioners in the form of many assessments, including checklists used to identify interests as well as strengths and problem areas in performance of play and leisure activities (Suto, 1998). For example, the Play History (Bryze, 2008), the Revised Preschool Play Scale (Knox, 2008), and the Pediatric Interest Profiles (Henry, 2008) provide taxonomies of play and leisure activities. A drawback to this view is lack of consideration of the clients' experience of the activities themselves (Hurd & Anderson, 2011; Primeau, 1996; Suto, 1998).

Play and Leisure as Experience

The category of play and leisure as experience views them as the overall experience of a client's engagement in play and leisure. The subjective experience, or the client's state of mind while participating in play and leisure, is of primary importance (Lee, Dattilo, & Howard, 1994). Personal meanings of play and leisure arise from these subjective experiences (Primeau, 1996). Several qualities of play and leisure as experience have been identified in the literature, including freedom, enjoyment/fun, adventure, relaxation, spontaneity, companionship, creative expression, involvement, aesthetic appreciation, intrinsic motivation, perception of control, timelessness, suspension of reality, and positive mood states (Byunggook, 2008; Edginton et al., 2006; Lee, 1999; Lee et al., 1994; Skard & Bundy, 2008). Of all these qualities, perceived freedom (freedom from obligations/constraints and freedom of choice), intrinsic motivation (influence of internal factors on the leisure experience), perceived competence (belief in skills related to challenge of leisure experience), and positive affect (feelings of enjoyment related to sense of choice and control over the process of the leisure experience) are most often identified as defining characteristics of play and leisure as experience (Edginton et al., 2006; Hurd & Anderson, 2011). Practitioners recognize the importance of evaluation of play and leisure as experience by gathering data on clients' experiences through interviews, participant observations, and specific formal assessments.

The view of play and leisure as experience holds the most promise for occupational therapy practice (Bundy, 1993; Primeau, 1996; Suto, 1998). Although evaluation of play and leisure as time, context, and activity are necessary, they are not sufficient to understand clients' participation in play and leisure. Best practice dictates that evaluation of play and leisure as experience must also be conducted to obtain the clearest picture of clients' engagement in play and leisure.

Evaluation of Play and Leisure

Guidelines for Evaluation of Play and Leisure

Evaluation of play and leisure should be client-centered and should follow a top-down approach. Client-centered evaluation is a collaborative process that combines the perspectives, expertise, and experiences of clients and practitioners to determine what is evaluated, how it is evaluated, and what will be the focus of intervention (Pollock & McColl, 1998). For practitioners who work with children, clients can "include the child, parents, siblings, other family members, peers, teachers, and other adults who are responsible for the child" (Primeau & Ferguson, 1999, p. 470). Best practice evaluation of play and leisure is guided by the principle that evaluation takes place in everyday life, including natural environments and settings (AOTA, 2010). As the practitioner considers the child in each environment and setting, a new group of individuals may become central to the collaborative process.

A top-down approach to evaluation begins with the client's occupational profile, including the client's participation in play and leisure in home, school, work, and community settings (AOTA, 2008; Stewart, 2010). The client and the practitioner collaboratively identify what the client wants and needs to do (AOTA, 2008) and the extent to which the client is able to engage in play and leisure in these settings (Coster, 1998; Law, Baum, & Dunn, 2005). Analysis of the client's occupational performance follows, with a specific focus on performance in the areas of occupation that were identified in the occupational profile (AOTA, 2008). Evaluation of play and leisure addresses the following issues: (1) how the client's contexts and environments facilitate or inhibit his or her engagement in play and leisure, (2) how the client's performance in the areas of occupation of play and leisure is enhanced or limited by the types of play and leisure activities in which he or she engages and his or her experience of these activities, and (3) how limitations or impairments in performance skills and client factors affect the client's ability to engage in play and leisure activities.

Parameters for Evaluation of Play and Leisure

Client-centered and top-down approaches to evaluation guide practitioners in the process of evaluation, or *how* to evaluate play and leisure. The client's overall pattern of participation in play and leisure across home, school, work, and community settings is the content, or *what* needs to be evaluated. The four definitions of play and leisure described previously provide parameters for evaluation that are aligned with the two substeps of the evaluation process: occupational profile and analysis of occupational performance (AOTA, 2008). Play and leisure as time aligns with the substep of the occupational profile, whereas play and leisure as context, as activity, and as experience are addressed in the substep of analysis of occupational performance. Specifically, play and leisure as context aligns with the domain aspect of context and environment, and play and leisure as activity and as experience align with the domain aspect of areas of occupation (AOTA, 2008). Also evaluated during the analysis of occupational performance are the domain aspects of performance skills and client factors; however, parameters for evaluation of these areas are drawn from general occupational therapy assessments used to evaluate clients in these areas and are not necessarily specific to play and leisure assessments. Table 50.1 lists assessments that can be used to develop the client's occupational profile (participation) and to evaluate play and leisure in the areas of contexts and environments, performance in areas of occupation (activity), performance skills, and client factors.

Occupational Profile: Play and Leisure

When developing an occupational profile, occupational therapy practitioners gather information about the client's past, current, and future play and leisure participation (AOTA, 2008). Play and leisure participation is defined as the client's engagement in play and leisure occupations that are typically expected of and available to a person of the same age and culture in home, school, work, and community settings (Coster, 1998; Primeau & Ferguson, 1999). This profile is used to determine clients' ***characteristics of play and leisure participation*** (nature, quality, frequency, and duration) in these settings.

Play and leisure participation may be restricted in nature, quality, frequency, or duration. Restrictions are relative to typical participation in each setting. Practitioners compare their clients' participation to that of individuals without participation restrictions to determine the clients' degree of participation or participation restriction (World Health Organization, 2001). They draw from their knowledge base about play and leisure as it occurs naturally in home, school, work, and community settings and from their observations of a typical person engaged in play and leisure in a particular setting to understand the play and leisure of people without restrictions in that setting (Dunn, 1998; Law et al., 2005). Then they may interview their clients and/or observe them to gather data on their participation in play and leisure (Stewart, 2010) and compare this information to that of a person without participation restrictions.

The focus of evaluation is on the nature, quality, frequency, and duration of clients' play and leisure participation. The nature and quality of participation can be addressed by answering the following questions (Coster, 1998): Is the client's participation in play and leisure positive? Does it support the client's physical, cognitive, and psychosocial growth? Is it personally satisfying? Does the client have access to the same opportunities for play and leisure as others of the same age and culture do? Is the client's participation in play and leisure acceptable to others in his or her settings? Frequency and duration of participation are related to definitions of play and leisure as time. Does the client participate in play and leisure to the same extent as others in that setting? Research on children with developmental coordination disorder (DCD) (see Appendix I) demonstrates how physical coordination, perceived freedom in leisure, and perceived self-efficacy affected their participation in playground activities and leisure-time social-physical activities as well as their preferences for participation in leisure activities (Engel-Yeger & Hanna Kasis, 2010; Poulsen, Ziviani, & Cuskelly, 2007; Smyth & Anderson, 2000). These studies found that children with DCD spent less time engaged in physical and social play and leisure activities, both while at school and outside of school, and had a lower preference for participation in play and leisure activities when compared to children without DCD. These findings indicate a gap between typical participation and that of children with DCD. When gaps in nature, quality, frequency, or duration of participation are found, practitioners must evaluate the client's play and leisure contexts to identify ways to bridge these gaps (Dunn, 1998).

Analysis of Occupational Performance: Play and Leisure

Evaluation of Play and Leisure Contexts and Environments. Evaluation of play and leisure contexts and environments is related to definitions of play and leisure as context. Contexts are interrelated conditions that may be external or internal to clients and may include internalized beliefs and values (AOTA, 2008, 2010). They may be cultural (customs, beliefs, behavior standards/expectations, political aspects), personal (age, gender, socioeconomic status, educational status), temporal (time of day/year, stage of life), and virtual (e-mail/text messaging, chat rooms, simulated environments). Environments are external to clients and surround them while they are engaged in play and leisure activities (AOTA, 2008, 2010). Environments include physical (built and natural environments, objects) and social (individuals, groups, organizations, systems).

Practitioners identify ***contextual and environmental features*** in their clients' settings of interest and then determine whether these features facilitate or hinder participation in play and leisure in those settings. Gathering objective data on contextual and environmental features is not sufficient; practitioners must assess the impact of these features on their clients' engagement in play and leisure (Dunn, 1998). Interviewing and observing clients in natural settings are optimal methods for doing this (Stewart, 2010). For example, the socioeconomic feature of the personal context was found to hinder participation in commercially based, organized leisure activities of children living in low socioeconomic areas when compared to their peers living in medium and high socioeconomic

TABLE 50.1 Assessments for Play and Leisure[a]

Assessment	Areas of Occupation		Quality of Life	Client Factors		Performance Skills	Performance Patterns	Activity Demands	Environmental Factors/Context and Environment
	Activity	Participation		Body Structures and Functions	Values, Beliefs, Spirituality				
Activity Card Sort	X	X							
Activity Index & Meaningfulness of Activity Scale	X	X							
Adult Playfulness Scale	X								
Assessment of Ludic Behaviors (ALB)	X			X		X			
Children's Assessment of Participation and Enjoyment (CAPE)	X	X							
Child Behaviors Inventory of Playfulness	X								
Interest Checklist	X								
Leisure Boredom Scale	X								
Leisure Competence Measure	X	X				X			
Leisure Diagnostic Battery	X					X			X
Leisure Interest Profile for Adults	X	X							
Leisure Interest Profile for Seniors	X	X							
Leisure Satisfaction Scale	X								
Pediatric Interest Profiles	X	X							
Playform	X					X			X
Play History	X	X				X			X
Preferences for Activities of Children (PAC)	X								
Qualitative Methods[b] (Interview, Observation)	X	X		X	X	X	X	X	X
Revised Knox Preschool Play Scale	X					X			
Self Directed Search—The Leisure Activities Finder	X								
Test of Environmental Supportiveness (TOES)									X
Test of Playfulness (ToP)	X								
The Experience of Leisure Scale (TELS)	X								
Transdisciplinary Play-Based Assessment-II	X			X		X			

[a]For more details about these assessments, see Appendix II, Table of Assessments.

[b]See Bundy, 1993, p. 220; Burke, Scaaf, & Hall, 2008, pp. 203–205; and Florey & Greene, 2008, p. 293 for samples of interview and observation guides.

areas (Ziviani et al., 2008). Conversely, the social environment, in the form of caregivers, facilitated the play participation of children with disabilities through the caregivers' provision of assistance to the child to participate (Bourke-Taylor, Law, Howie, & Pallant, 2009).

Evaluation of Performance in Areas of Occupation: Play and Leisure. Definitions of play and leisure as activity and as experience are central to evaluation of performance in these areas of occupation. Evaluation focuses on clients' play and leisure performance (what they actually do and their experience while doing it). Practitioners assess clients' play and leisure activities and their experience while engaged in these activities to identify performance limitations and determine how to enhance performance. Evaluation of **play and leisure activity** considers **activity interests/preferences** and **activity choices**, whereas evaluation of play and leisure experience explores **subjective experience**, **personal meaning**, and **satisfaction with experience**.

Evaluation of Play and Leisure Activity

- **Activity Interests/Preferences.** Interests or preferences are major determinants of play and leisure participation (King et al., 2004). They refer to inner dispositions and self-knowledge related to finding pleasure, satisfaction, and enjoyment from participating in occupations (Henry, 2008; Kielhofner, 2008). Activity interests and preferences address clients' affective responses to play and leisure activities (often expressed as likes, dislikes, and indifferences), their perceptions and awareness of themselves and their environments (Matsutsuyu, 1969), and their motivation to participate in specific play and leisure activities (Henry, 2008; King et al., 2004). Assessments of play and leisure activity interests provide information in two areas: preferences and self-knowledge as they relate to play and leisure activities. Clients are asked to identify their preferences for a variety of play and leisure activities. On the basis of their responses, practitioners can determine the extent and quality of clients' self-knowledge and awareness of these interests. For example, using an activity preference assessment tool, an adolescent boy identifies that he enjoys walking and hiking and has a high preference for taking care of a pet. Although they have a dog, his mother reports that the boy has not shown any interest in walking the dog on a regular basis. The boy's self-identified preferences can be used to enhance his self-knowledge and awareness of his environment (he likes to walk; he wants to take care of pets; he has a dog that needs walking), leading to his increased participation in the leisure activity of walking the dog, which can lead to a stronger interest in future participation in similar leisure activities (King et al., 2004).
- **Activity Choices.** Activity choices consist of the activities in which the client engages during play and leisure. Assessments in this area examine what clients do, with whom, and how often. Play and leisure activities are characterized as general categories (e.g., creative activities, social activities, physical activities, sports, indoor/outdoor activities) or specific activities (e.g., play with toys, board games, going to the movies, soccer, hanging out with friends). Other areas to explore include whether the activity is done alone or with others, including friends, family, or others, and how often a particular play and leisure activity is performed (Henry, 2008; King et al., 2004). This indicator of frequency differs from that evaluated in the occupational profile because practitioners are concerned here with the client's individual performance of a specific play and leisure activity, regardless of the setting in which it occurs, as an indicator of the client's history and familiarity with it. Recall the studies of the children with DCD that demonstrated their decreased participation in physical and social play and leisure activities when compared to their peers without DCD. Evaluation of their activity choices would focus on their history and familiarity with specific physical and social play activities (whether they had participated in them before and, if so, what types, with whom, and how often) rather than on their overall participation in these play and leisure activities.

Evaluation of Play and Leisure Experience

- **Subjective Experience.** Subjective experience refers to two aspects of engagement in play and leisure activities: state of mind with which these activities are approached and the affective experience of engagement in them. State of mind, sometimes termed *playfulness*, is characterized by freedom from constraint/freedom of choice, intrinsic motivation, perception of control, perceived competence, and suspension of reality (Byunggook, 2008; Hurd & Anderson, 2011; Lee, 1999; Skard & Bundy, 2008). The affective experience of engagement in play and leisure is generally a positive one, marked by feelings of fun, enjoyment, happiness, satisfaction, and pleasure (Hurd & Anderson, 2001; Lee et al., 1994; Miller & Kuhaneck, 2008). Assessments of subjective experience explore these two areas: playfulness and affective experience. Practitioners must remember that the subjective experience of play and leisure transcends cultural definitions of play, leisure, work, and ADL (Primeau, 1996). For example, a mother describing her experience of playing with her children while doing housework as "play-work" stated, "It's like work with an attitude. It's my way to get things done in a fun way. . . . No, [it] isn't exactly what I want to do right now, . . . but I'm getting it done and we're all enjoying it at the same time" (Primeau, 1995). Although she recognizes that she is restricted in her choice of activity, her use of the words "attitude" and "fun way" demonstrate a playful approach; and her statement that "we're all enjoying it" refers to a positive affective experience, suggesting that her subjective experience is one of play and leisure.

- **Personal Meaning.** Personal meaning derives from the subjective experience of play and leisure performance. Satisfaction of conscious or unconscious needs and benefits attributed to this experience create personal meanings, which often become motivation for clients' future engagement in play and leisure activities. Personal meanings can be categorized as physiological (e.g., physical fitness, stress and anxiety reduction, relaxation, restoration), educational/cognitive (e.g., learning, intellectual stimulation), social (e.g., social interaction, companionship, friendship), psychological (e.g., self-identity, self-expression, sense of accomplishment), aesthetic (e.g., appreciation of beauty, arts, and symbolic systems of meaning), and spiritual (e.g., heightened awareness, transcendent experiences) (Beard & Ragheb, 1980; Driver, Brown, & Peterson, 1991; Heo, Lee, McCormick, & Pedersen, 2010; Hoppes, Wilcox, & Graham, 2001). Evaluation of personal meaning becomes particularly important when practitioners want to increase their clients' repertoire of play and leisure activities (Bundy, 2001) or substitute a new activity for one that is no longer viable (Bundy, 1993; O'Brien, Renwick, & Yoshida, 2008). Clients' identified personal meanings can be matched with play and leisure activities that provide those meanings in the form of benefits derived from them, offering new play and leisure options. For example, a study found that bingo, bowling, ceramics, dancing, and volunteer activities were all rated as providing high levels of the benefit of companionship by elderly adults living in the community (Driver, Tinsley, & Manfredo, 1991). Practitioners could suggest these activities, or others that provide a similar benefit, for their elderly clients who have expressed a desire for companionship.
- **Satisfaction with experience.** Satisfaction with experience refers to clients' overall feelings and perceptions related to their play and leisure experiences. Feelings and perceptions can be positive (contentment and satisfaction) (Beard & Ragheb, 1980) or negative (boredom and dissatisfaction) (Iso-Ahola & Weissinger, 1990). Satisfaction with play and leisure experience is thought to have powerful consequences for clients' physical health, mental health, life satisfaction, and personal growth (Driver, Tinsley, et al., 1991). Evaluation must capture clients' range of feelings and perceptions about their play and leisure satisfaction across all activities and settings in which they participate (Figure 50.2). For example, elderly clients' decreased participation in and access to leisure activities did not translate into dissatisfaction with their leisure experience, suggesting that, although their range of activity choices were restricted, even infrequent participation in valued activities added meaning and satisfaction to their lives (Griffin & McKenna, 1998). Similarly, a study examining leisure participation in adults following a lower limb amputation revealed that although they experienced a decrease in participation across all categories of leisure activities, satisfaction with their current levels of participation, including available leisure opportunities, was high, indicating that a decrease in leisure participation did not necessarily correspond with a decrease in leisure satisfaction (Couture, Caron, & Desrosiers, 2010).

Evaluation of Performance Skills and Client Factors. Practitioners can choose from many general occupational therapy assessments and some specific play and leisure assessments that are designed to assess performance skills (see Chapter 22) and client factors (see Chapter 19). Practitioners can also make informal observations during clients' engagement in play and leisure activities. Specific assessments and observations ensure that practitioners are examining clients' performance skills and body functions and structures that are actually used in play and leisure activities (Bundy, 2001), thereby increasing the likelihood that their intervention will be focused on outcomes related to clients' participation in play and leisure. For example, practitioners often observe children at play with their peers to assess how the children's performance skills (motor/praxis, sensory-perceptual, emotional regulation, cognitive, communication/social) as well as their physical, cognitive, and psychosocial abilities (client factors) affect their play with others.

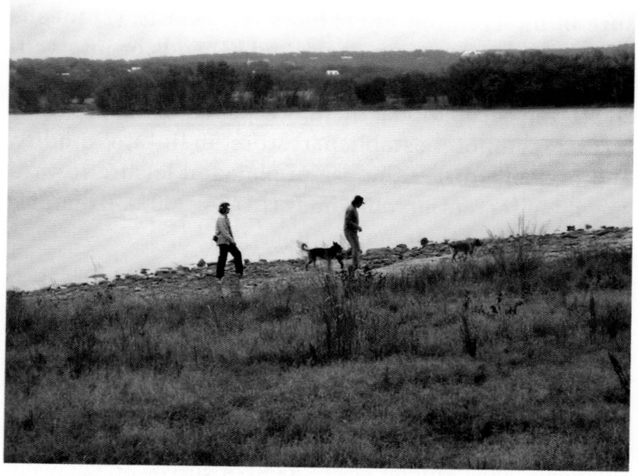

FIGURE 50.2 Participation in valued leisure activities, even if it is infrequent, adds meaning and satisfaction to people's lives.

Additionally, practitioners frequently use specific play and leisure assessments to assess children's developmental status, based on performance skills and client factors (Daunhauer, Coster, Tickle-Degnen, & Cermack, 2010; Knox, 2010). Specifically, the Revised Knox Preschool Play Scale (Knox, 2008) and the Transdisciplinary Play-Based Assessment (Linder, 2008) assess children's level of development in performance skills and client factors through observations of their play behaviors in natural settings.

Summary of Evaluation of Play and Leisure

Evaluation of play and leisure is guided by client-centered and top-down approaches and is focused on clients' overall patterns of participation in play and leisure across home, school, work, and community settings. The occupational profile gathers information related to clients' play and leisure participation, specifically characteristics of their participation (nature, quality, frequency, and duration). Analysis of occupational performance of clients' play and leisure consists of evaluation of their play and leisure contexts and environments and their performance in the areas of occupation of play and leisure, including play and leisure activity (activity interests/preferences, activity choices) and play and leisure experience (subjective experience, personal meaning, satisfaction with experience). Evaluation of performance skills and client factors related to play and leisure is conducted by using general occupational therapy assessments, specific play and leisure assessments, and observation. Practitioners who use this conceptual framework to evaluate play and leisure will be able to design and implement interventions that are directly related to their clients' participation in play and leisure in home, school, work, and community settings.

Play and Leisure Intervention

Occupational therapy practitioners use play and leisure in intervention as (1) lures or rewards, (2) means to achieve intervention goals, and (3) ends or intervention outcomes (Blanche, 2008; Munier, Myers, & Pierce, 2008). The occupational therapy intervention approaches (create/promote, establish/restore, maintain, modify, and prevent) direct the use of play and leisure toward specific intervention outcomes (AOTA, 2008). Examples below highlight their application.

Play and Leisure as Lures or Rewards

Practitioners use **play and leisure as lures or rewards** to motivate clients to participate in therapeutic activities or to reward them for their participation in intervention (Blanche, 2008; Munier et al., 2008). A survey of 222 occupational therapists working with preschool-aged children indicated that all respondents regarded play as important in motivating children to participate in intervention; 91% reported that it was very important (Couch, Deitz, & Kanny, 1998). Additionally, 75% of 103 occupational therapists reported using leisure assessments to plan their intervention; of these therapists, 32% reported using leisure activity to motivate their clients and facilitate their interest and participation in intervention (Turner, Chapman, McSherry, Krishnagiri, & Watts, 2000). The use of play and leisure in this manner corresponds to the therapeutic use of self (personality, attitude, tone of voice, body language) as a type of occupational therapy intervention (AOTA, 2008). For example, practitioners frequently use a playful attitude in their interactions with clients in order to draw them into intervention activities. Practitioners have historically attended to this affective aspect of therapy by creating intervention settings that are infused with feelings of cheerfulness, an esprit de corps, and hope (Kielhofner & Burke, 1983).

Play and leisure as rewards are also frequently employed in intervention. Of 203 occupational therapists working with preschool-aged children in school-based and non–school-based settings, 99% reported their use of play as a reinforcer during intervention; 40% indicated this use in over 50% of their caseload (Couch et al., 1998). Play as a reward or reinforcer is typically used when practitioners provide an opportunity for children to engage in free-play activities during, or at the conclusion of, an intervention session. Blanche (2008) urges those who use play to reinforce children's specific actions to allow time for play consistently at appropriate moments throughout a session rather than banishing it to the end of a session. The common practice of timing opportunities for free play at the end of a session leaves it open to interruption or postponement, suggesting that it is less important than other intervention activities and disregards children's view of play as one of primary importance (Blanche, 2008). Leisure is also used as a reinforcer, particularly when participation in specific leisure activities is the culmination of intervention sessions in which clients planned and organized these activities.

Play and Leisure as Means

Play and leisure as means refers to their use as a type of occupational therapy intervention, specifically therapeutic use of occupations and activities (AOTA, 2008), to achieve specific intervention goals. Clients' engagement in play and leisure is the method or process through which change occurs (Gray, 1998; Trombly, 1995). Practitioners employ play and leisure as means to target change in client factors and performance skills (underlying all areas of occupation) and performance in two specific areas of occupation (play and leisure).

Means to Address Client Factors and Performance Skills

Play and leisure as means are most often used to address impairments in client factors and limitations in performance skills. Using the intervention approach of *establish/restore* (AOTA, 2008), practitioners engage their

Commentary on the Evidence

The occupational therapy literature provides many rationales for the use of play and leisure in evaluation and intervention in occupational therapy practice (Bundy, 1993; CAOT, 1996; Kleiber, Reel, & Hutchinson, 2008; Majnemer, 2009, 2010; Parham, 2008; Primeau, 2008; Suto, 1998); however, direct evidence of their use and effectiveness in practice is limited. The majority of play and leisure studies in the occupational therapy literature describe how participation in play and leisure activities varies among specific population groups. Most of these studies provide descriptions of the characteristics of play and leisure participation of children and adults living with illnesses/disabilities, including how the illnesses/disabilities and contextual and environmental features facilitate or hinder their play and leisure participation. These descriptive studies are literature reviews or use qualitative, observational, survey, and/or mixed methods. Population groups examined by such studies include children with autism spectrum disorder (Desha, Ziviani, & Rodger, 2003; LaVesser & Berg, 2011; Ziviani, Rodger, & Peters, 2005), cerebral palsy (Imms, 2008; Pfeifer, Pacciulio, C. dos Santos, J. dos Santos, & Stagnitti, 2011; Shikako-Thomas, Majnemer, Law, & Lach, 2008), Down syndrome (Oates, Bebbington, Bourke, Girdler, & Leonard, 2011), and juvenile idiopathic arthritis (Hackett, 2003). Adult population groups studied include individuals living with acquired/traumatic brain injuries (Bier, Dutil, & Couture, 2009; Fleming et al., 2011), cerebral palsy and other congenital physical disabilities (Boucher, Dumas, Maltais, & Richards, 2010; Specht, King, Brown, & Foris, 2002), lower limb amputation (Couture et al., 2010), mental health problems (Pieris & Craik, 2004), rheumatoid arthritis (Reinseth & Espnes, 2007), spinal cord injury (O'Brien et al., 2008), post-stroke effects (McKenna, Liddle, Brown, Lee, & Gustafsson, 2009; O'Sullivan & Chard, 2010), and vision loss (Berger, 2010).

Less frequently, specific play and leisure assessments are used to describe the play and leisure participation as well as the play and leisure activity and experience of children living with illnesses/disabilities. Two assessments in particular, the Children's Assessment of Participation and Enjoyment (CAPE)/Preferences for Activities of Children (PAC) and the Test of Playfulness (ToP), are most frequently cited in the literature. For example, the CAPE and the PAC were used in studies of children with cerebral palsy to describe their participation in leisure activities, their leisure activity interests/preferences, and their leisure experience (Majnemer et al., 2008; Majnemer, 2009). Additional studies used the CAPE or the PAC to compare the play of children with acquired brain injury (Law, Anaby, DeMatteo, & Hanna, 2011), attention deficit hyperactivity disorder (ADHD; Shimoni, Engel-Yeger, & Tirosh, 2010), developmental coordination disorder (Engel-Yeger & Hanna Kasis, 2010), complex communication needs, and physical disabilities (Raghavendra, Virgo, Olsson, Connell, & Lane, 2011) to comparison groups of typically developing children. These studies reported differences in the characteristics of leisure participation, leisure activity interests/preferences, and leisure experiences of children living with illnesses/disabilities when compared to their typically developing peers. The ToP was also used to examine the play of children with ADHD (Cordier, Bundy, Hocking, & Einfeld, 2009, 2010; Leipold & Bundy, 2000), developmental disabilities (Hamm, 2006), and traumatic brain injury (Mortenson & Harris, 2006) with that of children without these disabilities. These studies demonstrated that the play experience (playfulness as defined by the ToP) of the children with disabilities was lower than that of their typically developing peers.

Studies that provide evidence of the use and effectiveness of play and leisure in occupational therapy practice can be organized according to their focus: (1) use of play and leisure as means in intervention, (2) use of play and leisure as ends of intervention, and (3) use of play and leisure as both means and ends of intervention. Literature supporting the use of play and leisure as means to address client factors and performance skills includes a study that examined the use of virtual reality play to enhance motivation (Harris & Reid, 2005), a systematic review of eight studies that investigated the effect of leisure activity on depression or self-esteem in elder adults, concluding that leisure activity has a positive effect on depression and self-esteem (Fine, 2000); and two correlational studies that found significant relationships between playfulness and coping skills in both preschool children and adolescents, suggesting that the use of play as means can positively affect coping skills in these groups (Hess & Bundy, 2003; Saunders, Sayer, & Goodale, 1999). Another correlational study demonstrated a moderate strength positive relationship between pre-kindergarten children's participation in play activities and their performance on a measure of school readiness skills, supporting the use of play as means to enhance developmental skill acquisition in young children (Long, Bergeron, Doyle, & Gordon, 2005).

Studies focused on use of play and leisure as ends through the use of means other than play and leisure participation are rare in the occupational therapy literature. One study compared the effects of the use of the education process to improve mother-child interactions with a neurodevelopmental treatment (NDT) session on playfulness of children with cerebral palsy and developmental delays (Okimoto, Bundy, & Hanzlik, 2000). Although the ToP scores of the children whose mothers participated in the education session were higher after the intervention than before, they were not significantly higher than those of the children who received direct NDT. These results suggest that interventions focused on enhancing mother-child interaction using the education process may have a positive effect on children's play experience (playfulness as defined by the ToP), especially when combined with direct intervention aimed at improving developmental motor skills.

Studies in the literature that focus on play and leisure as both means and ends of occupational therapy intervention include a study that examined the effects of virtual reality environments on the play experience (playfulness as defined by the ToP) of school-aged children with cerebral palsy (Reid, 2004). Seven of nine virtual reality environments were found to produce various levels of playfulness in the children, with three environments in particular producing the highest playfulness ratings. This study provides support for the use of virtual contexts to address play as ends in children with cerebral palsy. The effect of the social environment (play partners' interactions during play) on young children's play was explored in two separate studies. When preschool-aged children with social play delays were paired with peers, who had either lower or higher developmental play skills, during free play

(continued)

Commentary on the Evidence (*continued*)

dyad sessions, play with peers with higher developmental play skills resulted in increased initiations of and response to social play interactions than did play with peers with lower developmental play skills (Tanta, Deitz, White, & Billingsley, 2005). Similarly, young children institutionalized in an Eastern European orphanage were found to demonstrate more developmentally competent play when engaged in interactive play with caregivers than when playing independently (Daunhauer et al., 2010). The use of play and leisure as means on a school playground, when the physical environment was changed by the introduction of new objects and materials, demonstrated positive effects on the play experience (increased playfulness as defined by the ToP) of typically developing, school-aged children (Bundy et al., 2008). In summary, these studies suggest that occupational therapy interventions using play as means can enhance play as ends (children's participation in play activities), particularly when occupational therapy practitioners consider the impact of contextual (virtual) and environmental (social, physical) features on children's settings. Currently, the evidence in the literature for the use of play and leisure in occupational therapy evaluation and intervention consists mainly of rationales for their use in practice and descriptive studies of play and leisure participation, activity, and experience in a variety of population groups typically seen by occupational therapists. Direct evidence of the effectiveness of the use of play and leisure as means, as ends, or as both means and ends within the literature is limited. The current state of the evidence indicates a need for systematic and methodologically rigorous studies that examine the use of play and leisure in evaluation and intervention in occupational therapy.

clients in play and leisure activities that are designed to facilitate their achievement of intervention goals related to these impairments and limitations. Survey results indicated that 100% of 212 occupational therapists working with preschool-aged children in school-based and non–school-based settings used play as a therapeutic modality to enhance motor, sensory, or psychosocial outcomes; 92% indicated this use in over 50% of their caseload (Couch et al., 1998). These results resonate with occupational therapy literature in which play is typically described as means to facilitate children's development of their physical, cognitive, and psychosocial abilities and their acquisition of motor/praxis, sensory-perceptual, emotional regulation, cognitive, and communication/social skills (Blanche, 2008; CAOT, 1996; Knox, 2010; Long, Bergeron, Doyle, & Gordon, 2005; Munier et al., 2008; Parham, 2008).

Descriptions of leisure as means in the occupational therapy literature are limited (Bundy, 1993; Majnemer, 2010; Pereira & Stagnitti, 2008; Suto, 1998). A variety of responses to the use of leisure as means within occupational therapy practice has been reported, including promoting its use to address clients' needs in intervention, acknowledging its usefulness without applying it in practice, delegating it to secondary status to other areas of occupation (ADL, work, education), and choosing not to consider it or use it in practice at all (Majnemer, 2010; Pereira & Stagnitti, 2008). Nevertheless, occupational therapy practitioners often employ leisure activities, such as games or crafts, as means to increase their clients' strength, range of motion, endurance, standing tolerance; improve their manual dexterity and grasp; foster development of cognitive and psychosocial skills; and enhance their feelings of self-efficacy, self-worth, and self-expression (Blacker, Broadhurst, & Teixeira, 2008; Creek, 2008; Fenech, 2008; Hoppes, Wilcox, & Graham, 2001). Among 75% of 103 occupational therapists who reported using leisure assessments to plan their intervention, 38% of these therapists said that they used their clients' leisure interests to address their clients' development of skills (Turner et al., 2000).

Means to Enhance Performance in Areas of Occupation: Play and Leisure

Play and leisure as means can target change in performance in two specific areas of occupation: play and leisure. They are used to address limitations in clients' play and leisure performance (what they actually do and their experience while doing it). Practitioners engage their clients in play and leisure activities to achieve intervention goals related to their competence in and experience of these activities. Intervention provides opportunities for clients to practice specific play and leisure activities, explore new ones, facilitate their ability to perform them, and enhance their experience while engaged in them (Blacker et al., 2008; Bundy & Clemson, 2009; Fenech, 2008; Gray, 1998; Majnemer, 2010; Morrison & Metzger, 2001). For example, a Saturday morning group called Kids' Club, an occupational therapy intervention focusing on play and social participation, uses play as means in the form of games with rules to provide opportunities for children with developmental disorders to practice playing familiar games with their peers, explore games that are new to them, and experience fun and enjoyment during their participation in these games (Box 50.1).

When clients demonstrate problems with competence in their chosen play and leisure activities, practitioners can provide opportunities for them to practice play and leisure activities in a positive and safe environment or to explore alternate play and leisure activities in which they can experience higher levels of competence. For example, intervention for a boy with DCD who has difficulty playing soccer with his peers can include therapy sessions in which he and the occupational therapy practitioner actually play soccer so that he can practice the skills and tasks required for success in a safe and positive

BOX 50.1 Craig and Thomas

The occupational therapist uses play as means in the form of a game with rules in an intervention session with Craig and Thomas (Figure 50.3). Client factors/body functions (e.g., orientation, attention, motivation, and muscle power) and motor/praxis, sensory-perceptual, emotional regulation, cognitive, and communication/social performance skills (e.g., stabilizes, aligns, coordinates, calibrates, grips, attends, handles, heeds, gazes, orients, shares, sustains, focuses, and responds) are all addressed through their engagement in this game. Additionally, the boys' performance in the area of occupation of play is enhanced by the opportunity to play this game in a safe environment and by their positive and enjoyable experience of it.

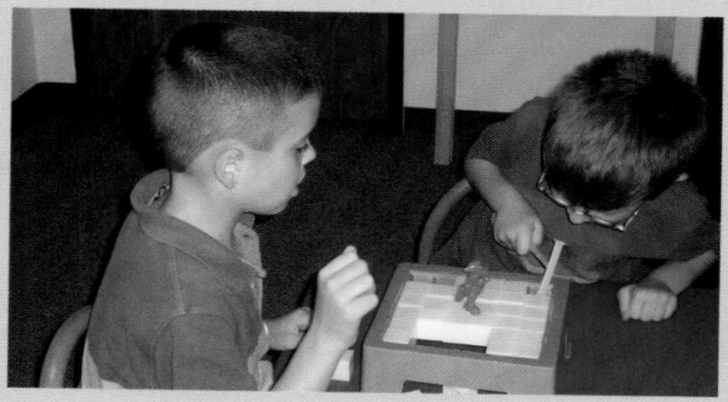

FIGURE 50.3 Play as means is used to address these boys' client factors and performance skills and to enhance their performance in the area of occupation of play.

environment with no serious consequences for failure (Morrison & Metzger, 2001). In addition, on the basis of evaluation of this boy's activity interests and activity choices, the practitioner can address the mismatch between his interest in and choice of soccer and his limited competence in it by engaging him in other sport activities that might provide a better match. Here, the practitioner uses the intervention approach of *prevent* to mitigate the effects of the boy's feelings of incompetence in soccer, thereby enhancing his performance in sports activities and reducing his risk for restricted participation in play and leisure activities.

When clients cannot perform specific play and leisure activities or they report problems with their experience while engaged in them, practitioners can adapt play and leisure activities, including the activity demands and their contextual and environmental features (Blacker et al., 2008; Bundy & Clemson, 2009; Fenech, 2008; Majnemer, 2010; Morrison & Metzger, 2001). Practitioners' use of adapted procedures, assistive technology, environmental modifications, and virtual reality can facilitate clients' ability to perform specific play and leisure activities (Dietz & Swinth, 2008). Case studies in the literature support the use of these methods to allow adults with acquired brain injury, stroke, or other neurological disorders to perform identified play and leisure activities of interest (Blacker et al., 2008; Deitz & Swinth, 2008; Lancioni et al., 2011; Lewis, Woods, Rosie, & Mcpherson, 2011). Additionally, these methods can be used to enhance clients' experience of playfulness, positive affect, personal meaning, and overall satisfaction with their play and leisure experience. Reid (2004) found that virtual reality environments successfully fostered varying levels of playfulness in children with cerebral palsy.

Occupational therapy practitioners frequently use more low-tech methods, such as adapted procedures, to enhance clients' play and leisure experiences. Among 75% of 103 occupational therapists who reported using leisure assessments to plan their intervention, 11% of these therapists stated that they focused on developing ways to adapt leisure activities for clients' current skill levels (Turner et al., 2000). For example, an elderly woman reported that the leisure experience she had previously obtained through cooking was no longer satisfying and personally meaningful because of her physical impairments related to a stroke (Bundy & Clemson, 2009). Using the intervention approach of *modify,* the practitioner adapted the leisure activity of cooking to facilitate the client's performance in such a way that her leisure experience during cooking was enhanced. Specifically, the practitioner demonstrated and taught the client adapted procedures that she could use to compensate for the mild weakness and abnormal muscle tone in her affected arm, such as sliding pans onto and off the cooktop rather than lifting and carrying them. Instead of focusing intervention on her body functions and structures and performance skills in the context of remediation of motor control, the practitioner used the client's leisure activity of cooking as means to enable her to regain the experience of leisure.

Play and Leisure as Ends

Play and leisure as ends refers to clients' participation in play and leisure as the goal or outcome of intervention (Gray, 1998; Trombly, 1995). Intervention focuses on their ability to engage in play and leisure occupations that are typically expected of and available to people of the same age and culture in home, school, work, and community settings (Coster, 1998; Primeau & Ferguson, 1999). Practitioners who address clients' play and leisure as ends promote clients' play and leisure participation for its own sake, not as a means to some other end (Blanche, 2008; Bundy, 1993; Munier et al., 2008; Parham 2008). Occupational therapy practitioners who address play and leisure as ends are rare (Majnemer, 2010; Munier et al., 2008; Parham, 2008; Pereira & Stagnitti, 2008). A survey of 222 occupational therapists working with preschool-aged children found that only 2% of them reported that their main use of play in intervention was as an outcome of intervention (Couch et al., 1998). Among 75% of 103 occupational therapists who reported using leisure assessments to plan their intervention, 35% of these therapists said that they used leisure activity in intervention to promote their clients' future leisure participation (Turner et al., 2000).

Many client populations seen by occupational therapy practitioners demonstrate detrimental effects on their play and leisure participation in their daily life, including children with disabilities and/or developmental disorders (LaVesser & Berg, 2011; Majnemer, 2010; Poulsen, Barker, & Ziviani, 2010; Shimoni et al,. 2010) and adults living with illnesses/disabilities (Berger, 2010; Bier, Dutil, & Couture, 2009; McKenna et al., 2009; O'Sullivan & Chard, 2010; Reinseth & Espnes, 2007). Literature outside occupational therapy, dating back to the 1970s, demonstrates a high correlational relationship between leisure satisfaction and overall life satisfaction (Parker, Gladman, & Drummond, 1997). When compared to participation in ADL, leisure participation was demonstrated to be a stronger factor related to life satisfaction (Nilsson, Bernspång, Fisher, Gustafson, & Lofgren, 2007). Although issues of causality in these correlational studies are inconclusive (Headey, Veenhoven, & Wearing, 1991), they indicate that play and leisure participation is linked to overall life satisfaction and quality of life (Brown & Frankel, 1993; Lloyd, 1996; Marans & Mohai, 1991).

Focus on play and leisure as ends in intervention addresses occupational therapy outcomes (AOTA, 2008), specifically, improved play and leisure performance, satisfying leisure participation in daily life, enhanced quality of life (Beesley, White, Alston, Sweetapple, & Pollack, 2011; Nilsson et al., 2007), and adaptation to illness/disability (Blacker et al., 2008; Kleiber et al., 2008) and overall health/wellness, including subjective well-being (Heo et al., 2010; Pereira & Stagnitti, 2008; Reynolds, Vivat, & Prior, 2008). Given these relationships among play and leisure participation and occupational therapy outcomes, the need for occupational therapy practitioners to focus on play and leisure as ends is critical. Practitioners promote clients' play and leisure as ends through their use of the following types of occupational therapy intervention: therapeutic use of occupations and activities, the education process, the consultation process, and advocacy (AOTA, 2008).

Therapeutic Use of Occupations and Activities

Therapeutic use of occupations and activities (play and leisure as means) can be used to facilitate clients' play and leisure as ends (Box 50.2). As was described previously, they are also means to address client factors, including impairments and limitations in body functions and structures, performance skills, and performance in the areas of occupation of play and leisure. The ability of clients to engage in other areas of occupation, besides play and leisure, may also be means to enhance play and leisure as ends. For example, practitioners may engage their clients in ADL, such as dressing or toileting, or in instrumental ADL, such as driving or money management, to improve their ability to participate in play and leisure in home, school, work, and community settings. In fact, older people's ability to live active and healthy lives including leisure participation can be negatively affected by limitations in their community mobility (Iwarsson, Stahl, & Carlsson, 2003), especially their inability to drive (McKenna et al., 2009; O'Sullivan & Chard, 2009). Occupational therapy practitioners who work with their older clients to facilitate their community mobility can also enhance their ability to participate in leisure in community settings.

BOX 50.2 Kids' Club

An occupational therapist in private practice offers a Saturday morning program called Kids' Club, a group intervention for children with developmental disorders focusing on play as ends, that is, the children's engagement in play and social participation as the outcome of intervention. She uses play as means, in the form of games with rules, to address client factors, performance skills, performance in the area of occupation of play, and play as ends. The power of the use of occupation of play as means to facilitate play as ends is demonstrated by two children's stories as told by their mothers.

Fredrick, a 6-year-old boy who was adopted from an Eastern European country, is nonverbal and demonstrates physical and social delays. He had been coming to Kids' Club for a few weeks. His mother called the therapist one night during the week to tell her excitedly about Fredrick's behavior that night in the waiting area outside his sister's karate class. She stated that Fredrick had, for the first time ever, approached a peer (who was also waiting for a sibling) and took his hand to lead him over to the area where Fredrick had been playing. His mother was very happy to see Fredrick initiate play with a peer in this everyday setting, and she attributed it directly to his participation in Kids' Club.

Daryll, a 6-year-old boy diagnosed with pervasive developmental disorder-not otherwise specified (PDD-NOS), had been coming to Kids' Club for about 6 months when his mother told the therapist that she and her husband had gotten up that Saturday morning to find that Daryll was out of bed and fully dressed. He had also already gotten himself his breakfast of cold cereal and milk. He was ready to leave for Kids' Club, and he was waiting for them to get up and take him there. She said that he had never before shown this kind of motivation to go anywhere. Clearly, Daryll's experience in Kids' Club was more than a means to an ends. His behavior suggested that he enjoyed his participation in Kids' Club as an ends and for its own sake.

See **Appendix I, Common Conditions, Autism Spectrum Disorders**, for more information on PDD-NOS.

Education Process

The education process is a type of occupational therapy intervention that provides knowledge and information to clients, family members, friends, teachers, coworkers, or other people of significance to clients (AOTA, 2008). Practitioners frequently address children's play and leisure as ends by educating others (e.g., parents, other family members, teachers, and caregivers) on how to create supportive physical and social environments for play and leisure participation within home, school, and community settings (Rigby & Huggins, 2003). They may provide information on play materials and toys, how to structure physical spaces for play, the importance of play and its effects on children's development, and how to facilitate children's play by modeling playful interactions (CAOT, 1996; Bundy et al., 2008; Bundy, Waugh, & Brentnall, 2009; Hamm, 2006). Practitioners also teach clients and others how to use adaptive equipment in play and leisure, such as computer games, toys with switches, and adaptive sports equipment (Deitz & Swinth, 2008; Majnemer, 2010). Leisure education programs educate clients about leisure, its potential benefits, and personal and community resources for and barriers to leisure and how to access or overcome them (Bundy, 2009; Kleiber et al., 2008). These types of leisure education programs exemplify the occupational therapy intervention approach of *maintain* by supporting clients' continued participation in leisure in community settings.

Consultation Process

The consultation process is a type of occupational therapy intervention through which practitioners collaborate with clients and others in their home, school, work, and community settings to identify issues that affect their successful participation in play and leisure, plan solutions to address those issues, implement solutions, and alter them as necessary for optimal effectiveness (AOTA, 2008). The focus is on clients' participation in play and leisure outside of therapy in the context of their daily lives (Kielhofner, 1997). Leisure counseling is a specific form of consultation that helps clients to identify and clarify leisure values, interests, and attitudes; determine their abilities and skills for leisure participation; improve or refine their skills as needed; and locate and access community resources for leisure (Barris, Kielhofner, & Watts, 1988; Caldwell & Smith, 1988; Malley, Cooper, & Cope, 2008; Poulsen et al., 2010).

Advocacy

Advocacy is a type of occupational therapy intervention that focuses on empowering clients to find and access resources to enable them to participate fully in play and leisure activities (AOTA, 2008). As advocates, practitioners advise, coordinate, educate, and collaborate with clients and others to remove barriers and shape supportive environments that facilitate clients' access to and inclusion in play and leisure opportunities (CAOT, 1996; Rigby & Huggins, 2003). For example, using the intervention approach of *create/promote*, practitioners advocate for accessible community playgrounds and collaborate with parents, teachers, and other adults to facilitate children's inclusion in play with peers and ensure protected play time (Blanche, 2008; Rigby & Huggins, 2003). Additionally, practitioners use the intervention approach of *prevent* to advise employers on the requirement of the Americans With Disabilities Act of 1990 to include clients with disabilities in all employment-related activities, including holiday parties, sports events, and business trips (Figure 50.4) (Crist & Stoffel, 1992).

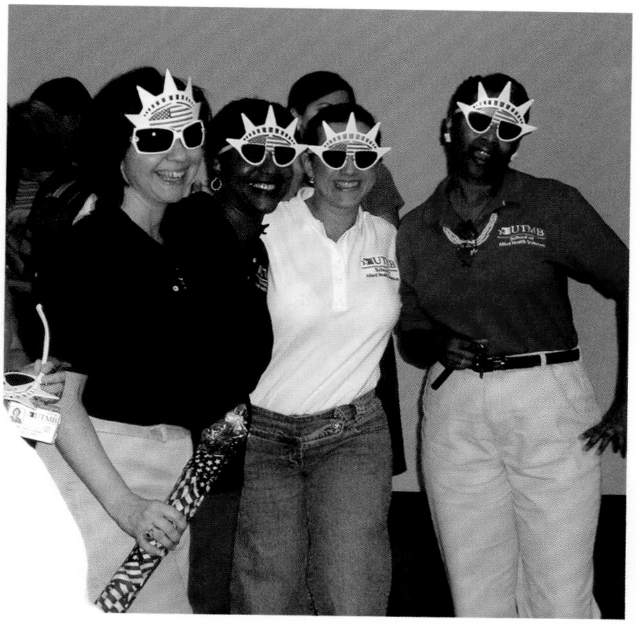

FIGURE 50.4 Play and leisure at work, such as participation in holiday parties and special events, is a significant feature of adults' participation in play and leisure.

Summary of Play and Leisure Intervention

Play and leisure in intervention may be lures or rewards, means, or ends. As lures, they motivate clients to engage in therapeutic activities; as rewards, they reinforce their participation in intervention. They are therapeutic means to achieve intervention goals related to clients' impairments and limitations in body functions and structures, performance skills, and play and leisure performance. Play and leisure as ends are the goals or outcomes of intervention when practitioners promote clients' play and leisure participation for its own sake, not as means to some other end. Therapeutic use of occupations and activities, the education process, the consultation process, and advocacy are types of occupational therapy intervention that facilitate clients' play and leisure as ends. Practitioners choose among these purposes of play and leisure as lures or rewards, means, or ends to design interventions that lead to outcomes directly related to clients' participation and occupational performance in home, school, work, and community settings.

Practice Dilemma

Leisure Counseling Program

You are an occupational therapy practitioner working on a mental health unit for adults with psychiatric disorders. You are asked to develop a leisure counseling program, focusing on leisure exploration and leisure participation (AOTA, 2008) for a group of adults with the following diagnoses:

- A 23-year-old woman with posttraumatic stress disorder
- A 35-year-old man with alcohol-related disorder
- A 28-year-old woman with major depression
- A 19-year-old woman with anorexia nervosa
- A 30-year-old man with panic disorder

Develop an intervention session plan for this group. Describe the activities that you would use and how you would present them to the group.

CASE STUDY 50.1 Putting It All Together: Evaluating and Designing Interventions for a Child's Participation in Play

Alvin is a 4 years and 6 months old boy with a diagnosis of autism. He has a fraternal twin brother who does not have autism. During the occupational therapy evaluation, the occupational therapist asks Alvin's parents about his play behaviors. They report that he essentially ignores other children and rarely engages in play with them. He prefers to play alone, choosing toys such as animal figurines or computer games. When he is around other children, he is likely to interact with those who are younger than him and is most comfortable interacting with others in structured play situations, such as preschool activities, and outdoor activities, such as tag, hide-and-seek, and jumping on the trampoline in their backyard. They also report that Alvin does not have any friends outside of structured play situations that occur in his preschool or that they set up for him at home. Although they state that he demonstrates playfulness, he rarely engages in the play behaviors that they observe in his twin brother's interactions with his peers. They report that Alvin is unable to make or keep friends, yet that is their wish for him: to have friends outside of the structured activities in which they involve him.

Questions and Exercises

1. What do you know about Alvin's characteristics of play participation, his play contexts, and his play activity and experience? Organize this information according to the parameters for evaluation of play and leisure provided in this chapter.
2. What do you need to know to develop and implement an intervention plan to address Alvin's performance in play and how will you obtain this information? Refer to Table 50.1 for specific assessments that you could use.
3. How could you use play in your intervention with Alvin and what types of intervention would you use?

References

American Occupational Therapy Association. (2008). Occupational therapy practice framework: Domain and process, 2nd edition. *American Journal of Occupational Therapy, 62*, 625–683.

American Occupational Therapy Association. (2010). Occupational therapy's perspective on the use of environments and contexts to support health and participation in occupations. *American Journal of Occupational Therapy, 64*, S57–S69. doi:10.5014/ajot.2010.64S57

Barris, R., Kielhofner, G., & Watts, J. H. (1988). *Occupational therapy in psychosocial practice*. Thorofare, NJ: SLACK Incorporated.

Beard, J. G., & Ragheb, M. G. (1980). Measuring leisure satisfaction. *Journal of Leisure Research, 12*, 20–33.

Beesley, K., White, J. H., Alston, M. K., Sweetapple, A. L., & Pollack, M. (2011). Art after stroke: The qualitative experience of community dwelling stroke survivors in a group art programme. *Disability and Rehabilitation, 33*, 2346–2355. doi:10.3109/09638288.2011.571333.

Berger, S. (2010). The meaning of leisure for older adults living with vision loss. *OTJR: Occupation, Participation and Health, 31*, 193–199. doi:10.3928/15394492-20101222-01.

Bier, N., Dutil, E., & Couture, M. (2009). Factors affecting leisure participation after a traumatic brain injury: An exploratory study. *Journal of Head Trauma Rehabilitation, 24*, 187–194.

Blacker, D., Broadhurst, L., & Teixeira, L. (2008). The role of occupational therapy in leisure adaptation with complex neurological disability: A discussion using two case study examples. *Neurorehabilitation, 23*, 313–319.

Blanche, E. I. (2008). Play in children with cerebral palsy: Doing with—not doing to. In L. D. Parham & L. S. Fazio (Eds.), *Play in occupational therapy for children* (2nd ed., pp. 375–393). St. Louis, MO: Mosby Elsevier.

Boucher, N., Dumas, F., Maltais, D. B., & Richards, C. L. (2010). The influence of selected personal and environmental factors on leisure activities in adults with cerebral palsy. *Disability and Rehabilitation, 32*, 1328–1338. doi:10.3109/09638280903514713.

Bourke-Taylor, H., Law, M., Howie, L., & Pallant, J. F. (2009). Development of the Assistance to Participate Scale (APS) for children's play and leisure activities. *Child: Care, Health and Development, 35*, 738–745. doi:10.1111/j.1365-2214.2009.00995.x

Brown, B. A., & Frankel, B. G. (1993). Activity through the years: Leisure, leisure satisfaction, and life. *Sociology of Sport Journal, 10*, 1–17.

Bryze, K. C. (2008). Narrative contributions to the play history. In L. D. Parham & L. S. Fazio (Eds.), *Play in occupational therapy for children* (2nd ed., pp. 43–54). St. Louis, MO: Mosby Elsevier.

Bundy, A. C. (1993). Assessment of play and leisure: Delineation of the problem. *American Journal of Occupational Therapy, 47,* 217–222.

Bundy, A. C. (2001). Measuring play performance. In M. Law, C. M. Baum, & W. Dunn (Eds.), *Measuring occupational performance: Supporting best practice in occupational therapy* (pp. 89–102). Thorofare, NJ: SLACK Incorporated.

Bundy, A. C., & Clemson, L. M. (2009). Leisure. In B. R. Bonder & V. Dal Bello-Haas (Eds.), *Functional performance in older adults* (3rd ed., pp. 290–310). Philadelphia, PA: F. A. Davis.

Bundy, A. C., Luckett, T., Naughton, G. A., Tranter, P. J., Wyver, S. R., Ragen, J., & Spies, G. (2008). Playful interaction: Occupational therapy for all children on the school playground. *American Journal of Occupational Therapy, 62,* 522–527.

Bundy, A. C., Waugh, K., & Brentnall, J. (2009). Developing assessments that account for the role of the environment: An example using the Test of Playfulness and Test of Environmental Supportiveness. *OTJR: Occupation, Participation and Health, 29,* 135–143. doi:10.3928/15394492-20090611-06

Burke, J. P., Schaaf, R. C., & Hall, T. B. L. (2008). Family narratives and play assessment. In L. D. Parham & L. S. Fazio (Eds.), *Play in occupational therapy for children* (2nd ed., pp. 195–215). St. Louis, MO: Mosby Elsevier.

Byunggook, K. (2008). Perceiving leisure: Humans view leisure through a lens tinted with experiences. *Parks & Recreation.* Retrieved from http://findarticles.com/p/articles/mi_m1145/is_5_43/ai_n53301707/

Caldwell, L. L., & Smith, E. A. (1988). Leisure: An overlooked component of health promotion. *Canadian Journal of Public Health, 79,* S44–S48.

Canadian Association of Occupational Therapists. (1996). Practice paper: Occupational therapy and children's play. *Canadian Journal of Occupational Therapy, 63,* 1–20.

Cordier, R., Bundy, A., Hocking, C., & Einfeld, S. (2009). A model for play-based intervention for children with ADHD. *Australian Occupational Therapy Journal, 56,* 332–340. doi:10.1111/j.1440-1630.2009.00796.x

Cordier, R., Bundy, A., Hocking, C., & Einfeld, S. (2010). Playing with a child with ADHD: A focus on the playmates. *Scandinavian Journal of Occupational Therapy, 17,* 191–199. doi:10.3109/11038120903156619

Coster, W. (1998). Occupation-centred assessment of children. *American Journal of Occupational Therapy, 52,* 337–344.

Couch, K. J., Deitz, J. C., & Kanny, E. M. (1998). The role of play in pediatric occupational therapy. *American Journal of Occupational Therapy, 52,* 111–117.

Couture, M., Caron, C. D., & Desrosiers, J. (2010). Leisure activities following a lower limb amputation. *Disability and Rehabilitation, 32,* 57–64. doi:10.3109/09638280902998797

Creek, J. (2008). Creative leisure opportunities. *NeuroRehabilitation, 23,* 299–304.

Crist, P. A., & Stoffel, V. C. (1992). The Americans With Disabilities Act of 1990 and employees with mental impairments: Personal efficacy and the environment. *American Journal of Occupational Therapy, 46,* 434–443.

Daunhauer, L. A., Coster, W. J., Tickle-Degnen, L., & Cermak, S. A. (2010). Play and cognition among young children reared in an institution. *Physical and Occupational Therapy in Pediatrics, 30,* 83–97.

Desha, L., Ziviani, J., & Rodger, S. (2003). Play preferences and behavior of preschool children with autistic spectrum disorder in the clinical environment. *Physical & Occupational Therapy in Pediatrics, 23,* 21–42.

Deitz, J. C., & Swinth, Y. (2008). Accessing play through assistive technology. In L. D. Parham & L. S. Fazio (Eds.), *Play in occupational therapy for children* (2nd ed., pp. 395–412). St. Louis, MO: Mosby Elsevier.

Driver, B. L., Brown, P. J., & Peterson, G. L. (Eds.). (1991). *Benefits of leisure.* State College, PA: Venture.

Driver, B. L., Tinsley, H. E. A., & Manfredo, M. J. (1991). The Paragraphs about Leisure and Recreation Experience Preference Scales: Results from two inventories designed to assess the breadth of the perceived psychological benefits of leisure. In B. L. Driver, P. J. Brown, & G. L. Peterson (Eds.), *Benefits of leisure* (pp. 263–286). State College, PA: Venture.

Dunn, W. (1998). Person-centered and contextually relevant evaluation. In J. Hinojosa & P. Kramer (Eds.), *Occupational therapy evaluation: Obtaining and interpreting data* (pp. 47–76). Bethesda, MD: American Occupational Therapy Association.

Edginton, C. R., DeGraaf, D., Dieser, R. B., & Edginton, S. R. (2006). *Leisure and life satisfaction: Foundational perspectives* (4th ed.). Chicago, IL: McGraw-Hill.

Engel-Yeger, B., & Hanna Kasis, A. (2010). The relationship between Developmental Co-ordination Disorders, child's perceived self-efficacy and preference to participate in daily activities. *Child: Care, Health and Development, 36,* 670–677. doi:10.1111/j.1365-2214.2010.01073.x.

Fenech, A. (2008). The benefits and barriers to leisure occupations. *NeuroRehabilitation, 23,* 295–297.

Fine, J. (2000). The effect of leisure activity on depression in the elderly: Implications for the field of occupational therapy. *Occupational Therapy in Health Care, 13,* 45–59.

Fleming, J., Braithwaite, H., Gustafsson, L., Griffin, J., Collier, A. M., & Fletcher, S. (2011). Participation in leisure activities during brain injury rehabilitation. *Brain Injury, 25,* 806–818. doi:10.3109/02699052.2011.585508

Florey, L. L., & Greene, S. (2008). Play in middle childhood. In L. D. Parham & L. S. Fazio (Eds.), *Play in occupational therapy for children* (2nd ed., pp. 279–299). St. Louis, MO: Mosby Elsevier.

Gray, J. M. (1998). Putting occupation into practice: Occupation as ends, occupation as means. *American Journal of Occupational Therapy, 52,* 354–364.

Griffin, J., & McKenna, K. (1998). Influences on leisure and life satisfaction of elderly people. *Physical & Occupational Therapy in Geriatrics, 15,* 1–16. doi:10.1300/J148V15n04_01

Hackett, J. (2003). Perceptions of play and leisure in junior school aged children with juvenile idiopathic arthritis: What are the implications for occupational therapy? *British Journal of Occupational Therapy, 66,* 303–310.

Hamm, E. M. (2006). Playfulness and the environmental support of play in children with and without developmental disabilities. *OTJR: Occupation, Participation and Health, 26,* 88–96.

Harris, K., & Reid, D. (2005). The influence of virtual reality play on children's motivation. *Canadian Journal of Occupational Therapy, 72,* 21–29.

Headey, B., Veenhoven, R., & Wearing, A. (1991). Top-down versus bottom-up theories of subjective well-being. *Social Indicators Research, 24,* 81–100.

Henry, A. (2008). Assessment of play and leisure in children and adolescents. In L. D. Parham & L. S. Fazio (Eds.), *Play in occupational therapy for children* (2nd ed., pp. 95–193). St. Louis, MO: Mosby Elsevier.

Heo, J., Lee, Y., McCormick, B. P., & Pedersen, P. M. (2010). Daily experience of serious leisure, flow, and subjective well-being of older adults. *Leisure Studies, 29,* 207–225. doi:10.1080/02614360903434092

Hess, L. M., & Bundy, A. C. (2003). The association between playfulness and coping in adolescents. *Physical & Occupational Therapy in Pediatrics, 23,* 5–17.

Hoppes, S., Wilcox, T., & Graham, G. (2001). Meanings of play for older adults. *Physical and Occupational Therapy in Geriatrics, 18,* 57–68.

Hurd, A. R., & Anderson, D. M. (2011). *Park and recreation professional's handbook.* Champaign, IL: Human Kinetics.

Imms, C. (2008). Children with cerebral palsy participate: A review of the literature. *Disability and Rehabilitation, 30,* 1867–1884. doi:10.1080/09638280701673542

Iso-Ahola, S., & Weissinger, E. (1990). Perceptions of boredom in leisure: Conceptualization, reliability, and validity of the Leisure Boredom Scale. *Journal of Leisure Research, 22,* 1–17.

Iwarsson, S., Stahl, A., & Carlsson, G. (2003). Accessible transportation: Novel occupational therapy perspectives. In L. Letts, P. Rigby, & D. Stewart (Eds.), *Using environments to enable occupational performance* (pp. 235–251). Thorofare, NJ: SLACK Incorporated.

Kielhofner, G. (1997). *Conceptual foundations of occupational therapy* (2nd ed.). Philadelphia, PA: F. A. Davis.

Kielhofner, G. (2008). Volition. In G. Kielhofner (Ed.), *A model of human occupation: Theory and application* (4th ed., pp. 32–50). Baltimore, MD: Lippincott Williams & Wilkins.

Kielhofner, G., & Burke, J. P. (1983). The evolution of knowledge and practice in occupational therapy: Past, present, and future. In G. Kielhofner (Ed.), *Health through occupation: Theory and practice in occupational therapy* (pp. 3–54). Philadelphia, PA: F. A. Davis.

King, G., Law, M., King, S., Hurley, P., Hanna, S., Kertoy, M., . . . Young, N. (2004). *Children's Assessment of Participation and Enjoyment (CAPE) and Preferences for Activities of Children (PAC).* San Antonio, TX: Harcourt Assessment, Inc.

Kleiber, D. A., Reel, H. A., & Hutchinson, S. L. (2008). When distress gives way to possibility: The relevance of leisure in adjustment to disability. *NeuroRehabilitation, 23,* 321–328.

Knox, S. (2008). Development and current use of the Revised Knox Preschool Play Scale. In L. D. Parham & L. S. Fazio (Eds.), *Play in occupational therapy for children* (2nd ed., pp. 55–70). St. Louis, MO: Mosby Elsevier.

Knox, S. H. (2010). Play. In J. Case-Smith & J. C. O'Brien (Eds.), *Occupational Therapy for Children* (6th ed., pp. 540–554). Maryland Heights, MO: Mosby Elsevier.

Lancioni, G. E., Singh, N. N., O'Reilly, M. F., Sigafoos, J., DePace, C., Chiapparino, & C., Spica, A. (2011). Technology-assisted programmes to promote leisure engagement in persons with acquired brain injury and profound multiple disabilities: Two case studies. *Disability and Rehabilitation: Assistive Technology, 6,* 412–419. doi:10.3109/17483107.2011.580899.

LaVesser, P., & Berg, C. (2011). Participation patterns in preschool children with an autism spectrum disorder. *OTJR: Occupation, Participation and Health, 31,* 33–39.

Law, M., Anaby, D., DeMatteo, C., & Hanna, S. (2011). Participation patterns of children with acquired brain injury. *Brain Injury, 25,* 587–595. doi:10.3109/02699052.2011.572945.

Law, M., Baum, C. M., & Dunn, W. (2005). Occupational Performance Assessment. In C. H. Christiansen, C. M. Baum, & J. Bass-Haugen (Eds.), Occupational therapy: Performance, Participation, and well-being (3rd ed., pp. 339–370). Thorofare, NJ: Slack.

Lee, Y. (1999). How do individuals experience leisure? *Parks & Recreation.* Retrieved from http//findarticles.com/p/articles/mi_m1145/is_2_34/ai_53984866/

Lee, Y., Datillo, J., & Howard, D. (1994). The complex and dynamic nature of leisure experience. *Journal of Leisure Research, 26,* 195–211.

Leipold, E. E., & Bundy, A. C. (2000). Playfulness in children with attention deficit hyperactivity disorder. *Occupational Therapy Journal of Research, 20,* 61–82.

Lewis, G. N., Woods, C., Rosie, J. A., & Mcpherson, K. M. (2011). Virtual reality games for rehabilitation of people with stroke: Perspectives from the users. *Disability and Rehabilitation: Assistive Technology, 6,* 453–463. doi:10.3109/17483107.2011.574310.

Linder, T. (2008). *Transdisciplinary Play-Based Assessment* (2nd ed.). Baltimore, MD: Brookes.

Lloyd, K. (1996). Planning for leisure: Issues of quality of life. *Social Alternatives, 15,* 19–22.

Long, D., Bergeron, J., Doyle, S. L., & Gordon, C. Y. (2005). The relationship between frequency of participation in play activities and kindergarten readiness. *Occupational Therapy in Health Care, 19,* 23–42. doi:10.1300/J003v19n04_03.

Majnemer, A. (2009). Promoting participation in leisure activities: Expanding role for pediatric therapists. *Physical and Occupational Therapy in Pediatrics, 29,* 1–5. doi:10.1080/01942630802625163.

Majnemer, A. (2010). Balancing the boat: Enabling an ocean of possibilities. *Canadian Journal of Occupational Therapy, 77,* 198–208. doi:10.2182/cjot.2010.77.4.2.

Majnemer, A., Shevell, M., Law, M., Birnbaum, R., Chilingaryan, G., Rosenbaum, P., & Poulin, C. (2008). Participation and enjoyment of leisure activities in school-aged children with cerebral palsy. *Developmental Medicine & Child Neurology, 50,* 751–758. doi:10.1111/j.1469.8749.2008.03068.x

Majnemer, A., Shikako-Thomas, K., Chokron, N., Law, M., Shevell, M., Chilingaryan, G. & Rosenbaum, P. (2009). Leisure activity preferences for 6- to 12-year old children with cerebral palsy. *Developmental Medicine & Child Neurology, 52,* 167–173.

Malley, D., Cooper, J., & Cope, J. (2008). Adapting leisure activity for adults with neuropsychological deficits following acquired brain injury. *NeuroRehabilitation, 23,* 329–334.

Marans, R. W., & Mohai, P. (1991). Leisure resources, recreation activity, and the quality of life. In B. L. Driver, P. J. Brown, & G. L. Peterson (Eds.), *Benefits of leisure* (pp. 351–363). State College, PA: Venture.

Matsutsuyu, J. S. (1969). The interest check list. *American Journal of Occupational Therapy, 23,* 323–328.

McKenna, K., Liddle, J., Brown, A., Lee, K., & Gustafsson, L. (2009). Comparison of time use, role participation and life satisfaction of older people after stroke with a sample without stroke. *Australian Occupational Therapy Journal, 56,* 177–188.

McMahon, F., Lytle, D. E., & Sutton-Smith, B. (Eds.). (2005). *Play: An interdisciplinary synthesis. Play & Culture Studies, Volume 6.* Lanham, MD: University Press of America.

Miller, E., & Kuhaneck, H. (2008). Children's perceptions of play experiences and play preferences: A qualitative study. *American Journal of Occupational Therapy, 62,* 407–415.

Morrison, C. D., & Metzger, P. (2001). Play. In J. Case-Smith (Ed.), *Occupational therapy for children* (4th ed., pp. 528–544). St. Louis, MO: Mosby-Year Book.

Mortenson, P. A., & Harris, S. R. (2006). Playfulness in children with traumatic brain injury: A preliminary study. *Physical and Occupational Therapy in Pediatrics, 26,* 181–198. doi:10.1080/J006v26n01_11.

Munier, V., Myers, C. T., & Pierce, D. (2008). Power of object play for infants and toddlers. In L. D. Parham & L. S. Fazio (Eds.), *Play in occupational therapy for children* (2nd ed., pp. 219–249). St. Louis, MO: Mosby Elsevier.

Nilsson, I., Bernspång, B., Fisher, A. G., Gustafson, Y., & Lofgren, B. (2007). Occupational engagement and life satisfaction in the oldest-old: The Umeå 85+ study. *OTJR: Occupation, Participation and Health, 27,* 131–139.

Oates, A., Bebbington, A., Bourke, J., Girdler, S., & Leonard, H. (2011). Leisure participation for school-aged children with Down syndrome. *Disability and Rehabilitation, 33,* 1880-1889. doi:10.3109/09638288.2011.553701

O'Brien, A., Renwick, R., & Yoshida, K. (2008). Leisure participation for individuals living with acquired spinal cord injury. *International Journal of Rehabilitation Research, 31,* 225–230. doi:10.1097/MRR.0b013e3282fb7d13

Okimoto, A. M., Bundy, A., & Hanzlik, J. (2000). Playfulness in children with and without disability: Measurement and intervention. *American Journal of Occupational Therapy, 54,* 73–82.

O'Sullivan, C., & Chard, G. (2010). An exploration of participation in leisure activities post-stroke. *Australian Occupational Therapy Journal, 57,* 159–166. doi:10.1111/j.1440-1630.2009.00833.x

Parham, L. D. (1996). Perspectives on play. In R. Zemke, & F. Clark (Eds.), *Occupational science: The evolving discipline* (pp. 71–80). Philadelphia, PA: F. A. Davis.

Parham, L. D. (2008). Play and occupational therapy. In L. D. Parham & L. S. Fazio (Eds.), *Play in occupational therapy for children* (2nd ed., pp. 3–39). St. Louis, MO: Mosby Elsevier.

Parham, L. D., & Fazio, L. S. (Eds.). (2008). *Play in occupational therapy for children.* St. Louis, MO: Mosby-Elsevier.

Parker, C. J., Gladman, J. R., & Drummond, A. E. (1997). The role of leisure in stroke rehabilitation. *Disability and Rehabilitation, 19,* 1–5.

Pereira, R. B., & Stagnitti, K. (2008). The meaning of leisure for well-elderly Italians in an Australian community: Implications for occupational therapy. *Australian Occupational Therapy Journal, 55,* 39–46. doi:10.1111/j.1440-1630.2006.00653.x

Pfeifer, L. I., Pacciulio, A. M., dos Santos, C. A., dos Santos, J. L., & Stagnitti, K. E. (2011). Pretend play of children with cerebral palsy. *Physical and Occupational Therapy in Pediatrics, 31,* 392–402. doi:10.3109/01942638.2011.572149

Pieris, Y., & Craik, C. (2004). Factors enabling and hindering participation in leisure for people with mental health problems. *British Journal of Occupational Therapy, 67,* 240–247.

Pollock, N., & McColl, M. A. (1998). Assessment in client-centred occupational therapy. In M. Law (Ed.), *Client-centered occupational therapy* (pp. 90–105). Thorofare, NJ: Slack.

Poulsen, A. A., Barker, F. M., & Ziviani, J. (2010). Personal projects of boys with developmental coordination disorder. *OTJR: Occupation, Participation and Health, 31*, 108–117. doi:10.3928/15394492-20100722-02

Poulsen, A. A., Ziviani, J. M., & Cuskelly, M. (2007). Perceived freedom in leisure and physical co-ordination ability: Impact on out-of-school activity participation and life satisfaction. *Child: care, health and development, 33*, 432–440. doi:10.1111/j.1365-2214.2007.00730.x

Primeau, L. A. (1995). Orchestration of work and play within families (Unpublished doctoral dissertation). University of Southern California, Los Angeles.

Primeau, L. A. (1996). Work and leisure: Transcending the dichotomy. *American Journal of Occupational Therapy, 50*, 569–577.

Primeau, L. A. (2008). AOTA's societal statement on play. *American Journal of Occupational Therapy, 62*, 707–708.

Primeau, L. A., & Ferguson, J. M. (1999). Occupational frame of reference. In P. Kramer & J. Hinojosa (Eds.), *Frames of reference for pediatric occupational therapy* (2nd ed., pp. 469–516). Philadelphia, PA: Lippincott Williams & Wilkins.

Raghavendra, P., Virgo, R., Olsson, C., Connell, T., & Lane, A. E. (2011). Activity participation of children with complex communication needs, physical disabilities and typically-developing peers. *Developmental Neurorehabilitation, 14*, 145–155. doi:10.3109/17518423.2011.568994.

Reid, D. (2004). The influence of virtual reality on playfulness in children with cerebral palsy: A pilot study. *Occupational Therapy International, 11*, 131–144.

Reilly, M. (1974). An explanation of play. In M. Reilly (Ed.), *Play as exploratory learning: Studies of curiosity behavior* (pp. 117–149). Beverly Hills, CA: Sage.

Reinseth, L., & Espnes, G. A. (2007). Women with rheumatoid arthritis: Non-vocational activities and quality of life. *Scandinavian Journal of Occupational Therapy, 14*, 108–115. doi:10.1080/11038120600994981

Reynolds, F., Vivat, B., & Prior, S. (2008). Women's experiences of increasing subjective well-being in CFS/ME through leisure-based arts and crafts activities: A qualitative study. *Disability and Rehabilitation, 30*, 1279–1288. doi:10.1080/09638280701654518

Rigby, P., & Huggins, L. (2003). Enabling young children to play by creating supportive play environments. In L. Letts, P. Rigby, & D. Stewart (Eds.), *Using environments to enable occupational performance* (pp. 155–176). Thorofare, NJ: SLACK Incorporated.

Rojek, C., Shaw, S. M., & Veal, A. J. (Eds.). (2007). *A handbook of leisure studies*. New York, NY: Palgrave Macmillan.

Rubin, K. H., Fein, G. G., & Vandenberg, B. (1983). Play. In P. H. Mussen (Series Ed.) & E. M. Hetherington (Vol. Ed.), *Handbook of child psychology: Vol. 4. Socialization, personality, and social development* (4th ed., pp. 693–774). New York, NY: John Wiley.

Saunders, E. B. (1922). Psychiatry and occupational therapy. *Archives of Occupational Therapy, 1*, 99–114.

Saunders, I., Sayer, M., & Goodale, A. (1999). The relationship between playfulness and coping in preschool children: A pilot study. *American Journal of Occupational Therapy, 53*, 221–226.

Scarlett, W. G., Naudeau, S., Salonius-Pasternak, D., & Ponte, I. (2005). *Children's play*. Thousand Oaks, CA: SAGE.

Shikako-Thomas, K., Majnemer, A., Law, M., & Lach, L. (2008). Determinants of participation in leisure activities in children and youth with cerebral palsy: Systematic review. *Physical and Occupational Therapy in Pediatrics, 28*, 155–169. doi:10.1080/01942630802031834

Shimoni, M., Engel-Yeger, B., & Tirosh, E. (2010). Participation in leisure activities among boys with attention deficit hyperactivity disorder. *Research in Developmental Disabilities, 31*, 1234–1239. doi:10.1016/j.ridd.2010.07.022

Skard, G., & Bundy, A. C. (2008). Test of Playfulness. In L. D. Parham & L. S. Fazio (Eds.), *Play in occupational therapy for children* (2nd ed., pp. 71–93). St. Louis, MO: Mosby Elsevier.

Slagle, E. C. (1922). Training aides for mental patients. *Archives of Occupational Therapy, 1*, 11–19.

Smyth, M. M., & Anderson, H. I. (2000). Coping with clumsiness in the school playground: Social and physical play in children with coordination impairments. *British Journal of Developmental Psychology, 18*, 389–413.

Specht, J., King, G., Brown, E., & Foris, C. (2002). The importance of leisure in the lives of persons with congenital physical disabilities. *American Journal of Occupational Therapy, 56*, 436–445.

Stebbins, R. A., (2008). Right leisure: Serious, casual, or project-based? *NeuroRehabilitation, 23*, 335–341.

Stewart, K. B. (2010). Purposes, processes, and methods of evaluation. In J. Case-Smith & J. C. O'Brien (Eds.), *Occupational Therapy for Children* (6th ed., pp. 193–215). Maryland Heights, MO: Mosby Elsevier.

Suto, M. (1998). Leisure in occupational therapy. *Canadian Journal of Occupational Therapy, 65*, 271–278.

Tanta, K. J., Deitz, J. C., White, O., & Billingsley, F. (2005). The effects of peer-play level on initiations and responses of preschool children with delayed play skills. *American Journal of Occupational Therapy, 59*, 437–445.

Trombly, C. A. (1995). Occupation: Purposefulness and meaningfulness as therapeutic mechanisms. *American Journal of Occupational Therapy, 49*, 960–972.

Turner, H., Chapman, S., McSherry, A., Krishnagiri, S., & Watts, J. (2000). Leisure assessment in occupational therapy: An exploratory study. *Occupational Therapy in Health Care, 12*, 73–85.

World Health Organization. (2001). *ICF: International Classification of Functioning, Disability, and Health*. Geneva: Author. Retrieved from http://www.who.int/icidh

Ziegler, L. H. (1924). Some observations on recreations. *Archives of Occupational Therapy, 3*, 255–265.

Ziviani, J., Rodger, S., & Peters, S. (2005). The play behaviour of children with and without autistic disorder in a clinical environment. *New Zealand Journal of Occupational Therapy, 52*, 22–30.

Ziviani, J., Wadley, D., Ward, H., Macdonald, D., Jenkins, D., & Rodger, S. (2008). A place to play: Socioeconomic and spatial factors in children's physical activity. *Australian Occupational Therapy Journal, 55*, 2–11. doi:10.1111/j.440-1630.2006.00646.x

For additional resources on the subjects discussed in this chapter, visit http://thePoint.lww.com/Willard-Spackman12e.

CHAPTER 51

Sleep and Rest

Jo M. Solet

OUTLINE

LEARNING OBJECTIVES

After reading this chapter, you will be able to:

1. Understand the elements of sleep architecture and sleep changes through the life cycle
2. Develop an epidemiological perspective on sleep deficiency
3. Relate sufficient sleep to individual health outcomes, memory, cognition, and occupational performance
4. Describe multiple factors that may influence sleep
5. Recognize common medical and psychiatric diagnoses treated by occupational therapists in which sleep may be implicated
6. Organize client options for sleep hygiene, including sleep habits and environments; relate these to self-care and occupational balance
7. Describe common primary sleep disorders
8. Provide basic client sleep education and screening assessment; anticipate need for specialized referrals and occupational therapy participation on the treatment team

Why Learn About Sleep?

We spend one-third of our lives asleep. Once thought of as a period of simple repose enforced by limited daylight, we now know sleep is a complex, dynamic state critical to growth and development. Many common medical and psychiatric disorders treated by occupational therapists affect client sleep or carry sleep-related signs and symptoms (Zee & Turek, 2006). Disordered sleep is a major public health concern affecting both genders, all races, and socioeconomic levels (Choi et al., 2006; Hale, 2005; Kim & Young, 2005) that increases with age (Ancoli-Israel & Cooke, 2005; Basner et al., 2007; Hale, 2005; Hale & Do, 2007; Patel et al., 2004). Sleep has documented impacts on health and safety, psychological well-being, learning and memory, and cognitive and occupational performance (Classen, 2011; Connor et al., 2002; Dorrian, Sweeney, & Dawson, 2011; Drake et al., 2010; Pizza et al.,

2010; Poe, Walsh, & Bjorness, 2010; Smith & Phillips, 2011; Van Dongen, Maislin, Mullington, & Dinges, 2003). Inadequate sleep has been implicated in performance deficits and can place individuals and those they are responsible for at risk. Excessive sleepiness has contributed to environmental disasters such as oil spills, air traffic control failures, medical errors, and auto and truck accidents. Sleep medicine is a dynamic, evolving field; research is underway at multiple levels, from genetic through epidemiological (Hobson, 2011; Shepard et al., 2005). New insights with clinical significance can be expected on a continuing basis. The 2008 "Occupational Therapy Practice Framework" (American Occupational Therapy Association, 2008) categorizes sleep as an occupation. This chapter provides a sleep foundation in this emerging area of practice for occupational therapists.

The Structure Of Sleep

Beginning in 1929 with the introduction of the **electroencephalogram (EEG)**, it was revealed that sleep consists of patterns of changing brain waves that present in cycles of about 90 minutes throughout the night. Within these cycles, different stages of sleep are identified by the frequency and amplitude of the brain waves. When comparing the EEG readings of waking and sleep stages, researchers and clinicians assess the frequency of the brain waves, measured in hertz (Hz), and the size, or amplitude, of the brain waves, measured in microvolts, which differ for various stages of wakefulness and sleep.

Sleep Stages and Architecture

The stages of sleep fall into two categories: **Rapid Eye Movement sleep** or **REM**, in which most dreaming occurs, and **nonrapid eye movement sleep,** called **NREM** or Non-REM, which displays progressively deeper stages identified as NREM1, NREM2, and NREM3. Infants and children have higher proportions of REM sleep than adults.

Transition from wakefulness begins with light sleep, known as stage 1 (NREM1), and deepens to stage 2 sleep (NREM2). In early cycles of the night, slow brain waves with low frequency and high amplitude characteristic of stage 3 or deep sleep (NREM3) are common. As morning approaches, the proportion of time in deep sleep drops, while the proportion in **REM** sleep—characterized by higher frequency and lower amplitude brain waves—increases. During REM sleep, there is diminished muscle tone, preventing the sleeper from acting out dream experiences. The map of a typical adult night's sleep showing the REM and NREM stages in 90-minute cycles through the night is called a **hypnogram** (Figure 51.1).

Current sleep medicine research explores the roles of REM and NREM sleep stages in contributing to specific functions, including emotional regulation, cognition, learning, and memory consolidation (American Academy of Sleep Medicine [AASM], 2009; Haack & Mullington, 2005; Poe et al., 2010; Stickgold, 2005; Walker & Stickgold, 2004).

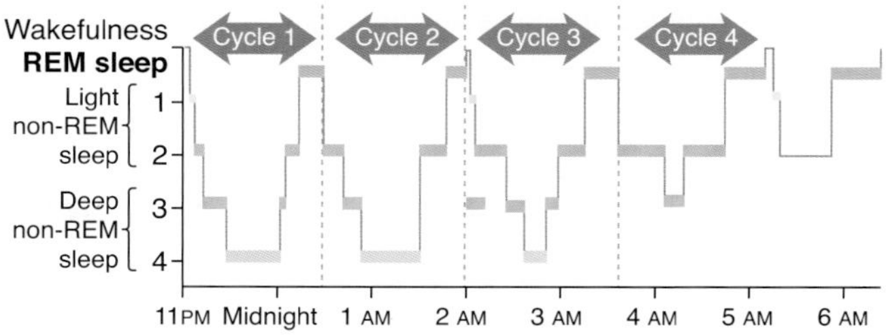

FIGURE 51.1 Sleep cycles across the night: "Hypnogram." *REM*, rapid eye movement.

Sleep Drives

Two processes interact to determine the drive for sleep: **sleep-wake homeostasis** and the **circadian biological clock**. The **homeostatic drive** increases with accumulated time awake. The circadian biological clock organizes a physiological cycle of body temperature and hormone release regulating the variability of sleepiness and wakefulness throughout the night and day. These two drives are not simply additive because with an increase in accumulated **sleep debt,** the circadian drive has been shown to exert greater impact on sleepiness (see Figure 51.2).

The **suprachiasmic nucleus (SCN)**, a group of cells in the hypothalamus that respond to light and dark, controls the circadian biological clock. Signals generated by light reaching the optic nerve through the eyes travel to the SCN, carrying the message to the internal clock for wakefulness. With exposure to morning light, the SCN orchestrates signals to other parts of the brain, raising body temperature and regulating certain hormone levels. Light delays the release of the hormone **melatonin**, which rises in the evening and stays elevated through the night, promoting sleep (Brendel, Florman, Roberts, & Solet, 2001; Edlund, 2003).

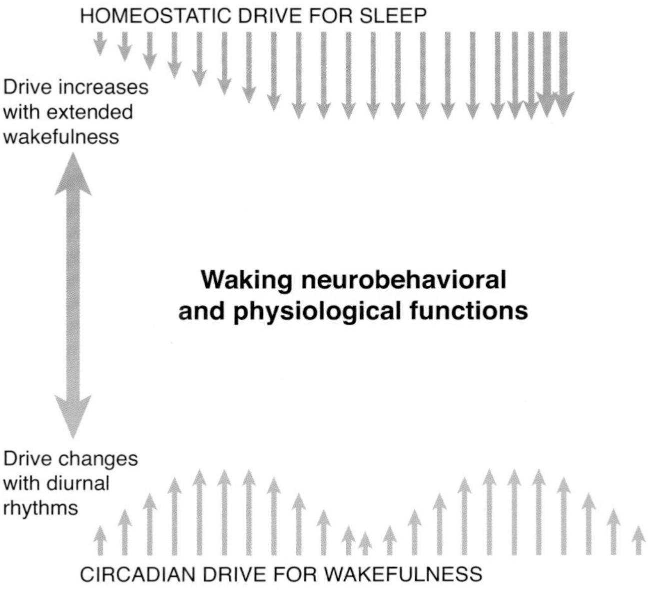

FIGURE 51.2 Sleep and wakefulness are regulated by two processes.

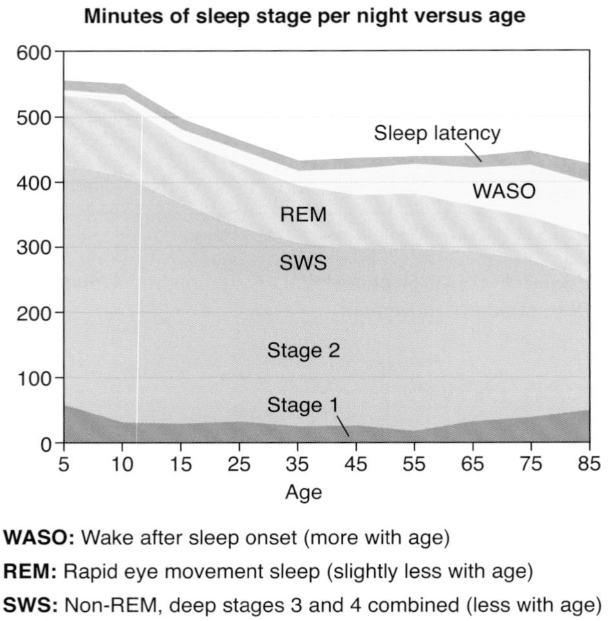

FIGURE 51.3 Sleep: less and lighter with aging. (*Source:* Reprinted with permission from Ohayon N. M., Carskadon, M. A., Guilleminault, C., & Vitiello, M. V. [2004]. Meta-analysis of quantitative sleep parameters from childhood to old age in healthy indviduals: Developing normative sleep values across the human lifespan. *SLEEP, 27,* 1255–1273.)

Sleep and the Life Cycle

Sleep changes through the life cycle, becoming shorter and lighter with aging (Figure 51.3). The period it takes to fall asleep, known as **sleep latency**, changes little over the life course, but the amount of time in restorative deep sleep drops off and the time spent **awake after sleep onset (WASO)** increases. The proportion of individuals with sleep-wake impairments also increases substantially with age (Hale, 2005; Ohayon, 2002; Ohayon & Vecchierini, 2005). As the baby boomers age, disordered sleep will require substantial attention and consumption of health care resources.

Sleep And Modern Life

Epidemiology

The average sleep time for Americans has dropped over the past 5 decades from 8.5 to 7 hours at the same time as obesity and diabetes rates have risen (Ayas, 2010; Flier & Elmquist, 2004; Hale, 2005; Patel & Hu, 2008; Quan, Parthasarathy, & Budhiraja, 2010; Watanabe, Kikuchi, Katsutoshi, & Takahashi, 2010; Watson, Buchwald, Vitiello, Noonan, & Goldberg, 2010. Furthermore, Centers for Disease Control and Prevention (CDC) overlay maps show an alarming congruence; states, especially in the Deep South, with populations having the most limited sleep also have the highest rates of obesity and diabetes (Figure 51.4) (see CDC Website). Not only does inadequate sleep increase appetite, lower satiation, and alter glucose metabolism, but as part of a dangerous cycle, obesity increases the risk for disordered sleep. Insufficient sleep is common even among children. Parents may not be aware of child sleep requirements and or may not enforce consistent sleep schedules (Owens & Mindell, 2005). Many believe that insufficient sleep is in part responsible for the alarming rise in childhood obesity.

Individual Health Impacts

The range of negative health impacts from insufficient or disrupted sleep includes elevated stress hormones, impaired glucose tolerance, diabetes (Zizi et al., 2011), obesity (Flier & Elmquist, 2004), cardiovascular disease, and stroke (Ayas et al., 2003a; Ayas et al., 2003b). In addition,

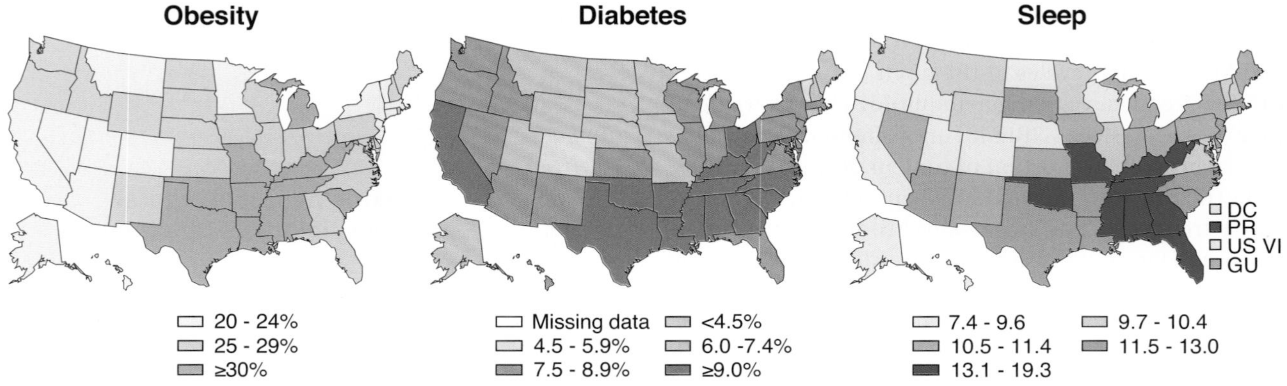

FIGURE 51.4 Intersecting epidemics. (Sources: Data from the following sources: Obesity: Centers for Disease Control and Prevention. [2012]. *Overweight and obesity: U.S. obesity trends.* Retrieved from http://www.cdc.gov/obesity/data/trends.html; Diabetes: Centers for Disease Control and Prevention, Division of Diabetes Translation. [2010]. *Maps of trends in diagnosed diabetes.* Retrieved from http://www.cdc.gov/diabetes/statistics/slides/maps_diabetes_trends.pdf; Insufficient sleep: Centers for Disease Control and Prevention, National Center for Chronic Disease Prevention and Health Promotion. [2012]. *Sleep and sleep disorders: Data and statistics.* Retrieved from http://www.cdc.gov/sleep/data_statistics.htm)

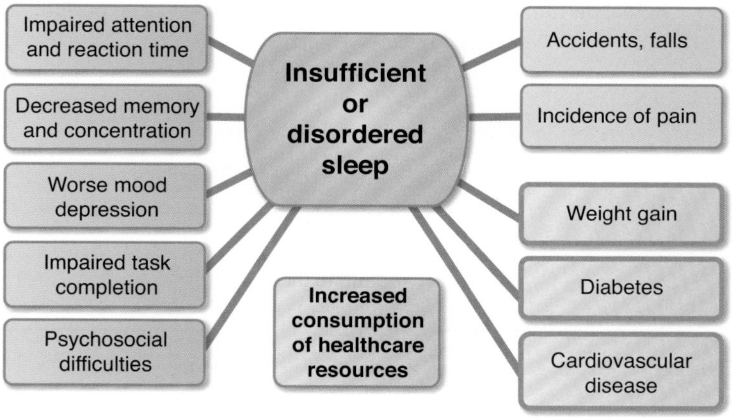

FIGURE 51.5 Insufficient or disordered sleep (Copyright Jo Solet, MS, EdM, PhD, OTR/L; Data from Ancoli-Israel, S., & Cooke, J. R. [2005]. Prevalence and comorbidity of insomnia and effect on functioning in elderly populations. *Journal of the American Geriatrics Society, 53*, S264–S271; Choi, S. W., Peek-Asa, C., Sprince, N. L., Rautiainen, R. H., Flamme, G. A., Whitten, P. S., & Zwerling, C. [2006]. Sleep quantity and quality as a predictor of injuries in a rural population. *American Journal of Emergency Medicine, 24*, 189–196; and Spiegel, K., Knutson, K., Leproult, R., Tasali, E., & Van Cauter, E. [2005]. Sleep loss: A novel risk factor for insulin resistance and Type 2 diabetes. *Journal of Applied Physiology, 99*, 2008–2019).

insufficient or disrupted sleep may be associated with **hyperalgesia** (Chhangani et al., 2009; Hamilton, Catley, & Karlson, 2007; Kristiansen et al., 2011; Roehrs, Hyde, Blaisdell, Greenwald, & Roth, 2006), lowered mood, irritability, aggressiveness, and psychosocial difficulties (AASM, 2009; Owens, Belon, & Moss, 2010). Decreased memory consolidation (Poe et al., 2010; Stickgold, 2005; Walker & Stickgold, 2004), impairments in concentration, impaired task completion, and decreased occupational performance have also been documented (Banks, Van Dongen, Mailsen, & Dinges, 2010; Cohen et al., 2010; Durmer & Dinges, 2005; Ohayon & Vecchierini, 2005). Industrial, truck and auto accidents are also associated with insufficient sleep (Classen, 2011; Connor et al., 2002; Drake et al., 2010; Pizza et al, 2010; Smith & Phillips, 2011; Tregear, Reston, Schoelles, & Phillips, 2009) (see Figure 51.5).

Sleep Requirements through the Life Cycle

Whereas newborns sleep as much as 16 hours a day, by 6 months, babies typically sleep 12 hours during the night, plus two naps during the day (Figure 51.6). Well-rested preschoolers may still take an afternoon nap while sleeping 12 consolidated hours at night. Elementary school children require as much as 10 to 12 hours. Teenagers are understood as a group to experience **delayed sleep phase**—their natural sleep inclinations, based on timing release of the sleep inducing hormone melatonin, are often toward later bedtime and later wake-up. This is in conflict with typical school schedules and may leave students who must awaken early feeling underslept and inattentive. Experiments with later high school start times showed improvements in multiple areas, including mood and academic performance as well as positive reactions from teachers (Owens et al., 2010). These findings are now driving policy initiatives to alter school schedules (Owens, 2011, personal communication). School-based occupational therapists are in the position to bring awareness of sleep impacts to parents, teachers, and administrators.

Along with changes during growth and development, there are individual differences in adult sleep requirements and schedule preferences. Ideally, individuals choose occupations that match their natural proclivities. However, it may be that many of us have become accustomed to a level of functioning that results from less than optimal sleep. In sleep restriction vigilance studies, subjects actually show limited insight into their deepening performance decrements over a 2-week period (Van Dongen et al., 2003) (Figure 51.7). Although 7.5 hours is frequently cited as adequate for healthy adults, recent sleep extension studies with college athletes showed performance enhancements at 10 hours of time in bed (TIB) (Mah, Mah, Kezerian, & Dement, 2011).

Although elderly people may sleep less, in part due to higher levels of medical disorders and pain, or because they lack a consolidated night sleep period, napping on and off during the day, there is no evidence to support the common belief that elderly people actually require less sleep.

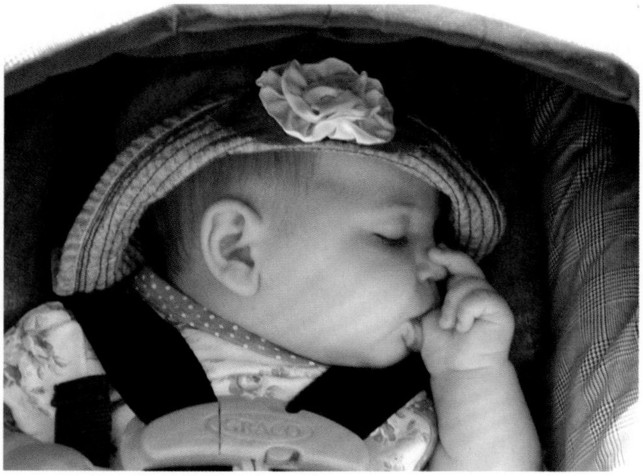

FIGURE 51.6 Infants have a faster sleep homeostasis, and a greater percentage of REM sleep than older children. *(Courtesy of Jo Solet, MS, EdM, PhD, OTR/L.)*

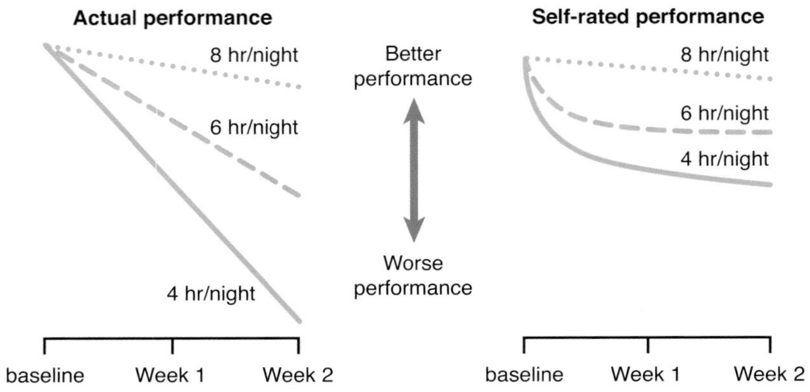

FIGURE 51.7 Restricting sleep impairs vigilance without parallel insight into increased deficits. (*Source:* Reprinted with permission from Van Dongen, H. P. A., Maislin, G., Mullington, J. M., & Dinges, D. F. [2003]. The cumulative cost of additional wakefulness: Dose-response effects on neurobehavioral functions and sleep physiology from chronic sleep restriction and total sleep deprivation. *SLEEP, 26*, 117–126. As redrawn by Orfeu Buxton.)

Influences On Sleep

As part of the clinical reasoning process and treatment planning, the occupational therapist is aware of multiple influences on sleep (see Figure 51.8), which fall into five realms of concern: (1) common medical conditions and psychiatric disorders, (2) health habits and behaviors, (3) stress and occupational balance, (4) sleep environments, and (5) sleep disorders. The next sections of the chapter will review each of these realms of concern with reference to these influences.

Sleep and Common Medical Conditions and Psychiatric Disorders

The majority of conditions and disorders treated by occupational therapists (see Appendix I: Common Conditions, Resources, and Evidence) may either impact client sleep, be exacerbated by insufficient or disordered sleep, or both (Stroe et al., 2010; Zee & Turek, 2006). The examples shown in Box 51.1 include possible mechanisms through which sleep may mediate functional disability.

Additional common medical conditions with sleep disrupting symptoms include **adenotonsillar hypertrophy** (breathing difficulties, especially in childhood), ulcers and gastroesophageal reflux disease, pain, **benign prostatic hypertrophy** (**nocturia**), and **atopic dermatitis** (itching). Pregnancy, especially the last trimester (discomfort, difficulty breathing, nocturia), postpartum (infant care), and menopause (autonomic instability, hot flashes) may compromise sleep for some women. Although it is beyond the scope of this chapter to fully describe sleep issues associated with each of these disorders, the occupational therapist becomes familiar with this information for the specific diagnostic categories that present in his or her clinical practice, using chapter references and other resources. The Practice Dilemma box describes a client with a sleep disorder.

Health Habits and Behaviors

Exercise for both adults and children is sleep enhancing (Buxton et al., 2003; Passos et al., 2010; Youngstedt & Buxton, 2003). Ideally, it is undertaken several hours before sleep. Following evening exercise, at least 2 hours are thought to be required for body temperature cooldown into sleep; a tepid shower may speed the process (see Figure 51.9).

Caffeine—as coffee, colas, or energy drinks—is very commonly used at "wake-up" and to fight fatigue and sleepiness. Caffeine can be an asset when used judiciously. Individuals develop tolerance for caffeine, needing more and more to provide the same effect. Especially when used to fight the midafternoon energy decline,

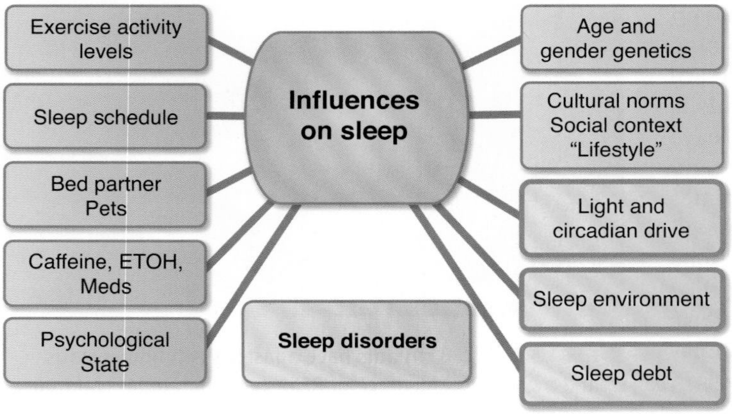

FIGURE 51.8 Influences on sleep: Many of these influences are open to modification as a part of occupational therapy collaborative treatment. *(Courtesy of Jo Solet, MS, EdM, PhD, OTR/L.)*

BOX 51.1 Mechanisms through Which Sleep May Mediate Functional Disability in Common Conditions and Disorders

- Acute or chronic pain
  - Arthritis
  - Burns
  - Low back pain
- Central nervous system disease or injury
  - Alzheimer's disease, dementias
  - Parkinson's disease
  - Head injury
  - Stroke
  - Spinal cord injury
- Reward system, appetite-satiation, or metabolic dysregulation
  - Substance abuse
  - Eating disorders
  - Obesity
  - Diabetes
- Respiratory compromise, disordered breathing
  - Chronic obstructive pulmonary disease
  - Asthma
  - Allergies
- Perceived lack of safety, insufficient environmental resources
  - Posttraumatic stress disorder, anxiety disorders
  - Poverty, homelessness
- Failure of self-care, isolation
  - Major mental illness
  - Developmental delays
  - Autism

See: Bondoc & Siebert, 2008; Braley & Chervin, 2010; Burton, Rahman, Kadota, Lloyd, & Vollmer-Conna, 2010; Buxton & Marcelli, 2010; Chandola, Ferrie, Perski, Akbaraly, & Marmor, 2010; Coelho, Georgsson, Narayansingh, Swartz, & Murray, 2010; Copinschi 2005; Epstein & Brown, 2010; Irwin et al., 2008; Johnson & Johnson, 2010; Luyster, Chasens, Wasko, & Dunbar-Jacob, 2011; McCall et al., 2009; Ownby et al., 2010; Parcell, Ponsford, Redman, & Rajaratnam, 2008; Redline, 2009; Sixel-Döring, Schweitzer, Mollenhauer, & Trenkwalder, 2011; Spiegel, Knutson, Leproult, Tasali, & Van Cauter, 2005; Spiegel, Tasali, Penev, & Van Cauter 2004; Watson, 2010; as well as comprehensive sleep textbook Kryger, Roth, & Dement, 2011.

caffeine may delay night sleep onset and reduce deep sleep (Roehrs & Roth, 2008). Depending on the planned sleep schedule, it is often recommended that the last caffeine be no later than early afternoon. Caffeine withdrawal can produce headache, fatigue, and drowsiness.

Though tobacco has multiple well-known negative health impacts, it remains among the chosen substances individuals use to manage mood and energy. Smokers are more likely to report problems falling asleep and staying asleep and may experience decreased REM sleep as compared with nonsmokers. Increased arousals from sleep may be reported with smoking cessation efforts (Roehrs & Roth, 2011a).

Alcohol is used by some to help bring on sleep. In healthy adults, alcohol has an initial sedative effect; but later during the night, following completed metabolism of alcohol, a rebound effect may actually interfere with sleep. In addition to effects on sleep initiation and sleep maintenance, alcohol also can also affect the proportion of the various sleep stages, including suppressing REM sleep. There is some evidence that alcohol may behave differently in insomniacs. Many questions remain, including whether insomniacs develop tolerance to alcohol's sedative effects and then increase intake (Roehrs & Roth, 2011b). A new category of beverage is one that combines caffeine and alcohol. These drinks are thought to be dangerous, since caffeine can produce a perception of wakefulness and mask insight into deficits caused by alcohol.

Numerous recreational drugs, over-the-counter and prescription medications, and herbs and "nutraceuticals" can impact sleep (Schweitzer, 2011). Chart review and careful history taking may identify these substances; information can be brought to the attention of the treating physician for review, including drug interactions and polypharmacy, the latter especially common in the elderly (Frazier, 2005).

Stress and Occupational Balance

The ideal sleep-wake pattern dedicates sufficient time for uninterrupted sleep, is congruent with natural circadian clock rhythms, and is regular and consistent.

Practice Dilemma

Celia is an occupational therapist called for a bedside activities of daily living (ADL) evaluation of Elvira, a 40-year-old naturalized citizen, following colostomy reversal surgery. Communicating with the help of a Spanish interpreter, Elvira complains that her pain is still "so so bad," that she is having "fears and visions" about her surgical experiences, and that "her legs are kicking and waking her up at night." Yet, in terms of ADL, Celia finds Elvira only requires minimal assistance.

1. How should Celia prioritize the multiple concerns which Elvira has raised?
2. Are there possible interactions between Elvira's pain report and her other complaints?
3. Which members of the clinical team should be called for consultation?
4. How might cultural competency help Celia and other team members address Elvira's complaints?

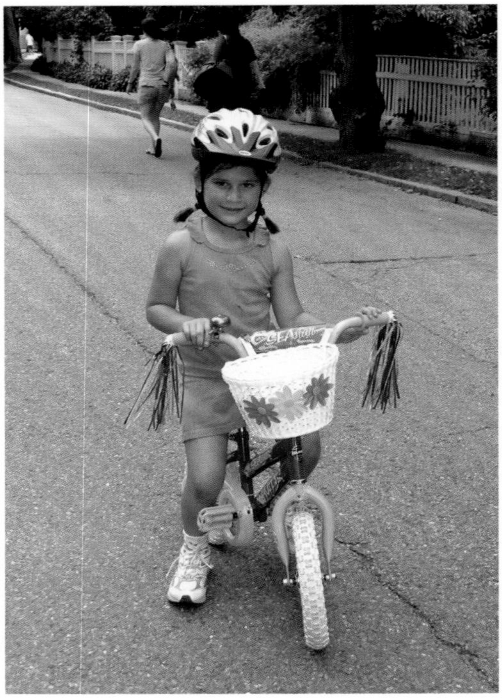

FIGURE 51.9 Exercise enhances sleep. *(Courtesy of Jo Solet, MS, EdM, PhD, OTR/L.)*

Yet, compelling opportunities and requirements for night activity, as well as situational stressors, at times override sleep needs. For some, these reflect lifestyle choices and leisure pursuits, with the option for easy reversal to increased TIB. For others, it is a challenge to complete work, school, family caregiving, and home responsibilities within a schedule that leaves adequate time for self-care and sleep (Berkman, Buxton, Ertel, & Okechukwu, 2010; Bibbs, 2011; Luckhaupt, Tak, & Calvert, 2010). For example, an increasing number of mothers of young children have joined the workforce and may struggle to maintain occupational balance (Anaby, Backman, & Jarus, 2010). Technologies bring work into the home setting, even well after normal work hours, demanding immediate attention. Occupations such as nursing, medicine, and air traffic controller must be accomplished around the clock, requiring night shift work (Edlund, 2003; Levine, Adusumilli, & Landrigan, 2010; Nurok, Czeisler, & Lehmann, 2010). Daytime sleep must then be undertaken against natural circadian rhythms. Travel to other time zones can disrupt natural sleep patterns, requiring alertness and high functioning during natural circadian sleep periods. This experience is colloquially known as jet lag (Youngstedt & Buxton, 2003). Finally, situations of grief, loss, and trauma, common in client populations that occupational therapy (OT) practitioners encounter, have ripple effects that can damage sleep.

The Ethical Dilemma box below illustrates some of the difficulties clients and occupational therapists can encounter while addressing sleep and occupational performance. The reader is urged to develop initial responses to the questions posed here and then to return to them after completing the chapter for discussion with colleagues.

Social Context

Eliciting the client's social context as part of the occupational profile and initial assessment can be particularly relevant with regard to sleep behaviors and occupational balance. For example, presleep stimulating computer use and video games and all-night texting are documented peer-driven sleep hazards for many young people (American College of Chest Physicians, 2010; Weaver, Gradisar, Dohnt, Lovato, & Douglas, 2010). Developing and maintaining balance in an environment where this is far from the norm, such as in a college dormitory, can be difficult.

A social context of emotional isolation experienced as loneliness has been identified as an independent risk factor for sleep problems (Hawkley, Cacioppo, & Preacher, 2011; Hawkley, Preacher, & Cacioppo, 2010; McHugh & Lawlor, 2011). In addition, individuals who have little contact with others, due to advanced age or disability, may have insufficient daily life structure. They may spend much of their time in bed, napping on and off. Providing for daily activities and companionship, which

Ethical Dilemma

Stanley is an occupational therapist working in an outpatient facility. During evaluation of Mr. Chevy, a 58-year-old overweight truck driver with high blood pressure (partially controlled by medication), he notices the client falling asleep midmorning.

Upon questioning, Mr. Chevy admits he sometimes "feels himself falling asleep" even while driving, especially on long hauls at night. In answering some basic screening questions about his sleep schedule, sleep experience, and sleep environment, he mentions that his wife gets angry with him on nights when he sleeps at home because his snoring wakes her up repeatedly at night.

Mr. Chevy has been referred to occupational by orthopedics for "energy conservation training and back school" to improve his driving comfort and lifting safety. He is afraid that any mention of sleep problems in his record could cause him to lose his job. He has just 2 years left before planned retirement. Mr. Chevy threatens to leave treatment entirely if Stanley will not agree to keep sleep problems off his record.

1. What should Stanley do in this situation?
2. What additional information should Stanley seek to help with his decision?
3. How might Stanley help educate Mr. Chevy about risks to himself and others?
4. Should Stanley reach out to Mrs. Chevy for help in supporting diagnosis or treatment?
5. Should Stanley make a referral for further assessment?

are common goals of OT intervention, may help to consolidate and improve sleep.

Naps and Safe Management of Fatigue

Naps have historically been part of occupational balance in some cultures, especially in the heat of midday. Even when brief, naps may have restorative effects. Like exercise, planned napping can be integrated into the daily routine to enhance health and well-being. There are times when the OT practitioner may recommend napping to manage fatigue and to improve safety and alertness, especially in anticipation of night performance requirements, such as driving, infant care, or medical **shift work**.

Short naps of 20 to 30 minutes, or longer naps of a full sleep cycle, 90 minutes, are more likely to allow for awakening without significant sleep inertia (Mednick & Ehrman, 2006). The sleep stage content of the nap is thought to affect the resulting enhancements, with REM containing naps shown to decrease negative emotional bias and amplify recognition of positive emotions (Gujar, McDonald, Nishida, & Walker, 2010). When naps are required even after adequate TIB, it can be a signal that further assessment is required. Chronic illnesses such as multiple sclerosis (MS) may increase fatigue levels for extended periods (Stout & Finlayson, 2011); under these circumstances, it may be useful to schedule naps and rest periods into the daily routine. In cases of excessive daytime sleepiness, safety must be given the highest priority, including arrangements for alternative transportation rather than driving and extra attention given to fall and accident prevention.

Sleep Environments

Along with healthy sleep habits, an optimal sleep environment is a component of **sleep hygiene**. The ideal sleep environment is *quiet, dark, cool, comfortable, clean,* and *safe*. As part of a home visit or review of a long-term care facility, the occupational therapist helps to adapt and organize the sleep environment (Figure 51.10).

Numerous studies document the disruptive effects of noise on sleep (Basner, Müller, Elmenhorst, 2011; Buxton et al., 2012; Hume, 2011; Solet, Buxton, Ellenbogen, Wang, & Carballiera, 2010). Ensuring quiet includes blocking disturbances from within the room, home, or building. This may include simple solutions such as closing doors and soliciting family and partner (or roommate) commitments to limit noisy activities after an agreed upon hour. Sometimes, external noise sources from the street-scape, such as truck deliveries and cycling air-handling equipment, disrupt sleep. Soothing sound and white noise machines or earplugs may be successful in blocking these disturbances. Be sure smoke alarms, phone signals, and other emergency alerts can penetrate.

Some communities have noise ordinances that limit decibel levels, especially during night hours. Night noise, from airplane overflights and truck traffic, for example,

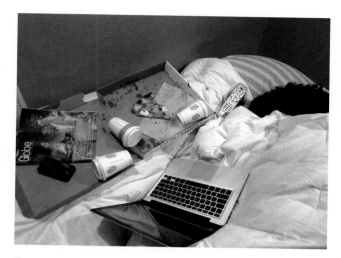

FIGURE 51.10 Inappropriate environment for sleep. *(Courtesy of Jo Solet, MS, EdM, PhD, OTR/L.)*

may be quite prevalent in some communities. Many American cities have homeless populations, limited shelter beds, and people sleeping on the streets. Availability of a safe, quiet place for sleep is an occupational justice issue. According to Blakeney and Marshall (2009), occupational justice rests on two important principles: that "occupational participation is a determinant of health" and the "principle of empowerment through occupation" (p. 47). Sleep qualifies on both counts. (See Chapter 41).

Ironically, some of the most difficult sleep environments are health care facilities, including critical care units (Busch-Vishniac et al., 2005; Dogan, Ertekin, & Dogan, 2005; Friese, Diaz-Arrastia, McBride, Frankel, & Gentilello 2003; Solet & Barach, 2012; Weinhouse & Schwab, 2006). Complaints of "noise around room" are among the most common in hospital quality-of-care surveys. In most states, since 2006, construction codes for new hospitals require single-bed patient rooms, preventing disturbance through roommates. Research demonstrating the sleep disruptive character of common hospital sounds has informed the most recent edition of *Design and Construction Guidelines for Healthcare Facilities*, which now includes acoustic guidelines for hospital rooms (Facility Guidelines Institute, 2010; Solet et al., 2010). Patient sleep disruption by hospital night staff led to the development of the Somerville Protocol, an evidence-based night routine solution that can be implemented by staff in health care settings to preserve patient sleep (Bartick, Thai, Schmidt, Altaye, & Solet, 2010).

Providing darkness in the sleep environment is an important sleep protector. Night shift workers who are required to sleep during the day are found to sleep more efficiently when true darkness is provided. Light has an alerting effect, especially during the natural circadian waking period (Edlund, 2003). Eye masks or "blackout" window shades can be used to block ambient light. Light sources within the room such as bright digital clocks should be dimmed or removed. The bedroom should be conditioned for sleep and sex, not meals, technology, and TV. Ideally, space allows the television and computers to be placed elsewhere; screens should be shut down well before sleep along with other compelling technology such as cell phones. A consistent "wind-down period" with a relaxing presleep ritual, such as a bath and reading or "story time" for children before bed is recommended.

Body temperature drops as part of the sleep cycle. A cool bedroom is thus most conducive to sleep. Most people report the mid to high 60s as quite comfortable. Conflicts between bed partners over room temperature are legendary. For this and other reasons, partners sometimes do not sleep well next to each other. Mismatched sleep schedules or even specific disorders in one partner (e.g., excessive movement during sleep, use of equipment to normalize breathing) may disturb the sleep of the other. Splitting into individual beds in the same room may be sufficient to preserve sleep; separate rooms, if available, may serve to protect sleep and ultimately preserve relationships. "Visits" can be planned.

A significant percentage of Americans responding to the U.S. census listed pets as family members. Pets are common bed partners. However, pets may have natural sleep cycles that are different from their owners', for example, becoming most active as the sun rises. Many people report that sleeping with their pets is a great comfort. However, this decision should be considered through balancing that comfort with the degree of sleep disruption and individuals' health status. A separate comfortable pet bed should be an option (see Figure 51.11).

A clean environment is especially important to those with allergies, who may experience breathing difficulties during sleep due to accumulated allergens, such as pet hair. HEPA air cleaning machines may be helpful. A clean environment is also safer, with clothes and other items off the floor. Any cords, equipment, or furniture that blocks the exit or the path to the bathroom should be relocated as part of fall prevention. Availability of a full set of fresh bedclothes should be assured, and a weekly room cleaning schedule put in place.

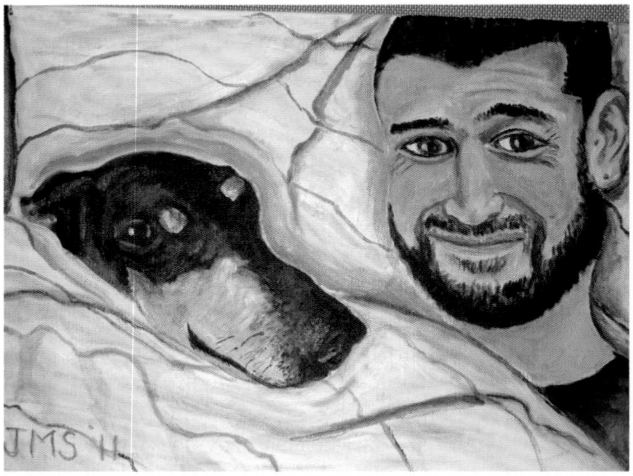

FIGURE 51.11 Sleeping with a pet may be comforting yet at times may disrupt sleep. *(Courtesy of Jo Solet, MS, EdM, PhD, OTR/L.)*

Sleep Disorders

While making a diagnosis of a sleep disorder is outside the professional expertise of occupational therapists, it is important to be aware of the ICSD-2, the International Classification of Sleep Disorders (available for download), to have access to criteria and standards as resources, and to recognize sleep disorders that are commonly diagnosed. The newest edition of the *Diagnostic and Statistical Manual of Mental Disorders, DSM V*, to be published in 2013, is anticipated to offer a revised categorization of sleep disorders (Grohol, 2010; Reynolds & Redline, 2010).

Sleep disorders can be understood through descriptions of the ways in which sleep is disturbed: inability to fall asleep, multiple awakenings, inability to fall back asleep, nonrestorative sleep, inadequate breathing during sleep (may be described as snoring and or gasping for breath), disruptive movements during sleep, non-sleep activities intruding into sleep, mistimed or uncontrolled sleep. Patients may describe significant distress related to safety and impairment in occupational and social functioning even when they have little insight into the cause of their difficulties.

Insomnias

The **insomnia**s are defined by repeated problems of sleep initiation, duration, consolidation, or quality that occur despite adequate time and opportunity for sleep and result in some form of daytime impairment (Haynes, 2009; Passos et al., 2010; Roth, Roehrs, & Pies, 2007; Vitiello, Rybarczk, Von Korff, & Stepanski, 2009). Using stringent criteria of sleep disturbance every night for two weeks or more, a consistent prevalence ranging between 9% and 17.7% of the adult population has been documented as affected (Ohayon, 2002). This translates into 30 to 40 million Americans. Historically, the insomnias have been organized into multiple subtypes with variable patterns at different phases of the life course: pediatric, pregnancy, menopause, and geriatric. Insomnia can be primary or **secondary insomnia** that is comorbid, at times related to pain, depression, posttraumatic stress disorder, and other medical conditions that should be identified and addressed in treatment planning.

Treatments may include use of the relaxation response such as meditation, progressive muscle relaxation, or **biofeedback**; cognitive behavioral therapy (especially addressing sleep-related anxieties and conditioning the bed for sleep only); improved sleep habits and environments; limits on caffeine and alcohol; and sometimes prescription medications.

Obstructive Sleep Apnea

Obstructive sleep apnea (OSA) is caused by partial or complete blockage of airway passages during sleep.

Diagnosis typically follows from laboratory sleep testing, frequently after the individual's roommate or sleep partner has reported hearing "loud snoring" or "gasping for breath" during the night. The index of OSA severity, called the **apnea/hypopnea index** or **AHI**, typically increases in untreated individuals with age and relates to the number of repeated awakenings per hour driven by decreased **oxygen saturation.** Awakenings may occur dozens or even hundreds of times a night; individuals may have no awareness, perhaps only reporting excessive daytime sleepiness. Morning headache is a common complaint (Vaughn & D'Cruz, 2011). Certain jaw, overbite, tongue and soft tissue proportions, and large neck girth as well as excessive weight, are recognized as anatomical risk factors. OSA can be a serious disorder, depriving the brain of oxygen leading to **hypertension** (high blood pressure) (O'Connor et al., 2009; Peppard, 2009), cardiovascular disease, weight gain, and cognitive impairments. Excessive sleepiness places these individuals at increased risk for auto and industrial accidents (Tregear et al., 2009).

Treatments include use of a **continuous positive airway pressure** system (**CPAP**) that pushes air through the nose (Tomfour, Ancoli-Israel, Loredo, & Dimsdale, 2011), sleep positioning to side-lying, dental devices, corrective surgery (Verse & Höormann, 2011) and weight loss. CPAP machines now include technology to monitor their use. Some individuals find the masks inconvenient or uncomfortable or feel the devices negatively impact intimate relationships. The consequences of untreated chronic OSA can be severe; support for seeking a comfortable CPAP mask fit and reinforcing treatment adherence through continuous monitoring are valuable therapeutic interventions (Cooke et al., 2009).

See instructional video http://healthysleep.med.harvard.edu/sleep-apnea

Restless Leg Syndrome and Periodic Limb Movement Disorder

Restless leg syndrome (RLS) is a sleep disorder in which there is an urge to move the legs in order to stop unpleasant leg sensations that may be described as "crawling" or "tingling." During sleep, involuntary leg movements can lead to awakenings and may occur repeatedly without being remembered (Bayard, Avonda, & Wadzinski, 2008; Kushida, 2007). Risk factors include peripheral neuropathy, chronic kidney disease, iron deficiency, Parkinson's disease, and side effects of certain medications; there is also higher prevalence among clients with a history of stroke (Coelho et al., 2010) and fibromyalgia (Viola-Saltzman, Watson, Bogart, Goldberg, & Buchwald, 2010). Genetic factors are implicated because certain families as well as populations, especially northern Europeans, show higher incidence. Some individuals experience movements without the sensations; upper extremities can also be involved. This is called **Periodic Limb Movement Disorder** or **PLMD.** Along with treatment of predisposing conditions, exercise, stretching, massage, and warm baths may provide some relief. In some cases, medications may be prescribed.

Parasomnias

Parasomnias are non-sleep behaviors that intrude during sleep. Sleepwalking and sleep-eating episodes can occur during deep sleep through partial awakening (Howell, Schenck, & Crow, 2009). Typically, individuals have no memory of these behaviors, which are reported to them by others or are discovered through evidence found in the morning. Sleep-walking is more common in children, who often outgrow the disorder. Organizing secure environments and alerting systems for parents or partners are practical safety measures.

Healthy REM sleep involves muscle paralysis—**atonia**. In **REM sleep behavior disorder (RBD),** this paralysis fails and the individual moves, as if acting out a dream. Most typical in men older than 50, recent research has suggested RBD may be a precursor to dementias or Parkinson's disease (Sixel-Döring et al., 2011). These individuals are easy to awaken and may remember their dreams. However, bed partners can be at risk of injury from these uncontrolled actions.

Other parasomnias include **night terrors**, ***rhythmic movement disorders in children***, **bruxism** (tooth grinding), and ***confusional arousals*** in adults. Secondary insomnia can result from an effort to block frightening parasomnia experiences by avoiding sleep.

Narcolepsy

Narcolepsy is characterized by an excessive uncontrollable daytime sleepiness even after adequate sleep at night. According to the National Institute of Health, it is estimated to be as common as Parkinson's disease or MS but is underdiagnosed. Experiences that affect some, but not all, narcoleptics include **cataplexy**: a sudden loss of muscle function ranging from weakness to full collapse, which may have an emotional trigger; inability to talk or move while falling asleep or waking up; and vivid, sometimes frightening images in transition to sleep, called **hypnagogic hallucinations**. In narcolepsy, the architecture of sleep is disturbed with REM rather than NREM occurring at sleep onset, and REM experiences actually intruding into waking periods. The main treatments are lifestyle adaptations to maintain safety, central nervous system stimulants, and antidepressant or other medications that suppress REM sleep.

Additional Resources for Sleep Disorders

Readers are also encouraged to visit

> http://healthysleep.med.harvard.edu/healthy/getting/treatment/an-overview-of-sleep-disorders. This is a section of online resources provided by the Division of Sleep Medicine at Harvard Medical School in collaboration with the WGBH (public television) Educational Foundation.

The National Institutes of Health also offers valuable online sleep disorder information: http://www.nhlbi.nih.gov/health/public/sleep

National Sleep Foundation: http://www.sleepfoundation.org/articles/sleep-disorders?

Also see the most comprehensive text currently available: Kryger, M. H., Roth, T., & Dement, W. C. (2011). *Principles and practice of sleep medicine* (5th ed.).St. Louis, MO: Elsevier Saunders.

Sleep Screening and Referral

Because the majority of medical and psychiatric disorders treated by occupational therapists may affect or be affected by sleep, and because sleep disorders are so common, brief sleep screening as part of initial OT assessment is valuable (Zee & Turek, 2006). The attuned occupational therapist will be alert to a history or current report of excessive daytime sleepiness and will probe for the degree to which sleep is experienced as nonrestorative and the extent to which daytime activities may be impaired. Some clients will report functional problems without recognizing any link to their sleep difficulties. Others, despite complaints of excessive sleepiness, may have little insight even into multiple night arousals, for example, due to OSA or RLS. Bed partners or family members of clients may be resources for supplying additional details and documentation, especially women (Umberson, 1992). As always, to protect privacy, clients' permission must be sought before these discussions.

Sleep History and Self-reports

Standardized client self-report questionnaires, such as the Epworth Sleepiness Scale, supplement the occupational profile and may be useful for screening and for tracking effectiveness of certain treatments (Box 51.2) (Johns, 1991). Many clinical settings make available preferred tools for sleep screening that have been validated for the specific treated population, such as school-age children (Owens, Spirito, & McGuinn, 2000).

When clients complain of ***excessive daytime sleepiness***, a **sleep diary** or a a wrist worn sleep-monitoring device, showing sleep timing and perceived refreshment, can be useful in collaborating to gain a picture defining sleep patterns (Figure 51.12). **Sleep inertia** is the normal period at awakening in which full alertness is not yet achieved. Diary rating of sleep should be completed after the individual is fully awake and through this transition period.

When diary or device results confirm insufficient time in bed or an erratic schedule, a critical OT sleep education and treatment goal is to evoke a cognitive shift: away from perceiving limited sleep as "no problem," "heroic," or "efficient," toward perceiving it as "a drain on well-being and performance," "an unwise health risk," or "a factor complicating recovery." Individuals suffering from certain medical, psychiatric, or sleep disorders can be doubly challenged and health risks raised further by poor sleep habits. This cognitive shift initiates readiness for a program to include sleep as a priority. The occupational therapist helps clients develop strategies to incorporate energy conservation and fatigue management techniques to cope with the extra demands associated with these conditions.

Recent research suggests that sleep symptoms are common but are not routinely screened for in primary care settings (Haponik et al., 1996; Senthilvel, Auckley, & Dasarathy, 2011; Sorscher, 2008). Although efforts are underway to enhance medical attention to sleep, an OT encounter could include the first sleep screening a client receives. Referral for follow-up, potentially including a home or laboratory sleep study, may be made to neurology, pulmonology, psychiatry, occupational health, or directly to sleep medicine, depending on comorbid diagnosis, potential severity, and available resources.

As part of the referral process and in follow-up team meetings, the occupational therapist takes the opportunity to make colleagues aware of his or her tools for addressing sleep problems and documents sleep interventions in care notes.

BOX 51.2 Epworth Sleepiness Scale

Used to determine the level of daytime sleepiness

A score of 10 or more is considered sleepy.

Use the following scale to choose the most appropriate number for each situation:

0 = would *never* doze or sleep
1 = *slight* chance of dozing or sleeping
2 = *moderate* chance of dozing or sleeping
3 = *high* chance of dozing or sleeping

Situations: Chance of dozing or sleeping

1. Sitting and reading ________
2. Watching TV ________
3. Sitting inactive in a public place ________
4. Being a passenger in a motor vehicle for an hour or more ________
5. Lying down in the afternoon ________
6. Sitting and talking to someone ________
7. Sitting quietly after lunch (no alcohol) ________
8. Stopped for a few minutes in traffic while driving ________

Total score (add the scores up) ________

Source: Johns, M. W. (1991). "A new method for measuring daytime sleepiness: The Epworth Sleepiness Scale." *SLEEP, 14*, 540–545.

SLEEP HEALTHCENTERS®
...better sleep. better health.

SLEEP DIARY

NAME: ______________________

WEEK OF: ______________________

Day	Duration of Naps (minutes)	Bedtime	Time to Fall Asleep (minutes)	Number of Awakenings	Duration of Awakenings (minutes)	Final Waketime	Out of Bed Time	Time Spent Asleep (hours)	Medications Taken	Next Day Alertness 1-10 (10=most alert)
Monday										
Tuesday										
Wednesday										
Thursday										
Friday										
Saturday										
Sunday										

- Please begin to complete the sleep diary on a daily basis. It will provide a subjective tracking of your sleep schedule for you and your sleep clinician to use as you work together to improve your sleep.
- Do not look at the clock to complete this form. You should complete this diary each morning with respect to your previous night of sleep. Do not complete it during the night or keep it in your bedroom.
- Use it only as a guideline and spend no more than 30 seconds filling it out in the morning.

BSM-DIRY-0002_1

Reviewed 3/05/10

FIGURE 51.12 Sleep diary. Source: Reprinted with permission from Sleep Healthcenters LLC, http://www.sleephealth.com

Sleep Evaluation

The technology used for sleep evaluation is evolving toward more complete home testing. **Actigraphy** is a wristband mounted accelerometer system that records periods of motion during sleep and indicates sleep latency, arousals, and time of awakening (Sadeh, 2011; Sánchez-Ortuño, Edinger, Means, & Almirall, 2010). Actigraphy systems for personal use can now be run through downloadable apps for smart phones. Consumer/home sleep tracking devices paired with smartphone apps, such as Lark, from Lark Technologies, provide a more accurate picture of sleep than diary recording alone.

Polysomnography is comprehensive testing that includes three simultaneously recorded parts: the electroencephalogram, which traces brain wave activity through scalp electrodes, recording differing frequencies identified as alpha, beta, delta, and theta rhythms; **electrooculograms,** which measure eye movements through electrodes placed on the skin around the eyes; and **electromyograms,** which measure motor activity through electrodes placed on the skin over muscles. As part of sleep evaluation, sensors may be used to track breathing and oxygen saturation in the blood. Video recordings are used for monitoring client positioning and movements during sleep, especially as coordinated with other readouts. Sleep stages (REM and NREM 1, 2, 3) have specific "fingerprints" based on brain activity and coordinated muscle and eye movements. Certain sleep disorders are more likely to occur during specific stages. Furthermore, alterations in architecture of sleep, as shown in the hypnogram, can be produced by environmental or medical conditions. Standardized scoring criteria are applied to analyze these recordings to identify stages, arousals, and anomalies supporting diagnoses (Chervin, 2010).

Summary: Sleep and Occupational Therapy Interventions

OT interventions to improve sleep and manage fatigue are based in client education, self-care and health habits, occupational balance, and optimal environments. As part

CASE STUDY 51.1 Alberta

Alberta is a 15-year-old private high school student who complains of "being so tired." Although she showed early academic ability, the high school "scene" has posed increasing problems. A large girl at 5 ft 9 in, 170 lb, her athletic activities are restricted due to asthma, which she has suffered since early childhood. She recently had an experience of social network bullying, which left her isolated from and unable to trust her female classmates. Her strong interest in math and science has allowed her to forge some friendships with boys in the class. Her mother has described her as "depressed." Alberta has been referred to a group private occupational therapy (OT) practice by her long-time pediatrician for help with "fatigue, fitness, and fitting-in."

1. What information should Alberta's OT seek from the pediatrician?
2. Describe components of a first OT meeting with Alberta?

   What could be helpful in establishing rapport?

   What screening and assessments might shed light on her fatigue?
3. Could bullying and isolation affect adolescent sleep?
4. Through what mechanisms might sleep affect fitness, mood?
5. Suggest possible components for an OT treatment program to improve adolescent self-care and sleep.

Case Discussion

1. The OT should ask for a developmental and medical history, information related to specific asthma symptoms and triggers, treatments, medications and their side effects, and restrictions.

   Any available information about mood and childhood sleep should be examined. Has the doctor discussed the referral with Alberta and has she agreed on specific goals? What kind of parental support can be anticipated?
2. The first meeting is critical for establishing rapport. Initial questions can include:

   "What do you hope to get out of our time together? How will we know that we are heading in the right direction? What will be different?

   Please describe your typical day. Are some times of day better/easier than others?

   When you are feeling your best, what are you doing?

of the continuum of care provided by occupational therapists, sleep-enhancing interventions may be adapted for primary prevention and health promotion, such work-based and school wellness programs (Beebe, Ris, Kramer, Long, & Amin, 2010; Gangwisch, Malaspina, Boden-Albala, & Heymsfield, 2005; Gangwisch et al., 2010, Quan et al., 2010); may address sleep problems related to aging, injury, illness, or disability; and may contribute to treatments directed specifically at sleep disorders. School and work wellness programs focus on life-cycle sleep requirements and schedules, health habits and behaviors that influence sleep, and adequate sleep environments.

OT treatments for common medical conditions and psychiatric disorders, many of which carry comorbid sleep difficulties, may be directed toward pain, anxiety, depression, limited mobility, poor self-care, respiratory compromise, substance abuse, insufficient resources, and/or social isolation. Broad components of treatment for these clients, which may also improve comorbid sleep difficulties, include (but are not limited to) cognitive behavioral therapy, relaxation response, graded exercise, activities to increase social integration, and resources for safety (Solet, 2012). Improvement in any of these complaint areas can also be expected to improve sleep; the effects are reciprocal (Zee & Turek, 2006).

Treatment components directed specifically at sleep either as a primary problem or a comorbidity include reinforcing consistent sleep schedules, sufficient TIB, conditioning bed for sleep only, and sleep environment modifications: quiet, dark, cool, safe, and clean. Sleep interventions also target related health habits including use of caffeine, alcohol, tobacco, or other substances; exercise; and support for treatment adherence such as use of CPAP equipment and weight loss programs (Barnes, 2009).

Although the primary focus of this chapter is sleep, occupational balance encompasses both patterns and cycles of activity, including periods of **rest.** Yoga, meditation, and other spiritual or relaxation practices, especially when undertaken consistently, may not only improve sleep by lowering autonomic arousal and bringing mindful attention to the present but may also have important independent adaptive and restorative qualities (Benson & Proctor, 2010; Solet, 2012). In *The Power of Rest*, Dr. Matthew Edlund (2010) offers an accessible, comprehensive review of the benefits of rest including through music and companionship.

Conclusion

Sleep medicine is a new frontier, an opportunity to enhance health, safety, well-being, performance, and even longevity. As occupational therapists, our unique perspective on daily living, together with the relationships we enjoy with our clients and colleagues, puts us in a unique position to contribute to this dynamic area of science and health care.

As part of your professional commitment, improve sleep awareness, evaluation, and treatment and sleep well!

Resources for more Information about Sleep and Rest

Websites

Center for Disease Control: http://www.cdc.gov/sleep/

Harvard Medical School, Division of Sleep Medicine: http://healthysleep.med.harvard.edu/portal/

Section on Sleep Disorders: http://healthysleep.med.harvard.edu/healthy/getting/treatment/an-overview-of-sleep-disorders

National Institute of Alcohol Abuse and Alcoholism: http://www.niaaa.nih.gov/

YMCA: http://www.ymca.net/healthy-family-home/sleep-well.html

Center for Health Design: http://www.healthdesign.org/chd/research/validating-acoustic-guidelines-healthcare-facilities

National Sleep Foundation: http://www.sleepfoundation.org/articles/sleep-disorders?

National Sleep Foundation Sleep in America Polls: http://www.sleepfoundation.org/category/article-type/sleep-america-polls

Additional Resources

American Academy of Sleep Medicine: http://www.aasmnet.org

SLEEP: http://www.journalsleep.org

Journal of Clinical Sleep Medicine: http://www.aasmnet.org/JCSM

SleepCenters.org: http://www.sleepcenters.org

Acknowledgments

I would like to thank the patients who have been my teachers for the more than 35 years I have been an occupational therapist as well as Jenny Lee Olsen, director of Library Services at Cambridge Health Alliance for help in the literature search, the chapter peer reviewers for their careful attention and thoughtful comments, and the editors for offering me the opportunity to contribute this chapter on sleep, an important emerging area of practice.

Disclosure: Author, Dr. Jo M. Solet serves as a science advisor to Lark Technologies.

References

American Academy of Sleep Medicine. (2009, June). Naps with rapid eye movement increase receptiveness to positive emotion. *ScienceDaily.* Retrieved from http://www.aasmnet.org/articles.aspx?id=1317

American College of Chest Physicians. (2010, November). *Electronic media taking its toll on teens.* Paper presented at the 76th CHEST annual meeting of American College of Chest Physicians, Vancouver, Canada. Retrieved from http://www.chestnet.org/accp/article/electronic-media-taking-its-toll-teens

American Occupational Therapy Association. (2008). Occupational therapy practice framework: Domain and process, 2nd edition. *American Journal of Occupational Therapy, 62,* 625–683.

Anaby, D. R., Backman, C. L., & Jarus, T. (2010). Measuring occupational balance: Theoretical exploration of two approaches to occupational balance. *Canadian Journal of Occupational Therapy, 77,* 280–288.

Ancoli-Israel, S., & Cooke, J. R. (2005). Prevalence and comorbidity of insomnia and effect on functioning in elderly populations. *Journal of the American Geriatrics Society, 53,* S264–S271.

Ayas, N. T. (2010). If you weigh too much, maybe you should try sleeping more. *SLEEP, 33,* 143–144.

Ayas, N. T., White, D. P., Al-Delaimy, W. K., Manson, J. E., Stampfer, M. J., Speizer, F. E., & Hu, F. B. (2003a). A prospective study of self-reported sleep duration and incipient diabetes in women. *Diabetes Care, 26,* 380–384.

Ayas, N. T., White, D. P., Manson, J. E., Stampfer, M. J., Speizer, F. E., Malhotra, A., & Hu, F. B. (2003b). A prospective study of sleep duration and coronary heart disease in women. *Archives of Internal Medicine, 163,* 205–209.

Banks, S.,Van Dongen, H. P. A., Mailsen, G., & Dinges, D. F. (2010). Neurobehavioral dynamics following chronic sleep restriction: Dose-response effects of one night for recovery. *SLEEP, 33,* 1013–1026.

Barnes, M., Goldsworthy, U. R., Cary, B. A., & Hill, C. J. (2009). A diet and exercise program to improve clinical outcomes on patients with obstructive sleep apnea—A feasibilty study. *Journal of Clinical Sleep Medicine, 5,* 409–421.

Bartick, M. C., Thai, X., Schmidt, T., Altaye A., & Solet, J. M. (2010). Decrease in as needed sedative use by limiting nighttime sleep disruptions from hospital staff. *Journal of Hospital Medicine: An Official Publication of the Society of Hospital Medicine, 5,* E20–E24.

Basner, M., Fomberstein, K. M., Razavi, F. M., Banks, S., William, J. H., Rosa, R. R., & Dinges, D. F. (2007). American time use survey: Sleep time and its relationship to waking activities. *SLEEP, 30,* 1085–1095.

Basner, M., Müller, U., Elmenhorst, E. M. (2011). Single and combined effects of air, road, and rail traffic noise on sleep and recuperation. *SLEEP, 34,* 11–23.

Bayard, M., Avonda, T., & Wadzinski, J. (2008). Restless legs syndrome. *American Family Physician. 78,* 235–240.

Beebe, D. W., Ris, D. M., Kramer, M. E., Long, E., & Amin, R. (2010). The association between sleep disordered breathing, academic grades, and cognitive and behavioral functioning among overweight subjects during middle to late childhood. *SLEEP, 33,* 1447–1457.

Benson, H., & Proctor, W. (2010). *Relaxation revolution: Enhancing your personal health through the science and genetics of mind body healing.* New York, NY: Scribner.

Berkman, L. F., Buxton, O., Ertel, K., & Okechukwu, C. (2010). Managers' practices related to work-family balance predict employee cardiovascular risk and sleep duration in extended care settings. *Journal of Occupational Health Psychology, 15,* 316–329.

Bibbs, M. (2011). A wake up call to sleepy workers. *Sleep Diagnosis and Therapy, 6,* 14.

Blakeney, A., & Marshall, A. (2009). Water quality, health, and human occupations. *American Journal of Occupational* Therapy, *63,* 46–57.

Bondoc, S., & Siebert, C. (2008). *The role of occupational therapy in chronic disease management.* Bethesda, MD: American Occupational Therapy Association.

Braley, T. J., & Chervin, R. D. (2010). Fatigue in multiple sclerosis: Mechanisms, evaluation, and treatment. *SLEEP, 33,* 1061–1067.

Brendel, D. H., Florman, J., Roberts, S., & Solet, J. M. (2001). "In sleep I almost never grope": Blindness, neuropsychiatric deficits, and a chaotic upbringing. *Harvard Review of Psychiatry, 9,* 178–188.

Burton, A. R., Rahman, K., Kadota, Y., Lloyd, A., & Vollmer-Conna, U. (2010). Reduced heart rate variability predicts poor sleep quality in a case-control study of chronic fatigue syndrome. *Experimental Brain Research, 204,* 71–78.

Busch-Vishniac, I. J., West, J. E., Barnhill, C., Hunter, T., Orellana, D., & Chivukula, R. (2005). Noise levels in Johns Hopkins Hospital. *The Journal of the Acoustical Society of America, 118,* 3629–3645.

Buxton, O. M., Ellenbogen, J. M., Wang, W., Carballeira, A., O'Connor S., Cooper D., . . . Solet, J. M. (2012). Sleep Disruption Due to Hospital Noises: A Prospective Evaluation. *Ann Intern Med.* Jun 11. [PMID: 22688839]

Buxton, O. M., Lee C. W., L'Hermite-Baleriaux, M., Turek, F. W., & Van Cauter, E. (2003). Exercise elicits phase shifts and acute alterations of melatonin that vary with circadian phase. *American Journal of Physiology. Regulatory, Integrative and Comparative Physiology, 284,* R714–R724.

Buxton, O. M., & Marcelli, E. (2010). Short and long sleep are positively associated with obesity, diabetes, hypertension, and cardiovascular disease among adults in the United States. *Social Science and Medicine, 71,* 1027–1036.

Chandola, T., Ferrie, J. E., Perski, A., Akbaraly, T., & Marmor, M. G. (2010). The effect of short sleep duration on coronary heart disease risk is greatest among those with sleep disturbance: A prospective study from Whitehall II cohort. *SLEEP, 33,* 739–744.

Chervin, R. D. (2010). Use of clinical tools and tests in sleep medicine. In M. H. Kryger, T. Roth, & W. C. Dement (Eds.), *Principles and practice of sleep medicine* (5th ed., pp. 666–679). St. Louis, MO: Elsevier Saunders.

Chhangani, B. S., Roehrs, T. A., Harris, E. J., Hyde, M., Drake, C., Hudgel, D. W., & Roth, T. (2009). Pain sensitivity in sleepy pain-free normals. *SLEEP, 32*, 1011–1017.

Chien, K. L., Chen, P. C., Hsu, H. C., Su, T. C., Sung, F. C., Chen, M. F., & Lee, Y. T. (2010). Habitual sleep duration and insomnia and the risk of cardiovascular events and all-cause death: Report from a community-based cohort. *SLEEP, 33*, 177–184.

Choi, S. W., Peek-Asa, C., Sprince, N. L., Rautiainen, R. H., Flamme, G. A., Whitten, P. S., & Zwerling, C. (2006). Sleep quantity and quality as a predictor of injuries in a rural population. *American Journal of Emergency Medicine, 24*, 189–196.

Classen, S., Levy, C., Meyer, D. L., Bewernitz, M., Lanford, D. N., & Mann, W. C. (2011). Simulated driving performance of combat veterans with mild traumatic brain injury and posttraumatic stress disorder: A pilot study. *AJOT, 65*(4), 419–427.

Coelho, F. M. S., Georgsson, H., Narayansingh, M., Swartz, R. H., & Murray, B. J. (2010). Higher prevalence of periodic limb movements of sleep in patients with history of stroke. *Journal of Clinical Sleep Medicne, 6*, 428–430.

Cohen, D. A., Wang, W., Wyatt, J. K., Kronauer, R. E., Dijk, D. J., Czeisler, C. A., & Klerman, E. B. (2010). Uncovering residual effects of chronic sleep loss on human performance. *Science Translational Medicine, 2*, 14ra3.

Connor, J., Norton, R., Ameratunga, S., Robinson, E., Civil, I., Dunn, R., . . . Jackson, R. (2002). Driver sleepiness and risk of serious injury to car occupants: Population-based case control study. *British Medical Journal, 324*, 1125.

Cooke, J. R., Ayalon, L., Palmer, B. W., Loredo, J. S., Corey-Bloom, J., Natarajan, L., . . . Ancoli-Israel, S. (2009). Sustained use of CPAP slows deterioration of cognition, sleep, and mood in patients with Alzheimer's disease and obstructive sleep apnea: A preliminary study. *Journal of Clinical Sleep Medicine, 5*, 305–309.

Copinschi, G. (2005). Metabolic and endocrine effects of sleep deprivation. *Essentials of Psychopharmacology, 6*, 341–347.

Dogan, O., Ertekin, S., & Dogan, S. (2005). Sleep quality in hospitalized patients. *Journal of Clinical Nursing, 14*, 107–113.

Dorrian, J., Sweeney, M., & Dawson, D. (2011). Modeling fatigue-related truck accidents: Prior sleep duration, recency and continuity. *Sleep and Biological Rhythms, 9*, 3–11.

Drake, C., Roehrs, T., Breslau, N., Johnson, E., Jefferson, C., Scofield, H., & Roth, T. (2010). The 10-year risk of verified motor vehicle crashes in relation to physiologic sleepiness. *SLEEP, 33*, 745–752.

Durmer, J. S., & Dinges, D. F. (2005). Neurocognitive consequences of sleep deprivation. *Seminars in Neurology, 25*, 117–129.

Edlund, M. (2003). *The body clock advantage: Finding your best time to succeed in love, work, play, and exercise.* Avon, MA: Adams Media.

Edlund, M. (2010). *The power of rest: Why sleep alone is not enough. A 30-day plan to reset your body.* New York, NY: HarperOne.

Epstein, J. E., & Brown, R. (2010). Sleep disorders in spinal cord injury. In V. W. Lin (Ed.), *Spinal cord medicine: Principles and practice* (2nd ed., pp. 230–240). New York, NY: Demos.

Facility Guidelines Institute. (2010). *Guidelines for design and construction of health care facilities – 2010 edition.* Chicago, IL: American Hospital Association Services.

Flier, J. S., & Elmquist, J. K. (2004). A good night's sleep: Future antidote to the obesity epidemic? *Annals of Internal Medicine, 141*, 885–886.

Frazier, S. C. (2005). Health outcomes and polypharmacy in elderly individuals: An integrated literature review. *Journal of Gerontological Nursing, 31*, 4–11.

Friese, R. S., Diaz-Arrastia, R., McBride, D., Frankel, H., & Gentilello, L. M. (2007). Quantity and quality of sleep in the surgical intensive care unit: Are our patients sleeping? *The Journal of Trauma, 63*, 1210–1214.

Gangwisch, J. E., Babiss, L. A., Malaspina, D., Turner, B., Zammit, G. K., & Posner, K. (2010). Earlier parental set bedtimes as a protective factor against depression and suicidal ideation. *SLEEP, 33*, 97–106.

Gangwisch, J. E., Malaspina, D., Boden-Albala, B., & Heymsfield, S. B. (2005). Inadequate sleep as a risk factor for obesity: Analyses of the NHANES I. *SLEEP, 28*, 1289–1296.

Grohol, J. M. (2010). *DSM 5 sleep disorders overhaul.* Retrieved from http://psychcentral.com/blog/archives/2010/06/07/dsm-5-sleep-disorders-overhaul/

Gujar, N., McDonald, S.A., Nishida, M., & Walker, M.P. (2010). A role for REM sleep in recalibrating the sensitivity of the human brain to specific emotions. *Cerebral Cortex, 21*, 115-23

Haack, G., & Mullington, J. M. (2005). Sustained sleep restriction reduces emotional and physical well-being. *Pain, 119*, 56–64.

Hale, L. (2005). Who has time to sleep? *Journal of Public Health, 27*, 205–211.

Hale, L., & Do, D. P. (2007). Racial differences in self-reports of sleep duration in a population-based study. *SLEEP, 30*, 1096–1103.

Hamilton, N. A., Catley, D., & Karlson, C. (2007). Sleep and affective response to stress and pain. *Health Psychology, 26*, 288–295.

Haponik, E. F., Frye, A. W., Richards, B., Wymer, A., Hinds, A., Pearce, K., . . . Konen, J. (1996). Sleep history is neglected diagnostic information. Challenges for primary care physicians. *Journal of General Internal Medicine, 11*, 759–761.

Hawkley, L. C., Cacioppo, J. T., & Preacher, K. J. (2011). As we said, loneliness (not living alone) explains individual differences in sleep quality: Reply. *Health Psychology, 30*, 136.

Hawkley, L. C., Preacher, K. J., & Cacioppo, J. T. (2010). Loneliness impairs daytime functioning but not sleep duration. *Health Psychology, 29*, 124–129.

Haynes, P. L. (2009). Is CBT-I Effective for pain? *Journal of Clinical Sleep Medicine, 5*, 363–364.

Hobson, J. A. (2011). *Dream life: An experimental memoir.* London, United Kingdom: MIT Press.

Howell, M. J., Schenck, C. H., & Crow, S. J. (2009). A review of nighttime eating disorders. *Sleep Medicine Reviews, 13*, 23–34.

Hume, K. I. (2011). Noise pollution: A ubiquitous unrecognized disruptor of sleep? *SLEEP, 34*, 7–8.

Irwin, M. R., Wang, M., Ribeiro, D., Cho, H. J., Olmstead, R., Breen, E. C., . . . Cole, S. (2008). Sleep loss activates cellular inflammatory signaling. *Biological Psychiatry, 64*, 538–554.

Johns, M. W. (1991). A new method for measuring daytime sleepiness: The Epworth Sleepiness Scale. *SLEEP, 14*, 540–545.

Johnson, K. G., & Johnson, C. D. (2010). Frequency of sleep apnea in stroke and TIA patients: A meta-analysis. *Journal of Clinical Sleep Medicine, 6*, 131–137.

Kim, H., & Young, T. (2005). Subjective daytime sleepiness: Dimensions and correlates in the general population. *SLEEP, 28*, 625–634.

Kristiansen, J., Perrson, R., Björk, J., Albin, M., Jakobsson, K., Ostergren, P. O., & Ardö, J. (2011). Work stress, worries, and pain intersect synergistically with modeled traffic noise on cross-sectional associations with self-reported sleep problems. *International Archives of Occupational and Environmental Health, 84*, 211–224.

Kushida, C. A. (2007). Clinical presentation, diagnosis, and quality of life issues in restless legs syndrome. *American Journal of Medicine, 120*, S4–S12.

Levine, A. C., Adusumilli, J., & Landrigan, C. P. (2010). Effects of reducing or eliminating resident work shifts over 16 hours: A systematic review. *SLEEP, 32*, 1043–1053.

Luckhaupt, S. E., Tak, S., & Calvert, G. M., (2010). The prevalence of short sleep by industry and occupation in the National Health Interview Survey. *SLEEP, 33*, 149–159.

Luyster, F. S., Chasens, E. R., Wasko, M. C. M., & Dunbar-Jacob, J. (2011). Sleep quality and functional disability in patients with rheumatoid arthritis. *Journal of Clinical Sleep Medicine, 7*, 49–55.

Mah, C. D., Mah, K. E., Kezerian, E. J., & Dement, W. C. (2011). The effects of sleep extension on the athletic performance of collegiate basketball players. *SLEEP, 34*, 943–950.

McCall, W. V., Kimball, J., Boggs, N., Lasater, B., D'Agostino, R. B., & Rosenquist, P. B. (2009). Prevalence and prediction of primary sleep disorders in a clinical trial of depressed patients with insomnia. *Journal of Clinical Sleep Medicine, 5*, 454–458.

McHugh, J., & Lawlor, B., (2011). Commentary: Living alone does not account for the association between loneliness and sleep in older adults: Response to Hawkley, Preacher, and Cacioppo, 2010. *Health Psychology, 30,* 135.

Mednick, S. C., & Ehrman, M. (2006). *Take a nap! Change your life.* New York, NY: Workman.

Nurok, M., Czeisler, C. A., Lehmann, L. S. (2010). Sleep deprivation, elective surgical procedures, and informed consent. *The New England Journal of Medicine, 36,* 2577–2579.

O'Connor, G. T., Caffo, B., Newman, A. B., Quan, S. F., Rapoport, D. M., Redline, S., . . . Shahar, E. (2009). Prospective study of sleep-disordered breathing and hypertension: The Sleep Heart Health Study. *American Journal of Respiratory Critical Care Medicine, 179,* 1159–1164.

Ohayon, M. M. (2002). Epidemiology of insomnia: What we know and what we still need to learn. *Sleep Medicine Reviews, 6,* 97–111.

Ohayon, M. M., Carskadon, M. A., Guilleminault, C., & Vitiello, M. V. (2004). Meta-analysis of quantitative sleep parameters from childhood to old age in healthy indviduals: Developing normative sleep values across the human lifespan. *SLEEP, 27,* 1255–1273.

Ohayon, M. M., & Vecchierini, M. F. (2005). Normative sleep data, cognitive function and daily living activities in older adults in the community. *SLEEP, 28,* 981–989.

Owens, J. A., Belon, K., & Moss, P. (2010). Impact of delaying school start time on adolescent sleep, mood, and behavior. *Archives of Pediatrics and Adolescent Medicine, 164,* 608–614.

Owens, J. A., & Mindell, J. A. (2005). *Take charge of your child's sleep: The all-in-one resource for solving sleep problems in kids and teens.* New York, NY: Marlowe & Company.

Owens, J. A., Spirito, A., & McGuinn, M. (2000). The Children's Sleep Habits Questionnaire (CSHQ): Psychometric properties of a survey instrument for school-aged children. *SLEEP, 23,* 1043–1051.

Owens, J. A., Spirito, A., McGuinn, M., & Nobile, C. (2000). Sleep habits and sleep disturbance in elementary school-aged children. *Journal of Developmental and Behavioral Pediatrics, 21,* 27–36.

Ownby, R. L., Saeed, M., Wohlgemuth, W., Capasso, R., Acevedo, A., Peruyera, G., & Sevush, S. (2010). Caregiver reports of sleep problems in non-Hispanic white, Hispanic, and African American patients with Alzheimer dementia. *Journal of Clinical Sleep Medicine, 6,* 281–289.

Parcell, D. L., Ponsford, J. L., Redman, J. R., & Rajaratnam, S. M. (2008). Poor sleep quality and changes in objectively recorded sleep after traumatic brain injury: A preliminary study *Archives of Physical Medicine and Rehabilitation, 89,* 843–850.

Passos, G. S., Poyares, D., Santana M. G., Garbuio, S., Tufik, S., & Mello, M. T. (2010). Effect of acute physical exercise on patients with chronic primary insomnia. *Journal of Clinical Sleep Medicine, 6,* 270–275.

Patel, S. R., Ayas, N. T., Malhotra, M. R., White, D. P., Schernhammer, E. S., Speizer, F. E., . . . Hu, F. B. (2004). A prospective study of sleep duration and mortality risk in women. *SLEEP, 27,* 440–444.

Patel, S. R., & Hu, F. B. (2008). Short sleep duration and weight gain: A systematic review. *Obesity, 16*(3), 643–653.

Peppard, P. E. (2009). Is obstructive sleep apnea a risk factor for hypertension?—Differences between the Wisconsin sleep cohort and the Sleep heart health study. *Journal of Clinical Sleep Medicine, 5,* 404–405.

Pizza, F., Contardi, S., Antognini, A. B., Zagoraiou, M., Borrotti M., Mostacci, B., . . . Cirignotta, F. (2010). Sleep quality and motor vehicle crashes in adolescents. *Journal of Clinical Sleep Medicine, 6,* 41–45.

Poe, G. R., Walsh, C. M., & Bjorness, T. E. (2010). Both duration and timing of sleep are important to memory consolidation. *SLEEP, 33,* 1277–1280.

Quan, S. F., Parthasarathy, S., & Budhiraja, R. (2010). Healthy sleep education—A salve for obesity? *Journal of Clinical Sleep Medicine, 6,* 18–19.

Redline, S. (2009). Does sleep disordered breathing increase hypertension risk? A practical perspective on interpreting the evidence. *Journal of Clinical Sleep Medicine, 5,* 406–408.

Reynolds, C. F., & Redline, S. (2010). The DSM-V Sleep-Wake Disorders nosology: An update and an invitation to the sleep community *SLEEP, 33,* 10–13.

Roehrs, T., Hyde, M., Blaisdell, B., Greenwald, M, & Roth, T. (2006). Sleep loss and REM sleep loss are hyperalgesic. *SLEEP, 29,* 145–151.

Roehrs, T., & Roth T. (2008). Caffeine: Sleep and daytime sleepiness. *Sleep Medicine Reviews, 12,* 153–162.

Roehrs, T., & Roth T. (2011a). Medication and substance abuse. In M. H. Kryger, T. Roth, W. C. Dement (Eds.), *Principles and practice of sleep medicine* (5th ed., pp. 1512–1523). St. Louis, MO: Elsevier Saunders.

Roehrs, T., & Roth, T. (2011b). *Sleep, sleepiness, and alcohol use.* Retrieved from http://pubs.niaaa.nih.gov/publications/arh25-2/101-109.htm

Roth,T., Roehrs, T., & Pies, R. (2007). Insomnia: Pathophysiology and implications for treatment. *Sleep Medicine Reviews, 11,* 71–79.

Sadeh, A. (2011). The role and validity of actigraphy in sleep medicine: An update. *Sleep Medicine Reviews, 15,* 259–267.

Sánchez-Ortuño, M. M., Edinger, J. D., Means, M. K., & Almirall, D. (2010). Home is where the sleep is: An ecological approach to test the validity of actigraphy for the assessment of insomnia. *Journal of Clinical Sleep Medicine, 6,* 21–29.

Schweitzer, P. (2011). Drugs that disturb sleep and wakefulness. In M. H. Kryger, T. Roth, W. C. Dement (Eds.), *Principles and practice of sleep medicine* (5th ed., pp. 542–562). St. Louis, MO: Elsevier Saunders.

Senthilvel, E., Auckley, D., & Dasarathy, J. (2011). Evaluation of sleep disorders in the primary care setting: History taking compared to questionnaires. *Journal of Clinical Sleep Medicine, 7,* 41–48.

Shepard, J. W., Buyesse, D. J., Chesson, A. L., Dement W. C., Goldberg, R., Guilleinault, C., . . . White, D. P. (2005). History of the development of sleep medicine in the United States. *Journal of Clinical Sleep Medicine, 1,* 61–81.

Sixel-Döring, F., Schweitzer, M., Mollenhauer, B., & Trenkwalder, C. (2011). Intraindividual variability of REM sleep behavior disorder in Parkinson's Disease: A comparative assessment using a new REM Sleep Behavior Disorder Severity Scale (RBDSS) for clinical routine. *Journal of Clinical Sleep Medicine, 7,* 75–80.

Smith, B., & Phillips, B. A. (2011). Truckers drive their own assessment for obstructive sleep apnea: A collaborative approach to online self-assessment for obstructive sleep apnea. *Journal of Clinical Sleep Medicine, 7,* 241–245.

Solet, J. M. (2012). Optimizing personal and social adaptation. In M. V. Radomski & C. A. Trombly (Eds.), *Occupational therapy for physical dysfunction* (7th ed.). Manuscript submitted for publication.

Solet, J. M., & Barach, P. (2012). Managing alarm fatigue in cardiac care. *Progress in Pediatric Cardiology, 33,* 85–90.

Solet, J. M., Buxton, O. M., Ellenbogen, J. M., Wang, W., & Carballiera, A. (2010). *Validating acoustic guidelines for healthcare facilities. Evidence-based design meets evidence-based medicine: The sound sleep study.* Concord, CA: The Center for Health Design. Retrieved from http://www.healthdesign.org/chd/research/validating-acoustic-guidelines-healthcare-facilities

Sorscher, A. J. (2008). How is your sleep: A neglected topic for health care screening. *Journal of the American Board of Family Medicine, 21,* 141–148.

Spiegel, K., Knutson, K., Leproult, R., Tasali, E., & Van Cauter, E. (2005). Sleep loss: A novel risk factor for insulin resistance and Type 2 diabetes. *Journal of Applied Physiology, 99,* 2008–2019.

Spiegel, K., Tasali, E., Penev, P., & Van Cauter, E. (2004). Brief communication: Sleep curtailment in healthy young men is associated with decreased leptin levels, elevated ghrelin levels, and increased hunger and appetite. *Annals of Internal Medicine, 141,* 846–850.

Stickgold, R. (2005). Sleep-dependent memory consolidation. *Nature, 437,* 1272–1285.

Stout, K., & Finlayson, M. (2011). Fatigue management in chronic illness: The role of occupational therapy. *OT Practice, 16*(1), 16–19.

Stroe, A. F., Roth, T., Jefferson, C., Hudgel, D. W., Roehrs, T., Moss, K., & Drake, C. L. (2010). Comparative levels of excessive daytime sleepiness in common medical disorders. *Sleep Medicine, 11,* 890–896.

Tomfohr, L. M., Ancoli-Israel, S., Loredo, J. S., & Dimsdale, J. E. (2011). Effects of continuous positive airway pressure on fatigue and sleepiness in patients with obstructive sleep apnea: Data from a randomized controlled trial. *SLEEP, 34,* 121–126.

Tregear, S., Reston J., Schoelles, K., & Phillips, B. (2009). Obstructive sleep apnea and risk of motor vehicle crash: A systematic review and meta-analysis. *Journal of Clinical Sleep Medicine, 5*, 573–581.

Umberson, D. (1992). Gender, marital status and the social control of health behaviors. *Soc. Sci. Med, 34*, 907–917.

Van Dongen, H. P. A., Maislin, G., Mullington, J. M., & Dinges, D. (2003). The cumulative cost of additional wakefulness: Dose-response effects on neurobehavioral functions and sleep physiology from chronic sleep restriction and total sleep deprivation. *SLEEP, 26*, 117–126.

Vasquez, M. M., Goodwin, J. L., Drescher, A. A., Smith, T. W., & Quan, S. F. (2008). Associations of dietary intake and physical activity with sleep disordered breathing in the Apnea Positive Pressure Long-term Efficacy Study (APPLES). *Journal of Clinical Sleep Medicine, 4*, 411–418.

Vaughn, B. V., & D'Cruz, O. (2011). Cardinal manifestations of sleep disorders. In M. H. Kryger, T. Roth, & W. C. Dement (Eds.), *Principles and practice of sleep medicine* (5th ed., pp. 647–657). St. Louis, MO: Elsevier Saunders.

Verse, T., & Hörmann, K. (2011). The surgical treatment of sleep-related upper airway obstruction. *Deutsches Ärzteblatt International, 108*, 216–221.

Viola-Saltzman, M., Watson, N. F., Bogart, A., Goldberg, J., & Buchwald, D. (2010). High prevalence of restless legs syndrom among patients with fibromyalgia: A controlled cross-sectional study. *Journal of Clinical Sleep Medicine, 6*, 423–427.

Vitiello, M. V., Rybarczk, B., Von Korff, M., & Stepanski, E. J. (2009). Cognitive behavioral therapy for insomnia improves sleep and decreases pain in older adults with co-morbid insomnia and osteoarthritis. *Journal of Clinical Sleep Medicine, 5*, 355–362.

Walker M. P., & Stickgold, R. (2004). Sleep-dependent learning and memory consolidation. *Neuron*, 44, 121–133.

Watanabe, M., Kikuchi, H., Katsutoshi, T., & Takahashi, M. (2010). Association of short sleep duration with weight gain and obesity at 1 year follow-up: A large-scale prospective study. *SLEEP, 33*, 161–167

Watson, N. F. (2010). Stroke and sleep specialists: An opportunity to intervene? *Journal of Clinical Sleep Medicine, 6*, 138–139.

Watson, N. F., Buchwald, D., Vitiello, M. V., Noonan, C., & Goldberg, J. (2010). A twin study of sleep duration and body mass index. *Journal of Clinical Sleep Medicine, 6*, 11–17.

Weaver, E., Gradisar, M., Dohnt, H., Lovato, N., & Douglas, P. (2010). The effect of presleep video-game playing in adolescent sleep. *Journal of Clinical Sleep Medicine, 6*, 184–185.

Weinhouse, G. L., & Schwab, R. J. (2006). Sleep in the critically ill patient. *SLEEP, 29*, 707–716.

Youngstedt, S. D., & Buxton, O. M. (2003). Jet lag and athletic performance. *American Journal of Medicine and Sports, 5*, 219–226.

Zee, P. C., & Turek, F. W. (2006). Sleep and health: Everywhere and in both directions. *Archives of Internal Medicine, 166*, 1686–1688.

Zizi, F., Jean-Louis, G., Brown, C. D., Ogedegbe, G., Boutin-Foster, C., & McFarlane, S. I. (2011). Sleep duration and risk of diabetes mellitus: Epidemiologic evidence and pathophysiologic insights. *Current Diabetes Reports, 10*, 43–47.

For additional resources on the subjects discussed in this chapter, visit http://thePoint.lww.com/Willard-Spackman12e.

CHAPTER 52

Social Participation

Mary Alunkal Khetani, Wendy J. Coster

LEARNING OBJECTIVES

After reading this chapter, you will be able to:

1. Describe how social participation has been defined
2. Evaluate the strengths and limitations of available assessments to develop participation profiles of clients seeking occupational therapy services
   a. Describe ways that you might appraise a client's participation using available measures
   b. Describe ways that you can incorporate information about environmental supports and barriers in your appraisal of a client's participation
3. Describe ways of intervening to promote social participation at the individual, group, or organizational level

OUTLINE

Introduction

Did you know that more than one billion people, or 15% of the world's population, live with some degree of disability? (World Health Organization [WHO] & World Bank, 2011). Disability estimates like this one from the recently published *World Report on Disability* are striking at face value, as well as when you consider the likelihood that this is an underestimate of the prevalence of disability because the estimates were based on the presence or absence of a select group of impairments. Current models of disability have supported a broader understanding of the construct. Disability is not conceptualized as a stable attribute of a person but rather as a state in which the individual experiences functional limitations (e.g., visual impairment) (Lollar & Andresen, 2011). *The International Classification of Functioning, Disability and Health* (ICF) and the *International Classification of Functioning, Disability and Health: Version for Children and Youth* (ICF-CY) identify that one way the impact of functional limitations can be described is by examining whether the person encounters difficulties participating in society on an equal basis with others (WHO, 2001, 2007). This definition of disability emphasizes the importance of knowledge about the contextualized experiences of individuals when they are meaningfully occupied (Cutchin, 2004). We need to understand the characteristics of individuals (e.g., age, gender, ethnicity, diagnosis) and their environments as they affect participation in everyday activities to fully determine the prevalence of and pathways to disability across the life course.

Information about participation is of particular importance for occupational therapists because a major focus of our profession is on promoting participation in everyday occupations that give meaning and purpose to people's lives (American Occupational Therapy Association [AOTA], 2008). As a student en route to a career in occupational therapy, this chapter is intended to provide you with an introduction to contemporary thinking about social participation—how it is currently understood, assessed, and promoted.

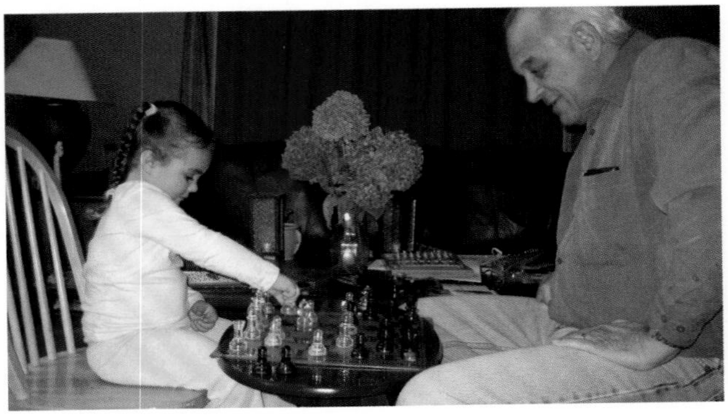

FIGURE 52.1 For children, life situations are organized sets and sequences of activities that typically involve the presence and engagement of others. These life situations may be directed toward development of skills and capacities as well as enjoyment.

Defining Social Participation

The Distinction between Participation and Social Participation

Participation and *social participation* are terms that are often used interchangeably. **Participation** is broadly defined in the ICF as "involvement in life situations" (WHO, 2001, 2007) without specific reference made to social participation as a separate concept. The ambiguity of the ICF definition of participation has led to scientific dialogue about how to define its key features. For children, McConachie, Colver, Forsyth, Jarvis, and Parkinson (2006) classified "life situations" as sets of activities that were pursued because they were essential for survival, supporting the child's development, discretionary, or educationally enriching. For young children as well as children and youth, life situations are organized sets and sequences of activities that typically involve the presence and engagement of others, are setting-specific, and are directed toward a personally or socially meaningful goal such as sustenance and physical health, development of skills and capacities, and enjoyment and emotional wellbeing (Coster & Khetani, 2008; Khetani, Cohn, Orsmond, Law, & Coster, 2011). Whiteneck and Dijkers (2009) proposed a definition of participation as performance or fulfillment of social roles that involve interacting with others. In each of these classification schemes, the social element of participation is noted in reference to the purpose of the activity (e.g., toward a socially meaningful goal) or in terms of how one might participate (e.g., interacting with others).

Alternatively, **social participation** has been defined as involvement in a subset of activities that involve social interactions with others (Bedell, in press) and that support social interdependence (Magasi & Hammel, 2004). For example, participating in services, potlucks, meetings, and fund-raising events are ways of belonging to a religious community. According to the "Occupational Therapy Practice Framework" (AOTA, 2008), social participation includes "organized patterns of behavior that are characteristic and expected of an individual or a given position within a social system" and encompasses the individual's engagement with family, peers and friends, and community members (p. 633) (see Figure 52.1).

There is no consensus about how useful any of these proposed definitions are in describing the participation patterns of our potential clients. Categorizing one's participation in occupations can be problematic because individuals can experience the same occupation in different ways, or an individual can pursue the same occupation for different reasons over time (see Chapter 46). For example, consider the situation of an infant or young child whose participation in almost every occupation is dependent on the presence and engagement of another person such as the child's caregiver (Lawlor, 2003; Olsen, 2004). The definition of social participation in reference to a subset of activities may be more relevant to children and youth but not in this instance where all activities that infants and young children engage in involve others. Similarly, the usefulness of defining participation in terms of social roles (Wade & Halligan, 2007; Whiteneck & Dijkers, 2009) is problematic when applied to children and youth whose participation in most activities is socially mandated by their families or educators and whose participation in some activities may not involve carrying out any prescribed role, such as when they are playing at the local playground (Coster & Khetani, 2008; Coster et al., 2011) (see Figure 52.2).

Given that there are age-related differences that influence how an individual participates in everyday life, it might be more useful to (1) assume that any life situation can be social and (2) classify areas of social

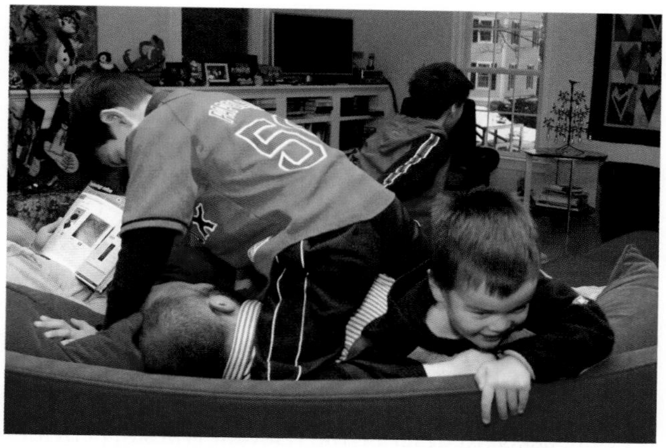

FIGURE 52.2 Social participation has been defined as involvement in a subset of activities that involve social interactions with others.

participation according to where they take place. Then we can identify contextual features of the setting or activity that influence participation, such as the availability and adequacy of resources to participate at home or one's access to a safe and supportive neighborhood to play basketball at the local playground after school (Heinemann, 2010). Thinking about social participation in this way will help us organize our thinking about participation in ways that are relevant across the life course. This approach also may enable us to identify standards for participation that are context specific. Recent evidence has suggested that participation is highly variable and that client standards may vary compared to others of the same age as well as across activities and settings (Khetani et al., 2011) and over time (Tamis-Monda et al., 2007). Even for adults, defining participation by degree of fit to a predefined social role may not be accurate if, for example, they have redefined caregiving to accommodate living with a mobility impairment (Jackson, 1998a, 1998b). As an example, Gloria Dickerson (see Chapter 11) describes how her lived experience as an adult with mental illness shaped her role as an educator:

> Dr. Spaniol mentored me and gave me a valued role facilitating recovery groups and cofacilitating statewide workshops . . . I now have a newly found identity of educator. This was a dream of mine when as a little girl. I played school with my childhood friends. These experiences allowed me a glimpse into the land of being accepted and well respected. And now, I am forever changed, and giving up is simply harder because of them. Their use of the universal concept that difficulties are caused by barriers took me out of the land of a defective human being failing to function and placed me squarely back in the land of human beings striving to overcome environmental obstacles without judgments about my intellect, character, or motivation. I was on an equal playing field with all others.

In the remainder of this chapter, we discuss ways to evaluate and intervene to achieve participation outcomes with reference to a broad range of activities that an individual client might engage in with others across the life course.

The Distinction between Social Participation and Quality of Life

Another important topic of discussion in the recent literature is how to differentiate the concepts of participation and quality of life. The WHO provides definitions of both concepts but does not clearly describe the relation between them. Whereas participation is defined as a person's "involvement in life situations," **quality of life** is defined as a measure of well-being and encompasses "individual's perceptions of their position in life in the context of the culture and value system where they live, and in relation to their goals, expectations, standards and concerns" (Quality of Life Assessment by World Health Organization Quality of Life [WHOQOL] Group as cited in WHO, 1998, p. 27). These definitions emphasize the objective aspect of participation and the subjective aspect of quality of life.

What we observe may be different from what an individual experiences. Therefore, several authors have argued that both the objective and subjective components of participation should be evaluated. The objective component of participation describes what an individual is doing, how often, and perhaps in what context. In contrast, the subjective component describes whether the person is doing what he or she wants to do and in a way that is satisfying to him or her. From an occupational therapy perspective, information about whether individuals are participating in the activities they would prefer may enable a more accurate determination of whether or not there is a problem with participation (Hemmingsson & Jonsson, 2005; Ueda & Okawa, 2003). Both objective and subjective aspects of participation were identified as important by parents of children with disabilities and the children themselves (Bedell, Khetani, Cousins, Coster, & Law, 2011) as well as by adults with disabilities (Hammel et al., 2008). Although some quality of life measures attempt to capture subjective well-being, most were developed without input from people with disabilities and therefore may not be appropriate to capture the subjective aspects of participation (Hays, Hahn, & Marshall, 2002). Based on this perspective, we can think about participation and quality of life as separate but closely related domains (Whiteneck, 2006). Participation can be considered to be one indicator of the individual's overall quality of life as described in the "Occupational Therapy Practice Framework" (AOTA, 2008,) and by McDougall, Wright, Schmidt, Miller, and Lowry (2011).

Evaluating Social Participation

We come to understand the social participation patterns of our clients by gathering information about their experiences engaging in the activities that comprise their everyday life. As defined, social participation is a *multidimensional* and *context-dependent* phenomenon. These key features of social participation imply that there is more than one way to ascertain whether or not our clients are participating (i.e., multidimensional) and that our clients' participation may, in fact, differ depending on what they are doing and where the activity takes place (i.e., context-dependent). Hence, the task of gathering useful information about how our diverse clients participate across the full range of relevant activities and settings is complex at best.

There is no single measure of social participation that is suitable for use with all of our potential clients across age groups, functional profiles, and activity contexts. In addition, measures can be more or less useful depending on whether we are using an assessment as it was intended to be used (e.g., for individualized service planning, program evaluation, intervention or population-based studies) (Bedell & Coster, 2008). In the next section, we describe the work that has been done to develop assessments of participation for individuals across the life course, with a focus on those approaches that can be used to guide our assessment of social participation to support individualized service planning.

Common Features of Social Participation Assessments

Evaluation approaches described in this section support the use of a top-down and client-centered approach to addressing our clients' occupational performance needs. When using a top-down approach, we first focus on obtaining the client's social participation profile by identifying what the client wants to do, needs to do, or is expected to do; and we then organize services to address impairments, functional limitations, and contextual factors that restrict their level of participation in a particular activity context. Assessments described in this section provide a way to systematically obtain clients' social participation profiles and more sharply focus our services toward those subsets of activities that they most want or need to participate in but are experiencing restriction(s).

We can gather information about what our clients want or need to participate in (i.e., their preferences) by asking them directly using an interview or survey format. Discussions about client-centered care typically focus on building a therapeutic alliance and partnering with clients in making decisions about services (see Chapter 33). Client-centeredness is also reflected by the extent to which the assessments themselves have been developed with consumer input about what to include in the measure so that we can be clear about whose voice is represented in the information we use to guide decision-making efforts with clients (Brown & Gordon, 2004; Coster, 2006). Consumers whose perspectives have been gathered on the topic of participation include those of adults with disabilities (Hammel et al., 2008), parents of children with and without disabilities (Bedell, Cohn, & Dumas, 2005; Bedell et al., 2011; Dunst, Hamby, Trivette, Raab, & Bruder, 2002; Khetani et al., 2011; Lawlor, 2003 Mactavish & Schleien, 1998), and children and youth with disabilities themselves (Heah, Case, McGuire, & Law, 2007; Kramer & Hammel, 2011; Majnemer et al., 2010; Shikako-Thomas et al., 2010). Participants in these studies were asked to describe the relevant types of activities that they or their child participate in. In some cases, they were also asked to describe the types of environmental factors that support or challenge their child's participation and how they evaluate the quality of their own participation or that of their child.

Overview of Selected Participation Measures

As mentioned earlier, we can gather information about our client's participation via interview or survey. Because participation is conceptualized as being strongly influenced by the environment, it is important to combine assessment of an individual's participation with assessment of how features of the environment support or challenge participation.

For this chapter, we build on what has been covered in other chapters and review a set of measures that explicitly address participation and that have some psychometric evidence to support their use in practice (McConachie et al., 2006; Morris, Kurinczuk, & Fitzpatrick, 2005). Most of these measures were developed within the past decade and offer ideas to think about and measure participation for individuals with disabilities across the life course. These measures vary in terms of their comprehensiveness, how they are administered, how long they take to complete, the target population they are designed for, and their intended purpose. In this section, we will describe 17 assessments of participation that have been developed for young children, children and youth, and adults and older adults (see Table 52.1). The following table provides an overview of what each assessment can help you gather information about as you begin the assessment process with your clients. For each measure selected for review in this chapter, we have indicated (1) whether its content addresses home, school, work and/or community participation; (2) whether objective or subjective approaches, or both, are used; (3) whether it includes an assessment of environment; and (4) its primary purpose.

More details about the psychometric properties of these assessments, visit **thePoint.lww.com/Willard&Spackman12e**.

TABLE 52.1 Overview of Participation Measures for Young Children, Children and Youth, and Adults and Older Adults

Assessment	Area(s) of Participation Addressed: Home	School or Work	Community	Dimensions Addressed: Objective Assessment	Subjective Assessment	Environmental Impact Addressed	Primary Purpose: Individualized Assessment (Practice)	Large-Scale Studies (Research)
Participation Measures for Young Children								
Preschooler Activity Card Sort (PACS)	✔	✔	✔	Frequency, Extent	Importance, Satisfaction	✔	✔	
Routines-Based Interview (RBI)	✔		✔	Engagement, Independence, Interaction	Satisfaction	✔	✔	
Asset-Based Context Matrix (ABC Matrix)	✔	✔	✔	Capabilities, Interactions	Interests	✔	✔	
Assessment of Preschool Children's Participation (APCP)	✔		✔	Diversity, Intensity			✔	
Children's Participation Questionnaire (CPQ)	✔	✔	✔	Diversity, Intensity	Enjoyment, Satisfaction	✔	❷	✔
Participation Measures for Children and Youth								
Pediatric Activity Card Sort (PACS)	✔	✔	✔	Frequency	Preference		✔	
Children's Assessment of Participation and Enjoyment (CAPE) and Preferences for Activities (PAC)	✔		✔	Diversity, Intensity, Where, With whom	Enjoyment, Preferences		✔	
School Function Assessment (SFA)		✔		Involvement		✔	✔	
Child and Adolescent Scale of Participation (CASP)	✔	✔	✔	Degree of restriction		✔	❷	✔
Assessment of LIFE-Habits for Children (LIFE-H)	✔	✔	✔	Accomplishment	Satisfaction	✔	❷	✔
Participation and Environment Measure for Children and Youth (PEM-CY)	✔	✔	✔	Frequency, Involvement	Desire for change	✔	❷	✔
Participation Measures for Adults and Older Adults								
Meaningful Activity and Participation Assessment (MAPA)	✔		✔	Frequency	Meaning		❷	✔
Engagement in Meaningful Activities Scale (EMAS)	✔		✔	Frequency	Meaning		❷	✔
Activity Card Sort (ACS)	✔		✔	% Maintained			✔	
Craig Handicap Assessment and Reporting Technique (CHART)		✔	✔	Time spent, No. of social contacts		✔	❷	✔
Participation Objective, Participation Subjective	✔	✔	✔	How often	Importance			✔
Community Integration Questionnaire (CIQ)	✔	✔		How often, With whom, Assistance			❷	✔

Selected Participation Measures for Young Children

Young children's participation is one of the four primary service outcomes addressed by occupational therapy practitioners working in early intervention (Guralnick, 2005) and is considered to be an important indicator of preschool inclusion. Although there has been extensive theoretical discussion on the concept of young children's participation, there is still no single measure of young children's participation available for use in service planning, multisite evaluation, and large-scale outcomes research within the early intervention field. All of the available instruments were initially designed for use in research and/or service planning and rely on parent report. Young children are typically in close contact with and guided by their parents or caregivers to participate in home and community-based activities. Due to this close proximity between parent and young child, parent-report measures are commonly used to make inferences about the qualities of young children's participation.

Preschooler Activity Card Sort

The Preschooler Activity Card Sort (Berg & LaVesser, 2006) is a semistructured interview for use with parents of children 3 to 6 years of age that is available in English and Spanish (Stoffel & Berg, 2008). The primary purpose of this tool is for intervention planning. In its current edition, the Preschooler Activity Card Sort contains 85 photographs of children engaged in one of seven types of activities: self-care, community mobility, leisure (both high physical demand and low physical demand), social interaction, domestic chores, and education. Parents are asked to view each of the 85 photographs and respond to the question "Does your child participate in this activity?" using one of the following response options: (1) yes, child participates; (2) yes, child participates but requires adult assistance beyond that typically required of preschoolers; (3) yes, with environmental assistance (e.g., can ride a bike on some surfaces—hard, smooth surfaces but not grass); (4) no (does not participate in the activity), for child reasons (e.g., due to pain, balance, vision); (5) no, for adult reasons (e.g., financial, fear, feels child is too young); or (6) no, for environmental reasons (e.g., community resources unavailable, neighborhood safety). Parents are then asked to identify five activities that they would like to be the focus of intervention and rate the relative importance of each activity, the frequency that the activity is performed, the extent of participation (from 0 = *currently not participating at all* to 10 = *fully participating*), and satisfaction with participation.

Routines-Based Interview

The Routines-Based Interview (RBI) (McWilliam, Casey, & Sims, 2009) is a semistructured interview designed for use with families of young children to obtain a rich picture of each routine within the child's day. The interviewer goes through a typical day for a family and for each routine (i.e., time of day or activity) that the parent identifies, the interviewer proceeds to ask the following questions: (1) What is everyone else doing? (2) What is the child doing? (3) What is the child's engagement like? (4) What is the child's independence like? (5) What are the child's social relationships like? and (6) How satisfactory is this time of day (from 1= *not at all* to 5 = *very satisfied*)? Afterward, the interviewer recaps concerns with the family and asks the parent or caregiver which of their reported concerns they would like to concentrate on, in order of importance. The RBI can be used together with the Scale for Assessment of Family Enjoyment within Routines (SAFER) (Scott & McWilliam, 2000) and the Scale for the Assessment of Teachers' Impressions of Routines and Engagement (SATIRE) (Clingenpeel & McWilliam, 2003) to obtain an estimate of the teacher's perceptions of the child's functioning within classroom routines. The RBI does not provide a score of the child's skills and abilities but can be used to obtain a narrative description of the child's functioning in cognitive, motor, adaptive, communication, and social skill areas.

Asset-Based Context Matrix

The Asset-Based Context Matrix (ABCM) (Wilson, Mott, & Batman, 2004) combines semistructured interview and observation to help practitioners identify the child's interests and abilities (i.e., assets) so that contextually based child outcomes can be developed. The information is gathered in an informal manner rather than by formally administering the scale. Parents are asked to describe a typical day and the everyday, weekly, and special activities and events in which the child and family participate. The ABCM focuses on activities and events that fall into one of three main contexts—family life, community life, and early childhood program—and the practitioner is guided to ask the parent about six characteristics of the child's behavior in each activity setting—the child's interests, the child's assets/capabilities, the child's functional/meaningful interactions with others, the amount of opportunity that the child has to participate in the activity or event, and the child's participation.

Assessment of Preschool Children's Participation

The Assessment of Preschool Children's Participation (APCP) scale (Law, King, Petrenchik, Kertoy, & Anaby, 2012) is a new measure that has been modeled after the Children's Assessment of Participation and Enjoyment (CAPE) and the Preferences for Activities of Children (PAC) (King et al., 2004) and is designed for use with children ages 2 to 5 years, 11 months. The APCP assesses young children's participation in voluntary, day-to-day activities outside of preschool. The APCP is a parent-report, paper-pencil survey that contains 45 drawings of activities across the areas of play (9 items); skill development (15 items); active physical recreation (10 items); and social activities (11 items). Parents are asked to identify activities that their child has participated in during the past 4 months (yes/no) and if yes, how often they did them (7-point scale). Similar to the CAPE/PAC, diversity and intensity scores can be generated for each of the four activity areas. Initial psychometric evidence of the APCP has been reported (Law et al., 2012) using baseline data from its use in a large-scale intervention study involving children with cerebral palsy (n = 128) (Law et al., 2011).

Children's Participation Questionnaire

The Children's Participation Questionnaire (CPQ) (Rosenberg, Jarus, & Bart, 2010) is a parent-report questionnaire that was designed for use with children with and without disabilities who are 4 to 6 years old. The CPQ contains 40 items that address six areas of participation: activities of daily living (5 items), instrumental activities of daily living (5 items), play (5 items), leisure (10 items), social participation (9 items), and education (11 items). For each activity, the parent is asked to report on the child's intensity (how often the child participates, from 0 = *never* to 5 = *every day*), the child's independence level (need for assistance, from 1 = *needs much assistance* to 6 = *fully independent*), the child's enjoyment (from 1 = *does not take pleasure* to 6 = *takes much pleasure*), and the parent's level of satisfaction with the child's performance (from 1 = *not at all satisfied* to 6 = *very satisfied*). Total summary scores and summary scores for each of the six participation areas can be computed for diversity (number of activities the child participates in), intensity (mean frequency), enjoyment (mean enjoyment), and satisfaction (mean satisfaction).

Selected Participation Measures for Children and Youth

We review six participation measures that were designed for school-aged children with and without disabilities.

Pediatric Activity Card Sort

The Pediatric Activity Card Sort (PACS) (Mandich, Polatajko, Miller, & Baum, 2004) is an adaptation of the Activity Card Sort (Baum & Edwards, 2008) that was developed for adults. The PACS uses Q-sort methodology and involves the use of pictures of children engaging in various activities to elicit the child's perspective of their level of occupational participation. The PACS includes 83 sorting cards that depict 75 activities addressing personal care, school/productivity, hobbies/social activities, and sports as well as 8 blank cards for additional activities that the child might report on during the course of the interview. The respondent is instructed to place the card in a "yes" or "no" pile based on whether he or she had participated in the activity within the last 4 months and if he or she participates, then it is asked how often he or she participates (daily, weekly, monthly, yearly). Scoring involves recording the five activities that are most important for the child to do and the activities that the child would like to do the most. The PACS can be administered to the parent or child and takes 20 to 25 minutes to complete with children who are between 5 and 14 years old.

Children's Assessment of Participation and Enjoyment

The CAPE (King et al., 2004) is a 55-item measure designed to obtain from the child or his or her parent a participation profile specific to leisure and recreation activities that take place outside of the school setting (e.g., hobbies, crafts, games, organized sports, clubs, groups, arts, and entertainment). The CAPE contains activity drawings on cards and visual response forms to help enable children to complete this assessment via self-report or interview. The CAPE assesses five dimensions of participation in reference to a 4-month time frame: (1) diversity of activities (whether child participates), (2) intensity or how often the child participates, (3) with whom the child participates, (4) where the child participates, and (5) extent of enjoyment in activities. The CAPE can be completed separately from the PAC and takes 30 to 45 minutes to complete. The primary purpose of the CAPE is individualized assessment although it has been employed in larger scale intervention studies.

School Function Assessment

The School Function Assessment (SFA) (Coster, Deeney, Haltiwanger, & Haley, 1998) includes a participation section that can be used to gather information about participation in the elementary school setting. The SFA participation scale examines six different school settings: (1) classroom (regular or specialized), (2) playground or recess, (3) transportation, (4) bathroom or toileting, (5) transitions, and (6) mealtime or snack time, with one item for each section. The SFA participation section consists of six items. Each item pertains to one of the six settings previously described and includes examples of tasks and activities that are typically part of that setting. Items are rated on a 6-point scale that reflects the extent to which the child participates in the tasks and activities compared to peers (from 1 = *extremely limited* to 6 = *child fully participates in all tasks and activities within each setting*). The SFA participation subscale can be completed by the child's teacher in about 5 to 10 minutes when used separately from the larger measure and has reported evidence of test–retest reliability and internal consistency. The SFA addresses the environment in terms of the use of human assistance and/or adaptations (modifications of equipment, environment, activity, program) to complete school tasks. The SFA was initially designed for individualized assessment but has been used in outcome studies. See Chapter 48 for more details.

Child and Adolescent Scale of Participation

The Child and Adolescent Scale of Participation (CASP) (Bedell, 2009) was developed as part of the Child and Family Follow-up Survey (CFFS) to monitor outcomes and needs of children with acquired brain injuries and subsequently has been used separately from the CFFS to assess children with other diagnoses (Bedell, 2004; Bedell, 2009; Bedell & Dumas, 2004). The CASP includes four subsections that address the extent to which children ages 5 years and older participate in broad types of home, school, and community activities compared to same-aged peers. All items are rated on a 4-point scale (from 1 = *unable* to 4 = *age expected*). The CASP includes open-ended questions that ask about effective strategies and supports and barriers that affect participation. The CASP alone takes about 10 minutes to complete and has reported evidence of test–retest reliability, internal consistency, and construct and discriminant validity (Bedell, 2004; Bedell, 2009; Bedell & Dumas, 2004). The 18-item Child and Adolescent Scale of Environment (CASE) is a separate but compatible measure that can be used with the CASP to obtain information about environmental barriers to participation (from 1 = *no problem* to 3 = *big problem*).

Assessment of Life Habits in Children

The Assessment of Life Habits (LIFE-H) (Noreau, Fougeyrollas, Post, & Asano, 2005; Noreau et al., 2007) was initially designed for adults but has been adapted for use as a parent-report survey for families of children ages 5 years and older. Its purpose is to identify disruptions in the accomplishment of 11 types of life habits that are described as "regular activities or social roles valued by the person or his/her sociocultural context according to his/her characteristics . . ." (Noreau et al., 2005). There are six categories of life habits that fall into the daily activities domain (communication, personal care, housing, mobility, nutrition, fitness) and five life habits that fall into the social roles domain (recreation, responsibility, education, community life, interpersonal relationships). The LIFE-H has a long form (197 items) that takes 1 to 2 hours to complete and a short form (64 items) that is estimated to take 30 to 45 minutes to complete. The LIFE-H assesses (1) level of accomplishment (according to level of difficulty and type of assistance) and (2) level of satisfaction. Level of accomplishment and satisfaction scores can be computed for items, life habit categories, and global scores.

Participation and Environment Measure for Children and Youth

The Participation and Environment Measure for Children and Youth (PEM-CY) (Coster, Law, & Bedell, 2010) is a caregiver-report instrument that combines assessment of participation and environment in a single measure. The PEM-CY contains 25 participation items reflecting broad types of activities that are typically done at home, at school, or in the community. Each participation item is rated in three ways: (1) frequency (from 0 = *never* to 7= *daily*), (2) involvement (from 1 = *minimally* to 5 = *very involved*), and (3) desire for change (Parents are asked if they want their child's participation to change [yes/no], and if yes, the parent is asked to indicate all of the ways in which change is desired [e.g., more or less frequency, more or less involvement, and/or more variety]). For each setting, parents are asked about whether features of the environment help or hinder their child's participation and whether there are available or adequate resources to support their child's participation. When administered online, the PEM-CY takes 20 to 30 minutes to complete and is a reliable and valid measure for children and youth ages 5 to 17 years, with and without disabilities (Coster et al., 2011). In its current version, the PEM-CY asks parents to identify up to three strategies for promoting their child's participation in each setting. The PEM-CY was originally designed for population-based assessment, although the use of a clinimetric approach (Coster et al., 2011) makes it possible to create composite or summary scores by administering a portion of the measure (e.g., home section) or by pulling items together to address a specific area of participation (e.g., participation in work-related activities that occur in the home, school, and community).

Selected Participation Measures for Adults and Older Adults

We report on five adult participation measures, some of which have been reviewed in greater detail in other chapters in this text.

Meaningful Activity Participation Assessment

The Meaningful Activity Participation Assessment (MAPA) is a survey checklist that was developed in the context of the USC Well Elderly 2 study and is designed to capture the meaningfulness of activity in older adults. The MAPA contains 28 activities ranging from using public transportation to physical exercise to musical activities to computer use. The respondent is asked to indicate how frequently they participate in each activity (from 0 = *not at all* to 7 = *every day*). The client is also asked to rate the meaningfulness of each activity, or "how much it matters or is personally fulfilling to you" (from 0 = *not at all meaningful* to 4 = *extremely meaningful*). The total score reflects the individual's overall level of meaningful activity participation by taking the frequency ratings and multiplying it by the meaning rating for each of the 28 activities. When summed, a total score is obtained such that higher scores indicate higher meaningful activity participation.

Engagement in Meaningful Activity Scale

The Engagement in Meaningful Activity Scale (EMAS) is a 12-item survey initially developed by Goldberg, Brintnell, and Goldberg (2002) and subsequently revised and validated (Eakman, 2007, 2011; Eakman, Carlson, & Clark, 2010a, 2010b). The EMAS also addresses meaningful participation and the respondent is asked to identify the accuracy of each statement to himself or herself (from 1 = *never* to 5 = *always*).

Activity Card Sort

The Activity Card Sort (ACS) (Baum & Edwards, 2008) is intended to help practitioners document the client's participation in instrumental, leisure, and social activities. The ACS uses Q-sort methodology that is a rank order procedure in which the client sorts a series of photographs into categories based on the question being posed by the person administering the assessment. There are 89 photographs that fall into one of the following domains: 20 instrumental activities, 35 low-physical-demand leisure activities, 17 high-physical-demand leisure activities, and 17 social activities. There are three versions of the ACS. The first version is for healthy older adults and involves having clients sort 80 photographs into the following 5 categories: never done, not doing as an older adult, do now, do less, and given up. The second version is intended for use with clients receiving services in a hospital, rehabilitation, or skilled nursing facility and uses the same 80 photographs that are sorted into two groups—done prior to illness or not done. The third version is intended for use with clients to record changes in activity patterns and the client sorts photographs into the following categories: not done in the last 5 years, gave up due to illness, beginning to do again, and do now. The score for each version of the ACS reflects the percentage of activities that the client maintains or retains.

Craig Handicap Assessment and Reporting Technique

The Craig Handicap Assessment and Reporting Technique (CHART) (Whiteneck, Charlifue, Gerhart, Overholser, & Richardson, 1992) was originally developed as a self-report instrument for persons with spinal cord injury, but it has since been used with other groups of individuals with physical disabilities. Content development was guided by the International Classification of Impairments, Disabilities, and Handicaps (ICIDH). There are 27 questions grouped into subscales addressing physical independence, mobility, occupation, social integration, and economic self-sufficiency. Questions focus on objective indicators such as time spent on a given activity or number of social contacts.

Participation Objective, Participation Subjective

The Participation Objective, Participation Subjective (POPS) (Brown, 2006; Brown et al., 2004) is a self-report survey that can be completed in about 10 to 20 minutes. It consists of 26 items that are situations of participation (e.g., going out, doing housework). Two types of questions are asked for each item, an objective question (e.g., "How often do you do this activity in a typical month?") and a subjective question (e.g., "How important is this activity?" "Are you satisfied with your level of participation?"). The items are grouped into five categories that reflect several chapters of the ICF: domestic life; major life activities; transportation; interpersonal interactions and relationships; and community, recreational, and civic life. Although it was developed in the context of traumatic brain injury, its content is broadly relevant to other adult populations.

Community Integration Questionnaire

The Community Integration Questionnaire (CIQ) (Corrigan & Deming, 1995; Sander et al., 2007; Willer, Rosenthal, Kreutzer, Gordon, & Rempel, 1993) is a brief semistructured phone interview that was developed for assessment of individuals after traumatic brain injury. The CIQ contains 15 items relevant to home integration, school integration, and productive activities. The respondent is asked how often the activity is performed and whether he or she performs the activity alone, with another person, or if performed by someone else. Subscores and a total community integration score can be computed based on frequency of performing activities or roles and whether or not activities are done jointly with others.

In summary, the measures reviewed in this section offer different approaches to gathering information about your client's participation. Even if initially designed for a purpose other than intervention planning, most of these selected measures could be used for intervention planning to describe a client's participation profile. When selecting the best measure for your information-gathering needs, it is important to first identify your clinical question and then identify those measures that best match that question in terms of the following considerations: (1) the characteristics of your target population (e.g., a 3-year-old child with developmental delay in which case only a subset of measures that have been validated on young children would be appropriate); (2) the type of information you are interested in gathering (e.g., areas where children are least satisfied in their participation in community activities, denoting an interest in gathering information about the subjective qualities of participation pertaining to a comprehensive set of activities within a specific setting); (3) whether it is important for you to obtain estimates of change in your client's participation, in which case you would want to identify measures that have some reported evidence of responsiveness to change or that have the potential to detect change, as is the case with measures that ask about participation in discrete activities vs. broader areas of activities; and (4) how much time you have to gather this information in the context of your daily practice.

Interventions to Promote Social Participation

Social participation is rather unique: it can simultaneously be viewed as a separate area of occupation (as defined in the "Occupational Therapy Practice Framework" [AOTA, 2008]) and as one aspect of engagement in other areas of occupation. Given that individuals have a strong motivation to be engaged with others, we suggest that social participation should always be considered when designing occupational therapy intervention, although the emphasis on social participation may differ according to the client's goals and current situation. For the purpose of this discussion, it is useful to distinguish two major ways in which social participation may be incorporated into intervention: (1) social participation as an *end goal* of intervention and (2) social participation as a *component* of a multifaceted intervention program.

There are numerous situations in which the primary target of occupational therapy intervention may be to improve clients' social participation, such as when interventions are designed to empower individuals who are socially isolated due to stigmatization, remove barriers that limit access to desired social activities, and/or help facilitate changes in an individual's major life roles following the onset of a chronic health condition. Although participation is inextricably linked to the environment, it is important to recognize the two-pronged approach to developing interventions that can promote social participation. By two-pronged approach, we mean that these types of interventions may involve an individual client or group of clients or they may be directed at a community agency, regulatory process, or environment. As support to this dual approach to intervention, Law and colleagues (2011) recently carried out a cluster randomized control trial in which they examined the relative efficacy of child-focused and context-focused intervention approaches for young children with cerebral palsy and found them to be equally effective.

Client-Centered Approaches to Promoting Social Participation as End Goal

Occupational therapists can intervene with individual clients to help them become participating members of a community, such as by linking the individual client to various services and supports before a crisis occurs and by helping them develop peer networks. As an example, Kramer and colleagues (in press) at Boston University have recently developed and pilot tested a TEAM intervention that applies a participatory action research approach to help youth with disabilities identify and advocate for removal of environmental barriers that prevent them from participating in school and community life. As another example, Schelly, Davies, and Spooner (2011) at the Center for Community Partnerships at Colorado State University are implementing a peer-mentored approach to help students with an ASD or Asperger's disorder develop strategies to navigate challenges associated with taking full advantage of college life such as time management and study skills, effective communication, forming relationships, and learning to advocate for themselves in the educational setting. As seen by these examples, the methods of intervention depend on the nature of the identified barriers limiting participation. Barriers related to lack of knowledge about available resources may be addressed through client education and guided exploration. On the other hand, barriers due to lack of accessibility may need to be addressed through advocacy with planning, building, and policy groups.

When social participation is the client's primary goal, it is important to ensure that the client's own definition of meaningful and satisfying participation guides the design of the intervention. Individuals have different preferences for different types of social engagement with others: some are "group" people, whereas others may be seeking a closer friendship with a few people; some enjoy and are comfortable with conversation as a main activity, others prefer to engage in the context of doing an activity together. Therefore, it is not enough to simply identify situations that offer social participation: the nature of the setting and their activities need to fit with individuals' values, interests, and preferences. The opportunity for choice is an important component to facilitating meaningful social participation, and clients may need a period of guided exploration to discover the options that offer the best fit.

Context-Based Interventions to Promote Social Participation as End Goal

Use of universal design principles to directly intervene on the environment have been applied by occupational therapy practitioners to promote social participation (see Chapter 18). For example, ensuring that residences have a single-level entrance and 32-in wide access to a bathroom on the main level are ways to ensure the "visitability" of a home (Maisel, 2006). The ACCESS project through the Center for Community Partnerships at Colorado State University builds on preliminary, successful implementation and dissemination of Universal Design for Learning (UDL) principles and strategies to improve the learning experience and persistence of college students with disabilities (Schelly et al., 2011). As yet another example of this environmentally focused approach to intervention, Cohn has been invited to consult for museums about how to increase access to and learning by visitors with and without disabilities (Silverman, Bartley, Cohn, Kanics, & Walsh, in press).

Although most of this discussion has focused on planned activities to facilitate social participation, spontaneous occurrences may offer unexpected opportunities.

Cohn (2001) provides an example in her description of the "waiting room," where parents whose children were attending therapy appointments began to connect with each other to share experiences. This example serves as a reminder of the important role the therapists can play in facilitating social participation simply by arranging the environments they work in. For example, one could experiment to see which arrangement of seating seems to facilitate social exchanges among clients in a waiting room area or among adults in a supported living environment. Evidence regarding the impact of color, lighting, organization of space, and selection of choice of play materials may be helpful to maximize the number of opportunities for spontaneous social participation within a particular clinic, school, or community setting.

Another focus of a context-based intervention approach is one that considers the human dimensions of environments, particularly in supported work and living situations such as group homes or assisted living facilities. Staff in these programs may view their primary role to be enabling clients to complete necessary daily tasks such as dressing, grooming, or eating and may not recognize the important role that meaningful social participation can play in supporting health and well-being. Educating staff in ways to facilitate client engagement in meaningful occupation in ways that also support social participation may be an important role for the occupational therapist in these settings. For example, studies have shown the positive impact of appropriate training of direct-care staff in group homes to increase the participation of residents with intellectual and developmental disabilities in social interactions and daily activities (Jones et al., 1999).

Interventions to Promote Social Participation as a Component of a Broader Program

Some interventions address social participation because it is believed to enhance the therapeutic value of the program. This is a key idea underlying various health promotion initiatives such as the Well Elderly Study 2 (Clark et al., 1997, 2011) and programs that apply concepts from this key study, including adult day programs (Horowitz & Chang, 2004) and older adults in senior housing (Matsuka, Giles-Heinz, Flinn, Neighbor, & Bass-Haugen, 2003). This is also the underlying premise of peer support groups, where it is believed that connecting with others who face similar challenges will decrease the sense of social isolation and provide additional emotional support and resources for managing the day-to-day impact of a health condition. Examples include self-management groups such as symptom self-management programs for people with multiple sclerosis (Finlayson, Preissner, Cho, & Plow, 2011) or Parkinson's disease (Tickle-Degnen, Ellis, Saint-Hilaire, Thomas, & Wagenaar, 2010). Some intervention programs may have more specific goals to provide positive social experiences as a component of an overall prevention effort. For example, Bazyk and Bazyk (2009) have been funded to develop social-skills groups for urban youth. Anti-bullying efforts share this goal of reducing risk by enhancing the overall social climate of the school community, as do programs designed to foster respect for diversity by engaging individuals from different groups in collaborative learning experiences. It is important to realize that simply incorporating social interaction into a group is not sufficient to ensure that meaningful social participation or participation that truly facilitates achievement of other group goals will occur. Just as activities need to be carefully selected to support achieving client skill development goals, the process and activities of the group also need to be carefully selected to facilitate meaningful social participation. Relevant considerations include the size and makeup of group, type of leadership and decision-making processes, and member roles and responsibilities.

Conclusions and Future Directions

Research to understand participation has been developing rapidly in the past decade and will continue to grow in the coming years. Most of the assessments and interventions described in this chapter were developed and tested within the past decade. Although most of the measures described were initially designed to support service planning to promote a client's participation, some of these assessments have been adapted for use in research studies to examine the participation patterns of clients according to such characteristics as their age, disability, or gender. The alternative uses of these measures have helped to develop a knowledge base about participation that can inform the implementation of evidence-based practice (see Chapter 31). Although participation in everyday occupations is the reason for occupational therapy, we expect that practitioners will want to stay abreast of developments in the following key areas and consider ways of contributing to them while situated in practice: (1) development and testing of new measures of social participation and/or development and validation of measures for alternative uses; (2) applying measures of social participation to identify participation patterns, profiles, and thresholds for individuals with or at risk for disabilities across the life course; and (3) the design and testing of new client-centered and context-based interventions to promote social participation.

Acknowledgments

We thank Colorado State University graduate occupational therapy students Sarah Pickle, Christina Alvord, and Anna Martin who have helped insert references and/or review earlier drafts of this chapter. We thank Karen Jacobs and Boston University graduate occupational therapy students whose photographic depictions of social participation across the life course have enhanced our mode of delivery on this important topic.

References

American Occupational Therapy Association. (2008). Occupational therapy practice framework: Domain and process, 2nd edition. *American Journal of Occupational Therapy, 62,* 625–683.

Baum, C., & Edwards, D. (2008). *Activity Card Sort* (2nd ed.). Bethesda, MD: American Occupational Therapy Association Press.

Bazyk, S., & Bazyk, J. (2009). Meaning of occupation-based groups for low-income urban youths attending after-school care. *American Journal of Occupational Therapy, 63,* 69–80.

Bedell, G. M. (2004). Developing a follow-up survey focused on participation of children and youth with acquired brain injuries after discharge from inpatient rehabilitation. *Neurorehabilitation, 19,* 191–205.

Bedell, G. M. (in press). Measurement of social participation. In V. Anderson & M. Beauchamp (Eds.), *Developmental social neuroscience and childhood brain insult: Implication for theory and practice.* New York, NY: Guilford.

Bedell, G. M. (2009). Further validation of the Child and Adolescent Scale of Participation (CASP). *Developmental Neurorehabilitation, 12,* 342–351.

Bedell, G. M., Cohn, E., & Dumas, H. (2005). Exploring parents' use of strategies to promote social participation of school-age children with acquired brain injuries. *American Journal of Occupational Therapy, 59,* 273–284.

Bedell, G. M., & Coster, W. (2008). Measuring participation of school-aged children with traumatic brain injuries: Considerations and approaches. *Journal of Head Trauma Rehabilitation, 23,* 220–229.

Bedell, G. M., & Dumas, H. M. (2004). Social participation of children and youth with acquired brain injuries discharged from inpatient rehabilitation: a follow-up study. *Brain Injury, 18,* 65–82.

Bedell, G. M., Khetani, M. A., Cousins, M. A., Coster, W. J., & Law, M. C. (2011). Parent perspectives to inform development of measures of children's participation and environment. *Archives of Physical Medicine & Rehabilitation, 92,* 765–773.

Berg, C., & LaVesser, P. (2006). The Preschool Activity Card Sort. *OTJR: Occupation, Participation and Health, 26,* 143–151.

Brown, M. (2006). Participation Objective, Participation Subjective. *The Center for Outcome Measurement in Brain Injury.* Retrieved from http://www.tbims.org/combi/pops

Brown, M., Dijkers, M., Gordon, W., Ashman, T., Charatz, H., & Cheng, Z. (2004). Participation Objective, Participation Subjective: A measure of participation combining outsider and insider perspectives. *The Journal of Head Trauma Rehabilitation, 19,* 459–481.

Brown, M., & Gordon, W. (2004). Empowerment in measurement: "muscle," "voice," and subjective quality of life as a gold standard. *Archives of Physical Medicine & Rehabilitation, 85,* S13–S20.

Clark, F. A., Azen, S. P., Zemke, R., Jackson, J. M., Carlson, M. E., Hay, J., . . . Lipson, L. (1997). Occupational therapy for independent-living older adults: A randomized controlled trial. *Journal of the American Medical Association, 278,* 1321–1326.

Clark, F. A., Jackson, J. M., Carlson, M. E., Chou, C. P., Cherry, B. J., Jordan-Marsh, M., . . . Azen, S. P. (2011). Effectiveness of a lifestyle intervention in promoting the well-being of independently living older people: Results of the Well Elderly 2 Randomised Controlled Trial. *Journal of Epidemiology and Community Health.* Advance online publication. doi:10.1136/jech.2009.099754

Clingenpeel, B. T., & McWilliam, R. A. (2003). *Scale for the Assessment of Teachers' Impressions of Routines and Engagement (SATIRE).* Vanderbilt University Medical Center: Center for Child Development.

Cohn, E. S. (2001). From waiting to relating: Parents' experiences in the waiting room of an occupational therapy clinic. *American Journal of Occupational Therapy, 55,* 168–175.

Corrigan, J. D., & Deming, R. (1995). Psychometric characteristics of the Community Integration Questionnaire: Replication and extension. *Journal of Head Trauma Rehabilitation, 10,* 41–53.

Coster, W. J. (2006). Guest editorial. The road forward to better measures for practice and research. *OTJR: Occupation, Participation & Health, 26,* 131.

Coster, W. J., Bedell, G. M., Law, M., Khetani, M., Teplicky, R., Liljenquist, K., . . . Kao, Y. (2011). Psychometric evaluation of the Participation and Environment Measure for Children and Youth. *Developmental Medicine & Child Neurology, 53,* 1030–1037.

Coster, W. J., Deeney, T., Haltiwanger, J., & Haley, S. M. (1998). *School Function Assessment.* San Antonio, TX: PsychCorp.

Coster, W. J., & Khetani, M. (2008). Measuring participation of children with disabilities: Issues and challenges. *Disability & Rehabilitation, 30,* 639–648.

Coster, W. J., Law, M., & Bedell, G. M. (2010). *Participation and Environment Measure for Children and Youth (PEM-CY).* Boston, MA: Boston University.

Coster, W. J., Law, M., Bedell, G. M., Khetani, M., Cousins, M., & Teplicky, R. (2012). Development of the participation and environment measure for children and youth: Conceptual basis. *Disability & Rehabilitation, 34,* 238–246.

Cutchin, M. (2004). Using Deweyan philosophy to rename and reframe adaptation-to-environment. *American Journal of Occupational Therapy, 58,* 303–312.

Dunst, C., Hamby, D., Trivette, C., Raab, M., & Bruder, M. (2002). Young children's participation in everyday family and community activity. *Psychological Reports, 91,* 875–897.

Eakman, A. (2007). Occupation and social complexity. *Journal of Occupational Science, 14,* 82–91.

Eakman, A. (2011). Convergent validity of the engagement in meaningful activities survey in a college sample. *OTJR: Occupation, Participation and Health, 31,* 23–32. doi:10.3928/15394492-20100122-02.

Eakman, A., Carlson, M., & Clark, F. (2010a). Factor structure, reliability, and convergent validity of the Engagement in Meaningful Activities Survey for older adults. *OTJR: Occupation, Participation & Health, 30,* 111–121.

Eakman, A. M., Carlson, M., & Clark, F. (2010b). The Meaningful Activity Participation Assessment: A measure of engagement in personally valued activities. *International Journal of Aging and Human Development, 70,* 339–357.

Finlayson, M., Preissner, K., Cho, C., & Plow, M. (2011). Randomized trial of a teleconference-delivered fatigue management program for people with multiple sclerosis. *Multiple Sclerosis, 17,* 1130–1140.

Goldberg, B., Brintnell, E., & Goldberg, J. (2002). The relationship between engagement in meaningful activities and quality of life in persons disabled by mental illness. *Occupational Therapy in Mental Health, 18,* 17–44.

Guralnick, M. J. (2005). Early intervention for children with intellectual disabilities: Current knowledge and future prospects. *Journal of Applied Research in Intellectual Disabilities, 18,* 313–324. doi:10.1111/j.1468-3148.2005.00270.x

Hammel, J., Magasi, S., Heinemann, A., Whiteneck, G., Bogner, J., & Rodriguez, E. (2008). What does participation mean? An insider perspective from people with disabilities. *Disability & Rehabilitation, 30,* 1445–1460.

Hays, R., Hahn, H., & Marshall, G. (2002). Use of the SF-36 and other health-related quality of life measures to assess persons with disabilities. *Archives of Physical Medicine & Rehabilitation, 83,* S4–S9.

Heah, T., Case, T., McGuire, B., & Law, M. (2007). Successful participation: The lived experience among children with disabilities. *Canadian Journal of Occupational Therapy, 74,* 38–47.

Heinemann, A. W. (2010). Measurement of participation in rehabilitation research. *Archives of Physical Medicine and Rehabilitation, 92,* 1729–1730.

Hemmingsson, H., & Jonsson, H. (2005). The issue is an occupational perspective on the concept of participation in the International Classification of Functioning, Disability and Health—some critical remarks. *American Journal of Occupational Therapy, 59*, 569–576.

Horowitz, B. P., & Chang, P. F. J. (2004). Promoting well-being and engagement in life through occupational therapy lifestyle redesign: A pilot study with adult day programs. *Topics in Geriatric Rehabilitation, 20*, 46–58.

Jackson, J. (1998a). Contemporary criticisms of role theory . . . part 1. *Journal of Occupational Science, 5*, 49–55.

Jackson, J. (1998b). Is there a place for role theory in occupational science? . . . part 2. *Journal of Occupational Science, 5*, 56–65.

Jones, E., Perry, J., Lowe, K., Felce, D., Toogood, S., Dunstan, F., . . . Pagler, J. (1999). Opportunity and the promotion of activity among adults with severe intellectual disability living in community residences: The impact of training staff in active support. *Journal of Intellectual Disability Research, 43*, 164–178.

Khetani, M. A., Cohn, E., Orsmond, G., Law, M., & Coster, W. (2011). Parent perspectives of participation in home and community life when receiving Part C early intervention services. *Topics in Early Childhood Special Education*. doi: 10.1177/0271121411418004

King, G. A., Law, M., King, S., Hurley, P., Rosenbaum, P., Hanna, S., . . . Young, N. (2004). *Children's Assessment of Participation & Enjoyment (CAPE) and Preferences for Activities of Children (PAC)*. San Antonio, TX: PsychCorp.

Kramer, J., Barth, Y., Curtis, K., Livingston, K., O'Neil, M., Smith, Z., . . . Wolfe, A. (in press). Involving youth with disabilities in the development and evaluation of a new advocacy training: Project TEAM. Disability and Rehabilitation.

Kramer, J., & Hammel, J. (2011). "I do lots of things": Children with cerebral palsy perceptions of competence for everyday activities. *International Journal of Disability, Development, and Education, 58*, 121–136.

Law, M., Darrah, J., Pollock, N., Wilson, B., Russell, D., Walter, S., . . . Galuppi, B. (2011). Focus on function: A cluster, randomized controlled trial comparing child- versus context-focused intervention for young children with cerebral palsy. *Developmental Medicine & Child Neurology, 53*, 621–629.

Law, M., King, G., Petrenchik, T., Kertoy, M., Anaby, D. (2012). The Assessment of Preschool Children's Participation: Internal consistency and construct validity. *Physical & Occupational Therapy in Pediatrics*. Advance online publication. doi: 10.3109/01942638.2012.662584

Lawlor, M. (2003). The significance of being occupied: The social construction of childhood occupations. *American Journal of Occupational Therapy, 57*, 424–434.

Lollar, D. J., & Andresen, E. M. (Eds.). (2011). Introduction. In *Public health perspectives on disability: Epidemiology to ethics and beyond* (pp. 3–12). New York, NY: Springer Publishing.

Mactavish, J., & Schleien, S. (1998). Playing together growing together: Parents' perspectives on the benefits of family recreation in families that include children with a developmental disability. *Therapeutic Recreation Journal, 32*, 207–230.

Magasi, S., & Hammel, J. (2004). Social support and social network mobilization in African American women who have experienced strokes. *Disability Studies Quarterly, 24*(4).

Maisel, J. L. (2006). Toward inclusive housing and neighborhood design: A look at visitability. *Community Development, 37*, 26–34.

Majnemer, A., Shikako-Thomas, K., Chokron, N., Law, M., Shevell, M., Chlingaryan, G., . . . Rosenbaum, P. (2010). Leisure activity preferences for 6–12 year old children with cerebral palsy. *Developmental Medicine & Child Neurology, 52*, 167–173.

Mandich, A., Polatajko, H., Miller, L., & Baum, C. (2004). *The Pediatric Activity Card Sort (PACS)*. Ottowa, ON: Canadian Association of Occupational Therapists.

Matsuka, K., Giles-Heinz, A., Flinn, N., Neighbor, M., & Bass-Haugen, J. (2003). Outcomes of a pilot occupational therapy wellness program for older adults. *American Journal of Occupational Therapy, 57*, 220–224.

McConachie, H., Colver, A., Forsyth, R., Jarvis, S., & Parkinson, K. (2006). Participation of disabled children: How should it be characterised and measured? *Disability & Rehabilitation, 28*, 1157–1164.

McDougall, J., Wright, V., Schmidt, J., Miller, L., & Lowry, K. (2011). Applying the ICF framework to study changes in quality-of-life for youth with chronic conditions. *Developmental Neurorehabilitation, 14*, 41–53.

McWilliam, R. A., Casey, A. M., & Sims, J. (2009). The Routines-Based Interview: A method for gathering information and assessing needs. *Infants & Young Children, 22*, 224–233.

Morris, C., Kurinczuk, J., & Fitzpatrick, R. (2005). Child or family assessed measures of activity performance and participation for children with cerebral palsy: A structured review. *Child: Care, Health and Development, 31*, 397–407.

Noreau, L., Fougeyrollas, P., Post, M., & Asano, M. (2005). Participation after spinal cord injury: The evolution of conceptualization and measurement. *Journal of Neurologic Physical Therapy, 29*(3), 147–156.

Noreau, L., Lepage, C., Boissiere, L., Picard, R., Fougeyrollas, P., Mathieu, J., & Nadeau, L. (2007). Measuring participation in children with disabilities using the Assessment of Life Habits. *Developmental Medicine & Child Neurology, 49*, 666–671.

Olsen, J. A. (2004). Mothering co-occupations in caring for infants and young children. In S. A. Esdaile & J. A. Olsen (Eds.), *Mothering occupations: Challenge, agency and participation* (pp. 28–51). Philadelphia, PA: F. A. Davis.

Rosenberg, L., Jarus, T., & Bart, O. (2010). Development and initial validation of the Children Participation Questionnaire (CPQ). *Disability & Rehabilitation, 32*(20), 1633–1644. doi:10.3109/09638281003611086

Sander, A. M., Seel, R. T., Kreutzer, J. S., Hall, K. M., High, W. M., & Rosenthal, M. (2007). Agreement between persons with traumatic brain injury and their relatives regarding psychosocial outcome using the Community Integration Questionnaire. *Archives of Physical Medicine and Rehabilitation, 78*, 353–357.

Schelly, C., Davies, P., & Spooner, C. (2011). Student perceptions of faculty implementation of universal design for learning. *Journal of Postsecondary Education and Disability, 24*, 17–28.

Scott, S., & McWilliam, R. A. (2000). *Scale for Assessment of Family Enjoyment within Routines (SAFER)*. Frank Porter Graham Child Development Center, University of North Carolina at Chapel Hill.

Shikako-Thomas, K., Lach, L., Majnemer, A., Nimignon, J., Cameron, K., & Shevell, M. (2009). Quality of life from the perspective of adolescents with cerebral palsy: "I just think I'm a normal kid, I just happen to have a disability." *Quality of Life Research, 18*, 825–832.

Silverman, F., Bartley, B., Cohn, E. S., Kanics, I. M., & Walsh, L. (in press). Occupational therapy partnerships with museums. *The International Journal of the Inclusive Museum*.

Stoffel, A., & Berg, C. (2008). Spanish translation and validation of the Preschool Activity Card Sort. *Physical & Occupational Therapy in Pediatrics, 28*, 171–189.

Tamis-Monda, C. S., Way, N., Hughes, D., Yoshikawa, H., Kalman, R. K., & Niwa, E. Y. (2007). Parents' goals for children: The dynamic coexistence of individualism and collectivism in cultures and individuals. *Social Development, 17*, 183–209.

Tickle-Degnen, L., Ellis, T., Saint-Hilaire, M. H., Thomas, C. A., & Wagenaar, R. (2010). Self-management rehabilitation and health-related quality of life in Parkinson's disease: A randomized controlled trial. *Movement Disorders, 25*, 194–204.

Ueda, S., & Okawa, Y. (2003). The subjective dimension of functioning and disability: What is it and what is it for? *Disability & Rehabilitation, 25*, 596–601.

Wade, D., & Halligan, P. (2007). Social roles and long-term illness: Is it time to rehabilitate convalescence? *Clinical Rehabilitation, 21*, 291–298.

Whiteneck, G. (2006). Conceptual models of disability: Past, present, and future. In M. J. Field & A. M. Jette (Eds.), *The future of disability in America* (pp. 50–64). Washington, DC: The National Academies Press.

Whiteneck, G., Charlifue, S., Gerhart, K., Overholser, J., & Richardson, G. (1992). Quantifying handicap: A new measure of long-term rehabilitation outcomes. *Archives of Physical Medicine and Rehabilitation, 73*, 519–526.

Whiteneck, G., & Dijkers, M. (2009). Difficult to measure constructs: Conceptual and methodological issues concerning participation and environmental factors. *Archives of Physical Medicine and Rehabilitation, 90*, S22–S35. doi:10.1016/j.apmr.2009.06.009

Willer, B., Rosenthal, M., Kreutzer, J. S., Gordon, W. A., & Rempel, R. (1993). Assessment of community integration following rehabilitation for traumatic brain injury. *Journal of Head Trauma Rehabilitation, 8*, 75–87.

Wilson, L., Mott, D. W., & Batman, D. (2004). The Asset-Based Context Matrix: A tool for assessing children's learning opportunities and participation in natural environments. *Topics in Early Childhood Special Education, 24*, 110–120.

World Health Organization. (1998). *Quality of life.* Retrieved from http://www.who.int/healthpromotion/about/HPR%20Glossary%201998.pdf

World Health Organization. (2001). *International classification of functioning, disability and health: ICF.* Geneva, Switzerland: Author.

World Health Organization. (2007). *International classification of functioning, disability and health: Version for children and youth.* Geneva, Switzerland: Author.

World Health Organization & World Bank. (2011). *World report on disability.* Retrieved from http://www.who.int/disabilities/world_report/en/index.html

For additional resources on the subjects discussed in this chapter, visit http://thePoint.lww.com/Willard-Spackman12e.

UNIT XII

Theory Guided Interventions: Examples from the Field

"Individuals have characteristics that support their participation; professionals have the responsibility to focus on their strengths as the foundation for of service programs and satisfying outcomes."

—Winnie Dunn

CHAPTER 53

Overview of Theory Guided Intervention

Barbara A. Boyt Schell, Glen Gillen

OUTLINE

LEARNING OBJECTIVES

After reading this chapter, you will be able to:

1. Discuss the importance of client subjective experiences in considering therapy approaches
2. Explore the limitations of deficit-oriented theories in light of the strength-based models
3. Critically examine both the benefits and limitations of restorative approaches in improving client participation
4. Examine opportunities for improving participation by attending to client preferences, occupational needs, and the timing and duration of theoretical approaches focused on client impairments

Introduction

Occupational therapy is a profession that demands much of its practitioners. Excellence in occupational therapy practice presumes that practitioners appreciate the complexity of occupation and are committed to helping those we serve be able to participate meaningfully in society. As discussed in many previous chapters in this text, occupation is seen as having curative powers as a therapeutic medium, but it is also seen as an end in itself. For those seeking to use occupation in a way that restores bodily impairments or promote improved bodily function, extensive knowledge of a range of scientifically based information from medical, educational, social, and psychological sciences is required. Occupational therapy researchers and expert practitioners blend knowledge from these fields with occupational therapy theories, and as a result, develop evaluation and intervention methods that are informed by these interdisciplinary perspectives. In this unit, we introduce you to some of the major theoretical perspectives that are commonly used in occupational therapy practice and have growing bodies of evidence indicating that they are effective approaches. Topics addressed include motor function, cognition and perception, sensory processing, emotional regulation, and communication/social interaction. Note that each chapter addresses these in the context of occupational performance and participation. Chapters include in-depth summaries of current practice theories and models that guide intervention, examples of standardized assessments used to document change, and available evidence to guide practitioners using these approaches.

Before moving on to these chapters, it is important to gain a sense of perspective about how these theories "fit" within effective occupational therapy practice. Important perspectives drawn from philosophy, disability studies, and from leaders within the profession are provided as guides on how to think about and use the theories discussed in this unit. Although all of these perspectives are addressed in other ways throughout this text, we feel it is especially important to consider in a unit such as this, where attention to the vast array of important information about each aspect of performance can threaten to overshadow the focus on each person and the uniqueness of each person as an occupational being. Therefore, this chapter is designed to help the reader approach the theories and practices covered in this unit in light of the core knowledge of occupation that guides the profession.

The "I" and the "It"

Perhaps the most therapeutic action that occupational therapy practitioners can do is to always hold in mind each person's hopes, dreams, and experiences while at the same time understanding all the many person and environmental factors that affect that person and his or her occupations. As discussed earlier in Chapter 30, therapists have to use many different perspectives to pull off this therapy tall order. Adding to the complexity, much of the practice of occupational therapy occurs within systems of health care and education, which are focused on measurable results (see for instance Merry & Crago, 2001). These efforts are intended to guide policy makers on how to efficiently parcel out social resources—in other words, to figure out what is worth paying for. Unfortunately, a focus on these results can either intentionally or unintentionally depersonalize the person receiving services.

Renowned leader and scholar, Dr. Elizabeth "Betty" Yerxa (2009) provided an effective metaphor for appreciating the dualing perspectives which challenge occupational therapy in her discussion entitled "Infinite Distance Between the I and the It" (p. 490). In the abstract of this article, she notes that

> Traditional science and medical practice in the 21st century often separates the *I* consciousness, the person who experiences daily life, from the *it* of an object that can be probed, tested, and fixed. This separation may also influence the development of occupational science and the practice of occupational therapy to the detriment of the profession.

Attention to theories focused on restoring bodily functions run the risk of creating therapy situations in which practitioners lose track of their clients as individuals who have unique desires and needs. The caution here is not to avoid using effective theoretical approaches to restore function but rather to be very mindful that these theories are used in service of the "I." The purpose of working on motor control is not to "fix" someone's arm; it is to help that person who wants to move her arm in order to fix her hair. The purpose of understanding theories of cognition is not to focus on someone's problems with memory that are affecting his ability to work but rather to figure out how to help him get back to work on a job he really cares about. The purpose of understanding how we all vary in our neurological processes is not to classify a child into a particular category. It is to find the best way for that child and her family to play, learn, and do all the things that child and her family want to do.

Strength-Based Approaches

Winnie Dunn (2011), another renowned occupational therapist and scholar, raises an additional important set of issues to consider, and that is the need to focus on strengths as the basis for effective intervention. She notes that although professions and programs logically develop out of an attempt to respond to needs, she goes on to say

> There is certainly a place for finding out what is interfering with participation.... However, what has happened is that, in doing the detective work to identify needs, professionals have gotten caught up in the empty places and have forgotten to consider what is working! (p. 7)

In many instances, the chapters that follow discuss adaptive approaches, strategy training approaches, and/or environmental modifications as effective interventions that indeed tap into our client's strength to overcome performance deficits. The theories provided in this unit provide a rich wealth of resources to notice what is working for the individuals being served. Dr. Dunn's (2011) advice can be taken as a call to document the "full" places as well as to notice the empty ones. When combined with Dr. Yerxa's (2009) advice to stay focused on the *I*, the opportunities to use these theories to support participations in occupation become even more visible.

Challenging Assumptions about Learning Transfer and Skills

Beyond the need to deal with people as unique individuals and to consider their strengths as the basis for improving performance, there is another perspective to consider. In many aspects of modern society, there are pervasive assumptions about the presumed sequencing of development and learning. The saying, "You must crawl before you can walk," presumes a developmental sequence to the process. Likewise, in some universities, one must have an algebra course as a prerequisite to a statistics course. Once again, the presumption is that there are foundation skills on which higher level performance is required. Yet, many of us likely know children who went right from sitting to walking, with little "crawling" involved. Likewise, there are many students who have successfully taken college level statistics without a prior college level algebra course. In spite of these examples to the contrary, there appears to be a durable assumption that one must have certain skills or abilities in order to engage in higher level activities. Therefore, it is not surprising that this assumption underlies clinical decisions that focus on the need to remediate impairments and build component skills in preparation for engaging in occupations. Even the American Occupational Therapy Association's (AOTA) "Occupational Therapy Practice Framework, 2nd Edition" (2008) adopts the term "preparatory" for one category of interventions.

It is important that practitioners not lose focus when managing these impairments. A recent study of occupational therapy practice patterns for stroke survivors clearly demonstrates potential pitfalls when we "can't see the forest through the trees." Smallfield and Karges (2009) investigated the specific type of occupational therapy intervention used by occupational therapists during inpatient stroke rehabilitation to determine the frequency of preparatory or prefunctional versus functional activity use. Of concern is that they found that most sessions (65.77%) consisted of activities that were prefunctional in nature compared with 48.26% that focused on activities of daily living. In other words, occupational therapists used prefunctional activities that aim to improve performance skills and body structures more often than occupation-based activities that incorporate meaningful activities into therapy sessions. This is clearly in contrast to our professions current philosophy (AOTA, 2008).

> The philosophy of occupational therapy includes the premise that meaningful activity is essential to occupational therapy intervention because occupation is the power of intervention. If occupational therapists believe in the use of occupation-based activities, it is contradictory for them to use prefunctional activities more often than functional activities with this diagnostic group. (Smallfield & Karges, 2009, p. 411)

There several studies across a wide variety of disciplines that are challenging these assumptions that you must "do this" before you can "do that." In Chapter 5, Humphrey and Womack provide a convincing summary of how the demands of the performance context (both physical and social) as well as engaging in the actual occupation itself explain performance variance in daily life. Consideration of sociological and ecological perspectives tempers our understanding of developmental hierarchies by acknowledging the power of actual performance to draw out needed skills. Likewise, educational scholars over the last several decades have challenged the reliance on learning transfer in schools (Detterman & Sternberg, 1996; Lave, 1988; Lave & Wegner, 1991). Mounting evidence suggests that learning transfer is unpredictable and is context and task

BOX 53.1 Is Restoration the Best Choice? Considerations for Practice.

Just because someone has an impairment, it doesn't necessarily follow that occupational therapy intervention focused directly on that impairment is the best approach. The following questions are intended to provoke careful reflection about the assumptions underlying the choice to use a restorative approach.

- What is the client interested in being able to do? If the client is focused on a bodily impairment, why does it matter? How does it affect the client's ability to live life?
- Why restore impairments versus choosing to work directly on the occupational areas the client wants to improve?
- Can engaging in relevant occupations serve to remediate an underlying impairment? If a person is engaged in housekeeping activities such as making a bed, don't our analysis skills lead us to think that we are simultaneously "working on" balance, strength, motor planning, attention skills, and so forth?
- How much evidence is there to suggest that an intervention aimed at a body function will actually result in improved occupational performance?
- If you choose remediation, how do you know which impairment to focus on to best improve performance?
- How do we know that the impairment is amenable to remediation?
- What strengths does the client have that can be marshaled to improve performance as well as restore bodily function?
- Can the bodily impairment be used to enhance performance (e.g., a woman with spasticity in her arm might be able to use the extra tension to hold a purse)?
- Have you chosen outcome measures that are indicative of improved occupational performance versus just a change in bodily function?
- How might your own cultural lenses, both your personal one and the ones imbedded in your workplace, affect the intervention options you present to your client?
- How open are you to exploring and negotiating differences with your clients over therapy goals and expectations?

(Note: Some questions adapted from Rosa & Hasselkus, 2005)

dependent. Similar findings in the motor control literature strongly suggest that practitioners should be moving away from impairment-based hierarchical approaches to approaches that are best described as task and context specific. These approaches are clearly better aligned with past and current philosophies of our profession (the reader is referred to Chapter 54 for more detail). These and other developments have influenced many occupational therapists to critically examine the assumption that improving an impairment will automatically transfer into the improvement of occupational performance and related social participation. See Box 53.1.

Blended Approaches and a Focus on Participation

Perhaps the best way for practitioners to use the focused theories designed to manage impairments is to blend them with theories that provide a broader understanding of human learning and motivation as it occurs within the context of occupation. There is promising evidence to suggest that by directly working on the occupational tasks that the client wants or needs to do, occupational participation is enhanced. The focused theories presented in this unit can be used *in the context of assisting the client to perform actual occupations.* That is different than trying to "fix" the person. Rather, it involves harnessing sound focused therapy techniques to enhance the likelihood of success while at the same time doing the "real thing." Furthermore, working on occupational participation directly, almost automatically, ensures opportunities to recognize and build on strengths and further serves to reinforce the identity of the client as one who can participate as a valued member of society.

References

American Occupational Therapy Association. (2008). Occupational therapy practice framework: Domain and process, 2nd edition. *American Journal of Occupational Therapy, 62,* 625–683.

Detterman, D. K., & Sternberg, R. J. (1996). *Transfer on trial: Intelligence, cognition, & instruction.* Norwood, NJ: Ablex.

Dunn, W. (2011). *Best practice occupational therapy for children and families in community settings* (2nd ed.). Thorofare, NJ: Slack.

Lave, J. (1988). *Cognition in practice: Mind, mathematics and culture in everyday life.* Cambridge, United Kingdom: Cambridge University Press.

Lave, J., & Wenger, E. (1991). *Situated learning: Legitimate peripheral participation.* Cambridge: Cambridge University Press.

Merry, M. D., & Crago, M. G. (2001). The past, present and future of health care quality. Urgent need for innovative, external review processes to protect patients. *Physician Executive, 27,* 30–35.

Rosa, S. A., & Hasselkus, B. R. (2005). Finding common ground with patients: The centrality of compatibility. *American Journal of Occupational Therapy, 59,* 198–208.

Smallfield, S., & Karges, J. (2009). Classification of occupational therapy intervention for inpatient stroke rehabilitation. *American Journal of Occupational Therapy, 63,* 408–413.

Yerxa, E. J. (2009). The infinite distance between the I and the it. *American Journal of Occupational Therapy, 63,* 490–497.

For additional resources on the subjects discussed in this chapter, visit http://thePoint.lww.com/Willard-Spackman12e.

CHAPTER 54

Motor Function and Occupational Performance

Glen Gillen

OUTLINE

LEARNING OBJECTIVES

After reading this chapter, you will be able to:

1. Understand how motor function supports occupational performance throughout the life course
2. Explain how impairments related to motor function limit occupational performance across the life course
3. Compare and contrast the approaches that are used to guide the occupational therapy process related to improving occupational performance for those with motor impairments
4. Become familiar with assessments that are used to measure motor function across the life course
5. Begin to construct evidence-based intervention plans that improve occupational performance for those living with motor impairments

Introduction: Motor Function and Everyday Living

This morning you may have rolled over in bed, reached over to your nightstand to turn off the alarm, transitioned to a seated position on your bed, followed by a transition to a standing posture prior to walking to the bathroom. On your way to the bathroom, you might step into your slippers by shifting your weight from one foot to the other. Your **postural control** system combined with your trunk and limb function work together to support your functional mobility and activities of daily living (ADL).

Samuel is taking care of his child. As he lifts his child from the crib, he must generate enough force in his upper limbs to move his child, calibrate this force as to not harm his child with too much pressure in his hands, maintain his balance as he lifts his child toward him, and coordinate/plan his movements so that his hand supports his child's head as he lifts. Samuel's parenting role is being supported by various motor functions.

Danielle is going ice-skating for the first time today at the age of 4 years. To be successful, she will need to learn to maintain her center of gravity, use various postural reflexes (e.g., righting and equilibrium responses) to maintain an upright position, learn that she can integrate her upper limbs to maintain her balance, and coordinate her limbs to glide over the ice. In addition, she requires enough strength and endurance to complete the task. Danielle's ability to engage in play is supported by multiple systems and structures related to motor function. To be successful, Danielle must also process and adapt to incoming information from her sensory systems (e.g., vestibular, proprioception, vision) (see Chapter 56 for more details).

Most of the day (and night albeit to a much lesser extent) is spent engaging in occupations that require motor functions to support performance. Occupational therapy practitioners treat various conditions (see Appendix I) that result in limited motor function and loss of motor control. As you can infer from the examples earlier, any change in motor function has a tremendous impact on our ability to engage in meaningful occupations. The following two cases will illustrate these points.

Approaches That Guide Therapy

Various approaches may be used when working with clients with motor deficits. Many times, approaches are combined and/or the therapist may switch from one to another based on the client's response or preference (see Chapter 26).

Client-Centered Approach

"**Client-centered practice** refers to collaborative approaches aimed at enabling occupation with clients who may be individuals, groups, agencies, governments, corporations, or others. Occupational therapists demonstrate respect for clients, involve clients in meeting clients' needs, and otherwise recognize clients' experience and knowledge" (Law, 1998, p. 3). Use of this approach involves collaboration with clients to set goals and prioritize the focus of intervention (Law, Baptiste, & Mills, 1995; Law & Mills, 1998). Recent reviews (Maitra & Erway, 2006; Phipps & Richardson, 2007) of the literature related to this approach have revealed that the

CASE STUDY 54.1 Jacob: Limited Occupational Performance due to Hemiparesis

Jacob is an 8-year-old boy with a hemiparetic right upper limb secondary to cerebral palsy. See Appendix I for more details on cerebral palsy. Jacob's parents are frustrated because he does have minimal movement in his arm and hand. They report constantly "nagging" Jacob to use his arm when he is outside of a structured therapy session. They also describe that his arm appears "useless" when he is at school or play. Both Jacob and his parents are getting frustrated with therapy. Specifically, his parents would like to see "carryover" from his present therapy. Jacob's occupational therapist (OT) informed the parents that there was a local therapeutic camp held during school holidays. Jacob was enrolled in this camp that incorporated an intervention called **constraint-induced movement therapy** (CI therapy).

The OT at the camp evaluated Jacob via observing his arm use during unstructured play in addition to two standardized assessments of motor function (the speed and dexterity subtest of the Bruininks-Oseretsky Test and the Jebsen-Taylor Test of Hand Function). Jacob's goals were established as (1) Jacob will use his right hand to drink without cues; (2) Jacob will be able to apply paste to his toothbrush using his right hand; and (3) Jacob will swing a bat using both hands.

The CI therapy intervention consisted of the following components (Gordon, Charles, & Wolf, 2005; Morris, Taub, & Mark, 2006):

- Restraint of Jacob's less involved extremity (left) using a sling.
- Encouraging the involved side to be active via engaging Jacob in unimanual activities with the involved extremity (right) 6 hours a day for 10 days (60 hours).
- Repetitive practice embedded in play and functional activities. Examples of activities include arts and crafts, board games, card games, puzzles, cleaning a table after a meal, etc.
- The technique of **shaping** was used. Shaping involves approaching a behavioral objective (task) in small steps by successive approximation. As Jacob's performance improved, the task was made more challenging, taking into consideration his abilities. The OT graded the tasks accordingly to target movements he wanted Jacob to achieve.
- Adherence-enhancing behavioral strategies ("the transfer package") such as a caregiver contract, home diary, home practice, etc.

Following the therapy, Jacob's parents reported that he was using his involved arm more spontaneously and automatically. Jacob was able to meet his goals. ■

CASE STUDY 54.2 Samuel: Limited Occupational Performance due to a Musculoskeletal Injury

Samuel (as discussed in the opening paragraphs) fell while jogging. He landed on his dominant right shoulder and returned home complaining of weakness and excruciating pain. Samuel's orthopedist diagnosed him with a full thickness tear of his rotator cuff. See Appendix I for more details on orthopedic injuries. Surgery was scheduled and the tear was repaired. Postoperatively, Samuel was referred for occupational therapy. The occupational therapist (OT) performed evaluations focused on Samuel's impairments and activity limitations related to areas of occupation. Various standardized measures were used. A Visual Analogue Scale documented that his pain was rated as 8 on a 1 to 10 scale. His **active range of motion** and strength, as tested by a manual muscle test, were intact with the exception of his right shoulder. These tests were deferred for his injured shoulder because the medical orders allowed only passive motion until the repair site began to heal. **Passive range of motion** of his involved shoulder was limited by pain as expected. Samuel reported and demonstrated difficulty with both basic and instrumental activities of daily living (ADL), stating, "I am very right dominant." The OT administered the Disabilities of the Arm, Shoulder, and Hand (DASH) Outcome Measure including the work module because Samuel was employed as a grocery store manager. The DASH is a 30-item, self-report questionnaire designed to measure physical function and symptoms in people with any of several musculoskeletal disorders of the upper limb. The DASH provided the OT with specific information regarding how Samuel's shoulder injury was impacting his daily functioning. Samuel's long term goals were defined as (1) independent in all basic ADL, (2) independent in child care, and (3) return to work part-time.

The OT used various interventions that were graded as Samuel's tendons healed over time. The interventions were based on both rehabilitative and biomechanical approaches. These included the following:

- ADL retraining using one-handed techniques and assistive devices. This was an early focus because Samuel was not allowed to actively move his right shoulder for several weeks. While he lived with his wife, he did not want to be a burden as she was taking care of their newborn. Therefore, he was highly motivated to be as independent as possible. These techniques were only employed temporarily.
- Physical agent modalities such as ice (**cryotherapy**) for pain control
- Education related to sleep postures
- Progressive mobilization of Samuel's shoulder (passive range of motion, active assisted range of motion, active range of motion, and strengthening)
- Physical agent modalities such as therapeutic heat to increase flexibility prior to therapy
- Engaging Samuel's right arm to support performance of occupations that were graded over time. The OT began with low-height activities such as reaching into cabinets under the sink, followed by medium height activities (e.g., applying deodorant), and followed by overhead reach activities such as hanging up clothing and putting groceries away on to high shelves.
- Resumption of bilateral ADL
- Simulated work activities

Using the aforementioned approaches and interventions, Samuel was able to meet his goals and soon after resumed full-time duties at work.

use of a client-centered approach may result in the following:

- Greater engagement and motivation on the part of the client
- Improved client satisfaction
- Improved intervention outcomes
- Increases in perceived performance efficacy
- Increased client adherence to and compliance with treatment programs
- Decreased length of stay in rehabilitation facility
- Improved functional outcomes

Maitra and Erway (2006) remind us that the success of client-centered practice depends on two principle components. These include (1) the desire and ability of the clients to take part in the decision-making processes and (2) the desire and ability of the occupational therapists (OTs) to include clients in the decision-making process (see Chapter 33 for further details about this approach).

Biomechanical Approach

The **biomechanical approach** is considered a remediation approach. It is focused at the client factor/impairment level when these said impairments are limiting occupational performance. Examples of impairments that are addressed by this approach include weakness, limitations in joint **range of motion**, edema, pain, low endurance, sensory changes, joint instability, poor coordination, etc. Clients living with cardiopulmonary diseases, various forms of arthritis, burns, cumulative trauma disorders/repetitive strain injuries, tendon tears or lacerations, fractures, etc. may be appropriate for interventions based on the biomechanical approach. See Appendix I for more details on these diagnoses.

More recently, components of this approach (e.g., **strengthening**) have been applied to those living with acquired brain injuries such as a stroke (Harris & Eng, 2010). Further research is recommended to determine the appropriate candidate (e.g., the Harris and Eng paper included those with mild spasticity) as well as the ability to generalize to improved occupational performance.

This approach is based on several assumptions:

- The underlying impairment is amenable to remediation.
- Engagement in occupation and various other therapeutic activities has the potential to remediate the underlying impairment(s).
- This remediation will result in improved occupational performance.

The key to successfully using this approach is linking the underlying impairment to the occupational performance deficit. This linking must occur in both the intervention planning process as well as in goal writing. See Box 54.1 for examples of goal writing for those with motor deficits. See Tables 54.1–54.4 for examples of assessments/evaluations and interventions that are commonly used when the biomechanical approach is adopted. See Table 54.2 for examples of evidence that supports interventions used in the biomechanical approach.

Rehabilitative Approach

The **rehabilitative approach** includes the concepts of adaptation, compensation, and environmental modifications

BOX 54.1 Keeping an Occupation-Based Perspective when Using the Biomechanical Approach during Goal Writing for Reimbursement

Goal 1 incorrectly focused on the impairment: *Client will demonstrate improved grip strength of 15 lb.*

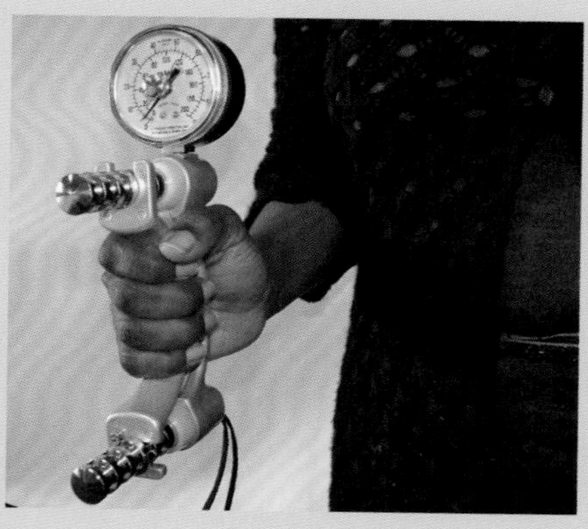

Goal 1 rewritten to reflect the change in performance: *Client will demonstrate improved grip strength of 15 lb in order to independently open a previously unopened jar.* It is assumed that the therapist has documented this client's difficulties with meal preparation in relation to her pattern of weakness. The goal should reflect an improvement in areas of occupation not an isolated change in impairment.

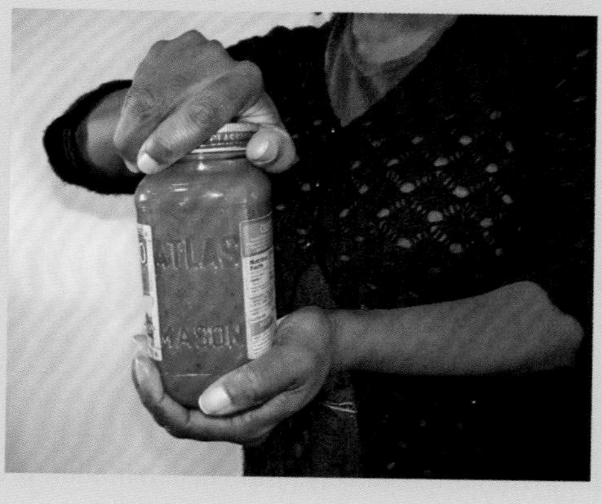

Goal 2 incorrectly focused on impairment: *Client will demonstrate a 20-degree increase in shoulder external rotation.*

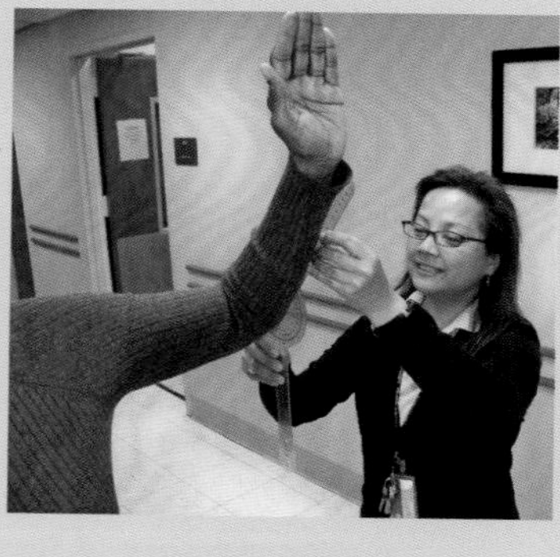

Goal 2 rewritten to reflect the change in performance: *Client will demonstrate a 20-degree increase in shoulder external rotation in order to comb the back of her hair with minimal assistance.* It is assumed that a self-care evaluation has been documented to demonstrate the impact of the loss of range of motion on basic activities of daily living.

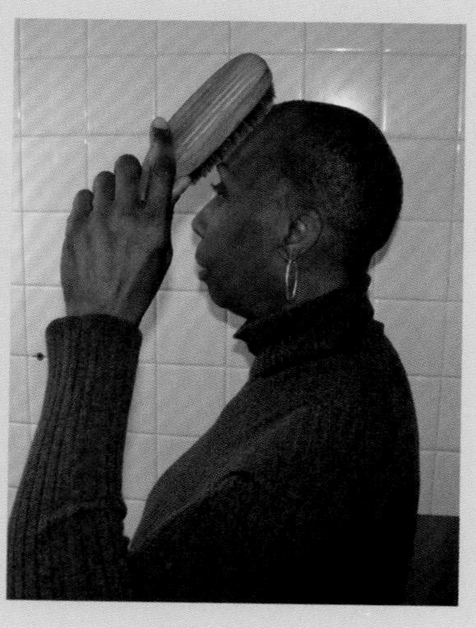

TABLE 54.1 Assessments/Evaluations and Interventions Commonly Associated with the Biomechanical Approach

Assessments/Evaluations[a]	Sample Interventions
• Standardized objective tests of occupational performance (see Unit XI) • Self-report measures of how impairments limit occupational performance (e.g., DASH, Manual Ability Measure) • Goniometry: active and passive range of motion • Manual muscle tests • Dynamometry (grip and pinch strength testing) • Sensory testing (e.g., Semmes Weinstein Monofilament Examination, 2-point discrimination) • Coordination testing • Provocative tests (tests used to provoke underlying symptoms) • Circumferential or volumetric measures to quantify edema • Pain scales • Examination of skin integrity/wounds • Borg Rating of Perceived Exertion Scale (endurance) • Ergonomic evaluations	• ADL retraining • Work hardening • Active, **active assistive**, passive **range of motion** exercises • High-load brief stretch • Low-load prolonged stretch • Orthoses (static and dynamic) (see Figures 54.1 and 54.2) • Strengthening • Endurance training • Joint protection techniques • Physical agent modalities (see Table 54.3) • Therapeutic exercise (see Table 54.4) • Edema control techniques (e.g., massage and mobilization, positional elevation, wrapping techniques) • Desensitization for hypersensitivity • Sensory retraining • Scar management • Joint mobilization • Tendon gliding • Nerve gliding

[a]See Table 54.11 and Appendix II for more details on standardized assessments for this population.

ADL, activities of daily living; DASH, disabilities of the arm, shoulder, and hand.

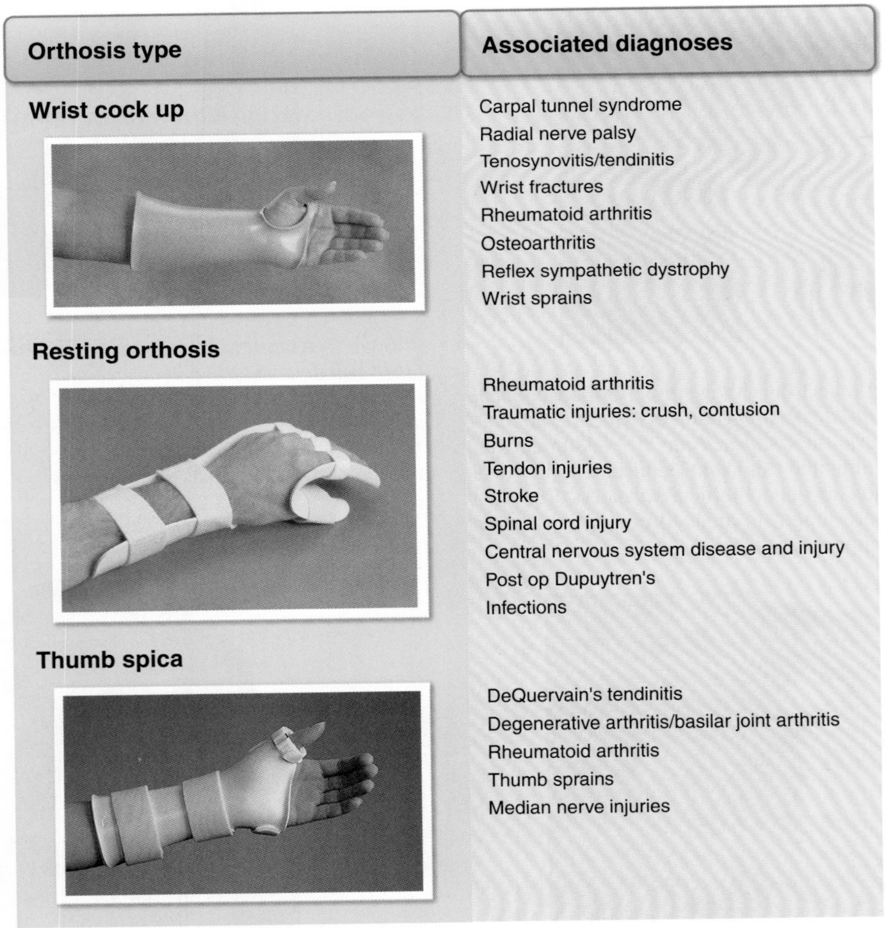

Orthosis type
Associated diagnoses
Wrist cock up
Carpal tunnel syndrome
Radial nerve palsy
Tenosynovitis/tendinitis
Wrist fractures
Rheumatoid arthritis
Osteoarthritis
Reflex sympathetic dystrophy
Wrist sprains
Resting orthosis
Rheumatoid arthritis
Traumatic injuries: crush, contusion
Burns
Tendon injuries
Stroke
Spinal cord injury
Central nervous system disease and injury
Post op Dupuytren's
Infections
Thumb spica
DeQuervain's tendinitis
Degenerative arthritis/basilar joint arthritis
Rheumatoid arthritis
Thumb sprains
Median nerve injuries

FIGURE 54.1 Common static orthoses associated with diagnostic conditions. (Photos courtesy of the Rehabilitation Division of Smith & Nephew, Germantown, WI.)

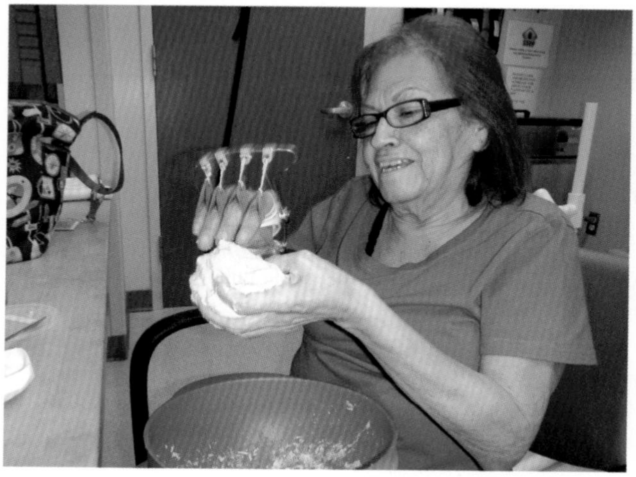

FIGURE 54.2 Using a dynamic orthosis to support engagement in occupation. (Photo courtesy of Lauro A. Munoz, OTR, MOT.)

(see Chapter 26 for more details). It may be used in conjunction with other approaches or in isolation. This approach places an emphasis on the client's strengths as opposed to their limitations. The ultimate goal is to maximize independence despite the presence of persistent impairments. This approach may be most appropriate for client's who are living with impairments that are permanent, including both static and progressive impairments. This approach may also be useful when an underlying impairment is potentially amenable to remediation but the client is not motivated to participate in the sometimes long and difficult process of remediation. Contextual factors such as limited therapy visits may also lead therapists to adopt this approach because some may argue that functional independence is achieved quicker.

Clients living with the following diagnoses may be candidates for the rehabilitative approach in isolation or in conjunction with the other approaches discussed: multiple sclerosis, amyotrophic lateral sclerosis, severe stroke, advanced arthritis, advancing Parkinson's disease, spinal cord injuries, etc. See Appendix I for more details on these diagnoses. Readers should note that the rehabilitative approach is used for various impairments beyond motor deficits.

In many cases, the OT takes on the role of "teacher" when using this approach and must consider the following questions:

1. What is the client's potential to learn?
2. Is the client motivated to learn?
3. What is the client's optimal learning style?

TABLE 54.2 Sample Evidence that Supports Interventions Used when Adopting the Biomechanical Approach

Author/Year	Objective	Conclusion
Egan & Brousseau, 2007	To review the evidence regarding the effectiveness of splinting for carpometacarpal osteoarthritis.	Research to date indicates that splinting may help relieve pain in persons with carpometacarpal osteoarthritis.
Guzelkucuk, Duman, Taskaynatan, & Dincer, 2007	To compare the efficacy of therapeutic activities that mimic the activities of daily living (ADL) with that of traditionally used therapeutic exercises in the management of injured hands in young adult patients.	The results showed that therapeutic activities that mimic ADL improve the functions of the hand more effectively. The authors suggest that therapeutic activities that mimic the ADL may be more beneficial than the standard rehabilitation activities in the management of an injured hand.
Harris & Eng, 2010	To evaluate the effects of strengthening on upper limb function after stroke via a meta-analysis.	There is evidence that strength training can improve upper limb strength and function without increasing tone or pain in individuals with stroke.
Muller et al., 2004	To determine the effectiveness of therapy interventions for carpal tunnel syndrome (CTS).	Current evidence demonstrates a significant benefit from splinting, ultrasound, nerve gliding exercises, carpal bone mobilization, magnetic therapy, and yoga for people with CTS.
Robinson et al., 2002	To evaluate the effectiveness of different physical agent modalities applications on objective and subjective measures of disease activity in patients with rheumatoid arthritis.	Superficial moist heat and cryotherapy (ice) can be used as a palliative therapy. Paraffin wax baths combined with exercises can be recommended for beneficial short-term effects for arthritic hands.
Werner, Franzblau, & Gell, 2005	To determine whether night splinting of workers identified through active surveillance with symptoms consistent with CTS would improve symptoms and median nerve function as well as impact medical care.	The results suggest that a short course of nocturnal splinting may reduce wrist, hand, and/or finger discomfort among active workers with symptoms consistent with CTS.

TABLE 54.3 Physical Agent Modalities

Modality	Indications	Contraindications/Precautions
Superficial heat: • Hot packs, heating pads • Paraffin wax • Fluidotherapy • Whirlpool	Prior to active exercise, passive stretching, and joint mobilization Before traction and soft tissue mobilization Reduce pain and muscle spasms After acute inflammation to increase tissue healing	Decreased circulation Decreased sensibility Altered cardiorespiratory status Open wounds or recently healed burns (paraffin) Significant areas of edema Over tissue during acute inflammation
Deep heat: • Ultrasound and phonophoresis	Soft tissue tightness Subacute and chronic inflammation (e.g., tendinitis) Bone fracture Wound healing	Do not use over or near the eyes, ears, heart, pregnant uterus, testes, known or expected malignant tumor, pacemaker, joint replacements or metal implants, or insensate areas
Therapeutic cold: • Cold packs and cold baths • Ice massage	Minimize acute inflammation associated with therapeutic intervention Reduce edema and bleeding Reduce spasticity	Temperature sensation deficits Circulation deficits Altered cardiorespiratory status Cold hypersensitivity such as Raynaud's phenomenon
Contrast baths	Promotes tissue healing and may control edema	Cardiovascular problems as fluctuations in pulse and blood pressure may occur Peripheral vascular diseases Loss of sensation Pregnancy Cold hypersensitivity such as Raynaud's phenomenon
Electrotherapy: • Functional electrical stimulation (neuromuscular electrical stimulation • Transcutaneous electrical nerve stimulation • Iontophoresis	Modulate pain Decrease inflammation (e.g., bursitis, tendinitis) Reduce edema Improve motor control Improve strength	Do not use over or near the eyes, ears, chest of person with cardiac disease, pregnant uterus, wounds or skin breaks, known or expected malignant tumor, pacemaker, blood vessels susceptible to hemorrhage, thrombosis or embolus, or insensate areas

Adapted from Poole, J. L. (2008). Musculoskeletal factors. In E. B. Crepeau, E. S. Cohn, & B. A. B. Schell (Eds.), *Willard & Spackman's occupational therapy* (11th ed.). Baltimore, MD: Lippincott Williams & Wilkins.

Motor learning principles to promote skill acquisition will be discussed later in this chapter. See Table 54.5 for a summary of assessments/evaluation and interventions used when adopting this approach.

Task-Oriented Approaches

Task-oriented approaches—also described as task-specific training, repetitive task practice, goal-directed training, and functional task practice—are considered the most current approach related to impaired motor function and **motor control** for those living with brain damage. Timmermans, Spooren, Kingma, and Seelen (2010) describe the components of task oriented training (see Box 54.2). In this approach, movement emerges as an interaction between many systems in the brain and is organized around a goal and constrained by the environment (Shumway-Cook & Woollacott, 2012). Rensink, Schuurmans, Lindeman, and Hafsteinsdottir (2009) describe **task-oriented training** as including a wide range of interventions such as walking training on the ground, bicycling programs, endurance training and circuit training, sit-to-stand exercises, and reaching tasks for improving balance. A major focus of task-oriented training is on arm training using functional tasks, such as grasping objects, and constraint-induced movement therapy (CI therapy) (Wolf et al., 2006). This approach is task and client focused and not therapist focused (Rensink et al., 2009). See Table 54.6 for examples of evidence that supports the use of a task-oriented approach.

Training components of the task-oriented approach have been described (adapted from Timmermans et al., 2010).

1. *Functional movements*: A movement involving task execution that is not directed toward a clear ADL goal.
2. *Clear functional goal*: A goal that is set during everyday life activities and/or hobbies (e.g., washing dishes, grooming activity, dressing oneself, playing golf).

TABLE 54.4 Therapeutic Exercise Programs

Type	Definition	Resistance	Muscles Grades	Precautions
Passive exercise	Involves passive range of motion and passive stretch, usually done by a practitioner	None Stretch may be held 15–30 seconds	Zero Trace	Inflammation Limited sensation for pain Prolonged immobilization
Isotonic active assistive exercise	Client moves the joint as far as possible, then an outside force such as a practitioner or equipment assists with moving the joint through the rest of the range	None	Trace Poor minus Fair minus	None
Isotonic active exercise	Client moves the joint through available range of motion without any assistance. The muscle shortens and lengthens.	None	Poor Fair	Poor muscles: Move in gravity eliminated plane Fair muscles: Move in against gravity plane
Isometric without resistance	Client contracts the muscle, increasing the tension, and holds the position for 5 seconds. Used when motion of a joint is prohibited.	None	Trace Poor Fair Good	Clients with cardiac conditions and high blood pressure
Isotonic resistive exercise	An isotonic contraction against resistance	Resistance provided by wrist weights, dumbbells, Thera-Band, Theraputty, elastic bands, springs, weights	Fair plus Good	Inflammation Unstable joint Recent or unhealed fracture Use with caution with conditions that are exacerbated by fatigue
Isometric resistive exercise	An isometric contraction against a load	Resistance could be an immovable surface (e.g., pushing the palm against a wall).	Fair plus Good	Clients with cardiac conditions and high blood pressure
Isokinetic exercise	Exercise that uses a machine that controls the speed of contraction within the range of motion	Resistance controlled by machine and is variable in proportion to the change in muscle length throughout the range of motion	Fair plus Good	Inflammation Unstable joint Recent or unhealed fracture Use with caution with conditions that are exacerbated by fatigue

Reprinted from Poole, J. L. (2008). Musculoskeletal factors. In E. B. Crepeau, E. S. Cohn, & B. A. B. Schell (Eds.), *Willard & Spackman's occupational therapy* (11th ed.). Baltimore, MD: Lippincott Williams & Wilkins.

3. *Client-centered patient goal*: Therapy goals that are set through the involvement of the patient himself or herself in the therapy goal decision process. The goals respect patients' values, preferences, and expressed needs and recognize the clients' experience and knowledge.
4. *Overload*: Overload is determined by the total time spent on therapeutic activity, the number of repetitions, the difficulty of the activity in terms of coordination, muscle activity type and resistance load, and the intensity, that is, number of repetitions per time unit.
5. *Real-life object manipulation*: Manipulation that makes use of objects that are handled in normal everyday life activities (e.g., cutlery, hairbrush).
6. *Context-specific environment*: A training environment (supporting surface, objects, people, room, etc.) that equals or mimics the natural environment for a specific task execution in order to include task characteristic sensory/perceptual information, task-specific context characteristics, and cognitive processes involved.
7. *Exercise progression*: Exercises with an increasing difficulty level that is in line with the increasing abilities of the patient in order to keep the demands

TABLE 54.5 Assessments/Evaluations and Interventions Commonly Associated with the Rehabilitative Approach as It Relates to Motor Deficits

Assessments/Evaluations[a]	Sample Interventions
• Standardized objective tests of occupational performance (see Unit XI) • Self-report measures of occupational performance • Ergonomic evaluations • Evaluations to determine client's strengths: – Cognitive evaluations (to evaluate learning potential) – Range of motion and strength testing of non-affected limbs – Balance testing • Evaluations of environmental and social contexts to determine supports and limitations.	• Energy conservation • Work simplification • Recommending and training with assistive devices to support occupational performance • Recommending and training with durable medical equipment • Recommending and training with assistive technology • Home modifications • Work modifications • Wheeled mobility and seating recommendations • Fabrication of orthoses that support function

[a]See Table 54.11 and Appendix II for more details on standardized assessments for this population.

TABLE 54.6 Sample Evidence that Supports Interventions Used when Adopting the Task-Oriented Approach

Author/Year	Objective	Conclusion
Almhdawi, 2011	To evaluate the functional and the impairment effects of the Occupational Therapy Task-Oriented Approach on upper limb function via a randomized clinical trial using a crossover design.	The results supported the approach as indicated by significant and clinically meaningful changes in the Canadian Occupational Performance Measure, the Motor Activity Log, and the time scale of the Wolf Motor Function Test. The author concluded that the approach is an effective upper extremity (UE) poststroke rehabilitation approach in improving the UE functional abilities.
Kwakkel, Wagenaar, Twisk, Lankhorst, & Koetsier, 1999	To investigate the effects of different intensities of arm and leg rehabilitation training on the functional recovery of activities of daily living (ADL), walking ability, and dexterity of the paretic arm in a single-blind randomized controlled trial.	Greater intensity of leg rehabilitation improved functional recovery and health-related functional status, and greater intensity of arm rehabilitation resulted in improvements in dexterity.
Peurala et al., 2012	To examine the effect of constraint-induced movement therapy (CI therapy) and modified CI therapy on activity and participation of patients with stroke by reviewing the results of randomized controlled trials.	CI therapy and modified CI therapy proved to be effective on affected hand mobility and to some extent self-care on the World Health Organization's *International Classification of Functioning, Disability, and Health* activity and participation component, but further studies are needed to find out the optimal treatment protocols for CI therapy.
Rensink et al., 2009	To examine the effectiveness of task-oriented training after stroke via a systematic review.	"Studies of task-related training showed benefits for functional outcome compared with traditional therapies. Active use of task-oriented training with stroke survivors will lead to improvements in functional outcomes and overall health-related quality of life" (p. 737). The authors recommended "creating opportunities to practise meaningful functional tasks outside of regular therapy sessions" (p. 737).
Wolf et al., 2010	To compare functional improvements between stroke participants randomized to receive CI therapy within 3–9 mo (early group) to participants randomized on recruitment to receive the identical intervention 15–21 mo after stroke (delayed group).	CI therapy can be delivered to eligible patients 3–9 mo or 15–21 mo after stroke. Both groups achieved approximately the same level of significant arm motor function 24 mo after enrollment.

of the exercises and challenges optimal for motor learning.

8. *Exercise variety*: Various exercises are offered to support motor skill learning of a certain task because of the person experiencing different movement and context characteristics (within task variety) and problem-solving strategies.
9. *Feedback*: Specific information on the patient's motor performance that enhances motor learning and positively influences patient motivation.
10. *Multiple movement planes*: Movement that uses more than one degree of freedom of a joint, therefore occurring around multiple joint axes.
11. *Patient-customized training load*: A training load that suits the individualized treatment targets (e.g., endurance, coordination, or strength training) as well as the patient's capabilities.
12. *Total skill practice*: The skill is practiced in total, with or without preceding skill component training (e.g., via chaining).
13. *Random practice*: In each practice session, the tasks are randomly ordered.
14. *Distributed practice*: A practice schedule with relatively long rest periods.
15. *Bimanual practice*: Tasks where both arms and hands are involved.

Occupational Therapy Task-Oriented Approach

In the early 1990s, Mathiowetz and Bass Haugen (1994) argued for a shift away from the traditional neurophysiologic approaches that were being used in occupational therapy. They proposed the Occupational Therapy Task-Oriented Approach that continues to develop (Mathiowetz, 2011; Mathiowetz & Bass Haugen, 2008). The approach is based on current understandings of motor control, recovery and development as well as contemporary motor learning principles. See Box 54.2 and 54.3. See Chapter 37 for more details on the Occupational Therapy Task-Oriented Approach.

Motor Relearning Program

The Motor Relearning Program (Carr & Shepherd, 1987, 2003) is specific to the rehabilitation of patients following stroke. The program is based on four factors that are thought to be essential for the learning of motor skill and assumed to be essential for the relearning of motor control: (1) elimination of unnecessary muscle activity, (2) feedback, (3) practice, and (4) the interrelationship of postural adjustment and movement. In this program, treatment is directed toward relearning of control rather than to activities incorporating exercise or to facilitation or inhibition techniques. Treatment is directed toward enhancing motor performance; and the emphasis is on the practice of specific tasks, the training of controllable muscle action, and control over the movement components of these tasks. The major assumptions about motor control underlying this approach are listed in Box 54.4. A four-step sequence is followed for skill acquisition (Carr & Shepherd, 1987):

1. Analysis of the task, including observation
2. Practice of missing components, including goal identification, instruction, practice, and feedback with some manual guidance
3. Practice of the task with the addition of reevaluation and encouraging of task flexibility
4. Targets transfer of training

Motor Learning

Motor learning is a key component of many of the earlier described intervention approaches. *Motor learning* is defined as "a set of processes associated with practice or experience leading to relatively permanent changes in the capability for skilled movement" (Schmidt & Lee, 2011, p. 327). Schmidt and Lee (2011) describe three stages of motor learning:

1. *Cognitive*: The learner is figuring out *what* is to be done; determining appropriate strategies to complete the task. Effective strategies are maintained

BOX 54.2 Assumptions of the Occupational Therapy Task-Oriented Approach Based on a Systems Model of Motor Behavior

- Functional tasks help organize behavior.
- Personal and environmental systems, including the central nervous system, are heterarchically organized.
- Occupational performance emerges from the interaction of persons and their environment.
- Experimentation with various strategies leads to optimal solutions to motor problems.
- Recovery is variable because patient factors and environmental contexts are unique.
- Behavioral changes reflect attempts to compensate and to achieve task performance.

Adapted from Mathiowetz, V., & Bass Haugen, J. (2008). Assessing abilities and capacities: Motor behavior. In M. V. Radomski & C. A. Trombly-Latham (Eds.), *Occupational therapy for physical dysfunction* (6th ed.). Baltimore, MD: Lippincott Williams & Wilkins.

BOX 54.3 Evaluation Procedures and Interventions Based on the Occupational Therapy Task-Oriented Approach

Occupational Therapy Task-Oriented Approach Evaluation Framework

There are five main areas to assess using this approach.

1. Role performance (social participation)

Roles: Worker, student, volunteer, home maintainer, hobbyist/amateur, participant in organizations, friend, family member, caregiver, religious participant, other.

- Identify past roles and whether they can be maintained or need to be changed.
- Determine how future roles will be balanced.

2. Occupational performance tasks (areas of occupation)

- Activities of daily living: bathing, feeding, bowel and bladder management, dressing, functional mobility, and personal hygiene and grooming
- Instrumental activities of daily living: home management, meal preparation and cleanup, care of others and pets, community mobility, shopping, financial management, and safety procedures
- Work and/or education: employment seeking, job performance, volunteer exploration and participation, retirement activities, and formal and informal educational participation
- Play/leisure: exploration and participation
- Rest and sleep: preparation and participation

3. Task selection and analysis

- What client factors, performance skills and patterns, and/or contexts and activity demands limit or enhance occupational performance?

4. Person (client factors; performance skills and patterns)

- Cognitive: orientation, attention span, memory, problem solving, sequencing, calculations, learning, and generalization
- Psychosocial: interests, coping skills, self-concept, interpersonal skills, self-expression, time management, and emotional regulation and self-control
- Sensorimotor: strength, endurance, range of motion, sensory functions and pain, perceptual function, and postural control

5. Environment (context and activity demands)

- Physical: objects, tools, devices, furniture, plants, animals, and built and natural environment
- Socioeconomic: social supports: family, friends, caregivers, social groups, and community and financial resources
- Cultural: customs, beliefs, activity patterns, behavior standards, and societal expectations

Intervention Principles

- Interventions are occupation based and client focused.
- Keep clients active during treatment.
- Use natural objects and environments.
- Help patients adjust to role and task performance limitations.
- Create an environment that uses the common challenges of everyday life.
- Practice functional tasks or close simulations to find effective and efficient strategies for performance.
- Provide opportunities for practice outside of therapy time.
- Structure practice of the task to promote motor learning.
- Minimize ineffective and inefficient movement patterns.
- Remediate a client factor (impairment) if it is the critical control parameter.
- Adapt the environment, modify the task, use assistive technology, and/or reduce the effects of gravity.
- For persons with poor control of movement, constrain the degrees of freedom.
- For persons who do not use returned function in their involved extremities, use constraint-induced movement therapy (CI therapy).

Adapted from Mathiowetz, V., & Bass Haugen, J. (2008). Assessing abilities and capacities: Motor behavior. In M. V. Radomski & C. A. Trombly-Latham (Eds.), *Occupational therapy for physical dysfunction* (6th ed.). Baltimore, MD: Lippincott Williams & Wilkins and Bass Haugen, J., Mathiowetz, V., & Flinn, N. (2008). Assessing abilities and capacities: Motor behavior. In M. V. Radomski & C. A. T. Latham (Eds.), *Occupational therapy for physical dysfunction* (6th ed.). Baltimore, MD: Lippincott Williams & Wilkins.

and ineffective ones are discarded. Performance is inconsistent because the learner is trying out multiple strategies. High cognitive demands are placed on the learner. The therapist uses instructions, models, feedback, etc. to assist in learning the task at hand.

2. *Fixation*: During this stage, the learner has already determined the effective strategy. The learner now makes adjustments related to *how* the task is performed. Performance becomes more consistent at this stage.
3. *Autonomous*: At this stage, the skill is *automatic*. The task can be performed with less interference by other activities or distractions. An example of this is dual tasking ability, being able to engage in a conversation while performing the task or memorizing a grocery list while walking. The task is performed with less attentional demands.

See Table 54.7 for a summary of motor learning principles and Table 54.8 for examples of evidence that supports the use of motor learning principles in clinical populations.

As our clients are learning or relearning skills, they must first acquire the skill (acquisition phase). This occurs during initial instruction on and practice of a skill or task. This usually occurs in the initial occupational therapy sessions. Following acquisition, the client must retain the skill (retention phase); this refers to *persistence of*

BOX 54.4 Assumptions Underlying the Motor Relearning Approach

- In regaining motor control, learning is required. This learning follows the same principles and factors as those incurred in normal learning. Therefore, practice, receiving feedback, and understanding the goal are essential for treatment.
- Motor control is exercised in both anticipatory and ongoing modes.
- Sensory input is related to motor output and helps to modulate action.
- Control of a specific task can be effectively regained by practice of that specific motor task in various contexts.
- Conscious practice of tasks builds up awareness of the ability to elicit motor control activity.
- Progression of practice is from conscious awareness to practice at a more automatic level in order to ensure that a skill is learned.
- Cognitive function is emphasized. If the client is to learn, then the environment must encourage the learning process.
- When clients can perform a task effectively and efficiently without thinking about it in a variety of contexts, learning has occurred.
- Contemporary theories of motor control emphasize distributed control rather than a top-down or bottom-up approach. Therefore, in the Motor Relearning Program, recovery is directed to relearning control through many systems.
- The client is defined as an active participant in the treatment process. The major goal in rehabilitation is to relearn effective strategies for performing functional activities.
- The role of the therapist is to prevent the use of inefficient strategies by the client.
- The program addresses seven categories of functional daily activities: upper limb function, orofacial function, sitting up over the side of the bed, balanced sitting, standing up and sitting down, balanced standing, and walking.

Adapted from Carr & Shepherd (1987, 2003). Reprinted from Giuffrida, C. G., & Rice, M. S. (2008). Motor skills and occupational performance: Assessments and interventions. In E. B. Crepeau, E. S. Cohn, & B. A. B. Schell (Eds.), *Willard & Spackman's occupational therapy* (11th ed.). Baltimore, MD: Lippincott Williams & Wilkins.

performance. This occurs after the initial practice period and the client is asked to demonstrate how he or she performs the newly acquired skill. Clients must then be able to transfer their performance (transfer phase). *Transfer of learning* refers to the gain in capability for performance in one task as a result of practice on another task. The individual can use the skill in a new context. Our clients can generalize the strategies learned in the therapy setting and use them in real-life situations (Sabari, 2011; Schmidt & Lee, 2011) (see Figure 54.3).

Sabari (2011) summarized the literature about skill acquisition and therapeutic interventions that promotes generalization of learning. These concepts can be categorized into three major groups: type of feedback, development of underlying strategies, and practice conditions (see Figure 54.4).

An Overview of Motor Development

Motor development is a process during which a person acquires skills and movement patterns. Malina (2004) has described motor development as "a continuous process of modification that involves the interaction of several factors:

1. Neuromuscular maturation;
2. The physical growth and behavioral characteristics of the child;
3. The tempo of physical growth, biological maturation, and behavioral development;
4. The residual effects of prior movement experiences;
5. The new movement experiences" (p. 50).

Although many consider motor development a process specific to children, it is in fact a lifelong process that should be considered from a life course perspective. Typical developmental changes that occur in infancy and childhood are considered positive when milestones are met and new skills are acquired. Maximum performance may be reached in adolescence and adulthood. As the aging process continues, there comes a decline in performance with loss of speed, accuracy, and precision of movement. That being said, "a progression to regression" of skills description of motor development may not be completely accurate. Older adults have the potential to acquire quite intricate new motor skills as well. Think of older adults in your life who have mastered new leisure activities such as knitting and/or ballroom dancing (see Figure 54.5).

Although neurodevelopment follows a predictable course, it is important to understand that intrinsic and extrinsic forces produce individual variation, making each child's developmental path unique. Intrinsic influences include genetically determined attributes (e.g., physical characteristics, temperament) as well as the child's overall state of wellness. Extrinsic influences during infancy and childhood originate primarily from the family. Parent and sibling personalities, the nurturing methods used by caregivers, the cultural environment, and the family's socioeconomic status with its effect on resources of time and

TABLE 54.7 Summary of Motor Learning Principles/Considerations

Principles/Considerations	Examples
Classification of tasks to be learned: Learning is contingent on the type of task that is being learned.	
• Discrete tasks: Tasks with a recognizable beginning and end.	Kick a ball, push a button
• Continuous tasks: There is no recognizable beginning and end. Tasks are performed until they are arbitrarily stopped.	Jogging, driving, swimming
• Serial tasks: Comprised a series of movements linked together to make a "whole."	Play an instrument, dressing, light a fireplace
• Closed tasks: Performed in a predictable and stable environment. Movements can be planned in advance.	Oral care, signing a check, bowling
• Open tasks: Performed in a constantly changing environment that may be unpredictable.	Driving in traffic, catching an insect, soccer
• Variable motionless tasks: Involve interacting with a stable and predictable environment, but specific features of the environment are likely to vary between performance trials.	Performance of ADL outside of the usual home environment.
• Consistent motion tasks: An individual must deal with environmental conditions that are in motion during activity performance; the motion is consistent and predictable between trials.	Stepping onto an escalator, assembly line work, retrieving luggage from an airport baggage carousel
Practice conditions: The law of practice refers to performance changing linearly with the amount of time spent in practice.	
• Massed practice: Rest time is much less than practice time.	Constraint-Induced Movement Therapy
• Distributed practice: Practice time is equal to or less than rest time.	Practice sessions of a tub transfer are spaced to include rest breaks.
• Blocked practice: Repetitive practice of the same task, uninterrupted by practice of other tasks.	Practicing moving from sit to stand multiple times in a row. Practice sequence of tasks "A," "B," and "C": AAAAABBBBBBBCCCCC.
• Random or variable practice: Tasks being practiced are ordered randomly. Attempt multiple tasks or variations of a task before mastering any one of the tasks.	Practice transferring to multiple surfaces (couch, toilet, bench, chair, stool, car) in one occupational therapy session. Practice sequence of tasks "A," "B," and "C": ACBACABCCBACABCACABBACCACB.
• Whole practice: The task is practiced in its entirety and not broken into parts.	Practicing dressing.
• Part practice: The task is broken down into its parts for separate practice.	Don/doff shirt.
Feedback: A key feature of practice is the information the learner receives about their attempts to learn a skill.	
• Inherent (intrinsic) feedback: Feedback normally received while performing a task.	Knowing you made an error as you spill water when trying to pour from a pitcher to a cup.
• Augmented feedback: Information about task performance that is supplemental to inherent feedback.	A therapist provides feedback related to task performance. "You need to lock your wheelchair brakes."
• Concurrent feedback: Given during task performance	While practicing reaching, the therapist says, "Don't hike your shoulder."
• Terminal feedback: Given after task performance.	After practice of reaching, the therapist says, "You didn't open your hand wide enough."
• Immediate feedback: Given immediately after performance.	Right after an attempt at a tub transfer the therapist says, "That was perfect."
• Delayed feedback: Feedback is delayed by some amount of time.	The OT says, "You did better this morning but keep checking your brakes."
• Knowledge of results (KR): Feedback given after task performance about the outcome.	The OT says, "Your shirt is on backwards" or "You dropped the cup."
• Knowledge of performance (KP): Feedback given after task about the nature of performance.	The OT says, "Next time, dress your right arm first" or "Your elbow was bent."

ADL, activities of daily living; OT, occupational therapist.

Data from Schmidt, R. A., & Lee, T. D. (2011). *Motor control and learning: A behavioral emphasis* (5th ed.). Champaign, IL: Human Kinetics; Sabari, J. (2011). Activity-based interventions in stroke rehabilitation. In G. Gillen (Ed.), *Stroke rehabilitation: A function-based approach* (3rd ed., pp. 80–99). St. Louis, MO: Mosby; and Zwicker, J. G., & Harris, S. R. (2009). A reflection on motor learning theory in pediatric occupational therapy practice. *Canadian Journal of Occupational Therapy*, 76, 29–37.

TABLE 54.8 Sample Evidence That Supports Motor Learning Based Interventions

Author/Year	Objective	Conclusion
Bar-Haim et al., 2010	To evaluate effectiveness of motor learning coaching on retention and transfer of gross motor function in children with cerebral palsy	In higher functioning children with cerebral palsy, the motor learning coaching treatment resulted in significantly greater retention of gross motor function and transfer of mobility performance to unstructured environments than neurodevelopmental treatment.
Giuffrida, Demery, Reyes, Lebowitz, & Hanlon, 2009	To determine how acquisition, retention, and transfer of skills differed among groups of participants with traumatic brain injury (TBI) who originally learned by using either a randomly ordered practice schedule (i.e., high contextual interference) or a blocked ordered practice schedule (i.e., low contextual interference)	Both groups showed a significant increase in performance during skill acquisition and maintained this performance. Only the random-practice group, however, was able to transfer this learning to another task. The findings provide evidence that people with TBI can improve their everyday skills with randomly structured practice.
Nilsen, Gillen, & Gordon, (2010)	To determine whether mental practice is an effective intervention to improve upper limb recovery after stroke	This systematic review revealed that most studies have shown that mental practice reduces impairments and improves functional recovery of the upper limb. Thus, it appears to be an appropriate intervention strategy to be used during poststroke rehabilitation.
Ste-Marie, Clark, Findlay, & Latimer, 2004	To examine whether introducing high levels of **contextual interference** is useful in handwriting skill acquisition	Overall, the results showed that the random practice schedule leads to enhanced retention and transfer performance of handwriting skill acquisition.
Subramanian, Massie, Malcolm, & Levin, 2010	To determine if the provision of extrinsic feedback results in improved motor learning in the upper limb poststroke	The author's systematic review "found strong evidence supporting the provision of explicit feedback for implicit motor learning in the upper limb of stroke survivors." The results suggest that "stroke survivors are able to use explicit feedback and preserve motor learning abilities despite having underlying upper limb motor control deficits. An important consideration is that the ability to use explicit feedback applies to both the less- and more-affected sides" (p. 121).
Timmermans et al., 2010	To investigate the influence of each task-oriented arm training component on the functional outcome, that is, skill or activity level	There was no correlation between the number of task-oriented training components used in a study and the treatment effect size. "Distributed practice" and "feedback" were associated with the largest post-intervention effect sizes. "Random practice" and "use of clear functional goals" were associated with the largest follow-up effect sizes.

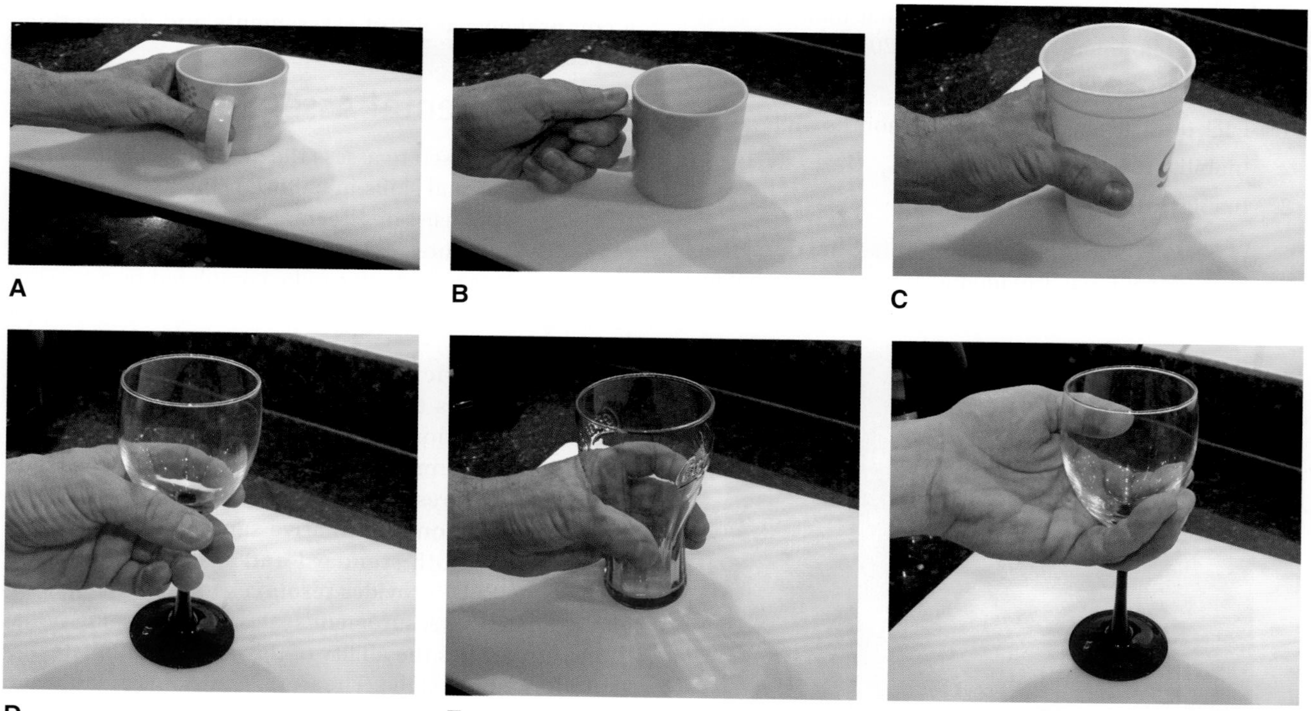

A B C D E F

FIGURE 54.3A–F. Variability in practice promotes both generalization and learning.

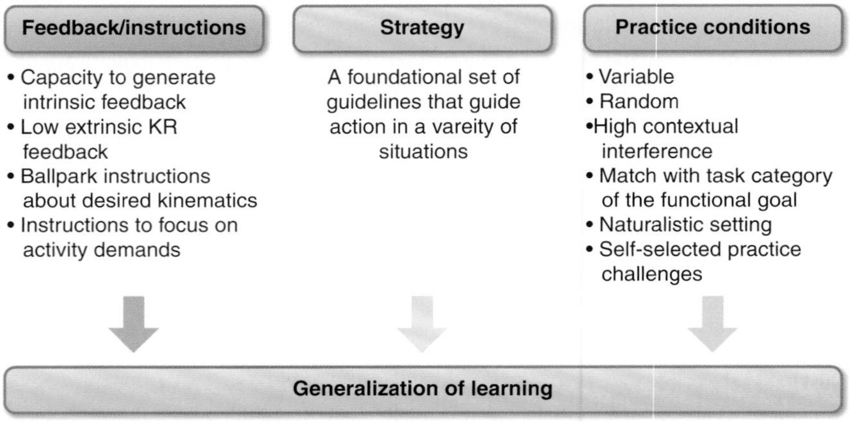

FIGURE 54.4 Factors that contribute to generalization of learning. *KR*, knowledge of results. (Reprinted with permission from Sabari, J. [2011]. Activity-based interventions in stroke rehabilitation. In G. Gillen [Ed.], *Stroke rehabilitation a function-based approach* (3rd ed., pp. 80–99). St. Louis, MO: Mosby.)

> money all play a role in the development of children. Developmental theory has, itself, developed as clinicians have tried to grapple with which influence is more predominant. (Gerber, Wilks, & Erdie-Lalena, 2010, p. 267)

Although there is a typical order of motor development that is commonly discussed and described (see Table 54.9), it is important to remember that individuals may achieve their developmental milestones in various orders, may skip a milestone step, may achieve them within different time periods (see Figure 54.6), etc. For example, Gerber et al. (2010) note that crawling is not a prerequisite to walking; pulling to stand is the skill infants must develop before they take their first steps.

It is of critical importance that therapists and parents are aware of the warning signs that indicate delays in motor development. Gerber et al. (2010) discuss three key "red flags":

1. Lack of steady head control at 4 months while sitting.
2. Inability to sit by 9 months.
3. Inability to walk by 18 months.

As part of their "Act Early" initiative, the Centers for Disease Control have provided a summary of behaviors that may be indicative of delays in motor development (see Table 54.10).

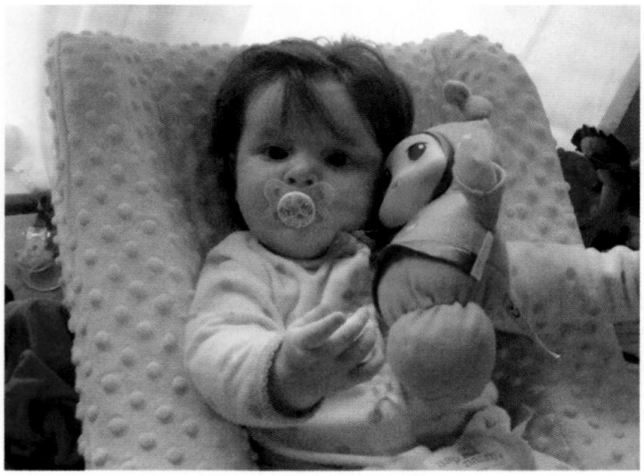

FIGURE 54.5 Development of motor control.

As will be discussed next, there are various standardized tools that OTs can use to monitor motor development.

Evaluation and Assessment of Motor Function

Many tools and procedures are available to document our client's level of motor function. These include developmental assessments, neurological screening methods, self-report measures, assessments of postural control, assessments of limb function, and assessments performed in natural contexts. The following paragraphs will give examples of each. See Table 54.11 and Appendix II for a comprehensive list of assessments and descriptions respectively.

Developmental Assessments

These tools are used to assess the development and capability of functional skills in children. The assessments in this category consist of screening instruments, criterion-referenced measures, rating scales, and norm-referenced measures, some of which can be completed by a teacher or caregiver or through direct interaction with the child being assessed.

The Pediatric Evaluation of Disability Inventory (PEDI) examines three categories: self-care, mobility, and social function. This test is designed for use with children, ages 6 months to 7 years, who have various disabilities that result in functional problems. The PEDI is standardized on a normative sample; therefore, one can calculate both standard and scaled performance scores. The PEDI provides resources to assess a child on three different measurement scales. The first, Functional Skills, establishes the ability of the child to complete discrete functional skills. The Caregiver Assessment scale determines the amount of assistance that the child is provided with during complex functional skills. And finally, the Modification Skills scale assesses what types of

TABLE 54.9 Examples of Developmental Motor Milestones

Age	Gross Motor	Fine Motor
1 mo	Chin up in prone position. Turns head in supine position.	Keeps hands fisted near face.
2 mo	Can hold head up and begins to push up when lying prone. Makes smoother movements with arms and legs.	Hands not fisted 50% of the time. Retains rattle if placed in hand. Holds hands together.
4 mo	Holds head steady, unsupported. Pushes down on legs when feet are on a hard surface. May be able to roll over from prone to supine. Brings hands to mouth. When lying on stomach, pushes up to elbows.	Hands held predominately open. Clutches at clothes. Reaches persistently. Can hold a toy and shake it and swing at dangling toys.
6 mo	Rolls over in both directions (front to back, back to front). Begins to sit without support. When standing, supports weight on legs and might bounce. Rocks back and forth, sometimes crawling backward before moving forward.	Transfers hand to hand. Rakes pellet. Takes a second cube in hand and holds on to first. Reaches with one hand.
9 mo	Stands, holding on. Can get into sitting position. Sits without support. Pulls to stand. Crawls.	Radial-digital grasp of cube. Bangs two cubes together.
1 y	Gets to a sitting position without help. Pulls up to stand, walks holding on to furniture ("cruising"). May take a few steps without holding on. May stand alone.	Scribbles after demonstration. Fine pincer grasp of pellet. Holds crayon. Attempts tower of two cubes.
18 mo	Walks alone. May walk up steps and run. Pulls toys while walking. Can help undress himself or herself.	Drinks from a cup. Eats with a spoon. Makes a four cube tower. Crudely imitates vertical stroke.
2 y	Stands on tiptoes. Kicks a ball. Begins to run. Climbs onto and down from furniture without help. Walks up and down stairs holding on. Throws ball overhand. Makes or copies straight lines and circles.	Makes a single-line "train" of cubes. Imitates circle. Imitates horizontal line.
3 y	Climbs well. Runs easily. Pedals a tricycle. Walks up and down stairs, one foot on each step.	Copies circle. Begins to cut awkwardly with scissors. Strings small beads well. Imitates bridge of cubes.
4 y	Hops and stands on one foot up to 2 s. Catches a bounced ball most of the time. Pours liquid.	Cuts food with supervision and mashes own food. Copies square. Ties single knot. Cuts 5-in circle. Uses tongs to transfer. Writes part of first name.
5 y	Stands on one foot for 10 s or longer. Hops; may be able to skip. Can do a somersault. Can use the toilet on his or her own. Swings and climbs.	Uses a fork and spoon and sometimes a table knife. Copies triangle. Puts paper clip on paper. Can use clothespins to transfer small objects. Cuts with scissors. Writes first name. Builds stairs from model.

Data from Centers for Disease Control and Prevention, National Center on Birth Defects and Developmental Disabilities "Learn the Signs. Act Early." campaign; Gerber, R. J., Wilks, T., & Erdie-Lalena, C. (2010). Developmental milestones: Motor development. *Pediatrics in Review*, *31*, 267–277.

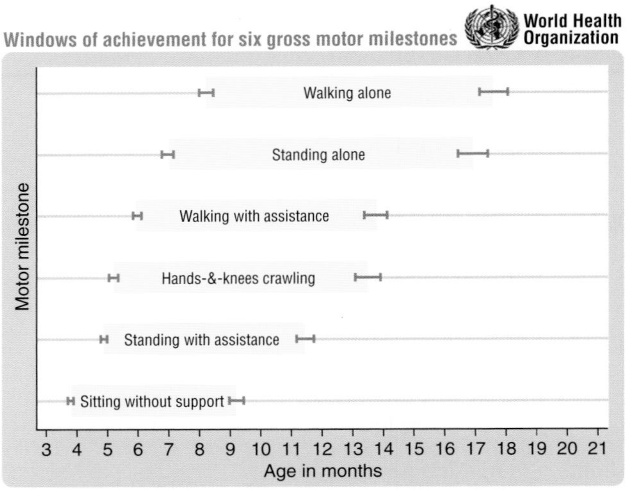

Reference: WHO Multicentre Growth Reference Study Group. WHO Motor Development Study: Windows of achievement for six gross motor development milestones. Acfa Paediatrica Supplement 2006;450:86-95.

FIGURE 54.6 Windows of achievement for six gross motor milestones.

TABLE 54.10 Delays in Motor Development

Age	Examples of Signs of Potential Delay in Motor Development
2 mo	Doesn't bring hands to mouth. Can't hold head up when pushing up when prone.
4 mo	Can't hold head steady. Doesn't bring things to mouth. Doesn't push down with legs when feet are placed on a hard surface. Has trouble moving one or both eyes in all directions.
6 mo	Doesn't try to get objects that are in reach. Has difficulty getting things to mouth. Doesn't roll over in either direction. Seems very stiff with tight muscles (increased tone). Seems very floppy like a rag doll (low tone).
9 mo	Doesn't bear weight on legs with support. Doesn't sit with help. Doesn't transfer toys from one hand to the other.
1 y	Doesn't crawl. Can't stand when supported. Doesn't learn gestures like waving or shaking head. Doesn't point to things. Loses skills he or she once had.
18 mo	Doesn't point to show things to others. Can't walk. Doesn't know what familiar things are for. Doesn't copy others. Loses skills he or she once had.
2 y	Doesn't know what to do with common things like a brush, phone, fork, or spoon. Doesn't copy actions and words. Doesn't walk steadily. Loses skills he or she once had.
3 y	Falls down a lot. Has trouble with stairs. Drools or has very unclear speech. Can't work simple toys (such as peg boards, simple puzzles, turning handle). Loses skills he or she once had.
4 y	Can't jump in place. Has trouble scribbling. Loses skills he or she once had.
5 y	Doesn't draw pictures. Can't brush teeth, wash and dry hands, or get undressed without help. Loses skills he or she once had.

Data from Centers for Disease Control and Prevention, National Center on Birth Defects and Developmental Disabilities "Learn the Signs. Act Early." campaign.

modifications the child requires to complete and support his or her function. The scales can be used concurrently or independently of one another depending on the domain of interest for each individual child (Haley, Coster, Ludlow, Haltiwanger, & Andrellos, 1992).

The Peabody Gross Motor Scale (2nd Edition) compares fine and gross motor skills to normally developing children ages 0 to 5 years. There are 170 activities that are assessed regarding reflexes, stationary skills, locomotion, object manipulation, grasping, and visual motor integration. Results from these subtests are used to generate the three composite scores: Gross Motor Quotient, Fine Motor Quotient, and Total Motor Quotient. Scores are presented as percentiles, standard scores, and age equivalents. Norms, based on a nationally representative sample of more than 2,000 children, are stratified by age (Folio & Fewell, 2000).

The Erhardt Developmental Prehension Assessment was designed to measure components of arm and hand development in children of all ages and cognitive levels who have cerebral palsy, multiple disabilities, and developmental delays. It can be used to identify intervention needs, modify programs with ongoing assessment, and provide accountability with retesting. Three hundred forty-one items are divided into three sections: (1) positional-reflexive: involuntary arm-hand patterns; (2) cognitively directed: voluntary movements of approach, grasp, manipulation, and release; and (3) prewriting skills: pencil grasp and drawing (Erhardt, 1994).

Neurological Screening Methods

Various procedures are used tests to document the presence of atypical motor performance and movements. These screening procedures related to motor function are outlined in Table 54.12.

TABLE 54.11 Standardized Assessments of Motor Function[a]

Assessment	Areas of Occupation: Activity	Areas of Occupation: Participation	Quality of Life	Client Factors: Body Structures and Functions	Client Factors: Values, Beliefs, and Spirituality	Performance Skills
ABILHAND Questionnaire and ABILHAND-Kids	X					
Action Research Arm Test				X		X
Activities-Specific Balance Confidence (ABC) Scale	X					
Arm Motor Ability Test	X					
Ashworth Scale				X		
Assessment of Motor and Process Skills	X	X				X
Assisting Hand Assessment	X					X
Bayley Scales of Infant Development, Second Edition				X		X
Bennett Hand-Tool Dexterity Test	X					X
Berg Balance Scale (adult and pediatric versions)	X			X		X
Box and Block Test				X		X
Bruininks-Oseretsky Test of Motor Proficiency, Second Edition	X			X		
Chedoke Arm and Hand Activity Inventory	X					
Clinical Observations of Motor and Postural Skills-Second Edition				X		
Complete Minnesota Dexterity Test				X		X
Crawford Small Parts Dexterity Test				X		X
Disabilities of the Arm, Shoulder, and Hand (DASH)	X	X				
Dynamometry				X		
Erhardt Developmental Prehension Assessment	X					X
Evaluation Tool of Children's Handwriting	X					X
FirstSTEp: Screening Test for Evaluating Preschoolers	X			X		
Frenchay Arm Test	X					X
Fugl-Meyer Sensorimotor Assessment				X		
Functional Reach Test and Multi-Directional Functional Reach Test						X
Goniometry				X		
Grooved Pegboard Test				X		
Gross Motor Function Measure	X					
Infant Neurological International Battery (INFANIB)				X		
Jebsen-Taylor Test of Hand Function	X					
Manual Ability Measure	X					
Manual Muscle Testing				X		

(continued)

TABLE 54.11 Standardized Assessments of Motor Function[a] (*Continued*)

Assessment	Areas of Occupation			Client Factors		
	Activity	Participation	Quality of Life	Body Structures and Functions	Values, Beliefs, and Spirituality	Performance Skills
Melbourne Assessment of Unilateral Upper Limb Function	X					X
Miller Assessment for Preschoolers	X			X		
Miller Function and Participation Scales	X	X		X		
Minnesota Rate of Manipulation Test				X		
Modified Ashworth Scale				X		
Motor Activity Log (adult and pediatric versions)	X					
Motor Assessment Scale	X			X		X
Motricity Index			X			X
Movement Assessment Battery for Children (Movement ABC)				X		X
National Institutes of Health (NIH) Pain Scales				X		
Nine-Hole Peg Test				X		
O'Connor Dexterity Tests				X		X
Peabody Developmental Motor Scales, Second Edition				X		X
Pediatric Evaluation of Disability Inventory	X	X				
Postural Assessment Scale for Stroke Patients	X					
Purdue Pegboard Test				X		
Quick Neurological Screening Test (QNST)				X		
Reflex Testing				X		
Rivermead Motor Assessment	X			X		
Sensory Organization Test				X		
School Assessment of Motor and Process Skills	X	X				X
School Function Assessment	X	X				
Tardieu Scale				X		
Tinetti's Balance and Gait Evaluation	X			X		
Timed Up and Go Test	X					
Trunk Control Test	X					
Upper Extremity Performance Test for the Elderly or *Test d'Evaluation des Membres Supérieurs de Personnes Agées* (*TEMPA*)	X					
Wolf Motor Function Test	X					X

[a]See Appendix II for more details related to these tools.

TABLE 54.12 Neurological Disorders and Their Stereotypical Coordination Patterns

Category	Description	Test
CEREBELLAR DYSFUNCTION		
Intention tremor	• Occurs during voluntary movement, is less apparent or absent during rest, and intensifies at the termination of the movement. • Evident in multiple sclerosis.	• Finger-to-finger test, finger-to-nose test. • May have trouble performing tasks that require accuracy and precision of limb placement (e.g., drinking from a cup or inserting a key in a lock).
Essential familial tremor	• Inherited as an autosomal-dominant trait, visible when client is carrying out a fine precision and accuracy task.	• Have the person reach for an item. Positive if tremors are present during the reach.
Adiadochokinesis	• Inability to perform rapid alternating movements (e.g., pronation/supination, elbow flexion/extension).	• Tests by counting how many cycles of alternating movements in 10-second time frame. Best to test unaffected/less affected side first, then compare performance to affected side.
Dysdiadochokinesia	• Decreased ability to perform rapid alternating movements smoothly.	• Supinate/pronate, flex/extend elbow, grasp/release hand, alternating bilateral tasks. Number of alternations within a time period and the differences between extremities are noted.
Dysmetria	• Inability to control muscle length results in overshooting when pointing to target objects. • Inability to estimate range of motion necessary to reach a target. Two types include hypermetria (overshoot) and hypometria (undershoot).	• Finger-to-finger or finger-to-nose tests.
Dyssynergia	• Movements are broken up into their component parts and appear jerky. Jerky movements are due to lack of synergy between agonist/antagonist. • Can cause problems in articulation and phonation.	• Alternating movement, finger-to-nose, finger-to-finger tests.
Ataxia	• Delayed initiation of movement responses, errors in range and force of movement, errors in rate and regularity of movement. Poor agonist/antagonist coordination, results in jerky, poorly controlled movements, poor postural stability.	• When reaching for object, shortest distance between the client and object is not a straight line.
Ataxic gait	• Unsteady, wide-based gait, tendency to veer or fall toward side of lesion. • Staggering, wide-based gait with reduced or no arm swing, uneven step length and tendency to fall.	• Observation of walking, turning quickly, walking toe to heel along straight line.
Rebound phenomenon of Holmes	• Lack of a check reflex. • Inability to stop a motion quickly to avoid striking something.	• Therapist releases resistance to client's elbow flexion unexpectedly, client's hand hits his or her own chest if unable to check motion.
Hypotonia	• Decreased muscle tone, decreased resistance to passive movement	• Can observe clinically and perform a quick stretch.
Nystagmus	• Involuntary (oscillating) movement of eyes. Interferes with head control and balance. Can occur as result of vestibular system, brainstem, or cerebellar lesions.	• Can observe by having the person look at a fixed object. Is positive if the eyes make small rapid oscillations (tremorlike movements).

(continued)

TABLE 54.12 Neurological Disorders and Their Stereotypical Coordination Patterns (*Continued*)

Category	Description	Test
Dysarthria	• Explosive or slurred speech caused by incoordination of the speech mechanism. • Speech may vary in pitch, seem nasal or tremulous.	• Can observe if ability to articulate words due to the oral-motor and/or larynx musculature. This is a motor problem, not due to aphasia.
POSTERIOR COLUMN DYSFUNCTION		
Ataxia	• Wide-based gait results from loss of proprioception, but client can self-correct using vision by watching their feet (compare with cerebellar dysfunction).	• Can observe in any part of the body. Is characterized by "large" tremors.
Romberg sign	• Inability to maintain standing balance with feet together and eyes closed.	• The test is the same as the definition.
BASAL GANGLIA DYSFUNCTION		
Athetoid movements	• Continuous, slow, wormlike, arrhythmic movements that primarily affect the distal portions of the extremities. Occur in the same patterns in the same subject, not present during sleep. Co-occurrence with athetosis = choreoathetosis.	• Therapist should note proximal or distal involvement extremities involved, pattern of motions, and which stimuli increase/decrease abnormal movements. Its occurrence can be documented through observation.
Dystonia	• A form of athetosis that causes twisting movements of the trunk and proximal muscles of the extremities, distorted postures, and torsion spasms. • Persistent posturing of the extremities (e.g., hyperextension of hyperflexion of the wrist and fingers) often with concurrent torsion of the spine and twisting of the trunk. Movements are often continuous and seen in conjunction with spasticity. Subtypes included segmental, generalized, focal, and multifocal.	• Its occurrence can be documented through observation.
Chorea	• Irregular, purposeless, involuntary, coarse, quick, jerky, and dysrhythmic movements of variable distribution. May occur in sleep.	• Its occurrence can be documented through observation.
Ballism	• A rare symptom produced by continuous, abrupt contraction of axial and proximal musculature of the extremity. Causes the limb to fly out suddenly. Occurs on one side (hemiballism) and is caused by lesions of the opposite subthalamic nucleus.	• Its occurrence can be documented through observation.
Resting tremors	• Stop at the initiation of voluntary movement, resume during holding phase of motor task (e.g., pill rolling tremor of Parkinsonism). • Occurs at rest and subsides when voluntary movement is attempted. Seen in Parkinson's disease.	• Have the person reach for an item. Positive if tremors are present before initiation of the reach but stop when the reach begins.
Bradykinesia	• Movement is very slow or even nonexistent, with accompanying rigidity.	• Ask the person to move; on attempting to move, the person's motions are extremely slow, if at all. Tone appears to be high.

Reprinted from Giuffrida, C. G., & Rice, M. S. (2008). Motor skills and occupational performance: Assessments and interventions. In E. B. Crepeau, E. S. Cohn, & B. A. B. Schell (Eds.), *Willard & Spackman's occupational therapy* (11th ed.). Baltimore, MD: Lippincott Williams & Wilkins.

Self-Report Measures

Several measures are available that allow clients to report their level of motor function. The DASH, as described in Case Study 54.1, is an example of this level of measurement that is typically used by therapists. The Motor Activity Log is also a self-report questionnaire (report by patient or family) related to actual use of the involved upper extremity outside of structured therapy time. It uses a semistructured interview format. Quality of movement ("How well" scale) and amount of use ("How much" scale) are graded on a 6-point scale. At present, there are 30, 28, and 14 item versions of the tool. Sample items include hold book, use a towel, pick up a glass, write/type, steady myself, etc. (Uswatte, Taub, Morris, Light, & Thompson, 2006; Uswatte, Taub, Morris, Vignolo, & McCulloch, 2005). The Pediatric Motor Activity Log is a structured interview intended to examine how often and how well a child uses his or her involved upper extremity in his or her natural environment outside the therapeutic setting. The child's primary caregiver is asked standardized questions about the amount of use of the child's involved arm and the quality of the child's movement during the functional activities specified in the instrument (e.g., point to a picture, turn pages in a book) (Uswatte et al., 2012; Wallen, Bundy, Pont, & Ziviani, 2009).

The 36-item Manual Ability Measure (MAM-36) is a new Rasch-developed, self-report disability outcome measure. It contains 36 gender neutral, commonly performed everyday hand tasks. The patient is asked to report the ease or difficulty of performing such items. It uses a 4-point rating scale, with 1 indicating *unable* ("I am unable to do the task all by myself"), 2 indicating *very hard* ("It is very hard for me to do the task and I usually ask others to do it for me unless no one is around"), 3 indicating *a little hard* ("I usually do the task myself, although it takes longer or more effort now than before"), and 4 indicating *easy* ("I can do the task without any problem"). Item examples include zip a jacket, turn a key, and take things/cards out of a wallet. The MAM-36 can be accessed (Chen, Kasven, Karpatkin, & Sylvester, 2007). A lookup table from raw scores to converted 0 to 100 Rasch measures is available (Chen & Bode, 2009).

The ABILHAND questionnaire asks clients to use a 3-point scale (0 = *impossible*, 1 = *difficult*, 2 = *easy*) to rate how difficult it would be to complete 23 bimanual (e.g., hammering a nail, wrapping a gift, thread a needle, file nails, cut meat, peel onions, open jar, etc.) (Penta, Tesio, Arnould, Zancan, & Thonnard, 2001). The ABILHAND-Kids comprised 21 mainly bimanual daily activities. The difficulty experienced by the child to perform the required tasks is scored on a 3-point ordinal scale (Arnould, Penta, Renders, & Thonnard, 2004).

Assessments of Postural Control

Various postural control measures are available based on client status. Examples follow. The Trunk Control Test examines four functional movements: roll from supine to the weak side, roll from supine to the strong side, sitting up from supine, and sitting on the edge of the bed for 30 seconds (feet off the ground). Each task is scored as follows: 0, unable to perform with assistance; 12, able to perform but in an abnormal manner; and 25, able to complete movement normally. The range of scores is 0 to 100 (Collin & Wade, 1990).

The Postural Assessment Scale for Stroke Patients contains 12 4-point items graded from 0 to 3 (Benaim, Perennou, Villy, Rousseaux, & Pelissier, 1999). Higher scores indicate better performance. Items include sitting without support, standing with and without support, standing on the nonparetic leg, standing on the paretic leg, supine to affected side, supine to unaffected side, supine to sit, sit to supine, sit to stand, stand to sit, and standing and picking up a pencil from the floor.

The Berg Balance Scale (BBS) was developed to measure balance among older people with impairment in balance function by assessing the performance of functional tasks. It is a valid instrument used for evaluation of the effectiveness of interventions and for quantitative descriptions of function in clinical practice and research. It includes 14 items such as sit to stand, transfers, and retrieving an object from the floor (Berg, Wood-Dauphinee, Williams, & Gayton, 1989).

Assessments of Limb Function

Assessments of limb function are usually composed of items that are best described as simulated ADL or movements that mimic those required to engage in daily activities. The Arm Motor Ability Test has been used to determine the effectiveness of interventions and includes 13 unilateral and bilateral tasks. Sample items include tying a shoe, opening a jar, wiping up spilled water, using a light switch, using utensils, and drinking. The therapist times task performance and rates movement quality on a 6-point scale. The test is appropriate for evaluating motor skills in high-level clients with active wrist and finger extension (Kopp et al., 1997).

The Wolf Motor Function Test has been used to document the outcomes related to CI therapy and other interventions and includes various tasks such as basic reaching tasks (e.g., lifting arm from lap to table, extending elbow with and without a weight attached) as well as more functional activities that involve fine motor control (e.g., picking up a pencil, turning a key in a lock). All tasks but one are unilateral and appropriate for both the dominant and nondominant arm. Because many tasks do not require distal control, it is appropriate for people with a more involved upper extremity. The therapist times task performance and qualitatively grades movement (Wolf et al., 2001).

The Jebsen Test of Hand Function includes the performance of seven test activities: writing a short sentence, turning over index cards, picking up small objects and placing them in a container, stacking checkers, simulating eating, moving empty large cans, and moving weighted large cans during timed trials. The original paper is based on data collected from 360 normal subjects and patients, including patients with hemiparesis resulting from a stroke. The mean times and standard deviations for normal subjects (with their dominant and nondominant hand) are published in the paper. The test is standardized and reliable and does not have a practice effect. Therapists must be aware that some of the tasks are simulated activities and some tasks cannot be considered ADL tasks (Jebsen, Taylor, Trieschmann, Trotter, & Howard, 1969).

The Melbourne Assessment of Unilateral Upper Limb Function measures quality of unilateral upper limb movement in children with neurological conditions aged 5 to 15 years. The assessment is designed to provide general information about levels of ability/disability rather than specific diagnostic information. The tool consists of 16 items that involve reach, grasp, release, and manipulation. A child's performance is recorded on videotape for subsequent scoring. Each test item has an individual scoring system so that various aspects of the movement can be considered such as range of movement, accuracy of reach and placement, fluency of reach and release, and developmental level of grasp. The test items and scoring system aim to be representative of the most important components of upper limb function (Randall, Johnson, & Reddihough, 1999).

The Assisting Hand Assessment (Krumlinde-Sundholm & Eliasson, 2003) examines how effectively a child's hemiplegic hand is actually used in bimanual activities. The spontaneous use is evaluated during a semi-structured play session with toys requiring bimanual handling. The items that are scored include general use, arm use, grasp and release, fine motor adjustments, and coordination and pace. All items are scored from 0 (*does not do*) to 4 (*effective use*).

The Chedoke Arm and Hand Activity Inventory (CAHAI) is an upper-limb measure that uses a 7-point quantitative scale in order to assess functional recovery of the arm and hand after a stroke. The tool is used to evaluate the functional ability of the paretic arm and hand to perform tasks that have been identified as important by individuals following a stroke. The CAHAI is a performance test using functional items. The tool is designed to measure the client's ability and encourage bilateral function (Barreca, Stratford, Lambert, Masters, & Streiner, 2005).

Assessments Performed in Natural Contexts

There are a limited number of tools that measure motor skills in a naturalistic context. The Assessment of Motor and Process Skills (AMPS) and School AMPS are two examples. The therapist evaluates motor and process skills within the context of basic ADL and instrumental ADL. The quality of the person's ADL performance is assessed by rating the effort, efficiency, safety, and independence of 16 ADL motor and 20 ADL process skill items while the person is doing chosen, familiar, and life-relevant ADL tasks. There are more than 100 tasks to choose from thus promoting a client-centered approach to assessment. Evaluated motor skills include skills related to body position (stabilizes, aligns, positions), obtaining and holding objects (reaches, bends, grips, manipulates, coordinates), moving self and objects (moves, lifts, walks, transports, calibrates, flows), and sustaining performance (endures, paces) (Fisher & Bray Jones, 2010). See Chapter 22 for more details.

The School AMPS is a naturalistic, observation-based assessment that is administered in the natural classroom setting while the student performs schoolwork tasks assigned by the teacher. No disruption of the normal classroom routine occurs during its administration. The School AMPS helps an OT answer the following questions:

What is the quality of this student's schoolwork task performance?
How does the quality of this student's task performance compare with that of his or her same-age peers?
Which school motor and/or school process skills are most impacting this student's occupational performance in the classroom?
What intervention strategies will have the most impact on this student's performance in the classroom?
Was there a change in this student's quality of schoolwork task performance since the last School AMPS evaluation?

The School AMPS examines the transaction between a student, a schoolwork task, and a classroom environment and evaluates the quality of the student's schoolwork task performance, measured at the level of complex activity and participation, not body functions (Fingerhut, Madill, Darrah, Hodge, & Warren, 2002; Fisher, Bryze, & Atchison, 2000; Fisher, Bryze, Hume, & Griswold, 2005).

Examples of Evidence-Based Interventions

Since the last edition of this book, there has been a substantial increase and focus on testing interventions for those with limitations in motor function. When using evidence to guide practice, it is important to reflect on the type of outcomes measures used as described previously. One should consider the following questions when interpreting evidence:

1. Is the population that was tested similar to my client?
2. Has the intervention been shown to be effective related to measures of activity and participation (areas of occupation) in addition to impairment measures (measurement of client factors)?

Although interventions have been discussed throughout this chapter (orthoses, strengthening, **physical agent modalities**, task oriented training, motor learning techniques such as mental practice, etc.), the following paragraphs will provide the reader with further examples of contemporary evidence-based interventions.

Constraint-Induced Movement Therapy

The term **learned nonuse** was coined by Taub et al. (1993). The learned nonuse phenomenon originally was identified in animal studies and later was applied to chronic stroke survivors and others. Taub et al. (1993) hypothesized that the nonuse or limited use of an affected upper extremity in human beings after a neurologic event results from a phenomenon of learned suppression. CI therapy is an intervention developed to reverse the effects of learned nonuse. This intervention is quickly becoming the gold standard to improve daily use of neurologically impaired upper extremities in both the adult population (stroke) and children with cerebral palsy who meet the motor inclusion criteria. Refer back to Case Study 54.2 for a description of pediatric applications. Box 54.5 and Box 54.6 provide more details related to how to implement this intervention.

Bilateral Arm Training/Bimanual Training

Bilateral arm training is emerging as a promising intervention to improve arm function after stroke. Stoykov, Lewis, & Corcos (2009) summarized that the technique

- Has been shown to be efficacious not only with stroke survivors who are only mildly impaired but also those with moderate and severe motor impairments;
- Protocols reported in the literature are diverse and can be categorized as categories: repetitive reaching with hand fixed, isolated muscle repetitive training, and whole arm functioning; and
- May be combined with rhythmic auditory cueing and is coupled with repetitive reaching with hand-fixed activities.

Examples of treatment activities include opening and closing two identical drawers, wiping a table with both arms using both arms symmetrically, bilateral reaching and placing objects, etc. Stoykov et al. (2009) compare the effectiveness of bilateral training with unilateral training for individuals with moderate upper limb hemiparesis. They concluded that both bilateral and unilateral

BOX 54.5 Summary of Constraint-Induced Movement Therapy

- Use to counteract learned nonuse. Hypothesized causes of learned nonuse include therapeutic interventions implemented during the acute period of neurologic suppression after stroke or other neurologic event, an early focus on adaptations to meet functional goals, negative reinforcement experienced by the patients as they unsuccessfully attempt to use the affected limb, and positive reinforcement experienced by using the less involved hand and/or use of successful adaptations.
- Motor inclusion criteria. Control of the wrist and digits is necessary to engage in this type of intervention. Current and past protocols have used the following inclusion criteria: 20 degrees of extension of the wrist and 10 degrees of extension of each finger; or 10 degrees extension of the wrist, 10 degrees abduction of the thumb, and 10 degrees extension of any two other digits; or able to lift a wash rag off a table using any type of prehension and then release it. It is clear that distal function (particularly wrist and digit extension) is a critical factor in being a candidate for the intervention. Therapists should focus on these movements early and intensely. Potential interventions to regain this motor control included electrical stimulation, mental practice, and activities that require distal extension such as reaching for large objects.
- Main therapeutic factor. Massed practice and shaping of the affected limb during repetitive functional activities appears to be the therapeutic change agent.
- Activity choices and therapist's interventions. Select tasks that address the motor deficits of the individual patient; assist the patient to carry out parts of a movement sequence if they are incapable of completing the movement on their own at first, providing explicit verbal feedback and verbal reward for small improvements in task performance, use modeling and prompting of task performance, use tasks that are of interest and motivating to the patient, ignore regression of function, and use tasks that can be quantified related to improvements.
- Outcome measures. The Motor Activity Log (actual use outside of structured therapy or "real-world use"), Arm Motor Ability Test, Wolf Motor Function Test, and the Action Research Arm Test have been used to document outcomes.
- Cortical reorganization. Constraint-induced movement therapy is the first rehabilitation intervention that has been demonstrated to induce changes in the cortical representation of the affected upper limb.
- The continued rigorous research that has been and continues to be carried out to demonstrate the effectiveness/efficacy of constraint-induced movement therapy should be used as a gold standard for other rehabilitation interventions that are used traditionally (e.g., neurodevelopmental therapy) but have little or no research support.
- Based on available evidence, constraint-induced movement therapy appears to be an effective intervention for those who have learned nonuse and who fit the motor inclusion criteria.

Reprinted with permission from Gillen, G. (Ed.). (2011). Upper extremity function and management. In *Stroke rehabilitation: A function-based approach* (3rd ed.). St. Louis, MO: Elsevier.

BOX 54.6 Constraint-Induced Movement Therapy Protocols

Traditional Protocol	Modified Protocols
The EXCITE trial defined the intervention as: "Participants in the intervention group were taught to apply an instrumented protective safety mitt and encouraged to wear it on their less-impaired upper extremity for a goal of 90% of their waking hours over a 2-week period, including 2 weekends, for a total of 14 days. On each weekday, participants received shaping (adaptive task practice) and standard task training of the paretic limb for up to 6 hours per day. The former is based on the principles of behavioral training that can also be described in terms of motor learning derived from adaptive or part-task practice. Standard task practice is less structured (i.e., repetition of tasks is not conducted as individual trials of discrete movements); it involves functional activities performed continuously for a period of 15 to 20 minutes (e.g., eating, writing)." (Wolf et al., 2006)	Page et al., (2008) described the following protocol consisting of 2 components. "The first component consisted of half-hour, one-on-one sessions of more affected arm therapy occurring 3 days per week during a 10-week period. This component included shaping in which operant conditioning was applied in such a way that subjects received positive verbal encouragement to more fully perform selected motor skills with their more affected arm. Shaping was applied with 2 or 3 upper-limb activities (e.g., writing, using a fork) chosen by the subjects with help from their therapist. In the second component of the mCIT intervention, during the same 10-week period, subjects' less affected arms were restrained every weekday for 5 hours identified as a time of frequent arm use, as identified by the subjects with assistance from the therapist. Their arms were restrained using a cotton hemi-sling, while their hands were placed in mesh, polystyrene-filled mitts with Velcro straps around the wrist." Lin et al. (2009) defined their protocol as "restraint of the less affected limb combined with intensive training of the affected limb for 2 hours daily 5 days per week for 3 weeks and restraint of the less affected hand for 5 hours outside of the rehabilitation training". Sterr et al. (2002) defined their protocol as 14 consecutive days; constraint of unaffected hand for a target of 90% of waking hours, with 3 hours of shaping training with the affected hand per day. To note, they concluded that: "The 3-hour CIMT training schedule significantly improved motor function in chronic hemiparesis, but it was less effective than the 6-hour training schedule."

CIMT, constraint induced movement therapy; EXCITE, Extremity Constraint-Induced Therapy Evaluation; mCIT, modified constraint induced movement therapy.
Reprinted with permission from Gillen, G. (2011). Upper extremity function and management. In G. Gillen (Ed.), *Stroke rehabilitation: A function-based approach* (3rd ed.). St. Louis, MO: Elsevier.

training are efficacious for moderately impaired chronic stroke survivors and that bilateral training may be more advantageous for proximal arm function.

Gordon, Charles, Schneider, and Chinnan (2007) developed a bimanual intervention, Hand-Arm Bimanual Intensive Therapy (HABIT), which is specifically aimed at upper extremity impairments in congenital hemiplegia. The authors describe HABIT as

- A form of functional training,
- Focusing on intensive practice,
- Focused on improving coordination of the two hands using structured task practice embedded in bimanual play and functional activities,
- Using principles of motor learning (practice specificity, types of practice, feedback), and
- Using principles of neuroplasticity (practice-induced brain changes arising from repetition, increasing movement complexity, motivation, and reward).

The authors conducted a randomized trial to examine the effectiveness of this intervention. Children were engaged in play and functional activities that provided structured bimanual practice 6 hours per day for 10 days. They concluded that for this carefully selected subgroup of children with hemiplegic cerebral palsy, HABIT appears to be efficacious in improving bimanual hand use.

Of note is that Gordon et al. (2011) conducted a randomized trial comparing CI therapy and HABIT that maintains the intensity of practice associated with CI therapy but where children are engaged in functional bimanual tasks. The children received 90 hours of CI therapy or HABIT. They concluded that both CI therapy and bimanual training lead to similar improvements in hand function. They note that a potential benefit of bimanual training is that participants may improve more on self-determined goals.

Use of Cognitive Strategies to Improve Performance

The use of cognitive strategies is emerging as an effective intervention for children with *developmental coordination disorder* (DCD). This term is used to describe children with motor skill impairment who experience problems with the performance of various motor-based tasks, such as catching/throwing a ball, playing on a jungle gym, dressing, feeding, riding a bicycle, and handwriting (see Appendix I for more details).

Hyland and Polatajko (2011) describe the Cognitive Orientation to daily Occupational Performance (CO-OP) approach as a multifaceted top-down approach that combines elements from various disciplines such as behavioral and cognitive psychology, health, and human movement science. They further describe it as a verbally based individualized approach that focuses on teaching children to use self-talk and problem-solving strategies to solve their motor-based performance problems. The children choose their own goals, and problem-solving strategies are used to identify and address performance issues.

> The CO-OP therapist guides the child in the learning of a global problem solving strategy and the discovery of domain specific cognitive strategies that improve motor performance. The global cognitive strategy is a problem-solving strategy, taken from the work of Meichenbaum (1977), which provides a structure within which the child can learn to talk through occupational performance problems. Domain specific strategies (DSS) are used in specific tasks or situations to help achieve specific occupational performance goals. (Sangster, Beninger, Polatajko, & Mandich, 2005, p.70)

Sangster et al. (2005) argue that it is the development of skills in using cognitive strategies that has supported the reported improvement in occupational performance. They state that the CO-OP approach has two hypotheses: (1) that children with DCD do not independently generate effective cognitive strategies to solve performance problems; and (2) that cognitive strategy use changes with the CO-OP intervention. Examples of strategies that are employed include verbal guidance, feeling the movement, attention to doing, practice, etc. Indeed, the author's pilot work has support the use of a cognitively based approach such as CO-OP in assisting children with DCD in developing cognitive strategies when solving occupational performance problems.

Cognitive strategies have also been used to enhance motor skill acquisition poststroke. McEwen, Huijbregts, Ryan, & Polatajko (2009) examined the literature and concluded that

- Research investigating cognitive strategies to improve motor skill acquisition in people with stroke is emerging in the peer-reviewed literature.
- The cognitive strategies studied included three general strategies (those that are applicable in many different situations) and four task-specific strategies: motor imagery (MI) (also known as *mental practice*); Feldenkrais Attention to Movement, goal setting with assigned, high, specific goals and preparatory arousal.
- None of the strategies have been studied exhaustively.
- There is strong evidence that general strategy training combined with MI during practice improves and maintains performance in both trained and untrained ADL compared to traditional functional training in people in the early rehabilitation phase after a stroke.
- There is strong evidence that general strategy training improves performance in untrained ADL compared to traditional occupational therapy in people with apraxia as a result of stroke (see Chapter 55 for more information on apraxia).

Postural Control/Balance Interventions

Adding purpose to daily occupations has been shown to improve standing balance (Hsieh, Nelson, Smith, & Peterson, 1996) in those with hemiplegia. Hsieh et al. (1996) examined three types of standing balance interventions. They hypothesized that the two added-purpose occupations would elicit more exercise repetitions than a rote exercise. They examined a dynamic standing balance exercise that involved bending down, reaching, standing up, and extending the arm. One condition of added purpose involved the use of materials (small balls and target); a second added-purpose condition involved the subjects' imagination of the small balls. The third condition was the rote exercise without added purpose. The subjects did significantly more exercise repetitions in the added-materials condition and in the imagery-based condition than in the rote exercise condition. The authors concluded that this study demonstrates how added purpose can enhance motor performance in persons with hemiplegia. They demonstrated that purpose may be effectively added to an exercise through the use of materials or imagery.

The concept of using reaching activities has also been shown to be effective in retraining seated postural control (Dean & Shepherd, 1997). As technology continued to be more and more common place, games such as the Wii are being used in rehabilitation settings to address multiple impairments including improving balance (Gil-Gomez, Llorens, Alcaniz, & Colomer, 2011).

Physical Agent Modalities

Electrical stimulation and electromyography (EMG)-triggered electrical stimulation are being used for those with impaired motor function. Electrical stimulation has been used in poststroke upper extremity rehabilitation for many years. Potential uses have included reduction of shoulder subluxation, reduction of pain, improved motor control, and increasing use of the involved extremity. In general, the effects of electrical stimulation

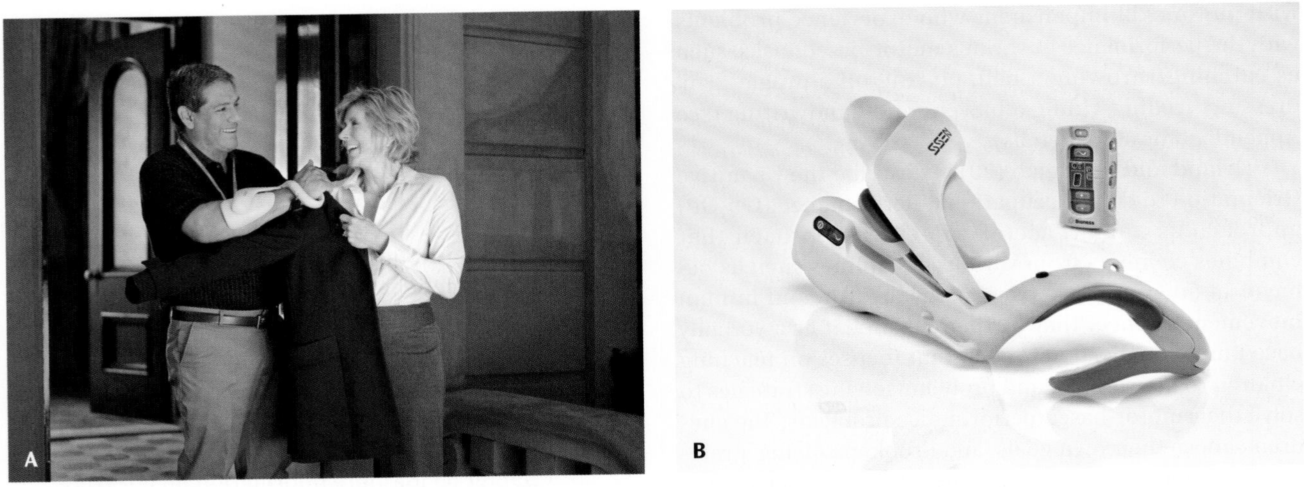

FIGURE 54.7A–B A neuroprosthesis (H200 Wireless) used to support occupational performance. This device combines a wrist/hand orthosis (to provide stabilization) with integrated surface electrodes to activate muscles of a paralyzed forearm and hand. (Photo courtesy of Bioness, Inc., Valencia, California.)

have been the most consistent at improving limb impairments such as range of motion and reducing pain. The effects on function and ADL have received less attention and have been inconsistent. Electrical stimulation can be triggered by voluntary movement or nontriggered. EMG-triggered stimulation detects underlying muscle activity when it reaches a threshold level prior to providing the stimulation. The stroke survivor must voluntarily activate the correct muscles prior to the stimulation facilitating the motor response. This type of stimulation assures that the intervention is not passive in nature. Triggered electrical stimulation may be more effective than nontriggered electrical stimulation in facilitating upper extremity motor recovery following stroke (de Kroon, Ijzerman, Chae, Lankhorst, & Zilvold, 2005). This intervention has been shown to be effective at improving wrist extension, a key movement to be considered a candidate for some task-oriented approaches such as CI therapy. Findings from systematic reviews and meta-analyses have been inconsistent. However, there is enough evidence to continue to integrate these modalities with other task oriented training activities. Further investigation is warranted (see Figure 54.7A–B).

Conclusion

Motor function and control is a multifaceted concept that relies on multiple body structures and functions, performance skills, etc. Successful rehabilitation is based on the adoption of a clear therapeutic approach or approaches; the interpretation of standardized, valid, and reliable assessments; and the adoption of evidence-based interventions. Remember, the goal of motor-based interventions is to improve overall occupational performance and *not* only reduce motor impairment.

References

Almhdawi, K. (2011). *Effects of occupational therapy task-oriented approach in upper extremity post-stroke rehabilitation* (Unpublished doctoral dissertation). University of Minnesota, Twin Cities.

Arnould, C., Penta, M., Renders, A., & Thonnard, J. L. (2004). ABILHAND-Kids: A measure of manual ability in children with cerebral palsy. *Neurology, 63*, 1045–1052.

Bar-Haim, S., Harries, N., Nammourah, I., Oraibi, S., Malhees, W., Loeppky, J., . . . Lahat, E. (2010). Effectiveness of motor learning coaching in children with cerebral palsy: a randomized controlled trial. *Clinical Rehabilitation, 24*, 1009–1020.

Barreca, S., Stratford, P., Lambert, C., Masters, L., & Streiner, D. (2005). Test-retest reliability, validity, and sensitivity of the Chedoke Arm and Hand Activity Inventory: A new measure of upper-limb function for survivors of stroke. *Archives of Physical Medicine and Rehabilitation, 86*, 1616–1622.

Benaim, C., Perennou, D. A., Villy, J., Rousseaux, M., & Pelissier, J. Y. (1999). Validation of a standardized assessment of postural control in stroke patients. *Stroke, 30*, 1862–1868.

Berg, K., Wood-Dauphinee, S., Williams, J. I., & Gayton, D. (1989). Measuring balance in the elderly: Preliminary development of an instrument. *Physiotherapy Canada, 41*, 304–311.

Carr, J. H., & Shepherd, R. B. (1987). *A motor relearning program for stroke* (2nd ed.). Rockville, MD: Aspen.

Carr, J. H. & Shepherd, R. B. (2003). *Stroke rehabilitation: Guidelines for exercise and training to optimize motor skill.* New York: Butterworth-Heinemann.

Centers for Disease Control and Prevention. (2012). *Learn the signs. Act early.* Retrieved from: http://www.cdc.gov/ncbddd/actearly/index.html

Chen, C. C., & Bode, R. K. (2009, April). *MAM-36: Psychometric properties and differential item functioning in neurologic and orthopedic patients.* Paper presented at the AOTA 88th Annual Conference, Long Beach, CA.

Chen, C. C., Kasven, N., Karpatkin, H. I., & Sylvester, A. (2007). Hand strength and perceived manual ability among patients with multiple sclerosis. *Archives of Physical Medicine and Rehabilitation, 88*, 794–797.

Collin, C., & Wade, D. (1990). Assessing motor impairment after stroke: A pilot reliability study. *Journal of Neurology, Neurosurgery, and Psychiatry, 53*, 576–579.

Dean, C. M., & Shepherd, R. B. (1997). Task-related training improves performance of seated reaching tasks after stroke. *Stroke, 28*, 722–728.

de Kroon, J., Ijzerman, M., Chae, J., Lankhorst, G., & Zilvold, G. (2005). Relation between stimulation characteristics and clinical outcome in studies using electrical stimulation to improve motor control of the upper extremity in stroke. *Journal of Rehabilitation Medicine*, *37*, 65–74.

Egan, M. Y., & Brousseau, L. (2007). Splinting for osteoarthritis of the carpometacarpal joint: A review of the evidence. *American Journal of Occupational Therapy*, *61*, 70–78.

Erhardt, R. (1994). *Developmental hand dysfunction: Theory, assessment, and treatment* (2nd ed.). Austin, TX: Pro-Ed.

Fingerhut, P., Madill, H., Darrah, J., Hodge, M., & Warren, S. (2002). Classroom-based assessment: Validation for the school AMPS. *American Journal of Occupational Therapy*, *56*, 210–213.

Fisher, A. G., & Bray Jones, K. (2010). *Assessment of Motor and Process Skills. Vol. 1: Development, standardization, and administration manual* (7th ed.). Fort Collins, CO: Three Star Press.

Fisher, A. G., Bryze, K., & Atchison, B. T. (2000). Naturalistic assessment of functional performance in school settings: Reliability and validity of the School AMPS. *Journal of Outcome Measurement*, *4*, 504–522.

Fisher, A. G., Bryze, K., Hume, V., & Griswold, L. A. (2005). *School AMPS: School Version of the Assessment of Motor and Process Skills* (2nd ed.). Fort Collins, CO: Three Star Press.

Folio, M. R., & Fewell, R. R. (2000). *Peabody Developmental Motor Scales: Examiner's Manual* (2nd ed.). Austin, TX: Pro-ED.

Gerber, R. J., Wilks, T., & Erdie-Lalena, C. (2010). Developmental milestones: Motor development. *Pediatrics in Review*, *31*, 267–277.

Gil-Gomez, J.-A., Llorens, R., Alcaniz, M., & Colomer, C. (2011). Effectiveness of a Wii balance board-based system (eBaViR) for balance rehabilitation: A pilot randomized clinical trial in patients with acquired brain injury. *Journal of Neuroengineering & Rehabilitation*, *8*, 30.

Gillen, G. (Ed.). (2011). Upper extremity function and management. In *Stroke rehabilitation: A function-based approach* (3rd ed.). St. Louis, MO: Elsevier.

Giuffrida, C. G., Demery, J. A., Reyes, L. R., Lebowitz, B. K., & Hanlon, R. E. (2009). Functional skill learning in men with traumatic brain injury. *American Journal of Occupational Therapy*, *63*, 398–407.

Giuffrida, C. G., & Rice, M. S. (2008). Motor skills and occupational performance: Assessments and interventions. In E. B. Crepeau, E. S. Cohn, & B. A. B. Schell (Eds.), *Willard & Spackman's occupational therapy* (11th ed.). Baltimore, MD: Lippincott Williams & Wilkins.

Gordon, A. M., Charles, J., Schneider, J. A., & Chinnan, A. (2007). Efficacy of hand-arm bimanual intensive therapy (HABIT) for children with hemiplegic cerebral palsy: A randomized control trial. *Developmental Medicine and Child Neurology*, *49*, 830–838.

Gordon, A. M., Charles, J., & Wolf, S. L. (2005). Methods of constraint-induced movement therapy for children with hemiplegic cerebral palsy: Development of a child-friendly intervention for improving upper-extremity function. *Archives of Physical Medicine and Rehabilitation*, *86*, 837–844.

Gordon, A. M., Hung, Y. C, Brandao, M., Ferre, C. L., Kuo, H.-C., Friel, K., . . . Charles, J. R. (2011). Bimanual training and constraint-induced movement therapy in children with hemiplegic cerebral palsy: A randomized trial. *Neurorehabilitation and Neural Repair*, *25*, 692–702.

Guzelkucuk, U., Duman, I., Taskaynatan, M. A., & Dincer, K. (2007). Comparison of therapeutic activities with therapeutic exercises in the rehabilitation of young adult patients with hand injuries. *Journal of Hand Surgery*, *32*, 1429–1435.

Haley, S., Coster, W., Ludlow, L., Haltiwanger, J., & Andrellos, J. (1992). Pediatric Evaluation of Disability Inventory (PEDI). Boston, MA: Trustees of Boston University.

Harris, J. E., & Eng, J. J. (2010). Strength training improves upper limb function in individuals with stroke. *Stroke*, *41*, 136–140.

Hsieh, C. L., Nelson, D. L., Smith, D. A., & Peterson, C. Q. (1996). A comparison of performance in added-purpose occupations and rote exercise for dynamic standing balance in persons with hemiplegia. *American Journal of Occupational Therapy*, *50*, 10–16.

Hyland, M., & Polatajko, H. J. (2011). Enabling children with developmental coordination disorder to self-regulate through the use of dynamic performance analysis: Evidence from the CO-OP approach. *Human Movement Science*. Advance online publication. doi:10.1016/j.humov.2011.09.003

Jebsen, R. H., Taylor, N., Trieschmann, R. B., Trotter, M. J., & Howard, L. A. (1969). An objective and standardized test of hand function. *Archives of Physical Medicine and Rehabilitation*, *50*, 311–319.

Kopp, B., Kunkel, A., Flor, H., Platz, T., Rose, U., Mauritz, K. H., . . . Taub, E. (1997). The Arm Motor Ability Test: Reliability, validity, and sensitivity to change of an instrument for assessing disabilities in activities of daily living. *Archives of Physical Medicine and Rehabilitation*, *78*, 615–620.

Krumlinde-Sundholm, L., & Eliasson, A. C. (2003). Development of the Assisting Hand Assessment, a rash-built measure intended for children with unilateral upper limb impairments. *Scandinavian Journal of Occupational Therapy*, *10*, 16–26.

Kwakkel, G., Wagenaar, R. C., Twisk, J. W., Lankhorst, G. J., & Koetsier, J. C. (1999). Intensity of leg and arm training after primary middle-cerebral-artery stroke: A randomised trial. *Lancet*, *354*, 191–196.

Law, M. (Ed.). (1998). *Client-centered occupational therapy*. Thorofare, NJ: Slack.

Law, M., Baptiste, S., & Mills, J. (1995). Client-centered practice: What does it mean and does it make a difference? *Canadian Journal of Occupational Therapy*, *62*, 250–257.

Law, M., & Mills, J. (1998). Client-centered occupational therapy. In M. Law (Ed.), *Client-centered occupational therapy* (pp. 1–18). Thorofare, NJ: Slack.

Lin, K. C., Wu, C. Y., Liu, J. S., Chen, Y. T., & Hsu, C. J. (2009). Constraint-induced therapy versus dose matched control intervention to improve motor ability, basic/extended daily functions, and quality of life in stroke. *Neurorehabilitation & Neural Repair*, *23*, 160–165.

Maitra, K. K., & Erway, F. (2006). Perception of client-centered practice in occupational therapists and their clients. *American Journal of Occupational Therapy*, *60*, 298–310.

Malina, R. (2004). Motor development during infancy and early childhood: Overview and suggested directions for research. *International Journal of Sport and Health Science*, *2*, 50–66.

Mathiowetz, V. (2011). Task-oriented approach to stroke rehabilitation. In G. Gillen (Eds.), *Stroke rehabilitation a function-based approach* (3rd ed., pp. 80–99). St. Louis, MO: Mosby.

Mathiowetz, V., & Bass Haugen, J. (1994). Motor behavior research: Implications for therapeutic approaches to central nervous system dysfunction. *The American Journal of Occupational Therapy*, *48*(8), 733–745.

Mathiowetz, V., & Bass Haugen, J. (2008). Assessing abilities and capacities: Motor behavior. In M. V. Radomski & C. A. Trombly-Latham (Eds.), *Occupational therapy for physical dysfunction* (6th ed., pp. 186–211). Baltimore, MD: Lippincott Williams & Wilkins.

McEwen, S. E., Huijbregts, M. P., Ryan, J. D., & Polatajko, H. J. (2009). Cognitive strategy use to enhance motor skill acquisition post-stroke: A critical review. *Brain Injury*, *23*, 263–277.

Morris, D. M., Taub, E., & Mark, V. W. (2006). Constraint-induced movement therapy: Characterizing the intervention protocol. *Europa Medicophysica*, *42*(3), 257–268.

Muller, M., Tsui, D., Schnurr, R., Biddulph-Deisroth, L., Hard, J., & MacDermid, J. C. (2004). Effectiveness of hand therapy interventions in primary management of carpal tunnel syndrome: A systematic review. *Journal of Hand Therapy*, *17*, 210–228.

Nilsen, D. M., Gillen, G., & Gordon, A. M. (2010). Use of mental practice to improve upper-limb recovery after stroke: A systematic review. *American Journal of Occupational Therapy*, *64*, 695–708.

Page, S. J., Levine, P., Leonard, A., Szaflarski, J. P., & Kissela, B. M. (2008). Modified constraint-induced therapy in chronic stroke: Results of a single-blinded randomized controlled trial. *Physical Therapy*, *88*, 333–340.

Penta, M., Tesio, L., Arnould, C., Zancan, A., & Thonnard, J.-L. (2001). The ABILHAND questionnaire as a measure of manual ability in chronic stroke patients: Rasch-based validation and relationship to upper limb impairment. *Stroke*, *32*, 1627–1634.

Peurala, S. H., Kantanen, M. P., Sjogren, T., Paltamaa, J., Karhula, M., & Heinonen, A. (2012). Effectiveness of constraint-induced movement therapy on activity and participation after stroke: A systematic review and meta-analysis of randomized controlled trials. *Clinical Rehabilitation, 26*, 209–223.

Phipps, S., & Richardson, P. (2007). Occupational therapy outcomes for clients with traumatic brain injury and stroke using the Canadian Occupational Performance Measure. *American Journal of Occupational Therapy, 61*, 328–334.

Poole, J. L. (2008). Musculoskeletal factors. In E. B. Crepeau, E. S. Cohn, & B. A. B. Schell (Eds.), *Willard & Spackman's occupational therapy* (11th ed.). Baltimore, MD: Lippincott Williams & Wilkins.

Randall, M., Johnson, L., & Reddihough, D. (1999). *The Melbourne Assessment of Unilateral Upper Limb Function: Test administration manual.* Melbourne, Australia: Royal Children's Hospital.

Rensink, M., Schuurmans, M., Lindeman, E., & Hafsteinsdottir, T. (2009). Task-oriented training in rehabilitation after stroke: Systematic review. *Journal of Advanced Nursing, 6*,737–754.

Robinson, V., Brosseau, L., Casimiro, L., Judd, M., Shea, B., Wells, G., & Tugwell, P. (2002). Thermotherapy for treating rheumatoid arthritis. *Cochrane Database of Systematic Reviews*, (2), CD002826.

Sabari, J. (2011). Activity-based interventions in stroke rehabilitation. In G. Gillen (Ed.), *Stroke rehabilitation: A function-based approach* (3rd ed., pp. 80–99). St. Louis, MO: Mosby.

Sangster, C. A., Beninger, C., Polatajko, H. J., & Mandich, A. (2005). Cognitive strategy generation in children with developmental coordination disorder. *Canadian Journal of Occupational Therapy, 72*, 67–77.

Schmidt, R. A., & Lee, T. D. (2011). *Motor control and learning: A behavioral emphasis* (5th ed.). Champaign, IL: Human Kinetics.

Shumway-Cook, A., & Woollacott, M. (2012). *Motor control: Translating research into clinical practice* (4th ed.). Baltimore, MD: Lippincott Williams & Wilkins.

Ste-Marie, D. M., Clark, S. E., Findlay, L. C., & Latimer, A. E. (2004). High levels of contextual interference enhance handwriting skill acquisition. *Journal of Motor Behavior, 36*, 115–126.

Sterr, A., Elbert, T., Berthold, I., Kolbel, S., Rockstroh, B., & Taub, E. (2002). Longer versus shorter daily constraint-induced movement therapy of chronic hemiparesis: an exploratory study. *Archives of Physical Medicine & Rehabilitation, 83*, 1374–1377.

Stoykov, M. E., Lewis, G. N., & Corcos, D. M. (2009). Comparison of bilateral and unilateral training for upper extremity hemiparesis in stroke. *Neurorehabilitation and Neural Repair, 23*, 945–953.

Subramanian, S. K., Massie, C. L., Malcolm, M. P., & Levin, M. F. (2010). Does provision of extrinsic feedback result in improved motor learning in the upper limb poststroke? A systematic review of the evidence. *Neurorehabilitation and Neural Repair, 24*, 113–124.

Taub, E., Miller, N. E., Novack, T. A., Cook, E. W., III, Fleming, W. C., Nepomuceno, C. S., . . . Crago, J. E. (1993). Technique to improve chronic motor deficit after stroke. *Archives of Physical Medicine and Rehabilitation, 74*, 347–354.

Timmermans, A. A. A, Spooren, A. I. F, Kingma, H., & Seelen, H. A. M. (2010). Influence of task-oriented training content on skilled arm-hand performance in stroke: A systematic review. *Neurorehabilitation & Neural Repair, 24*, 858–870.

Uswatte, G., Taub, E., Griffin, M. A., Vogtle, L., Rowe, J., & Barman, J. (2012). The Pediatric Motor Activity Log-revised: Assessing real-world arm use in children with cerebral palsy. *Rehabilitation Psychology, 57*, 149–158.

Uswatte, G., Taub, E., Morris, D., Light, K., & Thompson, P. A. (2006). The Motor Activity Log-28: Assessing daily use of the hemiparetic arm after stroke. *Neurology, 67*, 1189–1194.

Uswatte, G., Taub, E., Morris, D., Vignolo, M., & McCulloch, K. (2005). Reliability and validity of the upper-extremity Motor Activity Log-14 for measuring real-world arm use. *Stroke, 36*, 2493.

Wallen, M., Bundy, A., Pont, K., & Ziviani, J. (2009). Psychometric properties of the Pediatric Motor Activity Log used for children with cerebral palsy. *Developmental Medicine and Child Neurology, 51*, 200–208.

Werner, R. A., Franzblau, A., & Gell, N. (2005). Randomized controlled trial of nocturnal splinting for active workers with symptoms of carpal tunnel syndrome. *Archives of Physical Medicine and Rehabilitation, 86*, 1–7.

Wolf, S. L., Catlin, P. A., Ellis, M., Archer, A. L., Morgan, B., & Piacentino, A. (2001). Assessing Wolf Motor Function Test as outcome measure for research in patients after stroke. *Stroke, 32*, 1635–1639.

Wolf, S. L, Thompson, P. A, Winstein, C. J, Miller, J. P., Blanton, S. R., Nichols-Larsen, D. S., . . . Sawaki, L. (2010). The EXCITE stroke trial: Comparing early and delayed constraint-induced movement therapy. *Stroke, 41*, 2309–2315.

Wolf, S. L., Winstein, C. J., Miller, J. P., Taub, E., Uswatte, G., Morris, D., . . . Nichols-Larsen, D. (2006). Effect of constraint-induced movement therapy on upper extremity function 3 to 9 months after stroke: The EXCITE randomized clinical trial. *The Journal of American Medical Association, 296*, 2095–2104.

Zwicker, J. G., & Harris, S. R. (2009). A reflection on motor learning theory in pediatric occupational therapy practice. *Canadian Journal of Occupational Therapy, 76*, 29–37.

For additional resources on the subjects discussed in this chapter, visit http://thePoint.lww.com/Willard-Spackman12e.

CHAPTER 55

Cognition, Perception, and Occupational Performance

Joan Pascale Toglia, Kathleen M. Golisz, Yael Goverover

LEARNING OBJECTIVES

After reading this chapter, you will be able to:

1. Define cognition and describe its association with activity limitation and participation
2. Discuss the role of occupational therapy practitioners in cognitive rehabilitation
3. Describe the key characteristics and process of a comprehensive approach to evaluate cognition and perception.
4. Discuss the difference among models of intervention
5. Discuss the factors that need to be considered when choosing evaluation and intervention approaches, including the evidence that supports decisions
6. Define specific cognitive and perceptual skills, identify possible assessments to evaluate these skills, and discuss the different approaches for therapy that are described for each cognitive and perceptual skill

"Thinking, remembering, reasoning, and making sense of the world around us are fundamental to carrying out everyday living activities" (Unsworth, 1999, p. 3). **Cognition** consists of interrelated processes, including the ability to perceive, organize, assimilate, and manipulate information to enable the person to process information, learn, and **generalize** (Abreu & Toglia, 1987). Because so much of rehabilitation in general requires learning and generalization, the principles of intervention that are discussed in this chapter are important to consider with a wide spectrum of clients and are not limited to those who are typically identified with cognitive impairments. Cognitive impairments may be seen as a result of developmental or learning problems, brain injury or disease, psychiatric dysfunction, or sociocultural conditions (American Occupational Therapy Association [AOTA], in press).

OUTLINE

Cognitive impairments can result in significant activity limitations and participation restrictions in all aspects of the client's life, potentially compromising safety, health, and well-being. For example, decreased abilities to recognize potential hazards, anticipate consequences of actions and behaviors, follow safety precautions, and respond to emergencies are often major factors that interfere with independence. Cognitive limitations can also diminish one's sense of competence, self-efficacy, and self-esteem, further compounding difficulties in adapting to the demands of everyday living. The influence of cognitive symptoms can be observed across all aspects of the domain of occupational therapy practice. The aim of occupational therapy intervention for people with cognitive-perceptual impairments is to decrease activity limitations, enhance participation in everyday activities, and assist individuals to gain the abilities they need to take control over their lives and develop healthy and satisfying ways of living. Although the ultimate goal of intervention with this population is clear, there are different perspectives and rehabilitation approaches to accomplish the goal.

Overview of Models and Theories of Cognition

Models and theories of cognitive rehabilitation and recovery incorporate different perspectives on learning and the ability to generalize information. Each model incorporates several approaches; however, they differ in the areas targeted for change or emphasized in intervention. Although some models emphasize change in the task or environment (e.g., functional cognitive models), others emphasize change in the person's skills (e.g., remedial). Evaluation and treatment guidelines reflect these different areas of focus. Various models, theories, and intervention approaches to cognition are explored in this section. Factors that are critical in application of theory to the selection of an intervention approach as well as methods for systematically integrating them are also discussed.

Cognitive Functional Models: Functional Skill Training and Task or Environmental Adaptations

Cognitive functional models emphasize the ability to successfully perform everyday tasks and routines by capitalizing on the person's assets or residual skills. Activity limitations and participation restrictions are reduced by changing the task and environment or enhancing specific task performance rather than remediating or restoring impaired skills (Figure 55.1). Common approaches used within cognitive functional models include environmental adaptation (Allen, 1985); use of task modifications and compensatory methods; caregiver education and training (Gitlin, Hodgson, Jutkowitz, & Pizzi, 2010); task specific methods such as errorless learning, vanishing cues, or spaced retrieval; and use of everyday technologies such as mobile phones, iPads, or computers to support cognitive abilities (Katz, Baum, & Maeir, 2011; Page,Wilson, Sheil, Carter, & Norris, 2006). The effectiveness of these methods has been demonstrated in persons with schizophrenia (Velligan et al., 2009), brain injury (Giles, Ridley, Dill, & Frye, 1997), dementia (Bier et al., 2008; Gitlin, Jacobs, & Earland, 2010), and autism (Green, 2001). It is important to recognize that functional methods can require different levels of learning, environmental supports, and awareness. For example, adaptations, task modifications, or technologies may be set up, implemented, and monitored by others or practiced repeatedly to capitalize on automatic learning. On the other hand, the person may be taught methods to modify or adapt activities themselves. This latter approach requires higher levels of learning and is integrated with strategy approaches that are discussed later.

The Cognitive Disability Model

Allen (1985) developed a Cognitive Disability Model (CDM) that provides guidelines for matching and adapting the individual's functional cognitive capacities with activity demands and contexts. In this model, function is organized into six ordinal levels of global functional cognitive capacities ranging from normal (level 6) to profoundly disabled (level 1). Modes of performance within each level further qualify behavior variations and allow for more sensitive measurement of the person's global functional capacity. To obtain a comprehensive description of the Allen Cognitive Levels, refer to Allen (1985) and Levy and Burns (2011).

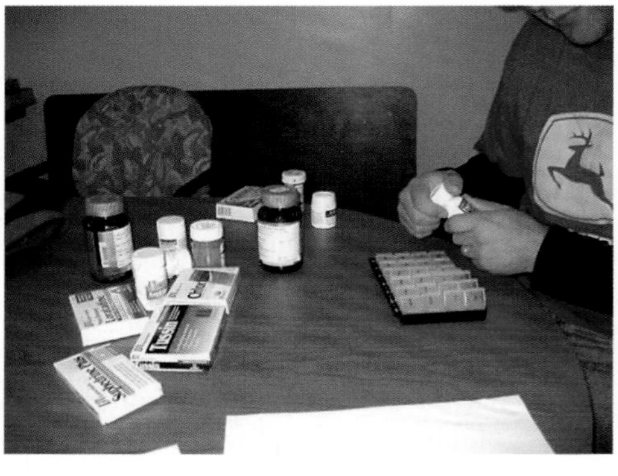

FIGURE 55.1 A pillbox organizer can be an important contextual cue to help those with memory impairments to safely self-administer medications.

More details about the CDM and Allen's levels are available at **http://thePoint.lww.com/Willard-Spackman12e.**

Environmental Skill Building Program

Gitlin, Winter, Dennis, Hodgson, and Hauck (2010a, 2010b) developed an environmental skill-building program (ESP) for persons with dementia that was influenced by the CDM and includes a system of matching environmental demands with the individual's capabilities. The ESP is a home based, individually tailored, client-centered program implemented by occupational therapists. It includes collaboration with caregivers to identify concerns and strategies that are practiced within the home environment. Studies have found that the ESP reduces frequency of behavioral symptoms and functional dependence in dementia clients, caregiver upset, and need for assistance from others and improves caregiver skill, efficacy, and mood (Gitlin et al., 2009; Gitlin et al., 2010a, 2010b).

Cognitive Adaptation Training

Another approach that shares some similarities with the CDM is cognitive adaptation training. Velligan et al. (2006) collaborated with occupational therapists to create a systematic approach for the use of environmental supports and compensatory strategies for persons with schizophrenia. Velligan et al. (2006) found that cognitive adaptation training improved functional behaviors for patients with schizophrenia; however, supports were not likely to be used unless they were customized for individual clients and set up in the home environment. Persons with different cognitive behaviors (e.g., decreased initiation versus disinhibition) were found to benefit from different types of adaptations (Velligan et al., 2009). This confirms it is important that adaptations and supports directly address the problems and needs that have been identified by the client or significant other as well as be appropriate to the client's cognitive symptoms.

Functional Task Training: The Neurofunctional Approach

Giles (2011) describes a neurofunctional approach (NFA) initially designed for persons with chronic or severe cognitive impairments as a result of traumatic brain injury. NFA emphasizes the use of task-specific training or rote repetition of specific task or routines within natural contexts to develop habits or functional behavioral routines. Repetitive practice reduces demands on cognitive resources needed for task performance and increases automaticity of performance. Emphasis is on the mastery of functional task performance through practice of "doing" meaningful activities. Intervention involves systematically breaking down a functional task into essential subcomponents for the person (Giles, 2011; Glisky, Schacter, & Butters, 1994). Behavioral techniques including feedback, reinforcement, and chaining are incorporated into structured practice sessions. Key techniques such as goal setting, task analysis, repetition, practice, cue experimentation, errorless learning, feedback, and reinforcement methods (Giles, 2011) may be used to promote skill acquisition. In errorless learning, the person is prevented from making incorrect or inappropriate responses during the learning process.

Functional task training capitalizes on procedural or implicit memory of "how to" do something rather than verbal memory for facts and events. Electronic cueing devices including pagers or PDAs can be used to promote internalization of habits and routines during task-specific training. Functional task training can produce significant changes in activities of daily living (ADL) and work tasks in people with severe or long-term cognitive impairments (Giles, 2011; Giles, Ridley, Dill, & Frye, 1997; Giles & Shore, 1989; Glisky et al., 1994; Hallgren & Kottorp, 2005; Kottorp, Hallgren, Bernspang, & Fisher, 2003).

Remedial Models

Remedial models place an emphasis on evaluating and restoring impaired cognitive-perceptual skills (Unsworth, 2007). The emphasis is on identifying and targeting the person's underlying deficits or skills rather than on manipulating the activity demands or context (Neistadt, 1990; Zoltan, 2007).

In traditional cognitive-perceptual remedial approaches, cognitive skills are conceptualized in terms of higher cortical skills, which are divided into a hierarchy of discrete subskills such as attention, discrimination, memory, sequencing, categorization, concept formation, and problem solving. The lower level skills provide the foundation for more complex skills and behaviors (Toglia, 2011). For example, attention skills are addressed before higher level cognitive skills such as problem solving. Cognitive remedial training has been applied to diverse populations; however, treatment appears to be most successful with those who have mild and discrete deficits, particularly in the area of working memory (Klingberg, 2010; Vallat et al., 2005), and demonstrate strong motivation for improvement.

Improvement in underlying cognitive or perceptual deficits is thought to promote recovery or reorganization of the impaired skill. Information on functional reorganization and adult brain plasticity supports this view.

More details about adult brain plasticity are available at **http://thePoint.lww.com/Willard-Spackman12e.**

Targeted and intense training of discrete skills using new technology that automatically adjusts challenge level based on the person's ability level and response is different than use of repetitive memory drills, logic games, or general cognitive stimulation activities.

In addition, remedial interventions have been criticized because a person can show changes in specific cognitive exercises without changes in everyday function (Cicerone et al., 2011). Remedial interventions have been found to be more effective when combined with other intervention techniques such as coaching, goal setting, peer support (Johansson & Tornmalm, 2012), self-monitoring techniques, strategy training, or when used to enhance a rehabilitation program. Although remedial cognitive activities can supplement comprehensive programs that address meaningful activities and motivational or affective components, the isolated use of computer-based tasks is not recommended because of limited evidence of generalization to function (Cicerone et al., 2011).

Cognitive Strategy Models

Models that emphasize the use of cognitive strategies view such strategies as part of normal cognition. Strategies are described as methods or tactics that we use to increase information processing, learning, or performance. Cognitive strategies can be internal and include self-talk, self-cues, self-questions, or use of mental practice, or they can be external and include the use of a checklist. They can also be situational or specific to certain tasks or environments, or general and used across a wide variety (Toglia, 2011). Rather than focusing on discrete cognitive skills, strategy models focus on methods or approaches to enhance learning and performance. Typically healthy people use multiple strategies simultaneously to cope with cognitively challenging situations. Use of strategies typically requires metacognitive skills such as the ability to anticipate challenges, monitor performance, detect errors, and self-evaluate performance. Models that focus on strategies, therefore, also emphasize metacognitive skills. Cognitive strategy approaches have been used with both children and adults. Examples of models and approaches that use strategies include Goal Management Training, the Occupational Goal Intervention (OGI) (Katz & Keren, 2011), the Multicontext Approach (Toglia, 2011), and the Cognitive Orientation to Occupational Performance (CO-OP) approach (Polatajko, Mandich, & McEwen, 2011). The latter two models are discussed in detail later.

The Dynamic Model of Cognition

The Dynamic Interactional Model of cognition was the first to draw on dynamic systems theory to explain the dynamic nature of cognitive functioning. It integrates information on learning from cognitive and educational psychology with occupational therapy practice. The Dynamic Interactional Model explains how cognitive symptoms and occupational performance change depending on the interaction between personal factors as well as activity and environmental demands. Personal characteristics that influence learning and performance include the person's lifestyle, beliefs, self-efficacy, emotional status, and motivation. Self-awareness and processing strategies are identified as key components of cognitive function. The ability to effectively use strategies and monitor performance varies with external factors such as activity demands and the social, cultural, or physical environment, as well as personal characteristics. Assessment, therefore, uses dynamic interactive methods to determine how external variables such as activity demands, alterations in the environment, and mediation from others influence a person's strategy use and self-awareness during task performance.

Because dynamic assessment examines *how* performance can be facilitated, it is naturally linked to intervention. During an evaluation, the therapist intervenes to change, guide, or improve the person's performance by using guided questioning, suggesting strategies, facilitating error detection, or modifying the activity (Tzuriel, 2000). This information directly relates to intervention planning. For example, if performance cannot be modified through dynamic procedures, then an intervention approach that seeks to change the environment or train caregivers might be more appropriate than an approach that focuses on changing a person's abilities or behaviors. Intervention may address the person's self-awareness and use of strategies, modification of the task or environment, or a combination of all three to optimize the fit between the person's abilities and the task and environment. The dynamic model of cognition provides a broad view of cognition that accommodates multiple intervention approaches.

The Multicontext Approach

The multicontext approach is based on the Dynamic Model of Cognition but provides a more specific framework for facilitating awareness and strategy use within activities or environments that may need to be adapted so that they are at a "just right" challenge level for the client (i.e., activities that are not too difficult but also not too easy). The key features of the multicontext approach include (1) consideration of personal context, (2) structured methods to promote self-monitoring and self-awareness, (3) strategy self-generation and training, and (4) practice across multiple activities and contexts using a transfer continuum. The strategies that are addressed in treatment vary depending on the client and their cognitive symptoms. Examples of the wide range of internal and external strategies that might be addressed in treatment are provided by Toglia (2011). There is a focus on assisting the client in anticipating challenges and generating strategies themselves. The ability to apply and transfer use of strategies across different situations is a focus of this approach.

For example, in the multicontext approach, the person practices application of a targeted strategy such as the use of a checklist, mental rehearsal, or self-cues across purposeful and occupation-based activities that systematically differ in appearance yet remain at a similar level of difficulty. This places gradual demands on the ability to transfer learning because the more two situations or activities are physically similar, the easier it is to transfer strategies learned in one situation to another (Davidson & Sternberg, 1998; Toglia, 1991b). Table 55.1 shows an

TABLE 55.1 The Transfer Continuum

Strategy emphasized in all activities: Use a checklist to gather and keep track of items to:							
Very Similar		**Somewhat Similar**		**Different**		**Very Different**	
Make vegetable salad (6–8 items)	Make fruit salad (6–8 items)	Set a table for dinner (for 6–8)	Pack 6–8 items in a lunchbox	Pack 6–8 items in a bag for an overnight stay	Put a list of 6–8 appointments in a calendar	Use a list to complete 6–8 party invitations	Use a list to complete 6–8 errands

example of intervention activities presented along the transfer continuum. Activity demands are not graded in difficulty until evidence of spontaneous strategy use along the entire transfer continuum is observed. The use of awareness and metacognitive training techniques to facilitate self-monitoring skills and self-evaluation is deeply embedded throughout intervention.

The multicontext approach was originally developed for use with adults with traumatic brain injury (Toglia, 2011); however, it has been applied to persons with schizophrenia (Josman, 2011), adults with lupus and multiple sclerosis, as well as with children and adolescents (Cermak & Maeir, 2011; Josman & Rosenblum, 2011).

The Cognitive Orientation to Occupational Performance Approach

The CO-OP approach was originally developed in 2001 to enhance skill acquisition in children with developmental coordination disorder (DCD; Polatajko, Mandich, Miller, & Mcnab, 2001) and subsequently applied to children with autism (Rodger & Vishram, 2010), cerebral palsy (Mandich, Polatajko, & Zilberbrant, 2008), and pervasive developmental disorder (Phelan, Steinke, & Mandich, 2009) as well as adults with stroke (Henshaw, Polatajko, McEwen, Ryan, & Baum, 2011) and brain injury (Dawson, Gaya et al., 2009). The CO-OP approach highlights the use of cognitive strategies in the development and acquisition of motor skills and daily living skills. It draws on dynamic systems theory as well as literature in motor performance, educational or cognitive psychology, and occupational therapy. Key components of the CO-OP approach include (1) client-centered goals, (2) dynamic performance analysis, (3) cognitive strategy use, (4) guided discovery, (5) enabling principles that include methods for promoting client engagement and learning, (6) parent or significant other involvement, and (7) a structured intervention format (preparation phase, acquisition phase, and check verification phase). The CO-OP approach is embedded within a client-centered framework and uses several techniques to ensure that the skills to be acquired are goals that the client wants, needs, or is expected to acquire. Evaluation uses several different tools to establish and assess client goals. In addition, dynamic performance analysis (DPA) is used as a top-down, structured method of observation to identify performance problems or breakdowns within activities that are chosen by the client and performed in context. The CO-OP approach uses a combination of a global strategy (Goal, Plan, Do, Check) as well as task-specific strategies to acquire skills that will support the person's daily functioning. For example, Rodger and Vishram (2010) describe the use of the CO-OP approach with two children with Asperger's syndrome. Goals for one child included getting organized for school in the morning, managing anger in the playground, and managing time to complete homework. The global "goal, plan, do, check" strategy was used as an overall problem-solving framework throughout intervention. Domain-specific strategies such as visual charts or lists as well as walking away, counting to 10, or punching a bag when feeling angry to manage specific tasks or situations were facilitated through the use of guided discovery and enabling principles. The children created and wrote their own goals and plans, reward charts, and time logs and were encouraged to discover their own solutions through the use of coaching, modeling, or feedback.

The Cognitive Rehabilitation Model

Averbuch and Katz (2011) describe a comprehensive occupational therapy cognitive rehabilitation model for adolescents and adults with neurological disabilities that integrates remedial principles with strategy use and awareness of abilities to broaden the capacity for learning. The model draws on neurophysiological, neurobiological, and neuropsychological theories to provide a framework for cognitive learning. Different approaches may be emphasized at various stages of the injury. Training is directed at initially enhancing remaining abilities and improving functional task performance within the context of client or family goals. Cognitive training is structured according to different levels and involves a gradual increase in the amount and complexity of information presented. Intervention involves systematic and structured activities that involve visual scanning, categorization or classification, sequencing, planning, or thinking operations but at the same time, there is an emphasis on teaching new learning strategies (e.g., systematic visual scanning strategy) to perform skills related to the different areas of cognitive function. Once clients learn to use strategies in various activities within the clinic, strategies are practiced in real-life situations. The authors use a combination of paper-and-pencil exercises, tabletop and computer activities, functional activities, compensatory methods, and virtual reality. If the client is incapable of using learning strategies, procedural strategies that focus on training the component parts of a task are used to promote the ability to perform ADL (Katz & Hartman-Maeir, 2005).

More details about applying various intervention models to specific cases are available at **http://thePoint.lww.com/Willard-Spackman12e.**

Selecting Intervention Approaches

Given the wide ranges of severity, symptoms, ages, populations, and performance challenges that can be observed with persons with cognitive perceptual dysfunction, there is not one model or approach that would be expected to fit all clients. Intervention approaches may result in different outcomes, depending on client characteristics such as age, severity of injury, etc.

In planning intervention, the clinician considers the following questions: How much change is expected from the person? How much learning and generalization are expected? How much do the activity demands or context need to be changed or altered to meet the person's capabilities? Is the person responsive to cues? Is the person aware of his or her difficulties? If the person is completely unaware of his or her difficulties, is unresponsive to cues, has severe global deficits, and does not show potential for change within the intervention time frame, a treatment approach that targets changes in strategy use such as the multicontext approach, CO-OP approach, or the cognitive retraining approach might not be appropriate. The CDM or the ESP that focuses on teaching others to change the environment or activity rather than the person may result in greater functional outcomes. The NFA, which uses repetitive practice to change performance on a specific task, might also be indicated to increase functional performance. On the other hand, a person that is highly motivated with focal cognitive deficits who is well aware of weaknesses and is able to engage in intense and consistent practice may show benefits from a remedial approach that targets specific cognitive skills. Another client who shows only partial or incomplete self-awareness, task error patterns that affect performance across situations, and decreased use of strategies might benefit from a cognitive strategy approach.

Considerations of the severity of the cognitive and functional deficits as well as assumptions regarding awareness and learning and the type of change expected within intervention models need to be carefully considered in planning intervention (Toglia, 2011). This is reflected in the scenarios described in Case Study 55.1.

CASE STUDY 55.1 Cognition and Performance Contexts

Scenario 1

Mr. James is a 24-year-old man with a 10-year history of attention and memory problems related to a head trauma that he sustained at age 14. He has difficulty in recalling conversations and events that occurred just hours before. During performance of a task, he easily loses track of the steps and repeats some steps twice while omitting other steps altogether. Mr. James denies any difficulty with his concentration or memory and would like to return to school. He currently lives with his parents, who care for him.

Scenario 2

Mr. Cornwall is a 64-year-old man with attention and memory problems related to a head trauma that he sustained 3 weeks ago. He has difficulty in recalling conversations and events that occurred just hours before. During performance of a task, he easily loses track of the steps and repeats some steps twice while omitting other steps altogether. Mr. Cornwall is well aware of his difficulties and is depressed by them. For example, he states, "I can't even remember what I ate for breakfast. What good am I? If I have to give up my business, my life is over." Mr. Cornwall was recently widowed and lived alone before his accident.

Questions

The two scenarios describe the same clinical symptoms but the performance contexts are different.

1. How do the differences in context influence the emphasis in intervention that you would use?
2. What influenced your selection?

Discussion

There are no absolute right or wrong answer to these questions. In scenario 1, Mr. James is 10 years postinjury, so the potential for change in the underlying cognitive skills is assumed to be minimal. A remedial approach that focuses on improving memory and attention skills would not be warranted unless there was some evidence of potential for further improvement. Compensatory strategies such as the use of a memory notebook or a checklist could be considered. However, Mr. James denies any difficulty in memory or attention. This lack of self-awareness will present a major obstacle to independent initiation and the use of compensatory strategies.

Caregiver training, task and environmental adaptation, and the possibility of functional skill training to increase performance on a specified task appear to be the most appropriate areas for intervention. Techniques to increase awareness may

CASE STUDY 55.1 Cognition and Performance Contexts (*Continued*)

be attempted as a prerequisite for using compensatory aids. External memory aids such as memory notebook training may be introduced by using task-specific training methods in combination with maximum prompts and external cues for their use; however, success likely depends on Mr. James's ability to gain some awareness and acceptance of his disability.

In scenario 2, Mr. Cornwall is only 3 weeks postinjury, so that the potential for change in the underlying skills is presumably present. In addition, Mr. Cornwall is well aware of his problems. This would appear to make him a potential candidate for remedial techniques. However, he is also depressed by his difficulties. He might not be able to cope emotionally with an approach that focuses on the underlying client factors.

An approach that will provide greater opportunities for success and control over his environment could be the initial intervention emphasis. For example, adaptive techniques in which the caregiver or practitioner presents directions one step at a time might make it easier for Mr. Cornwall to follow task instructions. Training in the use of compensatory strategies such as the use of a memory notebook to keep track of daily events and conversations and the use of a checklist to assist in keeping track of task steps that have already been completed might enhance task performance. As Mr. Cornwall gains self-confidence and control, remedial tasks that focus on improving attention may be gradually introduced if he is able to tolerate them. ■

Evaluation

This section provides detailed information about cognitive evaluation issues that are necessary for practitioners to understand before choosing and performing appropriate assessments. We present the importance of the evaluation process, its goals, and considerations in choosing an assessment.

Comprehensive cognitive evaluations are used for two primary reasons. First, evaluations provide evidence and information about the presence of impairments and performance competencies. Such information can be used to establish baselines, to plan discharge, and to measure intervention effectiveness (e.g., rehabilitation outcomes). Second, evaluations gather information for intervention planning.

The Cognition Evaluation Process

Occupational therapists approach the evaluation process with the goal of identifying cognitive challenges to occupational performance as well as the cognitive strengths that can support clients' engagement in their everyday life. Using a Cognitive Functional Evaluation Process (Hartman-Maeir, Katz, & Baum, 2009), therapists intentionally select and sequence evaluations that provide information about a client's cognitive capabilities. Initial interviews along with cognitive and functional screenings may be followed by more domain-specific assessments, specific cognitive measures in occupation-based tasks, and an environmental assessment. When combined, the data from the cognitive evaluation process provides the therapist with a comprehensive perspective of the potential interaction of the person-occupation-environment and the influence of cognitive symptoms. See Table 55.2 for detailed information about cognitive and perceptual assessments.

The role of the occupational therapist in evaluating cognition and perception is to provide clear, comprehensive information on the effect of cognitive-perceptual impairments on ADL, instrumental activities of daily living (IADL), education, work, play and leisure, and social participation. All team members need to consider that other factors besides cognitive impairments may impact the client's performance. The client's true cognitive abilities may be masked by language impairments, pain, fatigue, low motivation, depression, anxiety, or psychological distress.

Interviews—The Perspective of the Client and Others

The occupational therapist typically begins the evaluation process by gathering information directly from the client and/or family members. A structured interview that considers the client's typical routines and occupations helps the therapist develop an occupational profile of the client's past functioning and goals for the future (AOTA, 2008). The client is usually asked to identify everyday activities that he or she is most concerned about or would like to be able to do with greater ease (see Table 55.2).

Interviews with community-dwelling clients to identify current levels of participation and desired changes may involve the use of participation scales such as the Mayo-Portland Adaptability Inventory (MPAI-4; Malec & Lezak, 2008), the Community Integration Questionnaire (CIQ; Willer, Ottenbacher, & Coad, 1994), or the Participation Objective, Participation Subjective (POPS; Curtin et al., 2011). These scales typically ask the client to rate the frequency and satisfaction of their current participation in various tasks, most of which can be impacted by the presence of cognitive symptoms.

Because people with cognitive impairments often have limited awareness of their impairments and limited understanding of the implications of these impairments (Goverover, Chiaravalloti, & DeLuca, 2005), a close relative or friend should participate in identifying concerns and priorities for intervention. In acute or rehabilitation

TABLE 55.2 Cognitive Perceptual Assessments

Interview—Perspective of Client and Others	**Occupational Profile** Canadian Occupational Performance Measure (COPM) (Law et al., 2005) Activity Card Sort (ACS) (Baum & Edwards, 2001) Pediatric version (PACS) (Mandich, Polatajko, Miller, & Baum, 2004) **Awareness Assessments** Assessment of Awareness of Disability (AAD) (Tham, Bernspang, & Fisher, 1999) Awareness Questionnaire (AQ) (Sherer, Bergloff, Boake, High, & Levin, 1998) Patient Competency Rating Scale (PCRS) (Prigatano, 1986) Self-Awareness of Deficits Interview (SADI) (Fleming, Strong, & Ashton, 1996)
Cognitive Screening Instruments	**Mental Status Exams** Blessed Dementia Rating Scale (BDRS) (Blessed, Tomlinson, & Roth, 1968) Galveston Orientation and Amnesia Test (GOAT) (Levin, O'Donnell, & Grossman, 1979) Pediatric version: Children's Orientation and Amnesia Test (COAT) (Ewing-Cobbs, Levin, Fletcher, Miner, & Eisenberg, 1990) Mini-Mental State Exam (MMSE) (Folstein, Folstein, & McHugh, 1975) Modified Mini-Mental State Examination (3MS) (Teng & Chui, 1987) Montreal Cognitive Assessment (MoCA) (Nasreddine et al., 2005) Saint Louis University Mental Status (SLUMS) (Tariq, Tumosa, Chibnall, Perry, & Morley, 2006) **Comprehensive Cognitive Screenings** Brief Test of Head Injury (BTHI) (Helm-Estabrooks & Hotz, 1991) Cognitive Assessment of Minnesota (CAM) (Rustad et al., 1993) Cognistat (Kiernan, Mueller, & Langston, 2011) Dynamic Loewenstein Occupational Therapy Cognitive Assessment (DLOTCA) (Katz, Livni, Bar-Haim Erez, & Averbuch, 2011). Pediatric version available (DOTCA-Ch; Katz, Parush, & Traub Bar-Ilan, 2005) Lowenstein Occupational Therapy Cognitive Assessment (LOTCA) (Katz, Itzkovich, Averbuch, & Elazar, 1990) Geriatric version available Middlesex Elderly Assessment of Mental State (MEAMS) (Golding, 1989) Repeatable Battery for the Assessment of Neuropsychological Status (RBANS) (Randolph, 1998) Safe at Home (Robnett, Hopkins, & Kimball, 2003)
Functional Assessments of Cognition	**Assessments Measuring Competency or Assistance Required:** Independent Living Scales (ILS) (Loeb, 1996) Kettle Test (Hartman-Maeir, Harel, & Katz, 2009) Kitchen Task Assessment (KTA) (Baum & Edwards, 1993); Pediatric version available: Children's Kitchen Task Assessment (CKTA) (Rocke, Hays, Edwards, & Berg, 2008) Performance Assessment of Self-Care Skills, Version 3.1 (Holm & Rogers, 1999) Rabideau Kitchen Evaluation-Revised (RKE-R) (Neistadt, 1992b) Revised Observed Tasks of Daily Living (OTDL-R) (Diehl, 1998) Texas Functional Living Scale (TFLS) (Cullum, Weiner, & Saine, 2009) **Assessments Observing Factors Interfering with Performance** Actual Reality Task (Goverover, O'Brien, Moore, & DeLuca, 2010) ADL-focused Occupation-based Neurobehavioral Evaluation (A-ONE; formerly, Árnadóttir OT-ADL Neurobehavioral Evaluation) (Arnadottir, 1990) Allen Cognitive Level Test (ACL) (Allen, Earhart, & Blue, 1992) Assessment of Motor and Process Skills (AMPS) (Fisher, 1993a, 1993b) Cognitive Performance Test (CPT) (Allen et al., 1992) Do-Eat Assessment for Children (Josman, Goffer, & Rosenblum, 2010) Executive Function Performance Test (EFPT) (Baum, Edwards, Morrison, & Hahn, 2003) Instrumental Activities of Daily Living (IADL) profile (Bottari, Gosseli, Guillemette, LaMoureux, & Ptito, 2011) Routine Task Inventory-Expanded (RTI-E) (Katz, 2006)

TABLE 55.2 Cognitive Perceptual Assessments (*Continued*)

Functional Assessments of Cognition (*Continued*)	**Performance Assessments Measuring Error Patterns** Naturalistic Action Test (NAT) (Schwartz, Segal, Veramonti, Ferraro, & Buxbaum, 2002) Multiple Errands Test (MET) (Shallice & Burgess, 1991) Profile of Executive Control System (PRO-EX) (Branswell et al., 1992) Test of Adaptive Behavior in Schizophrenia (TABS) (Vanbellingen et al., 2010) Test of Grocery Shopping Skills (TOGSS) (Hamera & Brown, 2000) University of California, San Diego Performance-Based Skills Assessment-Brief (UPSA-Brief) (Mausbach, Harvey, Goldman, Jeste, & Patterson, 2007) Weekly Calendar Planning Task (WCPT) (Toglia, in press)
Cognitive Tests for Specific Domains	**Orientation Assessments** Orientation Log (O-Log) (Jackson, Novack, & Dowler, 1998) Test of Orientation for Rehabilitation Patients (TORP) (Deitz, Beeman, & Thorn, 1993) **Attention Assessments** Comprehensive Trail-Making Test (CTMT) (Reynolds, 2002) Paced Auditory Serial Addition Test (PASAT) (Gronwall, 1977) Test of Everyday Attention (TEA) (Robertson, Ward, Ridgeway, & Nimmo-Smith, 1994) Pediatric version available (TEA-CH) **Spatial Neglect Assessments** The Baking Tray Test (Tham & Tegner, 1996) The Balloons Test (Edgeworth, Robertson, & McMillan, 1998) Behavioral Inattention Test (BIT) (Wilson, Cockburn, & Baddeley, 1987) The Bells Test (Gauthier, Dehaut, & Joanette, 1989) Indented Paragraph Test (Caplan, 1987) Line Cancellation (Albert, 1973) Verbal and Nonverbal Cancellation Tasks (Mesulam, 2000) **Memory Assessments** Cambridge Prospective Memory Test (CAMPROMPT) (Shiel et al., 2005) Contextual Memory Test (CMT) (Toglia, 1993b) Hopkins Verbal Learning Test-Revised (HVLT-R) (Brandt & Benedict, 2001) Memory for Intentions Test (MIST) (Raskin & Buckheit, 2010) Prospective Memory Screening (PROMS) (Sohlberg & Mateer, 1989b) Rivermead Behavioral Memory Test-Extended version (RBMT-E) (Wilson, Clare, Baddeley, Watson, & Tate, 1998); Pediatric version available (RBMT-C) **Visual Perception Assessments** Brain Injury Visual Assessment Battery for Adults (biVABA) (Warren, 1998) Motor-Free Visual Perception Test (MVPT-3) (Colarusso & Hammill, 2002) Occupational Therapy Adult Perceptual Screening Test (OT-APST) (Cooke, McKenna, & Fleming, 2005) **Executive Function Assessments** Behavioral Assessment of Dysexecutive Syndrome (BADS) (Wilson, Alderman, Burgess, Emslie, & Evans, 1996) Behavioral Assessment of Dysexecutive Syndrome for Children (BADS-C) (Emslie, Wilson, Burden, Nimmo-Smith, & Wilson, 2003) Executive Function Route-Finding Task (EFRT) (Boyd & Sautter, 1993) Perceive, Recall, Plan, and Perform (PRPP@WORK) (Bootes & Chapparo, 2010) Plan-a-Day Test (Holt et al., 2011) Toglia Category Assessment (TCA) (Toglia, 1994) University of California, San Diego Sorting Test (U-SORT) (Tiznado, Mausbach, Cardenas, Jeste, & Patterson, 2010)

(*continued*)

TABLE 55.2 Cognitive Perceptual Assessments (*Continued*)

Cognitive Tests for Specific Domains (*Continued*)	**Motor Planning Assessments** Benton Constructional Praxis Test (Benton, Hamsher, Varney, & Spreen, 1983) Test of oral and limb apraxia (TOLA) (Helm-Estabrooks, 1992) Test of upper limb apraxia (TULIA) (Vanbellingen et al., 2010) Test of Ideational Praxis (TIP for children) (May-Benson & Cermak, 2007)
Ratings of Everyday Cognitive Symptoms and Behaviors	APT-2 Attention Questionnaire (Sohlberg & Mateer, 2001) Behavior Rating Inventory of Executive Function-Adult Version (BRIEF-A) (Roth, Isquith, & Gioia, 2005) Brief Assessment of Prospective Memory (BAPM) (Man, Fleming, Hohaus, & Shum, 2011) Catherine Bergego Scale (CBS) for Unilateral Neglect (Azouvi et al., 2003) Cognitive Failures Questionnaire (CFQ) (Broadbent, Cooper, FitzGerald, & Parkes, 1982; Wilhelm, Witthöft, & Schipolowski, 2010) Everyday Memory Questionnaire (EMQ) (Sunderland, Harris, & Baddeley, 1983; Prospective and Retrospective Memory Questionnaire (PRMQ) (Crawford, Smith, Maylor, Della Sala, & Logie, 2003)
Environmental Assessments	Analysis of Cognitive Environmental Support (ACES) (Ryan et al., 2011) Home Environmental Assessment Protocol (HEAP) (Gitlin et al., 2002) Home Occupational-Environmental Assessment (HOEA) (Baum & Edwards, 1998) Safety Assessment of Function and the Environment for Rehabilitation (SAFER tool) (Chui et al., 2006)

inpatient settings where clients' daily occupations are often structured and limited in nature, client's relatives may also be unaware of the presence of mild cognitive impairments. Subtle cognitive symptoms tend to be apparent only in higher level activities such as driving, social participation, shopping, or using public transportation. A clearer picture of the impact of the client's cognitive impairments may emerge when the client is discharged home to his or her community and resumes these higher level activities (Toglia & Golisz, in press).

Interview and rating scales for self-awareness (see Table 55.2) generally evaluate awareness of limitations and strengths, the ability to generalize the impact of limitations on functional tasks, and concerns regarding disability judgment (intellectual awareness). Typically, the person's self-ratings are compared to those of a relative or clinician (Bogod, Mateer, & MacDonald, 2003). Alternatively, some scales such as the Self-Awareness of Deficits Interview (Fleming et al., 1996) use a semistructured interview in which the clinician directly rates the person's level of awareness, depending on the response to questions. Both of these methods of assessing awareness examine intellectual awareness outside the context of an activity.

Although interviews and rating scales are the most common method of assessing awareness, it can also be assessed within the context of an activity by asking the client to estimate his or her performance before (i.e., anticipatory awareness) and immediately after (i.e., emergent awareness) performing a task. Differences between estimated performance and actual performance are compared. Task estimation including normative comparison is used within the Contextual Memory Test (Toglia, 1993b) and the Assessment of Awareness of Disability (Tham et al., 1999). Recently, a task-specific awareness scale was developed that asked the clients to identify challenges prior to task performance (Toglia, Goverover, Johnston, & Dain 2011; Toglia, Johnston, Goverover, & Dain, 2010). Changes in awareness that may occur during the experience of an activity can be examined by comparing responses to awareness questions before, during, and immediately after performance.

Cognitive Screenings

Cognitive-screening assessments are a type of standardized assessments designed to identify problems that need special or further attention. Mental status exams provide an overall score or diagnostic cutoff score that differentiates normal from suspect or impaired cognitive functioning. In choosing a screening, the published sensitivity (i.e., persons correctly identified as having cognitive impairment) and specificity (i.e., correct identification of persons without cognitive impairment) needs to be considered within the population that is being tested. Typically, mental status exams are 5- to 10-minute assessments that do not require equipment other than paper and pencil, making them convenient to bedside and office testing. In addition, many of these exams are in the public domain or freely available on the Internet. Mental status exams such as the popular Mini-Mental State Exam (MMSE; Folstein et al., 1975) were originally developed for clients with dementia of the Alzheimer's type but have been used and validated in other populations (Bour, Rasquin, Boreas, Limburg, & Verhey, 2010; Mackin, Ayalon, Feliciano, & Areán, 2010; Swirsky-Sacchetti et al., 1992; Toglia, Fitzgerald, O'Dell, Mastrogiovanni, & Lin, 2011). Most mental status exams provide global ratings of the client's orientation, attention, memory, language, and judgment. The more recent Montreal Cognitive Assessment (MoCA; Nasreddine et al., 2005) includes an executive function component to the mental status exam and has been shown to be more predictive of functional status and improvement than the MMSE in acute inpatients with stroke and mild cognitive impairment (Toglia, Fitzgerald et al., 2011). Mental status screenings generally identify the types of cognitive impairments that may be present; however, results need to be examined in combination with direct observation of functional performance to provide a complete picture of the client. Results of cognitive standardized assessments do not always translate clearly to functional performance.

Mental status exams have some additional disadvantages because they rely heavily on verbal skills, can be culturally biased (owing to comparison to normative populations), and have substantial false-negative rates (i.e., missing possible cognitive impairments). The deficits of clients with focal lesions, particularly right-hemisphere lesions, or mild diffuse cognitive disorders are often missed (Nelson, Fogel, & Faust, 1986). In general, cognitive-screening assessments may miss more subtle impairments that are displayed by higher level clients because the breadth and depth of item content are limited (Doninger, Bode, Heinemann, & Ambrose, 2000) (see Table 55.2).

Functional Assessment of Cognition

Direct observation of functional performance is another method used to identify cognitive-perceptual impairments. Clients with agitation or severely limited attention may be unable to engage in a standardized evaluation process. A task analysis system such as the Perceive, Recall, Plan, and Perform (PRPP) system may be used to assess information processing during functional or everyday tasks of clients in this phase of recovery (Nott & Chapparo, 2008; Nott, Chapparo, & Heard, 2009). The PRPP approach requires the occupational therapist to analyze the behavioral steps and typical cognitive processing strategies (i.e., sensory processing [Perceive], memory [Recall], response planning and evaluation [Plan], and performance monitoring [Perform]) used to successfully complete the task. Any functional task may be selected for observation and systematic rating of the efficacy of the information processing strategy demonstrated by the client. This method has been validated in adults with schizophrenia (Aubin, Chapparo, Gélinas, Stip, & Rainville, 2009), dementia (Steultjens, Voigt-Radloff, Leonhart, & Graff, 2011), and brain injury (Nott & Chapparo, 2008).

Some direct performance assessments such as the Kettle Test (Hartman-Maeir et al., 2009) rate the degree of assistance required for each substep of an IADL task within a functional context. This information may help determine the level of assistance needed for discharge planning. Other functional assessments are also designed to identify the cognitive and perceptual impairments that interfere with successful performance on such tasks. For example, in the ADL-focused Occupation-based Neurobehavioral Evaluation (A-ONE; formerly, Árnadóttir OT-ADL Neurobehavioral Evaluation) (Arnadottir, 1990), a client is observed performing a basic ADL (e.g., putting on a shirt) for possible cognitive impairments such as spatial relation difficulties, spatial or body neglect, and the like. The Executive Function Performance Test (Baum et al., 2003; Goverover et al., 2005) is a functional performance test that analyzes the need for assistance in executive components such as initiation, organization, and safety by observing client performance on IADL such as making a phone call. The Naturalistic Action Test (Schwartz et al., 2002) scores the accuracy of steps completed and types of error made (e.g., omissions, perseveration, spatial estimation, reversals, substitutions, quality) during the completion of three functional tasks (e.g., making toast and coffee, gift wrapping a present, and packing a child's lunchbox and schoolbag) under standardized conditions. Pediatric assessments such as the DO-Eat (Josman et al., 2010) and the Children's Kitchen Task Assessment (CKTA; Rocke et al., 2008) also consider the impact of executive function components on task performance. The development of cognitive domain assessments that use real-world objects or tasks has enabled therapists to make clearer links between observed functional task performance and the underlying cognitive impairments. The area of executive functioning is particularly robust with assessments that use function-based tasks. Tests such as the Multiple Errands Test (Shallice & Burgess, 1991) and Plan-a-Day Test (Holt et al., 2011) provide more specific information on client's performance of tasks requiring executive functioning skills. The occupational therapist must keep in mind that functional assessments simulating performance in a treatment setting may not be predictive of performance in natural **contexts** in which the person has to set goals, plan, initiate, problem-solve, and deal with subtle and complex environmental cues. Questionnaires or rating scales such as the Behavior Rating Inventory of Executive Function (BRIEF; Roth et al., 2005) or the Brief Assessment of Prospective Memory (BAPM; Man et al., 2011) can be completed by the client, clinician, and/or significant other. Although these assessments do not require actual performance of the functional task, they provide additional insight into how the cognitive symptoms impact everyday occupational performance (see Table 55.2).

Domain-Specific Cognitive Assessments

When the client's performance in either cognitive or occupation-based screenings indicates the potential for cognitive impairments, the occupational therapist may administer more specific standardized cognitive assessments. Comparing the client's performance to normative data can determine whether a cognitive impairment exists and quantify the severity of such impairments. This step in the evaluation process provides a more in-depth understanding of the client's cognitive impairments. Standardized cognitive assessments are typically static in nature, evaluating "here and now" performance and providing a baseline against which changes in condition or ability can be measured over time.

Cognitive impairments may also be assessed more specifically with assessments that simulate functional tasks or use functional objects (see Table 55.2). Many of these assessments have versions specifically designed for children and several assessments have been validated in individuals with schizophrenia.

Assessments based on the dynamic model of cognition such as the Contextual Memory Test (CMT; Toglia, 1993b) or the Toglia Category Assessment (TCA; Toglia, 1994) can provide information about underlying impairments and the ability to change the client's performance with cues or task modifications. Dynamic assessment methods have been applied to a wide range of ages and people with cognitive disabilities. However, research applications and specific tools are limited.

Environmental Assessment of Cognition Supports and Barriers

The environment in which cognitive tasks are performed may either support or hinder the client's occupational performance. Situations that require higher level cognitive-perceptual skills are difficult to capture in structured treatment environments. In addition, contextual factors can increase or decrease cognitive demands of performance, so it is important to consider the context in which an activity is performed. For example, Hamera and Brown (2000) developed the Test of Grocery Shopping Skills as a real-world measure of community function for people with chronic schizophrenia. Clients are asked to shop for a list of 10 grocery items in a natural context. In hospital-based treatment settings, the occupational therapist, however, might not be able to create a close enough approximation of a real-world environment. The contextual influence on performance needs to be kept in mind; and if feasible, performance should be observed across real-world contexts.

Occupational therapists may use one of several environmental assessments to specifically analyze the supports or barriers contributed by the environment to the performance of cognitive-based tasks. These assessments do not measure occupational performance or quantify the presence or severity of a cognitive impairment. They only provide additional information on how the environment influenced the client's performance. The Analysis of Cognitive Environmental Support (ACES; Ryan et al., 2011) assesses the cognitive supports and barriers with the environment, the client's awareness of the cognitive supports/barriers to performance, who introduced the support/barrier (e.g., client or someone else), and how recent is the support/barrier in relation to the client's cognitive impairment. The ACES is an expansion of the Home Occupational-Environmental Assessment (HOEA) developed by Baum and Edwards (1998).

Other environmental assessments such as the Safety Assessment of Function and the Environment for Rehabilitation (SAFER; Chui et al., 2006) focus on the client's ability to safely perform functional tasks within the home. Risks within the physical environment are rated in severity and environmental modifications are suggested. Some environmental assessments were designed for specific cognitively impaired populations, such as the Home Environmental Assessment Protocol (HEAP; Gitlin et al., 2002), which was developed for the dementia population.

Choosing the Most Appropriate Type of Assessment

Even within a structured cognitive evaluation process, there are numerous assessments that an occupational therapist can choose from to evaluate his or her client. In selecting the most appropriate type of assessment, an occupational therapist must first decide what questions need to be answered. The therapist can then select the assessment that will most effectively address such questions. Some factors to consider before choosing an assessment include questions such as the following:

1. *Does the therapist need to screen for the presence of cognitive impairments?* To answer this type of question, the therapist may use an assessment with normative comparison or cut-off scores with diagnostic-based sensitivity and specificity. The extent to which the person's scores deviates from expected performance identifies the presence and/or severity of cognitive impairments. In clients with moderate-to-severe impairments, occupational therapists may also use functional assessments such as the A-ONE to confirm the presence of deficits. If possible cognitive deficits are identified, the client may be referred to a neuropsychologist for a more comprehensive cognitive-perceptual assessment.
2. *Does the occupational therapist need to perform a comprehensive evaluation on a client who is confused, disoriented, and unable to identify common objects?* A client that presents with disorientation and possible agnosia will most likely be unable to follow the instructions of a standardized assessment. The therapist should monitor the client's orientation level and ability to appropriately identify and use common objects within functional tasks. If or when the confusion clears and the client can follow simple commands, the therapist may engage in more formal evaluation of the client's cognitive perceptual skills.
3. *Does the therapist need to understand the effect of cognitive-perceptual impairments on occupational performance (i.e., the activity limitation and participation restrictions from the International Classification of Function [ICF] [World Health Organization, 2001])?* When the existence of impairments has been validated by neuropsychological testing, the occupational therapist's role in evaluation usually focuses on describing the impact of cognitive dysfunction on functional

performance or analysis of the influence of different activity demands and contexts on everyday activities.

4. *Does the therapist need to be concerned about cognitive-perceptual deficits in a patient who scores within normal range on cognitive screenings and demonstrates no difficulty when completing self-care or routine activities?* Although the patient appears to be doing well in routine activities, the therapist also needs to consider complex activities or IADL tasks that the patient may need to perform as well as the ability to resume former roles and lifestyle. Testing the patient's ability to perform within unstructured IADL tasks and crowded environments requiring multitasking or executive skills will enable the therapist to identify any subtle impairment that may benefit from outpatient intervention. Participation measures may also identify difficulties in everyday life that may reflect subtle cognitive impairments.
5. *Does the therapist need information to guide intervention?* The model of cognitive intervention that the therapist is using often guides the selection of evaluation tools. Dynamic assessments emphasize the processes that are involved in learning and change (Grigorenko & Sternberg, 1998) and may provide information that is needed to plan and guide intervention that focuses on changing skills or behaviors.
6. *Does the therapist need to establish a baseline as a measurement of change or outcome of intervention?* To answer this question, the therapist needs to take into consideration short-term and long-term intervention goals. In documenting outcomes, it is important to take into consideration the three levels of disability described by the ICF: impairment, activity limitation, and participation restriction. Therefore, a cognitive perceptual evaluation that includes these three components will provide a more comprehensive view of the person's functioning.

Cognitive Impairments: Definitions, Evaluations, and Interventions

In this section, the main constructs involved in cognition will be discussed in terms of their definitions, evaluation, and treatment. Self-awareness will be discussed first because lack of awareness can affect the motivation, effort, and sustained participation that are needed for intervention (Toglia, 2011).

Following discussion of self-awareness, the areas of **orientation**, attention, memory, executive functions, **motor planning**, **spatial neglect**, and visual processing will be reviewed. Although these areas are discussed separately for the purposes of description, it should be kept in mind that cognitive problems are interrelated and rarely occur in isolation. Similarly, examples of intervention strategies and task or environmental adaptations for specific cognitive perceptual domains will be discussed; however, in clinical practice, various intervention methods are used in combination with each other and within the context of different models. The context of the person's life needs to be considered in planning and choosing intervention activities (Johnston, Goverover, & Dijkers, 2005). This includes the person's occupations, personality, interests, premorbid level of functioning, culture, values, external supports, and resources. Interventions that address cognitive impairments need to be blended with those that address interpersonal skills, social participation, and everyday activities, routines, and roles (Abreu & Peloquin, 2005).

More details about clinical signs and functional observations are available at **http://thePoint.lww.com/Willard-Spackman12e.**

Self-Awareness

Impaired self-awareness includes lack of knowledge about one's own cognitive-perceptual limitations and/or his or her functional implications as well as deficiencies in metacognitive skills such as the ability to anticipate difficulties, recognize errors, or monitor performance within the context of an activity (Toglia & Kirk, 2000). Impaired self-awareness presents obstacles to adjustment, collaborative goal setting, and active participation in intervention (Gillen, 2009). Decreased awareness results in poor motivation and compliance, lack of sustained effort, unrealistic expectations, incongruence between goals of the client and family, impaired judgment and safety, and inability to adopt the use of compensatory strategies (Hartman-Maeir, Soroker, Oman, & Katz, 2003; Sherer, Oden, Bergloff, Levin, & High, 1998; Toglia & Kirk, 2000). Several studies support the association between awareness and functional outcome (Ekstam, Uppgard, Kottorp, & Tham, 2007; Erickson, Jaafari, & Lysaker, 2011; Fischer, Gauggel, & Trexler, 2004; Goverover, 2004; Goverover, Chiaravalloti, Gaudino-Goering, Moore, & DeLuca, 2009; Griffen, Rapport, Bryer, Bieliauskas, & Burt, 2011; Hoofien, Gilboa, Vakil, & Barak, 2004; Noe et al., 2005; Tham, Ginsburg, Fisher, & Tegner, 2001; Verdoux, Monello, Goumilloux, Cougnard, & Prouteau, 2010).

Unawareness may be related to psychological or neurological sources. Denial is a psychological defense mechanism that is related to premorbid personality traits and is characterized by over-rationalization, hostility, resistance to feedback, and an unwillingness to confront problems (Prigatano, 1999). A person who has a history of denying inadequacies and resisting help from others and a strong desire to be "in control" is more likely to use denial as a coping strategy. Impaired self-awareness resulting from neurological lesions represents a lack of access to information regarding one's cognitive state and is characterized by surprise, indifference, or perplexity in response to feedback (Prigatano, 1999). In many cases, the neurological and psychological sources of unawareness coexist and cannot be easily differentiated. If denial is the predominant source of unawareness, methods of awareness training might not be effective (Lucas & Fleming, 2005).

Crosson et al. (1989) described a hierarchical pyramid model of awareness that distinguishes between intellectual awareness, emergent awareness, and anticipatory awareness. Clients with *intellectual awareness* verbally describe limitations in functioning whereas clients with *emergent awareness* recognize a problem only when it is actually happening. Clients with *anticipatory awareness* are able to anticipate that an impairment will likely cause a challenge before performing a given activity (Crosson et al., 1989). The hierarchical nature of this model has not been empirically demonstrated and there is some indication that the interrelationship between these concepts is complex and nonhierarchical (Abreu et al., 2001).

Toglia and Kirk (2000) proposed a dynamic model of awareness that includes self-knowledge or beliefs about knowledge and abilities that exists prior to an activity (i.e., intellectual awareness) and "online" awareness that includes self-monitoring and self-regulatory processes that are activated within the context of an activity. This view of awareness is nonhierarchical and proposes that levels of awareness vary across different tasks and contexts within the same domain. It implies that awareness needs to be assessed both outside and inside the context of an activity (Toglia & Kirk, 2000). In addition, it suggests that awareness involves both an interplay between neurological mechanisms as well as the task, the context, and personal factors such as personality, coping mechanisms, and culture.

A comprehensive evaluation of awareness plays a key role in guiding and selecting methods of intervention. Self-awareness training is a key component of the multicontext approach but not of other approaches such as the NFA. For example, in some cases, potential for changes in awareness may be limited, particularly within the intervention time frame or because of the disease course (e.g., Alzheimer's disease). In these situations, intervention methods that do not require awareness, such as functional skill training, errorless learning, or adaptation of the environment, might be most appropriate in facilitating occupational performance. If a lack of understanding of one's own strengths and limitations prevents a person from choosing goals that are realistic and attainable, the therapist should assist the client in focusing on skills or tasks that are needed for the "here and now."

Models that focus on helping persons to learn to monitor performance and increase understanding about their own strengths and limitations include the Cognitive Retraining approach, Multicontext approach, and the CO-OP approach. The two latter approaches stress the importance of helping a person discover his or her own errors and generate his or her own solutions; however, the multicontext approach places a greater emphasis on enhancing awareness of limitations across different activities, whereas the CO-OP approach focuses on discovering errors in specific tasks. Toglia and Kirk (2000) emphasize that directly pointing out errors or telling clients that they have problems is least effective in increasing awareness as this approach tends to elicit defensive reactions. They recommend a therapeutically supportive context, use of familiar activities at the "just right challenge level," and structured experiences to enhance the emergence of awareness. Initial studies indicate that direct intervention for awareness can be effective in some groups of clients (Fleming, Lucas, & Lightbody, 2006; Fleming, Shum, Strong, & Lightbody, 2005). For example, Goverover, Johnston, Toglia, and DeLuca (2007a, 2007b) found that compared to a control group, a structured occupation-based intervention based on Toglia and Kirk's self-awareness model significantly improved IADL performances and self-regulation in persons with acquired brain injury. Recently, a systematic review related to the use of feedback for impaired self-awareness concluded that feedback intervention was moderately effective in treatment of self-awareness (Schmidt, Lannin, Fleming, & Ownsworth, 2011). Following are descriptions of specific techniques that can be used in a wide range of activities to enhance awareness. These techniques are often used in combination with one other.

Self-Prediction

Self-prediction involves asking the person to anticipate difficulties or predict his or her performance on a task. The client might be asked to indicate on a rating scale whether the activity will be easy or hard or to identify the type of challenges or obstacles that one might encounter before actual performance of an activity. Immediately following performance, the actual results are compared with predicted results and any discrepancies are discussed (Toglia, 1991a; Toglia, 2011; Goverover et al., 2007a, 2007b).

Specific Goal Ratings

Daily or weekly self-ratings of clearly defined behaviors or targeted strategies can be used to help a person focus on what he or she can do in the present. Goal attainment scales offer a concrete, individualized focus that can increase self-awareness and realistic goal orientation (Malec, Smigielski, & DePompolo, 1991; Rockwood, Joyce, & Stolee, 1997). Client self-ratings of goal attainment can be compared to the ratings of the therapist or of a significant other and any discrepancies can be discussed. Self-ratings can be charted or graphed over time and tracked to improve awareness (Sohlberg & Mateer, 2001).

Videotape Feedback

A videotape of a client that illustrates difficulties in performing an activity may be used to enhance awareness.

Videotape feedback is concrete and it allows clients to re-experience their performance and evaluate their difficulties as they are occurring rather than simply discussing them after the fact. Videotape feedback has been used successfully in treating people with stroke and brain injury (Fleming et al., 2006; Liu, Chan, Lee, Li, & Hui-Chan, 2002; Ownsworth, Fleming, Desbois, Strong, & Kuipers, 2006; Ownsworth, Quinn, Fleming, Kendall, & Shum, 2010; Tham & Tegner, 1997).

Self-Evaluation

The practitioner provides a structured system such as a set of questions, a checklist, or a rating system that the client uses as a guide to evaluate his or her own performance (Toglia, 1991a, 2011; Goverover et al., 2007a, 2007b). Sample self-evaluation questions might include "Have I attended to all the necessary information?" and "Did I check over my work?"

Self-Questioning

Questions that are designed to cue the client to monitor his or her behavior may be written on an index card or memorized. At specific time intervals during the task, the client is expected to stop and answer the same two or three questions such as "Am I sure that I am looking all the way to the left?" "Am I paying attention to the details?" and "Am I going too quickly?" (Fertherlin & Kurland, 1989).

Journaling

The client keeps a journal in which he or she records activity experiences and performance results. The client is encouraged to reflect on and interpret activity experiences, think about what he or she has learned about himself or herself, and summarize strengths and weaknesses (Goverover et al., 2007a, 2007b; Tham et al., 2001; Ylvisaker & Feeney, 1998).

Awareness training techniques can be blended with strategy training and incorporated into all treatment sessions. The multicontext approach provides additional guidelines for simultaneously addressing awareness and strategy use (Toglia et al., 2010; Toglia et al., 2011).

Orientation

Orientation is the ability to understand the self and the relationship between the self and the past and present environment. Orientation depends on the integration of several mental activities that are represented in different areas of the brain. Disorientation is indicative of significant impairments in attention and memory (Lezak, Howieson, & Loring, 2004).

Evaluation

Evaluation of orientation traditionally includes the client's orientation to person, place, and time. Orientation to person involves both the self and others. Is the client able to report personal facts and events and describe his or her previous lifestyle? Does the client recognize people and associate them with their role and name? Orientation to place is demonstrated by the client's ability to understand the type of place he or she is in (e.g., a hospital), to report the name and location of the place, and to appreciate distance and direction. Orientation to time requires an ability to report the current point in time (e.g., day, month, and year), to show understanding of the continuity and sequence of time (i.e., estimation), and to associate events with time.

Topographical orientation, often considered a component of orientation to place, is the ability to follow a familiar route or a new route once given an opportunity to become familiar with it. Functionally, the person might not be able to find his or her way from the therapy area to his or her room or describe and draw the layout of a familiar room or route (Unsworth, 2007). Difficulties with the visual-spatial and memory aspects of topographical orientation need to be distinguished during evaluation (Brunsdon, Nickels, & Coltheart, 2007; Unsworth, 2007).

Orientation assessments are traditionally covered in **mental status examinations**. Table 55.2 provides a list of standardized screening tools for orientation. However, occupational therapists frequently use nonstandardized measures of orientation such as interviews with open-ended questions asked in a conversational or informal manner. Most practitioners use cues to determine the severity of the disorientation. If the client is unable to answer the questions independently, the practitioner might offer a multiple choice array or verbal cues. Cues usually move from general or abstract to more concrete, as determined by the severity of disorientation (e.g., "Today is the beginning of the work week" versus "Today is the day after Sunday"). The number and type of cues offer a method for scoring and monitoring progress. Fluctuations in orientation during the day should be noted because clients might experience **sundowning**, in which they become confused in the evening because of fatigue.

Intervention

Adaptations of Task or Environment. Adaptations that include increasing the saliency of external cues can be used to help a person feel less confused. For example, an information poster that contains orientation facts and pictures of family members can be placed on a wall or a key location within the room. As an alternative, an audiotape or videotape can be created by a family member to review orientation information at set times during the day or used whenever the person feels confused. Care must be taken to match the amount of information presented at one time with the person's processing abilities.

A calendar posted on the wall or closet may be helpful in orienting the person to time. If the client has poor selective attention, a single piece of paper with the day and date written daily rather than a monthly calendar might be needed. Electronic devices such as a talking clock or watch can also be preset to automatically announce the day and time on an hourly basis.

To assist the client in finding his or her room, directional arrows can be placed in the hallway and tape indicating the route to his or her room can be placed on the floor. Key landmarks can be pointed out and made more salient with arrows or colored tape and a special sign with the person's picture can be placed on the door of his or her room.

These adaptations are key characteristics of functional cognitive models and can be used directly with clients or as part of caregiver training programs. Task-specific training techniques used within the NFA such as errorless learning or spaced retrieval techniques can also be used to train use of specific external aids such as referring to a daily calendar through structured repetition and practice. Spaced retrieval involves systematically lengthening the period of retention and recall. There is evidence that this technique is more effective than cueing hierarchies in treating people with dementia (Bourgeois et al., 2003).

Attention

Attention is a multidimensional capacity that involves several components:

1. *Detect/react:* the ability to detect and react to gross changes in the environment such as a telephone ringing, a name being called, or a ball that is thrown.
2. *Sustained attention:* the ability to consistently engage in an activity over time such as reading for 15 minutes without losing concentration. Repetitive and predictable activities such as stuffing envelopes or folding letters place less demands on sustained attention.
3. *Selective attention:* the ability to attend to relevant stimuli while inhibiting distractions or irrelevant information. Examples include selecting specific locations on a map, finding items within a certain price range on a menu, choosing all the red or even playing cards, and finding specific ingredients in a closet. Selective attention demands are increased as the number of items presented simultaneously is increased and as the saliency of the target stimuli is decreased.
4. *Shifting of attention:* the ability to shift or alternate attention between tasks with different cognitive and/or motor requirements. Examples include the ability to shift between adding and subtracting when balancing a checkbook, answering the telephone and typing, and making a salad while cooking something on the stove.
5. *Mental tracking:* the ability to simultaneously keep track of two or more stimuli during ongoing activity. Examples include keeping track of what has already been done in a multistep cooking task and listening to the radio while cooking a meal.

During evaluation (see Table 55.2) and intervention, it is important to keep these different aspects of attention in mind.

Evaluation

Because attention is a multidimensional skill, therapists should ensure that they evaluate all components for potential impairments. More severe impairments in components such as sustaining attention may be easily observable in functional performance; however, more subtle impairments might be missed. Assessments such as the Test of Everyday Attention (Robertson et al., 1994) evaluate multiple components of attention.

Intervention

Strategy Training for Attention. Attention strategy training involves helping a person learn to control, monitor, or prevent the emergence of attentional symptoms. For example, awareness training techniques described earlier, including self-prediction, self-questioning, specific goal setting, and self-evaluation, can be embedded within strategy training to help a client monitor and regulate attentional lapses. Embedding attention strategy training in combination with self-awareness strategies is a key component of multicontext approach. As awareness of attentional lapses emerges, the person can be encouraged to generate strategies to help maintain attention. Strategy training can be integrated into a wide range of simulated or occupation-based activities, during which the practitioner assists the client in monitoring and recording the frequency with which the targeted strategy or behavior is initiated and used. Examples of simulated functional activities include looking through a random stack of greeting cards for a particular holiday card; looking through a stack of recipe cards for recipes that match ingredients on a list; and looking up information in a telephone directory, calendar, or TV guide while keeping track of the items found or while listening to the radio.

Strategies that may be emphasized include the following:

- Taking a time-out from a task when concentration begins to fade
- Remembering to get a sense of the whole situation before attending to the parts
- Monitoring a tendency to become distracted by internal thoughts or external stimuli
- Monitoring the ability to stay on task
- Remembering to look all over and actively search for additional information before responding
- Self-instruction or saying self-cues or each step of a task (aloud and then to self)
- Time pressure management techniques (Fasotti, Kovacs, Eling, & Brouwer, 2000)

Strategy training for attention deficits during postacute rehabilitation for people with traumatic brain injury (TBI) has been recommended as a practice standard based on a review of evidence. Successful interventions included strategy training and self-awareness techniques such as training participants to recognize when they are experiencing information overload or when they are off task (Cicerone et al., 2011). Similarly, Silverstein et al. (2005) demonstrated that attention training for people with schizophrenia combined with shaping techniques including specific goal setting and feedback regarding on task behaviors was more effective than attentional exercises alone. Recently, an attentional strategy training program has been applied to children ages 6 to 15 years with various neurological deficits. Children were taught strategies such as key phrases or "magic words" to help alert and prepare themselves for focusing. They were also taught to re-state task directions in their own words and write down or draw visual cues to remind them what to do. The strategy program was associated with improvement in several aspects of parent-reported attention and children's performance on tasks measuring attention (Luton, Reed-Knight, Loiselle, O'Toole, & Blount, 2011).

Adaptations of Task or Environment. Adaptations can be used to minimize attention demands within everyday activities. Techniques that include increasing saliency of items that require attention and reducing or limiting the amount of information presented to the client at one time can be used. Examples include the following (Toglia, 1993a):

- Modifying the environment to reduce visual clutter, interruptions, and auditory distractions
- Simplifying task instructions so that only one step is presented at a time
- Reducing the number of items or choices presented to the client at one time
- Preselecting relevant objects needed for tasks
- Task segmentation (e.g., presenting only one component of a task at a time) (Moulton, Taira, & Grover, 1995; Toglia, 1993a)
- Placing colored tape on house keys or on operating buttons of appliances

The enhancement of salient cues in the environment can be used to promote desired behaviors, as emphasized in the environmental adaptation component of the NFA. In the task of brushing teeth, for example, unnecessary items should be removed from the sink and the items that are required for use should be made salient with contrasting colors. The contrasting colors of the toothbrush, toothpaste, and cup provide a cue to assist the client in attending to the different items.

Remedial Training. Recent evidence suggests that attention, especially in relation to processing speed, may be strongly related to functional abilities in healthy older adults (Ball, Edwards, & Ross, 2007). Therefore, Ball et al. (2007) developed a training protocol based on the remedial approach. The training tasks involve at least three basic levels of complexity that are similar to the three subtests of the Useful Field of View (UFOV) assessment (for details on the UFOV test, see Edwards et al., 2005; Edwards et al., 2006). Treatment is delivered on a computer screen and involves many practice repetitions of at least 18 different tasks that are presented at 10 different display speeds and at graded difficulty. The researchers found that benefits were maintained for 2 years and translated to improvements in everyday abilities including efficient performance of IADL and safer driving performance (Ball et al., 2007). It is important to keep in mind that these results have not yet been replicated in persons with brain injury or other neurological impairments. An evidence-based review recommended that computer-based interventions for attention may be considered as an adjunct to treatment after TBI or stroke but did not recommend computer-based attentional tasks without some involvement and intervention by a therapist (Cicerone et al., 2011).

Spatial Neglect

Spatial neglect is a failure to orient to, respond to, or report stimuli that are presented on the side contralateral to the cerebral lesion in clients who do not have primary sensory or motor impairments (Heilman, Watson, & Valenstein, 2003). Because spatial neglect is more common after right hemisphere lesions, the left side of space is typically neglected. The term *neglect* connotes a volitional component to the disorder, but this is a misnomer. The client with spatial neglect is unaware of the incompleteness of his or her perception and responses to the environment. He or she often behaves as though one-half of the world does not exist (Corben & Unsworth, 1999). For example, following right hemisphere strokes, clients often begin scanning on the right side and miss or fail to explore most of the stimuli on the left. Asymmetry may be observed in functional activities, drawing tasks, reading, or writing. In severe cases, clients may eat food on one side of their plate, shave half their face, or dress half of their body without recognizing that anything is wrong. In milder cases, they may misread the first letter of a particular word or fail to attend information while crossing a street, shopping, or driving. Many clients with spatial neglect also exhibit anxiety or flattened affect.

Spatial neglect has been identified as a major factor impeding functional recovery in clients who have sustained strokes (Di Monaco et al, 2011; Gillen, 2009; Viken, Samuelsson, Jern, Jood, & Blomstrand, 2012). Those with spatial neglect have more difficulty resuming ADL, have longer hospital stays (Gillen, Tennen, & McKee, 2005; Katz, Hartman-Maeir, Ring, & Soroker, 1999), and are at increased risk for accidents (Webster et al., 1995).

Spatial neglect has been described as a heterogeneous disorder that includes different clinical subtypes and behavioral components (Barrett et al., 2006; Pierce & Buxbaum, 2002). Spatial neglect can involve one or more modalities, may vary with the nature of the stimuli (e.g., verbal versus nonverbal), and can encompass single objects or different spatial frames of space: extrapersonal or large space, peripersonal or space within reach, and personal or body space (Mesulam, 2000; Plummer, Morris, & Dunai, 2003). For example, some clients demonstrate neglect symptoms in large spaces, such as a room (extrapersonal neglect), but do not have reduced awareness of their body (personal neglect) or difficulty on paper-and-pencil tasks (peripersonal neglect). Neglect subtypes have also been proposed that involve internal mental images (representational neglect), decreased movement into or toward the contralesional space (motor neglect), or decreased ability to perceive sensory stimuli in contralesional space (sensory neglect) (Barrett et al., 2006).

Evaluation

Occupational therapists evaluating clients with spatial neglect must first distinguish between hemianopsia and spatial neglect. Visual field cuts (hemianopsia) are hemiretinal, whereas neglect is hemispatial. Clients with visual field cuts typically have awareness of their visual field loss and make compensatory head movements and turns. Spatial neglect may exist with or without hemianopsia, and one syndrome does not cause the other. Assessment of spatial neglect typically involves cancellation tasks that require detection of target stimuli, distributed on both sides of space (see Table 55.2). Typically, most targets on the contralesional side of space are missed. The complexity of spatial neglect symptoms is not fully captured by traditional tests of neglect. Therefore, it is important not to rely completely on test instruments in identifying spatial neglect. The tasks currently employed to assess neglect consist mainly of paper and pencil type of assessment and suffer from two main limitations. First, some of the most commonly used tests such as the cancellation task do not provide information regarding different forms of neglect. The cancellation test provides information of spatial biases in attention in peripersonal space but not on personal neglect. Second, the traditional paper-and-pencil tests may be insensitive to mild forms of neglect. Azouvi et al. (2003) found that a 10- item behavioral assessment of neglect called the Catherine Bergego Scale, which involves rating neglect in everyday tasks, was more sensitive than conventional tests. Neglect symptoms that are not observed in structured or quiet environments may emerge under busy, real-world environments, therefore environmental conditions need to be considered in assessment (Barrett et al., 2006). The different behavioral manifestations and subtypes of neglect also need to be kept in mind during observation of performance (Appelros, Nydevik, Karlsson, Thorwalls, & Seiger, 2003; Barrett et al., 2006; Plummer et al., 2003).

Dynamic assessment of spatial neglect provides information about task conditions that increase or decrease the symptoms of spatial neglect as well as the person's ability to respond to different types of cues or implement and carryover learned strategies to different situations. Toglia and Cermak (2009) describe a dynamic object search task that analyzes the ability to learn and apply a strategy across a series of search tasks in people with spatial neglect.

Intervention

Remedial Training. Evidence exists to support the use of visual scanning training, prisms, patching, and vibration to remediate disorders of spatial neglect.

In spatial neglect, clients demonstrate decreased eye movements to the affected side. This decrease in eye movements reflects a decrease in attention to one side of the environment (Antonucci et al., 1995; Toglia, 1991b). Scientific literature reviews by Cicerone et al. (2011) concluded that there is Level I evidence to support the use of visuospatial interventions that include practice in visual scanning because it improves compensation for spatial neglect and generalizes to everyday activities. Therefore, they recommended visuospatial rehabilitation with visual scanning as a practice standard for clients with visual neglect after right hemisphere stroke. The combination of forced limb activation or movements of the left arm or hand on the left side of space in conjunction with visual scanning also shows positive results (Cicerone et al., 2011; Robertson, Hogg, & McMillan, 1998). Intervention appears to be most effective when a wide combination of intervention activities, including everyday tasks, is used (Antonucci et al., 1995; Pizzamiglio et al., 1992). Programs with greater levels of intensity have generally produced more positive outcomes. However, even with intensive training, it has been demonstrated that people with spatial neglect have poorer functional outcome than do other people with stroke (Paolucci, Antonucci, Grasso, & Pizzamiglio, 2001).

Weinberg et al. (1977) designed systematic training techniques that incorporated a combination of remedial worksheets and strategy training techniques during reading and scanning tasks. Systematic training in visual scanning that gradually increases the amount and complexity of information presented but, at the same time, teaches new strategies to improve impaired functioning is in the basis of the CDM (Averbuch & Katz, 2011). For example, they used graded anchoring, pacing the speed of scanning, feedback, and decreasing the density of the stimulus. Anchoring, or teaching the person to use a spatial reference point, such as a colored line on the left side, is a common strategy in visual scanning training.

Gross motor activities involving vestibular input and whole-body movement in space increase general arousal and alertness and have been used in combination with visual scanning activities to increase gaze and attention to the affected side (Cappa, Sterzi, Vallar, & Bisiach, 1987). Bilateral activities such as balloon volleyball, with the client hitting the balloon with his or her hands clasped together, are encouraged to incorporate the use of the affected side of the body. Also, the use of neck muscle vibration for 5 minutes before occupational therapy was been found to be beneficial for reducing the symptoms of neglect (Kamada, Shimodozono, Hamada, & Kawahira, 2011).

Other intervention techniques that have been recommended for clients with spatial neglect include the use of prisms and visual occlusion techniques (Pierce & Buxbaum, 2002). Partial visual occlusion methods attempt to force the person to use the neglected visual field by patching the eye ipsilateral to the lesion, patching the non-neglected half field of eyeglasses (Ianes et al., 2012; Tsang, Sze, & Fong, 2009), or darkening the non-neglected half field of eyeglasses (hemispatial sunglasses) (Arai, Ohi, Sasaki, Nobuto, & Tanaka, 1997). Prism adaptation has been shown to alleviate the symptoms of spatial neglect following stroke. Prisms cause an optical deviation of the visual field to the right so that objects appear to be moved farther to the right than they actually are (Redding & Wallace, 2006). Recently, Turton, O'Leary, Gabb, Woodward, and Gilchrist (2010) assessed the impact of prism adaptation on self-care using a single blinded pilot randomized controlled trial. They found that prism adaptation treatments had no effect on everyday behavior. On the other hand, Shiraishi, Muraki, Ayaka Itou, and Hirayama (2010) found that the sustainability of the prism training effect lasted for 2 to 3.5 years and caused positive changes in basic and IADL.

Computer-assisted training programs for street crossing and wheelchair navigation have also been described. Trained subjects with spatial neglect performed better on real-life tasks after virtual reality training than control subjects did. The use of virtual reality–based technology appears to show potential for clients with spatial neglect (Katz et al., 2005; Webster et al., 2001).

Strategy Training. Strategies for spatial neglect can be practiced within everyday tasks such as setting a table for several people, dealing a deck of cards to six people, identifying appointments on a wall calendar, reading a newspaper, addressing envelopes of different sizes, or identifying all the pictures or chairs in the room. Because spatial neglect symptoms vary with the size of space, arrangement of space, and amount and density of information presented, these activity parameters need to be matched with the neglect symptoms, and systematically varied and graded in treatment to match the task to the "just right level" is especially emphasized in the multicontext approach. In some cases, treatment activities should emphasize large space activities; in other situations, activities should focus on tabletop tasks that involve visual detail. In general, activities that are unpredictable or involve stimuli randomly scattered on a table or page are more sensitive to the symptoms of spatial neglect than the activities that are arranged in a predictable, structured, or horizontal array (Ferber & Karnath, 2001). Intervention should include practice in identifying situations in which neglect symptoms are most likely to occur such as filling multiple bowls with salad, placing cookie dough on a baking sheet, or arranging photographs in a picture album.

Individuals with spatial neglect do not always know when they are attending to the left side. Intervention needs to assist clients in finding external cues that will provide feedback about when they are indeed attending to the left. An emphasis in intervention should be teaching the client to find the edges of a page or a table or the periphery of stimuli before beginning a task and to mark it with spatial point of reference such as colored tape, a colored highlighter, a bright object, or placement of his or her arm on the left border. Auditory cueing using a beeper or alarm device can be combined with strategy training to remind the person to use a strategy or visual cue. The alarm device can require the client to scan space and attend to the left to turn off the sound (Seron, Deloche, & Coyette, 1989). Alternatively, devices with vibrating or auditory cues can be placed in left pockets, clipped on the left side of a belt, or placed on a wrist to encourage attention to the left side of the body (personal neglect). These are examples of combining compensation with environmental adaptation approaches. Thus, even if in previous sections we highlight each method of intervention, sometimes, when appropriate (based on clinical reasoning), combination of approaches are beneficial for patients.

Other intervention strategies for spatial neglect include tactile search, use of mental imagery, and general alerting techniques. Tactile search includes teaching the client to feel the left side of space with eyes closed or to feel the left edges of objects before visual search. Visual imagery teaches imagining and describing familiar scenes or routes and using mental images during movement of limbs or visual scanning (Niemeier, 1998; Smania, Bazoli, Piva, & Guidetti, 1997). For example, reduction in neglect symptoms and increased performance on functional tasks were reported after a mental imagery program that involved teaching people with neglect to imagine their eyes as sweeping beams of a lighthouse from left to right across the visual field. Clients were cued to use this mental image during functional and therapy training tasks (McCarthy, Beaumont, Thompson, Pringle, 2002; Niemeier, 1998; Niemeier, Cifu, & Kishore, 2001). Recently, Welfringer, Leifert-Fiebach, Babinsky, and Brandt (2011) found that mentally imagined practice of positions and movements of the affected upper extremity lead to improvements in the perception of the body and space (personal neglect). In addition to strategies specifically aimed at facilitating attention to the left side, strategies that focus on the general ability to sustain attention have also been found to reduce spatial neglect. For example, Robertson, Tegner, Tham, Lo, and Smith (1995) taught clients with chronic spatial neglect to mentally tell themselves to "pay attention" and to tap loudly on a table.

It has been observed that response to strategy training depends on whether people with spatial neglect show improvements in their awareness (Robertson & Halligan, 1999; Tham et al., 2001). This observation directly supports the use of the multicontext approach in the treatment of neglect. It underscores the importance of deeply embedding awareness training techniques, such as those described earlier, into all intervention activities. In addition, intervention activities that are meaningful and functional in nature have more effect on the discovery of disability and developing self-awareness (Tham et al., 2001; Toglia et al., 2010).

Adaptations of Task or Environment. Adaptation of the task or the environment to enhance functional performance even in the presence of neglect is a key element of the functional cognitive approaches. To minimize the need to attend to the left, it has been suggested that the environment be rearranged so that key items (e.g., the telephone, the nurse call button) are on the unaffected side. However, a study by Kelly and Ostreicher (1985) found no significant difference in functional outcome in clients whose hospital rooms were rearranged in this way. Lennon (1994) described the successful use of large colored paper markings on the edges of tables, corners, and elsewhere to prevent collision for clients with spatial neglect. The client was trained to look for these markers. Markers were gradually faded. Performance improved and was maintained with removal of markers; however, effects did not generalize to other environments. Calvanio, Levine, and Petrone (1993) described the use of an adapted plate to increase feeding skills in a client with a severe case of left inattention and a dense left hemianopsia. The plate was mounted on a lazy Susan so that it could be rotated. As the client pushed the food with a fork, the plate rotated so that all the food eventually came into view, thus eliminating the need for scanning to the left. Other environmental adaptations include placing red tape on the client's wheelchair brakes or placing brightly colored objects such as a napkin or cup on the left side (Golisz, 1998).

Visual Processing and Visual Motor

Visual perceptual impairments are associated with difficulties in ADL and mobility in adults (Gillen, 2009). They are frequently observed after stroke, acquired brain injury, Parkinson's disease and other neurological disorders and have also been identified in adults with schizophrenia (Butler, Silverstein, & Dakin, 2008). Visual perceptual impairments are also a key feature of nonverbal learning disorders and have been hypothesized to contribute to difficulties in interpreting facial expressions and mathematics (Liddell & Rasmussen, 2005).

Visual perception can be viewed on an information-processing continuum involving the reception, organization, and assimilation of visual information. On one end of the continuum, simple visual-processing tasks such as matching shapes or objects occur quickly and automatically with minimal effort. On the opposite end of the continuum, complex visual tasks that include unfamiliar stimuli or subtle discriminations within visually crowded arrays require slower and effortful processing. In this conceptualization, visual-processing dysfunction is defined as a decrease in the amount that the visual system is able to assimilate at any one time (Toglia, 1989). To understand the client's **visual perceptual** skills and the effects of impairments on functioning, we need to analyze the activity conditions (complexity, amount, familiarity, and predictability) and context.

Problems in simple visual processing include difficulty in discriminating between objects, pictures of objects, and basic shapes; difficulty in detecting gross differences in size, position, direction, angles, and rotations; decreased ability to visually locate single visual targets in space or judge gross distance between two objects; and decreased ability to detect simple part–whole relationships in objects or basic shapes. The person may have difficulty in familiar and routine activities and may easily misinterpret or misidentify objects. Failure to recognize an object is labeled visual **agnosia**. Toglia (1989) proposes that labels such as visual agnosia are too broad for the purposes of intervention because there are many different underlying reasons for object recognition difficulties. For example, a person might fail to attend to the critical feature of an object or the part of the object that tells what it is (e.g., prongs of a fork). Attention might be captured by salient but irrelevant aspects of the object (e.g., the utensil's decorative handle). There might be an inability to process the overall shape and the details simultaneously, so the person might miss important details.

Complex visual processing skills are required in visually confusing environments; when there is abstract, unfamiliar, or detailed visual information; or in conditions under which the distinctive visual features are partially obscured (e.g., the object is rotated and partially hidden on a crowded desk). Dysfunction of complex visual perceptual skills may include decreased ability to detect subtle differences in shapes, features, objects, angles, size, location, distance, and position. A client might have difficulty recognizing and interpreting facial expressions or making sense out of ambiguous, incomplete, fragmented, or distorted visual stimuli. The client might misinterpret an object when it is in an unusual position or partially hidden. The person might experience increased difficulty in visually confusing, crowded, or dynamic environments. Everyday tasks such as finding items in a crowded closet, drawer, desk, or supermarket shelf; locating key information on a bill, map, or schedule; and copying or following a diagram might present difficulty. On these tasks, the person might misinterpret information, miss key visual details, or become sidetracked by irrelevant visual stimuli.

Visual motor skills include writing, copying or drawing tasks (e.g., drawing a map, copying a design), or construction of tasks that involve assembling pieces into a whole (e.g., assembling a coffeepot). Clients may demonstrate difficulty on visual motor tasks for many reasons. For example, a client might have difficulty copying a diagram of a room because of a poor ability to scan, locate, align, position, or rotate items accurately; decreased planning and organization; spatial neglect; or impaired discrimination of size and angle. The term *constructional apraxia* is used to refer to difficulty with drawing or assembly tasks that cannot be attributed to primary motor or sensory impairment, ideomotor apraxia, or general cognitive impairments (Farah, 2003). Constructional abilities are closely related to ADL performance (Neistadt, 1992a; Warren, 1981). Clients may have difficulty dressing (dressing apraxia), orienting clothes correctly on a hanger, or assembling a sandwich or coffeepot. People with left-hemisphere parietal lesions tend to omit individual pieces or details in constructional tasks, whereas those with right-hemisphere lesions demonstrate spatial disorganization of the pieces and lose the overall gestalt (Kramer, Kaplan, & Blusewicz, 1991). Constructional apraxia is not a unitary syndrome. Impairments in different types of perceptual processing or spatial relations are thought to underlie constructional apraxia in both right- and left-hemisphere lesions (Laeng, 2006).

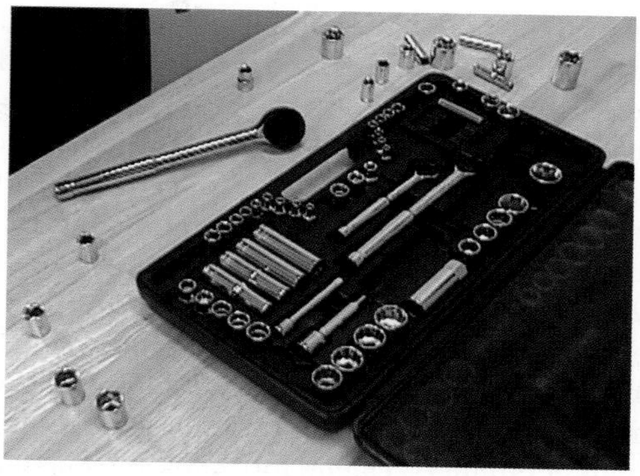

FIGURE 55.2 Organizing the components of a ratchet tool kit requires perception of size and shape as well as organizational skills.

Evaluation

Evaluation for people with visual perceptual impairments should examine visual foundations skills, visual abilities without a motor response, and visual motor skills. Visual foundation skills including visual acuity, ocular alignment, visual pursuits or smooth tracking of moving objects, saccades or quick eye movements to place an object of interest in view, and visual fields should be evaluated prior to a visual processing evaluation to screen out visual problems that will interfere with the accuracy of perceptual testing (Cate & Richards, 2000). Several clinical observations during functional tasks can alert occupational therapists to the need for a formal visual assessment: compensatory head movements and tilting, squinting, shutting of one eye, or a tendency to lose one's place while reading. The Brain Injury Visual Assessment Battery for Adults (biVABA) (Warren, 1998) is an example of an evaluation that includes screening of visual foundation skills. Any disruptions of foundational skills can affect interpretations of higher level visual processing assessments (Warren, 1993).

Standardized non-motor assessments of visual perception (see Table 55.2) categorize visual perception into specific skills such as figure–ground, position in space, form constancy, spatial relations, and visual recognition. Persons with visual perceptual impairments may have difficulty performing various types of visual processing tasks for similar reasons (e.g., a tendency to overfocus on parts, a tendency to miss visual details, failure to simultaneously attend to the details as well as the whole, difficulty in keeping track of what was just seen). Therefore, Toglia (1989) recommends an approach that conceptualizes visual processing on a continuum and evaluates both conventional and unconventional objects under a variety of different activity conditions. In a dynamic approach to visual perception, the therapist systematically manipulates activity parameters and analyzes responses to cues to understand why a client is having difficulty accurately discriminating objects or visual stimuli (Kline, 2000; Toglia, 1989; Toglia & Finkelstein, 1991). Visual perceptual assessment should examine responses to activities with and without a motor response to examine differences in performance. Visual motor skills are typically evaluated with contrived tasks such as block designs, puzzles, or copying designs; however, observation of everyday tasks provides the opportunity to analyze visual motor performance. The A-ONE standardized assessment (Arnadottir, 1990) identifies the effect of visual spatial impairments on self-care tasks such as grooming, feeding, and dressing (Gillen, 2009). Informal observations in tasks such as copying a map route, assembling a coffeepot or woodworking project, wrapping a package, packing a lunchbox, or folding clothes can provide additional information on visual motor abilities (Figure 55.2). Symptoms may include angular deviations; improper position, location, spacing, or alignment of parts; and spatial distortions. The client's ability to recognize and correct errors in alignment or position should be investigated. For example, some clients do not recognize visual spatial errors even when attention is directed to the problem area, whereas other clients recognize errors but are unable to correct them.

Intervention

Interventions may address visual foundation skills or visual processing skills with or without a motor response.

Visual Foundation Skills. Treatment of visual foundation skills such as visual acuity and contrast sensitivity, oculomotor skills, and visual fields generally involves adaptations such as large-print reading materials; magnifiers; talking devices; increasing contrast of edges, borders, or backgrounds; and changes in lighting. However, remedial exercises may be recommended for individuals with oculomotor or visual field deficits. For example, range-of-motion eye exercises to the involved muscle have been advocated for individuals with eye muscle paresis. Occlusion of the intact visual field with eye patching has been used to force use of the impaired visual field (Warren, 1993). These remediation treatments involve repetitions of graded activities and are linked directly to the remedial deficit specific approach.

Strategy Training. Strategies that maximize the client's ability to process visual information can include getting a sense of the whole before looking at the parts; teaching the person to partition space before localizing details; using one's finger to scan, trace visual stimuli, or focus on details; covering or blocking visual stimuli when too much information is presented at once; verbalizing salient visual features or subtle differences; and mentally visualizing a particular item before looking for it (Toglia, 1989, 2011). These strategies can be trained within everyday activities that involve choosing among objects that are similar in shape and size (e.g., matching socks, sorting teaspoons and soupspoons); locating information within supermarket circulars, calendars, maps, or schedules; arranging information within grids or spreadsheets; copying patterns in arts and craft activities; or finding information in crowded draws, shelves, tables, or bulletin boards.

Intervention involves careful manipulation of activity parameters. Activities that involve familiar items or contexts, high contrast (e.g., red socks and white socks), distinctive features, little detail, and solid colors or backgrounds require less attention, effort, and visual analysis than do activities that involve choosing among items that have low contrast (e.g., light beige and white socks), are in unusual positions, are embedded within crowded or distracting visual backgrounds, or are partially obscured. Changes in the familiarity, number of items, and degree of detail can place greater demands on visual processing. In addition, verbal mediation, including repeating a list of step-by-step instructions during a functional activity such as dressing, capitalizes on strengths in verbal abilities and can be effective in facilitating functional performance (Sunderland, Walker, & Walker, 2006). Strategies can be trained within a multicontext paradigm, where activities are graded within the "just right challenging level" for each client, or within a compensational paradigm where strategy is trained within a specific task context.

Adaptation of Task or Environment. The key guideline in minimizing the effects of visual perceptual difficulties is to make the distinctive features of objects more salient with color cues. An example is placing colored tape on buttons to operate appliances or using salient color cues on objects to make them easier to locate and discriminate (e.g., bright pink tape on a medication bottle). Cues such as colored marks or tape at spatial landmarks (e.g., tape recorder, wheelchair footrests, or label of a shirt) reduce spatial demands and make it easier to orient and align parts of an item. Visual stimuli such as items on a shelf or sentences on a page that are large and arranged in an organized manner with large spaces between items are easier to perceive. Consistent locations for objects in the refrigerator, closet or drawer, or a countertop increase predictability and provide contextual cues for recognition. Significant others should be instructed to decrease visual distractions in the room or within a task by limiting designs and patterns and by using solid colors with high contrast. Patterns, designs, and decorations make it harder to select and recognize critical features of an object. Significant others should also be trained to introduce only a small amount of visual information at one time.

Motor Planning

Motor planning, or praxis, is the ability to execute learned and purposeful activities. **Apraxia** is defined as a disorder of skilled movement that cannot be adequately explained by primary motor or sensory impairments, visual spatial problems, language comprehension difficulties, or cognitive problems alone (Heilman & Rothi, 2003). It has been suggested that apraxia is primarily a disorder of *learned* movement, whereas developmental dyspraxia or DCD represents difficulties in the *acquisition* of motor skills in the absence of a physical or neurological disorder in children (Tempest & Roden, 2008). Decreased motor learning, however, has also been observed in adults with apraxia (Poole, 1998). A study comparing adults with apraxia and children with dyspraxia found that both groups made similar types of errors suggesting similarities in behavioral manifestations (Poole, 2000).

Apraxia occurs most commonly after stroke; however, it can also be seen in persons with dementia, Parkinson's disease, or movement disorders such as Huntington's chorea (Vanbellingen & Bohlhalter, 2011). Apraxia may be seen after lesions in either hemisphere, although it is more frequently in clients who have sustained a left-hemisphere lesion. Aphasia is often associated with apraxia because the left hemisphere is also dominant for language (Heilman & Rothi, 2003). Apraxia can significantly impact ADL, functional outcome, and the ability to engage in meaningful activities (Gillen, 2009; Vanbellingen & Bohlhalter, 2011). Wetter, Poole, and Haaland (2005) found that limb apraxia is a better predictor of functional motor skills after left hemisphere damage than aphasia. Apraxia can persist over time and persons can continue to have significant functional limitations in both the learning of new motor tasks, such as one-handed shoe tying (Poole, 1998), and in the efficiency and accuracy of actions to verbal command or demonstration (Poole, 2000). Similarly, children with dyspraxia or DCD may present with functional difficulties in writing, riding a bike, self-care tasks, and engaging in sports (Kirby, 2011).

Roy (1978) identifies two major subsystems in apraxia: the conceptual and the production subsystems. Difficulties in motor planning may reflect disorders in one or both of these subsystems. The production aspect of motor planning, traditionally called *ideomotor apraxia*, involves generating the action plan, sequencing and organizing the appropriate elements, and carrying out the plan (e.g., reaching for a glass of water to take a drink). The greatest difficulty is observed when the client is asked to pretend to use a tool or object or to perform limb gestures. Some improvement may be seen when the client is asked to imitate the motion or perform the motion with the actual object, but the movement is still imprecise. These clients know what they want to do, but actions are carried out in an awkward, inefficient, or clumsy manner. Errors of preservation, sequencing, or omissions may be observed.

The conceptual aspect of motor planning (Roy, 1978) includes knowledge about the functional properties of an object, the object action, and the sequence of action. Conceptual or ideation errors, traditionally called *ideational apraxia*, involve object function, action knowledge, and knowledge of sequence. Clients might be able to accurately identify and match objects, but difficulties in sequencing or choosing appropriate objects or tools may be observed. For example, the client might try to brush his or her hair with a toothbrush. Although object recognition may be intact, the person might be unable to associate the object with its correct action plan. Dressing apraxia and constructional apraxia are additional subtypes of apraxia, previously described in the section on visual processing. Traditional labels of apraxia are narrow in scope and do not account for the wide range of skills that underlie motor planning and constructional abilities.

Evaluation

Motor planning involves an integration of multiple skills including visual spatial, executive functions, language, and somatosensory skills, as well as knowledge and understanding of object properties and sequences. The clinician is urged to analyze error patterns and underlying reasons contributing to difficulties in performance rather than attempting to classify clients within traditional categories. If aphasia and apraxia coexist, information on the client's language skills should be obtained from the speech-language pathologist or be screened for by testing for "yes" or "no" comprehension and ability to follow one-step commands.

In evaluating apraxia, the clinician typically observes the client's performance of different types of functional movements and tasks, noting the method of evocation (e.g., command, imitation, or object use), quality of movement, type of errors made, and the influence of familiarity and context (Haaland, 1993). Error patterns can be generally categorized into errors of production or errors of ideation. Assessments for apraxia are listed in Table 55.2. An observational method for assessing apraxia in ADL, adapted from the A-ONE, has been validated for people with stroke (van Heugten et al., 2000). May-Benson and Cermak (2007) developed the Test of Ideational Praxis (TIP) to objectively assess conceptual or ideational abilities in children. The CO-OP method has described DPA to identify breakdowns in task performance in children with DCD. In addition, Toglia (2011) has described a dynamic assessment approach for adults with aphasia and apraxia that analyzes response to cues across functional tasks with increasing number of steps.

Intervention

For an elaborated information about up-to-date treatment for limb apraxia with adults, we refer the readers to Gillen (2009) and Cermak and Larkin (2002), or Missiuna (2001) for children. Interventions to overcome motor planning deficits may emphasize either the production aspect or the conceptual aspect of motor planning (Roy, 1985). Techniques that address the orientation of an object or limb in space or the timing, sequence, and organization of the motor elements aim to enhance the production aspect of motor planning. For example, the practitioner might provide physical contact (i.e., hand-over-hand assistance or light touch) to limit inappropriate or extraneous movements while using guiding methods to facilitate a smooth motor pattern or to guide the manipulation of objects within functional tasks. Through repeated practice in different tasks using task-specific methods or errorless learning, the client begins to learn the movement patterns that feel "right," and the practitioner gradually withdraws assistance. Gillen (2009) provides detailed suggestions for guiding limbs during functional activities including guidance of both sides of the body when possible, providing changes in resistance during the activity, and keeping talking to a minimum.

Familiar tasks that are performed in context are easier for people with motor planning disorders because the context provide cues that facilitate the desired action (Ferguson & Trombly, 1997). Interventions can be graded by gradually increasing the number of tools and distractors, increasing the degrees of freedom (Gillen, 2009), or introducing activities and environments that have less stability and predictability such as negotiating around obstacles in a crowded store.

Intervention addressing the conceptual aspect of motor planning focuses on facilitating the client's understanding of how an object is used or how a gesture is performed (Helm-Estabrooks, 1982; Pilgrim & Humphreys, 1994; Smania et al., 2006; Smania, Girardi, Domenicali, Lora, & Aglioti, 2000).

Strategy Training. Clients may be taught to generate or use verbal, visual, or tactile cues to enhance movement. For example, before performing an activity, the client might mentally practice or imagine the task performance such as making tea, or the client might imagine how an object should look in his or her hand before picking it up. Audiotapes or verbal scripts can be used to guide mental practice (Wu, Radel, Hanna-Pladdy, 2011). Incorrect patterns of movement, such as holding an object in the wrong way, can also be visualized with an emphasis on having the client solve the problem and mentally practice correcting the movement. Talking to a client through action sequences or use of step-by-step written lists or illustrations can be useful in facilitating functional performance in tasks such as drinking from a cup (Butler, 1999). The person can be taught to verbally rehearse an action sequence or associate the movement with a rhyme, rhythm, or musical tune with a gradual fading of the verbalization. Self-monitoring strategies can be used to teach a client to monitor unnecessary contraction, incomplete actions, or difficulty in switching direction of movements. Treatment can also focus on a task analysis of the movements and articulation of goal-directed tasks. The treatment begins with physical manipulation plus verbalization of task elements (e.g., "reach the cup, grab the cup, carry to my lips, drink, stop"), and those cues are systematically withdrawn as performance improved (Pilgrim & Humphreys, 1994). Note that the use of strategies typically requires metacognitive skills. Models that focus on strategies therefore, also typically emphasize metacognitive skills (as in the compensatory approach or multicontextual approach). Preliminary studies indicate that strategy training is effective in improving everyday function (Donkervoort, Dekker, Stehmann-Saris, & Deelman, 2001; Geusgens et al., 2006; van Heugten et al., 1998). For example, in a randomized study design, changes on nontrained-ADL were greater in a group of people with stroke who had received strategy training as compared with those receiving usual occupational therapy. This suggests that the strategies are generalized to everyday activities (Geusgens et al., 2006). Similarly, the CO-OP approach, which emphasizes strategy use, has been demonstrated to be effective in enhancing task performance in children with DCD (Miller, Polatajko, Missiuna, Mandich, & Macnab, 2001).

Adaptation of Task or Environment. Simple adaptations to objects that draw attention to the critical features of the object or activity can facilitate action and motor planning (e.g., colored tape on the knife handle or toothbrush handle). Patterns and designs on utensils or clothing might draw attention to the wrong detail and result in an inappropriate motor response.

Tool use should be minimized (Poole, 2000) and adaptive equipment should be selected with caution for the client with apraxia. For example, some adaptations such as a button hook, one-handed shoe tying, or a one-arm-drive wheelchair might be confusing for clients with apraxia and place greater demands on motor planning abilities. Other adaptations, such as adaptive clothing closures, may simplify the task or motor pattern required to manipulate or hold objects, reduce the number of steps, and facilitate function in the client with apraxia.

Training caregivers to modify instructions so that the activity is broken into one command at a time (Unsworth, 2007) and to use simple whole commands (e.g., "Get up") can put the activity on an automatic level and effectively enhance motor planning (Zoltan, 2007). Another treatment that goes in line with this approach is the multiple-cues treatment method (Maher, Rothi, & Greenwald, 1991). It uses presentation of multiple cues including tools, objects, visual models, and feedback. Errors are corrected using imitation and physical manipulation. As performance improves, cues are systematically withdrawn. This method of treatment is based on the NFA that emphasizes mastery of functional task performance through practice rather than on the underlying skills that are needed to perform the task. Intervention involves breaking down a functional task into small subcomponents and provides reinforcement and chaining when needed (Giles, 2011; Glisky et al., 1994).

Memory

Memory gives us the ability to draw on past experiences and learn new information (Toglia, 1993a). This provides us with a sense of continuity in the environment and frees us from dependency in here-and-now situations. Memory is conceptualized as a multistep process involving encoding (i.e., input of information), storage (i.e., holding information), and retrieval (i.e., getting information) (Levy, 2011b). There are different types of memory. Working memory is the temporary storage of information while one is working with it or attending to it. It includes the ability to recall information immediately after exposure. It allows one to focus conscious attention and keeps track of information as one is performing an activity. Declarative memory is one aspect of long-term memory and includes conscious memory for events, knowledge, or facts. Procedural (nondeclarative) memory involves the ability to remember how to perform an activity or procedure without conscious awareness. Prospective memory involves the ability to remember intentions or activities that will be required in the future (Levy, 2011b).

Evaluation

It is important to distinguish whether everyday memory problems are due to failures to keep track of a conversation or what was just said (e.g., working memory) or recall of past events or conversations from the day before (e.g., declarative, event-based memory) or failures in carrying out future activities (e.g., prospective memory). A comprehensive evaluation of memory, whether static or dynamic, must address the different types of memory and methods of retrieval (Table 55.2). Assessments must consider factors such as the modality in which the information is presented (auditory or visual), the type of instructions (general or specific), the amount of stimuli presented, the familiarity and meaningfulness of the information, the presence of contextual cues during recall phases, the type of information to be remembered (factual or skill related), and the length of retention. Dynamic assessment of memory such as Toglia's (1993b) Contextual Memory Test evaluates awareness of memory capabilities and use of strategies.

Intervention

Memory impairments can be closely related to other cognitive impairments, particularly attention. Some investigators have suggested that an indirect approach that addresses other cognitive skills such as attention, organization, or processing speed (Chiaravalloti, Christodoulou, Demaree, & DeLuca, 2003; Leavitt, Lengenfelder, Moore, Chiaravalloti, & DeLuca, 2011) rather than memory may be effective. For example, Sohlberg and Mateer (1989a) reported improvement in memory function after attentional training using a remedial approach. Interventions for memory impairments include memory strategy training, external aids and devices, and adaptations as well as techniques of errorless learning, vanishing cues, and spaced retrieval that were discussed earlier in this chapter.

Strategy Training. Training of internal memory strategies is most appropriate for people with mild memory deficits or those in whom other areas of cognition are intact (Cicerone et al., 2011). The client practices one or two targeted memory strategies in various different tasks such as remembering telephone numbers, news headlines, a sequence of errands, items that need to be bought in a store, or instructions to an activity. During practice on different memory tasks, various awareness training techniques are used if the therapist selects the multicontext approach to guide intervention. The client may be trained on a specific strategy to facilitate performance of one specific task or the treatment could emphasize learning several strategies and determining which works best based on the content to be remembered and the task. Memory strategies may be directed primarily at encoding operations (i.e., getting information in) or the retrieval phase of memory (i.e., getting information out).

More details about encoding and retrieval memory strategies are available at **http://thePoint.lww.com/Willard-Spackman12e.**

Memory External Strategies and Aids. External aids such as mobile phones, smartphones, notebooks, tape and/or digital recorders, tablets, and computers store information that the person might have difficulty remembering. Other aids such as alarm watches or signals serve to remind a person to perform an action (prospective memory) (Toglia, 1993a). The success of an intervention program that used a combination of external aids and strategies with awareness training to improve prospective memory was recently described by Fleming, Shum, Strong, and Lightbody (2005). External memory aids include the following: timers, tape recorders, devices with preprogrammed alarms or alarm messages, electronic devices such as pillbox organizers, lists, daily planners and notebooks, and commercially available applications for mobile/smart phones, palm pilots, and computers (Figure 55.3). Studies have documented the effectiveness of external aids (Kim, Burke, Dowds, Boone, & Parks, 2000; McKerracher, Powell, & Oyebode, 2005; Wade & Troy, 2001; Wilson, Emslie, Quirk, & Evans, 2001). Intervention is most effective when the client is motivated, involved in identifying the memory problem, and fairly independent in daily function (Cicerone et al., 2011).

Evidence obtained from case studies supports the use of memory notebooks and other external aids in reducing everyday memory failures for people with moderate-to-severe memory impairments (Cicerone et al., 2011; McKerracher et al., 2005; Wade & Troy, 2001; Wilson et al., 2009; Wilson et al., 2001). However, the successful use of an external memory aid may require extensive training. The client may need to practice initiating and using the aid in various different situations. The use of external aids might need to be graded. In the initial stages, the client might be expected to use the aid only when it is initiated by another person. Gradually, the client might be trained to initiate the use of the aid independently. Errorless learning, spaced retrieval, and other task-specific training methods that capitalize on procedural memory and are core components of the NFA may be used in training clients with moderate or severe memory impairments to use an external aid. Recently, researchers started to turn their focus to how memory aids can be adapted and developed for other users such as the older adult (Thöne-Otto & Schulze, 2003). These technologies are more concerned with supporting the users' abilities rather than strengthening them. Compensation systems that have been developed for older adults range from simple reminder systems to home robotic support systems (LoPresti, Mihailidis, & Kirsch, 2004).

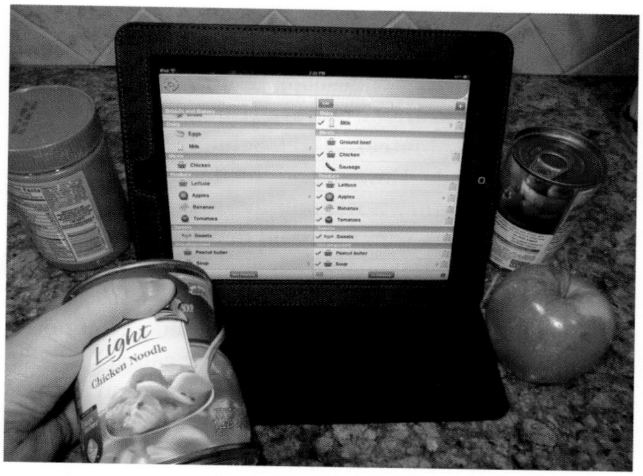

FIGURE 55.3 Use of an iPad app to aid organizing grocery shopping for clients with memory and executive function impairments.

The most commonly used external memory strategy is the memory notebook. The memory notebook needs to be designed with the person's needs and lifestyle in mind (McKerracher et al., 2005). Sample sections in a memory notebook are as follows: personal facts, names of people to remember, calendar and schedule, things to do/important events (daily, within the next week), daily log of important events, conversations, summary of readings (articles, newspaper), medication schedule, and directions to frequently traveled places. Initially, the notebook should begin with one or two sections and gradually increase.

Memory notebook training needs to take place in the context of various everyday activities. Therapy sessions should include role-playing and practice in the use of the notebook. In addition, the client may be asked questions that involve reviewing and rereading the memory notebook. Specific memory notebook training protocols have been described in the literature (Donaghy & Williams 1998; Sohlberg & Mateer, 2001). Schmitter-Edgecombe, Howard, Pavawalla, Howell, and Rueda (2008) examined the use of a memory notebook following a group program with patients who had mild dementia. They found that participants with dementia demonstrate improved posttreatment memory scores because of increased note-taking behavior and more frequent referencing of notes. Use of notebook as an external strategy can actually be used as another form of processing information again—something that increase processing of information into long-term memory.

There has been an enormous development in the field of electronic memory aids such as mobile/smart phones, iPads, or organizers. Some of the current trends in the use of technology in rehabilitation include:

- Home-based electronic memory aid with sensors for persons with memory impairments as support to carry out everyday activities in their own home environments. This "smart home" support system also includes individually spoken reminders (Boman, Bartfai, Borell, Tham, & Hemmingsson, 2010).
- Application for smartphones and tablets: for example, clients and/or caregivers can record all items that they need to be reminded about at any time. The playback time for when reminders need to be heard can be set and played through the day.
- Some applications for grocery shopping already exist, where information is categorized and arranged in a logical manner for the client (see Figure 55.3).
- Recently, population-based applications (i.e., apps) for smartphones were generated such as apps that could calm or engage the person with dementia of the Alzheimer's type and caregiver apps, which include tools that can ease treatment and care.

Adaptations of Task or Environment. A therapist applying the principles of the CDM may rearrange tasks and environments so that they place fewer demands on memory:

- Cue cards or signs in key places (e.g., a sign on door where it will be seen before leaving: "Take keys and . . .")
- Labeling the outside of drawers or closets to minimize the need to recall the location of items
- Providing step-by-step directions to reduce memory demands
- Providing checklists to assist in keeping track of task steps

Significant others can be trained to use methods that increase the likelihood that the client will remember material, such as asking the client to repeat any instructions or important information in his or her own words; encouraging the client to ask questions; and presenting material in small groups, clusters, or categories (Levy, 2011a).

Executive Functions, Organization, and Problem Solving

Executive functions are a broad band of skills that allow a person to engage in independent, purposeful, and self-directed behavior. Higher level cognitive skills including planning, cognitive flexibility, organization, problem solving, and self-regulation, are fundamental components of executive function (Katz & Hartman-Maeir, 2005). Lezak et al. (2004) identifies four primary components of executive functions: volition, planning, purposeful action, and self-awareness and self-monitoring. Impairments are associated with prefrontal lesions and may be seen in all of these components, with one or two areas of impairment especially prominent (Lezak et al., 2004). Volition is the capacity to formulate an intention or goal and to initiate action. Planning involves the ability to efficiently organize the steps or elements of a behavior or activity and includes the ability to look ahead, anticipate consequences, weigh and make choices, conceive of alternatives, sustain attention, and sequence the activity. Purposeful action is the translation of an intention into an activity, requiring the ability to initiate, switch, and stop sequences (flexibility), as well as self-regulation. Self-regulation involves the ability to monitor, self-correct, and evaluate performance.

Executive function impairments significantly influence social participation, daily activity, and functional outcome (Goverover, 2004; Reeder, Newton, Frangou, & Wykes, 2004; Voelbel et al., 2011). Clients who display executive dysfunction may be able to verbalize plans but have difficulty carrying them out. There is often a dissociation between stated intentions and actions. This creates gaps between what a person needs to do or wants to do and what the person actually does (Eriksson, Tham, & Borg, 2006). Decreased initiation, flexibility, impulsivity, or **perseveration** may be observed during performance. Often, the client's approach is haphazard or consists of trial and error, and there is decreased ability to maintain goal-directed actions and to monitor or modify behaviors. For example, when grocery shopping, the client might proceed in an unorganized manner, not using a list or the aisle headings and reentering the same aisle multiple times. The client might have difficulty deciding on appropriate substitute items, buy items that are not needed, and forget items that were needed (Sohlberg & Mateer, 2001). Rempfer, Hamera, Brown, and Cromwell (2003) found that grocery shopping accuracy and efficiency were significantly associated with measures of executive functions in people with chronic schizophrenia. In addition, limitations in the ability to view information from different perspectives, generate alternative solutions, and respond flexibly can reduce the ability to cope, adapt to everyday demands, and relate to others.

Executive functions impairments represent a distinct challenge because they can be masked within familiar ADL or routines but are most apparent when the client is required to function in situations that are less structured, require multitasking, or require dealing with novelty and unexpected situations (Burgess et al., 2006; Katz & Hartman-Maeir, 2005). Examples of activities that might present difficulty include following directions to a new location; selecting and ordering a gift from a catalogue; organizing a day's activities; planning a menu, lunch, picnic, vacation, or social gathering; investigating and comparing prices for delivery of flowers; mailing a package; or purchasing an electronic device.

More details about the evidence related to executive functions and participation are available at **http://thePoint.lww.com/Willard-Spackman12e.**

Evaluation

Most standardized cognitive assessments are structured and do not adequately examine the area of executive functions (Sohlberg & Mateer, 2001) (see Table 55.2). Newer ecologically valid evaluations for executive function have been designed such as the Multiple Errands Test (Dawson, Anderson et al., 2009; Maeir, Krauss, & Katz, 2011) and the Executive Function Performance Test (Baum et al., 2008). Although these assessments appear more "ecologically valid" (i.e., able to predict behavior in everyday situations) than previous assessments were, further research data on the reliability and validity of these assessment tools are needed.

Intervention

Remedial Deficit Specific Training. It is assumed in the remedial approach that improvement in underlying cognitive perceptual skills will have a greater influence on behavior than will direct training of functional task training because learning will spontaneously generalize to a wider range of activities. For example, Wang, Chang, and Su (2011) adopted the breakfast cooking task of Craik and Bialystok (2006) into a multitasking training task for elderly adults. Participants were required to constantly switch, update, and plan in order to control the cooking of several foods and concurrently perform a table-setting task. Training gains were exhibited on task-related measures and transfer was limited.

Strategy Training. Strategies that maximize executive functioning can be practiced in various unstructured tasks that require initiation, planning, organization, and decision making such as organizing medications according to a schedule, planning an overnight trip and packing a suitcase, obtaining and organizing a list of local business phone numbers, and organizing tools. Strategy training can be learned using the multicontext approach (Toglia et al., 2010; Toglia et al., 2011). Toglia et al. (2011) examined through a case study design the application of the multicontext approach in the treatment of clients with brain injury and executive deficits. They demonstrated that a checklist strategy combined with self-awareness training and practice across multiple tasks improved the occupational performance of clients with executive functions. Verbal mediation has been reported to be an effective strategy in improving executive function and self-regulation deficits. For example, Cicerone and Wood (1987) reported the successful use of a self-instructional procedure in a client with impaired planning ability and poor self-control secondary to brain injury. Intervention involved requiring the client to verbalize a plan of action before and during execution of a task. Gradually, the client was instructed to whisper rather than talk aloud. Generalization to real-life situations was observed after an extended period of time that included training in self-monitoring.

Training in problem-solving strategies involves teaching the person to break down complex activities into smaller, more manageable steps. Strategies may also aim to help the person to maintain the focus of goals and intentions (Katz & Hartman-Maeir, 2005). For example, Levine et al. (2000, 2007) studied a goal management training procedure where participants had to (1) "stop" and define what they are going to do, (2) "define" the main task, (3) "list" the steps, (4) "learn" the steps and *do* it, and (5) "check" if am I doing what I planned to do. They studied this strategy with both functional and nonfunctional tasks. An evidence-based review (Cicerone et al., 2011) concluded that there is evidence to support the use of formal problem-solving training with application to everyday activities. The authors recommended such training as a practice guideline for people with stroke or brain injury during postacute rehabilitation. The intervention goal is to replace an impulsive, disorganized approach with a systematic and controlled approach to planning activities, maintaining goal intentions, and solving problems. The steps of the problem-solving process are reinforced with the use of self-questioning techniques. For example, self-questioning cue cards with the following types of questions can be used during problem-solving tasks: What do I need to do? Do I need more information? What do I have to do next? Have I identified all the critical information? Do I understand the problem? What are all the possible solutions? Did I choose the best one? (e.g., Chan & Fong, 2011).

Broad checklists or task guidance systems are commonly used to assist the client in initiating, planning, and carrying out an activity systematically (e.g., Levine et al., 2000, 2007). Checklists may be specific to a particular activity (e.g., following steps to operate a computer program) or they may be designed broadly so that they can be used in various similar activities (e.g., a checklist for food preparation or cooking activities). Interventions should incorporate practice in identifying the situations or activities in which the use of a checklist could be helpful, as described in the multicontext approach (Toglia et al., 2010; Toglia et al., 2011). The client may be given the opportunity to practice the same activity with and without the use of a checklist to enhance awareness. Initially, the goal might be to have a client follow a checklist established by the practitioner or significant other. Eventually, the client might be given checklists with missing steps and be asked to review the lists to identify the missing components. Finally, the client might be required to create a checklist independently. Burke, Zencius, Wesolowski, and Doubleday (1991) describe four cases of individuals with executive dysfunction for whom checklists were successfully used to improve the ability to carry out routine vocational tasks.

Another example of intervention directed at enhancing strategy use is provided by a pilot study that examined the applicability of the CO-OP approach for use with adults with executive dysfunction arising from TBI. The intervention entailed guiding participants to use a meta-cognitive problem-solving strategy to perform self-identified daily tasks that they needed and wanted to do and with which they were having difficulties (Dawson, Gaya et al., 2009). The CO-OP approach was also applied successfully for patients with stroke (Henshaw et al., 2011).

Decreased initiation, one of the hallmark features of executive dysfunction, can significantly interfere with the ability to use and apply a learned strategy. For example, a person with deficits in executive functions might use a strategy effectively when cued but not use the strategy spontaneously because of a failure to initiate its use. External cues such as alarm signals can be used to prompt the client to initiate a task, switch to a different task component, or use a particular strategy within an activity (Evans, Emslie, & Wilson, 1998; Manly, Hawkins, Evans, Wodlt, & Robertson, 2002).

Adaptations of Task or Environment. Adaptations that minimize demands on executive functions include training a significant other to preorganize an activity or activity materials. For example, all the items needed for grooming can be prearranged on the sink in the sequence in which they are used. As an alternative, one task step can be introduced at a time. These adaptations limit the need for planning and organization (Sohlberg & Mateer, 2001).

People who have difficulty with initiation, organization, and decision making require structure. Open-ended questions such as "What do you want to eat" should be avoided. Clients who have difficulty in initiation will have a great deal of difficulty in answering open-ended questions. Questions should provide a limited number of choices whenever feasible.

A predictable and structured daily routine enhances the client's ability to initiate tasks and should be established and monitored by a significant other. Audiotape instructions that cue the client to initiate an activity and perform each step at a time in its proper sequence have been reported to be successful within the context of daily routines (Schwartz, 1995).

Group Interventions

Cognitive rehabilitation principles and strategies can be incorporated within group programs and combined with psychosocial or psychoeducational interventions. The group format can be used to target specific cognitive skills, train the use of compensatory task methods, or facilitate the use of cognitive strategies (Revheim & Marcopulos, 2006; Schwartzberg, 1999; Stuss et al., 2007). In addition, the group format can be used with various diagnoses such as patients with multiple sclerosis, TBI, lupus, psychiatric illnesses, attention deficit hyperactivity disorder (ADHD), and other diagnoses. Group activities can emphasize interpersonal skills within cooperative tasks such as planning a bake sale, publishing a newsletter, or role-playing scenarios involving interviews, conflicts, or on-the-spot problem solving. Strategies that include monitoring the tendency to respond impulsively become stuck in one viewpoint or wander off task can be practiced within social contexts (Toglia, 2011). Group programs that center on teaching self-monitoring techniques and strategies for paying attention, remembering, organization, or problem solving can be applied to a wide spectrum of clients such as multiple sclerosis (Shevil & Finlayson, 2010), mental illness (Revheim & Marcopulos, 2006), lupus (Harrison et al., 2005), or ADHD (Hahn-Markowitz, Manor, & Maeir, 2011). Activities such as remembering names and facts about group members, recalling directions for operating a new electronic device, or creating a checklist for a complex task can provide opportunity to practice different strategies and share experiences within a group context. Group members can be encouraged to reflect on performance and identify strategies that would be useful in their everyday activities. Group interventions that simultaneously address subtle cognitive difficulties and emotional issues have demonstrated value in improving self-awareness, self-efficacy, coping skills, psychosocial skills, and perceived daily functioning (Harrison et al., 2005; Huckans et al., 2010; Rath, Simon, Langenbahn, Sherr, & Diller, 2003; Revheim & Marcopulos, 2006; Shevil & Finlayson, 2010; Toglia, 2011). See Chapter 34 for more information on Group Process and Intervention.

Occupational Therapy Role within the Rehabilitation Team

A strong interdisciplinary approach is needed to address the complex of issues that arise from cognitive-perceptual problems. Team goals should be identified as well as specific discipline goals. The family and client are also members of the team and should be involved in team discussions and provide input into the overall intervention plan. Once the targeted behaviors for intervention have been clearly identified, the occupational therapist and occupational therapy assistant collaborate to choose various activities that can be used to reinforce the desired behaviors. The work environment in which the therapist practices may determine the depth of the occupational therapy practitioner's involvement because of the nature of the practice setting and the client's length of stay.

An interdisciplinary intervention program should emphasize the same major goals during treatment rather than working on separate skills. For example, the speech-language pathologist might address attention problems within the context of language material such as listening to tapes or conversations; the neuropsychologist might use remedial attentional exercises; the physical therapist might reinforce attention through motor tasks; and the occupational therapy practitioner might address attentional strategies within the context of self-care, leisure, community, or work activities. An integrated approach that assists the person in seeing patterns of behaviors across different activities is strongly advocated rather than one that reinforces the fragmentation that the client already perceives.

Summary

Recently, there is increasing evidence that supports the use of comprehensive cognitive rehabilitation programs that address a combination of cognitive, emotional, functional, and social participation skills in people with brain injury (Cappa et al., 2005; Cicerone et al., 2011; Cicerone, Mott, Azulay, & Friel, 2004; Sarajuuri et al., 2005; Tiersky et al., 2005). The need to blend cognitive interventions with those that address interpersonal and real-world functioning has been emphasized in recent literature; however, the outcome of cognitive rehabilitation is most commonly measured at the impairment level. As occupational therapists return to more community-focused intervention, we need to widen our perspective on the influence that cognitive-perceptual impairments have on our clients' ability to engage in the occupations they need or want to do within the contexts of their lives. We need to explore the effect of cognitive rehabilitation on occupational engagement and social participation because even subtle cognitive impairments can decrease satisfaction, participation, and quality of life, preventing our clients from leading enriching lives (McDowd, Filion, Pohl, Richards, & Stiers, 2003).

The outcome or benefit of cognitive rehabilitation needs to be examined broadly across different populations including effects on changing existing habits, routines, or increasing productive activity patterns; increasing the frequency and quality of social participation; decreasing caregiver assistance, stress, or burden; improving subjective well-being including self-efficacy, self-esteem, satisfaction, and quality of life; and preventing functional decline.

References

Abreu, B. C., & Peloquin, S. M. (2005). The quadraphonic approach: A holistic rehabilitation model for brain injury. In N. Katz (Ed.), *Cognition and occupation across the life span* (2nd ed., pp. 73–112). Bethesda, MD: AOTA.

Abreu, B. C., Seale, G., Scheibel, R. S., Huddleston, N., Zhang, L., & Ottenbacher, K. J. (2001). Levels of self-awareness after acute brain injury: How patients' and rehabilitation specialists' perceptions compare. *Archives of Physical Medicine and Rehabilitation, 82*, 49–55.

Abreu, B. C., & Toglia, J. P. (1987). Cognitive rehabilitation: A model for occupational therapy. *American Journal of Occupational Therapy, 41*, 439–448.

Albert, M. L. (1973). A simple test of visual neglect. *Neurology, 23*, 658–665.

Allen, C. K. (1985). *Occupational therapy for psychiatric diseases: Measurement and management of cognitive disabilities.* Boston, NY: Little Brown.

Allen, C. K., Earhart, C. A., & Blue, T. (1992). *Occupational therapy treatment goals for the physically and cognitively disabled.* Rockville, MD: AOTA.

American Occupational Therapy Association. (2008). Occupational therapy practice framework: Domain and process, 2nd edition. *American Journal of Occupational Therapy, 62*, 625–683.

American Occupational Therapy Association. (in press). Management of occupational therapy services for persons with cognitive impairments (statement).

Antonucci, G., Guariglia, A., Magnotti, L., Paolucci, S., Pizzamiglio, L., & Zoccolotti, P. (1995). Effectiveness of neglect rehabilitation in a randomized group study. *Journal of Clinical and Experimental Neuropsychology, 17*, 383–389.

Appelros, P., Nydevik, I., Karlsson, G. M., Thorwalls, A., & Seiger, A. (2003). Assessing unilateral neglect: Shortcomings of standard test methods. *Disability and Rehabilitation, 25*, 473–479.

Arai, T., Ohi, H., Sasaki, H., Nobuto, H., & Tanaka, K. (1997). Hemispatial sunglasses: Effect on unilateral spatial neglect. *Archives of Physical Medicine and Rehabilitation, 78*, 230–232.

Arnadottir, G. (1990). *The brain and behavior: Assessing cortical dysfunction through activities of daily living.* St. Louis, MO: Mosby.

Aubin, G., Chapparo, C., Gélinas, I., Stip, E., & Rainville, C. (2009). Use of the Perceive, Recall, Plan and Perform System of Task Analysis for persons with schizophrenia: A preliminary study. *Australian Occupational Therapy Journal, 56*, 189–199.

Averbuch, S., & Katz, N. (2011). Cognitive rehabilitation: A retraining model for clients with neurological disabilities. In N. Katz (Ed.), *Cognition, occupation, and participation across the life span: Neuroscience, neurorehabilitation, and models of intervention in occupational therapy* (3rd ed., pp. 277–298). Bethesda, MD: AOTA.

Azouvi, P., Olivier, S., Montety, G., Samuel, C., Louise-Dreyfus, A., & Luigi, T. (2003). Behavioral assessment of unilateral neglect: Study of the psychometric properties of the Catherine Bergego Scale. *Archives of Physical Medicine Rehabilitation, 84*, 51–57.

Ball, K., Edwards, J. D., & Ross, L. A. (2007). The impact of speed of processing training on cognitive and everyday functions. *Journals of Gerontology: Psychological Sciences and Social Sciences, 62B*, 19–31.

Barrett, A. M., Buxbaum, L. J., Coslett, H. B., Edwards, E., Heilman, K. M., Hillis, A. E., . . . Robertson, I. H. (2006). Cognitive rehabilitation interventions for neglect and related disorders: Moving from bench to bedside in stroke patients. *Journal of Cognitive Neuroscience, 18*, 1223–1236.

Baum, C. M., Connor, L. T., Morrison, T., Hahn, M., Dromerick, A. W., & Edwards, D. F. (2008). Reliability, validity, and clinical utility of the Executive Function Performance Test: A measure of executive function in a sample of people with stroke. *American Journal of Occupational Therapy, 62*, 446–455.

Baum, C. M., & Edwards, D. F. (1993). Cognitive performance in senile dementia of the Alzheimer's type: The Kitchen Task Assessment. *American Journal of Occupational Therapy, 47*, 431–436.

Baum, C., & Edwards, D. F. (1998). *Home Occupational Environmental Assessment: An environmental checklist for treatment planning.* Unpublished manuscript, University School of Medicine, St Louis, MO.

Baum, C., & Edwards, D. F. (2001). *Activity Card Sort (ACS). Program in occupational therapy.* St. Louis, MO: Washington University School of Medicine.

Baum, C., Edwards, D. F., Morrison, T., & Hahn, M. (2003). *Executive Function Performance Test.* St. Louis, MO: Washington University School of Medicine.

Benton, A. L., Hamsher, K. de S., Varney, N. R., & Spreen, O. (1983). *Contributions to Neuropsychological Assessment: Clinical manual.* New York, NY: Oxford University Press.

Bier, N., Provencher, V., Gagnon, L., van der Linden, M., Adam, S., & Desrosiers, J. (2008). New learning in dementia: Transfer and spontaneous use of learning in everyday life functioning. Two case studies. *Neuropsychological Rehabilitation, 18*, 204–235.

Blessed, G., Tomlinson, B. E., & Roth, M. (1968). The association between quantitative measures of dementia and of senile change in the cerebral gray matter of elderly subjects. *British Journal of Psychiatry, 114*, 797–811.

Bogod, N. M., Mateer, C. A., & MacDonald, S. W. S. (2003). Self-awareness after traumatic brain injury: A comparison of measures and their relationship to executive functions. *Journal of the International Neuropsychological Society, 9*, 450–458.

Boman, I. L., Bartfai, A., Borell, L., Tham, K., & Hemmingsson, H. (2010). Support in everyday activities with a home-based electronic memory aid for persons with memory impairments. *Disability and Rehabilitation: Assistive Technology, 5*, 339–350.

Bootes, K., & Chapparo, C. (2010). Difficulties with multitasking on return to work after TBI: A critical case study. *Work, 36*, 207–216.

Bottari, C., Gosselin, N., Guillemette, M., LaMoureux, J., & Ptito, A. (2011). Independence in managing one's finances after traumatic brain injury. *Brain Injury, 25*, 1306–1317.

Bour, A., Rasquin, S., Boreas, A., Limburg, M., & Verhey, F. (2010). How predictive is the MMSE for cognitive performance after stroke? *Journal of Neurology, 257*, 630–637.

Bourgeois, M. S., Camp, C., Rose, M., White, B., Malone, M., Carr, J., & Rovine, M. (2003). A comparison of training strategies to enhance use of external aids by persons with dementia. *Journal of Communication Disorders, 36*, 361–378.

Boyd, T. M., & Sautter, S. W. (1993). Route-finding: A measure of everyday executive functioning in the head-injured adult. *Applied Cognitive Psychology, 7*, 171–181.

Brandt, J., & Benedict, R., H. B. (2001). *The Hopkins Verbal Learning Test–Revised (HVLT-R).* Lutz, FL: Psychological Assessment Resources.

Branswell, D., Hartry, A., Hoornbeek, S., Johansen, A., Johnson, L., Schultz, J., . . . Sohlberg, M. (1992). *The Profile of Executive Control System.* Puyallup, WA: Association for Neuropsychological Research and Development.

Broadbent, D. E., Cooper, P. F., FitzGerald, P., & Parkes, K. R. (1982). The Cognitive Failures Questionnaire (CFQ) and its correlates. *British Journal of Clinical Psychology, 21*(Pt. 1), 1–16.

Brunsdon, R., Nickels, L., & Coltheart, M. (2007). Topographical disorientation: Towards an integrated framework for assessment. *Neuropsychological Rehabilitation, 17*, 34–52.

Burgess, P. W., Alderman, N., Forbes, C., Costello, A., Coates, L. M., Dawson, D. R., . . . Channon, S. (2006). The case for the development and use of "ecologically valid" measures of executive function in experimental and clinical neuropsychology. *Journal of the International Neuropsychological Society, 12*, 194–209.

Burke, W. H., Zencius, A. H., Wesolowskis, M. D., & Doubleday, F. (1991). Improving executive function disorders in brain injured clients. *Brain Injury, 5*, 241–252.

Butler, J. A. (1999). Evaluation and intervention with apraxia. In C. Unsworth (Ed.), *Cognitive and perceptual dysfunction* (pp. 257–298). Philadelphia, PA: F. A. Davis.

Butler, P. D., Silverstein, S. M., & Dakin, S. C. (2008). Visual perception and its impairment in schizophrenia. *Biological Psychiatry, 64*, 40–47.

Calvanio, R., Levine, D., & Petrone, P. (1993). Elements of cognitive rehabilitation after right hemisphere stroke. *Neurologic Clinics, 11*, 25–57.

Caplan, B. (1987). Assessment of unilateral neglect: A new reading test. *Journal of Clinical and Experimental Neuropsychology, 9*, 359–364.

Cappa, S. F., Benke, T., Clarke, S., Rossi, B., Stemmer, B., & van Heugten, C. M. (2005). EFNS guidelines on cognitive rehabilitation: Report of an EFNS task force. *European Journal of Neurology, 12*, 665–680.

Cappa, S. F., Sterzi, R., Vallar, G., & Bisiach, E. (1987). Remission of hemineglect and anosognosia during vestibular stimulation. *Neuropsychologia, 25*, 775–782.

Cate, Y., & Richards, L. (2000). Relationship between performance on tests of basic visual functions and visual-perceptual processing in persons after brain injury. *American Journal of Occupational Therapy, 54*, 326–334.

Cermak, S. A., & Larkin, D. (Eds.). (2002). *Developmental coordination disorder.* Albany, NY: Delmar/Thompson Learning.

Cermak, S. A., & Maeir, A. (2011). Cognitive rehabilitation of children and adults with attention-deficit hyperactivity disorder. In N. Katz (Ed.), *Cognition, occupation, and participation across the life span: Neuroscience, neurorehabilitation, and models of intervention in occupational therapy* (3rd ed., pp. 249–276). Bethesda, MD: AOTA.

Chan, D. Y., & Fong, K. N. (2011). The effects of problem-solving skills training based on metacognitive principles for children with acquired brain injury attending mainstream schools: A controlled clinical trial. *Disability Rehabilitation, 33*, 2023–2032.

Chiaravalloti, N., Christodoulou, C., Demaree, H., & DeLuca, J. (2003). Differentiating simple vs. complex processing speed: Influence on new learning and memory performance. *Journal of Clinical and Experimental Neuropsychology, 25*, 489–501.

Chui, T., Oliver, R., Ascott, P., Choo, L. C., Davis, T., Gaya, A., . . . Letts, L. (2006). *Safety Assessment of Function and the Environment for Rehabilitation (SAFER) version 3.* Toronto, ON: COTA Health. Retrieved from http://www.cotahealth.ca

Cicerone, K. D., Langenbahn, D. M., Braden, C., Malec, J. F., Kalmar, K., Fraas, M., . . . Ashman, T. (2011). Evidence-based cognitive rehabilitation: Updated review of the literature from 2003 through 2008. *Archives of Physical Medicine and Rehabilitation, 92*, 519–530.

Cicerone, K., Mott, T., Azulay, J., and Friel, J. (2004). Community integration and satisfaction with functioning after intensive cognitive rehabilitation for traumatic brain injury. *Archives of Physical Medicine and Rehabilitation, 85*, 943–950.

Cicerone, K. D., & Wood, J. C. (1987). Planning disorder after closed head injury: A case study. *Archives of Physical Medicine and Rehabilitation, 68*, 111–115.

Colarusso, R. P., & Hammill, D. D. (2002). *Motor-Free Visual Perception Test (MVPT-3).* Austin, TX: PRO-ED.

Cooke, D. M., McKenna, K., & Fleming, J. (2005). Development of a standardized occupational therapy screening tool for visual perception in adults. *Scandinavian Journal of Occupational Therapy, 12*, 59–71.

Corben, L., & Unsworth, C. (1999). Evaluation and intervention with unilateral neglect. In C. Unsworth (Ed.), *Cognitive and perceptual dysfunction* (pp. 357–392). Philadelphia, PA: F. A. Davis.

Craik, F. I., & Bialystok, E. (2006). Planning and task management in older adults: Cooking breakfast. *Memory & Cognition, 34*, 1236–1249.

Crawford, J. R., Smith, G. V., Maylor, E. A. M., Della Sala, S., & Logie, R. H. (2003). The Prospective and Retrospective Memory Questionnaire (PMRQ): Normative data and latent structure in a large non-clinical sample. *Memory, 11*, 261–265.

Crosson, C., Barco, P. P., Velozo, C., Bolesta, M. M., Cooper, P. V., Werts, D., & Brobeck, T. C. (1989). Awareness and compensation in postacute head injury rehabilitation. *Journal of Clinical and Experimental Neuropsychology, 2*, 355–363.

Cullum, C. M., Weiner, M. F., & Saine, K. (2009). *Texas Functional Living Scale.* San Antonio, TX: Pearson.

Curtin, M., Jones, J., Tyson, G. A., Mitsch, V., Alston, M., & McAllister, L. (2011). Outcomes of Participation Objective, Participation Subjective (POPS) measure following traumatic brain injury. *Brain Injury, 25,* 266–273.

Davidson, J. E., & Sternberg, R. J. (1998). Smart problem solving: How metacognition helps. In D. J. Hacker, J. Dunlosky, & A. G. Graesser (Eds.), *Metacognition in educational theory and practice* (pp. 47–68). Mahwah, NJ: Lawrence Erlbaum Associates.

Dawson, D. R., Anderson, N. D., Burgess, P., Cooper, E., Krpan, K. M., & Stuss, D. T. (2009). Further development of the Multiple Errands Test: Standardized scoring, reliability, and ecological validity for the Baycrest version. *Archives of Physical Medicine and Rehabilitation, 90*(11, Suppl.), S41–S51.

Dawson, D. R., Gaya, A., Hunt, A., Levine, B., Lemsky, C., & Polatajko, H. J. (2009). Using the cognitive orientation to occupational performance (CO-OP) with adults with executive dysfunction following traumatic brain injury. *Canadian Journal of Occupational Therapy, 76,* 115–127.

Deitz, T., Beeman, C., & Thorn, D. (1993). *Test of Orientation for Rehabilitation Patients.* Tucson, AZ: Therapy Skill Builders.

Diehl, M. (1998). Everyday competence in later life: Current status and future directions. *The Gerontologist, 38,* 422–433.

Di Monaco, M., Schintu, S., Dotta, M., Barba, S., Tappero, R., & Gindri P. (2011). Severity of unilateral spatial neglect is an independent predictor of functional outcome after acute inpatient rehabilitation in individuals with right hemispheric stroke. *Archives of Physical Medicine and Rehabilitation, 92,* 1250–1256.

Donaghy, S., & Williams, W. (1998). New methodology: A new protocol for training severely impaired patients in the usage of memory journals. *Brain Injury, 12,* 1061–1076.

Doninger, N. A., Bode, R. K., Heinemann, A. W., & Ambrose, C. (2000). Rating scale analysis of the Neurobehavioral Cognitive Status Examination. *Journal of Head Trauma Rehabilitation, 15,* 683–695.

Donkervoort, M., Dekker, J. Stehmann-Saris, F. C., & Deelman, B. G. (2001). Efficacy of strategy training in left hemisphere stroke patients with apraxia: A randomised clinical trial. *Neuropsychological Rehabilitation, 11,* 549–566.

Edgeworth, J. A., Robertson, I., H., & McMillan, T. M. (1998). *The Balloons Test.* Bury St. Edmunds, United Kingdom: Thames Valley Test Company.

Edwards, J. D., Ross, L. A., Wadley, V. G., Clay, O. J., Crowe, M. Roenker, D. L., & Ball, K. K. (2006). The Useful Field of View test: Normative data. *Archives of Clinical Neuropsychology, 21,* 275–286.

Edwards, J. D., Vance, D. E., Wadley, V. G., Cissell, G. M., Roenker, D. L., & Ball, K. K. (2005). Reliability and validity of the Useful Field of View test scores as administered by personal computer. *Journal of Clinical and Experimental Neuropsychology, 27,* 529–543.

Ekstam, L., Uppgard, B., Kottorp, A., & Tham K. (2007). Relationship between awareness of disability and occupational performance during the first year after a stroke. *American Journal of Occupational Therapy, 61,* 503–511.

Emslie, H., Wilson, F. C., Burden, V., Nimmo-Smith, I., & Wilson, B. A. (2003). *Behavioural Assessment of the Dysexecutive Syndrome for Children (BADS-C).* London, United Kingdom: Harcourt Assessment/The Psychological Corporation.

Erickson, M., Jaafari, N., & Lysaker, P. (2011). Insight and negative symptoms as predictors of functioning in a work setting in patients with schizophrenia. *Psychiatry Research, 189,* 161–165.

Eriksson, G., Tham, K., & Borg, J. (2006). Occupational gaps in everyday life 1–4 years after acquired brain injury. *Journal of Rehabilitation Medicine, 38,* 159–165.

Evans, J. J., Emslie, H., & Wilson, B. A. (1998). Case study: External cueing systems in the rehabilitation of executive impairments of action. *Journal of the International Neuropsychological Society, 4,* 399–408.

Ewing-Cobbs, L., Levin, H. S., Fletcher, J. M., Miner, M. E., & Eisenberg, H. M. (1990). The Children's Orientation and Amnesia Test: Relationship to severity of acute head injury and to recovery of memory. *Neurosurgery, 27,* 683–691.

Farah, M. J. (2003). Disorders of visual-spatial perception and cognition: Visuoperceptual, visuospatial, and visuoconstructive disorders. In K. M. Heilman & E. Valenstein (Eds.), *Clinical neuropsychology* (4th ed., pp. 146–160). New York, NY: Oxford University Press.

Fasotti, L., Kovacs, F., Eling, P., & Brouwer, W. H. (2000). Time pressure management as a compensatory strategy training after closed head injury. *Neuropsychological Rehabilitation, 10,* 47–65.

Ferber, S., & Karnath, H. (2001). How to assess spatial neglect: Line bisection or cancellation tasks? *Journal of Clinical and Experimental Neuropsychology, 23,* 599–607.

Ferguson, J. M., & Trombly, C. A. (1997). The effect of added purpose and meaningful occupation on motor learning. *American Journal of Occupational Therapy, 51,* 508–515.

Fertherlin, J. M., & Kurland, L. (1989). Self-instruction: A compensatory strategy to increase functional independence with brain injured adults. *Occupational Therapy Practice, 1,* 75–78.

Fischer, S., Gauggel, S., & Trexler, L. E. (2004). Awareness of activity limitations, goal setting and rehabilitation outcome in patients with brain injuries. *Brain Injury, 18,* 547–562.

Fisher, A. G. (1993a). Functional measures: Part 1. What is function, what should we measure and how should we measure it? *American Journal of Occupational Therapy, 46,* 183–185.

Fisher, A. G. (1993b). Functional measures: Part 2. Selecting the right test, minimizing the limitations. *American Journal of Occupational Therapy, 46,* 278–281.

Fleming, J. M., Lucas, S. E., & Lightbody, S. (2006). Using occupation to facilitate self-awareness in people who have acquired brain injury: A pilot study. *Canadian Journal of Occupational Therapy, 73,* 44–55.

Fleming, J. M., Shum, D., Strong, J., & Lightbody, S. (2005). Prospective memory rehabilitation for adults with traumatic brain injury: A compensatory training programme. *Brain Injury, 19,* 1–13.

Fleming, J. M., Strong, J., & Ashton, R. (1996). Self-awareness of deficits in adults with traumatic brain injury: How best to measure? *Brain Injury, 10,* 1–15.

Folstein, M. F., Folstein, S. E., & McHugh, P. R. (1975). Mini-mental state: A practical method for grading the cognitive state of patients for the clinician. *Journal of Psychiatric Research, 12,* 189–198.

Gauthier, L., Dehaut, F., & Joanette, Y. (1989). The Bells Test: A quantitative and qualitative test for visual neglect. *International Journal of Clinical Neuropsychology, 11,* 49–54.

Geusgens, C., van Heugten, C., Donkervoort, M., van den Ende, E., Jolles, J., & van den Heuvel, W. (2006). Transfer of training effects in stroke patients with apraxia: An exploratory study. *Neuropsychological Rehabilitation, 16,* 213–229.

Giles, G. M. (2011). A neurofunctional approach to rehabilitation after brain injury. In N. Katz, (Ed.), *Cognition, occupation, and participation across the life span: Neuroscience, neurorehabilitation, and models of intervention in occupational therapy* (3rd ed., pp. 351–382). Bethesda, MD: AOTA.

Giles, G. M., Ridley, J. E., Dill, A., & Frye, S. (1997). A consecutive series of adults with brain injury treated with a washing and dressing retraining program. *American Journal of Occupational Therapy, 51,* 256–266.

Giles, G. M., & Shore, M. (1989). A rapid method for teaching severely brain injured adults how to wash and dress. *Archives of Physical Medicine and Rehabilitation, 70,* 156–158.

Gillen, G. (2009). *Cognitive and perceptual rehabilitation: Optimizing function.* St. Louis, MO: Mosby.

Gillen, R., Tennen, H., & McKee, T. (2005). Unilateral spatial neglect: Relation to rehabilitation outcomes in patients with right hemisphere stroke. *Archives of Physical Medicine and Rehabilitation, 86,* 763–767.

Gitlin, L. N., Hodgson, N., Jutkowitz, E., & Pizzi, L. (2010). The cost-effectiveness of a nonpharmacologic intervention for individuals with dementia and family caregivers: The tailored activity program. *The American Journal of Geriatric Psychiatry, 18,* 510–519.

Gitlin, L. N., Jacobs, M., & Earland, T. V. (2010). Translation of a dementia caregiver intervention for delivery in homecare as a reimbursable Medicare service: Outcomes and lessons learned. *Gerontologist, 50,* 847–854.

Gitlin, L. N., Schinfeld, S., Winter, L., Corcoran, M., Boyce, A. A., & Hauck, W. W. (2002). Evaluating home environments of persons with dementia: Interrater reliability and validity of the home environmental assessment protocol (HEAP). *Disability and Rehabilitation, 24*, 59–91.

Gitlin, L. N., Winter, L., Dennis, M. P., Hodgson, N., & Hauck, W. W. (2010a). A biobehavioral home-based intervention and the well-being of patients with dementia and their caregivers: The COPE randomized trial. *JAMA: The Journal of the American Medical Association, 304*, 983–991.

Gitlin, L. N., Winter, L., Dennis, M. P., Hodgson, N., & Hauck, W. W. (2010b). Targeting and managing behavioral symptoms in individuals with dementia: A randomized trial of a nonpharmacological intervention. *Journal of the American Geriatrics Society, 58*, 1465–1474.

Gitlin, L. N., Winter, L., Vause Earland, T., Adel Herge, E., Chernett, N. L., Piersol, C. V., & Burke, J. P. (2009). The tailored activity program to reduce behavioral symptoms in individuals with dementia: Feasibility, acceptability, and replication potential. *The Gerontologist, 49*, 428–439.

Glisky, E. L., Schacter, L. D., & Butters, A. M. (1994). Domain-specific learning and remediation of memory disorders. In M. J. Riddoch & G. W. Humphreys (Eds.), *Cognitive neuropsychology and cognitive rehabilitation* (pp. 527–548). East Sussex, United Kingdom: Lawrence Erlbaum Associates.

Golding, E. (1989). *The Middlesex Elderly Assessment of Mental State*. Bury St. Edmunds, United Kingdom: Thames Valley Test Company.

Golisz, K. M. (1998). Dynamic assessment and multicontext treatment of unilateral neglect. *Topics in Stroke Rehabilitation, 5*, 11–28.

Goverover, Y. (2004). Categorization, deductive reasoning and self-awareness: Association to everyday competence in persons with acute brain injury. *Journal of Clinical and Experimental Neuropsychology, 26*, 737–749.

Goverover, Y., Arango, J. C., Hillary, G. M., Chiaravalloti, N., & DeLuca, J. (2009). Application of spacing effects to improve learning and memory for functional activities in traumatic brain injury: A pilot study. *American Journal of Occupational Therapy, 63*, 543–549.

Goverover, Y., Basso, M., Wood, H., Chiaravalloti, N., & DeLuca, J. (2011). An examination of the benefits of combining two learning strategies on memory of functional information in persons with multiple sclerosis. *Multiple Sclerosis, 17*, 1488–1497.

Goverover Y., Chiaravalloti, N., & DeLuca, J. (2005). The relationship between self-awareness of neurobehavioral symptoms, cognitive functions and emotional symptoms in multiple sclerosis. *Multiple Sclerosis, 11*, 203–212.

Goverover, Y., Chiaravalloti, N., Gaudino-Goering, E., Moore, N. B., & DeLuca, J. (2009). The relationship among performance of instrumental activities of daily living, self-report of quality of life, and self-awareness of functional status in individuals with multiple sclerosis. *Rehabilitation Psychology, 54*, 60–68.

Goverover, Y., Johnston, M. V., Toglia, J., & DeLuca, J. (2007a). Treatment to improve self-awareness for persons with acquired brain injury. *Brain Injury, 21*, 913–923.

Goverover, Y., Johnston, M. V., Toglia, J., & DeLuca, J. (2007b, February). *Treatment to improve self-awareness and functional independence for persons with TBI: A pilot randomized trial.* Paper presented at the Neuropsychological Society 35th Annual Meeting, Portland, OR.

Goverover, Y., O'Brien, A., Moore, N., & DeLuca, J. (2010). Actual reality: A new functional assessment in persons with multiple sclerosis. *Archives of Physical Medicine and Rehabilitation, 91*, 252–260.

Green, G. (2001). Behavior analytic instruction for learners with autism: Advances in stimulus control technology. *Focus on Autism and Other Developmental Disabilities, 16*, 72–85.

Griffen, J. A., Rapport, L. J., Bryer, R. C., Bieliauskas, L. A., & Burt, C. (2011). Awareness of deficits and on-road driving performance. *Clinical Neuropsychologist, 25*, 1158–1178.

Grigorenko, E. L., & Sternberg, R. J. (1998). Dynamic testing. *Psychological Bulletin, 124*, 75–111.

Gronwall, D. M. A. (1977). Paced Auditory Serial Addition Task: A measure of recovery from concussion. *Perceptual and Motor Skills, 44*, 367–373.

Haaland, K. Y. (1993, March). *Assessment of limb apraxia.* Paper presented at the AOTA Neuroscience Institute Treating Adults with Apraxia, Baltimore, MD.

Hahn-Markowitz, J., Manor, I., & Maeir, A. (2011). Effectiveness of cognitive-functional (cog-fun) intervention with children with attention deficit hyperactivity disorder: A pilot study. *American Journal of Occupational Therapy, 65*, 384–392.

Hallgren, M., & Kottorp, A. (2005). Effects of occupational therapy intervention on activities of daily living and awareness of disability in persons with intellectual disabilities. *Australian Occupational Therapy Journal, 52*, 350–359.

Hamera, E., & Brown, C. E. (2000). Developing a context-based performance measure for persons with schizophrenia: The test of grocery shopping skills. *American Journal of Occupational Therapy, 54*, 20–25.

Harrison, M. J., Morris, K. A., Horton, R., Toglia, J., Barsky, J., Chait, S., & Robbins, L. (2005). Results of an intervention for lupus patients with self-perceived cognitive difficulties. *Neurology, 65*, 1325–1327.

Hartman-Maeir, A., Harel, H., & Katz, N. (2009). Kettle Test: A brief measure of cognitive functional performance. Reliability and validity in stroke rehabilitation. *American Journal of Occupational Therapy, 63*, 592–599.

Hartman-Maeir, A., Katz, N., Baum, C. M. (2009). Cognitive Functional Evaluation (CFE) process for individuals with suspected cognitive disabilities. *Occupational Therapy in Health Care, 23*, 1–23.

Hartman-Maeir, A., Soroker, N., Oman, S. D., & Katz, N. (2003). Awareness of disabilities in stroke rehabilitation: A clinical trial. *Disability and Rehabilitation, 25*, 35–44.

Heilman, K. M., & Rothi, L. J. (2003). Apraxia. In K. M. Heilman & E. Valenstein (Eds.), *Clinical neuropsychology* (4th ed., pp. 215–245). New York, NY: Oxford University Press.

Heilman, K. M., Watson, R. T., & Valenstein, E. (2003). Neglect and related disorders. In K. M. Heilman & E. Valenstein (Eds.), *Clinical neuropsychology* (4th ed., pp. 296–346). New York, NY: Oxford University Press.

Helm-Estabrooks, N. (1982). Visual action therapy for global aphasics. *Journal of Speech and Hearing Disorders, 47*, 385–389.

Helm-Estabrooks, N. (1992). *Test of Oral and Limb Apraxia (TOLA).* Chicago, IL: Riverside.

Helm-Estabrooks, N., & Hotz, G. (1991). *Brief Test of Head Injury (BTHI).* Chicago, IL: Riverside.

Henshaw, E., Polatajko, H., McEwen, S., Ryan, J. D., & Baum, C. M. (2011). Cognitive approach to improving participation after stroke: Two case studies. *American Journal of Occupational Therapy, 65*, 55–63.

Holm, M. B., & Rogers, J. C. (1999). Performance Assessment of Self-Care Skills. In B. J. Hemphill-Pearson (Ed.), *Assessments in Occupational Therapy Mental Health: An integrative approach* (pp. 117–124). Thorofare, NJ: SLACK Incorporated.

Holt, D. V., Rodewald, K., Rentrop, M., Funke, J., Weisbrod, M., & Kaiser, S. (2011). The plan-a-day approach to measuring planning ability in patients with schizophrenia. *Journal of the International Neuropsychological Society, 17*, 327–335.

Hoofien, D., Gilboa, A., Vakil, E., & Barak, O. (2004). Unawareness of cognitive deficits and daily functioning among persons with traumatic brain injuries. *Journal of Clinical and Experimental Neuropsychology, 26*, 278–290.

Huckans, M., Pavawalla, S., Demadura, T., Kolessar, M., Seelye, A., Roost, . . . Storzbach, D. (2010). A pilot study examining effects of group-based Cognitive Strategy Training treatment on self-reported cognitive problems, psychiatric symptoms, functioning, and compensatory strategy use in OIF/OEF combat veterans with persistent mild cognitive disorder and history of traumatic brain injury. *Journal of Rehabilitation Research and Development, 47*, 43–60.

Ianes, P., Varalta, V., Gandolfi, M., Picelli, A., Corno, M., Di Matteo, A., . . . Smania N. (2012). Stimulating visual exploration of the neglected space in the early stage of stroke by hemifield eye-patching: A randomized controlled trial in patients with right brain damage. *European Journal of Physical and Rehabilitation Medicine, 48*, 189–196.

Jackson, W. T., Novack, T. A., & Dowler, R. N. (1998). Effective serial measurement of cognitive orientation in rehabilitation: The orientation log. *Archives of Physical Medicine and Rehabilitation, 79*, 718–720.

Johansson, B., & Tornmalm, M. (2012). Working memory training for patients with acquired brain injury: Effects in daily life. *Scandinavian Journal of Occupational Therapy, 19*, 176–183. doi:10.3109/11038128.2011.603352

Johnston, M. V., Goverover, Y., & Dijkers, M. (2005). Community activities and individuals' satisfaction about them: Quality of life in the first year after traumatic brain injury. *Archives of Physical Medicine & Rehabilitation, 86*, 735–745.

Josman, N. (2011). The dynamic interactional model in schizophrenia. In N. Katz, (Ed.), *Cognition, occupation, and participation across the life span: Neuroscience, neurorehabilitation, and models of intervention in occupational therapy* (3rd ed., pp. 203–222). Bethesda, MD: AOTA.

Josman, N., Goffer, A., & Rosenblum, S. (2010). Development and standardization of a "Do–Eat" activity of daily living performance test for children. *American Journal of Occupational Therapy, 64*, 47–58.

Josman, N., & Rosenblum, S. (2011). A metacognitive model for children with atypical brain development. In N. Katz, (Ed.) *Cognition, occupation, and participation across the life span: Neuroscience, neurorehabilitation, and models of intervention in occupational therapy* (3rd ed., pp. 223–248). Bethesda, MD: AOTA.

Kamada, K., Shimodozono, M., Hamada, H., & Kawahira, K. (2011). Effects of 5 minutes of neck-muscle vibration immediately before occupational therapy on unilateral spatial neglect. *Disability and Rehabilitation, 33*, 2322–2328.

Katz, N. (2006). *Routine Task Inventory—Expanded (RTI-E) manual, prepared and elaborated on the basis of Allen, C. K. (1989 unpublished).* Unpublished manuscript. Retrieved from http://www.allen_cognitive_network.org

Katz, N., Baum, C. M., & Maeir, A. (2011). Introduction to cognitive intervention and cognitive functional evaluation. In N. Katz, (Ed.), *Cognition, occupation, and participation across the life span: Neuroscience, neurorehabilitation, and models of intervention in occupational therapy* (3rd ed., pp. 3–12). Bethesda, MD: AOTA.

Katz, N., & Hartman-Maeir, A. (2005). Higher-level cognitive functions: Awareness and executive functions enabling engagement in occupation. In N. Katz (Ed.), *Cognition and occupation across the life span* (2nd ed., pp. 3–25). Bethesda, MD: AOTA.

Katz, N., Hartman-Maeir, A., Ring, H., & Soroker, N. (1999). Functional disability and rehabilitation outcome in right hemisphere damaged patients with and without unilateral spatial neglect. *Archives of Physical Medicine & Rehabilitation, 80*, 379–384.

Katz, N., Itzkovich, M., Averbuch, S., & Elazar, B. (1990). *Lowenstein Occupational Therapy Cognitive Assessment (LOTCA) manual.* Pequannock, NJ: Maddak.

Katz, N., & Keren, N. (2011). Effectiveness of occupational goal intervention for clients with schizophrenia. *American Journal of Occupational Therapy, 65*, 287–296.

Katz, N., Livni, L., Bar-Haim Erez, A., & Averbuch, S. (2011). *Dynamic Loewenstein Occupational Therapy Cognitive Assessment (DLOTCA).* Pequannock, NJ: Maddak.

Katz, N., Parush, S., & Traub Bar-Ilan, R. (2005). *Dynamic Occupational Therapy Cognitive Assessment for Children (DOTCA-Ch).* Pequannock NJ: Maddak.

Katz, N., Ring, H., Naveh, Y., Kizony, R., Feintuch, U., & Weiss, P. L. (2005). Interactive virtual environment training for safe street crossing of right hemisphere stroke patients with unilateral spatial neglect. *Disability and Rehabilitation, 27*, 1235–1243.

Kelly, M., & Ostreicher, H. (1985). Environmental factors and outcomes in hemineglect syndromes. *Rehabilitation Psychology, 30*, 35–37.

Kiernan, R. J., Mueller, J., & Langston, J. W. (2011). *Cognistat and Cognistat assessment system manual.* Fairfax, CA: Cognistat.

Kim, H. J., Burke, D. T., Dowds, M. M., Boone, K. A. R., & Parks, G. J. (2000). Electronic memory aids for outpatient brain injury: Follow-up findings. *Brain Injury, 14*, 187–196.

Kirby, A. (2011). Dyspraxia series: Part one. At sixes and sevens. *The Journal of Family Health Care, 21*(4), 29–31.

Kline, N. K. (2000). Validity of the modified Dynamic Visual Processing Assessment. *The Israel Journal of Occupational Therapy, 9*, 69–88.

Klingberg, T. (2010). Training and plasticity of working memory. *Trends in Cognitive Sciences, 14*, 317–324.

Kottorp, A., Hallgren, M., Bernspang, B., & Fisher, A. G. (2003). Client-centered occupational therapy for persons with mental retardation: Implementation of an intervention programme in activities of daily living tasks. *Scandinavian Journal of Occupational Therapy, 10*, 51–60.

Kramer, J. H., Kaplan, E., & Blusewicz, M. J. (1991). Visual hierarchical analysis of block design configural errors. *Journal of Clinical and Experimental Neuropsychology, 13*, 455–465.

Laeng, B. (2006). Constructional apraxia after left or right unilateral stroke. *Neuropsychologia, 44*, 1595–1606.

Law, M., Baptiste, S., Carswell, A., McColl, M. A., Polatajko, H., & Pollock, N. (2005). *Canadian Occupational Performance Measure* (3rd ed., Rev. ed.). Toronto, ON: CAOT.

Leavitt, V. M., Lengenfelder, J., Moore, N. B., Chiaravalloti, N. D., & DeLuca, J. (2011). The relative contributions of processing speed and cognitive load to working memory accuracy in multiple sclerosis. *Journal of Clinical and Experimental Neuropsychology, 33*, 580–586.

Lennon, S. (1994). Task specific effects in the rehabilitation of unilateral neglect. In M. J. Riddoch & G. W. Humphreys (Eds.), *Cognitive neuropsychology and cognitive rehabilitation* (pp. 187–203). East Sussex, United Kingdom: Lawrence Erlbaum Associates.

Levin, H. S., O'Donnell, V. M., & Grossman, R. G. (1979). The Galveston Orientation and Amnesia Test: A practical scale to assess cognition after head injury. *The Journal of Nervous and Mental Diseases, 167*, 675–684.

Levine, B., Robertson, I. H., Clare, L., Carter, G., Hong, J., Wilson, B. A., . . . Stuss, D. T. (2000). Rehabilitation of executive functioning: An experimental–clinical validation of goal management training. *Journal of the International Neuropsychological Society, 6*(3), 299–312.

Levine, B., Stuss, D. T., Winocur, G., Binns, M. A., Fahy, L., Mandic, M., . . . Robertson, I. H. (2007). Cognitive rehabilitation in the elderly: Effects on strategic behavior in relation to goal management. *Journal of the International Neuropsychological Society, 13*, 143–152.

Levy, L. L. (2011a). Cognitive aging. In N. Katz (Ed.), *Cognition, occupation, and participation across the life span: Neuroscience, neurorehabilitation, and models of intervention in occupational therapy* (3rd ed., pp. 93–116). Bethesda, MD: AOTA.

Levy, L. L. (2011b). Cognitive information processing. In N. Katz (Ed.), *Cognition, occupation, and participation across the life span: Neuroscience, neurorehabilitation, and models of intervention in occupational therapy* (3rd ed., pp. 117–142). Bethesda, MD: AOTA.

Levy, L. L., & Burns, T. (2011). The cognitive disabilities reconsidered model: Rehabilitation of adults with dementia. In N. Katz (Ed.), *Cognition, occupation, and participation across the life span: Neuroscience, neurorehabilitation, and models of intervention in occupational therapy* (3rd ed., pp. 407–442). Bethesda, MD: AOTA.

Lezak, M. D., Howieson, D. B., & Loring, D. W. (2004). *Neuropsychological assessment* (4th ed.). New York, NY: Oxford University Press.

Liddell, A., & Rasmussen, C. (2005). Memory profile of children with nonverbal learning disability. *Learning Disabilities Research and Practice, 20*, 137–141.

Liu, K. P. Y., Chan, C. C. H., Lee, T. M. C., Li, L. S. W., & Hui-Chan, C. W. Y. (2002). Self-regulatory learning and generalization for people with brain injury. *Brain Injury, 16*, 817–824.

Loeb, P. A. (1996). *Independent Living Scales.* San Antonio, TX: Psychological Corporation.

LoPresti, E. F., Mihailidis, A., & Kirsch, N. (2004). Assistive technology for cognitive rehabilitation: State of the art. *Neuropsychological Rehabilitation, 14*, 5–39.

Lucas, S. E., & Fleming, J. M. (2005). Interventions for improving self-awareness following acquired brain injury. *Australian Occupational Therapy Journal, 52*, 160–170.

Luton, L. M., Reed-Knight, B., Loiselle, K., O'Toole, K., & Blount, R. (2011). A pilot study evaluating an abbreviated version of the cognitive remediation programme for youth with neurocognitive deficits. *Brain Injury, 25*, 409–415.

Mackin, R. S., Ayalon, L., Feliciano, L., & Areán, P. A. (2010). The sensitivity and specificity of cognitive screening instruments to detect cognitive impairment in older adults with severe psychiatric illness. *Journal of Geriatric Psychiatry and Neurology, 23*, 94–99.

Maeir, A., Krauss, S., & Katz, N. (2011). Ecological validity of the Multiple Errands Test (MET) on discharge from neurorehabilitation hospital. *OTJR: Occupation, Participation and Health, 31*(Suppl), S38–S46.

Maher, L., Rothi, L., & Greenwald, M. (1991). Treatment of gesture impairment: A single case. *American Speech and Hearing Association, 33*, 195.

Malec, J. F., & Lezak, M. D. (2008). *Manual for the Mayo-Portland Adaptability Inventory (MPAI-4) for adults, children and adolescents.* Retrieved from http://www.tbims.org/combi/mpai/manual.pdf

Malec, J. F., Smigielski, J. S., & DePompolo, R. W. (1991). Goal attainment scaling and outcome measurement in postacute brain injury rehabilitation. *Archives of Physical Medicine and Rehabilitation, 72*, 138–143.

Man, D. W., Fleming, J., Hohaus, L., & Shum, D. (2011). Development of the Brief Assessment of Prospective Memory (BAPM) for use with traumatic brain injury populations. *Neuropsychological Rehabilitation, 21*, 884–898.

Mandich, A., Polatajko, H. J., Miller, L., & Baum, C. (2004). *The Paediatric Activity Card Sort (PACS).* Ottawa, ON: Canadian Association of Occupational Therapists.

Mandich, A. D., Polatajko, H., & Zilberbrant, A. (2008). A cognitive perspective on intervention. In A. C. Eliasson & P. Burtner (Eds.), *Improving hand function in children with cerebral palsy: Theory, evidence and intervention.* London, United Kingdom: Mac Keith Press.

Manly, T., Hawkins, K., Evans, J., Wodlt, K., & Robertson, I. H. (2002). Rehabilitation of executive function: Facilitation of effective goal management on complex tasks using periodic auditory alerts. *Neuropsychologia, 40*, 271–281.

Mausbach, B. T., Harvey, P. D., Goldman, S. R., Jeste, D. V., & Patterson, T. L. (2007). Development of a brief scale of everyday functioning in persons with serious mental illness. *Schizophrenia Bulletin, 33*, 1364–1372.

May-Benson, T. A., & Cermak, S. A. (2007). Development of an assessment for ideational praxis. *American Journal of Occupational Therapy, 61*, 148–153.

McCarthy, M., Beaumont, J. G., Thompson, R., & Pringle, H. (2002). The role of imagery in the rehabilitation of neglect in severely disabled brain-injured adults. *Archives of Clinical Neuropsychology, 17*, 407–422.

McDowd, J. M., Filion, D. L., Pohl, P. S., Richards, L. G., & Stiers, W. (2003). Attentional abilities and functional outcomes following stroke. *Journal of Gerontology, Series B, Psychological Sciences and Social Sciences, 58*, 45–53.

McKerracher, G., Powell, T., & Oyebode, J. (2005). A single case experimental design comparing two memory notebook formats for a man with memory problems caused by traumatic brain injury. *Neuropsychological Rehabilitation, 15*, 115–128.

Mesulam, M. M. (2000). Attentional networks, confusional states and neglect syndromes. In: M. Mesulam (Ed.), *Principles of behavioral neurology* (2nd ed., pp. 174–256). New York, NY: Oxford University Press.

Miller, L. T., Polatajko, H. J., Missiuna, C., Mandich, A. D., & Macnab, J. J. (2001). A pilot trial of a cognitive treatment for children with developmental coordination disorder. *Human Movement Science, 20*, 183–210.

Missiuna, C. (Ed). (2001). *Children with developmental coordination disorder: Strategies for success.* Binghamton, NY: Haworth Press.

Moulton, H. J., Taira, E. D., & Grover, R. (1995, November). *Utilizing occupational therapy and families at mealtimes with nursing home residents with dementia.* Paper presented at Gerontological Society on Aging Annual Conference, Los Angeles, CA.

Nasreddine, Z. S., Phillips, N. A., Bédirian, V., Charbonneau, S., Whitehead, V., Collin, I., . . . Chertkow, H. (2005). The Montreal Cognitive Assessment, MoCA: A brief screening tool for mild cognitive impairment. *Journal of the American Geriatrics Society, 53*, 695–699.

Neistadt, M. E. (1990). A critical analysis of occupational therapy approaches for perceptual deficits in adults with brain injury. *American Journal of Occupational Therapy, 44*, 299–304.

Neistadt, M. E. (1992a). Occupational therapy treatments for constructional deficits. *American Journal of Occupational Therapy, 46*, 141–148.

Neistadt, M. E. (1992b). The Rabideau Kitchen Evaluation–Revised: An assessment of meal preparation skill. *The Occupational Therapy Journal of Research, 12*, 242–255.

Nelson, A., Fogel, B. S., & Faust, D. (1986). Bedside cognitive screening instruments: A critical assessment. *Journal of Nervous and Mental Disease, 174*, 73–83.

Niemeier, J. P. (1998). The lighthouse strategy: Use of a visual imagery technique to treat visual inattention in stroke patients. *Brain Injury, 12*, 399–406.

Niemeier, J. P., Cifu, D. X., & Kishore, R. (2001). The lighthouse strategy: Improving the functional status of patients with unilateral neglect after stroke and brain injury using a visual imagery intervention. *Topics in Stroke Rehabilitation, 8*(2), 10–18.

Noe, E., Ferri, J., Caballero, M. C., Villodre, R., Sanchez, A., & Chirivella, J. (2005). Self-awareness after acquired brain injury: Predictors and rehabilitation. *Journal of Neurology, 252*, 168–175.

Nott, M. T., & Chapparo, C. (2008). Measuring information processing in a client with extreme agitation following traumatic brain injury using the perceive, recall, plan and perform system of task analysis. *Australian Occupational Therapy Journal, 55*, 188–198.

Nott, M. T., Chapparo, C., & Heard, R. (2009). Reliability of the perceive, recall, plan and perform system of task analysis: A criterion-referenced assessment. *Australian Occupational Therapy Journal, 56*, 307–14.

Ownsworth, T., Fleming, J., Desbois, J., Strong, J., & Kuipers, P. (2006). A metacognitive contextual intervention to enhance error awareness and functional outcome following traumatic brain injury: A single-case experimental design. *Journal of the International Neuropsychological Society, 12*, 54–63.

Ownsworth, T., Quinn, H., Fleming, J., Kendall, M., & Shum, D. (2010). Error self-regulation following traumatic brain injury: A single case study evaluation of metacognitive skills training and behavioural practice interventions. *Neuropsychological Rehabilitation, 20*, 59–80.

Page, M., Wilson, B. A., Sheil, A. Carter, G., & Norris, D. (2006). What is the locus of the errorless learning advantage? *Neuropsychologia, 44*, 90–100.

Paolucci, S., Antonucci, G., Grasso, M. G., & Pizzamiglio, L. (2001). The role of unilateral spatial neglect in rehabilitation of right brain-damaged ischemic stroke patients: A matched comparison. *Archives of Physical Medicine and Rehabilitation, 82*, 743–749.

Phelan, S., Steinke, L., & Mandich, A. (2009). Exploring a cognitive intervention for children with pervasive developmental disorder. *Canadian Journal of Occupational Therapy, 76*, 23–28.

Pierce, S. R., & Buxbaum, L. J. (2002). Treatments of unilateral neglect: A review. *Archives of Physical Medicine and Rehabilitation, 83*, 256–268.

Pilgrim, E., & Humphreys, G. W. (1994). Rehabilitation of a case of ideomotor apraxia. In M. J. Riddoch & G. W. Humphreys (Eds.), *Cognitive neuropsychology and cognitive rehabilitation* (pp. 271–315). East Sussex, United Kingdom: Lawrence Erlbaum Associates.

Pizzamiglio, L., Antonucci, G., Judica, A., Montenero, P., Razzano, C., & Zoccolotti, P. (1992). Cognitive rehabilitation of the hemineglect disorder in chronic patients with unilateral right brain damage. *Journal of Clinical Experimental Neuropsychology, 14*, 901–923.

Plummer, P., Morris, M., & Dunai, J. (2003). Assessment of unilateral neglect. *Physical Therapy, 83*, 732–740.

Polatajko, H. J., Mandich, A., & McEwen, S. E. (2011). Cognitive orientation to daily occupational performance (CO-OP): A cognitive-based intervention for children and adults. In N. Katz (Ed.), *Cognition, occupation, and participation across the life span: Neuroscience, neurorehabilitation, and models of intervention in occupational therapy* (3rd ed., pp. 299–322). Bethesda, MD: AOTA.

Polatajko, H. J., Mandich, A. D., Miller, L. T., & Macnab, J. J. (2001). Cognitive orientation to daily occupational performance (CO-OP): part II—the evidence. *Physical & Occupational Therapy in Pediatrics, 20*, 83–106.

Poole, J. L. (1998). Effect of apraxia on the ability to learn on-handed shoe tying. *Occupational Therapy Journal of Research, 18*, 99–104.

Poole, J. L. (2000). A comparison of limb praxis abilities of persons with developmental dyspraxia and adult onset apraxia. *Occupational Therapy Journal of Research, 20*, 106–120.

Prigatano, G. P. (1986). *Neuropsychological rehabilitation after brain injury.* Baltimore, MD: Johns Hopkins University Press.

Prigatano, G. P. (1999). *Principles of neuropsychological rehabilitation.* New York, NY: Oxford University Press.

Randolph, C. (1998). *Repeatable Battery for the Assessment of Neuropsychological Status (RBANS).* San Antonio, TX: Psychological Corporation.

Raskin, S., & Buckheit, C. (2010). *Memory for Intentions Test (MIST)*. Lutz, FL: Psychological Assessment Resources.

Rath, J. F., Simon, D., Langenbahn, D. M., Sherr, R. L., & Diller, L. (2003). Group treatment of problem solving deficits in outpatients with traumatic brain injury: A randomized outcome study. *Neuropsychological Rehabilitation, 13*, 461–488.

Redding, G. M., & Wallace, B. (2006). Prism adaptation and unilateral neglect: Review and analysis. *Neuropsychologia, 44*, 1–20.

Reeder, C., Newton, E., Frangou, S., & Wykes, T. (2004). Which executive skills should we target to affect social functioning and symptom change?: A study of cognitive remediation therapy program. *Schizophrenia Bulletin, 30*, 87–100.

Rempfer, M. V., Hamera, E. K., Brown, C. E., & Cromwell, R. L. (2003). The relations between cognition and the independent living skill of shopping in people with schizophrenia. *Psychiatry Research, 117*, 103–112.

Revheim, N., & Marcopulos, B. A. (2006). Group treatment approaches to address cognitive deficits. *Psychiatric Rehabilitation Journal, 30*, 38–45.

Reynolds, C. R. (2002) *Comprehensive Trail-Making Test (CTMT)*. Austin, TX: PRO-ED.

Robertson, I. H., & Halligan, P. W. (1999). *Spatial neglect: A clinical handbook for diagnosis and treatment*. East Sussex, United Kingdom: Psychology Press.

Robertson, I. H., Hogg, K., & McMillan, T. M. (1998). Rehabilitation of unilateral neglect: Improving function by contralesional limb activation. *Neuropsychological Rehabilitation, 8*, 19–29.

Robertson, I. H., Tegner, R., Tham, K., Lo, A., & Smith, N. I. (1995). Sustained attention training for unilateral neglect: Theoretical and rehabilitation implications. *Journal of Clinical Neuropsychology, 17*, 416–430.

Robertson, I. H., Ward, T., Ridgeway, V., & Nimmo-Smith, I. (1994). *The Test of Everyday Attention (TEA)*. Bury St. Edmunds, United Kingdom: Thames Valley Test Company.

Robnett, R. H., Hopkins, V., Kimball, J. G. (2003). The Safe at Home: A quick home safety assessment. *Physical Occupational Therapy in Geriatrics, 20*, 77–101.

Rocke, K., Hays, P., Edwards, D., & Berg, C. (2008). Development of a performance assessment of executive function: The Children's Kitchen Task Assessment. *American Journal of Occupational Therapy, 62*, 528–537.

Rockwood, K., Joyce, B., & Stolee, P. (1997). Use of goal attainment scaling in measuring clinically important change in cognitive rehabilitation patients. *Journal of Clinical Epidemiology, 50*, 581–588.

Rodger, S., & Vishram, A. (2010). Mastering social and organization goals: Strategy use by two children with Asperger's syndrome during cognitive orientation to daily occupational performance. *Physical & Occupational Therapy in Pediatrics, 30*, 264–276.

Roth, R. M., Isquith, P. K., & Gioia, G. A. (2005). *Behavior Rating Inventory of Executive Function—adult version*. Lutz, FL: Psychological Assessment Resources.

Roy, E. A. (1978). Apraxia: A new look at an old syndrome. *Journal of Human Movement Studies, 4*, 191–210.

Roy, E. A. (1985). *Neuropsychological studies of apraxia and related disorders*. Amsterdam, The Netherlands: Elsevier Science.

Rustad, R. A., DeGroot, T. L., Jungkunz, M. L., Freeberg, K. S., Borowick, L. G., & Wanttie, A. M. (1993). *The cognitive assessment of Minnesota*. Tucson, AZ: Therapy Skill Builders.

Ryan, J. D., Polatajko, H. J., McEwen, S., Peressotti, M., Young, A., Rummel, K., . . . Baum, C. M. (2011). Analysis of Cognitive Environmental Support (ACES): Preliminary testing. *Neuropsychological Rehabilitation, 21*, 401–427.

Sarajuuri, J. M., Kaipio, M. L., Koskinen, S. K., Neimela, M. R., Servo, A. R., & Vilkki, J. (2005). Outcome of a comprehensive neurorehabilitation program for persons with traumatic brain injury. *Archives of Physical Medicine and Rehabilitation, 86*, 2296–2302.

Schmidt, J., Lannin, N., Fleming, J., & Ownsworth, T. (2011). Feedback interventions for impaired self-awareness following brain injury: A systematic review. *Journal of Rehabilitation Medicine, 43*, 673–680.

Schmitter-Edgecombe, M., Howard, J. T., Pavawalla, S. P., Howell, L., & Rueda, A. (2008). Multidyad memory notebook intervention for very mild dementia: A pilot study. *American Journal of Alzheimer's Disease and Other Dementias, 23*, 477–487.

Schwartz, M. F., Segal, M., Veramonti, T., Ferraro, M., & Buxbaum, L. J. (2002). The Naturalistic Action Test: A standardised assessment for everyday action impairment. *Neuropsychological Rehabilitation, 12*, 311–339.

Schwartz, M. S. (1995). Adults with traumatic brain injury: Three case studies of cognitive rehabilitation in the home setting. *American Journal of Occupational Therapy, 49*, 655–668.

Schwartzberg, S. (1999). Use of groups in rehabilitation of persons with head injury: Reasoning skills used by the group facilitator. In C. Unsworth (Ed.), *Cognitive and perceptual dysfunction* (pp. 455–471). Philadelphia, PA: F. A. Davis.

Seron, X., Deloche, G., & Coyette, F. (1989). A retrospective analysis of a single case of neglect therapy: A point of theory. In X. Seron & G. Deloche (Eds.), *Cognitive approaches in neuropsychological rehabilitation*. Hillsdale, NJ: Lawrence Erlbaum Associates.

Shallice, T., & Burgess, P. (1991). Deficits in strategy application following frontal lobe damage in man. *Brain, 114*, 727–741.

Sherer, M., Bergloff, P., Boake, C., High, W., & Levin, E. (1998). The Awareness Questionnaire: Factor structure and internal consistency. *Brain Injury, 12*, 63–68.

Sherer, M., Oden, K., Bergloff, P., Levin, E., & High, W. M. (1998). Assessment and treatment of impaired awareness after brain injury: Implications for community re-integration. *NeuroRehabilitation, 10*, 25–37.

Shevil, E., & Finlayson, M. (2010). Pilot study of a cognitive intervention program for persons with multiple sclerosis. *Health Education Research, 25*, 41–53.

Shiel, A., Wilson, B. A., Emslie, H., Foley, J., Evans, J. J., Hawkins, K., . . . Groot, Y. (2005). *Cambridge Prospective Memory Test*. San Antonio, TX: Pearson.

Shiraishi, H., Muraki, T., Ayaka Itou, Y. S., & Hirayama, K. (2010). Prism intervention helped sustainability of effects and ADL performances in chronic hemispatial neglect: A follow-up study. *Neurorehabilitation, 27*, 165–172.

Silverstein, S. M., Hatashita-Wong, M., Solak, B. A., Uhlhaas, P., Landa, Y., Wilkniss, S. M., . . . Smith, T. E. (2005). Effectiveness of a two-phase cognitive rehabilitation intervention for severely impaired schizophrenia patients. *Psychological Medicine, 35*, 829–837.

Smania, N., Aglioti, S. M., Girardi, F., Tinazzi, M., Fiaschi, A., Cosentino, A., & Corato, E. (2006). Rehabilitation of limb apraxia improves daily life activities in patients with stroke. *Neurology, 67*, 2050–2052.

Smania, N., Bazoli, F., Piva, D., & Guidetti, G. (1997). Visuomotor imagery and rehabilitation of neglect. *Archives of Physical Medicine and Rehabilitation, 78*, 430–436.

Smania, N., Girardi, F., Domenicali, C., Lora, E., & Aglioti, S. (2000). The rehabilitation of limb apraxia: A study in left-brain-damaged patients. *Archives of Physical Medicine and Rehabilitation, 81*, 379–388.

Sohlberg, M. M., & Mateer, C. A. (1989a). *Attention process training*. San Antonio, TX: Psychological Corporation.

Sohlberg, M. M., & Mateer, C. A. (1989b). *Introduction to cognitive rehabilitation: Theory and practice*. New York, NY: Guilford Press.

Sohlberg, M. M., & Mateer, C. A. (2001). *Cognitive rehabilitation: An integrative neuropsychological approach*. New York, NY: Guilford Press.

Steultjens, E. M., Voigt-Radloff, S., Leonhart, R., & Graff, M. J. (2011). Reliability of the Perceive, Recall, Plan, and Perform (PRPP) assessment in community-dwelling dementia patients: Test consistency and inter-rater agreement. *International Psychogeriatrics, 14*, 1–7.

Stuss, D. T., Robertson, I. H., Craik, F. I., Levine, B., Alexander, M. P., Black, S., . . . Winocur, G. (2007). Cognitive rehabilitation in the elderly: A randomized trial to evaluate a new protocol. *Journal of the International Neuropsychological Society, 13*, 120–131.

Sunderland, A., Harris, J. E., & Baddeley, A. D. (1983). Do laboratory tests predict everyday memory? A neuropsychological study. *Journal of Verbal Learning and Verbal Behavior, 22*, 727–738.

Sunderland, A., Walker, C. M., & Walker, M. F. (2006). Action errors and dressing disability after stroke: An ecological approach to neuropsychological assessment and intervention. *Neuropsychological Rehabilitation, 16*, 666–683.

Swirsky-Sacchetti, T., Field, H. L., Mitchell, D. R., Seward, J., Lublin, F. D., Knobler, R. L., & Gonzalez, C. F. (1992). The sensitivity of the Mini-Mental State Exam in the white matter dementia of multiple sclerosis. *Journal of Clinical Psychology, 48*, 779–786.

Tariq, S. H., Tumosa, N., Chibnall, J. T., Perry, H. M., & Morley, J. E. (2006). The Saint Louis University Mental Status (SLUMS) examination for detecting mild cognitive impairment and dementia is more sensitive than the mini-mental status examination (MMSE)—a pilot study. *American Journal of Geriatric Psychology, 14*, 900–910.

Tempest, S., & Roden, P. (2008). Exploring evidence-based practice by occupational therapists when working with people with apraxia. *British Journal of Occupational Therapy, 71*, 33–37.

Teng, E., & Chui, H. (1987). The Modified Mini-Mental State (3MS) Examination. *Journal of Clinical Psychiatry, 48*, 314–318.

Tham, K., Bernspang, B., & Fisher, A. G. (1999). Development of the Assessment of Awareness of Disability. *Scandinavian Journal of Occupational Therapy, 6*, 184–190.

Tham, K., Ginsburg, E., Fisher, A., & Tegner, R. (2001). Training to improve awareness of disabilities in clients with unilateral neglect. *American Journal of Occupational Therapy, 55*, 46–54.

Tham, K., & Tegner, R. (1996). The baking tray task: A test of spatial neglect. *Neuropsychological Rehabilitation, 6*, 19–25.

Tham, K., & Tegner, R. (1997). Video feedback in the rehabilitation of patients with unilateral neglect. *Archives of Physical Medicine and Rehabilitation, 78*, 410–413.

Thöne-Otto, A. J., & Schulze, H. (2003). *MEMOS: Mobile Extensible Memory and Orientation System.* Retrieved from http://www.memosonline.de/contact_en.html

Tiersky, L. A., Anselmi, V., Johnston, M. V., Kurtyka, J., Roosen, E., Schwartz, T., & Deluca, J. (2005). A trial of neuropsychologic rehabilitation in mild-spectrum traumatic brain injury. *Archives of Physical Medicine and Rehabilitation, 86*, 1565–1574.

Tiznado, D., Mausbach, B. T., Cardenas, V., Jeste, D. V., & Patterson, T. L. (2010). UCSD SORT test (U-SORT): Examination of a newly developed organizational skills assessment tool for severely mentally ill adults. *The Journal of Nervous and Mental Disease, 198*, 916–919.

Toglia, J. P. (1989). Visual perception of objects: An approach to assessment and intervention. *American Journal of Occupational Therapy, 43*, 587–595.

Toglia, J. P. (1991a). Generalization of treatment: A multicontextual approach to cognitive perceptual impairment in the brain injured adult. *American Journal of Occupational Therapy, 45*, 505–516.

Toglia, J. P. (1991b). Unilateral visual inattention: Multidimensional components. *Occupational Therapy Practice, 3*, 18–34.

Toglia, J. P. (1993a). Attention and memory. In C. B. Royeen (Ed.), *AOTA self-study series: Cognitive rehabilitation* (pp. 4–72). Rockville, MD: AOTA.

Toglia, J. P. (1993b). *The Contextual Memory Test.* Tucson, AZ: Therapy Skill Builders.

Toglia, J. P. (1994). *Toglia Category Assessment (TCA).* Pequannock, NJ: Maddak.

Toglia, J. P. (2011). A dynamic interactional model of cognition in cognitive rehabilitation. In N. Katz (Ed.), *Cognition, occupation, and participation across the life span: Neuroscience, neurorehabilitation, and models of intervention in occupational therapy* (3rd ed., pp. 161–202). Bethesda, MD: AOTA.

Toglia, J. (in press). Examiner guidelines for the Weekly Calendar Planning Test.

Toglia, J. P., & Cermak, S. (2009). Dynamic assessment of unilateral neglect. *American Journal of Occupational Therapy, 64*, 569–579.

Toglia, J. P., & Finkelstein, N. (1991). *Manual for the Dynamic Visual Processing Assessment.* Unpublished manuscript.

Toglia, J. P., Fitzgerald, K. A., O'Dell, M. W., Mastrogiovanni, A. R., & Lin, C. D. (2011). The Mini-Mental State Examination and Montreal Cognitive Assessment in persons with mild subacute stroke: Relationship to functional outcome. *Archives of Physical Medicine and Rehabilitation, 92*, 792–798.

Toglia, J. P., & Golisz, K. M. (in press). Therapy for activities of daily living: Theoretical and practical perspectives. In N. D. Zasler, D. I. Katz, & R. D. Zafonte (Eds.), *Brain injury medicine* (2nd ed). New York, NY: Demos Medical.

Toglia, J. P., Goverover, Y., Johnston, M. V., & Dain, B. (2011). Application of the multicontextual approach in promoting learning and transfer of strategy use in an individual with TBI and executive dysfunction. *OTJR: Occupation, Participation and Health, 31*, S53–S60.

Toglia, J. P., Johnston, M. V., Goverover, Y., & Dain, B. (2010). A multicontext approach to promoting transfer of strategy use and self regulation after brain injury: An exploratory study. *Brain Injury, 24*, 664–677.

Toglia, J. P., & Kirk, U. (2000). Understanding awareness deficits following brain injury. *NeuroRehabilitation, 15*, 57–70.

Tsang, M. H. M., Sze, K. H., & Fong, K. N. K. (2009). Occupational therapy treatment with right half-field eye patching for patients with subacute stroke and unilateral neglect: A randomized controlled trial. *Disability & Rehabilitation, 31*, 630–637.

Turton, A. J., O'Leary, K., Gabb, J., Woodward, R., & Gilchrist, I. D. (2010). A single blinded randomised controlled pilot trial of prism adaptation for improving self-care in stroke patients with neglect. *Neuropsychological Rehabilitation, 20*, 180–196.

Tzuriel, D. (2000). Dynamic assessment of young children: Educational and intervention perspectives. *Educational Psychology Review, 12*, 385–435.

Ucok, A., Cakir, S., Duman, Z. C., Discigil, A., Kandemir, P., & Atli, H. (2006). Cognitive predictors of skill acquisition on social problem solving in patients with schizophrenia. *European Archives of Psychiatry and Clinical Neuroscience, 256*, 388–394.

Unsworth, C. (Ed.). (1999). Introduction to cognitive and perceptual dysfunction: Theoretical approaches to therapy. In *Cognitive and perceptual dysfunction: A clinical reasoning approach to evaluation and intervention* (pp. 1–41). Philadelphia, PA: F. A. Davis.

Unsworth, C. (2007). Cognitive and perceptual dysfunction. In S. B. O'Sullivan & T. J. Schmitz (Eds.), *Physical rehabilitation* (5th ed., pp. 1151–1188). Philadelphia, PA: F. A. Davis.

Vallat, C., Azouvi, P., Hardisson, H., Meffert, R., Tessier, C., & Pradat-Diehl, P. (2005). Rehabilitation of verbal working memory after left hemisphere stroke. *Brain Injury, 19*, 1157–1164.

Vanbellingen, T., & Bohlhalter, S. (2011). Apraxia in neurorehabilitation: Classification, assessment and treatment. *NeuroRehabilitation, 28*, 91–98.

Vanbellingen, T., Kersten, B., Hemelrijk, B. V., Van de Winckel, A., Bertschi, M., Müri, R., . . . Bohlhalter, S. (2010). Comprehensive assessment of gesture production: A new Test of Upper Limb Apraxia (TULIA). *European Journal of Neurology, 17*, 59–66.

van Heugten, C. M., Dekker, J., Deelman, B. G., van Dijk, A. J., Stehmann-Saris, J. C., & Kinebanian, A. (1998). Outcome of strategy training in stroke patients with apraxia: A phase II study. *Clinical Rehabilitation, 12*, 294–303.

van Heugten, C. M., Dekker, J., Deelman, B. G., van Dijk, A. J., Stehmann-Saris, J. C., & Kinebanian, A. (2000). Measuring disabilities in stroke patients with apraxia: A validation study of an observational method. *Neuropsychological Rehabilitation, 10*, 401–414.

Velligan, D. I., Diamond, P., Glahn, D. C., Ritch, J., Maples, N., Castillo, D., & Miller, A. L. (2007). The reliability and validity of the Test of Adaptive Behavior in Schizophrenia (TABS). *Psychiatry Research, 151*, 55–66.

Velligan, D. I., Diamond, P., Mueller, J., Li, X., Maples, N., Wang, M., & Miller, A. L. (2009). The short-term impact of generic versus individualized environmental supports on functional outcomes and target behaviors in schizophrenia. *Psychiatry Research, 168*, 94–101.

Velligan, D. I., Mueller, J., Wang, M., Dicocco, M., Diamond, P. M., Maples, N. J., & Davis, B. (2006). Use of environmental supports among patients with schizophrenia. *Psychiatric Services, 57*, 219–224.

Verdoux, H., Monello, F., Goumilloux, R., Cougnard, A., & Prouteau, A. (2010). Self-perceived cognitive deficits and occupational outcome in persons with schizophrenia. *Psychiatry Research, 178*, 437–439.

Viken, J. I., Samuelsson, H., Jern, C., Jood, K., & Blomstrand, C. (2012). The prediction of functional dependency by lateralized and non-lateralized neglect in a large prospective stroke sample. *European Journal of Neurology, 19*, 128–134.

Voelbel, G. T., Goverover, Y., Gaudino, E. A., Moore, N. B., Chiaravalloti, N., & DeLuca, J. (2011). Assessment of impairment and activity of executive dysfunction in multiple sclerosis. *OTJR: Occupation, Participation and Health (special issue of Executive Functions), 31*, 30–37.

Wade, T. K., & Troy, J. C. (2001). Mobile phones as a new memory aid: A preliminary investigation using case studies. *Brain Injury, 15*, 305–320.

Wang, M. Y., Chang, C. Y., & Su, S. Y. (2011). What's cooking?—cognitive training of executive function in the elderly. *Frontiers in Psychology, 2*, 228.

Warren, M. (1981). Relationship of constructional apraxia and body scheme disorders to dressing performance in CVA. *American Journal of Occupational Therapy, 35*, 431–442.

Warren, M. (1993). Visuospatial skills: Assessment and intervention strategies. In C. B. Royeen (Ed.), *AOTA self-study series: Cognitive rehabilitation* (pp. 6–76). Rockville, MD: AOTA.

Warren, M. (1998). *The Brain Injury Visual Assessment Battery for Adults.* Lenexa, KS: visABILITIES Rehab Services.

Webster, J. S., McFarland, P. T., Rapport, L. J., Morrill, B., Roades, L. A., & Abadee, P. S. (2001). Computer-assisted training for improving wheelchair mobility in unilateral neglect patients. *Archives of Physical Medicine and Rehabilitation, 82*, 769–775.

Webster, J. S., Roades, L. A., Morrill, B., Rapport, L. J., Abadee, P. S., Sowa, M. V., . . . Godlewski, M. C. (1995). Rightward orienting bias, wheelchair maneuvering, and fall risk. *Archives of Physical Medicine and Rehabilitation*, 76, 924–928.

Weinberg, J., Diller, L., Gordon, W. A., Gerstman, L. J., Lieberman, A., Lakin, P., . . . Ezrachi, O. (1977). Visual scanning training effect on reading-related tasks in acquired right brain damage. *Archives of Physical Medicine and Rehabilitation, 58*, 479–486.

Welfringer, A., Leifert-Fiebach, G., Babinsky, R., & Brandt, T. (2011). Visuomotor imagery as a new tool in the rehabilitation of neglect: A randomised controlled study of feasibility and efficacy. *Disability and Rehabilitation, 33*, 2033–2043.

Wetter, S., Poole, J. L., & Haaland, K. Y. (2005). Functional implications of ipsilesional motor deficits after unilateral stroke. *Archives of Physical Medicine & Rehabilitation, 86*, 776–781.

Wilhelm, O.,Witthöft, M., & Schipolowski, S. (2010). Self-reported cognitive failures: Competing measurement models and self-report correlates. *Journal of Individual Differences, 31*, 1–14.

Willer, B., Ottenbacher, K. J., & Coad, M. L. (1994). The Community Integration Questionnaire. A comparative examination. *American Journal of Physical Medicine & Rehabilitation, 73*, 103–111.

Wilson, B. A., Alderman, N., Burgess, P., Emslie, H., & Evans, J. (1996). *Behavioural Assessment of the Dysexecutive Syndrome.* Bury St. Edmunds, United Kingdom: Thames Valley Test Company.

Wilson, B. A., Clare, L., Baddeley, A. Watson, P., & Tate, R. (1998). *The Rivermead Behavioral Memory Test–Extended version (RBMT-E).* Bury St. Edmunds, United Kingdom: Thames Valley Test Company.

Wilson, B. A., Cockburn, J., & Baddeley, A. (1987). *Behavioral Inattention Test (BIT).* Bury St. Edmunds, United Kingdom: Thames Valley Test Company.

Wilson, B. A., Emslie, H. C., Evans, J. J., Quirk, K., Watson, P., & Fish, J. (2009). The NeuroPage system for children and adolescents with neurological deficits. *Developmental Neurorehabilitation, 12*, 421–426.

Wilson, B. A., Emslie, H. C., Quirk, K., & Evans, J. J. (2001). Reducing everyday memory and planning problems by means of a paging system: A randomised control crossover study. *Journal of Neurology, Neurosurgery & Psychiatry, 70*, 477–482.

World Health Organization. (2001). *ICIDH-2: International classification of functioning, disability and health.* Geneva, Switzerland: Author.

Wu, A. J., Radel, J., & Hanna-Pladdy, B. (2011). Improved function after combined physical and mental practice after stroke: A case of hemiparesis and apraxia. *American Journal of Occupational Therapy, 65*, 161–168.

Ylvisaker, M., & Feeney, T. J. (1998). *Collaborative brain injury intervention.* San Diego, CA: Singular.

Zoltan, B. (2007). *Vision, perception and cognition: A manual for the evaluation and treatment of the adult with acquired brain injury* (4th ed.). Thorofare, NJ: Slack.

For additional resources on the subjects discussed in this chapter, visit http://thePoint.lww.com/Willard-Spackman12e.

CHAPTER 56

Sensory Integration and Processing

Theory and Applications to Occupational Performance

Shelly J. Lane, Susanne Smith Roley, Tina Champagne

OUTLINE

LEARNING OBJECTIVES

After reading this chapter, you will be able to:

1. Describe the significance of sensory integration and processing to learning and behavior
2. Identify concepts that are central to sensory integration theory
3. Describe the mechanisms of receiving, organizing, and using sensory input and identify the major features of sensory systems
4. Explain the alerting and discriminating aspects of each sensory system
5. List ways to assess sensory integrative dysfunction
6. Define the principles of Ayres Sensory Integration®
7. Explain the use of sensory-based interventions
8. Conceptualize the application of sensory integration and processing constructs to multiple disorders and across the life course
9. Appreciate the significant contribution of sensation and sensory processing to one's ability to function during occupational performance
10. Recognize the evidence that supports and guides the use of sensory integration theory and principles in occupational therapy practice

Sensation: Our Window on the World

Sensation is everywhere. What we do with sensation and how we process it contribute to how we define ourselves. Sensation influences what we do and how we interact, our states of attention and arousal, and our ability to interpret the world around us. As such, processing and integration of sensation are intimately tied to occupation, participation, and health. Given that these constructs are essential to us as occupational therapy (OT) practitioners, it is crucial that we understand sensation; how sensation from the body and the environment is received, integrated, and processed; how it is used in everyday interactions with people and objects; how sensory integration (SI) and processing underlie our ability to produce an adaptive response; and ultimately, how sensory processing and integration support occupational performance and participation in desired activities.

Theoretical and Conceptual Background

The foundation for SI theory and practice was developed by Dr. A. Jean Ayres (1920–1988). In the 1960s, Ayres, an occupational therapist and educational psychologist, recognized and described hidden disabilities, referring to them as dysfunction in sensory integrative processes (Ayres, 1968) and later as sensory integrative dysfunction (Ayres, 1979, 2005;[1] Blanche-Keiffer & Surfas, 2011). Her insights and subsequent theory development were made through keen observation of behavior; review of the neurophysiological underpinnings of behavior; synthesis of literature from neurology, psychology, neurophysiology, and education; ongoing research on assessment; and statistical analysis of patterns of dysfunction (Ayres, 1972a, 1972b, 1974).

Since its inception, SI theory has been an evolving, dynamic, and ecological theory that specifies the critical influence of sensory processing on human development, function, and occupational participation. Building on the work of Sherrington (1951) and other neuroscientists, Ayres developed this theory that emphasizes a person's ability to appropriately process sensory information from his or her body and integrate it with information about what is going on around him or her so that he or she can effectively act on the environment. Ayres's theory of SI contributes to our understanding of how sensation impacts learning, social-emotional development, and neurophysiological processes that support occupations such as motor performance, attention, and arousal. Dynamic systems theories have emerged that provide an understanding of the complexity of development (Smith & Thelen, 1993) and help to explain the dynamic way in which this intervention affects change across the life course (Ikiugu, 2007; Spitzer, 1999). Advances in neuroscience continue to expand and support Ayres's original hypotheses, contributing to evidence-based practice (Bauman, 2005; Schneider, 2005). Ongoing review and expansion of dynamic systems theories and neuroscience continues to inform therapeutic practice (Bundy, Lane, & Murray, 2002; Ikiugu, 2007; McLaughlin, Kennedy, & Zemke, 1996; Royeen, 2003; Schaaf et al., 2009; Smith Roley, Blanche, & Schaaf, 2001).

In addition to her contributions to the professional world, Ayres (1979, 2005) published *Sensory Integration and the Child*, in which she sought "to help parents recognize sensory integrative problems in their child, understand what is going on, and do something to help their child" (p. 12). She anticipated that as our understanding of the central nervous system (CNS) advanced, our understanding of the neurological basis of SI theory, assessment, and intervention would become more refined. The basic premises of her work stand today. In a 25th anniversary edition of *Sensory Integration and the Child: Understanding Hidden Sensory Challenges* (2005),[1] Ayres has been described as a "developmental theorist" (Knox, 2005, p. 171), a "pioneer in affective neuroscience" (Schneider, 2005, p. 169), a "pioneer in our understanding of developmental **dyspraxia**" (Cermak, 2005, p. 175), "one of the original perceptual-motor theorists" (Smith Roley, 2005, p. 179), and "an astute observer of human behavior and neurological development" (Bauman, 2005, p. 180). Her work made major inroads into our understanding of clinical neuroscience, the importance of experience in brain development, the role of **tactile defensiveness** and **sensory modulation** disorders as contributors to behavioral disorders, and the impact of **sensory registration** in autism.

The term "sensory integration" is not unique to OT literature. It is a term used to refer to a theory, a neurological process, a disorder, and an intervention approach (Bundy, 2002; Mulligan, 2003). Neurophysiologically, SI describes a nonlinear process of multisensory information (Rolls, 2004). Perception, action, and emotional regulation are significantly shaped by SI. To distinguish the work originated by Ayres, the term *Ayres Sensory Integration®* (ASI) was trademarked (Smith Roley, Mailloux, Miller-Kuhaneck, & Glennon, 2007). Inclusive of various frameworks and theories emerging in OT, the terms *sensory processing* and *sensory integration* are often used together or interchangeably (Watling, Koenig, & Davies, 2011). In this chapter, we will use the term *sensory integration and processing* to refer to broad concepts of SI and sensory processing and ASI, when referring specifically to the frame of reference used in therapeutic fields as originated by Ayres (see Figure 56.1).

Occupational therapists commonly use SI theory in their clinical practice. The theoretical propositions guide both assessment and intervention with people who have sensory integrative and processing

[1]Throughout this chapter, references to Ayres, 1979 and Ayres, 2005 refer to *Sensory Integration and the Child.*

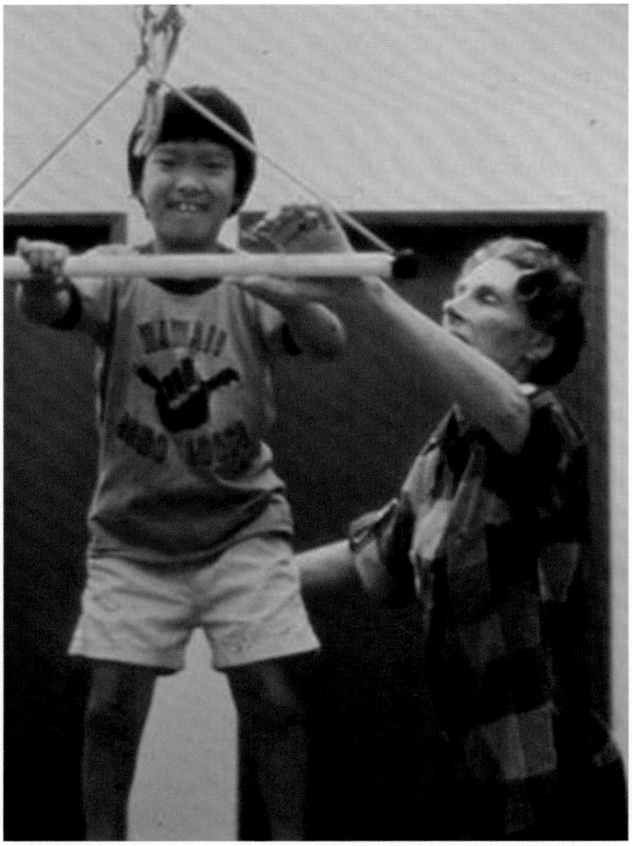

FIGURE 56.1 Dr. Ayres applied her theories through precise evaluation, which guided the intervention that is characterized by playful, self-motivated, motor engagement in sensory activities.

dysfunction that adversely impacts function, occupational performance, and participation (Parham & Mailloux, 2010). As noted earlier, the theoretical propositions supporting the focus on SI and processing in practice draw on evidence from neuroscience as Ayres recognized that behavior, emotions, and perceptions are regulated by brain mechanisms. SI and processing difficulties are present in individuals with and without other diagnoses (Goldsmith, Van Hulle, Arneson, Schreiber, & Gernsbacher, 2006; Kinnealey & Fuiek, 1999; Kinnealey, Oliver, & Wilbarger, 1995; Reynolds & Lane, 2007; Smith Roley et al., 2001). In fact, sensory differences are now considered ubiquitous in the population of individuals with autism spectrum disorder (ASD) (Marco, Hinkley, Hill, & Magarajan, 2011) and are highly common in children with attention deficit hyperactivity disorder (ADHD) as well (Bar-Shalita, Vatine, & Parush, 2008; Dunn & Bennett, 2002; S. J. Lane, Reynolds, & Thacker, 2010; Yochman, Parush, & Ornoy, 2004). Specific evaluation of SI and processing concerns allow practitioners to determine the nature and severity of the difficulties and the impact that the difficulties have on arousal, attention, praxis, and ultimately on occupational performance and participation in desired activities.

SI evaluation and intervention methods are used by practitioners throughout the world in various settings (e.g., hospitals, schools, clinics, and community settings) and with various populations (e.g., learning disabilities, ASD, attentional disorders, mental health disorders). A survey conducted by Case-Smith & Miller (1999) indicated that 95% to 99% of occupational therapists working with individuals with ASD routinely employ SI theory and intervention methods. Evidence for the use of ASI intervention methods has varied in rigor and in fidelity to the structure and process elements of this method; the outcomes have generally indicated that this intervention is as effective as are other interventions (Parham et al., 2007). However, May-Benson & Koomar (2010) concluded in their systematic review of intervention effectiveness studies that overall, the evidence suggests positive outcomes in "sensorimotor skills and motor planning; socialization, attention, and behavioral regulation; reading-related skills; participation in active play; and achievement of individualized goals" (p. 403). Current evidence of treatment effectiveness, from the studies that include the use a fidelity measure to insure adherence to ASI intervention principles, is emerging as promising (Pfeiffer, Koenig, Kinnealey, Shepherd, & Henderson, 2011; Schaaf, 2011). In a pilot study for the purpose of preparation for the implementation of a randomized control trial, Schaaf, Benevides, Kelly and Mailloux-Maggio (2012) reported that this intervention is safe, feasible, well accepted by therapists and parents, and could be implemented with fidelity to ASI methods.

Ayres Sensory Integration®: Theoretical Propositions

Five basic propositions form the theoretical basis for Ayres's thinking:

1. The remarkable potential for change of the developing brain or **neuroplasticity** throughout the life course (for reviews, see Buonomano & Merzenich, 1998; Cruikshank & Weinberger, 1996; Gross, 2000);
2. Interactions between the "higher order" (cortical) areas of the brain and "lower order" subcortical areas as fundamental to adequate SI;
3. Neurophysiological development of sensory integrative functions that occur in a natural order and follow a basic sequence;
4. An **adaptive response**, defined as "the ability to adjust one's action on environmental demand" (Ayres, 1972a, p. 8) and promotes a higher level of integration as a consequence of the **feedback** to the CNS; and
5. The presence of an **inner drive** to meet and master a challenge, which fosters the development of SI.

Neuroplasticity

Ayres's appreciation of the importance of experience as a major determinant of cortical organization and resulting function remains a bedrock principle in the field of neuroscience today. This "experience-dependent plasticity in the cerebral cortex reflects the importance of learning in our mental life and behaviors" (Miller, 2000, p. 1067). During the period when Ayres studied neuroplasticity, researchers thought that the brain's ability to be modified was robust during childhood but, after a critical period of development, was quite limited. It is now known that the brain has the capacity to be modified throughout the life course (Bear, Connors, & Paradiso, 2006; Galvan, 2010; Gilbert & Wiesel, 1992; Kerr, Cheng, & Jones, 2011). Given this knowledge, ASI interventions are being modified and increasingly used with diverse populations across the life course (Smith Roley et al., 2001).

Organization of the Brain

Although our nervous systems are almost constantly being bombarded by sensation, not all of this sensation reaches the cortex. If the cortex had to process every sensation a person experienced, it would not be able to do higher level tasks, such as thought and action. Neuroscientists have long explored hierarchical organization of the brain. Ayres understood that higher order brain regions, as they develop, remain dependent on lower order brain regions (Ayres, 1972a, 1979, 1989, 2004, 2005).[1] Before many of the incoming sensory messages ascend, or somewhere along their ascent toward the thalamus and then the cortex, other neurons act on them to either dampen their activity (**inhibition**) or, in some cases, enhance their activity (**facilitation**). Ayres (1979, 2005) described this process of inhibition and facilitation as a CNS process of self-organization. In this way, the subcortical structures are seen as important mediators of the information on which the higher cortical levels may act.

Based on her understanding that perception of any sensation requires facilitation of some input and inhibition of other input, Ayres designed interventions that would incorporate these mechanisms and promote more integrated functioning of the brain as a whole. For instance, use of meaningful stimuli that have an inhibitory effect on the CNS, coupled with a purposeful activity that elicits an adaptive response, were proposed by Ayres as early therapeutic propositions to advance CNS organization. For example, multisensory activities that involve active movement while engaged in a swinging activity couple organizing proprioceptive sensations with alerting vestibular sensations. These propositions remain today as core elements of OT when using ASI.

To date, there is no change in our appreciation of the role of the subcortical structures to provide the foundation for efficient functioning. However, there is currently a greater understanding and focus on the reciprocal interdependence between higher order and lower order brain regions (Middleton & Strick, 2000; Wall, Xu, & Wang, 2002). This interplay of activity between cortical and subcortical structures (in particular, the thalamus) further contributes to the self-organizing processes of the brain. In this way, the brain is able to develop perceptions that impart deeper meaning than is provided by the multisensory information alone. For example, an object that is orange and round (vision), has a citrus scent (olfaction), and a slight bumpiness along its surface (tactile) contributes to our ability to identify it as an orange; integrating these sensory features with emotion and memory lead many of us to fondly recall eating oranges on the back porch with our friends.

Ayres believed that the therapeutic use of appropriate, multisensory, and client-driven activities was the most effective way to promote sensory integration and thereby occupational performance and participation. The research that guided her thinking suggested that there were common integrating sites within the CNS where information from separate sensory sources converged onto neurons that had the potential to respond to inputs from multiple sensory sources. These were referred to as "convergent" or "polysensory" neurons (Ayres, 1972a). Over the past 25 years, there has been extensive research into cross-modality or multisensory convergence, and findings demonstrate that this process takes place at sites in the midbrain, thalamus, and cortex (for review, see Calvert, Spence, & Stein, 2004; Stein & Meredith, 1993). At every such site, there is the opportunity for cross-modality or multisensory integration.

One of the best-studied groups of multisensory neurons is in the superior colliculus (SC) (Alvarado, Stanford, Rowland, Vaughan, & Stein, 2009; Cuppini, Stein, Rowland, Magosso, & Ursino, 2011; Sparks & Groh, 1995; Wallace, Meredith, & Stein, 1993). This midbrain structure is classically divided into superficial layers predominantly containing visual neurons and deep layers containing multisensory (visual, somatosensory, and/or auditory) and premotor neurons. Investigation into the SC has demonstrated how signals from the different senses are combined and used to guide adaptive motor responses, such as hearing a sound and turning to visually locate the source (King & Palmer, 1985; Stein, Huneycutt, & Meredith, 1988; Stein & Meredith, 1993; Stein, Meredith, Huneycutt, & McDade, 1989; Wallace et al., 1993). In this example of the orienting response, when the auditory and visual stimuli occur close together in space and time, their combination enhances the ability to detect and identify the external stimuli. Conversely, cross-modality cues that are significantly discordant (e.g., spatially disparate) can have the opposite effect and depress responses (Stein et al., 1989). Whether the response is enhanced or depressed, an important behavioral consequence of the synthesis (or discordance) of the sensory information is closely related to changes in attention (Stein et al., 1989).

Recent studies exploring multisensory integration demonstrate that the cortex plays an important role in mediating convergence of sensory inputs at the level of the SC (Cuppini et al., 2011; Stein & Rowland, 2011). By temporarily deactivating the information flow from the cortex to SC neurons, response enhancement is compromised. As a consequence, the ability to use cross-modal stimuli to enhance SC-mediated behavioral performance is also compromised. As Ayres suspected and as the ongoing research has confirmed, the process of multisensory integration is highly adaptive, "knitting together information from different sensory channels to better detect, identify and respond to environmental events. . . . Sensory integration is critical to perception and behavior" (Stein et al., 1989, p. 12).

We have come to recognize that primary sensory pathways, rather than merely transmitting sensation in an inflexible manner, are sending impulses that are being constantly adjusted in relation to attention, arousal, emotion, and anticipation, as well as thought and planning. Eide (2003) notes that "when the sensory system is working effectively, cross-modality improves our responsiveness and interaction with our environment. However, when sensory systems are under-responsive (low registration) or over-responsive (sensory defensiveness), attention becomes inappropriately directed or diverted" (pp. 1–2). Eide (2003) proposes that therapeutic interventions focused on environmental adaptations and appropriate sensory strategies "are often children's best hope of reducing bodily 'distractions' so that they can focus on learning and socialization" (p. 2).

Over the past two decades, findings from neuroscience research indicate that sensory information (such as the information which allows us to perceive an object as an "orange") is distributed as serial and parallel streams of information (Felleman & Van Essen, 1991; Pons, Garraghty, Friedman, & Mishkin, 1987; for review, see Mesulam, 1998). Even though this distributed processing model of brain structure and function was not specified at the time, in 1972, Ayres (1972a) wrote, "[o]rganization must and does occur vertically among the levels of the brain as well as horizontally between two structures at the same level" (p. 27), demonstrating an understanding of the integrative and reciprocal complexity of the brain that is both hierarchical and heterarchical. Bundy and Murray (2002) comment that a system's approach to nervous system organization, in which "systems interact, and both cortical and subcortical structures contribute to sensory integration" (p. 11) is consistent with ASI.

Developmental Progression

Applying the developmental process to our understanding of the CNS, Ayres (1972a) noted that "each child's brain is designed to follow an orderly, predictable, interrelated sequence of development that results in the capacity for learning" (p. 4). Given an enriched, supportive environment, children will grow and develop sensory and motor memories that will help them adapt to their own growth and interests in the context of an ever-changing environment. Although Ayres focused on the first 7 years of life as the time frame in which this occurred, we now know that the brain continues to develop throughout the life course (Bear et al., 2006; Galvan, 2010; Gilbert & Wiesel, 1992; Kerr et al., 2011). A critical aspect of this process is that the child experiences various sensations, placing a demand on the brain to organize the incoming stimuli into increasingly more complex **perceptions**. Depending on the meaning of and context in which the stimuli are experienced, the child might focus and attend to the input or, if it is not relevant, the stimuli might be ignored (S. J. Lane, Miller, & Hanft, 2000; Miller & Lane, 2000). For example, a child who is riding a bicycle typically attends to visual and auditory inputs along the ride while ignoring the feel of the shirt as it is blown by the wind. If the child's brain is unable to efficiently organize incoming sensation, these "filtering out" and "attending to" processes may be inadequate. In this example, the child who is unable to tolerate the tactile input from the shirt's movement against the body will have difficulty attending to the important multisensory information in the environment (visual, auditory) that are necessary for both safety and skill. Until the tactile sensation is interpreted as "safe" and comfortable, the child may respond in a more primitive "fight-or-flight" mode. In general, this primitive state is thought to undermine both the development of skills and emotions, because it is through the ability of the brain to organize sensations that "the child gains control over his emotions" (Ayres, 2005, p. 14).

Adaptive Response

Our ability to make adaptive responses to ever-changing environmental demands and challenges allows us to learn something new and, in turn, change our actions, behaviors, and the environment (Ayres, 1972a, 1979, 2005). Spitzer (1999) discusses the congruence between the concept of self-organization in dynamic systems theory and Ayres's concept of the adaptive response in SI theory. In both theories, feedback from the individual's spontaneous, active adjustments contributes to self-organization of the brain (Ayres, 1979, 2005; Smith & Thelen, 1993). Ayres (1972a) stressed the importance of "organizing adaptive responses to increasing complexity" (p. 128) as a key component of intervention. She was guided by neuroscience research suggesting that inefficiency in **synaptic activity** along anatomical pathways might contribute to poor integration of sensory information and proposed that focusing on eliciting a response that was not yet well developed might enhance **synaptic function** (Ayres, 1972a; Katz & Shatz, 1996; Schlaug, 2001). Thus, for an individual with difficulty with motor coordination, an adaptive response is often most clearly observable during a motor task; however, it is also apparent with demands arising in emotional regulation, cognition, and social interactions. For instance, a child with difficulties planning and executing motor tasks might throw a "transformer" toy in frustration when unable to get it to properly transform. An adaptive response consistent with a higher level of emotional regulation would have the child asking for help in figuring out the transformation.

Ayres (2005) designed SI intervention strategies to engage the client in natural play activities. She stated that if the child is unable to integrate his or her nervous system successfully in typical environments, "[h]e needs a highly specialized environment, tailor-made for his nervous system" (Ayres, 2005, p. 141). This style of therapy requires that the OT practitioner designs a rich set of sensory-based activities and, in conjunction with the child, cofacilitate the child's self-organization and physical engagement with the environment. Although intervention using ASI in a classic setting is provided in a carefully designed clinic setting (Parham & Mailloux, 2010), SI and processing principles and activities can be adapted to be used in various sensory-based activities in settings such as at home, in the community, or at school (Ruzzano, Smith Roley, & Mailloux, 2003). A defining feature of ASI intervention, however, is that the individual has a room to safely move, jump, and crash and rearrange the objects in order to interact in new or novel ways.

Inner Drive

Although a therapist can help provide activities and environments to support participation and SI, the individual is the change agent, whose response to experiences impacts his or her ability to self-regulate and generate an adaptive response. It is the drive for mastery or the motivation to explore that elicits in the individual the willingness to participate. "Organizing and evincing an adaptive response which is more mature and complex than any emitted before requires effort—the kind of effort that a client gladly summons when he is emotionally involved in the task and believes he can cope with it" (Ayres, 1972a, p. 127). Embedded in this statement are two important concepts of intervention. One is the concept of the "**just-right challenge**," whereby the task is beyond what the client is already capable of achieving yet sufficiently demanding to promote CNS integration. The other concept is the client-led nature of ASI intervention, during which the therapist supports the client's freedom to choose and engage in activities as long as they are safe, appropriately challenging, foster increasingly complex adaptive behaviors, and generally further the development of sensory integration (Parham et al., 2007; Parham et al., 2011).

Other Models of Sensory Integration and Processing

As is the case for many pioneer theories, OT scientists and clinicians have developed additional models with variations in the interpretation and application of Ayres's theory of SI. In this section, we will look at three such models of SI and processing.

Dunn's Model

Dunn (1997a) proposed a model based on interactions between neurological threshold and behavioral responses to sensation, which is defined in her assessment tool, the *Sensory Profile* (Dunn, 1999). In this model, **neurological threshold** is seen as a reflection of the intensity or duration of a sensory stimulus required to activate a response; *behavioral response* is the observable response (of the young client in the original model) to his or her threshold. A *high* neurological threshold is present when intense sensation, or sensation delivered over a prolonged period of time, is needed to elicit a behavioral response; a *low* neurological threshold is present when minimal sensation elicits a response.

Behaviorally, Dunn (1999) identifies responses that are *passive* and *active*. When a client responds passively to sensation, they do nothing to alter intensity or duration. In contrast, an active response indicates that the client either actively seeks sensation in order to satisfy a high threshold or actively avoids sensation in the face of a low threshold. As an example, a child, we will call her Madeline, has a low threshold to auditory input and a high threshold to movement. An active response to her auditory environment would be reflected in covering her ears or moving away from a sound source because she is very sensitive to sound; an active response in the movement domain would find Madeline engaging in high intensity movement activities such as swinging very high or spinning very fast on the merry-go-round on the playground. In contrast, a passive response to sound would be reflected in Madeline becoming distressed with sounds but doing nothing to diminish sound intensity; a passive response to her movement threshold would have Madeline do nothing to meet her movement needs, resulting in low **arousal** and seeming lack of awareness of her environment. Dunn (1999) indicated that the thresholds represent continua, capturing thresholds that range from low to high and behaviors that range from very passive to very active.

Dunn (1999) defines the four categories of poor sensory processing challenges depicted in a quadrant

TABLE 56.1 Dunn's Sensory Processing Model

	Passive Behavioral Response	Active Behavioral Response
High Neurological Threshold	**Poor registration**	**Sensory seeking**
Low Neurological Threshold	**Sensory sensitivity**	**Sensory avoiding**

Adapted from Dunn, W. (1999). *Sensory profile.* San Antonio, TX: Therapy Skill Builders.

(Table 56.1). *Poor registration* reflects a high neurological threshold matched with a passive behavioral response; *sensory seeking* reflects a high threshold coupled with an active response. *Sensory sensitivity* is seen when a low neurological threshold is paired with a passive behavioral response, and *sensory avoiding* is seen when a low neurological threshold is paired with an active behavioral response.

Dunn (1999) suggested that this model could guide practitioners toward a better understanding about how sensory processing problems affected participation in and performance of everyday activities. Current neurophysiological research examining this model further seeks to identify the psychophysiological processes linked to sensory modulation difficulties, particularly over-responsiveness (Bar-Shalita et al., 2008).

Bundy and Murray Model of Sensory Integration

As an extension of Ayres' model of SI, Bundy and Murray (2002) created a model in which the sensory systems were depicted at the model core and their relationship to disorders of praxis and modulation shown on either side. Where Ayres' model defined functions associated with adequate processing and integration of sensation, the Bundy and Murray model defines SI deficits and associated behaviors, separating those constructs linked with modulation from those linked with dyspraxia. The model was organized such that constructs closer to the core represented more clear neurophysiologic relationships to basic sensory system integration and processing, while constructs more distant from the core represent observable behaviors. Separating behaviors linked with modulation from those linked with dyspraxia was intended to clarify the manifestations of these disorders.

Ecological Model of Sensory Modulation Disorder

Miller, Reisman, McIntosh, and Simon (2001) define both *external* (culture, environment, relationships, and tasks) and *internal* (sensation, emotion, and attention) dimensions in their Ecological Model of Sensory Processing. Their model, which focuses on sensory modulation, emphasizes that the response of an individual with a SI and processing disorder can be understood only within the context of his or her own life by examining the interaction between internal and external dimensions.

External dimensions include societal mores and expectations (cultural), physical and sensory surroundings (environment), interactions with other people and their meaning to the individual (relationships), and the things the individual does or wishes to do (tasks). Internal dimensions include the ability to generate the needed focus and activity level to accomplish a task or have a successful interaction (attention), the ability to give and receive emotional cues and regulate affective behavior (emotion), and the ability to take in and process environmental sensory stimuli (sensation). Internal dimensions are considered multifaceted (i.e., sensation includes tactile, vestibular, proprioceptive, visual, auditory, olfactory, and gustatory sensory systems) and seen as reflecting a continuum of responsiveness, much like Dunn (1999) defined. Miller and colleagues (2001), however, also included fluctuating responsivity wherein an individual might appear to have over-responsiveness at one point in the day and under-responsiveness at another. Internal and external dimensions interact with and influence each other, and internal dimensions themselves are interactive.

This model emphasizes the interaction between sensory processing, emotions, and attention relative to interactions with variable factors outside the individual. Individuals who have difficulty modulating sensation will have difficulty interacting with people and things in their environment. When there is a mismatch between what is expected within one or more external dimensions and the capabilities of individuals with regard to their internal dimensions, individuals will have difficulty regulating their responses. For instance, with a task such as going to the grocery store, the adult expectation would be that the child will come along, sit in the grocery cart or walk close by, and tolerate the multisensory stimuli (e.g., sounds and sights) of the grocery store. For a child with a very sensitive auditory system, the sounds in the grocery store might quickly become overwhelming. And, although this child may wish to retreat to the quiet of the car, this is not possible because Mom needs to get the shopping done. Thus, a mismatch is created between environmental (parental) expectations and the child's sensory processing capabilities. This child might cover his or her ears to reduce the sound but will likely soon start whining, ignoring his or her mother's requests to just sit still for a few minutes. This mismatch may result in overarousal, diminished attention, and ultimately, an emotional outburst (e.g., temper tantrum) for the child and frustration for the mother.

Sensory Processing Nosology

In consultation with professionals revising the *Diagnostic Classification of Mental Health and Developmental*

Disorders of Infancy and Early Childhood, Revised (*DC: 0–3R*) (Zero to Three, 2005) and the *Diagnostic Manual for Infancy and Early Childhood* of the Interdisciplinary Council on Developmental and Learning Disorders (ICDL) (2005), a team of occupational therapists developed a taxonomy reflecting what was termed *sensory processing disorder* in 2004 (Miller, Anzalone, Lane, Cermak, & Osten, 2007; Miller, Cermak, Lane, Anzalone, & Koomar, 2004). The long-term intent was to propose one or more subtypes of sensory processing for the developing revision of the *Diagnostic and Statistical Manual of Mental Disorders, (4th ed., text rev.; DSM-IV-TR)* of the American Psychiatric Association (APA) (2000). This taxonomy is firmly rooted in the historical work of Ayres, but the authors sought to include the additional work that had been done as well as the new evidence. The diagnostic categories proposed were based on work by several theorists and researchers (e.g., Ayres, 1972a, 1979; DeGangi, 2000; Dunn, 2001; Mulligan, 1998b). The terminology in the nosology was conceived as a tool that would guide practitioners toward greater clinical reasoning when using the multitude of terms that reflected the integration and processing of sensation for use in environmental interaction. Within the nosology, "sensory processing disorder" (SPD) was suggested as the term to be used for the diagnosis of sensory-based processing challenges to differentiate the disorder from ASI theory and intervention as well as to differentiate the disorder from the neurophysiologic process of integrating sensation. The nosology (Figure 56.2) generated a great deal of controversy in its promotion of this terminology shift and in the reorganization of concepts originally proposed and researched by Ayres.

In this conceptualization, SPD comprised sensory modulation disorder (SMD), sensory discrimination disorder (SDD), and sensory-based motor disorder (SBMD). Within each of the categories are subcategories of SI and processing concerns. SMD is reflected in sensory over-responsitivity (SOR), sensory under-responsivity (SUR), and/or sensory seeking; it can be seen in any sensory system, although that is not reflected in the figure. The SMD categories roughly map onto those depicted in the Dunn (1999) quadrant table where SUR parallels poor registration and SOR is reflected in both sensory avoidance and sensory sensitivity. SDD is a disorder of sensory perception or discrimination (e.g. visual perception, tactile perception), and this disorder can be seen in any sensory system. Ayres (1971) had also identified SDDs, most notably poor tactile discrimination and poor visual perception. Although discrimination is separated from both modulation and motor disorders in this model, it was recognized that discrimination disorders are often seen with SBMD as well as with modulation disorders. For instance, the link between poor tactile discrimination and dyspraxia is well established (Ayres, 1989; Mailloux et al., 2011; Mulligan, 1998a, 1998b, 2000). Disorders of discrimination in one or more sensory system should be viewed as underlying SBMD; and potentially coexisting with disorders of modulation. The category of SBMD is subdivided into dyspraxia and postural disorders. Dyspraxia in this typology is consistent with **somatodyspraxia** and **postural disorder** and parallels **vestibular bilateral integration and sequencing disorder**. Both somatodyspraxia and vestibular bilateral integration and sequencing disorder are factors that emerged via research by Ayres (1989) in a confirmatory factor analysis by Mulligan (2000) and again a more recent factor analysis by Mailloux et al. (2011). These factor analysis studies revealed consistent patterns of sensory integrative dysfunction including visual praxis and sensory modulation difficulties, in addition to somatodyspraxia and vestibular bilateral integration and sequencing disorder. These terms will be defined in later sections of this chapter.

Neuroscience of Sensation

Although there are some basics in the mechanics of intake and processing of sensation that are consistent person to person, sensory processing and integration

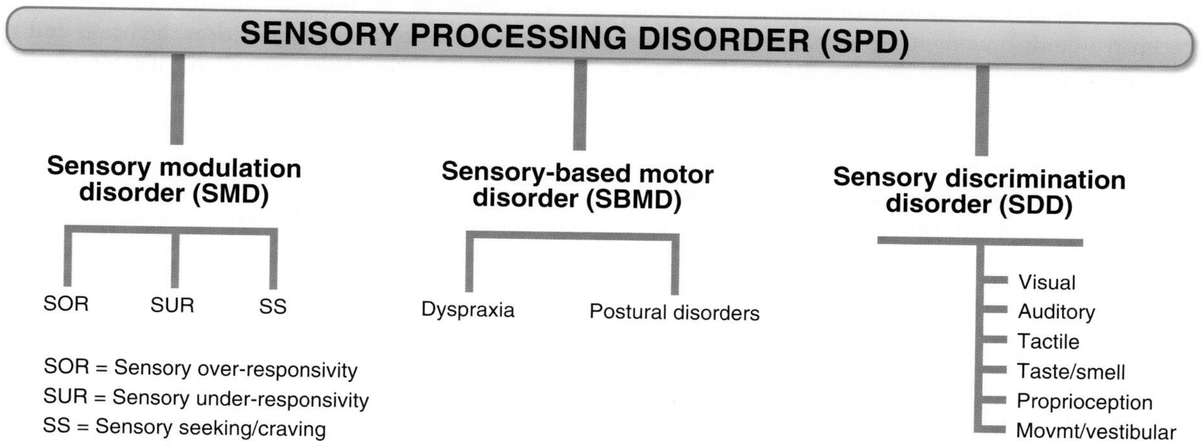

FIGURE 56.2 Proposed nosology for sensory processing disorder.

are also highly personal. How we process sensory information from our bodies and from outside of our bodies and the effect this has on our individual nervous systems significantly influences how we interact with people and things in the environment. When focusing on SI and processing as part of the OT process, we need to understand sensory system function in order to understand dysfunction.

The Mechanics of Processing Sensation

Sensory intake begins at the receptor. Sensory receptors for touch lie in the skin and deeper tissues; for proprioception, they lie in muscles, tendons, and joints. Vestibular receptors are hair cells in the vestibular apparatus of the inner ear; auditory receptors are also hair cells, residing in the cochlea of the inner ear. Rods and cones compose the receptors for the visual system, taste buds for the gustatory system, and olfactory cilia for our sense of smell. Each of these receptors responds best to a specific form of environmental energy (e.g. light energy for the cones of the retina) and changes the environmental energy into something the CNS can understand. The processing of changing environmental energy into a neural signal is called **transduction**. Transduction allows information from the environment to be interpreted by the brain.

Looking at some of the features of neural transmission that apply to the receptor, the sensory or afferent fiber that carries this information to the brain and to central processing will help us understand the impact of sensation on behavior. The following information was gleaned from several neuroscience texts. Interested readers might refer to Siegel and Sapru (2011), Patestas and Gartner (2006), or Purves et al. (2012) for more detailed information.

Within each sensory system are receptors with varying sizes of **receptive fields**. A receptive field is the area served by one sensory neuron. Some receptive fields are large, others are small, some overlap a great deal, and others do not. Areas of the body with small and overlapping receptive fields have dense innervations or multitudes of sensory receptors and sensory (afferent) fibers to carry the information to the CNS. Thus, with smaller receptive fields, the brain receives information about more limited areas, balanced by the fact that there are many fibers carrying the information. The end result of smaller receptive fields paired with higher density of receptors and afferent fibers is greater detail. In the tactile system, for instance, the brain compares the receptive fields of all the active neurons to detect the location of the touch; so when the receptive fields are small, dense, and overlap a lot, we know exactly where touch occurs; and when they are larger, less dense, and overlap little, we can tell only the general area of touch. When we have an itch on a high-density area such as our nose, we can get right to the spot to scratch, but when we have an itch on our back, we have to feel around a little to find the right spot.

As a general rule of thumb, sensory systems are designed to inform the CNS about two aspects of sensation: ongoing background status and stimulus change. These functions are related to the **adaptation rate** of the receptor. For instance, receptors in the tactile system are always receiving input about what you are touching or what is touching you. Some of these are designed to turn on and turn off quickly (rapidly adapt), providing information to the brain about a change in what has touched the skin. Others are designed to turn on and stay on for longer periods of time (slowly adapt), providing the brain with background information on what is touching the skin in a more constant manner. We need the combination of these inputs as a foundation for interaction in and with people and things in the environment.

Signal strength varies between stimuli. At the periphery, we find that some sensations are of sufficient strength that the neural signal generated will reach the CNS and be further processed. Other sensory inputs must be summed, or added together to reach sufficient strength that they will be sent, or propagated to the CNS. The receptor threshold must be reached in order for a response to be triggered. Summation may be either temporal or spatial. **Temporal summation** occurs when a stimulus of limited strength is repeated in quick succession, such that the strength of the second stimulus is "added to" the strength of the first stimulus, and so forth, until threshold is reached and the signal is sent forward. This is rather like someone is tapping you on the shoulder; you may not feel the first light tap, but if the tapping continues in fast enough succession, threshold will be reached and the tapping will get your attention.

Spatial summation involves activating several receptors and summing the excitation from each to produce a response. Think about this as the difference between being touched lightly by the tip of a pin as opposed to by the tip of a finger. The finger is larger and has the potential to activate more surface receptors; summing activation of the receptors results in threshold being reached and a response on your end. Summation, both temporal and spatial, also takes place within the brain and spinal cord. And, centrally, the sum may be of excitatory inputs, inhibitory inputs, or a combination of the two.

Sensory receptors are attached to sensory or afferent fibers. **Fiber diameter** will influence the speed by which the sensation is perceived by the brain. Large fibers conduct faster than small fibers. If you think of a fiber as though it is a straw and consider drinking a milk shake through this straw, it is clear that you will finish your milk shake faster if the straw diameter is bigger. There is simply less resistance in the straw to the flow of the milk shake. For nerve fibers, it is the same, bigger fibers offer lower resistance to the flow of ions and generation and propagation of the action potential so the information travels faster. In the somatosensory system, the afferent largest fibers carry proprioceptive information from muscle spindles and the smallest fibers carry pain sensation.

Habituation to sensory input is defined as a decrease in response strength following repeated exposure. On a cellular level, habituation can be seen at peripheral receptors as well as within cells in the brain and spinal cord. Cellular habituation is reflected behaviorally when we stop attending to background sounds (like soft music) in the environment. Habituation is an essential function of the brain because it helps us tune out sensation in the environment that is not pertinent to current tasks. The ability to habituate to sensation is personal, like many aspects of SI and processing. Some of us do well with background music when we are trying to concentrate; we habituate to the rise and fall of the sounds and this becomes our "white noise," supporting our concentration. Others cannot do this; they need perfect silence for concentration.

Progressive increases in response to a stimulus with repeated exposure is called **sensitization**. This, too, occurs both peripherally and centrally. For instance, if you repeatedly rub a spot on your arm, initially, you will feel the touch; but eventually, the rubbing will elicit pain as the receptors become increasingly responsive. Central sensitization has been associated with mental health disorders such as anxiety and posttraumatic stress disorder (PTSD); in both cases, the behavioral response seems to exceed what you might expect given the sensory "trigger."

Divergence is the brain's ability to transmit sensory input to many parts of the brain so that the input can affect multiple places at once. When a person is in danger, a mild stimulus (e.g., the faint smell of smoke) needs to recruit lots of activity; we refer to these high activity levels as a *fight-or-flight response*. In contrast, **convergence** is the phenomenon of bringing input together from many sources. It is as if the brain is seeking confirmation by getting information from several sensory systems and is being careful to act only when there is enough input to tell a clear story. Convergence prevents us from reacting inappropriately when only partial stimuli are available and keeps us from reacting to every stimulus that comes along. In the sensory systems, inputs from multiple sensory inputs converge so that the brain can create a more organized response.

The brain depends on a balance of excitation and inhibition to mediate input and output. These concepts were discussed earlier in this chapter. With too much excitation, we overreact; and with too much inhibition, we will fail to notice and respond to the world around us. At each synapse and within neuron systems, there is a continuous negotiation between the excitation and inhibition messages that are available. When inputs converge on a neuron or group of neurons, the output will be the sum of excitatory and inhibitory inputs. There has to be enough excitation to override the inhibition in order to get an action and, when needed, enough inhibition to override excitation. When we consider this dynamic process from a systems level, we also see the power of the complementary functions of the brain as a whole. Some parts of the brain are responsible for increasing our attention, whereas others are responsible for scanning the environment. These systems remain "balanced" because of the excitation and inhibition patterns between these parts of the brain. When brain injury disrupts typical function, people experience a *release phenomenon*. This means that one function is set free from the excitatory and inhibitory controls of its complementary parts of the brain. Heightened or dampened reactions occur when there is a release phenomenon. Another way to balance excitation and inhibition is through **feed forward** and feedback mechanisms. The brain has connections that enable it to "listen in" to input and reactions. This allows the brain to monitor itself and make adjustments in plans for acting. Feed forward circuits send a message ahead of the primary sensory message either to alert higher centers about incoming input (i.e., "pay attention") or to create an inhibitory path so that the sensory message gets stronger (i.e., "notice only THIS"). Feedback circuits send a message back to modulate the strength of a response. For example, feedback occurs after you have completed a movement and allows the brain to evaluate how effective that movement was to reaching your goal. On the basis of feedback (action-perception-action), the system will make adjustments in how the message gets sent the next time (e.g., "a little more of those muscles, a little less of these muscles").

The Sensory Systems: Intake, Processing, and Integration

Sensation occurs from inside the body, from the body's position and movement, and from outside of the body. The five exteroceptive senses provide us with information about the external world; vision, hearing, touch, smell, and taste allow individuals to be actively engaged in tasks and with people in the environment. We also need to have ongoing information about body position in space and movement through space; this input comes from our proprioception and vestibular systems. ASI theory highlights the "hidden" sensory systems (vestibular and proprioception) as well as the tactile system as the "powerhouses," considering that this body-centered information interacts with information from internal systems and the external world to provide an "integrated" perception and response to the world. These "body senses" then are placed at the heart of sensory integration and processing approaches. The body-centered senses are most mature at birth and play an important role in early development. The distance senses of vision and hearing, our exteroceptive senses, play an increasingly important role as the CNS matures. Our chemical senses, taste and smell, although crucial in their own rights, have been less well studied from an ASI theoretical perspective. Interoceptors, providing sensory information relative to events within the body, are of increasing interest, given the multisensory interactions between interoceptors, proprioceptors, and exteroceptors (Calvert, Spence, & Stein, 2004).

The Body Senses: Touch and Our Proprioceptors

Body senses provide the CNS with a dynamic map of ourselves and of our encounters with the physical environment. The somatosensory system, which includes receptors for both touch and proprioception, provides information on what we touch, what touches us, and the movement and position of our muscles and joints. This information is crucial to our ability to develop a body map or scheme. The vestibular system, considered a "special proprioceptor," contributes to our knowledge of position in space by responding to movement through space; this system provides ongoing information about our relationship with gravity.

The Somatosensory System. Somatosensation includes both touch and proprioception. Thinking first about touch, there are various touch receptors that together provide us with deep knowledge of what we touch and what touches us. All receptors in this system respond to mechanical deformation; the receptor must be "deformed" in order for the sensation to be transmitted to the CNS.

Our skin is rich with tactile receptors and broadly conceptualizing the skin as being the receptor for touch can put into perspective the pervasive nature of this sensory system. There are receptors that are very superficial and those that are deep in the layers of the skin, receptors that are easily activated, and receptors that require more intense stimuli before they fire. This later point relates to the concept of threshold for activation, discussed earlier in this chapter. This combination of receptor types and threshold means that this system responds to an array of tactile sensations including light and deep touch, pinpoint-sized and large surface touch, hot and cold temperatures, vibration, and pain. In fact, in a typical nervous system, the tactile receptors are firing all the time, providing an ongoing array of input to the CNS about what is touching the skin, where, how intense, how long, and in what direction. It is easy to see that if the brain cannot organize and filter this vast array of input, it could pose clear problems for participation in a variety of occupations.

In addition to skin receptors, the somatosensory system has receptors in muscles and joints responding to muscle contraction and joint movement. These are our proprioceptors responsible for our knowledge of the position of our body and limbs in space. Muscle spindles respond to changes in muscle length and provide information about the speed and direction of movement as well as information about static position of the arms and legs. The muscle spindles are the source of the sensory component of the stretch reflex that supports **muscle tone** or the resting level of tension in a muscle. Muscle tone is important because it allows the muscle to respond optimally to central commands or reflex actions. When the system is working well, quickly stretching a muscle leads to its contraction; this is what you see when a tendon is tapped with a reflex hammer; the tap stretches the muscle and the spindle responds, leading to muscle contraction (Purves et al., 2012). The motor centers of the brain control the actions of the muscles by dampening the activity of the reflex arcs. When the motor centers of the brain are damaged, the reflex arc continues to activate without inhibitory control; this mechanism creates spasticity (Crenna & Frigo, 1985; Sheean & McGuire, 2009).

Muscle tension is detected by the Golgi tendon organs (GTO); joint receptors provide information about joint position. Interestingly, these receptors may be of high importance for fine control of finger movement (Purves et al., 2012). The action of the GTO is important in cramp relief. During cramping, the muscle contains a high degree of tension. When you slowly and consistently stretch a cramped muscle, you pull on the tendon, which activates the GTO. This sensory message creates increased inhibition to the muscle, enabling the muscle to relax. This is the mechanism that we are harnessing when we use sustained stretch with people who have spasticity (Crenna & Frigo, 1985; Sheean & McGuire, 2009).

Our proprioceptors provide information about where our muscles and joints are in space and how they move relatively to each other and relatively to resistance. Imagine not knowing where your arms and legs are as you attempt to move through space, avoid objects, pick things up, and put things down. The absence of proprioceptive input makes interaction with the environment a nearly insurmountable challenge.

Somatosensory information travels to the brain stem, the thalamus, and then the sensorimotor cortex, specifically the parietal lobe. Traditionally, neuroscientists divided this system into the posterior and anterolateral systems; the posterior portion being responsible for touch pressure and proprioception and the anterolateral portion being responsible for light touch, pain, and temperature reception. We now understand that those divisions provide general guidance and recognize that individual experiences are unique. Generally, the posterior system, called the *dorsal column-medial lemniscal pathway*, carries specific information about the surface of the skin and about the muscles and joints. In reference to Tables 56.2 and 56.3, this system transmits the discriminating and mapping information. The input that travels through the dorsal columns goes directly to the thalamus and on to the parietal lobe in a very specific pattern, creating the sensory homunculus (a map of the body from a sensory point of view). Recall that some areas of the body are very densely populated with sensory receptors; the receptor density is reflected in the size of this region at the sensory homunculus; larger peripheral receptor

TABLE 56.2 Arousal/Alerting and Discrimination/Mapping Descriptors of the Sensory Systems

Sensory System	Arousal/Alerting Descriptors[a]	Discrimination/Mapping Descriptors[b]
For all systems	*Unpredictable*: The task is unfamiliar; the child cannot anticipate the sensory experiences that will occur in the task.	*Predictable*: Sensory pattern in the task is routine for the child, such as diaper changing—the child knows what is occurring and what will come next.
Somatosensory	*Light touch*: gentle tapping on skin; tickling (e.g., loose clothing making contact with skin) *Pain:* brisk pinching; contact with sharp objects; skin pressed in small surface (e.g., when skin is caught in between chair arm and seat). *Temperature*: Hot or cold stimuli (e.g., iced drinks, hot foods, cold hands, cold metal chairs). *Variable*: Changing characteristics during the task (e.g., putting clothing on requires a combination of tactile experiences). *Short duration stimuli*: Tapping, touching briefly (e.g., splashing water). *Small body surface contact*: Small body surfaces, as when using only fingertips to touch something.	*Touch pressure*: Firm contact on skin (e.g., hugging, patting, grasping). Occurs both when touching objects or persons, or when they touch you. *Long duration stimuli*: Holding, grasping (e.g., carrying a child in your arms). *Large body surface contact*: Large body surfaces include holding, hugging; also includes holding a cup with the entire palmar surface of hand.
Vestibular	*Head position change*: The child's head orientation is altered (e.g., pulling the child up from lying on the back to sitting). *Speed change*: Movements change velocity (e.g., the teacher stops to talk to another teacher when pushing the child to the bathroom in his wheelchair). *Direction change*: Movements change planes, such as bending down to pick something up while carrying the child down the hall. *Rotary head movement*: head moving in an arc (e.g., spinning, turning head side to side).	*Linear head movement*: Head moving in a straight line (e.g., bouncing up and down, going down the hall in a wheelchair). *Repetitive head movements*: Movements that repeat in a simple sequence (e.g., rocking in a rocker).
Proprioception	*Quick stretch*: Movements that pull on the muscles (e.g., briskly tapping on a muscle belly).	*Sustained tension*: Steady, constant action on the muscles pressing or holding on the muscle (e.g., using heavy objects during play). *Shifting muscle tension*: Activities that demand constant change in the muscles (e.g., walking, lifting, moving objects).
Visual	*High intensity*: Visual stimulus is bright (e.g., looking out a window on a bright day). *High contrast*: A difference between the visual stimulus and surrounding environment (e.g., cranberry juice in a white cup). *Variable*: Changing characteristics during a task (e.g., a TV program is a variable visual stimulus).	*Low intensity*: Visual stimulus is subdued (e.g., finding objects in the dark closet). *High similarity*: Small differences between visual stimulus and its surrounding environment (e.g., oatmeal in a beige bowl). *Competitive*: The background is interesting or busy (e.g., the junk drawer, a bulletin board).
Auditory	*Variable*: Changing characteristics during a task (e.g., a person's voice with intonation). *High intensity*: The auditory stimulus is loud (e.g., siren, high volume radio). *Competitive*: The environment has a variety of recurring sounds (e.g., the classroom, a party).	*Rhythmic*: Sounds repeat in a simple sequence/beat (e.g., humming; singing nursery songs). *Constant*: The stimulus is always present (e.g., a fan noise). *Noncompetitive*: The environment is quiet (e.g., the bedroom when all is ready for bedtime). *Low intensity*: The auditory stimulus is subdued (e.g., whispering).
Olfactory/ gustatory	*Strong intensity*: The taste/smell has distinct qualities (e.g., spinach).	*Mild intensity*: The taste/smell has nondistinct or familiar qualities (e.g., cream of wheat).

[a]Arousal/alerting stimuli tend to generate "noticing" behaviors. The individual's attention is at least momentarily drawn toward the stimulus (commonly disrupting ongoing behavior). These stimuli enable the nervous system to orient to stimuli that may require a protective response. In some situations, an arousing stimulus can become part of a functional behavior (e.g., when the arousing somatosensory input from putting on shirt becomes predictable, a discriminating/mapping characteristic).

[b]Discriminatory/mapping stimuli are those that enable the individual to gather information that can be used to support and generate functional behaviors. The information yields spatial and temporal qualities of body and environment (the content of the maps), which can be used to create purposeful movement. These stimuli are more organizing for the nervous system.

Adapted with permission from Dunn, W. (1991). The sensorimotor systems: A framework for assessment and intervention. In F. P. Orelove & D. Sobsey (Eds.), *Educating children with multiple disabilities: A transdisciplinary approach* (2nd ed., pp. 33–78). Baltimore, MD: Paul H. Brookes.

TABLE 56.3 Reasons for Incorporating Various Sensory Qualities into Integrated Intervention Programs

Sensory System	Arousal/Alerting Descriptors	Discrimination/Mapping Descriptors
For all systems	*Unpredictable*: To develop an increasing level of attention to keep the child interested in the task/activity (e.g., change the position of the objects on the child's lap tray during the task).	*Predictable*: To establish the child's ability to anticipate a programming sequence or a salient cue; to decrease possibility to be distracted from a functional task sequence (e.g., use the same routine for diaper changing every time).
Somatosensory	*Light touch*: To increase alertness in a child who is lethargic (e.g., pull cloth from child's face during peek-a-boo). *Pain*: To raise from unconsciousness; to determine ability to respond to noxious stimuli when unconscious (e.g., flick palm of hand or sole of foot briskly). *Temperature*: To establish awareness of stimuli; to maintain attentiveness to task (e.g., use hot foods for spoon eating and cold drink for sucking through a straw). *Variable*: To maintain attention to or interest in the task (e.g., place new texture on cup surface each day so child notices the cup). *Short duration*: To increase arousal for task performance (e.g., tap child on chest before giving direction). *Small body surface contact*: To generate and focus attention on a particular body part (e.g., tap around lips with fingertips before eating task).	*Touch pressure*: To establish and maintain awareness of body parts and body position; to calm a child who has been overstimulated (e.g., provide a firm bear hug). *Long duration*: To enable the child to become familiar, comfortable with the stimulus; to incorporate stimulus into functional skill (e.g., grasping the container to pick it up and pour out contents). *Large body surface contact*: To establish and maintain awareness of body parts and body position; to calm a child who has been overstimulated (e.g., wrap child tightly in a blanket).
Vestibular	*Head position change*: To increase arousal for an activity (e.g., position child prone over a wedge). *Speed change*: To keep adequate alertness for functional task (e.g., vary pace while carrying the child to new task). *Direction change*: To elevate level of alertness for a functional task (e.g., swing child back and forth in arms prior to positioning him or her at the table for a task).	*Linear head movement*: To support establishment of body awareness in space (e.g., carry child around the room in fixed position to explore its features). *Repetitive head movement*: To provide predictable and organizing information; to calm a child who has been overstimulated (e.g., rock the child).
Proprioception	*Quick stretch*: To generate additional muscle tension to support functional tasks (e.g., tap muscle belly of hypotonic muscle while providing physical guidance to grasp).	*Sustained tension*: To enable the muscle to relax, elongate, so body part can be in more optimal position for function (e.g., press firmly across muscle belly while objects are being manipulated). *Shift muscle tension*: To establish functional movements that contain stability and mobility (e.g., prop and reach for a top; reach, fill, and lift spoon to mouth).
Visual	*High intensity*: To increase opportunity to notice object; to generate arousal for task (e.g., cover blocks with foil for manipulation task). *High contrast*: To enhance possibility of locating object and maintaining attention to it (e.g., place raisins on a piece of typing paper for prehension activity). *Variable*: To maintain attention to or interest in the task (e.g., play rolling catch with a clear ball that has moveable pieces inside).	*Low intensity*: To allow visual stimulus to blend with other salient features; to generate searching behaviors, because characteristics are less obvious (e.g., find own cubbyhole in back of room). *High similarity*: To establish more discerning abilities; to develop skills for naturally occurring tasks (e.g., scoop applesauce from beige plate). *Competitive*: To facilitate searching; to increase tolerance for natural life circumstances (e.g., obtain correct tools from equipment bin).

TABLE 56.3 Reasons for Incorporating Various Sensory Qualities into Integrated Intervention Programs *(Continued)*

Sensory System	Arousal/Alerting Descriptors	Discrimination/Mapping Descriptors
Auditory	*Variable*: To maintain attention to or interest in the task (e.g., play radio station after activating a switch). *High intensity*: To stimulate noticing the person or object, to create proper alerting for task performance (e.g., ring a bell to encourage the child to locate the stimulus).	*Rhythmic*: To provide predictable/organizing information for environmental orientation (e.g., sing a nursery rhyme while physically guiding motions). *Constant*: To provide a foundational stimulus for environmental orientation, especially important when other sensory systems (e.g., vision, vestibular) do not provide orientation (e.g., child recognizes own classroom by fan noise and calms down). *Competitive*: To facilitate differentiation of salient stimuli; to increase tolerance for natural life circumstances (e.g., after child learns to look when his or her name is called, conduct activity within busy classroom). *Noncompetitive*: To facilitate focused attention for acquiring a new and difficult skill; to calm a child who has been overstimulated (e.g., move child to quiet room to establish vocalizations). *Low intensity*: To allow the auditory stimulus to blend with other salient features; to generate searching behaviors because stimulus is less obvious (e.g., give child a direction in a normal volume).
Olfactory/gustatory	*Strong intensity*: To stimulate arousal for task (e.g., child smells spaghetti sauce at lunch).	*Low intensity:* To allow the olfactory stimulus to blend with other salient features in the environment; to generate searching behaviors since stimulus is less obvious (play a game where the child finds an item/location by scent). *Mild intensity:* To facilitate exploratory behaviors; to stimulate naturally occurring activities (e.g., smell of lunch food is less distinct, so child is encouraged to notice textures, smells, colors). *Competitive:* To facilitate searching; to increase tolerance for natural circumstances where there are competing stimuli (e.g., to stand in lunch line with many food options and make food choices).

Adapted with permission from Dunn, W. (1991). The sensorimotor systems: A framework for assessment and intervention. In F. P. Orelove & D. Sobsey (Eds.), *Educating children with multiple disabilities: A transdisciplinary approach* (2nd ed., pp. 33–78) Baltimore; MD: Paul H. Brookes.

density parallels a larger region in the sensory homunculus. As a result, although the homunculus *resembles* a body, it appears quite out of proportion.

The *anterolateral system* is actually a collection of pathways, transmitting information about light touch, pain, and temperature to regions of the brain responsible for arousal, alerting, and emotional regulation (Patestas & Gartner, 2006) (see Tables 56.2 and 56.3 for examples). This input travels into the spinal cord and from there projects to the reticular formation of the brain stem, to regions of the limbic system, and to other brain stem regions. The reticular formation is responsible for generalized arousal of the brain, so these connections are less specific and more diffuse; the projections to other regions attach such things as emotional significance to the sensation. These connections may underlie the calming feeling we get with a warm hug or the startle and discomfort sensation generated when we perceive something to be crawling on our skin. The anterolateral input is important when people need more arousal to participate, and it is the input to be avoided when people are already agitated or have heightened responsiveness.

Proprioceptive input also, and importantly, projects to the cerebellum. The cerebellum receives proprioception directly before it is processed in the higher brain centers. This raw sensory input enables the cerebellum to be very precise in how it organizes motor actions. The cerebellum makes adjustments on the basis of what is actually happening (input from the muscle spindles and GTO), which is why our motor planning can be so accurate. The cerebellum also gets information from the brain about the proposed movement plans and compares the plan with the sensation to determine whether an alteration must occur. We can make just the right step because the cerebellum is fine-tuning the plan just before we need to act. The links with the cerebellum are crucial for knowing position in space.

The Vestibular System. Vestibular receptors are categorized as "special proprioceptors." This system functions as a gravity and movement detector and is responsible for our orientation in space, balance and equilibrium, and the coordination of head and eye movements, enabling coordinated movement through space. The vestibular labyrinth, as it is sometimes called, houses the two groups of receptor structures: the semicircular canals responding to angular movement such as swinging, spinning, and rolling and the otolith organs responding to static head position relative to gravity and linear acceleration, such as what happens with jumping and running. The receptors in this system are hair cells, which are activated when the projections (hairs) at the top of the cell are bent. Bending of the hairs is caused by movement of fluid through the semicircular canals during head rotation or by shifting the membrane into which the hair cells project in the otolith organs. We understand movement direction based on the direction in which the hair cells are bent. Together, these structures record direction, angle, and speed of movement, with particular attention to the position of the head (Purves et al., 2012).

The vestibular system sends sensory information directly to vestibular nuclei located in the brain stem and to the cerebellum. Of note, the vestibular nuclei receive bilateral vestibular inputs, along with information from the visual and somatosensory system, making these nuclei important integrative centers (Purves et al., 2012). Projections from the vestibular nuclei go to brain stem and midbrain nuclei that control eye movements; to neck motor neurons, playing a role in head-righting reflexes; and to trunk extensor motor neurons, playing a role in postural control. We don't see the world as bobble heads because of these links; instead, we are able to coordinate head and trunk and eye and head movements within a stabilized visual field.

Vestibular-visual interactions are designed to maintain a stable visual field when the head and body are moving. Cranial nerves III, IV, and VI, motor nerves for the eye muscles, receive complex vestibular projections, which support the coordination of eye and head movements. Head position and eye position have to be in concert with each other to stay oriented in space. These connections enable us to determine whether our eyes are moving, our head is moving, or the world is moving. People who have motion sickness have more difficulty resolving this potential conflict.

Vestibular inputs to the cerebellum join with proprioceptive inputs to provide this structure with an ongoing stream of sensory input from head movement and body movement, contributing to postural control. Postural control is a basic building block for human behavior; although it is easy to only think of postural control as a motor operation, it is important to remember that postural control is built on accurate sensory input. Sometimes, poor postural stability is due to weakness of muscles or poor biomechanical positioning, but equally likely is the possibility that inaccurate or unreliable sensory input makes it impossible to create postural control. When sensory integration and processing disorders are the source of the problem, our interventions must involve sensory-based strategies in order for postural control to improve. Without postural control, all other actions will be poorly orchestrated because there will be no stability on which to build movements. The sensory systems are the silent partners during occupational performance, creating a background on which to build purposeful movement (Horak, Henry, & Shumway-Cook, 1997).

Descending projections from vestibular nuclei connect with motor neurons in the cervical region of the spinal cord. These projections have their origin in the semicircular canals and as such regulate head position during rotary or angular movement. Other descending projections, originating in the otolith organ known as the *utricle*, activate motor neurons for trunk extensors directly and inhibit motor neurons for trunk flexors indirectly, leading to strong postural extension in response to a change in the relationship with gravity. These connections are crucial for our ability to maintain upright posture and balance (Purves et al., 2012).

The vestibular system also projects to the thalamus and on to the cortex. The cortical cells responding to vestibular inputs also respond to proprioceptive and visual inputs, suggesting a role in body orientation in and movement through space.

Exteroception: Vision and Hearing

Vision and hearing allow perceptions of events and objects in the world around us and distant from us. They inform us about the objects and people around us in a temporal-spatial context, contributing heavily to verbal and nonverbal language. The visual system is enormously complex, providing information about size, shape, color, and placement. The auditory system is concerned with distance, intensity, and range. These senses work in concert with the chemical and body senses by providing the maps about where we are so that we can understand what our bodies might need to do in response to environmental demands.

The Visual System. The visual system is responsible for mapping the spatial relationships in the world for us. Receptors are contrast (edge) and movement detectors (Purves et al., 2012). Receptor cells are rods and cones; rods are active during dimmed lighting, whereas cones are active in bright light. Shape and space are defined by these receptors based on a comparison between focal point and visual surround contrast. Rods, working in dim light, allow us to use any and all ambient light to define our visual world. In the dim world, we can see something but precision is missing because rods trade specificity for sensitivity. Cones, on the other hand, provide high acuity, color perception in lighted conditions. In order to capture our entire visual environment, the eye scans the visual environment, taking in contours and color, and sending this information to the brain for integration. In the absence of these quick and continual eye movements, or saccades, the visual scene "grays out."

Movement detection is a basic visual function and it is among the oldest of visual skills; movement within the environment draws the eye and enhances detection (Siegel & Sapru, 2011). Have you ever wished your car keys would just wiggle a little so you could see them? We often see things better once they begin to move; and for some visual systems, object movement is essential for vision.

Projections from the retina, the location of rods and cones, to the brain begin with the optic nerves. Some fibers in each optic nerves cross at the optic chiasm, merging to carrying information from left and right visual fields on to the optic tracts. The optic tracts contain fibers from both eyes—the fibers in the left optic tract transmit information from the right visual world and the fibers in the right optic tract transmit information from the left visual world. This pattern of fibers converging and reorganizing leads to specific visual losses with brain damage; occupational therapists must understand these patterns so that they can hypothesize about what functional challenges an individual might face with particular losses. For example, without use of the left eye (close your left eye to see what it is like), the person cannot fully capture visual input to the left side. The right eye's visual span covers part of the space in front of the left eye so the person does not lose all vision to the left (see Figure 56.3).

As we have seen with other sensory systems, visual information projects to the thalamus and on to the primary visual cortex. Here, we are able to process some

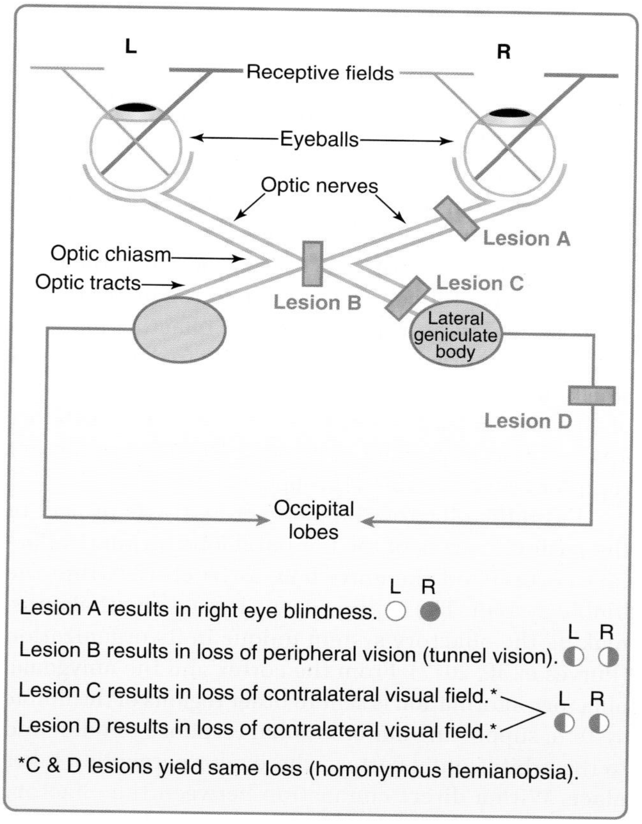

FIGURE 56.3 Neural lesions of visual field deficits. (Reprinted with permission from Dunn, W. [1997b]. Implementing neuroscience principles to support habituation and recovery. In C. Christiansen & C. Baum [Eds.], *Occupational therapy: Enabling function and well-being* [2nd ed.]. Thorofare, NJ: Slack.)

basics of visual orientation, motion, direction, and speed. From this point, visual information is further processed within other regions of the visual cortex and subsequently "streamed" forward along two pathways, one dorsal and the other ventral, both leading to the prefrontal cortex. The dorsal stream, which goes through the parietal cortex, is associated with movement detection. This projection may be important in our ability to navigate through the environment, direct eye movements to follow objects, and interpret objects as they move through space. The ventral stream, projecting through the temporal cortex, is important in color and form perception and, interestingly, facial recognition (Purves et al., 2012).

OT practitioners are well known for our expertise in visual motor skills. Attending to the complexity of the contributions of vision including ocular motor, visual perceptual, and visual motor control allows the therapist to determine the best strategies for supporting development of visually related skills and abilities. The visual system is most challenged by lack of contrast (e.g., misty, homogeneous environments) and also by overly busy environments (e.g., the contents of the junk drawer). Knowing this, therapists can be attentive to the contrasts in the visual environment to increase the chances that the person can detect important cues. For example, we can place a dark cloth on the work table to highlight white paper and writing utensils. We can also offer organizing strategies (e.g., sectioning off drawers) to increase the chances of finding things when they are needed. Working in concert with visual specialists, such as optometrists and ophthalmologists, is important for OT practitioners who have clients with these concerns.

The Auditory System. The auditory system processes sounds by detecting distance, direction, and sound quality; this enables us to orient within the environment. Receptors for this system are hair cells located in the cochlea of the inner ear. Through an interplay between structures in the outer and middle ear, sound waves create movement in fluid in the cochlea (endolymph). The cochlea is spiral shaped, such that it resembles a snail. Uncoiled, it is roughly triangular in shape with a membrane, the basilar membrane, running through the center. Sitting on top of this basilar membrane are the hair cells—the hairs of which are embedded in a second membrane, the tectorial membrane. Fluid movement creates movement of the basilar membrane and, consequently, the hair cells. Embedded in the tectorial membrane, the hairs bend, starting the process of neural transmission. Tone frequency differences are reflected in endolymph and basilar membrane movement differences; low-frequency sounds generate endolymph waves and basilar membrane movement from base to apex; high-frequency sounds will result only in movement at the base of the basilar membrane.

Information from the hair cells is projected to brain stem cochlear nuclei; from this point, the system gets increasingly complex. With connections in the pons, midbrain, and thalamus, auditory information eventually finds its way to the primary auditory cortex. A unique characteristic of the auditory system is the bilateral connections within the nervous system. Other sensory system input crosses to the opposite side of the brain when traveling to the cortex. When auditory input reaches the brain stem, information travels bilaterally to the cortex. This is important because bilateral connections create a safeguard for auditory input; both sides of the brain receive sounds from both sides of the world. When some auditory input is lost, we lose the ability to localize sounds but the brain continues to receive input bilaterally. The auditory system also has a feedback loop that sends information back to the cochlea; this feedback loop dampens the actions of some noises so that other sounds can be processed more clearly. This process, called *auditory figure-ground perception*, enables people to focus on the important sounds (e.g., the musician) and dampen the potentially interfering sounds (e.g., the person whispering next to you).

OT practitioners consider the impact of processing auditory information within context. The way in which clients perceive various sounds may contribute to their ability to attend such as being distracted by the hum of the lights while trying to listen to instructions. Practitioners may choose to suggest accommodations such as the use of noise-reduction head phones, changing context such as working in a quieter environment, and increasing volume such as the use of amplification systems if the individual has difficulty understanding. For example, we might suggest that a worker use earphones with music during work hours to increase focus on work and decrease distraction from other environmental sounds. We might suggest that a teacher give a student easier seatwork when working in the classroom and send the student to do more challenging work in the library. Working in concert with audiologists and speech and language pathologists who specialize in auditory processes is important for OT practitioners who have clients with these concerns.

The Chemical Senses

The chemical senses, taste (gustatory) and smell (olfactory), are tightly linked. These systems function together to enable us to perceive flavor; they are crucial to our ability to meet the needs of such physiologic drives as thirst and hunger and to our ability to avoid potentially harmful environmental chemicals.

The Gustatory System. We identify tastes by how the chemicals break down within our systems in the well-known categories of sweet, salty, sour, and bitter and the less well-known *umami*, sometimes likened to savory (Purves et al., 2012). We have an innate preference for sweet and an innate distrust of bitter. Giving consideration to the fact that breast milk is sweet, whereas many poisons are bitter adds some logic to this fact. Interestingly, taste preferences can be influenced by experience to overcome these innate tendencies; black coffee anyone? Still, our tastes are not so categorically simple, and we are able to determine a wealth of different tastes based on the combination of taste buds activated by the chemicals in our food.

Taste buds house our taste receptor cells. A typical person would be expected to have 2,000 to 5,000—more in younger and less in older people. Taste goes from the taste buds to the brain stem, then to the thalamus, and on to the sensory homunculus in the parietal lobe. Taste is compromised when there is brain stem trauma and with degenerative diseases that affect the thalamic and cortical regions that serve taste. Taste on the tongue has been mapped many times; but functionally, food appeals to us because of the overall experience we have with the food, including not only the taste but also the texture, temperature, and smell (i.e., intersensory integration of other senses with taste). People do not have universal reactions to tastes; for example, researchers have reported that some people taste caffeine and others do not (Reed, Toshiko, & McDaniel, 2006). Older adults often complain about foods being bland; this is because the reduction of taste receptor viability. Because the taste receptors recover in about 10 seconds, changing the flavors in the mouth during the meal (e.g., salty then sweet) can keep food interesting.

The Olfactory System. As noted earlier, smell and taste mingle, enabling us to enjoy the foods we eat. Like taste, smell also serves as a warning system, preventing us from eating things like rotten food or ingesting toxins. According to some reports, we can detect over 100,000 smells, of which only 20% are pleasant (Purves et al., 2012). We identify smells from the environment through a chemical reaction with the cells at the top of the nose. Olfactory receptor cells are located in the upper part of the nose, and they project first to the olfactory bulb in a highly precise organization. Our ability to detect various smells noted earlier comes from the activation of an array of olfactory bulbs, much like we saw within the gustatory system. Also in parallel with taste receptors, olfactory receptor cells are created throughout life.

From the olfactory bulb, olfactory tracts project to the piriform cortex of the temporal lobe (primary olfactory cortex) and the amygdala, a structure within the limbic system. These projections bypass the thalamus, making the olfactory system unique in its organization (Purves et al., 2012). From the cortex and the amygdala, olfactory information is sent to other regions of the limbic system, supporting our emotional response to odor, and to the orbitofrontal cortex, where odor perception takes place. With a direct connection between the olfactory and the limbic systems, smells are strongly associated with our emotions and memories. An odor can be comforting and triggering and bring back very vivid images of the past (positive and negative associations). Thus, the olfactory system is also directly linked to arousal mechanisms, which is why it can be so helpful in getting a response from people who are comatose. It is this powerful influence on our emotions and memories that we must keep in mind in practice. Clients might react strongly to smells that we are not even aware of, including personal hygiene products that we use. An acutely ill person, a person with severe disabilities, or someone with a limited sensory acuity in other sensory systems might recognize people and things by their smells as well, providing grounding and comfort in a confusing world. We must also be aware of the unfamiliar odors of a sterile environment and the comfort of familiar odors even if those odors are unpleasant to us. Entering a family's home can expose the therapist to pleasant and unpleasant odors that are differently perceived by family members.

Interoception

Although interoception historically has been primarily linked specifically to sensations generated within the viscera, the term can be more broadly interpreted to include the physiological condition of the entire body and the ability of visceral afferent information to reach awareness and affect behavior. Interoceptors do provide information about the physiological condition of the body and lay the foundation for maintenance of an optimal internal state (Purves et al., 2012). This is accomplished by monitoring events such as stomach distention (pain and discomfort) when we overeat; they also serve chemoreceptor functions such as monitoring and responding to changes in blood pH and detect temperature changes. These sensations serve to support local reflexes modulating ongoing visceral activity and to provide integrative regions of the CNS with information that supports higher level behavior and action. Direct activation of interoceptors elicits no noticeable sensation under normal circumstances. However, three distinct visceral sensations have been identified: no awareness (our typical state), awareness without pain (parasympathetic), and awareness with pain (sympathetic and parasympathetic). Input from interoceptors permits only vague discrimination of pain, and this underlies our difficulty pinpointing visceral discomfort and pain.

Sensory input from interoceptors is transmitted via fibers that project to lamina 1 of the spinal cord, joining the anterolateral system along with other tactile input. Lamina 1 fibers project to spinal cord and brain stem regions associated with both sympathetic and parasympathetic nervous systems. Lamina 1 fibers are also projected to the hypothalamus, an autonomic control center. Brain stem nuclei project interceptive input to regions of the thalamus and on to the dorsal insular cortex (primarily on the right or nondominant side), a region associated with the sense of physiological well-being (Andrew & Craig, 2002). The physiological state of the body is neurologically "rerepresented" in regions associated with limbic functions, a relationship that investigators link with our ability to have physical self-awareness. William James (1884) first proposed that visceral responses to biologically relevant sensory inputs were fundamental to our ability to experience emotion. This perspective coincides with that put forth by more recent theorists (Craig, 2002). Investigators are just beginning to unravel possible links between abnormal visceral function and conditions such as autism, warranting further consideration.

Summary

Although it is useful to examine each sensory system independently, it is crucial to appreciate the integration and interaction that occur within and between these systems. We alluded to the impact of multisensory integration earlier in this chapter; functions of the sensory systems are not fully understood when each is view as a separate entity. Although initial processing of sensation may be system specific, very little complex behavior can be traced to a single system because our experience is multimodal. For instance, although it is important to know that tactile shape perception is a function of activating the receptors that transmit over the dorsal column-medial lemniscal system and that visual shape perception is associated with the ventral stream projection of the visual system, tactile perception also lays a foundation for visual perception, largely through interactions within the parietal lobe. Likewise, knowledge of position of and movement through space requires the interaction of proprioceptive, vestibular, and visual systems.

Although our assessment may begin at the sensory system level, for instance, when we assess visual perception or vestibular responses to rotation, our interpretation of findings must consider multisystem interactions. Tools such as the Sensory Integration and Praxis Tests (SIPT) offer us the ability to assess the functions of some of our sensory systems, and interpretation leads us to examine the interface between sensory and motor systems. Ayres (1979) stated, "It is [not] appropriate to think in terms of isolated sensory modality development or function. That is not the major means by which the brain functions. It functions as a whole" (p. 31). Our ability to interact with people and things in our environments and to participate in the occupations that make up our daily lives require integration and processing of sensation, both within and across sensory systems. When integration and processing of sensation is inadequate, participation and occupational performance are at risk; when we do not adequately integrate and process sensation, we cannot interact adaptively with the environment.

Sensory Processing, Integration, and Occupation

SI and processing are fundamental to interpreting information from the environment and to learning. Ayres (2004) defined *sensory integration* as "the neurological process that organizes sensations from one's body and from the environment and makes it possible to use the

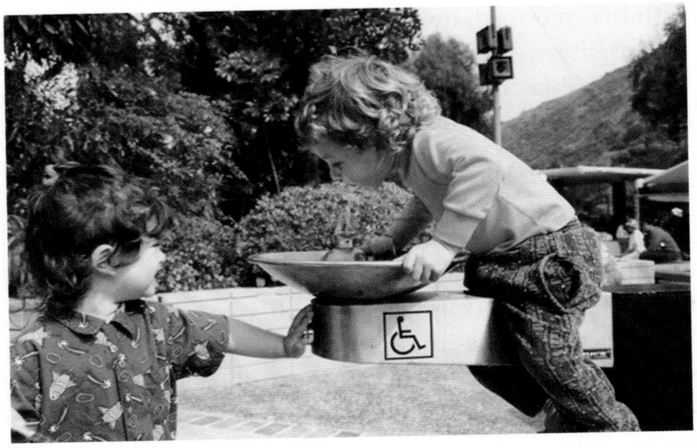

FIGURE 56.4 Children need various experiences to learn how to use their bodies in novel ways and how to balance, adjust, and coordinate their actions with the way things feel and come up with new and novel ways to interact with the environment. Interacting cooperatively with other people may require the most adaptive responses of all these skills.

body effectively in the environment" (p. 9). Sensation is used to guide an individual's engagement with people and objects in the environment—in other words, to engage in needed and desired occupations (see Figures 56.4 and 56.5).

Defining the Constructs Underlying Sensory Integration Processes

Research identifying the types and patterns of sensory integrative dysfunction is strong (Ayres, 1989; Mailloux et al., 2011; Mulligan, 1998a, 1998b, 2000). Ayres used various performance tests and clinical observations to assess individuals suspected of underlying sensory deficits. She conducted multiple factor and cluster analyses on the test results of children with learning disabilities to empirically identify patterns of dysfunction. Mulligan (1998a, 1998b, 2000) conducted confirmatory factor and cluster analyses that supported Ayres's original patterns of dysfunction. Using a current sample of children referred for OT evaluations, Mailloux et al. (2011) conducted a factor analysis using SIPT and sensory responsiveness data, again confirming the patterns of SI dysfunction originally identified by Ayres. These patterns include visual dyspraxia (difficulty with visual form and space perception and visual construction), somatodyspraxia (poor motor planning associated with poor tactile discrimination), **vestibular-related bilateral integration and sequencing difficulties** (poor processing of vestibular and proprioceptive information such that it interferes with bilateral integration and the

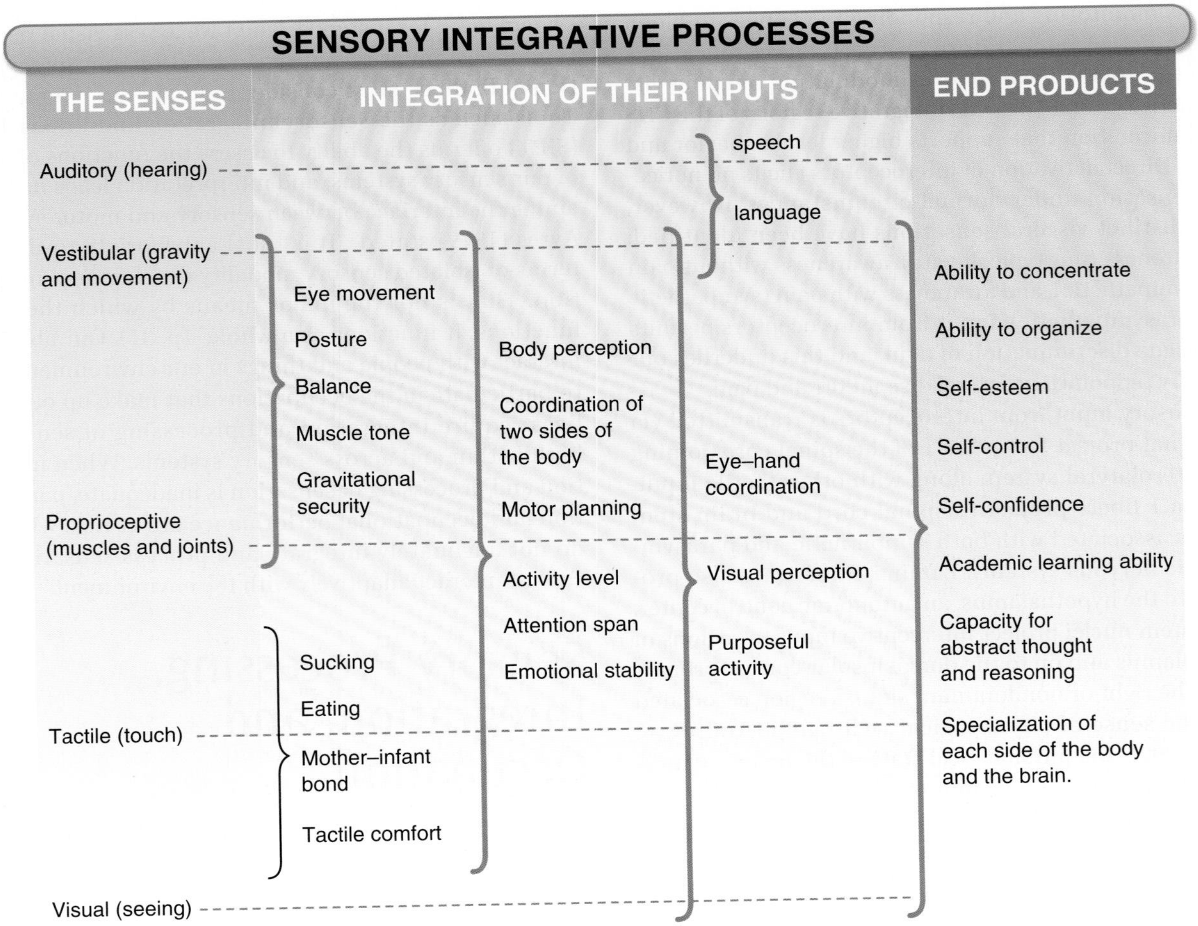

FIGURE 56.5 Ayres's flowchart.

ability to sequence tasks), tactile and visual discrimination, and tactile defensiveness with attention difficulties (Mulligan, 1998b, 2000; Mailloux et al., 2011). Subtypes of sensory responsiveness or modulation difficulties have also been identified through analysis of questionnaire and nonstandardized data (Ayres & Tickle, 1980; Brown & Dunn, 2002; Dunn, 1999, 2002b; Dunn & Bennet, 2002; Liss, Saulnier, Fein, & Kinsbourne, 2006; Miller et al., 1999). These studies suggest that sensory integrative dysfunction is not a single disorder but is a spectrum of disorders (Parham & Mailloux, 2010) related to the processes described in the following section.

Sensory Responsiveness and Modulation

Ayres (2005) proposed that the "combination of facilitatory and inhibitory messages produces modulation, which is the nervous system's process of self-organization" (p. 36). These modulatory processes are essential to **self-regulation**. Sensory responsiveness provides a means by which to determine the way in which an individual manages the intensity of changing sensory conditions from the body and the environment. Each individual will have unique thresholds for sensations or combinations of sensations that are pleasurable, neutral, or aversive.

Difficulties with sensory responsiveness are often observed as unusual, fluctuating, or extreme responsiveness (either over or under) to the intensity of one or more sensations during everyday activities that most individuals find pleasurable or neutral, such as grooming, eating, and social interactions. Specific behaviors may include auditory hyperacusis (oversensitivity to certain frequency ranges of sound); tactile defensiveness; gravitational insecurity (excessive emotional reactions in response to changes in movement or head position); aversion to movement, visual, or light sensitivity; feeling overwhelmed in high-stimulus environments, such as shopping malls; and under-responsiveness to touch, sound or movement (Koomar, 1995; May-Benson & Koomar, 2007; Weisberg, 1984). Unusual sensory responsiveness is often observed in concert with physiological regulation, external regulation, or self-regulation issues including colic, poor rhythmic respiration, digestion, and elimination; arousal and attention deficits; hyperactivity; anxiety and other signs of emotional instability; and social problems (DeGangi, 2000; DeGangi & Greenspan, 1988; Schaaf & Anzalone, 2001; Schaaf, Miller, Seewal, & O'Keefe, 2003; Williamson & Anzalone, 2001).

Sensory responsivity and modulation disorders have been identified as a feature of ASD for many years. As such, the basic science research on ASD can be examined to guide our understanding of these disorders. Early investigations capitalized on postmortem examination of the brain structure of individuals with an ASD. These studies identified reduced cell size and increased cell density in areas of the limbic system (i.e., hippocampus, amygdala) and the cerebellum (Purkinje cells) (Fatemi et al., 2002; Kemper & Bauman, 1998; Ritvo et al., 1986). Investigators have suggested that the structural differences reflect brain immaturity (Verhoeven, DeCock, Lagae, & Sunaert, 2010). It can be hypothesized that aspects of SOR seen in individuals with ASD are linked with the structural limbic system deficits; similarly, the cerebellar abnormalities may help explain the praxis difficulties often seen. However, it is important to emphasize that these differences reflect overall changes identified in the adult and associated with the full range of behaviors associated with ASD, not just related to SI and processing.

Other interesting investigations have involved neuroimaging of children with ASD. These studies document increased overall brain volume, most evident between ages 2 and 4.5 years and leveling off during adolescence (Courchesne et al., 2001; Tate, Bigler, McMahon, & Lainhart, 2007). It is hypothesized that this difference is related to increased neurogenesis, diminished cell pruning, or growth of nonneuronal tissue. Younger children with ASD also show reduced size in some regions of the cerebellum and enlarged amygdala (Verhoeven et al., 2010), which may impact function of systems elsewhere in the brain, including those involved in sensory and motor processing (Courchesne et al., 2001). Enlargement of one basal gangliar nucleus may also have some bearing on sensory modulation (Brambilla et al., 2003).

Cortisol is often referred to as the "stress" hormone because it is released in times of stress, allowing us to mount an effective response to the stressor. Considering poor sensory modulation, for instance, sensory over-responsiveness, to be a stressor suggests that examining cortisol in populations with sensory modulation deficits may shed light on SI and processing. Although there is some inconsistency in findings, evening values of cortisol, which is low in typical children, are elevated in children with ASD. This interesting finding is suggested to be due to greater response to the events of the day (Corbett, Mendoza, Wegelin, Carmean, & Levine, 2008). Further, children with ASD show great variability in the typical diurnal pattern, perhaps reflecting compromised ability to regulate stress response throughout the day. Corbett and colleagues (2008) suggest that sensory sensitivity may make children with ASD more susceptible to events of the day. In addition to examining cortisol in children with ASD, it has been studied in children with ADHD. For this group of children, sensitivity to sensory stimuli may influence the cortisol response to sensory challenge (Reynolds, Lane, & Gennings, 2010). It therefore appears that cortisol will be of continuing interest as we seek to learn more about SMD.

The autonomic nervous system (ANS) carries afferent information from our viscera and organs, connects to centers in the medulla and brain stem, and carries efferent signals back to the heart, the vascular system, and other body organs. Composed of the **parasympathetic** and **sympathetic nervous systems**, the ANS mediates our responses to such things as changes in posture, environmental conditions, and stressful experiences. It therefore makes sense to examine ANS functions as we try to understand the impact of

SMD. Research on ANS functions has indicated that some children with ASD show increased sympathetic activity in response to sensation (Ming, Juluc, Brimacombed, Connore, & Daniels, 2005) and others show diminished response patterns (Miller et al., 2001; Schoen, Miller, Brett-Green, & Hepburn, 2008); other patterns of modulation have also been recognized (Schoen, Miller, Brett-Green, Reynolds, & Lane, 2008; Schoen, Miller, Brett-Green, & Nielsen, 2009). In contrast, children with fragile X syndrome show strong sympathetic responses and recover from sensory challenge less well. Children with ADHD may have greater responses to sensory challenge (Mangeot et al., 2001); but in this population, it is possible that responsivity is related to anxiety (Lane, Reynolds, & Dumenci, in press; S. J. Lane et al., 2010). It has been suggested that SOR be considered in examining ADHD subtypes because it may contribute to many of the behaviors associated with the diagnosis (S. J. Lane et al., 2010; Parush, Sohmer, Steinberg, & Kaitz, 2007). Reduced baseline parasympathetic activity and less effective parasympathetic response mediation has also been found in children with SMD in response to sensory challenge (Ming et al., 2005; Schaaf et al., 2010; Schaaf et al., 2003). Diminished vagal tone, a reflection of reduced parasympathetic activity, has been linked with stress vulnerability and reactivity. Thus, poor sensory modulation appears to be linked with altered function of the ANS, and this warrants continued investigation.

Other investigators have examined brain wave response to sensation (event-related potential [ERP] or sensory-evoked potential [SEP]). These studies can inform us about how quickly a sensory stimulus reaches the brain and, to some extent, how the brain handles the sensory input. SEP can be investigated in the CNS at the cortical, brain stem, and spinal cord levels. Children with SPD show less effective sensory filtering (Brett-Green, Miller, Schoen, & Nielsen, 2010; Davies & Gavin, 2007) and more difficulty registering and processing brief auditory stimuli than either typical peers or adults (Davies, Chang, & Gavin, 2010). It has been suggested that these differences reflect difficulties discriminating and organizing sensations and result in difficulties using sensory input to interact with the environment (Gavin et al., 2011). In addition, the integration and processing of sensation at the brain stem (Hitoglou, Ververi, Antoniadis, & Zafeiriou, 2010) and cortical levels (Seri, Pisani, Thai, & Cerquiglini, 2007) has been shown to be disrupted in children with ASD.

Our understanding of the neural mechanisms underlying sensory responsivity and modulation is in its infancy. There is much to learn and much to be done in this area.

Sensory Discrimination

Sensory discrimination is information processing from one or more sensory channels that allows the individual to rapidly and accurately know the position of the body, relative distance to other people, details about the body and what is on the body, and details about the surrounding environment. *Sensory discrimination deficits* are a result of slow and inaccurate processing of one or more types of sensory information, under-responsiveness to sensation, inadequate perception formation, and poor sensory associations.

Consistent with findings from Ayres (1989), Mulligan (1998b), and Mailloux et al. (2011) factor analyses, sensory discrimination difficulties impact skilled environmental interactions. Vestibular-proprioceptive deficits will impact skilled body-centered interactions such as anticipatory and reactive postural control, lateralized skills, bilateral motor control, and sequencing. Discrimination difficulties with exteroceptors and chemical senses will affect interaction with objects and people. Tactile discrimination deficits are associated with poor fine motor skills and praxis. Visual perceptual deficits are associated with poor visual construction ability and visual motor skills. Auditory perceptual deficits often contribute to poor auditory language skills and the ability to figure out what to do based on verbal commands.

Praxis

Praxis is the ability to conceptualize, plan, and execute skilled tasks; it is a goal-directed motor action, supported through the processing of sensation (Blanche, 2001; Cermak, 2011). It involves coming up with an idea and problem-solving how to do it in context (May-Benson & Cermak, 2007). Sensation is seen as crucial to praxis during the processes of ideation, planning, and execution of action, and also in the sensory feedback we use to comprehend the impact of our actions on the environment. Ayres (1972a, 1972b) had hypothesized that sensory discrimination, particularly of tactile, visual, and auditory perception, provided the foundation for praxis and later, through several factor analyses, found a consistent relationship particularly between the tactile system and praxis.

Praxis requires somatosensory awareness of what one's body can do, exploration of people and things in the environment to know what they can do, and the urge to interact in new and novel ways based on needed and desired engagement. Each interaction has the potential to demand some level of praxis depending on the novelty of the situation and difficulty of the task. The child learning how to dive stands at the water's edge, positions his arms over his head, shifts his weight forward, tucks his chin against his chest, and then propels his body head first into the water. This series of sequential actions requires a cognitive understanding of the depth and property of the water in the pool; the ability to organize the time and space for the action and to predict the consequences of his actions, spatially locating the appropriate space in which to perform the dive; and the timing of the effort so that no one else is below or in front of him. The resulting sensory motor experiences from the activity are processed by the brain and this further informs the child about his body in relation to itself as well as to other people and objects in the environment. Importantly, the whole experience is then stored in memory for future reference; it will be used again when aspects of this skilled performance are needed to accomplish another task (Ayres, 1989, 2004).

There are many facets of praxis and thus various problems that can be identified, including poor ideation of creative activities. For example, the child in the sandbox who shovels sand into the pail and then pours it out and repeats the process but does not come up with the idea that she can "make a cake" by filling the pail with sand and a little water, and then turning the pail over to form a mound that she can then "decorate" shows poor ideation. Other praxis problems include somatodyspraxia, or poor use of the body to motor plan action sequences; poor use of language for sequencing and planning; poor ability to modify an action while in motion to enhance skill and precision; poor visual construction (e.g., difficulty replicating a block design); and poor ability to organize a task by breaking down the steps and organizing them in a proper sequence in future time and space.

Conceptualizing an action, or forming the idea about *what* one wants to do, is a critical aspect of praxis because it requires that we understand the **affordances** of objects in the context of their environment. This is ideation and it is a cognitive function (May-Benson, 2001; May-Benson & Cermak, 2007). Planning *how* one intends to engage in the task is also cognitive. A typical child observing a newly constructed playground with swings, slides, tree house, poles, and sand will have 101 ideas about what to do and will be able to develop plans to do them all. Similarly, a typical adult desiring to learn a new sport (i.e., golf) will likely have many ideas on how to begin the process and will be able to develop plans for action. The child or adult then sequences his or her ideas into motor actions: swinging, sliding, and digging for the child or approaching the ball, holding the club, and the mechanics of the golf swing for the adult. As the activity unfolds, both child and adult can modify the sequence of action or the challenge of the activity so that it is more fun and successful. The actual execution of the activity is the part of praxis that we can observe, and this is the part that we can assess to determine the individual's skills.

Significant overlap has been identified between the terms *dyspraxia* and *developmental coordination disorder* (DCD). In the end, many investigators and publications favor the use of the diagnosis "developmental coordination disorder" to cover the broad category of children with disorders in motor coordination that results in difficulties with activities of daily living (ADL). DCD is considered an appropriate term if the motor difficulties are developmental and not due to other medical condition or to intellectual disability (Gibbs, Appleton, & Appleton, 2006). The SI theory framework would add to this definition that children with dyspraxia must also be shown to have a deficit in the processing and use of sensation in the production of a motor response (Ayres, 1972a, 1979). See Appendix I for more details on DCD.

Many neuroscience investigations of deficits in praxis and the related diagnosis of DCD have focused on functions related to poor balance and postural control. Children with DCD have poor balance, although whether this is due to less than optimal processing of somatosensory, visual, or vestibular inputs remains controversial (Cermak & Larkin, 2002; Fong, Lee, & Pang, 2011; Grove & Lazarus, 2007; Inder & Sullivan, 2005). Investigations have been directed toward the cerebellum because postural control and motor coordination are both linked with this structure. Multiple cerebellar functions have been identified as problematic in children with DCD including postural control, anticipatory movement, timing of muscle recruitment, and motor adaptation (Cantin, Polatajko, Thach, & Jaglal, 2007; Kagerer, Contreras-Vidal, Bo, & Clark, 2006; Polatajko & Cantin, 2006). Further, children with DCD do poorly on tests of cerebellar function such as finger-to-nose touching and diadokokinesis (O'Hare & Khalid, 2002). Difficulties with the use of mental imagery, also identified in children with DCD, may be the result of inadequate cerebellar activation (Deconinck et al., 2008), inadequate parietal lobe processing (Katschmarsky, Cairney, Maruff, Wilson, & Currie, 2001), or both.

More current work using functional magnetic resonance imaging suggests that children with DCD use different regions of the brain when performing a tracing task when compared to typical children. Zwicker, Missiuna, Harris, and Boyd (2010) found that although motor performance was not substantially different between the two groups of children, children with DCD showed greater activation of brain areas associated with the processing of spatial information. These regions were in the parietal lobe and the cerebellum. Children with DCD appeared to rely heavily on visual information, perhaps because the somatosensory feedback from joint and muscle movement did not provide a sufficient motor reference for movement. Of additional interest, children with DCD activated many more regions of the brain than did typical children when engaging in the same motor challenge. Children with DCD often experience physical fatigue as they engage in motor tasks; this new finding suggests that they may also experience cognitive fatigue in the planning and execution of movement (Zwicker et al., 2010).

There is a wealth of research being conducted on praxis and DCD, and it will enrich our understanding of dyspraxia as we learn more about how the processing of sensation underlies ideation, planning, and execution of movement.

Assessment of Sensory Integration and Processing

Although some education in SI theory and intervention principles is part of the entry-level curricula for OT practitioners, postgraduate training is recommended when specializing in the assessment and intervention of sensory processing and integration in practice. Occupational therapists with certification in SI and mentorship with a master clinician are best prepared to evaluate and provide ASI intervention. OT assistants may provide intervention using ASI principles with appropriate supervision from an occupational therapist (Miller-Kuhaneck & Smith Roley, 2005).

Sensory integration and processing cannot be observed directly, which is why Ayres (2005) used the term "hidden disabilities" when referring to sensory integrative dysfunction. The practitioner must rely on information from interviews, direct observations, and structured and unstructured assessments of skills and abilities related to occupational performance in order to understand the way in which the individual is processing information (Windsor, Smith Roley, & Szklut, 2001).

Ayres (1989) provided a model for observing SI and praxis that culminated in a series of standardized tests, nonstandardized clinical observations, and questionnaires about sensory responsiveness. The SIPT (Ayres, 1989) include 17 tests that assess visual perception; visual motor control; two and three dimensional construction; tactile discrimination; kinesthesia; vestibular-related functions, including postrotary nystagmus and balance; bilateral motor coordination and sequencing; and praxis, including following unfamiliar verbal directions, imitation of body and oral-facial gestures, and visual-motor planning.

It is recommended that practitioners augment standardized assessment with clinical observations of neuromotor functions, play, responses to sensation, and ideation and praxis during structured and unstructured activities (Blanche, 2002; Blanche & Reinoso, 2008; May-Benson & Cermak, 2007; Mutti, Martin, Sterling, & Spalding, 2010; Reisman & Hanschu, 1992; Wilson, Pollock, Kaplan, & Law, 2000). Client, parent, and teacher questionnaires, such as the *Sensory Profile* series (Brown & Dunn, 2002; Dunn, 1999) and the Sensory Processing Measure (Parham et al., 2007) are created for use with clients of varied age ranges and contexts (home, school). Additional assessments are available that provide insights into sensory processing, integration, and praxis. For a list of assessment tools that may be used to assess many aspects of SI and processing, refer to Table 56.4 as well as Appendix II for more details.

Intervention Planning and Implementation

OT, using a sensory integrative approach, is guided by the evaluation data obtained using tools specific to the sensory integration theory and coupling this with information obtained from a client's occupational profile (American Occupational Therapy Association [AOTA], 2008). Assessment specific to SI and processing skills and abilities provides essential knowledge about client strengths and weaknesses in the use of sensation in everyday life. Based on the information from the occupational profile, the therapist considers the identified occupationally related outcomes that are important to the client, family and caregivers, and the reimbursement agency. The analysis of performance provides detailed information on client factors, performance skills, and patterns that contribute to the development of interventions customized specifically to the client, therapeutic activities, and environmental modifications.

Direct intervention most often involves provision of services within a specialized therapeutic environment that includes various equipment designed to address needs in the areas of sensory modulation, perception, and praxis. Intrinsic to direct intervention is the impact of the practitioner on the intervention. The therapeutic use of self, a crucial aspect of any OT intervention, is an essential element in the application of the SI and processing theoretical propositions; the way therapists use their body and tone of their voice, how they pace and create flow within the session, the activities they create with the client and involved caregivers, and the contextual framework around activities and interactions all significantly impact the ability to develop and maintain a therapeutic relationship (Ayres, 1979). In conjunction with direct therapy, additional therapeutic activities characteristically include regulatory strategies such as a "sensory diet" that can be implemented throughout the day and environmental modifications or accommodations that capitalize on the **sensory-related affordances** available. Strategies and environmental modifications are designed to meet the sensory needs of the individual in various contexts. Additionally, education and consultation is required to support the family and caregivers so that the team understands the relationship of the individual's sensory integrative functions to participation in daily life activities.

Central to intervention using SI principles is a unique philosophy that reflects Dr. Ayres's sense of trust, compassion, and respect for individuals (Spitzer & Smith Roley, 2001). Ayres originally developed SI methods for children, adolescents, and adults with sensory perceptual disorders. Although most of its use is in the area of pediatrics, the theoretical foundation is relevant to people of all ages. Ayres proposed that intervention delivered in a playful style at the client's level could elicit his or her "inner drive" to learn and develop; the need to tap into inner drive is no less important for adolescents or adults. When we engage a client according to the needs of his or her own nervous systems, the activity serves as its own reward. In this way and in parallel with changes reported on use of enriched environments (Diamond, Rosenzweig, Bennett, Lindner, & Lyon,1972; Kempermann & Gage, 1999), Ayres (1972a) anticipated that intervention would facilitate enhanced neuronal growth and development leading to increased skills in daily life activities.

Research on sensory deprivation and investigations relative to the lack of the appropriate amounts and types of stimulation during critical developmental periods demonstrates that sensory input does in fact play a role

TABLE 56.4 Assessments Useful in Identifying Strengths and Needs in Sensory Integration and Processing[a]

Assessment Tool	Application
Assessment of Preterm Infant Behavior	Assesses function and integration of five systems: physiological, motor, state, attention/interactive, and regulatory
Bayley Scales of Infant and Toddler Development, 3rd Edition (Bayley-III)	Assesses adaptive behavior, cognition, language, motor development, and social-emotional development; behaviors relative to sensory integration and processing can be inferred.
Beery-Buktenica Developmental Test of Visual-Motor Integration for Children, 6th Edition (Beery VMI)	Assesses visual motor skills; inference can be made relative to visual praxis.
Bruininks-Oseretsky Test of Motor Proficiency, 2nd Edition (BOT-2)	Assesses gross and fine motor skill, including balance and bilateral skills; observation of performance can provide information on motor planning.
Checklist of environmental factors	Qualitative data about physical, emotional, and social aspects of the environment; may be useful for examining environmental "fit" for children with sensory integration and processing needs
DeGangi-Berk Test of Sensory Integration	Screens postural control, bilateral motor integration, and reflex integration
Developmental Test of Visual Perception, 2nd Edition Developmental Test of Visual Perception—Adolescent and Adult	Visual perception and visual-motor integration; inferences can be drawn relative to visual praxis.
Dynamic Occupational Therapy Cognitive Assessment for Children Dynamic Loewenstein Occupational Therapy Cognitive Assessment Dynamic Loewenstein Occupational Therapy Cognitive Assessment—Geriatric	Dynamic assessment of cognitive abilities and learning potential
Early Coping Inventory	Coping effectiveness across three categories: sensorimotor organization, reactive behavior, and self-initiated behavior
Family Environment Scale	Family's assessment of social-environmental characteristics, family relationships (support, expression of feelings, and conflict), personal growth of family and family members, and system maintenance (organization and control of family life)
Family Needs Scale	Assists families in clarifying concerns and defining nature of their needs
First STEP (Screening Test for Evaluating Preschoolers)	Identifies preschool children at risk for developmental delays across five domains: cognitive, communication, motor, social/emotional, and adaptive behavior; inferences can be drawn about sensory integration and processing.
Functional Emotional Assessment Scale	Examination of sensory integration and processing reflected in parent/child play with toys: symbolic play toys, tactile-play toys, and vestibular situations
Home Observation for Measurement of the Environment (HOME)-Revised	Examines quality and quantity of social, emotional, and cognitive support available to children in the home environment and factors that facilitate or limit play; can help in examination of environmental/child goodness of fit
Imitation of gestures	Examines body scheme and motor planning
Impact on Family Scale	Examines impact of a child's chronic illness on financial, social/family, personal strain, mastery, sibling strain relative to family functioning
Infant/Toddler Symptom Checklist	Examines predispositions towards developing sensory integration disorders, attention deficits, emotional behavioral problems, and learning difficulties
Miller Assessment for Preschoolers	Screening for sensory integration and processing and impact on motor skills and behaviors
Miller Function & Participation Scales	Examines development in fine, gross, and visual motor skills, functional, play, and school-based activities

Continued

TABLE 56.4 Assessments Useful in Identifying Strengths and Needs in Sensory Integration and Processing[a] *(Continued)*

Assessment Tool	Application
Mullen Scales of Early Learning	Five scales provide a complete picture of cognitive and motor ability including: Gross Motor, Visual Reception, Fine Motor, Expressive Language, and Receptive Language.
Newborn Individualized Developmental Care and Assessment Program (NIDCAP) (Revised)	Naturalistic observation of infant in the nursery or home relative to response to environmental input and caregiver routine
Parent Needs Survey	Information regarding the needs of families in areas such as treatment for the child, formal and informal support for family, eliminating competing family needs, and needs for information
Parenting Stress Index	Identifies specific parenting stress factors; helps parents understand importance of creating positive environment
Questionnaire on Resources and Stress for Families	Measures stress and coping in families caring for ill relatives; covers three domains: personal problem for responders, family problems, and problems for patient/ill family member
School Observation-Environment	Observation of general environment, sensory environment, and a particular environment
Sensory Integration and Praxis Tests (SIPT)	Assesses praxis and sensory integration and processing of vestibular, proprioceptive, tactile, kinesthetic, and visual systems
Sensory Integration Observation Guide	Parent reports regarding infant sensory responsiveness on four factors: tactile-kinesthetic, vestibular-proprioceptive, adaptive motor, and regulatory
Sensory Profile	Measures response to routine sensation across the following eight categories: auditory, visual, taste/smell, movement, body position, touch, activity level, and emotional/social
Sensory Processing Measure	Identifies sensory concerns; helps determine if sensory integration difficulties influence a child's behaviors in school, at home, and in the community
Test of Ideational Praxis	Score based on assessment of a child's ability to demonstrate awareness of object affordances
Test of Sensory Functions in Infants	Measures sensory processing responsivity in five domains: tactile deep pressure, visual-tactile integration, adaptive motor, ocular motor, and responsivity to vestibular stimuli

[a]See Appendix II for more details.

in the developmental process (Cermak & Daunhauer, 1997; Lin, Cermak, Coster, & Miller, 2005; Thelen & Smith, 1994). This research supports Ayres's assumption that sensations impact dynamic human systems. Further, the research indicates that SI and processing theories help to explain why OT practitioners propose the need for the use of skilled and nurturing sensory supportive interventions.

Hallmark Features of Ayres Sensory Integration® Intervention

SI methods, as originally proposed by Ayres (1972a), are showing promising evidence (Pfeiffer et al., 2011; Schaaf, 2011). In an effort to be able to accurately identify the use of these methods from other methods, the ASI Fidelity Measure© was created (Parham et al, 2007). The structural and process elements of ASI intervention outlined in this measure are indicated in Box 56.1 (Parham et al., 2011).

Basic Tenets of Ayres Sensory Integration®

The basic tenets of ASI include the following:

- *Integrated sensation* is "nourishment for the brain" (Ayres, 1979).
- *Adaptive responses* are required to successfully meet challenges essential for growth and development (Ayres, 1972a). The adaptive response is essential to increased SI.
- The *inner drive* of the human being invites the experience of life. It is this motivation to enjoy life that Dr. Ayres wished to engage during intervention.

BOX 56.1 Structural and Process Elements of Ayres Sensory Integration® Intervention

Structural elements include the following:

- Professional qualification and expertise—A qualified therapist with an understanding of therapeutic methods and neurobiological principles of SI theory and its methods; postgraduate certification in SI is available for occupational therapists, speech and language pathologists, and physical therapists only.
- Appropriate evaluation as previously discussed.
- Communication with family and other related professionals.
- Therapeutic environment—The therapeutic environment designed by Ayres was unique in its ability to safely provide opportunities for vestibular, proprioceptive, and tactile sensations and adaptive motor responses. Although commercially available equipment is now readily available, Ayres used simple and readily available objects such as tires and ropes, wood boards, hula hoops, and rocker boards and created unusual obstacle courses and games with them. She used ceiling beams and devices so that she could suspend equipment that allowed the client to swing safely through space. She invented this equipment as the need arose for individual clients.

Process elements include the following:

1. Safe environment—The therapist scaffolds success emotionally, physically, cognitively, and socially.
2. Environmental affordances—Providing environmental affordances (the opportunities that the environment affords individuals to do things) that invite interactions with the environment including space to move and jump and crash and items that stimulate creativity and engagement.
   a. The use of sensory opportunities that feature varied and appropriate vestibular, tactile, and proprioceptive sensations including thick mats, large overstuffed pillows, swings, ramps, ladders, ropes, targets, manipulatives, balls, vibrating toys, various textures such as stretchy soft or furry fabrics, brushes, props, and materials used during daily routines.
   b. The environment has flexible arrangement of equipment and space to move and swing and crash.
3. Therapist-client interactions (scaffolding).
   a. Collaborates with client in activity choices (child directed): The therapist does not predetermine the type and quantity of activities in which the client will engage but cocreates the activities according to the needs and interests of the client and his or her ability to be adaptive. Intervention based on SI theory is *child directed* in that the therapist vigilantly observes the child to understand the current capabilities, structures the activities around the interests and abilities of the child, and engages the child by eliciting his or her *intrinsic motivation* to play. "When the therapist is doing her job effectively and the child is organizing his nervous system, it looks as if the child is merely playing" (Ayres, 2005, p. 142).
   b. Creates, encourages, and ensures child's success.
   c. Supports child's intrinsic motivation to play. The therapist is a partner in play themes and activities and a source of pleasure and assistance.
4. Facilitates the adaptive response.
   a. Modifies activities for the "just-right challenge".
   b. Supports sensory modulation and responsiveness for more regulated arousal, emotion, attention, and activity level.
   c. Supports postural, ocular, oral, and bilateral motor control.
   d. Supports ideation, motor planning, and organization of behavior: assisting in organization of behavior relative to physically interacting with objects and people in time and space including the opportunity to rearrange the environment and the way in which it is used (Parham et al., 2007).
5. Provided within professional practice towards relevant outcomes.
   a. Health and participation.
   b. Creation of identity through engagement in activities.
   c. Building sense of self, creativity, and exploration.
   d. Builds performance skills and patterns.
   e. Assists in occupational performance generalized across settings.
   f. Builds foundation for future occupations.

- *Active participation* promotes organization.
- Artful vigilance is essential on the part of the therapist in order to facilitate the *just-right challenge.*

Therapeutic activities to address the identified deficits are designed with specific attention to the contribution of the tactile, proprioceptive, and vestibular sensations to function (see Figures 56.6, 56.7, and 56.8).

- Special consideration is given to include proprioception in the form of active movement and heavy work activities. Heavy work activities are those that require effort and provide enhanced proprioceptive feedback about action; pulling or pushing a big mat into place or other activities that provide resistance to movement are examples of heavy work. Proprioception exerts a regulatory influence on other sensations (Blanche & Schaaf, 2001).
- Vestibular activities are especially important so that the client can develop the capacity to hold the body upright against gravity while holding still and while moving (Ayres, 1972a). Processing vestibular information is important for the development of the sense of space and navigation (Berthoz, 2000).
- Tactile information is essential for refined interactions with the external, social, and physical environment (Ayres, 1972a, 2005; Montegue, 1986).

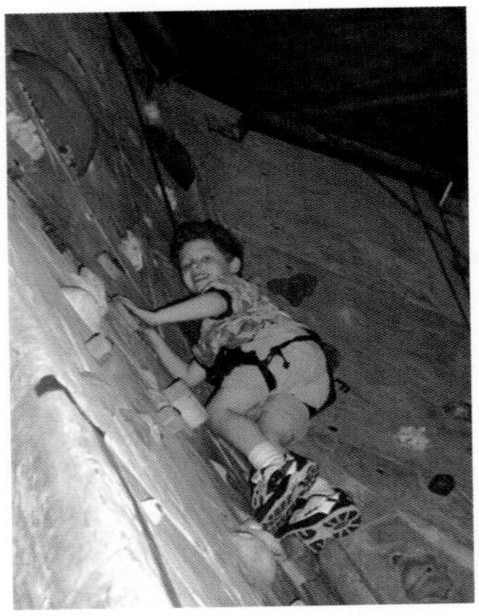

FIGURE 56.6 Rock climbing is a heavy-work, proprioceptive activity requiring muscular exertion, body awareness, and resisting the pull of gravity, helping him stay organized and alert while concentrating on his foot and hand placement.

Tables 56.5, 56.6, and 56.7 provide information on the various considerations when grading sensory-based activities.

When using SI intervention strategies, the practitioner will provide a balance of structure and freedom so that clients will have opportunities to problem-solve and make some of their own choices. Some essential characteristics that differentiate SI methods from other approaches are freedom within the structure of a sensory-rich environment, the ability to physically move through space and move objects in space, and the assistance of the practitioner so that the client can learn to use his or her body in new and novel ways, thus increasingly more complex possibilities for physical engagement will emerge. Interventions using ASI are not to be confused with those that use sensory stimulation due to the imperative of the adaptive response and modification of the activity based on the client's response (Anzalone & Murray, 2002). It is not practitioner planned and designed, but rather, the practitioner sets up the structure and possibilities in which the client's interests and ability to cope with the sensory, motor, and organization demands dictate the level of challenge and intensity of the activities. Therefore, the equipment does not stay in the same place each time and the therapy does not follow an orderly and predictable sequence, making each session somewhat novel. The intervention is not provided with the expectation of a subsequent reward. The activities are intended to be fun and inviting and therefore are rewarding in and of themselves. Play is one of the most important and powerful features of the process of intervention using SI strategies and one that facilitates the intrinsic reward of occupational engagement (Bundy, 2002).

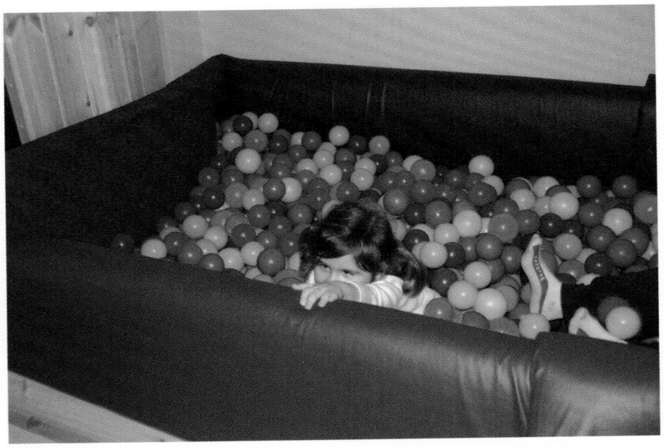

FIGURE 56.7 Playing in a ball pool provides transient and deep pressure tactile stimulation and resistance to movement, increasing the child's body awareness.

Sensory integrative and processing deficits commonly occur in individuals with diagnoses such as ASD, fragile X syndrome, and cerebral palsy; both clinical experience and research indicate that these children will benefit from various approaches in addition to SI methods (Mailloux, 2001; Mailloux & Smith Roley, 2010; Schaaf & Smith Roley, 2006; Smith Roley et al., 2001). During a typical OT session, SI methods are often used in conjunction with complementary methods such as play-based approaches (Burke & Mailloux, 1997; Knox & Mailloux, 1997), developmental and behavioral approaches (Anzalone & Murray, 2002), and cognitive approaches such as the Alert Program for Self-Regulation (Williams & Shellenberger, 1996). This is especially true for children with multiple impairments.

Goals of Occupational Therapy Using Sensory Strategies

The principles of ASI applied within OT practice result in improved occupational engagement and social participation for clients (Case-Smith & Bryant, 1999; Linderman & Stewart, 1999; Miller, Coll, & Schoen, 2007; Miller, Schoen, James, & Schaaf, 2007; Roberts, King-Thomas, & Boccia, 2007). To accomplish the overarching goals of OT, SI intervention strategies are used to facilitate adaptive responses in various domains. In addition to the somatomotor adaptive response described by Ayres (1972a), Parham and Mailloux (2010, p. 393) described the following potential outcomes from intervention using SI strategies:

- Increase in the frequency or duration of adaptive responses
- Cognitive, language, and academic skills

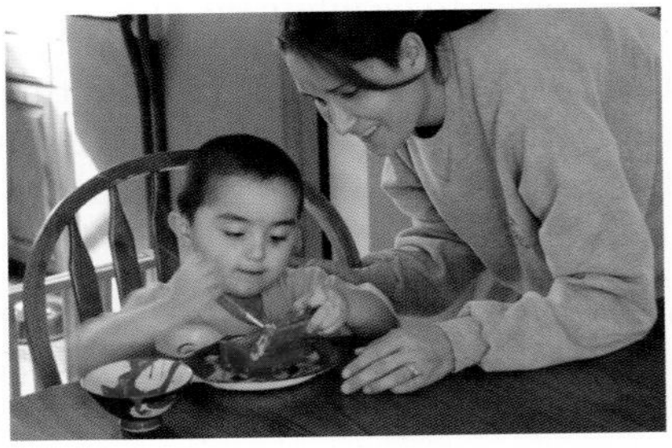

FIGURE 56.8 Following vigorous play, this client more easily engages in this activity with his mother that involves tactile media, spatial organization, and visual motor control.

TABLE 56.5 Variables Related to Vestibular Sensations

Client Factors	Types of Vestibular Sensations	Environmental Condition
Head Position		**Visual Field**
Prone	Linear (vertical and horizontal)	Stable
Supine	Rotary (around in circles)	Moving
Vertical and Upright	Axial (around the body)	
Quadruped	Orbital (in an axis outside of the body)	
Head tilted	Arc	
Side lying	Coriolis (three types at once)	
Inverted		
Head Movement		
Static		
Transient		
In motion		
Body Status		**Physical Environment**
Static	Speed, intensity	Stable
Moving	Duration, rhythmicity	Moving
Passive	Stop and start	
Active	Changes in direction	

- Gross and fine motor skills
- Self-confidence and self-esteem
- Enhanced occupational performance and social participation
- Enhanced family life

The diverse array of possibilities makes it difficult to exactly predict the areas of life that may change as a result of intervention using SI strategies (Mailloux et al., 2007). Traditionally, effectiveness of pediatric OT intervention has focused on skills such as improved handwriting or improved balance or ball skills. These outcomes alone are insufficient to capture the dynamic and pervasive changes in an individual's quality of life. Reports from parents include comments such as the following:

"My child and family are happier."
"My life is easier."
"My child now has friends."
"I can actually cook dinner without disruption."
"My kids play together longer without needing me to intervene."
"I feel like I am brave enough to try a family vacation."
"Occupational therapy is the first place I've been where I feel like they understood what I'm going through."

TABLE 56.6 Variables Related to Proprioceptive Sensations

Client Factors	Types of Proprioceptive Sensations	Environmental Condition
Muscles	Stretch	Distance/size/dimension
Tendons	Traction—pull	With or against gravity
Joints	Compression—push	Time
At rest	Coactivation—cocontraction	Physical environment
Transient	Isometric/isotonic	Stable
In motion	Speed, intensity	Moving
Static/dynamic	Duration/rate/rhythm	
Active/passive	Direction	
Effort exerted	Resistance	
Motivation or purpose	Tension/weight-bearing load	

TABLE 56.7 Variables Related to Tactile Sensations

Client Factors	Types of Tactile Sensations	Environmental Condition
Head	Light touch	Familiar versus unfamiliar object
Face including cheeks, mouth, tongue, and ears	Deep pressure	Familiar versus unfamiliar person
Hands	Texture	Intensity of other stimuli in the environment
Feet	Temperature	Task demands
Limbs	Sharp/dull/pain/numbness	Intention of person touching
Front	One and two point	Time of day
Back		Cultural norms
Avoid ventral midline		
While stressed or relaxed (existing arousal level and arousability)	Transient	
Amount of surface area	Sustained	
Anticipated versus expected	Intermittent	
Unanticipated versus unexpected	Duration	
Self versus other initiated	Rhythm	
Prior experiences	Frequency	

"It is nice to see someone playing with my child, and it showed me another way to view my child in a more positive light."

"I wish that I knew about this when I was younger, but at least now (as an adult), I can understand myself better and work with my occupational therapist to address these issues."

Cohn, Miller, and Tickle-Degnen (2000) found that parents of children with sensory modulation disorders who brought their children to OT using an SI approach hoped that intervention would enable their child's participation in school, home, and community contexts and support their parenting role. In this study, the parents reported a desire to learn strategies to help their child achieve increased social participation, self-regulation, and competence. In a subsequent study focused on valued outcomes after receiving intervention for their children, Cohn (2001a) found that parents valued an increased understanding of their child's behavior as well as the validation of their parenting efforts and being able to advocate for services for their children. Cohn (2001b) also identified that the ritual of waiting for their children in the waiting room at the clinic site afforded the parents the opportunity to share resources, validate their experiences, and engage in social dialogue with others. In fact, this naturally occurring support for parents helped them to reframe their views and expectations of their children. This work broadens the potential outcomes related to OT using a sensory integrative approach to include family perspectives and consider participation and quality of life as meaningful outcomes.

Structured and unstructured observations of occupational performance continue to be useful ways to measure progress. For children such as those with ASD, progress is often not reflected on formalized measures. Mailloux et al. (2007) suggest using Goal Attainment Scaling (GAS) to measure valued outcomes. GAS is a method of setting achievable goals in conjunction with the family that may prove to be useful in capturing significant changes as the result of intervention. Mailloux et al. (2007) gives the following example:

CONCERN: Inability to participate in a family dinner due to oversensitivity to textures, tastes, smells, and sounds.

GOAL: To be able to participate in a family meal at home, at friends' and relatives' homes, and at a restaurant by decreasing oversensitivity to textures, smells, tastes, and noises.

Once defined, behaviors that reflect scaled goal attainment are defined, with scaling that may range from −2 (much less than expected level: tolerates the family eating area during mealtime without signs of discomfort or distress [e.g., crying, gagging, whining, or leaving the table or room], four of five opportunities) to 2+ (much better than expected level: eats multiple bites of two new foods without signs of discomfort or distress [e.g., crying, gagging, whining, or leaving the table or room], four of five opportunities) (Mailloux et al., 2007).

CASE STUDY 56.1 Larissa

Referral

Larissa is an energetic 4-year-old girl who loves to play but does not seek out play with other children. She does not seem to mind them, but she is happy playing alone or alongside others. She has good attachment to her mother and relies on her for guidance and nurturing, which her mother readily and effectively provides. Larissa is happiest if she is close to her mother day and night. Household routines are difficult for the family. Larissa loves to take a bath and often does not want to get out. Larissa does not want to stop playing to do general hygiene tasks, making routine activities such as toothbrushing difficult. Errands, shopping, or spontaneous outings are problematic because Larissa is overly active and tires easily when she has to stand in line or wait. Larissa's mother has learned to provide her three children a time to prepare for transitions; otherwise, Larissa or one of her older brothers, ages 5 and 8 years, may have tantrums. Larissa is not currently attending preschool due to excessive crying and poor interactions including aggression with peers.

Larissa's mother requested an occupational therapy evaluation to determine if there were services available that provided assistance with parenting and support to her child's development. She reported that her life is very difficult. She always had difficulty organizing herself; and now with three children and a husband, sometimes she feels that her life is unmanageable. She decided to focus on services for the youngest child first but feels that all of her children and herself need assistance to varying degrees.

Occupational Profile:

When asked what Larissa likes to do during the day, her mother replied:

If I'm not in the room when she wakes up, she will cry or whine "mommy" until I come in. She then wants to nurse until she is completely awake. I usually carry her downstairs and she starts playing with little toys. It's a little hard to stop playing but she usually climbs into her chair for breakfast and eats neatly. When she's done she sometimes puts her hands in her warm cereal and smears it on herself, the table, her head . . . and has a good time with it. She likes to touch everything wherever we go. She LOVES to play out back with water, dirt, and mud. She usually gets herself all wet with the hose and has several changes of clothes a day. She likes to play in the sand, lie in the sand with her face in the sand, and eat the sand. She loves the bath but I usually have to take her out early for hitting her brothers or pouring water out of the tub. Then she screams, cries, and tries to get back in the bath. Eventually she calms down and lies down or jumps on the bed. She never wants to put her clothes on, but when she is very tired, she will.

Through the process of creating an occupational profile for Larissa, the therapist also determined that Larissa's mother has organizational difficulties and possibly dyspraxia. Mom's strengths and difficulties played a role in determining the next steps in this process. Larissa's high activity level, anxiety, and sensory-seeking behaviors interfered with her ability to cope with and engage in typical daily occupations and attend preschool. Additionally, her behaviors created situations in which her mother was unable to carry out her daily activities without upset, contributing to family stress. The therapist recommended direct intervention for Larissa and consultation for the family especially her mother to support her management of daily routines. The therapist recommended a standardized evaluation using the Sensory Integration and Praxis Tests (SIPT). The following scores indicate a subtle but significant problem in sensory integration (see Figure 56.9).

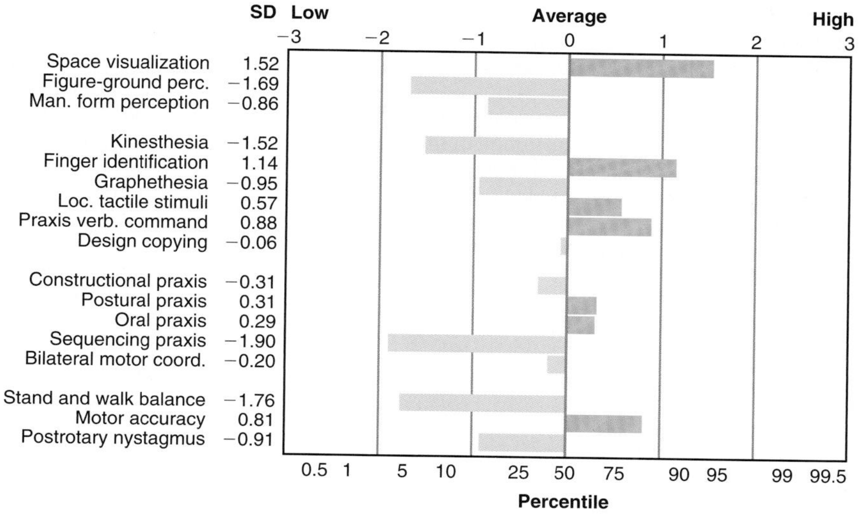

FIGURE 56.9 Larissa. Sensory Integration and Praxis Tests (SIPT) scores at age 4 years.

(continued)

CASE STUDY 56.1 Larissa (*Continued*)

CASE INFORMATION

Child's First Name: Larissa
Child's Year in School: Preschool
Child's Age: 4 years 0 months
Parent/Guardian(s) Name: Jamie

EVALUATION

Reasons for Referral (include the occupational concerns/desires for the child and family):
Clingy, tantrums easily, fights with siblings, difficulty taking her to grocery store, not interested in playing with other children.

Background Information

Medical History: OK
Developmental History: Normal milestones. Concerns regarding balance, activity level, self-regulation, and social skills
Educational History: N/A
Occupational History/Profile: (see the aforementioned narrative)

Evaluation of Occupational Performance

Interview data:

- Teacher report:
- Guardian Report:
  (see the aforementioned)
- Others:

Observation data:

Strengths:
Bright
Affectionate
Good attachment with parents
Good fine motor
Enjoys tactile play

Challenges:
Does not seek interactions with other children
Sensitivity to sounds
Excessively seeks tactile play
Poor interactions with other children
Inattention to task
Poor sustained sitting
Difficulty adapting to transitions and high-stimulus environments

Test data:

Structured assessments:
See SIPT scores

Unstructured assessment:
Mildly low muscle tone
Difficulty imitating movement sequences

Interpretation:
Vestibular and bilateral integration and sequencing issues

INTERVENTION

Goals and Objectives

By (date): To demonstrate improved fine motor and self-care skills, Larissa will use two hands to independently don and doff socks and shoes when given minimal physical assistance, 4 of 5 opportunities.

By (date): To demonstrate improved organization of behavior during social interactions, Larissa will engage in play with another child, for 10 minutes of turn-taking interaction, when given no more than 3 prompts, 4 of 5 opportunities.

By (date): To demonstrate improved balance and postural/protective reactions for increased participation, Larissa will execute smooth and efficient movement patterns with her trunk and upper extremities (i.e., imitating motions to songs, etc. . . .) while maintaining a cross-legged sitting posture on the floor for 5 minutes with minimal verbal and/or visual prompting, 4 of 5 opportunities.

OT Intervention Plan includes the following:

Setting: Specialized clinic two times a week

Duration: 6 months with reevaluation at that time to determine the need for further therapy

Discharge plan: Create enriched sensory environment in home and at school with a sensory diet in place that is adjusted as needed or at least every 6 months.

Referrals: Psychoeducational testing

OT Intervention Process and Strategies:

Therapeutic Activities:
In the process of play include
Vigorous swinging using flexion swing, platform swing
A variety of textures along with vibration toys and messy materials
Stereognosis games
Static and dynamic balance activities
Obstacle courses that include gross motor sequences

Environmental Modifications:
Provide picture/word schedule of daily routines
Provide swinging equipment in the home
Enrich the tactile play by including interactive and shape or object-identifying games
Mobile seating devices such as a peanut ball during mealtimes

CASE STUDY 56.1 Larissa (*Continued*)

OUTCOMES

Expected or Reported Outcomes:

- Occupational Performance: Improve social skills, dressing skills, grooming activities, and participation in daily events without emotional outbursts. Participation at school is good.
- Client Satisfaction: Mother report on usefulness of the information and strategies provided by the OT/OTA.
- Adaptability/Generalized skills: Improve tolerance to outings that include shopping, increased harmony in home due to acceptance of routine and changes in routine.
- Impact on Family Life (including the occupations of other family members): Mother report of improved life satisfaction, stress reduction, improved coping, and organization. ■

Sensory-Based Modalities

Understanding the theory and principles of SI and processing provides a foundation for using sensation as a modality in intervention. A modality is a therapeutic agent, tool, or object that is used for a specific therapeutic purpose (Brienes, 2006). OT practitioners often use sensory-based modalities in interventions. Examples of sensory-based modalities include things such as sound therapy and listening programs, Wilbarger's deep pressure proprioceptive technique (DPPT), the use of dynamic seating (Schilling, Washington, Billingsley, & Deitz, 2003), and the use of weighted modalities (weighted vests, blankets, wraps, stuffed animals, hats, belts). Our knowledge of SI and processing guides the use of these modalities and enables the practitioner to identify sensory stimuli that may be arousing or alerting to the client or those stimuli that support the development of discrimination and the generation of functional behaviors (Dunn, 2009). For instance, a person who engages in a self-injurious behavior for apparent "centering" purposes may be guided to use a cold cloth to the face or a weighted wrap to feel more oriented and centered. The use of intense tastes (e.g., biting into a lemon) or scented items (clinical aromatherapy) may help distract someone from negative thoughts and urges. Modalities may also be used for calming or grounding purposes (e.g., use of clay, essential oils, weighted blanket). There is limited evidence available on the use of many of these approaches; however, the evidence base for some is growing (Bazyk, Cimino, Hayers, Goodman, & Farrell, 2010; Hall & Case-Smith, 2007; Kimball et al., 2007; Moore & Henry, 2002; Mullen, Champagne, Krishnamurty, Dickson, & Gao, 2008; Vandeberg, 2001). See Table 56.8 for an example of how a sensory modality can be used in various ways. Table 56.9 demonstrates additional ways on how therapeutic activity and modality intervention approaches may be used to meet OT outcomes with individuals across the life course.

Use of Sensation in Daily Life: The Sensory Diet

A "sensory diet" is a metaphor for a sensory menu of individualized, structured activities and/or modalities

TABLE 56.8 Occupational Therapy Intervention Types (American Occupational Therapy Association, 2008) and Weighted Blanket Applications (Champagne, 2010b)

Intervention Type	Intervention Definition	Weighted Blanket (WB) Example
Preparatory	Methods or techniques that prepare a client for occupational engagement	The client is provided with a WB to decrease anxiety or arousal in order to increase the ability to engage in self-care and milieu activities during an acute inpatient psychiatric hospitalization.
Purposeful activity	Client engages in specifically selected activities that allow the development of skills, which enhance occupational engagement.	The client practices changing the amount of weight in the WB and trials in at each weight to determine his or her preferences in the optimal amount of weight for rest and sleep.
Occupation based	Client engages in client-directed occupations that match identified goals.	After learning how to use a WB under therapeutic guidance, the client uses a WB, along with other sheets and blankets at night at home as part of his or her general sleep routine. The WB is no longer a novel intervention, it is self-initiated at this point and is part of one's habitual sleep routine.

TABLE 56.9 Sensory-Based Interventions: Applications across the Life Course

Client	Intervention	Outcome
22-year-old male with tactile over-responsivity	Co-create a sensory diet to implement the consistent use of sensory modalities and activities addressing sensory over-responsivity	Decreased sensory over-responsivity, supports the ability to work at his job requiring close proximity to others
26-year-old female with PTSD	Co-create a sensory kit to keep sensory modulation strategies organized and readily available for use as needed for prevention and crisis intervention purposes	Increased ability to maintain active participation in meaningful roles
58-year-old male with paranoid schizophrenia	Co-create sensory supportive modifications to the bedroom to allow for a more relaxing physical space	Increased ability to fall sleep and stay asleep at night
75-year-old woman with dementia and agitation	Use of a weighted wrap to prevent agitation and the need for the use of PRN medications	Increased social participation (ability to engage in visits with family and group sessions with peers)

PRN, as needed (when necessary or needed); PTSD, posttraumatic stress disorder.

used as part of one's daily routine to meet the individual's values, needs, and occupational performance goals (P. Wilbarger, 1984; J. Wilbarger & Wilbarger, 2002). A sensory diet may be used within an overall OT intervention to meet the sensory needs of individuals throughout their daily activities (J. Wilbarger & Wilbarger, 2002). Individuals may benefit from the use of a sensory diet that provides the amount and type of sensory input needed to support arousal, attention, emotion, cognition, behavior regulation, social participation, or overall health and well-being. When it is determined that a sensory diet is warranted as part of the intervention plan, it is collaboratively created with the client and involved caregivers and used for specific therapeutic purposes. Sensory diets are used to help to facilitate changes in occupational performance skills (e.g., sensory perceptual skills), patterns (e.g., rituals, routines), and contexts in order to meet specific occupational goals.

Sensory Diet: Individuals. OT practitioners are skilled in grading activities to meet specific therapeutic goals. Intensity of sensory input is influenced by frequency, duration, speed, rhythm, body position, context, and complexity of the experience. It is important to be sure that interventions are meaningful, age and culturally appropriate, and provide the "just right" amount of intensity to match the individual's specific needs. For instance, for one client, the use of a stress ball when anxious may be a just right fit; but for another individual, this may not meet the intensity demands and may ultimately feel invalidating to the person.

Although a sensory diet is one aspect of an approach initially introduced for the treatment of sensory defensiveness (J. Wilbarger & Wilbarger, 2002), the concept has been adapted for broader use to address specific SI and processing problems and for prevention, health and wellness, and crisis de-escalation purposes. To be effective, a sensory diet must be practical and part of the daily routine; often they involve the adaptation of routines or environmental modifications. Individualized sensory kits can be created with clients and used to assist in keeping helpful strategies organized and accessible for use for prevention, maintenance, and crisis de-escalation purposes (Champagne, 2011b). A sensory kit is a container filled with sensory items; and whenever possible, the theme of each kit should be chosen by the person using it. Sensory kits often contain items that are used for focusing, distraction, self-soothing, stress management, mindfulness, prevention, and de-escalation purposes (Champagne, 2011b).

Sensory stories, adapted by Marr and Nackley (2005) from Gray's Social Stories (Gray, 2000), may be part of a sensory diet created to help children with SI and processing difficulties create a story about a particular area of difficulty (e.g., hair brushing) that include strategies to help enable occupational participation. Sensory stories can be used to help children and caregivers implement parts of the sensory diet in various contexts (Marr, Gal, & Nackley, 2007; Marr, Mika, Miraglia, Roerig, & Sinnott, 2007).

Sensory Diet: Programmatic Applications. Although sensory diets are often considered for individuals, programmatic applications are also beneficial (e.g., schools, day programs, residential programs, hospital settings). Table 56.10 provides examples.

Sensory-Based Individual and Group Sessions

Sensory-based interventions may be implemented through the use of individual and/or group sessions and combined with other therapeutic methods. Examples of Annabelle and Daniel in the following section will demonstrate the use of sensory-based interventions during individual sessions, and George's case will illustrate both participation in both sensory-based individual and group sessions.

TABLE 56.10 Sensory Diet and Varied Contextual Applications

Context	Intervention Example	Occupational Performance
Home	A 6-year-old child rolls up in a warm blanket, with his mother's assistance, before beginning bath and bedtime routines. This may help reduce his arousal level, defensiveness to touch, and to prepare him for sleep.	Decreased tactile defensiveness may support the ability to engage more fully in routines.
School	Movement breaks (yoga poses, gym, wall/chair push-ups, changing classrooms) are strategically built into the structure/routine of the day and before transition times that may help support self-regulation, social skills, and the capacity to learn.	Building movement breaks into the daily routine may help to support the child's ability to stay alert and focused in school in order to have a positive impact on academic performance and social participation.
Acute inpatient mental health setting	The hospital's group schedule is modified to include activities to help people wake up in the morning (stretching/exercises), to stay alert and focused in group sessions, to cope with change of shift (leisure activities, go for a walk, spend time in sensory room, pet therapy), to start to wind down in the evening (use of sensory cart items for calming, relaxation groups, art expression), and to make available strategies to facilitate rest/sleep (weighted blanket, aromatherapy).	Availability and use of strategies, built into the daily routine, may help to facilitate the ability to participate in self-care, social, and therapeutic activities. It may also be used on a programmatic scale for prevention and crisis de-escalation purposes to decrease the need for the use of seclusion/restraint.

Sensorimotor Groups. Ross and Burdick (1981) were the first occupational therapists to publish on the formalized use of the five-stage sensorimotor group (Ross, 1997; Ross & Burdick, 1981). The approach was designed to be SI informed and incorporate group process principles with people with mental illness and dementia. In 2005, Moore (2005) published a variation of the five-stage group, expanding on Ross and Burdick's (1981) work. Champagne (2012) has developed group curriculums combining psychotherapy and OT models with a focus on SI and processing in her groups for varied age ranges: Movin' & Groovin' (ages 4 to 6 years), Sensory Mod Squad (ages 7 to 12 years), and the Regulators (teens). While research is needed to examine the effectiveness of interventions that combine the theory bases of SI and processing with that of psychotherapy, the models provide a starting place. See Chapter 34 for information on group work and group process.

Yoga. Yoga is also used as an OT group or individual intervention with various populations and across practice contexts (e.g., schools, residential programs, day programs, outpatient clinics). Many variations to yoga practices have evolved to assist OT practitioners in providing yoga as a therapeutic intervention. Recently, Stoller, Greuel, Cimini, Fowler, and Koomar (2012) demonstrated the effectiveness of the integration of a sensory-enhanced hatha yoga group intervention among 35 military personnel on deployment in Iraq. The sensory-enhanced yoga group helped to reduce state and trait anxiety and to improve 16 out of 18 mental health and quality of life indicators for the participants, leading investigators to conclude that sensory-enhanced hatha yoga served as a proactive stress management intervention for this population. More research is necessary to examine how modifications to existing yoga practices (e.g., trauma-informed yoga) as well as other proprioceptive and vestibular-rich interventions such as tai chi and dance may be effective modes of intervention for varied populations.

Environmental Modifications

Environmental modifications may be subtle or substantial and as noted earlier in this chapter may be included as part of OT intervention. For instance, moving someone's desk so that it is in a quieter, less well-traveled part of the room may be recommended for an individual who is sensitive to sounds and touch; using a sit disc on a desk seat may be recommended for a child who requires more vestibular-proprioceptive input throughout the day in order to pay attention in class.

Specialized rooms have been designed for their sensory enrichment or calming effects for individuals across their life course (Champagne, 2006, 2011b). Active engagement in environments that provide multiple opportunities for calming and alerting sensation is consistent with SI and processing constructs. Environmental areas that emphasize sensory modulation offer various tools, equipment, and furnishings that support a sense of feeling calm, uplifted, and organized (e.g., sensory modulation rooms). Enriched environments offer affordances for enhanced vestibular, proprioceptive, and tactile interactions with equipment and objects with enough variety to offer novelty and problem solving to support organizational skills and praxis (e.g., SI clinic).

Environments that provide more passive sensory experiences are inconsistent with many core elements of ASI but may be used for sensory stimulation. Multisensory rooms, previously called Snoezelen rooms, were created for use with people with severe and profound developmental and intellectual delays and dementia (American Association of Multi-sensory Environments, 2010). Multisensory environments are created to promote leisure, relaxation, and social participation and often include some of the following types of equipment: interactive switches, projectors, bubble lamps, comfortable furnishings, and various lighting options. It has been suggested that the therapeutic use of multisensory rooms may help to delay neuronal loss or slow down progression of sensory processing difficulties (R. Baker et al., 2001; Bower, 1967); promote a sense of happiness; and calm and decrease sadness, fear, and negative behaviors (Cornell, 2004; Minner, Hoffstetter, Casey, & Jones, 2004). As we have seen with many of the other sensory-based modalities discussed thus far, additional research is needed to substantiate the effectiveness of these interventions.

Additionally, although many settings have created sensory rooms and spaces to support and promote occupational performance and participation, the use of sensory carts and sensory-based enhancements, such as sensory gardens, may also be advantageous. Home modifications are also helpful for those who benefit from sensory integration and processing approaches. OT practitioners must assist clients, caregivers, and organizations with creating the types of therapeutic physical environments that are most appropriate to the populations served.

Sensory-Based Curriculums

In order to help operationalize the use of sensory-based approaches in varied settings and with different age groups, sensory-based curriculums may be considered. In using each of the following, note the intended client group and modify for other clients as is appropriate. Some examples of sensory-based curriculums include the following:

- ***D****evelopmental,* ***I****ndividual Difference,* ***R****elationship-Based Model*/Floortime (DIR®/Floortime™) Model is an interdisciplinary and developmental framework created to help clinicians, caregivers, and educators to provide a comprehensive assessment process and to develop intervention programs unique to each child's strengths and barriers. This model is specifically created for use with children with ASD and developmental challenges. The objectives of the DIR®/Floortime™ Model are to build the foundational capacity for social, emotional, and intellectual abilities rather than focusing on specific skills and problematic behaviors (Greenspan & Wieder, 2006).
- *How Does Your Engine Run?* (The Alert Program) was created by Williams & Shellenberger (1996) and it is sometimes also referred to as the Alert Program. This curriculum was created primarily to help children, caregivers, clinicians, and educators choose appropriate strategies to assist the child in maintaining optimal levels of alertness for a given activity, context, or environment. It is intended for home and school use and may be adapted for use with adults.
- *Sensation, Task, Environment, Predictability, Self-Monitoring, and Interactions* (STEP-SI) is a principle-based, clinical reasoning model that breaks down assessment and intervention approaches into easily understandable components. Initially conceptualized for use with children with sensory modulation dysfunction, it may also be adapted for use with children with other SI and processing problems as well (Miller, Wilbarger, Stackhouse, & Trunnell, 2002).
- *Sensory Modulation Program* (SMP) was created in 2003 by Champagne (2011b) to assist interdisciplinary staff in operationalizing the use of sensory modulation approaches when working with people with mental health symptoms and diagnoses across various settings. The SMP provides a framework guiding the use of sensory modulation, trauma, and attachment-informed approaches as part of mental health care services. The SMP components include an emphasis on the therapeutic use of self, sensory-based assessments, sensorimotor activities, sensory-based modalities, programming, and environmental modifications. The SMP is not meant to be used to the exclusion of other assessments or therapeutic activities. It is to be used in a client-centered manner, supporting the ability to meet the client's goals.
- *Sensory Motor Arousal Regulation Treatment* (SMART) is a model created by and for psychotherapists and occupational therapists working in mental health practice. The SMART model is designed to support arousal regulation with individuals with trauma symptoms and diagnoses by providing a framework for the integration of psychotherapy and sensory integration and processing approaches when working with individuals with trauma symptoms and diagnoses (Warner, Cook, Westcott, & Koomar, 2011). The SMART model is a treatment approach organized to support arousal regulation in children who have been traumatized. It also integrates approaches from SI, trauma and attachment frames of reference, and sensorimotor psychotherapy.

Sensory Integration and Processing Considerations for Individuals with Specific Diagnoses

Throughout this chapter, we have presented information on the application of SI theory, assessment, and intervention methods throughout the life course and with various populations (Schaaf & Smith Roley, 2006; Smith Roley et al., 2001). The following section will demonstrate specific application of SI propositions for those living with an ASD, mental health diagnoses, and older adults.

Sensory Integration and Processing in Children with Autism Spectrum Disorder

Although sensory and motor concerns are not currently identified as core features of ASD, many researchers think they should be. There is research to suggest that sensory symptoms may contribute to some of the atypical behaviors, academic difficulties, and functional delays often seen in this population, and that motor deficits are highly prevalent in both boys and girls with ASD.

Sensory Modulation Disorders in Children with Autism Spectrum Disorders

As noted in other sections of this chapter, ASD is defined by features of social communication disorders and the presence of stereotyped behaviors; disordered integration and processing of sensory inputs are considered one aspect of repetitive behaviors and are not currently central to the diagnosis. Nonetheless, SI and processing difficulties have been identified in up to 95% of children with ASD (Tomchek & Dunn, 2007); and over-responsiveness and under-responsiveness , as well as sensory seeking, have been identified with differences across sensory systems; both over-responsivity and under-responsivity have been identified in the same individual (Baranek, 2002; Baranek, David, Poe, Stone, & Watson, 2006; Harrison & Hare, 2004). Clear characterization of deficits in SI and processing, and their relationship to core features of ASD remains elusive.

Investigations of SI and processing differences in individuals with ASD are not a new phenomenon. Differences in processing sensation have been reported to occur across tactile, vestibular, auditory, and visual sensory domains (Harrison & Hare, 2004); but clear characterization of deficits in SI and processing and their relationship to core features of ASD remains elusive.

Behavioral responses to sensation provide a mixed picture of responsivity in children with ASD. Regardless of age, children with ASD show both SOR and SUR (Ben-Sasson, Carter, & Briggs-Gowan, 2009; Liss et al., 2006). There is some evidence that younger children with ASD do not show sensory seeking, whereas older children do (Ben-Sasson et al., 2009; Dunn & Bennett, 2002), and that younger children show stronger responses to sensations that they find challenging (Baranek, Boyd, Poe, David, & Watson, 2007). Further, extremes of over-responsivity and under-responsivity are seen when there is a high frequency of either SOR or SUR (Ben-Sasson et al., 2009).

Generally, aspects of the modulation disorder are seen with other behaviors characteristic of ASD. For instance, Liss and colleagues (2006) found that over-responsivity was seen with overfocused and perseverative behavior along with exceptional memory, whereas under-responsivity was seen with impairments in communication and poor social interaction. In the absence of sensory problems, Liss and colleagues (2006) found that their population of school-aged children had minimal symptoms of ASD and were relatively high functioning. Maladaptive behavior has been linked with a global SMD that emphasizes movement sensitivity and taste/smell sensitivity with more general SI and processing deficits with poor social communication across a wide age range of children with ASD (A. E. Baker, Lane, Angley, & Young, 2008; A. E. Lane, Young, Baker, & Angley, 2010). Auditory filtering differences were also noted in a large percentage of children with ASD; it is important to note that the auditory filtering parameter on the Sensory Profile encompasses both over-responsiveness and under-responsiveness.

Examining studies published through 2007 in which parents reported on the SI and processing of their child with ASD, Ben-Sasson, Carter, and Briggs-Gowan (2010) concluded that children with ASD showed different patterns relative to typical children and children with developmental disabilities. The different patterns encompassed greater under-responsivity, over-responsivity, and sensory seeking, depending on the investigation. Further, SI and processing difficulties appeared to be moderated by many factors, including comorbidities, ASD severity, and chronological age. Differences were greater when groups were matched on chronological age as opposed to mental age or children with developmental disabilities, suggesting that modulation differences are not unique to ASD and may be modulated by the presence of disability. Chronological age was identified as a moderating variable in this study in that infants tend not to show sensory seeking, whereas children aged 6 to 9 years showed the greatest SI and processing differences relative to comparison groups. Further, ASD severity was related to severity of SMD but not to the type of SMD.

Thus, while SI and processing disorders are a commonly identified behavioral aspect of ASD, patterns of over-responsiveness, under-responsiveness, and sensory seeking have all been reported and they appear to be modified by the child's age, the severity of ASD, and coexisting conditions. When SI and processing difficulties are extreme, there also appears to be a high incidence of the repetitive behaviors prevalent in those with an ASD diagnosis. Further, over-responsiveness and under-responsiveness are often seen in the same child, such that there may be over-responsiveness to sensation in one domain, with under-responsiveness to sensation in a different domain. The exact pattern of sensory integrative and processing disorder and the relationship between these concerns and other features of the ASD diagnosis varies among studies. It is likely that subgroups will be identified that will link SI and processing deficits with other specific characteristics of ASD. Research is needed to further define these relationships.

Atypical behaviors seen in the ASD population include behavioral rigidity; motor stereotypies; and repetitive movements, vocalizations, or thought patterns. Among the more commonly seen stereotypies and repetitive behaviors are observable actions such as turning on/off lights or electronics, hand or object flapping, lining up toys, body rocking, skin picking, and finger flicking. As noted earlier in this chapter, these behaviors may be linked with altered SI and processing, as means to either (1) seek out sensation in order to combat a low level of arousal or (2) calm a nervous system that has become over-aroused from sensations in the environment. For instance, Baranek, Foster, and Berkson (1997) found a significant relationship between levels of tactile defensiveness and rigid or inflexible behaviors, repetitive verbalizations, visual stereotypies, and abnormal focused affections in children with ASD and developmental disabilities (Baranek et al., 1997). Additionally, in a small sample of children with ASD and intellectual disabilities, Gal, Dyck, and Passmore (2002) found that children initiated stereotyped movements immediately following the onset of aversive sensory stimuli, terminated or decreased stereotyped movements following the onset of an attractive stimulus, and initiated or increased stereotyped movements during periods of neutral stimulus. Although this study included only four children, it suggests that stereotypies may occur in children who are both under-responsive and over-responsive and may be significantly dependent on general levels of arousal and overall context.

Academic challenges for children with ASD vary greatly based on the child's innate cognitive abilities, attention capacity, and motor coordination and praxis abilities. Given that the primary modes of learning in the United States are through visual and auditory methods (e.g., listing to a lecture, reading from slides or a book), it is important to consider how the ability to modulate sensory information may also impact academic performance in children with ASD. Ashburner, Ziviani, and Rodger (2008) identified associations between cognitive problems or inattention and sensory domains of tactile sensitivity, auditory filtering, and under-responsivity or sensation seeking. Overall academic performance was also associated with auditory filtering and under-responsivity or sensation seeking. This suggests that children with ASD may have a difficult time filtering out unimportant sensory information such as unpleasant tactile input or background noise and registering or prioritizing important information such as the teacher's voice or the task at hand.

The diagnosis of ASD is often preceded by parental reports of functional delays in their child's development; the child cannot do what his or her same-age peers can do or what his or her older siblings could do at the same age. Daily living skills often provide ongoing challenges for children with ASD, and these challenges may persist into adulthood. *Activities of daily living* are defined as daily activities designed to take care of one's own body (AOTA, 2008); they are considered key tasks, which an individual must master in order to become an independent member of society. Most children have mastered basic ADL by the time they enter first grade, including the ability to bathe and dress themselves, independent toothbrushing, toilet trained and able to manage toilet hygiene, use of utensils for feeding and establishment of regular rhythms of eating, and sleeping. Many parent and self-report items on questionnaires related to sensory responsivity relate to ADL activities, such as behavior during grooming activities (e.g., nail clipping, haircutting) and limitations in what the child will eat (e.g., will only eat certain foods or textures). There seems to be a logical connection between SOR and mastery of self-care tasks in that a child who finds a task unpleasant will be more likely to find ways to avoid it (e.g., throwing a tantrum before bath time, refusal to allow a toothbrush and certain foods to enter the mouth). Supporting this assumption, Jasmin et al. (2009) found significant correlations between the sensory avoiding quadrant of the *Sensory Profile* (Dunn, 1999) and the self-care section of the Functional Independence Measure for Children (WeeFIM®) and the Daily Living Skills section of the Vineland Adaptive Behavior Scales-Second Edition.

Sleep is an occupation in which children with ASD and, secondarily, their families may struggle (see Chapter 51). Although typical children often have difficulty with sleep as well, children with ASD show a much higher incidence (Souders et al., 2009). Children with ASD with poor sleep patterns have been found to have higher scores related to affective problems and more difficulty with reciprocal social interaction (Malow et al., 2006). Further, exploration of the causes of sleep disturbance in this population is warranted. It has been proposed that some sleep problems may be related to difficulties with sensory modulation, particularly when children tend to be easily over-aroused by sensory stimuli (Reynolds, Lane, & Thacker, 2012; Shani-Adir, Rozenman, Kessel, & Engel-Yeger, 2009; Shochat, Tzischinsky, & Engel-Yeger, 2009). Electroencephalogram (EEG) research supports the notion that sensory gating impairments (P50 sensory gating reflects sensory filtering) are present in poor sleepers during presleep wakefulness in those with difficulty with sleep (Milner, Cuthbert, Kertesz, & Cote, 2009). These authors note that "good sleepers can initiate and maintain sleep by disengaging from the environment in an automatic and effortless manner and can successfully gate irrelevant stimuli" (Milner et al., 2009, p. 335). This suggests that for individuals with SMD, sleep may be a more effortful process and that intervention may be needed to develop regular sleep patterns, which may prevent secondary behavioral problems from occurring.

Sensory Integration and Praxis and Children with Autism Spectrum Disorders

In addition to SMD, it is well established that both boys and girls with ASD demonstrate various sensory perceptual and praxis difficulties with ideation, planning, and motor execution—all aspects of what Ayres termed as *dyspraxia* (Ayres, 1979). Using the SIPT and clinical observations, Ayres (1989) identified tactile, proprioceptive, and vestibular sensory processing deficits along with praxis deficits in children with ASD.

Although there is some discrepancy in the literature regarding characterization of motor performance difficulties, the evidence indicates that children on the autism spectrum have poorer motor coordination and ability than typical peers (Fournier et al., 2010; Kopp, Beckung, & Gillberg, 2010). Analysis of early motor development has revealed head lag (Flanagan, Bauman, & Landa, in press) and motor asymmetries (Teitelbaum, Teitelbaum, Nye, Fryman, & Maurer, 1998). Aspects of motor performance that have been shown to be problematic include an array of difficulties, including general coordination and motor performance, balance and postural control, gait, speed of timed movements, gesture and imitation, planning and execution of movement, and overflow of movements. General motor delays, toe walking, and hypotonia are often reported (Ming et al., 2005). Further, when an intellectual disability complicates the diagnosis of ASD, the motor problems have been shown to be both more common and more severe (Green et al., 2009; Kopp et al., 2010). The motor concerns identified encompass both praxis and basic motor functions. However, even when basic motor function deficits are taken into account, high-functioning children with ASD have difficulty with praxis (Dziuk et al., 2007). Dziuk and colleagues (2007) speculate that noted cerebellar differences, or links between the cerebellum and the frontal and parietal cortices, may underlie deficits in the development of motor skills. These investigators further suggest that the impaired performance of skilled gestures (including social gestures), an aspect of praxis, may underlie another core feature of ASD: impaired social interaction and functional communication. It is feasible that both dyspraxia and impaired social interaction and communication share a common neurological basis that is disrupted in autism.

Imitation is one aspect of praxis and an aspect with which children with ASD have been shown to have deficits, although the exact nature of these deficits varies between studies. The type of imitation (hand gestures versus facial gesture, for example) and symbolic content (presence or absence of meaning in the gesture), and whether or not imitation is directed or self-initiated, appear to influence performance (see Sevlever & Gillis, 2010 for reviews). There is some suggestion that imitation is important for the development of social communication skills and a predictor of language development in children with ASD (Carpenter, Tomasello, & Striano, 2005) as well as the development of symbolic play (Ingersoll, 2008). A recent finding suggests that the development of imitation may be delayed not only in young children with ASD but also in young children with other developmental delays (Young et al., 2011). Although this means that imitation may not differentiate between children with ASD and other delays, it does not diminish the fact that children with ASD show delayed imitation development. Looked at from the perspective of the OT practice framework, poor imitation, an aspect of praxis, interferes with social participation and at least symbolic play, both areas of occupation (AOTA, 2008). As such, praxis concerns in children with ASD go beyond motor control and impact the child at several levels of function.

CASE STUDY 56.2 Kline

Kline is a sensitive and curious 10-year-old who loves talking about space and space travel. He tends to enjoy being alone and is quite content reading about things related to space travel and playing computer games that include things about space ships, planets and stars, and astronauts. He has just begun fourth grade in a regular education class. He has an aide for academic tasks due to his difficulty staying in his seat and completing his assignments. He has a diagnosis of autism spectrum disorder and attention deficit hyperactivity disorder.

At school, Kline shows needs for personal space that have led to placement of his desk out of classroom traffic patterns; lining up for lunch, recess, and to move to a different class are all problematic if Kline is not allowed to be at the end of the line. Kline bounces rather than walks most of the time and, when standing in line, will also bounce on his toes as he waits to move. On the playground, at recess, his favorite activity is to climb to the top of the slide and jump to the ground, something he has been told not to do because of safety concerns. When he gets upset in the classroom, he will run to the corner of the room, put his back against the wall, and bang his torso repeatedly on the wall. At times, he flaps his hands at the side of his face as he withdraws to the corner of the room.

Kline's teacher requested consultation with an occupational therapist to better understand his classroom behavior. The occupational therapist asked the teacher to complete a Sensory Processing Measure Main Classroom Form; she also

(continued)

CASE STUDY 56.2 Kline (*Continued*)

called to speak with Kline's mother and learned a great deal about his behavior at home. The occupational therapist learned that Kline is highly avoidant of many forms of touch: he wears only very soft, cotton/synthetic blend shirts and refuses to wear them once they get "balls" on them; his pants must have an elastic waist; and his socks must fit tight enough that they do not move when he puts his shoes on. Kline eats only smooth textured foods (creamy peanut butter, blended yogurt) and prefers foods that are white. He has great difficulty accepting hugs from individuals aside from his Mom but can be coaxed into this when necessary. The occupational therapist requested that Kline's mother complete a Sensory Processing Measure (Parham & Ecker, 2007) checklist related to his behaviors at home.

Both the teacher and his mother identified behaviors consistent with tactile over-responsivity and proprioceptive seeking with no significant difference between Home and School checklists. Both teacher and mother indicated that Kline's senory-based behaviors were interfering with his ability to fully participate. This lead the occupational therapist to identify Kline as having sensory modulation difficulties and recommend intervention. It was also recommended that Kline be given a Sensory Integration and Praxis Test to provide a full picture of his sensory integration and processing strengths and weaknesses and further refine recommendations for treatment.

Kline's mother requested services outside of classroom time. As such, Kline will begin receiving therapy at a local private practice clinic. Additionally, the occupational therapist has consulted with the teacher to develop sensory-regulatory strategies to use in the classroom, in addition to those she is already using. Placing his desk in a nontraffic area and allowing him to be last in line are both excellent strategies to help him avoid the tactile input that seems to be very distressing. The occupational therapist also talked with Kline, and together, they discovered that having a rubber band in his pocket that he could pull out and stretch between his hands sometimes helped him stay in his desk. Although the teacher was somewhat worried about the safety of having this (concerned that it would be shot at another student), she was willing to give it a try. In addition to these strategies, the teacher and Kline were able to define a space at the back of the classroom where he could pace if he needed to do so; she offered this "moving-thinking" option to other children as well. A mini-trampoline was placed on the playground, away from the other play structures, for Kline and the other children.

Sensory activities such as vigorous physical play before, during, and after school assisted in Kline's ability to regulate his attention and activity level. At home, the occupational therapist suggested that Kline make use of a mini-trampoline routinely before going to school, once he gets home, and periodically during homework. A chewy tube was also suggested, used mostly during homework time, to provide Kline with some oral proprioceptive input that might help him stay seated longer. Kline has indicated that it helps him to settle down for work.

Work with the occupational therapist in the clinic has not yet begun. This therapist suspects that Kline has significant difficulty with vestibular-related postural and bilateral skills and somatosensory based dyspraxia, both affecting his performance as well. It is likely that his poor organization and some of the motor behaviors observed may be related to poor praxis. ■

Sensory Integration and Processing Considerations in Mental Health

There has been a significant increase in the awareness of SI and processing disorders within the field of mental health care; this has led to the rising demand for sensory-based assessments, interventions, and research for its use with clients across the life course (Chalmers, Harrison, Mollison, Molloy, & Gray, 2012; Champagne, 2011b). And, although SI and processing disorders are often evident without the presence of other mental health diagnoses, it is becoming increasingly evident that the two groups of disorders coexist. Recent studies by Van Hulle, Schmidt, and Goldsmith (2011) and Carter, Ben-Sasson, and Briggs-Gowan (2011) that used large samples identified SMD in children with and without comorbid psychiatric conditions.

OT practitioners have a significant leadership role to play in helping clients and interdisciplinary teams in mental health care practice to collaboratively recognize, plan, and provide interventions to address SI and processing issues impacting participation. Problems with SI and processing, as part of or in addition to other mental health symptoms and diagnoses, often lead to difficulties such as occupational alienation (isolation) and occupational deprivation (poor sleep, poor hygiene), which compromise the recovery process (Champagne, 2010a). OT practitioners are advocating to include SI and processing approaches as part of many of the national mental health care initiatives (e.g., recovery movement, trauma-informed care, seclusion and restraint reduction) (Champagne, 2011b; Champagne & Stromberg, 2004; LeBel & Champagne, 2010; Massachusetts Department of Mental Health [MA DMH], 2010; National Association of State Mental Health Program Directors [NASMHPD], 2003; U.S. Department of Health and Human Services [USDHHS], Substance Abuse and Mental Health Services Administration, 2003a, 2003b). The following section provides an overview of some of the ways in which mental health symptoms and diagnoses often coincide with SI and processing symptoms and disorders.

Trauma

Trauma is an experiential process, and variables that impact the perception of trauma include some of the following: degree of perceived control over the situation, predictability, expectancy, supports available, and the adaptability of the individual at the time of the experience(s) (APA, 2000). In addition, the effects of and responses to trauma are specific to each individual's perceptions. For example, what is perceived to be traumatic by one individual may or may not be considered traumatic to another. Currently, the only trauma disorder in the *DSM-IV-TR* is PTSD. Within the *DSM-IV-TR*, PTSD is categorized under the anxiety disorders (APA, 2000). PTSD may emerge when an individual "experienced, witnessed, or was confronted with an event or events that involved actual or threatened death or serious injury, or a threat to the physical integrity of self or others" (APA, 2000, p. 467). Thalamic dysfunction is evident in people with PTSD (Bremner et al., 1999a; Liberzon, Taylor, Fig, & Koeppe, 1996–1997), which can interfere with the relay of sensory information to the limbic and neocortical systems. Thus, for people with PTSD, sensory processing–related fragmentation and thalamic dysfunction are some of the variables that impact the ability to recall one's experiences as an integrated whole (e.g., unexplained somatic symptoms, dissociated memory fragments) (Ogden, Minton, & Pain, 2007). Annabelle, presented in the following section, provides an example of the link between PTSD and SI and processing challenges.

CASE STUDY 56.3 Annabelle

Annabelle is a tall, lanky 16-year-old who likes hanging out with friends individually rather than in groups. She studies hard and, when it is quiet in her study and learning environment, does well with course work. Annabelle has a diagnosis of posttraumatic stress disorder (PTSD) and has severe affect dysregulation; she also has sensory modulation disorder (SMD). One of the sensory modulation challenges that have negatively impacted her school performance and ability to sleep is sensory over-responsivity (SOR) to auditory stimulation. For example, when in music class, she cannot sing along and appears to find the sounds in the music room intolerable. Annabelle cringes and covers her ears during class; sometimes she also demonstrates behavioral outbursts. She also complains about the noise in the cafeteria and the gymnasium; sometimes, the loud voices and banging lockers in the hallways bother her to the point that she screams for quiet. Initially, her teachers had great difficulty understanding why Annabelle reacts this way and why she did not participate more fully in her classes. An occupational therapist was consulted and determined that Annabelle's SOR to sounds in the environment, especially those over which she did not have control, was part of why she demonstrated difficulty participating in school. The occupational therapist introduced the option of wearing earplugs—or when the teachers deemed it

(continued)

appropriate, ear buds connected to an mp3 player—so that environmental sounds might become more tolerable. In class, earplugs (which dampened the sound) were most appropriate but also cut down on how much Annabelle could hear when the teacher was giving instruction. Therefore, the occupational therapist recommended sitting closer to the teacher and the necessary adjustments were made in the classroom. These simple strategies significantly improved Annabelle's participation and behavior in class. Given the success in school, ear plugs, ear buds, or the use of a fan for constant background noise were also suggested for use at home to help her when doing homework and to fall asleep and stay asleep at night. Annabelle preferred the use of the fan, which she reported significantly helped her with studying and with her sleep. And, although these environmental strategies did not "fix" her PTSD or SMD symptoms, they helped her to feel more comfortable and thereby reduced outbursts at school and allowed her to study and sleep better at home. These strategies also gave Annabelle the ability to have greater control over her experiences in school and home environments. ■

The term *complex trauma* is used in the traumatic stress field when referring to "the experience of multiple, chronic and prolonged developmentally adverse traumatic events most often of an interpersonal nature (e.g., physical, emotional or sexual abuse, domestic violence, war, bullying) and early-life onset" (van der Kolk, 2005, p. 402). When trauma occurs in childhood prior to the ability to develop one's core—cohesive sense of self—the pervasive impact differs from that of trauma occurring in adulthood (van der Kolk, 2005, 2006). Amount and type of cumulative trauma experiences have been linked with increased trauma symptom complexity in a large sample of college students ($n = 2{,}543$) (Briere, Kaltman, & Green, 2008) and were shown to be a predictor of trauma symptom complexity in children and adults (Cloitre et al., 2009). Further, adverse childhood experiences (ACEs) are linked with many physical (e.g., obesity) and mental health symptoms and diagnoses (e.g., depression), self-injurious behaviors (e.g., suicide attempts, substance abuse), and high-risk behaviors (e.g., sexual promiscuity, domestic violence) (Felitti et al., 1998).

Many leaders in the field of trauma science advocated for the inclusion of *developmental trauma disorder* (DTD) into the next edition of the *DSM* (Ford & Kidd, 1998; van der Kolk, 2005, 2006). DTD emphasizes the pervasive, developmental impact of complex trauma during critical developmental phases of childhood, which often leads to the onset of mental health symptoms (e.g., chronic depression, anxiety, dissociation); affect dysregulation; and sensory perceptual, physiological, attachment, and personality disorders (Atchinson, 2007; Hughes, 2004; Schore, 1994; van der Kolk, 2005, 2006). Within OT, it is well understood that early sensory, motor, and perceptual development provides the foundational base supporting higher order occupational performance skills (Ayres, 1979). Van der Kolk (2005) emphasizes

> The PTSD diagnosis does not capture the developmental effects of childhood trauma: the complex disruptions of affect regulation; the disturbed attachment patterns; the rapid behavioral regressions and shifts in emotional states; the loss of autonomous strivings; the aggressive behavior against self and others; the failure to achieve developmental competencies; the loss of bodily regulation in the areas of sleep, food and self-care; the altered schemas; the anticipatory behavior and traumatic expectations; the multiple somatic problems, from gastrointestinal to headaches; the apparent lack of awareness of danger and resulting self endangering behaviors; the self-hatred and self-blame; and chronic feelings of ineffectiveness. (p. 406)

Specific links between SI and processing disorders and trauma have not been well delineated, but we can draw some inferences from clinical practice and the literature. Integrative capacity requires the synthesis of cognitive, emotion, sensory processing, bodily sensations, motor performance, and one's sense of self as differentiated from the experiences of others (van der Kolk, 2005, 2006). One's locus of control (degree of control over thoughts, emotions, behaviors) is significantly impacted by "differentiation" and "presentification"—both parts of one's integrative capacity. *Differentiation* is the ability to differentiate between self and other people, places, things, and between one's own experiential processes. *Presentification* is the awareness of the present moment while realizing its relevance to the past and potential future implications; this includes the awareness of whether one's sensations, postures, and movements are appropriate to a given experience or situation (Van der Hart & Steele, 1997).

Further, having a trauma history increases the probability of engagement in self-injurious behavior (e.g., self-mutilation, starving one's self, self-poisoning, substance abuse, suicidal acts) and the development of attachment and personality disorders (Boriskin, 2004; Bowlby, 1988; Saxe, Chawla, & van der Kolk, 2002). Based on these early theories, sensory approaches are being used not only to address specific SI and processing disorders in mental health OT practice but also the intense neurophysiological and psychosocial manifestations of traumatic sequelae (e.g., affect dysregulation, self-regulation, and attachment disorders) (LeBel, Champagne, Stromberg, & Coyle, 2010; NASMHPD, 2003, 2009).

Affect Regulation

The capacity for affect regulation begins with the attachment formation between a child and a primary caregiver (Bowlby, 1988). This capacity is expected to increase as individuals mature, supporting the ability to tolerate and cope with daily life stressors, real, and perceived threats (e.g., separation from loved ones, loss of relationships, job loss, relationship conflicts). Given that affect regulation is a higher order occupational performance skill (e.g., emotion regulation), problems in early childhood development, including trauma or problems with SI and processing, often contribute to difficulty with affect regulation (DeGangi, Breinbauer, Doussard-Roosevelt, Stephen, & Greenspan, 2005; van der Kolk, 2005, 2006). Like disorders of sensory modulation, affect dysregulation has recently received growing concern regarding the role it plays in developing or furthering psychopathology (Bradley, 2000). Difficulty with affect regulation is often included as a common issue among many psychiatric disorders in the *DSM-IV-TR* (APA, 2000); these include, but are not limited to, some of the following: anxiety disorders (including trauma), attachment disorders, ADHD, DCD, learning disorders (e.g., ADHD, nonverbal learning disorder), mood disorders (major depressive disorder, bipolar disorder), conduct disorders (e.g., oppositional defiant disorder), regulatory disorders, Tourette's and tic disorders, and personality disorders (Cheng & Boggett-Carsjens, 2005). Furthermore, it is very common to see people with SI and processing disorders have difficulty with affect regulation as well, which impacts occupational performance and participation (see Chapter 57).

Attachment Disorder

Attachment disorder often arises from pathological caregiving in infancy and early childhood and is often evident among individuals with trauma histories (APA, 2000). Attachment styles are often viewed as being on a continuum and include secure, insecure-avoidant, insecure-ambivalent, and insecure-disorganized type. Interestingly, the only attachment disorder listed in the *DSM-IV-TR* is reactive attachment disorder (APA, 2000), which is considered the most severe. In addition to the literature proposing that attachment disorders arise from pathological or inadequate parenting or caregiving, Kraemer (1992) proposes a psychobiological etiology for attachment disorder. Kraemer emphasized that attachment disorders may arise when a caregiver is nurturing but the child has or is at risk for having developmental delays that may negatively impact the ability to attune and bond with the caregiver. Thus, within OT practice, it is necessary to help caregivers identify whether developmental difficulties such as difficulty with SI and processing problems may be impacting a person's ability to develop healthy attachment formation, which ultimately impacts social relationships and social participation.

SI and processing disorders are common among those with PTSD, complex trauma, DTD, and attachment disorders (Ayres, 1979; Ogden et al., 2007; van der Kolk, 2005, 2006). Ayres (2005) explained that problems with SI often interfere with attachment, which she referred to as the "primary level of integration" (p. 56). Sensory-based approaches are used to help alter SI and processing patterns, modify activities and routines (sensory diet), modify physical environments (sensory rooms), in order to support occupational participation. When working with clients with attachment disorders, it is essential to include the primary caregiver(s) in the therapeutic process. SI and processing assessment and intervention of both the primary caregiver(s) and client helps to identify strengths and barriers to the ability to attune, bond, and develop a close interpersonal relationship. Difficulty with relationship formation between primary caregiver(s) and the child impacts feelings of safety, security and the development of healthy attachments, the capacity for self-regulation, and higher order capacities (Bowlby, 1988; Champagne, 2011a; Hughes, 2004; Kinninburgh & Blaustein, 2005; Koomar, 1995; Schore, 1994). Ayres's (1979) flowchart (Figure 56.5) of the senses, integration of inputs, and end products further demonstrates the role of SI and processing as part of the developmental process also leading to such higher order capacities. Sabine, described in the following section, is a child challenged by a combination of SI and processing and mental health concerns.

CASE STUDY 56.4 Sabine

Sabine is 5 years old; she loves swinging at the playground, singing, and listening to music. Sabine has been in foster care since age 3 due to severe parental abuse and neglect in infancy and early childhood. She has had significant difficulty bonding with her primary caregiver, her foster mother, demonstrating an insecure-disorganized attachment style. Additionally, Sabine often becomes dissociative (out of touch with reality) when distressed or triggered. Complicating her attachment difficulties, Sabine has a gastrostomy tube for feeding and complex sensory integration and processing concerns including sensory over-responsivity (SOR), poor body awareness, gravitational insecurity, and poor fine motor skills. This combination of problems has resulted in difficulty with school performance in kindergarten and significantly contributes to her difficulty with regulating how she feels. Sabine tends to engage in parallel play versus interacting with her peers in an age-appropriate manner. SOR patterns (tactile and auditory) impact Sabine's ability to tolerate dressing, toothbrushing, different food textures, and for being touched or held. Problems with sensory discrimination impact safety awareness (e.g., poor gravitational awareness on playground equipment). Problems with fine motor skills impact the ability to write, color, and cut with scissors in an age-appropriate manner. At times, she becomes so frustrated she bites herself, head bangs, has tantrums, and may dissociate. The occupational therapist used clinical reasoning skills to provide an integrative approach combining sensory integration

(continued)

and processing and attachment-focused therapeutic interventions with Sabine and her foster mother to target her sensory, trauma, and attachment concerns. These interventions were used to ultimately address her occupational performance and participation goals. One example of a therapeutic session was the client-directed and family-centered use of the sensory integration gym during sessions with both Sabine and her foster mother as active, collaborative participants. The equipment available, typical of that in a room designed for sensory integrative intervention, fostered positive, safe, successful play, and relational experiences to support the bonding and sensory integrative needs necessary to help target some of the therapy goals. Modeling by the occupational therapist and encouraging the foster mother's active participation as the child initiated the use of the cuddle swing, ball pit, and weighted blanket with Sabine were some of the initial interventions explored together following the occupational therapy evaluation process. ■

Anxiety Disorders

Although PTSD is listed in the *DSM-IV-TR* under the category of anxiety disorders (APA, 2000), other anxiety disorders include social phobia, panic disorder with or without agoraphobia, obsessive-compulsive disorder (OCD), acute stress disorder, generalized anxiety disorder, and several others. Globally, research supports the links between problems with SI and processing, anxiety disorders, and other mental health issues in children and adults (Atchison, 2007; Brown, Tollefson, Dunn, Cromwell, & Filion, 2001; Kinnealey & Fuiek, 1999; Kinnealey et al., 1995; S. J. Lane, Reynolds, & Thacker, 2010; McIntosh, Miller, Shyu, & Hagerman, 1999; Moore & Henry, 2002; Reynolds et al., 2010).

Several investigations have focused on the relationship between anxiety and balance. Early work demonstrated that clients with panic disorder and agoraphobia had more vestibular abnormality than clients with panic disorder but without agoraphobia, depressive disorders, other anxiety disorders, or healthy controls (Jacob & Furman, 1996). Balaban (2002) developed a neurological model that takes into account the mutually excitatory relationship between anxiety-related systems and balance-related systems. Along this line, adults with generalized social anxiety disorder have been shown to demonstrate SOR patterns along with agoraphobic avoidance and harm avoidance patterns (Hoffman & Bitran, 2007). Further, when examining the role of balance function in the development of agoraphobia in adults with panic disorder, Perna et al. (2001) documented abnormalities of static posture with eyes open and eyes closed. The noted balance dysfunction has been speculated to result in increases in the sensitivity to visual or proprioceptive balance cues thus facilitating the development of fear of heights or agoraphobia (Furman & Jacob, 2001). In a study of children ages 7 to 14 years being seen for a primary diagnosis of generalized or separation anxiety disorder, significantly lower scores on static and dynamic balance tests were evident (Erez, Gordon, Sever, Sadeh, & Mintz, 2004). Plus a higher incidence of fear was reported in a large sample of 7- to 18-year-old children with cerebellar-vestibular dysfunction compared to the general population (Levinson, 1989).

Intervention studies also provide further support for a link between vestibular dysfunction and anxiety. Bart et al. (2009) demonstrated the comorbidity of anxiety and balance disorders among children ages 5 to 7 years. After administering interventions focused primarily on balance for 12 weeks, the children had lower anxiety and increased self-esteem and self-acceptance. Further, vestibular rehabilitation was shown to significantly decrease anxiety levels in the clients with anxiety, presumably maintained by vestibular dysfunction.

The first line of intervention for people referred for anxiety is often psychotherapy and psychopharmacology, although occupational therapists working with people with symptoms of anxiety and anxiety disorders often employ the use of sensory-based approaches in addition to others (Champagne, 2011b, 2011c; Champagne, Koomar, & Olson, 2010; Moore, 2005). Outside of OT practice, the comorbidity between anxiety and balance or other SI and processing–related disorders is rarely a focus in general mental health care practice. In addition, rehabilitation professionals must recognize and address the emotional (e.g., anxiety, self-esteem) and cognitive components of balance-related symptoms and disorders as well.

Schizophrenia

Historically, schizophrenia has not been viewed as a disorder of developmental origin; however, recent research proposes that schizophrenia be reconceptualized as a neurodevelopmental disorder that causes psychiatric symptoms (Twamley, Salva, Zurhellen, Heaton, & Jeste, 2008). Additionally, increased research supports the need to include the consideration of SI and processing disorders as part of what is addressed during OT assessments and therapeutic interventions with people with schizophrenia (Champagne & Frederick, 2011). Much of the research in this area has focused on sensory discrimination and the impact on cognition. Butler et al. (2009) stated, "deficits in visual processing are well documented in schizophrenia" and may be related to cognitive deficits and functional performance outcomes (p. 1085).

Martinez et al. (2008) further propose that impaired functioning of the magnocellular visual pathways (sensory discrimination problem), which project to the amygdala, is evident in schizophrenia and may contribute to problems with higher order cognitive performance skill issues (e.g., attention, executive functioning, working memory). Interestingly, problems with magnocellular processing are also evident in individuals with dyslexia and ASD (Demb, Boynton, Best, & Heeger, 1998; McCleery, Allman, Carver, & Dobkins, 2007). Morey, Mitchell, Inan, Lieberman, and Belger (2008) found that problems with sensory discrimination of auditory processing and cognitive processing are present in people with schizophrenia. Javitt (2009a, 2009b) also reports that problems in early visual and auditory processing leads to higher order impairment (e.g., auditory emotion recognition, object recognition, perceptual closure). Research reveals that difficulty in visual perception contributes to difficulty with emotion identification and understanding social cues in people with schizophrenia, which often has a significant impact on occupational participation (e.g., social, leisure, vocational) (Butler et al., 2009).

Examining aspects of sensory modulation, Brown, Cromwell, Filion, Dunn, and Tollefson (2002) found that people with schizophrenia demonstrated higher scores in low registration and sensation avoiding and lower scores in the area of sensation seeking on the Adolescent/Adult Sensory Profile (A/ASP) (Brown & Dunn, 2002). Olson (2010) suggested that to best understand the SI and processing challenges that people with schizophrenia face, we must begin to address other variables such as diagnosis type (e.g., paranoid type, schizoaffective, disorganized type), illness phase, possible correlations to positive and negative symptoms, and correlations to occupational performance and participation. Daniel provides one example of the interaction between schizophrenia and SI and processing difficulties.

CASE STUDY 56.5 Daniel

Now 26 years old, Daniel was diagnosed with schizophrenia, paranoid type. In early childhood, he had multiple developmental delays; difficulty with proprioceptive, vestibular, tactile, and auditory discrimination; emotion dysregulation; and difficulty understanding emotional and social cues. As he grew older, he also reported a high threshold for pain, difficulty with attention, concentration, and high sensitivity to smell and taste. In his early 20s, Daniel began to demonstrate slowed responses during conversation and would often stare for long periods of time before responding. He became more isolated, was unable to hold a job, and demonstrated decreased self-care (poor hygiene, wearing unclean clothes) and home management skills (apartment was in disarray, not paying bills). At age 24 years, he had his first psychotic break and was admitted to an acute inpatient hospital for assessment and psychopharmacology. During the admission, he began expressing paranoid and delusional thoughts. When

CASE STUDY 56.5 Daniel (*Continued*)

working with the occupational therapist on the acute inpatient unit, Daniel first expressed the need to feel "less anxious" during an individual session. He was introduced to various potentially calming therapeutic options. Daniel first explored these items and equipment in the unit's sensory modulation room (rocking chair, weighted wrap) as preparatory interventions. At the time, Daniel was having difficulty with participating in self-care, sleep/rest, and group sessions and found the initial use of sensory modulation interventions to be helpful in reducing his anxiety. After the session, he reported feeling more safe on the unit and was able to shower and attend his first group session. By day 2 of the admission, he was able to begin engaging in the formal assessment of sensory integration and processing patterns by completing the Adolescent/Adult Sensory Profile (A/ASP) with the occupational therapist. The results of the A/ASP revealed that he had low registration, sensory sensitivity, and sensation-avoiding patterns that were much more than most people in his age range but sensory seeking patterns that were similar to most people in his age range.

Having developed a trusting relationship with the occupational therapist, they worked collaboratively to help Daniel to better understand how these sensory integration and processing patterns manifested in his life. He was able to express the belief that, in addition to his symptoms of paranoia, his sensory sensitivity and avoidance patterns played a role in his difficulty with being around others. He identified with low registration patterns as well and stated that he often does not notice things in his environment, which interferes with his work, self-care participation, and home management abilities. With this knowledge, Daniel and the occupational therapist first explored sensory-based interventions to help support his occupational performance needs and goals while on the unit. Throughout the admission, they co-created a sensory diet to be used at home after discharge. The occupational therapist recommended that Daniel continue to work with an occupational therapist in the community upon discharge and provided a discharge summary with his assessment results and intervention recommendations to assist with continuity of care.

Other Mental Health Disorders

Problems with SI and processing have been identified in individuals with other mental health disorders aside from those mentioned previously. Notably, work has documented SI and processing concerns in many people with ADHD (DeGangi et al., 2005). SI and processing problems for children with ADHD include tactile SOR (Parush, Sohmer, Steinberg, & Kaitz, 1997), vestibular and proprioceptive SUR, and dyspraxia (Mulligan, 1996; Reynolds et al., 2010). Cheng and Boggett-Carsjens (2005) explain that some of the frequently observed patterns among those with ADHD may include the following:

- Sensory overload when in busy environments (e.g., classrooms, restaurants, playgrounds, large stores, or shopping malls)
- Auditory and tactile SOR
- High sensory seeking of proprioceptive and vestibular (movement-based) stimulation
- Visual distractibility including difficulty with screening out irrelevant visual stimuli (e.g., easily overwhelmed by visual stimuli) and poor eye coordination when visually focusing (e.g., visual scanning when reading)

Several studies on mood found correlations between sensory sensitivity, anxiety, and depression (Kinnealey & Fuiek, 1999; Liss, Timmel, Baxley, & Killingsworth, 2005; Meyer, Ajchenbrenner, & Bowles, 2005; Neal, Edelmann, & Glachan, 2002). Moore and Henry (2002) also demonstrated that people with borderline personality disorder have decreased pain perception, which may be why there is a higher tolerance for pain experienced during engagement in self-injurious behavior. Sensory-based interventions have been shown to play a significant positive role in the disturbances of motor control (e.g., deficits in the feed forward mechanism) in clients with ASD, schizophrenia, and Alzheimer's disease (Velasques et al., 2011).

A new arena of interest and an area in need of investigation is in pediatric autoimmune neuropsychiatric disorder associated with strep (PANDAS), pediatric infection-triggered autoimmune neuropsychiatric disorder (PITAND), and pediatric acute neuropsychiatric syndrome (PANS). In each of these disorders, children experience sudden-onset tics, OCD behaviors, and attention problems when having an infection such as strep throat (PANDAS) or other bacterial or viral infections (PITAND, PANS) (Jenike & Dailey, 2011; Murphy, Kurlan, & Leckman, 2010) followed by a slow return of function. Sensory defensiveness is reported in up to 40% of children with PANDAS; 36% experience deterioration in handwriting and 60% show changes in school performance (Swedo et al., 1998). A loss of motor coordination and executive function leading to functional deficits in daily living activities is also reported (Moretti, Pasquini, Tarsitani, Blondi, & Mandarelli, 2008; Swedo et al., 1998). These symptoms also appear suddenly and slowly diminish. Symptom onset is thought to be due to an autoimmune reaction in the basal ganglia in which antibodies meant to deactivate the infection mistakenly target neuronal tissue, interfering with neurochemical production, including production of dopamine (Kirvan, Swedo, Snider, & Cunningham, 2006).

Neurochemical changes during symptom exacerbation may prevent the children from benefitting from interventions designed to improve sensory and motor functioning. During exacerbation, OT practitioners may best serve these children and families by using compensatory techniques and sensory tools such as a sensory diet to help children and families cope with the exacerbated symptoms. ASI intervention and motor retraining may be appropriate once the exacerbation has subsided to address any residual deficits. Tona and Posner (2011) suggest specific compensatory accommodations and remedial interventions that have been anecdotally reported to be successful; empirical evidence for OT intervention in this new arena is lacking. The National Institutes of Mental Health (NIMH) has taken a strong interest in PANDAS/PITAND recently, with the director calling this a "frontier" in mental health (Insel, 2010). Given the applicability to OT and the paucity of research on OT intervention for these children, these autoimmune neuropsychiatric disorders are an emergent area for OT research, evaluation, and intervention.

Summary

In mental health care practice, understanding the correlation between sensory integration and processing in mental health symptoms and disorders and the impact on occupational performance and participation will aid occupational therapists in the ability to help clients identify and target these issues as part of the OT process. In addition, the introduction of sensory integration and processing assessments and interventions has helped to significantly expand on the therapeutic approaches available to support emotion regulation, stress management, and other mental health–related issues impacting participation in meaningful life roles and occupations. Treatment for sensory integration and processing disorders coupled with mental health diagnoses is likely to include both ASI and sensory-based approaches. Research is needed to better define the relationship between sensory integration and processing disorders and mental health diagnoses and to identify optimal treatment.

Sensory Integration and Processing and Aging

Although information is available on the neurophysiology of the aging brain and aging sensory systems, no empirical studies exist examining these functions from the perspective of SI theory. Nonetheless, the literature does provide food for thought. Peripheral sensory receptor thresholds for activation increase with age, the number and shape of receptors change, and nerve conduction slows. As a result, a much higher intensity stimuli or stimuli of longer duration may be required to activate receptors and send information to the CNS (Dinse, 2006; Kalisch, Tegenthoff, & Dinse, 2008). However, central sensory processing appears to remain highly plastic, such that new processing strategies can be developed as the gradual decline in function takes place (Greenwood, 2007; Greenwood & Parasuraman, 2010). This means that in a typically aging nervous system, the challenge of physiologic change can be met by the construction of new processing strategies. Of further interest is that sensorimotor processes and cognitive processes become increasingly linked in aging, such that changes in one can accommodate for changes in the other. The changes may be reflected as neural reorganization or resource reallocation (Li & Lindenberger, 2002).

Moving from these findings to SI theory requires research to determine its applicability and appropriateness. However, things to consider when working with older adults include (1) awareness of the natural decline in peripheral sensory functions; this decline begins in middle adult years and is quite gradual, possibly requiring altering some or all qualities of sensory input used in any therapy; and (2) understanding that there is a link between SI and processing and cognition. As this link strengthens, with aging, in working with older individuals experiencing cognitive decline, this may become an issue. And it is common for OT practitioners to use sensory supportive interventions with older persons to support alertness, sleep, pain regulation, increased social and leisure participation, and much more (Champagne, 2011b; Moore, 2005; Ross, 1997). George, presented in the following section, provides a case example that demonstrates a potential link between issues of aging and issues of SI and processing correlations within OT practice.

CASE STUDY 56.6 George

George, at age 87 years, currently lives in a skilled nursing unit at the local Veterans Administration hospital. He has been identified as having posttraumatic stress disorder, anxiety, and dementia. George also becomes highly agitated when he is asked to lean back to have his hair washed, lay down to aid in donning pants, or engage in any transfer that involves a change in head position. Because he is dependent on the staff to assist him with activities of daily living (ADL), leisure, and social participation, these later issues are of great concern. Although generally quiet, George yells and strikes out at staff when they try to transfer him during ADL activities. He is often resistant to participating in leisure and social activities if they involve leaning over (as in bowling or the morning exercise group) or moving from one seat to another (as he is asked to do to enter a card game). Staff requested that an occupational therapist evaluate George to help them determine if his behavioral outbursts might be due to causes other than anxiety and confusion. After spending time with George and talking with available caregivers, the occupational therapist presented the idea that George may be experiencing gravitational insecurity—that he is deeply afraid of moving his head out of an

CASE STUDY 56.6 George (*Continued*)

upright position. The occupational therapist provided training to staff on gravitational insecurity and how they might help people like George to feel safer and more secure during ADL, which would also decrease the probability of striking out. Approaching him from the front; the use of a slow pace, providing something for him to hold onto; and wrapping or holding him very securely during transfers were just some of the general recommendations for staff to use during ADL. The occupational therapist also worked with the activities staff to help identify leisure and social activities that George would not find anxiety producing. This required looking at the sensory integration and processing aspects of the activities and understanding how certain types of sensation can often feel overwhelming. Together, the occupational therapist and activities staff worked to modify the activities and physical environment to support more active participation. In addition, the occupational therapist offered a sensorimotor group daily to help George and other clients engage in active movements each day to feel more reality oriented, safe, and secure and to ultimately facilitate occupational participation (Moore, 2005; Ross, 1997).

There is much more to understand and research about sensory integration and processing and the aging adult population.

Summary and Conclusion

SI theory has a long background that begins with the work of Ayres. Concepts related to sensory integration and processing can be used to guide us in using ASI, and in weaving sensory-based approaches into OT interventions. Knowledge of assessment and intervention for sensory-based concerns comprises one of the unique contributions of the profession. Increasingly, sensory integration and processing approaches are more widely understood and applied to help foster the developmental and recovery processes and to promote health and participation in meaningful roles and activities across the life course. Given the growing body of evidence and the rise in the application of the use of sensory integration and processing approaches across age ranges and practice areas, occupational therapists must continue to take a leadership role in researching and advancing this body of work. Expanding and integrating the evidence base in neuroscience and OT practice, such as sensory integration and processing frameworks, will help occupational therapists provide more cutting edge and evidence-based options to persons, organizations, and populations.

Acknowledgments

We wish to acknowledge our mentors, Dr. A. Jean Ayres and Ginny Scardina, along with the many outstanding colleagues with whom we have collaborated. We wish to acknowledge the contributions of Dr. Winnie Dunn as we included and expanded on some of her work from the 11th edition of this text.

References

Alvarado, J. C., Stanford, T. R., Rowland, B. A., Vaughan, J. W., & Stein, B. E. (2009). Multisensory integration in the superior colliculus requires synergy among corticocollicular inputs. *Journal of Neuroscience, 29*, 6580–6592.

American Association of Multi-Sensory Environments. (2010). *Research*. Retrieved from http://www.aamse.us/research.php

American Occupational Therapy Association. (2008). Occupational therapy practice framework: Domain and process, 2nd edition. *American Journal of Occupational Therapy, 62*, 625–683.

American Psychiatric Association. (2000). *Diagnostic and statistical manual of mental disorders* (4th ed., text rev.). Washington, DC: Author.

Andrew, D., & Craig, A. (2002). Quantitative responses of spinothalamic lamina I neurones to graded mechanical stimulation in the cat. *Journal of Physiology, 545*, 913–931.

Anzalone, M. E., & Murray, E. A. (2002). Integrating sensory integration with other approaches to intervention. In A. C. Bundy, S. J. Lane, & E. A Murray (Eds.), *Sensory integration: Theory and practice* (pp. 371–394). Philadelphia, PA: F. A. Davis.

Ashburner, J., Ziviani, J., & Rodger, S. (2008). Sensory processing and classroom emotional, behavioral, and educational outcomes in children with autism spectrum disorder. *American Journal of Occupational Therapy, 62*, 564–573.

Atchison, B. (2007). Sensory modulation disorders among children with a history of trauma: A frame of reference for speech-language pathologists. *American Speech-Language-Hearing Association, 38*, 109–116.

Ayres, A. J. (1968). Sensory integrative processes and neuropsychological learning disability. *Learning Disorders, 3*, 41–58.

Ayres, A. J. (1971). Characteristics of types of sensory integrative dysfunction. *American Journal of Occupational Therapy, 25*, 329–334.

Ayres, A. J. (1972a). *Sensory integration and learning disorders*. Los Angeles, CA: Western Psychological Services.

Ayres, A. J. (1972b). Types of sensory integrative dysfunction among disabled learners. *American Journal of Occupational Therapy, 26*, 13–18.

Ayres, A. J. (1974). *The development of sensory integrative theory and practice: A collection of the works of A. Jean Ayres*. Dubuque, IA: Kendall/Hunt.

Ayres, A. J. (1979). *Sensory integration and the child*. Los Angeles, CA: Western Psychological Services.

Ayres, A. J. (1989). *Sensory Integration and Praxis Tests*. Los Angeles, CA: Western Psychological Services.

Ayres, A. J. (2004). *Sensory Integration and Praxis Tests manual: Updated edition*. Los Angeles, CA: Western Psychological Services.

Ayres, A. J. (2005). *Sensory integration and the child: Understanding hidden sensory challenges* (Rev. ed.). Los Angeles, CA: Western Psychological Services.

Ayres, A. J., & Tickle, L. S. (1980). Hyper-responsivity to touch and vestibular stimuli as a predictor of positive response to sensory integration procedures by autistic children. *American Journal of Occupational Therapy, 34*, 375–381.

Baker, A. E. Z., Lane, A., Angley, M. T., & Young, R. L. (2008). The relationship between sensory processing patterns and behavioural responsiveness in autistic disorder: A pilot study. *Journal of Autism and Developmental Disorders, 38*, 867–875.

Baker, R., Bell, S., Baker, E., Gibson, S., Holloway, J., Pearce, R., . . . Wareing, L. A. (2001). A randomized controlled trial of the effects of multi-sensory stimulation (MSS) for people with dementia. *British Journal of Clinical Psychology, 40*(Pt. 1), 81–96.

Balaban, C. (2002). Neural substrates linking balance control and anxiety. *Physiology & Behavior, 77*(4–5), 469–475.

Baranek, G. T. (2002). Efficacy of sensory and motor interventions for children with autism. *Journal of Autism and Developmental Disorders, 32*, 397–422.

Baranek, G. T., Boyd, B. A., Poe, M. D., David, F. J., & Watson, L. R. (2007). Hyperresponsive sensory patterns in young children with autism, developmental delay and typical development. *American Journal on Mental Retardation, 112*, 233–245.

Baranek, G. T., David, F. J., Poe, M. D., Stone, W. L., & Watson, L. R. (2006). Sensory experiences questionnaire: Discriminating sensory features in young children with autism, developmental delays, and typical development. *Journal of Child Psychology and Psychiatry, 47*, 591–601.

Baranek, G. T., Foster, L. G., & Berkson, G. (1997). Tactile defensiveness and stereotyped behaviors. *American Journal of Occupational Therapy, 51*, 91–95.

Bar-Shalita, T., Vatine, J. J., & Parush, S. (2008). Sensory modulation disorder: A risk factor for participation in daily life activities. *Developmental Medicine and Child Neurology, 50*, 932–937.

Bart, O., Bar-Haim, Y., Weizman, E., Levin, M., Sadeh, A., & Mintz, M. (2009). Balance treatment ameliorates anxiety and increases self-esteem in children with comorbid anxiety and balance disorder. *Research in Developmental Disabilities, 30*, 486–95.

Bauman, M. L. (2005). Commentary—Chapter 9: The child with autism. In A. J. Ayres (Ed.), *Sensory integration and the child: Understanding hidden sensory challenges* (p. 180). Los Angeles, CA: Western Psychological Services.

Bazyk, S., Cimino, J., Hayers, K., Goodman, G., & Farrell, P. (2010). The use of therapeutic listening with preschoolers with developmental disabilities: A look at the outcomes. *Journal of Occupational Therapy, Schools, & Early Intervention, 3*, 124–138.

Bear, M. F., Connors, B. W., & Paradiso, M. A. (2006). *Neuroscience: Exploring the brain* (3rd ed.). Baltimore, MD: Lippincott Williams & Wilkins.

Ben-Sasson, A., Carter, A. S., & Briggs-Gowan, M. J. (2009). Sensory over-responsivity in elementary school: Prevalence and social-emotional correlates. *Journal of Abnormal Child Psychology, 37*, 705–716.

Ben-Sasson, A., Carter, A. S., & Briggs-Gowan, M. J. (2010). The development of sensory over-responsivity from infancy to elementary school. *Journal of Abnormal Child Psychology, 37*, 705–716.

Berthoz, A. (2000). *The brain's sense of movement*. Boston, MA: Harvard University Press.

Blanche, E. I. (2001). The evolution of the concept of praxis in sensory integration. In S. Smith Roley, E. I. Blanche, & R. C. Schaaf (Eds.), *Understanding the nature of sensory integration with diverse populations* (pp. 125–162). Philadelphia, PA: Harcourt Health Sciences.

Blanche, E. I. (2002). *Observations based on sensory integration theory*. Torrance, CA: Pediatric Therapy Network.

Blanche, E. I., & Reinoso, G. (2008). The use of clinical observations to evaluate proprioceptive and vestibular functions. *OT Practice, 13*, 17, CE1–CE7.

Blanche, E. I., & Schaaf, R. C. (2001). Proprioception: A cornerstone of sensory integrative intervention. In S. Roley, E. I. Blanche, & R. C. Schaaf (Eds.), *Understanding the nature of sensory integration with diverse populations* (pp. 109–122). San Antonio, TX: Therapy Skill Builders.

Blanche-Keiffer, D., & Surfas, S. (2011). *A. Jean Ayres: The pioneer behind sensory integration* [DVD]. Torrance, CA: Pediatric Therapy Network.

Boriskin, J. (2004). *PTSD and addiction: A practical guide for clinicians and counselors*. Center City, MN: Hazelden.

Bower, H. M. (1967). Sensory stimulation and the treatment of senile dementia. *Medical Journal of Australia, 1*, 1113–1119.

Bowlby, J. (1988). *A secure base: Clinical application of attachment therapy*. London, United Kingdom: Routledge.

Bradley, S. (2000). *Affect regulation and the development of psychopathology*. New York, NY: Guilford Press.

Brambilla, P., Hardan, A., di Nemi, S. U., Perez, J., Soares, J. C., & Barale, F. (2003). Brain anatomy and development in autism: review of structural MRI studies. *Brain Research Bulletin, 61*, 557–569.

Bremner, J. D., Narayan, M., Staib, L., Southwick, S., McGlashan, T., & Charney, D. (1999). Neural correlates of memories of childhood sexual abuse in women with and without posttraumatic stress disorder. *American Journal of Psychiatry, 156*, 1787–1795.

Brett-Green, B. A., Miller, L. J., Schoen, S. M., & Nielsen, D. M. (2010). An exploratory event-related potential study of multisensory integration in sensory over-responsive children, *Brain Research, 1321*, 67–77. doi:10.1016/j.brainres.2010.01.043

Brienes, E. (2006). Therapeutic outcomes and modalities. In H. M. Pendleton & W. Schultz-Krohn (Eds.), *Pedretti's occupational therapy: Practice skills for physical dysfunction* (6th ed., pp. 658–684). St. Louis, MO: Mosby.

Briere, J., Kaltman, S., & Green, B. L. (2008). Accumulated childhood trauma and symptom complexity. *Journal of Traumatic Stress, 21*, 223–226.

Brown, C., Cromwell, R., Filion, D., Dunn, W., & Tollefson, N. (2002). Sensory processing in schizophrenia: Missing and avoiding information. *Schizophrenia Research, 55*, 187–195.

Brown, C., & Dunn, W. (2002). *Adolescent/Adult Sensory Profile*. San Antonio, TX: The Psychological Corporation.

Brown, C., Tollefson, N., Dunn, W., Cromwell, R., & Filion, D. (2001). The Adult Sensory Profile: Measuring patterns of sensory processing. *American Journal of Occupational Therapy, 55*, 75–82.

Bundy, A. C. (2002). Play theory and sensory integration. In A. C. Bundy, S. J. Lane, & E. A. Murray (Eds.), *Sensory integration: Theory and practice* (pp. 227–240). Philadelphia, PA: F. A. Davis.

Bundy, A. C., Lane, S. J., & Murray E. A. (Eds.). (2002). *Sensory integration: Theory and practice* (2nd Ed.). Philadelphia, PA: F. A. Davis.

Bundy, A. C. & Murray, E. A. (2002). Sensory integration: A. Jean Ayres's theory revisited. In A. C. Bundy, S. J. Lane, & E. A. Murray (Eds.) *Sensory integration: Theory and practice* (2nd Ed.). Philadelphia: F. A. Davis.

Buonomano, D. V., & Merzenich, M. M. (1998). Cortical plasticity: From synapses to maps. *Annual Review of Neuroscience, 21*, 149–186.

Burke, J. P., & Mailloux, Z. (1997). Play and the sensory integrative approach. In L. D. Parham & F. S. Fazio (Eds.), *Play in occupational therapy for children* (pp. 112–125). St. Louis, MO: Mosby-Year Book.

Butler, P. D., Abeles, I. Y., Weiskopf, N. G., Tambini, A., Jalbrzikowski, M., Legatt, M. E., . . . Javitt, D. C. (2009). Sensory contributions to impaired emotional processing in schizophrenia. *Schizophrenia Bulletin, 35*, 1095–1107.

Calvert, G., Spence, C., & Stein, B. E. (Eds.). (2004). *The handbook of multisensory processes*. Cambridge, MA: MIT Press.

Cantin, N., Polatajko, H. J., Thach, W. T., & Jaglal, S. (2007). Developmental coordination disorder: Exploration of a cerebellar hypothesis. *Human Movement Science, 26*, 491–509.

Carpenter, M., Tomasello, M., & Striano, T. (2005). Role reversal imitation and language in typically developing infants and children with autism. *Infancy, 8*, 253–278.

Carter, A. S., Ben-Sasson, A., & Briggs-Gowan, M. J. (2011). Sensory over-responsivity, psychopathology, and family impairment in school-aged children. *Journal of the American Academy of Child and Adolescent Psychiatry, 5012*, 1210–1219.

Case-Smith, J., & Bryant, T. (1999). The effects of occupational therapy with sensory integration emphasis on preschool-age children with autism. *American Journal of Occupational Therapy, 53*, 489–497.

Case-Smith, J., & Miller, J. (1999). Occupational therapy with children with pervasive developmental disorder. *American Journal of Occupational Therapy, 53*, 506–513.

Cermak, S. A. (2005). Commentary—Chapter 6: Developmental dyspraxia. In A. J. Ayres (Ed.), *Sensory integration and the child: Understanding hidden sensory challenges* (Rev. ed., p. 175). Los Angeles, CA: Western Psychological Services.

Cermak, S. A. (2011). Twenty five years of research in developmental dyspraxia. In A. J. Ayers (Ed.), *Ayres dyspraxia monograph (25th anniversary edition)*. Torrance, CA: Pediatric Therapy Network.

Cermak, S., & Daunhauer, L. (1997). Sensory processing in the postinstitutionalized child. *American Journal of Occupational Therapy, 51*, 500–507.

Cermak, S., & Larkin, D. (Eds.). (2002). *Developmental coordination disorder*. Albany, NY: Delmar.

Chalmers, A., Harrison, S., Mollison, K., Molloy, N., & Gray, K. (2012). Establishing sensory-based approaches in mental health inpatient care: A multidisciplinary approach. *Australasian Psychiatry, 20*, 35–39.

Champagne, T. (2006). Creating sensory rooms: Essential enhancements for acute inpatient mental health settings. *Mental Health Special Interest Newsletter, 29*, 1–4.

Champagne, T. (2010a). Occupational therapy in special situations including high-risk. In M. Scheinholtz (Ed.), *Occupational therapy in mental health: Considerations for advanced practice* (pp. 179–198). Bethesda, MD: American Occupational Therapy Association.

Champagne, T. (2010b). Weighted blanket competency-based training program. Doctoral Manuscript. Proquest. Retrieved from http://udini.proquest.com/view/the-weighted-blanket-competency-goid:577642570/

Champagne, T. (2011a). Attachment, trauma and occupational therapy practice. *OT Practice, 16*, CE1–CE8.

Champagne, T. (2011b). *Sensory modulation and environment: Essential elements of occupation*. (3rd ed., Rev. ed.). Sydney, Australia: Pearson Assessment.

Champagne, T. (2011c). The influence of posttraumatic stress disorder, depression, and sensory processing patterns on occupational engagement: A case study. *WORK: A Journal of Prevention, Assessment, & Rehabilitation, 38*, 67–75.

Champagne, T. (2012). Creating groups for children and youth in community-based mental health occupational therapy practice. *OT Practice, 17*:14, 13–18.

Champagne, T., & Frederick, D. (2011). Sensory processing research advances in mental health: Implications for occupational therapy. *OT Practice, 16*, 7–8.

Champagne, T., Koomar, J., & Olson, L. (2010). Sensory processing evaluation and intervention in mental health. *OT Practice, 15*(5), CE1–CE8.

Champagne, T., & Stromberg, N. (2004). Sensory approaches in inpatient psychiatric settings: Innovative alternatives to seclusion and restraint. *Journal of Psychosocial Nursing, 42*, 35–44.

Cheng, M., & Boggett-Carsjens, J. (2005). Consider sensory processing disorders in the explosive child: Case report and review. *Canadian Academy of Child and Adolescent Psychiatry, 14*, 44–48.

Cloitre, M., Stolbach, B. C., Herman, J. L., van der Kolk, B., Pynoos, R., Wang, J., & Petkova, E. (2009). A developmental approach to complex PTSD: Childhood and adult cumulative trauma as predictors of symptom complexity. *Journal of Traumatic Stress, 22*, 399–408. doi:10.1002/jts.20444

Cohn, E. S. (2001a). Parent perspectives of occupational therapy using a sensory integration approach. *American Journal of Occupational Therapy, 55*, 285–294.

Cohn, E. S. (2001b). From waiting to relating: Parents' experiences in the waiting room of an occupational therapy clinic. *American Journal of Occupational Therapy, 55*, 167–174.

Cohn, E. S., Miller, L. J., & Tickle-Degnen, L. (2000). Parental hopes for therapy outcomes: Children with sensory modulation disorders. *American Journal of Occupational Therapy, 54*, 36–43.

Corbett, B. A., Mendoza, S., Wegelin, J. A., Carmean, V., & Levine, S. (2008). Variable cortisol circadian rhythms in children with autism and anticipatory stress. *Journal of Psychiatry & Neuroscience, 33*, 227–234.

Cornell, B. D. (2004). The superior colliculus: New approaches for studying sensorimotor integration. *Quarterly Review of Biology, 79*, 457.

Courchesne, E., Karns, C. M., Davids, H. R., Ziccardi, R., Carper, R. A., Tigue, Z. D., . . . Yeung-Courchesne, R. (2001). Unusual brain growth patterns in early life in patients with autistic disorder. *Neurology, 57*, 245–254.

Craig, A. D. (2002). How do you feel? Interoception: the sense of the physiological condition of the body. *Nature Reviews Neuroscience, 3*, 655–666.

Crenna, P., & Frigo, C. (1985). Hindered muscle relaxation in spasticity: Experimental evidence suggesting a possible pathophysiological mechanism. *Italian Journal of Neurological Science, 6*, 481–489.

Cruikshank, S. J., & Weinberger, N. M. (1996). Evidence for the Hebbian hypothesis in experience-dependent physiological plasticity of neocortex: A critical review. *Brain Research Reviews, 22*, 191–228.

Cuppini, C., Stein, B. E., Rowland, B. A., Magosso, E., & Ursino, M. (2011). A computational study of multisensory maturation in the superior colliculus (SC). *Experimental Brain Research, 213*, 341–349.

Davies, P. L., Chang, W. P., & Gavin, W. J. (2010). Middle and late latency ERP components discriminate between adults, typical children, and children with sensory processing disorders. *Frontiers in Integrative Neuroscience, 4*, 16.

Davies, P. L., & Gavin, W. J. (2007). Validating the diagnosis of sensory processing disorders using EEG technology. *American Journal of Occupational Therapy, 61*, 176–189.

Deconinck, F. J., De Clercq, D., Van Coster, R., Ooostra, A., Dewitte, G., Savelsbergh, G. J., . . . Lenoir, M. (2008). Sensory contributions to balance in boys with developmental coordination disorder. *Adaptive Physical Activity Quarterly, 25*, 17–35.

DeGangi, G. (2000). *Pediatric disorders of regulation in affect and behavior: A therapist's guide to assessment and treatment*. San Diego, CA: Academic Press.

DeGangi, G., Breinbauer, C., Doussard-Roosevelt, J., Stephen, P., & Greenspan, S. (2005). Prediction of childhood problems at three years in children experiencing disorders of regulation during infancy. *Infant Mental Health Journal, 21*, 156–175.

DeGangi, G., & Greenspan, S. (1988). The development of sensory functioning in infants. *Physical & Occupational Therapy in Pediatrics, 8*, 21–33.

Demb, J., Boynton, G., Best, M., & Heeger, D. (1998). Psychophysical evidence for a magnocellular pathway deficit in dyslexia. *Vision Research, 38*, 1555–1559.

Diamond, M. C., Rosenzweig, M. R., Bennett, E. L., Lindner, B., & Lyon, L. (1972). Effects of environmental enrichment and impoverishment on rat cerebral cortex. *Journal of Neurobiology, 3*, 47–64. doi:10.1002/neu.480030105

Dinse, H. R. (2006). Cortical reorganization in the aging brain. *Progress in Brain Research, 157*, 57–80.

Dunn, W. (1991). The sensorimotor systems: A framework for assessment and intervention. In F. P. Orelove & D. Sobsey (Eds.), *Educating children with multiple disabilities: A transdisciplinary approach* (2nd ed., pp. 33–78). Baltimore, MD: Paul H. Brookes.

Dunn, W. (1997a). The impact of sensory processing abilities on the daily lives of young children and families: A conceptual model. *Infants and Young Children, 9*(4), 23–35.

Dunn, W. (1997b). Implementing neuroscience principles to support habituation and recovery. In C. Christiansen & C. Baum (Eds.), *Occupational therapy: Enabling function and well-being* (2nd ed., pp. 183–232). Thorofare, NJ: Slack.

Dunn, W. (1999). *Sensory Profile*. San Antonio, TX: Therapy Skill Builders.

Dunn, W. (2001). The sensations of everyday life: Theoretical, conceptual and pragmatic considerations. *American Journal of Occupational Therapy, 55*, 608–620.

Dunn, W. (2002a). *Infant/Toddler Sensory Profile*. San Antonio, TX: Therapy Skill Builders.

Dunn, W. (2002b). *The Adolescent/Adult Sensory Profile*. San Antonio: TX: Therapy Skill Builders.

Dunn, W. (2009). Invited commentary on "sensory sensitivities of gifted children." *American Journal of Occupational Therapy, 64*, 296–300.

Dunn, W., & Bennett, D. (2002). Patterns of sensory processing in children with attention deficit hyperactivity disorder. *Occupational Therapy Journal of Research, 22*, 4–15.

Dziuk, M. A., Gidley Larson, J. C., Apostu, A., Mahone, E. M., Denckla, M. B., & Mostofsky, S. H. (2007). Dyspraxia in autism: Association with motor, social, and communication deficits. *Developmental Medicine & Child Neurology, 49*, 734–39.

Eide, F. F. (2003). Sensory integration: Current concepts and practical implications. *Sensory Integration Special Interest Section Quarterly, 26*(3), 1–3.

Erez, O., Gordon, C., Sever, J., Sadeh, J., & Mintz, M. (2004). Balance dysfunction in childhood anxiety: Findings and theoretical approach. *Journal of Anxiety Disorders, 18*, 341–356.

Fatemi, S. H., Halt, A. R., Realmuto, G., Earle, J., Kist, D. A., Thuras, P., & Merz, A. (2002). Purkinje cell size is reduced in cerebellum of patients with autism. *Cellular and Molecular Neurobiology, 22*, 171–175.

Felleman, D. J., & Van Essen, D. C. (1991). Distributed hierarchical processing in the primate cerebral cortex. *Cerebral Cortex, 1*, 1–47.

Felitti, V. J., Anda, R. F., Nordenberg, D., Williamson, D. F., Spitz, A. M., Edwards, V., . . . Marks, J. S. (1998). Relationship of childhood abuse and household dysfunction to many of the leading causes of death in adults: The adverse childhood experiences (ACE) study. *American Journal of Preventive Medicine, 14*, 245–258.

Flanagan, J., Bauman, M., & Landa, R. (in press). Head lag in infants at risk for autism: A preliminary report. *American Journal of Occupational Therapy*.

Fong, S. S. M., Lee, V. Y. L., & Pang, Y. C. (2011). Sensory organization of balance control in children with developmental coordination disorder. *Research in Developmental Disabilities, 32*, 2376–2382.

Ford, J., & Kidd, P. (1998). Early childhood trauma and disorders of extreme stress as predictors of treatment outcome with chronic posttraumatic stress disorder. *Journal of Traumatic Stress, 11*, 743–761.

Fournier, K. A., Hass, C. J., Sagar, K. N., Lodha, N., & Cauraugh, J. H. (2010). Motor coordination in autism spectrum disorders: A synthesis and meta-analysis. *Journal of Autism and Developmental Disorders, 10*, 1227–1240.

Furman, J., & Jacob, R. (2001). The interface of balance disorders and anxiety. *Journal of Anxiety Disorders, 15*, 9–26.

Gal, E., Dyck, M. J., & Passmore, A. (2002). Sensory differences and stereotyped movements in children with autism. *Research in Developmental Disabilities, 30*, 342–352.

Galvan, A. (2010). Neural plasticity of development and learning. *Human Brain Mapping, 31*, 879–890.

Gavin, W. J., Dotseth, A., Roush, K., Smith, C., Spain, H. & Davies, P. L. (2011). Electroencephalography in children with and without sensory processing disorders during auditory perception. *American Journal of Occupational Therapy, 65*, 370–377. doi: 10.5014/ajot.2011.002055

Gibbs, J., Appleton, J., & Appleton, R. (2006). Dyspraxia or developmental coordination disorder/unravelling the enigma. *Archives of Disabilities in Childhood, 92*, 534–539.

Gilbert, C. D., & Wiesel, T. N. (1992). Receptive field dynamics in adult primary visual cortex. *Nature, 356*, 150–152.

Goldsmith, H. H., Van Hulle, C. A., Arneson, C. L., Schreiber, J. E., & Gernsbacher, M. A. (2006). A population-based twin study of parentally reported tactile and auditory defensiveness in young children. *Journal of Abnormal Child Psychology, 34*, 393–407.

Gray, C. (2000). *The new social story book*. Arlington, TX: Future Horizons.

Green, D., Charman, T., Pickles, A., Chandler, S., Loucas, T., Simonoff, E., & Baird, G. (2009). Impairment in movement skills of children with autistic spectrum disorders. *Developmental Medicine & Child Neurology, 51*, 311–316.

Greenspan, S., & Wieder, S. (2006). Engaging autism: Using the floortime approach to help children relate, communicate, and think. *Adolescence, 41*, 399.

Greenwood, P. M. (2007). Functional plasticity in cognitive aging: Review and hypothesis. *Neuropsychology, 21*, 657–673.

Greenwood, P. M., & Parasuraman, R. (2010). Neuronal and cognitive plasticity: A neurocognitive framework for ameliorating cognitive aging. *Frontiers of Aging Neuroscience, 2*, 150.

Gross, C. G. (2000). Neurogenesis in the adult brain: Death of a dogma. *National Review of Neuroscience, 1*, 67–73.

Grove, C. R., & Lazarus, J. A. C. (2007). Impaired re-weighting of sensory feedback for maintenance of postural control in children with developmental coordination disorder. *Human Movement Science, 26*, 457–476.

Hall, L., & Case-Smith, J. (2007). The effect of sound-based intervention on children with sensory processing disorders and visual-motor delays. *American Journal of Occupational Therapy, 61*, 209–215.

Harrison, J., & Hare, D. J. (2004). Brief report: Assessment of sensory abnormalities in people with autistic spectrum disorders. *Journal of Autism and Developmental Disorders, 34*, 727–730.

Hitoglou, M., Ververi, A., Antoniadis, A., & Zafeiriou, D. I. (2010). Childhood autism and auditory system abnormalities. *Pediatric Neurology, 42*, 309–314.

Hoffman, S., & Bitran, S. (2007). Sensory processing sensitivity in social anxiety disorder: Relationship to harm avoidance and diagnostic subtypes. *Journal of Anxiety Disorders, 21*, 944–954.

Horak, F. B., Henry, S. M., & Shumway-Cook, A. (1997). Postural perturbations: New insights for treatment of balance disorders. *Physical Therapy, 77*, 517–533.

Hughes, D. (2004). An attachment-based treatment of maltreated children and young people. *Attachment & Human Development, 6*, 263–278.

Ikiugu, M. (2007). *Psychosocial conceptual practice models in occupational therapy: Building adaptive capacity*. St. Louis, MO: Mosby.

Inder, J. M., & Sullivan, S. J. (2005). Motor and postural response profiles of four children with developmental coordination disorder. *Pediatric Physical Therapy, 17*, 18–29.

Ingersoll, B. (2008). The effect of context on imitation skills in children with autism. *Research in Autism Spectrum Disorders, 2*, 332–340. doi:10.1016/ j.rasd.2007.08.003

Insel, T. (2010). *NIMH Director's Blog. Microbes and mental illness*. Retrieved from http://www.nimh.nih.gov/about/director/index-ocd .shtml

Interdisciplinary Council on Developmental and Learning Disorders. (2005). *Diagnostic manual for infancy and early childhood: Mental health, developmental, regulatory-sensory processing and language disorders and learning challenges (ICDL-DMIC)*. Bethesda, MD: Author.

Jacob, R. G., & Furman, J. M. (1996). Panic, agoraphobia, and vestibular dysfunction. *American Journal of Psychiatry, 153*, 503.

James, W. (1884). What is emotion? *Mind, 9*, 188–205.

Jasmin, E., Couture, M., McKinley, P., Reid, G., Fombonne, E., & Gisel, E. (2009). Sensori-motor and daily living skills of preschool children with autism-spectrum disorders. *Journal of Autism and Developmental Disorders, 39*, 231–241.

Javitt, D. (2009a). Sensory processing in schizophrenia: Neither simple nor intact. *Schizophrenia Bulletin, 35*, 1059–1064.

Javitt, D. C. (2009b). When doors of perception close: Bottom-up models of disrupted cognition in schizophrenia. *Annual Review of Clinical Psychology, 5*, 249–275.

Jenike, M., & Dailey, S. (2011). *Sudden and severe onset OCD (PANS/ PANDAS)—Practical advice for practitioners and parents*. Retrieved from http://www.ocfoundation.org/PANDAS

Kagerer, F. A., Contreras-Vidal, J. L., Bo, J., & Clark, J. E. (2006). Abrupt, but not gradual visuomotor distortion facilitates adaptation in children with developmental coordination disorder. *Human Movement Science, 25*, 622–633.

Kalisch, T., Tegenthoff, M., & Dinse, H. R., (2008). Improvement of sensorimotor functions in old age by passive sensory stimulation. *Clinical Interventions in Aging, 3*, 673–690.

Katschmarsky, S., Cairney, S., Maruff, P., Wilson, P. H., & Currie, J. (2001). The ability to execute saccades on the basis of efference copy: Impairments in double-step saccade performance in children with developmental co-ordination disorder. *Experimental Brain Research, 136*, 73–78.

Katz, L. C., & Shatz, C. J. (1996). Synaptic activity and the construction of cortical circuits. *Science, 274*, 1133–1138.

Kemper, T. L., & Bauman, M. (1998). Neuropathology of infantile autism. *Journal of Neuropathology and Experimental Neurology, 57*, 645–652.

Kempermann, G., & Gage, F. H. (1999). Experience-dependent regulation of adult hippocampal neurogenesis: Effects of long-term stimulation and stimulus withdrawal. *Hippocampus, 9*, 321–332. doi:10.1002/ (SICI)1098-1063(1999)9:3,321::AID-HIPO11.3.0.CO;2-C

Kerr, A. L., Cheng, S. Y., & Jones, T. A. (2011). Experience-dependent neural plasticity in the adult damaged brain. *Journal of Communication Disorders, 44*, 538–548.

Kimball, J. G., Lynch, K. M., Stewart, K. C., Williams, N. E., Thomas, M. A., & Atwood, K. D. (2007). Using salivary cortisol to measure the effects of a Wilbarger protocol-based procedure on sympathetic arousal: a pilot study. *American Journal of Occupational Therapy, 61*, 406–413.

King, A. J., & Palmer, A. R. (1985). Integration of visual and auditory information in bimodal neurons in the guinea-pig superior colliculus. *Experimental Brain Research Journal, 60*, 492–500.

Kinnealey, M., & Fuiek, M. (1999). The relationship between sensory defensiveness, anxiety, depression and perception of pain in adults. *Occupational Therapy International, 6*, 195–206.

Kinnealey, M., Oliver, B., & Wilbarger, P. (1995). A phenomenological study of sensory defensiveness in adults. *American Journal of Occupational Therapy, 49*, 444–451.

Kinninburgh, K., & Blaustein, M. (2005). Attachment, self-regulation and competency: A comprehensive intervention framework for children with complex trauma. *Psychiatric Annals, 35*, 424–430.

Kirvan, C. A., Swedo, S. E., Snider, L. A., & Cunningham, M. W. (2006). Antibody-mediated neuronal cell signaling in behavior and movement disorders. *Journal of Neuroimmunology, 179*, 173–179.

Knox, S. H. (2005). Commentary—Chapter 2: Watching sensory integration develop. In A. J. Ayres (Ed.), *Sensory integration and the child: Understanding hidden sensory challenges* (Rev. ed., p. 171). Los Angeles, CA: Western Psychological Services.

Knox, S., & Mailloux, Z. (1997). Play as treatment and treatment through play. In B. E. Chandler (Ed.), *The essence of play: A child's occupation* (pp. 175–204). Bethesda, MD: The American Occupational Therapy Association.

Koomar, J. (1995). *Vestibular dysfunction is associated with anxiety rather than behavior inhibition or shyness* (Unpublished doctoral dissertation). Boston University, Boston, Massachusetts.

Kopp, S., Beckung, E., & Gillberg, C. (2010). Developmental coordination disorder and other motor control problems in girls with autism spectrum disorder and/or attention-deficit/hyperactivity disorder. *Research in Developmental Disabilities, 31*, 350–361.

Kraemer, G. W. (1992). A psychobiological theory of attachment. *Behavioral and Brain Sciences, 15*, 493–541.

Lane, A. E., Young, R. L., Baker, A. E. Z., & Angley, M. T. (2010). Sensory processing subtypes in autism. *Journal of Autism and Developmental Disorders, 40*, 112–122.

Lane, S. J., Miller, L. J., & Hanft, B. E. (2000). Toward a consensus in terminology in sensory integration theory and practice: Part 2: Sensory integration patterns of function and dysfunction. *Sensory Integration Special Interest Section Quarterly, 23*(2), 1–4.

Lane, S. J., Reynolds, S., & Dumenci, L. (in press). Sensory over-responsivity and anxiety in typical children and children with autism and attention deficit hyperactivity disorder: Cause or co-existence? *American Journal of Occupational Therapy.*

Lane, S. J., Reynolds, S., & Thacker, L. (2010). Sensory over-responsivity and ADHD: Differentiating using electrodermal responses, cortisol, and anxiety. *Frontiers in Integrative Neuroscience, 4*, 1–18.

LeBel, J., & Champagne, T. (2010). Integrating sensory and trauma-informed interventions: A Massachusetts state initiative, part 2. *Mental Health Special Interest Quarterly, 33*(2), 1–4.

LeBel, J., Champagne, T., Stromberg, N., & Coyle, R. (2010). Integrating sensory and trauma-informed interventions: A Massachusetts state initiative, part 1. *Mental Health Special Interest Section Quarterly, 33*(1), 1–4.

Levinson, H. (1989). A cerebellar-vestibular explanation for fears/phobias: Hypothesis and study. *Perceptual and Motor Skills, 68*, 77–84.

Li, K. Z. H., & Lindenberger, U. (2002). Relations between aging sensory/sensorimotor and cognitive functions. *Neuroscience and Biobehavioral Reviews, 26*, 777–783.

Liberzon, I., Taylor, S., Fig, L., & Koeppe, R. (1996–1997). Alteration of corticothalamic perfusion ratios during a PTSD flashback. *Depression and Anxiety, 4*, 146–150.

Lin, S. H., Cermak, S., Coster, W. J., & Miller, L. (2005). The relation between length of institutionalization and sensory integration in children adopted from Eastern Europe. *American Journal of Occupational Therapy, 59*, 139–147.

Linderman, T. M., & Stewart, K. B. (1999). Sensory integrative-based occupational therapy and functional outcomes in young children with pervasive developmental disorders: A single-subject study. *American Journal of Occupational Therapy, 53*, 207–213.

Liss, M., Saulnier, C., Fein, D., & Kinsbourne, M. (2006). Sensory and attention abnormalities in autistic spectrum disorders. *Autism, 10*, 155–172.

Liss, M., Timmel, L., Baxley, K., & Kilingsworth, P. (2005). Sensory processing sensitivity and its relation to parental bonding anxiety and depression. *Personality and Individual Differences, 39*, 1429–1439.

Mailloux, Z. (2001). Sensory integrative principles in intervention with children with autistic disorder. In S. Roley, E. I. Blanche, & R. C. Schaaf (Eds.), *Understanding the nature of sensory integration with diverse populations* (pp. 365–384). San Antonio, TX: Therapy Skill Builders.

Mailloux, Z., May-Benson, T. A., Summers, C. A., Miller, L. J., Brett-Green, B., Burke, J. P., . . . Schoen, S. A. (2007). Goal attainment scaling as a measure of meaningful outcomes for children with sensory integration disorders. *American Journal of Occupational Therapy, 61*, 254–259.

Mailloux, Z., Mulligan, S., Smith Roley, S., Cermak, S., Blanche, E., Bodison, S., . . . Lane, C. (2011). Verification and clarification of patterns of sensory integrative dysfunction in a retrospective clinical sample. *American Journal of Occupational Therapy, 65*, 143–151.

Mailloux, Z., & Smith Roley, S. (2010). Sensory integration. In H. Miller & R. Watling (Eds.), *Autism* (3rd ed., pp. 469–507). Bethesda, MD: The American Occupational Therapy Association.

Malow, B. A., Marzec, M. L., McGrew, S., Wang, L., Henderson, L. M., & Stone, W. L. (2006). Characterizing sleep in children with autism spectrum disorders: A multidimensional approach. *Sleep, 29*, 1563–1571.

Mangeot, S. D., Miller, L. J., McIntosh, D. N., McGrath-Clarke, J., Simon, J., Hagerman, R. J., & Goldson, E. (2001). Sensory modulation dysfunction in children with attention-deficit-hyperactivity disorder. *Developmental Medicine and Child Neurology, 43*, 399–406.

Marco, E. J., Hinkley, L. B. N., Hill, S. S., & Magarajan, S. S. (2011). Sensory processing in autism: A review of neurophysiologic findings. *Pediatric Research, 69*, 48R–54R.

Marr, D., Gal, E., & Nackley, V. L. (2007). Sensory stories: Improving participation for children with sensory modulation dysfunction (SMD). *The Israeli Journal of Occupational Therapy, 15*, E41–E55.

Marr, D., Mika, H., Miraglia, J., Roerig, M., & Sinnott, R. (2007). The effect of sensory stories on targeted behaviors in preschool children with autism. *Physical and Occupational Therapy in Pediatrics, 27*, 63–79.

Marr, D., & Nackley, V. L. (2005). Sensory stories: A new tool to improve participation for children with over-reproductive sensory modulation. *SI Focus*, 8–9.

Martinez, A., Hillyard, S. A., Dias, E. C., Hagler, D. J., Jr., Butler, P. D., Guilfoyle, D. N., . . . Javitt, D. C. (2008). Magnocellular pathway impairment in schizophrenia: Evidence from functional magnetic resonance imaging. *Journal of Neuroscience, 28*, 7492–7500.

Massachusetts Department of Mental Health. (2010). *Seclusion/restraint reduction initiative*. Retrieved from http://www.mass.gov/eohhs/gov/departments/dmh/restraintseclusion-reduction-initiative.html

May-Benson, T. A. (2001). A theoretical model of ideation in praxis. In S. Smith Roley, E. I. Blanche, & R. C. Schaaf (Eds.), *Understanding the nature of sensory integration with diverse populations* (pp. 163–181). New Mexico, NM: Therapy Skill Builders.

May-Benson, T. A., & Cermak, S. A. (2007). Development of an assessment for ideational praxis. *American Journal of Occupational Therapy, 61*, 148–153.

May-Benson, T. A., & Koomar, J. A. (2007). Identifying gravitational insecurity in children: A pilot study. *American Journal of Occupational Therapy, 61*, 142–147.

May-Benson, T. A., & Koomar, J. A. (2010). Systematic review of the research evidence examining the effectiveness of interventions using a sensory integrative approach for children. *American Journal of Occupational Therapy, 64*, 403–414.

McCleery, J., Allman, E., Carver, L., & Dobkins, K. (2007). Abnormal magnocellular pathway visual processing in infants at risk for autism. *Biological Psychiatry, 62*, 1007–1014.

McIntosh, D. N., Miller, L. J., Shyu, V., & Hagerman, J. L. (1999). Sensory-modulation disruption, electrodermal responses, and functional behaviors. *Developmental Medicine and Child Neurology, 41*, 608–615.

McLaughlin, J., Kennedy, B., & Zemke, R. (1996). Dynamic systems theory: An overview. In R. Zemke & F. Clark (Eds.), *Occupational science: The evolving discipline* (pp. 297–308). Philadelphia, PA: F. A. Davis.

Mesulam, M. M. (1998). From sensation to cognition. *Brain, 121*, 1013–1052.

Meyer, B., Ajchenbrenner, M., & Bowles, D. P. (2005). Sensory sensitivity, attachment experiences, and rejection responses among adults with borderline and avoidant features. *Journal of Personality Disorders, 19*, 641–658.

Middleton, F. A., & Strick, P. L. (2000). Basal ganglia and cerebellar loops: Motor and cognitive circuits. *Brain Research Reviews, 31*, 236–250.

Miller, E. K. (2000). Organization through experience. *Nature Neuroscience, 3*, 1066–1068.

Miller, L. J., Anzalone, M. A., Lane, S. J., Cermak, S., & Osten, E. T. (2007). Concept evolution in sensory integration: A proposed nosology for diagnosis. *American Journal of Occupational Therapy, 61*, 135–140.

Miller, L. J., Cermak, S., Lane, S., Anzalone, M., & Koomar, J. (2004). Position statement on terminology related to sensory integration dysfunction. *S.I. Focus*, 6–8.

Miller, L. J., Coll, J. R., & Schoen, S. A. (2007). A randomized controlled pilot study of the effectiveness of occupational therapy for children with sensory modulation disorder. *American Journal of Occupational Therapy, 61*, 228–238.

Miller, L. J., & Lane, S. J. (2000, March). Toward a concensus [sic] in terminology in sensory integration theory and practice: Part 1: Taxonomy of neurophysiological processes. *Sensory Integration Special Interest Section Quarterly, 23*(1), 1–4.

Miller, L. J., McIntosh, D. N., McGrath, J., Shyu, V., Lampe, M., Taylor, A. K., . . . Hagerman, R. (1999). Electrodermal responses to sensory stimuli in individuals with fragile X syndrome: A preliminary report. *American Journal of Medical Genetics, 83*, 268–279.

Miller, L. J., Reisman, J. E., McIntosh, D. N., & Simon, J. (2001). An ecological model of sensory modulation: Performance of children with fragile X syndrome, autistic disorder, attention-deficit/hyperactivity disorder, and sensory modulation dysfunction. In S. Smith Roley, E. I. Blanche, & R. C. Schaaf (Eds.), *Understanding the nature of sensory integration with diverse populations* (pp. 57–88). Philadelphia, PA: Harcourt Health Sciences.

Miller, L. J., Schoen, S. A., James, K., & Schaaf, R. C. (2007). Lessons learned: A pilot study on occupational therapy effectiveness for children with sensory modulation disorder. *American Journal of Occupational Therapy, 61*, 161–169.

Miller, L. J., Wilbarger, J. L., Stackhouse, T. M., & Trunnell, S. L. (2002). Use of clinical reasoning in occupational therapy: The STEP-SI model of treatment of sensory modulation dysfunction. In A. C. Bundy, S. J. Lane, & E. A. Murray (Eds.), *Sensory integration: Theory and practice* (2nd ed., pp. 435–451). Philadelphia, PA: F. A. Davis.

Miller-Kuhaneck, H., & Smith Roley, S. (2005). A kindergartner with sensory integration dysfunction. In K. Sladyk (Ed.), *Ryan's occupational therapy assistant* (pp. 139–154). Thorofare, NJ: Slack.

Milner, C. E., Cuthbert, B. P., Kertesz, R. S., & Cote, K. A. (2009). Sensory gating impairments in poor sleepers during presleep wakefulness. *Neuroreport, 20*, 331–336.

Ming, X., Juluc, P. O. O., Brimacombed, M., Connore, S., & Daniels, M. L. (2005). Reduced cardiac parasympathetic activity in children with autism. *Brain and Development, 27*, 509–516.

Minner, D., Hoffstetter, P., Casey, L., & Jones, D. (2004). Snoezelen activity: The good shepherd nursing home experience. *Journal of Nursing Care Quality, 19*, 343–348.

Montegue, A. (1986). *Touching: The human significance of the skin*. New York, NY: Harper and Row.

Moore, K. (2005). *The sensory connection program: Activities for mental health treatment. Manual and handbook*. Framingham, MA: Therapro.

Moore, K., & Henry, A. (2002). Treatment of adult psychiatric patients using the Wilbarger protocol. *Occupational Therapy in Mental Health, 18*, 43–63.

Moretti, G., Pasquini, M., Tarsitani, L., Blondi, M., & Mandarelli, G. (2008). What every psychiatrist should know about PANDAS: A review. *Clinical Practice and Epidemiology in Mental Health, 4*(13), 1–9. doi:10.1186/1745-0179-4-13

Morey, R., Mitchell, T., Inan, S., Lieberman, J., & Belger, A. (2008). Neural correlates of automatic and controlled auditory processing in schizophrenia. *The Journal of Neuropsychiatry and Clinical Neurosciences, 20*, 419–430.

Mullen, B., Champagne, T., Krishnamurty, S., Dickson, D., & Gao, R. (2008). Exploring the safety and therapeutic effects of deep pressure stimulation using a weighted blanket. *Occupational Therapy in Mental Health, 24*, 65–89.

Mulligan, S. (1996). An analysis of score patterns of children with attention disorders on the Sensory Integration and Praxis Tests. *American Journal of Occupational Therapy, 50*, 647–654.

Mulligan, S. (1998a). Application of structural equation modeling in occupational therapy research. *American Journal of Occupational Therapy, 52*, 829–834.

Mulligan, S. (1998b). Patterns of sensory integration dysfunction: A confirmatory factor analysis. *American Journal of Occupational Therapy, 52*, 819–828.

Mulligan, S. (2000). Cluster analysis of scores of children on the Sensory Integration and Praxis Tests. *Occupational Therapy Journal of Research, 20*, 256–262.

Mulligan, S. (2003). Examination of the evidence for occupational therapy using a sensory integration framework with children: Part two. *Sensory Integration Special Interest Section Quarterly, 26*(2), 1–5.

Mutti, M. C., Martin, N. A., Sterling, H. M., & Spalding, N. V. (1998). Quick Neurological Screening Test manual (3rd ed.). Novato, CA: Academic Therapy.

Murphy, T. K., Kurlan, R., & Leckman, J. (2010). The immunobiology of Tourette's disorder, pediatric autoimmune neuropsychiatric disorders associated with streptococcus, and related disorders: A way forward. *Journal of Child and Adolescent Psychopharmacology, 20*, 317–331. doi:10.1089/cap.2010.0043

National Association of State Mental Health Program Directors. (2003). *National Executive Training Institute: Training curriculum for the reduction of seclusion and restraint*. Alexandria, VA: Author.

National Association of State Mental Health Program Directors. (2009). *Training curriculum for creation of violence-free, coercion-free treatment settings and the reduction of seclusion and restraint* (7th ed.). Alexandria, VA: National Association of State Mental Health Program Directors, Office of Technical Assistance.

Neal, J., Edelmann, R. J., & Glachan, M. (2002). Behavioural inhibition and symptoms of anxiety and depression: Is there a specific relationship with social phobia? *British Journal of Clinical Psychology, 41*, 361.

O'Hare, A., & Khalid, S. (2002). The association of abnormal cerebellar function in children with developmental coordination disorder and reading difficulties. *Dyslexia, 8*, 234–248.

Ogden, P., Minton, K., & Pain, C. (2007). *Trauma and the body: A sensorimotor approach to psychotherapy*. New York, NY: W. W. Norton.

Olson, L. (2010, March). Examining schizophrenia and sensory modulation disorder: A review of the literature. *Sensory Integration Special Interest Section Quarterly, 33*(1), 1–3.

Parham, L. D., Cohn, E. S., Spitzer, S., Koomar, J., Miller, L. J., Burke, J. P., . . . Summers, C. A. (2007). Fidelity in sensory integration intervention research. *American Journal of Occupational Therapy, 61*, 216–227.

Parham, L. D., & Ecker, C. J. (2007). *Sensory Processing Measure—Home form*. Los Angeles, CA: Western Psychological Services.

Parham, L. D., & Mailloux, Z. (2010). Sensory integration. In J. Case-Smith (Ed.), *Occupational therapy for children* (6th ed., pp. 325–372). St. Louis, MO: Mosby.

Parham, L. D., Smith Roley, S., May-Benson, T., Koomar, J., Brett-Green, B., Burke, J. P., . . . Schaaf, R. C. (2011). Development of a fidelity measure for research on effectiveness of Ayres sensory integration intervention. *American Journal of Occupational Therapy, 65*, 133–142.

Parush, S., Sohmer, H., Steinberg, A., & Kaitz, M. (1997). Somatosensory functioning in children with attention deficit hyperactivity disorder. *Developmental Medicine and Child Neurology, 39*, 464–468.

Parush, S., Sohmer, H., Steinberg, A., & Kaitz, M. (2007). Somatosensory function in boys with ADHD and tactile defensiveness. *Physiology & Behavior, 16*, 553–558.

Patestas, M., & Gartner, L. P., (2006). *A textbook of neuroanatomy*. Oxford, United Kingdom: Wiley-Blackwell.

Perna, G., Dario, A., Caldirola, D., Stefania, B., Cesarani, A., & Bellodi, L. (2001). Panic disorder: The role of the balance system. *Journal of Psychiatric Research, 35*, 279–286.

Pfeiffer, B. A., Koenig, K., Kinnealey, M., Sheppard, M., & Henderson, L. (2011). Effectiveness of sensory integration interventions in children with Autism Spectrum Disorders: A pilot study. *American Journal of Occupational Therapy, 65*, 76–85.

Polatajko, H. J., & Cantin, N. (2006). Developmental coordination disorder (dyspraxia): An overview of the state of the art. *Seminars in Pediatric Neurology, 12*, 250–258.

Pons, T. P., Garraghty, P. E., Friedman, D. P., & Mishkin, M. (1987). Physiological evidence for serial processing in somatosensory cortex. *Science, 237*, 417–420.

Purves, D., Augustine, G. J., Fitzpatrick, D., Hall, W. C., LaMantia, A.-S., & White, L. E. (2012). *Neuroscience* (5th ed.). Sunderland, MA: Sinauer Associates.

Reed, D.R., Toshiko, T., McDaniel, A.H.. 2006. Diverse tastes: genetics of sweet and bitter perception. *Physiology & Behavior, 88*: 215–226.

Reisman, J., & Hanschu, B. (1992). *Sensory Integration Inventory User's Guide.* Stillwater, MN: PDP Press.

Reynolds, S., & Lane, S. J. (2007). Diagnostic validity of sensory over-responsivity: A review of the literature and case reports. *Journal of Autism and Developmental Disabilities, 38*, 516–529.

Reynolds, S., Lane, S. J., & Gennings, C. (2010). The moderating role of sensory over-responsivity in HPA activity. *Journal of Attention Disorders, 13*, 468–478.

Reynolds, S., Lane, S. J., & Thacker, L. (2012). Sensory processing, physiological stress, and sleep behaviors in children with and without autism spectrum disorder. *Occupation, Participation and Health, 31*, 246–257.

Ritvo, E. R., Freeman, B. J., Scheibel, A. B., Duong, T., Robinson, H., Guthrie, D., & Ritvo, A. (1986). Lower Purkinje cell counts in the cerebella of four autistic subjects: Initial findings of the UCLA-NSAC autopsy research report. *American Journal of Psychiatry, 143*, 862–866.

Roberts, J. E., King-Thomas, L., & Boccia, M. L. (2007). Behavioral indexes of the efficacy of sensory integration therapy. *American Journal of Occupational Therapy, 61*, 555–562.

Rolls, E. T. (2004). Multisensory neuronal convergence of taste, somatosensory, visual, olfactory, and auditory inputs. In G. Calvert, C. Spence, & B. E. Stein (Eds.), *The handbook of multisensory processes* (pp. 311–332). Cambridge, MA: The MIT Press.

Ross, M. (1997). *Integrative group therapy: Mobilizing coping abilities with the five-stage group.* Bethesda, MD: American Occupational Therapy Association.

Ross, M., & Burdick, D. (1981). *Sensory integration: A training manual for therapists and teachers for regressed, psychiatric and geriatric patient groups.* Thorofare, NJ: Slack.

Royeen, C. (2003). Chaotic occupational therapy: Collective wisdom for a complex profession. *American Journal of Occupational Therapy, 57*, 609–624.

Ruzzano, S., Smith Roley, S., & Mailloux, Z. (2003). *Applying Sensory Integration Where Children Live, Learn, and Play (DVD).* Torrance, CA: Pediatric Therapy Network.

Saxe, G., Chawla, N., & van der Kolk, B. (2002). Self-destructive behavior in patients with dissociative disorders. *Suicide Life Threatening Behavior, 32*, 313–320.

Schaaf, R. C. (2011). Interventions that address sensory dysfunction for individuals with autism spectrum disorders: Preliminary evidence for the superiority of sensory integration compared to other sensory approaches. In B. Reichow, P. Doehring, D. V. Cichetti, & F. R. Volkmar (Eds.), *Evidence-based practices and treatments for children with autism* (pp. 245–273). New York, NY: Springer.

Schaaf, R. C., & Anzalone, M. A (2001). Sensory integration with high risk infants and toddlers. In S. Smith-Roley, E. I. Blanche, & R. C. Schaaf (Eds.), *Understanding the Nature of Sensory Integration with Diverse Populations* (pp. 275–312). San Antonio, TX: Harcourt Assessment.

Schaaf, R. C., Benevides, T., Blanche, E. I., Brett-Green, B. A., Burke, J. B., Cohn, E. S., . . . Schoen, S. A. (2010). Parasympathetic functions in children with sensory processing disorder. *Frontiers in Integrative Neuroscience, 4*, 4. doi:10.3389/fnint.2010.00004

Schaff, R. C., Benevides, T., Kelly, D., & Mailloux-Maggio, Z. (2012). Occupational therapy and sensory integration for children with autism: a feasibility, safety, acceptability and fidelity study. *Autism, 16*, 321–327.

Schaaf, R. C., Miller, L. J., Seewal, D., & O'Keefe, S. (2003). Children with disturbances in sensory processing: A pilot study examining the role of the parasympathetic nervous system. *American Journal of Occupational Therapy, 57*, 442–449.

Schaaf, R. C., Schoen, S., Smith Roley, S., Lane, S., Koomar, J., & May-Benson, T. (2009). A frame of reference for sensory integration. In P. Kramer & J. Hinojosa (Eds.), *Frames of reference for pediatric occupational therapy* (3rd ed., pp. 99–186). Baltimore, MD: Lippincott Williams & Wilkins.

Schaaf, R. C., & Smith Roley, S. (2006). *Clinical reasoning: Applying sensory integration principles to practice with diverse populations.* San Antonio, TX: Psychological Corporation.

Schilling, D. L., Washington, K., Billingsley, F. F., & Deitz, J. (2003). Classroom seating for children with attention deficit hyperactivity disorder: Therapy balls versus chairs. *American Journal of Occupational Therapy, 57*, 534–541.

Schlaug, G. (2001). The brain of musicians. A model for functional and structural adaptation. *New York Academy of Sciences, 930*, 281–299.

Schneider, M. (2005). Commentary—Chapter 1: What is sensory integration? In A. J. Ayres (Ed.), *Sensory integration and the child: Understanding hidden sensory challenges* (pp. 169–170). Los Angeles, CA: Western Psychological Services.

Schoen, S. A., Miller, L. J., Brett-Green, B., & Hepburn, S. L. (2008). Psychophysiology of children with autism spectrum disorder. *Research in Autism Spectrum Disorders, 2*, 417–429.

Schoen, S. A., Miller, L. J., Brett-Green, B., & Nielsen, D. M. (2009). Physiological and behavioral differences in sensory processing: A comparison of children with autism spectrum disorder and sensory modulation disorder. *Frontiers in Integrative Neuroscience, 3*, 29. doi:10.3389/neuro.07.029.2009

Schoen, S. A., Miller, L. J., Brett-Green, B., Reynolds, S., & Lane, S. J. (2008). Arousal and reactivity in children with sensory processing disorder and autism spectrum disorder. *Psychophysiology, 45*, S102.

Schore, A. (1994). *Affect regulation and the origin of the self: The neurobiology of emotional development.* Hillsdale, NJ: Lawrence Erlbaum Associates.

Seri, S., Pisani, F., Thai, J. N., & Cerquiglini, A. (2007). Pre-attentive auditory sensory processing in autistic spectrum disorder: Are electromagnetic measurements telling us a coherent story? *International Journal of Psychophysiology, 63*, 159–163.

Sevlever, M., & Gillis, J. M. (2010). An examination of the state of imitation research in children with autism: Issues of definition and methodology. *Research in Developmental Disabilities, 31*, 976–984.

Shani-Adir, A., Rozenman, D., Kessel, A., & Engel-Yeger, B. (2009). The relationship between sensory hypersensitivity and sleep quality of children with atopic dermatitis. *Pediatric Dermatology, 26*, 143–149.

Sheean, G., & McGuire, J. R. (2009). Spastic hypertonia and movement disorders: Pathophysiology, clinical presentation, and quantification. *Physical Medicine and Rehabilitation, 19*, 827–833.

Sherrington, C. S. (1951). *Man on his nature.* Garden City, NY: Doubleday.

Shochat, T., Tzischinsky, O., & Engel-Yeger, B. (2009). Sensory hypersensitivity as a contributing factor in the relation between sleep and behavioral disorders in normal children. *Behavioral Sleep Medicine, 7*, 53–62.

Siegel, A., & Sapru, H. N., (2011). *Essential neuroscience* (2nd ed.). Philadelphia, PA: Lippincott Williams & Wilkins.

Smith, L. B., & Thelen, E. (Eds.). (1993). *A dynamic systems approach to development.* Cambridge, MA: MIT Press.

Smith Roley, S. (2005). Commentary—Chapter 8: Visual perception and auditory-language disorders. In A. J. Ayres (Ed.), Sensory integration and the child: Understanding hidden sensory challenges (pp. 169–170). Los Angeles, CA: Western Psychological Services.

Smith Roley, S., Blanche, E. I., & Schaaf, R. C. (Eds.). (2001). *Understanding the nature of sensory integration with diverse populations.* San Antonio, TX: Therapy Skill Builders.

Smith Roley, S., Mailloux, Z., Miller-Kuhaneck, H., & Glennon, T. (2007). Understanding Ayres sensory integration. *OT Practice, 12*(17), CE1–CE8.

Souders, M. C., Mason, T. B. A., Valladares, O., Bucan, M., Levy, S. E., Mandell, D. S., . . . Pinto-Martin, J. (2009). Sleep behaviors and sleep quality in children with autism spectrum disorders. *Sleep, 32*, 1566–1578.

Sparks, D. L., & Groh, J. M. (1995). The superior colliculus: A window to problems in integrative neuroscience. In M. S. Gazzaniga (Ed.), *The cognitive neurosciences* (pp. 565–584). Cambridge, MA: MIT Press.

Spitzer, S. L. (1999, June). Dynamic systems theory: Relevance to the theory of sensory integration and the study of occupation. *Sensory Integration Special Interest Section Quarterly, 22*(2), 1–4.

Spitzer, S., & Smith Roley, S. (2001). Sensory integration revisited: A philosophy of practice. In S. Smith Roley, E. I. Blanche, & R. C. Schaaf (Eds.), *Understanding the nature of sensory integration with diverse populations* (pp. 3–23). San Antonio, TX: Therapy Skill Builders.

Stein, B. E., Huneycutt, W. S., & Meredith, M. A. (1988). Neurons and behavior: The same rules of multisensory integration apply. *Brain Research, 448*, 355–358.

Stein, B. E., & Meredith, M. A. (1993). *The merging of the senses.* Cambridge, MA: MIT Press.

Stein, B. E., Meredith, M. A., Huneycutt, W. S., & McDade, L. (1989). Behavioral indices of multisensory integration: Orientation to visual cues is affected by auditory stimuli. *Journal of Cognitive Neuroscience, 1*, 12–24.

Stein, B. E., & Rowland, B. A. (2011). Organization and plasticity in multisensory integration: Early and late experience affects its governing principles. *Progress in Brain Research, 191*, 145–163.

Stoller, C., Greuel, J., Cimini, L., Fowler, M., & Koomar, J. (2012). Effects of sensory-enhanced yoga on symptoms of combat stress in deployed military personnel. *American Journal of Occupational Therapy, 66*, 59–68.

Swedo, S. E., Leonard, H. L., Garvey, M., Mittleman, B., Allen, A. J., Perlmutter, S., . . . Dubbert, B. K. (1998). Pediatric autoimmune neuropsychiatric disorders associated with streptococcal infections: Clinical description of the first 50 cases. *American Journal of Psychiatry, 155*, 264–271.

Tate, D. F., Bigler, E. D., McMahon, W., & Lainhart, J. (2007). The relative contributions of brain, cerebrospinal fluid-filled structures, and non-neural tissue volumes to occipital-frontal head circumference in subjects with autism. *Neuropediatrics, 38*, 18–24.

Teitelbaum, P., Teitelbaum, O., Nye, J., Fryman, J., & Maurer, R. G. (1998). Movement analysis in infancy may be useful for early diagnosis of autism. *Proceedings of the National Academy of Science, 95*, 13982–13987.

Thelen, E., & Smith, L. B. (1994). *A dynamic systems approach to the development of cognition and action.* Cambridge, MA: MIT Press.

Tomchek, S. D., & Dunn, W. (2007). Sensory processing in children with and without autism: A comparative study using the Short Sensory Profile. *American Journal of Occupational Therapy, 61*, 190–200.

Tona, J., & Posner, T. (2011). Pediatric autoimmune neuropsychiatric disorders: A new frontier for occupational therapy intervention. *OT Practice, 16*(20), 14.

Twamley, E. W., Salva, G. N., Zurhellen, C. H., Heaton, R. K., & Jeste, D. V. (2008). Development and pilot testing of a novel compensatory cognitive training intervention for people with psychosis. *American Journal of Psychiatric Rehabilitation, 11*, 144–163.

U. S. Department of Health and Human Services, Substance Abuse and Mental Health Services Administration (2003a). *A national call to action: Eliminating the use of seclusion and restraint.* Rockville, MD: USDHHS.

U. S. Department of Health and Human Services, Substance Abuse and Mental Health Services Administration. (2003b). *National consensus statement on recovery.* Retrieved from http://mentalhealth.samhsa.gov/publications/allpubs/sma05-4129/

Vandeberg, N. (2001). The use of a weighted vest to increase on-task behavior in children with attention difficulties. *American Journal of Occupational Therapy, 55*, 621–628.

Van der Hart, O., & Steele, K. (1997). Time distortions in dissociative identity disorder: Janetian concepts and treatment. *Dissociation: Progress in the Dissociative Disorders, 10*, 91–103.

Van der Kolk, B. (2005). Developmental trauma disorder: Toward a rational diagnosis for children with complex trauma histories. *Psychiatric Annals, 35*, 401–408.

Van der Kolk, B. (2006) Clinical implications of neuroscience research and PTSD. *Annals of the New York Academy of Science, 1071*, 277–293.

Van Hulle, C., Schmidt, N., & Goldsmith, H. (2011). Is sensory over-responsivity distinguishable from childhood behavior problems? A phenotypic and genetic analysis. *Journal of Child Psychology and Psychiatry, 53*, 64–72.

Velasques, B., Machado, S., Paes, F., Cunha, M., Sanfim, A., Budde, H., . . . Ribeiro, P. (2011). Sensorimotor integration and psychopathology: Motor control abnormalities related to psychiatric disorders. *The World Journal of Biological Psychiatry, 12*, 560–573.

Verhoeven, J. S., DeCock, P., Lagae, L., & Sunaert, S. (2010). Neuroimaging of autism. *Neuroradiology, 52*, 3–14.

Wall, J. T., Xu, J., & Wang, X. (2002). Human brain plasticity: An emerging view of the multiple substrates and mechanisms that cause cortical changes and related sensory dysfunctions after injuries of sensory inputs from the body. *Brain Research Reviews, 39*, (2–3), 181–215.

Wallace, M. T., Meredith, M. A., & Stein, B. E. (1993). Converging influences from visual, auditory, and somatosensory cortices onto output neurons of the superior colliculus. *Journal of Neurophysiology, 69*, 1797–1809.

Warner, E., Cook, A., Westcott, A., & Koomar, J. (2011). *SMART: Sensory motor arousal regulation treatment.* Brookline, MA: Trauma Center at JRI.

Watling, R., Koenig, K., & Davies, P. (2011). *Occupational therapy practice guidelines for children and adolescents with challenges in sensory processing and sensory integration.* Bethesda, MD: AOTA Press.

Weisberg, A. (1984). The role of psychophysiology in defining gravitational insecurity: A pilot study. *Sensory Integration Special Interest Section Newsletter, 7*(4), 1–4.

Wilbarger, P. (1984, September). Planning an adequate sensory diet: Application of sensory processing theory during the first years of life. *Zero to Three*, 7–12.

Wilbarger, J., & Wilbarger, P. (2002). Clinical application of the sensory diet. In A. C. Bundy, S. J. Lane, & E. A. Murray (Eds.), *Sensory integration theory and practice* (2nd ed., pp. 339–341). Philadelphia, PA: F. A. Davis.

Williams, M. S., & Shellenberger, S. (1996). *How does your engine run?: A leader's guide to the alert program for self-regulation.* Albuquerque, NM: TherapyWorks.

Williamson, G. G., & Anzalone, M. E. (2001). *Sensory integration and self-regulation in infants and toddlers: Helping very young children interact with their environment.* Washington, DC: Zero to Three.

Wilson, B. N., Pollock, N., Kaplan, B. J., & Law, M. (2000). *Clinical Observations of Motor and Postural Skills (COMPS).* Framingham, MA: Therapro.

Windsor, M., Smith Roley, S., & Szklut, S. (2001). Assessment of sensory integration and praxis. In S. Roley, E. I. Blanche, & R. C. Schaaf (Eds.), *Understanding the nature of sensory integration with diverse populations* (pp. 215–245). San Antonio, TX: Therapy Skill Builders.

Yochman, A., Parush, S., & Ornoy. A. (2004). Responses of preschool children with and without ADHD to sensory events in daily life. *American Journal of Occupational Therapy, 58*, 294–302.

Young, G. S., Rogers, S. J., Rozga, A., Ozonoff, S., Hutman, T., & Sigman, M. (2011). Imitation from 12 to 24 months in autism and typical development: A longitudinal Rasch analysis. *Developmental Psychology, 47*, 1565–1578.

Zero to Three. (2005). *Diagnostic classification of mental health and developmental disorders of infancy and early childhood, revised (DC: 0–3R).* Arlington, VA: National Center for Clinical Infant Programs.

Zwicker, J. G., Missiuna, C., Harris, S. R., &. Boyd, L. A. (2010). Brain activation of children with developmental coordination disorder is different than peers. *Pediatrics, 126*, e678–e686. doi:10.1542/peds.2010-0059

For additional resources on the subjects discussed in this chapter, visit http://thePoint.lww.com/Willard-Spackman12e.

CHAPTER 57

Emotion Regulation

Marjorie E. Scaffa

LEARNING OBJECTIVES

After reading this chapter, you will be able to:

1. Describe the neurophysiological and developmental aspects of emotion regulation
2. Discuss the relationship between emotion regulation and trauma
3. Understand how emotion regulation supports or limits occupational performance
4. Identify assessments that are used to measure emotion regulation
5. Develop intervention plans that address the needs of persons with emotion dysregulation and improve occupational performance
6. Discuss a strength-based approach to emotion regulation

OUTLINE

Introduction

Emotions are an essential component of being human. It is impossible to be alive and not experience emotions. According to Mahoney (2005), "emotional processes are among the most powerful and primitive of human self-organizing processes" (p. 747). Although the term **emotion** is difficult to define, there is consensus that emotions are evaluative mental states that occur in the present moment and consist of neurobiological arousal, perceptual-cognitive processes, subjective experience, and affective expression (Izard, 2010). Emotions arise when a situation appears that has relevance to one's goals. Situations that are likely to enhance goal attainment elicit pleasurable emotions, whereas situations that are likely to inhibit goal attainment elicit negative or unpleasant feelings. Emotions provide us with qualitative information on which to make decisions that result in adaptive responses in our everyday lives. Emotions serve various functions including "motivating and focusing individual endeavors, social interactions, and the development of adaptive and maladaptive behavior" (Izard, 2010, p. 368).

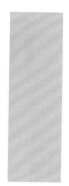

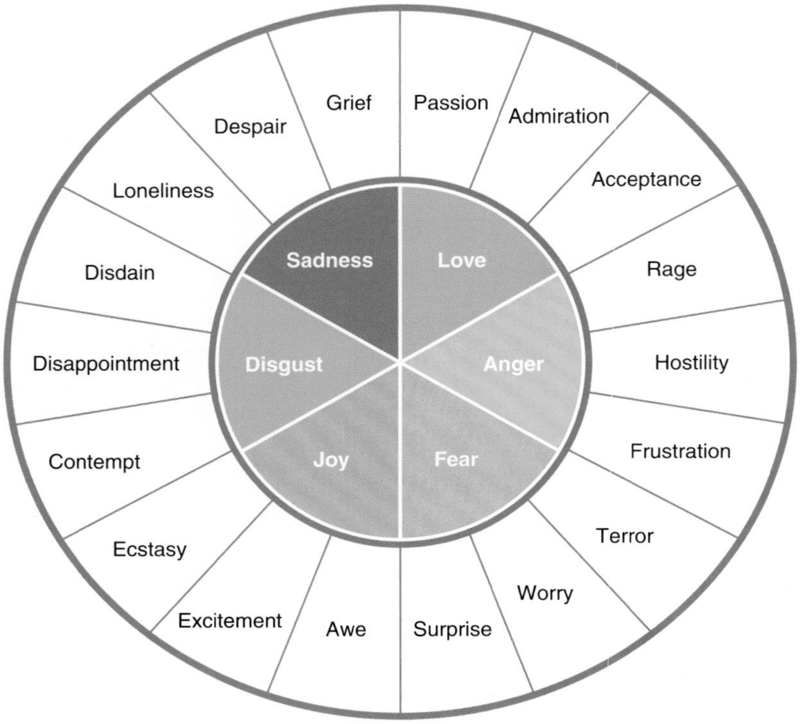

FIGURE 57.1 Emotions wheel.

Some emotions are ubiquitous and experienced by all human beings, for example, love, anger, grief/sadness, fear, joy, and disgust. Other emotions are often melds of these primary emotions. For example, surprise could be conceived of as a melding or combination of joy and fear, whereas contempt is a melding of anger and disgust. Emotions vary in intensity. For example, disappointment, frustration, and rage are varying intensities of anger, whereas anticipation, happiness, and ecstasy are varying intensities of joy (Nussbaum, 2001). One way to illustrate the variety and intensities of emotion is through an emotions wheel (see Figure 57.1).

Emotions can affect health directly and indirectly, and that impact can be either positive or negative. Emotions can influence health directly through their impact on the immune, endocrine, cardiovascular, and nervous systems. Emotions affect health indirectly through adherence to medical regimens and participation in healthy or unhealthy behaviors (Kiecolt-Glaser, McGuire, Robles, & Glaser, 2002).

An Overview of Emotion Regulation

Emotions are rarely obligatory or automatic and are therefore subject to self-regulation and response modulation. Eisenberg and Spinrad (2004) define *emotion-related self-regulation* as

> the process of initiating, avoiding, inhibiting, maintaining, or modulating the occurrence, form, intensity, or duration of internal feeling states, emotion-related physiological, attentional processes, motivational states, and/or the behavioral concomitants of emotion in the service of accomplishing affect-related biological or social adaptation or achieving individual goals. (p. 338)

More simply, *emotion regulation processes* are those behaviors, skills, and strategies that monitor, evaluate, modulate, modify, inhibit, or enhance emotional experiences in the pursuit of one's goals. **Emotion dysregulation** refers to actions or behaviors related to emotional experience that interfere with goal-directed pursuits, interpersonal relationships, or healthy adaptation (Schore, 2003). Individuals who are referred for occupational therapy services with diagnoses of traumatic brain injury, cerebrovascular accident (CVA), autism spectrum disorders, dementia, diabetes, cancer, chronic obstructive pulmonary disease (COPD), heart disease, progressive neurological disorders, attention deficit disorder, eating disorders, addictions of all types, depression, bipolar disorder, posttraumatic stress disorder, and other psychiatric diagnoses often present with emotion dysregulation problems that interfere with their occupational performance and participation.

Emotion regulation occurs along a continuum from fully automatic, effortless, and subconscious to conscious, effortful, and voluntary. Emotion regulation may be intrinsic or extrinsic. *Intrinsic* refers to factors within the person that contribute to emotion regulation, for example, temperament, cognitive processes, and neurological, and physiological functions. *Extrinsic* refers to social and contextual influences that affect emotion regulation, for example, interactions with caregivers, sibling and peer relationships, and cultural context (Fox & Calkins, 2003). Although typically focused on reducing negative or painful emotions, emotion regulation can also involve heightening positive emotions (Eisenberg & Spinrad, 2004).

The modal model of emotion consists of five components: the situation, attention to the situation, appraisal of the situation, the emotional and behavioral response to the situation based on the appraisal, and feedback on the effects of the response. Emotions can be regulated before (antecedent focused), during, and after (response focused) they occur. Although these regulatory mechanisms will be described separately, they are often employed in combination. Antecedent-focused emotion regulation involves selecting and modifying situations that typically give rise to emotional response tendencies. Situation selection involves taking actions that increase or decrease the likelihood that one will end up in a situation that evokes desirable or undesirable emotional reactions. Situation modifying involves consciously altering external environmental conditions to reduce or enhance the likelihood of evoking specific emotions (Gross & Thompson, 2007).

Regulating emotions in the midst of experiencing them may take the form of attentional deployment or cognitive change. *Attentional deployment* refers to "how individuals direct their attention within a given situation to influence their emotions" and includes distraction, or focusing attention away from the situation, and concentration, or focusing on the emotional aspects of the situation in order to gain control over them (Gross & Thompson, 2007, p. 13). *Cognitive change*, sometimes referred to as cognitive reappraisal, involves changing one's evaluation of a situation, its consequences, or one's ability to manage the consequences in order to alter its emotional significance or modify its impact.

Response-focused emotion regulation, also called response modulation, involves modifying the physiological effects, the experiential aspects, and/or the behavioral expression of emotion. Emotional responses are not adaptive or maladaptive in and of themselves but rather are adaptive or maladaptive depending on the context. For example, crying may be adaptive in one situation and maladaptive in another. Cultural values also determine emotional response modulation and the interpretation of what is socially appropriate, desirable, and adaptive (Gross & Thompson, 2007).

Neurophysiological Aspects of Emotion Regulation

Research has demonstrated that the areas of the brain most involved in emotion regulation are the sensory thalamus, amygdala, the hippocampus, and the prefrontal cortex (PFC) (Davidson, Fox, & Kalin, 2007). The amygdala is the primary brain structure involved in the generation of normal and pathological emotional behavior and is responsible for directing attention to salient stimuli and determining if further processing is needed. The PFC is often considered the locus of cognitive control, but it also has a role in affective processing. The PFC develops and stores goals and the means to their achievement. Therefore, the PFC appraises the situation to determine if it is a facilitator or threat to one's goals. In stressful situations, threat stimuli are registered in the sensory thalamus and are almost instantaneously relayed to the amygdala, which is the emotional center responsible for fight-or-flight responses. From there, the message travels to the hippocampus and PFC. The hippocampus applies context to the threat situation and regulates the amygdala, whereas the cortex incorporates memory (Davidson et al., 2007).

Trauma exposure compromises neurological function particularly in the hippocampus, which is responsible for learning and memory, and in the frontal-limbic systems, which are responsible for emotion regulation (Karl et al., 2006). There is evidence to suggest that at least half of the psychiatric disorders described in the *Diagnostic and Statistical Manual of Mental Disorders* (4th ed., text rev.; *DSM-IV-TR*; American Psychological Association [APA], 2000) are characterized by emotion dysregulation, possibly as a result of dysfunction of the prefrontal-amygdala pathway (Drevets, 2000; Mennin, Heimberg, Turk, & Fresco, 2005; Ochsner & Gross, 2007; Suveg & Zeman, 2004).

Developmental Aspects of Emotion Regulation

The biological foundations for emotion regulation develop prenatally. For example, stress during pregnancy has been associated with "problematic outcomes such as hyperactivity, deficits in attention, and maladaptive social behavior, all of which are characterized by deficits in self-regulation and emotion regulation in particular" (Calkins & Hill, 2007, p. 238). The ability to self-regulate emotional states begins to develop in infancy. Research on infant temperament has demonstrated biologically based tendencies toward the experience and expression of particular emotions. *Temperament* refers to the speed and intensity of emotional reactivity and the ability to modify, or self-regulate the intensity and duration of the emotional experience. Babies and toddlers self-regulate using strategies such as gaze aversion, self-sucking, and seeking proximity to their caregiver (Cole, Martin, & Dennis, 2004).

Young children learn to self-regulate through their relationships with their primary caregivers (see Figure 57.2).

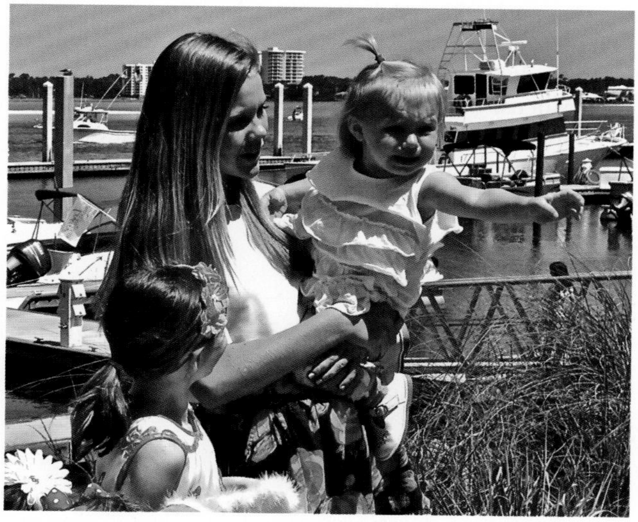

FIGURE 57.2 Learning emotion regulation through relationships with caregivers.

Mothers influence their child's emotional states by interpreting the infant's emotional signals, modulating the baby's level of physiological arousal, and reinforcing the child's efforts at self-regulation. For example, when an infant cries, the caregiver often tries to calm and soothe the child through gentle, rhythmic rocking. Cole et al. (2004) postulate that the "quality of these emotional exchanges . . . is an important precursor of the developing child's ability to regulate his or her own emotions" (p. 324).

Toddlers and preschoolers learn to incorporate these caregiver-directed strategies into their behavioral repertoires for self-regulation of emotion. Children at this age typically demonstrate a decrease in self-soothing strategies and an increase in more complex emotion regulation approaches using objects and interpersonal interactions (Cole et al., 2004). These emotion regulation skills can then be applied across various situations in both deliberate and automatic ways. Failure to develop these early emotion self-regulatory skills may constrain the development of more complex emotional skills later and can lead to poor school adjustment and a low level of social competence (Calkins & Hill, 2007).

For older children, "learning to tolerate distress, correctly label uncomfortable situations, and develop appropriate ways to respond to emotions is central to healthy development" (Scheinholz, 2011, p. 347). This is accomplished through the development of effortful control. **Effortful control** refers to a volitional ability to shift attention, inhibit the tendency to enact a dominant response, and/or activate an alternative response as needed (Rothbart & Bates, 1998). Other factors that impact the development of adaptive emotion regulation are the maturation of language skills that enable the labeling and expression of emotions, observation of the expression of emotions by others in various contexts, and cultural values and mores (Gross & Thompson, 2007). Neurophysiological processes continue to mature during adolescence, enabling teenagers to develop self and other awareness, empathy, impulse control, mastery over the environment, and self-regulation of emotion.

Among healthy adults, emotional experience and emotion regulation are well maintained into late adulthood and typically do not deteriorate with aging. However, the frequency of use of different modes of regulation may change. In middle adulthood, suppression of emotion may be used more frequently to succeed in higher education and work, whereas in older adulthood, there appears to be more of a tendency to use cognitive reappraisal to lessen unpleasant emotional experiences and heighten positive emotional states (Gross & Thompson, 2007). Older adults perceive daily stressors as less threatening and therefore report less negativity as a result when compared to their younger counterparts (Birditt, Fingerman, & Almeida, 2005).

Relationship between Emotion Regulation and Trauma

Many children and adults have been impacted by trauma. The effects of exposure to trauma are dependent, in part, on the developmental stage of the individual when the trauma occurs. Trauma early in life has a negative effect on a child's ability to establish and maintain healthy interpersonal attachments and his or her capacity for emotional self-regulation (Hughes, 2004). This results in poorly moderated affect and impulse control; distrust of others and problems with intimacy; and the lack of a stable, predictable sense of self (van der Kolk, 2003).

Children and adolescents exposed to trauma, in the form of neglect and child abuse in all its forms, as well as witnessing domestic violence, war, and violent crime, have difficulty identifying and describing internal arousal states, labeling and expressing emotions, and making their needs and wants known. Childhood trauma increases the risk of major depressive disorder later in life often with earlier onset and longer duration. The presence of a competent, emotionally supportive caregiver can mitigate these effects. There appear to be three critical factors in a caregiver's response to his or her child's trauma experience that facilitate adaptive emotional functioning. These are believing and validating the child's experience, accepting and understanding the child's affect, and managing the caregiver's own emotional reactions (Cook et al., 2005).

Even mentally healthy, competent adults demonstrate significant declines in cognitive and emotional functioning when traumatized. Adults with posttraumatic stress disorder experience persistent arousal (e.g., sleep difficulties, concentration problems, irritability, and exaggerated startle responses) and continue to reexperience the traumatic event after it is over through flashbacks, nightmares, and intrusive thoughts, which produce emotional distress (APA, 2000). In their attempts to regulate these distressing emotions, persons exposed to trauma may exhibit externalizing and/or internalizing behaviors. These are listed in Box 57.1.

BOX 57.1 Externalizing and Internalizing Behaviors

Acting Out—Externalizing Behaviors

- Anger
- Violence toward others
- Truancy
- Criminal acts

Acting In—Internalizing Behaviors

- Denial, repression
- Substance abuse (self-medicating)
- Eating disorders
- Self-injury
- Dissociation

There is clearly a relationship between trauma and emotion regulation. In fact, Luxenberg, Spinazzola, and van der Kolk (2001) suggest that "affect dysregulation may be the core dysfunction that results from psychological trauma" (p. 377). As a result, occupational therapy practitioners should be alert to the presence of emotion dysregulation in children, adolescents, adults, and older adults who have experienced trauma.

Impact of Emotional Dysregulation on Occupational Performance

Poorly regulated emotions can impair occupational functioning and are therefore important considerations in occupational therapy evaluation and intervention. In the "Occupational Therapy Practice Framework" (American Occupational Therapy Association [AOTA], 2008), **emotional regulation skills** are defined as "actions or behaviors a client uses to identify, manage, and express feelings while engaging in activities or interacting with others" (p. 640). In the framework, examples of emotional regulation skills included are the following:

- Responding to the feelings of others
- Controlling anger
- Coping with stressful events
- Expressing emotions appropriately
- Recovering from hurt or disappointment
- Tolerating frustration and persisting in the performance of tasks (AOTA, 2008)

Gratz and Roemer (2004) suggest emotion regulation skills also include the ability to

- Accept unpleasant, negative emotional experiences as an inevitable aspect of living;
- Redirect and focus one's attention in the presence of intense emotion;
- Soothe oneself in response to emotion-related physiological arousal;
- Inhibit inappropriate behaviors related to intense emotional experiences; and
- Initiate, organize, and persist in goal-directed activity regardless of mood state.

Under healthy conditions, these skills are acquired as part of the normal developmental process. However, some children demonstrate impairment in self-regulation as a result of emotional hyperreactivity and a poorly organized stress response system. This reflects an excessive reaction of the autonomic nervous system to relatively low levels of stress that results in intense reactions to emotional stimuli and a slow return to baseline or homeostasis. Linehan (1993a) believes that emotion

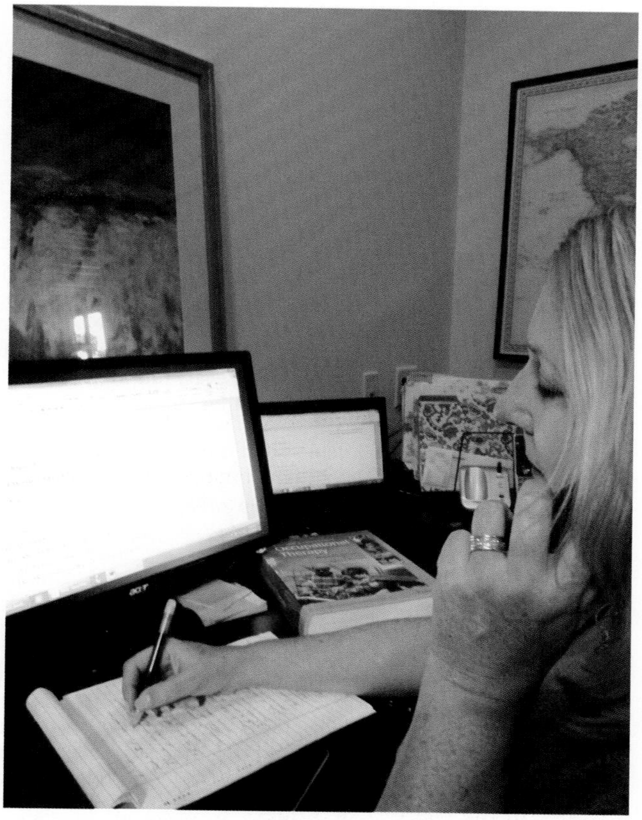

FIGURE 57.3 The workplace can be very stressful and challenge one's ability to self-regulate emotions.

dysregulation results when a child with high emotional vulnerability is exposed to an invalidating, neglectful, or abusive environment. These children demonstrate affective instability, impulsiveness, irritability, and distractibility all of which interfere with school performance, play, and family and peer relationships. Box 57.2 presents a day in the life of Henry, a child with emotional dysregulation.

In adults, affective instability and the accompanying behavior patterns interfere with the development and maintenance of healthy habits and routines and the ability to perform occupational roles effectively. Persons with emotion regulation deficits typically have occupational performance problems in work, instrumental activities of daily living, leisure, and social participation (see Figure 57.3) (Scheinholz, 2011). Box 57.3 presents a day in the life of Rebecca, an adult with emotional dysregulation.

Evaluation and Assessment of Emotion Regulation

Despite the importance of emotion regulation to overall health and well-being, there are few validated assessments to measure emotional regulation skills and none are specific to occupational therapy. The social history interview and occupation-based interview assessment

BOX 57.2 The Dynamics of Dysregulation: A Day in the Life of a Child with Emotion Dysregulation

Henry: Henry is a 7-year-old child who struggles with emotion regulation. Although he has not been formally diagnosed, his parents and teachers agree that many things in life are more difficult for Henry than for his siblings and his peers.

Morning mayhem: *Activities of daily living (ADL)*	Henry has little trouble awakening in the morning, although he is somewhat grouchy. The first thing Henry must do as part of his morning routine is discreetly throw away his "pull-up," being careful not to let any of his siblings see, even though he knows that they know. At 7 years old, Henry is not fully potty trained and bedwetting continues to be a problem despite all of his parent's efforts. Henry feels embarrassed every morning because his 2-year-old brother wears regular underwear to sleep. "What is wrong with me?" He worries and he wonders.
Bad luck on the bus: *Work*	Henry's dad is responsible for making sure that he gets to the bus stop on time. His father makes sure that the morning routine is kept structured to reduce anxiety for Henry and assist with the family's busy morning routine. But today, when Henry climbs on to the bus and attempts to sit down in his assigned seat, a new child is sitting where he is supposed to sit. The bus driver asks Henry to please be seated so that she can continue. Henry's eyes well up with tears because he doesn't know how to explain that someone is sitting in his seat. One of the older boys on the bus sees Henry crying and says tauntingly, "Cry baby!"
Suffering through school: *Education*	At school, Henry's teacher is working with the children on writing paragraphs from a prompt. The class has formed paragraphs together for weeks, and today, the teacher will give the students a prompt and ask the students to write a paragraph on their own. The teacher notes that Henry participates verbally when the class works together but notices that it takes Henry longer to copy the class paragraph from the board to his paper. Today, the teacher notes that as the other children are attempting to write their paragraph, Henry is off-task, playing in his desk. She quietly asks him to please get started, and he appears to be compliant. But when she collects the paragraphs, Henry has only written three sentences, whereas the other children have produced more than double the amount of sentences.
Cafeteria crisis: *Social participation*	Henry has several close friends; most of them are people he has known for a long time because they attended the same preschool as he did. One of the boys is in Henry's class. Henry usually sits next to his friend at the lunch table. But today, his friend is absent from school. Henry sits at the same table but eats his lunch in solitude because he is too shy to talk to any of the other children.
"It's not fair." *Play and leisure*	Henry has three siblings. He usually makes good choices when it comes to following the rules of games. But he gets overly angry when other people do not follow the rules. Often, he storms out in the middle of games with both siblings and peers if he thinks something is "unfair." His peers have difficulty with this pattern of behavior, which often results in them not wanting to include Henry in play.
Homework hostility: *Work*	One of Henry's parents' most difficult tasks is helping Henry complete his homework. They report that Henry has a difficult time focusing, often becomes distracted, and must have a quiet environment with no disruptions to complete even simple assignments. In a busy household, this is seldom possible. Henry also often cries if he cannot quickly figure out new material, and he is sensitive about even gentle corrections from his parents.
Medication complication: **"I can't sleep."** *Rest and sleep*	Recently, the pediatrician has recommended medication for Henry to help alleviate some of his noted anxiety and to improve his level of concentration. Henry's mother feels uncertain but decides to agree with her husband and try the medication. At times, the medication seems to be helping. But at night, Henry cannot sleep. This side effect bothers his parents and they feel that this sleep disruption may erase any benefit of the medication.

tools are useful in identifying occupational performance issues related to emotion dysregulation. However, naturalistic observation of emotion regulation skills in various contexts may be the most informative.

One assessment developed for adults, the Difficulties in Emotion Regulation Scale (DERS), has demonstrated "high internal consistency, good test-retest reliability, and adequate construct and predictive validity" (Gratz & Roemer, 2004, p. 41). The DERS was designed to measure the following dimensions of emotion regulation:

- Awareness and acceptance of emotions
- Ability to persist in goal-directed behavior when experiencing negative emotions, and
- Access to emotion regulation strategies that are perceived to be efficacious.

BOX 57.3 The Dynamics of Dysregulation: A Day in the Life of an Adult with Emotion Dysregulation

Rebecca: Rebecca is a 36-year-old adult who struggles with emotion regulation. Rebecca is married and has one child. She works as a legal secretary in a large law practice. Rebecca is the adult child of an abusive mother who abandoned the family when she was 14 years old. Rebecca was expected to take over the often overwhelming role of helping to raise her siblings after her mother left.

Mad already and it's only morning: *Rest and sleep*	The alarm goes off everyday at 5:30 a.m.; and everyday, Rebecca hits the snooze button because she dreads getting out of bed. Today, she doesn't have the opportunity to hit the snooze button; she has forgotten to set her alarm the night before. Instead, she awakens to her husband who says, "Rebecca, the alarm didn't go off, hurry up, get up, we've overslept." As is frequently the case, her misdirected anger causes her to snap at both her husband and her daughter repeatedly before leaving for work. Her husband, fed up with this treatment looks at her and says, "It's only morning, and you are already mad. I'm starting to wonder if you wake up this way?"
Breakfast on the run; life on the run: *Activities of daily living (ADL)*	Even though Rebecca considers herself an organized person, she often rushes through tasks because she has so many responsibilities. Most of her life, she has been expected to complete more than the reasonable amount of activities. She has come to believe that if she doesn't get it all done, she will not be valued. She also has difficulty saying, "no" when people ask her for help. She feels that her self-worth is dependent on task completion. Throughout her life, her ADL and personal care have taken a backseat to other people's needs. This morning is no different. In her hurry, after oversleeping, Rebecca skips breakfast and hurries out the door, forgetting also the lunch in the refrigerator her husband had packed for her.
"Never mind, I will do it myself." *The world of work*	At work, the firm has hired an additional legal secretary because of expansion. Rebecca feels threatened by the new legal secretary because she is younger and performs many tasks more quickly than Rebecca. Rebecca knows that she should ask the new secretary to share some of her workload; and today, she decides to ask for help because she is running late. After greeting the new coworker, she asks if she can complete the morning summaries for her while Rebecca moves on to the next item. Morning summaries are an area that the new secretary has not done before, and so she agrees to do the work but says she will need to ask a few questions. Before her new colleague can ask the first question, Rebecca snatches the papers from her hand and says, "Never mind, I will just do it myself." Her coworker comments later to their mutual supervisor that, "Rebecca seems a bit passive-aggressive to me." She follows with details of their earlier interaction.
Stop the stress: *Health promotion and maintenance*	Rebecca's job is busy and stressful. A trip to her doctor earlier that month confirmed that Rebecca has extremely high blood pressure, placing her at risk for various illnesses. He had insisted that she begin taking blood pressure medication but also told her that she must find other ways to reduce her stress and anxiety.
Finding friends, no time for play: *Social participation/ play and leisure*	Rebecca has difficulty trusting other people and therefore feels that she has little peer support. She had even been to counseling during adulthood to try to cope with the rejection, loneliness, fear of abandonment, and depression that she has experienced since her mother left. Because she had to help raise her siblings and even now takes on more than a reasonable share of responsibility at home and work, Rebecca has little opportunity to pursue hobbies. Also, she has few opportunities for social participation.
Taking care of everything and everyone: *Instrumental activities of daily living (IADL) overload*	Rebecca is still taking care of her siblings in addition to her responsibilities to her spouse and child. As a result, she manages several households and supplements her siblings financially as well. This causes marital stress because Rebecca is unable to say no to her siblings, and her spouse and child suffer as a result. When her spouse and/or child express their concerns or displeasure, Rebecca either retreats into isolation or becomes angry and verbally abusive toward them.
"I can't rest, I can't relax, and I can't SLEEP!" Turning off the emotionally dysregulated brain: *Rest and sleep*	Most nights, Rebecca lays in her bed; and she cannot stop thinking about how many things that she didn't finish that day, worried about how she will finish the next day's responsibilities, and feels that she cannot quiet her brain or her emotions. Rebecca sometimes uses alcohol to "quiet her mind." Her husband worries because this is a pattern that seems to be happening more frequently.

The DERS consists of 36 items that make up the following six subscales with higher scores indicating deficits in emotion regulation:

1. Acceptance of emotional responses
2. Engagement in goal-directed behavior
3. Impulse control
4. Emotional awareness
5. Access to emotion regulation strategies
6. Emotional clarity

Recently, the DERS was validated on a community sample of adolescents (Neumann, van Lier, Gratz, & Koot, 2010).

Other assessments, although not directly measuring emotion regulation, that may be useful to measure affective states include the Profile of Mood States 2 (POMS 2) and the Positive and Negative Affect Schedule (PANAS). The POMS 2, a self-report instrument, measures transient and enduring affect states. The total mood disturbance score is made up of six subscales: anger-hostility, confusion-bewilderment, depression-dejection, fatigue-inertia, tension-anxiety, and vigor-activity. There are two versions: one for youth aged 13 to 17 years and one for adults. The assessment has norms and is easily scored and interpreted (Heuchert & McNair, n.d.). The PANAS is a 20-item assessment that measures positive and negative affective dispositions. High negative affect scores indicate the presence of subjective distress and unpleasant engagement, whereas low negative affect scores represent the absence of these feeling states. High positive affect scores indicate enthusiasm and pleasurable engagement with the environment, whereas low positive affect scores represent a lack of pleasurable engagement and lethargy. Using a large sample of the general adult population, the PANAS demonstrated adequate to good reliability and validity (Crawford & Henry, 2004).

Another assessment that might provide an insight on emotional regulation is the Mayer-Salovey-Caruso Emotional Intelligence Test, Version 2.0 (MSCEIT V2.0). This tool is designed as a performance-based assessment of the ability to reason using emotional information, including the capacity to access, perceive, and understand emotions; to use emotional knowledge; and to regulate emotions. It can be administered individually or in groups and presents the client with eight tasks that require emotional problem solving. The test has norms based on data from over 5,000 participants in various countries and has demonstrated acceptable reliability and validity (Mayer, Salovey, Caruso, & Sitarenios, 2003).

Because coping skills are related to emotion regulation, the *Early Coping Inventory* (Zeitlin, 1985) may be a useful assessment for some clients. The *Early Coping Inventory* is available in two forms: an observation-based assessment for children aged 3 years and older and a self-rating form for adolescents and adults. The inventory measures two categories of coping behaviors (self and environment) on three dimensions including active-passive, flexible-rigid, and productive-nonproductive coping strategies (Zeitlin, 1985). The *Early Coping Inventory* is designed to be used with young children from 4 to 36 months of age. It is an observation-based instrument that measures coping-related behavior in three categories including sensorimotor organization, reactive behaviors, and self-initiated behaviors (Zeitlin, Williamson, & Szczepanski, 1988). Other assessments related to emotional function are listed in Table 57.1.

TABLE 57.1 Other Emotion-Related Assessments

Name of Assessment	Authors (Date Published)	Source
Adult Manifest Anxiety Scale	Reynolds, Richmond, & Lowe (2003)	Western Psychological Services Los Angeles, CA
Beck Depression Inventory-II (BDI-II)	Beck, Steer, & Brown (1996)	Psychological Corporation San Antonio, TX
Carey Temperament Scales	Carey, McDevitt, & Medoff-Cooper, B. (2007)	Behavioral Development Initiatives Scottsdale, AZ
Children's Depression Rating Scale-Revised (CDRS-R)	Poznanski & Mokros (1996)	Western Psychological Services Los Angeles, CA
Depression and Anxiety in Youth Scale (DAYS)	Newcomer, Barenbaum, & Bryant (1994)	Pro-Ed Inc. Austin, TX
Functional Emotional Assessment Scale (FEAS)	Greenspan, DeGangi, & Weider (2001)	Interdisciplinary Council on Developmental and Learning Disorders Bethesda, MD
Geriatric Depression Scale (GDS)	Sheikh & Yesavage (1986)	Stanford University www.stanford.edu/~yesavage/GDS.html
Multidimensional Anxiety Scale for Children (MASC)	March (1997)	Pearson Education, Inc. San Antonio, TX

Interventions to Enhance Emotion Regulation

There are few psychological interventions designed specifically for emotion regulation published in the literature, and only one, Dialectical Behavior Therapy (DBT), has an extensive evidence base. DBT will be described briefly and its applicability to occupational therapy will be discussed. Two other approaches, social and emotional learning (SEL) and sensory-based interventions, will also be described.

Dialectical Behavior Therapy

DBT is based on cognitive behavioral principles. Cognitive-behavioral intervention approaches are based on evidence that suggests that cognitive processes influence emotional states. These cognitive processes occur when people use situational cues, judgment, and memory to identify the source of their physiological arousal, to recognize other people's emotions, and to interpret and respond effectively to emotionally charged situations (Nussbaum, 2001).

Developed by Linehan (1993a, 1993b), DBT was originally designed as an outpatient psychotherapy protocol to treat persons with borderline personality disorder but has been adapted for use with a variety of populations. The DBT philosophy is based on the following principles and assumptions, which are critical to the effectiveness of the approach:

- The client wants to change and is trying but may not always appear so.
- The client's emotional responses and behaviors are best understood in the context of personal history and present circumstances.
- The client is not to blame for their current situation but is responsible for making changes in his or her life.
- Blaming and labeling the client as manipulative, deceptive, etc. will not enhance the therapeutic intervention.
- A client does not fail at DBT, it is the intervention that is not working and needs to be modified (Linehan, 1993a).

DBT combines individual psychotherapy with group-based skills training. Although occupational therapists are not qualified to provide psychotherapy, we are adequately prepared to implement aspects of the skills training component.

Skills taught include mindfulness, interpersonal effectiveness, emotion modulation, and distress tolerance (Linehan, 1993b). Mindfulness training facilitates the awareness of emotional states without judgment and thereby decreases the arousal associated with negative mood states. Mindfulness also encourages living in the moment; observing, interpreting, and experiencing emotions in productive ways to satisfy one's own needs and to meet the demands of the environment. Interpersonal effectiveness training facilitates the development of effective communication skills, social skills, and interpersonal problem solving. Participants learn how to meet their needs in interpersonal encounters without damaging their relationships with their significant others.

Emotion modulation training is designed to help clients understand their emotions, reduce emotional suffering, and increase emotional resilience. Skills taught include identifying emotions, expressing emotions appropriately, and responding to the feelings of others. Distress tolerance training facilitates the ability to cope with stressful events, self-soothe, and persist in tasks despite frustration. This requires the capacity to accept the current reality, experience negative emotions without judgment, and thoughtfully determine a course of action.

Miller, Wyman, Huppert, Glassman, and Rathus (2000) have pioneered the use of DBT with adolescents. An early study evaluated the use of DBT with 27 adolescents with suicidal ideation. Suicidal adolescents typically demonstrate four characteristic problems: (1) emotional instability, (2) impulsivity, (3) confusion about self, and (4) difficulties with interpersonal relationships. The study intervention consisted of skill modules on mindfulness, distress tolerance, emotion regulation, and interpersonal effectiveness. Based on the *Life Problems Inventory* (Rathus & Miller, 1995), statistically significant improvements were noted in all four problem areas (Miller et al., 2000).

Miller and Smith (2008) described the application of DBT for teens who demonstrate nonsuicidal self-injurious (NSSI) behavior. From a DBT perspective, NSSI behavior is "considered to be a maladaptive solution to overwhelming and intensely painful negative emotions" (Miller & Smith, 2008, p. 180) and a manifestation of emotion dysregulation. They concluded that DBT is a promising intervention for this population, but more research is needed. DBT has also been used effectively with adolescents with eating disorders (Safer, Lock, & Couturier, 2007; Salbach-Andrae, Bohnekamp, Pfeiffer, Lehmkuhl, & Miller, 2008) and adults with substance dependence (Dimeff, Rizvi, Brown, & Linehan, 2000; Wagner, Miller, Greene, & Winiarski, 2004).

Anger management programs are typically based on cognitive behavioral principles. Tang (2001), an occupational therapist, designed an anger management intervention for persons with mental disorders that, like DBT, included skills training sessions. This anger management intervention consisted of ten 90-minute group meetings in which participants learned and practiced anger management and relaxation strategies. Homework was assigned, which included readings, journaling, and recording situations that evoked anger in a hassle log. Over a period of 2 years, 64 clients participated in cohorts of 7 to 10 persons per group. A quasi-experimental pretest and posttest study demonstrated declines in the participants' overall experience of angry feelings, anger intensity, and anger duration. Significant reductions in maladaptive cognition and maladaptive behaviors were also noted (Tang, 2001).

The effectiveness of DBT for improving emotion regulation has been validated through research for a variety of populations. Occupational therapists who wish to infuse their practice with DBT principles and strategies should participate in continuing education in order to gain knowledge and skills regarding the science and practice of DBT.

Social and Emotional Learning

SEL is a strategy to teach children, adolescents, and adults the skills needed for self-management and the establishment of healthy relationships. These skills include, but are not limited to, identifying and managing one's emotions, initiating and maintaining interpersonal relationships, handling challenges effectively, and making responsible decisions. The overall goal of SEL is to reduce risk factors and enhance resiliency factors for positive adjustment. The five core competencies in SEL are the following:

1. Self-awareness
2. Self-management
3. Social awareness
4. Relationship skills
5. Responsible decision making (Collaborative for Academic, Social and Emotional Learning [CASEL], 2011).

A large-scale meta-analysis indicated that SEL programs are effective for racially and ethnically diverse students at the elementary, middle, and high school levels and can be implemented successfully in both school and after-school settings. The outcomes identified by this study included higher achievement test scores and improved social-emotional skills, prosocial behavior, and attitudes toward self, others, and school for students who participated in SEL. In addition, a reduction in conduct problems and emotional distress were noted (Durlak, Weissberg, Dymnicki, Taylor, & Schellinger, 2011).

The most effective SEL programs incorporated four best practices. These programs were sequenced (S), active (A), focused (F), and explicit (E). This has become known as the SAFE approach to SEL. The interaction of these practices produces greater results than any single factor alone. *Sequenced* means breaking down complex skills into smaller steps and mastering them sequentially within a developmental perspective. *Active learning* involves incorporating opportunities to experiment and practice the skills being taught in various contexts, for example, through role-play and behavioral rehearsal. *Focused* means that sufficient time and attention are allotted for the development of specific skills, and *explicit* refers to the importance of specific, rather than general, learning objectives (Durlak et al., 2011).

Sensory-Based Approaches

Sensory-based approaches to intervention are based on the biological aspects of emotion regulation and are neuroregulatory in nature. The underlying concept, although not well researched, is by managing and/or controlling physiological responses, it is possible to regulate emotional states.

Sensory integration as a therapeutic approach is designed to help children develop the ability to self-regulate. Self-regulation involves various processes of which emotion regulation is just one. Sensory integration theory posits that some developmental problems in children are due in part to hyposensitivity or hypersensitivity to sensory stimuli. This undersensivity or oversensitivity results in emotional hypoarousal or hyperarousal. Hypoarousal may manifest as flat affect, detachment, withdrawal, depression, and passive-aggressive behavior. Hyperarousal may appear in the form of emotional tantrums, hypervigilance, anxiety, fear, and overreaction to perceived threats (Champagne, 2011). Sensory-based interventions include therapeutic sensorimotor groups, sensory activities, sensory diet, and environmental enhancements such as multisensory rooms (Champagne, Koomar, & Olson, 2010).

Champagne (2006) describes the use of multisensory rooms as an intervention that addresses the emotion regulation needs of adults with psychiatric disorders. Multisensory rooms are designed to reduce a client's exposure to chaotic, sensory overload and thereby elicit a relaxation response. This is typically accomplished through the use of muted, soft paint colors; a variety of comfortable seating options; soothing music; and visually appealing imagery. For more information about sensory integration evaluation and intervention, see Chapter 56.

Future Directions

Most research in emotion regulation focuses on decreasing and/or managing negative emotions and behaviors. An alternative approach is to focus on enhancing positive emotions, strengths, and resilience. The health benefits of positive emotion are being documented in the literature. For example, greater optimism predicted better health outcomes among persons with heart disease (Scheier et al., 1999). The mechanisms through which positive emotion impacts health are not yet clear but are likely to involve endocrine and immune system functions (Kiecolt-Glaser et al., 2002). Two intervention models will be described briefly, the Broaden and Build Model (Fredrickson, 2001) and the Four-Branch Model of Emotional Intelligence (Salovey, Mayer, & Caruso, 2002).

Fredrickson's (2001) Broaden and Build Model provides a framework for enhancing positive emotions and resilience. She asserts that negative, distressing emotions narrow an individual's attention and focus to the problem or source of dissatisfaction, whereas positive emotion broadens the field of attention. The broader field of attention facilitates creative problem solving that builds personal resources and resilience (Fredrickson, 2001). As a result, *broadening* a person's range of attention, cognition, and action and *building* his or her physical, intellectual, emotional, and social resources can enhance

BOX 57.4 Aspects of Emotional Intelligence

- Knowledge that an individual possesses regarding how and when emotions can be regulated
- Knowledge of strategies for emotion regulation and when to deploy them
- Ability to implement emotion regulation strategies
- Ability to identify and describe one's emotional experience
- Ability to express one's feelings in words or some other symbolic expression

resilience and improves physical and mental health. Positive affect, especially curiosity, also encourages exploration and mastery (Peterson & Seligman, 2004).

The ability to access positive emotion is an important aspect of coping. **Coping** can be described as "conscious, volitional efforts to regulate emotion, cognition, behavior, physiology, and the environment in response to stressful events or circumstances" (Compas, Connor, Saltzman, Thomsen, & Wadsworth, 2001, p. 89). Eliciting positive emotions reduces stressful reactions and returns the body to a more balanced state. For example, prompting positive emotions such as gratitude and joy in response to stressful situations resulted in reduced heart rate, blood pressure, and vasoconstriction (Fredrickson & Levenson, 1998).

The concept of emotional intelligence, first introduced into the popular media by Goleman (1995), has received a great deal of attention over the past decade. The Four-Branch Model of Emotional Intelligence (Salovey et al., 2002) posits that a person's emotional quotient (EQ) consists of four skill sets: perceiving emotions in self and others, understanding emotional information, incorporating emotions into one's thought processes, and managing or regulating one's emotions. Emotion management or regulation in this model consists of the ability to

- Be open to both pleasant and unpleasant emotional experiences;
- Monitor and reflect on emotional states;
- Access, reduce, or prolong an emotional response;
- Manage one's own emotions; and
- Respond to the emotions of others (Salovey et al., 2002).

Other aspects of emotional intelligence are presented in Box 57.4.

Although there are many studies that have linked emotional intelligence to overall health and well-being, academic and occupational success, quality of life, and resilience, little attention has been paid thus far to the development of interventions that enhance EQ. One experimental study consisting of 37 participants (19 in the intervention group and 18 in the control group) evaluated the effectiveness of a psychoeducational approach based on the four-branch model of emotional intelligence. The intervention consisted of four weekly sessions of 2.5 hours each. The sessions consisted of mini lectures, role-play, group discussions, readings, and homework. Results indicated positive changes in trait emotional intelligence, emotion identification, and emotion management for the intervention group but not for the control group; and the changes were sustained at the 6-month follow-up (Nelis, Quoidbach, Mikolajczak, & Hansenne, 2009).

Other intervention-based studies in worksites have demonstrated some effectiveness in improving emotional intelligence of managers and resulted in improved health and well-being (Slaski & Cartwright, 2003). Although interventions designed to enhance emotional intelligence skills are valuable, Salovey and Grewal (2005) caution that in order to be effective, such interventions should "address the contextual and motivational factors affecting the use of these skills" (p. 285). More intervention studies are clearly needed.

Conclusion

Effective occupational therapy interventions focus on helping clients participate in meaningful occupations. For some individuals, emotional dysregulation impairs occupational performance and limits participation. It is for this reason that occupational therapists must attend to and attempt to enhance the emotional regulation and emotional intelligence of their clients. However, emotion regulation skills cannot be considered in isolation. They must be addressed in the context of the client's desired and meaningful occupations; his or her habits, roles, and routines; and his or her values and beliefs. In addition, emotion regulation is a complex phenomenon that requires attention to be paid to the physiological, cognitive, affective, behavioral, and motivational aspects of the client. Our unique role as occupational therapy practitioners is to help clients manage emotions within the context of occupational performance and identify the appropriate contextual supports that are needed to enhance emotion regulation and thereby facilitate occupational participation.

Although research in this area is limited, there are indications of the effectiveness of various approaches including sensory-based interventions, dialectical behavior therapy, social-emotional learning, and strengths-based approaches to enhancing emotional intelligence. Occupational therapy practitioners and researchers are in a unique position to develop and evaluate occupation-based assessment tools and interventions related to emotion regulation and emotional intelligence.

CASE STUDY 57.1 Maria: Struggling with the Emotion Dysregulation Associated with Bipolar Disorder

I first met Maria when she began participating in a program at the local high school for teenage mothers who were without a high school diploma. At the time, I was teaching and facilitating a grant-based program that provided adult basic education, high school completion, English language literacy services, and parenting classes. Maria was 15 years old at the time, and she had a 6-month-old daughter named Rosie. Maria had limited English language skills and very little family support.

Maria could attend classes 3 days per week for 4 hours each day, and childcare was provided for her daughter. What I remember the most about Maria was that despite her circumstances, she always tried to make everyone else happy. Generally, she would entertain her peers by telling funny jokes (translated by peers and sometimes made even funnier with the attempts at translation). Maria had days of flourishing, with the support of peers, demonstrating the positive effects of social and emotional learning. But sometimes, she would have days where neither her peers nor the teachers recognized her because of her sullen and withdrawn affect and apparent unwillingness to participate.

I also remember that sometimes, Maria and Rosie just wouldn't show up for a week or even several weeks at a time. Because Maria lived near enough to the facility where the classes were taught, she would walk to the classes, bringing her daughter in a stroller. When Maria didn't attend, one of my coteachers immediately assumed and often verbalized that she felt that Maria's missing class was the result of "laziness, irresponsibility, and lack of motivation." Whereas I and another teacher, although we didn't realize it at the time, consistently chose to focus on what Maria was doing well when she did attend classes. We also factored into our consideration the environmental, social-emotional, and language barriers that were the more likely reasons for her absences.

When Maria had progressed academically, she signed up to take the General Education Development (GED) test. I remember all of us waiting anxiously for her exam results. Unfortunately, Maria did not pass the test on her initial attempt. After that, Maria's attendance to the classes began to wane. When she did attend, she would often express tearful regret about many of the life choices that she had made, was sometimes deeply upset, and especially self-deprecating about her failed attempt at the GED exam. Although the staff made frequent home visits and phone calls to encourage Maria to continue through the classes, she eventually displayed anger about "being bothered" and soon stopped attending classes completely.

Changes in my life led to a change in my career, and today I am an occupational therapist practicing in a variety of settings. Now nearly a decade later, last week, as I sat to provide a group intervention at a hospital-based inpatient psychiatric unit where I sometimes work, I noticed a young girl sitting in the corner. I knew that she looked familiar; and although we made eye contact, and although I invited her to join the group, I couldn't place her. But as I left, I turned back and asked her name, explaining that she looked familiar to me. And before she even had time to answer, I knew who she was. I knew it was Maria.

I sat and talked with her. In our conversation she told me that she was at the hospital because she had attempted suicide. She disclosed to me that she had been diagnosed with bipolar disorder not long after she left our program. She also let me know that her daughter was doing well, but she tearfully expressed that " . . . life just doesn't seem to ever get any easier for me."

The *Comprehensive Occupational Therapy Evaluation* (COTE) and *Coping Inventory* were administered. The COTE indicated strengths in reality orientation, cooperation, sociability, following directions, and interest in accomplishments. Deficits identified included problem solving, decision making, and organization. Maria becomes easily overwhelmed with complex tasks and has a low frustration tolerance. Her COTE score indicated moderate impairment in general behaviors and task behaviors; however, she was functional in the category of interpersonal behaviors. Many of the identified problems are directly related to her diagnosis of bipolar disorder. The *Coping Inventory* indicated that Maria has a rigid coping style and a limited repertoire of strategies to reach a goal or solve a problem. She tends to be passive, making little or no effort to initiate or sustain action in response to stressful situations. In addition, Maria demonstrates little resilience in response to disappointment or setbacks. Her adaptive coping behaviors include her ability to talk to others about personal needs, her desire and effectiveness in being liked and accepted by others, and her socially appropriate behavior in various situations.

Intervention goals included increasing Maria's frustration tolerance, improving her ability to problem-solve, expanding her repertoire of coping skills, and enhancing her ability to manage her medications. Maria participated in two individual and five occupational therapy group sessions. However, her length of stay was only 5 days for medication stabilization; and as a result, many of her occupational therapy goals were not realized.

1. Describe the elements of emotional regulation that are demonstrated in this case.
2. What principles and assumptions of the Dialectical Behavior Therapy philosophy apply to this case?
3. Discuss which emotional regulation intervention or approach would be most successful for Maria. Provide a rationale for your choice.
4. Describe the occupational therapy theoretical approach(es) that most closely support(s) your emotional regulation intervention.
5. What discharge recommendations would you make for this client?

Source: Case Study courtesy of Courtney Sasse.

References

American Occupational Therapy Association. (2008). Occupational therapy practice framework: Domain and process, 2nd edition. American Journal of Occupational Therapy, 62, 625–683.

American Psychiatric Association. (2000). *Diagnostic and statistical manual of mental disorders* (4th ed., text rev.). Washington, DC: Author.

Beck, A. T., Steer, R. A., & Brown, G. K. (1996). *Beck Depression Inventory Manual* (2nd ed.). San Antonio, TX: Psychological Corporation.

Birditt, K. S., Fingerman, K. L., & Almeida, D. M. (2005). Age differences in exposure and reactions to interpersonal tensions: A daily diary study. *Psychology and Aging, 20*, 330–340.

Calkins, S. D., & Hill, A. (2007). Caregiver influences on emerging emotion regulation: Biological and environmental transactions in early development. In J. J. Gross (Ed.), *Handbook of emotion regulation*. New York, NY: Guilford Press.

Carey, W. B., McDevitt, S. C. & Medoff-Cooper, B. (2007). *Carey Temperament Scales*. San Antonio, TX: Pearson.

Champagne, T. (2006, December). Creating sensory rooms: Environmental enhancements for acute inpatient mental health settings. *Mental Health Special Interest Section Quarterly, 29*(4), 1–4.

Champagne, T. (2011). *Sensory modulation & environment: Essential elements of occupation* (3rd ed.). San Antonio, TX: Pearson.

Champagne, T., Koomar, J., & Olson, L. (2010). Sensory processing evaluation and intervention in mental health. *OT Practice, 15*(5), CE1–CE7.

Cole, P. M., Martin, S. E., & Dennis, R. A. (2004). Emotion regulation as a scientific construct: Methodological challenges and directions for child development research. *Child Development, 75*, 317–333.

Collaborative for Academic, Social and Emotional Learning. (2011). *What is social and emotional learning?* Retrieved from http://casel.org/why-it-matters/what-is-sel/

Compas, B. E., Connor, J. K., Saltzman, H., Thomsen, A. H., & Wadsworth, M. E. (2001). Coping with stress during childhood and adolescence: Problems, progress, and potential in theory and research. *Psychological Bulletin, 127*, 87–127.

Cook, A., Spinazzola, J., Ford, J., Lanktree, C., Blaustein, M., Cloitre, M., . . . van der Kolk, B. (2005). Complex trauma in children and adolescents. *Psychiatric Annals, 35*(5), 390–398.

Crawford, J. R., & Henry, J. D. (2004). The Positive and Negative Affect Schedule (PANAS): Construct validity, measurement properties, and normative data in a large non-clinical sample. *British Journal of Clinical Psychology, 43*, 245–265.

Davidson, R. J., Fox, A., & Kalin, N. H. (2007). Neural bases of emotion regulation in nonhuman primates and humans. In J. J. Gross (Ed.), *Handbook of emotion regulation*. New York, NY: Guilford Press.

Dimeff, L., Rizvi, S. L., Brown, M., & Linehan, M. M. (2000). Dialectical behavior therapy for substance abuse: A pilot application to methamphetamine-dependent women with borderline personality disorder. *Cognitive and Behavioral Practice, 7*, 457–468.

Drevets, W. C. (2000). Neuroimaging studies of mood disorders. *Biological Psychiatry, 48*(8), 813–829.

Durlak, J. A., Weissberg, R. P., Dymnicki, A. B., Taylor, R. D., & Schellinger, K. B. (2011). The impact of enhancing students' social and emotional learning: A meta-analysis of school-based universal interventions. *Child Development, 82*, 405–432.

Eisenberg, N., & Spinrad, T. L. (2004). Emotion-regulated regulation: Sharpening the definition. *Child Development, 75*, 334–339.

Fox, N. A., & Calkins, S. D. (2003). The development of self-control of emotion: Intrinsic and extrinsic influences. *Motivation and Emotion, 27*, 7–26.

Fredrickson, B. L. (2001). The role of positive emotions in positive psychology: The broaden-and-build theory of positive emotions. *American Psychologist, 56*, 218–226.

Fredrickson, B. L., & Levenson, R. W. (1998). Positive emotions speed recovery from the cardiovascular sequelae of negative emotions. *Cognition and Emotion, 12*, 191–220.

Goleman, D. (1995). *Emotional intelligence: Why it can matter more than IQ*. New York, NY: Bantam.

Gratz, K. L., & Roemer, L. (2004). Multidimensional assessment of emotion regulation and dysregulation: Development, factor structure, and initial validation of the Difficulties in Emotion Regulation Scale. *Journal of Psychopathology and Behavioral Assessment, 26*, 41–54.

Greenspan, S. I., DeGangi, G. A., & Weider, S. (2001). *The Functional Emotional Scale (FEAS) for infancy and early childhood: Clinical and research applications*. Bethesda, MD: Interdisciplinary Council on Developmental and Learning Disorders.

Gross, J. J., & Thompson, R. A. (2007). Emotion regulation: Conceptual foundations. In J. J. Gross (Ed.), *Handbook of emotion regulation*. New York, NY: Guilford Press.

Heuchert, J. P., & McNair, D. M. (n.d.). *Profile of Mood States 2nd edition (POMS 2)*. Retrieved from http://downloads.mhs.com/poms/POMS2_US_InfoSheet.pdf

Hughes, D. (2004). An attachment-based treatment of maltreated children and young people. *Attachment & Human Development, 6*, 263–278.

Izard, C. E. (2010). The many meaning/aspects of emotion: Functions, activation and regulation. *Emotion Review, 2*, 363–370.

Karl, A., Schaefer, M., Malta, L. S., Dörfel, D., Roleder, N., & Werner, A. (2006). A meta-analysis of structural brain abnormalities in PTSD. *Neuroscience and Biobehavioral Reviews, 30*, 1004–1031.

Kiecolt-Glaser, J. K., McGuire, L., Robles, T., & Glaser, R. (2002). Emotions, morbidity and mortality: New perspectives from psychoneuroimmunology. *Annual Review of Psychology, 53*, 83–107.

Linehan, M. M. (1993a). *Cognitive behavioral treatment for borderline personality disorder*. New York, NY: Guilford Press.

Linehan, M. M. (1993b). *Skills training manual for treating borderline personality disorders*. New York, NY: Guilford Press.

Luxenberg, T., Spinazzola, J., & van der Kolk, B. A. (2001). *Complex trauma and disorders of extreme stress (DESNOS) diagnosis, part one: Assessment*. Retrieved from http://www.aisjca-mft.org/desnos.pdf

Mahoney, M. J. (2005). Constructivism and positive psychology. In C. R. Snyder & S. J. Lopez (Eds.), *Handbook of positive psychology*. New York, NY: Oxford University Press.

March, J. S. (1997). *Manual for the Multidimensional Anxiety Scale for Children*. Toronto, Ontario, Canada: Multi-Health Systems

Mayer, J., Salovey, P., Caruso, D., & Sitarenios, G. (2003). Measuring emotional intelligence with the MSCEIT V2.0. *Emotion, 3*, 97–105.

Mennin, D. S., Heimberg, R. G., Turk, C. L., & Fresco, D. M. (2005). Preliminary evidence for an emotion dysregulation model of generalized anxiety disorder. *Behaviour Research and Therapy, 43*, 1281–1310.

Miller, A. L., & Smith, H. L. (2008). Adolescent non-suicidal self-injurious behavior: The latest epidemic to assess and treat. *Applied and Preventative Psychology, 12*, 178–188.

Miller, A. L., Wyman, S. E., Huppert, J. D., Glassman, S. L., & Rathus, J. H. (2000). Analysis of behavioral skills utilized by suicidal adolescents receiving dialectical behavior therapy. *Cognitive and Behavioral Practice, 7*, 183–187.

Nelis, D., Quoidbach, J., Mikolajczak, M., & Hansenne, M. (2009). Increasing emotional intelligence: (How) is it possible? *Personality and Individual Differences, 47*, 36–41.

Neumann, A., van Lier, P. A. C., Gratz, K. L., & Koot, H. M. (2010). Multidimensional assessment of emotion regulation difficulties in adolescents using the Difficulties in Emotion Regulation Scale. *Assessment, 17*, 138–149.

Newcomer, P. L., Barenbaum, E. M., & Bryant, B. R. (1994). *Depression and anxiety in youth scale*. Austin, TX: Pro-Ed.

Nussbaum, M. C. (2001). *Upheavals of thought: The intelligence of emotions*. Cambridge, United Kingdom: Cambridge University Press.

Ochsner, K. N., & Gross, J. J. (2007). The neural architecture of emotion regulation. In J. J. Gross (Ed.), *Handbook of emotion regulation*. New York, NY: Guilford Press.

Peterson, C., & Seligman, M. E. P. (2004). *Character strengths and virtues: A handbook and classification*. New York, NY: Oxford University Press.

Poznanski, E. O., & Mokros, H. B. (1996). *Children Depression Rating Scale, Revised* (CDRS-R). Los Angeles, CA: Western Psychological Services.

Rathus, J. H., & Miller, A. L. (1995). *Life Problems Inventory*. Unpublished manuscript, Montefiore Medical Center, Albert Einstein College of Medicine, Bronx, NY.

Reynolds, C. R., Richmond, B. O., & Lowe, P. A. (2003). *The Adult Manifest Anxiety Scale: Professional manual*. Los Angeles, CA: Western Psychological Services.

Rothbart, M. K., & Bates, J. E. (1998). Temperament. In W. Damon & N. Eisenberg (Eds.), *Handbook of child psychology, Vol. 3. Social, emotional, personality development* (pp. 105–176). New York, NY: Wiley.

Safer, D. L., Lock, J., & Couturier, J. L. (2007). Dialectical behavior therapy modified for adolescent binge eating disorder: A case report. *Cognitive and Behavioral Practice, 14,* 157–167.

Salbach-Andrae, H., Bohnekamp, I., Pfeiffer, E., Lehmkuhl, U., & Miller, A. L. (2008). Dialectical behavior therapy of anorexia and bulimia nervosa among adolescents: A case series. *Cognitive and Behavioral Practice, 15,* 415–425.

Salovey, P., & Grewal, D. (2005). The science of emotional intelligence. *Current Directions in Psychological Science, 14,* 281–285.

Salovey, P., Mayer, J. D., & Caruso, D. (2002). The positive psychology of emotional intelligence. In C. R. Snyder & S. J. Lopez (Eds.), *Oxford handbook of positive psychology* (2nd ed.). New York, NY: Oxford University Press.

Scheier, M. F., Matthews, K. A., Owens, J. F., Schulz, R., Bridges, M. W., Magovern, G. J., & Carver, C. S. (1999). Optimism and rehospitalization after coronary artery bypass graft surgery. *Archives of Internal Medicine, 159,* 829–835.

Scheinholz, M. (2011). Emotion regulation. In C. Brown & V. C. Stoffel (Eds.), *Occupational therapy in mental health: A vision for participation*. Philadelphia, PA: F. A. Davis.

Schore, A. (2003). *Affect dysregulation and disorders of the self.* New York, NY: Norton.

Sheikh, J. I., & Yesavage, J. A. (1986). Geriatric Depression Scale (GDS): Recent evidence and development of a shorter version. *Clinical Gerontologist, 5,* 165–173.

Slaski, M., & Cartwright, S. (2003). Emotional intelligence training and its implications for stress, health and performance. *Stress & Health, 19,* 233–239.

Suveg, C., & Zeman, J. (2004). Emotion regulation in children with anxiety disorders. *Journal of Clinical Child and Adolescent Psychology, 33,* 750–759.

Tang, M. (2001). Clinical outcome and client satisfaction of an anger management group program. *Canadian Journal of Occupational Therapy, 68,* 228–236.

Van der Kolk, B. A. (2003). The neurobiology of childhood trauma and abuse. *Child and Adolescent Psychiatric Clinics of North America, 12,* 293–317.

Wagner, E. E., Miller, A. L., Greene, L. I., & Winiarski, M. G. (2004). Dialectical behavior therapy for substance abusers adapted for persons living with HIV/AIDS with substance use diagnoses and borderline personality disorder. *Cognitive and Behavioral Practice, 11,* 202–212.

Zeitlin, S. (1985). *Coping Inventory: A measure of adaptive behavior*. Bensenville, IL: Scholastic Testing Service.

Zeitlin, S., Williamson, G. G., & Szczepanski, M. (1988). *Early Coping Inventory: A measure of adaptive behavior*. Retrieved from http://ststesting.com/COPI.html

For additional resources on the subjects discussed in this chapter, visit http://thePoint.lww.com/Willard-Spackman12e.

CHAPTER 58

Social Interaction and Occupational Performance

Lou Ann Griswold, C. Douglas Simmons

LEARNING OBJECTIVES

After reading this chapter, you will be able to:

1. Understand the importance of addressing social interaction skills as critical for engagement in all areas of occupation
2. Compare assessment approaches evaluating social interaction
3. Consider different intervention approaches to support social interaction skills
4. Consider factors that influence the quality of social interaction
5. Discuss how to support the quality of social interaction during a person's occupational engagement

OUTLINE

Introduction to Social Interaction and Occupational Performance

People are social beings, and many occupations in which people engage involve social interaction with others. Although social participation is considered a separate area of occupation within the "Occupational Therapy Practice Framework" (OTPF) (American Occupational Therapy Association [AOTA], 2008), work, leisure, play, education, and instrumental activities of daily living are often social. Children interact with one another as they play together, do school projects, and share information about their day with their families. Teens spend a large amount of their time interacting with their peers inside and outside of school as they participate in music groups, theater, team sports, and other youth activities. Adults interact with others at work, at home, and in the community. Depending on the circumstances, personal activities of daily living and rest and sleep might also involve social interaction with others. It appears, therefore, that social participation supports one's engagement in the many areas of occupation and is not a distinct or separate area of occupation.

Regardless of age, interacting with others requires decision making, collaborating, sharing information, gathering information, and conversing socially—intended purposes of social interaction. All social exchanges require similar skills to support interaction (see social interaction skills discussed in Chapter 22). People initiate interaction or respond to another person's greeting to begin an interaction. They communicate using words (i.e., speech, augmentative device, or sign language) and gestures. They ask questions, respond to a social partner, and take turns to support the interaction. A person also responds to messages sent by a social partner, empathizing, clarifying, and encouraging the other person to sustain interaction. Specific expectations and demands for skills may vary with the context of the social exchange, yet all of these skills are required for social interaction.

Because most occupations require social interaction, having difficulty interacting with others potentially influences all areas of occupation, significantly limiting full occupational engagement. In fact, difficulty with social interaction skills may be *the* limiting factor for full participation in work, leisure, or instrumental activities of daily living. Furthermore, a lack of social interaction skills may have long-lasting negative consequences, particularly for children (Elliott, Sheridan, & Gresham, 1989). Hartup (1992) emphasized the importance of social skills claiming, "the single best childhood predictor of adult adaptation is not school grades, and not classroom behavior, but rather, the adequacy with which the child gets along with other children" (p. 1). More details on the inclusion of social interaction skills in occupational therapy theory are available at http://thePoint.lww.com.

Assessment of Social Interaction

Assessments of social interaction have been primarily developed by psychologists and have taken two forms: report by the person or others and observation. According to Sheridan, Hungelmann, and Maughan (1999), report by self or others indicates a person's *social competence*, reflecting judgment of the person's behavior. Commonly used assessments based on report include the Social Skills Rating System (SSRS) (Gresham & Elliott, 1990), the Behavior Assessment System for Children (BASC) (Reynolds & Kamphaus, 1992), and the Matson Evaluation of Social Skills for Individuals with Severe Retardation (MESSIER) (Matson, 1995). Sheridan et al. (1999) argued that evaluation based on the perspective of another person is limited to that individual's perspective of the person's social interaction within a specific context. For example, when a parent or teacher completes a questionnaire on a child's social interaction, their reports are based on specific settings and situations, such as interacting during activities that occur at home, school, or on a playground and also social partners with whom the child interacts in a given environment (McCabe & Marshall, 2006; McConnell & Odom, 1999; Wight & Chapparro, 2008). Additionally, the persons completing the report may not have a clear understanding of the terms used in the rating scale (McCabe & Marshall, 2006) and may in fact be rating other constructs including psychopathology, self-esteem, adaptive behavior, and academic performance (for children) or work skills (for adults) (Matson & Watkins, 2009).

Although rating scales of social competence completed by others may be limited to a given context, they indicate the result of a person's quality of social interaction and how the person's social interaction skills interfere with work, education, leisure, and play. Such information may contribute to an occupational profile (the first phase of evaluation in OTPF) and may guide the occupational therapist to select an appropriate assessment tool for further evaluation. Assessments based on report by the person or others are easy to administer, convenient for the therapist, and require minimal training to give and interpret; and as result, Matson and Watkins (2009) claimed they will continue to be used. However, it is important for occupational therapists to know the type and extent of information gained from any assessment. Although assessment tools of social interaction based on report by the person or others provide information on one's social competence, they do not identify specific problems in social interaction to guide intervention planning to support improvement in social interaction skills (Elliott et al., 1989).

Observation is the second form of evaluation of social interaction and provides information on behaviors during a social exchange that can guide intervention. Occupational therapists frequently include observation of a person in their evaluation process. Assessments based on observation may be contrived or "set up" to elicit certain behaviors or may be conducted in a natural context. Assessments based on role-play reflect contrived situations based on social situations that are believed to be important to people. Because the role-play situations are predetermined, they allow for a standardized observation. Assessments using role-play are used particularly in mental health settings. An example of such an assessment was developed by Tsang and Pearson (2000) to evaluate social skills to prepare persons with mental illness for work. Their evaluation included two work-related role-play situations: a job interview and requesting time off from work. Tsang and Pearson's assessment also included a self-report. Bellack, Brown, and Thomas-Lohrman (2006) believed that assessments based on role-play provide information on a person's "behavioral capacity," rather than "real life performance" (p. 350).

Doble and Magill-Evans (1992) and later many others (Case-Smith, 2005; Coster 2008; Law, 2002; Lord et al., 2005; McConnell, 2002; Wight & Chapparo, 2008) advocated for evaluating social interaction in the natural context to gather information that will guide intervention to support participation in the contexts that are relevant for clients. Case-Smith (2005) referred to assessments based on observation in natural context as "authentic" assessments (p. 110). She claimed that observing in natural context enables the occupational therapist to understand how a person's performance is influenced by the context. Furthermore, assessment that occurs in a natural context during occupational engagement logically leads to intervention supporting enhanced occupational engagement (Fisher, 2009; Law, 2002). More details on evaluating social interaction in a natural context are available at http://thePoint.lww.com.

Occupational Therapy Assessment of Social Interaction

Two assessment tools have been developed by occupational therapists to evaluate social interaction skills: the Assessment of Communication and Interaction Skills (ACIS) (Forsyth, Salamy, Simon, & Kielhofner, 1998) and the Evaluation of Social Interaction (ESI) (Fisher & Griswold, 2009, 2010). For both of these assessments, therapists rate the social interaction skills using a four-point criterion-referenced scale indicating the person's level of competence.

When the ACIS is administered, the person evaluated is observed during more than one situation. Options for situations include interacting during (1) one-on-one conversations with another person to discuss a topic, (2) parallel tasks in which people work individually on tasks but near others, (3) cooperative groups in which several people interact to complete a task or play a game, and (4) open interactions without a preplanned agenda or limited number of persons (e.g., a break room or party) (Forsyth et al., 1998). Using the ACIS, the person can be observed during either naturalistic situations or in simulated situations in which the occupational therapist might become the social partner. The ACIS evaluates 20 skills in categories of (1) physicality, (2) information exchange, and (3) relations (Forsyth et al., 1998).

The psychometric properties of the ACIS were determined primarily with persons with psychiatric diagnoses (81 of the 117 subjects) (Forsyth, Lai, & Kielhofner, 1999, p. 72). Subsequent studies using the ACIS have also included that same client population (Bonsaksen, Myraunet, Celo, Granå, & Ellingham, 2011; Haglund, & Thorell, 2004; Hsu, Pan, & Chen, 2008).

Occupational therapists using the ESI only observe the person during social interactions in natural contexts with typical social partners (Fisher & Griswold, 2010). The person and occupational therapist determine what social interactions the occupational therapist will observe by discussing social interactions that are relevant to the person's daily life and are also challenging for the person. The ESI evaluates 27 skills related to (1) initiating and terminating social interaction, (2) producing social interaction, (3) physically supporting social interaction, (4) shaping content of social interaction, (4) maintaining flow of social interaction, (5) verbally supporting social interacting, and (5) adapting social interaction (Fisher & Griswold, 2010).

The ESI has been used with persons of all ages without a diagnosis and with those with various diagnostic conditions, including children with autism, learning disabilities, and anxiety disorders (Griswold & Townsend, in press); adults with traumatic brain injury (TBI) (Simmons, Griswold, & Berg, 2010); and adults with psychiatric disorders or neurological disorders (Søndergaard & Fisher, 2012).

CASE STUDY 58.1 Bethany

Evaluating Quality of Social Interaction

Background: Referral and Occupational Therapy Interview

Bethany is 31 years old and a survivor of two traumatic brain injuries (TBIs) (see Appendix I for more details on TBI). She currently lives in an apartment associated with an independent living organization and attends a community-based program for adults with acquired brain injury (ABI). It was in this setting that Bethany sought the services of occupational therapy. The occupational therapist, Steve, met with Bethany, at which point he gathered information about Bethany as a person and learned about her goals (see Figure 58.1)

Bethany told Steve about herself and her two accidents that resulted in two TBIs. Bethany identified herself as an artist since childhood. She loved painting and had been studying fine arts in college in a large urban area, with plans to become a studio artist and continue living in the city with her friends. On her way to class, she was crossing a busy intersection and was struck by a car by a driver who was texting and not aware of people in the crosswalk. Bethany was thrown 20 ft down the road and sustained

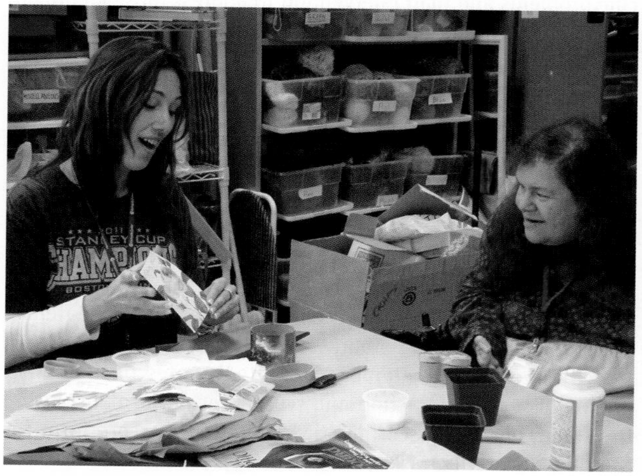

FIGURE 58.1 Bethany practicing social skills in an occupational therapy group.

(continued)

CASE STUDY 58.1 Bethany (*Continued*)

a TBI as well as orthopedic injuries. After 10 weeks of rehabilitation, Bethany was discharged to her parents' home where she lived for 1 year and then moved back to the city to pursue an art degree. Bethany reported that she continued to have minimal issues with balance and after a night of clubbing decided to return to her apartment alone. She was on the second flight of stairs up to her third floor apartment when she had a dizzy spell and fell down a flight and a half of stairs, sustaining a second head injury. She was again discharged to her parents' home post rehabilitation. After living with her parents for about a year and a half, she moved into her apartment associated with an independent living organization in the city where her parents live.

At the time of her discharge from rehabilitation services, Bethany had no identified options for employment and had few friends with whom she had contact. She had difficulty speaking and was given an augmentative communication device, which she did not use regularly. She felt isolated. When she learned about a community-based program for adults with ABI, she eagerly attended in hopes of meeting people and finding meaningful activities. In the program, Bethany began exploring new art media and had joined a cake decorating group, both of which she enjoyed. However, she stated that while she enjoyed the activities, she really missed having a strong social network. She recognized that her brain injuries had resulted in difficulty interacting with others.

Bethany's desires were to establish social networks and to use her art talents in some way to supplement her income. Steve and Bethany discussed that improved social interaction skills would be essential in supporting both of Bethany's goals. Bethany stated that when she was engaged in an activity with another program member, she usually did not interact a great deal and they usually worked side by side, not working together or talking. She knew this type of experience was important for her to practice using her augmentative communication device in a productive manner and to become more social again, but she did not know how to begin working in this direction.

Steve suggested using the Evaluation of Social Interaction (ESI) to evaluate Bethany's social interaction skills to identify specific problems and plan intervention to address those identified. Bethany agreed and together they identified two possible social exchanges that naturally occurred in the community program that Bethany reported were relevant and challenging for her. Bethany agreed to have Steve observe her as she (1) created a bulletin board with another program member and (2) decorated a cake with a different program member.

Evaluation Results

Steve followed the steps of implementing a standardized performance analysis using the ESI (refer to Chapter 22 for details of performance analysis and the definition of the 27 ESI items). Steve quietly observed Bethany as she engaged in the two tasks that involved social interaction. He took notes on Bethany's quality of social interaction and scored her performance using the standardized ESI scoring criteria. Bethany's score form for the cake decorating task is shown in Figure 58.2.

Steve entered Bethany's raw ESI scores into his copy of the ESI computer-scoring software (Fisher & Griswold, 2010) to generate a linear measure of the quality of social interaction. Bethany's quality of social interaction measure is reported on the computer-generated ESI Graphic Report (see Figure 58.3).

Bethany's ESI measures can be interpreted from a criterion-based interpretation and norm-based perspective. The arrow to the left of the scale indicates the location of Bethany's ESI measure along the scale at −0.52 logit. At this level, well below the criterion-referenced cutoff point of competent performance (at 1.0 logit, indicated by a heavy black line on the ESI scale), persons commonly have *moderately to markedly ineffective social interaction skills*. When making a norm-referenced interpretation, Steve compared the location of Bethany's ESI measure to the bar to the left of the scale that indicates the range (±2 *SD*) of quality of social interaction of typical adults between the ages of 22 and 59 years. The black dot in the middle of the bar indicates the mean quality of social interaction for typical adults.

Steve began his documentation with a global baseline statement reflecting Bethany's overall quality of social interaction:

> When Bethany was engaged in two social interactions, one with a program member to create a bulletin board for the program's hallway and another interaction with a different member to decorate a cake, the quality of her social interaction was moderately to markedly ineffective for both tasks. Bethany chose not to use her augmentative communication device and she did not collaborate with her social partners during either task.

Steve identified clusters of interrelated social interaction skills and wrote the following summary statements to document Bethany's social interaction and support her baseline statement (refer to Chapter 22 for details on clustering interrelated skills). Because Bethany's observed social interaction skills were similar in both social exchanges, creating a bulletin board and decorating a cake, Steve described them together.

- ***Produces Speech, Speaks Fluently, and Matches Language:*** Bethany spoke very little (two to three words per social exchange); and when she did, her speech was almost always unintelligible, with frequent pauses between words.
- ***Times Response, Times Duration, Takes Turns, and Clarifies:*** Bethany did not respond to most of her social partners' questions or comments; and when she did, she gave one-word responses, resulting in her partners asking for clarification, to which Bethany did not respond.
- ***Expresses Emotion and Empathizes:*** Bethany demonstrated little emotion throughout the two social exchanges and did not empathize with her partners' feelings when they were jovial or frustrated when they could not understand what Bethany was saying.
- ***Questions, Acknowledges/Encourages, and Heeds:*** Bethany did not ask her social partners any questions during either task and did not acknowledge or encourage her social partners to continue the social interaction. The result was that she did not collaborate with her partners when they were to work together to make the bulletin board and decorate the cake.

CASE STUDY 58.1 Bethany (*Continued*)

EVALUATION OF SOCIAL INTERACTION SCORE FORM (Page 1)

Name: Bethany

Occupational therapist: Steve

Gender: ___ Male X Female

Date of evaluation: ____________

Date of birth: ____________ **Age:** 31

Major diagnosis: Traumatic brain injury

Secondary diagnosis: ____________

Observation number: ___ 1 X 2 ___ 3 ___ 4

Intended purpose of social interaction:
- ___ Gathering information (GI)
- ___ Sharing information (SI)
- ___ Problem solving/Decision making (PD)
- X Collaborating/Producing (CP)
- ___ Acquiring goods and services (AG)
- ___ Conversing socially/Small talk (CS)

Social interaction code: CP-1

Detailed task description: Decorating a cake

Time of day: ___ Morning X Afternoon ___ Evening

Familiarity of the physical environment:
- X Familiar
- ___ Somewhat familiar
- ___ Unfamiliar

Degree of expected structure:
- ___ High structure
- X Relaxed structure
- ___ "Free" structure

Noise level:
- ___ Quiet
- X Moderate noise
- ___ Extreme noise

Number of social partners: 1

Primary social partner: KL

Familiarity of primary the social partner:
- X Familiar
- ___ Somewhat familiar
- ___ Unk…

Status of pri…
- ___ Exp…
- ___ Rec…
- X Frie…
- ___ Fam…
- ___ Othe…

Age of prim…
- ___ Chil…
- ___ Adol…
- X Adul…
- ___ Olde…

Social partn…
- ___ App…
- ___ Que…
- ___ Mini…
- X Mod…
- ___ Mar…

Overall com…
- ___ Gen…
- ___ Que…
- ___ Unc…
- X Very…

Person's ov…
- ___ Appr…
- ___ Que…
- ___ Mini…
- ___ Mod…
- X Mark…

EVALUATION OF SOCIAL INTERACTION SCORE FORM (Page 2)

ITEM RAW SCORES

Initiating and Terminating Social Interaction

1. Approaches/Starts 4 3 2 (1) — Did not respond to partner's greeting
2. Concludes/Disengages 4 3 (2) 1 — Ended somewhat abruptly

Producing Social Interaction

3. Produces Speech 4 3 2 (1) — Produced very little intelligible speech
4. Gesticulates 4 3 (2) 1 — Minimal gestures to support interaction
5. Speaks Fluently 4 3 2 (1) — Very little intelligible speech

Physically Supporting Social Interaction

6. Turns Toward 4 3 (2) 1 — Did not turn face toward partner
7. Looks 4 3 (2) 1 — Looked at partner out of corner of eye
8. Places Self 4 3 (2) 1 — Placed self far away from partner
9. Touches (4) 3 2 1
10. Regulates (4) 3 2 1

Shaping Content of Social Interaction

11. Questions 4 3 2 (1) — Did not ask partner questions
12. Replies 4 3 2 (1) — Did not reply to questions and comments
13. Discloses (4) 3 2 1
14. Expresses Emotion 4 3 2 (1) — Did not express emotion matching partner's messages
15. Disagrees 4 3 2 (1) — Did not respond to partner's suggestions
16. Thanks 4 3 (2) 1 — Did not thank partner for frosting tip

Maintaining Flow of Social Interaction

17. Transitions (4) 3 2 1
18. Times Response 4 3 2 (1) — Long delay to respond and no response
19. Times Duration 4 3 2 (1) — Spoke briefly -- partner needed clarification
20. Takes Turns 4 3 2 (1) — Did not take social turn

Verbally Supporting Social Interaction

21. Matches Language 4 3 2 (1) — Said very little and used simple language
22. Clarifies 4 3 2 (1) — Did not clarify when partner questioned
23. Acknowledges/Encourages 4 3 2 (1) — Did not encourage partner to engage
24. Empathizes 4 3 2 (1) — No support when partner was frustrated

Adapting Social Interaction

25. Heeds 4 3 2 (1) — Did not heed intended purpose: collaborate
26. Accommodates 4 3 2 (1) — Did not prevent problems from occurring
27. Benefits 4 3 2 (1) — Social interaction problems persisted

Additional comments:

FIGURE 58.2 Bethany's evaluation of social interaction (ESI) score form for her social interaction supporting decorating a cake with another person. (Fisher, A. G., & Griswold, L. A. [2010]. *The Evaluation of Social Interaction*. Fort Collins CO: Three Star Press. Reprinted with permission.)

(continued)

CASE STUDY 58.1 Bethany (*Continued*)

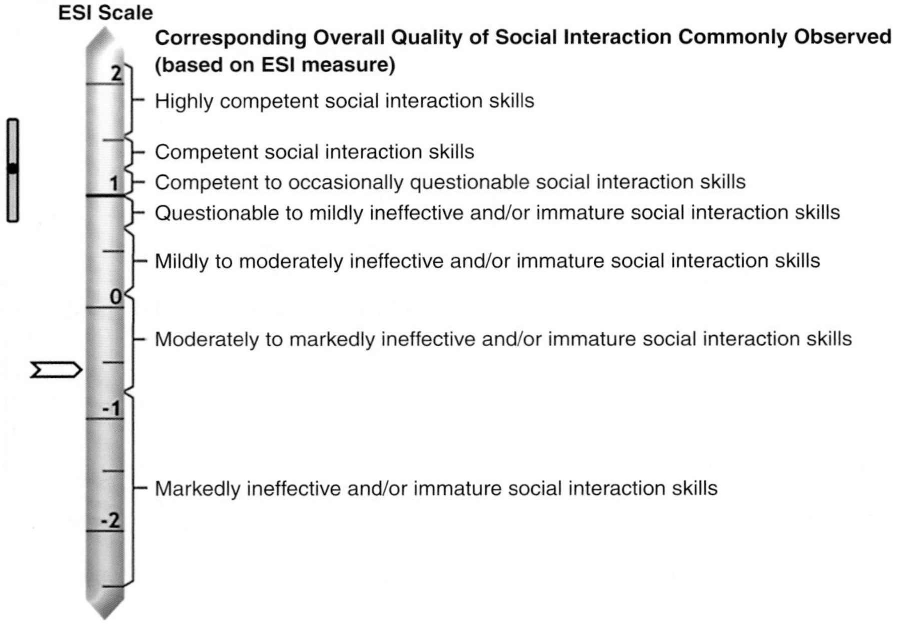

FIGURE 58.3 The evaluation of social interaction (ESI) scale illustrating Bethany's ESI measure, indicated by the arrow to the left. (Fisher, A. G., & Griswold, L. A. [2010]. *The Evaluation of Social Interaction*. Fort Collins CO: Three Star Press. Reprinted with permission.)

Steve's documentation included a description of Bethany's global baseline quality of social interaction, followed by a series of specific baseline statements that described behaviorally her specific problems with social interaction. Overall, her quality of social interaction was markedly ineffective.

Steve shared the results of his observations with Bethany so that they could use the information to refine Bethany's goal of improving her interaction with others. Steve's documentation clearly identified skills that Bethany might work on as a means to reaching her overarching goal.

Because Bethany had difficulty with several social interaction skills, Steve and Bethany had to determine which of these to address first. Steve knew that they had two approaches to use: (1) reflect on the skills that seemed to most interfere with Bethany's overall quality of social interaction or (2) address the skills that are relatively easier. The ESI manual (Fisher & Griswold, 2010) includes a hierarchy of the relative difficulty of all ESI skills, based on Rasch analysis of all evaluations for the ESI standardization sample. Steve and Bethany used a combination of these two approaches and decided to focus first on skills of *Clarifies, Questions, and Replies.* Steve reasoned that whereas *Replies* was a relatively more difficult skill on the ESI skill hierarchy, Bethany's lack of responding to her social partners had a very large impact on her overall quality of social interaction. Steve also reasoned that if Bethany improved her ability to reply to her social partner even somewhat, her overall social interaction would be enhanced.

Bethany and Steve wrote the following goals:

1. In a collaborative task (e.g., cooking, art project), Bethany will consistently answer her social partner's questions using five or more words.
2. In a collaborative task (e.g., cooking, art project), Bethany will clarify what she had said when prompted by her social partner, responding with five or more words.
3. In a collaborative task (e.g., cooking, art project), Bethany will ask her social partner at least two questions to seek his or her perspective on the task and/or how to proceed.

The measurable goals allow Bethany to know what she is working toward and provide her with objective benchmarks against which to measure progress. Most importantly, Bethany set her own goals with Steve, using the results from her observed performance.

Intervention to Enhance Social Interaction Skills

Research on Intervention Strategies

Intervention strategies to support social interaction skills found in the literature differ based on the age and diagnostic condition. Research typically has focused on one age group and one diagnosis at a time. Odom et al. (1999) organized intervention approaches described throughout the literature to promote social competence in young children with disabilities into four strategies: (1) adapting the environment, which included structuring play activities to promote social interaction, arranging and limiting materials, and matching socially competent peers with children with difficulty with social interaction; (2) teaching social skills to small groups of children and providing opportunity for them to practice the skills in play activities; (3) teaching peers who have good social skills how to support their peers who are having difficulty with social skills; and (4) combining the three other strategies. When Odom et al. (1999) compared the four approaches in a study with 92 preschool-age children with disabilities, they found that having one's peers support social interaction is most effective for improving proxy-reported competence of social interaction. They further found the improved social competence to be maintained 1 year later.

Intervention studies with adult populations have focused on the social interaction needs for people with mental illness, primarily schizophrenia. A dominant frame of reference used in these studies is social learning theory, originally described by Bandura (Kurtz & Mueser, 2008). Specific strategies include goal setting, role modeling, practice, and reinforcement. Kurtz and Mueser (2008) conducted a meta-analysis of 23 randomized controlled studies with a total of 1,599 persons with schizophrenia. Although the studies targeted social interaction, Kurtz and Mueser found that only eight of these studies focused on social interaction skills during intervention. Kurtz and Mueser reported that in spite of a lack of focus on social interaction skills, analysis of the studies revealed a strong effect size for self-reported improvements in social interaction.

Simmons and Griswold (2010) used the ESI to evaluate the quality of social interaction for a group of 10 survivors of TBI. The ESI provided a pretest measure of quality of social interaction, served as a guide for an 8-week occupational therapy intervention program, and was used as a posttest to measure intervention effectiveness. The difference between pre- and post-ESI measures was significant for the group of study participants. Their study demonstrated the utility of the ESI in guiding intervention and measuring change.

Intervention Planning

After setting goals, together the occupational therapist and person plan intervention. The occupational therapist brings his or her clinical reasoning, experience, theory, and evidence from research to the discussion and the person contributes suggestions related to activities, strategies, and locations in which intervention might occur naturally. Having evaluation results based on observation in a natural context enables the occupational therapist and person to logically plan well-targeted intervention to promote social interaction during occupations that are relevant and meaningful.

Intervention Guided by Theory

Occupational therapists use theory in their clinical reasoning to guide the planning of intervention. The *Occupational Therapy Intervention Process Model* (OTIPM; Fisher, 1998, 2009) guides the evaluation and intervention process in a true top-down model by first understanding the client as a person, the client's performance context, and occupations that are meaningful for the client, followed by observing the client perform meaningful tasks and conducting performance analyses. As discussed in detail in Chapter 22, performance analyses involve determining what specific goal-directed actions are effective and ineffective. This process was illustrated earlier with Bethany. The problems identified in the performance analysis provide the basis for goals and the focus of intervention.

Based on OTIPM, after conducting a performance analysis in which the occupational therapist determines which actions (e.g., social interaction skills) most limit the person's social interaction, the occupational therapist considers the cause of the problem (Fisher, 2009). Considering cause after implementing a performance analysis is the hallmark of true top-down reasoning. Using a top-down reasoning process also keeps the occupational therapist focused on occupations that are important to the client, reflecting client-centered and occupation-based practice (Fisher, 2009; and see Chapter 22).

Conceptual Model of Social Interaction and Factors That Impact Quality of Social Interaction. Fisher and Griswold (2010) proposed a conceptual model of social interaction and identified factors believed to influence a person's quality of social interaction (see Figure 58.4). Factors that support or hinder a person's quality of social interaction include societal and cultural influences, demands of the social exchange, environmental demands, and influences of person factors and body functions. Because each of the identified factors can impact a person's quality of social interaction, they can also contribute to the "cause" of the person's problems with social interaction. The many factors that influence the quality of one's social interaction can also provide the occupational therapist with options to consider when planning interventions to promote or support a person's quality of social interaction. Refer to http://thePoint.lww.com for a detailed discussion of the conceptual model of social interaction by Fisher and Griswold.

Based on Fisher and Griswold's (2010) conceptual model, the following assumptions regarding the quality of social interaction could be used to guide intervention.

Overall quality of social interaction is supported by the following:

1. Social and cultural influences that are explicit and/or well understood by the person
2. Social exchanges that have clear expectations for performance
3. Social exchanges that have less challenging intended purposes
4. Physical arrangement of objects and persons in the space

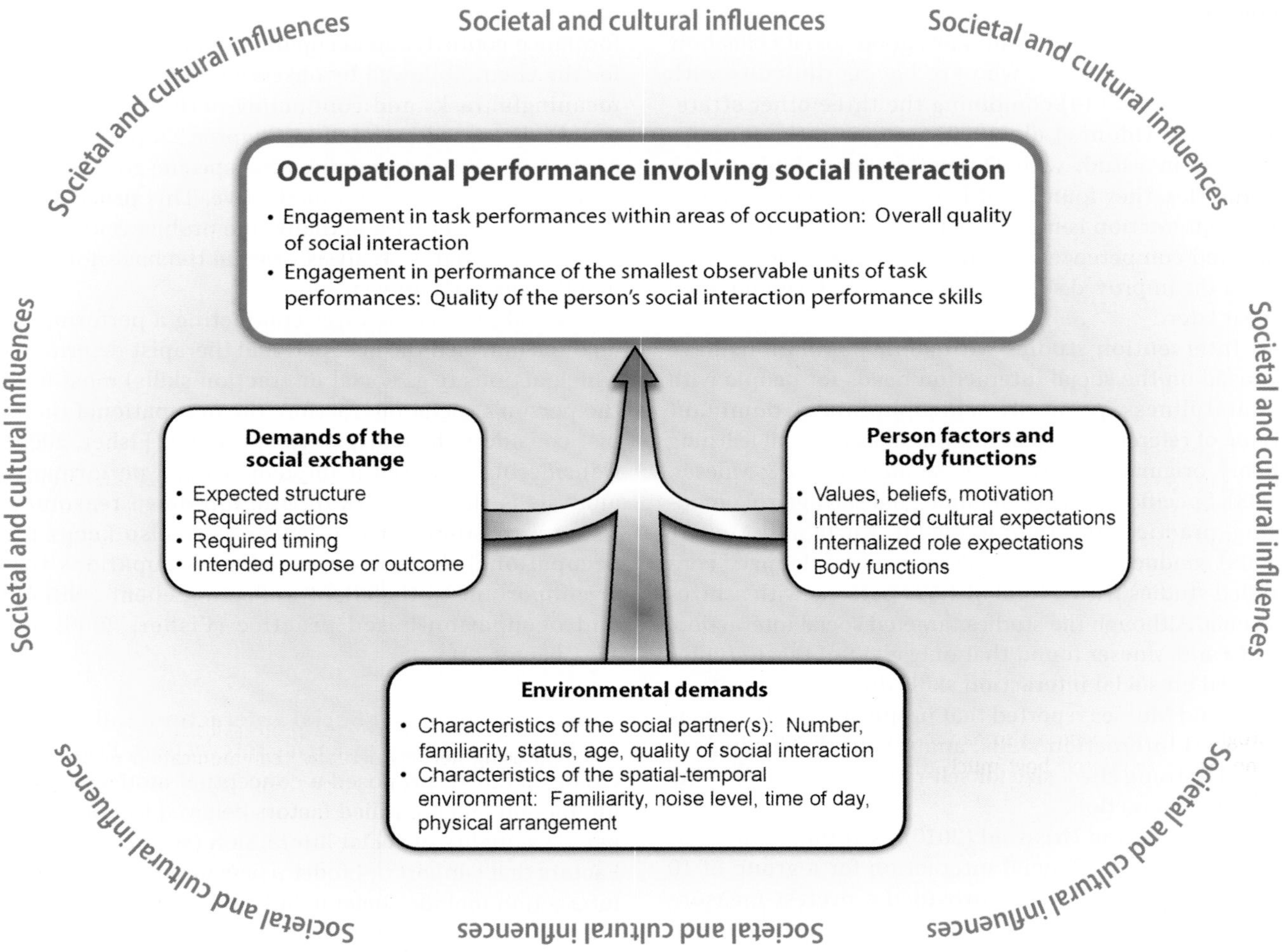

FIGURE 58.4 Schematic representation of the quality of social interaction influenced by transaction among societal and cultural influences, demands of the social exchange, environmental demands, and person factors and body functions. (Adapted from Fisher, A. G., & Griswold, L. A. [2010]. *The Evaluation of Social Interaction*. Fort Collins CO: Three Star Press. Reprinted with permission.)

5. Minimal to moderate noise level in the environment
6. The person having values, beliefs, and internalized role expectations that are consistent with prevailing social and cultural values and beliefs regarding social interaction
7. The person being motivated to engage in good quality social interaction
8. The person having underlying body functions and person factors that support good quality social interaction (e.g., ability to produce clear speech, ability to hear social partner, and having insight/awareness to abilities and problems)
9. Social partners who have a higher quality of social interaction
10. Social partners who are familiar with the person and have a higher status relative to the person

When a person has a goal related to improving social interaction to support his or her participation in desired occupations, an occupational therapist can use these assumptions to guide intervention to improve a person's quality of social interaction.

Models for Intervention. Once the occupational therapist and the person have considered factors that limited the person's quality of social interaction, they need to select an intervention approach to address the identified concerns and work towards the person's goals. According to OTIPM (Fisher, 2009), there are four models for intervention: ***adaptive occupation***, using adapted methods such as adaptive equipment or assistive technology or modifications of the environment or task demands to support performance; **acquisitional occupation**, using occupations to promote the person to develop or reacquire skills; **restorative occupation**, using occupations to facilitate restoring person factors and/or body functions; and ***occupation-based education programs***, providing education to large groups of people related to common problems and strategies to address problems. The occupational therapist uses the identified cause(s) of the problems to determine the most appropriate intervention model. The case study illustrates Steve's reasoning process in planning intervention for Bethany.

Effectiveness of Intervention

After intervention, it is essential that the occupational therapist reevaluate the person to determine if occupational therapy was effective. Again, using observation in natural context provides information that is relevant to the person's daily needs. A reevaluation might indicate that the person had made significant changes and no longer needs occupational therapy. Reevaluation might also reveal new areas of concern, in which case the occupational therapist and person would use the same top-down reasoning process to consider the cause of newly identified problems of social interaction in occupational performance, to identify appropriate intervention models and strategies, and to enhance quality of social interaction.

CASE STUDY 58.2 Bethany

Planning Intervention to Support Social Interaction

Steve considered how demands of the social exchange contributed to Bethany's quality of social interaction. Specifically, he thought that the challenge of the intended purpose of collaborating with another person was challenging for Bethany. Steve was aware that collaborating with another person requires many social interaction skills. Steve also recognized that both social exchanges did not offer much structure. Steve considered the environmental demands of the two social exchanges. Bethany had two different social partners from the community program, both of whom also had difficulty with social interaction. Steve wondered how much the partners' lack of social skill influenced Bethany's quality of social interaction. Steve was aware that both interactions had occurred in the natural environments of the hallway (for the bulletin board task) and the kitchen, where other members were passing through or also engaged in a task. Steve considered the influence of the noise from other people on Bethany's quality of social interaction. Steve then considered person factors and body functions. Bethany was motivated to engage with other people and to engage in both of the tasks. Discussion with Bethany about how well she thought she had interacted with her partners led Steve to reason that Bethany had internalized the expectations, as she reported that she knew her partners had asked questions and made comments, but she had chosen not to respond because it was "too hard." When Bethany did speak, her speech was slow, slurred, and not well articulated, making her speech unintelligible—all factors of body functions. Steve recalled that Bethany reported that she did not use her augmentative communication device because she thought it had not been programmed to include phrases that she commonly needed, so she did not find it helpful. Steve realized that there were many factors contributing to Bethany's ineffective quality of social interaction. Although limitation in body function was evident, Steve knew that Bethany was not likely to improve her ability to articulate her words more clearly, at least not very quickly.

As Steve and Bethany discussed the causes of Bethany's difficulty in social interaction, they began considering ways to address many of these factors. Steve considered the first three intervention models from OTIPM. Together, they determined that restoring body function around oral motor control was not going to be fruitful because Bethany had already received a great deal of speech therapy with little to no improvement. They decided that using the augmentative communication device would enable other people to better understand Bethany, provided the right phrases and words were programmed into the device. Steve agreed to program Bethany's augmentative communication device with phrases that Bethany thought she would need. For example, including the question, "Do you know what I mean?" would help Bethany ensure that her social partners where understanding her and allow her to clarify as needed. Bethany suggested that adding the question, "What do you think?" would promote her to encourage her partners in interactions that were collaborative. Steve knew that Bethany and he had just selected the *adaptive occupation* model of intervention.

Bethany was eager to reacquire skills around social interaction using her augmentative communication device, the *acquisitional occupation* model for intervention. However, Bethany stated that she needed assistance to identify when she might use her augmentative device to engage in interaction more successfully. Steve and Bethany discussed the use of a subtle cuing system in which Steve could prompt Bethany to ask questions or respond to her social partner. They practiced the cuing system briefly and then tried it later that day when Bethany engaged in casual conversation with other program members during lunch. Steve explained that he could support Bethany as she acquired skills through practice in the natural opportunities while she attended the community program.

Bethany and Steve concluded that a combination of using two models for intervention would provide the basis to enhance Bethany's social interaction skills: adaptive occupation, using the augmentative communication device; and acquisitional occupation, to acquire social interaction skills.

The natural context of the community-based program included many opportunities for Bethany to practice the skills she wanted to acquire. Bethany realized that Steve would not be with her throughout the day and suggested that a few of the other staff also be shown the subtle cues to prompt her as needed. Steve knew that many of the program members wanted to work on social interaction to support their desired occupational participation. Therefore, Steve decided to offer an in-service training session to all staff using another model of intervention—*occupation-based education program* (Fisher, 2009). During the training session, Steve shared the conceptual model for social interaction and led the staff in a discussion of natural strategies for the program to better support social interaction by adapting the environment. The staff and Steve discussed promoting more face-to-face opportunities for members to socially interact with one another, monitoring noise in areas in which social interactions frequently occurred, and pairing members so that they were

(continued)

CASE STUDY 58.2 Bethany (*Continued*)

better suited to support one another's social interaction. Steve suggested strategies to provide more structure to the activities with clear social interaction demands. For example, when cooking together, members might be organized into small groups of three persons with each person having a defined role for interacting, such as one person reading directions and the other two sharing the actual cooking task. Last, Steve introduced a simple universal system of cuing to prompt members on skills that many wanted to acquire. The in-service training session resulted in support of natural opportunities to acquire and practice social interaction skills throughout the day for all program members.

Determining Effectiveness of Occupational Therapy Intervention

After 8 weeks of working on improving her social interaction skills in the program, Bethany believed that she was meeting her goals. She requested that Steve see how she was doing by observing her again. Bethany and Steve again determined two social exchanges for Steve to observe and score using the Evaluation of Social Interaction (ESI). For this evaluation, Bethany taught another member how to use a digital camera that the program had recently purchased and then how to enhance the pictures using a computer. Steve again observed the two interactions, scored them, and entered Bethany's scores into the ESI computer software program. The results revealed that Bethany's overall quality of social interaction was now at 0.6 logits. Criterion-referenced interpretation indicated that her overall quality of social interaction was *mildly to moderately ineffective*, a significant improvement from the first evaluation. Steve verified the change by comparing Bethany's ESI measures for both evaluations, finding that the difference in the two measures was greater than the sum of the mean standard error of measurement for each assessment, according to the ESI manual (Fisher & Griswold, 2010). The ESI Progress Report, obtained from the computer-scoring software, includes the ESI scale indicating Bethany's ESI measure for the first and second assessment, marked with a number 1 and 2 for each respective assessment (see Figure 58.5). Using a standardized assessment such as the ESI enabled Steve to confirm that Bethany had indeed made significant progress in the quality of her social interaction skill. The ESI scale in the ESI Progress Report provided an understandable visual aid. Bethany was eager to further improve her social interaction skills and set new goals based on the last evaluation results.

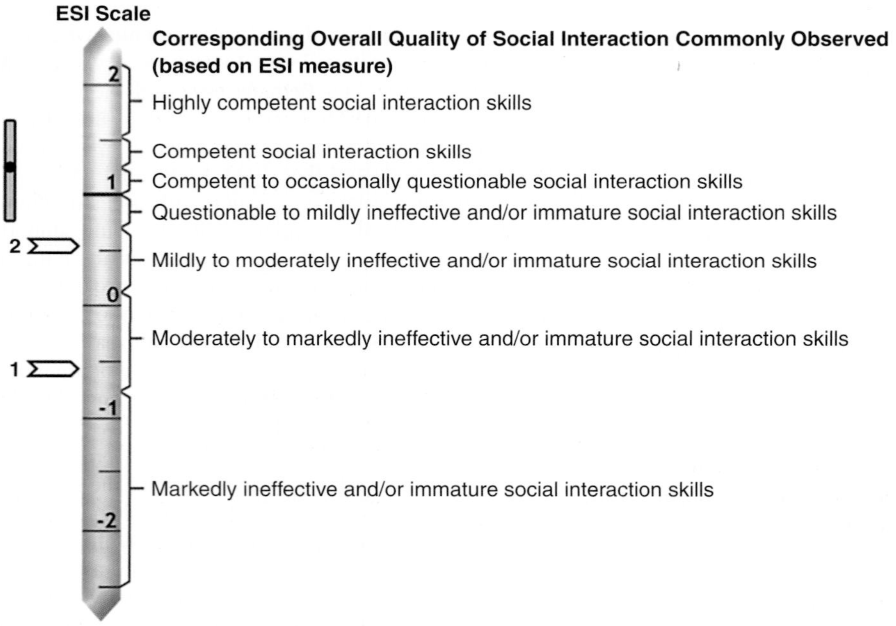

FIGURE 58.5 The evaluation of social interaction (ESI) scale illustrating Bethany's ESI measure for her first and second evaluation, indicated by arrows to the left. (Fisher, A. G., & Griswold, L. A. [2010]. *The Evaluation of Social Interaction*. Fort Collins CO: Three Star Press. Reprinted with permission.)

Conclusion

The case study illustrated how the occupational therapist listened to his client as she expressed a desire to interact with others. As Doble, Bonnell, and Magill-Evans (1991) reported, occupational therapists working in all areas of practice reported that their clients had a need to improve their social interaction. In the case study, Steve determined that Bethany had difficulty with social interaction skills and evaluated her social interaction using a standardized assessment. He then used the assessment results to guide intervention. Furthermore, Steve worked with Bethany to select various intervention models and specific strategies based on a conceptual model. Most importantly, Steve provided intervention in natural context to support Bethany's occupational participation.

References

American Occupational Therapy Association. (2008). Occupational therapy practice framework: Domain and process, 2nd edition. *American Journal of Occupational Therapy, 62*, 625–683.

Bellack, A. S., Brown, C. H., & Thomas-Lohrman, S. (2006). Psychometric characteristics of role-play assessments of social skill in schizophrenia. *Behavior Therapy, 37*, 339–352.

Bonsaksen, T., Myraunet, I., Celo, C., Granå, K. E., & Ellingham, B. (2011). Experiences of occupational therapists and occupational therapy students in using the assessment of communication and interaction skills in mental health settings in Norway. *British Journal of Occupational Therapy, 74*, 332–338.

Case-Smith, J. (2005). Contextual evaluation to support participation. In P. Kramer, J. Hinojosa, & P. Crist (Eds.), *Evaluation: Obtaining and interpreting data* (2nd ed., pp. 101–124). Bethesda, MD: American Occupational Therapy Association.

Coster, W. J. (2008). Embracing ambiguity: Facing the challenge of measurement [Eleanor Clarke Slagle Lecture]. *American Journal of Occupational Therapy, 62*, 743–752.

Doble, S. E., Bonnell, J. E., & Magill-Evans, J. (1991). Evaluation of social skills: A survey of current practice. *Canadian Journal of Occupational Therapy, 58*, 241–249.

Doble, S. E., & Magill-Evans, J. (1992). A model of social interaction to guide occupational therapy practice. *Canadian Journal of Occupational Therapy, 59*, 141–150.

Elliott, S. N., Sheridan, S. M., & Gresham, F. M. (1989). Assessment and treating social skill deficits: A case study for the scientist-practitioner. *Journal of School Psychology, 27*, 197–222.

Fisher, A. G. (1998). Uniting practice and theory in an occupational framework. 1998 Eleanor Clarke Slagle Lecture. *American Journal of Occupational Therapy, 52*, 509–521.

Fisher, A. G. (2009). *Occupational therapy intervention process model: A model for planning and implementing top-down, client-centered, and occupation-based occupational therapy interventions.* Fort Collins, CO: Three Star Press.

Fisher, A. G., & Griswold, L. A. (2009). *The Evaluation of Social Interaction.* Fort Collins, CO: Three Star Press.

Fisher, A. G., & Griswold, L. A. (2010). *The Evaluation of Social Interaction* (2nd ed.). Fort Collins, CO: Three Star Press.

Forsyth, K., Lai, J., & Kielhofner, G. (1999). The Assessment of Communication and Interaction Skills (ACIS): Measurement properties. *British Journal of Occupational Therapy, 62*, 69–79.

Forsyth, K., Salamy, M., Simon, S., & Kielhofner, G. (1998). *The Assessment of Communication and Interaction Skills (ACIS).* Chicago, IL: Model of Human Occupation Clearinghouse, University of Illinois.

Gresham, F. M., & Elliott, S. N. (1990). *Social Skills Rating System.* Circle Pines, MN: American Guidance Service.

Griswold, L. A., & Townsend, S. (in press). Assessing the sensitivity of the evaluation of social interaction: Comparing social skills for children with and without disabilities. *American Journal of Occupational Therapy.*

Haglund, L., & Thorell, L. (2004). Clinical perspective on the Swedish version of The Assessment of Communication and Interaction Skills: Stability of assessments. *Scandinavian Journal of Caring Sciences, 18*, 417–423.

Hartup, W. W. (1992). Having friends, making friends, and keeping friends: Relationships as educational contexts. ERIC Digest (ED345854), Champaign, IL: ERIC Clearinghouse on Elementary and Early Childhood Education.

Hsu, W., Pan, A., & Chen, T. (2008). A psychometric study of the Chinese version of the Assessment of Communication and Interaction Skills. *Occupational Therapy in Health Care, 22*, 177–185.

Kurtz, M. M., & Mueser, K. T. (2008). A meta-analysis of controlled research on social skills training for schizophrenia. *Journal of Consulting and Clinical Psychology, 76*, 491–504.

Law, M. (2002). Participation in the occupations of everyday life. *American Journal of Occupational Therapy, 56*, 640–649.

Lord, C., Wagner, A., Rogers, S., Szatmari, P., Aman, M., Charman, T., . . . Yoder, P. (2005). Challenges in evaluating psychosocial interventions for autistic spectrum disorders. *Journal of Autism and Developmental Disorders, 35*, 695–708.

Matson, J. L. (1995). *The Matson Evaluation of Social Skills for Individuals with Severe Retardation* (MESSIER). Baton Rouge, LA: Disability Consultants, LLC.

Matson, L., & Watkins, J. (2009). Psychometric testing methods for children's social skills. *Research in Developmental Disabilities, 30*, 249–274.

McCabe, P. C., & Marshall, D. J. (2006). Measuring the social competence of preschool children with specific language impairment: Correspondence among informant ratings and behavioral observations. *Topics in Early Childhood Special Education, 26*, 234–246.

McConnell, S. R. (2002). Interventions to facilitate social interaction for young children with autism: Review of available research and recommendations for educational intervention and future research. *Journal of Autism and Developmental Disorders, 32*, 351–372.

McConnell, S. R., & Odom, S. L. (1999). A multimeasure performance-based assessment of social competence in young children with disabilities. *Topics in Early Childhood Special Education, 19*, 67–74.

Odom, S., McConnell, S. R., McEvoy, M. A., Peterson, C., Ostrosky, M., Chandler, L. K., . . . Favazza, P. C. (1999). Relative effects of interventions supporting the social competence of young children with disabilities. *Topics in Early Childhood Education, 19*, 75–91.

Reynolds, C. R. M., & Kamphaus, R. W. (1992). *Behavior assessment system for children.* Circle Pines, MN: American Guidance Service.

Sheridan, S. M., Hungelmann, A., & Maughan, D. P. (1999). A contextualized framework for social skills assessment, intervention, and generalization. *School Psychology Review, 28*, 84–103.

Simmons, C. D., & Griswold, L. A. (2010). Using the evaluation of social interaction in a community-based program for persons with traumatic brain injury. *Scandinavian Journal of Occupational Therapy, 17*, 49–56.

Simmons, C. D., Griswold, L. A., & Berg, B. (2010). Evaluation of social interaction during occupational engagement. *American Journal of Occupational Therapy, 64*, 10–17.

Søndergaard, M. & Fisher, A. G. (2012). Sensitivity of the Evaluation of Social Interaction Measures Among People With and Without Neurologic or Psychiatric Disorders. *American Journal of Occupational Therapy, 66*, 356–362.

Tsang, H., & Pearson, V. (2000). Reliability and validity of a simple measure for assessing the social skills of people with schizophrenia necessary for seeking and securing a job. *Canadian Journal of Occupational Therapy, 67*, 250–259.

Wight, M., & Chapparo, C. (2008). Social competence and learning difficulties: Teacher perceptions. *Australian Occupational Therapy Journal, 55*, 256–265.

For additional resources on the subjects discussed in this chapter, visit http://thePoint.lww.com/Willard-Spackman12e.

The Practice Context: Therapists in Action

UNIT XIII

"The true expert, then, is someone who knows something of what lies beneath the surface of his or her practice, and spends time and effort not just understanding it but developing it further, and who can then talk about it more publicly too."

—DELLA FISH & COLIN COLES

CHAPTER 59

Continuum of Care

Pamela S. Roberts, Mary E. Evenson

OUTLINE

LEARNING OBJECTIVES

After reading this chapter, you will be able to:

1. Describe occupational therapy's typical roles in acute care, inpatient, outpatient, and community-based settings as illustrated in vignettes
2. Value the importance of client-centered care through the collaborative goal-setting process to guide the professional reasoning process and influence the intervention plan throughout the continuum of care
3. Recognize how client factors and contexts featured in the vignettes influence discharge recommendations and disposition through the continuum
4. Be aware of key health care system regulations within the United States that effect a client's eligibility for services and length of stay in various settings along the continuum
5. Acknowledge the opportunities for emerging practice areas to meet the needs of populations with varying access to health care

This chapter describes an overview of the **continuum of care** that are part of the U.S. health care system. Case vignettes are featured as examples to illustrate how different services can meet an individual client's needs and goals, depending on the level of care and the client's personal factors and occupational performance. A table at the end of the chapter provides an organizing structure to help understand dimensions of the different levels of the continuum at a glance (see Table 59.1). This chapter is a preface to the following chapters in this unit that more comprehensively address selected populations and occupational therapy's role to support optimal function and participation.

Introduction

Occupational therapy practitioners work in facilities that provide a range of services to address the occupational performance needs and concerns of children and adults across the life course (Roberts & Evenson, 2009). The reasons why individuals seek occupational therapy evaluation and interventions are often a result of a diagnosis/condition that requires medical, surgical, psychiatric, or rehabilitative intervention. As a consequence, individuals experience difficulty performing daily life habits and activities and participating in social roles within their homes and communities (World Health Organization [WHO], 2001).

As part of the occupational therapy process, practitioners collaborate with clients and their caregivers to identify goals that will influence the intervention plan and subsequent delivery of services to support the individual's optimal functioning, recovery, and desired outcomes (see Chapters 23, 24, and 33). In addition to the client's goals, the evaluation process ideally encompasses a biopsychosocial perspective, addressing safety, client factors, occupational performance, social support, and environmental contexts. In doing so, analysis of client functioning for areas of occupation, activities of daily living (ADL), instrumental activities of daily living (IADL), education, work, play and leisure, rest and sleep, and social participation is assessed throughout the various settings within the continuum of care (American Occupational Therapy Association [AOTA], 2008) (see Unit XI).

Types of Facilities

Hospitals are the largest employer of occupational therapy practitioners (AOTA, 2010), with more than 5,795 registered facilities in the United States (American Hospital Association [AHA], 2011a). Various levels of care may be available at an individual hospital, including **acute care**, **long-term acute care**, **inpatient rehabilitation**, and **outpatient rehabilitation**. Schools and **long-term care/skilled nursing facilities** also provide a substantial percentage of job opportunities within the field (AOTA, 2010). Administratively, facilities may be for-profit, not-for-profit, or governmental. Hospital-based health care is a labor-intensive industry operating on a 24 hours per day, 7 days per week basis, facing complex issues related to finances, workforce, and information technology (AHA, 2011b).

Once a client's condition is medically stable or in the case that inpatient medical services are not needed or indicated, occupational therapy practitioners also work in freestanding outpatient/ambulatory care services, **community agencies**, **private practices**, and home-based services, such as **early intervention** and **home health care**. Community-based settings often afford practitioners the opportunity to work in the client's natural environment, such as home or school, and to focus on authentic occupation, in comparison to the focus on medical stabilization as the priority for inpatient settings.

Dependent on the client's needs, an individual may receive occupational therapy services in different types of settings within the **continuum of care**, spanning **emergency**/acute care, inpatient and outpatient rehabilitation, skilled nursing and/or extended care, **partial hospital** or **day programs**, community-based services, home care, and/or **hospice**. Balancing the client's needs, resources, personal factors, and occupational performance in consideration of one's future goals also involves review and use of the best available evidence. This complex decision-making process requires practitioners to use their professional reasoning to make appropriate and meaningful recommendations to support and facilitate a client's progression through the continuum of care (see Chapters 30). Individual personal factors and levels of occupational performance, along with the contexts and environments in which one participates, greatly influence the options for discharge both between the levels of care and toward a final discharge disposition, ultimately enabling the client to be in a residential or home context. These individual client dimensions of care combine with legislative and funding/payment parameters to determine a client's eligibility for the frequency and duration of receiving occupational therapy services (see Table 59.1).

Continuum of Care Vignettes

The following vignettes illustrate examples of typical levels of the continuum of care as relevant to an individual's occupational profile, performance, needs, and goals.

Physical Disabilities: Adult with Cerebral Vascular Accident

See **Appendix I, Common Conditions, Resources, and Evidence**, for more information about cerebrovascular accident (stroke).

Jack is a mid–70-year-old male who had a sudden onset of right-sided weakness as well as aphasia at 10 p.m. Jack's wife immediately drove him to the local hospital, which had a certified stroke center. Within an hour of the onset of Jack's symptoms, he was assessed by the triage nurse and emergency room physician who consulted the neurologist on call. Jack was taken to imaging for a computed tomography (CT) scan, which showed no evidence of hemorrhage and a left middle cerebral artery infarct. The neurologist determined that Jack was a candidate for tissue plasminogen activator (tPA). tPA, if provided within an established time frame, can significantly reduce the effects of stroke and permanent disability. Risks and benefits were discussed with Jack and his wife, who consented. Jack was then transferred to the neuro intensive care unit where he was continuously monitored.

While in the neuro intensive care unit, occupational therapy (OT) was consulted. The occupational therapist performed an occupational therapy evaluation, which included an occupational profile and learned of Jack's active lifestyle prior to admission to the hospital. Jack lived with his wife in a one-story home with five steps to enter. Jack is a retired lawyer. He is active with guest lecturing at a local law school and in volunteering at the animal shelter in his community. Jack loves to cook for his wife, two children, and four grandchildren. Additionally, Jack enjoyed driving and going to the theater and out to restaurants at least two times per week. Jack's goals are to be able to return to his previous active lifestyle, especially being able to cook for his family.

Jack's past medical history is significant for coronary artery disease, osteoarthritis, and borderline renal insufficiency. The occupational therapy assessment revealed right hemiparesis and expressive aphasia, resulting in activity limitations in daily activities requiring maximum assistance for eating, grooming, dressing, bathing, toileting, and mobility. Further, Jack is dependent on others to perform instrumental activities of daily living (IADL). Occupational therapy started in the intensive care unit and continued on the acute stroke floor, with the focus on improving Jack's participation in daily activities and functional mobility. In order to assess for continued services at the next level of care, the inpatient rehabilitation admission coordinator and physical medicine and rehabilitation physician determined that Jack met admission criteria for inpatient rehabilitation (see Table 59.1). Jack's diagnosis of stroke is included in the Centers for Medicare and Medicaid Services thirteen qualifying diagnoses for inpatient rehabilitation. Additionally, Jack required intervention from multiple therapies, including physical therapy (PT), OT, and speech-language pathology (SLP). During his acute care hospitalization, Jack was actively participating in therapies (PT, OT, and SLP) and it was determined that he would benefit from an intensive therapy program with supervision by a rehabilitation physician. After 4 days in the acute hospital, Jack was admitted to the inpatient rehabilitation unit with the focus on restoration of function for eventual return to home with his wife.

The OT practitioner performed the facility's evaluation, including the Functional Independence Measure (FIM™) (Hamilton, Granger, Sherwin, Zielezny, & Tashman, 1987) and the Canadian Occupational Performance Measure (COPM) (Law et al., 2005), which revealed that Jack's goals were to be independent in self-care, cooking, and, eventually, to return to his community activities. Within the first week, the interdisciplinary team had a team conference that included Jack and his wife. During the team conference, Jack's functional status, barriers, and goals were discussed. This collaboration provided the foundation for the interdisciplinary treatment plan with focus on Jack's goals to increase his independence for self-care, functional mobility, and IADL. Jack's wife was not able to provide the necessary physical care; therefore, she hired a personal care attendant for 12 hours per day. Jack demonstrated significant improvement throughout his inpatient stay and was able to perform his daily activities with minimal assistance and cook simple meals with moderate assistance. He was able to eat a regular diet; however, he required assistance with cutting his food. Discharge planning included an evaluation of the home environment, ordering of durable medical equipment, and provision of referrals for community resources and support groups. After discharge, Jack plans to continue his therapy at home with home health services until he is no longer homebound; when he will then plan to transition to outpatient rehabilitation to support his goals of increased independence for home and community reintegration, including eventual return to driving. See Figure 59.1.

Physical Disabily: Adult with Total Hip Replacement

See **Appendix I, Common Conditions, Resources, and Evidence**, for more information about orthopedics (joint replacements).

Marion is an early 90-year-old Asian female who has severe osteoarthritis. Prior to the hospitalization, Marion was having increasing pain in her right hip, which was limiting her ability to perform her daily activities including walking. She failed conservative treatment including analgesic medications and physical therapy and had an elective right total hip arthroplasty. The orthopedic surgeon ordered post-surgery precautions with toe touch weight bearing on the right lower extremity. Marion's past medical history was significant for hypertension and congestive heart failure, which were controlled with medications. Prior to admission, Marion lived alone in an assisted living community. She was active within this community, participating in the daily social activities. Marion has three sons who are grown and have their own families and do not live locally.

One day after surgery, the acute care occupational therapist was consulted. The occupational profile revealed that Marion's goal was to eventually return to her assisted living residential community. At the time of occupational therapy evaluation, Marion required maximum assistance for functional mobility using a walker and for lower body activities of daily living. Marion also had pain and intermittent confusion since surgery, which

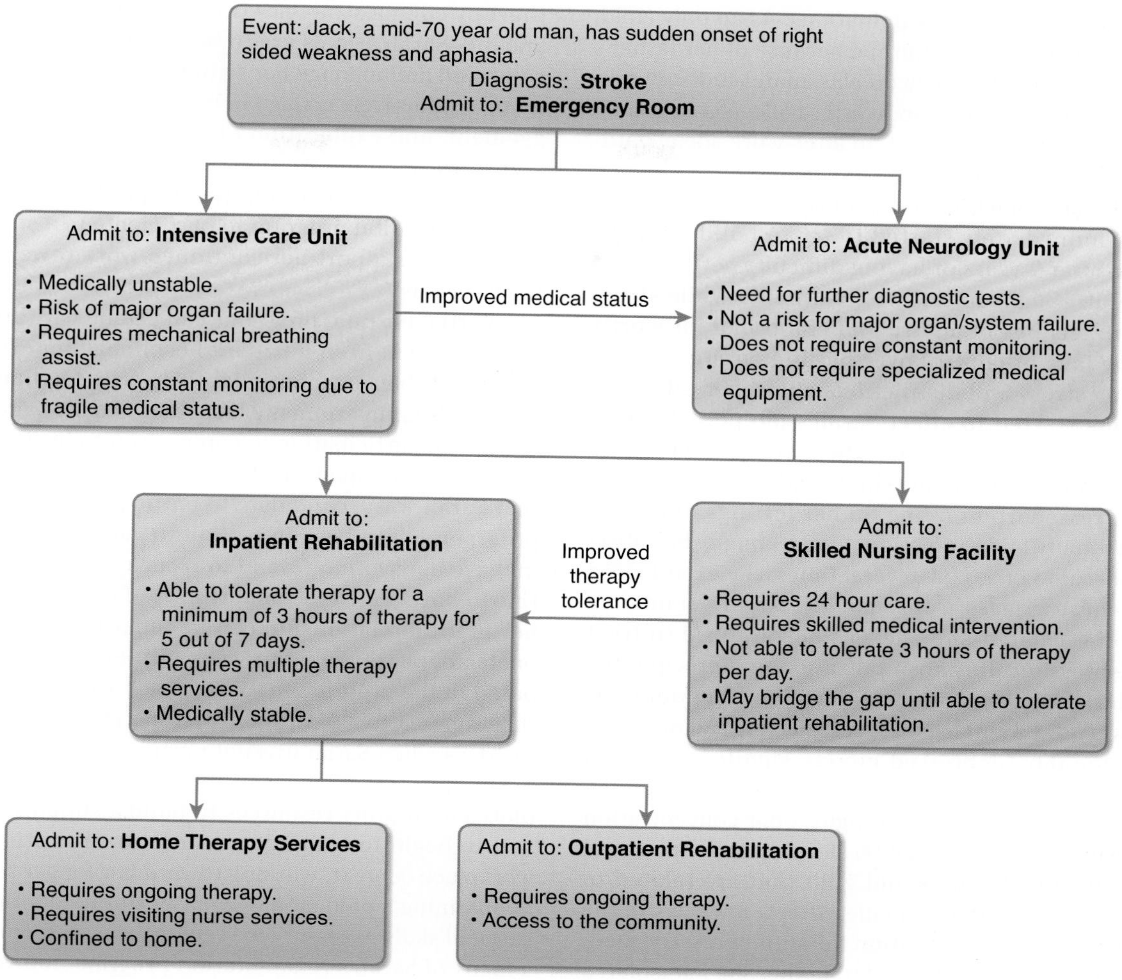

FIGURE 59.1 Example of transitioning through the continuum of care.

limited her ability to participate in therapy. It was determined that Marion would continue her rehabilitation at the local skilled nursing facility because she required skilled intervention but did not require an intensive therapy program of 3 hours daily.

The occupational therapy practitioner performed the facility's initial evaluation including, the Minimum Data Set (MDS, n.d.) and the Canadian Occupational Performance Measure (COPM) (Law et al., 2005). The COPM revealed Marion's desire to be independent in self-care and to return to her assisted living community. Intervention at the skilled nursing facility focused on self-care and functional mobility retraining. Within 20 days, Marion was independent in self-care except for minimal assistance for seated bathing in the shower and functional mobility using a front-wheeled walker. The occupational therapy practitioner provided caregiver training to the hired personal care attendant, ordered appropriate equipment for bathroom adaptations, and arranged for continued therapy in Marion's assisted living community to support her optimal recovery.

Mental Health: Adult with Depression and Anxiety

See **Appendix I, Common Conditions, Resources, and Evidence**, for more information about mood disorders (depression).

Sarah is a Caucasian female in her early 30s who has experienced a history of minor depression and anxiety beginning when she was in college. Initially, her symptoms were most noticeable at the end of the semester, stemming from the pressures of final examinations and fatigue that were associated with staying up late to study, resulting in irregular sleep patterns. Typically, Sarah managed her symptoms through social drinking of alcohol and partying with friends to celebrate finishing up their academic responsibilities after an exam and sometimes binge drinking. On a few occasions, Sarah sought out behavioral health counseling services offered by the university when she faced trouble focusing her attention or feeling panicky before examinations. As an only child, with her parents living in Europe because of her father's job, Sarah has relied heavily on classmates and coworkers for her social support. Soon after college graduation, she met her husband-to-be at an after-work social gathering featuring alcoholic drinks and dancing.

Sarah married within a year of meeting her husband and they immediately started to try to build a family. However, after 2 years of having difficulty getting pregnant, Sarah sought infertility treatments while struggling with feelings of failure and emotional insecurity about the lack of control over her life circumstances. Increasing stress and distractions about her infertility treatments started to affect Sarah's job performance. Ultimately, she was laid off when her company was downsizing personnel and she found herself increasingly distressed, ruminating on her feelings of failure, both personally and professionally. Although she subsequently became pregnant several times, she experienced multiple miscarriages. Consequently, Sarah's emotional condition escalated and she was hospitalized to treat major depression. This hospitalization was precipitated by Sarah experiencing many of the following symptoms nearly every day for at least 2 weeks: feeling sad or empty most of the day (depressed mood), significant loss of interest or pleasure in activities that used to be enjoyable, significant weight gain, fatigue, poor concentration and slowing down of thoughts, sleeping too much, and feelings of worthlessness and guilt that are related to thoughts about death or suicide. After a few days in the hospital and a new prescription for antidepressant medications, Sarah was discharged to home. She felt isolated and alone while her husband was at work and started to drink alcohol during the day, with her husband often finding her still in her pajamas and intoxicated when he got home from work. Her alcohol abuse further compromised her ability to cope with her feelings of depression and anxiety, impacting her ability to consistently perform basic self-care and home management daily activities. Frustrated with Sarah's debilitating symptoms, her marital relationship became significantly strained and her husband moved out of their apartment, asking for a separation and possibly a divorce if Sarah does not make an effort to change her situation.

Struggling to manage her symptoms, this change in her marital relationship triggered Sarah's contemplation of suicide along with the recognition that she needed to make a significant life change if she has any hope of salvaging her marriage. Consequently, Sarah sought voluntary readmission to an inpatient psychiatric hospital unit to treat her **dual diagnosis** of major depression and alcohol abuse. This hospitalization, covered under her husband's private health insurance benefits from his employer, addressed adjustment of her medication regimen, along with Sarah's participation in an occupational therapy evaluation and group interventions focusing on the use of **cognitive behavioral therapy** coping strategies (Ellis, 1992) (see Chapters 43 and 45). Sarah's goals are to be able to more effectively cope with and manage her symptoms; to regain her ability to productively engage in basic self-care, home management, and exploration of job search opportunities; and to work on her marital relationship. After a week, Sarah was discharged from the hospital and referred to a partial hospital program to participate in a structured program to support her continued work toward meeting her goals.

Partial hospital programs can extend care and serve as a transition from inpatient hospitalization. This level of care enables occupational therapists to support clients' goals for instrumental activities of daily living, work, and social participation in comparison to inpatient care that focuses on medical stabilization. It was determined that Sarah was a candidate to participate in this type of program due to her motivation to gain coping skills to manage her symptoms and to reengage in her daily routine to have a realistic opportunity of exploring whether her marital relationship can be repaired and her prospects about returning to work. Initially, Sarah participated in the program for 5 days each week for a month, then tapered to 3 days a week for her continued care. On the days when Sarah was not participating in the partial hospital program, she was able to take initiative to explore community resources to build a support network and to begin to volunteer in order to transition into a workplace context, working toward her longer term goal of obtaining a paid employment position. Identifying vocational skills necessary to reenter the workforce became a focus of Sarah's rehabilitation program and volunteer experience. This skill set capitalized on her work experience and included practicing communication skills to foster effective peer and supervisory relationships, sustaining concentration and using problem-solving skills, and regaining confidence and self-reliance for beginning a job search.

Pediatrics: Child with Traumatic Brain Injury, Orthopedic Fracture, and Amputation

See **Appendix I, Common Conditions, Resources, and Evidence**, for more information about traumatic brain injury, orthopedics (fractures), and amputations.

Joshua is a sixth-grade African-American male who experienced a traumatic brain injury (TBI) along with multiple fractures and a severe crush injury as a result of being hit by a truck when riding his bike home from a nearby friend's house after a soccer game. Joshua was not wearing his bike helmet because he forgot to bring it along with his soccer gear. Unconscious at the scene of the accident, emergency medical personnel transported Joshua to the nearest Children's Hospital Emergency Services via medic flight. Joshua underwent extensive orthopedic surgery to stabilize his left humeral fracture with an open reduction internal fixation (ORIF) and to amputate his right lower extremity below the knee due to the severe nature of his ankle and foot crush injury. Following surgery, Joshua was treated in the hospital's pediatric intensive care unit (PICU) to closely monitor his status while in a comatose state for 5 days. In the PICU, occupational therapist performed an initial evaluation and found that Joshua responded to localized stimuli before he eventually emerged from the coma. At first signs of consciousness, Joshua was sluggish and complained of feeling tired. He was disoriented, not knowing where he was or what had happened—common symptoms of posttraumatic amnesia.

After a week, Joshua became emotionally agitated, trying to get out of the hospital bed and repeatedly yelling, "It hurts . . . I want to go home!" After a few days, Joshua's confusion and agitation started to subside, and he began to more cooperatively participate in all of his nursing care and therapy sessions. This medical stabilization enabled Joshua to be transferred from the PICU to the hospital's pediatric ward and eventually, to the inpatient rehabilitation unit. Once on the rehabilitation unit, the occupational therapy practitioner worked closely with his mother and the nursing staff to engage Joshua in participating in his basic self-care such as eating, brushing his teeth, and dressing his upper and lower body. Nursing, occupational therapy, and physical therapy provided collaborative interventions to assist Joshua with his functional mobility in getting in and out of bed, building up his sitting tolerance, and toileting and bathing with adaptive equipment and assistance. Joshua tended to be impulsive and impatient with the extra time and effort required for getting from one place to another, requiring step-by-step verbal cueing and moderate physical assistance to support his safe performance. Joshua relied on the use of a wheelchair and practiced standing pivot functional transfers using his left leg for weight bearing. Part of therapy involved teaching Joshua and his mother important safety precautions to prevent falls and to adhere to his orthopedic precautions. Another aspect of care that was addressed during inpatient rehabilitation was coordination with Joshua's school. The interdisciplinary team obtained Joshua's school records and was able to address skills necessary for eventual return to school in the rehabilitation program. These skills included improving attention and concentration as well as other executive functioning activities. After 2 weeks on the inpatient rehabilitation unit, Joshua progressed to needing only minimal assistance from his mother or nursing staff for his basic self-care and functional transfers and he was discharged to home. The left distal humerus ORIF was still healing, and he was using a wheelchair for functional mobility until his right lower extremity prosthetic training progressed.

Initially, Joshua received home care occupational and physical therapy to assist with the discharge transition from the hospital. However, once the left upper extremity ORIF was fully healed, Joshua started outpatient occupational and physical therapy 3 days a week with his mother driving him to the hospital. Joshua's goals focused on "being able to do what I did before," requiring the support of the health care team and his mother to help him accept that he will need to find some new ways to do things after his accident. Because his accident was in the summer, Joshua will be returning to his middle school, an old building without an elevator, facing some personal performance challenges in addition to environmental barriers. Joshua's mother is very concerned about him going back to school and being frustrated with the challenges that he will face because of his injuries, especially ambulating with his new prosthesis and crutches while needing to determine a strategy for carrying his books between classrooms. Although the neuropsychological testing in the hospital revealed Joshua's performance to be at the low end of normal for his age, it is unknown to what extent his cognitive deficits as a result of his traumatic brain injury might pose to his academic performance in returning to school. Therefore, Joshua's outpatient rehabilitation program focused on transition to school-based occupational therapy (see chapter 48). The school-based therapists (physical therapy, occupational therapy, speech-language pathology, and neuropsychology) collaborated with the outpatient rehabilitation therapists to determine the skills and adaptations that would be necessary in order to have a smooth transition back to school in the fall. One of the aspects of continued care in the school system will be adaptive physical education and other identified strategies for taking notes and test taking since Joshua's brain injury. Coping and adaptation to disability within the educational setting is another transitional aspect that will need to be addressed through individual therapy and/or participation in a support group.

Emerging Practice

Emerging practice is commonly viewed as expanding service delivery models and contexts, often beyond traditional medical and health services. An important guiding rationale for emerging practice has been identified as "the successful promotion of participation in occupations among individuals, groups, or communities through the development of occupational therapy services to underserved or unserved clients" (Holmes & Scaffa, 2009, p. 196). However, a common barrier for emerging practice is the lack of third-party reimbursement for populations of all ages, including, but not limited to, children and adults with chronic disabilities, those who are homeless, and at-risk elderly. Opportunities for emerging occupational therapy practice are evolving through work in day programs, transitional housing and employment programs, and specialized services such as low vision and ergonomics.

Some specific examples of occupational therapy's contributions in emerging areas of practice involve consultation (see Chapter 73), program development, health promotion education, and grant-funded demonstration projects. Once young adults reach the age of 21 or 22 years, most are no longer eligible for school-based special education services. For this population, parents and guardians are responsible to assume a full-time caregiving role. **Group homes** provide residential options for young adults with disabilities to transition from living with parents/guardians into the community. **Centers for independent living** provide consumer services and resources to promote independent living skills. Occupational therapists can influence the quality of life for this population by offering consultation services to group homes or centers for independent living. Such services may address making recommendations for activity adaptations and environmental modifications and training clients in self-advocacy and support staff in approaches to provide quality care.

For adults with chronic conditions such as HIV/AIDS, fibromyalgia, arthritis, chronic fatigue syndrome, multiple sclerosis, etc., performance of desired occupations is often experienced in conjunction with pain and/or fatigue. For these populations, occupational therapists have collaborated and partnered with professional organizations that provide consumer services, resources, and support. Development of educational self-management programs that outline strategies to control and cope with symptoms and to simplify daily activities have been enhanced by occupational therapy's unique perspective. Furthermore, occupational therapists have participated in the development of fall prevention programs, targeting at-risk elderly populations, with interventions to promote wellness through active lifestyles and healthy habits for exercise as well as to assess home safety risks and to offer assistance with home modifications. The following vignette describes an example of occupational therapy–emerging practice in the area of low vision.

Older Adults: Community-Based Adult with Low Vision

See **Appendix I, Common Conditions, Resources, and Evidence**, for more information about vision problems (low vision, glaucoma).

Mr. Gonzales is a Spanish-speaking male in his late 70s who immigrated to the United States from Mexico more than 40 years ago with his wife and brother. When his wife died, he relocated to a subsidized housing development for elderly individuals where he has been living for the past 10 years. Mr. Gonzales has a history of diabetes mellitus with associated visual impairment as a result of glaucoma. He does not seek regular medical care and has not had an ophthalmological examination since before his wife passed away. He is aware that some of his neighbors have taken advantage of free vision screenings that are offered through a grant-funded mobile van service. Mr. Gonzales has told some of his neighbors that his glasses do not work as well as they used to, and his neighbors have encouraged him to go to the mobile van for a vision screening the next time that it comes to the housing development where he lives.

Mr. Gonzales voluntarily participated in a low-vision screening that was administered by an occupational therapist with specialty certification in low-vision rehabilitation. Besides recommending and referring him to an ophthalmologist, the therapist suggested that she could also visit his apartment and help to adapt the environment for safety and improved vision. Mr. Gonzales agreed and the therapist conducted a home safety assessment to identify risks and to recommend environmental adaptations, such as installing an overhead light in both his kitchen and bathroom.

Conclusion

Today's health care environment is ever changing and complex. Occupational therapy practice needs to be focused on the client based on where he or she is receiving services within the continuum of care as well as ensuring coordinated transitions of care. Other factors that may affect the client's transition through the continuum and ultimate outcome are the severity of the disability as well as the client's social and financial support systems. Care within the continuum requires teamwork, which can be informal and/or formal. Occupational therapists have the opportunity to advocate for the client in order to identify necessary transitions and resources at the next level within the continuum of care. This goal can be accomplished by collaborating with and exchanging information between providers to ensure that the client's needs and preferences for care are understood and to enhance the quality of care provided. It is important for occupational therapy practitioners to keep in mind the client's priorities as related to satisfaction and participation in life roles. Whether transitioning from acute care or long-term care, the role of occupational therapy is to support our clients' successful reintegration into the home and community environments.

Acknowledgments

Mary Evenson would like to acknowledge Dean Gloria Waters, Boston University College of Health and Rehabilitation Sciences, and Dr. Wendy Coster, chair of the Department of Occupational Therapy, for support in writing this chapter.

TABLE 59.1 Practice Settings

Setting	Requirements for Admission to Setting	Typical Setting	Typical Services	Type of Occupational Therapy	Role of Occupational Therapy Service	Legislation and Funding/Payment
Acute medical/ surgical care	• Need for medical or surgical diagnosis or intervention • Admitted from emergency room, direct admission, or transfer from another facility	• Private hospital • Community hospital • Academic hospital • Veteran's Administration hospital • Specialty hospital	• Trauma services • Intensive care unit • Monitored unit • Medical services • Surgical services • Consultations by allied health care providers	• Direct • Consultation	• Occupational therapy role for trauma services and ICU may be direct or consultation including positioning, range of motion, splinting/casting, and ADL • Occupational therapy role for monitored, medical, and surgical services may be direct or consultation including safety assessment, assessment of client's abilities, roles, habits, and routines; and functional survival skills such as eating/dysphagia, grooming, dressing, bathing, and toileting • Recommendations for continued services at next level of care • Discharge planning	• Prospective payment system • Private insurance or self-pay • Managed care (PPO or HMO) • Indemnity • Workers' compensation • Medicare • Medicaid • Unfunded
Inpatient rehabilitation	• Transfer from a hospital, nursing home, or home • 60% of clients must have a diagnosis within Centers for Medicare and Medicaid Services (CMS) 13 diagnostic groups.[a] • Must be able to tolerate intensive therapy for a minimum of 3 h of therapy for 5 out of 7 d • Must require active and ongoing intervention of multiple therapies, one of which must be physical therapy or occupational therapy • Must actively participate in and benefit from an intensive therapy program • Patient is stable at time of admission • Requires supervision by a rehabilitation physician, with face-to-face visits at least three times per week • Therapy treatments must begin within 36 h of admission.	• Freestanding rehabilitation center • Unit within hospital • Veteran's Administration rehabilitation unit	• Rehabilitation physician • Rehabilitation nursing • Physical therapy • Occupational therapy • Speech-language pathology • Recreational therapy • Neuropsychology or psychology • Social services • Respiratory therapy • Dietary • Pharmacy • Other services by consultation	• Direct	• Comprehensive evaluation • Participation in functional outcomes such as the Inpatient Rehabilitation Facility-Patient Assessment Instrument (IRF-PAI) • Self-care skills • Functional mobility • Functional communication • Social cognition • IADL • Community reintegration • Discharge planning • Recommendations for continued services at the next level of care	• Prospective payment system • Private insurance or self-pay • Managed care (PPO or HMO) • Indemnity • Workers' compensation • Medicare • Medicaid • Unfunded

(continued)

TABLE 59.1 Practice Settings *(Continued)*

Setting	Requirements for Admission to Setting	Typical Setting	Typical Services	Type of Occupational Therapy	Role of Occupational Therapy Service	Legislation and Funding/Payment
	• Therapy to be provided in 1:1 treatment sessions; group therapies are to be used as an adjunct. • Must include progress toward rehabilitation goals, problems, or barriers to discharge and any changes in rehabilitation goals or treatment plan • Interdisciplinary weekly team conferences directed by the rehabilitation physician					
Skilled nursing/ transitional care	• Require 24-h care for either a short or extended period of time • Bridge the gap with another level of care • Admitted from acute care hospital • Skilled intervention such as intravenous medication, wound care, etc. • Disability with new functional deficit	• Unit in a hospital • Freestanding nursing home	• Physician • Nursing • Social services • Activity therapy • Physical therapy • Occupational therapy • Speech-language pathology • Other services by consultation	• Direct • Consultation	• Short-term care is more intensive with specified frequency • Long-term care is by consultation • Self-care skills such as eating/ dysphagia, grooming, upper and lower body dressing, bathing, and toileting • Mobility skills during ADL such as bed, chair, and wheelchair transfers; toilet and tub/shower transfers; and locomotion activities • IADL and community skills such as car transfers, homemaking activities, public dining, care of pets, etc.	• Prospective payment system • Private insurance or self-pay • Managed care (PPO or HMO) • Indemnity • Workers' compensation • Medicare • Medicaid • Unfunded
Outpatient rehabilitation	• Medical/surgical diagnosis with functional limitation that interferes with abilities to participate in activities and roles • Admitted from a variety of places, including institutional care or home	• Part of a freestanding rehabilitation center • Within a hospital • Within the Veteran's Administration hospital • Satellite clinic (affiliated with a health care institution) • Independent, privately owned clinic	• Physician referral • Self-referral for self-pay services	• Direct	• Self-care skills such as eating/ dysphagia, grooming, upper and lower body dressing, bathing, and toileting • Mobility skills during ADL such as bed, chair, and wheelchair transfers; toilet and tub/shower transfers; and locomotion activities • IADL skills • Social participation such as student, worker, and caregiver roles	• Prospective payment system • Private insurance or self-pay • Managed care (PPO or HMO) • Indemnity • Workers' compensation • Medicare • Medicaid • Unfunded

Inpatient psychiatry	• Require 24-h care for either a short or extended period of time • Need for psychiatric diagnosis or intervention • Admitted from the emergency room • Direct admit • Transfer from another facility • Person requires 24-h monitoring for safety • May be court ordered as in the case of forensic cases in which clients require secured (locked) units due to safety risk to self or others	• Freestanding hospital • Private hospital • Unit within hospital • State hospital • Veteran's Administration hospital	• Psychiatry • Psychology • Nursing • Mental health workers • Social services • Occupational therapy • Recreational therapy • Art therapy • Expressive or music therapy • Behavior management • Other services by consultation	• Direct • Consultation	• Assessment of client's abilities, roles, habits, and routines • Safety assessment • Recommendations for continued services at next level of care • Discharge planning • Individual and/or group treatment • Functional skills such as self-care, home, and community function • Reinforce behavioral or therapeutic plan	• Private insurance • Self-pay • Medicare • Medicaid • SSI • Unfunded
Partial hospitalization	• Require episodic focused psychiatric intervention • Transition from inpatient or as an alternative to acute psychiatric hospitalization • Structured program	• Freestanding hospital • Private hospital • Unit within hospital • State hospital • Veteran's Administration hospital	• Psychiatry • Psychology • Nursing • Mental health workers • Social services • Occupational therapy • Recreational therapy	• Direct • Consultation	• Assessment of client's abilities, roles, habits, and routines • Continuity of care for self-management goals with emphasis on productive living for home, community, and work • Individual and/or group treatment • Recommendations for continued services at next level of care	• Private insurance • Self-pay • Medicare • Medicaid • SSI • Unfunded
Long-term care (physical and mental health)	• Require 24-h care for an indefinite period of time • When functional recovery may not be possible • Lack of resources to be safe at home • Transfer from a hospital, nursing home, or home • Bridge gap between inpatient setting and home versus determine need for permanent placement	• Freestanding hospital • Private hospital • State hospital • Veteran's Administration hospital • Freestanding nursing home • Private nursing home • Custodial care such as eating/dysphagia, grooming, and bathing	• Physician/psychiatrists • Nursing • Mental health workers • Therapy consultation as indicated for safety, assessment, self-care skills and routines, positioning, functional mobility during ADL, adaptations, and caregiver training	• Direct • Consultation	• Individual assessment and interventions as indicated • Consultant to program for ADL, environmental adaptations, and behavior management	• Medicare Part B • Medicaid • Private insurance or self-pay supplement

(continued)

TABLE 59.1 Practice Settings *(Continued)*

Setting	Requirements for Admission to Setting	Typical Setting	Typical Services	Type of Occupational Therapy	Role of Occupational Therapy Service	Legislation and Funding/Payment
Hospice	• Eligible for Medicare Part A • Physician and hospice medical director certify terminal illness, and the patient has 6 m or less to live if illness runs normal course • Sign statement choosing hospice care instead of other Medicare-covered benefits to treatment of terminal illness • Care from Medicare-approved hospice program	• Short-term inpatient care • Short-term respite care • Home	• Physician • Nursing • Counselors • Social services • Occupational therapy • Physical therapy • Speech-language pathology • Hospice aides • Homemakers • Volunteers • Dietician • Grief and loss counseling	• Direct • Consultation	• Assessment (living skills, work, leisure) • Home visits, environmental changes • Provision of aids and adaptations • Training in the use of equipment • Work simplification • Energy conservation, time management • Group activities • Group therapy (touch, role-play, psychodrama) • Education in coping with change (patient and family) • Relaxation and stress management • Therapeutic activities (arts, crafts, poetry, music) • Reminiscence therapy	• Medicare
Early intervention	• Developmental delay in one or more area of development or has diagnosis likely to result in developmental delay • Identified disability or condition or be at risk for developing a disability • Demonstrate atypical behaviors • Circumstances that place child and/or parent that places the child at risk for developmental delay • Each state has its own specific eligibility criteria	• Home • Hospital • Clinic • Child care	• Physician • Occupational therapy • Focus on family-centered model for service delivery	• Direct • Consultation	• Services to promote development • Promotion of parent–child interaction, ADL especially feeding, and play skills • Sensorimotor development • Gross motor skills • Fine motor skills • Self-help skills • Social-emotional development	• Individuals with Disabilities Education Act (IDEA) • Private insurance • Medicaid
Preschool	• Children who are 3 y and older (until enter elementary school) • Fit one of the categories under IDEA	• Public school setting • Childcare • Preschool setting	• Occupational therapy • Preschool teacher	• Direct • Consultation	• Carrying out or suggesting activities that promote the child's overall development and ability to fully participate in preschool activities • Sensorimotor development • Gross motor skills • Fine motor skills • Social-emotional development	• IDEA • Private insurance • Medicaid

School	• Identified disability that fits one of the categories under IDEA • All eligibility and service decision is made by a student's individual educational program.	• Public school • Private school	• Occupational therapy • School teacher	• Direct • Consultation • Supportive service	• Supports student's education program and ability to fully participate in school activities including recess • Organizing the student's daily schedule and materials • Negotiating cafeteria • At the point of planning for transition out of the school system, focus broadens to include independent living and community participation	• IDEA • Private insurance • Medicaid • No Child Left Behind legislation
Private practice	• Children of all ages • Decreased performance in daily tasks or desired activities	• Private clinic	• Occupational therapy	• Direct • Consultation	• Addressing the child's needs that may not be met at school • Focus on body functions such as sensory processing, motor planning, and visual perception that provide foundation skills needed in school, ADL, and play	• Private insurance • Medicaid • Federal grants • Private pay
Adult day services (social, medical, dementia)	• Provide social/medical programming to increase the quality of life and health status of participants • Social: day programs to provide social/recreational activities, meals, and some health supports • Medical: provides rehabilitation and medical services to provide sufficient supports to forestall nursing home placement • Dementia: programs designed to focus on providing programming with cognitive supports that improve the quality of life	• Freestanding • Associated with other community programs or health agencies such as senior centers, mental health centers, rehabilitation centers, nursing homes, or hospitals	• Personnel from adult day services • Occupational therapy • Physical therapy • Speech-language pathology	• Direct • Consultation	• Assistance with modifying and adapting activity programming for social, medical, and dementia programs • Assessment of ADL, IADL, safety, cognition, etc. • Educational services to staff and family members regarding ADL, IADL, safety, fall prevention, etc.	• Federal, state, county, city, or town budgets • Funded through churches or other charitable organizations • Medicaid • Long-term care policies • Scholarships • Sliding fees
Assisted living	• Residential care for elders who can no longer live independently but do not require medical services of a nursing home • Provides supportive care that enhances autonomy and choice • Provides supervision and support for ADL, IADL, safety, etc. caused by dementia, neurological impairment, or other medical problems • Provides activity programming to foster social engagement and participation	• Assisted living facilities	• Personnel from assisted living • Occupational therapy • Physical therapy • Speech-language pathology	• Direct • Consultation	• Consultation to ensure that program engages residents in occupations of their choice and assist facility personnel to modify the physical/social environment to promote safety and independence • Direct services including evaluation and intervention to increase independence in ADL and IADL, prevent falls, and enhance participation in social activities • Education or direct service regarding issues related to aging, occupation, and health promotion	• Private pay • Medicare and Medicaid for people with dementia • Long-term insurance

(continued)

TABLE 59.1 Practice Settings *(Continued)*

Setting	Requirements for Admission to Setting	Typical Setting	Typical Services	Type of Occupational Therapy	Role of Occupational Therapy Service	Legislation and Funding/Payment
Community mental health programs	• Provide ongoing support and structure to people who have mental health diagnoses to live in the community by promoting daily routine and sense of belonging to the program community and community at large • Participants may come and go based on program interests.	• Freestanding • Community health facility	• Personnel from community mental health programs • Occupational therapy • Social services • Recreational therapists • Art therapists • Dance movement therapists	• Direct • Consultation	• Establish or restore performance skills or work, self-care, and leisure including coping strategies, interpersonal skills, time management, and decision making • Strategies to support participants' behavior and ability to cope with challenges in social environments and adapt tasks for participant success	• State money • Medicaid
Group homes	• Adults with chronic mental or medical illness, cognitive dysfunction, or developmental disabilities who require 24-h residential care • Foster development of social networks	• Residential facilities designed to create support, structure, and stability in a homelike setting	• Personnel from group home • Occupational therapy	• Direct • Consultation	• Behavioral management techniques • Development of social and recreational programs in the home • Facilitate independence in ADL and IADL by establishing performance patterns or modifying environment or activity demands • Evaluation to identify skills and develop behavioral plans and involvement in social, recreational, and work-related injuries	• State money • Medicaid
Sheltered workshops and vocational training	• Provide support to workers as they perform work tasks such as parts assembly, packing, sorting, etc. Workers paid at percent of work output based on their performance in relation to typical work performance • Provide social opportunities for workers during the day and after work hours. • Goal setting and supports for transition to supported or independent employment in the community	• Freestanding facility	• Personnel from sheltered workshops and vocational training • Occupational therapy	• Direct • Consultation	• Evaluate workers' performance skills to match the activity demands of various possible jobs • Consultants to others to modify the work environment or activity demands for more efficient performance • Establish performance patterns and new performance skills • Maintain performance skills that workers have acquired	• Revenue from contracting company for which being done • State funding • Grants from nonprofit agencies

Supported employment	• Provide supported employment for people with severe chronic mental illness, mental retardation, learning disabilities, traumatic brain injury, and other severe disabilities who desire to work but have disabilities sufficient to preclude employment in traditional settings without ongoing support to perform job	• Work environments in the community	• Personnel from supported employment • Occupational therapy	• Direct • Consultation	• Consultation with worksites to ensure integration of the employee and to provide education regarding adaptation to worksite environment and activity demands • Direct services in the role of job coach to assist the employee to adapt to the worksite and to function effectively by learning job skills and interacting appropriately with other employees at worksite • Involved in matching prospective worker to potential worksites	• Vocational rehabilitation through state funding • Vocational rehabilitation through private funding
Work-related programs	• Serve people with acquired disability who require rehabilitation to return to workforce either on job or new one	• Freestanding • Part of other facilities such as hospital, rehabilitation center, or community program	• Employment specialists • Occupational therapy • Physical therapy • Certified vocational evaluation	• Direct • Consultation	• Provide rehabilitation services to enable the client to return to work • Evaluation of work tolerance • Development of work-related skills primarily using purposeful activities such as work simulation and preparatory methods such as work conditioning, work hardening, and exercise programs • Modification of job demands when necessary and possible to better match the current skills	• Vocational rehabilitation • Workers' compensation • Income from litigation • Private insurance

[a]These include (1) stroke; (2) spinal cord injury; (3) congenital deformity; (4) amputation; (5) major multiple trauma; (6) fracture of femur; (7) brain injury; (8) neurological disorders; (9) burns; (10) active polyarticular rheumatoid arthritis, psoriatic arthritis, and seronegative arthropathies; (11) systematic vasculitides with joint inflammation; (12) severe or advanced osteoarthritis; and (13) knee or hip replacement if one of the following conditions are met: (*a*) Patient underwent bilateral knee or bilateral hip joint replacement surgery immediately preceding the IRF admission, (*b*) patient is extremely obese with a body mass index of at least 50 at the time of admission to the IRF, and (*c*) patient is age 85 years or older at the time of the admission to the IRF.

ADL, activities of daily living; HMO, health maintenance organization; IADL, instrumental activities of daily living; ICU, intensive care unit; IRF, inpatient rehabilitation facility; PPO, preferred provider organization; SSI, supplemental security income.

Data from Medicare Benefit Policy Manual. (n.d.). Inpatient hospital stays for rehabilitation care, Chapter 1, Section 110.1 -110.5. Retrieved from http://www.cms.hhs/gov/manuals/downloads/bp102c13.pdf; Medicare Hospice Benefits. (n.d.). Retrieved from http://www.medicare.gov/Publications/Pubs/pdf/02154.pdf; Minimum Data Set. (n.d.). Retrieved from http://www.cms.gov/NursingHomeQualityInits/45_NHQIMDS30TrainingMaterials.asp#TopOfPage

References

American Hospital Association. (2011a). *AHA fast facts on US hospitals*. Retrieved from http://www.aha.org/aha/resource-center/Statistics-and-Studies/fast-facts.html

American Hospital Association. (2011b). *Reports and studies*. Retrieved from http://www.aha.org/research/rc/stat-studies/Studies.shtml

American Occupational Therapy Association. (2008). Occupational therapy practice framework: Domain and process, 2nd edition. *American Journal of Occupational Therapy, 62*, 625–683.

American Occupational Therapy Association. (2010). *Occupational therapy compensation and workforce study*. Retrieved from http://www.nxtbook.com/nxtbooks/aota/2010salarysurvey/index.php#/0

Ellis, A. (1992). Group rational-emotive and cognitive-behavioral therapy. *International Journal of Group Psychotherapy, 42*, 63–80.

Hamilton, B. B., Granger, C. V., Sherwin, F. S., Zielezny, M., & Tashman, J. S. (1987). A uniform national data system for medical rehabilitation. In M. J. Fuhrer (Ed.), *Rehabilitation outcomes: Analysis and measurement* (pp. 137–147). Baltimore, MD: Paul H. Brookes.

Holmes, W. M., & Scaffa, M. E. (2009). The nature of emerging practice in occupational therapy: A pilot study. *Occupational Therapy in Health Care, 23*, 189–206.

Law, M., Baptiste, S., Carswell, A., McColl, M., Polatajko, H., & Pollock, N. (2005). *The Canadian Occupational Performance Measure*, (4th ed.). Ottawa, Canada: CAOT Publications ACE.

Medicare Benefit Policy Manual. (n.d.). Inpatient hospital stays for rehabilitation care, Chapter 1, Section 110.1–110.5. Retrieved from http://www.cms.hhs/gov/manuals/downloads/bp102c13.pdf

Medicare Hospice Benefits. (n.d.). Retrieved from http://www.medicare.gov/Publications/Pubs/pdf/02154.pdf

Minimum Data Set. (n.d.). Retrieved from http://www.cms.gov/NursingHomeQualityInits/45_NHQIMDS30TrainingMaterials.asp#TopOfPage

Roberts, P., & Evenson, M. E. (2009). Occupational therapy resource summaries: Practice settings. In E. B. Crepeau, E. S. Cohn, & B. A. B. Schell (Eds.), *Willard and Spackman's occupational therapy* (11th ed., pp. 1070–1083). Philadelphia, PA: Lippincott Williams & Wilkins.

World Health Organization. (2001). *International classification of functioning, disability, and health (ICF)*. Geneva, Switzerland: Author.

For additional resources on the subjects discussed in this chapter, visit http://thePoint.lww.com/Willard-Spackman12e.

CHAPTER 60

Occupational Therapy in a Comprehensive Intervention Program for Individuals with Autism Spectrum Disorder

Early Intervention to Supported Employment

Scott D. Tomchek

LEARNING OBJECTIVES

After reading this chapter, you will be able to:

1. Identify the role of occupational therapy related to those living with an autism spectrum disorder (ASD) and their families
2. Understand the components of a comprehensive intervention program for individuals with an ASD across the life course and common roles of occupational therapy in that program
3. Have an understanding of the components of occupational therapy evaluation and intervention for this population

OUTLINE

Introduction

Autism is a neurodevelopmental disorder with onset prior to age 3 years characterized by qualitative impairments in social interactions and communication skills along with a restricted repetitive and stereotyped pattern of behavior, interests, and activities. It is identified in the *Diagnostic and Statistical Manual of Mental Disorders* (4th ed., text rev.; *DSM-IV-TR*) (American Psychiatric Association, 2001) as one of the five pervasive developmental disorders: autism, pervasive developmental disorder not otherwise specified (PDD-NOS), Asperger syndrome, childhood disintegrative disorder, and Rett syndrome (refer to Table 60.1 for a summary of autism symptoms across the life course and corresponding occupational therapy service continuum).

See **Appendix I, Common Conditions, Resources, and Evidence**, for details related to the presentation of autism.

This chapter will outline a comprehensive intervention program for an individual with autism using a case study approach. Although a team approach is highlighted, the occupational therapy intervention will serve

TABLE 60.1 Autism Spectrum Disorder Symptoms and Service Continuum across the Life Course

Age	Social	Communication	Behavior	Service Continuum	Roles and Goal Areas	Funding Options
Toddler/ preschool	• Lack of use of eye contact; looks through people • Decreased awareness of others • Lack of joint attention or shared enjoyment • Unable to read facial expressions and not sensitive to the feelings of others • Limited initiation and interaction with others • Poor imitation • Lack of imaginative and pretend play	• Delayed verbal language • Impaired nonverbal communication (eye gaze, pointing, gestures) • Communicative attempts limited to protesting and requesting only • Echolalic speech • Regression in language • Nonresponsive to language	• Repetitive interests (lines up toys, watches only certain part of movies, stuck on one show or one character from a show) • Difficulty with transitioning between tasks or activities • Motor stereotypes (hand or finger mannerisms, toe walking) • Unusual responsiveness to sensory input	Diagnostic center	• Function on a multidisciplinary or interdisciplinary team • Assist in differential diagnosis of an ASD or other developmental condition • Provide recommendations for appropriate intervention services	• Private insurance • Medicaid programs • IDEA Part C (EI)/ B(School)
				Early intervention program	• Service as primary service provider on or consultant to an IFSP team • Collaborate with the family and others in the client's natural environment(s) to facilitate IFSP goals	• IDEA Part C • Medicaid matching funds
				Preschool program	• Provide direct services to the child or consult with preschool staff • Facilitate relevant IEP outcomes • Address motor, social, behavioral, and/or sensory processing impairments causing functional limitations in pre-academic and ADL occupations	• IDEA Part B
				Private clinic/ practice	• Function independently or in co-treatment (e.g., speech therapist or psychologist) • Address motor, social, behavioral, and/or sensory processing impairments causing functional limitations in play, academic and ADL occupations	• Medicaid programs • Private insurance • Self-pay/fee-for-service
School	• Difficulty relating to both adults and peers • Inability to engage in cooperative play with peers • Unable to understand or follow rules of a classroom • Decreased awareness of social norms during interaction (e.g., touch, eye gaze/contact, personal space)	• Abnormal prosody of speech • Persistent echolalia • Developed verbal language, although limited use for social purposes • Errors with pronoun use	• Routine-based behavior; insistence on sameness • Difficulty with cognitive flexibility and generalization of skills across environments • Failure to see the gestalt (i.e., hyper-focus on one detail)	School-based related service	• Provide direct services to the child and/ or consult with educational staff • Facilitate relevant IEP outcomes • Address motor, social, behavior regulation, and/or sensory processing impairments causing functional limitations in school and ADL occupations	• IDEA, Part B programs including Response to Intervention • Section 504 Rehabilitation Act
				Private clinic/ practice	• Function independently in co-treatment (e.g., speech therapist or psychologist) or intervention group • Address motor, social, behavioral and/or sensory processing impairments causing functional limitations in play, school, ADL, or IADL occupations	• Medicaid programs • Private insurance • Self-pay/fee-for-service

Adolescence into adulthood	• Poor social judgment • Anxious in social situations • Continued lack of awareness of social norms during interaction • Inability to learn group rules • Difficulty with establishing and maintaining peer relationships, although greater ease with adults	• Prosody abnormalities persist • Pragmatic (social use) language deficits • Concrete interpretation of language and a lack of understanding of sarcasm or metaphors • Inability to coordinate nonverbal (e.g., eye contact, body proximity) with language	• Deficits with executive functions leading to decreased simultaneous processing • Some have a refinement of their special interest and develop a more discrete special interest • Routine-based behavior; insistence on sameness	School-based related service	• Provide direct services to the child and/or consult with educational staff • Facilitate relevant IEP outcomes • Address motor, social, behavior regulation, and/or sensory processing impairments causing functional limitations in school and ADL occupations	• IDEA, Part B programs including Response to Intervention • Section 504 Rehabilitation Act
				Driving rehab	• Function independently or on a team within a driving program • Evaluate physical, visual, and behavioral/mental abilities required for safe driving • Develop and implement intervention programs to allow for safe driving • Recommend, obtain and train in use of adaptive equipment to facilitate safe driving	• Private insurance • Self-pay/fee-for-service
				Transitional services	• Participate on Transitional Planning Team to support positive transitions and facilitate functional independence and community integration (e.g., employment, independent living, further education, adult services) • Assess physical, cognitive, communication, social, emotional, and behavioral skills necessary for planned transitions; identify resources as part of this process • Develop and implement intervention programs that promote self-advocacy and address areas impacting participation in planned transition contexts	• IDEA, Part B programs including Response to Intervention • Section 504 Rehabilitation Act • Community-based work transition programs • Supports for community living and other waiver programs • Department of Education RSA programs • State vocational rehabilitation programs

(continued)

TABLE 60.1 Autism Spectrum Disorder Symptoms and Service Continuum across the Life Course *(Continued)*

Age	Social	Communication	Behavior	Service Continuum	Roles and Goal Areas	Funding Options
				(Supported) Employment	• Function independently with a client or employer, consult as part of a vocational rehabilitation program • Assess physical, cognitive, communication, social, emotional, and behavioral skills necessary for engagement in work-related occupations; may include review of vocational interests and aptitudes • Conduct job analysis to include contextual factors supporting employment • Provide intervention services to increase the ability of the client to participate in and manage productive work, adhere to safe work practices and prevent work-related injuries	• Medicaid • Home and community-based services programs • Supports for community living and other waiver programs • Department of Education RSA programs
				Group home	• Provide direct intervention or consult with residential staff for functional limitations in ADL, IADL, and/or vocational occupations	• Medicaid programs • Private insurance • Self-pay/fee-for-service
				Post–secondary education	• Provide direct intervention or consult with a client to support social and community participation, daily living skill independence, or work occupations	• Supports for Community Living and other Waiver Programs • Department of Education RSA Programs • State Vocational Rehabilitation Programs
				Adult care	• Provide direct intervention or consult with residential staff for functional limitations in ADL, IADL, vocational and/or leisure occupations	• Medicaid programs • Private insurance • Self-pay/fee-for-service

ADL, activities of daily living; EI, early intervention; IADL, instrumental activities of daily living; IDEA, Individuals with Disabilities Education Act; IEP, individualized education programs; IFSP, Individual Family Service Plan; RSA, Rehabilitation Service Administration.

BOX 60.1 Therapist Narrative—The Author's Guiding Principles

Constant . . . family. . . context . . . engagement . . . words have multiple meanings. Many of these meanings are very relevant and fundamental to guiding interventions with individuals on the autism spectrum. As you will read summarized in this chapter, there are common themes across evidence-based interventions for individuals with an autism spectrum disorder (ASD). These themes relate to developing interventions that are individualized, structured, and consistent; offered over intense schedules; and that facilitate engagement socially, in activity and occupations. The constant in all of these is the "family." As an interventionist, I am only a small piece of the individual's day, week, month, and year(s). The *family*, used here in a broad sense to represent the client and those in context(s) facilitating engagement in occupations, is present on a consistent basis to address the daily struggles relating to the social communication and behavioral manifestations seen in individuals with an ASD. Therefore, the family is an integral active participant in all aspects of providing services to an individual with an ASD, from the occupational profile, to evaluation, to intervention planning and implementation, to outcome review, and to discharge. They drive the therapeutic train and determine which tracks the train stays on! Concerns, priorities, goals, and dreams of the family guide intervention planning. The context of intervention (i.e., home, school, workplace) often shapes those addressed across the continuum of services, but the family often carries the role of implementing interventions across these contexts to facilitate the intense schedules of intervention that need to be implemented to increase participation.

Also fundamental to all interventions and implementation of interventions is the concept of engagement. The key component to the active engagement construct is the ability to sustain attention to an activity or person (de Kruif & McWillam, 1999; McWilliam & Bailey, 1992). Engagement goes beyond measurement of the amount of time a child spends in an activity to capture important behaviors for learning (de Kruif & McWillam, 1999), such as the child's motivation for mastery and the extent of goal-directed behavior. Active engagement is a stable construct that appears to be related to internal child factors (temperament or diagnosis), observable child behaviors (level of play skill), and environmental factors (type of classroom activity) (de Kruif & McWilliam, 1999; McWilliam & Bailey, 1992; McWilliam, Trivette, & Dunst, 1985). Given the magnitude of core social, communication, and play impairments in ASDs and their impact on participation and engagement, all interventions are developed to facilitate engagement of the individual. This is what makes working with individuals with an ASD so challenging and at the same time rewarding. Finding these motivations that facilitate engagement socially, in occupations and in activity makes each client unique and keeps me fresh. What some see as repetitive behavior, I see as the gift(s) that the client provides. These gifts are often "unwrapped" during the occupational profile and/or assessment and imbedded to a degree throughout intervention to enhance motivation and in turn engagement.

If I have effectively followed my guiding principles of working with families to facilitate engagement in context, the outcomes are naturally reinforcing. The client is more socially interactive and able to meet the demand of his or her daily contexts to participate in occupations. These changes ease the daily routines of my clients, their families, and others in their environments. And where we once had impairments in engagement, we now have yet another gift.

as the primary emphasis of the comprehensive program (see Box 60.1 for the author's narrative).

Comprehensive Intervention Program Components

When the studies on interventions for children with autism are examined together, certain characteristics of interventions are consistently linked to positive outcomes. Critical reviews of intervention programs for individuals with autism spectrum disorder (ASD) have identified central aspects and common themes of comprehensive, effective intervention programs for children with autism (Horner et al., 2002; Mastergeorge, Rogers, Corbett & Solomon, 2003; Myers, & Johnson, 2007; National Research Council, 2001; Reichow & Volkmar, 2010; Simpson, 2005; Tomchek & Case-Smith, 2009). Important principles and themes that emerge from the research evidence include the following:

- Effective intervention programs are developed from individualized analysis that includes functional assessment of the physiological basis for behaviors and the environment's influence on behavior.
- The child's family is central to the intervention program and services should include family support and education.
- Intervention services need to be intensive, structured, and comprehensive while addressing all core features (i.e., functional communication, social skill, cognitive development, and adaptive behavior).
- Facilitating active engagement of the child is the essential priority for all interventions.

These evidence-based themes then guide the development of the individualized intervention plan for the client with an ASD. The case presented here will apply these principles within a comprehensive interdisciplinary program that includes multiple intervention methods across several contexts.

Collaborative Intervention

Given impairments in both communication and sensorimotor development, intervention by both speech-language pathologists and occupational therapists is often warranted. These interventions may be most beneficial if collaborative (Geis & Tomchek, 2000). In joint intervention sessions, the occupational therapy practitioner provides structured activities to foster improved bilateral motor integration, facilitate application of fine motor skills to functional tasks, and promotes appropriate sensory processing and responsivity. Within this array of therapeutic activities, the speech-language pathologist facilitates development of functional communication skills and play interaction. These intervention activities and sessions are grounded in principles of both Floortime (Greenspan & Wieder, 2006) and Social Communication/Emotional Regulation/Transactional Support (SCERTS) (Prizant, Wetherby, Rubin, Laurent & Rydell, 2006) approaches.

It has been predicted that the ability to use both speech and language is dependent on central nervous system (CNS) organization of sensory input (Windeck & Laurel, 1989). Use of visual, tactile, and vestibular input helps the child focus and participate in communication exchanges. Further, motor planning aspects of sensory integration are important for both fluent speech and nonverbal communication functions (e.g., gestures, coordination of eye gaze). Therefore, using principles of sensory integration therapy in collaboration with speech-language therapy promotes full use of gross and fine motor abilities and adds purpose and meaning to movement (see Chapter 56). The principles and strategies to facilitate social communication during collaborative intervention are summarized in Table 60.2 (also see Chapter 58).

TABLE 60.2 Principles and Strategies to Facilitate Social Communication during Collaborative Intervention

Principle	Strategies
Helping the child to understand communication	• In order for the child to understand communication, he or she must understand the cause and effect relationship. • Children with autism are usually better able to process static or repetitive visual information than the ever-changing acoustic signal. Consequently, using visual supports builds on their area of relative strength. Visual supports can be objects, line drawings, or photographs that give the child information about his environment and, in turn, can be used by him or her to give others information.
Giving the child something to talk about	It is no surprise that people are more likely to attend to and to communicate about what interests or affects them. It is no different with the children with whom we work. Therefore, • Incorporate motivating materials and themes into activities to create communication topics. For example, going down the ramp during a scooter board activity becomes riding *Thomas the Tank Engine*. • Also, build language concepts and vocabulary into the activities.
Giving the child a means of communication	Because many children that we see initially have limited or no functional communicative speech or gestures, they are significantly compromised in their ability to communicate appropriately and effectively with others. Therefore, • Provide augmentative or alternative forms of communication to give the child a mechanism to communicate. • One widely used picture communication system is the Picture Exchange Communication System (PECS) (Frost & Bondy, 1994). • In addition to picture communication systems, sign language and use of the written word may also be effective. • The understanding and use of conventional communicative gestures are also taught.
Giving the child a reason to communicate	Expand communicative functions of the child beyond protesting and requesting objects and actions. These functions regulate the behavior of others, as opposed to regulating social interaction (e.g., greeting and calling) or joint attention (e.g., commenting and requesting or providing information). Encourage by the following: • Providing the child with choices. The sensory needs of a child with autism may vary greatly from one moment to the next. Consequently, choices of activities are made available to the child via a picture choice board to address a variety of sensory needs. The choice board provides the structure for the child to initiate desired activities to meet her sensory need. • Violate routines and entice the child to communicate. • Providing opportunities for social interaction. These social interaction and joint attention functions of communication are more challenging. Greeting, calling, requesting social routine, commenting, requesting information, and providing information are examples of these functions.

Behavior Management/Family Counseling Interventions

Multiple interventions are often used to target problem behaviors for children with ASDs. Intensive behavioral, positive behavior supports, and behavior management counseling interventions will be briefly highlighted here.

Intensive Behavioral

Behavioral interventions that use applied behavioral analysis with discrete trial training are often used in intervention programs for children with ASDs. Occupational therapists often provide intervention to children who receive intensive behavioral intervention and consult with the psychologists and behavioral therapists directing the behavioral program. Intensive behavior intervention is often provided in the family home for 30 to 40 hours per week. The discrete trial program is typically implemented by four to six paraprofessionals (often students) who are trained and closely supervised. In some programs, parents and relatives participate in the training. The primary strategy of the program is highly structured, one-on-one, discrete trial training. Developmental appropriate goals are established, and skill components are identified to be taught step by step. The skills are taught by presenting the task, allowing the child to respond to the instruction or to imitate the action, and reinforcing/shaping the child's response. The task and reinforcement are repeated for three to eight trials to ensure that the child has mastered the skill. Skill mastery in discrete trials is defined as 90% accuracy across 2 days of intervention (Cohen, Amerine-Dickens, & Smith, 2006). Developmental skills across all domains are taught, with emphasis on language and cognitive skills but including self-care skills and play competency (Figure 60.1). The phases that follow the home-based, 30 to 40 hours a week program are designed to help the child generalize his or her skills to other contexts. The program systematically decreases the one-on-one treatment to enable the child to practice skills in a more natural environment (e.g., school, community, church). A recent meta-analysis suggested that long-term, discrete trial intervention leads to medium to large positive effects in intellectual functioning, language development, acquisition of activities of daily living skills, and social functioning of children with an ASD (Virues-Ortega, 2010).

Positive Behavioral Support

Positive behavioral support intervention is widely implemented and has a strong base of research supporting its effectiveness (National Research Council, 2001). Because this type of intervention is based on an individual analysis of the child's behavior to determine the underlying causes for the behavior and is implemented in the natural environment, occupational therapists frequently design and use this intervention. The goal of positive behavioral support is to prevent problem behaviors, and its pivotal element is functional assessment. In functional assessment, the team analyzes the underlying cause of the problem behavior in order to determine why it occurred and what is reinforcing the behavior. The activities that occurred prior to the behavior (i.e., antecedents) and the consequences of the behavior are evaluated to determine how these influence the occurrence or nonoccurrence of the behavior. Once the team determines the antecedents to a problem behavior, they design strategies to control it, such as modifying the environment, the child's schedule, or the classroom activities. Similar to occupational therapy approaches, the goal is to design an environment that matches the child's behaviors. When the demands placed on the child are consistent with the child's capabilities, he or she no longer needs to use problem behaviors.

Positive behavioral support is a comprehensive intervention that includes (1) using the functional assessment

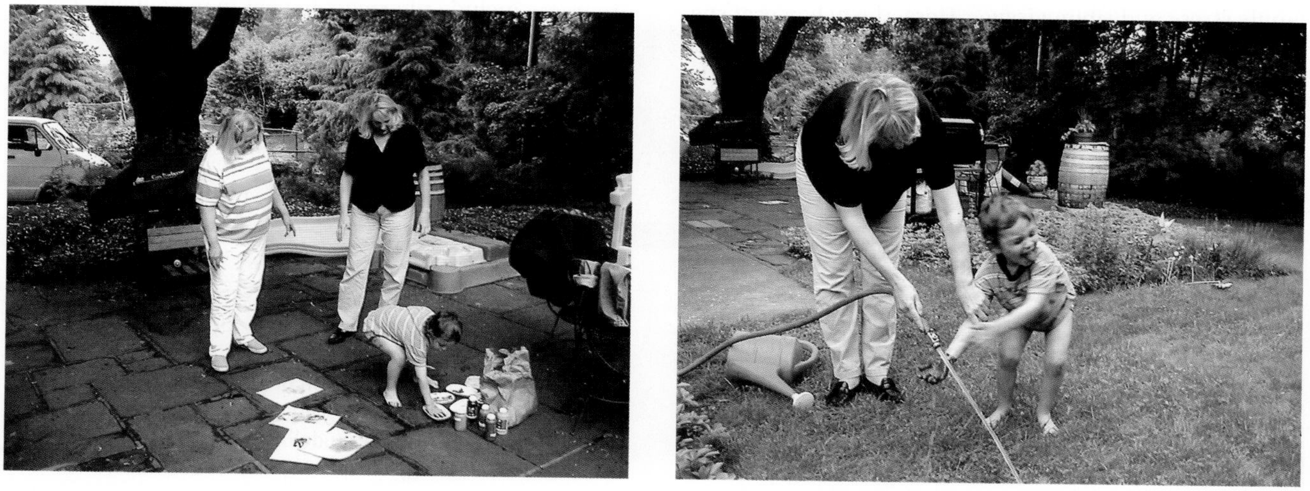

A B

FIGURE 60.1 **A.** Will, a 3-year-old boy with Asperger syndrome, fingerpaints while grandmom and mom supervise. Will's occupational therapist recommended fingerpainting as a good activity for Will to help him with sensory issues and to improve hand function. **B.** Will still needed help cleaning up!

to identify causative factors, (2) incorporating multiple behavioral interventions throughout the day, and (3) consistently applying the procedures developed by the team (Horner et al., 2002). Targeted behaviors include aggression toward others, self-injury, tantrums, and disruptive behaviors. A wide range of behavioral approaches are used, depending on how the child responds and what is most appropriate to the problem and the setting. Horner and colleagues listed five common procedures applied with children with ASDs, all based in behavioral theory: (1) stimulus based (altering the antecedent), (2) instruction based (direct instruction regarding appropriate behavior), (3) extinction based (withholding or minimizing delivery of reinforcers), (4) reinforcement based (rewards to increase behaviors), and (5) punishment based (may be positive or negative, i.e. intervention procedures designed to reduce problem behavior via contingent delivery of aversive stimuli versus contingent removal of positive stimuli). The team decides which of these procedures to use and in which context and activity they should be implemented. These procedures need to be implemented consistently by all adults who interact with the child to be optimally effective.

Behavior Management Counseling

Behavior management counseling focuses on assisting the family with ongoing behavioral issues that may be presenting problems in the home or at school. These sessions provide direction and support to the family by outlining behavior plan(s) to address specific and targeted behavioral issues. This intervention will also likely incorporate some of the previously discussed positive behavior supports to outline expectations, reinforcers, and rewards of the program to assist the child's understanding. For instance, a child is having tantrums when transitioning from the house. The family wishes to target this behavior because they find themselves leaving the home less and less to avoid the tantrums, which is causing significant family stress and sibling issues. Here, the behavioral specialist (e.g., psychologist) may develop a visual schedule to prepare the child to leave the house and transition to the car. Additionally, a reinforcer (e.g., favorite toy) may be incorporated to enhance motivation (Figure 60.2).

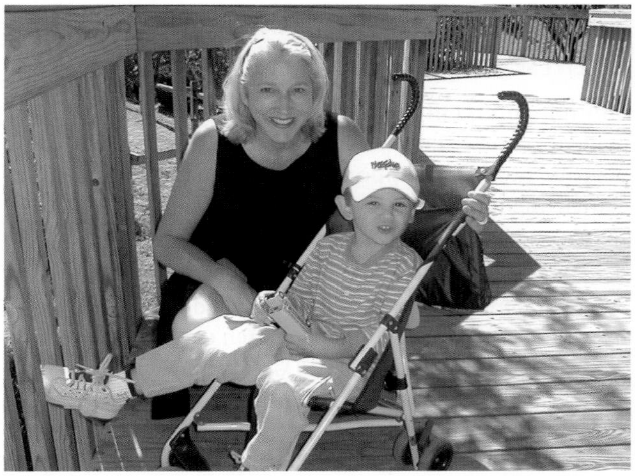

FIGURE 60.2 Will, at age 4 years, carried a favorite toy school bus with him on a trip to the park. Taking a favorite toy along was a motivator for Will.

Educational/Academic Programming

The U.S. Department of Education, Office of Special Education Programs, and National Research Council formed the Committee on Educational Interventions for Children with Autism (National Research Council, 2001) and charged the committee to integrate scientific, theoretical, and policy literature and create a framework for evaluating scientific evidence concerning the features and effects of educational programming for young children with autism. The primary focus of the charge was to define the effective programs for children younger than the age of 8 years with autism (see Chapter 48 for more details).

Pharmacological Management

Another component of many comprehensive intervention programs include pharmacological management. Please refer to a recent review of potential medications that have been found to be effective in addressing the secondary symptoms of ASDs (Canitano & Scandurra, 2011; Huffman, Sutcliffe, Tanner, & Feldman, 2011; Nazeer, 2011).

CASE STUDY 60.1 Cody

Referral

Cody, 2 years and 3 months of age, presented for a comprehensive evaluation at the request of his doctor and the early intervention program. He was having behavioral, social interaction, and communication difficulties at home and at preschool. Additionally, his development was noted to be delayed when compared to his twin sister's.

Diagnostic Evaluation

Individuals referred for evaluation because of suspected autism receive comprehensive interdisciplinary evaluations, a process consistent with best practice guidelines from both the American Academy of Neurology (Filipek et al., 1999) and American Academy of Child and Adolescent Psychiatry (Volkmar, Cook, Pomeroy, Realmuto, & Tanguay, 1999). Clinical specialists in

CASE STUDY 60.1 Cody (*Continued*)

each discipline use test administration procedures, methods, and measurements appropriate to individuals on the autism spectrum; data from the assessment were included in this study. As such, Cody and his parents participated in a comprehensive neurodevelopmental evaluation conducted by a developmental pediatrician, psychologist, speech-language pathologist, and occupational therapist.

Parent Concerns

Of primary concern to Cody's parents was his behavior and suspected developmental delays. His parents noted that his development was quite delayed in comparison to his twin sister's. Cody primarily used proximity to communicate his wants and needs. He often took his mother to what he wanted and waited or he used her hand as a tool and put her hand on the object he wanted. He used few gestures and he had few intelligible words. Socially, he did not interact with his older brother or his twin sister. His parents also described him as "being in his own little world." Difficulty with beginning toilet training was also noted. Behaviorally, concerns related primarily to overactivity and odd behavior. He was noted to have significant difficulty tolerating crowds. He spent much of his time engaged in repetitive behavior (e.g., opening and shutting doors, spinning, rubbing his head in a sandbox, eating dirt, dropping objects on his head). As such, play was also concerning in that Cody did not engage in reciprocal, pretend, or imaginative play.

Developmental Pediatric Evaluation

Birth history was reviewed and revealed that Cody was the 6 lb, 0 oz twin product of a 36-week pregnancy to his then 25-year-old mother. During the neurodevelopmental evaluation, Cody avoided interaction and ignored language directed to him. He spent much of his time climbing on tables, opening drawers and taking things out of them, and dumping boxes of blocks. Toe walking was noted during ambulation.

Psychological Evaluation

Cody was difficult to structure in the testing room, and he was noted to tune out language directed to him. He was in constant motion and perseverated on activities. He cried easily and frequently. Formal testing could not be completed, although development appeared globally delayed. Parent report measures were used to gauge developmental status.

Speech-Language Evaluation

From a communication standpoint, both receptive and expressive language delays were noted. Cody communicated primarily to request and protest and did so with primitive forms of nonverbal communication (e.g., tantrum, directing through the use of another's body, and limited eye gaze). He had a limited speech sound repertoire and few intelligible words.

Occupational Therapy Evaluation

At the time of the evaluation, Cody was noted to be active and unfocused. He presented with significant sensory modulation difficulties. In general, Cody was noted to be hyporesponsive to incoming sensory input, although he had paradoxical responses to tactile input. He frequently sought supplemental vestibular input in an attempt to self-regulate, spinning himself repeatedly for up to 10 minutes. He was also observed to frequently circle run (run in a tight circle). He also sought out tactile input, especially deep proprioceptive input to his head. He was observed to drop objects on his head (dump baskets of toys on his head, mouth/bite objects, rub sand in his hair, rub his head on the carpet, etc.). At the same time, he was reported to be hyperresponsive during grooming and hygiene tasks and to sticky substances that he came in contact with, especially on his hands. By report of his parents, Cody spent much of his day seeking proprioceptive and tactile sensory input, and, therefore, he rarely interacted purposefully with objects and had limited functional toy play. Given these deficits in play, Cody's fine motor skill development was delayed.

From this comprehensive evaluation, the skill levels and diagnoses shown in Table 60.3 were discussed with Cody's family.

Recommendations

At the conclusion of the diagnostic evaluation, the following recommendations were made:

1. To explore potential etiologies of Cody's delays, a complete neurobiologic work-up was recommended.
2. Given Cody's developmental presentation, a comprehensive intervention program was recommended. Active therapeutic intervention by speech pathology was recommended to address noted play and social communication deficits. Occupational therapy was recommended to address sensorimotor impairments. Additionally, behavior management/family counseling was recommended to assist the family with the many behavioral challenges they described in the home that were impacting the family. A component of the behavior management counseling would also likely include a sibling group for Cody's older brother and twin sister. Throughout these interventions, Cody's activity level and impulsivity would continue to be monitored by the developmental pediatrician to assess the need for psychopharmacological intervention.

(continued)

CASE STUDY 60.1 Cody (*Continued*)

TABLE 60.3 Initial Evaluation Diagnostic Impressions

Cody's Age: 2 y, 9 mo (33 mo)				
Speech-language evaluation	**Rossetti Infant Toddler Scale**	**Age Equivalent**		
	Receptive language	8–10 mo		
	Expressive language	8–10 mo		
Occupational therapy evaluation	**Peabody Developmental Motor Scales (Second Edition)**	**Scaled Score**	**Rank**	**Age Equivalent**
	Stationary	7	16	24 mo
	Locomotion	8	25	28 mo
	Object manipulation	7	16	23 mo
	Gross motor quotient	83	13	
	Grasping	3	1	11 mo
	Visual-motor integration	2	<1	10 mo
	Fine motor quotient	55	<1	
	Sensory regulatory difficulties			
Psychological evaluation	**Developmental Profile 3**	**Standard Score**		**Age Equivalent**
	Physical	61		16 mo
	Adaptive	50		12 mo
	Social-emotional	<50		10 mo
	Cognitive	<50		12 mo
	Communication	<50		10 mo
Developmental pediatric evaluation	Central nervous system dysfunction as manifested by muscular hypotonia and tremors			
Diagnoses (*ICD-9*):	Autistic disorder (299.00) Central nervous system dysfunction (349.9) Communication disorder (315.32) Muscular incoordination (781.3)			

Comprehensive Intervention Program Implementation

Functional Analysis, Strategies, and Reinforcer Assessment

The comprehensive program was initiated with studying Cody's behavior regulation further. Functional analysis of behavior was conducted across home, clinic, and preschool contexts. Of primary concern to the family and interventionists was Cody's activity level, his apparent seeking of sensory input (e.g., running, unusual visual inspection of objects, head banging, dropping of objects on his head), and the impact of these on his ability to sustain engagement with people and occupations. Data was collected over a 2-week period to allow for antecedent, consequence, communicative intent, and ecological analysis of the problem behaviors. The role of ensuring data was collected across environments and was assumed by the family. Analysis of the data revealed that across contexts, behavior regulation challenges were noted at times of transition between activities and likely related to his communication impairments and lack of understanding of routine. Additionally, it was noted that during periods of less activity, Cody tended to engage in activities that provided supplemental sensory input.

With a better understanding of the functions of Cody's behaviors, strategies were discussed to intervene. Positive behavior supports (e.g., visual schedules, task analysis visuals, activity progression indicators) for each context were discussed and developed to ensure consistency in implementation. Additionally, Cody needed a means to communicate; and given his strong visual skills, the Picture Exchange Communication System (PECS) (Frost & Bondy, 1994) was to be implemented.

Observations of play during the diagnostic assessment only provided a small picture of the qualitative aspects of play. Given the significant impact appropriate structuring of play can have on the overall success of the process, information about Cody's motivations needed to be gathered. A reinforcer assessment was used to define the activities Cody engaged in most often, along with his food, toy, video, and television preferences. Additionally, report of non-preferred activities, tasks, and items was gathered. This information was collected formally as a checklist and supplemented with insights from the interview during the occupational profile. Findings revealed that Cody preferred activities that incorporated movement. He disliked seated activities and often tantrummed when asked to sit still for prolonged periods (i.e., mealtimes, at church, small group activities). Increased engagement was noted when playing "chase" or when movement was allowed during an activity. He often stood, bounced in place, or spun in place while watching television. His favorite shows were *Thomas the Train* and *Speed Racer* and often chose clothing, mealtime materials, and toys related to these shows. Information gleaned from the reinforcer assessment was used to structure and adapt activities to facilitate increased engagement and participation from Cody.

Collaborative Intervention

Because many of Cody's social interaction and behavioral difficulties were felt to stem from noted impairments in communication and behavior regulation, it was thought that he would benefit from joint therapy with an occupational therapist and a speech-language pathologist. The primary emphasis of the occupational therapist was to develop structured activities to foster improved bilateral motor integration, facilitate application of fine motor skills to functional tasks, and facilitate enhanced sensory processing/responding. Recognizing Cody's seeking of supplemental vestibular and proprioceptive input, activities were built around these sensory characteristics (e.g., swing, scooter board, resistive activities). Within this array of activities, the speech-language pathologist facilitated development of functional communication skills and play interaction.

Initially, Cody was taught to use the PECS (Frost & Bondy, 1994) for requesting desired objects. The use of PECS was generalized across activities and used with a variety of toys to promote appropriate interaction and requesting. He quickly progressed to a point in which he was able to discriminate between pictures and exchange for desired objects. This awareness and inclusion of the object or task on a sentence strip was motivating to Cody, and through the use of a communication book, provided him the opportunity to communicate many of his wants and needs.

In addition to his PECS book, other visual supports (Bryan & Gast, 2000; Dettmer, Simpson, Myles, & Ganz, 2000; Massey & Wheeler, 2000) were used within an overall positive behavior support program (Horner et al., 2002) to provide Cody choices, direct his actions, and assist with transitions. An activity choice board was used to provide Cody with a selection of activities from which to choose during an intervention session. Prior to the session, therapists selected Polaroid pictures of activities to address specific sensorimotor skills (e.g., visual motor task, climbing, rolling in mat, and riding toys) that were components of the overall intervention program, goal areas, and naturally reinforcing to Cody.

Activity regulation boards and other visual supports were used to guide Cody and allow for choices within the chosen activity. The activity regulation board can serve to direct the child's actions or the child can use the board to direct the actions of others. For instance, when Cody was participating in a swing activity, the activity regulation board allowed him to select being spun or swung back and forth, continue the activity, or terminate the activity. Using this method also allowed Cody to direct the activity and facilitated development of vital self-regulation abilities. Within this activity, another activity board was used between periods of swinging to have Cody select individual pieces of a puzzle (e.g., one animal piece of a multipiece animal puzzle). This puzzle was also used as a visual support to show Cody how many times he would be performing the activity and to signal termination of the activity (i.e., when the puzzle is complete, the activity is finished).

In addition to the joint therapy, the occupational therapist also consulted with the family to improve tolerance for daily living activities. Here again, multiple methods were used. Social stories (Gray, 2000) were used prior to the tasks to outline expectations of a task. Visual and other positive behavioral supports were used to structure the tasks. Additionally, sensory-based calming strategies (i.e., proprioceptive deep pressure or movement) were used prior to, during, and following the activity if needed to support participation.

Pharmacology

Although making nice progress with respect to communication and sensorimotor aspects in the first 6 months of intervention, Cody continued to demonstrate significant impulsivity and a high activity level. Although he was responding nicely to collaborative and behavioral interventions, his activity level and inattention were felt to be interfering with making even more substantial gains. Therefore, a trial of Ritalin (stimulant) was also employed. Following dosage adjustments over a month period, Cody responded well to the drug and demonstrated prolonged period of attending without compromising social and play benefits seen following interventions. A significant improvement with behavior regulation was also noted with Cody requiring less sensory input to regulate his behavior.

Behavioral Intervention

In addition to the collaborative intervention, Cody participated in a brief 6-month period of intense discrete trial training. The goal of this intervention was to build an understanding of foundational responding, attending, and work-reward principles that could be readily applied to all other interventions and the teaching discrete skills. Cody participated in this intervention program in his home for 18 hours a week (6 days a week, 3 hours each day). Following initiation, ongoing team conferencing allowed the discrete trial interventionists to imbed positive behavior support and communication strategies into the program to facilitate generalization of concepts across intervention programs. The combination of interventions and level of intensity at the onset following diagnosis yielded rapid improvements in social communication awareness and responding, as well as an understanding of routines. Shaping techniques continued to be used to build appropriate responses to visual and verbal directives within task performance.

Initial behavioral difficulties in the home and community were also addressed through ongoing behavior management counseling with the family. Given his communication impairments, his parents had difficulty with structuring and setting clear expectations for Cody's behavior. For instance, Cody expressed significant anxiety to order. When his mother would clean and organize the house, Cody would immediately scatter toys and things around the house. The behavior program in this instance focused on providing visual supports to show Cody that it was acceptable to "organize" his own room how he wanted but not other areas of the house. If this expectation was violated, the behavior program outlined responses by the parents to foster consistency.

Reevaluation

After 18 months of involvement in the intensive intervention program, Cody's skills were formally reevaluated. The results of this evaluation at 4 years, 3 months of age demonstrated that his skill levels had improved both in the rate of development and overall. During that 18-month period, all aspects of development improved and he was developing social communication skills and using these skills across contexts. Table 60.4 displays the results of the reevaluation.

Program Continuation

Following this reevaluation, goals were reestablished to address deficit areas while using strength areas to accomplish the goals. Generally, communication goals continued to focus on increasing the sophistication of communicative means and purposes for communication. Sensorimotor goals focused more on teaching Cody self-regulation to enhance behavior regulation abilities while continuing to improve the functional application of his fine and visual motor skills during occupational

TABLE 60.4 Comprehensive Reevaluation after 18 Months of Intensive Intervention

Cody's Age: 4 yr, 3 mo (51 mo)				
Speech-language evaluation	**Preschool Language Scale-3**	**Age Equivalent**		
	Receptive language	33 mo		
	Expressive language	29 mo		
Occupational therapy evaluation	**Peabody Developmental Motor Scales (Second Edition)**	**Scaled Score**	**Rank**	**Age Equivalent**
	Grasping	5	5	37 mo
	Visual-motor integration	6	9	37 mo
	Fine motor quotient	73	3	
	Sensory regulatory difficulties			
Psychological evaluation	**Developmental Profile 3**	**Standard Score**		**Age Equivalent**
	Physical	90		42 mo
	Adaptive	85		40 mo
	Social-emotional	76		35 mo
	Cognitive	79		39 mo
	Communication	78		37 mo
	Leiter International Performance Scale-Revised	**Scaled Score (X = 10)**		
	Figure ground	6		
	Form completion	15		
	Matching	12		
	Classification	10		
	Developmental Test of Visual-Motor Integration	33 mo Standard score = 67 (X = 100)		
Developmental pediatric evaluation	Central nervous system dysfunction as manifested by muscular hypotonia			
Diagnoses (*ICD-9*):	Autistic disorder (299.00) Central nervous system dysfunction (349.9) Communication disorder (315.32) Muscular incoordination (781.3) Above average nonverbal intelligence			

performance. He continued to benefit from Ritalin. Discrete trial training was discontinued; and behavior management counseling was rarely needed to directly address behavioral concerns in that with the noted social communication and sensorimotor improvements, fewer behavioral concerns were noted.

Clinic-based collaborative intervention continued to supplement educational programming, although it was modified to create individual 30-minute periods around the 30-minute collaborative component. From an occupational therapy standpoint, intervention focused on improving performance skills and patterns that were limiting participation in self-help, play, and education occupations.

Cody accessed preschool services through the local public school district. Consultation between the clinic-based providers and the classroom teacher, instructional assistant, related service providers, and the district's autism specialist allowed for consistent applications of strategies that had been consistently implemented in the clinic and home to be generalized to the academic setting. Here, positive behavior supports and behavior regulation strategies became critical in facilitating the flow of the daily schedule and related transitions between activities. Activity progression indicators and structured teaching principles were incorporated into activities to maximize participation.

Cody continued to progress in the respective interventions during this period of time. Cody demonstrated at age level fine and visual motor performance on standardized measures when last evaluated. At that time, he was also noted to be independently accomplishing relevant activities of daily living. As a result, he was discharged from individual clinic-based occupational therapy intervention, although occupational therapy consultation at school continued to facilitate further development of written expression.

More details about Cody's progress and reevaluations are available at **http://thePoint.lww.com/Willard-Spackman12e**.

Pragmatic aspects of language were addressed with individual speech-language intervention as well as through a social skill group that included typical peers. The social skill group was a 12-week group facilitated by the speech pathologist and occupational therapist and created somewhat natural, age-appropriate social experiences for the individuals in the group (e.g., board games, Wii, card games) to allow for training of social responding in context (see Box 60.2 for a summary of Cody's occupational therapy beyond the services described in this case).

BOX 60.2 Case Life Course Perspective

Although Cody's case only followed him through school-age, as Table 60.1 demonstrates, occupational therapists work with this population throughout the life course in a myriad of settings. To highlight this aspect of the occupational therapy domain and process, the following section is a brief outline of occupational therapy supports Cody accessed given his developmental presentations. These services were provided for transition to post–secondary education and supported employment following completion of his degree. For additional aspects of the service continuum for individuals with an autism spectrum disorder (ASD) who may have greater limitations in participation, the reader is again referred to Table 60.1.

Transition and Driving

Transition planning began formally at age 15 years as a sophomore in high school. Given the fact that Cody was a good student with high academic achievement, all planning revolved around facilitating transition to post–secondary education and the skills need to be successful there. Cody's interests were explored to guide career planning throughout high school. Mathematics and science courses were his favorite classes and outside of school, he continued to have a strong interest in all things related to steam engine trains. When considered together, the family felt that exploring a career in engineering would be appropriate.

Another occupation targeted during the transition planning process was driving. An initial driver's education class at his high school revealed that Cody had some difficulties with processing and responding to the multiple factors associated with driving. Often, he became distracted by things seen while driving and would focus on these aspects instead of his speed and traffic pattern. Additionally, he had difficulty with understanding the global aspects of some of the driving laws. Because of these difficulties, he participated in a driving rehab program in which an occupational therapist participated. Factors limiting participation were addressed initially in a clinic setting through role-playing and computer-based methods and generalized to on-the-road occupational driving training.

Post–Secondary Education

Following the transition from high school, Cody enrolled at a local community college where he would have the benefit of smaller class sizes and better access to his professors. Without the support of his family, Cody struggled with organization and time management. Additionally, he wanted to make friends, so he was easily swayed by others and therefore was often pulled away from his studies and found himself in difficult situations. The occupational therapy program at the university provides some support to the counseling center. Cody visited the counseling center to seek assistance with time management and organization. An occupational therapist met with Cody; and as part of the occupational profile, they outlined his daily schedule and routines and reviewed course exams and projects. Together, they developed a structured visual schedule that included courses, study time, and social time. Additionally, social skills training was conducted within a group intervention program for other adults with an ASD. The group targeted social awareness and decision making in social situations.

Supported Employment

As Cody neared completion of college, occupational therapy consultation as part of a vocational rehabilitation program was provided to assist with the development of social skills in the workplace in preparation for his engineering internship placements. Additionally, interviewing skills were targeted through role-playing to prepare for the upcoming hiring process.

Conclusions

Given the wide-range of impairment seen in this population, a comprehensive integrated intervention program is often recommended but difficult to implement. This case review outlined one such program involving collaborative occupational and speech-language therapy, behavior management/family counseling, and pharmacological management. The case study is used to illustrate implementation of the intervention program following a comprehensive diagnostic assessment. As the case study demonstrates, successful implementation can address areas of difficulty to promote optimal outcomes and quality of life for the individual with autism and his or her family.

References

American Psychiatric Association. (2001). *Diagnostic and statistical manual of mental disorders* (4th ed., text rev.). Washington, DC: Author.

Bryan, L., & Gast, D. (2000). Teaching on-task and on-schedule behaviors to high functioning children with autism via picture activity schedules. *Journal of Autism and Developmental Disorders, 30*, 553–567.

Canitano, R., & Scandurra, V. (2011). Psychopharmacology in autism: An update. *Progress in Neuro-Psychopharmacology and Biological Psychiatry, 35*, 18–28.

Cohen, H., Amerine-Dickens, M., & Smith, T. (2006). Early intensive behavioral treatment: Replication of the UCLA model in a community setting. *Development and Behavioral Pediatrics, 27*, S145–S155.

de Kruif, R. E. L., & McWilliam, R. A. (1999). Multivariate relationships among developmental age, global engagement, and observed child engagement. *Early Childhood Research Quarterly, 14*, 515–536.

Dettmer, S., Simpson, R., Myles, B., & Ganz, J. (2000). The use of visual supports to facilitate transitions of students with autism. *Focus on Autism and Other Developmental Disabilities, 15*, 163–170.

Filipek, P. A., Accardo, P. J., Baranek, G. T., Cook, E. H., Jr., Dawson, G., & Gordon, B. (1999). The screening and diagnosis of autistic spectrum disorders. *Journal of Autism and Developmental Disorders, 29*, 439–484.

Frost, L. A., & Bondy, A. S. (1994). *The picture exchange communication system.* Cherry Hill, NJ: Pyramid Educational Consultants.

Geis, R., & Tomchek, S. D. (2000). Integration of sensorimotor and speech-language therapy. In R. A. Huebner (Ed.), *Autism: A sensorimotor approach to management.* Gaithersberg, MD: Aspen.

Gray, C. (2000). *The new social story book.* Arlington, TX: Future Horizons.

Greenspan, S. I., & Wieder, S. (2006). *Engaging autism: Using the floortime approach to help children relate, communicate, and think.* New York, NY: Da Capo Press.

Horner, R., Carr, E., Strain, P., Todd, A., & Reed, H. (2002). Problem behavior interventions for young children. *Journal of Autism and Developmental Disorders, 32*, 423–446.

Huffman, L. C., Sutcliffe, T. L., Tanner, I. S., & Feldman, H. M. (2011). Management of symptoms in children with autism spectrum disorders: A comprehensive review of pharmacologic and complementary-alternative medicine treatments. *Journal of Developmental and Behavioral Pediatrics, 32*, 56–68.

Massey, G., & Wheeler, J. (2000). Acquisition and generalization of activity schedules and their effects on task engagement in a young child with autism in an inclusive preschool classroom. *Education and Training in Mental Retardation and Developmental Disabilities, 35*, 326–335.

Mastergeorge, A. M., Rogers, S. J., Corbett, B. A., & Solomon, M. (2003). Nonmedical interventions for autism spectrum disorders. In S. Ozonoff, S. J. Rogers, & R. L. Hendren (Eds.), *Autism spectrum disorders: A research review for practioners* (pp. 133–160). Washington, DC: American Psychiatric Press.

McWilliam, R. A., & Bailey, D. B. (1992). Promoting engagement and mastery. In D. B. Bailey & M. Wolery (Eds.), *Teaching infants and preschoolers with disabilities* (pp. 229–255). Columbus, OH: Merrill.

McWilliam, R. A., Trivette, C. M., & Dunst, C. J. (1985). Behavior engagement as a measure of the efficacy of early intervention. *Analysis and Intervention in Developmental Disabilities, 5*, 59–71.

Myers, S. M., & Johnson, C. P. (2007). Management of children with autism spectrum disorders. *Pediatrics, 5*, 1162–1182.

National Research Council. (2001). *Educating children with autism.* Washington, DC: National Academy Press.

Nazeer, A. (2011). Psychopharmacology of autistic spectrum disorders in children and adolescents. *Pediatric Clinics of North America, 58*, 85–97.

Prizant, B. M., Wetherby, A. M., Rubin, E., Laurent, A. C., & Rydell, P. (2006). *The SCERTS Model: A comprehensive educational approach for children with autism spectrum disorders.* Baltimore, MD: Paul H. Brookes.

Reichow, B., & Volkmar, F. (2010). Social skill interventions for individuals with autism: Evaluation for evidence-based practices within a best evidence synthesis framework. *Journal of Autism and Developmental Disorders, 40*, 149–166.

Simpson, R. L. (2005). Evidence-based practices and students with autism spectrum disorders. *Focus on Autism and Other Developmental Disabilities, 20*(3), 140–149.

Tomchek, S. D., & Case-Smith, J. (2009). *Occupational therapy practice guideline for individuals with an autism spectrum disorder.* Bethesda, MD: American Occupational Therapists Association.

Virues-Ortega, J. (2010). Applied behavior analytic intervention for autism in early childhood: Meta-analysis, meta-regression and dose-response meta-analysis of multiple outcomes. *Clinical Psychology Review, 30*(4), 387–399.

Volkmar, F., Cook, E. H., Jr., Pomeroy, J., Realmuto, G., & Tanguay, P. (1999). American Academy of Child and Adolescent Psychiatry practice parameter for the assessment and treatment of children, adolescents, and adults with autism and other pervasive developmental disorders. *Journal of the American Academy of Child and Adolescent Psychiatry, 38*(Suppl), 32S–54S.

Windeck, S. L., & Laurel, M. (1989). A theoretical framework combining speech-language therapy with sensory integration treatment. *Sensory Integration Special Interest Section Newsletter, 12*(*1*), 1–4.

For additional resources on the subjects discussed in this chapter, visit http://thePoint.lww.com/Willard-Spackman12e.

CHAPTER 61

Providing Occupational Therapy for Individuals with Traumatic Brain Injury

Intensive Care to Community Reentry

Steven D. Wheeler

LEARNING OBJECTIVES

After reading this chapter, you will be able to:

1. Identify the role of occupational therapy throughout the full spectrum of traumatic brain injury (TBI) recovery
2. Appreciate the manner in which impairments, activity limitations, personal factors, and environmental barriers interact to impact successful and satisfying occupational performance following TBI
3. Understand the importance of therapeutic relationship building and occupation-based practice in facilitating optimal community reentry following TBI

OUTLINE

Introduction

Few conditions challenge the diverse knowledge base and skill set of occupational therapy (OT) practitioners like traumatic brain injury (TBI). TBI is a complex condition characterized by varying degrees of cognitive, physical, psychological, behavioral, and emotional impairment. These impairments contribute to a dramatic change in an individual's life course, profound disruption of the family, enormous loss of income or earning potential, and large expenses over a lifetime (McKinlay & Watkiss, 1999). One's presentation after TBI depends on the extent and location of damage to the brain mixed with that person's cultural background, personality, and life experiences. As a result, no two individuals presenting to the OT practitioner are exactly alike, necessitating a true client-centered approach to assessment and treatment (see Box 61.1 and Chapter 33).

Injuries of low severity (coma and posttraumatic amnesia less than 1 day) are generally associated with better work and social outcomes (Schutz & Schutz, 2010). With greater severity of injury comes increased likelihood of residual cognitive, psychosocial, behavioral, or physical impairment (Kersel, Marsh, Havill, & Sleigh, 2001). Although successful "community reentry" represents the ultimate goal of the TBI recovery process,

BOX 61.1 Therapist Narrative: The Importance of Therapeutic Relationship Building in TBI Rehabilitation

Although the phrase "risk-taking behaviors" is sometimes associated with actions and behaviors contributing to traumatic brain injury (TBI), taking risks is a necessary aspect of successful life functioning. Many of our greatest accomplishments and "self-esteem builders" come as a result of performing a task that carried with it the possibility of failure or rejection—asking someone out on a date, interviewing for a job, or even applying to college and pursuing occupational therapy studies. Those with a high self-esteem are better suited to taking such risks; failures are disappointments that fuel future attempts. If a decision doesn't work out, a high self-esteem can give you the strength and confidence necessary to pursue other avenues to reach your life goals.

Unsuccessful efforts to return to "normal" after TBI can be damaging to one's self-esteem and, subsequently, one's willingness to take chances and risk failure. This can pose a considerable challenge to occupational therapy practitioners responsible for encouraging clients to try new tasks necessary for the attainment of meaningful goals. Working within a client's comfort zone (i.e., doing activities that they're already competent at) can make a session manageable but may not be moving toward those meaningful occupations identified by the client and family in the early stages of therapy. Additionally, always keeping things "safe" also prevents the client from learning about their deficits, an important component in the development of self-awareness. The inability to recognize one's deficits interferes with the motivation to change behavior or adapt to one's environment (Fleming, Strong, & Ashton, 1998). Impaired self-awareness negatively impacts social participation and the ability to establish a productive daily routine (Trudel, Tryon, & Purdum, 1998).

The development of an unconditional, therapeutic relationship is central to building a climate of trust. Clients who believe that their therapist will remain supportive regardless of whether they succeed or fail at an activity are more likely to take those risks necessary to experience meaningful accomplishments and enhance self-esteem. Unfortunately, rapport building with many clients takes time and may even require the therapist to "prove" his or her commitment to the relationship by staying supportive with the client during periods of acting out, defiance, and other acts. Therapists who discharge or transfer clients to other therapists because of difficult behavior or "noncompliance" may be missing an opportunity to establish the therapeutic relationship needed to encourage clients risk taking and the attainment of major life accomplishments.

for most individuals, the road from intensive care to community reentry is a long and arduous one. In addition to injury severity, the presence of medical and nonmedical complications, preinjury health status, health insurance coverage, and the availability of services influence both the type and duration of services received.

Persons with TBI can receive medical care and/or rehabilitation in a variety of settings. Senelick and Dougherty (2001) summarize the possibilities for care and rehabilitation following TBI to include

1. Intensive care unit (ICU)/acute care,
2. Acute rehabilitation (inpatient),
3. Outpatient rehabilitation,
4. Skilled long-term care,
5. Skilled residential care, and
6. Transitional living/work.

There are many factors that influence the continuum of care following TBI. These are summarized in Figure 61.1 and discussed in Box 61.2. Regardless of the path following injury, OT is likely to play an important role.

Appendix I, Common Conditions, Resources, and Evidence of this text provides additional background information on TBI and summarizes common occupational therapy assessments and interventions used through the continuum of care.

Occupational Therapy in Action: Miles's Journey from the ICU to College Graduation

The case of Miles characterizes the complexity of TBI rehabilitation and the important impact of OT throughout the recovery spectrum. His experience following severe TBI also demonstrates the barriers to full community participation from the standpoint of both the individual and society.

Background Information

At the age of 22 years, Miles sustained a severe TBI in a motor vehicle accident while performing his job as a laborer with a local homebuilder. At the time of the injury, Miles was living with his mother, girlfriend, and infant daughter. He was a high school graduate who enjoyed sports, computers, and social events. Miles's injury was classified as severe. He remained in a coma for approximately 3 months, with computed tomography (CT) scan showing extensive brainstem damage and multiple contusions throughout his brain. OT at this stage focuses on both managing impairments resulting from the injury and preventing secondary impairments that can occur over periods of unconsciousness. Sensory stimulation programs may be implemented at

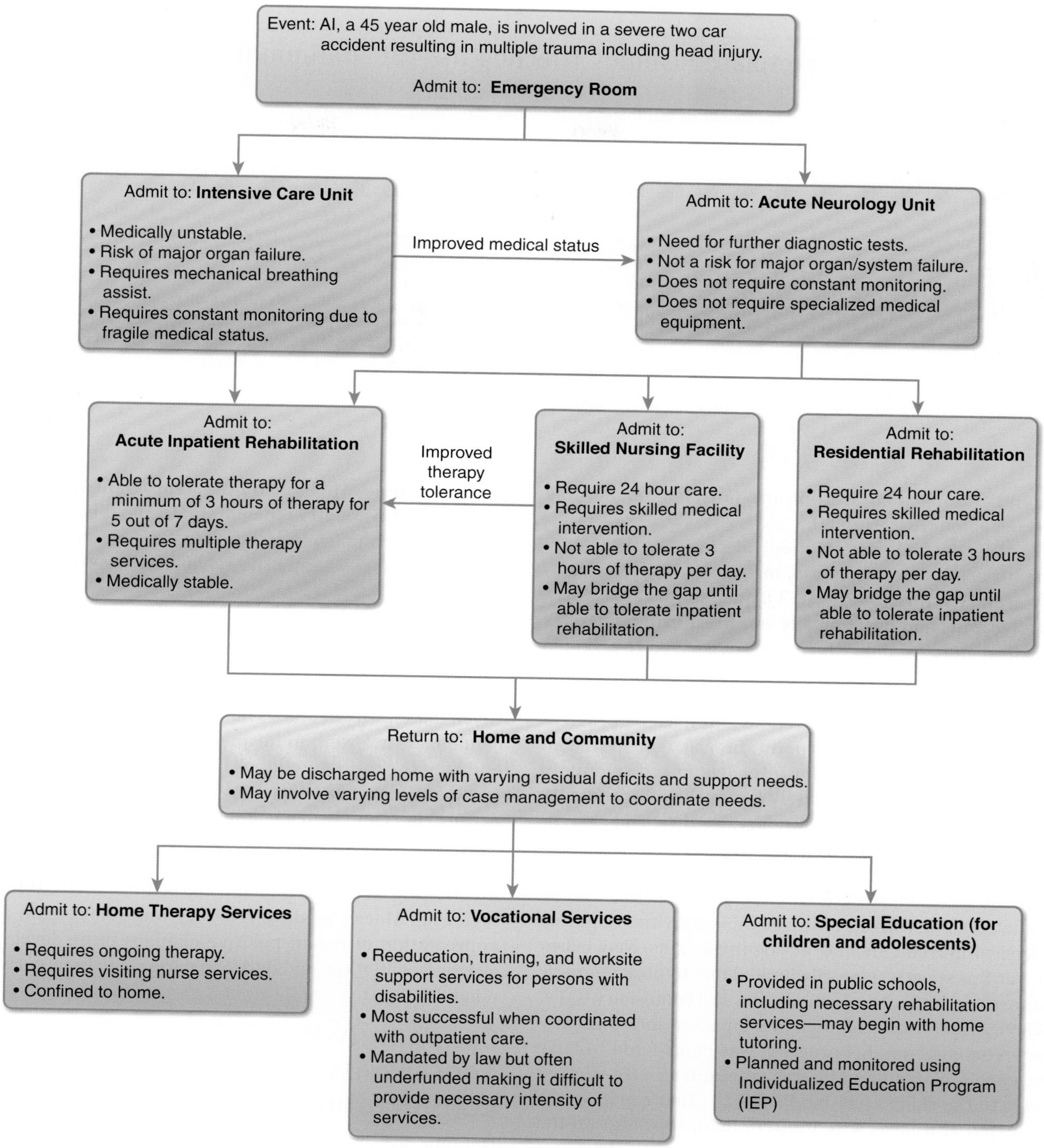

FIGURE 61.1 Potential continuum of care after traumatic brain injury.

this stage. They consist of team-coordinated sessions of brief applications of multimodal sensory stimulation with close observation of the patient for behavioral responses (American Occupational Therapy Association [AOTA], 2009). This approach typically involves stimulation of the visual, auditory, olfactory, gustatory, cutaneous, and/or kinesthetic system to promote awakening and enhance the rehabilitation potential of coma patients. Although used by various health professionals including OT practitioners, reliable evidence to support or rule out the effectiveness of sensory stimulation is lacking (Lombardi, Taricco, De Tanti, Telaro, & Liberati, 2002). Additionally, interventions such as passive range of motion (PROM), splinting, casting, and positioning are among the more "preparatory" methods used to either restore motor function or prevent secondary

BOX 61.2 Marketplace Realities Affecting the TBI Continuum of Care

The need to shift from the medical model of traumatic brain injury (TBI) rehabilitation to a more client-centered philosophy as an individual becomes medically stable is commonly cited in the literature (Brain Injury Association of America [BIAA], 2009). Unfortunately, the realities of the U.S. marketplace present considerable challenges to providing such care for many in need (Katz, Zasler, & Zafonte, 2007). For those fortunate enough to have health insurance, coverage for rehabilitation becomes incrementally more difficult across the continuum of care outlined in Figure 61.1—from inpatient to outpatient to residential and community services. For many, funding shifts from private to public sources such as Medicaid or Medicare for longer term care. The adequacy of public funding varies between states as some have developed Medicaid waivers to provide long-term home and community services that would otherwise be covered in institutional settings such as a nursing home (Katz et al., 2007). Understanding the complexities of reimbursement and sources of alternative funding is a challenging but essential element for clinicians, especially those providing services at the community level.

Numerous other factors exist that affect the availability of services during TBI recovery. These include a lack of transportation; a scarcity of appropriate, affordable housing; and limitations in resources for behavioral problems. Even if services are available, programs and professional providers may lack the knowledge and expertise to serve this population. According to Katz et al. (2007), the ability to provide a full scope of properly funded services to all age groups within a reasonable proximity "is an enormous challenge that may never be fully satisfied" (p. 5).

complications such as joint and muscle contractures during coma (AOTA, 2009).

Miles had numerous medical complications during his acute care admission, including a lower extremity deep vein thrombosis (DVT), pneumonia, atelectasis, bradycardia, and questionable seizure activity. When his medical status stabilized, he was transferred to a skilled nursing facility where he continued the coma recovery program as described earlier. He remained in this setting until he emerged from coma and became progressively more alert. At that point, he was transferred to a rehabilitation hospital for intensive interdisciplinary rehabilitation—approximately 6 months after the date of his injury. OT at this stage addresses the client's physical, cognitive, emotional, spiritual, communicative, and functional needs (AOTA, 2009). Depending on the client's level of agitation, structured basic self-care tasks can be initiated along with structured simple activities requiring physical movements and/or cognitive skills. New learning at this stage is generally limited due to posttraumatic amnesia, agitation, overstimulation, and confusion (AOTA, 2009). After 5 weeks of intensive, inpatient interdisciplinary rehabilitation, his progress was considered to have reached a plateau and he was subsequently transferred back to the skilled nursing facility. At that time, he was assessed at a Level V (confused, inappropriate) on the Rancho Los Amigos Levels of Cognitive Functioning Scale (Hagen, 1998). He continued to require assistance with all basic activities of daily living (ADL), had a percutaneous endoscopic gastrostomy (PEG) tube in place, was on a pureed diet with moderately thickened liquids, and was nonambulatory, dependent on others for wheelchair mobility. His verbal expression was described as "profoundly impaired" and he communicated via a communication board.

Referral

Approximately 2 months into his second admission to the skilled nursing facility, Miles was referred to a TBI postacute, residential rehabilitation program. As part of the community reentry rehabilitation team, I had the opportunity to complete a comprehensive assessment with Miles followed by an intensive rehabilitation program.

Evaluation

Initial Impressions

Given the severity of Miles's injury, I was very aware of the challenges that were to lie ahead for both of us. Schutz and Schutz (2010) noted that for injuries where coma is less than 1 day, most survivors regain independence and perform adequately in a competitive job. However, when coma is counted in months, as was the case for Miles, even the most intense therapy usually doesn't restore full functioning in any area (Schutz & Schutz, 2010). While reviewing Miles's medical record, I was able to gain an appreciation of recent positive changes in his level of alertness, initiation, and desire to participate in intensive rehabilitation.

Community-Based Occupational Therapy Assessment—Considerations

Helping people to be productive and satisfied in their least restrictive environment is central to OT regardless of treatment setting or medical diagnosis. McColl, Davies, Carlson, Johnston, and Minnes (2001) categorized meaningful aspects of community integration to include the following:

1. Activities to fill one's time
2. Independence in one's living situation
3. Relationships with other people

Additionally, I've found the constructs of the *International Classification of Functioning, Disability, and*

Health (ICF) (World Health Organization [WHO], 2001) to be particularly helpful in organizing my approach to both assessment and treatment. Both perspectives consider the interaction between person and environment and its impact on participation in meaningful occupations.

Assessment Priority No. 1—Therapeutic Relationship Building

If I were to name one thing that was essential to a positive outcome when working with persons with severe brain injury, it would be the establishment of a strong therapeutic relationship. That process begins with the very first interaction with the client. Standardized interview tools such as the Occupational Performance History Interview II (Kielhofner et al., 2004) and the Canadian Occupational Performance Measure (COPM) (Law et al., 2005) are excellent strategies for collecting important information and establishing client-centered goals. However, care should be taken to ensure that the interview isn't so structured that it hinders rapport building (refer back to Box 61.1). Additionally, for persons with a low frustration tolerance, moderate-to-severe cognitive deficits, and/or difficulty managing environmental stimulation, adaptations to the interview duration, wording of questions, and interview setting may be required in order to collect meaningful data. When initial rapport is established, the therapist is in a better position to encourage participation in home and community assessment tasks likely to be both challenging and frustrating for the client.

Assessment Results

Selected assessment strategies used to determine Miles's impairments, activity restrictions, and participation limitations as represented in the ICF are summarized in Table 61.1. Miles's initial assessment was completed over a period of approximately 1 week, a time frame that is longer than in many settings but necessary for community-based rehabilitation given the need to observe performance in both home and community settings.

During our initial interview, Miles presented as extremely motivated and eager to participate in assessment tasks. After collecting some background information, Miles was asked to identify long-term goals and areas of life that were most important to him. They included the following:

1. Getting reunited with his girlfriend and infant daughter who had relocated to her parents' home more than 1,000 miles away.
2. Being able to move more effectively and walk—"getting out of this wheelchair."
3. Being able to complete morning dressing, grooming, self-feeding, and toileting tasks without assistance from others—"taking care of myself and having some privacy."
4. Being able to communicate more effectively—"talking better without drooling so much."
5. Going back to school—wanted to attend college prior to injury
6. Being able to play sports—expressed a particular interest in basketball and running

Having Miles identify these areas was important. Clients who generate their own goals have been found to be more likely to want to work on them and feel that the goals are important (Doig, Fleming, Kuipers, & Cornwell, 2010). Given the gap between Miles's current and desired level of functioning, his full commitment to the program is especially essential.

Further impairment testing was carried out to determine which impairments limited occupational performance. Sensorimotor testing revealed severe ataxia affecting his ability to coordinate movements throughout the muscles of his extremities and trunk. Balance as evaluated through functional transfers from wheelchair to bed and toilet was poor. Generalized weakness and decreased endurance was also noted. Grip strength, evaluated using a dynamometer, was 20 lb on the dominant right side and 34 lb on the left. Range of motion was within normal limits, with the exception of right shoulder abduction and flexion, which were both limited to approximately 30 degrees actively and 90 degrees passively. It was noted in his medical record that Miles had sustained a severe fracture to his right forearm in his accident, resulting in prolonged immobilization of his right arm. Miles did not report discomfort with movement of his right upper extremity and no exercise restrictions were noted. Sensation was grossly intact.

In addition to the assessments listed in Table 61.1, Miles and I also completed a community living skills assessment (Angle & Buxton, 1991) that, as was hypothesized, demonstrated moderate-to-severe difficulty with all home and community tasks except money management and telephone use, which were mildly impaired. Although it appeared that physical impairments were the primary contributor to these functional difficulties, cognitive issues such as impulsivity and reduced awareness of deficits were also evident during observations. Such "executive cognitive functions" are commonly associated with damage to the brain's frontal lobes. These executive functions significantly influence other higher order cognitive skills such as decision making, goal setting, self-evaluation, and, ultimately, successful performance of the majority of life roles. Short-term memory impairments were also evident but appeared influenced by time of day and nature of the content to be remembered. Vision was tested prior to his admission and was determined to be consistent with preinjury acuity. Miles demonstrated functional vision during reading, computer keyboard access, and other evaluation activities.

TABLE 61.1 Community-Based Assessment Data Collection

Assessment Method	Rationale	Results	Interpretation
Initial interview	Rapport building, establish client goals and meaningful occupations, screen cognitive impairments and orientation	High motivation for therapy, goals to return with girlfriend and infant child, sports, and work/school; very concerned with physical impairments and impact on activities	Positive transition from skilled nursing; patient concerned about girlfriend and daughter relocating and not available to visit. Therapeutic relationship initiated with occupational therapy practitioners.
Functional Independence Measure (FIM™) (Keith, Granger, Hamilton, & Sherwin, 1987) Functional Assessment Measure (FAM) (Hall, 1997)	FIM™—Assesses dysfunction in the performance of basic activities of daily living; physical deficit based FAM—Addresses major functional areas less emphasized in the FIM to include cognitive, behavioral, communication, and community functioning	FIM™—Feeding, 2 Upper body dressing, 3 Lower body dressing, 2 Grooming, 2 Bathing, 2 Transfers (wheelchair to bed), 2 Transfers (wheelchair to bathtub), 1 FAM: Dependent (1) to Maximal assist (2) for home management and all instrumental activities of daily living	Moderate (client provides 50%–74% assistance) to maximum (client provides 25%–49% assistance) assist required for all aspects of basic self-care and functional transfers to bed and chair from wheelchair. Total assistance was required for transfer into a standard bathtub.
Community Integration Questionnaire (CIQ) (Willer, Ottenbacher, & Coad, 1994)	Brain injury specific measure to address actual participation in categories related to community integration 1. Integration into a homelike setting 2. Social integration 3. Integration into productive activities	Total score, 2 Home integration score, 0 Social integration score, 2 Productivity score, 0	A total CIQ score can range from 0 to 29, with higher scores indicating greater community integration. Miles's score reflects virtually no current participation in activities inside or outside home.
Satisfaction with Life Scale (SWLS) (Diener, Emmons, Larsen, & Griffin, 1985)	Measure of general life satisfaction, a factor of subjective well-being; quick administration, well established validity and reliability	Total score, 24	Scores on the SWLS range from 5 (very dissatisfied) to 35 (highly satisfied). Miles's score of 24 represented "mild satisfaction."
Neurobehavioral Functioning Inventory (Kreutzer, Seel, & Marwitz, 1999)	Completing patient form in concert with family caregiver form allows assessment of awareness of deficits, an important aspect of executive cognitive functioning and an area considered important to rehabilitation program compliance	*Miles* / *Caregiver* Depression 45 / 51 Somatic complaints 45 / 74 Memory 46 / 51 Communication 58 / 54 Aggression 39 / 44 Motor impairments 51 / 60	Comparison of patient and caregiver raw scores suggests possibility of deficit of self-awareness based on Miles reporting less severity of symptoms in all areas except communication.

Treatment Planning: Mapping Out Strategies to Turn Assessment Findings into Performance Outcomes

Assessment findings revealed a large performance discrepancy between Miles's current functioning and his stated goals. Overcoming the factors contributing to reduced community participation following TBI is generally much more challenging for OT practitioners than identifying them. My treatment plan with Miles was heavily influenced by the following:

1. The client-centered philosophy and the person-environment models of OT (see Chapters 33 and 38)
2. The ICF
3. The "Whatever it Takes" approach (Willer & Corrigan, 1994)

Whatever it Takes is a practical approach to fostering community integration after TBI that considers both environmental barriers and needed natural supports that may be necessary for long-term community functioning. The approach is based on the following principles:

- No two individuals with acquired brain injury are alike.
- Skills are more likely to generalize when taught in the environment where they can be used.
- Environments are easier to change than people.
- Community integration should be holistic.
- Life is a place-and-train venture (i.e., placing an individual in an environment of his or her choice and providing the necessary supports and coaching/training to facilitate success).
- Natural supports last longer than professionals.
- Interventions must not do more harm than good.
- The service system prevents many barriers to community integration.
- Needs of individuals last a lifetime; so should their resources.

To me, this model represents the "ideal" scenario for a community reentry OT plan because it integrates the client-centered, occupational-based focus of OT with what we've learned about the course of brain injury recovery. Unfortunately, the ability to fully implement the approach in most health care settings and systems is difficult, but clinicians should do all that is possible within the settings that they work. Working in Miles's favor was the fact that his health insurance case manager appeared supportive of intensive, long-term rehabilitation. More intensive rehabilitation following TBI has been linked to earlier functional gains (Turner-Stokes, Disler, Nair, & Wade, 2005). However, the chronic, complex, and evolving nature of TBI makes it very difficult to determine the optimal and most cost-effective amount of intervention for any particular individual (AOTA, 2009).

Given the gap between Miles's current functional level and desired goals, regular communication with him regarding his progress was essential so that he could see how small incremental goals were related to his long-term goals. Success experiences are essential to building self-esteem and self-confidence as well as fueling motivation. Encouragement and support from outside his treatment program would be negatively affected by the fact that his girlfriend and child relocated with her parents after his accident and were more than 1,000 miles away. Additionally, although his mother expressed a strong interest in helping Miles recover, both she and Miles acknowledged a turbulent and unstable family history that included little contact with his father. Miles's community-based rehabilitation program included a multidisciplinary treatment team that included, in addition to myself and a certified occupational therapy assistant (COTA), a psychologist, speech-language pathologist, physical therapist, nurse, and social worker. Key target areas of the interdisciplinary treatment program are described in Table 61.2.

Implementing the Treatment Plan

Miles's treatment program tested the strength of our therapeutic relationship right from the onset. His severe ataxia contributed to poor motor coordination and frequent frustration during our sessions. Despite his high drive to participate in tasks with me and the COTA, functional gains were slow, accompanied by growing self-awareness of the fact that getting physically stronger was not going to resolve his severe ataxic movements. Miles was less interested in compensatory strategies than being the person he was prior to his injury, and that contributed to resistance when it came to trying adaptive equipment and compensatory techniques.

OT treatment sessions used both home and community settings. In the home, ADL training and home management activities were in an actual bedroom, bathroom, kitchen, living room, and office area. Whenever possible, we practiced actual tasks at normal times in Miles's typical daily routine—dressing, grooming, transfers, meal preparation, using the computer, handwriting in his memory notebook, planning and participating in community outings, doing household chores, and doing leisure activities. Repetition during activities was used to strengthen muscles and improve performance in conjunction with daily upper extremity strengthening exercises. Although often considered an adjunct to occupation, Miles's upper extremity strengthening program

TABLE 61.2 Selected Target Areas of the Interdisciplinary Treatment Program

Occupational Therapy	Speech Therapy	Psychology	Physical Therapy
Basic ADL performance/functional transfers	Speech clarity	Counseling for adjustment to disability	Functional ambulation using walker
Handwriting skills to facilitate day planner/memory notebook use prevocational	Swallowing/oral-motor skills	Memory training and compensation	Strengthening exercises with home exercise program
Meal preparation/home management	Memory—recall of sentences and paragraphs	Family counseling	Balance training
Leisure and social community outings	Augmentative communication	Attention training	Transfers and bed/mat mobility
Prevocational preparation including computer access	Respiratory exercises	Comprehensive neuropsychological assessment	Family/caregiver training related to ambulation and exercises

ADL, activities of daily living.

was additionally important as exercising was meaningful occupation for him preinjury.

With repeated struggles, Miles gradually appeared more accepting of adaptive equipment to improve his independence in activities that were particularly important to him. For example, weighted feeding utensils with built-up handles, dishes with higher lips, and cups with a top were effective at improving motor function to improve his ability to feed himself and drink more efficiently without excessive spillage. Building up handles on writing and grooming utensils also improved quality of performance, although to a lesser degree. We attempted to use weighted wrist cuffs to improve movement efficiency during computer keyboard use. However, Miles insisted on a one-handed typing technique that involved stabilizing his wrist using the opposite hand (see Figure 61.2).

Miles had his first session in the community approximately 3 weeks into his program—a trip to a department store to purchase a music CD. From that point on, sessions in the community were a regular aspect of his program, occurring approximately two to three times a week. Community outings included visits to restaurants, visiting his mother at her home, and attending sporting events, including a wheelchair basketball game. During outings, OT focused on evaluating skills such as money management, functional mobility, planning, initiative, problem solving, and decision making in relation to his degree of independence for each task.

Although functional gains were positive, the rate of progress was inconsistent. Success was complicated by medical factors such as frequent medication changes attempting to manage upper extremity tremors and

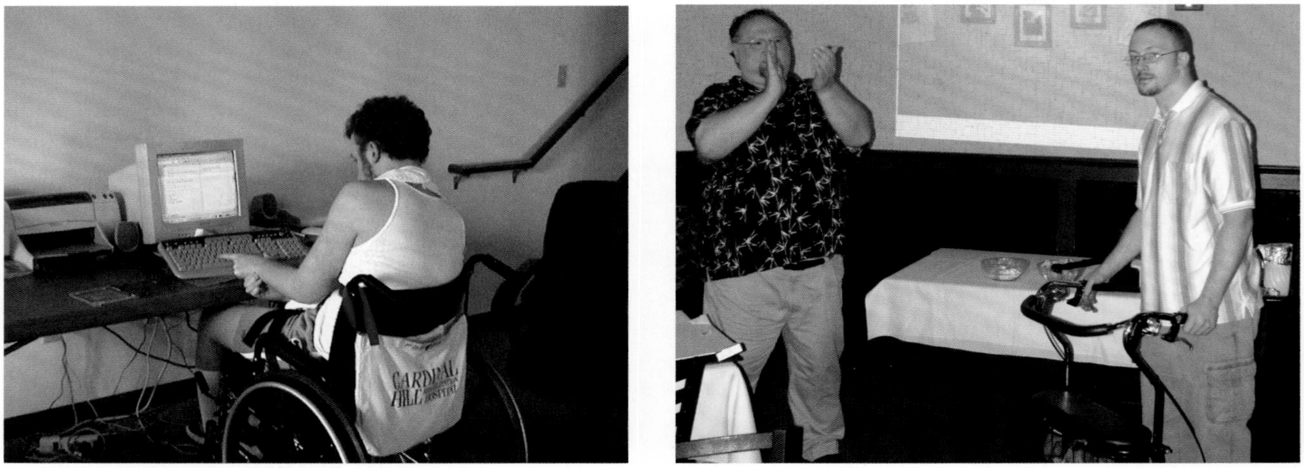

A B

FIGURE 61.2 Miles's educational program progressed from **(A)** basic computer keyboard access to **(B)** speaking to other survivors of brain injury.

TABLE 61.3 Selected Test Scores from 90-Day Evaluation

Evaluation	Baseline	90-Day Reassessment	Interpretation
Community Integration Questionnaire	Home integration, 0 Social integration, 2 Productive activity, 0	Home integration, 3 Social integration, 5 Productive activity, 0	Significant progress in home management and initiation and participation in social activities
FIM/FAM	Feeding, 2 Upper body dressing, 3 Lower body dressing, 2 Grooming, 2 Bathing, 2 Transfers (wheelchair to bed), 2 Transfers (wheelchair to bathtub), 1 Home management, 1	Feeding, 4 Upper body dressing, 5 Lower body dressing, 4 Grooming, 4 Bathing, 4 Transfers, 4 Home management, 2–3	Notable functional gains in ADL independence Assistance required for tasks requiring balance and fine motor coordination due to continued ataxia. Improved meal planning and money management
SWLS	24	12	Despite progress, significant reduction in self-reported life satisfaction

ADL, activities of daily living; FIM, Functional Independence Measure; FAM, Functional Assessment Measure; SWLS, Satisfaction with Life Scale.

severe esophageal reflux, which negatively impacted self-feeding and nutritional intake. His status 3 months after the onset of his postacute, residential program and 8 months from the date of his injury is summarized in Table 61.3. Despite his functional gains, Miles reported less satisfaction with life, frustration with his current situation, more frequent periods of agitation, and depressed mood. Additionally, he demonstrated increased self-awareness based on statements regarding the severity of his deficits and similarities between his and staff responses on the Neurobehavioral Functioning Inventory.

Revising the Treatment Plan: Expanding Occupations

With it becoming increasingly clear that Miles would have lifelong physical impairments, especially ataxia, aspects of Miles's program were modified to expand his occupations by putting greater emphasis on productivity and leisure goals. Up to this point in his treatment program, the occupations occupying Miles's typical day were almost entirely centered on self-care. The effort required for basic ADL and home management left little time and energy for other activities. That, combined with an increasing level of awareness of impairments, appeared to be negatively affecting life satisfaction. Although basic self-care and home management are necessary elements of successful community reentry, aspects of leisure and productivity, so central to Miles preinjury daily routine, were very limited and impacted his psychological well-being. It was hoped that by balancing self-care and home management goals with more productive activity and leisure, Miles would develop a greater sense of accomplishment and gain a more positive outlook in life in the face of residual disability.

The plan to increase Miles's productive occupations included two primary objectives, identified by Miles as being of primary importance:

1. Taking college courses to eventually obtain a degree
2. Taking greater responsibility of his finances to demonstrate capacity to become his own legal guardian

Additionally, OT continued working on self-care skills, home management, and community participation to help Miles and the clinical team make decisions on his least restrictive living environment after his discharge from the residential treatment program.

In addition to beginning college studies, planning was also initiated to look at options for community living. During family sessions, it became increasingly clear that Miles would not be residing with his parents, and his girlfriend had expressed an intention to break off their relationship. The therapeutic relationships established with many clinical team members served as a critical source of support during this period of social isolation and an uncertain future. Although supportive of Miles during his struggles, adherence to professional boundaries by the OT team and all staff was essential at all times. Purtilo and Haddad (1996) describe strategies to express genuine care for clients while maintaining some distance. Given Miles's emotional vulnerability, it would be understandable for him to misinterpret the nature of his relationships with health care providers (social friendships, intimacy, etc.). Strategies that the treatment team used to maintain professional boundaries included

- Having Miles participate in team meetings where issues about his progress were discussed,
- Dividing outings and activities between team members,
- Limiting visits/interactions to work hours,

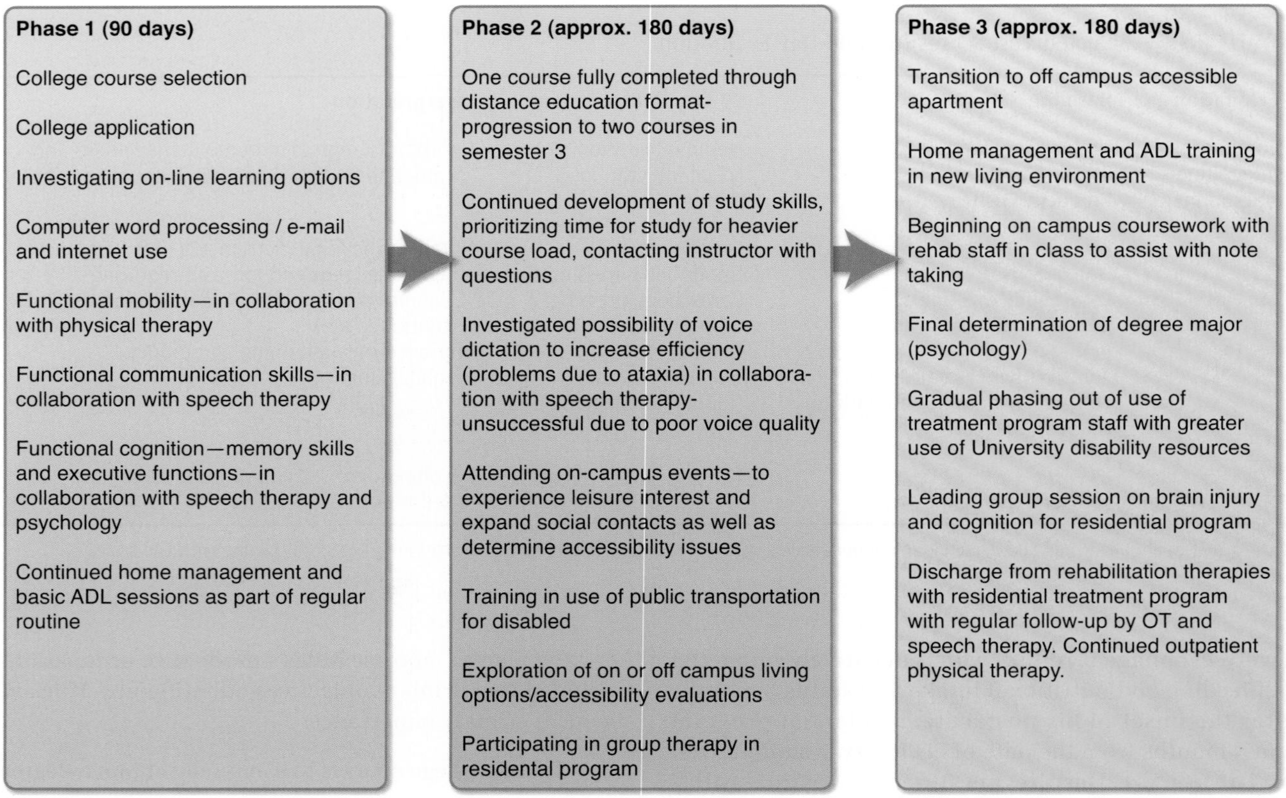
Phase 1 (90 days)
College course selection
College application
Investigating on-line learning options
Computer word processing / e-mail and internet use
Functional mobility—in collaboration with physical therapy
Functional communication skills—in collaboration with speech therapy
Functional cognition—memory skills and executive functions—in collaboration with speech therapy and psychology
Continued home management and basic ADL sessions as part of regular routine
Phase 2 (approx. 180 days)
One course fully completed through distance education format-progression to two courses in semester 3
Continued development of study skills, prioritizing time for study for heavier course load, contacting instructor with questions
Investigated possibility of voice dictation to increase efficiency (problems due to ataxia) in collaboration with speech therapy-unsuccessful due to poor voice quality
Attending on-campus events—to experience leisure interest and expand social contacts as well as determine accessibility issues
Training in use of public transportation for disabled
Exploration of on or off campus living options/accessibility evaluations
Participating in group therapy in residental program
Phase 3 (approx. 180 days)
Transition to off campus accessible apartment
Home management and ADL training in new living environment
Beginning on campus coursework with rehab staff in class to assist with note taking
Final determination of degree major (psychology)
Gradual phasing out of use of treatment program staff with greater use of University disability resources
Leading group session on brain injury and cognition for residential program
Discharge from rehabilitation therapies with residential treatment program with regular follow-up by OT and speech therapy. Continued outpatient physical therapy.

FIGURE 61.3 Stages of Miles's school/independent living progression with occupational therapy (OT) focus areas. *ADL*, activities of daily living.

- Working with Miles to expand his relationships beyond the rehabilitation setting, and
- Discreetly sharing with Miles personal incidents from everyday life.

According to Purtilo and Haddad (1996), such sharing can assist the occupational therapist in maintaining a "reality factor" that is beneficial to both client and professional.

The stages of Miles's education, independent living, and leisure goals are detailed in Figure 61.3. Each phase is characterized by significant clinical progress and incorporation of meaningful occupations into his daily routine. Each was also characterized by significant struggle and testing of the therapist–client relationship. On occasion, Miles would appear to sabotage his progress, acting out or refusing to participate in tasks that had been weeks, and sometimes months, in planning. The roles of OT changed throughout the phases, moving from predominantly direct skills teaching to advocate, working with landlords, builders, and professors to help Miles face environmental barriers in terms of accessibility and prejudice.

It took 8 years for Miles to receive his bachelor of arts degree in psychology (see Figure 61.4). At the time of graduation, he was living in the community with homemaker support and had successfully gained legal authority to manage his own finances. His outcomes defy the expected for persons with severe TBI. But despite these unlikely accomplishments, he also faces an uncertain future. Without secured employment, an absence of leisure activities, few friends, and residual motor impairments, it is likely that Miles will continue to require various rehabilitative and social services as future challenges present.

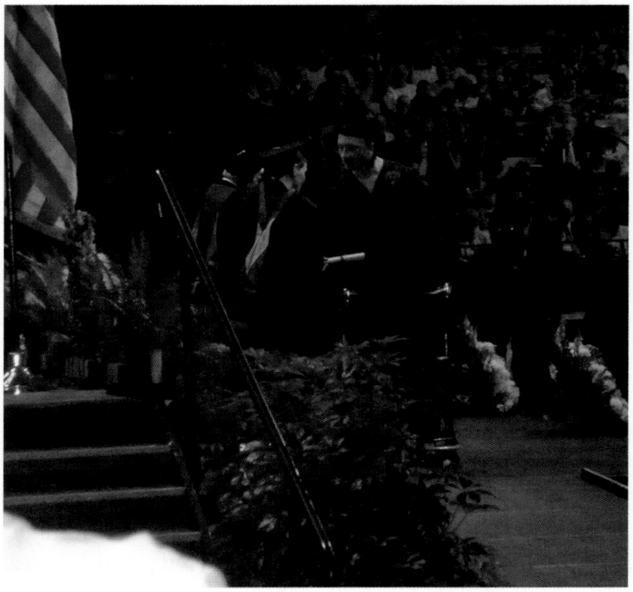

FIGURE 61.4 An intensive, occupation-based rehabilitation program helped Miles accomplish his goal of college graduation.

References

American Occupational Therapy Association. (2009). *Occupational therapy practice guidelines for adults with traumatic brain injury*. Bethesda, MD: AOTA Press.

Angle, D., & Buxton, J. (1991). *The community living skills workbook for the head injured adult*. New York, NY: Aspen.

Brain Injury Association of America. (2009). *The essential brain injury guide*. Vienna, VA: Author.

Diener, E., Emmons, R. A., Larsen, R. J., & Griffin, S. (1985). The Satisfaction with Life Scale. *Journal of Personality Assessment*, *49*, 71–75.

Doig, E., Fleming, J., Kuipers, P., & Cornwell, P. (2010). Clinical utility of the combined use of the Canadian Occupational Performance Measure and Goal Attainment Scaling. *American Journal of Occupational Therapy*, *64*, 904–914.

Fleming, J., Strong, J., & Ashton, R. (1998). Cluster analysis of self-awareness levels in adults with traumatic brain injury and relationship to outcome. *The Journal of Head Trauma Rehabilitation*, *13*, 39–51.

Hagen, C. (1998). Levels of cognitive functioning. In *Rehabilitation of the head injured adult: Comprehensive physical management* (3rd ed.). Dowey, CA: Professional Staff Association of the Rancho Los Amigos Hospital.

Hall, K. (1997). The Functional Assessment Measure (FAM). *Journal of Rehabilitation Outcomes Measures*, *1*, 63–65.

Katz, D., Zasler, N., & Zafonte, R. (2007). Clinical continuum of care and natural history. In N. Zasler, D. Katz, & R. Zafonte (Eds.), *Perspectives on rehabilitation care and research* (pp. 1–13). New York, NY: Demos.

Keith, R., Granger, C., Hamilton, B., & Sherwin, F. (1987). The Functional Independence Measure: A new tool for rehabilitation. *Advances in Clinical Rehabilitation*, *1*, 6–18.

Kersel, D., Marsh, N., Havill, J., & Sleigh, J. (2001). Neuropsychological functioning during the year following severe traumatic brain injury. *Brain Injury*, *15*, 283–296.

Kielhofner, G., Mallinson, T., Crawford, C., Nowak, M., Rigby, M., Henry, A., & Walens, D. (2004). *Occupational Performance History Interview—II* (version 2.1). Chicago, IL: MOHO Clearinghouse.

Kreutzer, J., Seel, R., & Marwitz, J. (1999). *Neurobehavioral Functioning Inventory*. San Antonio, TX: The Psychological Corporation.

Law, M., Baptiste, S., Carswell, A., McColl, M., Polatajko, H., & Pollock, N. (2005). *Canadian Occupational Performance Measure*. Ottawa, ON: CAOT.

Lombardi, F., Taricco, M., De Tanti, A., Telaro, E., & Liberati, A. (2002). Sensory stimulation for brain injured individuals in coma or vegetative state. *Cochrane Database of Systematic Reviews*, (2), CD001427.

McColl, M., Davies, D., Carlson, P., Johnston, J., & Minnes, P. (2001). The Community Integration Measure: Development and preliminary validation. *Archives of Physical Medicine and Rehabilitation*, *82*, 429–434.

McKinlay, W., & Watkiss, A. (1999). Cognitive and behavioral effects of brain injury. In M. Rosenthal, E. Griffith, J. Kreutzer, & B. Pentland (Eds.), *Rehabilitation of the adult and child with traumatic brain injury* (3rd ed., pp. 74–86). Philadelphia, PA: FA Davis.

Purtilo, R., & Haddad, A. (1996). *Health professional and patient interaction*. Philadelphia, PA: WB Saunders.

Schutz, L., & Schutz, M. (2010). *Head injury recovery in real life*. San Diego, CA: Plural.

Senelick, R., & Dougherty, K. (2001). *Living with brain injury*. Birmingham, AL: HealthSouth Press.

Trudel, T., Tryon, W., & Purdum, C. (1998). Awareness of disability and long-term outcome after traumatic brain injury. *Rehabilitation Psychology*, *43*, 267–281.

Turner-Stokes, L., Disler, P., Nair, A., & Wade, D. (2005). Multidisciplinary rehabilitation for acquired brain injury in adults of working age. *Cochrane Database of Systematic Reviews*, (3), CD004170. doi:1002/14651858.CD004170.pub2

Willer, B., & Corrigan, J. (1994). Whatever it takes: A model for community-based services. *Brain Injury*, *8*, 647–659.

Willer, B., Ottenbacher, K., & Coad, M. (1994). The Community Integration Questionnaire: A comparative examination. *American Journal of Physical Medicine and Rehabilitation*, *73*, 103–111.

World Health Organization. (2001). *International classification of functioning, disability, and health*. Geneva, Switzerland: Author.

For additional resources on the subjects discussed in this chapter, visit http://thePoint.lww.com/Willard-Spackman12e.

CHAPTER 62

Providing Occupational Therapy Services for Persons with Psychiatric Disabilities

Promoting Recovery and Wellness

Ruth Ramsey, Peggy Swarbrick

OUTLINE

LEARNING OBJECTIVES

After reading this chapter, you will be able to:

1. Describe the different settings in which occupational therapists deliver services to persons with serious mental illness/psychiatric disability
2. Understand the research basis and evidence-based rationale for the selection and application of occupational interventions for persons with serious mental illness/psychiatric disabilities
3. Define concepts of recovery, wellness, and peer support as they apply to persons with serious mental illness/psychiatric disability
4. Identify community supports for persons with serious mental illness that facilitate independence

Therapist Narrative

I was fortunate to have the opportunity to work with Sean, an intelligent, creative, 22-year-old man and observe him progress throughout his **recovery** process. His passions are music and art. He loves to paint and draw, is gifted musically, and plays guitar and drums. He lives with his parents and younger siblings who have converted their garage into a studio apartment for Sean so he can feel more independent from his family and have space to practice his music and art. He eats most of his meals with his family but will occasionally go out with friends or fix himself a sandwich in his mini kitchen.

Sean had a normal childhood and did well in school. He attended a high school for the arts and was admitted to the University of California, Santa Cruz as music major. In his sophomore year, he began to have difficulties, which included trouble concentrating, hearing voices, and problems sleeping. He became withdrawn from his small circle of friends and began to neglect his hygiene. His grades began to slide, and he started drinking and smoking marijuana heavily. He also started to draw strange pictures and was found singing loudly in the halls of his dorm several times at 3 a.m.

(*continued*)

Finally, one of his friends called his parents who came down and insisted Sean be seen by a physician. By this time, Sean was run down and sleep deprived and became angry and agitated when his parents told him their intention to have him hospitalized as a "danger to self." The police were called, and Sean was escorted to the psychiatric emergency room of a local community hospital. He was involuntarily committed and placed on a "72-hour hold," during which time the intended outcomes were for Sean to begin pharmacotherapy; reestablish normal sleeping and eating patterns; and, together with his team, make plans for future treatment.

Although Sean was initially upset at being in the hospital, he was able to recognize that he needed help and that his family and the staff wanted to help him. He agreed to sign himself involuntarily and committed to staying 10 days, at which time the treatment team would evaluate his progress and decide on next steps. His doctor diagnosed him as having **schizophrenia**, undifferentiated (*Diagnostic and Statistical Manual of Mental Disorders*, [4th ed., text rev.; *DSM-IV-TR*] Code 295.90; American Psychiatric Association, 2000) and characterized this episode as a "first break." Counseling was offered to help the family understand the implications of Sean's new diagnosis and how they could support him in his recovery. Sean's psychiatrist met with him daily to evaluate his response to medications and confer with the staff about Sean's progress. Sean was seen by other staff as needed to discuss issues of concern to him. Sean was referred to the dual diagnosis program to help him deal with his drug and alcohol use and asked to attend dual diagnosis meetings where he was introduced to the idea of self-help groups such as Alcoholics Anonymous.

I met with Sean for an initial occupational therapy (OT) evaluation within 48 hours of admission as required by third-party payers. The initial evaluation was a combination of an interview; an OT self-report functional assessment that was developed for the unit; and the Canadian Occupational Performance Measure, designed to help the client identify personally meaningful treatment goals (Law, Baum, & Dunn, 2001). Other assessments were considered but not performed due to the short length of stay anticipated for Sean.

I met with Sean to develop a daily grooming schedule and agreed to review it with him daily before morning meeting. We also made plans to meet individually twice weekly so he could learn some cognitive behavioral approaches to anger management, such as deep breathing and reframing the situation. Because Sean was very motivated to get better and go back to school, he attended groups and met with his therapists during the 10 days he was in the hospital. He adjusted well to the antipsychotic medication with few side effects and started sleeping better. He said that the voices in his head were diminished but not totally absent, so I taught him mindfulness meditation (Reid, 2009) to help him learn to relax, focus, and ignore the voices. We discussed his plans to attend a partial hospitalization program (PHP) and live with his parents while he continued his recovery. The treatment team felt that Sean had a good plan in place, so he was discharged and driven by his mother to the PHP for an intake interview.

The intake coordinator at the PHP, Kevin, explained that he was also an occupational therapist. Sean was given general information about the program and told that his insurance company (he was covered by private insurance under his father's policy) had approved him to attend the program 4 days a week for 2 weeks, with an evaluation of progress toward goals at the end of the second week. During the intake interview, Kevin shared with Sean that he was also a musician and played in a rock and roll band.

Sean was given the program schedule by Kevin, who told him that the program ran from 10 a.m. to 3 p.m. for clients, but staff had to be there at 9 a.m. to get ready and also used the time after clients left to complete documentation, meet individually with clients, explore community resources that might be of assistance to clients, and make sure that all needed materials and supplies would be ready for the next day. Kevin would also act as Sean's case manager, meeting with him individually to assess progress and communicating with other staff as needed.

Sean attended the PHP program 4 days a week for 2 weeks and then transitioned to the intensive outpatient program (IOP) in a "step-down" process, attending 3 days weekly for 1 week, then 2 days for 2 weeks, then 1 day for 2 weeks. During that time, he met with his psychiatrist to ensure that the medications were helping control his symptoms, talked in group therapy about the challenges of moving back in with his family and leaving school, and worked with Kevin to find a part-time job at a local art supply store and register for one class at a local community college. Kevin suggested he might be interested in a volunteer job teaching music to children, but Sean declined the offer, stating, "Kids make me nervous."

Sean was given information about a drop-in program for young adults experiencing mental health challenges, sometimes referred to as a *TAY*, or *Transition Age Youth* program (Osgood, Foster, & Courtney, 2010). At the program, he was offered opportunities to socialize with other young people his own age, use the computers at the center, attend outings, and take classes on topics such as computer graphics and Tai Chi. At his discharge meeting from the PHP/IOP, he thanked Kevin for asking him about his life goals and helping him develop some practical strategies to achieve them.

Introduction

Serious mental illness affects 11 million people, or one in five Americans, annually. In 2009, more than one in eight adults received treatment for mental disorders. Forty percent of people diagnosed with a serious mental illness such as schizophrenia, **major depressive disorder**, or **bipolar disorder** received no care at all (U.S. Department of Health and Human Services, Substance Abuse and Mental Health Administration, 2010). Mental illness takes a huge toll on the individual, the individual's family, and his or her loved ones. Persons with serious mental illness experience various cognitive, affective, and behavioral symptoms that make it very challenging to continue or resume normal life roles (see Box 62.1). The costs to society in lost wages, absent days from work, and disability payments are also very high (Kessler et al., 2008).

Mental health disorders co-occur at a significant rate with other conditions such as developmental disabilities, traumatic brain injury, rheumatoid arthritis, and chronic pain. Some therapists have noted the presence of sensory processing disorders, such as tactile defensiveness in adults with paranoid schizophrenia and schizoaffective disorder (Brown, Cromwell, Filion, Dunn, & Tollefson, 2002). Individuals with mental health disorders have shorter life spans and worse overall health than nondisabled individuals possibly due to increased vulnerability as a result of poverty, inadequate access to health care, and significantly higher rates of smoking, obesity and substance abuse than the overall population (Center for Mental Health Services, 2010).

BOX 62.1 Symptoms of Major Mental Illness

- Feeling sad or down over a long period of time with no reason
- Confused thinking that interferes with function
- Excessive fears or worries (anxiety)
- Withdrawal from friends and activities
- Persistent problems sleeping
- Detachment from reality (delusions) or hallucinations
- Inability to cope with daily problems or stress
- Alcohol or drug abuse
- Significant changes in eating habits
- Sex drive changes
- Excessive anger, hostility, or violence
- Suicidal thinking

Data from Mayo Foundation for Medical Education and Research. (2011). *Symptoms of mental illness.* Retrieved from http://www.mayoclinic.com/health/mental-illness/DS01104/DSECTION=symptoms

Fortunately, progress has been made in the treatment of persons with mental illness. New medications that are more effective at targeting symptoms and have fewer side effects have been developed (National Institute of Mental Health, 2010). Social understanding and awareness about mental illness and mental health have increased, and new approaches to helping people with serious mental illness are being used based on the belief that people can and do recover from serious mental illness (see Box 62.2). *Recovery* has been defined as

> a process of change through which individuals improve their health and wellness, live a self-directed life, and strive to reach their full potential (Substance Abuse and Mental Health Services Administration [SAMHSA], 2011, para. 3).

In addition to the recovery vision, community mental health practice has adopted a focus on wellness. Wellness is defined as a conscious, deliberate process that requires a person to become aware of and make choices for a more satisfying lifestyle. A wellness lifestyle includes a balance of health habits, including adequate sleep, rest, and good nutrition, productivity and exercise, participation in meaningful activity and connections with supportive relationships. Wellness views a person holistically, more than simply mental and emotional wellbeing, and includes physical, intellectual, social, environmental, occupational, financial and spiritual dimensions (Swarbrick, 1997; 2006).

Occupational therapists have a strong skill set to bring to serving persons with **serious mental illness** (SMI). The term **psychiatric disability** is also used to refer to those individuals whose illness is severe and persistent and has led to the inability to fulfill one or more life roles for a significant period of time (Center for Psychiatric Disability, 2011). Because occupational therapists have educational grounding in psychology, therapeutic use of self, task analysis, neuroscience, and the teaching of life skills, they can be effective members of teams treating persons with SMI. Persons with SMI might be seen by an occupational therapist in various settings, including inpatient units of a general hospital, partial hospitalization programs and intensive outpatient programs, supported employment programs, supported housing programs, and peer support programs (Table 62.1).

Occupational therapists can help facilitate the recovery process for persons with SMI, assisting them in identifying strengths and challenges, developing treatment/intervention goals, and providing skill building and resources development interventions in group and individual format.

BOX 62.2 Recovery Principles

Self-direction: Persons determine their own path of recovery through their choices.

Individualized and person centered: There are multiple personal paths to recovery.

Empowerment: People have the right to participate in all decisions that affect their lives.

Holistic: Recovery encompasses the mind, body, and spirit, and all aspects of life: housing, employment, social interactions, and community integration.

Nonlinear: Recovery is not a linear process, setbacks are normal, but progress is possible.

Strengths based: Recovery focuses on the talents and strengths of the person.

Peer support: Mutual support helps people learn from one another in recovery.

Respect: Self-acceptance and challenging mental illness stigmas are important parts of recovery.

Responsibility: Persons must take personal responsibility for their own recovery process.

Hope: Recovery provides the essential and motivating message of a better future.

Data from Substance Abuse and Mental Health Services Administration. (2006). *National consensus statement on mental health recovery* [Brochure]. Retrieved from http://download.ncadi.samhsa.gov/ken/pdf/SMA05-4129/trifold.pdf

TABLE 62.1 Mental Health Treatment Settings and Role of Occupational Therapist

Setting	Target Population	Average Length of Stay	Focus of Intervention	Occupational Therapy Role/Task
Inpatient acute general or psychiatric specialty hospital	People with acute symptoms—depression, psychosis, mania, alcohol or drug toxicity	3–7 d	Crisis stabilization, patient safety, start or adjust medication, comprehensive assessment	Participate in therapeutic milieu, initial functional assessment, and additional assessments as indicated; contribute to multidisciplinary treatment plan; lead therapeutic groups
Long-term care "locked" facilities—public or private	People who continue to experience severe symptoms or are considered dangerous after a short hospital stay	3 mo to many years	Secure placement, rehabilitation, community reintegration when possible	Assessments, group and individual sessions, community transition programs such as supported education or employment programs
Partial hospitalization and intensive outpatient	People who are no longer acute but still need daily supports to manage symptoms and begin recovery process	2–6 wk	Improve functional skills, resolve precipitants to recent hospitalization, refer to community resources	Individual assessment and intervention, therapeutic groups, case management, community reintegration
Community support/peer support programs	People with serious mental illness who need ongoing support to maintain community living	Indefinite, open-ended depending on client need	Ongoing support to maintain community living; assistance with jobs, housing, social skills, leisure activities, life management skills	Wellness and recovery planning tools; skill building; case management; therapy group leadership; staff training; social, educational, or recreational groups
Supported employment	People with serious mental illness who need ongoing support to maintain community living	Indefinite	Employment	Assisting clients to identify job skills and interests, help securing and keeping jobs, job development
Supported education	People with serious mental illness who need ongoing support to maintain community living	Indefinite	Education	Assisting clients to identify educational skills and interests, help entering the educational setting, referral to additional resources such as financial aid and tutoring as needed
Supported housing	People with serious mental illness who need ongoing support to maintain community living	Indefinite	Housing	Helping clients secure and maintain permanent housing through skill building, case management, and assessment of functional strengths and limitations; implementing of environmental modifications as needed

Institution-Based Services

Acute Inpatient Hospitalization

Persons with SMI often begin to display symptoms in early adulthood for various reasons. This can lead to an inpatient hospitalization if the individual is acutely psychotic, depressed, suicidal, manic, or displaying other behaviors that might pose a threat to self or others. Some individuals seek voluntary admission in order to receive evaluation, treatment, and medication that will enable them to stabilize and resume their lives in a safe environment. While in the hospital, the focus is brief intervention to stabilize symptoms and provide a comprehensive evaluation and diagnosis. At times, hospitalization is needed to start or change medications and monitor significant side effects. A multidisciplinary team of health care professionals, including physicians, nurses, social workers, and occupational therapists work together to facilitate recovery.

TABLE 62.2 Key Functional Assessments Used in Mental Health Occupational Therapy

Title	Author(s)
Adolescent/Adult Sensory Profile	Brown & Dunn, 2002
Allen Cognitive Level Screen (ACLS)	Allen, 1985
Assessment of Motor and Process Skills (AMPS)	Pan & Fisher, 1994
Canadian Occupational Performance Measure (COPM)	Law et al., 2001
Kohlman Evaluation of Daily Living Skills (KELS)	McGourty, 1999
Occupational Performance History and Interview (OPHI)	Kielhofner et al., 1997

Occupational therapists working in inpatient mental health services make valuable contributions to the multidisciplinary treatment team. Starting with a comprehensive functional evaluation, they provide practical and functional interventions to help clients establish or reestablish healthy habits of daily living while on the unit and plan for community reintegration after discharge (Table 62.2). Interventions may be offered in both group and individual format, and topics include activities of daily living skills, anxiety management skills, social interaction skills, community living skills, and leisure activities such as arts and crafts, fitness, and sports (Duffy & Nolan, 2005).

In inpatient settings, occupational therapists are also involved in the design, development, and therapeutic application of "sensory rooms" for people with mental illness. These sensorimotor or multisensory rooms have been developed as environmental enhancements in response to new evidence that many people with SMI experience sensory challenges, especially during times of crisis. The individuals may benefit from interventions designed to calm or stimulate their sensory systems and help them avoid seclusion and restraint (Champagne & Stromberg, 2004). Multisensory rooms can include calming elements such as weighted blankets for deep pressure, rocking chairs, calming music, and relaxing oils such as lavender or vanilla. Stimulating elements can include exercise equipment, peppermint or citrus oils, art materials, and energetic music.

The changing health care environment mandates shorter lengths of inpatient stay and thus more rapid treatment, which has been challenging for some occupational therapists (Lloyd & Williams, 2010). In order for occupational therapists to remain valued members of inpatient psychiatric treatment teams, they need to be clear about the core elements of their practice, which are individual functional assessment, individual occupation-focused treatment, therapeutic group facilitation, and participation in discharge planning (Lloyd & Williams, 2010).

Partial Hospitalization/Intensive Outpatient Programs

Partial hospitalization programs (PHPs) and intensive outpatient programs (IOPs) are both forms of ambulatory behavioral health care services. These programs typically use a medical model approach to the provision of services and are associated with a hospital or an established health care center (Association for Ambulatory Behavioral Healthcare, 2007). Ambulatory services are designed for people of all ages who do not require 24-hour care but do need psychiatric care that is more intense than can be provided by outpatient visits. Services include a comprehensive evaluation of client needs and a coordinated array of active treatment components, delivered in a manner that is least disruptive to and/or simulates daily functioning. Services are delivered in the least restrictive environment, rely on client strengths, and use existing family and community supports.

Partial hospitalization programs are intended to divert the person from hospitalization or serve as an intermediary step toward community living after an acute inpatient course of treatment. The goal is to reduce acute symptoms and provide crisis intervention. Persons at this level exhibit severe symptoms that cause significant functional disability, possibly resulting from an acute illness/episode or the exacerbation of a chronic illness. Services are usually provided on a full-time basis with attendance in a daylong program at least 4 days per week. Medicare specifically lists occupational therapy as a covered service in PHPs (U.S. Department of Health and Human Services, Centers for Medicare and Medicaid Services, 2005).

Occupational therapy practitioners in this setting focus on comprehensive and accurate assessment of function; preparation for community reintegration;

Practice Dilemma

Because Sean and his family may agree that he needs services beyond the initial 2-week authorization period for the partial hospitalization program, the occupational therapist will need to communicate both his progress and his continuing need for treatment in functional terms to the insurance case manager. Write a note attempting to use strengths-based recovery language and including what you know about ongoing functional challenges for people with serious mental illness.

Ethical Dilemma

At the end of the second week in the partial hospitalization program, Sean is expressing a desire to attend less frequently, saying that he is feeling better. Sean's mother contacts you and expresses her concern about Sean, saying that he sleeps all day when he is not in the program, sometimes neglects his hygiene, and often seem "internally preoccupied," talking to himself and singing snatches of songs. You are scheduled to talk to the insurance case manager tomorrow and need to decide whether you should ask for authorization for more days. What do you do first?

and teaching of coping, stress management, and community living skills. **Intensive outpatient programs** are designed as a step down from PHPs. Persons at this level may be functioning adequately in one or more of their occupational roles but need more support or therapy than traditional outpatient treatment.

Community-Based Services

Supported Housing

Having a positive living environment offers a place for healing and stability and is an important factor in mental health recovery. Over the years, various housing models for people with SMI have emerged, including transitional housing, congregate or group housing, and supported housing. The supported housing model provides access to permanent housing and service supports, such as case management, employment assistance, and linkages to other community resources. Housing is permanent, and individuals may remain as long as they adhere to the requirements of the lease. Housing can include single-room units, shared apartments, or scattered-site units. Some models include several people living in an apartment or house with professional services on site. In "scattered site" programs, people live in the community and a support team offers regular visits for social support and to help residents maintain tenancy. Services can include crisis intervention, medication monitoring support, wellness promotion, transportation, assistance with activities of daily living, and linkage to educational and employment opportunities (Swarbrick, 2009).

The supported housing model is different from traditional residential programs that congregate unrelated adults in supervised settings with rules and restrictions. Some traditional residential programs are transitional, requiring persons to move from place to place, which can cause instability and crisis. Supportive housing evolved from the consumer advocacy and recovery movements and fosters growth through support of risk taking and individual choice.

Occupational therapists can assume important roles in supported housing programs, including support team leader, case manager, and individual skills training for home management, money management, employment, education, and community engagement (Swarbrick, 2009).

Supported Education

Many individuals living with mental illness are undereducated, meaning they have not achieved their desired level of education. Onset of illness often occurs in early adulthood and can interfere with the completion of higher education goals. Limited education can have far-reaching effects impacting self-esteem and employment outcomes and can propel people into a life of poverty. Supported education is an evolving model considered an emerging best practice to help individuals succeed in higher education. Educational goals include completing a general equivalency diploma (GED), obtaining a technical training certificate, taking adult education courses at a community college, or attaining a college degree. It is only recently that interventions, specifically targeting adult education, have been developed, with supported education being the most widely accepted approach. The supported education model evolved to address the specialized support needs some students with psychiatric disabilities required for success in pursuing educational goals (Anthony & Unger, 1991).

Students with psychiatric disabilities often need additional support for things such as negotiating accommodations with faculty; discussing test anxiety; managing general anxiety, personal issues, and challenges related to symptoms including problems with memory and concentration; and learning how to cope with an academic environment. Although most colleges offer disability services for students with psychiatric disabilities, students report that they are often reluctant to disclose their disability in order to access those services (Mowbray et. al., 2005).

Supported education assists people in pursuing academic goals in integrated postsecondary education settings. Services are individualized and flexible with an emphasis on student choice, self-determination, and career development. People learn to engage and maintain the valued role of postsecondary student so they can achieve academic goals in order to gain meaningful employment. Supported education models include a **classroom model** where students attend closed classes on campus, an **onsite model** that provides individualized support sponsored by an educational institution, a **mobile support model** that meets students with psychiatric disabilities in the community to provide individualized educational support, and a **freestanding model** that provides support at the organization which sponsors program (Arbesman & Logsdon, 2011).

Supported education services focus on career/vocational counseling and planning; teaching coping skills for managing stressors and symptoms; providing assistance with locating and accessing resources including

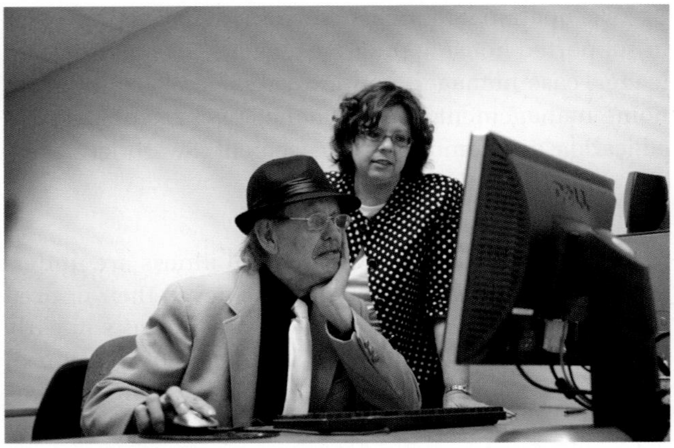

FIGURE 62.1 Learning to use the computer and Internet in a supported education program. (Photo courtesy of Christine Helfrich, PhD, OTR/L, FAOTA and Boston University Photography.)

financial aid, academic support, and applying for college; developing stress and time management skills; and referral and coordination with campus services as needed. Occupational therapists working in supported education programs may provide interventions and support in all of these areas.

An important role for occupational therapists working in supported education programs is to assist students with understanding their rights under the Americans with Disabilities Act, with securing reasonable accommodations in the classroom and with navigating disability support services to acquire them. Partnering with the office of disabilities should be an important function for these occupational therapists. They should also be aware of the many social variables that may prevent a student with a psychiatric disability from being successful at school, especially dealing with stigma and self-disclosure. Occupational therapists can be effective in helping students overcome challenges impacting school attendance, self-esteem issues, social awkwardness, and managing personal and family issues. Occupational therapists can offer assistance with stress and symptom management, such as the impact of medication on memory, retention, concentration, and problem solving. They can help students assess their needs, apply for reasonable accommodations, and learn coping skills to manage the daily stresses of academic life. Supported education programs can help people with psychiatric disabilities achieve college success, avoid unemployment, secure economic self-sufficiency, and improve their quality of life (see Figure 62.1).

Supported Employment

Supported employment is an approach to vocational rehabilitation that helps people with psychiatric disabilities to attain and succeed in competitive jobs (Becker & Drake, 2003). The Individual Placement and Support (IPS) model of supported employment ("Dartmouth IPS Supported Employment Center," n.d.) is an evidence-based approach to vocational rehabilitation for people with psychiatric disabilities (Box 62.3).

IPS-supported employment is a team-based model. The employment specialist joins one or more multidisciplinary teams: case management, assertive community treatment (ACT), intensive case management, supported housing, or other types of teams. The entire team is involved in helping the individuals select a good job match and securing employment. Occupational therapists often work on IPS teams as employment specialists, job coaches, or job developers, using their knowledge and skills in the areas of task analysis, grading of tasks, and modifying work environments to help clients achieve success. Based on a significant amount of research, IPS has been developed and refined for over two decades. The model has a clear procedural manual, a fidelity scale, and defined training procedures (Swanson & Becker, 2011). Extensive research on IPS includes 16 randomized controlled trials and numerous other notable international studies.

Peer-Operated Services

Peer-operated services are a part of the continuum of services available in the community for people with psychiatric disabilities and are based on the concept of peer support, a belief that people who have faced, endured, or overcome adversity can offer useful support, hope, and encouragement to others in similar situations. The peer-operated service model has been evolving throughout the world and in the United States is considered an essential ingredient in many people's mental health recovery.

BOX 62.3 Principles of Individual Placement and Support

Individual Placement and Support (IPS) principles include the following:

1. Zero exclusion—all clients who want employment are eligible
2. Competitive employment as the optimal goal
3. Client choice in all aspects of selecting, finding, and maintaining employment
4. Job development using a professional approach
5. Rapid job search, providing training on the job rather than prior to employment
6. Service integration—vocational plus housing, mental health, addiction, physical health services, and supports
7. Follow-along supports for as long as needed

CASE STUDY 62.1 Joseph

Joseph is a 51-year-old single male (never married) who has been in and out of the public mental health system during the past 30 years. During this time, he has been hospitalized many times and received numerous mental health diagnoses (schizophrenia, bipolar disorder). He is currently diagnosed with bipolar disorder and co-occurring alcohol dependence. About 9 months ago, he was referred to an assertive community treatment (ACT) team due to multiple short-term inpatient hospitalizations during a 14-month period of time. He was referred to the occupational therapist to review his strengths, needs, and goals and to develop a recovery plan. Joseph is the second of seven siblings. At age 9 years, he experienced a very stressful traumatic incident (sexual abuse by a relative). He was first diagnosed with mental illness at age 21 years, although records indicate that family reported signs of abnormal behavior as early as 10 years of age.

Physical Status

Joseph has a primary health care physician and schedules regular physical examinations. He recently was prescribed reading glasses and sometimes experiences blurred vision, which he believes is a side effect of the medication. He recently has been diagnosed with fibromyalgia and reports intense pain and bouts of sleeplessness. He reported that when he follows a regular sleep and wake schedule, he seems to feel better physically, emotionally, and socially. However, he has significant difficulty adhering to a regular routine because of many factors that he had difficulty clarifying. Joseph is currently taking prescribed psychiatric medications (Risperdal injections bimonthly and Depakote daily) that make him feel tired and he believes have contributed to recent weight gain. He is very concerned about his weight and periodically makes a conscious effort to eat a balanced diet and include exercise in his daily routine. He reports that he is negatively impacted when he consumes energy drinks such as Red Bull or when he consumes coffee or caffeinated beverages in the evening. He has been smoking for more than 30 years and is planning to quit smoking sometime soon as he feels it is starting to slow him down. Joseph acknowledges that alcohol has contributed to many negative events and losses in his life. He states that he realizes the needs to take medication to maintain mental and emotional stability, although he has major concerns regarding side effects (short and long term), especially how the medication slows him down and contributes to weight gain. This leads to struggles with health care providers and family over whether or not to take medication.

Psychosocial

Joseph reports that he frequently feels lonely and is disappointed that he has not achieved many of his life goals; this distress sometimes leads to drinking. He likes to offer support for peers, although he sometimes has become extremely vulnerable to peers who take advantage of his kindness, especially when he is under the influence of alcohol. During the past few years, he feels he has done a better job of creating better boundaries with such peers. He has developed the strength and confidence to assert clear boundaries; however, he does continue to report an intense sense of loneliness. He reports feeling very uncomfortable interacting with the ACT staff (especially the younger staff and nurses) because he feels they label him as a "hypochondriac" and tend to minimize his concerns. He realizes that he sometimes alienates people who care for him and sometimes harbors false suspicions in his mind. He states that due to the frequent turnover of staff in the programs he has attended in the past, he finds it difficult to trust staff members.

Vocational/Avocational/Financial

Joseph has had many jobs: lawn work/landscaping for older neighbors, caddy and painter, seasonal retail work, support work in mental health and developmental disability programs, maintenance worker, gas attendant, laborer, and school bus driver. He particularly feels proud of his work with adults with developmental disabilities and derives much satisfaction and pleasure from using his talents to help others. Eight years ago, he did some volunteer work with adults with Alzheimer's disease, developmental disabilities, and other cognitive problems. He liked this type of work but found that he becomes overly concerned and distressed regarding the conditions of people he was assisting. He desires to find volunteer or paid work opportunities to use his talents and skills so he can improve his sense of purpose and meaning. The ACT team and his family often discourage him from working because they believe it is too stressful for him. Joseph confided to the occupational therapist that this makes him feel angry because they don't believe he is capable of working, whereas he feels he is.

Joseph reads the newspaper, watches the news, and periodically goes to the local library. He is a high school graduate. Although he did not complete college, he has a tremendous ability to recall knowledge from his past educational and learning experiences. He did attend some various technical training programs and 1 year of college. He is interested in learning new information particularly in the areas of the environment and new technology such as computers. He likes to share what he learns. He appreciates receiving recognition and guidance from those with more knowledge and experience.

Joseph is currently living on a very limited budget ($820. 00 per month) and receives a housing subsidy to live in a studio apartment. He has the ability to manage money effectively, although at times, he becomes impulsive and spends his allocated money for the week too quickly. He has started reviewing supermarket circulars on weekends so he can plan his weekly spending to purchase important food and household items. Joseph takes pride in his appearance and apartment. He has determined a budget so he can do his wash at the Laundromat and purchase good food and household supplies. He wants a part-time job so he can eat out once in a while, purchase new clothing, and eventually plan to save for the future (a trip, or maybe a car).

The ACT team has encouraged Joseph to attend a peer program and a dual diagnosis of "double trouble" program for people with psychiatric disabilities and substance use issues. Joseph indicated he has tried those places, but the drop-in center tends to attract too many peers who are actively drinking or using drugs. Joseph states that he feels vulnerable to manipulation by others in these programs because of his intense loneliness.

(continued)

CASE STUDY 62.1 Joseph (*Continued*)

Role of the Occupational Therapist

The occupational therapist working in the ACT team will help Joseph with the following goals, which will help him develop an increased sense of purpose, become more self-sufficient, and move toward financial independence.

1. Maintain a daily healthy routine: wake up and go to sleep at set times, plan and eat healthy meals each day, and follow a moderate exercise routine.
2. Cut down or stop smoking.
3. Develop and maintain a monthly budget.
4. Set, list, and complete daily activities.
5. Find a part-time job or volunteer position at least three to four times a week (3 to 5 hours per day).
6. Develop an improved ability to effectively communicate his needs to the staff.

Occupational therapists link people to peer resources and also provide consultation and mentoring for the development and growth of peer programs (Swarbrick, 2009; Swarbrick & Pratt, 2006). "Clubhouse" programs are typically drop-in centers developed and run by people with psychiatric disabilities, offering a range of social, educational, and recreational opportunities (International Center for Clubhouse Development, 2011). Funding for clubhouse programs varies—some state Medicaid plans pay for this service but most do not. Clubhouses may be sponsored by a public or private mental health agency or they may be freestanding programs, and programs may be partially or completely peer operated. Additional programs such as member transportation, housing, homeless outreach, supported employment, supported education, physical health maintenance, and improvement may also be offered in clubhouse model programs.

There are a wide array of institutional and community support programs for people with SMI. Occupational therapists may be employed in any of these programs in various capacities, from direct service provider to case manager, consultant, program coordinator, or director.

Conclusion

Advances in research, public policy, and consumer advocacy have led to a systems transformation in treating people with SMI. Recovery from mental illness is now viewed as both possible and desirable. People living with mental illness should not be stigmatized or excluded from society but instead offered opportunities to flourish in communities of their choice. Treatment and services that range from short-term acute care through outpatient care and community-based services such as peer programs, supported housing, and supported employment are increasingly the norm. Occupational therapists can be key members of mental health treatment and service teams in all these programs, promoting occupation, wellness, and community integration.

In the last 10 years, the heart of psychosocial occupational therapy practice has shifted from institution to community. Occupational therapists can help foster client involvement in meaningful occupation, provide functional skills assessment, plan and implement wellness-focused interventions, train peers and professional staff, and participate in program development and leadership. At this time, occupational therapists can make meaningful contributions to improving the lives of people with SMI, especially in the areas of managing comorbid conditions and promoting wellness.

References

Allen, C. K. (1985). *Occupational therapy for psychiatric diseases: Measurement and management of cognitive disabilities.* Boston: Little, Brown & Company.

American Psychiatric Association. (2000). *Diagnostic and statistical manual of mental disorders* (4th ed., text rev.). Washington, DC: Author.

Anthony, W. A., & Unger, K. V. (1991). Supported education: An additional program resource for young adults with long-term mental illness. *Community Mental Health Journal, 27,* 145–156.

Arbesman, M., & Logsdon, D. (2011). Occupational therapy interventions for employment and education for adults with serious mental illness: A systematic review. *American Journal of Occupational Therapy, 65,* 238–246.

Association for Ambulatory Behavioral Healthcare. (2007). *Fast facts about partial hospitalization.* Retrieved from http://aabh.org/about-aabh-fast-facts/

Becker, D. R., & Drake, R. E. (2003). *A working life for people with severe mental illness.* New York, NY: Oxford Press.

Brown, C., Cromwell, R. L., Filion, D., Dunn, W., & Tollefson, N. (2002). Sensory processing in schizophrenia: Missing and avoiding information. *Schizophrenia Research, 55,* 187–195.

Brown, C., & Dunn, W. (2002). *Adolescent/adult sensory profile.* San Antonio, TX: Psychological Corporation.

Center for Mental Health Services. (2010). *The 10 by 10 campaign: A national action plan to improve life expectancy by 10 years in 10 years for people with mental illnesses. A report of the 2007 National Wellness Summit* (HHS Publication No. [SMA] 10-4476). Rockville, MD: Center for Mental Health Services, Substance Abuse and Mental Health Administration.

Center for Psychiatric Disability. (2011). *What is psychiatric disability and mental illness?* Retrieved from http://www.bu.edu/cpr/reasaccom/whatis-psych.html.

Champagne, T. (2006). *Sensory modulation and environment: Essential elements for occupation. General handbook and references* (2nd ed.). Southampton, MA: Champagne Conferences and Consultation.

Champagne, T. & Stromberg, N. (2004). Sensory approaches in inpatient psychiatric settings: innovative alternatives to seclusion and restraint. *Journal of Psychosocial Nursing, 42*(9), 35–44.

Dartmouth IPS Supported Employment Center. (n.d.). Retrieved from www.dartmouth.edu/~ips/

Duffy, R., & Nolan, P. (2005). A survey of the work of occupational therapists in inpatient mental health settings. *Mental Health Practice, 8*(6), 36–41.

International Center for Clubhouse Development. (2011). *International standards for clubhouse development.* Retrieved from http://www.iccd.org/quality.html

Kessler, R. C., Heeringa, S., Lakoma, M. D., Petukhova, M., Rupp, A. E., Schoenbaum, M., . . . Zaslavsky, A. M. (2008). Individual and societal effects of mental disorders on earnings in the United States: Results from the national comorbidity survey replication. *American Journal of Psychiatry, 165,* 663–665.

Kielhofner, G., Mallinson, T., Crawford, C., Novak, M., Rigby, M., Henry, A., & Walens, D. (1997). *A User's Guide to the Occupational Performance History II* (OPHI-II; Version 2.0). Chicago, IL: Model of Human Occupation Clearing House, Department of Occupational Therapy, College of Applied health Sciences, University of Illinois.

Law, M., Baum, C., & Dunn, W. (Eds). (2001). *Measuring occupational performance: supporting best practice in occupational therapy.* Thorofare, NJ: Slack.

Lloyd, C., & Williams, P. L. (2010). Occupational therapy in the modern acute mental health setting: A review of current practice. *International Journal of Therapy and Rehabilitation, 17,* 483–493.

Mayo Foundation for Medical Education and Research. (2011). *Symptoms of mental illness.* Retrieved from http://www.mayoclinic.com/health/mental-illness/DS01104/DSECTION=symptoms

McGourty, L. K. (1999). Kohlman evaluation of living skills. In B. J. Hemphill-Pearson (Ed.), *Assessments in occupational therapy mental health: An integrative approach* (pp. 231–242). Thorofare, NJ: Slack.

Medicare Benefit Policy Manual. (2011). *Chapter 15, covered medical and other health services, §§220 and 230.*

Mowbray, C. T., Collins, M. E., Bellamy, C. D., Megivern, D. A., Bybee, D., & Szilvagyi, S. (2005). Supported education for adults with psychiatric disabilities: An innovation for social and psychological rehabilitation practice. *Social Work,* 50(1),7–20.

National Institute of Mental Health. (2010). *Mental Health Medications.* NIH Publication No. 12-3929.

Osgood, D. M., Foster, D., & Courtney, M. (2010). Vulnerable populations and the transition to adulthood. *The Future of Children, 20*(1), 209–229. doi:10.1353/foc.0.0047

Pan, W. A. & Fisher, A. G. (1994). The Assessment of Motor and Process Skills of persons with psychiatric disabilities. *American Journal of Occupational Therapy, 48*(9), 775–780.

Reid, D. (2009). Capturing presence moments: The art of mindful practice in occupational therapy. *Revue Canadienne D'ergotherapie,* 76, 50–56.

Substance Abuse and Mental Health Services Administration. (2006). *National consensus statement on mental health recovery* [Brochure]. Retrieved from http://download.ncadi.samhsa.gov/ken/pdf/SMA05-4129/trifold.pdf

Substance Abuse and Mental Health Services Administration. (2011). *SAMHSA News Release: SAMHSA announces a working definition of "recovery" from mental disorders and substance use disorders.* Retrieved from www.samhsa.gov/newsroom/advisories/1112223420.aspx

Swanson, S. J., & Becker, D. R. (2011). *Supported employment: Applying the individual placement and support (IPS) model to help clients compete in the workforce.* Center City, MN: Hazelden.

Swarbrick, M. (1997). A wellness model for clients. *Mental Health Special Interest Section Newsletter, 20,* 1-4.

Swarbrick, M. (2006). A wellness approach. *Psychiatric Rehabilitation Journal, 29,* 311-314

Swarbrick, M. (2009). Does supportive housing impact quality of life? *Occupational Therapy in Mental Health, 25,* 352–366.

Swarbrick, M., & Pratt, C. (2006). Consumer-operated self-help services: Roles and opportunities for occupational therapy practitioners. *OT Practice, 11*(5), CE1–CE8.

U.S. Department of Health and Human Services, Centers for Medicare and Medicaid Services. (2005). *Medicare intermediary manual, part 3—Claims process.* Retrieved from https://www.cms.gov/Regulations-and-Guidance/.../R28GI.pdf

U.S. Department of Health and Human Services, Substance Abuse and Mental Health Administration. (2010). *Mental health, United States.* Rockville, MD: Author.

For additional resources on the subjects discussed in this chapter, visit http://thePoint.lww.com/Willard-Spackman12e.

CHAPTER 63

A Woodworker's Hand Injury

Restoring a Life

Karen Roe Garren

OUTLINE

LEARNING OBJECTIVES

After reading this chapter, you will be able to:

1. Describe the primary elements found in an evaluation for a person with a hand injury
2. Identify objective measures that might be used to evaluate a complex injury
3. Describe client-centered goal setting
4. Understand the use of functional activities to restore specific anatomical function and client-desired function
5. Describe the use of physical agent modalities to enhance healing and restoration of function

Therapist Narrative

Over years of practice, I have learned to incorporate methods such as physical agent modalities, manual therapy techniques, and wound care into hand therapy. However, occupational therapy methods and philosophy have always been the foundation of my therapeutic approach. Helping clients to achieve occupational goals requires more than tissue healing and joint mobility. I have learned that recovery is a fabric woven from psychological, spiritual, and physical pain. Hand therapy is about restoring meaning in client's lives as well as restoring tissue function.

Case Description: Don

It was a shock to hear that the father-in-law of a woman who worked in our building had cut his hand badly in a table saw. When he actually walked into the clinic, it was one of those moments when I could feel my heart sink. Don is a 58-year-old fine woodworker who built spectacular and complex crown moldings and built-ins in very upscale homes. He had indeed put his left hand through a table saw at work 10 days earlier. I had just gotten a call from the hand surgeon upstairs telling me that he was sending Don down to be seen immediately for splinting and to start therapy. This doctor had not done the surgery; Don had been rushed to a hospital near where he worked some distance away and was operated on there by a plastic surgeon. The operative report was not available, but from what the doctor was able to ascertain, Don had lacerated his hand through his proximal palm and severed both flexor tendons to his long and ring fingers, amputated his small finger at the metacarpal phalangeal joint (MP), and lacerated the nerves to all his fingers. The doctor was not sure about the involvement to Don's thumb and index fingers. Don had arrived in his office bandaged and protected only by a wrist support with the fingers free to move at the proximal interphalangeal joints (PIPs). This was not good. I brought Don in immediately and told him not to move anything. He said that the doctor had just told him that, but that the only thing he had been told at discharge from the hospital was to follow up in a week. He thought wiggling his fingers was good because they were not immobilized.

There are critical elements to consider in dealing with a patient who has recently undergone reconstructive surgery of tendons and nerves. The first and foremost concern is to protect the repair. I knew enough history from the brief discussion with the referring surgeon to know that I needed to get Don into a protective splint as quickly as possible to reduce the tension on the tendon and nerve repairs and to stop any active motion of the repaired tendons (Duran & Houser, 1975; Taras, Martyak, & Steelman, 2011). I also needed to assess the wound to determine the integument (skin) condition and, because no operative report was available, to visually assess the exact anatomical level of injury. During this process, I was monitoring his reactions to the situation. It can be an extremely emotional time, and patients often have not even looked at their wounds. I keep ammonia capsules and facial tissues readily available. Don seemed to be coping by focusing on the process and asking questions. At the same time, I needed to reassure Don that his zeal to get his fingers moving had probably not ruptured the repairs because he assured me that he could wiggle them. I do not deceive patients, but informing Don of all of the possible ramifications at that point would only have distressed him, and I needed him to be focused on where we were going and what he was going to need to do. Once Don's hand was bandaged in a dry dressing and he was safely tucked into a dorsal blocking splint that positioned his wrist in 30 degrees of flexion, his MPs in 70 degrees of flexion, and his PIPs and distal phalangeal joints (DIPs) in as much extension as he could actively produce (the ideal is full extension, but he was already contracted, and applying any force could compromise the repairs), I could safely continue his evaluation.

Note: Those with occupational performance limitations secondary to hand and/or upper extremity injuries, potentially interact with occupational therapists (OTs) and certified occupational therapy assistants (COTAs) in a variety of settings (see Box 63.1).

Don's Evaluation and Goal Setting

The evaluation consisted of the following:

Subjective examination and background

- Age, hand dominance
- Date and mechanism of injury
- Functional capability/work status
- Activities of daily living (ADL) status/help status
- Chief complaints: pain, loss of function, sensory changes, and/or sleep problems
- Rehabilitation expectations/goals
- Medical management and review of medical/surgical records, including available radiographic summaries.
- Awareness of pathology/precautions/contraindications/physician orders
- Past relevant medical history

Don was 58 years old at the time of the accident, right-handed, and married. He worked full time as a woodworker and loved his job. He wanted to return to his occupation as soon as it was possible to do so; he needed to be able to lift and carry wood supplies, hold and manipulate tools and hardware, and stabilize wood with his left hand. Secondary to being immobilized in the splint, Don was unable to use his left hand for any self-care; however, over the previous week, he had become sufficiently proficient with his right hand alone to manage to dress, feed, bathe, and even drive himself. His wife managed the meals and household tasks. Initially, his chief complaints were loss of function, inability to move his hand, and numbness in all of his fingers. Don could not describe exactly how the accident had happened except that he was cutting wood on the table saw and it caught, pulling his hand down on the blade. This is a familiar story. The blade spins at an incredible speed, and when things go wrong, it is too fast to actually see or react. A table saw blade does not cut like a knife but consists of teeth that are a series of angled chisels that are an eighth of an inch wide or more. It leaves a fairly wide slot when it cuts wood. The same happened to Don's hand. The blade had amputated his small finger and continued across his proximal palm in zone 3. When the tendons and nerves were cut, the result was that several millimeters of tissue were missing as well as skin and thenar and hypothenar muscle. It follows that when the ends of the tendons and nerves were sutured together, the result was shortening of the muscles, tendons, and nerves, creating additional tension on the repair.

Objective examination

- Integument
- Range of motion (ROM)
- Sensation
- Edema

BOX 63.1 Provision of Occupational Therapy: Clients with Performance Challenges Secondary to Hand and Upper Extremity Injuries

In many instances, these clients are treated by occupational therapists specializing in this practice area and who carry the additional credential of "certified hand therapist." The majority of these injuries are treated in outpatient hospital settings or private practices. However, the setting and progression through the settings is determined by the type and severity of injury, insurance coverage, and client preference (see Figure 63.1 for two examples).

A variety of sources of funding/reimbursement are available for these services. Examples include the following:

- Medicare Part A. Covers outpatient services. Clients may be seen two to three times per week for up to 3 months.
- Medicaid. Covers 20 visits per year. After this, an authorization request may be sent to the referring physician to continue intervention.
- Private insurance. Coverage varies greatly based on plan. If the plan covers the service, clients are usually seen two to three times per week for up to 3 months as needed.
- Private pay.
- Workmen's compensation. A case file must be opened, and authorization for services varies greatly based on insurance. For example, a client may be authorized for 6 to 12 visits. After this, further authorization is required.

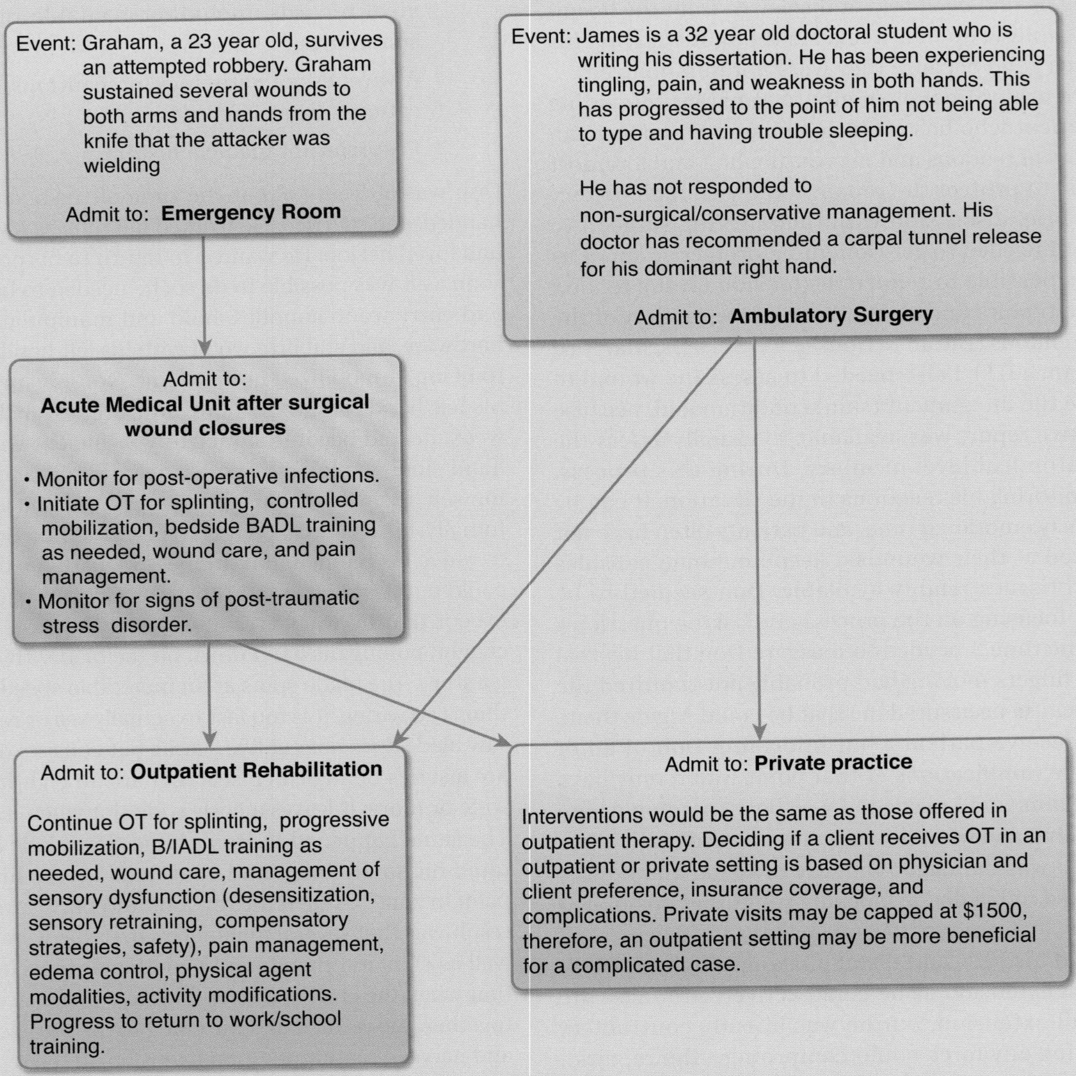
Event: Graham, a 23 year old, survives an attempted robbery. Graham sustained several wounds to both arms and hands from the knife that the attacker was wielding
Admit to: Emergency Room
Event: James is a 32 year old doctoral student who is writing his dissertation. He has been experiencing tingling, pain, and weakness in both hands. This has progressed to the point of him not being able to type and having trouble sleeping.
He has not responded to non-surgical/conservative management. His doctor has recommended a carpal tunnel release for his dominant right hand.
Admit to: Ambulatory Surgery
Admit to: Acute Medical Unit after surgical wound closures
• Monitor for post-operative infections.
• Initiate OT for splinting, controlled mobilization, bedside BADL training as needed, wound care, and pain management.
• Monitor for signs of post-traumatic stress disorder.
Admit to: Outpatient Rehabilitation
Continue OT for splinting, progressive mobilization, B/IADL training as needed, wound care, management of sensory dysfunction (desensitization, sensory retraining, compensatory strategies, safety), pain management, edema control, physical agent modalities, activity modifications. Progress to return to work/school training.
Admit to: Private practice
Interventions would be the same as those offered in outpatient therapy. Deciding if a client receives OT in an outpatient or private setting is based on physician and client preference, insurance coverage, and complications. Private visits may be capped at $1500, therefore, an outpatient setting may be more beneficial for a complicated case.

FIGURE 63.1 Two examples of progression through treatment settings. *BADL*, basic activities of daily living; *IADL*, instrumental activities of daily living; *OT*, occupational therapy.

To evaluate Don's hand, I needed to keep in mind the protocol that I would use to guide his physical recovery. There are multiple protocols to choose from, with extensive research supporting advantages and disadvantages. Most surgeons have a preferred pathway or protocol, and the therapist must be aware of these differences in preference. Pettengill (2005) has written a historical perspective on the research of tendon rehabilitation, with a comparison of the most recent early active motion protocols. My input is usually taken into consideration; however, it is the doctor who decides which protocol he or she wants to follow. The doctor who made this referral does not like to use any of the early active motion protocols because he thinks that research has shown that there is a greater risk of rupture. In Don's case, it was not an option because his was not a clean and simple wound, we were not starting therapy 3 days after surgery, and we had no knowledge of what suturing technique had been used to repair the tendons. In fact, we were beginning at the 10th day, which is when research has demonstrated that the tendon tissue actually softens and is at the highest risk of rupture. The doctor was concerned about the amount of trauma and the significant amount of scarring and wanted to minimize adhesions (bands of scar tissue that binds together two anatomic surfaces that are normally separated), so I used the modified Duran protocol (Duran & Houser, 1975) to begin early passive flexion with restricted active extension of the fingers but held any active motion until the sixth week. With his wrist and MPs splinted in flexion and his interphalangeal joints (IPs) in extension, I taught Don to passively flex his fingers into his palm and actively extend his fingers as far as the splint would allow. This allowed a few millimeters of tendon excursion with minimal resistance on the repair and has been shown by research to reduce tendon adhesions. On visual inspection, his hand was moderately swollen, indicative of inflammation, and he was not able to fully flex his fingers to his palm. Don had multiple system trauma involving not only the tendons but also nerves, muscle, palmar fascia, and skin. I tested his sensation with the Semmes-Weinstein Monofilament Test (Bell-Krotoski, 2002) because I was not sure whether all the digital nerve branches were severed. The test revealed loss of protective sensation or complete numbness in the median and ulnar nerves to his index, long, and ring fingers.

Setting goals for Don's therapy ultimately centered on what Don wanted to accomplish. The doctor always pushes for a perfect physical outcome, and usually the patient is in agreement; however, returning the patient to his or her previous job is not automatically a goal. I often do not set a return-to-work goal in the initial evaluation when there is a traumatic injury because it can be too early to determine what the patient wants and what the potential might be in terms of ability, time, and opportunity. Woodworking was Don's passion, not just his job. He had built something for each of his grandchildren, and he was anxious to build a rocking horse for his new grandchild.

For the next 5 weeks, the goals for Don were to understand the pathology, precautions, and home exercise program to increase his passive finger flexion; facilitate wound healing; and remodel scar to ensure necessary restoration of strength to the tendon tissues while safely allowing mobility through the adjacent tissues (Pettengill, 2011). The splint would not come off until the sixth week after surgery, so there could be no functional use of his hand. Don was diligent in his exercises and quickly recovered full passive finger flexion. He reported that he was keeping his hand elevated as much as possible to help decrease the swelling. The sutures were removed at 21 days with full skin closure. It was not until 4 weeks after his surgery that we finally got a copy of his original operative report revealing that there had been repair to his palmar arch, flexor pollicis longus to his thumb, and flexor digitorum superficialis (FDS) and flexor digitorum profundus (FDP) to his index finger, which had been only partially lacerated. The additional information helped me to anticipate what limitations there might be when the splint came off. Potential limitations included difficulty or inability to actively flex his thumb IP joint and index PIP and DIP joints due to scar adhesions or rupture from lack of protection in the first week postop.

Interventions and Ongoing Evaluation

Don's treatment initially consisted of manual ROM; dressing changes; and, when the sutures were removed, moist heat, low-intensity ultrasound, and manual scar massage to increase the soft tissue extensibility and remodel the scar. His treatment was a team effort with Erin (the other therapist in the clinic), Don, and me. This partnership required mutual attentiveness, the act of listening, and engaging in conversation in order for Don's feelings, needs, and desires to become part of the common understanding between Don, Erin, and myself (Crepeau, 1991; Crepeau & Garren, 2011; Rosendahl & Ross, 1982; Tickle-Degnen, 2008).

Six weeks after surgery was the next major hurdle for Don. The splint came off, and he was allowed to start moving his fingers (see Table 63.1). It was hard to prepare Don for the disappointment that he felt when his fingers did not actively flex into a fist. His hope was beyond realistic expectation, but Don just wanted to move forward and do whatever it took to be able to use his hand again. He still had no sensation in his fingers.

His goals were to increase the active range of motion (AROM) of his fingers and wrist to pull up his pants, button his pants, hold a washcloth to bathe, and eventually hold tools to return to work. This required heat modalities; low-intensity 3-MHz ultrasound (Michlovitz, 2005); and manual therapy to facilitate healing, increase soft tissue mobility, and remodel scar. We used occupational coaching (Clark, Ennevor, & Richardson, 1996) to teach Don the skills and strategies he needed for attaining the mutually agreed-on goals. Occupational coaching involves several techniques

TABLE 63.1 AROM (in Degrees) at 6 Weeks Post Surgery

6 Weeks Post Surgery	MP (0–90)	PIP (0–100)	DIP (0–80)
Index	0/60	−30/60	−10/30
Long	0/55	−30/45	−10/10
Ring	0/30	−35/45	−5/5
Thumb	−10/35		0/25
Wrist: 25/60			

AROM, active range of motion; DIP, distal interphalangeal joint; MP, metacarpal phalangeal joint; PIP, proximal interphalangeal joint.

TABLE 63.2 AROM (in Degrees) at 10 Weeks Post Surgery

10 Weeks Post Surgery	MP (0–90)	PIP (0–100)	DIP (0–80)
Index	0/80	−20/100	−10/65
Long	0/80	−35/92	−15/45
Ring	0/30	−35/70	0/25
Thumb	−10/50		−20/75
Wrist: 55/70			

AROM, active range of motion; DIP, distal interphalangeal joint; MP, metacarpal phalangeal joint; PIP, proximal interphalangeal joint.

aimed at moving Don toward a positive view of engagement in occupations. Examples of techniques include giving encouragement, making positive remarks, and teaching about occupation's role in recovery. We created a therapeutic alliance in which we worked in the presence of one another. Erin and I served a supportive function while guiding Don in an occupation-based intervention (Tickle-Degnen, 2008). As Don presented with a loss of protective sensation as measured by the Semmes-Weinstein Monofilament Test, we taught Don sensory loss precautions so that he would not accidentally burn or cut himself. His home program was expanded to include paraffin (to improve soft tissue extensibility) and a mini-vibrator (for scar remodeling and desensitization); however, he discovered that his hot tub water jets worked perfectly. Exercise and functional activities were initiated to increase his active motion and encourage grasp and pinch for pulling on clothes, holding utensils, and washing himself. He began desensitization for the scar and nerve hypersensitivity in his palm with particle immersion (submerging and moving the hand in rice and progressively more textured particles) and vibration (Pettengill, 2011).

For the next 6 weeks, Don used the dexerciser (a handheld wire maze that requires wrist and/or finger motion to move a washer along the wire), Chinese balls (2 to 2 ¾ in diameter smooth metal or enamel balls that are rotated around each other in the palm), pegboards, paper wadding, page turning, manipulating buttons, and pinching out beads in putty to regain active motion of his fingers. Experience guided the choice of these activities to promote tendon excursion through the very dense scar tissue in his palm and to train Don to begin to use his hand for light resistive functional activities. With this guided experience of how much pinch and grip force was safe, Don confidently began to try to use his hand safely at home for daily tasks. At 10 weeks, the tendons had healed sufficiently to add resistance using the hand gripper to pick up checkers (a strengthening device that uses graded rubber band resistance that when gripped separates two parallel bars held together by the rubber bands and when opened wide enough can fit and hold checkers, which can then be released into a container) and the BTE (work simulator/exercise machine) to increase the force against the scar adhesions that limited tendon excursion (Table 63.2). Sensation had begun to return in his distal palm, but his fingers remained numb.

His thumb, index, and long fingers progressed to full active flexion, but his ring finger had only 90 degrees of total motion. The loss of his small finger and severe limitation in active flexion of his ring finger due to adhesion of the FDP in his palm resulted in the syndrome of quadriga described by Verdan (1960), causing incomplete terminal flexion of his long and index fingers during grip. Quadriga is a phenomenon that results when one FDP tendon is tethered by proximal adhesions. This in turn will limit the remaining FDP tendons from proximal excursion and result in the inability to completely flex the fingers into a fist. It will also result in significant weakness in grip strength.

Don could not functionally grip a steering wheel or hold tools for work simulation. He was able to pinch and grip sufficiently to pull on clothes and bathe; however, buttoning and holding screws, boards, or nails were impaired by the sensory deficit.

Don's Second Surgery

At 12 weeks, the hand surgeon who had referred Don decided to take him back to surgery for a tenolysis (i.e., freeing the tendons from adhesions) or possible tendon repair depending on what he found when he opened Don's hand, so we discharged him to a home exercise program until he returned from surgery

Surgery revealed that the ulnar digital nerve to Don's ring finger was ruptured with a 2-cm defect between the proximal and distal ends. The proximal end of the digital nerve that had previously gone to his amputated small finger was in the immediate vicinity, so the surgeon connected that to the distal end of the ring finger ulnar digital nerve. On evaluation of the flexor tendons to the ring finger, it was discovered that both not only were extremely scarred down but also were attached only by pseudotendons (repaired tendons that fail to regenerate tendon tissue in the repair site but contain a section of scar tissue that lacks the tensile strength of tendon tissue). After tenolysis of both tendons, it was decided to leave the FDS alone and excise the pseudotendon to the FDP. A primary repair to the FDP was successfully performed with minimal loss of tendon excursion.

Don's Referral Back to Occupational Therapy

Don was referred to therapy 1 week after surgery for evaluation and initiation of treatment. His original splint was modified to free his index finger and thumb and his dressings were changed. Don was familiar with the Duran protocol and started passively ranging his long and ring fingers immediately. He required only one follow-up visit after the evaluation to achieve full passive range of motion (PROM) and was discharged to a home program until he came out of the splint to begin AROM. The biggest difference in the course of rehabilitation this time was that Don returned to work in a supervisory capacity as soon as the sutures were removed.

The doctor again decided to hold all active motion until the sixth week after surgery. Even though Don was ready this time for his finger not to move immediately, by the end of the first week of therapy, he was extremely frustrated and disappointed by the lack of progress. By the third week of therapy (9 weeks postoperative), Don was finally beginning to find it easier to do his self-care. Lack of sensation in the fingertips continued to be a problem, but Don was beginning to compensate. As patients progress through the healing process and therapy, they become more cognizant of their own physical and emotional capacity to return to previous occupations or accomplish their goals. Our goal at this juncture was to help Don begin to identify the problems that interfered with reentering or performing his occupation and to begin to plan possible solutions with him. Clark and colleagues (1996) identified this process as evoking insights in occupational storymaking. We chose many of the same activities to gain grip and pinch; however, we geared them as much as possible toward work using the nut and bolt board, pegs to simulate nails, and grasping of various-sized objects. Don had already learned how to use his hand safely for self-care tasks after the first surgery and expressed his desire to concentrate specifically on tasks that would restore function related to work.

At the 10th week, a dynamic PIP extension splint was added to reduce the flexion contracture in his ring finger and to mobilize the tendon distally through the scar adhesions by applying a low-load long duration force to manipulate the scar tissue (Pettengill, 2005). Don worked relentlessly at home, gripping putty in an attempt to force the tendon through the thick scar, but there was still no appreciable difference in flexion, and Don was devastated. At 12 weeks, the repair site had developed enough tendon tissue growth through the anastomosis to almost eliminate the possibility of rupture. On the basis of our experience, we decided to use iontophoresis with dexamethasone to reduce the inflammation and adhesions around the healing tendon. Within 1 week, Don had increased his ring finger flexion and was able to flex to his central palm (Table 63.3).

TABLE 63.3 AROM (in Degrees) at 12 Weeks Post Second Surgery

12 Weeks (Second Surgery)	MP (0–90)	PIP (0–100)	DIP (0–80)
Ring	WNL	−25/90	0/50

AROM, active range of motion; DIP, distal interphalangeal joint; MP, metacarpal phalangeal joint; PIP, proximal interphalangeal joint; WNL, within normal limits.

Don's therapeutic activities expanded to gripping tools and swinging a hammer into a pillow for

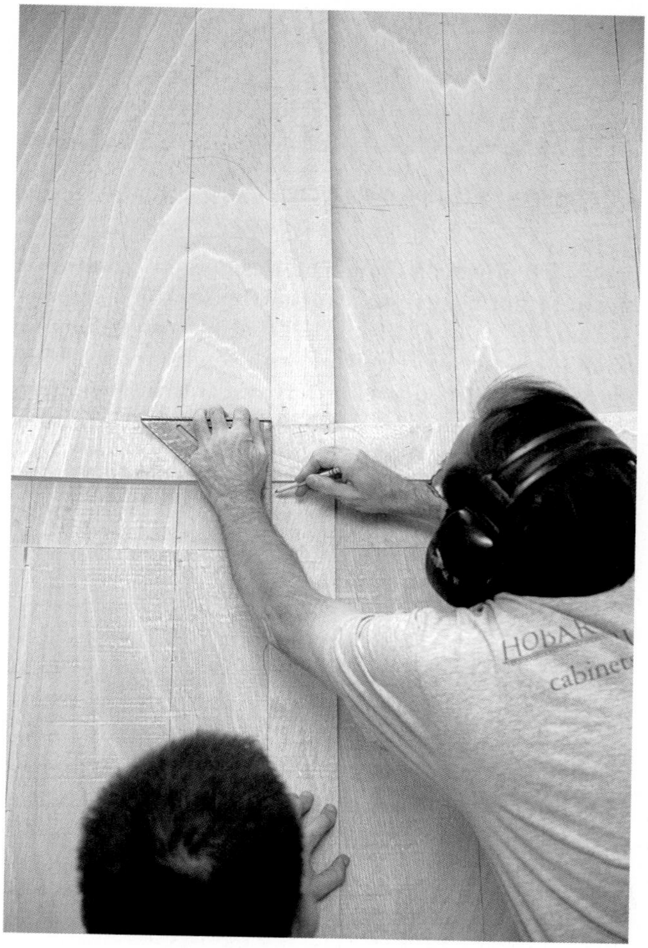

FIGURE 63.2 Don using a measuring triangle.

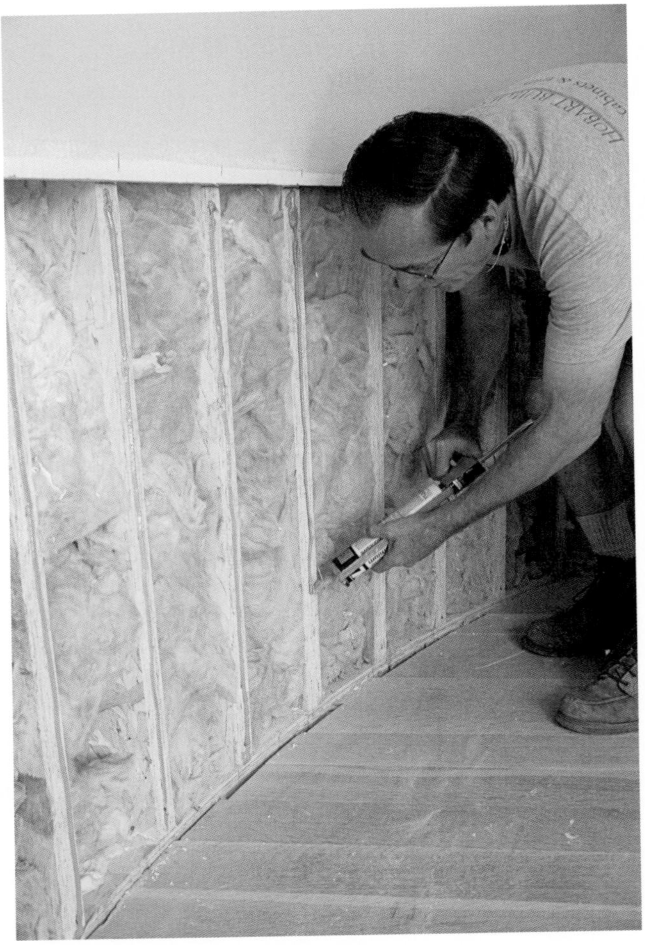

FIGURE 63.3 Don using a caulking gun.

controlled grip even though he was not left-handed. He began to notice a significant decrease in hypersensitivity in his palm and reported that he was picking up small pieces of wood at work with some success. At 15 weeks, he returned to full duty but was in a position to modify his activities when needed, lifting Sheetrock with his wrist instead of his fingers. At 18 weeks, he was discharged with L42/R130 lb of grip, L19/R27 lb of lateral pinch, and L12/R20 lb of three-point pinch; he was able to do his job and was working at home on his grandchild's rocking horse.

Epilogue

It has been a couple of years since Don left therapy, but he recently stopped by to drop off a *Fine Homebuilding* magazine in which there were pictures of him building complicated wainscot on a curved stairwell. Most notable in the pictures which Don proudly showed was his left hand holding a measuring triangle, holding a caulking

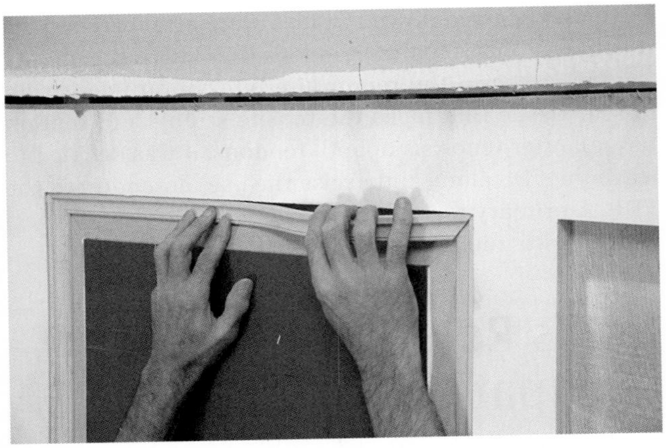

FIGURE 63.4 Don supporting molding against a wall.

gun, and supporting molding securely against the wall (Figures 63.2, 63.3, and 63.4).

References

Bell-Krotoski, J. A. (2002). Sensibility testing with the Semmes-Weinstein Monofilaments. In E. Mackin, A. Callahan, T. Skirven, L. Schneider, & A. Osterman (Eds.), *Rehabilitation of the hand and upper extremity* (5th ed., pp. 194–213). St. Louis, MO: Mosby.

Clark, F., Ennevor, B. L., & Richardson, P. L. (1996). A grounded theory of techniques for occupational storytelling and occupational storymaking. In R. Zemke & F. Clark (Eds.), *Occupational science: The evolving discipline* (pp. 373–392). Philadelphia, PA: F. A. Davis.

Crepeau, E. B. (1991). Achieving intersubjective understanding: Examples from an occupational therapy treatment session. *American Journal of Occupational Therapy, 45,* 1016–1025.

Crepeau, E. B., & Garren, K. R. (2011). I looked to her as a guide: The therapeutic relationship in hand therapy. *Disability and Rehabilitation, 33,* 872–881.

Duran, R., & Houser, R. (1975). Controlled passive motion following flexor tendon repair in zones 2 and 3. In *AAOS symposium on tendon surgery in the hand* (pp. 105–114). St. Louis, MO: Mosby.

Michlovitz, S. L. (2005). Is there a role for ultrasound and electrical stimulation following injury to tendon and nerve? *Journal of Hand Therapy, 18,* 292–296.

Pettengill, K. (2005). The evolution of early mobilization of the repaired flexor tendon. *Journal of Hand Therapy, 18,* 157–168.

Pettengill, K. (2011). Therapist's management of the complex injury. In L. Skirven, A. Osterman, J. Fedorczyk, & P. C. Amadio (Eds.), *Rehabilitation of the hand and upper extremity* (6th ed., pp. 1238–1251). St. Louis, MO: Mosby.

Rosendahl, P. P., & Ross, V. (1982). Does your behavior affect your patient's response? *Journal of Gerontological Nursing, 8,* 572–575.

Taras, J. S., Martyak, G.G., & Steelman, P.J. (2011). Primary care of flexor tendon injuries. In L. Skirven, A. Osterman, J. Fedorczyk, & P. C. Amadio (Eds.), *Rehabilitation of the hand and upper extremity* (6th ed., pp. 445–456). St. Louis, MO: Mosby.

Tickle-Degnen, L. (2008). Therapeutic rapport. In M. V. Radomski & C. A. Trombly Latham (Eds.), *Occupational therapy for physical dysfunction* (6th ed., pp. 402–420). Philadelphia, PA: Lippincott Williams & Wilkins.

Verdan C. (1960). Syndrome of the quadriga. *Surgical Clinics of North America, 40,* 425–426.

For additional resources on the subjects discussed in this chapter, visit http://thePoint.lww.com/Willard-Spackman12e.

CHAPTER 64

Providing Occupational Therapy for Older Adults with Changing Needs

Bette R. Bonder

LEARNING OBJECTIVES

After reading this chapter, the reader will be able to:

1. Discuss normal age-related changes that affect occupational performance
2. Describe health conditions and trajectories in later life as these affect occupational performance
3. Describe environmental factors that influence the experience of growing older
4. Discuss unique considerations in evaluating and intervening to support successful aging and minimize dysfunction in later life
5. Describe characteristics of health care systems that serve older adults
6. Describe social factors that support or impede successful aging
7. Discuss unique considerations in providing occupational therapy services to older adults throughout late life development
8. Analyze common ethical issues in providing occupational therapy services for older adults

OUTLINE

Introduction: Understanding the Life Course in Later Life

Older adults constitute the fastest growing segment of the population in the United States and in much of the world. At present, persons older than age 65 years constitute roughly 15% of the U.S. population; by 2050, it is expected that they will be more than 20% (U.S. Census Bureau, 2008). This rapid increase in older adults has significant implications for every aspect of life—workforce, education, economic development, and, of course, health care.

Although opinions vary about the precise consequences of an aging population for health care, there is no question that preventing health problems is both possible and desirable from an individual and a societal perspective. Researchers have increasingly focused on strategies for ensuring **successful aging**, maintaining positive quality of life as normal age-related physical and cognitive changes occur. Rowe and Kahn (1998) theorized that successful aging is based on three factors: avoiding disease and disability, maintaining mental and physical function, and maintaining active engagement with life. Although there have been several refinements and additions to this conceptualization, for example, noting that spirituality is a vital factor in successful aging (Crowther, Parker, Achenbaum, Larimore, & Koenig, 2002), there is general agreement that this model captures essential components of well-being in later life.

There are many actions that individuals of all ages can take to avoid disease and disability; however, to some extent, this is not within personal control. Likewise, it is possible to take several positive steps to maintain mental and physical function, although again, these do not guarantee that function will not decline. In fact, some degree of functional decline is a fact of life in later life (National Institutes of Health [NIH], 2007). The third factor, maintaining active engagement with life, is within individual control and is the central emphasis of occupational therapy (OT) (American Occupational Therapy Association [AOTA], 2008).

Therapist Narrative

One of my early experiences in working with older adults came when I was a research assistant on a study focused on the causes of falls. The study was undertaken in a low-income residential facility in an urban inner city. One of the questions posed to participants asked them to rate how happy they were. The researchers expected a low level of happiness because the participants were so economically disadvantaged. It was a surprise to learn that these individuals indicated they were very happy with their current lives, largely because they had the freedom to do what interested them, typically after many years earning a living at needed but unfulfilling work. Over the years that I have interacted with older adults, it has become increasingly evident to me that once basic needs for shelter and food are met, it is what one does and not what one has that makes for happiness in later life. There is no question that occupational therapists are central to promoting the ability of these individuals to do what matters most to them.

Occupational Therapy in Action: Mrs. Ramirez's Path through Later Life

In general, there has been a reduction in disabling health conditions in late life (Freedman, Schoeni, Martin, & Cornman, 2007). A common experience of aging is a gradual decline in aspects of body function and performance skills. Vision almost universally deteriorates; a condition known as *presbyopia* is readily accommodated using reading glasses. Hearing may worsen. Muscle mass decreases. These body function changes can affect motor and sensory-perceptual skills. Decline is often gradual for long periods of time, then punctuated by acute health problems that can accelerate functional loss. A bout of pneumonia may severely reduce cardiovascular endurance, a situation compounded by the fact that elders also take longer to recover and may never return to their pre-illness baseline.

Superimposed on this gradual decline with occasional acute episodes is the development of chronic health conditions such as arthritis, osteoporosis, and dementia, which have profound consequences for function and quality of life. Issues requiring special attention in later life include the following:

- Health conditions may have more benign (some cancers) or severe (pneumonia, influenza) consequences in late life.
- Decrements in sensory systems, cardiovascular and musculoskeletal function, and cognition are universal, although variable in degree.
- Multiple, sometimes conflicting, health conditions can complicate treatment choices (e.g., osteoporosis and arthritis).
- Social, economic, and environmental factors profoundly influence aging.

Background Information

Mrs. Estelle Ramirez is a 78-year-old widow when she first receives OT services. She lives alone in a third floor walk-up apartment in Brooklyn, New York—the apartment in which she raised her three daughters, now aged 56, 53, and 51 years. It is also where she and her husband lived together after the girls left home for college. Mrs. Ramirez and her husband moved to New York from Puerto Rico when Mr. Ramirez took a job in a factory. Mrs. Ramirez began working as an accountant when her girls were in high school. She retired at age 66 years to take care of her husband until in the late stages of Alzheimer's disease (AD). He died 4 years later.

Mrs. Ramirez believes herself to be in good health. She is of normal weight, and although she has joint pain that she characterizes as *artritis* (arthritis), it does not interfere very much with her function. She wears glasses, now trifocals, but sees reasonably well with them. She has noted lately that she has some difficulty seeing at night and as a result has chosen not to drive after sunset. She never drove much, preferring as do many New Yorkers to use public transportation but does not feel safe doing so after dark. These two factors have limited her evening activities, a fact that is causing her some distress. She has also begun to complain to her daughters about her memory. They note that she tends to repeat herself when speaking with them and that she sometimes forgets appointments.

Puerto Rican culture has a strong emphasis on *familismo*, a belief in the importance of strong family ties. In Mrs. Ramirez's case, this is reflected in the conversations that her daughters have had about whether Mrs. Ramirez should be living by herself, and there is growing tension regarding possible alternate arrangements. One daughter is adamant that Mrs. Ramirez should stay in her home with the three girls providing supportive care; one believes her mother should come live with her; and one is strongly in favor of moving her to an assisted living facility.

Since her husband's death, Mrs. Ramirez volunteers at the local elementary school reading to the children. She sees her daughters frequently because all three live in the New York City area. She takes great pleasure in spending time with her nine grandchildren and her first great-grandchild who was born last year; she particularly likes cooking traditional Puerto Rican meals and telling them about their heritage. She spends time at the local Hispanic Senior Center. She misses her husband and regrets that she had to stop working earlier than she would have liked, but she is reasonably satisfied with her current life and enjoys her apartment and neighbors.

First Encounter

Mrs. Ramirez was present when the consulting occupational therapist at the senior center made a presentation about home safety and provided a checklist for the participants so that they could assess their environments. As the therapist knows, falls are common among older populations and can have dire consequences (Tideiksaar, 2009), including significant disability or death. Mrs. Ramirez was very interested in the presentation, but because she does not have a current disability, there is no obvious source of funding for a therapist to come to her home to do an assessment. Funding for home safety interventions has been increasingly available for individuals with disabilities but there remains a significant gap in financial support for these efforts (Beattie & Peterson, 2007).

Reimbursement Issues and Ethical Dilemmas in Working with Older Adults

The funding difficulty that Mrs. Ramirez has encountered is not an unusual one for older adults. Although in the United States, individuals older than age 65 years benefit from being eligible for Medicare, a nearly universal form of health insurance for elders, Medicare has numerous—and frequently changing—limitations and regulations (Dal Bello-Haas & Tryssenaar, 2009). Medical services associated with preventive care (vaccinations, mammography, diabetes care) are covered, but preventive OT services are not. This is particularly unfortunate because there is strong research evidence that early intervention focused on lifestyle issues can maintain health and reduce costs (Clark et al., 2011).

Even when OT services are covered, there can be significant challenges providing needed care because of the regulations limiting reimbursement. This creates one of the many ethical dilemmas that confront occupational therapists working with elders. How can one ensure that vital services are made available in a reimbursement environment that regulates the kinds of goals that will be covered while also limiting providers' ability to impose charges for services not covered? Creativity in selecting goals and activities that address multiple goals can be an essential component of an effective intervention plan.

The involvement of family can also create ethical challenges for therapists. It is not unusual for family members to have divergent views regarding the best interests of the older adult. It is important for the occupational therapist to recognize that the elder is his or her client and to remain focused on what is best for that individual even in the face of sometimes intense lobbying by family. Mrs. Ramirez's family is supportive, but it is evident early on that they have different views about what is best for her.

Wellness and Prevention

Evaluation

As described previously, funding for **wellness** and **prevention** can be challenging. Most often, occupational therapists provide such services by consulting with organizations rather than caring for individual clients (Scaffa & Bonder, 2009). The process by which this occurs mirrors individual evaluation and intervention but requires focus on the needs and interests of groups of individuals as well as epidemiological data that suggest what kinds of problems are most common (Centers for Disease Control and Prevention and the Merck Company Foundation, 2007). Other sources of health indicators can also guide program planning (Vladeck, Segel, Oberlink, Gursen, & Rudin, 2010). These data demonstrate, for example, that smoking, poor diet, and physical inactivity are the root causes of a third of deaths in the United States. Such information would be useful in framing goals of senior center activities, educational programs, and health screenings. Further, data demonstrate that cognitive decline and falls are among the most common and, particularly in the case of falls, preventable health problems in later life.

Interventions to Support Successful Aging

In wellness and prevention services for older adults, the occupational therapist's most typical role is to assist in understanding the needs of clients and in design of programming that will be delivered by activity therapists, aides, and, often, volunteers. Based on the information gleaned from the participants and a review of literature about common health problems, the therapist generates a list of program goals and explores best practice about effective programming to address those goals. In the case of the Hispanic Senior Center that Mrs. Ramirez attends, one of the activities that participants most enjoy is the lunch, which includes typical Puerto Rican foods. They also enjoy listening to Hispanic music on the radio and watching the Spanish-language soap operas that air each day on television.

Thus, the therapist suggests that senior center programming focus on culturally relevant activities that encourage physical activity through meaningful and enjoyable activities such as dancing while listening to the music they enjoy, gardening, and nature hikes; maintain supportive social interaction and cognitive wellness through interactive, challenging activities such as a book club, lectures with discussion, creative writing, and discussion of the soap opera that they enjoy; encourage positive health promotion behaviors through nutrition and cooking demonstrations and discussions, safety awareness activities, and group discussion; and provide opportunities for altruistic activities such as visits to a local preschool to read to children, food drives, and care for program participants who become ill.

The occupational therapist attends team meetings during which the activity therapist, part-time nurse, nutritionist, and consulting physician discuss the needs of the center's participants. Along with the occupation-based programming, a series of wellness events is designed and implemented. These include blood pressure screening, vision and hearing screening, quarterly visits by a dentist, and an invitation to a physical therapist to plan an appropriate exercise program for participants. These activities are relevant to Mrs. Ramirez's situation because she has not had regular screenings for common health problems and has become increasingly sedentary.

Naturally Occurring Retirement Communities

One of the factors that is important in Mrs. Ramirez's life is the fact that her apartment building is now populated almost exclusively by individuals older than age 65 years. This occurred gradually over time because children of residents became adults and moved on, whereas Mrs. Ramirez and her age cohorts remained in place. The building now constitutes a naturally occurring retirement community (NORC; Naturally Occurring Retirement Communities Programs, 2012). The emergence of NORCs reflects the wish of many older adults to age in place; that is, to remain in their lifelong homes as they grow older. There are many advantages to doing so, including the familiarity of the surroundings, social support from longtime neighbors, and access to family and to health care professionals who know their histories and needs.

Recognizing the opportunity offered by NORCs to support successful aging, government and social agencies have begun to provide various wellness and health promotion services in these facilities. In 2008, the Administration on Aging (AoA; 2011) established a funding initiative designed to

- Enhance the ability of older adults living in a residential community to continue living independently;
- Increase healthy aging behaviors through exercise, recreation, socialization, education, and culturally appropriate activities; and
- Identify needs of at-risk residents, facilitate access to existing community/government resources, and create gap-filling supportive services.

This initiative and its goals offer significant opportunities for occupational therapists to serve community-residing, well older adults. In particular, offering evidence-based services such as lifestyle redesign (Jackson, Carlson, Mandel, Zemke, & Clark, 1998) can promote the goals of the AoA NORC program. Based on Mrs. Ramirez's current status, transportation services would be of particular value, as would evening activities in her apartment building to reduce her sense of loss as a result of her nighttime transportation difficulties.

Primary Care

Occupational therapists' involvement with traditional primary care for older adults is somewhat circumscribed. Although they have an important role to play in wellness, health promotion, and quality of life, their most typical involvement in primary care focuses on safety, as described earlier. Occupational therapists may also be consulted for counseling on joint protection for people with arthritis and energy conservation for older adults with various kinds of debilitating illnesses, but these interventions are most common in settings that will be described in the following section.

Inpatient Care

Several months after her first encounter with the occupational therapist, Mrs. Ramirez misses a week at the senior center. Concerned staff call her home and, when they cannot reach her, her oldest daughter. They discover to their dismay that she recently fell on the steps leading to her apartment and sustained a fracture of the femur.

Evaluation

Mrs. Ramirez is hospitalized, and a surgery to stabilize the fracture is performed. A metal plate with several screws is inserted, although the surgeon is somewhat concerned about the outcome, given the osteoporotic condition of her bones. The occupational therapist is involved immediately, both to help minimize any hospital-induced cognitive loss and to help Mrs. Ramirez prepare for the rehabilitation that will follow her surgery.

The occupational therapist spends some time talking with Mrs. Ramirez to get to know about her interests and her life before the accident. She is pleased when two of Mrs. Ramirez's daughters stop by to visit while she is in the room so that she can meet them and get a sense of the kind of support Mrs. Ramirez may have on her eventual return home. The therapist also administers the Mini-Cog (Borson, Scanlan, Brush, Vitaliano, & Dokmak, 2000), a quick screening instrument for cognitive impairment, and the Functional Independence Measure (FIM) (Heinemann, Linacre, Wright, Hamilton, & Granger, 1994) to evaluate Mrs. Ramirez's current physical capacity. She finds that Mrs. Ramirez has some memory loss but does not meet the standard for dementia. In addition, Mrs. Ramirez is struggling with basic self-care such as dressing, getting herself to and from the bed to a chair or wheelchair, and moving from the wheelchair to the toilet safely.

Interventions to Minimize Dysfunction

The therapist is aware that Mrs. Ramirez will be transferred very soon to a skilled nursing facility where she can receive rehabilitation services. In consultation with Mrs. Ramirez, she determines that the focus of intervention will be on planning for a smooth discharge to the rehabilitation setting. For the brief time that they are together, they work on safe transfers from bed to chair and from wheelchair to toilet. They also focus on dressing, in part because Mrs. Ramirez expresses unhappiness that she looks so disheveled.

The therapist makes a point of dropping in to Mrs. Ramirez's room several times a day, and she encourages some of the hospital volunteers to do likewise. The daughters have expressed concern that Mrs. Ramirez seems more confused than usual; and the therapist is aware that for an older adult who already has memory problems, hospital stays can lead to rapid deterioration (Boustani, Munger, Beck, Campbell, & Weiner, 2007). Thus, the treatment plan includes various strategies to provide stimulation and orientation to time and place. For example, the therapist ensures that Mrs. Ramirez receives a newspaper each day and talks with her about current events reported. The therapist and the volunteers make sure to ask Mrs. Ramirez about events happening in her own day: "What did you have for breakfast?" or "Have you had company today?" And they have a conversation each day about the events in the Spanish-language soap opera that Mrs. Ramirez likes to watch.

Skilled Nursing

Three days after her surgery, Mrs. Ramirez is transferred to a skilled nursing facility. She expresses relief at being out of the hospital but great concern about whether she will be able to go home. She is adamant that this is what she wants and expresses this wish to every staff member she meets as well as to her daughters.

Evaluation

Skilled nursing facilities are among the most highly regulated health care institutions with both federal and state guidelines about the nature of services, expectations for improvement, and requirements about length of stay (Centers for Medicare and Medicaid Services, 2007). Mrs. Ramirez will receive care from a comprehensive team as long as she shows improvement. If her condition stabilizes before she can safely go home, other arrangements will need to be made. Because of these guidelines, staff are pleased to discover that Mrs. Ramirez is highly motivated to regain function. The occupational therapist is involved early based on evidence that intensive OT is associated with shorter stay and better functional outcomes (Jette, Warren, & Wirtalla, 2005).

Medicare guidelines are quite specific about the services to be provided. The occupational therapist is aware that his evaluation and interventions must focus on Mrs. Ramirez's activities of daily living (ADL) and instrumental activities of daily living (IADL). He reviews the report from the occupational therapist at the inpatient facility and participates with others on the team in completing the Minimum Data Set (MDS) (Centers for Medicare and Medicaid Services, 2012). In addition, he repeats the FIM and interviews Mrs. Ramirez about her goals. He requests her permission to involve her family in the intervention process, to which Mrs. Ramirez readily agrees.

Intervention

Mrs. Ramirez wants to regain independence in self-care and to resume her usual activities. She and the therapist begin to practice fundamental skills like dressing, bathing, toileting, and grooming. One goal of their sessions is to identify ways to minimize the difficulties of some of these activities, using, where appropriate, modified clothing (especially for lower extremity dressing), assistive devices (reachers, bath seat), and task modification to reduce energy expenditure.

During these treatment sessions, the therapist inquires about Mrs. Ramirez's typical patterns at home and about the environment to which she wants to return. The therapist talks with the physical therapist about the challenges of a third floor apartment, and both agree this may be quite difficult for Mrs. Ramirez. They suggest to the social worker that she explore the possibility of moving Mrs. Ramirez to a first floor apartment in the same building, realizing that this may not be acceptable to Mrs. Ramirez or feasible in New York's tight housing market.

It becomes apparent to the therapist that Mrs. Ramirez's cognitive difficulties are interfering with her ability to master the changes in her typical occupational patterns that are required by her new physical status. He requests an evaluation by the psychologist who indicates that Mrs. Ramirez has amnestic mild cognitive impairment (MCI) (Kramer et al., 2006). Unlike AD and other frank dementias, MCI is characterized by forgetfulness and poor short-term memory. Well-learned functions tend to remain intact so that individuals with MCI can manage their daily activities in their accustomed environments. Function becomes much more challenging when the individual is in a new setting or when physical changes require new patterns for ADL and IADL. Mrs. Ramirez's hip fracture and subsequent stay in inpatient care and now in a skilled nursing facility has increased her confusion. The occupational therapist finds that her retention from session to session is poor so begins to focus on low-tech memory aids (lists, labeling, mnemonic strategies) that will support her function.

Transition to Home Care

Reimbursement rules from Medicare limit the amount of time that an individual can remain in skilled nursing. Very early in Mrs. Ramirez's stay, the social worker and the treatment team begin conversations with her and, with her permission, her daughters regarding a plan for her discharge. Although only one daughter supports her wish, Mrs. Ramirez remains determined to return to her home. Ultimately, one of the daughters agrees to stay with her for several weeks to help her readjust to the apartment. However, all three of them and the treatment team are concerned about her ability to manage the stairs.

A week before her scheduled departure, the social worker contacts a home health agency. Given Mrs. Ramirez's continued physical limitations and the fact that she has had inpatient care, she is eligible for home health services paid for by Medicare. All agree that these services will be very helpful to her, and the social worker arranges for the intake nurse from the home health agency to visit Mrs. Ramirez on her first full day at home.

Home Care

As is true for rehabilitation, Medicare coverage of home health care is based on very specific rules guiding the kinds of services that can be provided (Centers for Medicare and Medicaid Services, 2010). OT is a covered service, as is supportive care provided by a home health aide (although supportive care must be in concert with rehabilitation). A challenge for OT is that the guidelines specify that services must focus on either improvement or establishing a maintenance plan focused on ADL and IADL, not on other activities that focus on quality of life. This may create an ethical dilemma for the therapist who believes that she has an obligation to provide comprehensive services to meet client needs. One strategy for addressing this dilemma is to provide intervention that can generalize to multiple activities. So, for instance, efforts to improve Mrs. Ramirez's balance might incorporate a few minutes dancing the salsa rather than more straightforward balance exercises, and practice using the phone to report emergencies might also include a call to the senior center to reestablish contact.

Evaluation

Home health reimbursement guidelines require that there should be an initial intake assessment, typically completed by a nurse. The Outcomes and Assessment Information Set (OASIS) (Centers for Medicare and Medicaid Services, n.d.) must be administered, and the intake worker then determines what other services should be provided. These may include OT, physical therapy (PT), speech-language therapy, home aide services (but only in conjunction with therapeutic services), and nursing care. In Mrs. Ramirez's case, it is evident that OT is important to a positive outcome.

OT evaluation in the client's own environment is often the most meaningful in terms of occupational performance. Familiarity with the environment and the psychological comfort of being at home can enhance a client's ability. For Mrs. Ramirez, whose cognitive status has affected her performance greatly, this is particularly true. On her first visit, the occupational therapist asks Mrs. Ramirez to demonstrate her daily routine: getting out of bed, toileting, grooming, bathing, and dressing. Mrs. Ramirez is able to dress independently, sitting in a chair as she was shown during her rehabilitation. However, she struggles with bathing and is unsafe getting on and off the toilet. The therapist orders appropriate durable medical equipment (bath seat, grab bars, raised toilet seat) that may assist with safety and function. She also does a home safety evaluation (Beattie & Peterson, 2007), looking for unstable area rugs, inadequate lighting, and clutter.

In addition to ADL, Mrs. Ramirez will need to be able to manage some IADL for herself.

Her daughters are willing to stop by to help with laundry, grocery shopping, and light housecleaning, but Mrs. Ramirez will need to fix some meals for herself and read and respond to mail, including bills. The therapist asks her to demonstrate these activities.

As they are working on this assessment, the therapist takes the opportunity to learn more about Mrs. Ramirez's activities and interests. Although these cannot be a main focus of intervention, the therapist can keep these in mind when designing strategies for Mrs. Ramirez to build the endurance, problem solving, and the community mobility skills that will be needed.

Intervention

If Mrs. Ramirez is to be able to manage in her home, there is much to do. The therapist orders appropriate durable medical equipment (bath seat, grab bars, raised toilet seat) to assist with safety and function. She and Mrs. Ramirez reorganize the kitchen so that frequently used items are within easy reach (Figure 64.1). With Mrs. Ramirez's approval, she works with the daughters to remove safety hazards from the home. They continue

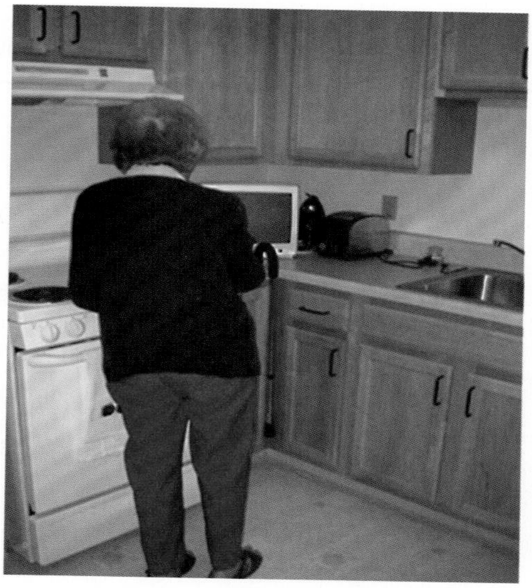

FIGURE 64.1 Mrs. Ramirez, with help from the occupational therapist, organizes her kitchen for ease of use.

to work on self-care skills, bathing in particular, that are giving Mrs. Ramirez difficulty.

As a way to address leisure and social activities, the therapist structures conversation while they work on self-care so that Mrs. Ramirez can identify what she would like to be able to do and can problem-solve about how to make those activities possible. She is eager to return to the Hispanic Senior Center as soon as possible, and the therapist helps her make the phone call that will arrange transportation.

Throughout their time together, the therapist notes that Mrs. Ramirez's increasing cognitive deficits create problems for her independent function. They work on organizing her space to help her find commonly used items, to lay out her grooming supplies in the bathroom, to label cabinets, and to use lists to help her remember important procedures and events; but the lists are frequently mislaid or forgotten, and the therapist is increasingly concerned about Mrs. Ramirez's safety. Mrs. Ramirez continues to be unsteady on her feet and seems unable to remember the precautions that the therapist showed her regarding standing carefully from a seated position, using her cane effectively to move around the apartment, and using the grab bars that have been installed in the bathroom.

Assisted Living

Although Mrs. Ramirez is very motivated to live on her own, ultimately, the challenges of her environment are simply too much. There are two daunting difficulties. One is the three steep flights of stairs leading to the apartment. Although Mrs. Ramirez is increasingly functional at home, leaving and returning are painful and exhausting. Using the stairs does not fall strictly within the goals for home health services (which are intended for individuals who are homebound, not to assist such individuals with return to their community activities), the therapist feels comfortable having Mrs. Ramirez practice as a way to regain strength and endurance. However, her progress is painfully slow. Mrs. Ramirez feels increasingly isolated and depressed.

The second dilemma is Mrs. Ramirez's failing memory, which causes concern for the therapist and for Mrs. Ramirez's daughters. The therapist arranges a visit from the social worker to discuss the options. The daughters are not in agreement, and there are several very intense sessions during which the therapist, with Mrs. Ramirez's permission, reviews her skills and abilities. Ultimately, they agree that an assisted living facility is the best solution.

Evaluation

For OT, Mrs. Ramirez's move to assisted living means coming full circle in terms of services. Occupational therapists typically serve as consultants to such facilities, advising on programming, environmental considerations, and staff training. Residents of assisted living facilities may be referred for outpatient OT as needed, but assisted living is not designed to provide such services within the facility. Their purpose is to provide a supportive environment where meals, housekeeping, and activities are provided and health care can be accessed easily. Thus, Mrs. Ramirez will not be formally evaluated by an occupational therapist at the assisted living facility.

Intervention

There is evidence that function-focused interventions are very helpful in assisted living facilities (Resnick, Galik, Gruber-Baldini, & Zimmerman, 2011). The occupational therapist encourages an array of activities that support wellness (physical activity, socialization at mealtime to encourage adequate nutrition) and quality of life (culturally appropriate, creative, spiritual, altruistic, and other meaningful and enjoyable occupations). In addition, the occupational therapist works with staff to assist in creating strategies for monitoring Mrs. Ramirez's well-being and for interacting with and supporting the family. Effective intervention and monitoring in assisted living can provide support for residents and families to prolong high quality and meaningful life.

Summary

OT practitioners have a well-defined and critical role in the care of older adults. Our roles and methods change based on the evolving needs of these clients. However, as shown in Table 64.1, our OT goals remain the same:

1. Prevent functional decline.
2. Maximize our client's performance in areas of occupation.
3. Decrease participation restrictions and maximize quality of life.

TABLE 64.1 Typical Areas of Emphasis in Prevention, Inpatient Care, Skilled Nursing, Home Health, and Assisted Living

Prevention	Inpatient Care	Skilled Nursing	Home Health	Assisted Living
Consult on design of programs to support meaningful activity	Evaluate ADL in preparation for discharge/transition planning	Evaluate ADL/IADL	Evaluate ADL/IADL	Design wellness programs
Consult on design of physical activities	Provide stimulation to prevent cognitive loss	As feasible, explore meaningful occupations	As feasible, explore meaningful occupations	Design leisure programs with an emphasis on function and meaning
Train staff	As appropriate, discuss needs with family/other informal caregivers	Provide interventions to increase functional ability in ADL/IADL, increase physical capacity	Provide interventions to increase functional ability in ADL/IADL	Consider development of day care programming
Advise on physical design of facilities	Low vision services	Provide assistive devices as appropriate and provide training in their use	Provide interventions to promote wellness	Train staff
			Complete safety assessment	Advise on physical design of facilities
			Support environmental modifications to enhance safety and function	
			Provide assistive devices as appropriate and provide training in their use	
			Low vision services	
			Fall prevention	

ADL, activities of daily living; IADL, instrumental activities of daily living.

References

Administration on Aging. (2011). *Naturally occurring retirement communities.* Retrieved from http://www.aoa.gov/AoARoot/AoA_Programs/HCLTC/NORC/index.aspx

American Occupational Therapy Association. (2008). Occupational therapy practice framework: Domain and process, 2nd edition. *American Journal of Occupational Therapy, 62,* 625–688.

Beattie, B. L., & Peterson, E. W. (2007). *Exploring practice in home safety for fall prevention: The creative practices in home safety assessment and modification study.* Washington, DC: National Council on Aging.

Borson, S., Scanlan, J., Brush, M., Vitaliano, P., & Dokmak, A. (2000). The mini-cog: A cognitive "vital signs" measure for dementia screening in multi-lingual elderly. *International Journal of Geriatric Psychiatry, 15,* 1021–1027.

Boustani, M., Munger, S., Beck, R., Campbell, N., & Weiner, M. (2007). A gero-informatics tool to enhance the care of hospitalized older adults with cognitive impairment. *Clinical Intervention in Aging, 2,* 247–253.

Centers for Disease Control and Prevention and the Merck Company Foundation. (2007). *The state of aging and health in America.* Whitehouse Station, NJ: The Merck Company Foundation.

Centers for Medicare and Medicaid Services. (2007). *Medicare coverage of skilled nursing facility care.* Retrieved from http://www.medicare.gov/Publications/Pubs/pdf/10153.pdf

Centers for Medicare and Medicaid Services. (2010). *Medicare and home health care.* Retrieved from http://www.medicare.gov/Publications/Pubs/pdf/10969.pdf

Centers for Medicare and Medicaid Services (2012). *Nursing home quality initiative.* Retrieved from http://www.cms.gov/Medicare/Quality-Initiatives-Patient-AssessmentInstrumentsNursingHomeQualityInits/index.html?redirect=NursingHomeQualityInits/

Centers for Medicare and Medicaid Services. (n.d.). *OASIS overview.* Retrieved from https://www.cms.gov/OASIS/01_Overview.asp

Clark, F., Jackson, J., Carlson, M., Chou, C., Cherry, B. J., Jordan-Marsh, M., . . . Azen, S. (2011). Effectiveness of a lifestyle intervention in promoting the well-being of independently living older people: Results of the Well Elderly 2 Randomised Controlled Trial. *Journal of Epidemiology and Community Health.* doi:10.1136/jech.2009.099754

Crowther, M. R., Parker, M. W., Achenbaum, W. A., Larimore, W. L., & Koenig, H. G. (2002). Rowe and Kahn's model of successful aging revisited: Positive spirituality—The forgotten factor. *Gerontologist, 42,* 613–620.

Dal Bello-Haas, V., & Tryssenaar, J. (2009). Rehabilitation. In B. R. Bonder & V. Dal Bello-Haas (Eds.), *Functional performance in older adults* (3rd ed., pp. 513–543). Philadelphia, PA: F. A. Davis.

Freedman, V. A., Schoeni, R. F., Martin, L. G., & Cornman, J. C. (2007). Chronic conditions and the decline in late-life disability. *Demography, 44,* 459–477.

Heinemann, A. W., Linacre, J. M., Wright, B. D., Hamilton, B. B., & Granger, C. (1994). Prediction of rehabilitation outcomes with disability measures. *Archives of Physical Medicine and Rehabilitation, 75,* 133–143.

Jackson, J., Carlson, M., Mandel, D., Zemke, R., & Clark, F. (1998). Occupation in lifestyle redesign: The well elderly study occupational therapy program. *American Journal of Occupational Therapy, 52,* 326–336.

Jette, D. U., Warren, R. L., & Wirtalla, C. (2005). The relation between therapy intensity and outcomes of rehabilitation in skilled nursing facilities. *Archives of Physical Medicine and Rehabilitation, 86,* 373–379.

Kramer, J. H., Nelson, A., Johnson, J. K., Yaffe, K., Glenn, S., Rosen, H. J., & Miller, B. L. (2006). Multiple cognitive deficits in amnestic mild cognitive impairment. *Dementia and Geriatric Cognitive Disorders, 22,* 306–311.

National Institutes of Health. (2007). *8 areas of age-related change.* NIH MedLine Plus. Retrieved from http://www.nlm.nih.gov/medlineplus/magazine/issues/winter07/articles/winter07pg10-13.html

Naturally Occurring Retirement Communities Programs. (2012). *NORC blueprint: A guide to community action.* Retrieved from http://www.norcblueprint.org/

Resnick, B., Galik, E., Gruber-Baldini, A., & Zimmerman, S. (2011). Testing the effect of function-focused care in assisted living. *Journal of the American Geriatric Society, 59,* 2233–2240.

Rowe, J. W., & Kahn, R. L. (1998). *Successful aging.* New York, NY: Dell.

Scaffa, M., & Bonder, B. R. (2009). Health promotion and wellness. In B. R. Bonder & V. Dal Bello-Haas (Eds.), *Functional performance in older adults* (3rd ed., pp. 449–467). Philadelphia, PA: F. A. Davis.

Tideiksaar, R. (2009). Falls. In B. R. Bonder& V. Dal Bello-Haas (Eds.), *Functional performance in older adults* (3rd ed., pp. 193–214). Philadelphia, PA: F. A. Davis.

U.S. Census Bureau. (2008). *U.S. population projections.* Retrieved from http://www.census.gov/population/www/projections/summarytables.html

Vladeck, F., Segel, R., Oberlink, M., Gursen, M. D., & Rudin, D. (2010). Health indicators: Aproactive and systematic approach to healthy aging. *Cityscape: A Journal of Policy Development and Research, 12*(2), 67–84.

For additional resources on the subjects discussed in this chapter, visit http://thePoint.lww.com/Willard-Spackman12e.

CHAPTER 65

Providing Occupational Therapy for Disaster Survivors

Theresa M. Smith, Marjorie E. Scaffa

OUTLINE

LEARNING OBJECTIVES

After reading this chapter, you will be able to:

1. Describe the impact of disasters on mental health including factors that may predispose a person to posttraumatic stress disorder
2. Discuss the role of occupational therapy practitioners in addressing the needs of individuals, families, and communities at various stages of disasters
3. Describe how occupational therapy practitioners might address the needs of special populations during disasters
4. Identify potential training needs of occupational therapy personnel in order to more effectively participate in disaster work

Introduction

I (Theresa Smith) first became interested in effects of disasters after being evacuated before Hurricane Katrina struck the Gulf Coast on August 29, 2005. At that time, I was working as a faculty member at Louisiana State University (LSU) Health Science Center (LSUHSC), New Orleans. After the storm, most parts of New Orleans were not accessible until October including residents' homes. Some residents were never able to move back into their homes including myself (Figure 65.1). The LSUHSC campus was heavily damaged and did not reopen until the summer of 2006. However, the students enrolled in the Occupational Therapy Program were adamant that they wanted classes to resume so some routine would be restored to them. The administration of LSU secured room in a research center in Baton Rouge, where the Occupational Therapy Program continued its program.

My interest in disaster effects intensified after I moved to Houston, Texas in August 2006 to escape the daily Katrina-related trauma in New Orleans. In Houston, I found many people living separated from other family members who had returned to New Orleans. I did my first research study on former New Orleans residents evacuated to and now living in Houston (T. M. Smith &

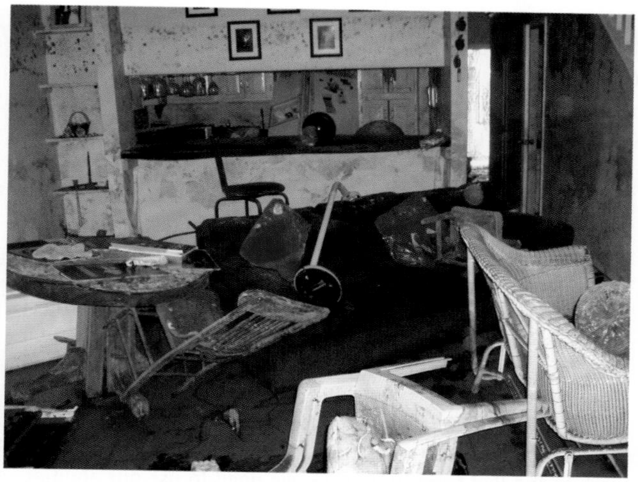

FIGURE 65.1 Theresa Smith's home after Hurricane Katrina.

Hessler, 2009). Participants from that study reported that engaging in new and old occupations produced new supportive routines and that their reliance on old routines facilitated their transition to their new context. After Hurricane Ike hit the Gulf Coast of Texas in September 2008, I was again displaced from my home and did a study on fieldwork students from a nearby university affected by Hurricane Ike (T. M. Smith, Dreyfus, & Hersch, 2011). In addition, 1 year after Hurricane Ike, the student participants were still engaged in three less valued roles than before the storm.

In writing this chapter, we have drawn on our own personal experiences; the occupational therapy and other literature on disaster preparation, response, and recovery; and from personal communication with other occupational therapists involved in disaster work (see the case study about Shannon Magnum, an occupational therapist who has been involved in disaster recovery for several years). Our intent is to help illuminate the complexity and need for occupation-based interventions after disasters.

CASE STUDY 65.1 Shannon Magnum

Shannon Magnum, MPS, LOTR, has been involved in disaster work over the past 7 years. She is an occupational therapist specializing in mental health practice and teaches the mental health, wellness, and community course content in the Occupational Therapy Department at Louisiana State University Health Sciences Center (LSUHSC) in New Orleans, Louisiana. In addition, Shannon owns a private practice on the north shore of Lake Pontchartrain.

Shannon's disaster work after Katrina began during the recovery period. She organized students and they gutted people's homes to prepare the houses for rebuilding. To foster recovery, she and the students made mirror and cross collages for the homeowners out of shards of china from their homes and those of other New Orleans residents' (Kim, 2006). This creative use of occupation allowed her and her students to feel that they were part of the rebuilding process. The mosaics were a tangible reminder of the meaning of place in people's lives (Figure 65.2).

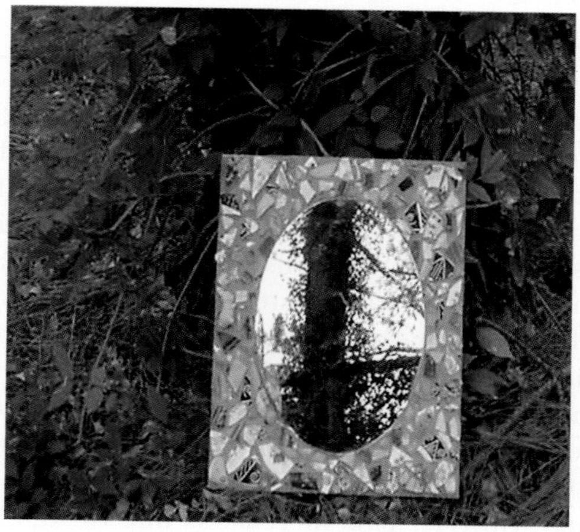

FIGURE 65.2 Mirror mosaic made by Shannon Magnum and her students.

Shannon and the occupational therapy faculty at LSUHSC continue to be involved in disaster work from Katrina, but this work is now at the reconstruction stage. Curriculum changes have been made as the faculty processed their "new" understanding of meaning of place and the impact that living in a recovery era holds at many levels. She has instituted a required leadership project in all the courses she teaches in which students foster community awareness and community contributions. Shannon and the occupational therapy faculty as well as the students' disaster work at the rebuilding and reconstruction stage includes educating at both the policy and at the resident level. They have urged the residents to rebuild with aging in place in mind and helped the city assess and rectify public transportation system issues to allow riders with disabilities to use services within the redeveloping neighborhoods.

After Katrina, Shannon saw a tremendous need to educate occupational therapy practitioners on the skills required in disaster work and she has presented locally, regionally, and nationally on this topic. In this time of increasing disasters, practitioners need to know about trauma-informed care (S. Magnum, personal communication, March 8, 2012). All occupational therapy practitioners have the basic mental health background to screen for depression and anxiety. They can assist individuals by decreasing the chaos of the situation and by fostering resilience needed to move forward (S. Magnum, personal communication, March 8, 2012). Clinicians can foster resilience by using narrative reasoning and listening to survivors' stories without forgetting their own personal stress management strategies. Although most occupational therapy practitioners are not skilled in specific mental health interventions, they should be alert for signs of clients stuck in a stage of grief and/or experiencing posttraumatic stress disorder and refer them for professional help (S. Magnum, personal communication, March 8, 2012). Finally, all occupational therapists would

CASE STUDY 65.1 Shannon Magnum (*Continued*)

benefit by formal education on grief work because this is a natural response to any loss and occupational therapists are directly treating the loss of function, health, roles, and dreams in their clients.

Directly after the British Petroleum oil spill occurred in 2010, Shannon and a group of students responded. They focused their efforts on an elementary school in a parish most impacted by the oil spill. Shannon and the occupational therapy students worked with the children, their parents, and the teachers using social-emotional learning to cope with the trauma (S. Magnum, personal communication, March 9, 2012). The students learned the importance of asking for support and also had an opportunity to act out a play about the oil spill, addressing third-graders issues with an age-appropriate intervention. In addition, resources were gathered for parents to assist their navigation and adjustment into a new context (Yamkovenko, n.d.). Shannon also engaged in a personal occupation at this time by becoming involved in bird rehabilitation efforts.

Shannon has recently attempted to intercede at the systems level and address disasters at the prevention stage. Despite the ongoing rebuilding of homes and businesses in New Orleans and the surrounding area, the suicide rate has risen to 30% on the North shore ("St. Tammany," 2011). To combat the rise in suicide rate, Shannon and her group of students developed an evidence-based suicide prevention awareness project and presented it to the St. Tammany School Board. Although their project was not implemented at this time, Shannon reports feeling reenergized with the writing of this case study about her experiences and left me with these words, "We [occupational therapy practitioners] can't just leave disaster work to the Red Cross and FEMA; we need to use our abilities. We are well trained and poised to support the resiliency of individuals while also impacting the environments in which they call home thus making a difference in our communities as well" (S. Magnum, personal communication, March 9, 2012).

Impact of Disasters

It is estimated that between 13% and 30% of the United States population have been exposed to one or more disasters in their lifetime (Briere & Elliott, 2000). The term **disaster** refers to dangerous accidental or uncontrollable situations or events that cause significant environmental destruction, loss of life, and disruption of social structure and normal daily life routines. Disasters overwhelm the local capacity to respond and necessitate requests for external assistance (Centre for Research on the Epidemiology of Disasters, 2009; Fritz, 1961).

Due to growing number of natural and technological disasters and continued terrorist threats, it can be expected that the number of individuals affected by disasters will rise. This increase is due to significant population density in flood plains and along vulnerable coasts and earthquake fault lines, an increase in climate-related disasters as evidenced by the average number of Atlantic hurricanes doubling in the last century (Holland & Webster, 2007), technological failures such as the Gulf Oil Spill and the subsequent use of dispersant to clean it up (Hollis, 2010), and international terrorist attacks resulting in thousands of fatalities (LaFranchi, 2010).

Disasters are not delineated as a singular event but rather conceptualized as progressing through a sequence of stages (American Occupational Therapy Association [AOTA], 2011). The five stages of pre-impact period, impact period, immediate post-impact period, recovery period, and reconstruction period require different responses.

Disasters can result in great personal loss, fragmented social support, and community destruction (Lowe, Chan, & Rhodes, 2010). Personal loss can include not only injury to oneself but also the injury or death of a loved one, property damage, and/or financial loss. Social support can be affected due to widespread evacuations, and lack of social connections has been determined to be a risk factor for the development of posttraumatic stress disorder (PTSD) (Hobfoll et al., 2007). The destruction of a community leads to loss of community support and the social structure where "individuals routinely, and habitually, enact and shape identity through doing within everyday social interactions" (Huot & Laliberte Rudman, 2010, p. 72).

Following disasters, most survivors experience acute stress reactions including emotional, physical, cognitive, and interpersonal effects (AOTA, 2011). Emotional reactions such as grief, fear, guilt, numbness, and despair (Rao, 2006) are usually more severe and last longer than physical effects (Carroll, Morbey, Balogh, & Araoz, 2008). In addition, disaster survivors have reported cognitive effects such as confusion and inability to concentrate and interpersonal problems secondary to avoidance of social interaction (AOTA, 2011). Health problems or injuries were evident in approximately one-third of the Katrina evacuees in Houston shelters (Brodie, Weltzien, Altman, Blendon, & Benson, 2006). Recent research has shown that the psychosocial and health effects of disasters can sometimes last for years (Te Brake et al., 2009).

Post-disaster distress is nearly universal and important to address among disaster survivors (North, 2010). However, psychosocial responses vary depending on the disaster, affected population and setting, so no one mental health model can adequately address all post-disaster scenarios (North, 2010). The range of people's reactions posttrauma will vary from a transient stress reaction needing support and provision of resources to those reactions that need psychological assessment and intensive intervention (Hobfoll et al., 2007).

Some survivors may develop psychiatric disorders including PTSD, depression, prolonged grief, or substance abuse (Rao, 2006). Rao (2006) lists the following predisposing and posttraumatic factors that may contribute to the development of these disorders.

Predisposing factors:

- Childhood sexual abuse
- Previous unresolved losses and traumas
- Substance use
- Previous psychiatric history
- Minority or disadvantage status (economic, social)
- Multiple life stressors

Posttraumatic factors:

- Severe and acute psychological reactions after the event
- Lack of social and family supports
- Extensive personal loss
- Adverse reactions from others (blame or rejection)
- Survivor guilt (p. 504).

Other factors that may predispose a person to a post-disaster psychiatric disorder include sustaining injuries (Norris, Sherrieb, & Galea, 2010), viewing upsetting events, the death of family or friend, displacement (Fullilove, 1996), property loss, and a perceived decrease in social support (Hobfoll et al., 2007; Lowe et al., 2010). Survivors with post-disaster psychiatric disorders require rapid mental health interventions and long-term continuation of services (North, 2010).

Not all effects from disasters are detrimental. **Posttraumatic growth** can occur when survivors find something positive in a tragedy and try to make sense of it (Kessler, Galea, Jones, & Parker, 2006). Personal growth may manifest as increased emotional closeness to loved ones, faith in the ability to reconstruct life, spirituality, meaning or purpose in life, and/or recognition of inner strength (Kessler et al., 2006). For example, in research studies, spouses reported growing closer and several participants reported increased spirituality (T. M. Smith et al., 2011; T. M. Smith & Hessler, 2009). One participant specifically mentioned finding a greater appreciation for life itself (T. M. Smith et al., 2011). Posttraumatic growth can be facilitated as an individual reflects through journaling, or talking with friends and establishes a support system or creates a positive vision of life (Cancer.net, 2011).

Addressing the Needs of Individuals and Families

During disaster work, occupational therapy practitioners can focus on supporting people's health and participation through engagement in occupation (AOTA, 2008). Many areas of occupation are essential in managing the ensuing disorder of a disaster. Disaster survivors commonly face disrupted habits, routines, and roles and participation in occupation can help restore these (AOTA, 2011).

Occupational therapy practitioners can contribute at every stage of a disaster and on an individual, family, or community level. They can assist in the pre-disaster stage by addressing evacuation plans with individuals and providing consultation for community agencies. In areas more susceptible to natural disasters, occupational therapists can assist with planning culturally sensitive shelter accommodations that provide equal access for all persons including those with disabilities. Post-disaster, occupational therapists can provide mental health services to mitigate acute stress reactions and facilitate adaptation to changed contexts. Some of the distress experienced in later stages of a disaster can be prevented or mitigated by being organized during the preparation and impact stages. Box 65.1 contains information on how to prepare individuals and families for the different disaster stages.

Addressing the Needs of Communities

Disasters impact whole communities, resulting in potential community-wide economic, environmental, governmental, social, and cultural disruptions that can themselves contribute to psychological distress (Norris et al., 2010). Occupational therapy practitioners can contribute at the community level during different disaster stages. However, if occupational therapy practitioners expect to work at this level, they should be involved in the community disaster response agencies prior to a disaster occurring (AOTA, 2011; Stone, 2006; Taylor, Jacobs, & Marsh, 2011).

Preparation Stage for Communities

In the preparation stage, Taylor et al. (2011) recommend that occupational therapists assist in planning evacuations and in advising communities on shelter accommodations for vulnerable individuals. It is especially central for occupational therapy practitioners to assist with planning shelter accommodations that support participation by those with disabilities. "It is important [for evacuees with disabilities] to have routine and have control. The planner must understand how to get them engaged in activity" (E. Garza, personal communication, July 14, 2011).

Many evacuees with disabilities who do not require medical support should not be moved far from their communities to specialized shelters. An occupational therapist in Texas determined that many of the individuals such as the elderly or those with well-managed chronic illnesses who were being sent to shelters with medical support did not need to be there (E. Garza, personal communication, July 14, 2011). Therefore, she developed

BOX 65.1 Individual and Family Needs at Different Stages of Disaster

Preparation Stage for Individuals and Family

Personal Items Needed

- A plastic container for legal documents (e.g., birth certificate, marriage certificate, passport, social security card)
- Monthly bills (e.g., utilities, mortgage) with phone numbers
- Insurance policies (e.g., homeowners, renters, flood)
- Pictures of your property
- Licensing information (e.g., license, continuing education certificates for professionals)
- Medications in pharmacy-issued bottles with recent refill if possible
- Hand sanitizer and antibacterial wipes
- Cash and debit/credit cards
- Give your contact information to someone outside the impact area
- Laptop with charged battery

Items Needed for the Home

- Rechargeable flashlight
- Candles and matches
- Charged cell phone
- Battery-operated radio with weather station
- Canned food and manual can opener
- Paper plates
- Bottled water
- Ice and cooler
- Put away all patio furniture, plants, hoses
- Close storm shutters or attach ply board as needed

Preparing the Car(s)

- Fill up gas tank
- Have a phone charger for the car
- Flashlight

Impact Stage for Individuals and Family: Evacuation and Shelter

	Needs Evacuation	Shelter in Place
Personal	Everything from the preparation stage Clothing for a week Pay monthly bills ahead if possible Toys and games for children	Everything from the preparation stage
Home	Arrange temporary housing	Everything from the preparation stage Fill bathtubs with water Prepare walk-in closets or bathtubs with bedding Have canned foods and bottled water
Car(s)	Everything from the preparation stage Drive all cars out of impact area Car radio for information on evacuation routes/shelters Pet carriers, food, and bedding	Park in the garage or a covered parking lot on at least the second level Know evacuation routes

Immediate Post-Impact Stage for Individuals and Family

Personal	Stay away from over-sensationalized news reports When safe to return, determine if protective clothing (face masks, rubber boots, and gloves) are needed. Buy items outside the impact area
Home	If necessary, continue in temporary housing and call insurance companies Assess damages, take pictures, and do not remove any damaged items until an insurance representative has arrived Determine through local news if the water is safe to drink before using from the tap If electricity has been off for quite a few hours, cook frozen food and discard refrigerated food
Cars	Assess for damages and call insurance company as needed

(continued)

BOX 65.1 Individual and Family Needs at Different Stages of Disaster (*Continued*)

Recovery and Reconstruction Stage for Individuals and Family

Personal	Return to routines (Te Brake et al., 2009) Institute stress management techniques (e.g., routine exercise, meditation, prayer, progressive relaxation) Ensure sleep quality through environmental and behavioral changes Participate in valued leisure activities (AOTA, 2011) Ventilation (e.g., talk about your experiences) (Rao, 2006) Restore social connections (Lowe et al., 2010) Reconnect with community
Home	If the area has been declared a disaster area, register with Federal Emergency Management Agency (FEMA) Remove damaged items such as wet wallboard or carpeting, which may cause further damage Save all receipts for any replacement items Organize insurance claims Rebuild to fit current lifestyle

refuges in the community where those individuals could come to escape vulnerable homes during the disaster. In these refuges, evacuees can participate in familiar routines and engage in organized activities.

Impact Stage and Post-Impact for Communities

Occupational therapy practitioners are experts in assisting people manage disruptions to their routines and could be among the essential personnel at shelters (Stone, 2006). Taylor et al. (2011) suggest that after disasters, occupational therapy practitioners can (1) assist vulnerable individuals' transition out of temporary and into permanent housing, providing comfort to children and respite to parents; (2) rebuild accessible housing through working with volunteer groups; and (3) provide mental health services. They recommend that mental health services focus on functional recovery such as problem solving, normalizing daily routines, and posttraumatic growth.

Addressing the Needs of Special Populations

Occupational therapy practitioners have skills that can address the needs of special populations before, during, and after disasters. These populations include evacuees in shelters, disaster relief workers (DRWs), children, and persons with disabilities.

Evacuees in Shelters

An occupational therapy supervisor described the work performed by the Harris County occupational therapy staff at the Astrodome and other buildings with Hurricane Katrina evacuees in Houston, Texas (P. Law, personal communication, July 10, 2011). He said that the largest focus was in developing a system to ensure that family members who had to be kept in isolation in separate buildings due to medical reasons would be reunited with other family members. Members of the occupational therapy staff also created a play area for children to help decrease their anxiety. Unfortunately, occupational therapists working in psychiatric settings were not considered certified mental health service providers in Texas and, therefore, were not permitted to address evacuees' mental health issues at the Astrodome. This is a barrier to the full participation of occupational therapists in many states. To better serve in future disasters, advocacy and education are needed if occupational therapists trained and experienced in psychiatric work are to be considered certified mental health service providers.

Disaster Relief Workers

DRWs work long, difficult hours under poor conditions and are often required to perform tasks that can potentially result in injury or even death. In addition, they can be exposed to horrifying images of people with significant injuries, observe grieving family members, and view body parts or corpses (Evans, Patt, Giosan, Spielman, & Difede, 2009). Occupational therapy practitioners working in disaster situations must be mindful of the need to prevent compassion fatigue for themselves and for other disaster responders.

Compassion fatigue, sometimes referred to as secondary traumatic stress reaction, occurs when the helper (volunteer or professional) becomes preoccupied with the suffering and distress being experienced by the recipients of care. This results in "a deep physical, emotional and spiritual exhaustion accompanied by acute emotional pain" (Pfifferling & Gilley, 2000, p. 39). Prevention of compassion fatigue requires personal self-care including good nutrition, adequate sleep, enjoyable physical activity, spending time with family and friends, prayer, and meditation.

Some DRWs are at risk for developing more severe psychological problems. Approximately 12% of utility DRWs cutting and restoring power at the World Trade Center disaster had substantial symptoms of PTSD (Evans et al., 2009). This percentage is consistent with data collected worldwide for DRWs (Marmar et al., as cited by Evans et al., 2009). Because each disaster site is unique, the psychological needs of DRWs at different disasters will vary. As Precin said of providing counseling to firefighters after 9/11, "There were no manuals or books written on how to do firehouse counseling in the wake of a devastating disaster of this magnitude" (2006, p. 47).

Children

Children in disaster zones are subject to the same tragedy observations and frightening media coverage as adults. In the chaos immediately after a disaster, they may be separated from family members and/or ultimately with their families; they may be displaced from a stable environment for years (Nadkarni & Leonard, 2007). It is estimated that at least 20,000 of the 160,000 children displaced by Hurricane Katrina have developed serious emotional or behavioral problems (Donnelly, 2010). These problems have been attributed to children not possessing the coping mechanisms adults do (Donnelly, 2010).

Researchers have suggested means to combat the fear and anxiety children experience from disasters. Therapeutic play can be initiated in shelters during the impact stage of a disaster or post-impact stage of a disaster (Nadkarni & Leonard, 2007). One play activity for which it is easy to transport supplies and that allows children to express their emotions is drawing (Nadkarni & Leonard, 2007). Goenjian et al. (as cited in Hobfoll et al., 2007) found that teaching children emotional regulation skills and enhanced problem-solving skills help them address adversities in a disaster's wake. Children also need to return to a normal routine as soon as possible and that means returning to school even if in a temporary setting (Rao, 2006).

An occupational therapist working in a school system in Japan, south of where the tsunami hit, spoke to me of her experience and frustrations (C. Haines, personal communication, July 16, 2011). She said students resumed school immediately so their lives could be normalized as much as possible. However, all of the children were "bouncing off the walls" and required calming, especially those with autism spectrum disorders. Children with sensory issues wanted to go to the gym and engage in proprioceptive or vestibular activities. Those with fine motor issues and older children wanted to play tag or games using the whole body. The children seemed relieved to be playing and not talking about "it."

Although this occupational therapist had a role to perform with the children in her charge, she felt that occupational therapy should play a much bigger role in disaster work. She knew of occupational therapists evacuated from the disaster site but social workers who were allowed to remain and help. She also has seen a growing number of displaced elders, homeless, and orphans from the tsunami, populations with which she believes occupational therapy practitioners could intervene. She said, "I am not saying that mental health is our role. I do feel we [occupational therapy practitioners] could play a bigger role if we were able to define the role of occupational therapy in disasters" (C. Haines, personal communication, July 16, 2011). She now feels a commitment to finding out how to best be involved as an occupational therapist in disaster work.

Persons with Disabilities

Persons with disabilities and activity limitations are at particular risk during emergency and disaster situations. Disasters pose "difficulties and challenges to daily life for all persons, especially for those with impairments and chronic illnesses" (Wisner, 2002, p. 2). Reduced abilities to see, speak, hear, walk, understand, learn, remember, and manipulate significantly affect a person's ability to respond in disaster situations. Due to the near limitless variety of potential activity limitations, there is no "one size fits all" when it comes to addressing the needs of people with disabilities before, during, and after disasters.

Certain characteristics of older adults with chronic health conditions and persons with disabilities may interfere with their ability to adequately prepare for disasters, leaving them vulnerable to increased morbidity and mortality. In addition, activity limitations may decrease a person's adaptability during disasters and predispose them to emotional trauma. After a disaster, lack of food and water, extremes of temperature, stress, interruptions in medication regimens, lack of access to medical care, and exposure to contaminants can contribute to the exacerbation of a chronic illness that was previously well managed (Aldrich & Benson, 2008).

The breakdown of infrastructure during and after disaster affects everyone, but it disadvantages persons with disabilities disproportionally, limiting their ability to access transportation, shelter, health care, and communication services (Priestley & Hemingway, 2007). It is important to incorporate "persons with disabilities and activity limitations into the fabric and the culture of emergency management services" (Kailes, 2005, p. 10). People with disabilities should be engaged as contributors and collaborators in the emergency response planning process and not seen merely as victims to be rescued. Through participation with disaster relief organizations, occupational therapy practitioners can participate in the design of shelters for persons with disabilities, training of shelter managers and staff, planning of accessible services after a disaster, and educating individuals and families on strategies for sheltering in place.

The Role of Occupational Therapy Organizations

On an international and national level, the profession of occupational therapy has contributed to emergency preparedness and disaster response (AOTA, 2011; Hasselkus, 2001; McColl, 2002; World Federation of Occupational Therapists [WFOT], 2009). The WFOT has developed and is updating an information package on disaster preparedness and response (WFOT, 2006). Proceeds from its sales allow the WFOT to send the information packet to countries that cannot afford it and to occupational therapists performing disaster work. The AOTA (2011) has a webpage of resources for emergency preparedness and response. It has facilitated communication from members affected by disasters in the past such as Hurricane Katrina and currently has a public forum on OT Connections entitled *Disaster Relief* (AOTA, 2008).

Occupational therapy practitioners and occupational therapy students (Persh, 2003; T. M. Smith et al., 2011;Taylor et al., 2011) are also victims and survivors of disasters (AOTA, 2011). Universities in disaster areas experience crisis; and their faculty, students, and infrastructures are forced to operate in survival mode (Morris, 2008). Whole communities and supporting institutions in disaster zones are unable to function, remain closed for extended periods of time, or never reopen. In these times, entities outside the impact zone must be prepared to respond. Given the growing likelihood of disasters and the number of occupational therapy practitioners and occupational therapy programs in areas of vulnerability, perhaps the time has come to consider a more formalized preparedness and response process on the part of occupational therapy organizations. The AOTA could publish a fact sheet on disaster work and have a volunteer disaster force that would provide education to the occupational therapy faculty, students, and programs, and practitioners in the impact zone as to what constitutes normal acute reactions to a disaster. Furthermore, the disaster force could help by suggesting to these individuals how to promote calming and a sense of efficacy, instill hope, and promote connectedness to the profession (Hobfoll et al., 2007). In addition, members of the disaster force can provide practical advice as to how affected occupational therapy programs can maintain Accreditation Council for Occupational Therapy Education (ACOTE) standards in a devastated environment.

There is an obvious disconnection between what occupational therapists believe are their abilities to serve in disaster situations and the credentials that the Red Cross expects of mental health service providers. This problem might best be addressed by the AOTA educating the Red Cross on occupational therapy practitioners' skills and determining how occupational therapy practitioners might best meet the Red Cross's criteria for mental health providers.

A Professional Responsibility

Occupational therapy practitioners have a professional responsibility to participate in disaster work on different fronts. First, by promoting access to occupation to ensure health and quality of life for individuals and populations affected by disasters, they can uphold the commitment of the profession to promote occupational justice (AOTA, 2011). Second, occupational therapy practitioners are obligated to facilitate the achievement of the AOTA Centennial Vision that requires occupational therapy practice to be evidence based and science driven. If disaster work by occupational therapy practitioners is to meet both criteria, then we must engage in research to determine the efficacy and effectiveness of occupational therapy services in disaster work. Although opportunities are growing for occupational therapy disaster practice and research, those in disaster work must remain mindful of the tragedies that clients have experienced and of the continued disaster effects they may suffer.

Training for Disaster Work

Education and training for occupational therapy practitioners in evidence-based, trauma-informed care is critical. **Trauma-informed care** refers to assessment and intervention that includes "a basic understanding of how trauma affects the life of an individual seeking services . . . so that these services and programs can be more supportive and avoid re-traumatization" (Substance Abuse and Mental Health Services Administration [SAMHSA], n.d., para. 1). It is a strengths-based approach that represents a paradigm shift from focusing on dysfunction and diagnosis to focusing on what happened to the person, recognizing that the individual's reaction may be a normal response to an abnormal situation.

Trauma-informed care has become the standard of care in mental health and is compatible with several occupational therapy theories and models, including the Model of Human Occupation, Occupational Adaptation, and the Canadian Model of Occupational Performance and Engagement. The Model of Human Occupation was found to be useful in evaluation of and intervention for older adults with a history of trauma in Israel "because of its emphasis on the ongoing possibility of people to maintain, reinforce, shape, and change their own capacities, beliefs, dispositions, and life stories through occupation" (Ziv & Roitman, 2008, p. 91). The theory of occupational adaptation is helpful in understanding and facilitating mature adaptive response behaviors, which in turn, allow "individuals to meet the demands of the environment, cope with the problems of everyday living, and fulfill age-specific roles" (Johnson, 2006, p.75). The Canadian model is valuable because it is a client-centered approach that incorporates spirituality (Law et al., 1997). Spirituality is often associated with better mental health outcomes because it can contribute to recovery by promoting hope and providing comfort during difficult times in one's life (Corrigan, McCorkle, Schell, & Kidder, 2003; B. W. Smith, Pargament, Brant, & Oliver, 2000).

In addition, occupational therapy practitioners can obtain training in disaster work by becoming a member of a disaster response team at the local, state, or national levels (AOTA, 2011). Prior to a disaster, practitioners should become involved with organizations like the American Red Cross, community emergency response teams, mental health crisis services, critical incident stress management teams, and employee assistance programs to increase the probability of being called on to serve during a disaster (AOTA, 2011). "We cannot wait until there is an emergency to volunteer as they [planners] cannot know what we do. We must make ourselves visible and become involved in our communities" (E. Garza, personal communication, July 14, 2011). Garza further recommends getting training and certification through Federal courses (http://www.citizencorps.gov/cert/, http://training.fema.gov/is/nims.asp). To ensure our participation in disaster work, it is incumbent on occupational therapy practitioners to educate the agency they have joined as to the scope and value of occupational therapy services (Taylor et al., 2011).

References

Aldrich, N., & Benson, W. F. (2008). Disaster preparedness and the chronic disease needs of vulnerable older adults. *Preventing Chronic Disease: Public Health Research, Practice and Policy, 5*(1), A27. Retrieved from http://www.cdc.gov/pcd/issues/2008/jan/07_0135.htm

American Occupational Therapy Association. (2011). *Emergency preparedness and response sources.* Retrieved from http://www.aota.org/Practitioners/Resources/Collections/Preparedness-Library/Emergency-Resources-.aspx

American Occupational Therapy Association. (2008). *Forums: Public forums.* Retrieved from http://otconnections.aota.org/forums/

American Occupational Therapy Association. (2011). *The role of occupational therapy in disaster preparedness, response, and recovery.* Retrieved from http://www.aota.org/Practitioners/Official/Concept/39464.aspx?FT=.pdf

Briere, J., & Elliott, D. (2000). Prevalence, characteristics, and long-term sequelae of natural disaster exposure in the general population. *Journal of Traumatic Stress, 13*, 661–679.

Brodie, M., Weltzien, E., Altman, D., Blendon, R., & Benson, J. (2006). Experiences of Hurricane Katrina evacuees in Houston shelters: Implications for future planning. *American Journal of Public Health, 96*, 1402–1408.

Cancer.net (2011). *Post-traumatic growth and cancer.* Retrieved from http://www.cancer.net/patient/All+About+Cancer/Cancer.Net+Feature+Articles/After+Treatment+and+Survivorship/Post-Traumatic+Growth+and+Cancer

Carroll, B., Morbey, H., Balogh, R., & Araoz, G. (2008). Flooded homes, broken bonds, the meaning of home, psychological processes and their impact on psychological health in disaster. *Health and Place, 15*, 540–547. doi:10.1016/j.healthplace.2008.08.009

Centre for Research on the Epidemiology of Disasters. (2009). *What's new.* Retrieved from http://www.cred.be/

Corrigan, P., McCorkle, B., Schell, B., & Kidder, K. (2003). Religion and spirituality in the lives of people with serious mental illness. *Community Mental Health Journal, 39*, 487–499.

Donnelly, B. (2010). *Katrina five years after: Hurricane left a legacy of health concerns.* Retrieved from http://www.foxnews.com/health/2010/08/27/katrina-years-hurricane-left-legacy-health-concerns/#ixzz1RLnhYn1G

Evans, S., Patt, I., Giosan, C., Spielman, L., & Difede, J. (2009). Disability and posttraumatic stress disorder in disaster relief workers responding to September 11, 2001 World Trade Center disaster. *Journal of Clinical Psychology, 65*, 684–694. doi:10.1002/jclp.20575

Fritz, C. E. (1961). Disasters. In R. K. Merton & R. A. Nisbet (Eds.), *Contemporary social problems* (pp. 651–694). New York, NY: Harcourt.

Fullilove, M. T. (1996). Psychiatric implications of displacement: Contributions from the psychology of place. *American Journal of Psychiatry, 153*, 1516–1523.

Hasselkus, B. R. (2001). From the desk of the editor—unspeakable occupations. *American Journal of Occupational Therapy, 5*, 606–607.

Hobfoll, S. E., Watson, P., Bell, C. C., Bryant, R. A., Brymer, M. J., Friedman, M. J., . . . Ursano, R. J. (2007). Five essential elements of immediate and mid-term mass trauma intervention: Empirical evidence. *Psychiatry, 70*, 283–315.

Holland, G., & Webster, P. (2007). Heightened tropical cyclone activity in the North Atlantic: Natural variability or climate trend? *Philosophical Transactions of the Royal Society*, 365 (1860), 2695–2716.

Hollis, P. (2010). *Gulf oil spill disaster latest example in list of technological blunders.* Retrieved from http://southeastfarmpress.com/gulf-oil-spill-disaster-latest-example-list-technological-blunders

Huot, S., & Laliberte Rudman, D. (2010). The performances and places of identity: Conceptualizing intersections of occupation, identity and place in the process of migration. *Journal of Occupational Science, 17*(2), 68–77.

Johnson, J. A. (2006). Describing the phenomenon of homelessness through the theory of occupational adaptation. *Occupational Therapy in Health Care, 20*(3/4), 63–80.

Kailes, J. I. (2005). *Disaster services and "special needs": Term of art or meaningless term?* Retrieved from http://www.nobodyleftbehind2.org/findings/pdfs/SpecialsNeeds.pdf

Kessler, R. C., Galea, S., Jones, R. T., & Parker, H. A. (2006). Mental illness and suicidality after Hurricane Katrina. *Community Advisory Group Bulletin of the World Health Organization, 84*, 930–939.

Kim, S. (2006). *"Shards ministry" transforms.* Retrieved from http://www.disasternews.net/news/article.php?articleid=2678&printthis=1

LaFranchi, H. (2010). *Last year, 10,999 terrorist attacks worldwide—a decline from 2008.* Retrieved from http://www.csmonitor.com/USA/Foreign-Policy/2010/0805/Last-year-10-999-terrorist-attacks-worldwide-a-decline-from-2008

Law, M. L., Cooper, B. A., Strong, S., Stewart, D., Rigby, P., & Letts, L. (1997). Theoretical contexts for practice of occupational therapy in C. Christiansen & C. Baum (Eds.), *Occupational therapy: Enabling function and well-being* (2nd ed.). Thorofare, NJ: SLACK.

Lowe, S. R., Chan, C. S., & Rhodes, J. E. (2010). Pre-hurricane perceived social support protects against psychological distress: A longitudinal analysis of low-income mothers. *Journal of Consulting and Clinical Psychology, 78*, 551–560. doi:10.1037/a0018317

McColl, M. (2002). Occupation in stressful times. *American Journal of Occupational Therapy, 56*, 350–353.

Morris, A. S. (2008). Making it through a traumatic life experience: Applications for teaching, research, and personal adjustment. *Training and Education in Professional Psychology, 2*(2), 89–95. doi:10.1037/1931-3918.2.2.89

Nadkarni, M., & Leonard, R. B. (2007). Immediate psychological support for children after a disaster: A concept. *The Internet Journal of Rescue and Disaster Medicine, 6*, 127–131.

Norris, F. H., Sherrieb, K., & Galea, S. (2010). Prevalence and consequences of disaster-related illness and injury from Hurricane Ike. *Rehabilitation Psychology, 55*, 221–230.

North, C. S. (2010). A tale of two studies of two disasters: Comparing psychosocial responses to disaster among Oklahoma City bombing survivors and Hurricane Katrina evacuees. *Rehabilitation Psychology, 55*, 241–246. doi:10.1037/a0020119

Persh, J. (2003). Coping with tragedy: A fieldwork student's experience with FEMA crisis counseling. In P. Precin (Ed.), *Surviving 9/11. Impact and experiences of occupational therapy practitioners* (pp. 129–151). New York, NY: Haworth Press.

Pfifferling, J. H., & Gilley, K. (2000). Overcoming compassion fatigue. *Family Practice Management, 7*(4), 39–44.

Precin, P. (2006). *Healing 9/11: Creative programming by occupational therapists.* New York, NY: Haworth Press.

Priestley, M., & Hemingway, L. (2007). Disability and disaster recovery: A tale of two cities? *Journal of Social Work in Disability & Rehabilitation, 5*(3–4), 23–42.

Rao, K. (2006). Psychosocial support in disaster-affected communities. *International Review of Psychiatry, 18*, 501–505. doi:10.1080/09540260601038472

Smith, B. W., Pargament, K. I., Brant, C., & Oliver, J. M. (2000). Noah revisited: Religious coping by church members and the impact of the 1993 Midwest flood. *Journal of Community Psychology, 28*, 169–186.

Smith, T. M., Dreyfus, A., & Hersch, G. (2011). Habits, routines and roles of graduate students: Effects of Hurricane Ike. *Occupational Therapy in Health Care, 24*(4). doi:10.3109/07380577.2011.600426

Smith, T. M., & Hessler, C. (2009). *Effects of Hurricane Katrina on displacees' routines and roles.* Unpublished manuscript.

Stone, G. V. M. (2006). Occupational therapy in times of disaster. *American Journal of Occupational Therapy, 60*, 7–8.

St. Tammany sees spike in suicide rate [Video file]. (2011). Retrieved from http://www.wwltv.com/news/northshore/St-Tammany-sees-spike-in-suicide-rate-124704709.html

Substance Abuse and Mental Health Services Administration. (n.d.). *Trauma-informed care and trauma services.* Retrieved from http://www.samhsa.gov/nctic/trauma.asp

Taylor, E., Jacobs, R., & Marsh, E. D. (2011). First year post-Katrina: Changes in occupational performance and emotional responses. *Occupational Therapy in Mental Health, 27*, 3–25. doi:10.1080/0164212X.2011.543454

Te Brake, H., Dückers, M., De Vries, M., Van Duin, D., Rooze, M., & Spreeuwenberg, C. (2009). Early psychosocial interventions after disasters, terrorism, and other shocking events: Guideline development. *Nursing & Health Sciences, 11*, 336–343. doi:10.1111/j.1442-2009.00491.x

Wisner, B. (2002). *Disability and disaster: Victimhood and agency in earthquake risk reduction.* Retrieved from http://onlinewomeninpolitics.org/sourcebook_files/Ref5/Disability%20and%20Disaster-%20Victimhood%20and%20Agency%20in%20Earthquake%20Risk%20Reduction.pdf

World Federation of Occupational Therapists. (2006). *Shop: CDROM: Disaster preparedness and response information package.* Retrieved from https://www.wfot.org/wfotshop/shopexd.asp?id=71

World Federation of Occupational Therapists. (2009). *News-WFOT disaster preparedness and response.* Retrieved from http://www.wfot.org/news.asp?state=&name=&id=&pagenum=3

Yamkovenko, S. (n.d.). *Gulf Coast way of life dramatically changed: OT can assist in recovery.* Retrieved from http://www.aota.org/news/consumer/oil.aspx

Ziv, N., & Roitman, D. M. (2008). Addressing the needs of elderly clients whose lives have been compounded by traumatic histories. *Occupational Therapy in Health Care, 22*(2–3), 85–93.

For additional resources on the subjects discussed in this chapter, visit http://thePoint.lww.com/Willard-Spackman12e.

UNIT XIV

Professional Development

"... it is increasingly clear that learning does not occur in any enduring fashion unless it is sparked by people's own ardent interest and curiosity."

—Peter Senge, Art Kleiner, Charlotte Roberts, Richard B. Ross, & Bryan J. Smith

CHAPTER 66

Fieldwork and Professional Entry

Mary E. Evenson

OUTLINE

LEARNING OBJECTIVES

After reading this chapter, you will be able to:

1. Comprehend how fieldwork is integral to the educational curriculum and one's own professional development
2. Realize the requirements and levels of fieldwork education in United States and international academic occupational therapy programs
3. Become familiar with traditional and innovative types of fieldwork settings and supervision models
4. Appreciate the roles and responsibilities of those stakeholders who are involved in the fieldwork education process
5. Gain an understanding of the process and types of competencies that are used to evaluate student fieldwork performance
6. Grasp the dynamic nature of the personal and professional transitions that are inherent in the role shifts from that of being a student to assuming the role of a professional
7. Be aware of responsibilities for meeting professional credentialing requirements for certification and licensure/registration
8. Understand the entry-level competencies for both occupational therapists and occupational therapy assistants

Introduction

This chapter addresses the purpose and goals of fieldwork along with various models. Roles and responsibilities of students and educators are identified. Shifts in the learning context and expectations related to the transition from student to professional are discussed in addition to special considerations for students with disabilities. Lastly, factors associated with professional entry into employment are described.

Fieldwork or **practice placements** are structured learning experiences that are formally administered by academic programs in partnership with facilities that offer supervised training experiences. Whereas hospitals have served as traditional fieldwork settings, increasing numbers of placements are occurring in skilled nursing and long-term care facilities, community health, schools, private practice, and home-based settings (Rodger et al., 2008). Fieldwork education provides students with opportunities to apply theoretical and scientific knowledge to address the occupational performance needs of individuals and/or groups in authentic practice contexts (American Occupational Therapy Association [AOTA], 2009). The consensus within the occupational therapy profession is that the fieldwork experience plays an integral role in professional development. Through progressively more challenging fieldwork requirements, designed as a part of each academic program's curriculum, students gain exposure to a "variety of clients across the lifespan and to a variety of settings" (Accreditation Council for Occupational Therapy Education [ACOTE], 2007a, 2007b, 2007c).

Participating in fieldwork affords students the opportunity to develop collaborative supervisory relationships that evolve and shift as competency grows. Both students and supervisors experience the rewards of effective communication to nurture the teaching-learning process within the dynamic context of real-life practice. Optimally, supervisors use teaching techniques such as grading and scaffolding to support students in taking an active role in providing client services. Doing so requires flexibility because the supervisor role releases responsibilities to the student, whereas the student builds confidence in taking risks that are inherent in new learning and skill development. These formative fieldwork experiences significantly influence each student's future career choices, as discussed later in this chapter with professional entry.

It is important to differentiate between fieldwork, volunteerism, and **service learning**. Guided by accreditation requirements, fieldwork differs from volunteerism and service learning with specific professional competencies targeted as learning outcomes. Volunteer experiences focus on the benefit of service to the community or sponsoring agency without formal evaluation of the volunteer. On the other hand, service learning tends to be aligned with academic course objectives (Hansen et al., 2007). Based on a community-identified need, various service learning activities involve more than one visit and may evolve during a semester or at multiple points across a curriculum in a programmatic approach. Level I fieldwork or a project-based practice placement in a community-based setting may be organized as a service learning experience (Hansen et al., 2007).

Purpose and Goals of Fieldwork

The purpose of fieldwork education is to provide students with opportunities to apply the knowledge, skills, and attitudes learned in the classroom by putting them into practice in the fieldwork setting (Costa, 2004). Fieldwork experiences are intended to provide students with opportunities to carry out professional responsibilities under supervision of professionals who also act as role models (ACOTE, 2007a, 2007b, 2007c). Working in the context of real-life practice enables students to develop a multitude of skills. The two main categories of skill development that are inherent in participating in fieldwork are (1) the core skills and techniques that are relevant to occupational therapy service delivery for a given setting and (2) the personal skills that evolve and transform one's level of professional behavior (Missiuna, Polatajko, & Ernest-Conibear, 1992). For example, fieldwork interactions with clients and team members from other disciplines provide significant learning opportunities in the development of one's therapeutic use of self (Taylor, Lee, Kielhofner, & Ketkar, 2009) and in gaining awareness of the impact of cultural diversity on service provision (Murden et al., 2008).

Fieldwork also provides a venue for enculturation into the field as the interplay between the student as a person, the profession, and the environment supports the development of a professional identity along with a set of basic professional competencies (Alsop & Donald, 1996). This component of education functions as the gateway into the profession because it enables students to establish the fundamental skills of the profession that will support them in transitioning from the practice context of fieldwork into employment. The ultimate goal of fieldwork is to prepare students who possess the necessary competencies to be able to enter the workforce as a generalist practitioner. Beyond establishing basic skills in service provision, fieldwork also enables students to engage in advocacy, leadership, and managerial/administrative learning activities that require critical thinking, communication and collaboration, and ethical reasoning.

Levels of Fieldwork: United States

The ACOTE (2007a, 2007b, 2007c) outline the general fieldwork requirements for doctoral-level degree and master's-level degree occupational therapy students and for occupational therapy assistant students. The requirements are divided into two classifications: Level I and Level II fieldwork.

Level I Fieldwork Experience

Level I fieldwork offers students practical experiences that are integrated throughout the academic program. The ACOTE standards describe **Level I fieldwork** as "experiences designed to enrich didactic course work through directed observation and participation in selected aspects of the occupational therapy process" (ACOTE, 2007a, p. 650, 2007b, p. 661, 2007c, p. 670). For both occupational therapy and occupational therapy assistant students, the goal of Level I fieldwork is to introduce students to the experience, "to apply knowledge to practice, and to develop understanding of the needs of clients" (ACOTE, 2007a, p. 650, 2007b, p. 661. 2007c, p. 670).

Through Level I fieldwork experiences, students are exposed to the values and traditions of occupational therapy practice and have the opportunity to examine their reactions to clients, systems of service delivery, related personnel, and potential role(s) within the profession. Because the academic Level I performance expectations and specific purposes of the Level I fieldwork experience vary in each occupational therapy curriculum, the timing, length, requirements, and specific focus of the experience are determined by each academic program on an individual basis (AOTA, Commission on Education, 1999). For example, schedule options may include full or half days throughout an academic term, a 1-week placement, or otherwise prearranged visits to fieldwork sites.

A study of contexts and perceptions of Level I fieldwork in current practice revealed that the number of placements in emerging practice is growing and that students generally rated their Level I fieldwork experiences as positive (Johnson, Koenig, Piersol, Santalucia, & Wachter-Schutz, 2006). In examining the types of learning opportunities that are afforded to Level I students, observation and communication skills were the most commonly practiced skills across all types of settings (Johnson et al., 2006). Practice of additional clinical skills during Level I fieldwork most frequently included fine and gross motor activities in pediatrics (94%), range of motion in physical disabilities (82%), interviewing in emerging practice settings (77%), and behavioral management in mental health settings (73%) (Johnson et al., 2006, p. 281). Overall, Level I fieldwork students can maximize their learning experiences by proactively seeking opportunities to practice skills and to experience occupation-based practice.

Level II Fieldwork Experience

The goal of **Level II fieldwork** for the occupational therapy and occupational therapy assistant student is "to develop competent, entry-level generalist" practitioners (ACOTE, 2007a, p. 650, 2007b, p. 661, 2007c, p. 670). Accreditation standards state that "Level II fieldwork must be integral to the program's curriculum design and must include an in-depth experience in delivering occupational therapy services to clients, focusing on the application of purposeful and meaningful occupation" (ACOTE, (2007a, p. 650, 2007b, p. 661, 2007c, p. 670). The goal of students participating in administration and management of occupational therapy services and research is differentiated for occupational therapy Level II fieldwork when applicable. Additional learning outcomes for occupational therapy Level II fieldwork are to "promote clinical reasoning and reflective practice; to transmit the values, beliefs, that enable ethical practice; and to develop professionalism and competence as career responsibilities" (ACOTE, 2007a, p. 650, 2007b, p. 661). For occupational therapy assistant students, the purpose of Level II fieldwork is to "promote clinical reasoning, appropriate to the occupational therapy assistant role" as well as to achieve professionalism and competence (ACOTE, 2007c, p. 670). For more information about duration of placements, settings, and supervisor qualifications, see Table 66.1.

Initially working under direct supervision, students test firsthand the theories and facts learned in academic study and have a chance to refine skills through interaction with clients across the life course, with clients' families, and with team members while working in various service delivery settings and systems. As students' abilities grow, supervision may become less direct as appropriate for the setting and the severity of the client's condition. A developmental model of supervision can be applied as an approach for planning, intervening, and evaluating the students' readiness for learning and participation throughout the trajectory of a fieldwork placement. Within a developmental framework,

TABLE 66.1 Educational Requirements for Level II Fieldwork

	Occupational Therapy (ACOTE, 2007a/b)	Occupational Therapy Assistant (ACOTE, 2007c)	WFOT (Hocking & Ness, 2002)
Duration	24 wk full time	16 wk full time	1,000 h, some placements—8 wk
Settings	Minimum of one setting if reflective of more than one practice setting; maximum of four settings	Minimum of one setting if reflective of more than one practice setting; maximum of four settings	Different levels of health care: acute care, rehab, disability, community, and wellness
Supervisor qualifications	OT with 1 y of experience	OT or OTA with 1 y of experience	OT with 1 y of experience

ACOTE, Accreditation Council for Occupational Therapy Education; OT, occupational therapist; OTA, occupational therapy assistant; WFOT, World Federation of Occupational Therapists.

Practice Dilemma

You are participating in an outpatient fieldwork placement finishing up your fourth week. Your skills and confidence are growing, and your supervisor has assigned you primary responsibilities for several individuals on your shared caseload. You are treating a woman who sustained a wrist fracture as a result of a fall (unknown etiology). You have established a friendly and open rapport in working with this client over the past couple of weeks. However, the client comes into the clinic for her intervention session noticeably distressed. It is apparent that she has been crying with red, puffy eyes and she is acting withdrawn, not making eye contact, and limiting her normal conversation with you to short answers. You notice that she has a bandage on her arm with a cut/wound that appears to need stitches. The client's cell phone continues to ring/buzz throughout the session. Finally, she tells you that is her boyfriend calling and that she is afraid to talk with him because they had a fight before her coming into the clinic. The client breaks down crying as she explains to you that she does not feel safe to go back home. Other clients in the clinic are noticing that there is a problem. What do you do?

the learner and supervisor relationship progresses through four different phases: directive, coaching, supportive, and delegation (Barnes & Evenson, 2000). Throughout the placement, the fieldwork educator is responsible to assess the level of student competency for engaging in direct care and retains legal obligations for service provision in the fieldwork setting. In all, supervision of students must meet existing local, state/provincial, and/or federal/national safety and health requirements for relevant policies, laws, and regulations for occupational therapy practice.

Fieldwork: International Perspectives

Educational Standards

Internationally, the World Federation of Occupational Therapists (WFOT) Minimum Standards for the Education of Occupational Therapists (Hocking & Ness, 2002) require that students complete fieldwork in different health care settings. Within these settings, fieldwork must provide students with the opportunity to work with people of different ages who have acute and chronic health needs, delivering interventions that focus on the person, the occupation, and the environment (Hocking & Ness, 2002). Targeted learning outcomes for graduates of WFOT-approved educational programs are to demonstrate knowledge, skills, and attitudes in the following competencies: the person-occupation-environment and its relationship to health, therapeutic and professional relationships, occupational therapy processes, professional reasoning and behavior, and the context of professional practice (Hocking & Ness, 2002).

Placements

For students who are interested in elective international placements, the WFOT Website lists "Country Profiles" with contact details for national occupational therapy associations. It is recommended that students and academic programs allow at least 18 months for advance planning, working through the resources of the WFOT member country association in order to understand the supervision requirements of the country of interest as well as to assess individual student qualifications (AOTA, International Fieldwork Ad Hoc Committee for the Commission on Education, 2009; WFOT, n.d.) (see Box 66.1). As an alternative, non-fieldwork experiences abroad may be more readily accessible with wider choices and greater flexibility for scheduling when organized through volunteer organizations, charitable mission trips, faculty initiatives, or university global center institutes. With any type of intercultural learning experience, it is important to explicitly acknowledge and address disparities between health care providers and recipients of services, including belief systems, political systems, social structures, health status, educational level, and wealth (Whiteford & McAllister, 2007). Internationally, health educators have identified a number of factors that are influencing clinical education (see Box 66.1).

BOX 66.1 Requirements and Qualifications for Foreign Fieldwork

- Language fluency
- Support on local dialects and customs
- Knowledge of health care regulations and practices
- Personal safety
- Insurance
- Criminal records/police checks
- Travel advisories
- Conflict areas
- Housing
- Finances
- Contract between academic program and training facility
- Presence of qualified supervisors
- Duration of placement (meets curricular/accreditation standards)

BOX 66.2 Commentary: International Trends in Health Clinical Education

A multitude of factors are influencing fieldwork and practice placements and expectations of students and educators. Increasingly, university educators are facing challenges in providing sufficient placements for students with a trend of rising enrollments (Rodger et al., 2008). Health care environments are experiencing significant issues with staffing and decreased funding that are contributing to increased workloads. Work demands involving care provision to individuals with more acute health conditions and growing documentation demands create time constraints. At the organizational level, these issues are resulting in training facilities that have diminishing resources to effectively support students. These workplace demands, along with new educational requirements/standards, have shaped increased expectations of students, especially in the areas of initiative, judgment, and taking responsibility for independent learning (Vogel, Grice, Hill, & Moody, 2004). Preparing students to be competent practitioners in an increasingly complex and culturally diverse global health environment requires evidence-based care, reflective professional reasoning skills, population-based and preventive services, interprofessional collaboration, and a commitment to lifelong learning (Rodger et al., 2008).

Models of Fieldwork: Placement Settings and Supervision

Traditionally, fieldwork has taken place in the context of a hospital or primary health care setting in which students spend 6 weeks to 3 months at one facility with a single supervisor. However, a number of factors such as increasing demand for occupational therapy services, personnel shortages, and increasing needs for student placements are influencing the profession to develop and expand innovative fieldwork opportunities (Box 66.2). Fieldwork is now taking place in settings such as community-based day treatment programs, senior centers, assisted living facilities, sheltered workshops, homeless shelters, after-school programs, home health care, rural settings, and international placements (AOTA, Commission on Education and Fieldwork Issues Committee, 2000; AOTA, Education Department, 1999; Johnson et al., 2006; Thomas, Penman, & Williamson, 2005). For a summary of various fieldwork models and their benefits and challenges, see Table 66.2.

Roles and Responsibilities of Students and Educators

Students are eligible to begin fieldwork experiences upon completion of the prerequisite academic coursework or concurrently aligned with specific course(s) within the curriculum. Academic fieldwork coordinators or designated faculty are responsible for administrative arrangements to support student participation in fieldwork experiences, commensurate with the goals of the curriculum and accreditation standards as well as with the policies of affiliated practice settings and health care systems (Figure 66.1). Clearly defined objectives and guidelines can help to organize student efforts toward achieving professional competence. Working toward mastery of the entry-level skills required for high-quality client care is a mutual undertaking between fieldwork educators in academic and professional practice and students. Fieldwork or practice educators assume primary responsibility for the process of evaluating student progress and modifying the learning experience within the environment, in consultation with the academic fieldwork coordinator, as appropriate. See Table 66.3 to gain insight into how each person contributes to and participates in the overall fieldwork process.

Fieldwork Educator Guidelines

The role for the people who are responsible for providing student supervision is formally titled **fieldwork educator**, although the terms *clinical educator*, *fieldwork supervisor*, *student supervisor* (AOTA, Commission on Education and Fieldwork Issues Committee, 2000), or *practice educator* (Turpin, Fitzgerald, & Rodger, 2011) are also commonly and interchangeably used. Although the minimum requirement is 1 year of experience, fieldwork educators should be competent practitioners who meet governmental practices acts and regulations and serve as good role models or mentors for future practitioners. Supervising students can be beneficial in keeping up to date with research evidence and professional theoretical frameworks to guide occupation-based interventions. Additionally, serving in the role as a fieldwork educator enables practitioners to hone their teaching skills in fostering the professional development of future colleagues.

Beyond training students, supervision is fundamentally viewed as underlying to the quality of service provision and development of the workforce (College of Occupational Therapists [COT], 2006). National initiatives are providing training to support the professional development of fieldwork educators in response to identified needs (Gaitskell & Morley, 2008). In the United States, AOTA has implemented a Fieldwork Education Certificate Program with the curriculum centered on the Self-Assessment Tool for Fieldwork Educator Competency (AOTA, Commission on Education, 2009) that addresses five areas: professional practice, education, supervision, evaluation, and administration. Regional

TABLE 66.2 Fieldwork Models

Fieldwork Model and Definition	Benefits/Opportunities	Challenges/Drawbacks
Same-site model of fieldwork (Evenson, Barnes, & Cohn, 2002) *Level I and Level II Fieldwork in the same site*	• Gain familiarity with site • Increase comfort, decrease anxiety • Preparation for Level II	• Decreased exposure to field • Negative Level I can increase anxiety
Part-time fieldwork (Adelstein, Cohn, Baker, & Barnes, 1990; Phillips & Legaspi, 1995) *Placement "in accordance with usual and customary personnel policies as long as it is at least 50% of a full-time equivalent at that site" (ACOTE)*	• May support students with special learning needs or social obligations • Longer duration can promote skill development and client rapport • Optimal in long-term care, schools, or community settings	• Longer time in academic program • Can be challenging in acute care settings due to discontinuity in therapeutic relationship
Project-focused/role-emerging models (Fisher & Savin Badin, 2002; Fortune, Farnworth, & McKinstry, 2006) *Placement in which there is no occupational therapist on site*	• Focuses on occupational needs of setting/population • Establishes OT's role • Students serve as ambassadors for profession • Often in collaboration with community agencies or industry settings	• Generally requires extra support from academic program • Alters the number of clinical/hospital-based fieldwork
– Primary care (Hunt, 2006)	• Three phases: academic, exploratory, implementation and evaluation	• Supported integration of theory to practice
– Evaluation of cohort (Thew, Hargreaves, & Cronin-Davis, 2008)	• Structured 1 per week for 5 wk, then 5 wk full-time weekly formal and informal supervision	• May be inconsistent expectations of students between academic and facility educators
Collaborative models (Cohn, Dooley, & Simmons, 2001; Ladyshewsky, 1995) *Placement may entail one or more supervisors working with multiple students "with all participants viewed as more equal partners in the learning process" (Thomas et al., 2005, p. 80)*	• Promotes: – Positive interdependence – Face-to-face interaction skills – Cooperative, group problem solving • Supports both collaborative and autonomous learning	• Interpersonal difficulties, random-pairing (collaborative assignments) • Requires established structure and practices along with advance orientation for all parties to support optimal outcomes
– Peer-assisted blog (Ladyshewsky & Gardner, 2008)	• Heightened learning • Built trust	• Detailed guidelines are needed • Consider size of group
– Intraprofessional OT-OTA (Jung, Salvatori, & Martin, 2008)	• Develops relationship • Facilitates understanding of roles • Recognize environmental influences on learning	• Coordinating schedule between OT and OTA programs • Additional tutorial once per week with resources binder
– Aggregate (Precin, 2007)	• Involves interdisciplinary training/intervention • Continuous student interns on-site	• Students may underestimate skills and knowledge until they orient the next cohort
– Multiple mentoring (Nelson, Copley, & Salama, 2010)	• Working with other students • Accessing multiple supervisors • Increased independence and development of a range of skills	• Preplanned structure and organization needed to support learning and supervision of the group and individuals

ACOTE, Accreditation Council for Occupational Therapy Education; OT, occupational therapist; OTA, occupational therapy assistant.

workshops are instructed by a team of a practice and an academic educator. Online training programs have been developed in Canada and Australia. The Preceptor Education Certification Program for Health Professionals and Students consists of seven modules to guide learning (Bossers et al., n.d.). Developed in Australia, an online training package is freely available to support the use of the Student Placement Evaluation Form–Revised (SPEF-R), including resources addressing the use of the tool, various assessment processes, and approaches for providing feedback (Turpin et al., 2011). Each of these training programs serve as tools to assist the fieldwork educators who strive to develop and provide the best opportunity for the implementation of theoretical concepts offered as part of the academic educational program while creating an environment that facilitates learning, inquiry, self-direction, and reflection on one's practice.

Evaluation of Student Performance

Both formal and informal mechanisms for providing feedback and evaluation of performance, judgment, and attitude are built into the fieldwork experience. These

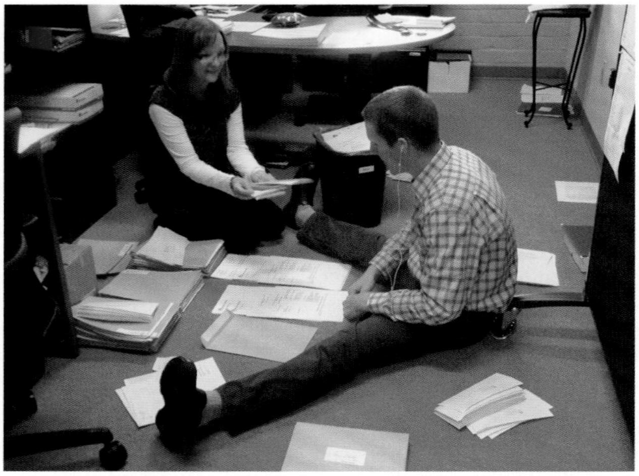

FIGURE 66.1 A fieldwork coordinator and her assistant sort through required paperwork.

evaluations have two distinct purposes, which are referred to as **formative** and **summative** processes. The formative process occurs throughout the fieldwork experience so that students and their fieldwork educators can compare perceptions, assess which learning activities are important and which are less so, review objectives, plan new learning opportunities, and make necessary modifications in behaviors and expectations. The summative process serves to document the level of skills attained. This cumulative review requires documentation of performance at the midpoint of the placement and upon completion of the fieldwork experience.

TABLE 66.3 Roles and Responsibilities in Fieldwork

Roles	Responsibilities
Academic fieldwork coordinator (AFWC)	• Serves as a liaison and collaborator with faculty and fieldwork educators to ensure integration of curricular goals with fieldwork (ACOTE, 2007a, 2007b, 2007c) • Selects training sites and assigns students • Oversees administrative requirements, such as contracts and student health records • Available for consultation to fieldwork educators and students
Fieldwork/practice educator	• Meets requisite eligibility for supervisory role as applicable (ACOTE, 2007a, 2007b, 2007c; CUFE-ACOTUP, 2011) • Engages in administrative collaboration with AFWC to determine and schedule assignments • Provides day-to-day student supervision • Completes evaluation of student performance as designated • Structures learning and create a positive learning environment
Student	• Fulfills all duties identified by the fieldwork educators and academic fieldwork coordinators within the designated time lines • Complies with the professional standards identified by the fieldwork facility, the education program, and the Occupational Therapy Code of Ethics (AOTA, 2010)

ACOTE, Accreditation Council for Occupational Therapy Education.

In the United States, the Fieldwork Performance Evaluation for the Occupational Therapy Student (FWPE/OTS) (AOTA, 2002b) and the Fieldwork Performance Evaluation for the Occupational Therapy Assistant Student (FWPE/OTAS) (AOTA, 2002a) are companion instruments, adopted by AOTA's Commission on Education in 2002 (Atler, 2003). Apart from a numeric rating system, the forms provide space for supervisors to add or qualify their scoring with written descriptions and comments (Atler, 2003). The intent of the fieldwork evaluation is not to differentiate between students but to measure one's achievement of specific entry-level competencies. A profession usually defines its boundaries by setting up criteria for entry. In occupational therapy, the fieldwork experience is an essential component of the entry criteria. Successful completion of Level II fieldwork is a requirement for certification as a registered occupational therapist (OTR) or certified occupational therapy assistant (COTA) (National Board for Certification in Occupational Therapy [NBCOT], n.d.). Future employers want assurance that students satisfy the entry-level requirements. The FWPE data may be synthesized to provide the foundation for employment references.

Internationally, there is a trend toward the use of standardized approaches for the evaluation of student fieldwork performance. The Competency Based Fieldwork Evaluation for Occupational Therapists (CBFE-OT) (Bossers, Miller, Polatajko, & Hartley, 2001), widely used across Canada and the United Kingdom, is designed for use in any level of fieldwork and within any placement area. This instrument is used in conjunction with a learning contract associated with each competency. In Australia, the Student Placement Evaluation Form–Revised (eSPEF-R) has been revised and included as part of an online package of resources (Allison & Turpin, 2004; Turpin et al., 2011; University of Queensland, Division of Occupational Therapy, 1998). A unique aspect of the SPEF-R tool is the option to select domains that relate to the streams of either direct service provision or project management/consultancy. It is noteworthy that each of these fieldwork evaluation tools is intended to be used across and within all practice settings. Furthermore, similar content and competency areas are evident among these tools, as noted in Table 66.4.

Student Evaluation of the Fieldwork Experience

Students also have the opportunity to provide their fieldwork educators and the fieldwork facility with feedback. AOTA, Student Evaluation of Fieldwork Experience Task Force (2006) recommends the Student Evaluation of Fieldwork Experiences (SEFWE) form. This form allows

TABLE 66.4 Fieldwork Evaluation in the United States, Australia, Canada, and the United Kingdom

	FWPE/OTS (United States)	FWPE/OTAS (United States)	SPEF-R; eSPEF-R (Australia)	CBFE-OT (Canada, United Kingdom)
Fieldwork evaluations and authors	(AOTA, 2002b)	(AOTA, 2002a)	(Turpin, Fitzgerald, & Rodger, 2011; University of Queensland, 1998)	(Bossers et al., 2001)
Purpose	To measure entry-level competence of the occupational therapy student	To measure entry-level competence of the occupational therapy assistant student	To assess student performance for professional practice and behavior	To evaluate a student's performance and learning
Content: Areas of competency	• Fundamentals of practice • Basic tenets • Evaluation/screening • Intervention • Management of OT services • Communication • Professional behavior	• Fundamentals of practice • Basic tenets • Evaluation/screening • Intervention • Communication • Professional behavior	• Professional behavior • Self-management skills • Coworker communication • Communication skills • Documentation • Information gathering • Service provision • Service evaluation	• Practice knowledge • Clinical reasoning • Facilitating change with a practice process • Professional interactions • Communication • Professional development • Performance management
Number of items	42	25	Variable; stream selected by practice educator; items vary for • direct client contact, including case management • project management/ consultancy	Variable; learning objectives are written by each fieldwork site as relevant to the setting
Rating scale	4 points	4 points	5 points	3 points
Evaluation	Midterm, final	Midterm, final	Midterm (halfway), final	Midterm, final

FWPE/OTS, Fieldwork Performance Evaluation for the Occupational Therapy Student; FWPE/OTAS, Fieldwork Performance Evaluation for the Occupational Therapy Assistant Student; SPEF-R, Student Placement Evaluation Form–Revised; CBFE-OT, Competency Based Fieldwork Evaluation for Occupational Therapists.

students to provide feedback about orientation, caseload, and occupational therapy process; theory, frames of reference, and models of practice; fieldwork assignments; supervisor interactions; aspects of the environment, such as team relationships; and how the entire learning experience related to the academic curriculum and to one's own professional development. In Canada and Australia, similar forms are used for students to provide feedback to fieldwork sites. Overall, documentation of students' feedback regarding their participation in fieldwork experiences provides valuable program evaluation information to both the training site and the academic program.

Transition from Classroom to Fieldwork

The shift from the academic setting to the fieldwork setting is an obvious, yet often underestimated, life change. As a student, this entails making the environmental transition from the classroom to the fieldwork setting while simultaneously emerging from the role of student into the role of occupational therapy practitioner (Figure 66.2). As with any transition, leaving academia triggers a process of change from one structure, role, or sense of self to another. The struggle to assimilate into a new environment and to develop a new role can jolt students into disequilibrium, and some students have trouble adjusting to the new role. As is true of all life changes, this disequilibrium can be an opportunity for growth, especially in the context of a supportive supervisory relationship.

This time of transition results in changes in assumptions about one's self and the world, requiring a corresponding change in behaviors, relationships, learning styles, and self-perceptions. In fieldwork settings, students may begin to reassess suppositions about occupational therapy, the theories learned in school, and their views of themselves as a practitioners, learners, and individuals. Because individuals differ in their ability to adapt to change and because each student is placed in a different fieldwork setting, these transitions have different effects on each student.

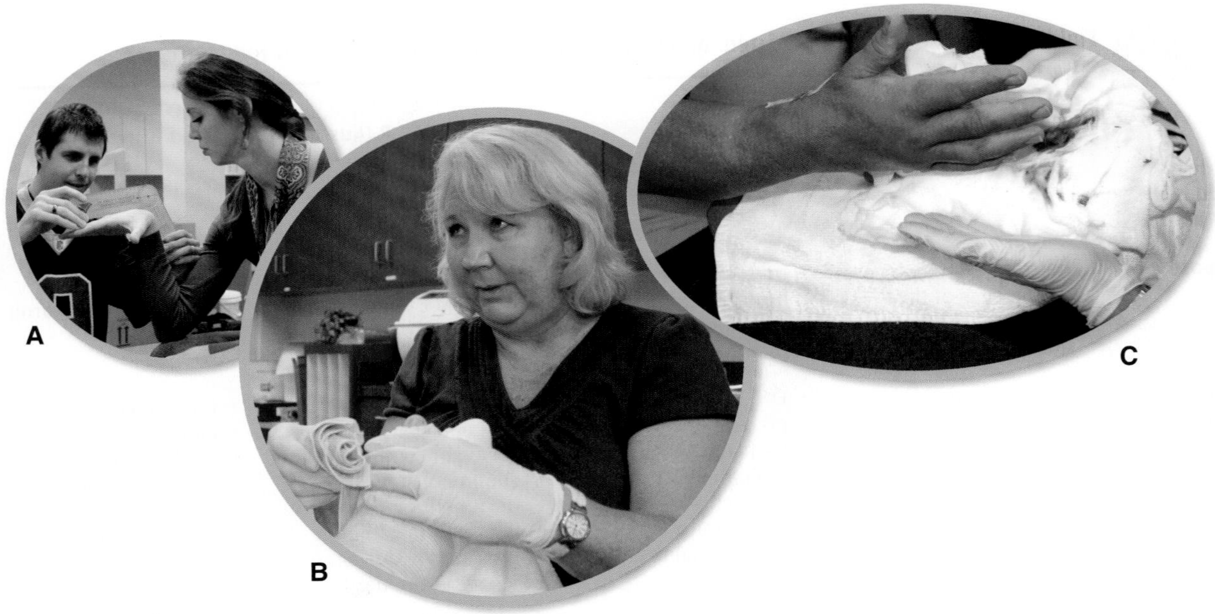

FIGURE 66.2 Moving from classroom to fieldwork: A lot to think about. Practicing techniques in the classroom can be very different than doing them with a client, as shown in these examples related to assessing wrist range of motion. **A.** The students are practicing how to measure wrist motion. **B.** The occupational therapist is unwrapping a man's hand during his first therapy session after hand surgery. This requires her to remove his dressings and manage any postoperative bleeding from his wound. **C.** The occupational therapist is observing how well he can move his wrist. She may eventually measure his wrist mobility using a similar technique as the students did during lab. Note how in the classroom, students can worry less about the client's fear and pain and focus on the technique. In practice, the therapist has to carefully monitor the client's response and postsurgical precautions while observing universal precautions and functional range of motion. Photos courtesy of Krisi Probert and Barbara Schell.

The nature of the fieldwork environment is fundamentally different from that of the academic environment. Knowing and acknowledging some of the distinctions between the two settings can ease the transition and provide support and insight to accept the challenges of fieldwork experiences (see Table 66.5). Within the fieldwork environment, the learning focus shifts to the application or implementation of therapy techniques in an applied interpersonal context. Techniques that were introduced in a simulated context now must be mastered and applied with attention to the client's emotional needs.

Abstract questions that are appropriate in the academic environment shift to pragmatic questions to reduce the possibility of error in one's thinking. For example, rather than thinking about a client's function in the kitchen from an abstract perspective, one has to think about the client's function in the context of a specific kitchen in a certain small apartment and attend to the client's concerns about his or her roles, activities, family, and home environment. Recognizing that actions have an influence on the client's life, supervisor tolerance for ambiguity or uncertainty declines during fieldwork.

In the academic setting, students are accountable primarily to self; and performance is evaluated on a summative basis through tests, assignments, and grades. Students can choose whether to disclose grades to family or peers, and performance has little effect on others. In the fieldwork placement, a student's performance is evaluated on a formative basis and may be observed by the entire health care team, especially at team meetings. Performance is no longer the private matter that it was at school but is publicly observed because it has direct and critical consequences for clients. Colleagues, clients, and their families may offer meaningful feedback. Although all these opportunities may create disequilibrium or tension, they also constitute new ways to learn about one's self and the profession. The broad and diverse experience within fieldwork settings presents challenges to redefine one's sense of self and evolving professional identity.

Fieldwork takes place in a situation over which fieldwork educators have little control. The organizational factors of the health care setting, combined with client care factors, such as the nature and complexity of the client's problem, the length of stay, and fluctuation in the client load, make planning difficult, especially in acute care settings. In settings that provide extended care for clients, however, the fieldwork educators are able to plan ahead because the client population is more constant and the fieldwork educator knows which clients will be available during student placements.

Fieldwork/professional practice educators' primary responsibility is client care; they have an ethical imperative to ensure the welfare of clients. This appropriate professional ethic may constrain activities that are desirable

TABLE 66.5 Distinctions between Academic and Fieldwork Settings

Characteristic	Academic Setting	Fieldwork Setting
Purpose	Dissemination of knowledge, development of creative thought, student growth	Provide high-quality client care
Faculty/supervisor accountability	To student, to university/college	To client and significant others, to fieldwork center and team, to student
Student accountability	To self	To clients and significant others, to supervisor and team, to fieldwork center
Pace	Depends on curriculum, adaptable to student and faculty needs	Depends on clients' needs, less adaptable, shaped by facility procedures
Student:educator ratio	Many students to one faculty member	One student to one supervisor, small group of students to one supervisor, one or two student(s) to two supervisors
Source of feedback	Summative at midterm or end of term, provided by faculty	Provided by clients and significant others, supervisor, and other staff; formative
Degree of faculty/supervisor control of educational experience	Able to plan, controlled	Limited control; various diagnoses and length of client stay, pace of setting, and size of caseload varies from setting to setting
Primary learning tool	Books, journal articles, lectures, audiovisual aids, case studies, simulations, technology, Internet	Situation of practice; clients, families, significant others, and staff; may be face to face or electronic (e.g., webcams, e-mail, -telehealth)
Conceptual learning	Abstract, theoretical	Pragmatic, applied in interpersonal context
Learning process	Teacher directed	Client, self, peer, supervisor-directed
Tolerance for ambiguity	High	Low
Lifestyle	Flexible, able to plan time around class schedule	Structured, flexible time limited to evenings and weekends or days-off
Contexts	University or college classroom, online learning	Hospitals, schools, nursing homes, day care centers, day treatment programs, community-based agencies, clients' homes

from the standpoint of education. However, the supervisory relationship allows fieldwork educators to adapt to the constraints of the setting. This unique relationship is a positive aspect of the fieldwork environment because fieldwork educators can adapt the fieldwork experiences to meet the learner's needs.

Examination of supervisors' perceptions of successful fieldwork students showed important themes of active experimentation as part of the learning process, including adaptability and doing as well as being flexible and engaging in teamwork (Herzberg, 1994). Specifically, successful students tend to take initiative to seek input from their supervisor(s), be more open to feedback, and work more independently (James & Musselman, 2005). A literature review on fieldwork success identifies a number of positive attributes to promote student participation (Sladyk, 2002, p. 8), as summarized in Box 66.3. Awareness of these attributes and characteristics, in addition to positive coping strategies, can aid students in preparing for and participating in their fieldwork placements.

Exploration of students' coping strategies and their perceptions of fieldwork has shown that a majority of students view the experience as important, while at the same time, more than half found the experience to be stressful (Mitchell & Kampfe, 1993). Level II fieldwork students invested significantly more effort in the positive coping strategies of being problem-focused, making a plan of action and following it, and seeking social support to obtain information, advice, or emotional support. These results verify healthy approaches and "coping skills for dealing with fieldwork transition and stress" (Mitchell & Kampfe, 1993, p. 537). Students less frequently used negatively regarded strategies such as blaming, wishful thinking, or avoidance—implying that students have healthy coping skills available to them to support their participation in the transitions associated with fieldwork.

An occupational adaptation model of professional development as applied to Level II fieldwork outlines three classes of adaptive response behaviors: primitive, transitional, and mature, which are typically demonstrated

BOX 66.3 Positive Attributes of Successful Fieldwork Students

- Showing interest in the area of practice and the profession
- Demonstrating concern for the client's needs and issues
- Regarding safety as a priority
- Taking responsibility for one's attitude and behaviors
- Managing time
- Adhering to time lines and due dates
- Seeking additional information
- Practicing skills
- Listening
- Using supervision time effectively
- Exchanging feedback with one's supervisor
- Accepting criticism
- Avoiding excuses
- Exploring new approaches or projects
- Engaging in creative problem solving

Sladyk, K. (Ed.). (2002). *The successful occupational therapy fieldwork student*. Thorofare, NJ: Slack.

among all students (Garrett & Schkade, 1995). When faced with situations that perceived as too difficult or too unfamiliar, students may tend to revert to lower level behaviors—see Box 66.4 for examples of at-risk behaviors that can jeopardize growth and success during fieldwork.

The occupational adaptation model can be a useful resource both for fieldwork students, to self-assess one's own behavior; and for supervisors, to help understand the implications and timing for increasing workload assignments and providing new learning challenges during fieldwork. Additionally, a student experiencing difficulty during fieldwork should communicate directly with his or her fieldwork supervisor and contact the academic program as a resource. Often, an action plan can be developed with specific strategies to address any identified challenges. The Fieldwork Experience Assessment Tool (FEAT) can be a useful method to help clarify which key components of fieldwork might be posing the greatest challenges, whether related to the student, the fieldwork educator, and/or the learning environment (AOTA, The Fieldwork Research Team, 2001).

Considerations for Students with Disabilities

Although occupational therapists are skilled in adaptation, the context of fieldwork education within practice environments presents legal, administrative, and emotional issues that impact supervision, especially for students with disabilities (Verma & Patterson, 1998). The demands of fieldwork are different from the classroom portion of academic programs and may push a student with disabilities past his or her ability to effectively compensate (AOTA, 2008). This realization may arise for students with an unknown or invisible disability that is uncovered through fieldwork challenges (Archer, 1999). Alternatively, students who are aware of their disabilities, whether visible or invisible to others, have the right to self-identify and work with the college or university administrative office to determine qualifications for accommodations. A student who chooses not to self-identify is not protected by the law and further risks compromising supervisory relationships with resentment and a lack of

BOX 66.4 Behaviors That Put Students at Risk

Affective Behaviors

- Making excuses or blaming others
- Being defensive, not receptive to feedback
- Allowing fear/anxiety to interfere with new learning and risk taking
- Making insensitive/unfiltered comments to others
- Difficulty upholding professional demeanor, appearing sleepy/sluggish, disinterested, distracted
- Becoming avoidant/passive or overwhelmed/shut down

Performance and Judgment Behaviors

- Arriving late in the morning to client sessions or to meetings
- Being disorganized or unprepared, such as misplacing schedule, documentation, etc.
- Failing to change behavior/performance after repeated feedback and redirection from supervisor
- Inconsistently maintaining your level of performance, "backsliding," regressing
- Violating facility policies, such as dress code, cell phone usage/texting
- Lacking ability to "think on your feet"
- Demonstrating poor safety awareness and adherence to precautions
- Breeching confidentiality by posting client or facility-related information to social networking Websites

respect (Kornblau, 1995; Llorens, Burton, & Still, 1999) and the possibility of failing fieldwork (Archer, 1999). Kornblau (1995) asserts that "students who fail to disclose their disabilities . . . create uncomfortable situations for all parties involved, including themselves" (p. 140).

Challenges described by educators provide evidence of the benefits of advance disclosure for students who have a disability. A pilot study of practice educators with experience supervising students with disabilities revealed important insights about setting demands and students' needs (Hirneth & Mackenzie, 2004). Practitioners working in rehabilitation and community settings described a higher degree of control in adapting time and organizational demands to facilitate student autonomy in comparison to those working in acute care. Furthermore, students who lacked initiative and confidence in acknowledging their strengths and limitations often caused a shift from a student–supervisor relationship to that of a client–therapist relationship, an approach that was perceived as less effective than an "educator" role (Hirneth & Mackenzie, 2004). The most difficulty described by educators was based on their experiences with students who had significant physical disabilities, rigid thinking, or lack of insight. Llorens et al. (1999) also reported the most challenges for students and faculty in determining accommodations for disabilities as a result of head trauma, learning disabilities, mental health conditions, and physical disabilities. It is hoped that the awareness of the experiences of these educators will help to motivate students with disabilities to be courageous and proactive in their communication to plan and prepare for participation in fieldwork.

Students who are aware of their disability have an opportunity to be self-advocates and disclose their status in advance of fieldwork to enable collaboration between themselves, the academic program and fieldwork coordinator, other health professionals, and the prospective fieldwork site(s) (Brown, James, & Mackenzie, 2006; Hirneth & Mackenzie, 2004). The decision to disclose can promote an open dialogue in exploring strategies and barriers and types of support available from the university, placement site, family and friends, and personal health care providers (Brown et al., 2006; Kornblau, 1995). Recommendations in advance of placements are to obtain a job description and to clarify the essential performance requirements. When possible, it can be useful for the student to also visit the fieldwork facility to plan ahead for accommodations and to explore what modifications may be necessary and those which are deemed reasonable by the training facility. In addition to these preparatory steps, key strategies identified by individuals with disabilities include setting personal goals, learning from prior experiences, identifying coping actions, and maintaining a positive attitude (Brown et al., 2006).

A qualitative study of practitioners with disabilities revealed themes related to having a unique therapeutic rapport and sensitivity to clients' needs, openly acknowledging and accepting personal strengths and limitations, and recognizing effective coping mechanisms (Velde, 2000). Resonating with these findings, a pilot study of health professional students with disabilities discovered that each individual reported a "unique experience" and the use of individual strategies were used to overcome individual barriers (Brown et al., 2006, p. 36). Overall, students identified the value of support during placements as an important component contributing to a positive educational experience (Brown et al., 2006; Hirneth & Mackenzie, 2004). Students who seek assistance in building confidence to take initiative in identifying and negotiating strategies and accommodations can plan for positive placement experiences and develop self-advocacy skills that will be needed in the future.

Transition from Fieldwork to Employment

For all students, the overarching purpose of the fieldwork experience is to gain mastery of occupational therapy clinical reasoning and techniques to develop entry-level competence. Effective oral and written communication of ideas and objectives that are relevant to the roles and duties of an occupational therapist or occupational therapy assistant, including professional interaction with clients and staff, is expected of all students. Students are responsible for demonstrating sensitivity to and respect for client confidentiality, establishing and sustaining therapeutic relationships, and working collaboratively with others. Another expectation, more internal to the students' development of positive professional identity, includes taking responsibility for maintaining, assessing, and improving self-competence. Students are responsible for articulating their understanding of theoretical information and identifying their abilities to implement evaluation or intervention techniques. Moreover, the ability to benefit from supervision as a resource for self-directed learning is *crucial* to professional development, establishing valuable habits that will support and sustain growth as a new practitioner.

Fieldwork has been described as a "road to employment," with students gaining important insights into practice demands, their preferences, and directions for the future (Simhoni & Andersen, 2002). Christie, Joyce, and Moeller (1985) highlighted that value by documenting the fieldwork experience as having the greatest influence on the development of a therapist's preference for a specific area of practice. Of the 131 therapists who were surveyed, 55% indicated that practice preferences were either formed or changed during the fieldwork experience, and another 24% noted that fieldwork experience expanded their interests to other areas of practice. Similarly, Crowe and Mackenzie (2002) examined the influence of fieldwork on preferred future practice areas of occupational therapy students. This study also demonstrated that "students use the fieldwork experience to guide their decision to enter an area of practice" (Crowe & Mackenzie, 2002, p. 25). Thus, the fieldwork experience can be rich and rewarding, and as such, it is likely to have a tremendous bearing on one's career choices.

Recruitment of students into paid employment positions has been identified as a benefit to organizations offering fieldwork placements (Rodger et al., 2007). However, in order to be eligible for employment, students must first apply for and successfully meet requirements for national certification and state licensure or registration, as applicable to laws and regulations for health care practitioners. Initial certification often involves successfully passing a national examination once all degree requirements are completed and verified by the university or college. New graduates must take responsibility to investigate and adhere to professional credentialing requirements and procedures. Once certification and licensure/registration, as applicable, have been granted, new graduates are ready to search for and accept a job position.

Studies report that new graduates may experience a range of feelings and stages of adjustment that are associated with entering the workforce. Hodgetts et al. (2007) identify that 6 months to 2 years of practice is often required for practitioners to feel competent. Tryssenaar and Perkins (2001) describe four stages associated with the first year of practice: "Transition, Euphoria and Angst, Reality of Practice, and Adaptation" (p. 19). Viewing the entry to employment as a time of predictable stress and rapid professional development can aid new graduates in seeking jobs that provide support and supervision to ease this transition. For example, the United Kingdom has implemented a 1-year preceptorship, whereby newly qualified NHS practitioners are paired with senior colleagues who serve as day-to-day role models and resources (Morley, Rugg, & Drew, 2007). Evaluation of this model revealed that new graduates sought out supervision for validating their clinical reasoning, addressing organizational and/or managerial situations, and fostering personal/professional development. Overall, these studies illustrate the importance of acknowledging that a transition period is normal for new practitioners entering employment.

This recognition is apparent in a survey of what attributes employers seek when hiring therapists, with less or modified expectations for new graduates (Mulholland & Derdall, 2004). Besides background experience, employers sought job candidates who possess attributes in teamwork, communication, interpersonal skills, and specific practice competencies. These findings can offer important insights to new graduates who are marketing themselves to prospective employers along with a realistic understanding of expectations for entry-level competencies.

Entry-level Competencies: OT and OTA

The outcome of successful classroom and fieldwork preparation is considered the achievement of **entry-level competence**. The occupational therapist and the occupational therapy assistant have different entry-level competencies when each begins practice. In the U.S., the occupational therapist receives a postbaccalaureate degree, which may either be a master's or entry-level doctorate degree, and the occupational therapist assistant typically receives an associate's degree. Although there are differences in the depth of learning, both practitioners receive education in the liberal arts; take prerequisites in the biological, physical, social, and behavioral sciences; and learn about the basic tenets of occupational therapy (ACOTE, 2007a, 2007b, 2007c). The occupational therapist comprehends and knows how to apply the various theoretical perspectives of occupational therapy and understands the evaluation process, which emphasizes the interpretation of assessments in terms of the underlying factors contributing to occupational performance needs and concerns as well as how the environment presents barriers to and supports for participation in daily life. The occupational therapy assistant may assist with the screening and assessment process through data collection depending on institutional regulations and policies.

The occupational therapist uses the interpretation of the assessment data to formulate an intervention plan—in collaboration with the client and the occupational therapy assistant—designed to improve occupational performance and daily life participation. Both practitioners may implement the intervention plan, but the occupational therapist is ultimately responsible for the entire occupational therapy process. The occupational therapist is trained in service management within various types of service delivery models. The occupational therapy assistant supports the occupational therapist in service management and understands the influence of these service delivery models, such as educational, medical, or community. Both practitioners read the professional literature, but the occupational therapist is able to determine how to use and apply research evidence for specific clients or populations. There is an emphasis in the education of both practitioners on advocacy, lifelong learning, professional ethics, values, and responsibilities. See Chapter 72 for more information about the roles responsibilities of occupational therapists and occupational therapy assistants.

Conclusion

Participating in fieldwork, successfully completing this component of an academic program, and entering employment are influential rites of passage in becoming an occupational therapy practitioner. Historically and in contemporary practice, fieldwork functions as a critical link between the academic world of theory, the scientific world of research, and the world of practice, now and in the future (Cohn & Crist, 1995; Lewis, 2005). Quality fieldwork involves an investment of all parties to promote successful experiences (Kirke, Layton, & Sim, 2007). The depth of the experience depends greatly on the degree to which students and fieldwork educators share the responsibility for teaching and learning. Today's rapidly changing health and human service delivery systems are providing new opportunities for occupational therapy practice and fieldwork education. Globally, the profession is giving attention to innovative approaches to improving the quality of fieldwork while taking into consideration each country's health, economic, educational, and social status (Bonello, 2001). To be successful in these dynamic and complex situations, practitioners must be able to make judgments based on thoughtful inquiry, analysis, and reflection on practice in order to support their clients in improving their participation in daily and social activities and overall quality of life.

Acknowledgments

A sincere thanks to Dr. Ellen S. Cohn for her longtime mentorship. I would like to acknowledge Dean Gloria Waters, Boston University College of Health and Rehabilitation Sciences, and Dr. Wendy Coster, Chair of the Department of Occupational Therapy, for support in writing this chapter. Also, I am grateful to the many fieldwork students, fieldwork educators, and colleagues who I have worked with, contributing to the value of fieldwork and recognizing the complexities of this learning experience.

References

Accreditation Council for Occupational Therapy Education. (2007a). Accreditation standards for a doctoral-degree level educational program for the occupational therapist. *American Journal of Occupational Therapy, 61*, 641–651.

Accreditation Council for Occupational Therapy Education. (2007b). Accreditation standards for a master's-degree level educational program for the occupational therapist. *American Journal of Occupational Therapy, 61*, 662–671.

Accreditation Council for Occupational Therapy Education. (2007c). Accreditation standards for an educational program for the occupational therapy assistant. *American Journal of Occupational Therapy, 61*, 652–661.

Adelstein, L. A., Cohn, E. S., Baker, R. C., & Barnes, M. A. (1990). A part-time level II fieldwork program. *American Journal of Occupational Therapy, 44*, 60–65.

Allison, H., & Turpin, M. (2004). Development of the student placement evaluation form: A tool for assessing student fieldwork performance. *Australian Occupational Therapy Journal, 51*, 125–132.

Alsop, A., & Donald, M. (1996). Taking stock and taking chances: Creating new opportunities for fieldwork education. *British Journal of Occupational Therapy, 59*(11), 498–502.

American Occupational Therapy Association. (2002a). *Fieldwork performance evaluation for the occupational therapy assistant student.* Bethesda, MD: Author.

American Occupational Therapy Association. (2002b). *Fieldwork performance evaluation for the occupational therapy student.* Bethesda, MD: Author.

American Occupational Therapy Association. (2008). *Ethical considerations for professional education of students with disabilities.* Retrieved from http://www.aota.org/Practitioners/Ethics/Advisory/Disabilities.aspx

American Occupational Therapy Association. (2009). Occupational therapy fieldwork education: Value and purpose. *American Journal of Occupational Therapy, 63*, 821–822.

American Occupational Therapy Association. (2010). Occupational therapy code of ethics. *American Journal of Occupational Therapy, 64*, 151–160.

American Occupational Therapy Association, Commission on Education. (1999). *Guidelines for an occupational therapy fieldwork experience: Level I.* Bethesda, MD: Author.

American Occupational Therapy Association, Commission on Education. (2009). *The AOTA Self-Assessment Tool for Fieldwork Educator Competency.* Bethesda, MD: Author. Retrieved from http://www.aota.org/Educate/EdRes/Fieldwork/Supervisor/Forms/38251.aspx?FT.pdf

American Occupational Therapy Association, Commission on Education and Fieldwork Issues Committee. (2000). *Guidelines for an occupational therapy fieldwork experience Level II.* Bethesda, MD: Author.

American Occupational Therapy Association, Education Department. (1999). *Innovative fieldwork annotated bibliography.* Bethesda, MD: Author. Retrieved from http://www.aota.org/Educate/EdRes/Fieldwork/38240.aspx

American Occupational Therapy Association, The Fieldwork Research Team. (2001). *Fieldwork Experience Assessment Tool (FEAT).* Bethesda, MD: Author. Retrieved from http://www.aota.org/Students/Current/Fieldwork/FEAT.aspx?FT=.pdf

American Occupational Therapy Association, International Fieldwork Ad Hoc Committee for the Commission on Education. (2009). *Recommended international fieldwork timelines for academic OT/OTA programs and fieldwork sites.* Retrieved from http://www.aota.org/Educate/EdRes/International/International-Fieldwork-Timelines.aspx?FT=.pdf

American Occupational Therapy Association, Student Evaluation of Fieldwork Experience Task Force. (2006). *Student evaluation of fieldwork experience.* Bethesda, MD: Author.

Archer, J. (1999). Essential functions: The journey of an OT student with learning disabilities. *Occupational Therapy in Health Care, 11*, 67–74.

Atler, K. (2003). *Using the fieldwork performance evaluation forms: The complete guide.* Bethesda, MD: American Occupational Therapy Association.

Barnes, M. A., & Evenson, M. E. (2000). Supervision and mentoring. In S. C. Merrill & P. A. Crist (Eds.), *Meeting the fieldwork challenge: A self-paced clinical course, Lesson 5* (pp. 9–12). Bethesda, MD: American Occupational Therapy Association.

Bonello, M. (2001). Fieldwork within the context of higher education: A literature review. *British Journal of Occupational Therapy, 64*, 93–99.

Bossers, A., Bezzina, M. B., Hobson, S., Kinsella, A., MacPhail, A., Schurrs, S., . . . & Jenkins, K. (n.d.). *Preceptor education program (PEP) for health professionals and students.* Ontario, Canada: University of Western Ontario. Retrieved from http://www.preceptor.ca

Bossers, A., Miller, L. T., Polatajko, H. J., & Hartley, M. (2001). *Competency based fieldwork evaluation for occupational therapists CFE-OT.* Albany, NY: Delmar Thomson Learning.

Brown, K., James, C., & Mackenzie, L. (2006). The practice placement education experience: An Australian pilot study exploring the perspectives of health professional students with a disability. *British Journal of Occupational Therapy, 69*, 31–37.

Christie, B. A., Joyce, P. C., & Moeller, P. L. (1985). Fieldwork experience 1: Impact on practice preference. *American Journal of Occupational Therapy, 39*, 671–674.

Cohn, E. S., & Crist, P. (1995). Back to the future: New approaches to fieldwork education. *American Journal of Occupational Therapy, 49*, 103–106.

Cohn, E. S., Dooley, N. R., & Simmons, L. A. (2001). Collaborative learning applied to fieldwork education. *Occupational Therapy in Health Care, 15*, 69–83.

College of Occupational Therapists. (2006). *Management briefing: Supervision.* London, United Kingdom: Author.

Committee on University Fieldwork Education, Association of Canadian Occupational Therapy University Programs. (2011). *Canadian guidelines for fieldwork education in occupational therapy (CGFEOT).* Retrieved from http://www.caot.ca/pdfs/Exam/June7.pdf

Costa, D. (Ed.). (2004). *The essential guide to occupational therapy fieldwork education: Resources for today's educators and practitioners.* Bethesda, MD: American Occupational Therapy Association.

Crowe, M. J., & Mackenzie, L. (2002). The influence of fieldwork on the preferred future practice areas of final year occupational therapy students. *Australian Occupational Therapy Journal, 49*, 25–36.

Evenson, M., Barnes, M. A., & Cohn, E. S. (2002). Brief report: Perceptions of level I and level II fieldwork in the same site. *American Journal of Occupational Therapy, 56*, 103–106.

Fisher, A., & Savin Badin, M. (2002). Modernizing fieldwork, part 2: Realizing the new agenda. *British Journal of Occupational Therapy, 65*, 275–282.

Fortune, T., Farnworth, L., & McKinstry, C. (2006). Project-focused fieldwork: Core business or fieldwork fillers? *Australian Occupational Therapy Journal, 53*, 233–236.

Gaitskell, S., & Morley, M. (2008). Supervision in occupational therapy: How are we doing? *British Journal of Occupational Therapy, 71*, 119–121.

Garrett, S. A., & Schkade, J. K. (1995). Occupational adaptation model of professional development as applied to level II fieldwork. *American Journal of Occupational Therapy, 49*, 119–126.

Hansen, A. W., Munoz, J., Crist, P. A., Gupta, J., Ideishi, R. I., Primeau, L. A., & Tupe, D. (2007). Service learning: Meaningful, community-centered professional skill development for occupational therapy students. *Occupational Therapy in Health Care, 21*, 25–48. doi:10.1300/J003v21n01_03

Herzberg, G. L. (1994). The successful fieldwork student: Supervisor perceptions. *American Journal of Occupational Therapy, 48*, 817–823.

Hirneth, M., & Mackenzie, L. (2004). The practice education of occupational therapy students with disabilities: Practice educators' perspectives. *British Journal of Occupational Therapy, 67*, 396–403.

Hocking, C., & Ness, N. E. (2002). *Minimum standards for the education of occupational therapists*. Forrestfield, Australia: World Federation of Occupational Therapists.

Hodgetts, S., Hollis, V., Triska, O., Dennis, S., Madill, H., & Taylor, E. (2007). Occupational therapy students' and graduates' satisfaction with professional education and preparedness for practice. *Canadian Journal of Occupational Therapy, 74*, 148–160.

Hunt, S. G. (2006). A practice placement education model based upon a primary health care perspective used in So. Australia. *British Journal of Occupational Therapy, 69*, 81–85.

James, K. L., & Musselman, L. (2005). Commonalities in level II fieldwork failure. *Occupational Therapy in Health Care, 19*, 67–81.

Johnson, C. R., Koenig, K. P., Piersol, C. V., Santalucia, S. E., & Wachter-Schutz, W. (2006). Level I fieldwork today: A study of contexts and perceptions. *American Journal of Occupational Therapy, 60*, 275–287.

Jung, B., Salvatori, P., & Martin, A. (2008). Intraprofessional fieldwork education: Occupational therapy and occupational therapy assistant students learning together. *Canadian Journal of Occupational Therapy, 75*, 42–50.

Kirke, P., Layton, N., & Sim, J. (2007). Informing fieldwork design: Key elements to quality fieldwork education for undergraduate occupational therapy students. *Australian Occupational Therapy Journal, 54*, S13–S22.

Kornblau, B. L. (1995). Fieldwork education and students with disabilities: Enter the Americans with Disabilities Act. *American Journal of Occupational Therapy, 49*, 139–145.

Ladyshewsky, R. K. (1995). Enhancing service productivity in acute care inpatient settings using a collaborative clinical education model. *Physical Therapy, 75*, 53–58.

Ladyshewsky, R. K., & Gardner, P. (2008). Peer assisted learning and blogging: A strategy to promote reflective practice during clinical fieldwork. *Australian Journal of Educational Technology, 24*, 241–257.

Lewis, L. M. (2005, September). Fieldwork requirements of the past, present, and future. *Education Special Interest Section Quarterly, 15*, 1–4.

Llorens, L. A., Burton, G., & Still, J. R. (1999). Achieving occupational role: Accommodations for students with disability. *Occupational Therapy in Health Care, 11*, 1–7.

Missiuna, C. A., Polatajko, H. I., & Ernest-Conibear, M. (1992). Skill acquisition during fieldwork placements in occupational therapy. *Canadian Journal of Occupational Therapy, 59*(1), 28–39.

Mitchell, M. M., & Kampfe, C. M. (1993). Student coping strategies and perceptions of fieldwork. *American Journal of Occupational Therapy, 47*, 535–540.

Morley, M., Rugg, S., & Drew, J. (2007). Before preceptorship: New occupational therapists' expectations of practice and experience of supervision. *British Journal of Occupational Therapy, 70*, 243–253.

Mulholland, S., & Derdall, M. (2004). Exploring what employers seek when hiring occupational therapists. *Canadian Journal of Occupational Therapy, 71*, 223–229.

Murden, R., Norman, A., Ross, J., Sturdivant, E., Kedia, M., & Shah, S. (2008). Occupational therapy students' perceptions of their cultural awareness and competency. *Occupational Therapy International, 15*, 191–203. doi:10.1002/oti

National Board for Certification in Occupational Therapy. (n.d.). *Online certification examination handbook*. Gaithersburg, MD: Author. Retrieved from http://www.nbcot.org/pdf/eligibility_01.pdf

Nelson, A., Copley, J., & Salama, R. (2010). Occupational therapy students' perceptions of the multiple mentoring model of clinical supervision. *Focus on Health Professional Education: A Multi-disciplinary Journal, 11*, 14–27.

Phillips, E. C., & Legaspi, W. S. (1995). A 12-month internship model of level II fieldwork. *American Journal of Occupational Therapy, 49*, 146–149.

Precin, P. (2007). An aggregate fieldwork model: Interdisciplinary training/intervention component. *Occupational Therapy in Health Care, 21*, 123–131.

Rodger, S., Thomas, Y., Dickson, D., McBryde, C., Broadbridge, J., Hawkins, R., & Edwards, A. (2007). Putting students to work: Valuing fieldwork placements as a mechanism for recruitment and shaping the future occupational therapy workforce. *Australian Occupational Therapy Journal, 54*, S94–S97. doi:10.1111/j.1440-1630.2007.00691.x

Rodger, S., Webb, G., Devitt, L., Gilbert, J., Wrightson, P., & McMeeken, J. (2008). Clinical education and practice placements in the allied health professions: An international perspective. *Journal of Allied Health, 37*, 53–62.

Simhoni, O., & Andersen, L. T. (2002). Fieldwork: A road to employment. *Occupational Therapy in Health Care, 16*, 37–43.

Sladyk, K. (Ed.). (2002). *The successful occupational therapy fieldwork student*. Thorofare, NJ: Slack.

Taylor, R. R., Lee, S. W., Kielhofner, G., & Ketkar, M. (2009). Therapeutic use of self: A nationwide survey of practitioners' attitudes and experiences. *American Journal of Occupational Therapy, 63*, 198–207.

Thew, M., Hargreaves, A., & Cronin-Davis, J. (2008). An evaluation of a role-emerging practice placement model for a full cohort of occupational therapy students. *British Journal of Occupational Therapy, 71*, 348–353.

Thomas, Y., Penman, M., & Williamson, P. (2005). Australian and New Zealand fieldwork: Charting the territory for future practice. *Australian Occupational Therapy Journal, 52*, 78–81.

Tryssenaar, J., & Perkins, J. (2001). From student to therapist: Exploring the first year of practice. *American Journal of Occupational Therapy, 55*, 19–27.

Turpin, M., Fitzgerald, C., & Rodger, S. (2011). Development of the student practice evaluation form revised edition package. *Australian Occupational Therapy Journal, 58*, 67–73.

University of Queensland, Division of Occupational Therapy. (1998). *Student placement evaluation and handbook*. Brisbane, Australia: Author.

Velde, B. P. (2000). The experience of being an occupational therapist with a disability. *American Journal of Occupational Therapy, 54*, 183–188.

Verma, S., & Patterson, M. (1998). Evaluating the marginal student: A workshop for clinical faculty. *Journal of Allied Health, 27*, 162–166.

Vogel, K. A., Grice, K. O., Hill, S., & Moody, J. (2004). Supervisor and student expectations of level II fieldwork. *Occupational Therapy in Health Care, 18*, 5–19. doi:10.1300/J003v18n01_02

Whiteford, G. E., & McAllister, L. (2007). Politics and complexity in intercultural fieldwork: The Vietnam experience. *Australian Occupational Therapy Journal, 54*, S74–S83.

World Federation of Occupational Therapists. (n.d.). *FAQ—International fieldwork*. Retrieved from http://www.wfot.org/faq.asp?name=Education

For additional resources on the subjects discussed in this chapter, visit http://thePoint.lww.com/Willard-Spackman12e.

CHAPTER 67

Competence and Professional Development

Patricia A. Hickerson Crist

LEARNING OBJECTIVES

After reading this chapter, you will be able to:

1. Discuss the professional expectation of and individual accountability for pursuing continuing competence and professional development
2. Differentiate the terms *competence* and *continuing competence* and explain the multiple variables influencing each concept
3. Describe the basic differences in competence expectations for occupational therapists and occupational therapy assistants
4. Understand how to demonstrate competence on an ongoing basis through self-assessment, individualized professional development, and portfolio preservation
5. Identify available resources and the steps in the process of creating a relevant professional development learning plan including beneficial learning activities for plan implementation
6. Consider the important role of certification, licensure, and advanced and specialty certifications for practice
7. Compare and contrast the merits of practice competence and practice excellence

OUTLINE

Introduction

Society insists that occupational therapy services are, at minimum, delivered competently. In reality, consumers, their families, those who pay for services, and the public expect occupational therapy practitioners to offer the highest quality services possible using competent delivery, reflecting best practice grounded in evidence. Applying ***best practice*** means consistently showing the most beneficial outcomes by "thinking about problems in imaginative ways, applying knowledge creatively to solve participation problems, and taking the responsibility for evaluating the effectiveness of the innovations to inform future practitioners" (Dunn, 2011, p. 2). Specifically in occupational therapy, doing best practice includes promoting participation in daily life activities that are important to our clients. This is done primarily through task modification, environmental adaptation, and customized therapeutic interventions designed to improve client's performance skills and to promote health (American Occupational Therapy Association [AOTA], 2010b). Excellence in practice requires each practitioner to establish, maintain, and update professional performance knowledge and skills to offer service delivery that is effective, safe, ethical, and accountable (AOTA, 2010a, 2010c, 2010d).

The foundation for competence is built on standards of practice that are established by a variety of entities, most importantly, the ones established by the profession of occupational therapy. Standards are the principles, rules, and ethics that are the components of delivering good practice consistently. Effective practitioners are expected to continuously reflect on their current competence in light of professional knowledge and standards. Commitment to *intentional, ongoing professional development activities* is expected in order to improve the quality of one's services (Figure 67.1).

This chapter discusses different aspects of competence as a professional responsibility. *Competence* refers to knowledge, critical thinking, motives, traits, characteristics, or skills to achieve a specific goal or perform job responsibilities. For all occupational therapy practitioners, competence is a generic principle regardless of where or how one practices. So although this chapter will primarily discuss the perspective in the United States, general concepts are likely to be relevant to various professional roles or settings as well as international perspectives regarding entry-level competency. First, expectations for entry-level competency are summarized because these form the foundation for building future competence as an occupational therapy practitioner. Next, approaches and resources to sustain professional competence are described, followed by a discussion of advanced certification and specialty certification. This chapter will close with reflections about viewing ideal or benchmark competency in the pursuit of practice excellence. Practice excellence is aspiring to more than the attendance of professional standards or evidence-based best practice.

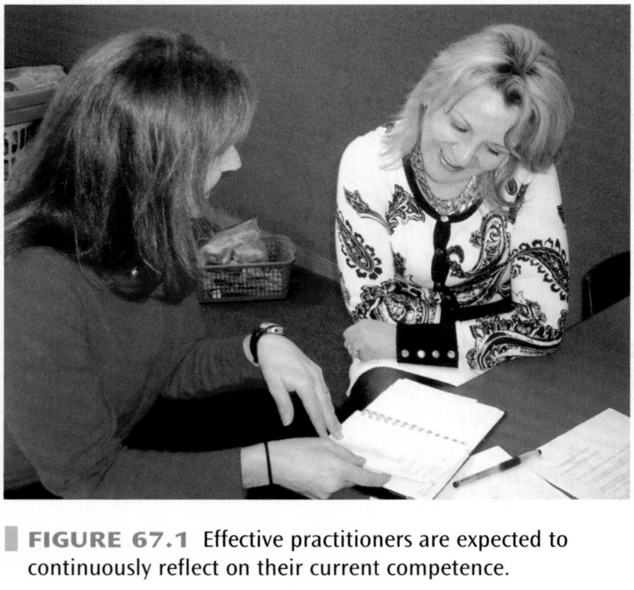

FIGURE 67.1 Effective practitioners are expected to continuously reflect on their current competence.

Entry-level Competencies

Occupational therapists (OTs) and occupational therapy assistants (OTAs) acquire the requisite knowledge, skills, and attitudes required for entry-level competence for the profession by completing both academic and fieldwork education (AOTA, 2011a). Table 67.1 provides a comparative summary of the expected standards of practice that practitioners are expected to demonstrate commencing with graduation from an entry-level academic program as an OT or OTA in the United States (AOTA, 2010c). For more detail, readers are referred to the official document and the AOTA's *Guidelines for Supervision, Roles, and Responsibilities during the Delivery of Occupational Therapy Services* (AOTA, 2009a). Readers from other countries are referred to the World Federation of Occupational Therapy for relevant resources (http://www.wfot.org). Upon graduation, all occupational therapy practitioners have acquired entry-level competence affecting these educational standards.

Continuous Learning and Improved Practice Performance

Occupational therapy practice is constantly changing in response to new practice evidence, advancements in technology, health policy modifications, institutional changes, and emerging areas of practice that create new employment options. In addition, practitioners may seek new employment opportunities requiring expansion of their knowledge of a new role, practice setting, or both. Clients, employers, third-party reimbursement resources, licensure boards, accreditation agencies, and society in general expect OTs and OTAs to assertively keep up with changes in practice by maintaining their abilities to skillfully deliver effective services in their specific service delivery contexts. Meeting these expectations can be challenging for several reasons (Moyers, 2009, p. 241):

- The skills and abilities of all practitioners fade with lack of practice, feedback, or administrative/systems support.
- The explosion of knowledge makes it challenging to focus learning and upgrade practice knowledge and skills.
- Significant sophistication is required to translate knowledge discoveries.

TABLE 67.1 Differences in Occupational Therapists and Occupational Therapy Assistant Standards of Practice—United States

Occupational Therapy Process	Occupational Therapist	Occupational Therapy Assistant
Education, Examination, and Licensure Requirements		
1. Graduated from an OT program accredited by ACOTE	x	x
2. Successfully completed a period of supervised fieldwork	Masters: 24 wk Doctors: 24 wk + 16 wk experiential	16 wk
3. Passed nationally recognized entry-level examination for OT	x	x
4. Fulfills state requirements for licensure, certification, or registration	x	x
Professional Standing and Responsibility		
1. Delivers occupational therapy services that reflect the philosophical base of occupational therapy and are consistent with the established principles and concepts of theory and practice	x	x
2. Knowledgeable about and delivers occupational therapy services in accordance with AOTA standards, policies, and guidelines and state, federal, and other regulatory and payer requirements relevant to practice and service delivery	x	x
3. Maintains current licensure, registration, or certification as required by law or regulation	x	x
4. Abides by the *Occupational Therapy Code of Ethics* (AOTA, 2010a)	x	x
5. Abides by the *Standards for Continuing Competence* (AOTA, 2010c) by establishing, maintaining, and updating professional performance, knowledge, and skills	x	x
6. Responsible for all aspects of occupational therapy service delivery and is accountable for the safety and effectiveness of the occupational therapy service delivery process	x	
7. Responsible for providing safe and effective occupational therapy services under the supervision of and in partnership with the occupational therapist and in accordance with laws or regulations and AOTA documents		x
8. Maintains current knowledge of legislative, political, social, cultural, societal, and reimbursement issues that affect clients and the practice of occupational therapy	x	x
9. Knowledgeable about evidence-based research and applies it ethically and appropriately to provide occupational therapy services consistent with best practice approaches	x	x- service implementation
10. Respects the client's sociocultural background and provides client-centered and family-centered occupational therapy services	x	x
Screening, Evaluation, and Reevaluation		
1. Responsible for all aspects of the screening, evaluation, and reevaluation process	x	
2. Accepts and responds to referrals in compliance with state laws or other regulatory requirements	x	
3. In collaboration with the client, evaluates the client's ability to participate in daily life activities by considering the client's capacities, the activities, and the environments in which these activities occur	x	
4. Initiates and directs the screening, evaluation, and reevaluation process and analyzes and interprets the data[a]	x	contributes
5. Uses current assessments and follows defined protocols when standardized assessments are used	x	x as delegated by OT
6. Completes and documents occupational therapy evaluation results[a]	x	contributes
7. Communicates screening, evaluation, and reevaluation results within the boundaries of client confidentiality to the appropriate person, group, or organization	x	

(continued)

TABLE 67.1 Differences in Occupational Therapists and Occupational Therapy Assistant Standards of Practice—United States (*Continued*)

Occupational Therapy Process	Occupational Therapist	Occupational Therapy Assistant
8. Recommends additional consultations or refers clients to appropriate resources when the needs of the client can best be served by the expertise of other professionals or services	x	
9. Educates current and potential referral sources about the scope of occupational therapy services and the process of initiating occupational therapy services	x	x
Intervention		
1. Has overall responsibility for the development, documentation, and implementation of the occupational therapy intervention based on the evaluation, client goals, current best evidence, and clinical reasoning	x	
2. Ensures that the intervention plan is documented within the time frames, formats, and standards[a]	x	contributes
3. Collaborates with the client to develop and implement the intervention plan based on the client's needs and priorities, safety issues, and relative benefits and risks	x	x
4. Coordinates the development and implementation of the occupational therapy intervention with the intervention provided by other professionals when appropriate	x	x
5. Selects, implements, and makes modifications to therapeutic activities and interventions	x	x-as delegated by OT
6. Modifies the intervention plan throughout the intervention process and documents the changes in the client's needs, goals, and performance	x	contributes
7. Documents the occupational therapy services provided within the time frames, formats, and standards[a]	x	x
Outcomes		
1. Selects, measures, documents, and interprets expected or achieved outcomes that are related to the client's ability to engage in occupations	x	
2. Documents changes in the client's performance and capacities and for transitioning the client to other types or intensities of service or discontinuing services when the client has achieved identified goals, reached maximum benefit, or does not desire to continue services	x	contributes
3. Prepares and implements a transition or discontinuation plan based on the client's needs, goals, performance, and appropriate follow-up resources.	x	contributes
4. Facilitates the transition or discharge process in collaboration with the client, family members, significant others, team, other professionals, and community resources when appropriate	x	x
5. Evaluates the safety and effectiveness of the occupational therapy processes and intervention within the practice setting	x	contributes

[a]In accordance with applicable federal and state laws; other regulatory, external accreditation programs and payer requirements; and AOTA documents as well as established time frame, formats, and standards established by practice settings and agencies.

ACOTE, Accreditation Council for Occupational Therapy Education; AOTA, American Occupational Therapy Association; OT, occupational therapy.

Adapted from American Occupational Therapy Association. (2010d). Standards of practice for occupational therapy. *American Journal of Occupational Therapy*, *64*, S106–S111; and American Occupational Therapy Association. (2009a). Guidelines for supervision, roles and responsibilities during the delivery of occupational therapy services. *American Journal of Occupational Therapy*, *63*, 173–179.

- The pressure from complex health care and social systems create barriers to practice enhancements.
- Rapid shifts in health policy and third-party reimbursement processes that modify intervention delivery and outcome expectations.

Each of the aforementioned mandates that the practitioner continuously engage in learning activities to ensure his or her continuing competency. This reflective process values competence as a dynamic interaction between acquired knowledge, practice skill efficacy, and critical reasoning (AOTA, 2010c).

In occupational therapy literature and professional discussions, competence and competency have become linked to professional discussions related to lifelong learning (Baum, 2000; Moyers & Hinojosa, 2003). Lifelong learning is advocated to promote practice scholarship that will assist with not only bridging education research and practice but also with developing the knowledge, skills, and abilities among OTs and OTAs to ensure competencies in the future (AOTA, 2007, 2010a, 2010c, 2010d).

What Does It Mean to Be Competent?

Competence refers to knowledge, critical thinking, motives, traits, characteristics, or skills to achieve a specific goal or perform job responsibilities. In the occupational therapy literature, competence is often related to the ability to use effective professional or clinical reasoning, which results in effective therapy (Moyers, 2009; Moyers & Hinojosa, 2003). **Competency** is the *actual performance* of competence. Competency is the result of comparing one's practice process and outcomes with a specific criterion such as using evidence-based practice. Substantiating competency implies internal self-determination coupled with external validation regarding one's effectiveness in performing certain skills or behaviors.

Ensuring competence and practicing competently is a dynamic and evolving process requiring lifelong learning. Determining the currency of one's competence requires self-evaluation of one's existing abilities according to criteria such as completing a self-development tool, a periodic peer review, a knowledge examination, a refresher course offered by the employer, or even recalibrating oneself against published standardized procedures published for an assessment tool or meeting continuing education (CE) requirements for licensing or certification. Also, one may seek out professional development opportunities to identify and enhance a skill set to ensure implementation of contemporary approaches during practice. Common approaches include pursuing post–professional education or workshops, reading scholarly publications and/or evidence-based practice briefs, securing specialty certifications, participating in local special interest practitioner groups, or attending focused in-service or conference presentations. At minimum, thoughtful engagement in these professional development activities is validation that one is engaging in expected practice standards.

Costs of Poor Competency

Competence is a core professional value because of the risks to clients when poor or substandard services are provided. The public perception of the profession is also harmed by poor practice, thus potentially discouraging the use of effective services by clients who could benefit from effective occupational therapy services. All stakeholders, including the client, their family, employers, payers, and social service agencies, expect at least minimally effective practice; and for the most part, the use of best practices grounded in evidence that suggests that intervention will lead to desired outcomes. For instance, consider possibilities such as new research describing an effective method of functional retraining for individuals after stroke, suggesting methods to significantly reduce the impact of autism on school performance, or explaining an intervention to support community-based independent living for individuals with persistent mental illness. Professional ethics and accountability requires the practitioner to be aware of such innovations to continually maintain high standards of competence. Not knowing about new evidence or seeking relevant training for practice approaches supported by evidence represents unethical and neglectful practice and may lead to charges of malpractice. Waiting for external funding from employers or others to be educated is not sufficient. An ethical, responsible occupational therapy practitioner needs to proactively advocate for and complete continuing competence activities to ensure contemporary practice competence. In some situations, self-funding is advised not only to honor one's professional responsibility to do one's best but also to prevent neglect or harm, which includes not delivering the most effective intervention available.

Incompetent or substandard evaluation, intervention planning, or intervention processes may harm the client, resulting in permanent functional limitations. Additionally, payment for services may be denied. Practitioners may be held legally liable for malpractice. Incompetent action resulting in harm may lead to censure by professional groups, such as AOTA or National Board for Certification in Occupational Therapy (NBCOT), or punitive actions by governmental bodies such as state regulators or external accreditors or third-party reimbursers. Actions such as these can significantly limit practice options or even terminate recognition as a qualified occupational therapy practitioner.

Professional Development and Resources in the United States

The continuing competency journey begins with becoming familiar with external guides and resources developed by organizations and agencies committed to ensuring a work force enabled to provide quality occupational therapy services. Professional organizations, certification agencies, institutional accreditation programs, and state regulatory groups each play a unique and pivotal role in defining and applying standards related to competence and continuing competence. For occupational therapy in the United States, the primary ones are AOTA, NBCOT, governmental programs, state regulatory agencies, and institutional accreditation bodies. All have vested interests in promoting quality service delivery that provides congruities between entities. On the other hand, each of their missions and purposes are very unique, and as a result, a healthy tension exists that supports quality service delivery, promotes the profession, honors all the stakeholders, and protects professional domains of concerns. Table 67.2 presents the major players addressing continuing competence in practice and their role.

TABLE 67. 2 Organizations and Focus Related to Continuing Professional Development in Occupational Therapy

	American Occupational Therapy Association (AOTA; state associations also)	National Board for Certification in Occupational Therapy (NBCOT)	State Regulatory Agencies	Institutional Accreditation Bodies
	AOTA http://www.aota.org (state associations parallel)	NBCOT http://www.nbcot.org	Check each state's government site[a]	Examples: CARF, JC[b]
Purpose	Support the profession by setting standards to assure high-quality services; represent the interests and concerns of occupational therapy practitioners, students, and educational programs to the public and to policy groups; improve consumer access to health care services; and promote the professional development of members.	Certification of occupational therapy practitioners; develop, administer, and continually review a certification process based on current and valid standards that provide reliable indicators of competence for the practice of occupational therapy.	Oversee implementation of laws or statutes enacted by legislators who are elected public officials; regulations specifically describe how the intent of the laws will be carried out.	Quality assurance; indicate service provider's commitment to continually improve services, encourage feedback, and serve the community.
Oversight responsibilities	Profession	Certificants (initial) and those who voluntarily recertify after initial certification.	State government regulators who are appointed public officials of various departments or boards in state government to enact state law.	Nonprofit agencies offering accreditation to institutions.
Responsible to	Members of the association	Consumers of practice or intervention	Citizens of the state	Consumers of services
OT Input	OT and OTA members elect key leaders and representatives who make decisions. Appointed or elected volunteer committees make recommendations to decision makers.	OTR and COTA representatives along with public representatives are appointed by the governing board. Working groups such as certification examination development have OT/OTAs.	Government-appointed board members oversee regulations (writing and ensuring implementation). OTs can be appointed to a board.	Experts invited by agency to set standards and accredit. Standards are developed independently but seek input from related professions such as OT. Can be trained as an evaluator.
Professional development	Provides standards and guidelines for practice, self-assessment tools, profession-focused continuing education, and advanced board and specialty certification processes	Certification renewal requires acquisition of professional development unit, self-assessment tools and verification documents	Requirements for continuing education established by each state	Standards related to continuing competency promote institutional supports
Value	Supports OT and OTA members by promoting the profession, educating the public, and advancing the profession	Public, regulatory groups, and employers by providing certification examination, verification of credentials, disciplinary actions, and oversight of ongoing general professional certification	Public health and welfare	Public health and welfare, including third parties who provide service reimbursement

[a]AOTA and NBCOT maintain current lists.

[b]The Joint Commission accredits nine types of health care settings, including hospitals, behavioral health care, home care, and long-term care (http://www.joint commission.org).

CARF, Commission on the Accreditation of Rehabilitation Facilities (http://www.carf.org); COTA, certified occupational therapy assistant; JC, The Joint Commission; OT, occupational therapist; OTA, occupational therapy assistant; OTR, occupational therapist, registered.

The promotion of the profession comes from each of these organizations being sufficiently well established and powerful enough to oversee and drive valuable change in response to challenges and opportunities. As stated earlier, continuing competency is complex and multifactorial. Thus, it benefits practitioners to have many sets of resources to guide and/or support professional development in occupational therapy.

The **American Occupational Therapy Association** (http://www.aota.org) is committed to ensuring quality service delivery and has several resources that are useful: "AOTA Standards for Continuing Competence" (AOTA, 2010c) and the "AOTA Standards of Practice" (AOTA, 2010d). Together, these outline core performance expectations that oversee all practice. The AOTA (2010c) describes continuing competency as multidimensional including the following required core competencies related to individual practitioner roles and responsibilities:

- *Knowledge* about multiple roles and responsibilities
- *Critical reasoning* processes as the basis for decision making
- *Interpersonal skills* for professional relationships and communication
- *Performance skill* capabilities reflecting expertise, aptitudes, proficiencies, and abilities
- *Ethical practice* responding responsibly to issues and dilemmas in the changing context

In addition, AOTA publishes various practice guidelines and related documents that are specific to practice with specific populations, conditions, and/or contexts. The AOTA (2003) *Professional Development Tool* provides a process for self-assessing professional development interests and needs then presents a guide for planning. Board and specialty certification provides validation for dedication to continuing competence and quality service delivery in advanced or specialty practice areas that exceed the profession's core expectations. For these, the competencies outlined serve as a guide for self-assessing as well as accumulating evidence regarding one's advanced or specialty practice competency (see Case Study 67.1, which describes initiating the professional development process). Due to the nature of the AOTA mission, CE opportunities are focused exclusively on "best practices" in occupational therapy to strengthen and promote this profession only.

CASE STUDY 67.1 An Entry-level Practitioner Initiates a Professional Development Plan

Tramar has just accepted his first position as an occupational therapy practitioner with very limited access to experienced practitioners. As part of the position negotiation, he obtained agreement for a consultant to mentor him and help him "come up to speed" in any areas he feels that his abilities need to be enhanced. At the end of the first 3 weeks on the job, he discusses his professional development needs with both his mentor and his manager regarding specific practice competency needs and expectations in this setting. He has used the current job description, his observations of practice in this setting, and standards of practice and practice guidelines published by the profession through American Occupational Therapy Association (AOTA) to complete the *AOTA Professional Development Tool*. During this process, he reflected on his prior experience in a similar fieldwork setting but also standards for practice specific to this setting in which he is seeing a mix of clients, some with acquired brain injuries (ABIs) and some with orthopedic conditions, including hand injuries. He feels reasonably competent in areas such as self-care retraining and basic use of adaptive devices as well as positioning devices such as static finger and hand splints.

Tramar has identified gaps in his knowledge and skills that need attention in order to be competent using best practice and to be safe in certain practice expectations. These include the effective integration of both cognitive and motor control theories in the context of occupation-based approaches for the patients he is seeing with ABIs. Additionally, he is uncomfortable managing the patients who have complex hand injuries. Using resources to identify gaps in knowledge and practice skills coupled with considering the large number of different ways to engage in continuing competency activities outlined both by National Board for Certification in Occupational Therapy and AOTA, Robert and his supervisor negotiate a beneficial professional development plan for him. In the meantime, he purposely and ethically self-manages by not engaging in practices where he does not feel currently competent. He does this by referring the patients with complex hand injuries to a private therapist to do the initial evaluation and splinting, and he then follows the intervention plan suggested by this colleague. His mentor helps him think through safe options for intervening with his clients with traumatic brain injury (TBI). His supervisor appreciates this self-monitoring and supports these decisions.

In the short term, he negotiated release from daily work in order to go to another facility to be mentored by an occupational therapist (OT) who is more experienced in how to integrate motor control approaches in the context of occupational therapy with individuals who have ABI. He also has identified several texts to review and some continuing education courses that are based on current innovation in occupational therapy for people with TBI that focus on improving motor function during activity. He recognizes that the facility would benefit from having someone who has advanced skills in hand therapy, so he also presents a long-term plan to become a certified hand therapist.

State professional associations provide similar activities as AOTA but are more parochial to state interests, particularly as desired by the state government agencies or programs. The goal of state professional associations is to represent and advocate for practice opportunities and challenges at the state level, whereas many require some form of continuing competence engagement. State associations also closely monitor, even provide suggestions regarding the state regulations regarding continuing competency.

The NBCOT (http://www.nbcot.org) is most known for its role in initial certification examination for OT and OTAs, which culminates in being awarded use of the occupational therapist, registered (OTR) or certified occupational therapy assistant (COTA©) credential. "NBCOT also serves the public interest by developing, administering, and continually reviewing a certification process that reflects current standards of competent practice in occupational therapy" (NBCOT, 2011, para. 1). The professional development requirement for NBCOT recertification is to be able to demonstrate continuing competency of the certificants to the public, be it consumers, employers, agencies, etc. To retain use of the OTR or COTA© professional certification designations, one must apply for certification renewal every 3 years and be able to present documentation regarding continuing competency activities. One of the goals regarding recertification is to engage certificants of all levels of experience in self-reflective assessment of one's current levels of proficiency or efficacy leading to ongoing, role-related engagement in continuing competency activities. Certification renewal requires assembling documentation of continuing competence activities called *professional development units* (PDUs). In addition, NBCOT provides self-assessment tools to self-identify professional developmental needs in the highest frequency practice areas for the OTR and COTA.

Some form of **government-based state regulation of practice** is present in all 50 states plus the District of Columbia, Puerto Rico, and Guam for occupational therapy practitioners in some capacity. The major purpose of regulation is to protect consumers in a state or jurisdiction from unqualified or unscrupulous practitioners (AOTA, 2011b). Different states have various types of regulation that range from licensure, the strongest form of regulation, to title protection or trademark law, the weakest form of regulation. State laws and regulations significantly affect the practice of occupational therapy. Eighty percent of the states have a continuing proficiency or education requirement requiring acquisition of continuing education units (CEUs). However, the types and amount of qualified professional development activities varies widely between states.

The expectation of continuing competency is universal, but the process to demonstrate this knowledge and skill is variant, and sometimes the value is questioned. For instance, does mere accumulation of PDUs or CEUs[1] really support competency? How does the quality of the provider and/or the program contribute to enhanced professional development? What evidence or critical analysis of knowledge is provided to support application of an approach? How effectively can learning from workshops be implemented into daily practice? AOTA provides a voluntary, approved CE provider screening and designating process called the AOTA Approved Provider Program (APP) that aligns with the professional association's mission. The International Association for Continuing Education and Training (IACET), who originated the CEU concept, is another prominent source overseeing quality through accrediting adult learning programs (http://www.iacet.com). Even so, the major responsibility still lies on each occupational therapy practitioner to constantly reflect on his or her practice outcomes; determine critical learning needs to ensure continuing competence; and thoughtfully engage in quality, meaningful learning activities to be competent in service delivery and related roles. This requires an ongoing process of skillfully integrating new learning into practice.

Factors Motivating Competency Assurance

Moyers (2009) described continuing competence as a dynamic, multi-factorial process. She notes that there can be multiple and overlapping roles in practice along with a variety of tasks performed in one or more contexts. The ongoing changes in these prompt professional development. Relevant professional development or career goals might include the following:

- Deepening one's knowledge and skill to move from one level of practitioner maturation to another in a specific practice area (e.g., moving from being competent to provide services for infants to becoming an expert in providing services in the neonatal intensive care unit).
- Expand current knowledge and skills to have a greater variety of approaches during practice for new work contexts, roles, or projects (e.g., developing increased skills in environmental assessment and modifications in order to provide home visits and support older adults in returning home after major illness or disabling conditions).
- Expanding, changing roles, or adding new roles and related abilities (e.g., adding a new role such as fieldwork educator, manager, consultant, entrepreneur, academic educator, or practice scholar).
- Considering the relevance and evidence for recent innovative or novel therapy approaches (e.g., introducing Smartphone apps as a therapeutic support or documentation device).
- Moving into unexpected roles or contexts to apply one's occupational therapy skill set (e.g.,

[1]One hour of professional development activity = one CEU and one PDU.

competence in emerging areas of practice or roles where occupational therapy skills are valuable but not essential such as being a practice manager for a physiatrist, a coordinator for a local government's programs for aging citizens, or the chief executive officer for a community, nonprofit agency).

Regardless, if the goal is to be a competent practitioner, engagement in thoughtful, continuous professional development processes is essential. A practitioner must also critically evaluate who determines competence when implementing a continuous, goal-directed competency development plan that is not only individually relevant but also judiciously and ethically reflects external practice demands.

Who Determines if Someone Is Competent?

Being competent to deliver practice is a responsibility that each practitioner must self-determine and, preferably, be able to document. In addition, the profession and public use credentials for practice as indicators that the practitioner has met minimal standards to provide safe, quality practice. The most common approaches to determining competency are entry-level education expectations, testing, credentialing, and requiring position-related CE (Moyers, 2009). Graduation from an accredited educational program, licensure, and/or professional certification is presumed to protect the public from incompetent practitioners.

State regulatory authorities and NBCOT protect the public by providing practice credentials to qualified individuals: this is referred to as *credentialing*. Not only do these groups credential individuals who have met their standards, they also remove credentials from individuals if the practitioner is either not able to or not willing to act according to established standards. Both groups actively share information about practitioners which includes the credentialing status, any practice violations of professional misconduct as well as any regulatory and certification renewal issues. This information is of particular interest to current or future employers. On finding significant misconduct or malpractice, one's practice credential will be removed, reprimanded, or censored. Most states have licensure portals that readily identify the current state-credentialed practitioners. For NBCOT, current verification is only available on request and includes a fee.

Planning and Engaging in Reflective Professional Development

Professional development is a career maturation process that supports competence and engaging in continuing competency activities. Continuing competence of a practitioner mirrors one's commitment to growth and self-improvement (Moyers, 2009). "The challenge of staying current with one's professional roles and responsibilities reflects:

1. Job analysis reflecting roles, responsibilities, and resulting tasks
2. Capacity for performing tasks competently (from novice to expert functioning)
3. Meeting professional development requirements to ensure quality improvement." (Moyers, 2009, pp. 242–243)

Professional development outcomes result from engaging in reflection of current competence for daily work and plans for future aspirations in a greater variety of roles, different settings, or future work with different or emerging areas of practice. Professional development planning guides career change into new roles, such as administrator, consultant, educator, or entrepreneur as well as changes in practice settings or different populations. Likewise, a practitioner can apply professional development processes to becoming an expert or leader in his or her current practice.

All professional development planning is based on continuous self-reflection and critical analysis regarding one's current practice competence and one's career aspirations coupled with sustained environmental scanning of practice standards and expectations. Formal tools currently available to support this reflective activity are presented in Table 67.3.

Attention to external accreditation standards are also advised, such as the Joint Commission (JC)–required competency assessment using various feedback methods, including the assessment of information from current and previous employers, collecting peer feedback, verifying certification and licensure, reviewing test results with a written or oral competency, and observation of skills. A thorough assessment includes focus on the particular competency needed for the assigned position (The Joint Commission, 2012).

Regardless of the external stakeholders and credentialing processes, the individual OT or OTA is always responsible for ensuring that he or she is competent to deliver current practice. The *Occupational Therapy Code of Ethics and Ethics Standards* states that the duty of occupational therapy practitioners is to "take responsibility for maintaining high standards and continuing competence in practice, education, and research by participating in professional development and educational activities to improve and update knowledge and skills" (AOTA, 2010c, S103–S105). The steps in engaging in continuing competency planning are outlined in Box 67.1.

Case Study 67.1 provides insight into a new practitioner beginning his first position and initiating this professional development process.

TABLE 67.3 Professional Development Reflection Tools

Professional Development Tool(s)	Tool Description
AOTA Professional Development Tool	To guide self-assessment regarding one's professional development needs and interests; to develop an individualized professional development plan; and to recommend the use of a portfolio to retain documentation of professional development activities. Source: AOTA (2003).
AOTA Self-Assessment Tool for Fieldwork Educator Competency	To support the development of skills necessary to be an effective fieldwork educator. Source: AOTA (2009b).
NBCOT online, entry-level self-assessment tools	Individual tools in the areas of general practice, mental health, pediatrics, and physical disabilities. Source: http://www.nbcot.org/index.php?option=com_content&view=article&id=6&Itemid=35
NBCOT OTR Self-Assessment Tool and *COTA Self-Assessment Tool*	Online tools to empower certificants of all levels of experience to engage in self-reflection with the goal of assessing current levels of proficiency with the domains of occupational therapy practice for general practice, physical disability, pediatrics, older adult, mental health, orthopedics, and community mobility (OTR only). Source: http://www.nbcot.org/index.php?option=com_content&view=article&id=218&Itemid=136
Guidelines for Reentry into the Field of Occupational Therapy (AOTA, 2010d) *Guidelines for Supervising Roles and Responsibilities during the Delivery of Occupational Therapy Services* (AOTA, 2009a) *AOTA Code of Ethics* (AOTA, 2010a) *AOTA Standards for Continuing Competence* (AOTA, 2010c) *NBCOT OTR & COTA Validated Domain, Task, Knowledge and Skill Statements*	Standards or guidelines related to area(s) of practice or current status within the profession. For instance, review professional publications, individual state regulatory agency rules Source: http://www.nbcot.org/pdf/OTR_Domain_Task_Knowledge_Skills_Roll-out.pdf?phpMyAdmin=3710605fd34365e380b9ab41a5078545

AOTA, American Occupational Therapy Association; COTA, certified occupational therapy assistant NBCOT, National Board for Certification in Occupational Therapy; OTA, occupational therapy assistant; OTR, occupational therapist, registered.

Competence assessment is dynamic and ongoing and many times is tied to the annual performance goals and review process by one's employer as well as certification and licensing responsibilities.

Choosing Effective Learning Approaches

Evaluating the quality of professional development opportunities is essential in order to develop a productive competence improvement plan. More than just acquiring or enhancing competence-related knowledge and skills are targeted; enhancing one's critical and ethical reasoning processes and requisite interactional skills as well as observing or modeling a highly competent practitioner are also present in higher quality. Observing closely a client's reactions and outcomes is indispensable as well. Today, audio- or video-taping practice is a great resource for experiential self-learning. One can either study the tape or digital media alone or share with another practitioner who can provide feedback allowing the use of virtual tools and time efficiencies. Numerous approaches and tools are available to engage in learning about desired practice competencies. One should remember that "being competent" is not based on attending a learning activity or what is stored in one's portfolio documentation regarding the learning activity. **Competence is continually enhancing "best practice" to achieve the highest potential or outcome for the client that is possible according to evidence and applied knowledge in the practice area.**

The outcomes from competency improvement processes are only as good as the quality of learning activities and the successful integration of the knowledge and skills into more competent practice. Because competence is usually not achieved on the first attempt, repeated practice including constantly reflecting on and comparing results to benchmark outcomes is expected. The

BOX 67.1 Planning for Professional Development and Continuing Competence

1. Identify indicators that prompt the need for or expectation to continuously engage in professional development such as new practice standards or policies, published evidence, or establishing professional development goals at work.
2. Self-assess using tools such as job descriptions, regulations, employment annual reviews, environmental scanning of practice-related developments, publications (standards and guidelines for practice and evidence), service delivery outcomes, and self-assessment tools.
3. Reflect on identification of educational needs or gaps in knowledge and skills for competent practice.
4. Develop a competence improvement plan.
5. Implement the competence improvement plan.
6. Document completed professional development activities in one's portfolio.
7. Integrate new learning into services and critically reflect on the results.
8. Critically analyze the outcomes resulting from using new practice competencies and fine-tune for better results.
9. Demonstrate continuing competence through one's daily practice habits and routines ever vigilant to reconsider all or part of the continuing competence assessment process when outcomes are not sufficient.

following questions guide individual reflection on the results of competency-based learning:

- What are my outcomes in relation to predicted ones?
- How can I improve effective, efficient competency use?
- When does the approach work best or worst?
- What are cues that I can use to move forward?
- When is use beneficial?
- When should I withhold use when cues suggest difficulty or failure in achieving desired results?

Selecting Effective Learning Activities

Attending valuable contemporary workshops or classes or doing reading from quality professional publications are the usual approaches to learning for professional development purposes. Any professional development workshop or seminar is only as good as the information that is shared. Both formal education and CE are highly variable in quality and the motives for offering the programs. Box 67.2 provides some considerations for evaluating the quality of both formal education and CE offerings. Workshops offered by associations are more likely to promote their mission as well as develop quality professionals. For instance, the AOTA, which offers APPs to promote the quality and relevance of CE for occupational therapy practitioners, has a review process for CE program objectives, content, and outcomes in order to use the AOTA APP designation. Independent CE programs are more variant because the profit motive to present "hot topics" may take the lead in offerings more so than quality of education.

Regardless of the educational program attended, learning will not be translated into practice competencies without practice to test and refine skills to guide future application (O'Brien et al., 2007). Evidence found in systematic reviews indicates that workshops that mix interactive components with didactic information are better

BOX 67.2 Strategies for Selecting Effective Educational Options

Formal Education

- Look for regional accreditation (Council for Higher Education Accreditation).
- Seek advice from potential future employers (i.e., if interested in a faculty position, speak to a curriculum director about program level and quality).
- Look at publication record of faculty.
- Get references from former students.

Continuing Education

- Look for quality endorsements (i.e., American Occupational Therapy Association–Approved Provider; continuing education (CE) units, National Board for Certification in Occupational Therapy Professional Development Registry).
- Check documented expertise of speaker.
- Examine integration of quality evidence.
- Notice inclusion of related perspectives and approaches.
- Look to see if assessments are used to improve programs.
- See if experiential post-CE essays or portfolios are included to facilitate critical thinking and demonstrate skill refinement.
- See if there are publications of outcomes from the CE event (more than just narrative quotes such as pretesting/posttesting of attendees to demonstrate learning).
- Seek recommendations from practitioners who are recognized for expertise in area.
- Ask for recommendations from online communities of interest.

integrated into intervention processes than educational meetings that only have didactic components. Experiential learning activities such as storytelling, case history reviews, and simulated practice photovoice adapted to self-study can all be effective. Problem-based learning in learning cells with practitioners can work through study groups, conference calls, and networking through LISTSERVs. Assistance from a more expert practitioner can include mentoring and structured observation of your practice in which newly acquired skills are used (O'Brien et al., 2007). Even role-playing with other staff can assist to effectively integrate learning into practice. The key in self-directed learning is to consider integrating any continuing competency into practice coupled with continuous feedback and reflection regarding practice results.

A multifactor approach to evaluating the quality of CE offerings would include doing a comparative review of options before investing in and selecting a CE program.

Specialty and Advanced Certification

Specialization refers to becoming proficient in a particular practice area, diagnostic procedure or evaluation tool, or intervention approach (Moyers, 2009). The use of advanced and specialty practice are often confused. According to Madill and Hollis (2003), an advanced health care professional that possesses breadth and depth of knowledge focuses on continuous learning and critical thinking as well as contributing to one's area of practice. The growing use of the words *advanced practice* and *advanced practitioner* raises the issue of what is meant by the term advanced. Advanced practitioners possess a higher level of practice expertise resulting from engagement in theory-informed, evidence-based practice, proactively planned continuing professional development with sustained focus on reflections, skill enhancement, applied ethics and strategically planning a career. This issue is debated globally within occupational therapy as well as other fields, such as nursing (Finlayson & Craik, 2009). A nurse is identified as an advanced nursing practitioner if one has acquired a specialty area of practice such as nurse practitioner or nurse midwife. For occupational therapy, advanced practice is defined as knowledge and skills regarding both the breadth and depth of a major practice category or major population engaged (mental health, pediatrics, gerontology, and physical rehabilitation), whereas specialty certification is in more precise or definitive intervention skill area (such as hand therapy or sensory integration or low vision), which is a subcomponent of larger practice.

AOTA provides both board certifications of advance practice (for OTs only) and specialty certifications (for OTs and OTAs). Additionally, post–professional credentialing is available from other groups invested in being able to document and attest to specific practitioner competencies. Table 67.4 lists advanced, specialty, and other post–professional certifications.

The list is not intended to be exhaustive. Today, with the public's requirement for public safety, competence assurance, and accountability, the growth of certification processes in type and numbers is ever increasing. All certification processes encourage, if not require, engagement in continuing professional development to retain certification.

Professional Sustainability: Mapping and Documenting

Sustainability is the capacity to persist. For occupational therapy practitioners, engagement in continuing professional development is sustainability. Responsible, long-term maintenance of one's knowledge and skills enables one to remain productive and effective over time. Professional development sustainability stems from a commitment not only to personal competence but also to upholding the social justice of providing the best practice possible coupled with the economic value associated with this promise and obligation. Sustaining professional competence reflects continuous, dynamic engagement in one's professional development.

Beneficial tools and resources to sustain professional development processes specific to occupational therapy are the following:

American Occupational Therapy Association:
Professional Development Tool (AOTA, 2003)
Self-Assessment Tool for Fieldwork Educator Competency (AOTA, 2009b)
Board and Specialty Portfolio Process for Certification (AOTA, 2012)
National Board for Certification in Occupational Therapy (Areas: physical disability, pediatrics, older adult, mental health, orthopedics, and community mobility [OTR only])
COTA Self-Assessment Tool (NBCOT, 2012a)
OTR Self-Assessment Tool (NBCOT, 2012b)

Integrating information from the professional development self-assessment process leads to the bases for the development of an individualized, professional development plan answering the following questions:

- Where are the gaps between my current competence and what is expected or possible?
- What new learning will fill these gaps in my practice competence to ensure best practice?
- What evidence can I accumulate to demonstrate my acquired competencies?

Reflection on the first two questions provides a personalized map or plan for professional development. The last one calls for the development of a reflective portfolio to collect ongoing activities and evidence of competence.

TABLE 67.4 Entry-level (Initial) and Post–Entry-level (Specialty) Certifications for Practice in the United States

Credentials		**Granting Organization**	
Entry-level Credentialing and Certification Renewal *Note that credentialing starts with graduation from ACOTE accredited educational program*			
OTR	Occupational therapist, registered (professional level)	NBCOT	http://www.nbcot.org/
COTA	Certified occupational therapy assistant (technical level)	NBCOT	http://www.nbcot.org/
AOTA Advanced Practice Certification (For OTs only)			
BCG	Board Certification in Gerontology	AOTA-BASC	http://www.aota.org/Practitioners/ProfDev/Certification.aspx#areas
BCMH	Board Certification in Mental Health	AOTA-BASC	http://www.aota.org/Practitioners/ProfDev/Certification.aspx#areas
BCP	Board Certification in Pediatrics	AOTA-BASC	http://www.aota.org/Practitioners/ProfDev/Certification.aspx#areas
BCPR	Board Certification in Physical Rehabilitation	AOTA-BASC	http://www.aota.org/Practitioners/ProfDev/Certification.aspx#areas
AOTA Specialty Certifications (For OTs & OTAs)			
SCDCM	Specialty Certification in Driving and Community Mobility	AOTA-BASC	http://www.aota.org/Practitioners/ProfDev/Certification.aspx#areas
SCEM	Specialty Certification in Environmental Modification	AOTA-BASC	http://www.aota.org/Practitioners/ProfDev/Certification.aspx#areas
SCFES	Specialty Certification in Feeding, Eating, and Swallowing	AOTA-BASC	http://www.aota.org/Practitioners/ProfDev/Certification.aspx#areas
SCLV	Specialty Certification in Low Vision	AOTA-BASC	http://www.aota.org/Practitioners/ProfDev/Certification.aspx#areas
Other Specialty Certifications (Professional level varies)			
ATP	Assistive Technology Practitioner	RESNA	http://resna.org/
CCM	Certified Case Managers	CCMC	http://www.ccmcertification.org/
CDRS	Certified Driver Rehabilitation Specialist	ADED	http://www.driver-ed.org/
CHT	Certified Hand Therapist	HTCC	http://www.htcc.org/
CLVT	Certification in Low Vision Therapy	ACVREP	http://www.acvrep.org/
CPE	Certified Professional Ergonomist	BCPE	http://www.bcpe.org/
CVE	Certified Vocational Evaluation Specialist	CRCC	http://www.crccertification.com/
PC or CC	Professional Coach Certification	ICF IAC	(PC) http://www.coachfederation.org/ (CC) http://www.certifiedcoach.org/
SMS	Seating and Mobility Specialist	RESNA	http://resna.org/certification/

ACOTE, Accreditation Council for Occupational Therapy Education; AOTA-BASC, American Occupational Therapy Association: Board and Specialty Certification; ACVREP, Academy for Certification of Vision Rehabilitation and Education Professionals; ADED, Association for Driver Rehabilitation Specialists; BCPE, Board of Certification in Professional Ergonomics; CCMC, Commission for Case Manager Certification; CCWAVES, Commission on Certification of Work Adjustment and Vocational Evaluation Specialists; CRCC, Commission on Rehabilitation Counselor Certification; HTCC, Hand Therapy Certification Commission; IAC, International Association of Coaching; ICF, International Coach Federation; NBCOT, National Board for Certification in Occupational Therapy; RESNA, Rehabilitation Engineering and Assistive Technology Society of North America.

A **transitional portfolio** is a dynamic, flexible, and reflective tool for one to self-direct and document professional development through thoughtful engagement with artifacts created and accumulated during one's career in relationship to professional goals and desired roles (Crist, Wilcox, & McCarron, 1998). A transitional portfolio contains three important sections that the occupational therapy practitioner maintains to ensure practice relevance and verification of continuing competency. The **references and resources section** contains information related to current practice or desirable future learning opportunities, such as information reading certification requirements, relevant evidence-based publications, workshop notes, etc., from a wide variety of learning activities to support competency. The **work-in-progress section** reflects current activities that are being completed to create new evidence regarding one's learning and/or competencies. Ongoing work artifacts might include gathering documentation needed to apply for advanced or specialty certification: notes to prepare a staff in-service, outlines for a new fieldwork program activity or drafts of a publication regarding an innovative program description, or an outcome report for a professional publication. The third component of a transitional portfolio is the **showcase section.** In this section, outstanding work, awards, annual performance reviews, recommendations, certificates, and other evidence of specific accomplishments are stored to attest to others the achievement of specific knowledge and exemplary practice competence. The transitional portfolio changes as the individual accumulates evidence documenting and archiving accumulated knowledge and skill acquisition and organizes the reference section for ongoing work.

Changing Areas of Practice, Pursuing Emerging Areas, or Reentering

Sometimes during one's career, the opportunity presents itself to take one's professional work in a new direction such as with changing practice focus, seeking a new emerging practice area, or reentering after a leave of absence from practicing—all which require professional development considerations (see Practice Dilemma for an example). Reentering OTs and OTAs are defined as individuals who have practiced in the field for a minimum of 1 year, who have not engaged in the practice of occupational therapy for a minimum of 18 months, and who wish to return to the profession in the capacity of delivering occupational therapy services to clients (AOTA, 2010e). Regardless of the reason for change, practitioners have the ethical accountability to ensure high standards of practice competency and skills. The AOTA's (2010e) "Guidelines for Re-entry into the Field of Occupational Therapy" contains procedural recommendations to follow for returning to practice after an extended absence. These strategies could be adapted to entering new areas of unfamiliar practice (Waite, 2011).

The plans for development for switching from one existing area of practice to another or reentering into well-established practice areas is easier to map because there are more supports readily available. Switching areas of practice or reentering benefits from mentoring and supervised practice. For occupational therapy practitioners who pursue an emerging area of practice, there is the added responsibility of being a pioneer because they are creating a mosaic of new structure and skills in order to develop and sustain occupational therapy in the new area. Jumping into emerging areas of practice requires more risk taking and creative thinking to discern the desirable learning activities to support competence and success (Holmes & Scaffa, 2009). Networking with others both within and outside the profession who hold some information of the knowledge or skills related to emerging practice expectations is valuable for these circumstances.

Practice Excellence

Valuing practice competence is a responsible, ethical professional attitude and position to enact as an occupational therapy practitioner. Mastery competence is meeting standards for best practice. The noble goal for professional development is to exceed standards. Some

Practice Dilemma

Starting a New Program

Marina works in a large rehabilitation center where many of the patients report reliance on being able to return to driving as a priority to be independent and stay in their homes. Right now, these individuals would have to go to another city to get these services. The rehabilitation manager is encouraging Marina to develop a program. She recalls a lecture that she had in school over 4 years ago about adapted driving, which prompts her to think that she will need some specialized skills. She wants not only to have the skills but she also wants to design a quality program to perform the related roles and responsibilities to be competent in offering this service.

1. Where should Marina look to get reliable resources on the skills she will need?
2. What are some key educational strategies she might consider?
3. How would you advise her to proceed?

might see specialty, advanced, or expert practice as a form of excellence, but are any of these?

Practice excellence is engaging in the highest quality of work as long as the work reflects social as well as ethical responsibility coupled with contemporary, evidence-based application. Our occupational therapy literature alludes to excellence but seldom specifies the parameters or details what is at minimum an aspiration and more likely an intricate merging of acquired skill, clinical reasoning, continuous reflective practice, and achievement motivation. Parham (1987) posited that excellence was an intertwining of researcher and theorist in the practitioner. This perspective would advocate for the role of practice scholar as the requisite groundwork leading to practice excellence (Crist, Muñoz, Hansen, Benson, & Provident, 2005).

Perhaps practitioner excellence is decoding the evidence to create an individualized approach to provide "best practice" by holding oneself to a higher standard than the fundamental understanding of competency alone can provide. In addition, commitment to other practitioners achieves this excellence through modeling as well as dissemination, publication, or presentation (Crist, 2010). Regardless, continuing to reach a shared definition and comprehension of what creates practice excellence across the profession of occupational therapy and the contribution of professional development to achieving this level of practice proficiency or competency will benefit both our clients and the profession. At minimum, professional development targeting excellence would include quality practice experiences steeped in both the arts and sciences, continuous reflection on practice process and outcomes, enacting awareness of limitations to one's knowledge and abilities, and commitment to ongoing, goal-oriented professional development related to specialized practice as the essential attributes (Courtney, 2005).

Conclusion

Rapid changes in health care, knowledge, and technology require constant reevaluation and modification of the role and functions of every occupational therapy practitioner. Our clients, their families, our employers, the profession, and the public expect OTs and OTAs to provide the highest quality services possible. Engaging in continuous professional development is an essential responsibility for every occupational therapy practitioner to ensure continuing competence and competency. Professional development results from continuous, reflective self-assessment accounting for client outcomes, job responsibilities, and context as well as future trends in practice (Moyers, 2009). Professional development is individualized goal-directed learning that not only responds to but also leads to incessant change in practice delivery and sustains practice competence.

The universal standard is to be able to deliver best practices with encouragement to strive for practice excellence. Self-responsibility for engaging in continuous professional development is primary. Seeking administrative support for continuing competency improvement activities is beneficial. Transitional portfolios are useful to collect evidence regarding competencies and continuing competency activities and recognitions.

References

American Occupational Therapy Association. (2003). *Professional development tool.* Bethesda, MD: Author. Retrieved from http://www.aota.org/pdt

American Occupational Therapy Association. (2007). *Create better linkages between education, research and practice: Ad hoc final committee report to the AOTA board of directors.* Retrieved from http://www.aota.org/News/Centennial/Background/AdHoc/2007/40991.aspx?FT=.pdf

American Occupational Therapy Association. (2009a). Guidelines for supervision, roles and responsibilities during the delivery of occupational therapy services. *American Journal of Occupational Therapy, 63,* 173–179.

American Occupational Therapy Association. (2009b). *Self-assessment tool for fieldwork educator competency.* Retrieved from http://www.aota.org/Educate/EdRes/Fieldwork/Supervisor/Forms/38251.aspx?FT=.pdf

American Occupational Therapy Association. (2010a). Occupational therapy code of ethics and ethics standards. *American Journal of Occupational Therapy, 64,* 517–526.

American Occupational Therapy Association. (2010b). Scope of practice. *American Journal of Occupational Therapy, 64,* S70–S77. doi:10.5014/ajot.2010.64S 7 0-64S77

American Occupational Therapy Association. (2010c). Standards for continuing competence. *American Journal of Occupational Therapy, 64,* S103–S105.

American Occupational Therapy Association. (2010d). Standards of practice for occupational therapy. *American Journal of Occupational Therapy, 64,* S106–S111.

American Occupational Therapy Association. (2010e). The guidelines for re-entry into the field of occupational therapy. *American Journal of Occupational Therapy, 64,* S27–S29.

American Occupational Therapy Association. (2011a). *2011 Accreditation Council for Occupational Therapy Education (ACOTE) standards and interpretation guide.* Retrieved from http://www.aota.org/Educate/Accredit/Draft-Standards/50146.aspx?FT=.pdf

American Occupational Therapy Association (2011b). *Licensure.* Retrieved from http://www.aota.org/Practitioners/Licensure.aspx

American Occupational Therapy Association (2012). *AOTA certification: Board and Specialty Portfolio Process for Certification.* Retrieved from http://www.aota.org/Practitioners/ProfDev/Certification.aspx

Baum, C. M. (2000). Occupations-based practice: Reinventing ourselves for the new millennium. *OT Practice, 5*(1), 12–15.

Courtney, M. (2005). The meaning of professional excellence for private practitioners in occupational therapy. *Australian Journal of Occupational Therapy, 52*(3), 211–217.

Crist, P. A. (2010). Adapting research instruction to support the scholarship of practice: Practice-scholar partnerships. *Occupational Therapy in Health Care, 24*(1), 39–55.

Crist, P., Muñoz, J. P., Hansen, A. M. W., Benson, J., & Provident, I. (2005). The practice-scholar program: An academic-practice partnership to promote the scholarship of "best practices." *Occupational Therapy in Health Care, 19*(1/2), 71–93.

Crist, P., Wilcox, B., & McCarron, K. (1998). Transitional portfolios: Orchestrating our professional competence. *American Journal of Occupational Therapy, 52,* 729–736.

Dunn, W. (Ed.). (2011). Best practice philosophy for community services for children and families. In *Best practice occupational therapy for children and families in community settings* (2nd ed., pp. 1–14). Thorofare, NJ: Slack.

Finlayson, M., & Craik, J. (2009, June). *Report and background discussion on advanced practice in occupational therapy*. Paper presented at the Advanced Practice Professional Issues Forum, Canadian Occupational Therapy Association Conference, Ottawa, Ontario, Canada.

Holmes, W. M., & Scaffa, M. E. (2009). An exploratory study of competencies for emerging practice in occupational therapy. *Journal of Allied Health, 38*(2), 81–90.

Madill, M. H. M., & Hollis, V. (2003). Developing competencies for advanced practice: How do we get from there to here? In G. Brown, S. A. Esdaile, & S. E. Ryan (Eds.), *Becoming an advanced health care practitioner*. New York, NY: Butterworth Heinemann.

Moyers, P. (2009). Occupational therapy practitioners: Competence and professional development. In E. B. Crepeau, E. S. Cohn, & B. A. B. Schell (Eds.), *Willard and Spackman's occupational therapy* (pp. 240–251). Philadelphia, PA: Lippincott Williams & Wilkins.

Moyers, P. A., & Hinojosa, J. (2003). Continuing competency. In G. L. McCormick, E. G. Jaffe, & M. Goodman-Levey (Eds.), *The occupational therapy manager* (pp. 463–489). Bethesda, MD: American Occupational Therapy Association.

National Board for Certification in Occupational Therapy. (2011). *Welcome*. Retrieved from http://www.nbcot.org/

National Board for Certification in Occupational Therapy. (2012a) *COTA Self-Assessment Tool Manual*. Retrieved from http://www.nbcot.org/pdf/cota-Self-Assessment-Manual.pdf?phpMyAdmin=3710605fd34365e380b9ab41a5078545

National Board for Certification in Occupational Therapy. (2012b). *OTR Self-Assessment Tool Manual*. Retrieved from http://www.nbcot.org/pdf/OTR-Self-Assessment-Manual.pdf?phpMyAdmin=3710605fd34365e380b9ab41a5078545

O'Brien, M. A., Rogers, S., Jamtvedt, G., Oxman, A. D., Odgaard-Jensen, J., Kristofferson, D. T., . . . Harvey, E. (2007). Educational outreach visits: Effects on professional practice and health care outcomes. *Cochrane Database Systematic Reviews*, (4), CD000409. doi:10:1002/14651858.CD000409.pub2

Parham, D. (1987). Nationally speaking: The reflective practitioner. *American Journal of Occupational Therapy, 41*(9), 555–561.

The Joint Commission. (2012). *Standards FAQs: Competency assessment*. Retrieved from http://www.jointcommission.org/standards_information/jcfaqdetails.aspx?StandardsFaqId=31&ProgramId=1

Waite, A. (2011, November). Switching areas of practice. *OT Practice Magazine* (pp. 10–13). Rockville, MD: American Occupational Therapy Association.

For additional resources on the subjects discussed in this chapter, visit http://thePoint.lww.com/Willard-Spackman12e.

CHAPTER 68

Occupational Therapy Professional Organizations

Shawn Phipps

LEARNING OBJECTIVES

After reading this chapter, you will be able to:

1. Describe the importance of lifelong membership and participation in occupational therapy professional organizations
2. Understand the structure and function of state, national, and international occupational therapy professional organizations
3. Describe the roles of National Board for Certification in Occupational Therapy (NBCOT) and state regulatory boards in the licensing, regulation, and credentialing of occupational therapy practitioners in the United States
4. Understand how professional and regulatory organizations serve the consumers of occupational therapy through standard setting and education
5. Appreciate the roles that both volunteer and paid staff members in professional organizations play in developing and supporting all aspects of the occupational therapy profession and the clients served by its members

OUTLINE

Introduction

When students and practitioners from a profession come together to discuss mutual challenges and opportunities, the nucleus of an association or professional organization is formed (Mata, Latham, & Ransome, 2010). **Professional organizations** offer the opportunity to collectively advance the profession in a way that cannot be achieved by an individual student or practitioner alone. Professional organizations are nonprofit organizations seeking to further the profession, the interests of individuals engaged in that profession, and the public interest by building a strong community of students and practitioners that collectively contribute power in numbers. Although the structure and function of professional organizations are evolving (Schneider

BOX 68.1 Common Acronyms in Occupational Therapy Professional Organizations

ACOTE	Accreditation Council for Occupational Therapy Education
AOTF	American Occupational Therapy Foundation
AOTPAC	American Occupational Therapy Political Action Committee
ASAP	Affiliated State Association Presidents
ASD	Assembly of Student Delegates
AOTA	The American Occupational Therapy Association, Inc.
CCCPD	Commission on Continuing Competence and Professional Development
COE	Commission on Education
COP	Commission on Practice
NBCOT	National Board for Certification in Occupational Therapy
OT	Occupational Therapist
OTA	Occupational Therapy Assistant
RA	Representative Assembly
EC	Ethics Commission
SIS	Special Interest Section
WFOT	World Federation of Occupational Therapists

& Somers, 2006), the roles of professional organizations include uniting the profession around a shared **mission** and **vision**, developing strategic initiatives to achieve this vision, advancing practice, safeguarding the public interest, providing opportunities for professional networking, and representing the interests of students and practitioners through legislative advocacy and public promotion of the profession. This chapter introduces the reader to the major state and national professional organizations in the United States as well as to the World Federation of Occupational Therapists (WFOT)—the major international occupational therapy organization. Refer to Box 68.1 to see a list of organizations and their acronyms.

Readers from countries other than the United States can use this information as a basis to explore comparable professional organizations in their own countries or regions.

Importance of Lifelong Professional Association Membership

Professional societies have made significant contributions as consultants to governments and academia and have played a major role in broadening the scope of practice and the scientific body of knowledge (Bickel, 2007). Meetings of the various professional organizations offer an opportunity for the exchange of ideas while providing a forum for discourse on the direction of education, practice, and research. As a result, higher standards of professionalism are continuously evolving to serve the profession through **professional development** activities, conferences, adherence to **core values**, and the profession's **code of ethics**.

The socialization of students and practitioners through guided interactions with mentors and professional peers is a central component of professional identity development (Greenwood, Suddaby, & Hinings, 2002). **Professional identity formation** is a socialization process that involves both the acquisition of specific knowledge and skills required for professional practice as well as the internalization of attitudes, dispositions, and self-identity that connect the individual to the larger profession. Members of a professional organization can choose which types of networks to join and can move in and out of these networks to pursue other professional interests and enrich their individual development and experiences as a professional. These networks are especially important when a student enters a profession or when pursuing a new area of professional interest. Through conferences, networking meetings, online practice communities, and reading professional journals, one can interact with colleagues to gain guidance and expertise that enhance professional development and ultimately contribute to the advancement of the profession.

The professional development that occurs through membership and active involvement in professional organizations illustrates the importance of being a lifelong member of your state, national, and international professional organizations (Ritzhaupt, Umapathy, & Jamba, 2008). Through active participation, members function as the "bosses" to the leaders and staff of professional associations. Active participation in professional associations also has the benefit of building leadership capacity, powerful and interconnected collegial networks, and the translation of those leadership skills into educational and practice settings. Professional leaders are more externally connected, interacting with a broader and more diverse range of stakeholders from both inside and outside the profession while scanning the larger environment for emerging trends and opportunities that can benefit occupational therapy and the clients served by the profession. Rather than seeing the future as a minor variation or logical extension of the present, professionals connected to professional organizations see the future as an invention that may require fresh thinking and innovative solutions very different than the current organizational norms.

Although each professional organization has its own unique benefits, most professional associations offer "members only" access to a variety of publications, resources, conferences, online communities, and professional development opportunities that are not available to nonmembers (Osborn & Hunt, 2007). Member dues provide the necessary resources to move the profession forward. Joining professional organizations and committing to lifelong membership can have the benefit of providing students and practitioners with access to knowledge, networks, and resources that can advance one's professional career through a modest investment in annual dues to support the important work of the professional organization. Employers see the value in membership to professional associations because it demonstrates that individual's dedication, commitment, and professionalism. Professional association membership also qualifies students and practitioners for the opportunity to apply for academic scholarships and research grants.

Occupational therapy students, occupational therapy assistants (OTAs), and occupational therapists (OTs) are—by virtue of their education, license, and/or certification—eligible to become members of their state, national, and international occupational therapy professional organizations (Mata et al., 2010). The formation of professional identity is a developmental process that begins at the point at which an individual chooses occupational therapy as a career path. This developmental process does not cease when the individual graduates and enters practice but continues to develop throughout his or her career. Professionals recognize and adhere to a code of ethics, practice within their legal scope, and contribute to the evolving development of knowledge and skills that are necessary to advance the profession. State, national, and international professional organizations provide the support needed for professional development, public awareness, **advocacy**, and **standard setting**, making lifelong membership and participation in professional organizations a key component to a successful occupational therapy career trajectory, beginning as an occupational therapy student. The following case study illustrates how occupational therapy professional organizations support professional development as an occupational therapy student enters the profession. As you read this chapter, refer back to this case.

CASE STUDY 68.1 Jennifer Enters the Occupational Therapy Profession

Jennifer is a new occupational therapy practitioner who recently graduated from an accredited occupational therapy program. Through her academic and fieldwork experiences, she decided to pursue a career as an occupational therapist working with children with special needs. This case highlights the many ways that a new professional benefits from active participation in professional organizations.

Jennifer as a Student

As an occupational therapy student, Jennifer decided to join as student member of the American Occupational Therapy Association (AOTA), World Federation of Occupational Therapists (WFOT), and her state association and continued her memberships when entering occupational therapy practice. She attended her first AOTA conference to attend workshops and courses on innovative occupational therapy practice for children with autism and how to make a successful transition from student to practitioner. She also found that the *American Journal of Occupational Therapy, OT Practice,* and the *Special Interest Section Quarterly* contained interesting articles that were relevant to her and which she used in various course assignments. Using *OT Connection*, a social media site accessible on the home page of the AOTA Website, her coordinator found other fieldwork coordinators in Florida and was able to locate an appropriate fieldwork placement. During her final Level II fieldwork placement, Jennifer contacted the National Board for Certification in Occupational Therapy (NBCOT) and applied to take her certification examination after completing her fieldwork. She could take the examination at a site that was close to her home.

Getting Ready to Work

Jennifer began to answer advertisements for occupational therapy positions. She was interviewed at several clinical sites and finally narrowed her choices down to a position in South Carolina and another site closer to her home in Texas. Because she was not sure which of the positions she would accept, she contacted the state regulatory boards in both states to apply for licensure. She asked NBCOT to send her examination results to both of them. She anxiously awaited her certification examination results from NBCOT and after a couple of weeks was thrilled to learn that she had passed the examination and was now a registered occupational therapist. She accepted the offer from a private pediatric practice group in Texas and began her new job working with children with autism.

When her student membership expired, she renewed her memberships with the AOTA, WFOT, and her state association and joined both the Developmental Disabilities and the School System Special Interest Sections so that she could communicate with other occupational therapists who worked with this population. Jennifer welcomed the information and resources provided by these therapists and by her supervisor and coworkers.

Practicing Abroad

Jennifer was also interested in international practice opportunities; and through her membership with WFOT, she discovered the Occupational Therapy International Outreach Network (OTION), which facilitated her involvement in occupational therapy practice in Haiti.

Networking and Advocating Back Home

After returning from Haiti, Jennifer learned that federal and state funding for occupational therapy services was at risk for children with autism. She immediately went to the AOTA

(continued)

CASE STUDY 68.1 Jennifer Enters the Occupational Therapy Profession *(Continued)*

Website to learn about the proposed cuts to occupational therapy services for children with autism. Jennifer used OT Connection to connect with other practitioners regarding concerns for declining reimbursement rates and coverage for occupational therapy services. She decided to donate to the American Occupational Therapy Political Action Committee (AOTPAC), which provides support to candidates for elected office who support occupational therapy and the coverage of occupational therapy services for children with autism. Jennifer also contacted the association to find out how she could get involved with advocating for fair reimbursement and coverage of occupational therapy services for children with autism.

Becoming Part of the Solution

Jennifer joined an ad hoc committee of practitioners to develop recommendations to the AOTA Board of Directors on strategic priorities for advocating for occupational therapy and children with autism. Jennifer also scheduled visits with her elected representatives to discuss her concerns regarding the proposed cuts to reimbursement and occupational therapy coverage for the children she served. She then invited her elected representatives and their legislative staff to tour her clinic to educate policymakers on the critical role of occupational therapy for children with autism. She followed up with each of the legislative representatives with a letter further advocating for fair reimbursement and coverage of occupational therapy services. She also worked with her state association leaders and fellow practitioners to organize a grassroots advocacy effort to promote access to occupational therapy services for children with autism.

Summary

Through active participation in her state, federal, and international professional associations, Jennifer witnessed the power of membership and participation in her professional organizations and committed to maintaining her lifelong state, national, and international professional organizational membership and to actively participate in shaping the future of the occupational therapy profession.

American Occupational Therapy Association

AOTA is the national professional organization in the United States that is responsible for guiding and developing professional standards, professional development, and advocacy on behalf of occupational therapy practitioners and the clients served by occupational therapy (Figure 68.1) (AOTA, 2011a). AOTA was incorporated in 1917 as the National Society for the Promotion of Occupational Therapy in New York. The name was eventually changed in 1927 to AOTA. AOTA's membership is composed of individual OTs, OTAs, and students from around the world. AOTA members develop and refine AOTA's mission, vision, practice standards, professional development, and code of ethics—all of which shape the future success of the occupational therapy profession. This is accomplished by individual members working together as volunteers serving the association in various leadership capacities. Members and volunteer leaders are supported by staff employed by AOTA. The staff is supervised by the AOTA executive director, who in turn is supervised by the AOTA board of directors (BOD).

Board of Directors

The AOTA BOD has the legal and financial responsibility for AOTA's strategic direction and business operations. AOTA has four officers on the board, all of whom are elected by all members; they include the president, the vice president, the secretary, and the treasurer. The president presides over the BOD and the annual business

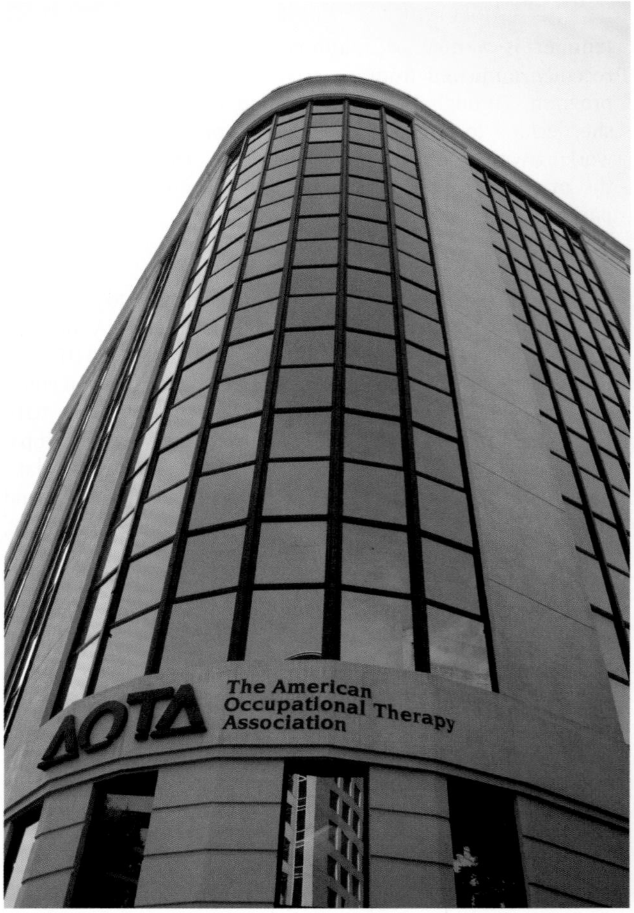

FIGURE 68.1 AOTA's national office building in Bethesda, Maryland.

meeting and is the primary spokesperson of the occupational therapy profession. The vice president's primary responsibility is to guide the development of the association's **strategic plan**. For instance, a major role of the AOTA vice president over the last decade has been to monitor the association's progress toward the AOTA Centennial Vision when the occupational therapy profession in the United States turns 100 years old in 2017. The secretary is responsible for tracking the official minutes and documents of the association, whereas the treasurer is responsible for ensuring fiscal effectiveness and guiding the budgetary processes. The BOD also consists of elected directors and appointed consumer and public advisors to the board. All board members have voice and vote during official meetings. The AOTA executive director (a full-time paid employee of the association) serves as nonvoting member of the board.

Representative Assembly

The largest body of AOTA, the Representative Assembly (RA), is the policy-making body of the association, often referred to as the "congress" of the occupational therapy profession (AOTA, 2011a). Each representative is elected either nationally or by the AOTA members who reside in a particular state or jurisdiction. Before these meetings, the representatives seek input from their members about important policy decisions facing the profession. Professional policy and practice issues, such as the move from a bachelor's degree to a graduate degree requirement for entry into the occupational therapy profession, are deliberated and approved by the assembly. Practice standards and positions on the role of occupational therapy in various specialty areas, such as driving and neonatal intensive care, are ultimately approved by the RA (refer to Box 68.2 for a look behind the scenes on the complex and sometimes controversial process of policy development).

Commissions

The AOTA commissions serve to develop specific guidelines for practice, education, ethics, and professional development (AOTA, 2011a). There are four commissions in AOTA, including the Commission on Practice (COP), the Commission on Education (COE), the Ethics Commission (EC), and the Commission on Continuing Competency and Professional Development (CCCPD). The COP is charged with developing practice guidelines that are related to and define the practice of occupational therapy. The COE generates education-related policy recommendations to the RA for deliberation. The COE identifies, analyzes, and provides recommendations for educationally relevant initiatives. The EC develops the association's code of ethics and provides recommendations for ethical standard setting in the occupational therapy profession. The EC also serves as an oversight body regarding complaints concerning unethical behavior of AOTA members.

BOX 68.2 Behind the Scenes

When you read a chapter such as this, it might seem that all these organizations and the policies that they promote "just happen." Nothing could be farther from the truth. Not only is there a great deal of work by volunteers and staff alike but there is also a lot of discussion, negotiation, and sometimes professional tension that occur in the making of policies and standards. One of the best ways to see this is to watch the discussions of the Representative Assembly in action. Hotly contested topics over the years have included the following:

- *Whether AOTA should reorganize the Representative Assembly to a model that is less regionally based and designed for members to actively participate via grassroots networks.* The discussion of how best to organize the American Occupational Therapy Association (AOTA) is still under review at the time this chapter was being written.
- *Whether AOTA should support state licensure of occupational therapists.* Many therapists thought that it would be better to maintain a national certification so that therapists would not be hampered when moving from state to state. However, over time, the argument for becoming licensed won, as therapists wanted a legally defined scope of practice in their states. Until therapists were licensed in their states, anyone could say that he or she was an occupational therapy practitioner whether the person had the professional credentials or not.
- *Whether the educational level for occupational therapists in the United States should move from a bachelor's to a master's level.* This discussion went on for more than 20 years until the move was made to postgraduate entry for occupational therapists. Those who were against the move were concerned that it would reduce the number of therapists, thus making access to services even more of a problem during times of shortage. Those who supported the move thought that many programs were requiring so many credit hours that it was like getting a postgraduate education without the degree. Although occupational therapists now must enter at the master's level, the dialogue about the appropriate standards and role of the occupational therapy doctorate is in development.
- *The scope of occupational therapy.* A perennial concern is related to guidelines for what sorts of evaluations and interventions are truly "occupational therapy" and which ones go beyond the scope of practice. For example, one question was whether it is appropriate for occupational therapists to use physical agent modalities or complementary and alternative interventions in their practice. Some of this has recently been resolved via state licensure changes, national statements, and modifications to educational standards.
- *The role of the Occupational Therapy Assistant (OTA).* Although AOTA policies are clear that the OTA functions under the supervision of an occupational therapist, the exact nature of that supervision is frequently reexamined as practice evolves and new arenas emerge.

The CCCPD is responsible for overseeing professional development standards and board and specialty certification. The CCCPD recommends continuing competence standards and develops tools to assist members in the development and implementation of continuing competence plans.

Special Interest Sections

In addition to the four commissions, there is a grassroots network of AOTA members representing special interest sections (SISs) (AOTA, 2011d). The SISs are designed to respond to emerging practice issues by focusing on specialized areas of occupational therapy practice. Each SIS provides its members with the opportunity for dialogue through its newsletters and through social media networks. These are invaluable tools for occupational therapy students and practitioners who want to communicate with colleagues who have similar practice interests and challenges. Members of the SIS often work collaboratively with the various commissions on projects such as defining the roles and functions of occupational therapy practitioners in a particular practice arena, guiding the development of advanced competencies and specialized skills and related educational materials, or developing standards for education of occupational therapy personnel.

Assembly of Student Delegates

Students are valued members of AOTA and belong to the Assembly of Student Delegates (ASD) (AOTA, 2011a). Each educational program may select a student as its delegate to the ASD meeting that takes place during the AOTA Annual Conference and Exposition. The ASD provides a platform for students to share their perspectives on student issues that affect the occupational therapy profession.

Accreditation Council for Occupational Therapy Education

Working under the umbrella of AOTA is the Accreditation Council for Occupational Therapy Education (ACOTE®) (AOTA, 2011b). Members of the council are OTs and OTAs who are AOTA members who represent both clinical and academic interests. The role of ACOTE is to develop and implement the standards for all occupational therapy and OTA educational programs. ACOTE standards are related to all aspects of the program, including the curriculum, the credentials of faculty and staff, the content of courses, the physical facilities and resources, and the administrative policies of the school that relate to the occupational therapy program. To become accredited and to maintain accreditation, every OT and OTA program is evaluated on a regular basis by ACOTE. Completion of an occupational therapy program that is accredited by ACOTE is an eligibility requirement for students taking the certification examination and who subsequently wish to be licensed to practice.

AOTA Staff

All of the efforts of AOTA's large volunteer network of members would not be possible without a highly competent and dedicated staff at the national headquarters housed in Bethesda, Maryland (AOTA, 2011a). The AOTA staff includes occupational therapy practitioners, attorneys, accountants, policy specialists, and administrative personnel. The national headquarters staff is led by an executive director who is responsible for all of the personnel and operations of the national headquarters. The purpose of the national headquarters is to support the efforts of the association by providing the personnel and expertise required to accomplish the association's mission and vision. Some of AOTA's key operations include supporting the work of the volunteer leadership groups, designing and delivering continuing education, compiling evidence-based practice information, monitoring and influencing public policy, maintaining sound business operations, and advocating for the profession and the clients served by occupational therapy practitioners.

Continuing Education and Professional Development

AOTA staff develop and coordinate continuing education and professional development opportunities, including live and online workshops, seminars, online courses, and self-paced clinical courses (AOTA, 2011a). Many of these educational opportunities are offered throughout the world and in varied formats designed to best meet the needs of the participants. The most widely publicized event is the AOTA Annual Conference and Exposition, which includes continuing education presentations, networking, and exhibit hall vendors and employers. AOTA members may attend the conference at a reduced cost. This conference and exposition is planned and implemented by staff from the national headquarters, although volunteer members perform peer reviews that are used to select which presentations are presented at conference. Volunteers also help provide the necessary human resources during conference.

Evidence for Practice

Another major initiative of the AOTA staff is researching the literature to locate and gather the data that provide evidence for the practice of occupational therapy (AOTA, 2011c). As data are collected, they are compiled into Evidence-Based Practice Briefs that therapists and students can use to support occupational therapy intervention. In addition to the Evidence-Based Practice Briefs, AOTA maintains a practice directory that provides links to various publications and virtual resources providing additional information that supports practice.

Public Policy and Advocacy

An important AOTA staff role is to represent and advocate for the interests of occupational therapy practitioners and their clients in the areas of public policy (AOTA,

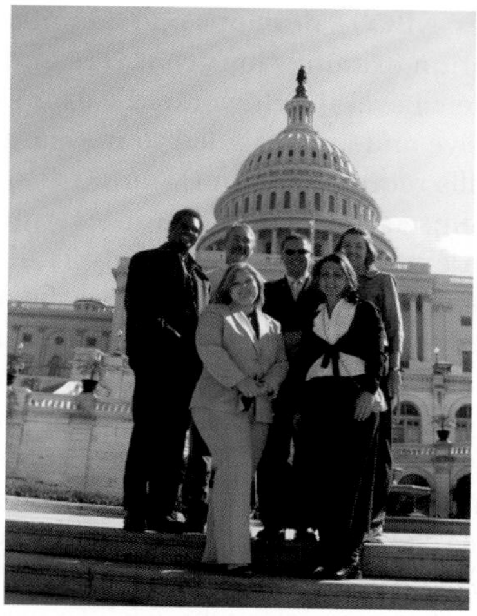

FIGURE 68.2 Students and practitioners advocating for occupational therapy on the Capitol.

2011a). This work involves lobbying with legislators regarding initiatives that are important to the profession and to the people who are served by occupational therapy (Figure 68.2). At the federal level, this may also involve working with the policymakers from the Office of Special Education, the Rehabilitation Services Administration, and other governmental agencies regarding eligibility for service as well as guidelines for reimbursement. AOTA staff members are often called on to provide information and testimony before congressional committees who make recommendations regarding the interpretation and implementation of legislation.

The State Affairs Department and the Federal Affairs Department also support the activities of state occupational therapy associations and licensure boards to ensure that language supportive of occupational therapy is included in state legislation and that occupational therapy is supported and not inappropriately restricted by encroachment by other professions (AOTA, 2011a). AOTA also provide educational materials and individual support to members and state associations to prepare them to effectively advocate for the profession and those who are served in their area by occupational therapy (Figure 68.3).

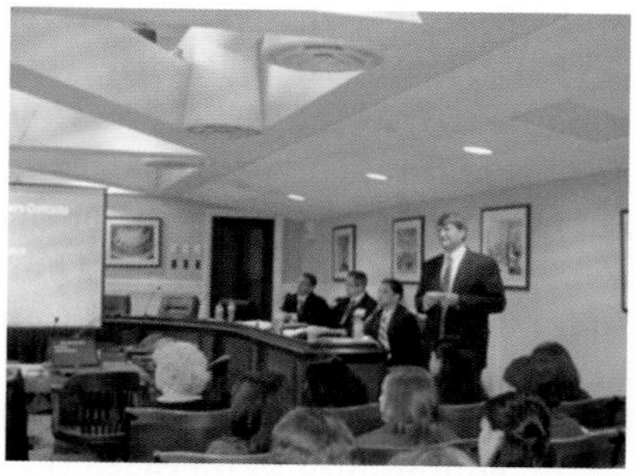

FIGURE 68.3 Speakers discuss legislative updates and advocacy opportunities to members at a state professional association conference.

American Occupational Therapy Political Action Committee (AOTPAC)

A **political action committee** is a committee that provides financial support to candidates that support a profession and its initiatives through private donations from members. AOTA members can voluntarily donate to the American Occupational Therapy Political Action Committee to support candidates for elected office that support occupational therapy and the clients served by occupational therapy.

Publications

The official publication of the association is the *American Journal of Occupational Therapy* (AJOT®) (AOTA, 2011c). This peer-reviewed journal is available to all association members and is included in their annual professional dues. The association also publishes *OT Practice*, a bimonthly magazine that includes informative articles about the profession. In addition to this magazine and the AJOT, AOTA publishes *Special Interest Section Quarterly*, newsletters on state policy initiatives, monthly updates on legislative issues, and biweekly e-mail updates on current events that are of interest to members of the profession. In addition to its periodical publications, AOTA Press publishes books, manuals, monographs, and consumer guides that address topics of concern to occupational therapy students, practitioners, and consumers. AOTA also maintains a marketplace or clearinghouse for these publications, videos, and other documents as well as items that are appropriate for marketing occupational therapy.

Affiliated State Associations

Each state has a professional organization that serves the local and regional needs of occupational therapy practitioners (AOTA, 2011a). These state organizations are independent from AOTA, and thus individuals join these state groups directly. State organizations are affiliated with AOTA to advance the profession in that particular state and to advocate for the clients who are served by occupational therapy. For example, AOTA provides model language for state laws and regulations, but the state professional organization must work with the state government directly to get this language into state laws and policies. The president of each state association belongs to the Affiliated State Association Presidents (ASAP), thus supporting a close synergy among state- and federal-level activities. All affiliated state associations can be accessed via the home page of the AOTA Website. Membership in state organizations is critical for maintaining local networks and for mobilizing advocacy efforts related to state government–funded programs and state policies, including professional licensure.

State Regulatory Boards

Each state or jurisdiction regulates occupational therapy in some way through a licensure board or regulatory agency (AOTA, 2011a). The definitions and guidelines are enacted by the legislature in that particular state and are intended to protect the citizens of that state. AOTA is a valued resource for these regulatory agencies, providing information about the profession and assisting with monitoring and advocating for occupational therapy in the state legislature. When students complete their Level II fieldwork and successfully pass the certification examination of the NBCOT, they are eligible to apply for licenses and certificates to practice. These applications are handled through state government bodies.

American Occupational Therapy Foundation

The American Occupational Therapy Foundation (AOTF) is a nonprofit organization that was established in 1965 to advance the science and increase public awareness of occupational therapy (AOTF, 2011). The AOTF is composed of occupational therapy practitioners, corporate partners, and sponsors that support occupational therapy education and research. The AOTF is financially supported by private contributions and through sponsors that value occupational therapy. Each year, the foundation holds special events at the AOTA annual conference and exposition to raise money to support its work on behalf of occupational therapy education and research.

As part of the AOTF mission to advance the science of occupational therapy, AOTF publishes a scholarly journal, *Occupational Therapy Journal of Research: Occupation, Participation and Health* (OTJR) (AOTF, 2011). The foundation also maintains the Wilma West Library, a national clearinghouse for occupational therapy information. In addition to the excellent library, the foundation maintains OT SEARCH, a comprehensive electronic search engine for literature related to occupational therapy.

AOTF supports students and scholars through educational scholarships and research grants (AOTF, 2011). Small grants are available to graduate students to fund their research. Larger amounts are granted to scholars to fund innovative studies that contribute to the occupational therapy body of knowledge and build an understanding of occupational science. Finally, the foundation partners with higher education to fund centers of scholarship and research.

National Board for Certification in Occupational Therapy

The occupational therapy profession is also supported through the work of the National Board for Certification in Occupational Therapy (NBCOT, 2011). NBCOT is the credentialing body for OTs and OTAs practicing in the United States. NBCOT develops and administers the initial certification examinations that OTs and OTAs take following their Level II fieldwork. The examinations are comprehensive and are designed to measure the knowledge and skills required for an OT or OTA to enter practice. The items in the certification examinations are based on an extensive practice analysis of entry-level occupational therapy practice. The certification examination includes items that reflect occupational therapy evaluation and intervention with diverse populations in a variety of practice environments. Examination results are shared with individual state licensure boards. Achievement of a passing score on the certification examination is required in almost every state to be eligible to obtain a license or certificate to practice. OTs and OTAs from other countries who wish to practice in the United States must successfully complete the certification examination.

World Federation of Occupational Therapists

Occupational therapy is a global profession and is actively expanding worldwide (WFOT, 2011). There are an estimated 600 million persons worldwide with disabilities who are restricted or denied access to meaningful participation in daily life. The WFOT was created in 1952 as the official international organization for the promotion of occupational therapy and has more than 70 member countries around the world and more than 6,000 individual members, representing more than 160,000 occupational therapy practitioners around the globe. WFOT membership is coordinated through each national association worldwide.

The WFOT is recognized as an official partner with the World Health Organization (WHO) and is recognized as a nonprofit nongovernmental organization (NGO) by the United Nations (UN) (WFOT, 2011). The WFOT promotes international cooperation for more than 70 national occupational therapy associations; advances the international standards for occupational therapy practice, education, and research; and coordinates with other international allied health organizations, such as Rehabilitation International (RI), the International Council on Disabilities (ICOD), the Asia Pacific Occupational Therapist Regional Group (APOTRG), La Confederación Latino Americana de Terapeutas Ocupacionales (CLATO), the Council of Occupational Therapists for the European Countries (COTEC), the Occupational Therapy Africa Regional Group (OTARG), and the World Confederation for Physical Therapy (WCPT).

The WFOT offers support to the international occupational therapy community to increase the number of educational programs relevant to each country's cultural uniqueness, increasing the number of occupational therapy practitioners to provide critical services to clients; to

BOX 68.3 Websites for Professional Organizations

To learn more about the profession of occupational therapy and the organizations that support it, refer to the following Websites:

American Occupational Therapy Association: http://www.aota.org

(Note: The AOTA home page also provides a link to all affiliated state associations.)

American Occupational Therapy Foundation: http://www.aotf.org

National Board for Certification in Occupational Therapy: http://www.nbcot.org

World Federation of Occupational Therapists: http://www.wfot.org

(Note: The WFOT home page provides a direct link to occupational therapy professional organizations in countries throughout the world.)

promote international standards for practice, education, and research; and to governmental support of occupational therapy (WFOT, 2011). The WFOT also publishes the WFOT Bulletin twice per year as the official peer-reviewed journal and organizes the WFOT Congress, an international conference that brings together OTs from around the globe every 4 years.

The Occupational Therapy International Outreach Network (OTION) provides volunteer and work opportunities for occupational therapy students and practitioners interested in international practice (WFOT, 2011). The OTION provides a forum for partnerships between occupational therapy practitioners in resource-rich countries serving persons with disabilities in resource-poor countries. With the increasing globalization of the occupational therapy profession, international cooperation is critical for spearheading responses to improving the health and well-being of individuals and groups throughout the world by responding to natural and human-made disasters and emphasizing the importance of participation in meaningful occupation to a global citizenry.

Conclusion

Occupational therapy professional organizations offer the opportunity to collectively advance the profession in a way that cannot be achieved by an individual student or practitioner alone (see Box 68.3 on how to find more information on these groups). Professional organizations are nonprofit organizations seeking to further the profession, the interests of individuals engaged in that profession, and the public interest. By building a strong community of students and practitioners that unite the profession around a shared mission and vision, strategies can be developed that advance practice and serve the public interest. These associations represent the interests of students and practitioners through legislative advocacy and public promotion of the profession.

As OTs, OTAs, and occupational therapy students, we are supported by our state, national, and international occupational therapy professional organizations that provide the resources and information that we need to practice effectively. As professionals, we also have the opportunity and responsibility to support and participate in our professional organizations so that we can work toward continually developing, shaping, and promoting the occupational therapy profession through lifelong membership and active participation.

References

American Occupational Therapy Association. (2011a). *Accreditation*. Retrieved from http://www.aota.org

American Occupational Therapy Association. (2011b). *Governance*. Retrieved from http://www.aota.org

American Occupational Therapy Association. (2011c). *Publications*. Retrieved from http://www.aota.org

American Occupational Therapy Association. (2011d). *Special interest sections*. Retrieved from http://www.aota.org

American Occupational Therapy Foundation. (2011). *Scholarships*. Retrieved from http://www.aotf.org

Bickel, J. (2007). The role of professional societies in career development in academic medicine. *Academic Psychiatry, 31*, 91–94.

Greenwood, R., Suddaby, R., & Hinings, C. R. (2002). Theorizing change: The role of professional associations in the transformation of institutionalized fields. *Academy of Management Journal, 45*, 58–80

Mata, H., Latham, T. P., & Ransome, Y. (2010). Benefits of professional organization membership and participation in national conferences: Considerations for students and new professionals. *Health Promotion Practice, 11*, 450–453

National Board for Certification in Occupational Therapy. (2011). *NBCOT*. Retrieved from http://www.nbcot.org

Osborn, R. N., & Hunt, J. G. (2007). Leadership and the choice of order: Complexity and hierarchical perspectives near the edge of chaos. *Leadership Quarterly, 18*, 319–340.

Ritzhaupt, A. D., Umapathy, K., & Jamba, L. (2008). Computing professional association membership: An exploration of membership needs and motivations. *Journal of Information Systems Applied Research, 1*, 1–22.

Schneider, M., & Somers, M. (2006). Organizations as complex adaptive systems: Implications of complexity theory for leadership research. *Leadership Quarterly, 17*, 351–365.

World Federation of Occupational Therapists. (2011). Retrieved from http://www.wfot.org

For additional resources on the subjects discussed in this chapter, visit http://thePoint.lww.com/Willard-Spackman12e.

UNIT XV

Occupational Therapy Management

"In turbulent times, an enterprise has to be managed both to withstand sudden blows and to avail itself of sudden unexpected opportunities. This means that, in turbulent times, the fundamentals have to be managed and managed well."

—Peter F. Drucker

CHAPTER 69

Management of Occupational Therapy Services

Brent Braveman

OUTLINE

LEARNING OBJECTIVES

After reading this chapter, you will be able to:

1. Analyze and explain the relationship and differences between administrators, managers, supervisors, and leaders in the oversight of work activities in organizations
2. Identify and explain examples of the common roles, functions, and responsibilities of managers
3. Identify and explain the areas of knowledge and skills necessary for a manager to demonstrate competency

Management Can Mean Many Things

Becoming an occupational therapy or interdisciplinary manager is just one of the many professional roles that an occupational therapy practitioner may assume over his or her career. Being a "manager" can mean many different things depending on the setting in which you practice, the scope of duties included in your job description, and the related roles and functions assumed by others in that setting. There is a wealth of information to guide management practice, including theory, research and other types of evidence, formal education, continuing education and training, publications, and other scholarly forms. Investigators and practitioners in a variety of disciplines such as organizational development, business psychology, business administration, and human resource management have contributed to this knowledge base over the past decades. Consequently, many resources to guide managers in their jobs are readily available on the Internet, in bookstores, and through educational courses offered at colleges and universities or at continuing education events, such as professional conferences. Resources are also available from the American Occupational Therapy Association (AOTA).

Similar to clinical practice within occupational therapy, demonstrating effective practice as an occupational therapy manager is dependent on familiarity with the relevant theories and the ability to apply these theories based on the most current evidence. Just as there are multiple clinical practice models that occupational therapy practitioners draw upon depending on the area of practice and the needs of the client, there are multiple theories and skill sets on which a manager draws to guide effective managerial practice. Becoming an effective occupational therapy manager is a complicated and time-intensive process. Therefore, this chapter will focus on introducing the reader to the scope of what an occupational therapy manager *is* and what an occupational therapy manager *does*. Chapter 72 provides a complementary discussion that focuses on supervision and the roles and functions that occupational therapy supervisors perform.

In order to truly understand and appreciate the variety of roles and functions that an occupational therapy manager can serve, it is critical to recognize that most managers function in ways often described as supervisors and leaders. Table 69.1 provides definitions of **administration**, **management**, **supervision**, and **leadership**.

An administrator may be defined as a member of a *governing body*, such as a board of directors of an organization; the top officials, such as the president or chief executive officer of an organization; or that official's leadership team. Together, administrators perform the key function of being responsible for the overall welfare and direction of the organization, including oversight of financial affairs, establishing the major policies that guide operations, and planning for the health and future of the organization. Administrators typically supervise others but usually are only indirectly responsible for the oversight of the day-to-day work of the organization. They frequently delegate authority for much of the day-to-day coordination of organizational functioning to managers.

Managers are responsible for oversight of work units (such as an occupational therapy department or a program for head injury survivors) and of their contributions to the organization's mission. Managers put the policies and directives of administration into action in measurable and visible ways. The specific responsibilities of a manager have been traditionally categorized according to four major functions, which are (1) **planning**, (2) **organizing**, (3) **directing**, and (4) **controlling**. Staffing is a management function that is sometimes grouped with organizing (e.g., organizing and staffing). These four functions are briefly defined in Table 69.1 and further discussed in the next sections of this chapter.

TABLE 69.1 Administration, Management, Supervision, and Leadership Defined

Administration	The process of guiding an organization through the authoritative control of others completed by the governing body of the organization
Management	The process of guiding a work unit by planning for future work obligations, organizing employees into functional units, directing employees in the process of completing daily work tasks, and controlling work processes and systems to ensure adequate quality of work output
Supervision	The control and direction of the work of one or more employees in a manner that promotes improved performance and a higher quality outcome
Leadership	The process of creating structural change where the values, vision, and ethics of individuals are integrated into the culture of a community as a means of achieving sustainable change

Supervisors are responsible for direct oversight of employees who perform the work of the organization. Although managers are typically given the ability to decide who becomes part of their work unit through the ability to hire and fire, there are many supervisory roles in organizations that do not perform this or many other functions of the manager. Understanding the important concept of **requisite managerial authority** can help us to further clarify how an occupational therapy manager is different from an organizational administrator or from an occupational therapy supervisor. Elliot Jaques (1998, p. 69) defined minimum requisite managerial authority as

> the level of control and discretion that a manager must have to be fairly held responsible for the outcomes of work groups.

For example, requisite managerial authority includes the authority to hire and fire employees and to determine within reason how rewards are distributed. However, in occupational therapy, it is not uncommon for a therapist to accept a formally named position within an organization in which he or she has supervisory responsibilities but does not have requisite managerial authority. An example of such a position would be that of a *senior therapist*—an individual who might have specialized or advanced skills and who might provide clinical supervision to other therapists but who does not have the full range of managerial responsibilities.

Administrators, managers, and supervisors may often be viewed as *leaders* by virtue of their formally named positions in an organization, although there are typically many informal leaders in organizations as well. One conceptualization of the relationship between management and leadership is that the role of a manager is to maintain stability in the organization, whereas a leader guides change. For example, Levey, Hill, and Green (2002) suggested that whereas management is conservative and maintenance directed, leadership is innovative, change oriented, and informed by vision. Similarly, Beech (2002) suggested that managers tend to rely primarily on strategy, structure, and systems, whereas leaders are inclined to use style, staff, skills, and shared goals to yield desired results. Effective leadership is a topic that has been the focus of much research, and several leadership theories have been investigated in depth. A brief description of five of the most commonly cited theories of leadership are presented in Table 69.2.

TABLE 69.2 Common Theories of Leadership

Supervisory Theories of Leadership	Primary Focus
Path–Goal	Leaders increase personal payoffs for subordinates for goal attainment and make the path to these payoffs easier to travel by reducing obstacles, thereby improving performance.
Transactional	Leaders promise rewards and benefits to subordinates for meeting work goals, and leaders and subordinates agree through transactions on what will lead to reward and how to avoid punishment.
Strategic Theories of Leadership	
Charismatic	Stresses the personal identification of followers with the leader who formulates an inspirational vision and impression that the leader's mission is extraordinary.
Transformational	Leaders achieve change by expressing the value associated with outcomes and by articulating a vision of the future, resulting in commitment, effort, and improved performance on the part of subordinates.
Situational	Leaders should adopt a leadership style that best fits the developmental level of their subordinates' competence and commitment.

Practice Dilemma

Brent Returns to Being a Manager

After working at a university as an occupational therapy faculty member for 10 years, Brent has returned to full-time job as a manager. He has accepted the position of director of Rehabilitation Services at a large, internationally recognized cancer research and treatment center and is now responsible for a staff of more than 90 employees. His direct reports include inpatient and outpatient supervisors for occupational therapy and physical therapy, a business manager, and a senior administrative assistant. Brent was hired because of his strong background in management, leadership, strategic planning, and organizational consulting, even though he had very little experience in oncology.

The first 6 months in his job were pretty overwhelming for Brent; and as he started month 7, he was just starting to feel like he knew what he was doing. He had established a good working relationship with his leadership team and was 3 months into the process of developing a strategic plan. He was leading his department through the process of updating its mission statement and developing a vision statement for a decade into the future. Several key positions had been filled, but some staff had resigned and it seemed clear that recruiting and retaining staff would be a constant challenge. Although he had managed a clinical department before and developed and managed budgets, he was now responsible for much larger sums of revenue and expenses and had more autonomy in decision making than he did in the past. There were many issues he was encountering for the first time, such as the need to make many decisions related to the department's electronic medical record, establishing new contracts with vendors, establishing credibility with the physical therapy staff he managed, and developing services at the organization's satellite centers.

Brent had been an occupational therapist for 26 years including 11 as a manager and had a wealth of knowledge and experience to draw upon. Still, he recognized the need to take advantage of the many resources available to him to help him grow as a professional and succeed in his new position. He was aware that there is a wealth of management theory, research, and other forms of evidence on effective management available from a variety of disciplines such as business, organizational psychology, and the health fields. Luckily, the organization recognized the need to help new executives develop, and Brent chose to take advantage of the training and educational opportunities made available to him by his employer. Brent recognized that he had taken on a big challenge but also knew he would be a success if he was open to continuing to learn as a professional.

Questions

As you read this chapter, consider Brent's situation and ask yourself the following questions:

1. What other sorts of challenges and new responsibilities do you think Brent is likely to encounter as he spends more time in his new job?
2. What types of managerial knowledge and skills does Brent need to develop to help him confront the challenges he is facing?
3. What would be examples of the traditionally identified management functions of planning, organizing, directing, and controlling that Brent is likely to perform?
4. What questions should Brent ask to guide him toward useful management theory and evidence to make his practice as a manager more effective?

Administrators, managers, and supervisors all perform various tasks related to the four functions of management described in Table 69.3, but the scope of these tasks varies for the different levels of leadership. Table 69.4 provides a comparison of sample functions of administrators, managers, and supervisors organized according to the traditional four functions of management.

TABLE 69.3 The Four Traditional Functions of Management

Planning	The process of deciding what to do by setting performance goals and identifying the specific objectives and activities that need to be carried out to accomplish these objectives
Organizing	Designing workable units, determining lines of authority and communication, and developing and managing patterns of coordination
Controlling	Providing guidance and leadership so that the work that is performed is congruent with goals
Directing	Establishing performance standards, measuring, evaluating, and correcting performance

The Four Functions of Management

Planning

Planning is the first of four critical functions that managers perform in an organization. As the pace of change in society and the rate of global information sharing have increased, planning has become more important today than ever. Planning is the process of establishing

TABLE 69.4 Comparisons of Sample Functions of Administrators, Managers, and Supervisors

Management Function	Organizational Administration	Occupational Therapy Managers	Occupational Therapy Supervisors
Planning	• Establishment of organizational mission and vision • Creation of an organizational culture • Strategic planning • Financial forecasting • Establishing organization policies and procedures	• Interpreting the organizational mission and vision for the staff • Aligning the departmental mission and vision with the organizational mission and vision • Establishing departmental objectives • Creating and implementing the departmental budget • Establishing departmental policies and procedures	• Integration of the mission and vision of the organization and department in the daily work of the department and staff • Oversight of work tasks related to achievement of departmental objectives • Ensuring that work is completed effectively and efficiently
Organizing and staffing	• Oversight of the organizational chart and determination of primary organizational structure • Establishing systems for staff functions such as human resources and marketing[a]	• Recruiting, hiring, orienting, and training staff • Appraising performance, determining rewards, and overseeing disciplinary actions	• Providing management with feedback related to the appropriateness of staffing levels • Provide daily supervision, coaching, and feedback to line staff
Directing	• Development of parameters for staff training, education, and development • Mentoring and coaching middle managers	• Mentoring and coaching supervisors • Implementing staff training, education, and development programs	
Controlling	• Establishing systems to measure organizational performance and achievement of key organizational goals • Setting expectations for performance for management	• Oversight and implementation of departmental continuous quality improvement and quality control systems • Establishing performance expectations and measures for department functions and outputs	• Ensuring compliance with policies and procedures • Measuring and recording quality indicators • Alerting management to systems problems

[a]Staff functions relate to the overall maintenance and management of an organization (e.g., human resources, housekeeping, or marketing). Line functions relate to carrying out the primary work of the organization (e.g., occupational therapy, physical therapy, or social work in medically oriented organizations).

short- and long-term goals, measurable objectives, and action plans that are both congruent with the mission of the organization and consistent with the vision that current organizational leaders have established. An organization's mission is typically established by its founders and remains relatively stable. It is often expressed in the form of a mission statement that sets forth the organization's purpose, products, and services. **Mission statements** succinctly describe (1) why an organization exists or the function the organization performs in society or in a community, (2) who the organization serves or who its customers are, and (3) an indication of how an organization goes about achieving its purpose.

A **vision statement**, by contrast, expresses an aspirational message about what a department or organization would like to become as it seeks to fulfill its mission. Vision statements are inherently future oriented and therefore are helpful management tools in long-term planning. Both missions and visions are often communicated in *statements*, but the process itself of developing a mission statement or vision statement can be of tremendous value to an organization.

One example of a mission statement and vision statement are those developed by the University of Texas MD Anderson Cancer Center in Houston, Texas. The mission of the University of Texas MD Anderson Cancer Center is to "eliminate cancer in Texas, the nation, and the world through outstanding programs that integrate patient care, research and prevention, and through education for undergraduate and graduate students, trainees, professionals, employees and the public" (MD Anderson Cancer Center, 2011, para. 1). The vision statement for MD Anderson reads, "We shall be the premier cancer center in the world, based on the excellence of our people, our research-driven patient care and our science. We are Making Cancer History" (MD Anderson Cancer Center, 2011, para. 2).

It is common to distinguish between strategic planning or long-range planning and the shorter term day-to-day planning that most managers complete. **Strategic planning** is "the process of ensuring that an organization's current purpose, aspirations, goals, activities and strategies connect to plans and support its mission" (Strickland, 2011, p. 103). Strategic plans are often developed with 3- to 5-year time frames in mind, although hopefully the top leadership of an organization (e.g., administration) is thinking much further into the future. The *goals* included in the strategic plan are a reflection of the scope of the desired outcomes such that they can be broad and encompass the full breadth of organizational activities or they can be more focused on critical segments of an organization. *Objectives* are the measurable steps that are taken to reach each goal. The discreet objectives for each goal are commonly based on a 1-year period that corresponds with an organization's financial cycle, or *fiscal year*. Fiscal years may correspond with a calendar year or may be reflective of some other time cycle such as an academic calendar. It is common for organizations to have fiscal years that begin on July 1st and end June 30th.

Operating in an environment in which change occurs frequently, such as the health care arena, may make long-term planning more difficult than in industries or environments that are more stable. When an organization experiences significant change, the processes of mission review and visioning previously discussed become even more important (Braveman, 2006c). The scholarship on change management has focused on four principal aspects: (1) theoretical models and frameworks that reveal and guide organization members' and researchers' thinking about organization change, (2) approaches and tools for creating and managing change, (3) factors that are important to successful change management, and (4) outcomes and consequences of the process of change management (Branch, 2002). It is strongly recommended that new managers become familiar with theories of change and strategies for promoting successful change. For example, Kurt Lewin (1997) proposed a prominent and relatively simple approach to understanding change still commonly employed today that includes three stages (Figure 69.1). These three stages are (1) unfreezing or recognizing the need to change, (2) changing, and (3) refreezing or standardizing new procedures or ways of behaving. Managers can apply this theory by identifying different strategies to use with employees during each of the three stages to facilitate the change process. Two other theories that are often used to understand change include the following:

- Prochaska and DiClemente's transtheoretical stages of change model, which conceptualizes change in five stages: (1) precontemplation, (2) contemplation, (3) preparation, (4) action, and (5) maintenance (Franche, Corbière, Lee, Breslin, & Hepburn, 2007).
- Social cognitive theory, which focuses on change in individuals who can learn by direct experiences, human dialogue and interaction, and observation (Cervone & Pervin, 2008).

Although the transtheoretical stages of change model and social cognitive theory have most often been applied to change as it relates to health behaviors, they can also be useful in understanding how humans interpret and respond to change in the workplace.

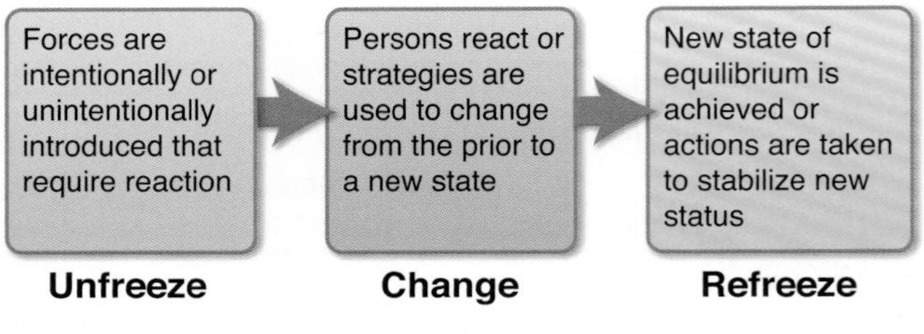

Forces are intentionally or unintentionally introduced that require reaction
Persons react or strategies are used to change from the prior to a new state
New state of equilibrium is achieved or actions are taken to stabilize new status
Unfreeze
Change
Refreeze

FIGURE 69.1 Lewin's three-stage model of change.

In addition to establishing goals and objectives, planning includes determining the needs for the human resources, materials, supplies, facilities, and equipment required to meet goals and objectives. Financial planning and budgeting and the writing of policies and procedures that guide the use of materials, supplies, facilities, and equipment are also commonly considered components of planning.

Organizing and Staffing

Typically, an organization's administration will determine the overall structure of the organization, including how line authority will be organized and how employees may be grouped into departments. Organizational structures can vary in complexity. An organizational chart helps to facilitate understanding of an organization's structure. Liebler and McConnell (2011) explain that an organizational chart is a management tool that visually depicts the following aspects of an organization:

- Major functions, usually by department
- Relationships of functions or departments
- Channels of supervision
- Lines of authority and of communication
- Positions by job title within departments or units

When one examines an organizational chart, one must keep in mind that it is a static picture of how the organization is structured at one point in time. It might not reflect recent changes, vacancies, or informal relationships because written charts typically indicate only formal lines of command. Earlier, it was noted that there are many informal leaders in organizations; and these sources of knowledge, power, and influence are not communicated in an organizational chart. The organizational charts of many large organizations support the notion that systems are often quite organic in how they grow and are restructured over time.

Although few large organizations fit the perfect theoretical profile of any formal organizational form or structure, there are a few basic structures commonly found in health care and service organizations and systems that are useful for a new manager or practitioner to understand. These structures include the dual-pyramid form of organizing, product line or service line organizations, and hybrid or matrix organizations.

The term *dual-pyramid* has been used to describe the common structure found in many medical model settings, such as acute and general hospitals. The pyramid structure is also commonly found in community-based organizations, although the second pyramid representing medical staff might be absent in these cases. A pyramid is typically used to represent an organization of personnel with upper management at the top and line staff at the bottom (Figure 69.2).

In the dual-pyramid form of organizing, the traditional relationship between medical staff and administration

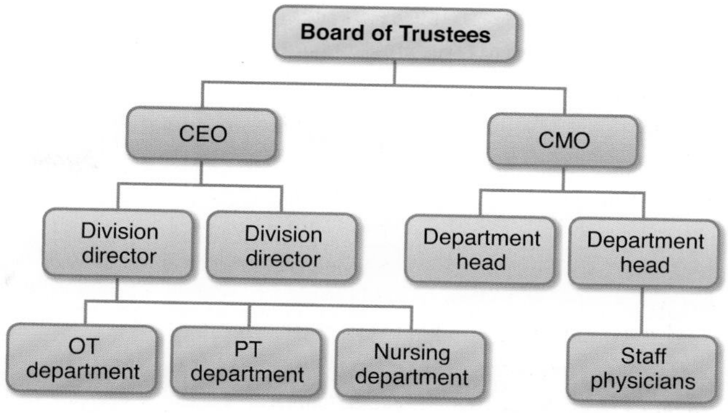

FIGURE 69.2 A sample dual-pyramid form of organizing. *CEO*, chief executive officer; *CMO*, chief medical officer; *OT*, occupational therapy; *PT*, physical therapy.

results in the structure shown in Figure 69.2, in which two supervisory pyramids are arranged side by side. One pyramid represents the structure of the professional staff that is organized in departments, including administration (with the chief executive officer at the top of the pyramid); health professionals such as occupational therapists, physical therapists, and social workers; and all support services such as engineering, housekeeping, and human resource personnel. A second pyramid mimics that structure but represents the organization of the medical staff with the chief medical officer at the top of the pyramid, department heads as middle management, and staff physicians as line employees (Braveman, 2006c). Although the medical staff, professional staff, and support staff all ultimately report to a board of trustees or board of directors, there are two distinct chains of command that result in the authority and accountability systems being separated. So, for example, physicians, nurses, occupational therapists, and physical therapists all work together as part of an interdisciplinary team. However, the physicians on a particular service (e.g., cardiovascular) report to a department head (also a physician) who reports to the chief medical officer, who in return reports to the chief executive officer. The other members of the team report to a supervisor and/or a department director who in turn may report to a vice president who reports to the same chief executive officer as the chief medical officer.

A second common form of organizational structure is the *product line*, or *service line*, structure. In a product line structure, personnel are organized according to the service or product that they provide rather than according to the specific function that they complete or their departments. A board of directors maintains ultimate authority, and the chief executive officer and chief medical officer often still maintain parallel but distinct responsibilities and authority. An example of the organizational chart for a product line form is provided in Figure 69.3. Additional ways of structuring organizations may combine elements of the dual-pyramid and product line structures and may function in a more *matrixed* manner with many interconnections between departments, dual reporting structures

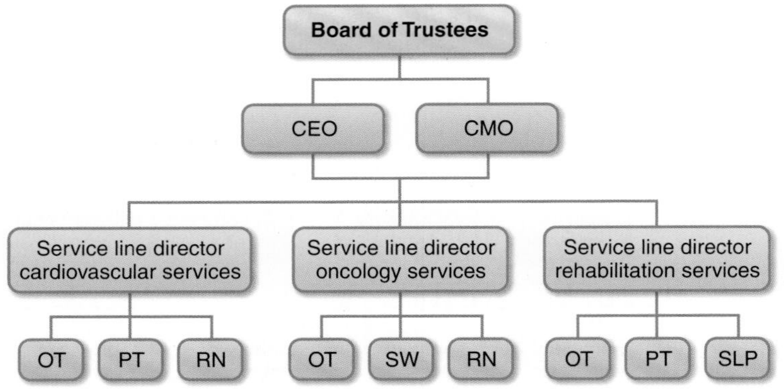

FIGURE 69.3 A sample product line management form of organizing. *CEO*, chief executive officer; *CMO*, chief medical officer; *OT*, occupational therapist; *PT*, physical therapist; *RN*, registered nurse; *SLP*, speech languange pathologist; SW, social worker.

where some employees report to more than one manager, and heavy use of internal consultants.

Each of the methods of organization has advantages and disadvantages, and understanding how structure influences the function of an organization can help one to capitalize on the system's benefits and compensate for its limitations. For example, health care organizations that have a dual-pyramid structure rely on departments structured by discipline or professional education and training to provide for strong supervision of staff and their clinical performance. Thus, communication within a professional discipline is facilitated, and the discipline-specific daily work of a unit may be completed more efficiently. Because a department manager or supervisor representing each discipline has direct access to staff and to the data related to routine processes and interventions, performance improvement and outcome measurement using these data may also be easier in a dual-pyramid organization. Nonetheless, in this form of organizing, communication across disciplines (e.g., from occupational therapy to nursing) might be more complicated, which can pose potential hazards for developing and managing new programs. Problem-solving and process improvement in existing programming can be cumbersome when staff members feel that it is necessary to communicate up through the chains of command. The advantages and disadvantages of the dual-pyramid and the product line forms of organizing are summarized in Table 69.5.

Once decisions have been made about how an organization or a department is to be structured, administrators and managers ideally work together to develop plans

TABLE 69.5 Advantages and Disadvantages of Common Forms of Organizing

	Pyramid	Product Line
Communication	• Communication within a discipline is facilitated.	• Communication between disciplines becomes harder.
Planning	• Planning for activities such as professional development and clinical supervision is facilitated, but program planning becomes harder.	• Program planning and planning for interdisciplinary activities such as program evaluation is facilitated, but planning functions within disciplines becomes harder.
Budgeting	• Tracking and planning for finances related to single-discipline costs are facilitated, but tracking and planning for interdisciplinary activities (e.g., cost per unit of care) are harder.	• Tracking and planning for finances related to programmatic costs are facilitated (e.g., cost per unit of care), but tracking and planning for discipline-specific activities are harder.
Staffing	• Some needs such as providing coverage for leaves or vacancies may be easier, but the need to communicate with other managers increases. Recruitment activities are facilitated.	• Staffing activities influenced by other disciplines such as scheduling programmatic elements may be facilitated, but coverage for leaves or vacancies becomes more difficult. Recruitment of staff may be more difficult, or you might need to rely on managers from other disciplines for assistance.
PI, program evaluation, and outcomes	• Improving discipline-specific processes is easier as is measuring single-discipline outcomes and indicators of program evaluation, but interdisciplinary programs require extra effort.	• Improving interdisciplinary or program processes is easier, as is measuring program outcomes and indicators of program evaluation, but discipline-specific elements require extra effort.
Professional development	• Development of discipline-specific skills related to assessment and intervention may be facilitated by the ease of access to disciplinary specialists.	• Development of interdisciplinary skills related to the needs of a population or program development or implementation may be facilitated.

PI, process improvement.

for staffing and human resources management. Functions related to recruitment and staffing, such as advertising job vacancies or the development of policies and procedures related to employment, may be performed by a human resources department. Occupational therapy managers are frequently involved in a number of other staffing-related activities. The following is a list of some of these activities:

- Human resources planning: collaborating with administrators and supervisors at all levels of the organization to forecast the short- and long-term personnel needs of the organization based on the organizational mission, leadership vision, and strategic plans
- Recruitment: seeking out and attracting adequate numbers of qualified personnel to meet ongoing organizational needs, including contingencies, such as resignations and leaves of absence for medical or personal reasons
- Hiring: selecting the appropriate personnel for vacant positions and activities related to the hiring process, such as benefits counseling and overseeing background and reference checks
- Orientation: introducing the new employee to organizational policies, benefits, procedures, values, personnel, and environments
- Training and development: meeting the short- and long-term educational and professional development needs of employees at all levels of the organization
- Separation: terminating the employment of personnel due to resignation or inadequate job performance or that which may come about as the result of a decrease in organizational resources

Maintaining a viable workforce by retaining a qualified and competent staff is perhaps one of the most important functions of the manager for an organization. Retention of staff can also be very difficult in professions such as occupational therapy and physical therapy where much of the workforce is young and mobile and the demand for staff far outnumbers the supply. Staff retention and satisfaction is another area where the occupational therapy manager can benefit from considerable research and evidence (Fisher, 2011). Similar to the topics of leadership and change, an in-depth discussion of theories related to staff retention and satisfaction are beyond the scope of this chapter, and managers would benefit from a thorough review of contemporary literature. A few examples of theories that have evolved regarding employee satisfaction and retention are the following:

- Self-determination theory, which explores the relationship of intrinsic and extrinsic motivators to work motivation (Gagne & Deci, 2005)
- Need theories such as Maslow's hierarchy of needs and McClelland's need theory that focus on identifying physiological and psychological needs of employees with the rationale that satisfying these needs will lead to employee satisfaction (Ramlall, 2004)
- Expectancy theory, which holds that people are motivated to behave in ways that produce expected and desired combinations of outcomes (Pinder, 2008)

Directing

Directing is the management function that involves giving guidance, instruction, and leadership to subordinates so that work that is performed is goal oriented and contributes to meeting organizational or departmental requirements. More specifically, a manager could assign and manage the workload, develop and implement policies and procedures to guide others in uniform completion of their work, provide mentoring and coaching for improved future performance, and appraise performance by providing feedback to employees about current performance.

Managing the workload is a complicated and multistep process that involves projecting the amount of work to be done, determining which resources are necessary to complete the work, and managing these resources to make certain that the appropriate person with the right skills and right equipment and space is available when needed. The workload is typically projected on a yearly basis as part of planning a departmental budget, but it may also be done on a week-to-week, day-to-day, or even hourly basis. Effective workload management requires flexibility, creativity, a commitment to planning, and advanced problem-solving skills.

Writing policies and procedures to guide staff in their daily tasks in a standardized manner, as well as their use of materials, supplies, facilities, and equipment in ways that are compliant with accreditation and other standards, is a specific aspect of directing that is typically the responsibility of a department manager. Policies are statements of values that are congruent with the organizational or departmental mission and justify the boundaries that govern the services provided. They set parameters for making decisions about day-to-day operations. Procedures outline the specific tasks that should be completed or that provide specific direction about how a policy should be implemented. A manager should not only be able to cite a policy or procedure but also be able to give the underlying logic for the policy's existence.

Most organizations follow a prescribed standard format that guides managers in deciding what to include in a department's policy and procedure manual. If a policy and procedures format is not provided, the organization may purchase existing customizable resources on the Internet. It is typical for managers to network with others both locally and nationally, and most managers will freely share nonproprietary information such as a policy and procedure. The basic components of a policy and procedure protocol are presented in Box 69.1.

BOX 69.1 Basic Components of a Policy and Procedure

(This is not for an entire manual but the components of a single policy and procedure statement that is typically one document within a manual.)

- Policy statement(s): Brief statements of the guiding principles to be communicated
- Purpose statement(s): Brief statements that outline the reasons for inclusion of the policies or procedures
- Applicability: Lists the employee groups to which the policy and procedure applies (e.g., all occupational therapy department staff members)
- Procedures: Statements outlining the specific actions to be taken by the identified employee groups and criteria for determining adherence to the policy
- Responsibility: Identifying the individuals who are responsible for oversight of the policy and procedure (e.g., all occupational therapy team leaders)
- Review period: Lists the date of the last review and update of the policy and procedures (typically, policies and procedures are reviewed on an annual basis)

Managers also serve as mentors, coaches, and appraisers of overall work performance; resources to develop the skills and knowledge necessary for these functions should be sought out both from within the profession of occupational therapy and from outside of it. AOTA has a number of resources related to supervisory tasks specific to occupational therapy assistants or to occupational therapy aides (http://www.aota.org). For more generic information on models of supervision, theories of motivating others, developing effective performance appraisal systems, or providing effective mentoring or coaching, managers should look outside the occupational therapy literature. For example, associations such as the American Management Association (http://www.amanet.org) or the National Association for Employee Recognition (http://www.recognition.org/) provide resources about how one may become an effective supervisor.

Controlling

Controlling is a management function that relates to the processes of establishing specific work performance standards and the measurement, evaluation, and correction of performance. A key responsibility of managers is to promote the delivery of appropriate intervention through the use of quality control (QC) mechanisms and performance improvement (PI), which is sometimes also called continuous quality improvement (CQI). QC and PI are related functions, but each serves a different purpose and relies on different philosophies, strategies, tools, and techniques. The focus of QC is to intervene when the quality or quantity of work output falls below predetermined measures (indicators). The focus of PI is to improve customer satisfaction by constantly striving to meet customer expectations through enhancing critical processes. A critical process is defined as any process that is performed to produce the work of an organization. Examples of occupational therapy critical processes include responding to referrals for service, administering assessments, fabricating adaptive equipment, and making postdischarge referrals.

PI is viewed both as a philosophy of management and as an approach to managing. A PI approach requires that managers develop a wide range of skills related to assessing tasks and people. PI projects may be complex and time intensive because they rely on decision making based on data and therefore require an organized and structured approach to gathering and analyzing data. Explaining PI in depth is beyond the scope of this chapter, but Figure 69.4 provides a brief overview of commonly identified steps to choose a critical process and implementing steps that improve its performance. The Plan, Do, Study, Act (PDSA) Cycle may be invoked under other names or acronyms, but the steps of the PI process remain constant (Figure 69.5). The most common tools and techniques and their uses are presented in Table 69.6.

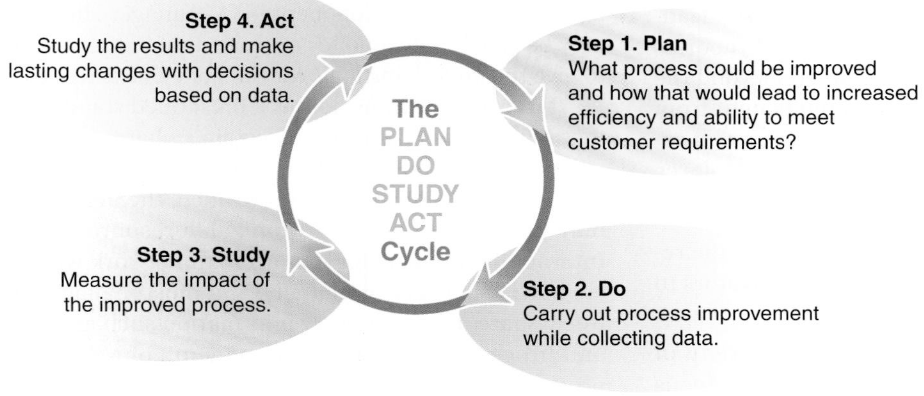

Step 4. Act
Study the results and make lasting changes with decisions based on data.
Step 1. Plan
What process could be improved and how that would lead to increased efficiency and ability to meet customer requirements?
The PLAN DO STUDY ACT Cycle
Step 3. Study
Measure the impact of the improved process.
Step 2. Do
Carry out process improvement while collecting data.

FIGURE 69.4 The Plan, Do, Study, Act (PDSA) Cycle.

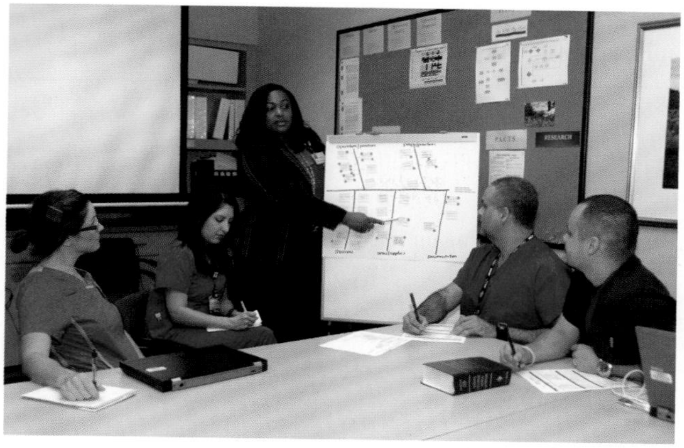

FIGURE 69.5 Staff members complete a cause-and-effect diagram to identify potential root causes of a problem as part of a formal performance improvement project.

Financial Management

An important function of most managers is the planning and controlling of a department budget. Budgets are typically planned for a calendar year or a fiscal year (e.g., many organizations operate on a fiscal year that runs from July 1 to June 30). The process of planning and managing a budget requires that a manager have a comprehensive understanding of the goals and objectives of the larger organization so that he or she can establish priorities for funding that support this mission over time.

Occupational therapy practitioners who want to become managers or directors of an occupational therapy department or to own and operate their own businesses are encouraged to learn financial planning and management and to become well versed in the use of information management technologies, such as spreadsheets or other financial management tools. Braveman (2006b) notes that effective financial planning and management requires a working knowledge of the following:

- Health care systems, including city, county, state, and national systems
- Payment and reimbursement structures, such as Medicare, Medicaid, Worker's Compensation, private insurance, and grants or foundation support
- Human resources systems and costs, including salary and benefit administration, training and educational costs and systems, and recruitment and retention structures
- Equipment and materials purchasing and management, including medical supplies such as splinting or assistive and adaptive equipment, office supplies, and other supportive supplies
- Facilities management, maintenance, and improvement protocols, including cleaning and maintenance of physical plant structures

Budgets may also include revenue and expenses, although it is not uncommon for a community-based organization manager to have oversight of only expenses with no control over direct sources of revenue. Typically, the revenues and expenses associated with each department in an organization are given some sort of marker or code in the organization's accounting system that indicates how the subset of revenues and expenses relate to that department. These subsets of revenues and expenses are commonly referred to as *cost centers.* They may represent the budget of a single department or of several related services. Common examples of revenues and expenses are shown in Table 69.7 and are further explained in the following section.

Forecasting revenue requires that the manager be able to accurately predict the volume of work that a department will deliver and how that work will happen. In some settings, almost all occupational therapy intervention is provided to consumers on a one-to-one basis, whereas in some settings, intervention is provided in groups and elsewhere there can be a combination.

Ethical Dilemma

Pressures to Increase Revenue and Service

Shammi is a new manager in a community hospital in a small town. The hospital provides acute care services and has a small rehabilitation unit that focuses on orthopedic patients and some patients who have had strokes. Staffing including recruitment and retention is an ongoing challenge because there are no academic programs near her community. Few therapists are willing to make the commute from the nearest large city even though her facility pays an excellent salary and a sign-on bonus.

Because of the problems she has in recruiting staff, it is difficult to provide patients on the rehabilitation unit the 3 hours of skilled therapy that is required by payers. Shammi realizes that if patients do not receive the required therapy, the hospital may receive denials for payment; but if she shifts staff to the rehabilitation unit, other patients on acute care units will not receive adequate attention. The prior manager directed staff to run a therapy group and to send all patients on the unit to the group even if they were not always appropriate for the focus of the group. Shammi discontinued this practice and directed staff members to only include patients in the group if the focus of the group was directly related to their plan of care. This has increased the pressure on her staff, and now this practice is being questioned by the case manager on the rehabilitation unit and her boss. For a moment, Shammi considered reversing her decision but instead decided that charging patients for therapy that was not appropriate violated the American Occupational Therapy Association Code of Ethics and the ethical practices laid out in her state practice act. Despite pressure, Shammi expressed her concern about ethical practice to her boss and set up a meeting with her human resources representative to brainstorm new recruitment strategies.

TABLE 69.6 Common Process Improvement (PI) Concepts, Tools, and Techniques

Core Concepts	Use/Importance/Summary
• The Plan, Do, Study, Act (PDSA) Cycle	• The overarching framework for guiding and ordering PI activities.
• Critical processes	• The important processes that are repeated again and again to complete the organization's or department's work.
• Operational definitions	• A quantifiable description of what to measure and the steps to follow to measure it consistently.
• Customers and customer requirements	• Identifying internal and external customers or individuals who receive the output of your work and their valid requirements.
• Quality indicators	• Quantitative measures of compliance to valid customer requirements.
• Variation	• The spread of process output over time. Discriminating between natural "common cause" variation that is inherent in a process and the uncommon "special cause" variation that you want to eliminate from a process or emulate if positive.
Strategies	
• Ground rules for meetings	• Explicit agreements about how a team will work together and behave as team members.
• Roles for effective meetings	• Assigning roles such as the leader, scribe, facilitator, and timekeeper can lead to more effective meetings.
• Consensus	• A method for reaching agreement whereby all members agree to fully support a decision even if it is not how they would act if they were acting alone.
Tools	
• Process flowcharts	• A visual representation of the steps in a process used to highlight redundancies, rework, or bottlenecks.
• Control charts	• A chart with statistically determined upper and lower control limits used to determine whether a process has changed and to highlight variation.
• Cause-and-effect diagrams	• A tool to assist in determining possible root causes to a problem.
• Proposed options matrix	• A tool for comparing possible options for action against a set of predetermined criteria.
Techniques	
• Data stratification	• Methods for categorizing collection of data; it is important to decide how to stratify data before you collect it.
• Designing an effective data collection tool	• Tools to gather facts on how a process works or its effectiveness that allows for accurate collection of data in the simplest manner.
• Balancing tasks and people	• Attending to both the needs of team members and the work to be completed to maintain team motivation.
• Icebreakers	• Short activities to help team members learn about each other or to become more comfortable interacting with each other.
• Brainstorming	• A method for creatively generating lists of possible causes of problems, solutions, or processes to improve.
• Multivoting	• A decision-making method to narrow a larger number of options to a number that can be reasonably discussed individually.

Regulations regarding group treatment or treating more than one patient at a time has changed over time, and managers must remain current in their understanding of regulations regarding billing and coding of services. By accurately predicting the total volume of work for a year, managers are able to predict the total gross revenue by multiplying the number of work units (e.g., a 15-minute unit of therapy) by the charge for each unit of service. It is important to note that in the current managed care environment, few payers reimburse at the full rate that is billed; and the net revenue, or the amount of revenue after all discounts to insurers and

TABLE 69.7 Examples of Revenues and Expenses

Revenues	Expenses
Individual 15 minutes: ADL treatment	Variable expense—salary
Individual 15 minutes: cognitive remediation	Variable expense—wages
Individual 15 minutes: community reintegration	Variable expense—office supplies
Individual 15 minutes: neuromuscular facilitation	Variable expense—splinting supplies
Group 15 minutes: home management	Fixed expense—phone
Group 15 minutes: communication skills	Fixed expense—rent
Group 15 minutes: community reintegration	Fixed expense—utilities

ADL, activities of daily living.

non-reimbursed charges are accounted for, is typically much less than gross revenue.

Expenses typically include costs associated with personnel, supplies, facilities management, and equipment. As part of the process of forecasting the expense budget, managers determine the number of full-time equivalent (FTE) employees that will be required to handle the projected work volume. Generally, an FTE represents an employee who will be paid 2,080 hours in a year (i.e., 40 hours × 52 weeks). Setting productivity standards (e.g., the amount of work a practitioner is expected to perform in a given period such as a day or week) and helping staff to meet such standards is a common challenge faced by occupational therapy managers. Personnel expenses can include salary expenses for professional staff that are exempt from the labor laws that require an organization to pay extra for overtime effort and wages for support staff that are nonexempt. Occupational therapists are often categorized as exempt, and occupational therapy assistants and occupational therapy aides are often categorized as nonexempt.

Nonpersonnel expenses such as supplies, equipment, food, phone, continuing education, or travel allowances must also be projected. In private businesses, expenses for utilities and rent must also be considered. These expenses are categorized as either fixed or variable expenses. Fixed expenses are costs that are not directly influenced by changes in client volume, such as expenses budgeted for employee continuing education, heating costs, or monthly rent if space is leased. Variable expenses are those that are directly influenced by changes in client volume. For example, you may use more of some types of office supplies, food used for meal preparation activities, or splinting or medical supplies if patient volumes rise and less if they are lower (Ellexson, 2011). Although there might not always be a direct correlation, over time, one will be able to estimate how an increase or decrease in volume might affect expenses.

To effectively plan and control a budget, managers must learn many useful concepts and strategies. Some organizations may provide training or orientation for new managers, but, most often, it is assumed that a new manager understands the basic information needed to develop and oversee a budget. People who are assuming their first management position would benefit from additional education or training in financial management and from networking with experienced managers. AOTA provides networking opportunities such as the professional networking site *OT Connection* and resources for managers through its Administration and Management Special Interest Section (AMSIS). More information on AMSIS, *OT Connection*, and other resources can be found at http://www.aota.org. Occupational therapy associations in other countries should be consulted for resources relevant to occupational therapy management in systems outside the United States.

Technology and Management

The technological advances in medicine, information management, communication, and related areas that have occurred over the last few decades are astounding. Managers must evaluate and integrate a wide range of technology into their departments, ranging from computer software programs to clinical equipment, such as driving simulators or environmental controls. Choosing and successfully integrating a new technology requires that managers synthesize information, including costs of initial purchase, maintenance, space, and training requirements and the rate at which the specific technology is advancing so that an estimate can be made of when the current technology may become outdated.

One major area of technology used by managers is that employed in information management, which includes the use of computers for documentation, billing, and financial management as well as data collection and analysis for outcomes management. Table 69.8 lists common types of data and information that must be collected and managed and their possible uses. Becoming skilled at the use of common software programs such as managing a spreadsheet to organize and analyze the large amount of data available to most managers has become a common expectation of most managers.

Marketing

Occupational therapy managers are often responsible for assessing the needs of the target populations served by their department or organization; determining programmatic strategies for meeting these needs; designing,

TABLE 69.8 Common Types of Data, Sources, and Possible Uses

Types of Data	Sources	Uses
Demographics (age, sex, educational level, etc.)	• Admissions records • Public data sets	• Program planning • Program evaluation
Revenue (payer source, rates, discounts)	• Accounting • Budget reports	• Budgeting • Program planning
Expense (accounts payable)	• Financial reports • Purchasing records	• Budgeting • Program planning and evaluation
Payroll (salary, benefits, leave usage)	• Accounting • Budget reports	• Staffing plans • Recruitment and retention
Productivity (visits, staff activity)	• Automated charge systems • Department billing records or productivity tracking sheets	• Staffing plans • Performance appraisal • Recruitment
Personnel (licensure, competencies, professional development, performance)	• Human resources • Departmental personnel files • Professional association data sets	• Accreditation visits • Staffing plan development • Professional development plans
Clinical (diagnosis, intervention, outcomes)	• Medical records • Outcome databases	• PI • Program evaluation
Legal (contracts, leases)	• Legal or grants and contracts department	• Facility planning

PI, process improvement.

implementing, and evaluating the interventions to meet identified needs; and promoting the intervention to consumers, payers, physicians, and others. These processes, collectively, are called *marketing*. Traditionally, the following four steps are identified in the marketing process:

- *Organizational assessment:* examination of the factors within an organization that will influence the development and promotion of a new product or service
- *Environmental assessment:* examination of the data and other forms of evidence, including the needs of the target population that will guide the development and promotion of a new product or service
- *Market analysis:* use of the information gained during organizational and environmental assessments to validate perceptions of the wants and needs of the target populations that will receive a new product or service
- *Marketing communications:* packaging and promoting a product so the target populations and other key stakeholders in the new product or service have a clear understanding of what the product or service is and how it may be accessed

In larger organizations, other professionals, such as members of a marketing department, often perform portions of the marketing process such as collecting demographic and other data about potential consumers or may be called on to collaborate with a manager to perform these functions. However, occupational therapy managers who are also business owners or who work in community-based, nonprofit organizations might need to learn the marketing process in greater depth. These managers benefit from establishing effective networks with other managers and becoming active in professional organizations, such as their state and national occupational therapy associations and business-oriented groups such as the local chamber of commerce.

Who Should Be a Manager?

Over the last two decades, numerous professions have addressed managerial competencies with increasing urgency and concern, emphasizing the need to determine the initial competence of health professionals, to assess specific job competencies as professionals are hired and begin to work, and to promote the professionals' continuing development of competence (Braveman, 2006a). The assessment of initial competency and facilitation of continuing development of staff competency is a function of the occupational therapy manager.

Before assuming a role as an occupational therapy manager, one should assess one's own level of preparedness to perform the tasks associated with the role. Although the assessment of competencies for managers has not received the same attention by certifying or regulatory bodies such as accrediting agencies, competency development and assessment have been addressed, and some empirical investigations of managerial competencies have been conducted by a number of professions (Braveman, 2006a).

BOX 69.2 Sample Areas for Assessment of Competency for Managers

- Planning
  - Use of goal setting
  - Financial management skills
  - Understanding the changing health care environment
- Organizing and staffing
  - Understanding team structure and flexible work design
  - Designing and leading effective teams
  - Applying coordination techniques
- Directing
- Interpersonal competencies
  - Communication skills
  - Communicating with the boss
  - Communicating with peers and others
  - Communicating with employees
  - Being politically astute
  - Managing conflict
  - Managing diversity
- Role model competencies
  - Demonstrating professionalism in conduct and demeanor
  - Enhancing technical competence
- Controlling
  - Empowering employees
  - Applying continuous quality improvement efforts

Some competencies might be considered "universal" for managers. One method of identifying managerial competence is to compare their performance against the "yardstick" of previously described traditional managerial functions (e.g., planning, organizing and staffing, directing, controlling). As a guide for this process, each of the management functions is listed subsequently with sample areas for assessment of competency provided for each. (See Box 69.2 for additional areas for development of competencies.)

Other managerial competencies will depend on the nature of the manager's job. Not all managers perform

Commentary on the Evidence

The State of Evidence Related to Management

Decades of evidence on management theory, effective managerial strategies, and practices has been produced by multiple disciplines and fields such as business, organizational development, organizational psychology, social work, and nursing. The topics that have been investigated are quite diverse; examples include effective leadership strategies, performance appraisal processes, factors affecting recruitment and retention, effective recognition and reward structures, change management, and performance improvement.

A variety of forms of evidence, including the results of empirical studies, program descriptions, and descriptions of managerial interventions, are published widely in a range of professional journals, Websites, and books. Although the body of evidence specifically related to management in health care organizations might be more limited, it is growing, and occupational therapy managers who wish to use an *evidence-based* approach to management will benefit from research and science conducted by other disciplines such as those mentioned.

Particularly in the last decade, there has been a movement toward discussions of *evidence-based management* as the role of evidence in guiding decision making has become more prevalent in health care and other industries. However, caution has been advised to address the worry that application of evidence can become too rote and prescriptive. For example, Arndt and Bigelow (2009) cautioned,

> Managers should use all available information and data when planning and implementing decisions, and evidence from research should play a role in that. At the same time, in a turbulent and uncertain environment, creativity and risk taking also will be important, and unanticipated outcomes may result from, among other factors, limits on human cognition, unknowable differences in initial conditions in organizations, and adaptive responses to change as it is implemented. (p. 206)

Current trends in management research include use of more qualitative methods such as grounded theory to understand organizational phenomena (Binder & Edwards, 2010). There continues to be a growing body of experimental management research such as a randomized controlled trial to examine whether an intervention designed to increase self-efficacy for transformational leadership results in more transformational leadership self-efficacy and a higher level of transformational leadership (Fitzgerald & Schutte, 2010).

Although occupational therapy managers can certainly make valuable judgments by generalizing from evidence produced in other disciplines, the profession would benefit from research specifically related to occupational therapy. Questions for investigation might include the following:

- How will health care reform and other societal influences affect the profession?
- How might occupational therapy managers influence the delivery of culturally relevant services as we become more globally connected?
- What are the most effective strategies for retaining occupational therapy practitioners within the profession across the life course to prevent attrition from the discipline?

the same tasks and functions, so it is important that, before accepting a management position, one understands what will be expected of one and have done a thorough assessment of readiness by identifying strengths and areas in which help might be needed.

Conclusion

This chapter has provided an overview of the numerous tasks, functions, and responsibilities that an occupational therapy manager may perform. Readers are encouraged to appreciate the variety and complexities of a manager's responsibilities and the need for a beginning manager to get appropriate training and education. Managers work closely with the administrators and supervisors in large organizations, but small business owners and entrepreneurs also function independently as managers. Fortunately, many resources are available that are specific to occupational therapy managers; and more resources may be found in other fields, including business, psychology, and organizational development, that are useful guides for a manager performing his or her job.

References

Arndt, M., & Bigelow, B. (2009). Evidence-based management in health care organizations: A cautionary note. *Health Care Management Review, 34*(3), 206–213.

Beech, M. (2002). Leaders of managers: The drive for effective leadership. *Nursing Standard, 16*, 34–36.

Binder, M., & Edwards, J. S. (2010). Using grounded theory method for theory building in operations management research: A study on inter-firm relationship governance. *International Journal of Operations & Production Management, 30*, 232–259.

Branch, K. M. (2002). *Change management.* Washington, DC: U.S. Department of Energy. Retrieved from http://library.monts.cc/cm.htm

Braveman, B. (Ed.). (2006a). Competency and the occupational therapy manager. In *Leading and managing occupational therapy services: An evidence-based approach* (pp. 169–195). Philadelphia, PA: F. A. Davis.

Braveman, B. (Ed.). (2006b). Roles and functions of managers. In *Leading and managing occupational therapy services: An evidence-based approach* (pp. 109–139). Philadelphia, PA: F. A. Davis.

Braveman, B. (Ed.). (2006c). Understanding and working within organizations. In *Leading and managing occupational therapy services: An evidence-based approach* (pp. 53–80). Philadelphia, PA: F. A. Davis.

Cervone, D., & Pervin, L. A. (2008). *Personality theory and research* (10th ed.). Hoboken, NJ: Wiley.

Ellexson, M. T. (2011). Financial planning and budgeting. In K. Jacobs & G. L. McCormack (Eds.), *The occupational therapy manager* (5th ed., pp. 113–125). Bethesda, MD: AOTA Press.

Fisher, T. F. (2011). Personnel management. In K. Jacobs & G. L. McCormack (Eds.), *The occupational therapy manager* (5th ed., pp. 209–216). Bethesda, MD: AOTA Press.

Fitzgerald, S., & Schutte, N. S. (2010). Increasing transformational leadership through enhancing self-efficacy. *Journal of Management Development, 29*, 495–505.

Franche, R., Corbière, M., Lee, H., Breslin, F. C., & Hepburn, C. G. (2007). The readiness for return-to-work scale: Development and validation of a self-report staging scale in lose-time claimants with musculoskeletal disorders. *Journal of Occupational Rehabilitation, 17*, 450–472.

Gagne, M., & Deci, E. L. (2005). Self-determination theory and work motivation. *Journal of Organizational Behavior, 26*, 331–362.

Jaques, E. (1998). *Requisite organization.* Arlington, VA: Cason Hall.

Levey, S., Hill, J., & Green, B. (2002). Leadership in health care and the leadership literature. *Journal of Advanced Nursing, 25*, 68–74.

Lewin, K. (1997). *Resolving social conflict and field theory in social sciences.* Washington, DC: American Psychological Association.

Liebler, J. G., & McConnell, C. R. (2011). *Management principles for health professionals* (6th ed.). Boston, MA: Jones and Bartlett.

MD Anderson Cancer Center. (2011). Retrieved from http://www.mdanderson.org/about-us/index.html

Pinder, C. (2008). *Work motivation in organizational behavior* (2nd ed.). New York, NY: U.S. Psychology Press.

Ramlall, S. (2004). A review of employee motivation theories and their implications for employee retention within organizations. *Journal of American Academy of Business, 5*, 52–63.

Strickland, R. (2011). Strategic planning. In K. Jacobs & G. L. McCormack (Eds.), *The occupational therapy manager* (5th ed., pp. 103–112). Bethesda, MD: AOTA Press.

For additional resources on the subjects discussed in this chapter, visit http://thePoint.lww.com/Willard-Spackman12e.

CHAPTER 70

Disability Rights and Advocacy

Partnering with Disability Communities to Support Full Participation in Society

Joy Hammel, Jim Charlton, Robin A. Jones, Jessica M. Kramer, Tom Wilson

LEARNING OBJECTIVES

After reading this chapter, you will be able to:

1. Compare and contrast different models of framing disability, key terms within each model, and implications of each model for occupational therapy practitioners and for disabled people
2. Describe the disability rights movement in the United States and its history as an example of a social movement's framing of the disability experience from within
3. Describe the sociopolitical and social justice advocacy issues that disabled people as a minority group face in the effort to realize rights and improve participation opportunities and access in society
4. Critically reflect on your practice as an occupational therapist, how you "treat" disability, and key points in the process of reflecting and incorporating sociopolitical, economic, and cultural perspectives into your practice
5. Develop innovative strategies to collaborate with disability communities on systems change advocacy and community and empowered consciousness building

OUTLINE

Introduction

How you think about and construct disability significantly influences how you experience disability in your own life as well as how you "treat" disability and disabled people as an occupational therapy practitioner and as a member of society. Notice that we put the term *treat* in quotation marks. Practitioners frequently use the term *treatment* to designate what therapists do to or do in collaboration with clients during therapeutic sessions. However, the term *treat* can also refer to how people are viewed and treated as a social group in society.

BOX 70.1 Initial Learning Activity

Take out a piece of paper and jot down what you think about when you hear the words *disability* and *independence*. What do these words mean to you? How are they defined and constructed in society (e.g., by the public or in the media)? How does the profession of occupational therapy view disability and independence?

This chapter focuses on this sociological framing of treatment by exposing you to different models and framings of disability and the disability experience using a critical theory stance. Critical theory involves stepping back to critically reflect on how disability is constructed in society and your role as a rehabilitation professional in that social construction. This chapter also introduces you to a sociological framing of the political, economic, social, and cultural issues that influence the disability experience of individuals and that of disabled people[1] as a collective minority group. Specifically, a critical theory framework will challenge you to reflect on every aspect of your evaluation and intervention as an occupational therapist to determine whether they authentically reflect the insider experiences, needs, priorities, issues, and goals of people with disabilities and what is most meaningful and relevant to them as a minority group. This framework also provides a strong framework for occupational therapists to partner and collaborate with the disability rights community to advocate for long-term systems change to address participation disparities and instead realize participation opportunities in society and in everyday life areas of community living, community engagement and citizenship, social participation, and learning/work participation.

Comparing and Contrasting Models of Disability

Individuals do not exist or operate in isolation from their social worlds, their communities, and the broader society with its expectations, norms, cultural beliefs, and sociopolitical and economic realities. Nor do occupational therapists operate in isolation from their own beliefs or from the values and economic interests of the systems within which they work and the broader society in which they live. Yet we often try to achieve this isolation within the therapeutic context; that is, we try to focus on individual rehabilitation goals, impairment remediation, or functional return without fully considering the holistic needs and desires of the individual as influenced by society.

We can look to different models and conceptual framings of disability to better understand this social phenomenon and to critically examine how rehabilitation professionals such as occupational therapists have situated themselves in relation to disability and to disabled people.

From a historical perspective, some of the earliest documented societal framings of disability are situated within religious and cultural constructions (for detailed history accounts, see Longmore & Umansky, 2001; Oliver, 1990, 1996). Although different religious sects and cultures treat disability differently, one of the most important influences in defining disability has been that of Western Christianity and the *moral model* of disability. In the moral model, disability is seen as a moral marking. In most cases, the mark is seen as a negative one—one that designates a sinner or an evil or unclean presence within the person. Historically, the mark was used to validate the separation of that person from the rest of society lest the evil spread or to justify the need to cleanse the person from the evil spirit—a type of early cure. At the same time, however, the moral model asserted the responsibility of the religious community to have pity on the less fortunate and to take care of them, thus extending into the *charity model*. Together, these beliefs led to the formation of institutions, asylums, sanitariums, and segregated communities to isolate yet take care of people with disabilities.

The charity model was also reified by Western-influenced societies, such as the United States and United Kingdom, and in turn extended beyond religion into a societal practice within the *welfare model*. In this model, society assumes responsibility over the welfare of the less fortunate, who are otherwise deemed not to be capable of supporting themselves (Oliver, 1990, 1996). Using a welfare model, groups of people, including people with diverse disabilities and those labeled as *sick*, *feeble*, *poor*, *criminals*, and the *underclass* were often grouped, housed, and "treated" together, separate from the rest of society.

Although they were framed within a charity model, conditions in these institutions were often less than charitable; and because these individuals were not deemed to be a valid part of the productive workforce, financial supports were often limited and were cut back even more during times of economic depression. This trend toward a *political economic* and *materialist framing* of

[1]Although the term *people with disabilities* often appears in the literature as recommended people-first language, *disabled people* and other "disability-centered" terms are increasingly preferred and used by many activists and scholars who promote positive disability identity as an act of resistance against disability oppression (e.g., the focus is not on the deficit in the individual but on the society that imposes disability on disabled people as a collective minority group).

disability focuses on labor economics and on surplus or deficit in the labor market to define and treat disability (Hahn, 1985; Oliver, 1990, 1996). In our capitalist society in the United States, the ability to work or not and the simultaneous value of independence have been central forces in defining and socially constructing disability and the treatment of disabled people.

Historically, as science and technology came to the fore and continued to progress within industrialized societies, we began to see the formulations of a more scientific approach to disability in the field of professionalized medicine (Foucault, 1973; Mechanic, 1974; Oliver, 1996). The scientific focus was based on a positivist framing that there are certain universal truths or facts that can be identified and proven. In this case, those truths relate to disability in the tenet that one can identify what is wrong, how it came to be wrong, and therefore how to treat and/or cure that wrong. In some branches of medicine, these tenets applied to treating physical ailments, conditions, and impairments. In psychology, similar tenets were applied to diagnosing and treating illnesses of the mind, such as psychiatric and cognitive conditions.

However, given the difficulties involved in trying to objectively explain social and psychological behaviors, other psychologists began to qualitatively examine how people interacted in the moment and how actions were shaped by and given meaning via social interactions with other people in everyday contexts (Blumer, 1969; Goffman, 1963). Concepts such as stigma, learned helplessness, self-efficacy, and social learning emerged, tying together the individual with the immediate social environment in an *ecological framing* (Bronfenbrenner, 1979). Sociologists and anthropologists challenged the focus on the individual, however, and began to focus on cultural and societal constructions of disability, pointing to the political, economic, and cultural influences of the society on individuals and groups of people in society. Concepts such as oppression, marginalization, and alienation were used to describe disabled people as a minority group. The *social model of disability* (Oliver, 1990, 1996) asserts that oppression occurs because of the political economy of societies that exclude disabled people and prevent them from moving out of welfare systems to the productive workforce, thus invalidating them as full citizens. The *minority group model of disability* (Hahn, 1985; Longmore, 1995) acknowledges the societal oppression of disabled people but, like other minority group social movements (e.g., by race, ethnicity, gender, or sexual identity), equally emphasizes the strengths, power, and pride of the group. Thus, the minority group model introduces concepts such as disability identity, culture, community, and pride as ways to reframe and own disability "from within." Feminist scholars further tie the individual and the society together via the slogan, "The personal is political and the political is personal," pointing to the need to recognize how the personal experience of disability and gender intersect and, in turn, are heavily influenced and constructed by societal beliefs, norms, and ideologies (Morris, 1992; Thomas, 1999). It is within these sociological and cultural framings that disabled people as a social group and as insiders to the disability experience continue to assume control and power over reframing disability from an insider perspective according to a critical theory stance.

Although it is beyond the scope of this chapter to comprehensively review the history of medicine, rehabilitation, disability, and sociology, this brief history leads us to a contemporary critical analysis of disability models as shown in Table 70.1 that you can use to inform your everyday practice. The table presents three key models of disability: the medical model, the rehabilitation model, and the closely related social and minority group models, which are ascribed to and framed from within disability-led groups and social movements.

What is important to note is the location and construction of disability, moving from

- A deficit or dysfunction within the individual to treat or cure within the medical model;
- To a negative interaction of the person with his or her immediate environment within a rehabilitation model, pointing to the need to remediate, compensate, or normalize the individual;
- To a societally constructed and imposed phenomena that can be addressed only through social and societal change within the social model; and
- To a collective social movement of empowered consciousness from within (e.g., disability culture and art, community building, identity, and pride) within a minority group cultural model.

Also note the shifts in power across the models, from the expert, professionally driven medical model to the professional–client relationship of the rehabilitation model (which can vary from professional led to client centered) to the disability constituency–led movements of social change and critical consciousness within the social and minority group models. Depending on which model you situate yourself within, terms such as *independence*, *participation*, and *empowerment* can take on different meanings as well. For example, *independence* can be defined as the individual ability to safely perform activities by oneself (as we frequently ascribe to in rehabilitation) or as a rights-based framing of freedom of choice, access, and opportunity in society and autonomy in managing one's life decisions (as framed in a minority group model).

It is important for occupational therapists to be aware of and responsive to the disability rights movement's conceptualizations and underlying philosophy of independent living as something that is not about the individual's impairment or independent function so much as about the individual's right to societal opportunities and the need to create environments and to change systems, rather than individuals, to support those rights. For example, an occupational therapist might focus

TABLE 70.1 Comparison of Disability and Independence Constructions

	Medical Model	Rehabilitation Model	Minority Group/Social Model
What is disability?	Disability is deficiency or abnormality.	Disability is loss or inability to functionally perform everyday activities independently or in a socially expected way (e.g., timely, safely, efficiently).	Disability is difference. (Some would argue for saying that *impairment* is difference, whereas *disability* occurs only when societally imposed barriers limit people.)
How is disability constructed?	Being disabled is negative.	Being disabled is negative and something to overcome or to accept/adjust or adapt to its negative consequences within one's life.	Being disabled is neutral; negative constructions occur when society imposes barriers and oppresses participation; positive constructions occur when the personal and social world own difference and support and validate people.
Where is disability located?	Disability is in the individual body.	Disability is in the individual or in the interaction between the individual and the immediate environment.	Disability derives from the interaction between the individual and society. Disability is located in societal structures and practices that oppress.
What is the mechanism for change?	The remedy for disability-related problems is cure or normalization.	The mechanism for change for disability-related problems is to rehabilitate or remediate to normal and/or to become as physically/cognitively independent in everyday activities as possible.	The mechanism for change is changing the interaction between the individual and society.
What are examples of change strategies?	Examples are surgery, medication, medical technology, and intervention.	Examples are individual remediation and person/environment compensation or adaptation.	Examples are systems and social action change; collective activism; and disability identity, pride, and culture.
Who/what are the agents of change?	The agent of remedy is the professional.	The agent of change is the professional in collaboration with the individual client and/or people in client's immediate social world (e.g., client-centered approach).	The agent of change can be the individual; an advocate or ally; any person or group of people that changes the interaction; the community; the society's sociopolitical structure and systems; and art, culture, and media.
What is independence?	Independence is individual physical, cognitive, and mental ability to perform and capacity to make decisions.	Independence is individual physical and cognitive ability to perform everyday activities safely and in a reasonable amount of time	Independence is the freedom to do what you want to do, when, where, and with whom you want; choice; power over life decisions; and control over everyday life and resources to support it.

Adapted by Joy Hammel and Access Living from Gill, C. (1999). *Models of disability*. Chicago, IL: Chicago Center for Disability Research; Linton, S. (1998). *Claiming disability: Knowledge and identity*. New York, NY: New York University Press; Longmore, P. K. (1995). The second phase: From disability rights to disability culture. *The Disability Rag and ReSource, 16*, 4–11; Oliver, M. (1996). *Understanding disability from theory to practice*. New York, NY: St. Martin's Press: Macmillan; Rioux, M. (1997). Disability: The place of judgment in a world of fact. *Journal of Intellectual Disability Research, 41*(2), 102–112.

exclusively on increasing a client's functional independence, that is, the client's ability to perform activities independently. If you assume a social or minority group model instead, disabled people would argue that independence to them means the freedom to make choices and to be in control of decisions regardless of whether they can perform an activity by themselves. So as an occupational therapist, you might consider spending equal time collaborating with the consumer on whether he or she might want to use a personal attendant and how to access and get funding for this supportive resource to remain "independent."

Summarizing the Early Years of Disability Politics: Linking Rights, Organization, and Consciousness

To better understand and apply these models, it is important to situate them within the history of the disability rights movement internationally. The history that follows represents a synthesis of accounts documented by disabled people with and about disabled people who were a part of this history (for detailed histories, see Charlton, 1998; Longmore, 1995; Longmore & Umansky, 2001).

The Organization of Empowerment

Out of the different and often hard realities of everyday life, organizations of people with disabilities have appeared in virtually every country in the world. Most of these organizations embrace the principles of empowerment and human rights, independence and integration, and self-help and self-determination, and these organizations form the core of the international disability rights movement. In a few places, people with disabilities have been politically active for many decades, but in most places, the disability rights movement is a recent phenomenon. Today, most activists locate the beginning of what constitutes the contemporary disability rights movement in the early 1970s.

Trying to pin any social movement down to a given period is complicated, but two periods stand out. It was during the early 1970s that people with disabilities in the United States and Europe, influenced by and directly involved in the civil rights, antiwar, and student movements, began to organize on disability-related issues. The year 1972 is associated with the founding of the Berkeley Center for Independent Living (CIL). It was also about then that the Boston Self-Help Center became interested in independent living as an alternative kind of organization. The independent living movement has been the linchpin of the disability rights movement (DRM) in the United States, and its leaders have had an influence on activists and leaders elsewhere. For example, the first disability rights–oriented group in Europe was established in England when Vic Finkelstein, Paul Hunt, and others initiated the Union of Physically Impaired Against Segregation in 1975. As activists in the United States and Europe began to take up major disability-related issues, the DRM began to develop and grow. Early on, these issues included the inaccessibility of public transportation; the lack of accessible, affordable housing; the institutionalizing of poor, young people with severe disabilities in nursing homes because of the prohibitive cost of personal assistance; the struggle for inclusion of students with disabilities in regular classrooms; and efforts to change the way in which the public relates to, perceives, and understands disability.

The first center, Berkeley CIL, began in 1973, but most CILs in the United States were set up in the early 1980s. There are now more than 350 in the United States. CILs are the most important organizations within the U.S. DRM for two reasons. First, most of the early disability rights leaders were identified with CILs, and the philosophy of independent living formed much of the basic philosophical underpinning of the larger DRM. Second, CILs were and still are cornerstones of the DRM because of the sheer numbers of paid staff. These centers have extensive resources. Out of the work of early activists, legislation and legal mandates concerning the "handicapped" appeared. This happened in North America and northern Europe and to a lesser extent in the Third World. The most important legislation in North America was the Rehabilitation Act of 1973.[2]

The first half of the 1980s was also crucial. The year 1981 was designated the International Year of Disabled Persons (IYDP) by the United Nations. The significance of this was not lost on most disability rights activists in the United States. The year 1981 was very important to the DRM on the international front. In many cases, it was the first time efforts had been made to involve people with disabilities in disability-related projects and programs. Indeed, a crucial event had taken place earlier than the IYDP, in late June 1980, when there was a split in Rehabilitation International (RI), the most significant disability-related international body. RI was a large membership organization composed primarily of rehabilitation professionals. Through efforts of people from Sweden and Canada, RI for the first time made an attempt to bring people with disabilities to its conference in Singapore. The largely token effort backfired. The few hundred participants who had disabilities demanded that RI mandate that 50% of its delegate assembly be composed of people with disabilities. This motion was overwhelmingly defeated by a vote of 61 to 37, a vote that probably represented the sentiments of the 3,000 other delegates at the convention. Those with disabilities and a few supporters led a split in RI, the outcome of which was the formation of Disabled Peoples' International (DPI).[3] DPI has seen impressive growth in the last 25 years. There are affiliated groups in dozens of countries and an international headquarters in Winnipeg, Canada.[4]

---

[2]It took a month long sit-in and office takeover at the San Francisco office of the U.S. Department of Health, Education, and Welfare to force Secretary Joseph Califano to mandate enforcement of the act. There are several interesting accounts of this action. "More than 150 people took over the federal building and remained for 28 days. Ed Roberts left his new office as director of the California Department of Rehabilitation to join the protest. Judy Heumann crossed the Bay from Berkeley to become one of the leaders of the takeover. Early in action, Heumann, in a statement reminiscent of freedom fighters of all ages, declared that 'we will no longer allow the government to oppress disabled individuals. . . . We will accept no more discussion of segregation.' . . . The Black Panthers and the Gray Panthers brought in food donated by Safeway and assisted with personal care needs. The siege remains the longest takeover of a federal building by any group in American history" (S. E. Brown, 1992, pp. 57–58).

[3]DianeDriedger's book, *The Last Civil Rights Movement: Disabled Peoples' International* (1989, especially pp. 28–57), is a good history of the split and the subsequent formation of DPI.

[4]RI remains much larger and more influential than DPI. In recent years, RI has added people with disabilities to its executive committee, but it is still dominated by rehabilitation "professionals" (doctors, therapists, social workers, psychologists, etc.). Since the split, several disability rights activists have worked with both RI and DPI. RI is headquartered in New York City.

The early 1980s was also a time when many of the leading disability rights organizations were founded, such as the National Council of Disabled Persons of Zimbabwe, the Organization of the Revolutionary Disabled in Nicaragua, the Self-Help Association of Paraplegics (Soweto) (SHAP), the Program of Rehabilitation Organized by Disabled Youth of Western Mexico (PROJIMO), DPI-Thailand, the Southern Africa Federation of the Disabled (SAFOD), and the American Disabled for Accessible Public Transportation (now known as ADAPT) (2006). At the same time, different disability constituency groups began to form and further assert their voice and their rights, including groups such as People First and Self-Advocates Becoming Empowered (SABE), representing people with intellectual disabilities, and groups such as MindFreedom and MadNation, representing people with psychiatric disabilities. From many disparate beginnings and places, networks began to form, and the disability movement, as owned and framed from within, began to go public.

Many of these organizations started as a response to the simple need for survival, and their goals were limited to economic self-help and self-sufficiency. Others started as political groups that wanted to mobilize people with disabilities in their communities, cities, countries, or regions. These groups and purposes have gradually merged. All seek to link their work with the struggle for self-determination and human rights. With few exceptions, this is their common denominator. All the organizations within the DRM have a few basic things in common. Most important, they are organizations that are controlled by people with disabilities. Each, in its own way and in its own circumstances, confronts the everyday realities of disability oppression. Another crucial similarity is that each embraces the general philosophical principle that people with disabilities must have their own voice and have control in their lives.

Empowered Consciousness

The emergence of disabled people's organizations, the concomitant promotion of independence and empowerment, and the recognition of the centrality and imperative of speaking for themselves spawned a whole new generation of disabled people who rejected the paternalistic, medical model notions regarding disability. As hundreds of thousands or even millions of disabled people worldwide have come to understand that the "problems" of disability have little to do with them and much to do with how society is organized, large numbers of political activists with disabilities have come forward.

Out of similar and divergent experiences, people with disabilities have acquired a consciousness about themselves and the world around them. This new understanding has affected their aspirations and responsibilities. They have come to a raised consciousness of themselves not only as people with disabilities but also as oppressed people. Moreover, they have become political activists because their raised consciousness has become empowered (see Figure 70.1 for images of collective activism and empowered consciousness). They no longer think of disability as a medical condition; instead, they see it as a human condition. They are no longer interested in the "welfare of the handicapped"; they are interested in the human rights of disabled people. They have joined a social movement to free people with disabilities from political, economic, and cultural oppression (Charlton, 1998).

For political activists, consciousness that resists the emasculation of the self by the dominant ideology, that is, raised consciousness, has been transformed into a consciousness of active opposition: empowered consciousness.[5] *Empowered consciousness* means acting collectively to empower an entire social group. This can mean educating people, creating disturbances, confronting institutions, and seeking group power in churches, schools, communities, and institutions. Empowered consciousness insists on the active, collective contestation for control over the necessities of life: housing, school, personal and family relationships, respect, independence, and more. People with empowered consciousness might still see only part of the larger world, but they understand that they can and should influence it. This does not mean that they insist on being leaders. It does mean that they want to empower others, especially other people who are experiencing disability. These people see the connections between themselves and others and begin to recognize a level of universality that was obscured in their consciousness. They begin to speak of "we" instead of "I" or "they." Some of these activists are motivated by personal experience (poverty, harassment, institutionalization, a personal loss, rape, indignity, etc.). Others are motivated by something they have learned by being exposed to injustice and oppression in school or out of an outraged sense of social injustice. Most people are politically active for a combination of these and other reasons. A consciousness of empowerment is growing among people with disabilities (see Figure 70.2 for symbols of this empowered consciousness created from within.).

Empowered consciousness is, in Cheryl Marie Wade's (1994) words, being passed around on notes, and it has to do with being proud of self and having a culture that fortifies and spreads that feeling:

> Disability culture. Say, what? Aren't disabled people just isolated victims of nature or circumstance? Yes and no. True, we are far too often isolated. Locked away in the pits, closets,

---

[5]Whenever and wherever this transformation occurs, it produces recognition of the self on both the personal and political levels. This transformation has been particularly important to feminist and multicultural studies. See Charles Taylor's "The Politics of Recognition" (Goldberg, 1994, pp. 81–85).

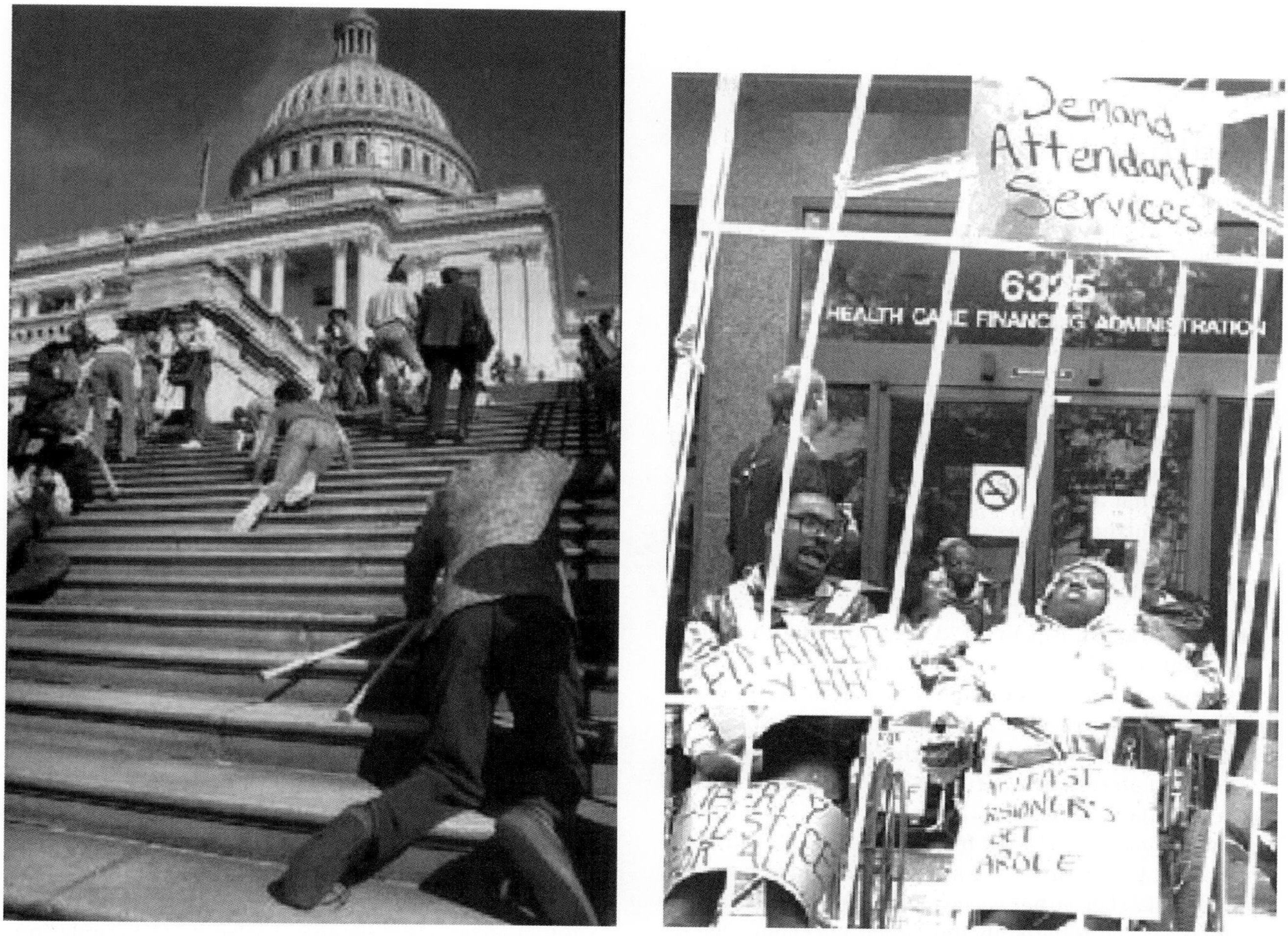

A B

FIGURE 70.1 Collective disability activism took disability public during the fight to pass the Americans with Disabilities Act (**A**) and continues to do so in the ongoing movement to mandate and fund community-based living options with supports (**B**). (Copyright Tom Olin, photographer.)

and institutions of enlightened societies everywhere. But there is a growing consciousness among us. . . . Because there is always an underground. Notes get passed among survivors. And the notes we are passing these days say, "There's power in difference. Power. Pass the word." Culture. It's about passing the word. And disability culture is passing the word that there's a new definition of disability and it includes power. (pp. 119–120)

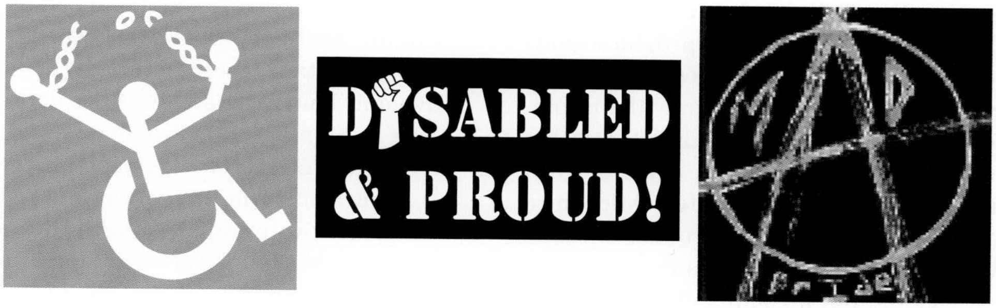

FIGURE 70.2 Symbols of disability identity, power, and pride. (Adapted from [from left to right] American Disabled for Accessible Public Transportation. [2006]. *ADAPT Home Page*. Retrieved from http://www.adapt.org/index1.html; Triano, S. [2007]. *Disabled and proud*. Retrieved from http://www.disabledandproud.com/; MadPride.[2007]. *MadPride home page*. Retrieved from http://www.ctono.freeserve.co.uk/)

Legislative and Social Policy Initiatives Experienced by Disabled People

The history of the disability rights movement has culminated in several key pieces of legislation that reify the values and rights of the movement. It is critical that occupational therapists be informed about this legislation and stay abreast of changes to it in reauthorizations because this information is essential to advocacy. Table 70.2 summarizes many of the primary social policies and legislation within the United States that influence the rights, choices, and control of disabled people. They correspond to major areas of societal participation (e.g., transportation, work) that also represent ongoing areas of disability activism to further increase societal opportunities.

Following is a brief overview of these policies, legislation, and systems:

- **Rehabilitation Act of 1973, Section 504:** A federal act that prohibits discrimination on the basis of disability in programs conducted by federal agencies, in programs that receive federal financial assistance, in federal employment, and in the employment practices of federal contractors. Section 504 states that "no qualified individual with a disability in the United States shall be excluded from, denied the benefits of, or be subjected to discrimination under" any program or activity that either receives federal financial assistance or is conducted by any executive agency or the U.S. Postal Service. Each federal agency has its own set of Section 504 regulations that apply to its own programs. Agencies that provide federal financial assistance also have Section 504 regulations covering entities that receive federal assistance. Requirements common to these regulations include reasonable accommodation for employees with disabilities, program accessibility, effective communication with people who have hearing or vision disabilities, and accessible facilities whether or not they are newly constructed or altered.
- **Individuals with Disabilities Education Act of 1990 (IDEA):** A federal program that provides funds to states and local education agencies (school districts) to support education for children with disabilities ages 3 to 21 years and supports early intervention services for children from birth to age 3 years. IDEA provides guidelines and protections for children to ensure their right to a free and appropriate public education. The principle of the law is that children with disabilities should not be denied the opportunities that are offered to everyone else; everyone gets access to public education and therefore children with disabilities should have the same access. Public school districts are obligated to prepare and implement an Individualized Education Program (IEP) for each disabled child that is designed to meet the child's unique needs. Transition services are required beginning at age 14 years to prepare a student for independent living, postsecondary education, and/or employment.
- **Americans with Disabilities Act of 1990 (ADA):** A comprehensive federal civil rights law that provides protections to individuals with disabilities similar to those provided to individuals on the basis of race, color, sex, national origin, age, and religion. This legislation was amended in 2008 (ADA Amendments Act [ADAAA]) to address the narrowing of the definition of who was "a person with a disability," which occurred over time due to court interpretations. The revised definition places less emphasis on proving the severity of impairment in order to have protections under the law and recognizes conditions that are episodic in nature or involve impairments to bodily systems. The three-prong definition of disability includes (1) individuals who have a physical or psychological impairment that limits them in one or more major life activities, (2) individuals who have a record of having such an impairment, and (3) individuals who are regarded as having such an impairment. The final regulations implementing the ADAAA were published by the Equal Employment Opportunity Commission in 2011. The ADAAA called amendments to the definition of disability in the Section 504 regulations to be amended so that they are consistent with the ADA's definition of disability as well. The U.S. Department of Justice issued sweeping changes to the regulations implementing Title II and Title III of the ADA on September 25, 2010. The purpose of the amended regulations was to reflect the policies of the agency based on a 20-year history of enforcing the ADA, update the technical standards to keep pace with the changes in the construction and design industry, and address immersing issues. The revised definition of disability as well as the updated regulations clarified accessibility guidelines for Title II (Nondiscrimination on the Basis of Disability in State and Local Government Services, 2011) and Title III (Nondiscrimination on the Basis of Disability by Public Accommodations and in Commercial Facilities, 2011) reflects key changes to this legislation. These reinforce the fact that this is a dynamic law. There are five titles under the ADA:

  Title I: Employment. Prohibits discrimination in all aspects of the employment process including recruitment, hiring, retention, and benefits of employment. Private employers with 15 or more employees and public employers with one or more employees are covered. The definition of "who is a person with a disability" was expanded via passage of the ADAAA of 2008.

  Title II: State and Local Government. Prohibits discrimination in all programs and services offered to the public and requires that all programs, services,

TABLE 70.2 Important Policies and Legislation Corresponding to Major Areas of Societal Participation and Occupational Therapy Practice

	Section 504	IDEA	ADA	HAVA	Medicaid/Medicare
Transportation	Requires transportation systems owned/operated by entities that receive federal financial assistance to be accessible	Requires appropriate transportation services to be provided to students with disabilities	Requires all public and the majority of private transportation systems to be accessible to individuals with disabilities		Provision of transportation for medically related services
Employment	Prohibits discrimination against qualified individuals with disabilities in all aspects of employment	Requires provision of a free appropriate public education for children with disabilities in the least restrictive environment	Prohibits discrimination against qualified individuals with disabilities by private employers of 15 or more employees and public employers with 1 or more employees		
Education	Requires entities that receive federal financial assistance to ensure equal access through architectural accessibility and provision of reasonable accommodations in K-12 and postsecondary education		Prohibits discrimination by public and private educational entities including architectural accessibility, provision of reasonable accommodations, and effective communication		
Voting	Requires entities that receive federal financial assistance to ensure equal access, including architectural accessibility, provision of reasonable accommodations, and effective communication		Requires nondiscrimination in voting as a program of state and local government	Requires equal access to voting facilities and the voting process	
Housing	Requires entities that receive federal financial assistance to ensure nondiscrimination in housing, including construction of accessible housing units and reasonable modification of policy and procedure		Requires transient housing (i.e., hotels/motels, dormitories, social service housing) to be constructed in accordance with the ADA accessibility guidelines, reasonable modification of policy and procedure, and effective communication		Provision of institutional care and/or use of available (state by state) Medicaid waiver program to finance community-based placement; may be used by states to meet their nonsegregation obligations under ADA
Health Care	Nondiscrimination in the provision of medical services offered by entities receiving federal financial assistance, including architectural accessibility, reasonable accommodations, and effective communication		Nondiscrimination in the provision of medical services, including architectural accessibility, reasonable accommodations, and effective communication		Financial support of basic medical services (dental, skilled nursing services, etc.)
Community Participation	Nondiscrimination in programs and services offered by entities receiving federal financial assistance including architectural accessibility, modification of policy and procedure, and effective communication		Nondiscrimination in access to goods and services offered by public and private entities, including architectural accessibility, modification of policy and procedure, and effective communication		Community Based Waiver Program can be used to support nonmedical services that enhance quality of life (e.g., environmental modifications)

ADA, American with Disabilities Act; HAVA, Help America Vote Act; IDEA, Individuals with Disabilities Education Act.

and facilities be readily accessible to and usable by people with disabilities, including transportation. Based on the Rehabilitation Act of 1973, the language in this section mandates service provision in the most "integrated setting possible," which was reinforced through interpretation by the courts in cases like *Olmstead v. L.C.* (1998). Exceptions to reasonable modification in policies and procedures or the provision of auxiliary aids and services necessary to ensure that individuals with disabilities have equal access and are served in the most integrated setting can be made if the public entity can show that the changes would "fundamentally alter" the service provided or result in an undue financial burden. It further extends coverage to all units of state and local governments even if they do not receive federal financial assistance. Public transportation when provided must be accessible including passenger rail service, mainline bus service, and any demand responsive systems. The transportation provisions of the ADA are phased in over a 30-year period with a mandate that all vehicles and rail cars purchased new must be accessible and all stations must be made accessible by 2020.

Title III: Places of Public Accommodation. Prohibits discrimination in the delivery of goods and services by places of public accommodation (identified as "serving the public"), including architectural accessibility, modifications in policies and procedures, and effective communication. Included are restaurants, retail establishments, movie theaters, private schools, day care centers, hotels and motels, recreational facilities, professional services (e.g., lawyers, accountants, hair dressers), medical facilities, museums and galleries, and any privately owned entity that is open to the public and affects commerce. Private clubs, federally recognized tribal entities, and religiously controlled and operated organizations are exempted. Private transportation services are covered including Amtrak, Greyhound, and similar over-the-road bus systems and shuttle bus services (hotels, rental cars, etc).

The regulations implementing several provisions within Title II and III were revised in 2010, with the majority of provisions going into effect on March 15, 2011. Some of the major revisions include (1) a new definition of service animal that only recognizes domestic dogs and creates an exception for miniature horses while clarifying that emotional support animals are not covered; (2) a new definition for "other power-driven mobility devices" and a requirement to modify policies and procedures to allow, when appropriate, individuals with mobility limitations to use devices other than the standard wheelchair, including Segways, golf carts, and all-terrain devices in public places; (3) modifications in ticketing policies to allow individuals with disabilities who want to sit with their family or friends to purchase up to four seats adjacent to an accessible seat in venues such as theatres, concert halls, and stadiums; and (4) establishes guidelines for the use of video remote interpreting to meet the communication needs of someone who is deaf or hard of hearing. The 2010 Accessibility Standards became enforceable on March 15, 2012 for all buildings newly constructed or altered thereafter. The 2010 Standards harmonize the ADA's provisions with other building codes and standards including the International Building Code (IBC) and the Architectural Barriers Act (ABA) to promote better compliance and consistency in how structures are built. The 2010 Standards contain new technical standards for playgrounds, facilities primarily designed for children, recreational facilities (e.g., golf courses, swimming pools and spas, bowling alleys, fishing and boating piers, exercise equipment), residential housing, correctional facilities, and court houses.

Title IV: Telecommunications. Requires access for people who have hearing or speech disabilities to the telecommunication services provided by private telecommunication companies through the provision of various services including but not limited to teletypewriter (TTY) relay services, voice-over services, video-relay services, third-party communication assistants, and so forth.

Title V: Miscellaneous. Provisions for nondiscrimination in areas including insurance, retaliation based on exercising rights under the statute, availability of attorney fees, and more.

- **Help America Vote Act of 2002 (HAVA):** A federal law that was enacted in 2002 to reform elections management and voter registration nationwide. The following issues are covered by HAVA:

1. The proper operation and maintenance of voting systems and technology
2. The rights of voters to cast provisional ballots, the proper processing and counting of those ballots, and how provisional voters can determine whether their votes were counted and, if not, why not
3. The nondiscriminatory application of HAVA's identification requirement for certain voters who register by mail
4. Identifying and assisting voters with disabilities, including psychiatric disabilities, in order that such voters can participate fully in the voting process independently and privately
5. The rights of minority language voters to receive language assistance at the polling place

- **Medicare:** A federal health insurance program for people aged 65 years or older. Certain people younger than age 65 years can qualify for Medicare, too, including those who have disabilities and those who have permanent kidney failure or amyotrophic lateral sclerosis (Lou Gehrig's disease). The program helps with the cost of health care, but it does not cover all medical expenses or the cost of most long-term care (LTC). The Centers for Medicare & Medicaid Services (CMS) (2011) is the agency in charge of the Medicare program. Of note, there are many ongoing changes and initiatives to restructure Medicare and Medicaid, including the Affordable Care Act, that point to the need to create and cover more community-based supports and programming, especially for the growing population of people with chronic conditions and long-term disabilities.

- **Medicaid:** A federal or state entitlement program established under Title XIX of the Social Security Act to pay for medical assistance for certain individuals and families with low incomes and resources. It is a cooperative venture funded jointly by the federal and state governments to assist states in furnishing medical assistance to eligible needy individuals. Medicaid is the largest source of funding for medical and health-related services for America's poorest people, including people with disabilities. Medicaid policies for eligibility, services, and payment are complex and vary considerably by state, even among states of similar size or geographic proximity. Thus, a person who is eligible for Medicaid in one state might not be eligible in another state; and the services that one state provides can differ considerably in amount, duration, or scope from services that are provided in a similar or neighboring state. Medicaid has been critical in reform efforts to authorize waiver and demonstration authorities to allow states flexibility in operating Medicaid programs. The waiver that is most commonly used by people with disabilities is the Home and Community-Based Services Waiver (commonly known as HCBW). This program allows for the waiver of Medicaid provisions to allow LTC services to be delivered in least restrictive community settings. This program is the Medicaid alternative to providing comprehensive long-term services in institutional settings. Recently, this initiative has also included Money Follows the Person (MFP) initiatives, which allow monies that would have been spent on institutional or nursing home care to "follow the person" into the community. Many states now have MFP programs with a more flexible, consumer-directed set of supports and options.

Despite the existence of this disability and civil rights legislation, the DRM continues to face many important social policy issues and challenges to advancing the equality of disabled people. The level of sheer desperation in parts of the disability community continues to be astounding. More than 1.8 million people with disabilities remain isolated in nursing homes and institutions. The minimal income supports available for people living on Social Security condemn people with disabilities to abject poverty. Sheltered workshops remain an established system to address unemployment among disabled people at wages much lower than the already low minimum wage. Transportation is difficult for many disabled people, given that there are few lift-equipped over-the-road buses in the nation's bus fleet. In many cities, paratransit systems are consistently late, require advance notice to book, have increasingly limited budgets, and suffer frequent service cutbacks; in rural areas, such systems often are not available at all.

According to the National Council on Disability (NCD), other social policy areas that have high priority among disabled people include access to affordable, accessible, and integrated housing; high-quality health care, education, work, telecommunications, and assistive technologies; voting rights; parenting rights; euthanasia or assisted suicide advocacy; and sexual identity and freedom (NCD, 2006a, 2006b, 2010). Every single day, people with disabilities face social policy issues that limit or completely bar their full participation (Kessler Foundation/National Organization on Disability, 2011). To illustrate what the DRM is doing to address ongoing isolation, discrimination, and impoverishment, this section will focus on one key social policy example: that of community living rights that cut across policies of LTC, housing, access to services, and provision of community-based supports.

LTC is an area of rapidly evolving change in concept, policy, and practice. As recently as 50 years ago, home care was mostly seen as a family responsibility with state-run institutions filling in, where families were unable or unwilling to respond. Although "Homes for the Feeble Minded," "County Farms," and "Institutions for Mental Disease" were at first seen as reform, it was not very long before journalists and whistleblowers were exposing the abuse and neglect that were common in these places. Despite this exposure, they continue to exist in various forms or are being replaced by other institutions such as nursing homes and intermediate-care facilities.

In 1965, Medicare and Medicaid were created, and the social policy for providing LTC changed. While the state-operated institutions continued to be funded, the private nursing home industry began to also widely expand because large sums of Medicaid dollars became available to place lower-income people into a system that had been previously used by private pay middle- and upper-class citizens. The medical system also played a role in convincing families that all parties were better off when disabled family members were placed in institutions, such as nursing homes, citing benefits of health care access, safety, and socialization. Existing research on nursing homes has documented abuse, neglect, crime, and rapid declines of quality of life and health that would challenge these assertions (DePoy & Werrbach, 1996; Henderson, 1995; NCD, 2003, 2005a, 2006b; Wright, Gronfein, & Owens, 2000). At the same time, emerging research on community-based alternatives has pointed to the high meaning of aging in place in the community and the positive outcomes of home- and community-based waiver programs that provide supports to live in community settings on emotional and physical health and well-being (CMS, 2011; Minkler et al., 2008; NCD, 2003, 2005a, 2005b, 2006a, 2006b). Despite this research, the struggle to rebalance LTC toward community-based alternatives continues, in large part because of the strength of the multibillion-dollar nursing home and institutional industry and its political lobbies.

Some of the first steps for affecting a paradigm shift in LTC involved advocating for the creation of new consumer-directed models and use of nonprofessionalized personal assistant services. The many forms of alternatives to institutional care are known as home- and community-based services. Critical steps in making this change in LTC social policy included the following:

1. The establishment of the Berkeley CIL with its experimentation with personal assistant services that resulted in the funding in 1980 of a national network of CILs as a base to build a broad advocacy campaign and recreate community-based alternatives (Resources for links to CILs in every state may be found online at http://thePoint.lww.com/Willard-Spackman12e).
2. The formation of People First, a national organization for and controlled by people with intellectual disabilities that was instrumental in filing court challenges to the forced institutionalization of their people.
3. The book and film (based on the book) *One Flew over the Cuckoo's Nest* and other literature, art, and films that promoted the liberation of people in LTC institutions in the public media, which also resulted in changes in public attitudes about disabled people.
4. The passage of the ADA, which defined unwanted institutionalization as a violation of the civil rights of people with disabilities.
5. The national campaign by ADAPT (2006), a national disability rights organization, to pass The Community First Choice Option (CFCO) initiative in many states, which calls for mandated funding of home- and community-based services at least as strong as the mandate to fund nursing homes and institutions (see CMS, 2011 for current status). If passed in states, CFCO would allocate significant amounts of money to help people move from institutions to home and community settings and allow people real choice in where they would receive their LTC. Many states are also now involved in a joint initiative by Medicaid and Housing and Urban Development (HUD) to implement innovative demonstration projects to coordinate housing voucher assistance (vouchers to live in integrated community settings and offset rent costs to do so) with community-based community living supports from Medicaid such as personal attendant care, technology, home modifications, and so forth.
6. The *Olmstead* decision, a Supreme Court case interpreting the ADA, which asserted that people with disabilities have a right to live in the most integrated setting that is appropriate to their needs. This decision has ignited activists and led to widespread systems change, particularly in Medicaid rules, regulations, formation of community-based waiver programs, and more recent MFP initiatives to rebalance LTC financing toward community-based options and away from institutional bias.

The rally across the street from the Supreme Court at the time the *Olmstead* case was being argued was one of the largest DRM rallies ever held in Washington, DC. Strikingly, this activism resulted in many states changing their opinions to side with the DRM on *Olmstead* least restrictive placement rights. However, the political systems in many states are still skewed toward an institutional bias; approximately 70% of LTC spending nationally still goes to segregated institutional settings such as nursing homes, state mental hospitals, nursing homes specific to people with psychiatric disabilities, and intermediate-care facilities specific to people with intellectual disabilities (CMS, 2011; NCD, 2003, 2005a, 2005b, 2006a, 2006b). Despite this institutional bias, many important steps were taken at the federal level to support *Olmstead* implementation under the umbrella policy and executive directive of the New Freedom Initiative. These actions included the following:

1. The CMS continues to send ongoing policy letters to all state Medicaid directors elaborating on what the states should be doing to be in compliance with *Olmstead* and to rebalance LTC financing toward community-based options.
2. CMS System Change Grants allowed states to apply for grant money that could be used to create home and community alternatives to segregated settings, to strengthen existing home and community infrastructure, and to experiment with consumer-directed programs to support community living. Some states have used the grants well and developed models that other states could learn from (see CMS, 2011).
3. In 2006, CMS appropriated $1.75 billion to establish MFP Demonstration Projects, which calls for consumer-directed management and choice in supports with the money that would otherwise have been spent on institutional placement to follow the person to the community. The MFP concept is one of the operative principles of the ongoing disability activism to federally support community living choice and resource provision for all disabled people, including within the Affordable Care Act and other ongoing health care reform advocacy. Since MFP was implemented in Texas, more than 10,000 people have left nursing homes to live in the community

with supports; this represents strong evidence for systems change (CMS, 2011).

4. In 2011, the Community First Choice was established under the Patient Protection and Affordable Care Act of 2010 to further rebalance funds toward community-based options and supports (CMS, 2011).

Now the battle for home- and community-based LTC is specifically focused at the state level in which policies and outcomes vary widely across the country. There are a few states such as Mississippi, Kentucky, Alabama, and Tennessee that rank in the bottom quartile for home- and community-based service spending. They can be contrasted with other states such as Oregon, Washington, and Minnesota that rank in the top quartile and spend more than 50% of their LTC dollars on home- and community-based services, including access to occupational therapy, assistive technology, and environmental modifications. (Reinhard, Kassner, Houser, & Mollica, 2011)

LTC is an issue that the DRM is winning, albeit slowly. The DRM is also closely collaborating to apply the same philosophy of least restrictive, community-based living and consumer direction with senior citizens, people with psychiatric disabilities, and people with developmental disabilities. Activists face a government that is trying to drop its responsibility to fund LTC for people who do not have resources to purchase it in the private marketplace and to limit available least restrictive community living options in times of significant state budgetary crises. Cuts to Medicaid—and therefore to states—further hinder progress and threaten return to institutional bias and care delivery, such as nursing homes. Nursing homes, other private providers, and unions will intensify their efforts to hold onto the lion's share of the funding. Change will require greater political empowerment by disabled people and senior citizens as a coalition to counter this political power; occupational therapists can be a powerful ally in this advocacy to promote full participation, choice, and control in society for disabled people.

Ongoing policy issues still include the need to build stronger home- and community-based infrastructure as baby boomers age. There is an increasing need to provide enough affordable, accessible housing that supports aging in place and can meet the demand that comes with increasing numbers of people moving out of institutions. Occupational therapists can play a key role in helping to design and create accessible, affordable, and integrated community living options that fully support aging in place over time. New models of services that support consumer control and meet the needs of people with cognitive and psychiatric disabilities also require creative exploration, demonstration, and study. Occupational therapists can play key roles in these policy initiatives as allies in the activism movement and as contributors in the design, implementation, and evaluation of new community living environments and programs in collaboration with the disability and aging communities.

How Models of Disability, History, and Policy Influence Intervention

Now that you have learned about disability models, disability rights history, key legislation, and some of the major social policy issues that affect disabled people as a minority group, the next step is one of praxis, that is, reflecting back on what you have learned and applying it to your everyday practice. Following are some key concerns and strategies to consider in trying to integrate social and minority group model approaches throughout the process of occupational therapy assessment and intervention.

- **Environmental management and contextual reasoning.** Throughout the assessment and intervention process, critically reflect on how the social, political, economic, and cultural environments are influencing an individual's choice, control, motivation, and self-efficacy. Embed new participation in context and environmental barriers and supports assessments and discussions into your assessment process (e.g., Hammel et al., 2008; Heinemann et al., 2011), including asking whether a person has access to economic resources to engage in certain activities or even to access his or her own home, school, and worksite; whether the person is given opportunities and supports to fully participate in these societal activities; or whether the person is aware of resources and supports such as waivers, vouchers, home services, adapted transportation services, assistive technology, and home modifications. Can you equally emphasize environmental management and contextual reasoning rather than focusing solely on your "clinical reasoning" during intervention; that is, can you collaboratively plan, strategize, and negotiate how the environment and the systems within it influence a person's occupational choice and control and how you can collaborate on building supportive environments as well as community living management skills?
- **Consumer direction.** To what extent are you supporting consumer direction throughout the rehabilitation process and in key decision making beyond it? As a profession, we consistently voice our commitment to client-centered practice. However, research has shown that in reality, this often does not happen, and the therapist instead leads the therapy process (Bowen, 1996; C. Brown & Bowen, 1998). In contrast, the policy trend within the disability and senior activism communities is to move away from professional-directed services and to promote consumer-directed choice and control with supports to do so. What are you doing as an occupational therapist to promote not only client centeredness but also consumer direction

and leadership in advocating for full participation in society? For example, can you incorporate time into your intervention so that the consumer can practice directing his or her own care, such as directing a personal attendant in how to support and communicate with him or her as employer, practicing how to communicate with a rehabilitation counselor to justify the need for supports to live in the community or seek employment, and applying for and managing a menu of community-based supports across different systems (e.g., medical, medication, housing, attendant care, home modifications, workplace, or school accommodations)? These are all occupational participation activities that disabled people have identified as critical to community living choice and control.

- **Risk with dignity versus individual safety.** A large part of occupational therapy involves determination of safety, as in safe performance of everyday activities. For example, a person might be deemed too unsafe to go back home and instead recommended for nursing home placement, even if temporarily. In contrast, disabled people are bringing to the fore the concept of risk with dignity, that is, being able to take risks as the rest of society does and instead focusing on providing environmental supports to minimize the risk yet still give least restrictive living choice. What can you do as an occupational therapist to strategize environmental supports that would enable a person to live in the community or the least restrictive setting of his or her choice? Can you anticipate potential safety risks and work to problem-solve these in the natural home and community contexts? For example, in a home-based environmental intervention program for older adults with Alzheimer's disease and their spouses, the occupational therapist did a full home audit; collaborated with the consumer/caregiver to identify any potential safety issues; and used a problem solving worksheet to list the issues, assign next steps to work on between occupational therapy visits, and revisit the situation to see what worked or did not work (see examples from Corcoran & Gitlin, 1992; Gitlin, Corcoran, Winter, Boyce, & Hauck, 2001). Such a program could support people to stay in their homes and communities of highest meaning for as long as possible. Another way to do this is to work with the consumer to advocate for needed supports for personal safety and security, such as personal attendants, community safety check-ins, environment modifications, assistive technology such as intercoms and emergency call systems, and access to information technologies such as cell phones, personal digital assistants, and GPS systems.
- **Disability identity.** How are you framing disability in every interaction with disabled people? Do you talk about people as diagnostic labels (e.g., refer to people as *paras*, *quads*, *stroke*, *LD*, *TBI*, and the like) or as deficits (e.g., *your bad arm* or *affected arm*) versus respecting the individual's personhood and dignity? Do you treat disability as a negative deficit within the person that needs to be remediated, compensated for, or normalized? Can you instead frame disability as difference, as a different way of being and of doing that is significantly influenced by the environment? Can you link consumers with other disabled people who have been through a similar disability experience who can serve as positive role models and mentors on how to own difference and maintain a high quality of life? For example, can you link someone who is new to disability with disability advocates and peer-mentoring activities at a local CIL or start a peer-mentoring program at your own facility by inviting prior clients back to serve as mentors to new clients? Some community programs have also started intergenerational groups in which adults with disabilities mentor youths with disabilities or disabled youths mentor older adults who become disabled later in life. With the booming growth of online social network tools such as Facebook and YouTube, disabled people can virtually network with disability rights and advocacy community members remotely, creating a strong support network that can build and sustain emotional and physical health and quality of life over time.
- **Social interdependence.** How are you framing "success" in the rehabilitation process? Are you focusing on functional independence, that is, cognitive and physical ability to perform activities by oneself (or more likely, the burden of care if not fully independent)? Many disabled people and feminist scholars as well would challenge this emphasis on individual independence. Instead, they point to the importance of social interdependence that is, relying on each other and on other people and, in turn, giving back and supporting others within reciprocal relationships (Hammel et al., 2008; Magasi & Hammel, 2004; Morris, 1992). This concept of interdependence and how to support it is critical for many disabled people. For example, during therapy, are you talking with consumers about prioritizing energies and options to use other supports and people, such as family, personal attendants, and homemakers? Are you strategizing with consumers about how to assertively ask for support without feeling helpless or dependent? Are you offering consumers information about options for support in the community, such as where to look for qualified personal attendants; how to hire, fire, and train them; and systems to fund them in the home, such as home- and community-based waiver programs and CIL attendant pools?
- **Social participation, support, networking, and capital.** The concept of social interdependence extends to many other areas of social participation. Active engagement and participation in social relationships and membership in any social community are increasingly being identified as positively contributing

to emotional and physical health outcomes and well-being (Barlow & Harrison, 1996; Barlow & Williams, 1999; Fawcett et al., 1994; Hernandez, 2005; Magasi & Hammel, 2004). Yet we often spend little, if any, time on these social issues within therapy, assuming that people will work on them after therapy or that it is not our role to do so, given current funding systems. However, we also know that many disabled people are socially isolated and report that they are not participating in social opportunities as much as the rest of society is (Hammel et al., 2008; Kessler Foundation/National Organization on Disability, 2011). We also know that in response to these societal disparities, funding and health care accreditation agencies are now prioritizing "full participation and access to it" as fundable mandates and indicators of quality care (Commission on Accreditation of Rehabilitation Facilities & National Stroke Association, 2007). Strategizing ways to "be a part of," to express and strategize social and intimate relationships, and to develop a social network to meet different needs, such as emotional, instrumental, and thriving needs (Hammel et al., 2008; Magasi & Hammel, 2004), is a valid focus for occupational therapy, given our emphasis on meaningful engagement as well as research pointing to the benefits of this social engagement. As an occupational therapist, you can help to facilitate this social network development by using assessments such as a role inventory or a social network map so that people can identify what their network looks like now versus what they want it to be and then working with consumers to link to community groups and organizations in which they can begin to create or recreate their networks of choice. For example, a consumer might identify the importance of participation in a religious community, and you as an occupational therapist could support the consumer in exploring how to do this and how to work with that community to make it a supportive and accessible environment to people with disabilities. As another example, you might invite in peer mentors during therapy sessions so that clients can meet other people with disabilities and determine whether they might want to establish a social network with the disability community or a local CIL as another way to build social capital in their lives.

- **Your role and power as a professional.** Are you aware of your own power as a professional therapist? Many therapists would reply that they work within a system that dictates what they can do and that they really do not have much power themselves. However, when you reflect on it, you have a great deal of power as a rehabilitation professional. You have power in determining whether a person is qualified to receive therapy services and the type and extent of therapy the person will receive, what goals are focused on in therapy and how therapy time is spent, discharge and transition planning and whether people are aware of and referred to follow-up services, information access and awareness of options and choices people have and how to advocate for needed supports, whether assistive technology is recommended and funding of it, and so on. You can passively abdicate your power or you can use it creatively to be an advocacy ally with disabled people throughout and beyond the rehabilitation context.
- **Advocacy as a life role and the development of an advocacy network.** It is critical that occupational therapists recognize the importance of advocacy as a life role and work collaboratively with consumers to develop advocacy skills (including how to access information and systems to advocate for supports). An equally important occupational skill is the development of an advocacy network of support that people can count on when they need it or when self-advocacy is too tiring or not enough to address the bigger societal barriers they are facing. For example, you might work with a consumer to identify a primary personal attendant who will support the consumer in his or her everyday activities as well as several emergency backup strategies (e.g., signing up for an attendant pool at a local CIL or having the phone number of an attendant service if the person's attendant does not show that day). Just connecting a person with community advocacy groups, such as CILs, the ADA centers, and Protection and Advocacy or Ombudsman programs (available across the country), can offer the person an important source of support on which he or she can call when it is needed rather than having to try to find them during a crisis or emergency or to try to advocate for self in situations that may be unsafe to the consumer. These groups can also link consumers to civil rights and legal assistance if needed, which can be particularly critical for someone who is living alone or in an institution.
- **Peer mentoring, support, and advocacy.** Recognizing your limitations and role as an occupational therapist is also important. Are you serving as a liaison or ally in linking consumers with other disabled people who can share their experiences and strategies or with disability-led community groups such as CILs that offer peer counseling and mentoring? Increasingly, research is showing the positive benefits of peer mentoring and social learning in supporting emotional and physical health, well-being, community living management, and advocacy skills (Balcazar et al., 1991; Barlow & Harrison, 1996; Barlow & Williams, 1999; Garcia-Iriarte, Kramer, Kramer, & Hammel, 2008; Hernandez, 2005; Lorig, Ritter, & Plant, 2005).
- **Collective and empowered consciousness.** One of the most powerful ways to develop self-advocacy is to become involved in collective activism; this is relevant for disabled people and for occupational therapy

as a profession. The disability rights community offers many opportunities for social action on behalf of disabled people as a minority group. Do not assume that you need to already have self-advocacy skills to participate in these actions; instead, participation in such collective activism can lead to the development of self-advocacy. Above and beyond fighting for rights, however, comes the added benefit of empowered consciousness when one becomes a part of a shared community that is creating disability identity, culture, community, and pride. Exposing people, including yourself and clients with whom you work, to this social movement and to the culture and art that are produced within it can be a transformative experience and, in turn, can build community and power from within.

Incorporating Disability Experience into Practice, Research, and Advocacy: Examples from Participatory Action Research

In this final section, we focus on opportunities to promote empowered consciousness via participatory action research (PAR). The disability community's history of interaction with researchers has led the community to distrust or be wary of the research process because of mistreatment, continued perpetuation of concepts of incompetence, or irrelevance of research findings and outcomes to their everyday lives (Kitchin, 2000; Zarb, 1992). As a result, the disability community has called for participatory and emancipatory research that is conducted by people with disabilities and that empowers people with disabilities (Zarb, 1992).

One way in which researchers and practitioners can engage in research that is more empowering is to collaborate with disabled people and disability-led community groups in PAR. PAR is an approach rather than a specific design or set of methods (Tewey, 1997). It involves a dynamic collaboration between researchers, community partners, disabled constituents, and key stakeholders using an agenda that is driven by social issues that have been identified from within the community. PAR can result in shared knowledge that the community can use as evidence to effect social action change and to build community and empowered consciousness from within (Reason & Bradbury, 2001). It is research that is done by and with disabled people rather than for them or on their behalf. Given this applied, community-driven focus, PAR can be a useful framework for occupational therapy collaborative programming (Hammel et al., 2008; Minkler et al., 2008; Taylor, Braveman, & Hammel, 2004) as well as a basis for collaborating on systems change to improve participation opportunities in society. Case Study 70.1 provides one example of a collaborative PAR project that focused on disability rights, social justice, and empowered consciousness building with a disability community.

CASE STUDY 70.1 Empowerment by People with Intellectual Disabilities

This is a story about a participatory action research project that was a collaboration between the Chicago chapter of People First; the staff of El Valor of Chicago (a local community agency offering services to people with intellectual disabilities); the Rehabilitation Research and Training Center on Aging with Developmental Disability (with Joy Hammel as principal investigator); and Edurne Garcia, John Kramer, and Jessica Kramer, former doctoral students in the Disability Studies Program at the University of Illinois at Chicago. People First, run by people with disabilities, is an international movement that promotes the self-advocacy of people with disabilities. More information about the self-advocacy movement in the United States can be found at http://www.sabeusa.org

The Issue

Community agency staff members, who were people without disabilities who provided support to the Chicago chapter of People First, expressed concerns that people with intellectual disabilities in the group were not demonstrating self-advocacy behaviors. The supporters wanted the members to speak up more in the meetings as well as be more involved in advocating for their needs and desires in the larger community. Group members also wanted to become more involved in advocacy and community participation activities.

The Community-Building Process

Disability studies and occupational therapy practitioners and researchers approached People First as a group to do a PAR project together. Together, the team decided to work on the goal of raising the community's awareness of the group through activities and advocacy. However, the practitioners and researchers did not want to "teach" the group how to be self-advocates. Instead, the practitioners and researchers hoped to develop the empowered consciousness of the group itself through supported engagement in activities the group found meaningful. This focus is aligned with the concept of empowerment as defined by Fawcett and colleagues (1994) as a process by which people gain some control over valued events, outcomes, and resources of importance.

Participatory Strategies

Several participatory strategies were used to recognize and tap into the wisdom and experience of the members with intellectual disabilities and to locate members in positions of power within

CASE STUDY 70.1 Empowerment by People with Intellectual Disabilities (*Continued*)

the group. Rather than imposing preset therapeutic goals, the researchers observed and participated in several People First meetings to evaluate the group dynamics and identify existing strengths and concerns within the group. The People First members then engaged in a participatory focus group discussion that sought to better articulate why they liked being People First members, how they made decisions in the group, and what activities they would like to do as a group. To facilitate the participation of members, various strategies were used, including the use of a circular room arrangement in which participants face each other (with staff positioned outside the circle), round-robin questioning in which each person in the circle takes a turn in offering his or her perspectives, passing a microphone to designate who has the floor, the use of a timer, and the inclusion of many pictures to support the generation of ideas and concrete action plans.

Actions and Lessons Learned

This group discussion resulted in two main actions. First, the members identified that many decisions and actions were carried out by staff supporters rather than members. Second, the members identified that they would like their community to know about People First and that they wanted to publish a newsletter as a first step toward this goal. Many participatory strategies were introduced to support these actions. For example, the group used pictures and questions (such as "what do we want" and "what do we need to do") to create a picture-based logic model, or visual process guide, to guide the newsletter creation (see Figure 70.3) (additional examples of logic models and how to use them in occupational therapy can be found in the work of Letts and colleagues, 1999). Group members took turns generating names and ideas for the newsletter and voted by placing a sticker next to their favorite name. They used the same strategies to break down tasks associated with writing a newsletter and to select positions (see Figure 70.4).

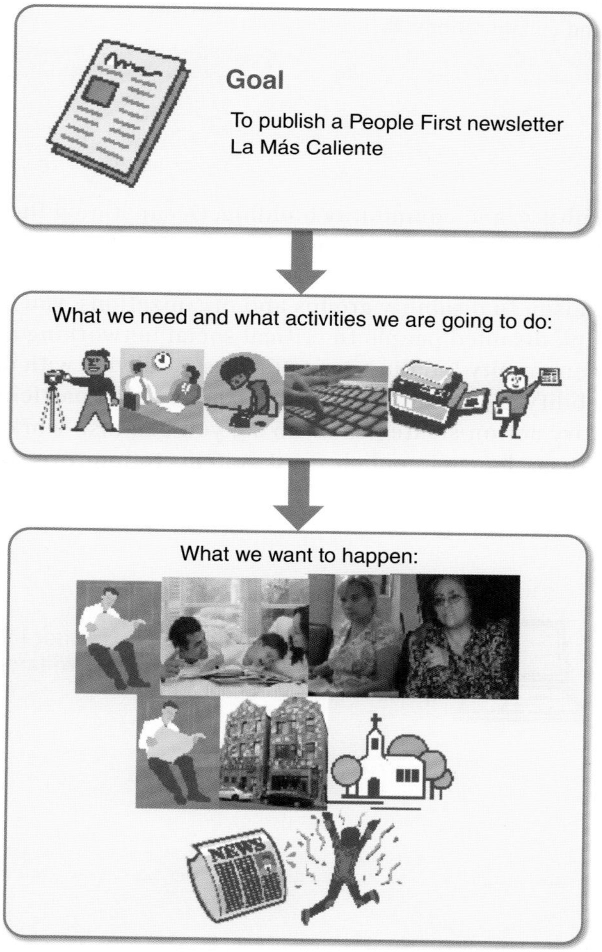

FIGURE 70.3 Picture-based logic model developed by People First group members to define their social group, membership in it, and actions they most want to do and direct.

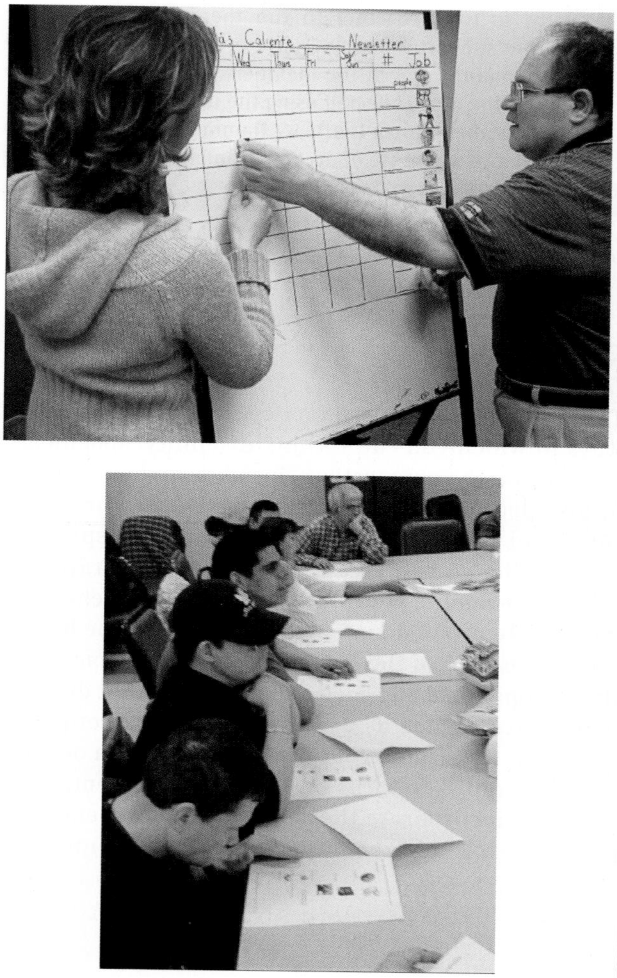

FIGURE 70.4 Examples of action research strategies to promote access to information, decision making, and control within the People First group and empowerment activities. Top: Flipchart of tasks for newsletter with picture voting on who will take lead on each task. Bottom: Use of picture-based meeting agendas developed by participants so that they can run their own meetings.

(continued)

CASE STUDY 70.1 Empowerment by People with Intellectual Disabilities (*Continued*)

With support, members then started to apply these strategies at every group meeting, slowly assuming control on a wider basis. To facilitate the group's reflection and growing empowerment, a checklist of meeting tasks was developed. At the end of each meeting, the whole group listened as a member read each checklist item out loud and decided who carried out each task during each meeting. Completing this checklist made the members realize supporters completed most meeting tasks. Several members spoke on behalf of the group and expressed a desire to have officers run all aspects of the meeting, from making the agenda to taking attendance. The practitioners and researchers then worked with the officers to develop tools, including an agenda template and a blank attendance log that would enable them to complete meeting tasks. Members were able to use their individual strengths to work together to run the meeting with little input from supporter (Garcia-Iriarte et al., 2008). At the end of the 22-month project, the members worked as a group to analyze all the data collected using the meeting task checklist (Kramer, Kramer, Garcia-Iriarte, & Hammel, 2011). The group expressed a strong sense of accomplishment when identifying the meeting tasks they most frequently performed. However, the group also expressed an appreciation for their supporters, who helped run some tasks and enabled the group to work toward their goals.

The actions taken on by this group illustrate the importance of three types of supports: peer support from within the group, advisor and system supports from outside the group, and strategy supports that use accessible formats to scaffold members' participation. Together, these supports not only enabled group members to develop self-advocacy but also group determination and power. Self-advocacy did not need to be taught on an individual basis or required as a prerequisite to group participation but could be learned and built on via a social group approach, with the added benefits of increased community activism and group-empowered consciousness (for more information on the project and resources developed, see Garcia-Iriarte et al., 2008 and Kramer et al., 2011). Many of the participatory strategies that are featured in this example could also be applied in community-based occupational therapy practice and collaborations. ■

Summary

This chapter has focused on exposing you to different ways in which you can rethink disability, specifically focusing on the perspectives, insights, and experiences of disabled people and disability advocacy organizations and communities. Many of these perspectives may challenge you as an occupational therapist to critically examine your own power and influence as a health care professional. By understanding the history and philosophy of the disability rights movement and the sociopolitical and social justice issues that disabled people experience as a collective social group, you can begin to reframe your own practice as an occupational therapist to focus on these environmental barriers and incorporate these visions of independence; participation; citizenship; and disability identity, culture, and community building. Occupational therapists can play a critical role in shaping a person's disability experience. By serving as a facilitator and a liaison to disability groups and organizations, you can link disabled people to critical social networking and community-building opportunities. By allying with disability groups and organizations and using participatory action strategies to do so, you can also work to effect change in policies and systems to improve societal opportunities and rights for disabled people as a societal group long term.

For a list of resources for disability activism and social justice, visit **thePoint.lww.com/Willard-Spackman12e**

BOX 70.2 Summative Learning Activity

Take out a piece of paper again and reflect back on your replies to the questions at the start of this chapter. How would you change your responses? How would you change your actions as an individual, as a member of society, and as an occupational therapist?

References

ADA Amendment Act of 2008 Regulations, 76 Fed Reg. 29 C.F.R. pt. 1630 (2011).

ADA Amendments Act of 2008, Pub. L. NO. 110-325, 122 Stat. 3553.

American Disabled for Accessible Public Transportation. (2006). *ADAPT Home Page*. Retrieved from http://www.adapt.org/index1.html

Americans with Disabilities Act of 1990, 42 U.S.C.A. § 12101 *et seq.*

Balcazar, F., Majors, R., Blanchard, K., Paine, A., Suarez-Balcazar, Y., Fawcett, S., . . . Meyer J. (1991). Teaching minority high school students to recruit helpers to attain personal and educational goals. *Journal of Behavioral Education, 1*, 445–454.

Barlow, J., & Harrison, K. (1996). Focusing on empowerment: Facilitating self-help in young people with arthritis through a disability organization. *Disability and Society, 11*(4), 539–552.

Barlow, J., & Williams, B. (1999). "I now feel that I'm not just a bit of left luggage": The experiences of older women with arthritis attending a personal independence course. *Disability and Society, 11*, 53–64.

Blumer, H. (1969). *Symbolic interaction: Perspective and method.* Englewood Cliffs, NJ: Prentice-Hall.

Bowen, R. (1996). Should occupational therapy adopt a consumer-based model of service delivery? *American Journal of Occupational Therapy, 50*(10), 899–902.

Bronfenbrenner, U. (1979). *The ecology of human development.* Cambridge, MA: Harvard University Press.

Brown, C., & Bowen, R. (1998). Including the consumer and environment in occupational therapy treatment planning. *Occupational Therapy Journal of Research, 18*, 44–62.

Brown, S. E. (1992). Creating a disability mythology. *International Journal of Rehabilitation Research, 15*, 227–233.

Centers for Medicare & Medicaid Services. (2011). *Balancing long-term services and supports.* Baltimore, MD: Author. Retrieved from http://www.medicaid.gov/Medicaid-CHIP-Program-Information/By-Topics/Long-Term-Services-and-Support/Balancing/Balancing-Long-Term-Services-and-Supports.html

Charlton, J. (1998). *Nothing about us without us.* Berkeley, CA: University of California Press.

Commission on Accreditation of Rehabilitation Facilities & National Stroke Association. (2007). CARF stroke specialty program standards. *Stroke Clinical Updates, Summer 2007, 7*(1).

Corcoran, M. A., & Gitlin, L. N. (1992). Dementia management: An occupational therapy home-based intervention for caregivers. *American Journal of Occupational Therapy, 46*(9), 801–808.

DePoy, E., & Werrbach, G. (1996). Successful living placement for adults with disabilities: Considerations for social work practice. *Social Work in Health Care, 23*(4), 21–34.

Driedger, D. (1989).*The last civil rights movement: Disabled Peoples' International.* New York, NY: St. Martin's Press.

Fawcett, S. B., White, G. W., Balcazar, F. E., Suarez-Balcazar, Y., Mathews, R. M., Paine-Andrews, A., . . . Smith, J. F. (1994). A contextual-behavioral model of empowerment: Case studies with people with physical disabilities. *American Journal of Community Psychology, 22*, 475–496.

Foucault, M. (1973). *The birth of the clinic: An archaeology of medical perception.* New York, NY: Vintage Books.

Garcia-Iriarte, E., Kramer, J. C., Kramer, J. M. & Hammel, J. (2008). "Who did what?": A participatory action research project to increase group capacity for advocacy. *Journal of Applied Research in Intellectual Disabilities, 22*(1), 10–22.

Gill, C. (1999). *Models of disability.* Chicago, IL: Chicago Center for Disability Research.

Gitlin, L. N., Corcoran, M., Winter, L., Boyce, A., & Hauck, W. W. (2001). A randomized, controlled trial of a home environmental intervention: Effect on efficacy and upset in caregivers and on daily function of persons with dementia. *Gerontologist, 41*(1), 4–14.

Goffman, E. (1963). *Stigma: Notes on the management of spoiled identity.* New York, NY: Simon & Schuster.

Goldberg, D. (Ed). (1994). *Multiculturalism: A critical reader.* Cambridge, MA: Blackwell.

Hahn, H. (1985). Disability policy and the problem of discrimination. *American Behavioral Scientist, 28*(3), 293–318.

Hammel, J., Magasi S., Heinemann, A., Whiteneck, G., Bogner, J., & Rodriguez, E. (2008). What does participation mean? An insider perspective from people with disabilities. *Disability and Rehabilitation, 30*(19), 1445–1460.

Heinemann, A. W., Lai, J., Magasi, S., Hammel, J., Corrigan, J. D., & Bogner, J. (2011). Measuring participation enfranchisement. *Archives of Physical Medicine & Rehabilitation, 92*(4), 564–571.

Help America Vote Act of 2002, Pub. L. No. 107-252, 116 Stat. 1666.

Henderson, J. N. (1995). The culture of care in a nursing home: Effects of a medicalized model of long-term care. In J. N. Henderson & M. D. Vesperi (Eds.), *The culture of long term care: Nursing home ethnography.* Westport, CT: Bergin & Garvey.

Hernandez, B. (2005). A voice in the chorus: Perspectives of young men of color on their disabilities, identities, and peer-mentors. *Disability & Society, 20*(2), 117–133.

Individuals with Disabilities Education Act of 1990, 20 U.S.C. § 1400 *et seq.*

Kessler Foundation/National Organization on Disability. (2011). *2010 gap survey of Americans with disabilities.* Washington, DC: Author. Retrieved from http://www.2010disabilitysurveys.org/

Kitchin, R. (2000). The researched opinions on research: Disabled people and disability research. *Disability and Society, 15*(1), 25–47.

Kramer, J. M., Kramer, J. C., Garcia-Iriarte, E., & Hammel, J. (2011). Following through to the end: The use of inclusive strategies to analyze and interpret data in participatory action research with individuals with intellectual disabilities. *Journal of Applied Research in Intellectual Disabilities, 24*, 263–273.

Letts, L., Law, M., Pollock, N., Stewart, D., Westmorland, M., Philpot, A., & Bosch, J. (1999). Developing a programme logical model as a basis for programme evaluation. In *A Programme Evaluation Workbook for Occupational Therapists: An evidence-based practice tool.* Ottawa, Canada: CAOT Publications.

Linton, S. (1998). *Claiming disability: Knowledge and identity.* New York, NY: New York University Press.

Longmore, P. K. (1995). The second phase: From disability rights to disability culture. *The Disability Rag and ReSource, 16*, 4–11.

Longmore, P., & Umansky, L (2001). *The new disability history: American perspectives.* New York, NY: New York University Press.

Lorig, K., Ritter, P. L., & Plant, K. (2005). A disease-specific self-help program compared with a generalized chronic disease self-help program for arthritis patients. *Arthritis & Rheumatism, 53*, 950–957.

MadPride. (2007). *MadPride home page.* Retrieved from http://www.ctono.freeserve.co.uk/

Magasi, S., & Hammel, J. (2004). Social support and social network mobilization in older African American women who have experienced strokes. *Disability Studies Quarterly, 24*, 4–19.

Mechanic, D. (1974). *Politics, medicine, and social science.* New York, NY: John Wiley & Sons.

Minkler, M., Hammel, J., Gill, C., Magasi, S., Breckwich Vásquez, V., Bristo, M., & Coleman, D. (2008). Community-based participatory research in disability and long-term care policy: A case study. *Journal of Disability Policy Studies, 19*(2), 114–126.

Morris, J. (1992). Personal and political: A feminist perspective on researching physical disability. *Disability, Handicap, and Society, 7*, 157–166.

National Council on Disability. (2003). *Olmstead: Reclaiming institutionalized lives.* Washington, DC: Author.

National Council on Disability. (2005a). *The civil rights of institutionalized persons act: Has it fulfilled its promise?* Washington, DC: Author.

National Council on Disability. (2005b). *Living independently and in the community: Implementation lessons from the United States: Quick reference guide.* Washington, DC: Author.

National Council on Disability. (2006a). *National disability policy: A progress report. December 2004–December 2005.* Washington, DC: Author.

National Council on Disability. (2006b). *The state of 21st century long-term services and supports: Financing and systems reform for Americans with disabilities.* Washington, DC: Author.

National Council on Disability. (2010). *The state of housing in America in the 21st century: A disability perspective.* Washington, DC: Author.

Nondiscrimination on the Basis of Disability by Public Accommodations and in Commercial Facilities, 76 Fed. Reg. 28 C.F.R. pt. 36 (2011).

Nondiscrimination on the Basis of Disability in State and Local Government Services, 76 Fed. Reg. 28 C.F.R. pt. 35 (2011).

Oliver, M. (1990). *The politics of disablement.* London, United Kingdom: Macmillan.

Oliver, M. (1996). *Understanding disability from theory to practice.* New York, NY: St. Martin's Press.

Olmstead v. L.C., 5279 U.S. 581 (1998).

Patient Protection and Affordable Act of 2010, Pub. L. No. 111-148, 124 Stat. 119.

Reason, P., & Bradbury, H. (2001). Introduction: Inquiry and participation in search of a world worthy of human aspiration. In P. Reason & H. Bradbury (Eds.), *Handbook of action research* (pp. 1–14). Thousand Oaks, CA: Sage.

Rehabilitation Act of 1973, 29 U.S.C. § 701 *et seq.*

Reinhard, S., Kassner, E., Houser, A., & Mollica, R. (2011). *Raising expectations: A state scorecard on long-term services and supports for older adults, people with physical disabilities, and family caregivers.* Washington, DC: AARP Foundation, the Commonwealth Fund, and the SCAN Foundation. Retrieved from http://www.longtermscorecard.org/

Rioux, M. (1997). Disability: The place of judgment in a world of fact. *Journal of Intellectual Disability Research, 41*(2), 102–112.

Taylor, R., Braveman, B., & Hammel, J. (2004). Developing and evaluating community-based services through participatory action research: Three case examples. *American Journal of Occupational Therapy, 58*, 73–82.

Tewey, B. P. (1997). *Building participatory action research partnerships in disability and rehabilitation research.* Washington, DC: National Institute on Disability and Rehabilitation Research.

Thomas, C. (1999). *Female forms: Experiencing and understanding disability.* Philadelphia, PA: Open University Press.

Triano, S. (2007). *Disabled and proud.* Retrieved from http://www.disabledandproud.com/

Wade, C. M. (1994). *Disability culture rap. tools for change: Disability identity and culture.* Santa Cruz, CA: Diversity World.

Wright, E. R., Gronfein, W. P., & Owens, T. J. (2000). Deinstitutionalization, social rejection, and the self-esteem of former mental patients. *Journal of Health & Social Behavior, 41*, 68–90.

Zarb, G. (1992). On the road to Damascus: First steps towards changing the relations of disability research production. *Disability, Handicap, and Society, 7*, 125–138.

For additional resources on the subjects discussed in this chapter, visit http://thePoint.lww.com/Willard-Spackman12e.

CHAPTER 71

Payment for Services in the United States

Helene Lohman

LEARNING OBJECTIVES

After reading this chapter, you will be able to:

1. Describe the historical impact of public policy related to health insurance on occupational therapy practice in the United States
2. Explain the key types of governmental and private pay insurance as well as other methods of payment that are accessed by clients in occupational therapy practice
3. Identify how occupational therapists can seek out and obtain grants
4. Discuss how occupational therapists can become advocates for third-party coverage

OUTLINE

Introduction: Overview of Payment

Payment issues are a major force affecting occupational therapy practice (Burke & Cassidy, 1991). When major changes occur with payment sources, practice is transformed. Federal and state legislation regulating payment strongly influences the direction of these practice shifts. For example, **Medicare**, Title XVIII of the Social Security Act enacted in 1965, enabled expansion of occupational therapy practice for older adults; and subsequent amendments that changed how the law was regulated resulted in shrinking practice in some areas. The passage of the Patient Protection and Affordable Care Act (P.L. 111-148) (PPACA) in 2010, as well as any other new legislation or regulations, will change future practice patterns.

In daily practice, the knowledge that practitioners have about payment is often based on the typical sources that cover their patients and clients. Some therapists who handle their own billing for services are very aware of the regulations affecting the payment that they receive. Others, like Patrice (case study 71.1) depend on their billing department or their manager to keep them abreast of payment policies and procedures.

CASE STUDY 71.1 Heather and Patrice

Heather and Patrice are two occupational therapists in their second year of practice. Their friendship goes back to when they attended the same occupational therapy professional program. Since graduating, they have made the effort to have occasional dinners at each other's homes. Their get-together serves as a time to continue their friendship as well as to discuss practice issues. During one get-together, their conversation centers on payment issues. Heather works in a school-based occupational therapy practice. Recently, Heather had a circumstance that awakened her to the realities of payment.

Heather found out that a change with **Medicaid** in her state required getting physician orders for all clients. That created a large amount of work for Heather because she had to do extensive research to find the children's physicians and get orders. Some of these clients had been followed for years and it was quite a challenge to get the required information. Up to that point, she had never considered the reimbursement sources for her clients.

Patrice shared that at her job in an acute care hospital in outpatient therapy, she never really thought much about payment because she considered that the billing department took care of it. Yet, when one of her clients did not show up for therapy, she found out from calling him that his last four therapy sessions had been denied and that the client did not want to continue therapy until his insurance situation was figured out. Patrice decided to research the claim denial. As a result, she became familiar with the billing department at the hospital (Figure 71.1). From talking with one of the staff at the billing department, she learned about the client's particular insurance and about other private and public insurance options commonly assessed by the clients she follows. She was surprised to learn how often denials occur and the behind-the-scenes work the billing department did to facilitate payment. Patrice decided to help her client advocate for continual therapy.

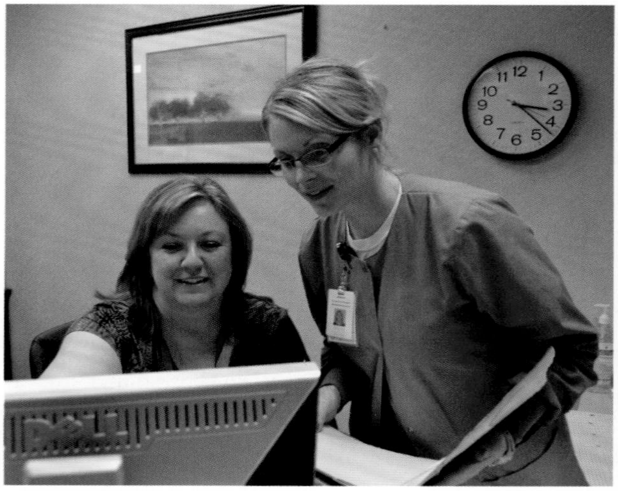

FIGURE 71.1 Therapist communicating with a staff person about a billing issue.

Patrice also shared with Heather that her mother recently was diagnosed with De Quervain's tenosynovitis, a condition that developed because of repetitive thumb motions. Her mother was ordered to have occupational therapy and she was motivated for the therapy, especially because of her awareness of its benefits. Her mother had a **consumer-directed health plan** (CDHP) with a **health savings account** (HSA) and a high deductible. Until she met her high deductible, she would be paying for most of the therapy out of pocket. Patrice wondered if others would be as willing to spend money out of pocket for therapy. As a result of these situations, both Heather and Patrice were motivated to be aware of payment sources for their clients and to educate and advocate for payment issues.

I suggest that it is important for all therapists, no matter where they work, to understand payment systems that affect practice and to be proactive by being aware of changes that may affect practice. Why? Because obtaining payment is the "bread and butter" of most practices, and therapists should be involved in obtaining optimal payment. This knowledge helps to support clients in their ability to access occupational therapy services.

This chapter provides a foundation about payment systems in the United States by first overviewing a brief history of insurance and then by reviewing the key payment sources that occupational therapists may encounter in practices. To fully understand payment systems, knowledge is required about the legislation that affects reimbursement and associated regulations. Public policy related to payment is discussed in this chapter, supplemented by some of the information mentioned earlier in Chapter 70. Documentation, which is directly related to receiving third-party reimbursement, is discussed in Chapter 36.

History of Health Insurance

Health insurance was introduced in the United States in the 1700s with the federal Marine Hospital Service (McCarthy & Schafermeyer, 2001). This insurance was an anomaly because most people self-paid for any health care they needed until the 20th century when the insurance industry grew (Patel & Rushefsky, 1999). During the 20th century, several types of insurance were introduced, which laid the foundation for insurance in the 21st century. Factors such as advances in medicine with expensive technological interventions, Americans wanting increased value for their medical care, and expansion of medical costs led to the development of the insurance industry (Shi & Singh, 2004). At the beginning of the 20th century, the first workers' compensation laws were enacted. These laws based on concerns for the well-being of injured workers brought about a system that remains today of state legislation regulating the care of injured workers.

Third-party Payment

In 1929, a model for hospital-based insurance, Blue Cross, and eventually a physician/medical services plan, Blue Shield, developed that laid the foundation for modern-day health insurance. Blue Cross/Blue Shield established a third-party payment system historically used as a benefit for employed Americans in which health care consumers paid a set monthly premium to receive medical services (Patel & Rushefsky, 2006). Providers were reimbursed a **fee-for-service** based on **"reasonable and necessary"** criteria, with minimal restrictions on the numbers and types of interventions that consumers accessed (Sandstrom, Lohman, & Bramble, in press). Fee-for-service type of payments occurred in **indemnity plans** in which payments were made retrospectively to the provider or insured person. With these plans, the insured person has the benefit of choosing the health care provider or facility without restrictions (Joseph, n.d.). Indemnity plans grew in the private employment-based market after a failed attempt for national health insurance by President Truman. Business and union leaders believed that building the private insurance market was a means to prevent government interference (Daschle, Greenberger, & Lambrew, 2008).

The 20th century also saw the growth of employer-based self-insurance plans as companies found them to be more cost effective (Daschle et al., 2008). With self-insurance, businesses established their own internally funded plans and determined what services to include. For example, businesses could choose to include or exclude occupational therapy as a service if the insurance company from which they contracted services offered therapy in its menu of options. In 1965, federalization of health care insurance was introduced with Medicare or Title XVIII of the Social Security Act and Medicaid or Title XIX of the Social Security Act. Provision of these plans paralleled the fee-for-service approach toward insurance payment at the time. During most of the remainder of the 20th century, health care insurance primarily remained a benefit of employment and was a fee-for-service system with indemnity plans.

Shifting from Fee-for-service to Managed Care

Legislation helped the health insurance industry grow. Because of public policies that included tax incentives for employers and provided protection of self-insurance plans from state laws (Employment Retirement Income Security Act of 1974), the insurance industry expanded, especially in the area of self-insurance. The passage of the Health Maintenance Organization Act of 1973 laid the foundation for the development and growth of **managed care** in the insurance industry. However, it was not until the 1980s and beyond that managed care came to dominate the insurance market (Raffel & Barsukiewicz, 2002). (Managed care will be discussed in more depth later in this chapter.)

With the advent of managed care, a paradigm shift occurred that influenced health care payment. The insurance industry no longer focused on providing unrestricted and unlimited coverage for health care services; rather, it focused on controlling costs and coverage. An analogy of this paradigm change is like a change from having unrestricted food at a cruise ship buffet without considering the costs or amount of food being eaten (fee-for-service/indemnity plans) to knowing the food allowance before the meal and being restricted to what you can order within that predetermined amount (managed care environment). Similarly, managed care restricted payment for health care services. One result was a movement away from retrospective payment for interventions, in which payment was made based on what was billed, to prospective payments, in which the amount to be paid for services was established before the intervention. In the mid-1980s, the advent of **diagnostic-related groups** (DRGs) for Medicare Part A patients in inpatient acute care hospitals reflected this prospective approach and the overall paradigm shift. Although DRGs were originally for Medicare beneficiaries, other insurance systems have adapted this approach. On the whole, these measures were intended to contain the spiraling costs that resulted from Americans using their health care insurance with no limitations and thus consuming services much like those eating at a cruise ship buffet. Although consumer demand did factor into the spiraling increase in health care costs, there were other significant contributing elements, such as high spending on technological advances and prescription drugs, the cost of managing chronic diseases, the aging of the American population, and administrative costs of insurance companies (Kimbuende, Ranji, Lundy, & Salganicoff, 2010).

Consumer-Driven Health Care and a Movement toward Community Partnerships

During the past several years, public policy trends have influenced payment options. One trend is consumer-driven health care, which was introduced during the George W. Bush presidency with the Medicare Prescription Drug Improvement and Modernization Act of 2003 (P.L. 108-173). This economically driven approach involves lowering health care expenditures while at the same time providing consumer control over their health plans. Thus, decision making about health care moves to the consumer instead of to the insurer. An example of consumer-driven health care is a **high-deductible health plan** (HDHP), which is often accompanied by a health savings account. These plans, also known as consumer-directed health plans (CDHPs), allow people to save and apply pretax dollars to health-related payments. Pretax dollars can be used to pay for deductibles, coinsurance,

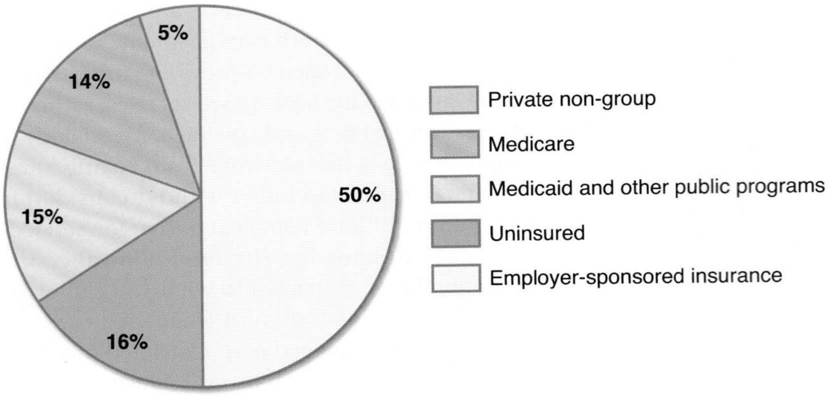

FIGURE 71.2 Approximate health insurance coverage in the United States, 2010.

co-payments, and health insurance premiums, which are traditionally paid for with after-tax dollars. The consumer can choose areas for health care intervention that are not always covered by some traditional insurance. Consumer plans are growing, with recent research indicating that between 14% and 20% of persons younger than 65 years old with private health insurance are enrolled in an HDHP and between 5% and 13% are enrolled in a CDHP (Cohen, Martinez, & Free, 2008; Fronstin, 2010; Kaiser Family Foundation [KFF], 2010a). Because these plans provide an incentive not to spend health care dollars, therapists need to strongly educate clients about therapy services so that they can see the value of spending their health dollars.

Another trend is a movement toward stronger coordination and integration between hospitals and the community. Numerous demonstration projects under Medicare and Medicaid, many of which were introduced with the PPACA, illustrate this trend. A Medicare example are **accountable care organizations** (ACOs). ACOs are made up of hospitals, physicians, specialists, and others, such as home health care (HHC). The ACO contracts to manage the quality and cost of care for a minimum of 5,000 Medicare beneficiaries for 3 years. Several cost-saving structures are part of ACOs, such as providing "bonuses when providers keep costs down and meet specific quality benchmarks" (Gold, 2011, p. 1). The hope is that ACOs will save Medicare money by managing care better. A Medicaid Waiver program for adults with disabilities is another example of hospital and community integration. These optional programs allow states to provide a variety of home and community services as a substitution for institutionalization (Maryland Medical Programs, n.d.). Medical Waiver programs can be a potential source of reimbursement for occupational therapy in community settings.

Types of Payment

This section briefly describes many different methods of payment for occupational therapy services. It helps to have an overall perspective of the current status of how Americans are insured, which is presented in Figure 71.2. This section includes several case studies that illustrate payment systems.

Grants

One aspect of the American Occupational Therapy Association's (AOTA, 2006) Centennial Vision involves "demonstrating and articulating our value to individuals, organizations, and communities" (p. 3). As Case Study 71.2 illustrates, assisting clients in community settings often entails obtaining grant funding. However, grant fund can also be employed in many other types of settings such as in medical settings, educational settings, and school settings. Grant writing is a learned skill set and an art that involves clear documentation along with understanding the focus of the granting agency. In most cases, grant proposals must follow strict guidelines, and, in all cases, proposals require careful documentation of the proposed program, service recipients, and expected outcomes (Braveman, 2006). Grant funding can be obtained from federal, state, or local government agencies and from private organizations. This type of "soft" payment provides funding for a prescribed time period, but when the grant is completed, practitioners need to find other payment sources for program support. Therapy practitioners can learn grant-writing skills from many sources including taking classes, participating in continuing education courses, using online resources, and receiving mentorship from faculty at universities. Practitioners can also network with the Small Business Administration or the American Association of Grant Professionals to help learn grant-writing skills.

Optional Sources for Government Funding in the Community

Another area that therapists can seek out funding for programs is through their State Vocational Rehabilitation Programs. These state/federally funded programs' focus on helping people with disabilities "prepare, gain, or retrain" for employment (Division of Vocational Rehabilitation, n.d.) are based on the Rehabilitation Act (P.L. 93-112, 87). Therapists can also work with other agencies funded through the federal or state government. For example, they might contract with their Area Office on Aging (AOA) to provide services, such as home modifications, or they might obtain a grant from the AOA to support a program.

CASE STUDY 71.2 Amy: Paying for Services for a Program Idea

Amy had a creative idea. She wanted to develop and administer a program to help single mothers with a disability living in homeless shelters develop life and job skills. She knew from her professional education that occupational therapy services can be provided in the community and had a passion for this project because of a personal story of having an unemployed sister with multiple sclerosis who was having difficulty finding a job due to not having the right job skills. Amy began the process of networking with people in her state and with professors at the local university. Through this networking, she located a state grant for which she wanted to apply to finance the program. Amy partnered with a therapist at the university, and together they wrote a proposal for a grant, which was funded for one year. Amy planned to continue working with the university to diversify funding sources. Amy later reflected that she would never have been able to create this program without the university partner's mentorship. Amy also acknowledged that it was her dream paired with her occupational therapy knowledge that ultimately provided women in this project with life and job skills.

Government Payment in the United States

Although we do not have universal health care in the United States as in other major industrial countries (e.g., Canada, the United Kingdom), government funding does account for a large percentage of our health care dollar in different systems such as hospitals, home health agencies, and skilled nursing homes, as Figure 71.3 illustrates. The following sections outline key government programs. Note that one is a federal program (Medicare), others are federal/state programs (Medicaid, ***Children's Health Insurance Program [CHIP]***, **Individuals with Disabilities Education Act [IDEA]**), and one is a state program (**Workers' compensation**).

Medicare

It is important to consider the history of Medicare because it remains the principal financier of health care in the United States (Sandstrom et al., in press), and changes with the Medicare law have influenced overall health care provision and occupational therapy practice. This section includes an overview of the history of Medicare followed by a discussion of what is included in the law and how it affects current occupational therapy practice.

History

Part of the impetus for the Medicare law was to provide a solution to a growing concern about providing

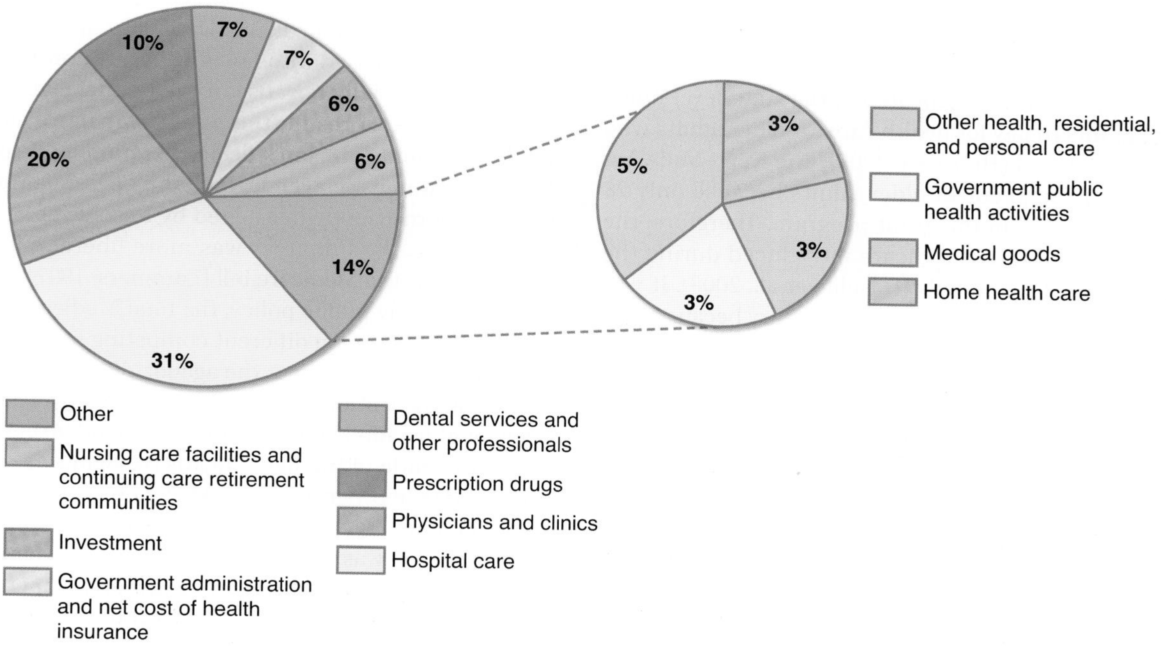

FIGURE 71.3 The nation's health dollar, 2009—where it went.

Practice Dilemma

Courtney: A Therapist Working with a Pediatric Client over the Years in Different Settings with Different Payment Issues

Courtney followed Joseph, a 10-year-old child with cerebral palsy, in therapy for most of his young life. Courtney found that during the time when she followed him for therapy intervention not only had her skills developed, but she has also learned about obtaining payment because of different issues. Courtney first saw Joseph when she was a therapist working in a neonatal intensive care unit (NICU) at an inpatient acute care hospital. The charge nurse mentioned to Courtney that Joseph could benefit from occupational therapy intervention and had communicated this with his physician. The physician, however, seemed reluctant to order occupational therapy because he was unfamiliar with the role of therapy in NICU. Therefore, Courtney clearly communicated with the physician the benefits of occupational therapy for Joseph's medical and developmental needs and received an order. Because Joseph's therapy was covered by a managed care organization, Courtney became familiar with the requirements for coverage. Five years later, Courtney saw Joseph again, this time through the school district where she contracted part time. Because Courtney was new to school-based practice, she had to learn to change her focus from working in a traditional medical model to working in an educationally based model. Joseph's insurance was now covered by Medicaid. Because Courtney was unfamiliar with the state Medicaid program and how it related to payment for Joseph's therapy in the school system, she decided to seek out education about Medicaid. When Joseph was 7-and-a-half years old, he fell and broke his wrist. Because Courtney still provided some contractual services at the hospital, she was able to follow Joseph in outpatient therapy; and his therapy remained reimbursed by Medicaid. A managed care approach was used by the state Medicaid program to guide and monitor therapy. Joseph's intervention goals were based on regaining the functional use of his upper extremity. Joseph was authorized to receive a set number of therapy visits from Medicaid, which Courtney felt were not adequate to meet Joseph's therapy goals.

Questions

1. Courtney's initial practice issue with Joseph was the need to advocate for occupational therapy services with the physician who was unfamiliar with therapy services in an NICU setting. Discuss how you would advocate with a physician to obtain therapy services.
2. Courtney's second practice issue was her identified need to learn more about the state Medicaid system and payment for Joseph's care. Discuss how you would learn more about Medicaid in your state and how it relates to school-based practice and practice in other settings.
3. Courtney's third practice issue was figuring out how to ask for additional therapy time beyond what was authorized by Medicaid for Joseph. Discuss how you would go about requesting more therapy visits.

health care coverage for all Americans. An earlier attempt during Harry Truman's presidency to amend the Social Security Act to include health insurance for all workers and their dependents as well as retired people had failed. During Eisenhower's presidency, the Kerr–Mills Act passed, which allocated at the state-level funds through grants to pay for health care for older adults who were impoverished (Hoffman, 2009). The Kerr–Mills Act did not meet the needs of older adults because only 28 states participated in the grant program. Therefore, the next proposed bill was Medicare introduced during the presidency of John Kennedy (Daschle et al., 2008). It was argued that the Medicare bill was necessary because only 15% of all older adults in the United States had health insurance (Bodenheimer & Grumbach, 2005) and that older adults with lower incomes were especially at risk for not having health insurance (Daschle et al., 2008). It was also acceptable to target older adults because the earlier Social Security Act of 1935 addressed this population and it was reasoned that everyone inevitably would age and need health care benefits (Fein, 1986; Patel & Rushefsky, 1999).

Medicare, however, did not pass into law during Kennedy's presidency because he was not politically strong enough to push forward a national health insurance plan, having won the election by a narrow margin (Patel & Rushefsky, 1999). Additionally, the American Medical Association (AMA) strongly lobbied against the bill, linking it with socialized medicine (Daschle et al., 2008).

Medicare passed into law during Lyndon Johnson's presidency partially because of the financial stability of the country. As a result, the public was more supportive of President Johnson's desire to complete President Kennedy's domestic agenda, including passing Medicare (Dorris Kearns Goodwin as cited by Daschle et al., 2008). Additionally, the Congress was more liberal, making it easier to pass the Medicare bill (Lammers, 1997).

As with any public policy, the final Medicare bill was a compromise among different competing factions. Thus, the final Medicare bill met the agenda of Johnson's democratic administration by including a national health insurance for older adults funded through payroll taxes. The bill met the agenda of the Republicans by including a voluntary insurance program called Medicare Part B for physician and other services (Starr, 2011), such as occupational therapy, which was funded through general revenues.

Much of therapy practice is directly linked to the Medicare law. Therefore, it is useful to understand an overview of key changes in the Medicare law since it was enacted in 1965. Table 71.1 highlights historical

TABLE 71.1 Historical Highlights of Changes in the Medicare Law Influencing Occupational Therapy Practice

Year	Amendment/Change	Impact on Occupational Therapy
1965	Medicare or Title XVIII of the Social Security Act was signed into law.	Encouraged the growth of OT practice.
1972	Medicare was extended to cover populations younger than 65 years old with disabilities and end-stage renal disease.	Extended OT services to those who were qualified to be disabled.
1980	The Omnibus Budget Reconciliation Act included OT as a qualifying service under Part B with home health and a provision established comprehensive outpatient rehabilitation facilities to be Part B providers.	Had the potential of expanding OT services in home health because OT solely could qualify a person for skilled home health services if the person was considered to be homebound. The second provision allowed occupational therapists to receive Part B reimbursement in freestanding rehabilitation outpatient settings, which expanded intervention coverage.
1981	The Budget Reconciliation Act eliminated OT as a qualifying service with home health.	This change required nursing, speech therapy, and physical therapy to qualify the patient for skilled care before OT. (To date, this provision remains unchanged.)
1982	In the Tax Equality and Fiscal Responsibility Act, hospice benefits were enacted on a temporary basis.	Occupational therapists began to work in hospice.
1983	Change from "reasonable cost" payment to a prospective payment system in hospitals (DRGs).	Resulted in shorter acute care hospital inpatient stays, with patients often transitioned to other settings, such as skilled nursing facilities (SNFs), for additional intervention. Occupational therapists began working in larger numbers in the settings to which patients were being discharged, such as SNFs and subacute care units.
1986	In the Consolidated Omnibus Budget Reconciliation Act of 1985, hospice benefit became permanent.	Occupational therapists work in hospice.
1992	Physician services paid for on a fee schedule.	Occupational therapists also bill Medicare from the fee schedule, using Physician's Current Procedural Terminology Codes for Part B services.
1997	The Balanced Budget Act (BBA) of 1997 included a prospective payment system for home health beginning in 2000. The act also included a prospective payment plan for Medicare Part A in SNFs beginning in 1998. The BBA also established "caps" on Part B outpatient rehabilitation services of $1,500 for OT and $1,500 for speech therapy and physical therapy combined. The Balanced Budget Refinement Act called for the establishment of a PPS in inpatient rehabilitation units.	Changed the approach of practice in SNFs. Several legislative attempts were made to suspend and repeal the outpatient cap. Occupational therapist work under the PPS system in inpatient rehabilitation units.
1999	The Medicare B $1,500 cap became effective in January 1999 for non–hospital-based clinics (SNF inpatient and outpatient therapy under Medicare Part B). The Medicare, Medicaid, and SCHIP Balanced Budget Refinement Act of 1999 passed, adding a 2-year moratorium on therapy caps in November 1999 (became effective in 2000). Increased payment for **resource utilization groups** (RUGs). Added regulations for medically complex patients.	Although the caps were on moratorium, OT practice with Part B remained the same.

(*continued*)

TABLE 71.1 Historical Highlights of Changes in the Medicare Law Influencing Occupational Therapy Practice (*Continued*)

Year	Amendment/Change	Impact on Occupational Therapy
2002	PPS was instituted in inpatient rehabilitation hospitals (Inpatient Rehabilitation Facility-Patient Assessment Instrument [IRF-PAI])	Occupational therapists assist in completing the IRF-PAI for the patient classification payment system.
2000–2005	Several acts placed moratoriums on the Medicare Part B therapy cap (2000, 2002). Several acts were introduced to repeal the cap (2001, 2002, 2003, and 2005). The cap again became effective (September 2003). Another 2-year moratorium was placed on the cap (December 2003).	Although the caps were on moratorium, OT practice with Part B remained the same. When the cap became effective, again it limited therapy services and patient access to therapy.
2006–2012	The therapy cap for hospital-based clinics was instituted. The passage of the Deficit Reduction Act of 2006 allowed for a temporary exemption process for the therapy cap for certain conditions in both hospital and nonhospital-based clinics. Each year, legislation continues to be reintroduced to repeal the therapy cap and for the exceptions process to remain.	With the exemptions process, occupational therapists can apply for continued intervention when required services are "reasonable and medically necessary." If the patient has "qualifying conditions or complexities," there is an automatic exceptions process (Medpac, 2010c, p.3).

DRG, diagnostic-related group; OT, occupational therapy; PPS, prospective payment system; SCHIP, State Children's Health Insurance Program.

Compiled from American Physical Therapy Association. (2007). *History of the therapy caps*. Retrieved from http://www.apta.org/FederalIssues/TherapyCap/History/; Medicare: Past, present, and future. (1999). *Caring, 18*(9), 16–17; Chartlinks. (2005). *Evolution of the inpatient rehabilitation facility prospective payment system*. Retrieved from http://www.chartlinks.com; Mallon, F. J. (1981). Nationally speaking: History of occupational therapy Medicare amendments. *American Journal of Occupational Therapy, 35*(4), 231–235; Medpac. (2010c). *Medicare payment basics: Outpatient therapy services payment system*. Retrieved from http://www.medpac.gov/documents/MedPAC_Payment_Basics_10_OPT.pdf; National Association for the Support of Long Term Care. (2005). *History of the Medicare Part B "therapy caps."* Retrieved from http://www.nasl.org/Advocacy_pages/Cap_History.htm

changes in the Medicare law over the years that have influenced occupational therapy practice. From the inception of Medicare in 1965 until 1983, changes in the law influenced occupational therapy practice in home health and hospice. In 1983, the introduction of the **prospective payment system (PPS)** using DRGs replaced the fee-for-service model in acute care hospitals, which forever changed the landscape of Medicare reimbursement and, along with it, of occupational therapy practice. With DRGs, hospitals received a fixed payment per stay for treatment of specific conditions. DRGs resulted in much shorter hospital stays with patients being discharged to other settings for additional care such as to outpatient therapy, inpatient rehabilitation units, HHC, or skilled nursing facilities (SNFs).

As a result of the DRGs, occupational therapists began working in larger numbers in other settings besides acute care hospitals, such as SNF (Swartz, 1998). The introduction of PPS in acute care hospitals also led to the development of new delivery settings. During the 1980s, subacute care units evolved to provide cost-efficient service to more acutely ill patients who had been discharged from hospitals with complex medical and rehabilitation needs (Griffin, 1998).

The establishment of a PPS as a cost-cutting measure spread over the next 20 years (between 1983 and 2003) into many other settings covered by Medicare reimbursement. Even as early as 1984, there was discussion about launching PPS in SNFs (Scott, 1984). However, most of the changes occurred in the late 1990s (in 1997, PPS in SNFs) or early into the next century (in 2000, HHC; in 2002, PPS in inpatient rehabilitation hospitals). In each of these settings, PPS is administered differently; but in all the systems, reimbursement for Medicare beneficiaries is allocated prospectively rather than retrospectively.

Other cost-cutting measures have been introduced, such as a cap on Part B Medicare outpatient therapy. As the large numbers of baby boomers age and qualify for Medicare coverage, one can anticipate continual cost-cutting measures. Issues of solvency are and will continue to be discussed. This has shown up in numerous cost-saving measures with the PPACA and in discussions in Congress related to health care and the federal budget.

How the Medicare System Works

Medicare Parts A and B

Medicare is a federal health insurance system overseen by the Centers for Medicare and Medicaid Services

TABLE 71.2 An Overview of Medicare Part A Payment in Different Settings

Facility Type	Payment Based On
Inpatient perspective payment system (IPPS hospital) acute hospital	Diagnostic-related group (DRG)
Inpatient rehabilitation facility	Case mix group based on patient assessment instrument
Critical access hospitals	Rehabilitation services are paid at cost
Inpatient psych hospitals	DRG
Part A skilled nursing facility	Resource utilization groups (RUGs) based on Minimum Data Set (MDS)
Home health	Case mix based on the Outcome and Assessment Information Set (OASIS)

(CMS, 2011d) that covers "people that are 65 and older, people under 65 with certain conditions and people of any age with End-Stage Renal Disease (ESRD) (permanent kidney failure requiring dialysis or a kidney transplant)" (p. 14). All Medicare beneficiaries are covered under Part A, and some elect to be covered under the voluntary program of Part B. Part A covers inpatient hospitalization and ***critical access hospitals***, SNFs, HHC, and hospice care. Medicare beneficiaries pay deductibles to supplement this coverage. (Refer to Table 71.2 for an overview of Medicare Part A payment in different settings.)

Generally, Medicare payments are based on the type of service provided, where services are rendered, and the portion that Medicare will pay for the service. With Part B, the beneficiary pays a set fee per month and 20% of costs after a yearly deductible has been met to cover physician and outpatient services such as diagnostic tests; outpatient surgery; physical, speech, and occupational therapy; HHC; blood tests; and some preventive tests. Part B also covers some durable medical equipment (CMS, 2011e). All Medicare beneficiaries under Medicare Part B are subject to a therapy "cap" covering rehabilitation services (occupational therapy, physical therapy, and speech therapy) for an established amount per year. In 2011, the amount was $1,870 for occupational therapy (CMS, 2011g). This means that costs for occupational therapy cannot go beyond the cap amount or the person will pay out of pocket. Physical therapy and speech therapy share the same cap amount.

In some cases for intervention that is "reasonable and medically necessary" with "qualifying medical conditions or complexities" (CMS, 2010, p. 3), there can be an extension of therapy services called the exceptions process (CMS, 2011g). Because Medicare does not fully pay for all services under Part A and Part B, some Medicare beneficiaries may have supplemental insurance called a **Medigap policy** or pay out of pocket (Planprescriber, 2012). (Refer to Table 71.1 for the history of the therapy cap.) Figure 71.4 illustrates the distribution of outpatient (Part B) spending by setting.

Payment for medically necessary outpatient occupational therapy (Part B) is computed with the Medicare Physician Fee Schedule (MPFS). All health care provision with Medicare are categorized and

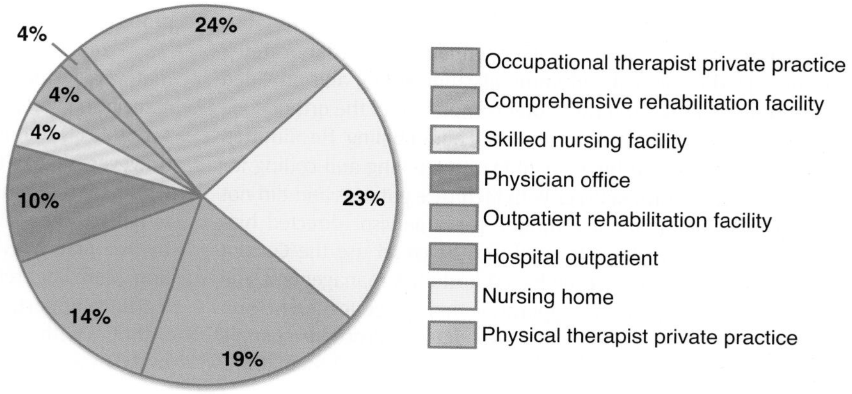

FIGURE 71.4 Distribution of Medicare outpatient therapy spending by setting. (From Medpac. [2010c]. *Medicare payment basics: Outpatient therapy services payment system*. Retrieved from http://www.medpac.gov/documents/MedPAC_Payment_Basics_07_OPT.pdf)

TABLE 71.3 Payment Terminology for Medicare Part B

Type	Definition	Application
Medicare Physician Fee Schedule (MPFS)	Fee schedule used for Medicare billing in outpatient settings. Each "unit of payment is for each individual service" and "services are classified and reported to CMS according to the Healthcare Common Procedure Coding System" (refer to subsequent definition) (Medpac, 2010c, p. 2)	Used by therapists and other qualified health care providers to bill Medicare Part B.
Level I Healthcare Current Procedural Terminology (CPT codes)	"Identifies medical services and procedures" (CMS, 2011b, para. 12)	Typically, therapists use codes from sections 97000 to 97999 or appropriate codes from other sections (Thomas, 2010). Can be timed codes based on an **8-min rule** (CMS, 2006a) or untimed codes billed once daily (Robinson, 2007)
Level II Healthcare Common Procedure Coding System (HCPCS codes)	"Identifies products, supplies, and services not included in the CPT-4 codes such as durable medical equipment, prosthetics, and orthotics" (CMS, 2011b, para. 13)	Used for payment of **durable medical equipment**, prosthetics, orthotics, and supplies (DMEPOS) (Medpac 2010a)
Correct Coding Initiative (CCI)	"National correct coding methodologies and to control improper coding leading to inappropriate payment in Part B claims" (CMS, 2011f, para. 2)	Used to review claims for improper bundling of pairs of CPT codes. There are specific requirements for billing certain codes together (Robinson, 2007).
International Statistical Classifications of Diseases codes or *ICD* codes	"Alphanumeric designations given to every diagnosis, description of symptoms and cause of death attributed to human beings" (Torrey, n.d., para. 1) These codes are found on billing claims forms.	Therapists select the most appropriate codes to explain the primary medical condition and primary and secondary therapy diagnoses.

documented with the Healthcare Common Procedure Coding System (HCPCS) or Current Procedural Terminology (CPT) codes (Medpac, 2010c). CPT codes developed by the AMA are updated annually, and each codes listed on the MPFS has a detailed payment amount. (Refer to Table 71.3 for an explanation of payment terminology for Medicare Part B.) Case Study 71.3 illustrates the importance of becoming familiar with different types of coding. Case Study 71.4 illustrates payment for low-vision services.

CASE STUDY 71.3 Marc Learning about Medicare Payments for Orthoses and Related Public Policy

Marc, a new graduate, is employed in an outpatient setting in the community. He was thrilled when he received an order to fabricate an orthotic for Henry, an older gentleman. Marc fabricated a resting hand orthotic (hand immobilization splint) and provided education on usage and care. After completion of the orthotic, he approached his supervisor for guidance about billing. He admitted to his supervisor that he was still learning billing and coding for occupational therapy services with Medicare patients and did not understand billing about orthotics. His supervisor directed him to resources where Marc learned that he could use the Current Procedural Terminology code 97760 (orthotics management and training) to bill for orthotic application and the education he provided. He researched the Healthcare Common Procedure Coding System (HCPCS) codes to bill his durable medical equipment (DME) carrier and he found the appropriate HCPCS "L" code for orthotic procedures and "A" code for supplies (AOTA, n.d.).

From further research, Marc even found out about a bill that was introduced by the American Orthotic and Prosthetic Association (Medicare Orthotics and Prosthetics Improvement Act of 2011) that initially might have restricted therapy practice. However, thanks to AOTA's efforts, an agreement was made to eliminate the requirement in the bill for occupational therapists to have additional certification to work with orthotics and prosthetics. Marc was relieved to discover this additional information. Marc later reflected to his supervisor that it was an excellent learning opportunity to find out not only about payment for orthotics with Medicare but also to learn about advocacy efforts by AOTA to protect occupational therapy scope of practice.

CASE STUDY 71.4 Michelle: Developing a Focus with Clients with Low Vision

Michelle worked with older adults in a skilled nursing facility and part time in a home health setting. Michelle enjoyed working with older adults and found it particularly rewarding to work with patients who had accompanying low-vision problems. After lengthy reflection, Michelle recognized that she wanted to specialize with adults who had low-vision deficits. Michelle made plans to achieve this goal and strategized to get further education and a mentor. She plans to eventually obtain an American Occupational Therapy Association specialty certification in low vision. She also recognized that to be successful, she would need to better understand payment and billing. So she researched Medicare payment under Medicare Part B for vision impairment and found the correct Current Procedural Terminology codes and diagnosis International Statistical Classification of Diseases (*ICD*) codes (eye-disease codes) on the MPFS to use in intervention. She was pleased to learn the history of Medicare, issuing a program memorandum specifically about rehabilitation of Medicare beneficiaries with vision impairment (CMS, 2002b), thus recognizing low vision in practice. She also considered the feasibility of having some private pay or self-pay clientele. She realized that some clientele would self-pay because of not having adequate insurance coverage for the low-vision service, not qualifying for Medicare, and wanting the service. ■

Medicare Parts C and D

The next part of Medicare is Medicare Part C, also commonly known as "Medicare Advantage." Medicare Part C is the private part of Medicare covering Parts A and B as well as some additional benefits (Medicare.gov, n.d.). Medicare Part D is a voluntary Medicare Prescription Drug Plan that involves beneficiaries paying a monthly premium, a yearly deductible, and partial co-payments depending on the amount that is spent out of pocket (CMS, 2011d). A major fix with the PPACA, if it remains as law, is gradually closing what was nicknamed the "donut hole." The donut hole is the large part of Medicare Part D that was not reimbursed.

As with any public policy, the original Medicare law was written very generally, with the interpretation of the law written into specific regulations, which health practitioners follow to receive payment. Although many regulatory changes have occurred with Medicare, such as adding the PPS in different systems, the same guidelines remain for determining occupational therapy coverage (see Box 71.1).

Therapists need to keep abreast of Medicare regulations related to therapy because they are constantly updated. Typically, the most current information is found on the Internet. Resources for Medicare regulations are also provided on the Willard and Spackman's Website.

PPS in Skilled Nursing Facilities

The PPS system in SNFs involves a mandated assessment structure (the Resident Assessment Instrument [RAI]) with periodic patient reviews. The Minimum Data Set (MDS)—the patient-screening form—considers the patient's status, includes quality measures (Thomas, 2010), and determines clinical care and payment. The MDS contains "extensive information on the resident's nursing needs, ADL impairments, cognitive status, behavioral problems, and medical diagnoses" (CMS, 2002a, p. 2) as well as "preferences and lifestyle wishes" (Thomas, 2010, p. 386). Sections of this instrument help to establish the classification categories for patients and ultimately the allocation of therapy time that patients can be seen.

Patients qualify to be admitted to an SNF under Medicare Part A by having enough days left for Medicare Part A coverage, having a 3-day hospital stay, being admitted to the SNF within 30 days of hospitalization, and obtaining a physician order. Patients must have a **"skilled"** need for being admitted to an SNF (CMS, 2007, p. 13). This skilled need means that the need for skilled nursing care and/or therapy and the skilled services provided must be "reasonable and necessary" (CMS, 2007, p. 14). The MDS screen is completed on each qualified patient. Results from the screen divide residents into six resource utilization groups (RUGs) ranging from

BOX 71.1 Guidelines for Determining Occupational Therapy Coverage

- Treatment must be completed by a qualified occupational therapist or occupational therapy assistant under the supervision of a qualified occupational therapist.
- Reimbursement for occupational therapy treatments requires a physician's order.
- Treatment must be of reasonable duration and amount and must be appropriate for the patient's condition.
- Treatment must "be furnished while under a plan of care (POC) certified by a physician or non-physician practitioner" (NPP) (CMS, 2010, p. 1).
- Treatment must result in practical improvements in the patient's functional performance.
- Therapist must follow Medicare policies (CMS, 1987, 2010).

ultrahigh to low and rehab plus extensive services. Each RUG group has a set total amount of therapy minutes that a patient receives in a week and the disciplines (ranging from one to three) that can follow the patient. In addition, RUGs establish the number of days to be followed. For example, a patient who qualifies to be in the "very high" RUG category is followed for 500 minutes by at least one discipline for 5 days per week (CMS, 2009a; Health Care Financing Administration, 1998). Specific regulations exist for payment for individual, group, and concurrent minutes. Therapists have learned to work effectively with the PPS by seeking out education to understand the regulations related to practice. Therapists also need to be very time efficient and have good communication skills with other disciplines (Brayford et al., 2002). It helps to find a mentor in learning the PPS system (Zellis, 2001).

Recent Changes in SNF

Regulations are constantly changing with Medicare, and therapists need to consistently monitor these changes. For example, newer versions were implemented with the MDS 3.0 in 2010 and RUGs IV in 2011. At the time of this writing, some of the key Medicare changes that impact therapy are with the coding of minutes and payment according to individual, concurrent, or group therapy (AOTA, 2009b).

PPS in Home Health Settings

Often, there are similarities between the different parts of the Medicare program. Thus, similar to the PPS system in SNF, which requires usage of the MDS as a screening tool, home health practice includes a screening tool for Part A patients called the Outcome and Assessment Information Set (OASIS). The OASIS is used to evaluate patient status and monitor outcomes for quality of patient care. Occupational therapists can consult with the nurse who completes the OASIS about the primary diagnosis for which HHC is needed and about the patient's functional status. Home health agencies are paid prospectively every 60 days, an established amount based on calculations (Medpac, 2010b). This calculation is derived from a case mix index and a clinical model from which patients are classified into groups called home health resource groups (HHRGs). Data from the OASIS, which may include therapy information, determine the patient's classification (CMS 2011a; Medpac, 2010b).

Other regulations that were made prior to the PPS remain intact, such as requiring **homebound** status for patients under Medicare Part A and the requirement that the other health care professions of nursing, physical therapy, or speech-language pathology must first skill-qualify a patient to receive the Medicare home health benefit before occupational therapy services can be provided. That means that "according to law, in order to receive services under the Medicare home health care benefit, a Medicare beneficiary must [initially] be in need of nursing, physical therapy, or speech therapy, in addition to being home bound" (Metzler, 2000, para. 1). However, once a patient is qualified for home health coverage, then occupational therapy can be initiated for medically necessary services and can continue to follow the patient even after other rehabilitation services have ended (Thomas, 2010).

The AOTA is lobbying to improve occupational therapy status in HHC. For the past few years, AOTA (2009a) has introduced a bill to "allow occupational therapists to open and provide the initial comprehensive assessment for Medicare rehabilitation cases when occupational therapy is listed on the physician's order along with a qualifying service" (para. 2).

PPS in Inpatient Rehabilitation Facilities

For acute inpatient rehabilitation facilities, the PPS includes an evaluation tool that is called the Inpatient Rehabilitation Facility-Patient Assessment Instrument (IRF-PAI). The IRF-PAI is based on the Functional Independence Measure™. Like the requirements in SNFs, patients are classified. However, in this system, patients are categorized in several ways: by impairment group code, by rehabilitation impairment category, by case mix group, and by the presence of comorbidities. Within this system, occupational therapy practitioners can play an important role in facilitating improved patient function from their interventions, as reflected by the scores on the IRF-PAI (Roberts, 2002).

There are specific regulations for inpatient rehabilitation that guide patient care. Regulations require that 60% of inpatient rehabilitation patients have 1 of 13 diagnoses (Medpac, 2010d). Patients must be able to tolerate 3 hours of therapy (Medpac, 2008) and are required to have "therapy from 2 disciplines (physical therapy, occupational therapy, speech-language pathology, or prosthetics/orthotics therapy) one of which must be physical or occupational therapy" (CMS, 2009b, p. 33).

Medicaid

Because of an unmet societal need to help low-income people, Medicaid, or Title XIX of the Social Security Act, was enacted in 1965. Medicaid insures older adults, children and parents of dependent children, pregnant women, and people with disabilities who meet the eligibility requirements. The majority of Medicaid recipients are children, and Medicaid covers one-quarter of all children in the United States. Yet, expenses for a small proportion of the Medicaid recipients, the older adults and disabled, account for two-thirds of Medicaid spending because of extensive use of acute and long-term care services (KFF, 2010b). Medicaid pays for two-thirds of all nursing home residents in the United States (Kaiser Commission on Medicaid and the Uninsured, 2010). It is not surprising that older adults need Medicaid services, especially for nursing home care, with the average cost of nursing home care in the United States being $80,000 to $83,585 per year (Consumer Health Ratings, 2010).

Medicaid also provides support to 4 in 10 children who have special needs. The Early and Periodic Screening, Diagnosis, and Treatment (EPSDT) benefit covers a large amount of services for children (Kaiser Commission on Medicaid and the Uninsured, 2011) up to the age of 21 years (Thomas, 2010). It addresses "screening and diagnosis" (Thomas, 2010, p. 385) of the health, mental health, and developmental needs of children that are low income (Health Resources and Services Administration [HRSA], n.d.).

Medicaid is a program jointly financed by federal and state governments that is regulated by each state. It is considered to be a *means tested* program as people qualify if their assets and income levels are below standards set by the program (Shi & Singh, 2004). States can choose to expand their baseline Medicaid coverage and income eligibility requirements beyond the federal minimal requirements. Medicaid programs vary as each state provides different services and different systems for delivery. Quite often, programs are administered with a managed care approach (CMS, 2006b). Each state has a plan that documents how the program is administered, eligibility requirements, and required and optional health services. Occupational therapy is one of the optional services; therefore, in some states, occupational therapy might not be a covered benefit. In 2008, 31 states included occupational therapy as a covered benefit; and in 19 states, occupational therapy was not a covered benefit (KFF, 2008). However, even in states where occupational therapy is included as an optional benefit, states have minimized the benefit by limiting the number of therapy visits or by cutting fee schedule rates for occupational therapy services (C. Willmarth, personal communication, June 13, 2011). Furthermore, because of the current economic environment, there are ongoing attempts to decrease state costs with other parts of the Medicaid program.

States are required to reimburse occupational therapy services for children covered under the EPSDT benefit if ordered by a physician and deemed to be medically necessary (M. Steiner, personal communication, June 8, 2007). It behooves occupational therapists to be aware of changes on a state level and advocate for therapy coverage in their state.

The PPACA enhances Medicaid benefits with the objective of improving insurance coverage for all Americans. With the Supreme Court decision on the PPACA on June 28, 2012, Medicaid expansion to childless adult citizens younger than 65 and for citizens with incomes below 133% of poverty (KFF, 2010b) became an optional state benefit. States choosing not to add the new Medicaid benefits do not lose existing funds and states including the new benefits receive federal support. In addition, as part of the PPACA, there are numerous pilot studies with Medicaid that emphasize focus on community care and better integrated care (Amerigroup, 2010). For example, the PPACA includes financial incentives for a "health home" for care coordination with Medicaid (KFF, 2010b).

Children's Health Insurance Program

A more recent federal/state health insurance program, the State Children's Health Insurance Program (SCHIP), or Title XXI, was created in 1997 as part of the Balanced Budget Act (the name was later changed to Children's Health Insurance Program or CHIP). This program provides health insurance to children and some parents in families that are ineligible for Medicaid and for whom health insurance is either unobtainable or cost prohibitive. Like Medicaid, CHIP is financed through the federal and state governments, and states administer their programs (Kaiser Commission on Medicaid and the Uninsured, 2011). CHIP is quite an expansive health insurance program, covering one-third of all children in the United States and one-half of all children with low incomes (Kaiser Commission on Medicaid and the Uninsured, 2011). Since its inception, CHIP has been successful in expanding health coverage and access to care as well as in decreasing the number of uninsured children in the United States (Kaiser Commission on Medicaid and the Uninsured, 2011). With the PPACA, if all goes as scheduled, funding for CHIP continues through 2015. The program is authorized with a federal match until 2019 when children in CHIP merge into Medicaid or exchange plans (KFF, 2010b). Thus, if the PPACA remains without changes, many of the children in the United States would be insured.

Individuals with Disabilities Education Act

As of 2010, the second highest percentage of occupational therapists (26.4%) was employed in school-based and early intervention practice (AOTA, 2010). In school-based practice, the Individuals with Disabilities Education Act (IDEA), a federal/state program, regulates and finances services, including occupational therapy. IDEA is for children with special needs to facilitate their optimal participation within the educational environment and to allow them a **Free and Appropriate Public Education** (FAPE). This law was most recently amended in 2004, and when it is reamended in the near future, therapists should carefully watch the bill to advocate for the best services for their clients. The specifics of school-based practice are beyond the scope of this chapter. Nevertheless, therapists working in school-based practice will need to have a strong knowledge of the regulations related to the IDEA and the focus of occupational therapy in the school system. It is beneficial for therapists to understand how IDEA finances services for children with special needs. Because it is a federal/state program, IDEA provided some federal funding, but most of the financing for IDEA comes from taxpayers in local school districts (Baumgartner, Berry,

Hojnacki, Kimball, & Leech, 2002). Thus, IDEA is really a federal, state, and school district partnership. As a result, there will be differences in services among school districts and across states. Beyond the IDEA, some financing for children in the school systems comes from Medicaid for educational services that are medically necessary (AOTA, 2007). States determine and regulate the payment rates for therapy and that amount can vary (S. Milliken, personal communication, June 6, 2007).

Workers' Compensation

Workers' compensation programs are state programs that pay for care of workers who have injuries or illnesses due to work-related causes. Each state has a governing body that determines the administration of the state program. Like other programs that have been discussed in this chapter (Medicaid, IDEA), workers' compensation programs vary from state to state, and their place within state governments vary. Programs generally pay for medical and rehabilitation services to get the person back to work, for partial repayment of lost wages, and short- and long-term disability. Programs also pay for partial as well as permanent disability. Permanent disability can be paid if the condition has long lasting outcomes and is related to employment (Social Security Administration, 2003/2004). Programs may include services such as vocational rehabilitation, medical rehabilitation, job placement for someone with a permanent disability, and social services. Many of these programs are instituted with a managed care approach. Funding for workers' compensation programs varies from state to state. Generally, programs are financed through employer insurance, state funds, or self-insured businesses. Programs control expenditures, such as employing treatment guidelines (Thomas, 2010).

Managed Care

Managed care has dominated the private health care market for several years (KFF, 2010a). There are many definitions for managed care. However, common to most definitions is the emphasis on controlling and reducing health care costs. Managed care "integrates the functions of financing, insurance, delivery, and payment within one organization" (Shi & Singh, 2004, p. 326). Most managed care organizations (MCOs) include primary and preventive care (Shi & Singh, 2004). Health maintenance organizations (HMOs), preferred provider organizations (PPOs), and point of service (POS) plans are examples of managed care options. (Please refer to the chart included on the Willard and Spackman's Website for more information about these plans.) In recent years, PPO plans, or plans in which the participants choose from a limited number of health care providers, have proven to be the most popular because of increased consumer choice (KFF, 2010b).

In order to receive payment, occupational therapy practitioners need to understand how each patient's plan works. As with any payer source, information about a patient's plan should be obtained or provided by the patient before the initiation of intervention. Some plans require preauthorization for beginning intervention. Plans may also require authorization for the number of treatments allowed and for continued intervention. Occupational therapists work with case managers who monitor care, and good communication is essential for coordination of care (Sandstrom et al., in press). Finally, managed care has not been without controversy with issues from consumers and health care providers alike (Lohman, 2003). As new systems evolve, such as CDHP, it is possible that managed care will have a decreased role in the private health care market place.

Consolidated Omnibus Budget Reconciliation Act of 1985 and Health Insurance Portability and Accountability Act of 1996

Some people who are at risk for being uninsured are those who change employment or have been laid off from their jobs. As a result, the **Consolidated Omnibus Budget Reconciliation Act** of 1985 (**COBRA**) was passed. COBRA allows employees additional months of continued insurance coverage after leaving a place of employment. COBRA is very costly because individuals pay more than their group rate to obtain this insurance. High costs of health insurance limit some people who cannot afford COBRA (Dalrymple, 2003).

Therapists should be familiar with the ***Health Insurance Portability and Accountability Act*** of 1996 (HIPAA, P.L. 104-191) because of the privacy regulations, claim implementation guidelines, and many other aspects of the law. Since 2003, the HIPAA Privacy Rules include regulations that speak to "the use and disclosure of individuals' health information" or "protected health information" (U.S. Department of Health and Human Services, 2003, p. 2). The HIPAA Privacy Rules include national standards for security with electronic health information and a Patient Safety Rule, which allows confidentiality with identifiable information from analysis of patient safety events (U.S. Department of Health and Human Services, n.d.). With electronic medical records, there are "national identifiers for providers, health plans, and employers" (CMS, 2011c, para. 1), including occupational therapists (AOTA, 2007). National standards for claim implementation allow for more standardized exchange of electronic data. Standards for security and uniformity with claims with electronic health information will be especially important as more documentation and billing move into electronic medical records.

The Patient Protection and Affordable Care Act

Throughout this chapter, several references have been made to the PPACA and how it might influence practice. The PPACA is the strongest attempt to date to change our health care system in both the public and private health markets. Factors behind the development of PPACA were the large numbers of uninsured and underinsured, the rising contribution of health care to the gross national product (GNP), and the inefficiencies in the health care market (Kohl, Nanof, & Metzler, 2011). At the time of this writing, the PPACA may be altered or even repealed based on court decisions, the composition of the Congress, or the residing president. It is this author's belief that regardless of what happens to this bill, many concepts planted in the marketplace, such as better coordination of care, will grow to influence practice.

Advocacy for Payment

Now let's return to the scenario of Patrice and Heather presented at the beginning of this chapter. You will recall that Patrice faced a challenge resulting from lack of coverage for her patient's occupational therapy services. Consequently, Patrice might become more aware of many chances to advocate for payment for her patients. She might consider advocacy on the state level with her state occupational therapy association or even on a national level (Sandstrom et al., in press). Using evidence with advocacy at any level enhances its credibility (Anderson et al., 2005; Sandstrom et al., in press). With Patrice's case, providing adequate documentation that demonstrates improvement in functional status, researching evidence of the efficacy of intervention (if available), and communicating with the insurance agency may increase the chances of payment coverage. If necessary, Patrice could find out the process for appealing a denied claim and then help her patient work within the insurance organization's system or possibly contacting the state insurance board.

As this discussion illustrates, every time practitioners experience problems with payment for services in their daily practice, they should critically consider how best to obtain and advocate for reimbursement. Sometimes, effective communication with case managers or other key people in an insurance system makes it possible to obtain payment. As discussed, providing evidence of the efficacy of the intervention is helpful. Other times, simply following through with the processes in place, such as an appeals system, can work. Sometimes, going beyond the traditional system to get funds through charitable, community organizations might be an option. For example, therapists might consider contacting an association that specializes in a patient condition, such as the Multiple Sclerosis Association, or might find that a client's friends, family, or faith group may donate needed funds.

The issue that Heather encountered illustrates the importance of becoming more aware of payment and regulatory changes. Some of Heather's best resources are available from being a member of her state and national professional organization (AOTA). On a state level, there is usually some type of structured committee or person, such as a legislative committee and a reimbursement chair, who can provide assistance with questions. On a national level, as a member of AOTA, Heather can access the resources about reimbursement on the AOTA Website. Awareness is the first step toward advocacy; and if Heather becomes passionate about changing a payment issue, she can then use her state and national resources to advocate for an issue.

Practice Dilemma

Advocating for Service Payment with a Policy Regulation

Larry was a newly employed occupational therapy practitioner practicing in a skilled nursing facility. He worked closely with physical therapy and speech therapy peers on the treatment team. Larry primarily followed patients under Medicare Part A. When Larry was asked to provide intervention to a Medicare Part B patient, he recognized that he was unfamiliar with the therapy cap. Larry communicated with Melissa, a physical therapist, and Jennifer, a speech therapist, to learn more about the therapy cap. Larry learned that at that time, the annual therapy cap per patient for occupational therapy was $1,880 and that speech therapy and physical therapy shared a combined therapy cap of $1,800. He also learned that historically, there had been several attempts to repeal the therapy cap and that legislative efforts continued. He found out about an exception process for more coverage for certain conditions. In fact, that year, he learned that the exceptions process had been extended for 2 months and a new bill had been introduced to repeal the therapy cap. Larry felt passionate about desiring better Medicare coverage with Part B and his practice dilemma was being unsure about how to begin with advocacy efforts.

Questions

1. What resources can Larry use to help advocate for a payment issue?
2. How should Larry begin his advocacy efforts?
3. How can Larry work with Melissa and Jennifer to advocate?
4. How can Larry use evidence with his advocacy efforts?

Conclusion

As the case examples and practice dilemmas in this chapter have illustrated, dealing with payment issues is a regular part of therapy practice. Practitioners may work with a variety of payment systems. On the surface, knowledge about payment systems might seem overwhelming because the financial system for health care and social services in the United States is very complex. Yet, it is every practitioner's professional duty to learn about these systems in order to be able to provide needed occupational therapy services and to advocate for payment when considered necessary (AOTA, Ethics Commission, 2010). Payment systems change, and these changes often occur because of new or amended legislation. Keeping current with policy and legislation that affect payment for one's area of practice is essential for successful practice.

References

American Occupational Therapy Association. (2006). *AOTA's centennial vision*. Retrieved from http://www.aota.org/nonmembers/area16/docs/vision.pdf

American Occupational Therapy Association. (2007). *Coding and billing FAQs*. Retrieved from http://www.aota.org/Practitioners/Reimb/Coding/37785.aspx#3

American Occupational Therapy Association. (2009a). *Help make OT an initiating service: AOTA's home health leave behind 2009*. Retrieved from http://www.aota.org/Practitioners/Advocacy/Federal/Home-Health.aspx

American Occupational Therapy Association. (2009b). *Medicare rules for concurrent therapy*. Retrieved from http://www.aota.org/Archive/ReimbursementArchive/2009/37784.aspx

American Occupational Therapy Association. (2010). *2010 occupational therapy workforce and compensation study*. Retrieved from http://www.nxtbook.com/nxtbooks/aota/2010salarysurvey/index.php#/24

American Occupational Therapy Association. (n.d.). *Health care reform: An OT perspective*. Retrieved from http://www.aota.org/Practitioners/Advocacy/Federal/Highlights/Reform.aspx

American Occupational Therapy Association, Ethics Commission. (2010). *Occupational therapy code of ethics and ethics standards*. Retrieved from http://www.aota.org/Practitioners/Ethics/Docs/Standards/38527.aspx?FT=.pdf

American Physical Therapy Association. (2007). *History of Medicare therapy caps*. Retrieved from http://www.apta.org/FederalIssues/TherapyCap/History/

Amerigroup. (2010). *Medicaid grant and demonstration programs: Helping states test new payment, quality and wellness models*. Retrieved from http://hcr.amerigroupcorp.com/wp-content/uploads/2011/02/Special-Focus-Edition-Medicaid-Pilots-and-Demonstrations.pdf

Anderson, L. M., Brownson, R. C., Fullilove, M., Teutsch, S. M., Novick, L. F., Fielding, J., & Land, G. (2005). Evidence-based public health policy and practice: Promises and limitations. *American Journal of Preventive Medicine, 28*(Suppl. 5), 226–230.

Baumgartner, F., Berry, J., Hojnacki, M., Kimball, D., & Leech, B. (2002). *Case overview: Individuals with Disabilities Education Act*. Retrieved from http://lobby.la.psu.edu/063_IDEA/summary_idea.htm

Bodenheimer, T. S., & Grumbach, K. (2005). *Understanding health policy: A clinical approach* (4th ed.). New York, NY: McGraw Hill.

Braveman, B. (Ed.). (2006). Communicating effectively in person and in writing. In *Leading and managing occupational therapy services: An evidence-based approach* (pp. 305–331). Philadelphia, PA: F. A. Davis.

Brayford, S., Muscatine, J., Dunbar, C., Frank, A., Nguyen, P., & Fisher, G. S. (2002). A pilot study of delivery of occupational therapy in long term care settings under the Medicare Prospective Payment System. *Occupational Therapy in Health Care, 15*, 67–76.

Burke, J. P., & Cassidy, J. C. (1991). Disparity between reimbursement-driven practice and humanistic values of occupational therapy. *American Journal of Occupational Therapy, 45*, 173–176.

Centers for Medicare and Medicaid Services. (1987). *Coverage of services, skilled nursing facility manual*. Retrieved from http://cms.hhs.gov.manuals/12/SNFs/SN00.asp

Centers for Medicare and Medicaid Services. (2002a). *Chapter 6: Medicare skilled nursing facility prospective payment system (SNF PPS)*. Retrieved from http://www.azdhs.gov/als/ltc/postmans/rai6a.pdf

Centers for Medicare and Medicaid Services. (2002b). *Program memorandum: Provider education article: Medicare coverage of rehabilitation services for beneficiaries with vision impairment*. Retrieved from http://www.cms.gov/Transmittals/Downloads/AB02078.pdf

Centers for Medicare and Medicaid Services. (2006a). *CMS manual system: Pub 100–04 Medicare claims processing (8 minute rule)*. Retrieved from https://www.cms.gov/transmittals/downloads/R1019CP.pdf

Centers for Medicare and Medicaid Services. (2006b). *Medicaid managed care overview*. Retrieved from http://www.cms.hhs.gov/MedicaidManagCare/

Centers for Medicare and Medicaid Services. (2007). *Medicare coverage of skilled nursing facility care*. Retrieved from http://www.medicare.gov/publications/pubs/pdf/10153.pdf

Centers for Medicare and Medicaid Services. (2009a). *Federal register*. Retrieved from http://edocket.access.gpo.gov/2009/pdf/E9-18662.pdf

Centers for Medicare and Medicaid Services. (2009b). *Medicare program: Inpatient rehabilitation facility prospective payment system for federal fiscal year 2010. Final rule*. Retrieved from http://edocket.access.gpo.gov/2009/pdf/E9-18616.pdf

Centers for Medicare and Medicaid Services. (2010). *Medicare learning network: Medicare outpatient therapy billing*. Retrieved from http://www.cms.gov/Outreach-and-Education/Medicare-Learning-Network-MLN/MLNProducts/Downloads/Medicare_Outpatient_Therapy_Billing_ICN903663.pdf

Centers for Medicare and Medicaid Services. (2011a). *CMS manual system Pub 100–20: One time notification*. Retrieved from http://www.cms.gov/transmittals/downloads/R824OTN.pdf

Centers for Medicare and Medicaid Services. (2011b). *HCPCS—General information*. Retrieved from http://www.cms.gov/medhcpcsgeninfo/

Centers for Medicare and Medicaid Services. (2011c). *HIPAA—General information*. Retrieved from http://www.cms.gov/hipaageninfo/

Centers for Medicare and Medicaid Services. (2011d). *Medicare & you 2011*. Retrieved from http://www.medicare.gov/publications/pubs/pdf/10050.pdf

Centers for Medicare and Medicaid Services. (2011e). *Medicare benefit policy manual. Chapter 15—Covered medical and other health services: Part B*. Retrieved from http://www.cms.gov/manuals/Downloads/bp102c15.pdf

Centers for Medicare and Medicaid Services. (2011f). *National corrective coding initiatives edits: Overview*. Retrieved from http://www.cms.gov/NationalCorrectCodInitEd/

Centers for Medicare and Medicaid Services. (2011g). *Therapy services, overview: Extension of therapy cap exceptions process*. Retrieved from http://www.cms.gov/therapyservices/

Chartlinks. (2005). *Evolution of the inpatient rehabilitation facility prospective payment system*. Retrieved from http://www.chartlinks.com

Cohen, R. A., Martinez, M. E., & Free, L. F. (2008). *Health insurance coverage: Early release of estimate from the national health interview survey, January–March 2008*. Retrieved from http://www.cdc.gov/nchs/data/nhis/earlyrelease/insur200809.htm

Consumer Health Ratings. (2010). *Nursing home, home health, assisted living—General average cost. Primary listings*. Retrieved from http://www.consumerhealthratings.com/index.php?action=showSubCats&cat_id=208

Dalrymple, M. (2003, October 9). Senators seek tax credit for unemployed. *Associated Press Online*.

Daschle, T., Greenberger, S. S., & Lambrew, J. M. (2008). *Critical: What we can do about the health-care crisis* (pp. 47–103). New York, NY: Thomas Dunne Books.

Division of Vocational Rehabilitation. (n.d.). *Vocational rehabilitation.* Retrieved from http://www.rehabworks.org/

Fein, R. (1986). *Medical care, medical costs: The search for a health insurance policy.* Cambridge, MA: Harvard University Press.

Fronstin, P. (2010). *Findings from the 2010 EBRI/MGA consumer engagement in health care survey.* Retrieved from http://www.ebri.org/pdf/briefspdf/EBRI_IB_12-2010_No352_CEHCS.pdf

Gold, J. (2011). *Accountable care organizations, explained.* Retrieved from http://www.npr.org/2011/04/01/132937232/accountable-care-organizations-explained

Griffin, K. M. (1998). Evolution of transitional care settings: Past, present, future. *AACN Clinical Issues, 9*398–408.

Health Care Financing Administration. (1998). *Federal register: Medicare program: Prospective payment system and consolidated billing for, final rule.* Retrieved from http://www.cms.hhs.gov/providers/SNFspps/fr12ma98.pdf

Health Resources and Services Administation. (n.d.). *EPSDT Program background.* Retrieved from http://mchb.hrsa.gov/epsdt/overview.html

Hoffman, C. (2009). *National health insurance—A brief history of reform efforts in the U.S.* Retrieved from http://www.kff.org/healthreform/upload/7871.pdf

Joseph, C. (n.d.). *Indemnity plans.* Retrieved from http://www.ehow.com/facts_7199028_health-insurance-indemnity-plans.html

Kaiser Commission on Medicaid and the Uninsured. (2010). *Medicaid: A primer.* Retrieved from http://www.kff.org/medicaid/7334.cfm

Kaiser Commission on Medicaid and the Uninsured. (2011). *Health coverage of children: The role of Medicaid and CHIP.* Retrieved from http://www.kff.org/uninsured/upload/7698-05.pdf

Kaiser Family Foundation. (2008). *Benefits by service: Occupational therapy services.* Retrieved from http://medicaidbenefits.kff.org/service.jsp?gr=off&nt=on&so=0&tg=0&yr=4&cat=4&sv=25

Kaiser Family Foundation. (2010a). *Employer health benefits: 2010 summary of findings* (pp. 1–8). Retrieved from http://www.keanecare.com/resources/files/RUG-IV.pdf

Kaiser Family Foundation. (2010b). *Medicaid and children's health insurance program provisions in the new health reform law.* Retrieved from http://www.kff.org/healthreform/upload/7952-03.pdf

Kimbuende, E., Ranji, U., Lundy, J., & Salganicoff, A. (2010). *U.S. health care costs.* Retrieved from http://www.kaiseredu.org/Issue-Modules/US-Health-Care-Costs/Background-Brief.aspx

Kohl, R., Nanof, T., & Metzler, C. (2011). *Health care reform: What's in, what's, out and what it means for occupational therapy* [PowerPoint Slides]. Retrieved from http://www.aota.org/Practitioners/Advocacy/Tools/Presentations/2011-PA.aspx

Lammers, W. W. (1997). Presidential leadership and health policy. In T. J. Litman & L. S. Robins (Eds.), *Health politics and policy* (3rd ed., pp. 11–35). Albany, NY: Delmar.

Lohman, H. (2003). Critical analysis of a public policy: An occupational therapist's experience with the patient bill of rights. *American Journal of Occupational Therapy, 57*, 468–472.

Mallon, F. J. (1981). Nationally speaking: History of occupational therapy Medicare amendments. *American Journal of Occupational Therapy, 35*, 231–235.

Maryland Medical Programs. (n.d.). *Waiver programs.* Retrieved from http://www.dhmh.state.md.us/mma/waiverprograms/

McCarthy, R. L., & Schafermeyer, K. W. (2001). *Introduction to health care delivery: A primer for pharmacists* (2nd ed.). Gaithersburg, MD: Aspen.

Medicare.gov. (n.d). *Medicare advantage: Part C.* Retrieved from http://www.medicare.gov/navigation/medicare-basics/medicare-benefits/part-c.aspx

Medicare: Past, present, and future. (1999). *Caring, 18*(9), 16–17.

Medpac. (2008). *Payment basics: Rehabilitation facilities (inpatient) payment system.* Retrieved from http://www.medpac.gov/documents/MedPAC_Payment_Basics_08_IRF.pdf

Medpac. (2010a). *Medicare payment basics: Durable medical equipment payment system.* Retrieved from http://www.medpac.gov/documents/MedPAC_Payment_Basics_10_DME.pdf

Medpac. (2010b). *Medicare payment basics: Home health care services payment system.* Retrieved from http://www.medpac.gov/documents/MedPAC_Payment_Basics_10_HHA.pdf

Medpac. (2010c). *Medicare payment basics: Outpatient therapy services payment system.* Retrieved from http://www.medpac.gov/documents/MedPAC_Payment_Basics_10_OPT.pdf

Medpac. (2010d). *Medicare payment basics: Rehabilitation facilities (inpatient) payment system.* Retrieved from http://www.medpac.gov/documents/MedPAC_Payment_Basics_10_IRF.pdf

Metzler, C. (2000). *Advocate for OT in home health.* Retrieved from http://www.aota.org/Pubs/OTP/1997-2007/Columns/CapitalBriefing/2000/cb-060500.aspx

National Association for the Support of Long Term Care. (2005). *History of the Medicare Part B "therapy caps."* Retrieved from http://www.nasl.org/Advocacy_pages/Cap_History.htm

Patel, K., & Rushefsky, M. E. (1999). *Health care politics and policy in America* (2nd ed.). Armonk, NY: M. E. Sharpe.

Patel, K., & Rushefsky, M. E. (2006). *Health care politics and policy in America* (3rd ed.). Armonk, NY: M. E. Sharpe.

Planprescriber. (2012). *Cost of Medicare—Understanding your out-of-pocket expenses in 2012.* Retrieved from http://www.planprescriber.com/medicare-insurance-news/medicare-costs/

Raffel, M. W., & Barsukiewicz, C. K. (2002). *The U.S. health system: Origins and functions* (5th ed.). Albany, NY: Delmar Thomson Learning.

Roberts, P. (2002, July). Navigating the inpatient rehabilitation facility prospective payment system (PPS). *OT Practice*, CE1–CE8.

Robinson, M. (2007). Medicare 101: Understanding the basics. *OT Practice, 12*(2), CE1–CE7.

Sandstrom, R. W., Lohman, H., & Bramble, J. D. (in press). *Health services: Policies and systems for therapists* (3rd ed.). Upper Saddle River, NJ: Prentice Hall.

Scott, S. J. (1984). The Medicare prospective payment system. *American Journal of Occupational Therapy, 38*, 330–334.

Shi, L., & Singh, D. A. (2004). *Delivering health care in America: A systems approach* (3rd ed.). Boston, MA: Jones and Bartlett.

Social Security Administration. (2003/2004). *Workers' compensation, social security disability insurance, and the offset: A fact sheet.* Retrieved from http://www.ssa.gov/policy/docs/ssb/v65n4/v65n4p3.html

Starr, P. (2011). *Remedy and reaction : The peculiar American struggle over health care reform.* New Haven, CT: Yale University Press.

Swartz, K. B. (1998). The history of occupational therapy. In M. E. Neistadt & E. B. Crepeau (Eds.), *Willard & Spackman's occupational therapy* (9th ed., pp. 884–865). Philadelphia, PA: Lippincott.

Thomas, J. V. (2010). Reimbursement. In K. Jacobs & G. L. McCormack (Eds.), *The Occupational Therapy Manager* (5th ed., pp. 385–405). Bethesda, MD: The American Occupational Therapy Association.

Torrey, T. (n.d.). *What are the ICD-9 or ICD-10 codes?* Retrieved from http://patients.about.com/od/medicalcodes/a/icdcodes.htm

U.S. Department of Health and Human Services. (2003). *Summary of the HIPAA privacy rule.* Retrieved from http://www.hhs.gov/ocr/privacy/hipaa/understanding/summary/privacysummary.pdf

U.S. Department of Health and Human Services. (n.d.). *Health information privacy.* Retrieved from http://www.hhs.gov/ocr/privacy/

Zellis, S. (2001). Occupational therapy and PPS: Let's take another look. *Gerontology Special Interest Section Quarterly*, 24(4), 1–3.

For additional resources on the subjects discussed in this chapter, visit http://thePoint.lww.com/Willard-Spackman12e.

CHAPTER 72

Supervision

Mary Jane Youngstrom

OUTLINE

LEARNING OBJECTIVES

After reading this chapter, you will be able to:

1. Understand the roles and functions of supervision
2. Differentiate types of supervision
3. Describe supervisory processes and implementation
4. Describe approaches to managing performance
5. Apply American Occupational Therapy Association (AOTA) guidelines for appropriate supervision of occupational therapy personnel in the United States

Supervision is an integral part of occupational therapy service provision. The supervisory process is consciously used in our profession to ensure that our clients receive safe and effective occupational therapy services. Although the ability to supervise skillfully is developed throughout one's practice career, the entry-level practitioner must be knowledgeable about the supervisory process and have a beginning understanding of how to give and receive supervision in a manner that is consistent with the profession's values and expectations. This chapter will provide you with an overview of what supervision is and introduce you to basic information you will need to develop positive and effective supervisory relationships. Supervisory expectations in general and supervisory standards specific to practice in the United States will be presented.

Supervision Embedded in Practice

The supervision process is an everyday feature of each practitioner's work experience. It is a process that supports effective job performance as well as personal growth. Read the case study about Marta, an occupational therapist (OT), and Kim, an occupational therapy assistant (OTA), which describes their career experiences with supervision.

CASE STUDY 72.1 Marta and Kim: Supervision Embedded in Practice

Marta began her career as an occupational therapist (OT) in a pediatric hospital. She worked with two other OTs and was supervised by Sarah, the senior OT in the setting. Although she met regularly with Sarah, Marta also sought and received feedback and guidance from the other OT, who was particularly experienced in working with children with head injuries. Marta used input from both OTs to expand her knowledge and develop her clinical reasoning skills. Six months after taking the job, she was given the responsibility of supervising volunteers who provided service in a playtime program for hospitalized children. She was responsible for orienting and training the volunteers. Periodically, she would observe their interactions with the children and was always available for questions. During her first year of practice, Marta was regularly involved in supervising both Level I OT and occupational therapy assistant (OTA) students. She found these experiences to be rewarding. At the end of her second year of work, she was assigned her first Level II clinical fieldwork student, whom she supervised on a daily basis. As the department's caseload expanded, an OTA, Kim, was hired, and Marta supervised Kim as they collaboratively worked to provide OT services to referred patients. Marta oriented Kim to the hospital and the department's policies and procedures. Initially, Marta closely observed Kim's treatments and/or cotreated with her. Kim came to the hospital with 3 years of experience with children, but her prior work had been in a school setting, so she was not as familiar with occupational therapy interventions involving acute medical conditions. Several months after Kim joined the department, she was given the responsibility for supervising the volunteers in the playtime program. She consulted with the recreational therapist, Terry, who worked on a different unit in the hospital, about strategies for expanding the play activities and improving volunteer participation.

In the case scenario, supervision was a regular feature of Marta's and Kim's daily work experience. Supervision provided feedback, direction, and support for Marta and Kim as they learned to carry out their responsibilities effectively and supported them in their personal professional development to gain additional competencies. Each practitioner had a designated formal supervisor, but both Marta and Kim received informal peer supervision from other therapists. The close-knit nature of the work group and everyone's interest in providing the best possible care allowed this type of supervision to occur naturally. Adding supervisory responsibilities to their jobs expanded both Marta's and Kim's job roles and offered opportunities for personal growth.

As the case study illustrates, practitioners are involved in giving as well as receiving supervision. Supervisory skills are an expected entry-level competency for OTs who are responsible for supervising OTAs (American Occupational Therapy Association [AOTA], 2009). Entry-level OTAs may be responsible for supervising OT aides and later may move into supervisory roles with other OTAs. Both OTs and OTAs should know how to effectively provide supervision and benefit from it. Before exploring how to best provide supervision, let's first look at what supervision is and how it fits into the overall management structure of a work setting.

Formal Supervision

Definition and Focus

Dictionaries trace the roots of the term *supervise* to the Latin roots *super-*, "over," + *videre-*, "to see" (McKean, 2005). Supervision is a process that involves "overseeing" or "watching" the work of another. The employer gives a supervisor formal authority to watch the work of others and ensure that the work meets the organization's goals and objectives. To effectively oversee the work of others, supervisors need to be familiar with the work of the positions they supervise. If individuals who move into supervisory positions do not have advanced knowledge or experience in the job positions they supervise, they are expected to familiarize themselves with the job tasks and responsibilities. This background allows them to provide the support and direction that supervisees need to solve work problems, to learn and grow in their jobs, and to better meet the organization's objectives (Figure 72.1).

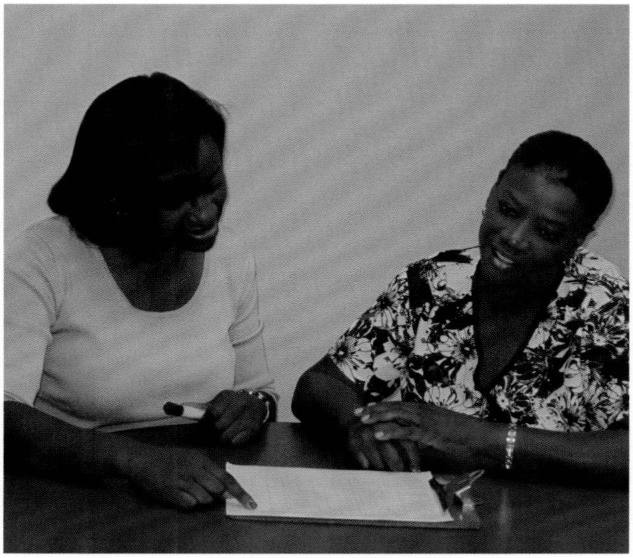

FIGURE 72.1 Discussing weekend coverage plans and how they will be implemented is a common supervisory task in hospital-based occupational therapy.

How does the supervisor fit in the management structure of an organization? Braveman (2006) offers insight into the relationship of the two by defining *supervision* as "the control and direction of the work of one or more employees in a manner that promotes improved performance and a higher quality outcome" (p. 142). Although supervisors may participate in all functions of management (planning, organizing, directing, and controlling), the majority of the supervisor's time is typically focused on the directing and controlling functions (Braveman, 2006, p. 142). (See Chapter 69 for a discussion of management functions.) When we consider the supervisor's placement within the management hierarchy, this becomes easier to understand (see Figure 72.2). Supervisors are placed closest to the staff level of the organization and typically do not supervise others who are in management positions. Supervisors are generally considered to be the first line of management. Although they have some management responsibilities, they are not considered to be managers.

The emphasis primarily on the directing and controlling functions of management rather than the planning and organizing functions does not diminish the importance of the supervisor's role. Formal supervisors, because of their placement within the organization, serve as a bridge between the staff and higher levels of management. In this position, the supervisor must support and interpret management decisions as well as relay staff concerns to higher management, which can influence planning and organizing functions. How well the supervisor can convey management concerns to staff and staff concerns to management can make or break the organization's effectiveness and ability to adapt to change.

Up to this point, we have been emphasizing the supervisor's responsibility to the organization—to oversee work to ensure the organization's success. Supervision takes on an added dimension and responsibility when people who are members of a profession (e.g., occupational therapy, nursing, psychology) take on responsibilities to supervise other members of their profession in a work setting. Providing professional supervision that is consistent with the profession's values and standards and supports the professional growth and development of the professionals who are being supervised is integrated with the supervisor's responsibility to meet the organization's needs. For example, the supervisor must not assign tasks and responsibilities that are outside of the supervisee's professional scope of practice. The supervisor must be cognizant of the profession's standards and guidelines regarding frequency of supervision and requirements for training and competency. Overall, the supervisor must manage and supervise work in a manner that respects the profession's scope and that supports the supervisee's development of continuing competence.

The supervisor who is providing professional supervision must continually ask two related but different questions, which will guide the supervisor's observations, analysis, decisions, and actions:

1. Is the supervisee successfully accomplishing the work?
2. Is the supervisee demonstrating continued professional growth and development?

Supporting the supervisees' efforts to maintain and develop continuing competence does not conflict with supporting the supervisee to successfully accomplish the work. As individuals develop new skills and abilities, clients receive better care and organizations benefit from workers' improved expertise. The supervisor should be concurrently providing feedback on performance and assessing the supervisee's learning and professional development needs.

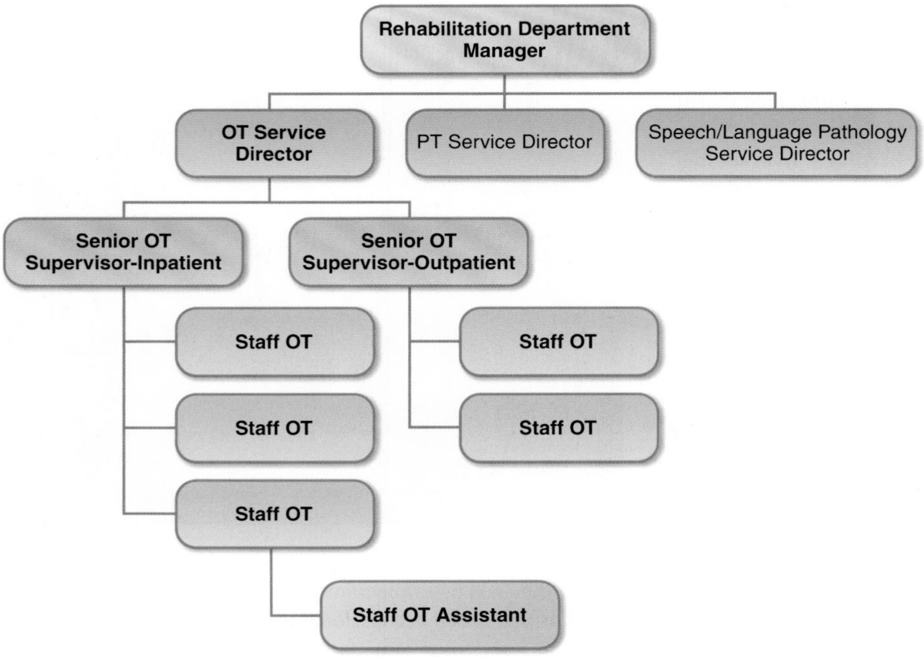

FIGURE 72.2 In this organization, the senior occupational therapists (OTs) are supervisors, and the occupational therapy service director is a manager. *PT*, physical therapist.

TABLE 72.1 Examples of Supervisory Tasks within Different Supervisory Functions

Administrative Function	Educational Function	Supportive Function
• Plan and assign workload • Make schedules • Set priorities for department's work activities • Check performance against work standards • Interpret policies and procedures • Delegate work • Provide written and verbal reports to managers	• Orient new staff • Identify training needs • Develop and provide training programs • Identify and provide educational resources • Assess performance and provide feedback • Discipline	• Hold group meetings to allow for expression of concerns • Meet individually with supervisee on a quarterly basis to check on progress toward work goals • Provide informal and formal support for performance

Functions of Supervision in a Professional Practice Setting

The supervisor's role in a professional practice setting encompasses three broad functions that are carried out under the broader management functions of directing and controlling. These functions are administrative, educational, and supportive functions (Kadushin, 1992). Table 72.1 lists examples of supervisory tasks for each function.

Administrative functions are directed toward managing the day-to-day work performance and process. Checking that all clients were seen and assigning clients to specific supervisees are examples of administrative tasks. Carrying out administrative functions ensures that the organization's day-to-day work is accomplished. The educational function is focused on the worker and is concerned with teaching and training, providing feedback about performance, and disciplining if necessary. Educational functions assist the supervisee to be effective in meeting job demands and also can help to promote the supervisee's own professional growth and development. The supportive function is directed toward relationships—both individual and group relationships within the workplace. This function focuses on developing harmonious relationships that will maintain a positive work environment in which people can be productive and successful.

Informal Supervision: Peer Supervision

Supervision is typically understood as a formalized process that occurs in a work setting in which a person's work is supervised by a formally designated supervisor. In a health care professional practice environment where all staff members are committed to providing the best quality of service, informal peer supervision may also occur. Peer supervision is oversight that is provided by another professional who has no formal authority to provide supervision. The peer supervisor provides feedback and shares knowledge with the intent of influencing the peer professional's practices to improve client outcomes.

Peer supervision is a natural extension of each professional's responsibility to ensure that clients receive the highest quality of care. It may or may not be solicited by the "supervisee" practitioner. In the case study, Marta did seek input from her peers as a way of continuing to learn and grow as a professional, but not all practitioners seek input from others. When a peer therapist provides peer supervision and feedback that is not requested, the intent is to improve client outcomes by offering information that could help other practitioners to improve their services.

In a professional and collegial work environment, peer supervision often occurs spontaneously and is seen as a benefit of working with others. Exchange and feedback among practitioners frequently occur as colleagues explore how to solve clinical problems and seek the best solutions for their clients. Such exchanges can be energizing for both parties. Engaging in peer supervision can be perceived as a method of mutual accountability and commitment to the profession's obligation to provide the best quality of services to clients.

Mentoring

Being mentored by another professional is often confused with supervision. Mentorship and supervision are different types of relationships. In a mentor relationship, the mentor's primary concern is the personal and professional growth of the mentee (Braveman, 2006). The mentor does not necessarily have any formal authority to oversee the mentee's work. Although the mentor is interested in the work the mentee is doing, direct observation of work does not regularly occur as part of the mentoring function, and discussion does not focus on work performance per se. Instead, discussions between the mentor and mentee center on career options and decisions, identification of personal and professional growth needs and resources, and feedback about the mentee's behaviors and choices. The mentor supports the mentee in overall professional development and offers support, praise, and encouragement. The mentor is focused solely on the mentee's personal growth.

TABLE 72.2 Comparison of Supervision, Mentorship, and Peer Supervision

	Supervision	Mentorship	Peer Supervision
Authority	Provided by the work organization	No formal authority	No formal authority; supported by professional responsibility
Nature of relationship and how it is established	Formal—established by the workplace	Personal, voluntary	Informal, spontaneous
Purpose	To support growth and development that will benefit the organization	To foster personal and professional growth and development that will benefit the mentee	To support growth and development that will ensure best outcomes for clients
How established	Assigned	Sought by the mentee and mutually agreed on	Offered by a peer or may be solicited by a practitioner
Accountability for performance	Organizational	Personal	Professional
Whose needs are met—outcomes expected	Needs of organization—work meets organizational objectives and needs	Needs of mentee—mentee achieves personal and professional growth	Needs of mentee and clients—clients receive best services

A mentor relationship may be sought by the mentee who is feeling the need of guidance and direction in professional growth and development. Sometimes mentor–mentee relationships occur spontaneously in a work environment or between two professionals who are attracted to each other. The mentee usually is attracted to the mentor's knowledge, skills, and accomplishments, and the mentor is attracted to the mentee's talent and potential as well as the opportunity to contribute to another professional's development. Generally, the mentor is an older and more experienced professional.

True mentoring relationships are acknowledged by both parties and require formal commitment of time and effort. Both parties discuss and agree on learning needs and goals for the relationship. A structure for the mentoring process is identified, whether it is periodic face-to-face meetings, written communication, or a combination of the two. Some work environments, recognizing the value of mentors, may formally assign a more experienced therapist who is not the employee's supervisor to function in a mentor role. The assigned mentor would provide support and guide the new employee in learning about and adjusting to new work situations. Less structured or more informal mentoring relationships can also develop during the course of a practitioner's professional life. These relationships are less intense and usually of shorter duration.

It is easy to see how a mentee–mentor relationship might develop within a supervisory relationship. When this happens, both parties need to be clear about the different purposes and responsibilities of the two types of relationships. It is possible that what the mentor might counsel would not be what the supervisor would counsel. For example, a person who is functioning in the role of a mentor might recognize that a mentee would benefit from staying in one clinical setting for several months to allow for solidification of learning. However, this same person, functioning as a supervisor, recognizes that staffing limitations require that the supervisee must be rotated to a new clinical setting each month. Holding both roles simultaneously can lead to role conflicts, highlighting the need to be very clear about the different responsibilities of each role. Table 72.2 offers a comparison of supervision, mentorship, and peer supervision.

Mentoring should not be confused with role modeling. A role model is usually watched and admired by a practitioner, but the role model does not have a reciprocating active interest in the person's development and might not even be aware that he or she is serving as a role model (Urish, 2004).

The Supervisory Process

The overseeing of work is an *ongoing* process: It occurs repeatedly across time and is embedded in the everyday work experience. A supervisor, both formally and informally, observes and checks on the work of supervisees by talking to them about their work as well as observing them on a regular basis. A supervisor who observes the work of supervisees only occasionally and meets with them only annually to discuss performance during an annual performance review is not providing appropriate supervision. Supervisors should be regularly present in the workplace and have regular contact with their supervisees.

Supervision is an *orderly* process. A good supervisor establishes a process in which the supervisee understands when regular contacts and meetings will occur. The supervisor is clear about performance expectations and consistent in providing feedback. The supervisee learns to trust and value the supervisory process as a tool that promotes personal growth and success in the job.

The supervisory process, although orderly and expected, is also *dynamic*. It changes as people grow and work demands shift. Upon initial hiring, the supervisor might observe an employee daily and meet weekly. However, after several weeks, the employee might practice more independently without daily observation.

Finally, the supervision is an *interactive* process. It is based on an exchange or communication between the supervisor and the supervisee. The exchange that occurs between the occupational therapy supervisor and supervisee is central to the development and maintenance of professional competence. The AOTA (2009) document "Guidelines for Supervision, Roles, and Responsibilities during the Delivery of Occupational Therapy Services" describes supervision as "a cooperative process in which two or more people participate in a joint effort to establish, maintain, and/or elevate a level of competence and performance" (p. 797).

Observe, in this description, that the profession sees supervision as a two-way street. The supervisee as well as the supervisor actively participates in the process. This is in sharp contrast to the common understanding of supervision as something that is done "to" a person and that the supervisee receives or accepts. In our profession, supervision is viewed as a cooperative process in which both parties have professional responsibility. This cooperative approach to supervision stems from the profession's ethical responsibility to demonstrate concern for the safety and well-being of their clients (e.g., see Principle 1: Beneficence, AOTA 2010a) and the profession's responsibility to abide by standards directed to developing and maintaining competent practice (AOTA, 2010b, 2010c)

The AOTA (2009) "Guidelines for Supervision, Roles, and Responsibilities during the Delivery of Occupational Therapy Services" describes the supervisory process as having two purposes that relate to these responsibilities: (1) to ensure safe and effective delivery of occupational therapy services and (2) to foster professional competence and development (p. 797). These objectives reflect the organizational duties of the supervisor as well as professional practice obligations. All OTs and OTAs have a common interest in providing the best possible care to their clients, and all practitioners are obligated to demonstrate continuing competence. The supervisory process is the tool that OTs and OTAs use to reach these goals.

Developing a Supervisory Relationship

The supervisory relationship is central to the supervisory process. An effective supervisory relationship is built on trust and integrity. To develop trust and integrity, the supervisor must be approachable and open to the supervisee's questions and concerns; the supervisee, likewise, must be open and willing to share his or her observations, perceptions, and ideas. Both must value and respect the input of the other. The supervisor must be responsive and follow through with actions that indicate that the supervisee's concerns were considered; the supervisee will feel valued and confident in his or her personal abilities, and commitment to the organization will increase. The supervisor must be clear about expectations and provide regular objective feedback about performance; the supervisee will understand what is expected and feel more comfortable in the job. The supervisor must be consistent in the application of rewards and punishments and not play favorites; the supervisee will develop a level of trust in how he or she will be treated. When communications and actions are clear, consistent, and fair, an environment of trust develops and anxiety about performance decreases. When the supervisor is approachable and responsive, the supervisory relationship can thrive. Box 72.1 provides some additional examples of supervisory behaviors that build trust and integrity.

BOX 72.1 Important Behaviors in Supervision

Key Positive Supervisory Behaviors

- Praises others
- Accepts criticism and suggestion without judging
- Tells the truth
- Is supportive of supervisee—goes to bat for supervisees
- Gives credit for accomplishments
- Abides by the same rules as expects others to abide by
- Gives clear and frequent feedback
- Is dependable
- Is loyal to organization—makes decisions that are in best interest of organization
- Is respectful of differences

Key Positive Supervisee Behaviors

- Accepts feedback
- Seeks feedback
- Provides information
- Asks for clarification
- Attempts to integrate feedback to improve performance
- Shares ideas and concerns in a direct but not critical manner
- Sensitive to feelings and needs of supervisor

Supervisor's Role in Building the Relationship

Both supervisee and supervisor bring their own values, beliefs, and attitudes about supervision to the relationship. Each brings past experiences with other supervisors and authority figures, which may have been positive or negative. It is the supervisor's responsibility to set the tone for the relationship in a job setting and to take actions that will support an ongoing positive relationship. The following four steps will help to ensure that a positive supervisory relationship is initiated and developed:

1. **Learn about the supervisee.** Remember that you are responsible for guiding the learning of this new employee. To do this effectively, you need to understand what your new supervisee knows and how he or she learns best. You will be particularly interested in how his or her knowledge and skills match with those that are needed for this job. Interviewing the new employee about past experiences and asking for his or her current strengths and learning needs sends the message that you are interested in building on what the person knows and you value the person's experiences. You might wish to develop a skills checklist that the employee can fill out to supplement the interview process. Although the supervisor never stops learning about the supervisee's abilities, gathering this information formally during orientation to use as you begin to design training and learning experiences is very helpful. Understanding not only *what* the supervisee knows but also *how* he or she learns is also important. Does the supervisee learn best by reading, demonstration, or both? Does the supervisee prefer to work more independently with periodic review, or would he or she like daily contact with you? What kind of feedback would the supervisee like, and how frequently would he or she like to receive it? Identifying the employee's learning styles and preferences can facilitate the learning process on the new job and avoid wasted time and effort for both parties.
2. **Be clear about job expectations.** During the initial orientation and training, the supervisor needs to clearly outline the performance expectations for the job. The job requirements and expectations should have been broadly discussed during the job interview and hiring process. Now is a good time to revisit this discussion and provide more specifics. Reviewing the job description is an objective method for beginning this discussion. Although job descriptions delineate major functions and lines of authority, they often do not specify in detail the quality and quantity of performance that are expected. Expectations about productivity and quality of work should be made clear to the employee. Be honest and open about consequences for various behaviors—rewards as well as punishments. In addition, organizational cultural expectations such as attitudes and behaviors employees are expected to exhibit in interdisciplinary, peer, and client/family interactions should be addressed. These expectations are often not included in a job description but are central to acceptable performance. Discuss your expectations regarding the supervisee's responsibility to learn and grow. Remember that one of your responsibilities as a professional supervising other members of your profession is to facilitate the supervisee's professional growth and competence. Share your commitment to this goal, and enlist the supervisee's commitment to it. Find out what the supervisee's personal professional goals and objectives are.
3. **Develop and implement a supervisory plan.** Our profession views the supervisory process as a collaborative one. Early in your new supervisee's employment, discuss how you view the supervisory process and work with the employee to develop a supervisory plan that will work for both of you. Discuss topics such as frequency of supervisory contact (e.g., daily, three times per week, weekly), types of contact (e.g., informal, spontaneous, formal scheduled meeting), methods of contact (e.g., face to face, e-mail, phone, written), and preferred supervisory methods (e.g., observation, cotreatment, dialogue, documentation review). Discuss the obligations of the supervisee as well as the supervisor in supervision; for example, explain that you expect the supervisee to initiate contact with you if more frequent feedback or supervision is needed and to share his or her concerns and ideas with you openly.
4. **Document supervision that is provided.** Document when you meet with your supervisee and what was discussed. A supervisory log or folder is a helpful tool that allows you to keep a record of incidents, observations, and meetings. If used routinely, the log allows you to track performance and see how it has changed. The log record provides concrete examples that can be used in your feedback and also in regular performance review meetings. Regulatory laws in some states require that supervisory logs be kept to document the supervisory process that occurs between an OT and an OTA to maintain current licensure.

Supervisee's Role in Building the Relationship

Supervision occurs as an ongoing process of involving the exchange of information about the job and feedback about performance. The feedback process is a two-way street, with both the supervisor and supervisee playing important roles. Feedback—both positive feedback and constructive criticism—should be provided on a regular basis by the supervisor as described in the next section. However, the supervisee also has a responsibility to regularly seek feedback as a way to validate work performance and identify areas for further professional development. In order to be effective, this is a reciprocal process. The supervisor needs to be skilled in delivering feedback, and the supervisee needs to be skilled in seeking and responding to feedback.

How does a supervisee respond effectively to feedback? First and most importantly, the supervisee needs to view the supervisory relationship positively and be open to receiving feedback. Feedback provided by a supervisor provides honest information about how work is to be done and behaviors and performance are perceived. This information can be used to develop new skills, refine current skills, and monitor personal growth and development. Sometimes hearing how others see you can be difficult to accept. You may be tempted to respond defensively by explaining your behavior or by discounting the feedback as uninformed. Neither strategy will promote the supervisory relationship nor lead to professional growth. If aspects of the information received are unclear because the feedback may not have been behaviorally specific enough, the supervisee should ask for clarification and/or concrete examples of the performance in question. If the feedback is based on incomplete information, the supervisee should provide more information in a calm and matter-of-fact manner. Exchanges that occur during supervisory sessions can help to clarify performance for both the supervisee as well as the supervisor and contribute to the collaborative supervisory relationship. Some general guidelines for receiving feedback are outlined in Box 72.2.

After feedback has been received, the supervisee needs to reflect on how he or she may respond to it. How can this new information be integrated into your daily work performance?

How might this new information influence your professional goals and skill development?

Perhaps your supervisor pointed out how your ability to communicate succinctly in team meetings has improved. Based on this feedback, you decide you would like to offer to more frequently attend team meetings when others cannot. Perhaps your supervisor has observed that your skill in wheelchair assessment and positioning are weaker. Based on this feedback, you decide to look for a continuing education opportunity in this skill area. Feedback can sensitize you to behaviors, attitudes, and skills that validate your abilities and can also help to provide direction for new learning and growth.

Performance Evaluation: A Supervisory Responsibility

All supervisory actions are directed toward managing the supervisee's work performance. The purpose of performance management is to encourage the supervisee to meet or exceed the established job performance standards and behave safely and appropriately at work (Newstrom, 2007, p. 319). Supervisors use a variety of methods in managing performance (e.g., incentives, job structure), but providing ongoing evaluation of performance by providing both formal and informal feedback is a central supervisory responsibility and skill.

Providing Feedback

Effective feedback is the supervisor's primary tool in influencing the employee's job performance. Employees need to know when they are meeting job performance standards and when they are not. When positive supervisory relationships have been established, feedback occurs naturally and informally throughout the work week. The supervisor comments on what he or she observes and uses the feedback to point out when performance needs to be changed as well as to verify and praise effective performance. Effective feedback needs to be descriptive rather than evaluative.

> **Evaluative:** Your initial interview was poorly done.
> **Descriptive:** Your initial interview used more "closed" yes/no answer questions than open-ended questions, limiting the amount of information you were able to gather.

Effective feedback also needs to be specific rather than general.

> **General:** Your productivity performance is below our standard.
> **Specific:** We expect our therapists to see nine clients each day, and you are seeing only six.

BOX 72.2 Guidelines for Receiving Feedback

- Listen openly. Assume feedback is being shared with positive intentions.
- Make sure you understand what is being said. Paraphrase what you have heard to check for accuracy.
- Ask for clarification or examples if feedback is unclear.
- Pause and think before you respond. If you want some time to consider feedback, ask for it.
- Acknowledge mistakes.
- Avoid interrupting or becoming defensive. Provide justification only if asked.
- Seek a solution to problems presented. Ask for examples of how you could perform better.
- Thank the person for providing you with the feedback.
- Make appropriate changes.
- Initiate a follow-up discussion to assure that needed changes have occurred as expected.

BOX 72.3 Guidelines for Giving Feedback

- Provide timely feedback—give feedback as close to when the behavior was observed as is possible.
- Provide balanced feedback—point out what is working as well as what needs to be changed.
- Provide feedback on behaviors that can be changed.
- Use "I" statements.
- Avoid the use of generalizations such as "always," "never," and "all."
- Ask the supervisee if he or she understood what you said; ask the supervisee to restate it in his or her own words.
- Ask for feedback about your feedback—how did you do?

Providing feedback that is descriptive and specific will help you to focus on the effectiveness of the supervisee's work behaviors and not on his or her personal characteristics or personality. This distinction is critical to the supervisee's being able to "hear" and respond to the feedback. Other suggestions for giving feedback are listed in Box 72.3.

Remember that the purpose of supervision is to support effective work performance. When supervisors evaluate employees, they are evaluating what employees do—how they behave, how they act, how effectively they are accomplishing the work. The focus of feedback in supervision—both informal and formal—is on the task, not the person. The purpose is to relay information about performance to the performer so that actions can be taken to maintain or improve performance.

Performance Evaluation and Appraisal

Newstrom (2007, p. 276) points out four basic reasons for appraising an employee's performance:

1. To encourage good behavior or to correct and discourage below-standard performance
2. To satisfy employee's curiosity to know how they are doing
3. To provide an opportunity for coaching to develop employee skills
4. To provide a firm foundation for later judgments that concern an employee's career such as promotions, pay raises, and transfers.

A supervisor should be regularly evaluating the supervisee's performance and providing feedback. However, at least once or twice a year, the supervisor should meet with the employer and provide a formal and systematic evaluation of how the person is performing, using a structured performance appraisal format. Most organizations have formal performance appraisal systems and appraisal forms. Appraisal methods and formats may vary and could include written narratives, behaviorally anchored rating scales, management by objectives, or 360-degree feedback. In a formal performance appraisal, the employee's performance is compared to established standards.

As a supervisor, you might be asked to develop job standards for occupational therapy personnel. Professional organizations such as the AOTA can help you to identify standards. For example, AOTA's "Standards of Practice" (AOTA, 2010c) and the "Guidelines for Supervision, Roles, and Responsibilities during the Delivery of Occupational Therapy Services" (AOTA, 2009) are important resources for supervisors practicing in the United States. The World Federation of Occupational Therapists (WFOT) (http://www.wfot.org) provides a listing of member occupational therapy professional organizations throughout the world, each of which are likely to have resources relevant to practice within that region. Refer to Chapter 68 for more information on professional organizations in occupational therapy. Equally important are worksite job descriptions. Standards will vary by workplace, but all standards should include *what* performance or behaviors are expected, *how* performance will be *measured*, and *when* performance is to occur. An example of a standard that includes all of these criteria is "Evaluations are completed and distributed within 24 hours of initial contact with the client."

In preparing a formal performance appraisal, the supervisor needs to complete three steps:

1. **Gather information about the employee's performance.** Review your supervisory logs, noting key incidents that you recorded. Record additional information that might have been overlooked. Review other employee records, such as attendance, training and educational records, and competency check-off completions. Review the previous year's performance appraisal. Talk to other members of the team both within and outside of your department to understand how the employee's performance is viewed by others. Ask the employee to perform a self-appraisal of his or her work, identifying accomplishments, strengths, and weaknesses. You can ask the employee to give this to you before the performance appraisal or have the employee bring it to the performance appraisal meeting.
2. **Compare current performance to standards.** Note areas of strength and areas in which improvement may be needed.
3. **Reflect on and synthesize information.** Consider the needs of the department as well as the professional growth needs of the supervisee. Provide

feedback about the effectiveness, efficiency, and safety of performance. Note how the employee has contributed to the department's achievements. Document your comments, including both positive feedback and constructive criticism. Be careful to avoid allowing an employee's positive or negative qualities in one area to influence your assessment in other areas. Be watchful of being overly lenient or strict. Be objective and balanced, and focus feedback on task performance. Numerous Websites offer information on how to perform effective performance evaluations and can alert you to additional factors to be aware of.

When the performance appraisal is completed, it is time to meet with the employee. The purpose of this meeting is to provide an opportunity for the supervisor and supervisee to discuss the employee's job performance and to collaborate on ways to improve it. Unfortunately, performance appraisal meetings are often viewed as anxiety-provoking events that focus on what the employee has done wrong. The common emphasis on the supervisor's rating of the employee tends to detract from a collaborative educational process during which supervisee and supervisor share perspectives and work together to identify barriers to improved performance. The supervisor can use several approaches to correct this problem:

4. **Demystify the process.** Make sure the employee is familiar with the evaluation process ahead of time. If a standard form is used, make sure the employee has seen it and understands any terminology or rating scales that are used. Make sure the employee is aware of the job expectations and standards. Involvement of staff members in establishing performance standards promotes adherence to and acceptance of standards. Involve the employee in the appraisal process by using a self-assessment.
5. **Plan ahead.** Notify the employee ahead of time as to when the meeting will be, and allow the employee time to prepare.
6. **Establish a comfortable climate for the exchange.** Meet in private. Avoid interruptions. Allow adequate time for discussion. Put the employee at ease in the beginning and explain that you view this time as an opportunity for mutual sharing on how to improve job performance for the benefit of the employee and the organization.

During the performance appraisal interview, be prepared to collaborate with the employee and exchange ideas. Share accomplishments, and review what has not been accomplished. If performance ratings are provided, be sure to provide reasons for your ratings that are based on actual job performance. If the employee is surprised by any of your ratings or comments, you probably have not provided enough regular feedback during the year. Take note and work to correct that. The appraisal interview offers another opportunity to realign expectations about job performance and to target goals for the future.

Handling Work Performance Problems

Although there are numerous types of performance problems in professional practice settings, the most common ones are behavior or conduct problems in which a rule is broken, performance that falls below the standard expected, and interpersonal issues that interfere with department morale and effectiveness. Each type of problem is handled differently, but in all situations, the actions that are taken are directed toward helping the employee to improve performance and meet job expectations.

Behavior or Conduct Problems

Behavior or conduct problems are handled by disciplining. Behavior or conduct problems may include absenteeism, chronic late arrival, intoxication, insubordination, negligence in following procedures, and falsification of records. These are all serious infractions and should not be allowed to persist. Although individual facilities may adopt their own specific procedures for disciplining a variety of infractions, disciplining is generally handled in a progressive manner. In a progressive discipline approach, the employee is counseled repeatedly if performance does not improve, and the penalties for noncompliance with the rules become increasingly harsh (see Figure 72.3).

In the first stage of progressive disciplining, the performance problem is discussed with the employee, clear expectations for acceptable performance are outlined, and consequences of not improving are described. In the second stage, the process is repeated, and this time, a written record of the exchange is documented. The employee signs it, and it is placed in his or her personnel file. If the behavior persists, in the third stage, the employee is laid off for a period of time and is told that when he or she returns to work, the behavior must be corrected

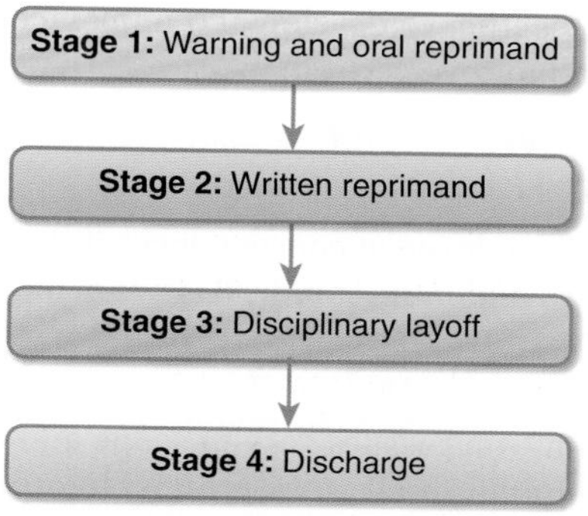

FIGURE 72.3 Using a standard sequence for dealing with performance problems is required in many formal organizations and is considered good practice in most settings.

or the employee will be discharged. The last stage occurs if the employee returns to work and another infraction occurs, at which time the employee is discharged.

A useful analogy for administering any discipline is the "red-hot stove" rule. The analogy likens the process of administering discipline to that of touching a red-hot stove and points out the four essential characteristics of a good disciplinary policy and practice. Discipline should be administered in the following manner:

- **With advance warning.** When you see a red-hot stove, you know that if you touch it, you will be burned. An employee should know what will happen if he or she breaks a rule or policy.
- **Immediately.** When you touch a red-hot stove, you will be burned right away. Administration of discipline should be done as soon after the occurrence of the behavior as possible.
- **Impartially.** No matter who touches a red-hot stove, the person will be burned. Supervisors should not play favorites in administering discipline. Everyone should receive the same penalty for the same infraction.
- **Consistently.** Every time you touch a red-hot stove, you get burned. Discipline should be administered the same way with each occurrence.

Performance Problems

Problems of substandard performance may occur in professional practice. When dealing with these types of problems, the supervisor needs to adopt an approach of collaborating with the supervisee and enlisting his or her help in resolving the problem. Typical steps in dealing with this type of problem after the performance problem is identified include the following:

1. Meet with supervisee and point out the performance problem. Review the standard and describe the expected performance.
2. Collaborate with the supervisee to determine reasons for the problem.
3. Work together to develop and implement an action plan to improve performance.
4. Monitor performance.
5. Repeat the process if needed.
6. Inform employee of consequences if the standard is achieved and if the standard is not achieved.

Interpersonal Work Issues

Interpersonal work issues vary in scope and complexity and are common in all work groups. In a professional practice environment in which teamwork is central to the department's effectiveness and to the achievement of positive client outcomes, problems among workers should not be ignored. Interpersonal issues can arise among practitioners in the occupational therapy department or among team members from different disciplines. These types of work problems often stem from miscommunication and/or differences in communication styles or personalities. Lack of clarity about job roles or about expectations can also lead to interpersonal problems.

Just because two people are different or disagree does not mean that they cannot work effectively together. The supervisor's role in resolving these types of performance issues should focus not on personalities, individuals, or differences but on the job tasks and mutual goals that need to be accomplished. The first approach to take when an employee complains to you about another employee is to listen carefully and encourage the person with the complaint to talk directly to the other individual. You should help the person to clarify his or her concerns and frame them in terms of how the other person's actions are affecting the person's ability to get his or her own job done. This approach often works and begins the process of opening communication.

When this approach does not work, you might need to take further action by talking to each of the parties involved. You might want to do this individually at first and then together, or you might want to approach the problem by talking to the parties at the same time. In either case, you will want to interview both to understand all of the facts and frame the issues or problems in terms of specific behavior and job performance expectations that are being affected. As the supervisor, you also must be clear about your expectations for job performance actions and attitudes and remind both of them about the department's expectations. During this discussion, each party should become more aware of his or her own behaviors as well as the behaviors of the other and how the interaction of their choices is affecting their work. Your goal in this exchange is for both parties to work out a solution that does not compromise the work of either and allows the work of the department to continue more effectively.

Supervision of Occupational Therapy Personnel

Effective supervision of OT personnel is necessary to ensure safe and effective delivery of services. As was mentioned at the beginning of this chapter, supervision is embedded within the OT process. However, OT practitioners work in a broad range of work environments (medical, educational, and community-based settings). To guide practitioners in developing effective supervisory practices in these different situations, professional organizations may develop supervisory guidelines that can be applied in all settings. These guidelines describe how the profession views the supervisory process, who needs to be supervised, the methods and frequency of supervision, and supervisory responsibilities of different occupational therapy personnel.

Occupational Therapists

The AOTA describes OTs as "autonomous practitioners who are able to deliver services independently" (AOTA, 2009, p. 797). Likewise, the WFOT endorses the autonomy of the profession (WFOT Council, 2007) and describes the minimum qualifications for OTs (WFOT, 2008). Entry-level OTs are qualified to practice without supervision. The therapist's preparation to deliver services independently is based on education and training, which in the United States includes a minimum of 6 months of supervised fieldwork experience and successful completion of the initial certification exam. Entry-level OTs are trained as generalists and are qualified to enter general practice settings as autonomous therapists. Although entry-level therapists do not require supervision, in the past, close supervision by an intermediate or advanced level OT was recommended by AOTA (1999). As the profession moved to entry-level master's degree preparation in the United States, thinking shifted; and responsibility is now placed on every therapist, at all levels of experience, to assess his or her personal need for supervision and seek it if needed. The current guidelines state that "occupational therapists are encouraged to seek supervision and mentoring to develop best practice approaches and to promote professional growth" (AOTA, 2009, p. 797). This statement underscores each therapist's professional responsibility to maintain the competencies that are needed to provide safe and effective services. The therapist who enters a work setting that does not provide professional supervision should carefully compare his or her current competencies with the demands of the work setting. When this comparison reveals that current knowledge and skills may need further support or development, the therapist should seek supervision or mentoring to ensure competent practice and professional growth. Although this is not required, many entry-level therapists seek first-time jobs in which supervision will be available. These positions allow them more time to solidify clinical skills and develop confidence. Therapists beyond entry level should continue to assess their need for professional supervision if it is not provided in their work setting. Career changes, such as switching practice settings (from school to nursing home) or types of clients treated (children with autism to adults with spinal cord injuries), may challenge the therapist's current competency and alert the therapist to the need to seek supervision or mentoring (AOTA, 2010b; Youngstrom, 1998).

In many occupational therapy practice settings, there may be no formal supervision by another OT. In situations such as these, OTs often seek informal peer supervision from OTs in similar settings. They ask for feedback from each other and share case information, often problem solving together to plan effective interventions. The advent of social networking and Web-based resources has expanded the informal consultation resources available to practitioners. This is a positive and proactive approach that helps to ensure effective professional practice and personal competence.

Occupational Therapy Assistants

Although OTAs are used in as many as 23 other countries throughout the world (WFOT, 2010), supervisory guidelines are better developed in the United States. Our discussion of OTA supervision will be based on current practice in the United States. OTs working with OTAs in other countries will want to contact the professional association in those countries to determine if supervision requirements are different.

In the United States, OTAs who deliver occupational therapy services must be supervised by an OT (AOTA, 2009, 2010c). OTAs are trained and educated in basic occupational therapy approaches and techniques, and their role is one of assisting the OT with the delivery of services. The OT is responsible for all aspects of service delivery and works in partnership and collaboration with the OTA to provide appropriate services to clients. Entry-level OTs are expected to be able to supervise OTAs and to be knowledgeable about the collaborative supervisory relationship that the profession values (Accreditation Council for Occupational Therapy Education [ACOTE], 2008a). Entry-level OTAs are expected to be knowledgeable of the supervisory partnership and to seek supervision appropriately. OTAs, by virtue of their training and education, are often well qualified to take on related work roles (e.g., assistive technologists, activity program directors). When they do take jobs in these related work positions, they are not providing occupational therapy services and consequently do not need to be supervised by an OT.

Fieldwork Students

Level II fieldwork students at the therapist and assistant level both must be supervised by occupational therapy practitioners. In the United States, OT students must be supervised by an OT who has at least 1 year of experience after being initially certified by the National Board for Certification in Occupational Therapy (ACOTE, 2008a). OTA students may be supervised by either an OT or an OTA, who also must have at least 1 year of experience after initial certification (ACOTE, 2008b). If an OTA is providing the Level II supervision for the OTA student, it is understood that the supervising assistant is supervised by an OT. According to ACOTE, personnel who are qualified to supervise Level I OT or OTA students include OTs and OTAs as well as individuals from other disciplines such as psychology, social work, and teaching (ACOTE, 2008a, 2008b).

To benefit from Level II fieldwork supervision, the OT student needs to seek and respond to feedback that is given. The supervisory relationship that is established

TABLE 72.3 Patterns of Supervision: Who Can Supervise Whom?

	Personnel to Supervise							
				OT Fieldwork Student		OTA Fieldwork Student		
Type of Supervisor	**OTA**	**OT Aide**	**Volunteer**	**Level I**	**Level II**	**Level I**	**Level II**	**OT**
Entry-level OT	X	X	X	X		X		
OT with more than 1 year of experience	X	X	X	X	X	X	X	X
Entry-level OTA		X	X					
OTA with more than 1 year of experience	X	X	X	X		X	X	

OT, occupational therapist; OTA, occupational therapy assistant.

during fieldwork is similar to a professional supervisory relationship. Chapter 66 discusses the nature of supervision in the fieldwork setting.

Other Personnel

Other types of personnel who may assist with the provision of OT services or the management of services delivery, such as office personnel, OT aides, or volunteers, may be supervised by either OTs or OTAs. Table 72.3 provides an overview of whom various personnel may supervise.

Types of Supervision: Overseeing Various Aspects of Work

Work is a complex activity. The responsibility for supervising various aspects of work is sometimes assigned to different people. It is not uncommon for an occupational therapy practitioner to receive supervision from more than one person for different aspects of their work performance. Discussion of three distinct aspects of work performance and the type of supervision used to oversee that performance will help you to see how supervision in some settings may require a multifaceted approach.

Administrative Supervision

Administrative supervision is focused on monitoring performance and making sure that the supervisee's work performance and professional development meet the objectives and standards of the employing organization. Administrative supervisors focus on the administrative aspects of job performance, such as attendance, schedules, benefit usage, and checking for appropriate completion of assigned job tasks. This type of supervision correlates closely with the administrative function of supervision discussed earlier.

Administrative supervision can be provided by an OT or an OTA to other OTs and OTAs or to members of other disciplines. Likewise, members of other disciplines can administratively supervise OTs and OTAs. This type of supervision commonly occurs in public school settings in which school principals or special education administrators are the designated supervisors for OTs. As the OT's supervisor, the principal or special education administrator would be supervising the administrative aspects of the OT's work. Similarly, in rehabilitation settings, an OT may function in a management role, and thus provide administrative supervision to members of other disciplines such as physical therapy or speech-language pathology.

Clinical or Professional Practice Supervision

Supervision that is aimed at providing support, training, and evaluation of a supervisee's professional performance and development is called **professional practice supervision** or **clinical supervision**. The term *clinical supervision* was the most commonly used term in the past to describe this type of supervision. However, as more OTs and OTAs have moved into work settings outside the clinical medical model (e.g., school settings), the term *clinical supervision* seems less appropriate than the broader term *professional practice supervision*. In professional practice supervision, the supervisor's responsibilities extend beyond the purely administrative aspects of job performance and are additionally aimed at assisting and supporting the supervisee's development of professional discipline-specific skills, such as interviewing skills, appropriate use of selected therapeutic techniques, and professional reasoning.

Professional practice supervision can appropriately be provided only by a member of the supervisee's discipline. Consequently, it would not be appropriate for a physical therapist to provide professional practice supervision or clinical supervision to an OT. Likewise, an OT cannot be expected to provide professional practice or clinical supervision for a physical therapist. Professional practice supervision is the type of supervision that is provided by fieldwork educators during OT and OTA Level II fieldwork experiences. (Fieldwork educators also provide administrative supervision to students.) An OT may provide professional practice supervision to other OTs and OTAs, and an OTA may provide professional practice supervision to other OTAs. This type of supervision correlates closely with the educational and supportive supervisory functions.

Functional Supervision

A third type of supervision that is seen in some occupational therapy practice environments is **functional supervision** (AOTA, 1993, p. 1088). In this type of supervision, a specific aspect of work or a "function" of clinical practice is delegated to a specified individual to provide training and oversight in that aspect of work. The supervisor who is providing only functional supervision generally has advanced knowledge, skill, and competence in the area being supervised. For example, an OT supervisor of a new employee might request that another OT who is experienced in wheelchair assessment and positioning provide functional supervision to the new employee in this area. When providing functional supervision the supervisor is not responsible for the entire supervisory process, but rather supervises the person's performance and development of specific skills or competency in only the selected job function area.

Methods of Supervision

A professional practice supervisor needs to consider what supervisory methods will be most effective in developing and monitoring performance. Supervisees have different learning styles. Worksites have varying caseload demands, administrative requirements for supervision, and time available to provide supervision. Supervisory methods need to be selected to meet the supervisee's needs and the demands of the worksite.

The supervisor is responsible for initially orienting and training the supervisee and then supporting the supervisee's professional growth and development. Careful thought should be given to the type of teaching methods that will be most effective in learning new information and developing work skills. Should information be presented verbally? In writing? Via video? How interactive should the learning be? Should the learner simply observe without demonstrating his or her own

Commentary on the Evidence

Supervision in Occupational Therapy

The majority of research in supervision has been conducted by business and management researchers. Within the health care professions, nurses, social workers, and counseling psychologists have been the primary contributors to the research on clinical supervision. In occupational therapy, direct empirical evidence to support effective supervisory practice is lacking. The research that is available in occupational therapy is often related to management issues and/or is descriptive in focus. For example, occupational therapy managers, concerned with employee satisfaction and retention, have shown that factors such as feedback and recognition of accomplishments, realistic workloads, and autonomy and opportunities for professional growth and skill development all influence job satisfaction (Barnes, 1998; Smith, 2000). Although these studies did not directly look at supervision, the factors that were identified are all factors that a supervisor can affect, so effective supervision should attend to these factors.

Two recent studies have provided some insight into current supervisory practices. Johnson, Koenig, Piersol, Santalucia, and Wachter-Schutz (2006) reported that more fieldwork educators who supervise Level I fieldwork students are not occupational therapists (OTs) than in the past. In April 2006, the National Board for Certification in Occupational Therapy reported the results of a 2005 online survey of OT and OTA certification exam candidates that included data on who the practitioner's primary supervisor was and the number of hours of direct supervision received per week (Bent & Conway, 2006). Thirty-eight percent of OTs and 23% of OTAs were supervised by members of other disciplines. Thirty-one percent of OTs and 18% of OTA received zero hours of direct supervision per week. Descriptive statistics such as these prompt us to ask other questions: How does being supervised by someone who is not an OT affect practitioners' professional growth and commitment to occupation-based practice? Does frequency of direct supervision affect the quality of services delivered and the rate of professional growth?

Research about supervision practices with OT fieldwork students is somewhat more prevalent. Some researchers have explored the supervisory experiences of fieldwork educators (Richard, 2008) to identify supervision issues. Others have studied the effectiveness of different models of supervision: use of non-OT supervisors for Level I fieldwork experiences (Heine & Bennett, 2003) and use of an aggregate fieldwork model (Precin, 2009).

Both descriptive and empirical studies of supervision in occupational therapy are needed. How do supervisory practices vary by setting? What is the most efficient and effective way to establish service competency with an OTA? What supervisory approaches are most effective in supporting professional growth and development with supervisees? These are only a few of the many questions that need to be answered to provide supervisors with the evidence they need to supervise effectively.

BOX 72.4 Examples of Learning Methods

- Provide written protocols or instructions.
- Have the learner report back on what he or she learned from reading.
- Provide articles or books to read or use as reference.
- Demonstrate and have the learner return the demonstration.
- Provide a verbal explanation or lecture that covers the content.
- Provide videotapes with questions about content to answer at end.
- Have the learner participate in small group discussion to problem-solve clinical situations.
- Discuss cases or problems presented, either one on one or in small groups.
- Role-play situations.
- Provide repeated practice opportunities to apply new knowledge and skills.
- Observe others carrying out tasks; ask the learner to describe what he or she observed.
- Model desired performance and behaviors.

skills? Should questions be encouraged? It is a good idea to vary methods and to select the ones that mesh with the learner's skill and comfort level. Involve the supervisee in the process by asking what learning approaches he or she prefers. Box 72.4 lists examples of various learning methods.

To monitor and evaluate performance, the supervisor can use direct and indirect approaches.

Direct or Line-of-Sight Supervision

In direct or line-of-sight methods of supervision, the supervisor is present when the employee is performing the job and actually observes performance. When we think of supervision methods, this approach is generally the first one that comes to mind. Direct observation gives firsthand information to the supervisor, but this approach is time consuming, and it is not always practical to use as the only method of supervision.

Indirect Supervision

Indirect methods allow the supervisor to ascertain how the job was performed by gathering this information after performance occurs. Indirect methods include communicating with the supervisee (via phone, e-mail, or written correspondence) after performance, looking at written records (attendance records, documentation), or receiving reports from others (clients, parents, other staff, or team members) about the supervisee's performance. Listening to what others say provides information about the employee's performance and provides feedback about how others perceive the performance. Supervising performance in a clinical setting by reading the supervisee's documentation is a frequently used indirect method in occupational therapy practice. Reading documentation tells the supervisor what happened when clients were seen and provides insight into the supervisee's clinical reasoning and documentation skills. However, using only the indirect method of supervision without also periodically observing performance would not give the supervisor a well-rounded picture of the employee's performance in areas such as interpersonal skill, technique application, adaptability in spontaneous clinical situations, and problem solving. Both indirect and direct methods need to be used to develop an accurate and complete picture of employee performance.

Frequency of Supervision

One of the first decisions a supervisor must make when developing a supervision plan is to determine how frequently to have contact with the supervisee to teach, train, monitor, and evaluate performance. The members of the profession have considered this question in relation to how frequency of supervision should be determined in supervising OTAs (see AOTA, 2009, p. 798). The factors that are outlined next can be considered in all supervisory situations. In determining frequency of supervisory contact, the supervisor should consider the following:

1. **His or her own supervisory skills.** Supervisors who are new and just developing their skills might require more frequent contact with the supervisee because they are less efficient in observing and analyzing performance. They might need more time to recognize possible performance issues and to provide supervisory interventions. The supervisor who has had more experience and/or who has previously supervised in a setting might be clearer about performance expectations and able to anticipate problems and provide guidance and direction sooner.
2. **The skills of the supervisee.** New employees who come to a job with background and experience in a similar job probably bring the needed skills to the new job. Generally, these employees will require less initial training and often move very quickly to a point at which they need less frequent supervision. The supervisor, however, must individually evaluate each employee because experience does not always guarantee effective performance. The employee's speed and style of learning will also affect the frequency of supervision needed.

TABLE 72.4 Continuum of Supervision

Frequency of Supervision	Definition
• Continuous	Supervisor is in sight of the supervisee who is working (AOTA, 1999, p. 592)
• Close supervision	Requires daily, direct contact at the site of work (AOTA, 1999, p. 592)
• Routine supervision	Requires direct contact at least every 2 weeks at the site of work, with interim supervision occurring by other methods, such as telephone or written communication (AOTA, 1999, p. 592)
• General supervision	At least monthly direct contact, with supervision available as needed by other methods (AOTA, 1999, p. 592)
• Minimal supervision	Provided only as needed and may be less than monthly (AOTA, 1999, p. 592)

3. **The nature of the work.** Work that is more varied and complex might require more frequent supervisory contact to allow the supervisor to observe performance at different times under various conditions and levels of complexity. The new OT working in a rehabilitation hospital whose caseload consists only of patients who had stroke might require less frequent supervision than the new OT who is working in an acute care setting seeing clients with orthopedic, neurological, and acute medical conditions.
4. **The expectations and requirements of the work setting.** In various work settings, standards and expectations may have developed, based on experience in that setting, that require certain levels of supervision. Although an experienced supervisor might think that weekly contact is sufficient, a worksite might require daily contact.
5. **The expectations and requirements of external regulatory or legislative agencies.** Federal or state laws and regulations and accrediting agencies may specify certain methods of oversight and contact that must occur between the OT and OTA.

Frequency of supervision is generally viewed as occurring on a continuum. At the high end of the continuum, the supervisor is continually in sight of the supervisee who is working. At the low end of the continuum, the supervisor contacts the supervisee only as needed. Table 72.4 provides a description of the various levels along the continuum. In the past, the profession recommended certain frequency levels of supervision for therapists and assistants who were at various experience levels. This approach has been replaced by a more flexible approach that recognizes the variety of factors needed to contribute to the supervisory frequency decision and allows for increased flexibility in dealing with the wide variety of practice setting and supervisory demands that exist within the profession. There are, however, two firm directives regarding need for supervision adopted by the profession:

1. Entry-level OTs do not *require* supervision. They are, however, "encouraged to seek supervision and mentoring to develop best practice approaches and promote professional growth" (AOTA, 2009, p. 797).
2. OTAs must *always* receive some level of regular supervision from an OT when they are providing occupational therapy services.

The OT/OTA Supervisory Relationship

In the United States, where the role of the OTA has been developed over a longer period of time, the profession perceives the supervisory relationship between the OT and OTA as a partnership. The discussion that follows describing the OT–OTA supervisory relationship is based on this partnership perspective.

Both levels of practitioners in the United States are trained and educated within the profession but at different levels. The OT is educated at the professional knowledge and skill level and receives an entry-level graduate degree. The OTA is educated at the technical level and receives an associate of arts degree. Each level of practitioner has complementary but distinct roles. The OT is responsible for overall service provision and can carry out all facets of service provision (i.e., evaluation, intervention planning, intervention implementation and review, and outcomes assessment). The OTA's primary role is in the implementation phase of service provision. OTAs may contribute to other aspects of service provision, such as performing selected assessments or recommending intervention changes under the supervision of the OT.

The "Guidelines for Supervision, Roles, and Responsibilities during the Delivery of Occupational Therapy Services" (AOTA, 2009) outlines the roles and responsibilities of each level of practitioner during the delivery of services. For the partnership to be successful, the OT and OTA each must have a clear understanding of each other's role and respect and value the contribution that each practitioner makes. When the OT and OTA work as a team, they are able to use and build on each other's skills and expand the number and kinds of services that can be provided to clients. When an OT

Practice Dilemma

Changing Practice Patterns: Taylor Supervises an OTA

Taylor recently started a new job as an occupational therapist (OT) at a large long-term care facility in her community. She works with a team of two other OTs and two occupational therapy assistants (OTAs). She is responsible for supervising Diane, one of the OTAs. Diane has been working at this facility for 5 years and considers herself very experienced in dealing with this population. When Taylor started the job, she met with Diane to discuss their supervisory relationship and to determine how they would conduct their OT–OTA partnership. Taylor spent time observing and working with Diane and found Diane to be very helpful in orienting her to the facility and familiarizing her with the patients and the typical occupational therapy interventions that were being used.

Taylor has now worked at the facility for more than 6 months and is more familiar with the clients and their individual needs. She is interested in developing intervention plans that are more individualized and that use intervention activities that relate to each patient's own needs and personal lifestyle choices, whether they will return home or remain in the nursing home's long-term care wing. Interventions in the past have been focused primarily on self-care issues, and Taylor, although not wanting to ignore these occupations, would like to emphasize more instrumental activities of daily living and leisure occupations in which patients will want to engage if they return home or that might allow them to increase their sense of self-efficacy and control if they remain in long-term care. She has communicated this goal to Diane, and when they develop intervention plans, individualized goals are developed in these areas. However, as she follows up with Diane and observes interventions and monitors patient progress, Taylor has noted that Diane is not choosing to address these goals and continues to use the routine types of tasks and activities that she was previously using.

Questions

1. How would you define the supervisory issues and problems in this situation?
2. As a supervisor in this scenario, what are Taylor's responsibilities?
3. As a supervisee in this scenario, what are Diane's responsibilities?
4. What do you think might be some of the reasons for Diane's behavior?
5. How would you suggest that Taylor approach Diane and address this problem?
6. What do you think might be some supervisory interventions that Taylor could take that would help to improve this situation?

partners with an OTA, the OT is often able to see more clients and to use the OTA's personal expertise in specific practice areas or techniques to improve client care. See the Practice Dilemma box for a discussion of dilemmas that can occur when supervising an OTA.

Service Competency

The purpose of the supervisory process is to ensure that safe and effective services are delivered and that professional competence is fostered. The OT who carries the responsibility for overall service delivery must ensure that the OTA is performing effectively. To ensure that services provided by both levels of practitioners are safe and effective, the OT establishes service competency with the OTA.

> Service competency is the process of teaching, training, and evaluating in which the occupational therapist determines that the occupational therapy assistant performs tasks in the same way that the occupational therapist would and achieves the same outcomes. (AOTA, 1999)

When the OT and OTA initially start working together, the OT will establish service competency for overall job performance. In the early stages of the work relationship, the OT will need to determine what knowledge and skills the OTA has. The establishment of service competency is integrated into the normal supervisory process as the supervisor orients and trains the new employee and begins comparing the employee's performance to the established professional and worksite standards and expectations. The OT should identify the primary job tasks and skills that are needed for the OTA's job. These tasks will vary by site and service setting. The OT will observe and train the OTA and note whether the OTA can perform the identified skills and tasks and whether intervention outcomes are similar to those normally achieved by the OT. Examples of job tasks or skills for which service competency may be established include reading the medical record, being able to record appropriate and pertinent information, and being able to appropriately grade an activity to increase its cognitive difficulty.

The concept of service competency is based on the assumption that the supervising OT is competent in the skills for which competency is being established.

Both levels of practitioners are responsible for being aware of each other's competent behaviors and providing feedback to inform each other of possible problem areas.

It is important that the supervisor establish an acceptable standard of performance or level of agreement for skills and tasks on which service competency is being established. For example, when observing client dressing performance, the OTA will rate the client's level of independence at the same level as the OT 95% of the time. The comparison of outcomes between practitioners is an approach that helps to ensure that services clients receive are of comparable quality. It supports the validity of delegating to the OTA and ensures consistency of services. The methods the OT can use while establishing service competency could include observation, cotreatment, return demonstration of techniques or skills, review of documentation, testing for knowledge and its application, and discussion of cases to ascertain clinical reasoning and judgment.

After initial service competency is established, the OT supervisor will need to periodically recheck service competency to ensure that it is maintained. The OT may also select new tasks and skills in which to establish service competency with the OTA. For example, the OT might decide to train the OTA in how to carry out and score a particular structured assessment tool. After service competency has been established, the OT can delegate the administration of this assessment to the OTA and be assured that the results of the OTA's giving the test will be comparable to the results that would be obtained if the OT administered the test. Service competency does not mean that the OTA will perform the task in exactly the same manner as the OTA would—only that the outcomes will be similar.

Frequency and Type of OTA Supervision

The decisions about frequency of supervision for the OTA will vary with practice setting and should be decided based on the five factors previously discussed: skills of the supervisor, skills of the supervisee, nature of the work, expectations and requirements of the work setting, and expectations and requirements of external regulatory or legislative agencies. The OTA's level of service competency and skill will influence the frequency of supervision needed. If service competency has already been established, the need for supervision might be less frequent. When service competency is being established in a new area or skill, the supervisor will need to change the frequency of supervision until competency is established.

Work factors that can affect frequency of supervision needed by an OTA include increased complexity of client's needs and diagnoses, rapidity of client change, more involved or complex types of interventions, and increased number and diversity of clients in the assistant's caseload. When the client population is complex and/or rapidly changing, frequent reevaluation and adjustment in types of interventions and implementation plans are needed, which require the clinical reasoning and evaluation skills of the OT. Frequency of supervision needs should be regularly reassessed as workplace demands, client needs, and supervisee skills change.

Because the supervisory process with the OTA is collaborative and both practitioners are responsible for providing safe and effective services, the OT and OTA should discuss the decision about the frequency of supervision. Supervision frequency and methods should be mutually decided upon.

Although frequency of supervision can vary, OTAs who are providing occupational therapy services will always need some level of regular supervision. Supervision of the OTA on an irregular, spontaneous, or as-needed basis is not appropriate. It does not demonstrate that the OT is providing the ongoing oversight required to ensure safe and effective services nor does it validate that high-quality occupational therapy is being provided. Many external regulatory and legislative agencies now specify the frequency and type of supervisory contact that must take place between OT and OTA. The Centers for Medicare and Medicaid Services (CMS) states that the OTA providing services to Medicare patients under an OT working in a physician's office must have direct or on-site (in the building but not in the line of sight) supervision on the day of treatment (U.S. Department of Health and Human Services & CMS, 2006). In February 2006, CMS also clarified that the OT is required to write a progress report every 10 treatment days or once every 30-day interval and requires that the OT perform or actively participate in treatments at this frequency level if the treatments have been delegated to an OTA (Thomas, 2006). This requirement necessitates that the OT have regular contact with the client and with the OTA who is providing services. Many state regulatory agencies outline specific supervision requirements in their laws for OTA supervision. Texas requires a minimum of 6 hours per month of frequent communication including review of patient/client progress plus a minimum of 2 hours of face-to-face interaction with the OT directly observing the OTA's treatment (Occupational Therapy Practice Act, 2011). Pennsylvania states that the OT supervisor shall have supervisory contact with the OTA equal to at least 10% of the time that the OTA works in direct patient care. Face-to-face contact must occur on site at least once a month and must include direct observation of the OTA performing occupational therapy (Professional and Vocational Standard, 1992).

Effective OTA Supervisory Relationship

The OT supervisor has the obligation and responsibility to supervise the OTA, and the OTA has the obligation and responsibility to seek supervision. Each is open to the other. In writing about their own collaborative relationship, Barbara Hanft and Barbara Banks (1999) identified six qualities that support the development of collaborative supervisory relationships:

- *Sensitivity*, for perceiving and responding to one another's professional and personal needs;
- *Dependability*, for keeping commitments and responding to unexpected situations;

BOX 72.5 Summary of Steps to Take in Supervising an OTA

1. Orient occupational therapy assistant (OTA) to worksite.
2. Share job and professional expectations.
3. Identify OTA's skill level.
4. Identify OTA's learning needs and methods of learning—ASK!
5. Establish service competency.
6. Collaborate with OTA to establish ongoing supervisory plan:
   a. Select methods.
   b. Select frequency.
7. Document ongoing supervision.

- *Attentiveness*, for actively listening to one another;
- *Respectfulness*, for appreciating one another's distinct knowledge, experiences and judgment;
- *Collaborativeness*, for working toward a common goal and representing occupational therapy services together as a unit; and
- *Reflection*, for an ability to use self-observation to review situations objectively from different perspectives. (p. 31)

In a collaborative relationship, both parties understand their unique roles and responsibilities and respect their differences and similarities (Sands, 1998). The process of supervising the OTA will include the OTA in the decision-making process and will be individually tailored to meet the needs of the OTA and the worksite. Box 72.5 presents a summary of the primary steps that should be taken in supervising an OTA.

Ethical Dilemma

Joel Supervises an Employee with Depression

Joel is a supervising occupational therapist (OT) in a large metropolitan acute care hospital. He oversees a group of three OTs and one occupational therapy assistant. Recently, one of his supervisees, Naomi, met with him and told him that she has been diagnosed with clinical depression. Joel is not surprised. He had noted that Naomi's work performance had changed, and he was even beginning to become concerned about the quality of Naomi's patient care decisions and her ability to handle the normally fast-paced caseload. Naomi has asked for Joel's help and support by decreasing her caseload so that she may continue to work in an effective manner.

Questions

1. Who are the different players in this scenario to whom Joel has an obligation or duty?
2. As a supervisor, what are Joel's obligations to each player?
3. How are the different needs of the players conflicting?

Supervising Occupational Therapy Aides

Occupational therapy aides are individuals with no formalized education in the provision of occupational therapy services who are hired to provide supportive services to OT practitioners. Aides are trained on the job to meet the specific needs of the individual department. Aides do not provide skilled occupational therapy services, and the types of activities they can perform with clients are clearly prescribed in the "Guidelines for Supervision, Roles, and Responsibilities during the Delivery of Occupational Therapy Services" (AOTA, 2009). Aides can perform two types of tasks within the department: They can carry out (1) non–client-related tasks such as clerical work, clinic maintenance tasks, and preparation of work areas and equipment and (2) selected client-related tasks that are routine and supervised by an OT or OTA (AOTA, 2009). For a task to be considered routine, it must meet the following four criteria:

1. The outcome anticipated for the delegated task is predictable.
2. The situation of the client and the environment is stable and will not require that judgments, interpretations, or adaptations be made by the aide.
3. The client has demonstrated some previous performance ability in executing the task.
4. The task routine and process have been clearly established (AOTA, 2009).

These criteria are based on the understanding that aides do not have the knowledge and skill to evaluate or make changes in an intervention activity but can be helpful in providing oversight or practice of selected activities when change and judgment are not anticipated.

Before a selected task can be delegated to an aide, the OT and/or OTA must be assured that the aide can carry out the task safely and effectively. They must instruct the aide and assess his or her competency in performing the delegated task. The aide also must be aware of all precautions and signs or symptoms that a particular client might demonstrate that would indicate that the aide needs to seek assistance (AOTA, 2009). Each of these requirements is intended to ensure that the aide's interaction with the client will be safe and effective. Practitioners can appropriately use aides to oversee clients who are practicing certain skills after the process has been set up (e.g., one-handed shoe tying and exercise routines). Aides can also provide another pair of hands during physical activities when additional help is needed to engage the client in an activity as when providing assistance to transfer a patient.

Aides can be supervised by either an OT or an OTA. However, when the OTA supervises the aide, the OT maintains overall responsibility for the process because of the OT's supervision of the OTA.

Frequency of supervision will vary with tasks assigned and the aide's skill. Client-related tasks may require closer supervision because of the importance of patient safety and intervention effectiveness. The supervisory plan and process need to be documented to demonstrate accountability.

Supervising Non-OT Personnel

The same basic guidelines and process for effective supervision should be followed in supervising non-OT personnel. The OT who assumes a supervisory or management role may supervise personnel from other disciplines who provide direct services to clients (e.g., physical therapists, psychologists, recreational therapists) as well as personnel who provide support services for the department (e.g., secretaries, reimbursement specialists, information technology specialists). The type of supervision the OT will provide to personnel from other disciplines will be administrative. OTs cannot provide professional practice supervision or clinical supervision because OTs are not trained in the other individuals' professions. Astute supervisors will ensure that their supervisees from other disciplines seek and have access to professional practice supervision and will consult with members of the supervisee's discipline to assist them in evaluating the supervisee's professional practice performance.

Conclusion

Supervision is a person-oriented process—much like occupational therapy. The OT supervisor must continually balance the needs of the organization with the needs of supervisees to provide safe and effective services to clients. Awareness of the basic functions of supervision and an understanding of the supervisory process make up the first step in preparing practitioners for the supervisory role.

References

Accreditation Council for Occupational Therapy Education. (2008a). Accreditation standards for a master's-degree-level educational program for the occupational therapist. *American Journal of Occupational Therapy, 61*, 67–83.

Accreditation Council for Occupational Therapy Education. (2008b). Accreditation standards for an educational program for the occupational therapy assistant. *American Journal of Occupational Therapy, 61*, 662–671.

American Occupational Therapy Association. (1993). Occupational therapy roles. *American Journal of Occupational Therapy, 47*, 1087–1099.

American Occupational Therapy Association. (1999). Guide for the supervision of occupational therapy personnel in the delivery of occupational therapy services. *American Journal of Occupational Therapy, 53*, 592–594.

American Occupational Therapy Association. (2009). Guidelines for supervision, roles, and responsibilities during the delivery of occupational therapy services. *American Journal of Occupational Therapy, 63*, 797–803.

American Occupational Therapy Association. (2010a). Occupational therapy code of ethics and ethics standards (2010). *American Journal of Occupational Therapy, 64*, 151–160.

American Occupational Therapy Association. (2010b). Standards for continuing competence. *American Journal of Occupational Therapy, 64*, 411–413.

American Occupational Therapy Association. (2010c). Standards of practice for occupational therapy. *American Journal of Occupational Therapy, 64*, 415–420.

Barnes, D. S. (1998). Job satisfaction and the rehabilitation professional. *Administration and Management Special Interest Section Quarterly, 14*(4), 1–2.

Bent, M. A., & Conway, S. (2006). *Results of a national study profiling the 2005 certification candidate population.* Retrieved from http://www.nbcot.org

Braveman, B. (2006). *Leading and managing occupational therapy services: An evidence based approach.* Philadelphia, PA: F. A. Davis.

Hanft, B., & Banks, B. (1999, June). Competent supervision: a collaborative process. *OT Practice, 4*(5), 32–34.

Heine, D., & Bennett, N. (2003). Student perceptions of level I fieldwork supervision. *Occupational Therapy in Health Care, 17* 89–97.

Johnson, C. R., Koenig, K. P., Piersol, C. V., Santalucia, S. E., & Wachter-Schutz, W. (2006). Level I fieldwork today: A study of contexts and perceptions. *American Journal of Occupational Therapy, 60* 275–287.

Kadushin, A. (1992). *Supervision in social work* (3rd ed.). New York, NY: Columbia University Press.

McKean, E. (Ed.). (2005). *The New Oxford American Dictionary* (2nd ed.). New York, NY: Oxford University Press.

Newstrom, J. W. (2007). *Supervision: Managing for results* (9th ed.). Boston, MA: McGraw Hill Irwin.

Occupational Therapy Practice Act, 40 TAC § 454–373.3 (1999 & Supp. 2011).

Precin, P. (2009). An aggregate fieldwork model: Cooperative learning, research, and clinical project publication components. *Occupational Therapy in Mental Health, 25*(1), 62–82.

Professional and Vocational Standard, 49 PA Code § 42.22 (1992).

Richard, L. F. (2008). Exploring connections between theory and practice: Stories from fieldwork supervisors. *Occupational Therapy in Mental Health, 24*(2), 154–175.

Sands, M. (1998). Practitioner's perspective of the occupational therapist and occupational therapy assistant partnership. In M. E. Neistadt & E. B. Crepeau (Eds.), *Willard and Spackman's occupational therapy* (9th ed., pp. 83–89). Philadelphia, PA: Lippincott.

Smith, V. (2000). Survey of occupational therapy job satisfaction in today's health care environment. *Administration and Management Special Interest Section Quarterly, 16*(4), 1–2.

Thomas, J. (2006, April). Interpreting Medicare's documentation requirements. *OT Practice, 11*(7), 8.

Urish, C. (2004, February). Ongoing competence through mentoring. *OT Practice, 9*(3), 10.

U.S. Department of Health and Human Services, & Centers for Medicare and Medicaid Services. (2006). *11 part B billing scenarios for PTs and OTs.* Retrieved from www.cms.gov/.../Billing/.../11_Part_B_Billing_Scenarios_for_PTs_and_OTs. pdf

World Federation of Occupational Therapists. (2008). *Occupational therapy entry-level qualifications CM2008.* Retrieved from http://www.wfot.org/ResourceCentre/positionstatements.aspx

World Federation of Occupational Therapists. (2010). *OT human resources project 2010-alphabetical.* Retrieved from http://www.wfot.org/ResourceCentre/humanresourceproject.aspx

World Federation of Occupational Therapists Council. (2007). Professional OT autonomy-revised 2007. Retrieved from http://www.wfot/ResourceCentre/positionstatements.aspx

Youngstrom, M. J. (1998). Evolving competence in the practitioner role. *American Journal of Occupational Therapy, 52,* 716–720.

For additional resources on the subjects discussed in this chapter, visit http://thePoint.lww.com/Willard-Spackman12e.

CHAPTER 73

Consultation

Wendy M. Holmes, Claudia Leonard

LEARNING OBJECTIVES

After reading this chapter, the reader will be able to:

1. Describe the role, scope, and process of service-related occupational therapy (OT) consultation services
2. Recognize the diverse opportunities for service-related consultation within the profession
3. Discuss the competencies essential for an OT consultant
4. Articulate the business aspects of consultation services
5. Analyze the challenges, rewards, and ethical considerations associated with the consultant role

OUTLINE

Amanda holds the position of lead occupational therapist within a rehabilitation department at a small regional hospital. This is her first position since completing her occupational therapy (OT) educational program 2 years ago. The rehabilitation department also employs one part-time occupational therapist, a full-time occupational therapy assistant (OTA), and is managed by a rehabilitation nurse. The director of nursing at a local assisted living facility (ALF) contacted Amanda to request her assistance in developing a fall prevention and education program for staff. During a meeting, Amanda's supervisor encouraged her to provide the services as a consultant to the ALF and stated that the hospital would develop a contract as needed. Amanda is uncertain about how to respond. She is confident in her skills and abilities within her OT role at the hospital but always thought of consultation as a possible future role when she had more skills and experience within the profession. However, she is intrigued by the opportunity and needs to make a decision. As she thought about her decision, she identified the following key questions:

- Do I have the knowledge, skills, and experience to be a consultant in this situation?
- What would be the extent of my services, and how would I fit consultation in my current position at the hospital?
- What information do I need to develop a contract for consultation services?

OT practitioners provide consultation services within a continuum of services and settings. Opportunities for consultation are at times unanticipated but may only require a time-limited provision of services. Alternatively, consultation services can be the primary role of an occupational therapist in a private practice with multiple and extended contracts. The purpose of this chapter is to discuss the role and scope of consultation options for the OT practitioner. It will focus primarily on the range of OT service–related consultation as opposed to management consultation.

An Overview of Consultation

What Is Consultation?

Consultation is a collaborative process that takes place between a practitioner and clients, families, other professionals, organizations, or communities. The purpose of consultation is to identify and solve problems with engagement in occupations, prevent future problems, or achieve identified goals (Figure 73.1) (American Occupational Therapy Association [AOTA], 2008; Doll, 2010; Jaffe & Epstein, 2011; Sabatino, 2009). As a consultant, OT practitioners employ their expertise to develop programs, provide training and education, identify resources, and facilitate relationships on behalf of the recipient of services. The consultant to client relationship is based on a mutually agreed-on plan that describes how the consultant will address the occupational needs of the client. Moreover, the OT consultant is considered an expert in some area of practice and may be external to the client's existing service system or structure (Jaffe & Epstein, 2011).

Consultation involves the ability to analyze situations comprehensively and objectively in order to develop strategies and provide services that address the needs (Fazio, 2008; Jaffe & Epstein, 2011). The consultation process is a type of OT intervention identified in the AOTA's "Occupational Therapy Practice Framework: Domain and Process, 2nd Edition" (AOTA, 2008). As well, consultation services are considered an entry-level skill for new OT practitioners. Preparation for this role is required by the educational standards established by the Accreditation Council for Occupational Therapy Education (ACOTE, 2007) and the World Federation of Occupational Therapists (WFOT, 2002).

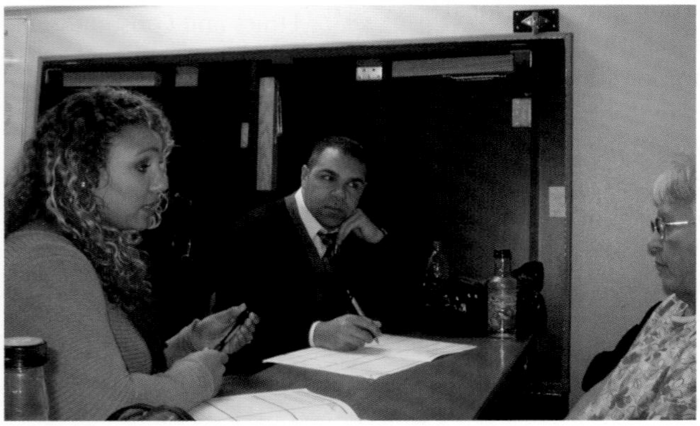

FIGURE 73.1 Consultation is a collaborative process with clients, families, other professionals, organizations, or communities to identify and solve problems with engagement in occupations, prevent future problems, or achieve identified goals.

There are different levels of consultation services: case centered, educational/collegial, and program/administration (Jaffe & Epstein, 2011, p. 524). These levels correspond to the potential recipients of OT services: persons, organizations, and populations included within the profession's domain and process (Framework II; AOTA, 2008). Providing consultation often involves elements of education and advocacy. However, the consultation process differs from direct OT services because as a consultant, the OT is not directly responsible for the outcome of the intervention (Framework II; AOTA, 2008). Service-related consultation differs from direct OT services because the consultant is helping other service providers address problems with participation rather than providing the services directly. The consultant typically does not have direct responsibility or authority to supervise or evaluate individuals unless that is specified within the consultation agreement (Sabatino, 2009).

The Consultation Role

The consultation role varies depending on the need for OT services and practice settings. It is a common role within school-based practice and in work-related programming (see Chapters 48 and 49). The ability to influence the desired change or achieve the targeted outcomes during the consultation process depends on numerous factors. For example, the relationship of the consultant to the client and others involved with the delivery of the OT services is a consideration. The OT consultant may be employed by the program or organization receiving services, as in school-based consultation. Or the consultant may be an independent contractor such as when hired by a local business to provide training for the prevention of work-related injuries. Examples of consultation services within specific practice settings will be discussed further in this chapter.

The Consultation Process

The consultation process can be thought of as occurring in progressive stages from initiation to termination of services, potentially with an opportunity for renegotiating ongoing services as needed (Golembiewski, 2000; Jaffe & Epstein 2011). However, the consultation process is organized, the fundamental steps share commonalities with the OT process (AOTA, 2008; Scaffa, 2001). Initially, the OT practitioner must become aware of the need for services. This may occur through a request for services (as with Amanda), the recognition of an opportunity to pursue (a community agency is developing a new skills program for individuals with mental illness), or from a strategic contact with a potential new client (a presentation to employees of a fitness center on health promotion for individuals with disabilities). Next, an agreement for services is reached, often in the form of a negotiated contract. The evaluative stage of the process requires the OT consultant to comprehensively assess the needs of the individual, group, or organization. Depending on the client and setting, the consultant may suggest completion of formal OT assessments or complete a comprehensive needs assessment. Frequently, interviews with family members, employees, volunteers, or others are required to fully understand the presenting problems and related factors. Once the issues or presenting problems are identified, the consultant collaboratively identifies the desired outcomes or goals with the client. It is then up to the OT consultant to design and develop a written plan of proposed services with time lines to submit to the client for consideration and a decision.

After the plan is accepted and services are delivered, the consultant must continuously gauge the progress toward the designated outcomes or goals, elicit feedback, and modify the services as needed with the permission of the client. Once the identified problems are addressed and resolved, the consultant communicates with the client in order to prepare for the termination of services. Depending on the type of consultation services, there may be an opportunity to renegotiate an agreement for continued services beyond the time specified in the initial contract or agreement. Throughout the process, the consultant provides written reports during each phase of the process: the evaluation and proposed plan, progress reports during the delivery of services, and a final report describing the outcomes achieved and further recommendations as appropriate. Figure 73.2 illustrates the typical stages and steps within the consultation process.

Assessing the Potential for Change

A consultant may provide services on a periodic, short- or long-term basis for client needs that vary in complexity. Furthermore, the consultant often has limited influence over the outcomes of the consultation process for problems that may involve significant behavioral changes from the individual client or other individuals. For those reasons, it is vital for the consultant to assess the client or organization's readiness for change. Borrowing from health behavior theories, the Transtheoretical or Stages of Change Model (DiClemente et al., 1991; National Cancer Institute, 2005; Prochaska & DiClemente, 1992) is one of several frameworks for evaluating and understanding the process of change useful to consultants. The Transtheoretical Model comprises six stages within the change process: precontemplation, contemplation, preparation, action, maintenance, and termination (Prochaska, Norcross, & DiClemente, 1994). According to the theory, individuals move within the stages of the change and may demonstrate repeated attempts to make a desired change. The consultant's task is to ask questions during interviews, gather comprehensive information about the past and current problems of concerns, and identify strategies to facilitate "movement or readiness for the next stages" (Reitz, Scaffa, Campbell, & Rhynders, 2010, p. 64), as services are being provided.

Systems Analysis

Consultants must possess the knowledge and skills to analyze and address a range of issues presenting within multiple, and often complex, systems. Consequently, understanding, incorporating, and applying OT practice models and additional theoretical frameworks are integral to the role. General and open systems theories (Braveman, 2006; Frankel & Gelman, 2004; McCormack, Jaffe, & Frey, 2003; von Bertalanffy, 1968) offer a useful perspective on families, organizations, agencies, and other systems. This theory views systems as cohesive, interrelated, and self-regulating entities that continuously process and respond to input from the environment. Through professional reasoning, the consultant uses this framework to systematically assess the internal and external factors of the contexts and environments during the evaluation phase of the process and when identifying potential solutions. The context is described within the

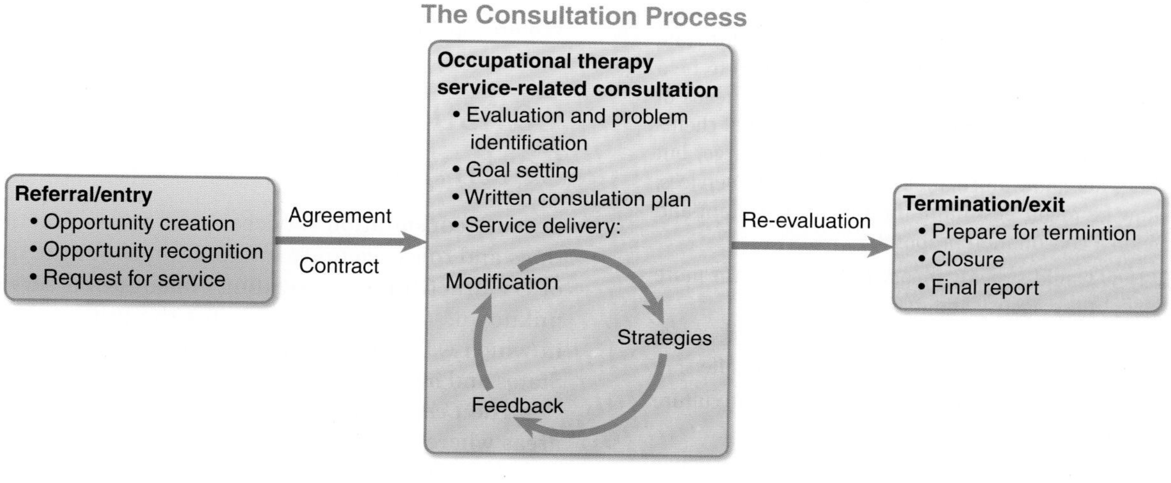

FIGURE 73.2 The consultation process.

"Occupational Therapy Practice Framework: Domain and Process" as the interrelated conditions within and surrounding the client that influence occupational performance such as cultural, personal, temporal, and virtual factors. The client's environment then includes the physical and social factors influencing the performance of occupations (AOTA, 2008, p. 670).

When applying systems theory to the analysis of client and the needs, it is also beneficial to consider a given situation from multiple levels in order to consider all of the internal factors and environment influences on the delivery of services (Frankel & Gelman, 2004; Reitz et al., 2010).

- The **micro level** considers the person and interpersonal factors in the scenario. The cultural and personal contexts of the individual receiving OT services along with those of other individuals within the social environment must be examined (AOTA, 2008).
- The **mezzo level** considers the factors of the environment external to the client including cultural, physical, temporal, and virtual elements.
- The **macro level** includes the broadest factors from the external environment, which affect policy, funding, services, and sociopolitical influences, which may be relevant to the identified need for services.

CASE STUDY 73.1 Considering a Consultation Opportunity

Peter is an occupational therapist employed by a rehabilitation hospital on a part-time basis. He also has a private practice focused primarily on consultation services for assistive technology evaluation, solutions, and training. He completed the requirements for his certification as an assistive technology professional (ATP) and provides consultation services to several school districts and an area independent living center. Recently, he received a request from his state Department of Vocational Rehabilitation (DVR) to be a consultant regarding the assistive technology needs of its clients. At the rehabilitation hospital, several clients were referred to DVR for services after discharge, but he does not know much about the agency, the services, or how he might best fulfill the role of consultant and develop a consultation proposal.

1. How would systems theory help Peter learn more about the agency and its services?
2. How might the micro, mezzo, and macro levels of DVR influence the OT consultation services Peter offers?
3. What questions about the organizational culture are pertinent for Peter to ask?
4. Is assessing the agency's readiness for change important in this scenario? Why or why not?

Success in the consultant role also requires an astute understanding and analysis of the related issues of individual and organizational culture, authority, and sources of power because these affect the ability to influence change and achieve the desired outcomes or goals. A tenet of all client-centered OT services is that the OT practitioner must understand the personal and cultural belief systems of the client and of the social context (AOTA, 2008; Crabtree, Royeen, & Benton, 2006). As a consultant, the development of an effective consultation plan depends on the exploration of the client's "cultural values, motivations, and expectations of the outcomes" (Crabtree et al., p. 4). From this exploration during the evaluation phase of the consultation process, the OT practitioner and client can more easily reach an accurate and realistic understanding regarding the type and scope of services to be provided.

Just as individuals and family members have values, beliefs, and attitudes influencing behavior and decisions, so do the employees or volunteers within organizations or agencies where consultants provide services. The culture of an organization encompasses the attitudes, experiences, beliefs, and values of that organization (Johnson, 2009). Ideas and expectations about how people should behave, how decisions are made, and who has the authority to make decisions are related to an organization's culture. Frequently, a consultant's plan for services may include recommendations for numerous changes within a family system or an organization. It is important for the consultant to recognize that the authority and power to ensure the recommended changes are made stems from the family member's or service provider's formal or informal position within the family system or organization and the degree of influence that individual has on other's beliefs, values, and behaviors (Ledlow & Coppola, 2011). Power can be thought as the ability to "stimulate productive action" and emerges from both individual characteristics and the organizational structure (Johnson, 2009, p. 138). The awareness of these elements allows the consultant to more effectively plan and deliver OT services. Refer to Case Study at http://thePoint.lww.com/Willard-Spackman12e for an illustration of these factors.

Consultation Practice Settings

Because consultation services occur across practice settings and roles, accurate information about the number of OT practitioners providing consultation services is unknown. Table 73.1 illustrates the practice settings in which OT consultation services occur in the United States and internationally.

The *Centennial Vision* (AOTA, 2006b) includes four areas where consultation is specifically identified. Also, the literature describes OT practitioners working in the areas of health and wellness, assistive technology, accessibility design and home modification, ergonomics, low

TABLE 73.1 Consulting Settings and Services: A Summary from the Evidence

Population	Type of Consultation Services	Payment Sources
Children	• Early intervention • School-based services	Government (regional or national)
	• Recreational programs	• Foundations
Adults	• Accessibility • ADA compliance • Assistive technology • Municipal health care	• Companies • Governmental organizations • Private pay
Workers	• Job analysis • Injury prevention • Ergonomics	• Companies • Governmental labor agencies • Worker unions
Older adults	• Aging in place • Home modification • Activity programs • Long-term care facilities	• Private pay • Insurance companies • Government agencies

ADA, Americans with Disabilities Act, 1991.

Sources: AOTA, 2010b; Banks, 2001; Cook & Hussey, 1995; Dunn, 1990, 2000; Furåker & Nilsson, 2011; Hanebrink & Parent, 2000; Mackersy, Robertson, & Mckay, 2003; Palisano, 1989; Pergrossi, 1999; Polichino & Scheer, 2006.

vision, and driver rehabilitation services (Dudgeon & Greenberg, 1998; Epstein, 1992; Gourley 2002; Jaffe, 1986, 1989; Siemsen, Bergstrom, & Hathaway, 2005). For OT practitioners in academic settings, consulting and pro bono work may be part of the culture to facilitate student supervision in Level 1 fieldwork and develop new experiences in Level II fieldwork or service learning opportunities. Case Study 73.2 describes a scenario common to consultation within school systems.

Knowledge, Skills, and Competencies for Consultation

Consultation requires a broad skill set and knowledge base in OT along with additional crucial areas of expertise. Both occupational therapists and OTAs may provide service-related consultation services. Because consultants are considered to have expertise in a particular area of OT practice, it is incumbent on the OT practitioners to carefully consider their knowledge, skills, and competencies for the consultation role and services requested. Continuing **competence** is an important focus for the profession, its leaders, and individual practitioners (AOTA, 2006a; AOTA, 2010c; Moyers Cleveland & Hinojosa, 2011). Chapter 67 offers information about the resources and processes for ongoing professional development within the profession. No matter the practice setting, when an OT practitioner is considering the role of consultant, an objective and careful evaluation of his or her readiness and ability to meet the recipient's needs are essential.

Before deciding whether to take on the role of consultant, an OT practitioner will need to review the profession's official documents. Important resources for U.S. practitioners include the *Standards of Practice for Occupational Therapy* (AOTA, 2010d) and the *Guidelines for Supervision, Roles, and Responsibilities During the Delivery of Occupational Therapy Services* (AOTA, 2009). It is also imperative to check legal factors such as licensure laws and regulations for OT practice. Additionally, practitioners must incorporate current research evidence and practice ethically. The depth of knowledge and level of skill for consulting is best determined by **service competency** based on performance within a practice setting. For example, a new graduate who has been working in a skilled nursing facility may have the competency level to provide consultation services regarding compliance training for the American with Disabilities Act (1991) and common environmental adaptations for individuals

CASE STUDY 73.2 Daniella: An Occupational Therapy Consultant in School Systems

Daniella is an occupational therapist in the western part of the United States. She provides services to a district that covers a broad geographic area, and most of her students are Native American. Due to the distances required, she can only travel to one of her elementary schools one day a week. She researched the evidence and appreciates the value of occupational therapy consultative services to teachers in classrooms. This approach seems especially appropriate because she has multiple children on caseload in one classroom.

Daniella knows that the combined first- and second-grade class teacher enjoys conducting story time with the children sitting cross-legged on the floor on traditional native rugs. Several of the children Daniella works with have difficulty with this position. One boy has attention deficit hyperactivity disorder (ADHD) and does not sit still through a story, which disrupts others and frustrates the teacher. Another student has cerebral palsy (CP), and her lower extremity spasticity decreases when she sits on a therapy ball or T-stool. Daniella requested a meeting with the teacher to consult on options for improved positioning during story time. She finds that the teacher is reluctant to give up the traditional rug usage but is willing to consider different positions.

1. What are the relevant issues for Daniella to consider in her consulting role?
2. What options would achieve the desired outcomes for supporting the desired sitting position and participation in story time for the students in the classroom?
3. What consultation skills and tools will help Daniella develop an effective response to the teacher?

with dementia. However, the same clinician would likely not have the competency level to consult regarding building a playground for children with disabilities due to limited experience, knowledge, and practice in this area.

For OTAs, an additional consideration is whether they are working under the supervision of an occupational therapist or if they are practicing outside of the OT role. For example, an OTA may work under the supervision of an occupational therapist to provide educational programs to consumer groups about durable medical equipment. Alternatively, by virtue of their education within the field, the OTA may independently provide consultation to activity therapists in skilled nursing facilities or work as a job coach for a developmental disabilities work transition program. When the OTA is not functioning in the OTA role, the level of supervision is not dictated by OT standards or state laws. (See Chapter 72 for further information about OT/OTA supervision).

For either the OT or the OTA practitioner, the identification of the line of supervision or authority, the recipient of the consultation services, and how the services are being reimbursed will all affect the roles assumed. The scope of the consultation may be limited to a single event or a short series of visits that results in a report. Consultations that continue for longer periods of time may require evolving roles by the OT practitioner to meet the needs of the consultation and setting.

Numerous authors suggest that the consultant role requires the demonstration of additional professional **competencies** based on diverse employment experiences (Fazio, 2008, Holmes & Scaffa, 2009; Jaffe & Epstein, 2011; McCormack, 2011; Scaffa, 2001; Scott, 2009). Additionally, authors propose that effective consultation requires the development of individual characteristics beyond those necessary for effectiveness in the direct service role. These are identified in Table 73.2.

TABLE 73.2 Additional Competencies and Characteristics Necessary for Consultants

Competencies and Characteristics	
Knowledge of:	Business ethics and behavior Systems theory and analysis Business principles Community systems and resources
Interpersonal skills & abilities for:	Personal resourcefulness Intercultural competence Strong active listening Strong oral and written communication skills Effective communication with various audiences Collaboration with diverse stakeholders Effective negotiation skills Conflict resolution skills Cultural competence
Performance skills to:	Envision OT services and roles Manage and prioritize time efficiently Advocate for client and needed services Educate and train effectively Monitor trends to identify opportunities for OT consultation services
Ethical practice to:	Suspend judgment—meet clients where they are Tolerate diverse points of view Able to establish and keep boundaries with recipients of services Practice self-assessment to identify needs for ongoing professional development
Individual traits, qualities, and characteristics demonstrated by:	Independence in generating and pursuing opportunities Self-confidence in skills and expertise for consultant role Tolerance of ambiguity for complex and unpredictable situations

OT, occupational therapy

Tools for Consultation

Contracts

Before agreeing to provide consultation services, an OT practitioner needs an understanding of the basic business aspects of this role. The degree of business acumen needed will depend on whether the consulting is done within a current work contract, such as school therapist consulting with a teacher, or through an independent contract. A general understanding of contracts, billing procedures, documentation, and marketing will benefit those starting out in independent consulting.

Contracts should be detailed enough to spell out who the participants are, what the terms of the consultation entail, and who is responsible for which actions within the consultation period. Including details of the type of written documentation expected at the conclusion of the consulting period and at any interim intervals that are deemed necessary is an excellent practice. Whether or not a **noncompete clause** needs to be included in a contract will depend on any potential overlap between the contracted services and the OT practitioner's other areas of practice. Confidentiality is usually expected in a contracted arrangement, and written, signed releases may be required if photographs or information are used for purposes other than agreed upon within the consultation contract. **Liability** and **tort law limits** can vary from state to state so unless the OT practitioner clearly understands the details and responsibilities of a contract, it is best not to sign the contract prematurely. Consulting a lawyer, or at minimum seeking out a template of a standard consulting contract, can be a good starting point. If the OT practitioner is using a contract developed and provided by the organization or agency receiving the consultation services, it is important to consider that the contract may not cover the practitioner for liability, and the protection of their assets will usually be their priority. An example of a sample contract that may be used for consultation is available on the Willard and Spackman's Website.

Billing and Reimbursement

For new consultants, understanding billing processes and determining how much to charge requires an understanding of the company's structure as well as an awareness of the supply and demand for OT services in the area. Some consultants charge by the hour. Hourly rates have the advantage of tracking time spent as a measure of work; however, for newer consultants, it may help to keep in mind that time incurred may be longer than anticipated until one understands the systems. Billing may need to be contained to reflect a maximum agreed-on limit of hours so that costs do not become exorbitant for the source being billed. Balancing out a fair rate is as much a factor of the perceived worth for your expertise because it is based on geographic considerations (Lahti & Beyerlein, 2000). Another option is to bill at the end of performed services, which can work well for a finite task such as ergonomic work station consulting. Yet another alternative for billing, practiced by lawyers and engineers more so than health service professionals, is to be placed on a retainer and ensure one is covered for services on a month-to-month or week-to-week basis. Retainers are more unpredictable for the source that is contracting and will likely only occur if OT practitioners demonstrate their worth and value as a consultant to a site.

Marketing

From a business perspective, the reputation of the consultant is what will earn a practitioner repeat business; therefore, it is very important to represent oneself well. Other ethical considerations follow in this chapter. Having an understanding of what unique services are being offered and a consultant's ability to market his or her knowledge and skill set separates one consultant from another (Lahti & Beyerlein, 2000). Numerous resources are available to assist the OT practitioner in marketing strategies, including local small business development centers, the U. S. Small Business Administration, and professional organizations such as AOTA and the American Marketing Association. Within the profession, resources are available for information on OT-specific marketing strategies (Braveman, 2006; Doll, 2010; Fazio, 2008; Richmond & Powers, 2004). Refer to the Willard and Spackman's Website for a comparative list of the benefits and challenges of the consultation process.

Ethics and Consultation

Consultants have an obligation to provide services that meet the standards for the profession around the world (AOTA, 2010d; WFOT, 2005). The role of expert advisor and practitioner can create situations where the pressure to provide services creates ethical problems or dilemmas (Purtillo, 2005). Examples of the type of ethical issues that consultants commonly face include lacking the appropriate knowledge, skills, experience, or time to provide the services clients require or being asked to provide services in a situation that may be a conflict of interest. The practitioner's professional reasoning is integral to making ethical decisions through the consultation process. Cherniss (2000) offered three key reflective questions for all consultants that may facilitate the reasoning process when considering the ethical dimensions of services (p. 183):

1. Should I consult in this situation?
2. If I do consult, whose interests will I serve?
3. What will be my primary focus?

It is important that practitioners understand ethical principles and related standards so that they are prepared to resolve ethical dilemmas that may occur (see Chapter 32). Because consultation is an inherently complex process, the practitioner's analytical skills are necessary to identify the underlying values and sources of conflict and separate the ethical issues from social or personal concerns (Arnold & Wilson Silver, 2003). An ethical dilemma common to OT practitioners is found in the following feature box.

Ethical Dilemma

Being Both an Employee and a Consultant

Jenna is a part-time staff occupational therapist for a rehabilitation center in the adult outpatient department in a small city. Her caseload includes adults with orthopedic, neurological, and chronic conditions, many of whom are older. Because of the prevalence of low vision within the aging population, Jenna completed a specialty certification in low vision offered by American Occupational Therapy Association. One month ago, she developed a consultation contract for occupational therapy (OT) services with the community-based agency serving adults with vision impairments, including blindness and low vision. The staff of the agency includes the director, a certified orientation mobility specialist (O & M), a certified low vision rehabilitation therapist (CVRT), and two rehabilitation teachers (Warren, 2011).

She received her first referral for consultation from the director for the community agency for an 82-year-old woman living alone with low vision from macular degeneration, rheumatoid arthritis, and symptoms from the early stages of dementia. After completing her consultation evaluation, Jenna developed a consultation plan including a limited number of OT sessions with the client and staff education on strategies for providing services to individuals with cognitive limitations.

During a routine meeting with her supervisor at the rehabilitation center, Jenna discussed her consultation practice in low vision. The supervisor expressed concerns about Jenna's consultation practice being a conflict of interest with her staff position at the rehabilitation center, stating that the client could receive all the needed services through the outpatient department at the rehabilitation facility.

1. What are the ethical considerations in this situation?
2. Which principles of the *Occupational Therapy Code of Ethics and Ethics Standards* (AOTA, 2010a) are relevant to consider?
3. Which professionals within the two systems of care would provide optimal services to meet this client's needs, and how could Jenna assure the client receives these services?
4. How should Jenna address the supervisor's concern about a potential conflict of interest?

BOX 73.1 Are You Ready to Be a Consultant?

- Do you have sufficient knowledge, skills, and experience with the client population to meet the needs?
- Do you need advanced or specialized certifications for this area of practice?
- Have you checked the state licensure law for information about your scope of practice?
- Do you have an understanding of occupational therapy models of practice and theoretical frameworks from other disciplines?
- Do you need mentoring or supervision to assist you in the role of consultant?
- Do you understand the business aspects of consultation and have resources to assist you as needed?
- Are you familiar with the *Occupational Therapy Code of Ethics and Ethics Standards* (AOTA, 2010a) and understand how to practice ethically as a consultant?
- Are you familiar with current research in order to practice with evidence?
- Are you able to communicate effectively in order to fulfill all aspects of the consultant role?

Conclusion

Providing OT services as a consultant offers the opportunity to address participation in occupations in diverse settings and situations. The potential to expand OT services and develop new skills exists. The consultation role is challenging yet can be rewarding and requires the OT practitioner to possess the necessary practice experience, knowledge, and competencies for providing services in an ethical and efficacious manner. For a checklist of your readiness to become a consultant, see Box 73.1.

Key to success in this role is the ability to develop collaborative relationships, pursue ongoing professional development, and seek out resources for the business and legal elements of the role. As the profession expands to meet its vision for the future, consultation services will continue to grow in importance and scope.

References

Accreditation Council for Occupational Therapy Education. (2007). Accreditation standards for the masters-degree-level educational program for the occupational therapist. *American Journal of Occupational Therapy, 61*, 652–661.

American Occupational Therapy Association. (2006a). *AOTA fact sheet: Continuing competence in the OT profession*. Bethesda, MD: Author.

American Occupational Therapy Association. (2006b). *Centennial vision*. Bethesda, MD: Author.

American Occupational Therapy Association. (2008). Occupational therapy practice framework: Domain and Process, 2nd edition. *American Journal of Occupational Therapy, 62*, 652–683.

American Occupational Therapy Association. (2009). *Guidelines for supervision, roles, and responsibilities during the delivery of occupational therapy services*. Bethesda, MD: Author.

American Occupational Therapy Association. (2010a). *Occupational therapy code of ethics and ethics standards*. Bethesda, MD: Author.

American Occupational Therapy Association. (2010b). *Occupational therapy compensation and workforce study*. Bethesda, MD: Author. Retrieved from http://www.aota.org/Practitioners.aspx

American Occupational Therapy Association. (2010c). *Standards for continuing competence*. Bethesda, MD: Author.

American Occupational Therapy Association. (2010d). *Standards of practice for occupational therapy*. Bethesda, MD: Author.

Americans with Disabilities Act of 1990. Pub. L. No. 101-336, § 2, 104 Stat 328 (1991).

Arnold, R. M., & Wilson Silver, M. H. (2003). Techniques for training ethics consultants: Why traditional classroom methods are not enough. In M. P. Aulisio, R. M. Arnold, & S. J. Youngner (Eds.), *Ethics consultation: From theory to practice* (pp. 70–87). Baltimore, MD: Johns Hopkins University Press.

Banks, F. M. (2001). Accessibility issues. In M. E. Scaffa (Ed.), *Occupational therapy in community-based practice settings* (pp. 119–136). Philadelphia, PA: F. A. Davis.

Braveman, B. (2006). *Leading and managing occupational therapy services: An evidence-based approach*. Philadelphia, PA: F. A. Davis.

Cherniss, C. (2000). Preentry issues revisited. In R. T. Golembiewski (Ed.), *Handbook of organizational consultation* (2nd ed., pp. 183–189). New York, NY: Marcel Dekker. Retrieved from http://web.ebscohost.com.ezproxy.brenau.edu:2048/ehost/ebookviewer/ebook/nlebk_44858_AN?sid=4577aa35-f19c-4dc7-b93a-f8e910a57085@sessionmgr104&vid=1&lpid=lp_COVER-0

Cook, A. M., & Hussey, S. M. (1995). *Assistive technologies: Principles and practice*. St. Louis, MO: Mosby.

Crabtree, J. L, Royeen, M., & Benton, J. (2006). Cultural proficiency in rehabilitation: An introduction. In M. Royeen & J. L. Crabtree (Eds.), *Culture in rehabilitation: From competency to proficiency* (pp. 1–16). Upper Saddle River, NJ: Pearson Prentice Hall.

DiClemente, C. C., Prochaska, J. O., Fairhurst, S. K., Velcier, W. F., Velasquez, M. M., & Rossi, J. A. (1991). The process of smoking cessation: An analysis of precontemplation, contemplation, and preparation stages of change. *Journal of Consulting and Clinical Psychology, 59*, 295–304.

Doll, J. (2010). *Program development and grant writing in occupational therapy: Making the connection*. Sudbury, MA: Jones and Bartlett.

Dudgeon, B. J., & Greenberg, S .L. (1998). Preparing students for consultation roles and systems. *American Journal of Occupational Therapy, 52*, 801–809.

Dunn, W. (1990). A comparison of service provision models in school-based occupational therapy services: A pilot study. *Occupational Therapy Journal of Research, 10*, 300–320.

Dunn, W. (2000). *Best practice occupational therapy: In community service with children and families*. Thorofare, NJ: Slack.

Epstein, C. F. (1992). Developing a consultation practice. In E. G. Jaffe & C. F. Epstein (Eds.), *Occupational therapy consultation: Theory, principles, and practice* (pp. 634–649). St. Louis, MO: Mosby Year Book.

Fazio, L. S. (2008). *Developing occupation-centered programs for the community* (2nd ed.). Upper Saddle River, NJ: Pearson Prentice Hall.

Frankel, A. R., & Gelman, S. R. (2004). *Case management: An introduction to concept and skills*. Chicago, IL: Lyceum Books.

Furåker, C., & Nilsson, K. (2011). The consultative work of occupational therapists working in municipal healthcare. *Scandinavian Journal of Occupational Therapy, 18*(2), 101–108.

Golembiewski, R. T. (2000). Six orientations for the reader: An interpretive introduction. In R. T. Golembiewski (Ed.), *Handbook of organizational consultation* (2nd ed., pp. 1–26). New York, NY: Marcel Dekker.

Retrieved from: http://web.ebscohost.com.ezproxy.brenau.edu:2048/ehost/ebookviewer/ebook/nlebk_44858_AN?sid=4577aa35-f19c-4dc7-b93a-f8e910a57085@sessionmgr104&vid=1&lpid=lp_COVER-0

Gourley, M. (2002). *Driver rehabilitation-a growing practice area for OTs. OT Practice online 3-25-02.* Retrieved from http://www.aota.org/Pubs/OTP/1997-2007/Features/2002/f-032502.aspx

Hanebrink, S., & Parent, B. B. (2000). ADA consulting opportunities. *OT Practice, 5*(17), 12–15.

Holmes, W., & Scaffa, M. (2009). An exploratory study of competencies for emerging practice in occupational therapy. *Journal of Allied Health, 38*(2), 81–90.

Jaffe, E. G. (1986). Prevention: "An idea whose time has come": The role of occupational therapy in disease prevention and health promotion. *American Journal of Occupational Therapy, 39*, 499–503.

Jaffe, E. G. (1989). Medical consumer education: Health promotion in the workplace. In J. A. Johnson & E. G. Jaffe (Eds.), *Occupational therapy: Program development for health promotion and preventive series* (pp. 5–24). Binghamton, NY: Haworth.

Jaffe, E. G., & Epstein, C. F. (2011). Consultation: Collaborative interventions for change. In K. Jacobs & G. L. McCormack (Eds.), *The occupational therapy manager* (5th ed., pp. 521–545). Bethesda, MD: AOTA Press.

Johnson, J. A. (2009). *Health organizations: Theory, behavior, and development.* Sudbury, MA: Jones and Bartlett.

Lahti, R., & Beyerlein, M. (2000). Knowledge transfer and management consulting: A look at "the firm." *Business Horizons, 43*(1), 65–74.

Ledlow, G. R., & Coppola, M. N. (2011). *Leadership for health professionals: Theory, skills, and application.* Sudbury, MA: Jones and Bartlett.

Mackersy, A., Robertson, L., & McKay, W. (2003). Implications of the health reforms for occupational therapy fieldwork education. *New Zealand Journal of Occupational Therapy 50*(2), 28.

McCormack, G. L. (2011). Common skill sets for occupational therapy managers and practitioners. In K. Jacobs & G. L. McCormack (Eds.), *The occupational therapy manager* (5th ed., pp. 17–35). Bethesda, MD: AOTA Press.

McCormack, G. L., Jaffe, E. G., & Frey, W. (2003). New organizational perspectives. In G. L. McCormack, E. G. Jaffe, & M. Goodman-Lavey (Eds.), *The occupational therapy manager* (4th ed., pp. 85–126). Bethesda, MD: AOTA Press.

Moyers Cleveland, P. A., & Hinojosa, J. (2011). Continuing competence and competency. In K. Jacobs and G. L. McCormack (Eds.), *The occupational therapy manager* (5th ed., pp. 485–501). Bethesda, MD: AOTA Press.

National Cancer Institute. (2005). *Theory at a glance: A guide for health promotion practice* (2nd ed.). Bethesda, MD: National Institutes of Health. Retrieved from https://cissecure.nci.nih.gov/ncipubs/home.aspx?js=1

Palisano, R. J. (1989). Comparison of two methods of service delivery for students with learning disabilities. *Physical and Occupational Therapy in Pediatrics, 9*, 79–100.

Pergrossi, J. C. (1999). Using activities for consulting in community mental health. *WFOT Bulletin, 11*, 44–49.

Polichino, J. E., & Scheer. J. (2006). Using AOTA ebp resources to enter pediatric practice in the context of public schools. *OT Practice Online.* Retrieved from http://aota.org/Pubs/OTP/1997-2007/Features/2006/f-082806.aspx

Prochaska, J. O., & DiClemente, C. C. (1992). Stages of change in the modification of behavior problems. In M. Hersen, R. M. Eisler, & P. M. Millers (Eds.), *Progress in behavior modification* (pp. 184–214). Sycamore, IL: Sycamore Press.

Prochaska, J. O., Norcross, J. C., & DiClemente, C. C. (1994). *Changing for good: A revolutionary six-stage program for overcoming bad habits and moving your life positively forward.* New York, NY: Harper Collins.

Purtillo, R. (2005). *Ethical dimensions in the health professions* (4th ed.). Philadelphia, PA: Elsevier Saunders.

Reitz, S. M., Scaffa, M. E., Campbell, R. M., & Rhynders, P. A. (2010). Health behavior frameworks for health promotion practice. In M. E. Scaffa, S. M. Reitz, & M. A. Pizzi (Eds.), *Occupational therapy in the promotion of health and wellness.* Philadelphia, PA: F. A. Davis.

Richmond, T., & Powers, D. (2004). *Business fundamentals for the rehabilitation professional.* Thorofare, NJ: Slack.

Sabatino, C. (2009). School social work consultation models and response to intervention: A perfect match. *Children & Schools, 31*(4), 197–206.

Scaffa, M. E. (2001). *Occupational therapy in community-based practice settings.* Philadelphia, PA: F. A. Davis.

Scott, J. B. (2009). Consultation. In E. B. Crepeau, E. S. Cohn, & B. A. B. Schell (Eds.), *Willard and Spackman's occupational therapy* (11th ed., pp. 964–972). Philadelphia, PA: Lippincott Williams & Wilkins.

Siemsen, D. W., Bergstrom, A. R., & Hathaway, J. C. (2005). Efficacy of a low vision patient consultation. *Journal of Visual Impairment & Blindness, 99*(7), 1–10.

von Bertalanffy, L. (1968). *General systems theory: Foundations, development, and application.* New York, NY: Braziller.

Warren, M. (2011). An overview of low vision rehabilitation and the role of occupational therapy. In M. Warren & E. A. Barstow (Eds.), *Occupational therapy interventions for adults with low vision* (pp. 1–26). Bethesda, MD: AOTA Press.

World Federation of Occupational Therapists. (2002). *Minimum standards for the education of occupational therapists.* Retrieved from http://www.wfot.org/Store/tabid/61/CategoryID/1/Default.aspx

World Federation of Occupational Therapists. (2005). *World Federation of Occupational Therapists code of ethics.* Retrieved from http://www.wfot.org/ResourceCentre/tabid/132/did/34/Default.aspx

For additional resources on the subjects discussed in this chapter, visit http://thePoint.lww.com/Willard-Spackman12e.

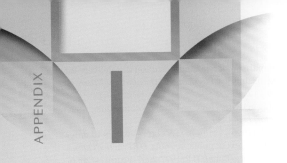

APPENDIX I

Common Conditions, Resources, and Evidence

Alzheimer's Disease

Emily Meibeyer

Description

Alzheimer's disease (AD), the most common form of dementia, is a progressively degenerative and irreversible disease that affects cognitive function, occurring most frequently in the elderly population. Dementia is characterized by the loss or decline in memory, along with aphasia, apraxia, agnosia, and loss of executive function (American Psychiatric Association [APA], 2000). AD has a tremendous impact on the person, the family, and his or her daily occupational and social functioning.

Incidence and Prevalence

Classification of AD is based on age of onset; *early*, or *younger onset*, is the presence of symptoms before age 65 years, and *late onset* occurs after age 65 years (Schaber & Lieberman, 2010). In 2010, it was estimated that there was 5.3 million Americans of all ages with AD. This figure includes 5.1 million individuals aged 65 years and older and approximately 200,000 under the age of 65 years. This is approximately 13% of people older than age 65 years, and the prevalence of AD is higher among women than men. At the current rate, the number of individuals with AD aged 65 years and older is estimated to reach 7.7 million in 2030 and between 11 and 16 million by 2050 (Alzheimer's Association, 2010).

Cause and Etiology

The etiology of AD is unknown, although genetics seem to play a major factor. Numerous other theories have been examined, including the development of abnormal structures called *plaques* and *tangles* in the brain (Alzheimer's Association, 2010; Schaber & Lieberman, 2010). Risk factors for AD consist of advancing age, family history, and heredity, but head trauma and vascular disease have also been theorized as having an associated risk (Alzheimer's Association, 2010). Extensive research on AD is being conducted to further examine the cause, treatment, and prevention.

Typical Course, Symptoms, and Related Conditions

Although the experience of symptoms and the time when symptoms may occur can differ greatly from one individual to the next, the progression of Alzheimer's symptoms can be categorized into three basic stages: early, middle or moderate, and severe or late stages.

Early Stage

- *Cognition*: mild memory deficits, particularly short-term memory (e.g., forgetting appointments, recent conversations, dates); lack of concentration and ability to learn new materials; mild language impairment; difficulty with novel and complex tasks
- *Behavioral/psychological*: personality changes; social withdrawal; increased depression, apathy, anxiety, or irritability
- *Activities of daily living (ADL)*: no significant changes; may still live independently with support for instrumental activities of daily living (IADL) or more complex tasks

Middle or Moderate Stage

- *Cognition*: severe impairment in recent memory and objective memory (e.g., loss of ability to spell or count), more obvious language impairments (e.g., aphasia, word-finding difficulties), apraxia, agnosia, disorientation, impaired judgment, impaired executive functioning
- *Behavioral/psychological*: increased aimless activities (e.g., wandering), disrupted sleep patterns, delusions, hallucinations, aggression/agitation, requires supervision
- *ADL*: requires supervision to extensive assistance with ADL, including dressing, bathing, toileting, and eating; fatigue

Severe or Late Stage

- *Cognition*: profound disturbances in orientation and memory, unable to recognize caregivers/family, severe intellectual deterioration, severely limited verbal communication, unaware of environment
- *Behavioral/psychological*: apathetic and unresponsive, except for facial grimacing and repetitive humming or moaning
- *Motor*: severe motor function impairments; progression to bedridden stage with pathological reflexes, loss of motor control, and limb rigidity
- *ADL*: complete loss of basic daily living abilities, incontinence of bowel and bladder, completely dependent on caregivers (APA, 2000; Hart et al., 2003; Schaber & Lieberman, 2010)

Precautions

Because the global functioning of an individual with AD changes and deteriorates with the progression of the disease, there becomes an increasing need to monitor and supervise the individual to ensure safety and optimal functioning.

- Avoid leaving individuals with AD alone and unsupervised secondary to tendency to wander, disorientation, impaired judgment, and increased fall risk.
- Avoid overstimulation of the individual because it may trigger or exacerbate behavioral or psychological symptoms.
- Avoid arguing with individuals with AD when they are disoriented to reality; this may also trigger behavioral problems, such as increased agitation.
- Minimize dangers in the environment; a safe environment enables persons with AD to experience increased security and mobility.

Interdisciplinary Interventions

Medication Therapy

Although current medications cannot cure AD or stop the progression of the disease, there are two types of prescription drugs presently approved to treat and lessen the symptoms: cholinesterase inhibitors (ChEIs) and memantine. ChEIs are prescribed to lessen symptoms related to memory, thinking, language, and other thought processes; they have been found to have a therapeutic effect associated with improved performance of ADL, reduced behavioral issues, stabilized cognitive impairment, and decreased caregiver stress (Alzheimer's Association, 2007; Hodgson, Gitlin, Winter, & Dennis, 2008). Common side effects are nausea, vomiting, loss of appetite, and increased frequency of bowel movements. Memantine is used to improve memory, attention, reason, language, and the ability to perform simple tasks with individuals in the moderate to severe stages (Alzheimer's Association, 2007). As the disease progresses, the use of psychotropic medications is often necessary for psychological symptom management (e.g., anxiety, agitation) (Hodgson et al., 2008).

Occupational Therapy Evaluations

The occupational therapy (OT) evaluation should be conducted with the client, caregiver or family member, or health care proxy to ensure that accurate information is exchanged. The client with AD should be encouraged to take an active role in the evaluation and interview process, with others providing additional information as needed. An occupational profile and observation of client engagement in functional tasks allow the practitioner to obtain information to determine the clients' needs and barriers to occupational performance (Schaber & Lieberman, 2010).

Activities of Daily Living or Instrumental Activities of Daily Living Assessments

- Assessment of Motor and Process Skills (AMPS): assesses motor and process skills in context of familiar functional tasks
- Disability Assessment for Dementia (DAD): scale to measure ADL/IADL in community-dwelling adults with dementia
- Functional Independence Measure (FIM): assesses functional status and assistance needs
- Kohlman Evaluation of Living Skills (KELS): evaluates ability to live independently
- Performance Assessment of Self-Care Skills (PASS): evaluates functional status
- Routine Task Inventory-Expanded (RTI-E): self-report or observation of functional behavior and self-awareness during typical tasks

Cognitive Assessments

- Allen Cognitive Level Screen-5 (ACLS-5)/Large Allen Cognitive Level Screen-5 (LACLS-5): screens global cognitive processing, capacities, and performance abilities
- Allen Diagnostic Module-2 (ADM-2): assesses cognitive processing and intervention needs
- Cognitive Performance Test (CPT): evaluates effect of cognitive processing on functioning
- Kitchen Task Assessment (KTA): measures level of cognitive support needed by individuals with dementia
- Mini-Mental State Examination (MMSE): evaluates orientation, attention, memory, and other cognitive skills

Occupation-Focused Assessments

- Activity Card Sort (ACS): clients describe instrumental, social, and leisure activities
- Adult Sensory Profile: assesses ability to process sensory input and effect on function
- Canadian Occupational Performance Measure (COPM): self-report of performance and satisfaction with occupations

Occupational Therapy Interventions

The primary goal of OT intervention for clients with AD is to maximize the quality of life and engagement in occupation and to promote safety. Intervention must occur at intervals over time given the progressive nature of the disease; the goals change based on the evolving needs of the client at each stage of the disease (Schaber & Lieberman, 2010). For a client in the early stage of AD, OT intervention might focus more on compensatory strategies for loss of cognitive abilities, and for a client in the later stages, the intervention will focus more on adaptation of the environment, safety, and caregiver training (American Occupational Therapy Association, 2007, 2010).

- *Task simplification*: diminish demands of ADL and other tasks through establishing daily routines or increasing visual, verbal, or tactile cues and support from caregivers; use of assistive technology or adaptive devices (e.g., pill boxes)

- *Environmental modification*: keep environments consistent to decrease confusion; increase lighting; adaptive equipment (e.g., grab bars, door alarms); provide a low-stimulus environment; labeling cupboards and doors with familiar pictures, names, or symbols as visual cues
- *Caregiver training/education*: provide resources for community support, such as respite care, in-home services, and caregiver support groups; education to increase knowledge of AD and the development of coping skills; enable caregivers to use routines, home modifications, and adaptive equipment; instruction on effective behavior management (e.g., calming strategies) and effective communication (e.g., validation)

Occupational Therapy and the Evidence

OT interventions focused on teaching compensatory strategies, environmental modifications, fall prevention and safety instruction, and balance and muscle exercises were shown to have a positive long-term effect on reducing functional decline and mortality in older adults (Gitlin et al., 2009). There is a strong evidence that environmental interventions for persons with AD, such as the use of visual cues and labeling, increases participation and ability to navigate home environment safely (Dooley & Hinojosa, 2004; Nolan, Matthews, & Harrison, 2001). Interventions that used step-by-step guidance, compensatory strategies, and alterations of the task demands by providing cueing and prompting were found to be effective for people in the early and middle stages of the disease with ADL performance, particularly at mealtimes (Dooley & Hinojosa, 2004; Graff et al., 2006; Watson & Green, 2006). Gitlin and colleagues (2008) support modifying activity demands to fit the skill level of the client because it can help reduce psychiatric behaviors and, in turn, caregiver burden. Hasselkus and Murray (2007) found that engagement in everyday occupation helped contribute to the relative well-being of both the caregiver and the care receiver and was an important source of satisfaction and a personal sign of good care. Caregiver training has been found to help decrease aggressive behavioral symptoms and promote independence in self-care for the person with AD and increase knowledge, coping skills, and sense of self-efficacy in the caregiver (Corcoran & Gitlin, 2001; Dooley & Hinojosa, 2004; Graff, Vernooij-Dassen, Hoefnagels, Dekker, & de Witte, 2003; Huang, Lotus Shyu, Chen, Chen, & Lin, 2003).

Resources

Organization

- Alzheimer's Association
  225 N. Michigan Ave., Fl. 17
  Chicago, IL 6061
  Telephone: 800-272-3900

- Alzheimer's Disease Education and Referral Center
  National Institute on Aging
  Building 31, Room 5C27
  31 Center Drive, MSC 2292
  Bethesda, MD 20892
  Telephone: 800-438-4380

- Alzheimer's Foundation of America
  322 8th Ave., 7th fl.
  New York, NY 10001
  Telephone: 1-866-232-8484

Books

- Cooney, E. (2003). *Death in slow motion: My mother's descent into Alzheimer's*. Pittsburgh, PA: HarperCollins.
  Cooney vividly described the everyday physical and emotional stresses on her as a caregiver to her mother diagnosed with AD.

- DeBaggio, T. (2003). *Losing my mind: An intimate look at life with Alzheimer's*. New York, NY: Free Press.
  A former journalist and professional gardener, DeBaggio depicts his life after being diagnosed with early onset AD at the age of 57 years.

- Genova, L. (2007). *Still Alice*. Bloomington, IN: iUniverse.
  Although a fictional account, Genova, a Harvard-educated neuroscientist, crafts a realistic portrait of life with early onset AD.

Journals

- *Alzheimer's Disease & Associated Disorders*
- *American Journal of Alzheimer's Disease & Other Dementias*
- *American Journal of Geriatric Psychiatry*
- *Topics in Geriatric Rehabilitation*

Websites

- Alzheimer's Association
  http://www.alz.org
  The Alzheimer's Association offers news, fact sheets, education, publications, support groups, and online message boards for those affected by AD and dementia.

- Alzheimer's Disease Education and Referral (ADEAR) Center
  http://www.nia.nih.gov/alzheimers/
  The ADEAR Center, a federal resource through the National Institute on Aging, provides free publications, fact sheets, research databases, clinical trials information, referrals to local services, training materials, and guidelines for health care professionals.

- Alzheimer's Foundation of America (AFA)
  http://www.alzfdn.org
  The AFA Website includes information about AD and related illnesses, caregiving strategies, and behavioral issues, as well as comprehensive educational materials, conferences and workshops, government programs, and current clinical trials.

- Family Caregiver Alliance (FCA)
  http://www.caregiver.org
  The FCA provides factsheets, publications, and newsletters related to caregiver issues, advice, public policy, and research. It also offers programs at the national, state, and local levels and online forums for caregivers to connect and share experiences.

References

Alzheimer's Association. (2007). *FDA-approved treatments for Alzheimer's*. Retrieved from http://www.alz.org/national/documents/topicsheet_treatments.pdf

Alzheimer's Association. (2010). Alzheimer's disease facts and figures. *Alzheimer's & Dementia, 6*, 1–70.

American Occupational Therapy Association. (2007). AOTA's societal statement on family caregivers. *American Journal of Occupational Therapy, 61*, 710.

American Occupational Therapy Association. (2010). *Alzheimer's disease FAQ*. Retrieved from http://www.aota.org/Practitioners/PracticeAreas/Aging/FAQ/37281.aspx

American Psychiatric Association. (2000). *Diagnostic and statistical manual of mental disorders* (4th ed., text rev.). Washington, DC: Author.

Corcoran, M. A., & Gitlin, L. N. (2001). Family caregiver acceptance and use of environmental strategies provided in an occupational therapy intervention. *Physical and Occupational Therapy in Geriatrics, 19*, 1–20.

Dooley, N. R., & Hinojosa, J. (2004). Improving quality of life for persons with Alzheimer's disease and their family caregivers: A brief occupational therapy intervention. *American Journal of Occupational Therapy, 58*, 561–569.

Gitlin, L. N., Hauck, W. W., Dennis, M. P., Winter, L., Hodgson, N., & Schinfeld, S. (2009). Long-term effect on mortality of a home intervention that reduces functional difficulties in older adults: Results from a randomized trial. *Journal of the American Geriatric Society, 57*, 476–481.

Gitlin, L., Winter, L., Burke, J., Chernett, N., Dennis, M., & Hauck, W. (2008). Tailored activities to manage neuropsychiatric behaviors in persons with dementia and reduce caregiver burden: A randomized pilot study. *American Journal of Geriatric Psychiatry, 16*, 229–239.

Graff, M. J. L., Vernooij-Dassen, M. J. M., Hoefnagels, W. H., Dekker, J., & de Witte, L. P. (2003). Occupational therapy at home for older individuals with mild to moderate cognitive impairments and their primary caregivers: A pilot study. *Occupational Therapy Journal of Research, 23*, 155–163.

Graff, M. J. L., Vernooij-Dassen, M. J. M., Thijssen, M., Dekker, J., Hoefnagels, W. H. L., & Rikkert, M. G. M. (2006). Community-based occupational therapy for patients with dementia and their caregivers: Randomized controlled trial. *British Medical Journal, 333*, 1196–1201.

Hart, D. J., Craig, D., Compton, S. A., Critchlow, S., Kerrigan, B. M., McIlroy, S. P., & Passmore, A. P. (2003). A retrospective study of the behavioral and psychological symptoms of mild and late phase Alzheimer's disease. *International Journal of Geriatric Psychiatry, 18*, 1037–1042.

Hasselkus, B. R., & Murray, B. (2007). Everyday occupation, well-being, and identity: The experience of caregivers in families with dementia. *American Journal of Occupational Therapy, 61*, 9–20.

Hodgson, N. A., Gitlin, L. N., Winter, L., & Dennis, M. (2008). Psychotherapeutic medications and dementia. *Consultant Pharmacist, 23*, 357–358.

Huang, H. L., Lotus Shyu, Y. I., Chen, M. C., Chen, S. T., & Lin, L. C. (2003). A pilot study on a home-based caregiver training program for improving caregiver self-efficacy and decreasing the behavioral problems of elders with dementia in Taiwan. *International Journal of Geriatric Psychiatry, 18*, 337–345.

Nolan, B., Matthews, R., & Harrison, M. (2001). Using external memory aids to increase room finding by older adults with dementia. *American Journal of Alzheimer's Disease and Other Dementias, 16*, 251–254.

Schaber, P., & Lieberman, D. (2010). *Occupational therapy guidelines for adults with Alzheimer's disease and related disorders*. Bethesda, MD: AOTA Press.

Watson, R., & Green, S. (2006). Feeding and dementia: A systematic literature review. *Journal of Advanced Nursing, 54*, 86–93.

Amputations

Pamela Vaughn

Description and Diagnosis

An *amputation* is the removal of a part of the body, a limb, or part of a limb via surgery. Types of amputation surgeries include the following:

- Primary—after a trauma, before infection has begun
- Secondary—after a trauma, after infection has begun
- Closed—in which flaps of tissue are retained and used to create a cover over the end of the bone
- Open—in which the amputation is temporarily left open while infection is cleared and surgical closure is completed at a later time
- Trans amputations (e.g., transhumeral)—an amputation made across the longitudinal axis of a long bone
- Disarticulation amputations (e.g., ankle disarticulation)—an amputation made at a natural joint, not involving the cutting of bone

Although individuals who were born with missing or partially developed limbs may experience the same or similar occupational barriers as those who have undergone surgical amputation, these clients are considered to have congenital developmental conditions and present with different needs—particularly psychological needs—than those with acquired amputations (*Mosby's Medical, Nursing, & Allied Health Dictionary*, 2002; Stubblefield & Armstrong, 2008).

Cause and Etiology

The most frequent causes of amputation are dysvascular disease, diabetes, and trauma (e.g., work-related accidents, motor vehicle accidents, war trauma) (Ziegler-Graham, MacKenzie, Ephraim, Travison, & Brookmeyer, 2008). Cancer and tumors are additional causes of amputation, but limb removal is often used only as a last resort in these cases.

Incidence and Prevalence

More than 1.6 million Americans are currently living with limb loss, and this figure is estimated to increase to more than 2.2 million by 2020 and 3.6 million by 2050 based on population projections (Ziegler-Graham et al., 2008). Males are significantly more affected than females. Lower extremity amputations (LEA; including hemipelvectomy, hip disarticulation, transfemoral, knee disarticulation, transtibial, ankle disarticulation, partial foot/toe amputation) are more common than upper extremity amputations (UEA; including scapulothoracic, transhumeral, elbow disarticulation, transradial, wrist disarticulation, partial hand/finger amputation); the leading cause of UEA is trauma (Kobayashi et al., 2011; Ziegler-Graham et al., 2008). The rate of nontraumatic LEA among people with diabetes has decreased in recent decades but is still at about 3.5 per 1,000 individuals with diabetes (DeFrances, Lucas, Buie, & Golosinskiy, 2008). Approximately 3.4%—5,283 individuals—of battle-injured U.S. military service members from the Vietnam War sustained traumatic limb loss. For the Operation Iraqi Freedom/Operation Enduring Freedom conflicts, approximately 2.6%, or 1,000 service members, had endured traumatic limb loss as of January 2010 (Reiber et al., 2010).

Typical Course, Symptoms, and Related Conditions

In the case of trauma, amputations occur when a limb or portion of a limb is surgically irreparable following the accident. In the case of disease, for example, diabetes or vascular disease, amputations may be necessary due to ischemia, ulcers, neuropathy, and so forth (Ziegler-Graham et al., 2008). Mortality rates are higher for clients with nontraumatic amputations than for those with traumatic amputations (Kratz et al., 2010).

Throughout recovery, clients with amputations may experience various psychological reactions such as shock, grief, anger, denial, helplessness, and depression (Stubblefield & Armstrong, 2008). Many are diagnosed with posttraumatic stress disorder (PTSD) as well (Epstein, Heinemann, & McFarland, 2010; Kratz et al., 2010). Phantom sensations or perceptions of pain, tingling, or other sensations in the missing limb are frequently reported by clients following amputation (Chapman, 2010). Particularly in the case of LEA, a decrease in physical activity may lead to a more sedentary lifestyle and result in health complications (Robbins, Vreeman, Sothmann, Wilson, & Oldridge, 2009). Additionally, clients may develop skin problems on their residual limb if proper hygiene is not maintained, especially if they use a prosthetic (Stubblefield & Armstrong, 2008).

Interdisciplinary Interventions

Orthopedics and Medicine

An orthopedic surgeon is typically the physician who performs amputation surgeries, although other medical specialties may be involved, particularly in the case of traumatic limb loss. Following the procedure, precautions to prevent infection are taken, that is, administration of antibiotics and proper cleaning by a nurse. Pain medication is frequently administered as well (Chapman, 2010).

Prosthetics

A prosthetist and/or an interdisciplinary team (including occupational therapist) discusses prosthetic options with the client and, if the client desires a prosthesis, helps prepare the client to use a prosthesis. This includes preparing the residual limb for proper prosthesis fit, desensitizing the residual limb, educating the client regarding limb and prosthesis hygiene, helping the client develop independence in activities of daily living (ADL) for times when they won't have use of the prosthesis, and providing psychological support throughout the transition and learning period (Stubblefield & Armstrong, 2008). There are several timelines for fitting and beginning to use a prosthetic device, but it is generally accepted that the sooner a prosthetic device can be used, the better the functional and psychological outcomes of the client (Robinson, Sansam, Hirst, & Neumann, 2010).

Physical Therapy

Physical therapists work with clients to maintain or increase strength and range of motion (ROM) of the residual limb and of the trunk. Exercises are designed to reduce swelling as well as prepare the limb for wearing and using a prosthetic device. Pain control modalities, such as heat and cold therapies, may be used. For LEA, physical therapy will work with the client on gait training with ambulation devices, for example, crutches, and to prepare for walking with a prosthesis (Robinson et al., 2010).

Psychology

Considering the implications of amputation, psychologists or counselors are often employed to assist clients with identifying and working through their emotions in a healthy and functional manner (Robinson et al., 2010).

Vocational Therapy

Depending on the nature of the amputation and the desires of the client, return to previous employment may not be an option. To specifically address this, vocational therapists may meet with clients to assist in identifying potential alternative modes of employment after acute rehabilitation.

Occupational Therapy Evaluations

The evaluation process focuses on what the client needs, wants, or is expected to do and analyzes what factors may impact desired occupational performance. The evaluation begins with occupation-focused assessments followed by specific evaluation of the potential impact of amputation on occupational performance.

Occupation-Focused Assessments

- Unilateral Upper Extremity Amputation: Activities of Daily Living Assessment (Atkins, 1989)
- Role Checklist (Oakley, Kielhofner, Barris, & Reichler, 1986)
- Occupational Performance History Interview II (OPHI-II) (Kielhofner et al., 2004)
- Assessment of Motor and Process Skills (AMPS) (Fisher & Jones, 2010)
- Activity Measure for Post-Acute Care (AM-PAC) (Jette, Hayley, Coster, & Ni, 2007)
- Performance Assessment of Self-Care Skills (PASS) (Holm & Rogers, 2008)
- Canadian Occupational Therapy Measure (COPM) (Law et al., 2005)
- Short Form-36 (SF-36) (Hays, Sherbourne, & Mazel, 1995)
- Activity Card Sort (ACS) (Baum & Edwards, 2008)

Client Factor Assessments

- Disabilities of the Arm, Shoulder, and Hand (DASH) Outcome Measure (Hudak, Amadio, Bombardier, & the Upper Extremity Collaborative Group, 1996)
- ROM
- Measures of pain (e.g., Visual Analog Scale [VAS])
- Measures of muscle strength
- Measures of edema

Occupational Therapy Interventions

The primary goal of occupational therapy intervention for clients with amputations is to facilitate a return to occupational functioning. This varies between clients depending on the type of amputation, their previous occupations, and their personal goals.

Acute Stages

Intervention during the acute stage of rehabilitation includes educating the client regarding wound care and residual limb hygiene, scar management, strategies to decrease swelling, exercises to increase and maintain ROM of the residual limb, and strategies to independently complete ADL (Smurr, Gulick, Yancosek, & Ganz, 2008; Stubblefield & Armstrong, 2008). With UEA, the client may have to change his or her dominant hand as well, so occupational therapist can assist in retraining fine motor skills of the intact limb. Pain management, including strategies to recognize and deal with phantom pain, should also be addressed during acute rehabilitation.

Prosthetic Devices

Occupational therapists are part of the prosthetic team, which prepares the client for wearing and use of a prosthetic device—this includes consultation regarding the prosthetic choice; preparing the client's body via strength and balance exercises; preparing the residual limb by desensitizing and shaping it; training the client to don, doff, and care for the prosthesis; and training the client in control and functional use of the prosthesis. Depending on the type of amputation and design of the prosthesis, adaptive and assistive devices may be recommended for the client to be able to perform occupations independently (Robinson et al., 2010; Smurr et al., 2008; Stubblefield & Armstrong, 2008).

Task and Environmental Adaptations

Depending on the needs of the client, occupational therapists can suggest strategies and methods for home, school, and workplace modifications in order to facilitate mobility and participation within these environments.

Consultation

Occupational therapist can assist clients in new and/or adapted occupations to participate in following amputation in order to maintain satisfaction, quality of life (QOL), and participation in meaningful occupations. As undergoing an amputation can be a very emotional process for clients, providing information regarding realistic post-rehabilitative goals and community supports can ease their adjustment (Smurr et al., 2008; Stubblefield & Armstrong, 2008).

Occupational Therapy and the Evidence

There is a correlation between satisfaction with prosthetic devices and a higher QOL among clients with amputations, and an increased need of assistance with ADL has been correlated with decreased QOL (Epstein, Heinemann, & McFarland, 2010). The use of assistive devices as well as task and environmental adaptations helped one client with bilateral finger amputations to independently perform most ADL, resume physical activity, and return to full-time work (Stapanian, Stapanian, & Staley, 2010). Community self-management programs for individuals with amputations that focus on developing problem solving, skill acquisition, and increasing activity and participation resulted in decreased levels of depression and functional limitations as well as increased QOL when compared to individuals who had not undergone the programs (Wegener, Mackenzie, Ephraim, Ehde, & Williams, 2009). Early mobilization of upper extremity joints via ROM exercises has been shown to be somewhat effective in decreasing pain and swelling and facilitating quicker return to previous occupations (Amini, 2011).

Caregiver Concerns

Family members, particularly parents, of individuals with amputations have reported experiencing an increase in expenditures related to medical expenses and having to quit jobs or decrease hours in order to care for their family members after amputation (Weir, Ephraim, & Mackenzie, 2010).

Resources

Organizations

- Amputee Coalition—an educational, support, and advocacy organization for individuals with limb loss; includes the National Limb Loss Information Center.
  900 East Hill Avenue, Suite 205
  Knoxville, Tennessee 37915-2566
  Telephone: (888) 267-5669
  Website: http://www.amputee-coalition.org/
- National Amputation Foundation—support program for veterans and civilians with amputations.
  40 Church Street
  Malverne, NY 11565
  Telephone: (516) 887-3600
  Fax: (516) 887-3667
  E-mail: amps76@aol.com
  http://www.nationalamputation.org/

Books

- Garrison, K. S. (2005). *It's just a matter of balance*. South Euclid, OH: Print Vantage.
- Sundquist, J. (2010). *Just don't fall: A hilariously true story of childhood, cancer, amputation, romantic yearning, truth, and Olympic greatness*. New York, NY: Viking.

References

Amini, D. (2011). Occupational therapy interventions for work-related injuries and conditions of the forearm, wrist, and hand: A systematic review. *American Journal of Occupational Therapy, 65*, 29–36. doi:10.5014/ajot.2011.09186

Atkins, D. J. (1989). Unilateral upper extremity amputation: Activities of daily living assessment. In D. J. Atkins & R. H. Meier (Eds.), *Comprehensive management of the upper-limb amputee* (p. 49). New York, NY: Springer-Verlag.

Baum, C. M., & Edwards, D. E. (2008). *Activity Card Sort* (2nd ed.). Bethesda, MD: AOTA Press.

Chapman, S. (2010). Pain management in patients following limb amputation. *Nursing Standard, 25*(19), 35–40.

DeFrances, C. J., Lucas, C. A., Buie, V. C., & Golosinskiy, A. (2008). *2006 National Hospital Discharge Survey* (National Health Statistics Reports No. 5). Hyattsville, MD: National Center for Health Statistics.

Epstein, R. A., Heinemann, A. W., & McFarland, L. V. (2010). Quality of life for veterans and servicemembers with major traumatic limb loss from Vietnam and OIF/OEF conflicts. *Journal of Rehabilitation Research & Development, 47*, 373–386. doi:10.1682/JRRD.2009.03.0023

Fisher, A. G., & Jones, K. B. (2010). *Assessment of Motor and Process Skills. Vol. 1: Development, standardization, and administration manual* (7th ed.). Fort Collins, CO: Three Star Press.

Hays, R. D., Sherbourne, C. D., & Mazel, R. M. (1995). *User's manual for Medical Outcomes Study (MOS) core measures of health-related quality of life*. Santa Monica, CA: RAND Corporation.

Holm, M. B., & Rogers, J. C. (2008). The Performance Assessment of Self-Care Skills (PASS). In B. Hemphill-Pearson (Ed.), *Assessments in occupational therapy mental health* (2nd ed., pp. 101–110). Thorofare, NJ: Slack.

Hudak, P. L., Amadio, P. C., Bombardier, C., & the Upper Extremity Collaborative Group. (1996). Development of an upper extremity outcome measure: The DASH (disabilities of the arm, shoulder and hand) [corrected]. *American Journal of Industrial Medicine, 29*, 602–608. Erratum in: *American Journal of Industrial Medicine, 30*, 372.

Kielhofner, G., Mallinson, T., Crawford, C., Nowak, M., Rigby, M., Henry, A., & Walens, D. (2004). *Occupational Performance History Interview II (OPHI-II)*. Chicago, IL: MOHO Clearinghouse.

Kobayashi, L., Inaba, K., Barmparas, G., Criscuoli, M., Lustenberger, T., Talving, P., . . . Demetriades, D. (2011). Traumatic limb amputations at a level I trauma center. *European Journal of Trauma and Emergency Surgery, 37*, 67–72. doi:10.1007/s00068-010-0011-3

Kratz, A. L., Williams, R. M., Turner, A. P., Raichle, K. A., Smith, D. G., & Ehde, D. (2010). To lump or to split? Comparing individuals with traumatic and nontraumatic limb loss in the first year after amputation. *Rehabilitation Psychology, 55*, 126–138. doi:10.1037/a0019492

Jette, A., Hayley, S. M., Coster, W., & Ni P. (2007). *Boston University Activity Measure for Post Acute Care: Instruction manual*. Retrieved from http://www.crecare.com/order/order.html

Law, M., Baptiste, S., Carswell, A., McColl, M., Polatajko, H., & Pollock, N. (2005). *Canadian Occupational Performance Measure* (4th ed.). Ottawa, Canada: CAOT Publications.

Mosby's medical, nursing, & allied health dictionary (6th ed.). (2002). St. Louis, MO: Harcourt Health Sciences.

Oakley, F., Kielhofner, G., Barris, R., & Reichler, R. (1986). The Role Checklist: Development and empirical assessment of reliability. *Occupational Therapy Journal of Research, 6*, 157–170.

Reiber, G., McFarland, L., Hubbard, S., Maynard, C., Blough, D., Gambel, J., & Smith, D. (2010). Servicemembers and veterans with major traumatic limb loss from Vietnam war and OIF/OEF conflicts: Survey methods, participants, and summary findings. *Journal of Rehabilitation Research & Development, 47*, 275–298. doi:10.1682/JRRD.2010.01.0009

Robbins, C. B., Vreeman, D. J., Sothmann, M. S., Wilson, S. J., & Oldridge, N. R. (2009). A review of the long-term health outcomes associated with war-related amputation. *Military Medicine, 174*, 588–592.

Robinson, V., Sansam, K., Hirst, L., & Neumann, V. (2010). Major lower limb amputation—What, why, and how to achieve the best results. *Orthopedics and Trauma, 24*, 276–285.

Smurr, L. M., Gulick, K., Yancosek, K., & Ganz, O. (2008). Managing the upper extremity amputee: A protocol for success. *Journal of Hand Therapy, 21*, 160–175. doi:10.1197/j.jht.2007.09.006

Stapanian, M. A., Stapanian, A. M. P., & Staley, K. E. (2010). Case report—Rehabilitation for bilateral amputation of fingers. *American Journal of Occupational Therapy, 64*, 923–928. doi:10.5014/ajot.2010.09153

Stubblefield, K., & Armstrong, A. (2008). Amputations and prosthetics. In M. V. Radomski & C. A. T. Latham (Eds.), *Occupational therapy for physical dysfunction* (6th ed., pp. 1265–1294). Philadelphia, PA: Lippincott Williams & Wilkins.

Wegener, S. T., Mackenzie, E. J., Ephraim, P., Ehde, D., & Williams, R. (2009). Self-management improves outcomes in persons with limb loss. *Archives of Physical Medicine & Rehabilitation, 90*, 373–380. doi:10.1016/j.apmr.2008.08.222

Weir, S., Ephraim, P., & Mackenzie, E. (2010). Effects of paediatric limb loss on healthcare utilisation, schooling and parental labour supply. *Disability & Rehabilitation, 32*(24), 2046–2055. doi:10.3109/09638288.2010.481028

Ziegler-Graham, K., MacKenzie, E. J., Ephraim, P. L., Travison, T. G., & Brookmeyer, R. (2008). Estimating the prevalence of limb loss in the United States: 2005 to 2050. *Archives of Physical Medicine and Rehabilitation, 89*, 422–429. doi:10.1016/j.apmr.2007.11.005

Amyotrophic Lateral Sclerosis

Christine M. Carifio

Description

Amyotrophic lateral sclerosis (ALS), also referred to as Lou Gehrig's disease, is a rare, progressive, degenerative condition that affects the motor neurons in the corticospinal pathways, the motor nuclei of the brain stem, and the anterior horn cells of the spinal cord. ALS causes decreased function of the nerve cells in the brain, brain stem, and spinal cord, which weakens and atrophies the muscles of the entire body, eventually leading to paralysis. ALS does spare personality and cognition. ALS currently has no known cure (Maddox, 2003).

Incidence and Prevalence

- ALS affects approximately 5 out of every 100,000 people in the world (*Amyotrophic Lateral Sclerosis*, 2010).
- About 5,600 people in the United States are diagnosed with ALS every year.
- In the United States, about 30,000 people currently have ALS.
- Most people develop ALS between the ages of 40 and 70 years.
- ALS is 20% more common in men than in women.
- ALS affects people of all races.
- 90% to 95% of cases occur at random with no known cause, whereas 5% to 10% are of genetic origin (*Amyotrophic Lateral Sclerosis Fact Sheet*, 2011).

Cause and Typical Course

The cause for ALS remains unknown. The onset is varied, asymmetrical, and usually begins in the lower extremities. ALS is characterized in three categories: upper motor, lower motor, and bulbar involvement. The major overarching sign of ALS is muscle weakness. As the disease progresses, ambulation, severe weakness, and speech and swallowing issues may arise, eventually leading to a complete decline in activities of daily living (ADL). Because the disease only affects the motor pathways, higher cortical processes of memory, insight, awareness, eye movement, bladder function, cognition, personality, and skin sensation remain intact. The median amount of life postdiagnosis ranges from 23 to 52 months; however, many individuals may live 5 years or more after being diagnosed. Death usually results from respiratory atrophy unless the individual is put on a ventilator (*Who gets ALS?*, 2008).

Symptoms

Motor Neuron Damage

- Damage to the lower motor neurons (spinal cord) may result in flaccid paralysis, decreased muscle tone and muscle weakness, and decreased reflexes.
- Damage to the upper motor neurons (in the brain) and to the corticospinal tract may lead to spasticity and hyperreflexia.
- Damage to the bulbar region includes symptoms of dysarthria and dysphagia (*Amyotrophic Lateral Sclerosis Fact Sheet*, 2011).

General Symptoms

- Muscle atrophy distal to proximal
- Muscle weakness
- Twitching (fasciculation) and cramping of the muscles
- Sialorrhea (excess drooling)
- Weight loss
- Loss of endurance, dexterity, and ADL function
- Fatigue
- Stumbling and falling due to lower extremity weakness (*Who gets ALS?*, 2008)

Interdisciplinary Interventions

There is not one specific assessment to diagnose ALS. Magnetic resonance imaging (MRI), electromyography, blood tests, nerve conduction velocity tests, and neurological examinations are conducted to rule out other diagnoses (*Amyotrophic Lateral Sclerosis Fact Sheet*, 2011). No known effective pharmacological treatment is available for ALS but riluzole (Rilutek), a U.S. Food and Drug Administration (FDA)–approved antiglutamate agent, which may extend survival for several months (*Riluzole*, 2008). Other medications can help manage some of the symptoms of ALS such as fasciculation, spasticity, anxiety, insomnia, and excessive saliva. Because ALS is progressive with a wide variety of symptoms, a multidisciplinary team of support including respiratory therapists, speech pathologists, physical therapists, occupational therapists, psychologists, and social workers is needed to sustain the individual's quality of life and support the family (Mitsumoto, 2009).

Precautions

- Pneumonia and pulmonary emboli
- Ventilator precautions (if applicable)
- Inability to cough/clear mucus from airway and other swallowing issues that present choking hazards
- Pressure sores due to decreased mobility
- Posture and balance instability may lead to fall risks
- Difficulty maintaining weight
- Shoulder subluxation
- Joint contractures (*Amyotrophic Lateral Sclerosis*, 2010)

Occupational Therapy Evaluations

Occupational therapy (OT) evaluations focus on individual daily functioning, the physical environment, social network, and quality of life for the client and their family or caregivers.

Comprehensive Evaluations

- ALS Functional Rating Scale: assesses the changes in physical functioning in persons with ALS
- Canadian Occupational Performance Measure (COPM): self-report of performance and satisfaction with occupations
- Activity Card Sort (ACS): helps clients describe instrumental and social activities
- Health Status Questionnaire (SF-36): assesses patient's perceptions of health and physical limitations
- Multidimensional Fatigue Inventory: self-report that measures fatigue

Activities of Daily Living or Instrumental Activities of Daily Living or Leisure Evaluations

- Function Independence Measure (FIM): measures function and assistance level
- Barthel Index: measures ADL performance
- Performance Assessment of Self-Care Skills (PASS): evaluates functional status

Upper Extremity Function/Strength/Balance Evaluations

- Purdue Pegboard: measures hand and finger dexterity
- Manual muscle testing: assesses a client's muscle strength
- Range of motion testing: measures range of movement for a joint
- Berg Balance Scale: measures balance through performance in functional tasks

Occupational Therapy Interventions

Education

- Energy conservation in client-preferred activities
- Compensatory strategies such as using gravity-eliminated devices
- Splints and orthotics to reduce pain, subluxation, and fatigue
- Adaptive devices
- Safety, positioning, safe transfers, and skin integrity
- Augmentative communication devices
- Continued participation in shifted life roles and meaningful occupations (Foley, 2004; Lyons, Orozovic, Davis, & Newman, 2002)

Adaptation

- Environmental modification to promote function
- Adaptive utensils or equipments (wheelchairs, self-care devices, grab bars) (Trail, Nelson, Van, Appel, & Lai, 2001)

Prevention

- Muscle deconditioning
- Contracture through active and passive range of motion exercises
- Pressure sores with proper positioning (Cazzolli, 1999)

Occupational Therapy and the Evidence

Although the outcomes of ALS appear hopeless, OT may offer the individual and his or her family the opportunity to seek meaningful occupations and participate in the mindfulness of living life to the fullest. The philosophy of OT is consistent with a quality of life construct that may be used with individuals that have ALS. In order to increase the well-being and quality of life for these individuals, occupational therapists may help them identify personal and meaningful occupations (Foley, 2004).

Occupational therapists provide a holistic approach of care for individuals with ALS with therapy that encompasses occupational performance, education, adaptation, coping strategies, leisure, social participation, and palliative care. The medical model is not sufficient to fulfill the needs of individuals with ALS (Matuz, Birbaumer, Hautzinger, & Kubler, 2010). OT is devoted to provide meaning to the client and family's unique needs in this new stage of life. According to some individuals with ALS, factors such as psychological well-being, social supports, and spirituality are more important than physical function in terms of quality of life. Therefore, occupational therapists help increase opportunities for those with ALS to participate in personally meaningful occupations (Roach,

Averill, Segerstrom, & Kasarskis, 2009; Robbins, Simmons, Bremer, Walsh, & Fischer, 2001).

Caregiver Concerns

Because of the rapid progression of ALS, caring for a loved one is extremely difficult and can be overwhelming at times. Life roles of the individual and his or her family often shift greatly. The individual with ALS may need to discontinue working, leading to financial concerns and loss of identity. Decrease in ADL or instrumental activities of daily living (IADL) function is not only physically demanding for caregivers but also symbolizes a loss of independence for the individual with ALS, which can also be psychologically draining. Learning more about the disease is essential for caregivers because the information can give all parties a stronger sense of control. It is important for individuals and family members to learn coping strategies with the disease and to still find solace in meaningful occupations. Caregiver support groups can be beneficial in providing answers, information, and support from others having similar experiences (see ALS Links).

Resources

Associations

- ALS Association (ALSA)
  27001 Agoura Road
  Suite 150
  Calabassas Hills, CA 91301-5104
  Telephone: 818-880-9007 or 800-782-4747
  Fax: 818-880-9006
  Website: http://www.alsa.org

- ALS Hope Foundation
  219 North Broad Street
  7th floor, PO Box 40777
  Philadelphia, PA 19107
  Telephone: 215-551-0967
  Fax: 215-762-8634
  Website: http://www.alshopefoundation.org

- ALS Therapy Development Institute (ALSTDI)
  215 First Street
  Cambridge, MA 02142
  Telephone: 617-441-7200
  Fax: 617-441-7299
  Website: http://www.als.net

- Les Turner ALS Foundation
  8142 North Lawndale Avenue
  Skokie, IL 60076-3322
  Telephone: 888-ALS-1107
  Fax: 847-679-9109
  Website: http://www.lesturnerals.org

Books

- Hanlan, A. J. (1979). *Autobiography about dying.* Garden City, NY: Doubleday.
  Through his diary entries, Allen Hanlan reveals his journey from being diagnosed with ALS to facing his impending death. His wife also writes a postscript that describes living with a husband with ALS.

- Rice, E. (2005). *If they could only hear me: A collection of personal stories about ALS and the families that have been affected.* Wakefield, MA: The Angel Fund.
  This collection of personal stories offers an inside perspective on ALS from individuals and families affected and depicts a fighting spirit and keeps hope alive.

- Simmons, P. (2000). *Learning to fall: The blessings of an imperfect life.* New York, NY: Bantam Dell.
  Depicts Philip Simmons spiritual journey with ALS. A thoughtful book that is humorous, poetic, and ironic.

- Wakefield, D. (2005). *I remember running: The year I got everything I ever wanted—And ALS.* New York, NY: Marlowe and Company.
  A meditative diary of a 33-year-old woman battling ALS where Wakefield shares her fears, triumphs, and frustrations. Despite her diagnosis, she is determined to still be a professor, a homeowner, and a mother.

Journals

- *Amyotrophic Lateral Sclerosis and Other Motor Neuron Disorders*
- *Journal of Neurology*
- *The World Federation of Neurology Research Group on Motor Neuron Diseases*

Websites

- ALS Links
  http://www.ALS-link.org
  This Website is an internet portal for the ALS community, including patients, doctors, and caregivers. It offers other informative resources and is very user friendly.

- National Institute of Neurological Disorders and Stroke
  http://www.ninds.nih.gov/disorders/amyotrophiclateralsclerosis
  This Website provides a comprehensive overview of ALS and gives useful information in a thorough yet simple format.

References

Amyotrophic Lateral Sclerosis. (2010). Retrieved from the U.S. National Library of Medicine website: http://www.ncbi.nlm.nih.gov/pubmedhealth/PMH0001708

Amyotrophic Lateral Sclerosis Fact Sheet. (2011). Retrieved from the National Institute of Neurological Disorders and Stroke website: http://www.ninds.nih.gov/disorders/amyotrophiclateralsclerosis/detail_ALS.htm

Cazzolli, P. (1999). *Preventing and treating complications of immobility in people with ALS.* Retrieved from the ALS Care Project website: http://www.alscareproject.org/phycare/immobility.pdf

Foley, G. (2004). Quality of life for people with motor neuron disorder: A consideration for occupational therapists. *British Journal of Occupational Therapy, 67,* 551–553.

Lyons, M., Orozovic, N., Davis, J., & Newman, J. (2002). Doing-being-becoming: Occupational experiences of persons with life-threatening illnesses. *American Journal of Occupational Therapy, 56,* 285–295.

Maddox, S. (Ed.). (2003). Amyotrophic lateral sclerosis. In *Paralysis resource guide* (pp. 3–6). Short Hills, NJ: Paralysis Resource Center.

Matuz, T., Birbaumer, N., Hautzinger, M., & Kubler, A. (2010). Coping with amyotrophic lateral sclerosis. *Journal of Neurology, Neurosurgery, and Psychiatry, 81*(8), 893–898.

Mitsumoto, H. (2009). *Amyotrophic lateral sclerosis: A guide for patients and families* (3rd ed.). New York, NY: Demos Medical.

Riluzole. (2008). Retrieved from the U.S. National Library of Medicine website: http://www.ncbi.nlm.nih.gov/pubmedhealth/PMH0000978/

Roach, A., Averill, A., Segerstrom, S., & Kasarskis, E. (2009). The dynamic of quality of life in ALS patients and caregivers. *Annals of Behavioral Medicine, 37,* 197–206.

Robbins, R., Simmons, Z., Bremer, B. A., Walsh, S. M., & Fischer, S. (2001). Quality of life in ALS is maintained as physical function declines. *Neurology, 56,* 442–444.

Trail, M., Nelson, N., Van, J. N., Appel, S. A., & Lai, E. C. (2001). Wheelchair use by patients with amyotrophic lateral sclerosis: A survey of user characteristics and selection preferences. *Archives of Physical Medicines and Rehabilitation, 82,* 98–102.

Who gets ALS? (2008). Retrieved from the ALS Association website: http://www.alsa.org/als/who.cfm?CFID=8034765&CFTOKEN=5274a1cfb538d089-45945068-188B-2E62-80631ADE35A68F5C

Anxiety Disorders

Pamela Vaughn

Description and Diagnosis

Anxiety disorders are the most common of psychiatric disorders and include a broad range of conditions, including, but not limited to, generalized anxiety disorder (GAD), obsessive-compulsive disorder (OCD), and posttraumatic stress disorder (PTSD). Anxiety itself is a normal response to stressful experiences, but when it is prolonged, inappropriate, and/or overwhelming to the point that it interferes with functioning, it becomes a pathological disorder (Davis, 2011).

The American Psychiatric Association's (APA; 2000) *Diagnostic and Statistical Manual of Mental Disorders* (4th ed., text rev.; *DSM-IV-TR*) lists the following criteria for each GAD, OCD, and PTSD:

Diagnosis and Description	Diagnostic Criteria (APA, 2000)
Generalized anxiety disorder (GAD): characterized by at least 6 mo of persistent and excessive anxiety and worry	A. Excessive anxiety and worry (apprehensive expectation), occurring more days than not for at least 6 mo, about a number of events or activities (such as work or school performance). B. The person finds it difficult to control the worry. C. The anxiety and worry are associated with three (or more) of the following six symptoms (with at least some symptoms present for more days than not for the past 6 mo). *Note*: Only one item is required in children. 1. Restlessness or feeling keyed up or on edge 2. Being easily fatigued 3. Difficulty concentrating or mind going blank 4. Irritability 5. Muscle tension 6. Sleep disturbance (difficulty falling or staying asleep or restless unsatisfying sleep) D. The focus of the anxiety and worry is not confined to features of an Axis I disorder. E. The anxiety, worry, or physical symptoms cause clinically significant distress or impairment in social, occupational, or other important areas of functioning. F. The disturbance is not due to the direct physiological effects of a substance (e.g., a drug of abuse, a medication) or a general medical condition (e.g., hyperthyroidism) and does not occur exclusively during a mood disorder, a psychotic disorder, or a pervasive developmental disorder.
Obsessive-compulsive disorder (OCD): characterized by obsessions (which cause marked anxiety or distress) and/or by compulsions (which serve to neutralize anxiety)	A. Either obsessions or compulsions: *Obsessions* as defined by the following: 1. Recurrent and persistent thoughts, impulses, or images that are experienced, at some time during the disturbance, as intrusive and inappropriate and that cause marked anxiety or distress 2. The thoughts, impulses, or images are not simply excessive worries about real-life problems. 3. The person attempts to ignore or suppress such thoughts, impulses, or images or to neutralize them with some other thought or action. 4. The person recognizes that the obsessional thoughts, impulses, or images are product of his or her own mind (not imposed from without as in thought insertion). *Compulsions* as defined by the following: 1. Repetitive behaviors (e.g., hand washing, ordering, checking) or mental acts (e.g., praying, counting, repeating words silently) that the person feels driven to perform in response to an obsession or according to rules that must be applied rigidly 2. The behaviors or mental acts are aimed at preventing or reducing distress or preventing some dreaded event or situation; however, these behaviors or mental acts either are not connected in a realistic way with what they are designed to neutralize or prevent or are clearly excessive. B. At some point during the course of the disorder, the person has recognized that the obsessions or compulsions are excessive or unreasonable. *Note*: This does not apply to children. C. The obsessions or compulsions cause marked distress; are time consuming (take more than 1 h a day); or significantly interfere with the person's normal routine, occupational (or academic) functioning, or usual social activities or relationships. D. If another Axis I disorder is present, the content of the obsessions or compulsions is not restricted to it. E. The disturbance is not due to the direct physiological effects of a substance or a general medical condition. Specify *with poor insight*, if for most of the time during the current episode, the person does not recognize that the obsessions and compulsions are excessive or unreasonable.
Posttraumatic stress disorder (PTSD): characterized by the reexperiencing of an extremely traumatic event accompanied by symptoms of increased arousal and by avoidance of stimuli associated with the trauma	A. The person has been exposed to a traumatic event in which both of the following were present: 1. The person experienced, witnessed, or was confronted with an event or events that involved actual or threatened death or serious injury or a threat to the physical integrity of self or others. 2. The person's response involved intense fear, helplessness, or horror. *Note*: In children, this may be expressed instead by disorganized or agitated behavior. B. The traumatic event is persistently reexperienced in one (or more) of the following ways: 1. Recurrent and intrusive distressing recollections of the event, including images, thoughts, or perceptions. *Note*: In young children, repetitive play may occur in which themes or aspects of the trauma are expressed.

(*continued*)

Diagnosis and Description	Diagnostic Criteria (APA, 2000)
	2. Recurrent distressing dreams of the event. *Note*: In children, there may be frightening dreams without recognizable content. 3. Acting or feeling as if the traumatic event were recurring (includes a sense of reliving the experience, illusions, hallucinations, and dissociative flashback episodes, including those that occur on awakening or when intoxicated). *Note*: In young children, trauma-specific reenactment may occur. 4. Intense psychological distress at exposure to internal or external cues that symbolize or resemble an aspect of the traumatic event 5. Physiological reactivity on exposure to internal or external cues that symbolize or resemble an aspect of the traumatic event C. Persistent avoidance of stimuli associated with the trauma and numbing of general responsiveness (not present before the trauma), as indicated by three (or more) of the following: 1. Efforts to avoid thoughts, feelings, or conversations associated with the trauma 2. Efforts to avoid activities, places, or people that arouse recollections of the trauma 3. Inability to recall an important aspect of the trauma 4. Markedly diminished interest or participation in significant activities 5. Feeling of detachment or estrangement from others 6. Restricted range of affect (e.g., unable to have loving feelings) 7. Sense of a foreshortened future (e.g., does not expect to have a career, marriage, children, or a normal life span) D. Persistent symptoms of increased arousal (not present before the trauma), as indicated by two (or more) of the following: 1. Difficulty falling asleep or staying asleep 2. Irritability or outburst of anger 3. Difficulty concentrating 4. Hypervigilance 5. Exaggerated startle response E. Duration of the disturbance (symptoms B, C, and D) is more than 1 mo. F. The disturbance causes clinically significant distress or impairment in social, occupational, or other important areas of functioning. Specify *acute*, if duration of symptoms is less than 3 mo; *chronic*, if duration of symptoms is 3 mo or more; *with delayed onset*, if onset of symptoms is at least 6 mo after the stressor.

Prevalence

Most recent prevalence estimates report that in a given year, approximately 40 million (~18%) of adults in the United States are affected by anxiety disorders. Approximate breakdowns by specific diagnosis are the following:

- 3% of U.S. adults have GAD
- 1% of U.S. adults have OCD
- 3.5% of U.S. adults have PTSD (Kessler, Chiu, Demler, Merikangas, & Walters, 2005)

Women are more at risk of developing an anxiety disorder than men, and anxiety disorders are seen in all cultures (Asnaani, Richey, Dimaite, Hinton, & Hofmann, 2010).

Cause and Etiology

Because there is such a wide variety of anxiety disorders, no single etiological factor can be identified. Each disorder is as unique as the individuals who develop the disorders are. Causal factors may include the following:

- Extreme or prolonged stress
- Genetic factors
- Neuroanatomical factors (e.g., reduction in the size of the hippocampus)
- Faulty neurotransmitter communication
- Cognitive and psychological factors (e.g., misinterpretation of stressful events as overwhelming, dysfunctional cognitive schemas)
- Environmental factors (e.g., traumatic event) (Davis, 2011)

Typical Course, Symptoms, and Related Conditions

Many anxiety disorders begin in childhood or adolescence, but they can also begin during adulthood (e.g., after a traumatic event). The course of the disorders also varies greatly by individual, as some disorders are addressed and controlled immediately, whereas others develop into disabling and chronic conditions that affect all areas of occupation. See diagnostic criteria for disorder-specific symptoms for GAD, OCD, and PTSD. General symptoms may include the following:

- Physical symptoms (e.g., rapid heartbeat, weakness, nausea, headaches) or impairments (e.g., poorer overall health, fatigue)
- Cognitive impairments based on excessive and irrational fear and/or dread, for example, difficulty focusing or following directions, poor memory, difficulty with processing
- Psychosocial impairments, for example, decreased number and/or quality of relationships, disruption of performance in school or at work, feeling hopeless (Davis, 2011; National Institute of Mental Health [NIMH], 2009)

Common comorbid conditions include depression, eating disorders, bipolar disorder, sleep disorders, and substance abuse; specifically with PTSD, physical injuries or conditions (e.g., amputation) may be present (APA, 2000).

Interdisciplinary Interventions

The most common approach to the treatment of anxiety disorders is to use medication, psychotherapeutic techniques, or a combination of the two.

Medication Therapy

Medication is used to control and alleviate the symptoms of anxiety disorders, but it cannot "cure" people of these disorders. Different medications are prescribed for different anxiety disorders, and dosages taken depend on the individual's needs and any experienced side effects. All health professionals working with clients with anxiety disorders should be aware of any medications that their clients are taking and any side effects, including withdrawal, which they are experiencing. The most common types of medication include the following:

- Antidepressants (selective serotonin reuptake inhibitors [SSRIs], tricyclics, monoamine oxidase inhibitors [MAOIs])
- Antianxiety drugs (benzodiazepines, azapirones)
- Beta-blockers—used to treat the physical symptoms of anxiety (NIMH, 2009)

Psychotherapy

Psychotherapeutic intervention "involves talking with a trained mental health professional, such as a psychiatrist, psychologist, social worker, or counselor, to discover what caused an anxiety disorder and how to deal with its symptoms" (NIMH, 2009, p. 17). The most common technique used is cognitive behavioral therapy (CBT), which helps clients change their thought processes surrounding their anxiety and develop individualized skills and strategies to change the way they react in situations that are anxiety inducing. Occupational therapists can be trained in CBT. Relaxation therapy, in which a client is taught to develop and use strategies such as deep breathing, meditation, muscle relaxation, and visualization before or during anxiety-inducing situations, is another psychotherapeutic approach (Davis, 2011).

Occupational Therapy Evaluations

The evaluation process focuses on what the client needs, wants, or is expected to do and analyzes what factors may impact desired occupational performance. The evaluation begins with occupation-focused assessments followed by specific evaluation of the potential impact of anxiety disorders on occupational performance.

Occupation-Focused Assessments

- Role Checklist (Oakley, Kielhofner, Barris, & Reichler, 1986)
- Occupational Performance History Interview II (OPHI-II) (Kielhofner et al., 2004)
- Assessment of Motor and Process Skills (AMPS) (Fisher & Jones, 2010)
- Occupational Self-Assessment (OSA) Version 2.2 (Baron, Kielhofner, Iyenger, Goldhammer, & Wolenski, 2006)
- Performance Assessment of Self-Care Skills (PASS) (Holm & Rogers, 2008)
- Canadian Occupational Performance Measure (COPM) (Law et al., 2005)
- Short Form-36 (SF-36) (Hays, Sherbourne, & Mazel, 1995)
- Activity Card Sort (ACS) (Baum & Edwards, 2008)
- Occupational Profile of Sleep (Pierce & Summers, 2011)
- Stress diary

Client Factor Assessments

- Beck Anxiety Inventory (BAI) (Beck, 1993)
- Revised Children's Manifest Anxiety Scale: Second Edition (RCMAS-2) (Reynolds & Richmond, 2008)
- Allen Cognitive Level Screen-Fifth Version (ACLS-5) (Allen et al., 2007)
- Adolescent/Adult Sensory Profile (Brown & Dunn, 2002)

Occupational Therapy Interventions

In addition to psychotherapeutic intervention techniques, specifically CBT, described previously, occupational therapy interventions for anxiety disorders may include the following:

- Modification of activities of daily living (ADL), instrumental activities of daily living (IADL), school, and/or work tasks and/or environments to decrease situations in which anxiety is triggered
- Development of coping strategies
- Time management and daily living routine development to increase participation in meaningful occupation
- Sleep regulation (Pierce & Summers, 2011)
- Sensory integration, particularly for clients with OCD or gravitational insecurity (Rieke & Anderson, 2009)
- Safe driving interventions

Occupational Therapy and the Evidence

Rieke and Anderson (2009) found that adults and adolescents with OCD have increased sensitivity to sensory stimuli, creating an opportunity for occupational therapists trained in sensory integration techniques to provide intervention for these clients. In recent years, many veterans have been diagnosed with PTSD, which has occupational implications including in the area of driving (Classen et al., 2011). CBT has been shown to be effective in decreasing symptoms of anxiety and even sometimes resulting in a remission of anxiety disorder diagnosis in both children/adolescents and adults with anxiety disorders (Hunot, Churchill, Teixeira, & Silva de Lima, 2007; James, Soler, & Weatherall, 2005).

Caregiver Concerns

Relatives of individuals with anxiety disorders have reported experiencing decreased physical and mental health (e.g., depression, anxiety) as a result of caring for their family member. Support groups and therapy for these family members and caregivers may be helpful in decreasing these negative impacts (Senaratne, Van Ameringen, Mancini, & Patterson, 2010).

Resources

Organizations

- Anxiety Disorders Association of America
  8730 Georgia Ave., Silver Spring, MD 20910
  Website: http://www.adaa.org/

- American Academy of Children and Adolescent Psychiatry
  3615 Wisconsin Avenue, N.W., Washington, DC 20016-3007
  Website: http://www.aacap.org

Books

- Ford, E., Liebowitz, M., & Andrews, L. W. (2007). *What you must think of me: A firsthand account of one teenager's experience with social anxiety disorder*. New York, NY: Oxford University Press.

- Yazzolino, K. (2010). *If seen . . . My journey living with anxiety*. Castroville, TN: Black Rose Writing.

Websites

- Freedom From Fear: http://www.freedomfromfear.org

- National Institute of Mental Health: http://www.nimh.nih.gov/health/publications/anxiety-disorders

- American Psychiatric Association: http://www.healthyminds.org/Main-Topic/Anxiety-Disorders.aspx

- American Psychological Association: http://www.apa.org/helpcenter/anxiety-treatment.aspx

- Mayo Clinic: http://www.mayoclinic.com/health/anxiety/DS01187

- Medline: http://www.nlm.nih.gov/medlineplus/anxiety.html#cat22

References

Allen, C. K., Austin, S. L., David, S. K., Earhart, C. A., McCraith, D. B., & Riska-Williams, L. (2007). *Manual for the Allen cognitive level screen-5 (ACLS-5) and large Allen cognitive level screen-5 (LACLS-5)*. Camarillo, CA: ACLS and LACLS Committee.

American Psychiatric Association. (2000). *Diagnostic and statistical manual of mental disorders* (4th ed., text rev.). Washington, DC: Author.

Asnaani, A., Richey, J. A., Dimaite, R., Hinton, D. E., & Hofmann, S. G. (2010). A cross-ethnic comparison of lifetime prevalence rates of anxiety disorders. *The Journal of Nervous & Mental Disease, 198*, 551–555. doi:10.1097/NMD.0b013e3181ea169f

Baron, K., Kielhofner, G., Iyenger, A., Goldhammer, V., & Wolenski, J. (2006). *Occupational Self-Assessment* (OSA; Version 2.2). Chicago, IL: MOHO Clearinghouse.

Baum, C. M., & Edwards, D. E. (2008). *Activity Card Sort* (2nd ed.). Bethesda, MD: AOTA Press.

Beck, A. T. (1993). *Beck Anxiety Inventory (BAI) manual*. San Antonio, TX: Psychological Corporation.

Brown, C. E., & Dunn, W. (2002). *Adolescent/adult sensory profile: User's manual.* San Antonio, TX: Psychological Corporation.
Classen, S., Levy, C., Meyer, D. L., Bewernitz, M., Lanford, D. N., & Mann, W. C. (2011). Simulated driving performance of combat veterans with mild traumatic brain injury and posttraumatic stress disorder: A pilot study. *American Journal of Occupational Therapy, 65*, 419–427. doi:10.5014/ajot.2011.000893
Davis, J. (2011). Anxiety disorders. In C. Brown & V. C. Stoffel (Eds.), *Occupational therapy in mental health: A vision for participation* (pp. 167–178). Philadelphia, PA: F. A. Davis.
Fisher, A. G., & Jones, K. B. (2010). *Assessment of Motor and Process Skills. Vol. 1: Development, standardization, and administration manual* (7th ed.). Fort Collins, CO: Three Star Press.
Hays, R. D., Sherbourne, C. D., & Mazel, R. M. (1995). *User's manual for Medical Outcomes Study (MOS) core measures of health-related quality of life.* Santa Monica, CA: RAND.
Holm, M. B., & Rogers, J. C. (2008). The Performance Assessment of Self-Care Skills (PASS). In B. Hemphill-Pearson (Ed.), *Assessments in occupational therapy mental health* (2nd ed., pp. 101–110). Thorofare, NJ: Slack.
Hunot, V., Churchill, R., Teixeira, V., & Silva de Lima, M. (2007). Psychological therapies for generalised anxiety disorder. *Cochrane Database of Systematic Reviews*, (1), CD001848. doi:10.1002/14651858.CD001848.pub4
James, A., Soler, A., & Weatherall, R. (2005). Cognitive behavioural therapy for anxiety disorders in children and adolescents. *Cochrane Database of Systematic Reviews*, (4), CD004690. doi:10.1002/14651858.CD004690.pub2
Kessler, R. C., Chiu, W. T., Demler, O., Merikangas, K. R., & Walters, E. E. (2005). Prevalence, severity, and comorbidity of 12-month DSM-IV disorders in the national comorbidity survey replication. *Archives of General Psychiatry, 62*, 617–627.
Kielhofner, G., Mallinson, T., Crawford, C., Nowak, M., Rigby, M., Henry, A., & Walens, D. (2004). *Occupational Performance History Interview II (OPHI-II).* Chicago, IL: MOHO Clearinghouse.
Law, M., Baptiste, S., Carswell, A., McColl, M., Polatajko, H., & Pollock, N. (2005). *Canadian Occupational Performance Measure* (4th ed.). Ottawa, Canada: CAOT Publications.
National Institute of Mental Health. (2009). *Anxiety disorders* (NIH Publication No. 09 3879). Retrieved from http://www.nimh.nih.gov/health/publications/anxiety-disorders
Oakley, F., Kielhofner, G., Barris, R., & Reichler, R. (1986). The Role Checklist: Development and empirical assessment of reliability. *Occupational Therapy Journal of Research, 6*, 157–170.
Pierce, D., & Summers, K. (2011). Rest and sleep. In C. Brown & V. C. Stoffel (Eds.), *Occupational therapy in mental health: A vision for participation* (pp. 736–754). Philadelphia, PA: F. A. Davis.
Reynolds, C. R., & Richmond, B. O. (2008). *Revised children's manifest anxiety scale: Second edition (RCMAS-2).* Torrance, CA: Western Psychological Services.
Rieke, E. F., & Anderson, D. (2009). Adolescent/adult sensory profile and obsessive-compulsive disorder. *American Journal of Occupational Therapy, 63*, 138–145.
Senaratne, R., Van Ameringen, M., Mancini, C., & Patterson, B. (2010). The burden of anxiety disorders on the family. *Journal of Nervous & Mental Disease, 198*, 876–880. doi:10.1097/NMD.0b013e3181fe7450

Arthritis

Pamela Vaughn

Description and Diagnosis

Arthritis is the inflammation of a joint and its surrounding tissues. It includes more than 100 diseases and conditions that affect the joint. Common forms include the following:

- Osteoarthritis (OA; also referred to as a *degenerative joint disease* [DJD])
- Rheumatoid arthritis (RA)
- Juvenile rheumatoid arthritis (JRA)
- Lupus
- Fibromyalgia
- Gout (Centers for Disease Control and Prevention [CDC], 2009)

Doctors perform physical exams and may use X-ray, magnetic resonance imaging (MRI), blood tests, and/or joint fluid analysis to diagnose arthritis and rule out other conditions that could be causing inflammation of the joint (CDC, 2009).

Incidence and Prevalence

Arthritis is the leading cause of disability in the United States with the following statistics:

- In 2009, more than 52.1 million (22%) U.S. adults reported having doctor-diagnosed arthritis.
- Women are more likely than men to be diagnosed with arthritis.
- Diagnosis of arthritis increases with age—54% of U.S. adults older than age 75 years versus 8% of U.S. adults aged 18 to 44 years reported having doctor-diagnosed arthritis in 2009.
- Asian adults and Hispanic adults are less likely to have arthritis than non-Hispanic White adults and non-Hispanic Black adults.
- Lower socioeconomic status is correlated with higher diagnoses of arthritis.
- Having Medicaid and/or Medicare insurance versus private health insurance is correlated with higher diagnoses of arthritis.
- It is projected that the incidence of arthritis will increase in coming years, reaching an estimated prevalence of 67 million U.S. adults by the year 2030.
- More than 9% of the U.S. adult population reports arthritis-attributable activity limitation (Cheng et al., 2010; Hootman & Helmick, 2006; Pleis, Ward, Lucas, & National Center for Health Statistics, Centers for Disease Control and Prevention, 2010).

According to the National Arthritis Data Workgroup (Helmick et al., 2008; Lawrence et al., 2008), U.S. prevalence of specific forms of arthritis is estimated at

- OA—27 million adults
- RA—1.3 million adults
- Juvenile arthritis, including JRA—294,000 children

Cause and Etiology

The precise cause of arthritis is unknown, but it is generally agreed on that both genetics and environment are factors. OA, or DJD, is caused by the gradual degeneration of the cartilage within a joint capsule (Yasuda, 2008).

Typical Course, Symptoms, and Related Conditions

The course of arthritis depends on the form and varies between individuals. Individuals diagnosed with arthritis report increased disability and a decreased quality of life (Poole, Chiappisi, Cordova, & Sibbitt, 2007). Depression is often a condition secondary to arthritis.

Osteoarthritis

OA—caused by a breakdown of cartilage within a joint often as a result of repetitive use, injury, and/or genetic factors—results in the bones rubbing together and producing pain and stiffness in the joint. When the bones rub together, bony growths called "spurs" may develop, and small pieces of bone may break off and float in the synovial fluid of the joint. Both of these aftereffects can lead to swelling of the joint, which is the characteristic symptom of arthritis. Commonly affected joints are the hips, knees, interphalangeal joints of the fingers, the first carpometacarpal joint (base of the thumb), and the spine (particularly the neck and the lower back). Symptoms include joint tenderness and pain that are often exacerbated by activity as well as limited joint movement and stiffness, particularly in the morning or after prolonged periods of rest. Obesity, as well as the repetitive use of joints, for example, at work, increase the likelihood of developing OA (Yasuda, 2008).

Rheumatoid Arthritis

RA is an autoimmune condition of unknown cause in which the lining of a joint—the synovial membrane—becomes inflamed and wears away at the bone and cartilage, resulting in destruction and deformation of joints. Many joints may be and often are affected at once, and RA is usually symmetrical. Onset can be gradual or sudden and generally begins with aching and soreness (sometimes flulike) followed by pain, tenderness, inflammation, and warmth in the joints. This results in a general overall stiffness, decreased movement and strength, and fatigue. Symptoms such as decreased strength, function, and appetite as well as increased fatigue and pain during movement persist and worsen as more joints are affected, whereas inflammation often decreases following the acute stage. Eventually, deformities (particularly in the distal extremities, e.g., swan-neck and boutonniere) and rheumatoid nodules (bumps under the skin) often appear. The systemic nature of RA indicates that multiple other physiological systems may be affected as well (e.g., swollen pulmonary and cardiac tissue). Depression is a common problem for individuals with RA due to the impact that the disease has on their everyday lives. Most clients have chronic RA, in which symptoms persist and/or flare up occasionally, although some enter remission. JRA is classified by a diagnosis at an age younger than 16 years; most children with JRA experience acute stages and symptoms between the ages of 1 and 6 years. Many children recover without lasting disability (Orchanian, 2007).

Interdisciplinary Interventions

Because arthritis is a chronic condition, intervention focuses on controlling symptoms and improving function.

Medical Management

- Medications: analgesics (e.g., acetaminophen or topical creams), nonsteroidal anti-inflammatory drugs (NSAIDs; e.g., ibuprofen), corticosteroid injections, biologics, and disease-modifying antirheumatic drugs (DMARDs), immunosuppressants
- Surgery: partial or total joint replacement

Physical Therapy

Physical therapy for arthritis focuses on strength maintenance and pain control. Methods of intervention may include strength training, heat and/or ice treatment, ultrasound, and the use of transcutaneous electrical nerve stimulation (TENS) machines (Paskins, Kamath, & Hassell, 2010).

Exercise and Weight Control

Exercise helps maintain joint health by preventing the degeneration of cartilage and maintaining strength, flexibility, and range of motion (ROM). It also increases the body's reparative processes and therefore helps control pain levels (Fitzcharles, Lussier, & Shir, 2010). Because individuals who are overweight or obese have a higher likelihood of developing OA, exercise as a means of losing weight can also alleviate OA symptoms. Several packaged exercise programs for individuals with arthritis are available (Brady, Jernick, Hootman, & Sniezek, 2009).

Complementary and Alternative Therapy

Many clients use complementary and alternative medicine (CAM) to alleviate symptoms associated with arthritis. Commonly used techniques include thermal springs, oral herbal therapies, hot and cold therapy, externally applied therapies, and massage. Many of these techniques—particularly heat therapy and massage—are perceived by clients as effective in reducing symptoms of arthritis (Unsal & Gozum, 2010).

Occupational Therapy Evaluations

The evaluation process focuses on what the client needs, wants, or is expected to do and analyzes what factors may impact desired occupational performance. The evaluation begins with occupation-focused assessments followed by specific evaluation of the potential impact of arthritis on occupational performance.

Occupation-Focused Evaluations

- Role Checklist (Oakley, Kielhofner, Barris, & Reichler, 1986)
- Occupational Performance History Interview II (OPHI-II) (Kielhofner et al., 2004)
- Assessment of Motor and Process Skills (AMPS) (Fisher & Jones, 2010)
- Activity Measure for Post-Acute Care (AM-PAC) (Jette, Hayley, Coster, & Ni, 2007)
- Performance Assessment of Self-Care Skills (PASS) (Holm & Rogers, 2008)
- Health Assessment Questionnaire (HAQ) (Ramey, Raynauld, & Fries, 1992)
- Canadian Occupational Performance Measure (COPM) (Law et al., 2005)
- Short Form-36 (SF-36) (Hays, Sherbourne, & Mazel, 1995)

Client Factor Evaluations

- Arthritis Hand Function Test (Backman & Mackie, 1997)
- Disability of Arm, Shoulder, and Hand (DASH) (Hudak, Amadio, Bombardier, & the Upper Extremity Collaborative Group, 1996)
- ROM
- Measures of pain (e.g., Visual Analog Scale [VAS])
- Manual muscle testing
- Measures of grasp and pinch strength

Occupational Therapy Interventions

The primary goal of occupational therapy (OT) intervention for arthritis is to restore clients to occupational functioning. This takes different forms depending on the diagnosis and individual needs of the client. The following interventions are common for use with clients with arthritis (Yasuda, 2008):

- Client education: Occupational therapists can assist other medical personnel in educating individuals with arthritis and their caregivers about arthritis, its symptoms, and its effect on occupation.
- Joint maintenance and protection: Help clients identify and apply techniques to preserve or improve current joint condition and decrease symptoms; may include strengthening, ROM exercises, hot/cold modalities to decrease pain and stiffness, ergonomic education, task modification, and so forth.
- Splinting: Particularly for the hands, splints can stabilize joints to reduce inflammation and pain, keep joints in proper positioning for maximal occupational performance, and prevent undesired motion or deformity.
- Fatigue management and energy conservation: Work with clients to identify fatiguing activities and determine alternative or modified activities to conserve energy and increase function and participation.
- Environmental modification: Identify and implement changes to the workplace, school, and home that will facilitate occupational performance while decreasing chances of exacerbating symptoms.
- Task modification: Alter tasks, potentially with the use of assistive devices, to increase client's ability to perform them satisfactorily (without fatigue, pain, etc.).
- Consultation for lifestyle changes: Collaborate with client to identify alternative occupations (for work, leisure, social participation, etc.) that will result in increased participation and satisfaction.
- Consultation regarding sexual relations: Educate client about potential barriers that arthritis can have on sexual participation; help identify strategies for communication with his or her sexual partner and for more comfortable sex.

Occupational Therapy and the Evidence

OT interventions (i.e., client education, joint protection training, use of splints and other adaptive devices) are effective in increasing function and participation in activities of daily living (ADL) with decreased pain among clients with RA (Steultjens et al., 2008). Hand, Law, and McColl

(2011) identified the following multiple OT interventions for clients with arthritis as beneficial:

- Joint protection groups led to improved ADL for adults with RA compared to controls; declines over time in ADL functioning were less for the intervention group than for the controls.
- In-home and telephone interventions increased self-efficacy and participation in ADL or instrumental activities of daily living (IADL) for clients with chronic conditions, including arthritis, when compared to controls.
- Multidisciplinary (including OT) interventions regarding employment can improve psychological health in clients with RA.

Mallinson, Fischer, Rogers, Ehrlich-Jones, and Chang (2009) suggest that the future of OT for clients with arthritis will experience a shift away from remediation interventions and begin to focus on increased health promotion on a public health level.

Caregiver Concerns

Martire et al. (2006) found that spouses of older adults with OA experience stress, burden, and irritation when they incorrectly estimate the levels of pain and functionality that their spouses have; those who have accurate perceptions report less burden, stress, and negative emotions in response to their spouses' condition.

Resources

Organizations

- Arthritis Foundation: a nonprofit research and educational association for professionals and clients.
  PO Box 7669
  Atlanta, GA 30357-0669
  Telephone: (800) 283-7800
  http://www.arthritis.org
- American College of Rheumatology: a resource for health professionals regarding education, research, practice, and advocacy of rheumatology.
  2200 Lake Boulevard NE
  Atlanta, GA 30319
  Telephone: (404) 633-3777
  Fax: (404) 633-1870
  http://www.rheumatology.org

Books

- Elton, K. (2010). *A resilient life: Learning to thrive, not just survive with rheumatoid arthritis.* Author.
- Guilbeaux, S. B. (2011). *In a good spot: My lifelong battle with rheumatoid arthritis.* Bloomington, IN: AuthorHouse.

Websites

- http://www.cdc.gov/arthritis/
- http://www.ra.com/
- Arthritis—PubMed Health: http://www.ncbi.nlm.nih.gov/pubmedhealth/PMH0002223/
- Mayo Clinic—Arthritis: http://www.mayoclinic.com/health/arthritis/DS01122

References

Backman, C., & Mackie, H. (1997). *Arthritis Hand Function Test: A standardized test for adults with arthritis.* Vancouver, BC: University of British Columbia.

Brady, T. J., Jernick, S. L., Hootman, J. M., & Sniezek, J. E. (2009). Public health interventions for arthritis: Expanding the toolbox of evidence-based interventions. *Journal of Women's Health, 18,* 1905–1917. doi:10.1089/jwh.2009.1571

Centers for Disease Control and Prevention. (2009). *Arthritis.* Retrieved from http://www.cdc.gov/arthritis/

Cheng, Y. J., Hootman, J. M., Murphy, L. B., Langmaid, G. A., Helmick, C. G., & Division of Adult and Community Health, National Center for Chronic Disease Prevention and Health Promotion, Centers for Disease Control and Prevention. (2010). Prevalence of doctor-diagnosed arthritis and arthritis-attributable activity limitation—United States, 2007–2009. *Morbidity and Mortality Weekly Report, 59*(39), 1261–1265.

Fisher, A. G., & Jones, K. B. (2010). *Assessment of Motor and Process Skills. Vol. 1: Development, standardization, and administration manual* (7th ed.). Fort Collins, CO: Three Star Press.

Fitzcharles, M., Lussier, D., & Shir, Y. (2010). Management of chronic arthritis pain in the elderly. *Drugs and Aging, 27,* 471–490.

Hand, C., Law, M., & McColl, M. A. (2011). Occupational therapy interventions for chronic diseases: A scoping review. *American Journal of Occupational Therapy, 65,* 428–436. doi:10.5014/ajot.2011.002071

Hays, R. D., Sherbourne, C. D., & Mazel, R. M. (1995). *User's manual for Medical Outcomes Study (MOS) core measures of health-related quality of life.* Santa Monica, CA: RAND.

Helmick, C. G., Felson, D. T., Lawrence, R. C., Gabriel, S., Hirsch, R., Kwoh, C. K., . . . National Arthritis Data Workgroup. (2008). Estimates of the prevalence of arthritis and other rheumatic conditions in the United States: Part I. *Arthritis & Rheumatism, 58,* 15–25. doi:10.1002/art.23177

Holm, M. B., & Rogers, J. C. (2008). The Performance Assessment of Self-Care Skills (PASS). In B. Hemphill-Pearson (Ed.), *Assessments in occupational therapy mental health* (2nd ed., pp. 101–110). Thorofare, NJ: Slack.

Hootman, J. M., & Helmick, C. G. (2006). Projections of U.S. prevalence of arthritis and associated activity limitations. *Arthritis and Rheumatism, 54,* 226–229.

Hudak, P. L., Amadio, P. C., Bombardier, C., & the Upper Extremity Collaborative Group. (1996). Development of an upper extremity outcome measure: The DASH (disabilities of the arm, shoulder, and hand) [corrected]. *American Journal of Industrial Medicine, 29,* 602–608. Erratum in: *American Journal of Industrial Medicine, 30,* 372.

Jette, A., Hayley, S. M., Coster, W., & Ni, P. (2007). *Boston University Activity Measure for Post Acute Care: Instruction manual.* Retrieved from http://www.crecare.com/order/order.html

Kielhofner, G., Mallinson, T., Crawford, C., Nowak, M., Rigby, M., Henry, A., & Walens, D. (2004). *Occupational Performance History Interview II (OPHI-II).* Chicago, IL: MOHO Clearinghouse.

Law, M., Baptiste, S., Carswell, A., McColl, M., Polatajko, H., & Pollock, N. (2005). *Canadian Occupational Performance Measure* (4th ed.). Ottawa, Canada: CAOT Publications.

Lawrence, R. C., Felson, D. T., Helmick, C. G., Arnold, L. M., Choi, H., Deyo, R. A., . . . National Arthritis Data Workgroup. (2008). Estimates of the prevalence of arthritis and other rheumatic conditions in the United States: Part II. *Arthritis & Rheumatism, 58,* 26–35. doi:10.1002/art.23176

Mallinson, T., Fischer, H., Rogers, J. C., Ehrlich-Jones, L., & Chang, R. (2009). The issue is—Human occupation for public health promotion: New directions for occupational therapy practice with persons with arthritis. *American Journal of Occupational Therapy, 63,* 220–226.

Martire, L. M., Keefe, F. J., Schulz, R., Ready, R., Beach, S. R., Rudy, T. E., & Starz, T. W. (2006). Older spouses' perceptions of partners' chronic arthritis pain: Implications for spousal responses, support provision, and caregiving experiences. *Psychology and Aging, 21,* 222–230. doi:10.1037/0882-7974.21.2.222

Oakley, F., Kielhofner, G., Barris, R., & Reichler, R. (1986). The Role Checklist: Development and empirical assessment of reliability. *Occupational Therapy Journal of Research, 6,* 157–170.

Orchanian, D. P. (2007). Rheumatoid arthritis. In B. J. Atchison & D. K. Dirette (Eds.), *Conditions in occupational therapy: Effect on occupational performance* (3rd ed., pp. 275–310). Philadelphia, PA: Lippincott Williams & Wilkins.

Paskins, Z., Kamath, S. N., & Hassell, A. B. (2010). Management of inflammatory arthritis in older people. *Reviews in Clinical Gerontology, 20,* 42–55. doi:10.1017/S095925980999044X

Pleis, J. R., Ward, B. W., Lucas, J. W., & National Center for Health Statistics, Centers for Disease Control and Prevention. (2010). *Summary health statistics for U.S. adults: National Health Interview Survey, 2009* (Department of Health & Human Services Publication No. [PHS] 2011–1577). Retrieved from http://www.cdc.gov/nchs/fastats/arthrits.htm

Poole, J. L., Chiappisi, H., Cordova, J. S., & Sibbitt, W., Jr. (2007). Quality of life in American Indian and White women with and without rheumatoid arthritis. *American Journal of Occupational Therapy, 61*, 280–289.

Ramey, D. R., Raynauld, J. P., & Fries, J. F. (1992). The Health Assessment Questionnaire 1992: Status and review. *Arthritis Care and Research, 5*, 119–129. doi:10.1002/art.1790050303

Steultjens, E. E. M. J., Dekker, J. J., Bouter, L. M., Schaardenburg, D. D., Kuyk, M. A. M. A. H., & Van den Ende, E. C. H. M. (2008). Occupational therapy for rheumatoid arthritis. *Cochrane Database of Systematic Reviews*, (1), CD003114. doi:10.1002/14651858.CD003114.pub2

Unsal, A., & Gozum, S. (2010). Use of complementary and alternative medicine by patients with arthritis. *Journal of Clinical Nursing, 19*, 1129–1138. doi:10.1111/j.13652702.2009.03111.x

Yasuda, Y. L. (2008). Rheumatoid arthritis, osteoarthritis, and fibromyalgia. In M. V. Radomski & C. A. T. Latham (Eds.), *Occupational therapy for physical dysfunction* (6th ed., pp. 1214–1243). Philadelphia, PA: Lippincott Williams & Wilkins.

Attention Deficit/Hyperactivity Disorder

Alaina Krumbach

Description and Diagnosis

Attention deficit/hyperactivity disorder (ADHD) is one of the most common childhood behavioral disorders and may continue into adolescence and adulthood. ADHD is characterized by persistent inattention, hyperactivity, and/or impulsivity (National Institute of Mental Health [NIMH], 2008). Individuals with ADHD have impairments in functioning and maintaining social relationships in multiple environments including home and school. ADHD is two to three times more frequent in boys than in girls (Centers for Disease Control and Prevention [CDC], 2007). Some children with ADHD experience sensory processing or sensory responsiveness difficulties when engaging in structured tasks and activities, resulting in limitations with sequencing and planning motor tasks and regulating emotions (Dunn & Bennett, 2002; Schaaf & Miller, 2005).

Incidence and Prevalence

According to the *Diagnostic and Statistical Manual of Mental Disorders* (4th ed., text rev.; *DSM-IV-TR*; American Psychiatric Association [APA], 2000), an estimated 3% to 7% of school-age children have ADHD. Approximately 9.5% or 5.4 million school-age children between the ages of 4 and 17 years have ever been diagnosed with ADHD (CDC, 2007).

Cause and Etiology

The cause and etiology of ADHD are unknown; however, studies suggest that genes play a significant role, especially in combination with environmental factors. Additional studies are looking at the contributions of nutrition, social environment, and brain injuries in ADHD (NIMH, 2008). Other possible factors may be premature birth, low birth weight, maternal body mass index (BMI) levels, and prenatal maternal smoking and/or alcohol use (NIMH, 2008; Rodriguez et al., 2007).

Typical Course, Related Conditions, and Symptoms

ADHD symptoms arise in early childhood between the ages of 3 and 6 years, unless they are associated with a brain injury later in life. Individuals with ADHD may continue to experience symptoms throughout life. Related conditions include sleep deprivation, depression, anxiety, learning disabilities, oppositional defiant disorder, and bipolar disorder (NIMH, 2008). Children with ADHD and sensory overresponsivity have significantly higher levels of anxiety than children with only ADHD and children without ADHD. Approximately 25% of children with ADHD are diagnosed with a comorbid anxiety disorder (Reynolds & Lane, 2009). A large percentage of individuals with ADHD also have developmental coordination disorder (Watemberg, Wasierberg, Zuk, & Lerman-Sagie, 2007).

ADHD is classified into three subtypes in the *DSM-IV-TR*:

1. ADHD predominantly inattentive type (ADHD-I): Individual may daydream, not seem to be listening, experience difficulty focusing on one task, be easily distracted by surroundings, and experience difficulty organizing work.
2. ADHD predominantly hyperactive-impulsive type (ADHD-HI): Individual may experience difficulty remaining seated or sitting still during tasks; may be impatient, interrupt others, or may talk excessively.
3. ADHD combined type (ADHD-C): Individual meets both sets of inattention and hyperactive-impulsive criteria; this is the most prevalent subtype of ADHD (APA, 2000).

Precautions

Individuals with ADHD may struggle in school and work with organizational skills, task completion, and time management. Individuals with ADHD are more prevalent to take risks, break rules, experience injury, and may have problems with substance abuse in adolescence and adulthood. Individuals on medication may experience undesirable or negative side effects including decreased appetite, sleep problems, and irritability (CDC, 2007; NIMH, 2008).

Interdisciplinary Interventions

Medication Therapy

Stimulants, including methylphenidate and amphetamine, are the most widely researched and most commonly prescribed medications because of their calming effects on individuals with ADHD (NIMH, 2008). Research has demonstrated that stimulants improve individual's behaviors and academic performance by reducing hyperactivity and impulsivity and improving focusing abilities (Biederman, Monuteaux, Spencer, Wilens, & Faraone, 2009).

Educational Management

Interventions for students with ADHD include tutoring and special education to maximize attention and concentration, counter impulsive behavior, improve self-esteem and socialization, assist in overcoming learning difficulties, and promote consistency of management between home and school (DuPaul, 2007; Reif, 2003). Common strategies include communication folders between parents and teachers, making clear assignment guidelines, and involving school psychologists or counselors in the intervention team (CDC, 2007; DuPaul, 2007).

Multimodal Treatment Study of Attention Deficit/Hyperactivity Disorder

The Multimodal Treatment of Attention Deficit Hyperactivity Disorder (MTA) study, conducted by the NIMH and cosponsored by the U.S. Department of Education, examined intervention effectiveness of medication therapy, behavioral therapy, combination therapy (medication and behavioral therapy), and routine community care for individuals with ADHD. Results indicated that a combination therapy significantly decreased symptoms of anxiety and improved academic performance, familial relations, and social skills (MTA Cooperative Group, 1999). A follow-up study conducted 3 years later showed no significant differences in the intervention groups of the MTA study. Possibilities for variations in results include alterations to medication regimens, age-related changes, familial factors, comorbid conditions, and initial symptom severity (Jenson et al., 2007).

Occupational Therapy Evaluations

Social Participation

- Children's Assessment of Participation and Enjoyment (CAPE) and Preferences for Activities of Children (PAC): social participation and enjoyment
- Children Helping Out: Responsibilities, Expectations, and Supports (CHORES): assessment of school-age children's participation in household activities

- Home Situations Questionnaire (HSQ): assesses impact of ADHD in the home on activities of daily living (ADL)
- Perceived Efficacy and Goal Setting System (PEGS): home, school, and community activities
- Social Skills Rating System (SSRS): teacher–student and peer relationships and academic performance

School Function

- Academic Performance Rating Scale: academic success, productivity, and impulse control
- School Function Assessment (SFA): performance of student's tasks and activities
- School Situations Questionnaire (SSQ): assesses impact of ADHD at school

Behavior

- Child Behavior Checklist: caregiver reports about child's behavior
- Adolescent Behavior Checklist: adolescent report to identify at-risk behavior
- ADHD Behavior Checklist for Adults: self-report questionnaire to diagnose ADHD

Self-Perception

- Child and Adolescent Social Perception Measure: aspects of nonverbal communication
- Self-Perception Profile for Children: self-esteem and perceived confidence in children
- Self-Perception Profile for Adolescents: self-esteem and perceived confidence in adolescents

Motor Coordination

- Bruininks-Oseretsky Test of Motor Proficiency (BOT-2): gross and fine motor function
- Peabody Motor Scales-2 (PDMS-2): motor development

Visual-Motor Integration

- Beery-Buktenica Developmental Test of Visual-Motor Integration (Beery VMI)
- Test of Visual-Perceptual Skills-3: visual-perceptual abilities without motor responses

Sensory and Sensory Motor Processing

- Sensory Integration and Praxis Tests (SIPT): praxis, sensory processing, and integration
- Sensory Profile: the ability to process sensory information and the effects on function
- Sensory Processing Measure (SPM): sensory processing abilities in the home or school

Marital Relationship and Family Functioning

- Dyadic Adjustment Scale (DAS): partners' perceptions of relationship adjustment
- Locke-Wallace Marital Adjustment Scale: marital adjustment

Occupational Therapy Interventions

Behavior Modification

Behavior modification includes creating routines, rewarding positive behavior, and communicating clear expectations. Using behavioral strategies in daily routines may result in improvements in social and academic functioning. The token system is one example of a positive reinforcement program that rewards and encourages specific positive behaviors (DuPaul, 2007).

Cognitive Strategy Training

Cognitive strategy training focuses on attention and working memory by repeating exposure to cognitive stimuli. Individuals with ADHD receiving cognitive strategy training and taking medication decreased their impulsivity on daily task performances (Toplak, Connors, Shuster, Knezevic, & Parks, 2008).

Cognitive Behavioral Therapy

Cognitive behavioral therapy (CBT) combines cognitive strategy training and behavioral modification; it is an action-oriented approach that integrates organization and planning strategies into daily life. CBT strategies include problem solving, self-reinforcement, self-redirection, modeling, role-playing, and self-instruction to manage behavior and increase self-control (Toplak et al., 2008). CBT is beneficial for individuals with ADHD because it provides a structured routine that incorporates client's goals (Knouse, Cooper-Vince, Sprich, Safren, 2008).

Sensory Integration

Sensory processing difficulties are often the basis of sensory integration therapy for children with ADHD, especially in addressing attention within the classroom (Dunn & Bennett, 2002; Schilling, Washington, Billingsley, & Deitz, 2003). Evidence demonstrates that sensory integration therapy can be effective in improving self-regulating strategies and enhancing academic performance, especially from a young age (Yochman, Parush, & Ornoy, 2004). Improvements in seated behaviors, attention skills, completion of class work, and regulation of aggressive behavior were observed as a result of sensory integration therapy (Schaaf & Miller, 2005; Schilling et al., 2003). Occupational therapy for children with sensory processing disorder enhances their ability to attend to higher level sensory information by decreasing interfering sensitivities to noxious stimuli (Schaaf & Miller, 2005).

Social Skills Training

Occupational therapists may use social skills training to promote effective coping strategies for interpersonal relationships. Current intervention approaches involve education and counseling through modeling, providing specific instructions, and rehearsing. By achieving success in social situations through these approaches, individuals with ADHD learn problem-solving strategies and methods to enhance their interpersonal relationships (Spence, 2003).

Occupational Therapy and the Evidence

Structure, organization, and routines are implemented to enhance an individual's functional performance in meaningful occupations by decreasing symptoms of inattention, hyperactivity, and impulsivity. Occupational therapists focus on the social, motor, behavioral, and sensory processing needs of individuals in the natural environments of the home, school, and social settings. Occupational therapists can also work with individuals to improve or enhance interpersonal relationships and social skills. Working with individuals to set personal goals shows significant improvements in the individual's performance (Schaaf & Miller, 2005; Schilling et al., 2003; Spence, 2003; Toplak et al., 2008).

Caregiver Concerns

Caregiver education should focus on providing structure and organization, managing environmental factors, and implementing a system around positive and negative reinforcement to help individuals become successful in every day routines (NIMH, 2008). Mornings and afternoons may be the most vulnerable times for families, especially if homework is involved (Firmin & Phillips, 2009; Segal & Hinojosa, 2006). Considerations to influence a child's performance should be individualized to each family's values and priorities and the expectations and perceptions of the child's abilities (Segal & Hinojosa, 2006). Family's financial resources and availability need to be considered before implementing strategies to enhance a child's task performance. Effective strategies can include enfolding occupations (completing more than one occupation at a time), temporal unfolding of occupations (completing one occupation at a time), or unfolding occupations by inclusion (completing occupations with different people) (Segal, 2000).

Resources

Organizations

- Children and Adults with Attention Deficit/Hyperactivity Disorder (CHADD)
  8181 Professional Place
  Suite 150
  Landover, MD 20785
  Telephone: 301-306-7070
  Website: http://www.chadd.org

- Attention Deficit Disorder Association
  PO Box 543
  Pottstown, PA 19464
  Telephone: 484-945-2101
  Website: http://www.add.org

Books

- Taylor, B. E. S. (2007). *ADHD & me: What I learned from lighting fires at the dinner table.* Oakland, CA: New Harrbinger Publications.
  This book shares the authors experiences of ADHD, including his perspectives about growing up and dealing with social, familial, and academic challenges.

- Taylor, J. F. (2006). *The survival guide for kids with ADD or ADHD.* Minneapolis, MN: Free Spirit.
  An advice guide written at a third to fifth grade reading level for students and families to discuss common experiences associated with ADHD.

- Monastra, V. J. (2004). *Parenting children with ADHD: 10 lessons that medicine cannot teach.* Washington, DC: American Psychological Association.
  The author explores various interventions individually and in combination with each other.

Websites

- ADHD Online Community
  http://www.adhd.com
  This website provides resources for family, adults with ADHD, and health care professionals.

- Focus on ADHD
  http://www.focus adhd.com
  This website provides information and guidelines about living with individuals with ADHD.

Journals

- *Journal of Attention Disorders*
- *Journal of Clinical Child and Adolescent Psychology*
- *Journal of Developmental & Behavioral Pediatrics*

References

American Psychiatric Association. (2000). *Diagnostic and statistical manual of mental disorders* (4th ed., text rev.). Washington, DC: Author.

Biederman, J., Monuteaux, M. C., Spencer, T., Wilens, T. E., & Faraone, S. V. (2009). Do stimulants protect against psychiatric disorders in youth with ADHD? A 10-year follow-up study. *Journal of Pediatrics, 124*, 71–78. doi:10.1542/peds.2008-3347

Centers for Disease Control and Prevention. (2007). *Attention-deficit/hyperactivity disorder (ADHD).* Retrieved from http://www.cdc.gov/ncbddd/adhd/

Dunn, W., & Bennett, D. (2002). Patterns of sensory processing in children with attention deficit hyperactivity disorder. *Occupational Therapy Journal of Research, 22*, 4–15.

DuPaul, G. J. (2007). School-based interventions for students with attention deficit hyperactivity disorder: Current status and future directions. *School Psychology Review, 36*, 183–194.

Firmin, M. W., & Phillips, A. (2009). A qualitative study of families and children possessing diagnoses of ADHD. *Journal of Family Issues, 30*, 1155–1174. doi:10.1177/0192513X09333709

Jenson, P. S., Arnold, L. E., Swanson, J. M., Vitiello, B., Abikoff, H. B., Greenhill, L. L., . . . Hur, K. (2007). 3-year follow up of the NIMH MTA study. *Journal of the American Academy of Child and Adolescent Psychiatry, 46*, 989–1002. doi:10.1097/CHI.0b013e3180686d48

Knouse, L. E., Cooper-Vince, C., Sprich, S., & Safren, S. (2008). Recent developments in the psychosocial treatment of adult ADHD. *Expert Review of Neurotherapies, 8*, 1537–1548.

Multimodal Treatment of ADHD Cooperative Group. (1999). A 14-month randomized clinical trial of treatment strategies for attention-deficit/hyperactivity disorder. *Archives of General Psychiatry, 56*, 1073–1086.

National Institute of Mental Health. (2008). *Attention deficit hyperactivity disorder (ADHD).* Retrieved from http://www.nimh.nih.gov/health/publications/attention-deficit-hyperactivity-disorder/complete-index.shtml

Reif, S. F. (2003). *The ADHD book of lists: A practical guide for helping children and teens with attention deficit disorders.* San Francisco, CA: Jossey-Bass.

Reynolds, S., & Lane, S. J. (2009). Sensory overresponsivity and anxiety in children with ADHD. *American Journal of Occupational Therapy, 63*, 433–440. doi:10.5014/ajot.63.4.433

Rodriguez, A., Miettunen, J., Henriksen, T. B., Olsen, J., Obel C., Taanila, A., . . . Järvelin, M. R. (2007). Maternal adiposity prior to pregnancy is associated with ADHD symptoms in offspring: Evidence from three prospective pregnancy cohorts. *International Journal of Obesity, 32*, 550–557. doi:10.1038/sj.ijo.0803741

Schaaf, R. C., & Miller, L. J. (2005). Occupational therapy using a sensory integrative approach for children with developmental disabilities. *Mental Retardation and Developmental Disabilities Research Reviews, 11*, 143–148. doi:10.1002/mrdd.20067

Schilling, D. L., Washington, K., Billingsley, F. F., & Deitz, J. (2003). Classroom seating for children with attention deficit hyperactivity disorder: Therapy balls versus chairs. *American Journal of Occupational Therapy, 57*, 534–541. doi:10.5014/ajot.57.5.534

Segal, R. (2000). Adaptive strategies of mothers with children with attention deficit hyperactivity disorder: Enfolding and unfolding occupations. *American Journal of Occupational Therapy, 54*, 300–306. doi:10.5014/ajot.54.3.300

Segal, R., & Hinojosa, J. (2006). The activity of homework: An analysis of three cases and implications for occupational therapy. *American Journal of Occupational Therapy, 60*, 50–59. doi:10.5014/ajot.60.1.50

Spence, S. H. (2003). Social skills training with children and young people: Theory, evidence and practice. *Child and Adolescent Mental Health, 8*, 84–96. doi:10.1111/1475-3588.00051

Toplak, M. E., Connors, L., Shuster, J., Knezevic, B., & Parks, S. (2008). Review of cognitive, cognitive-behavioral, and neural-based interventions for attention-deficit/hyperactivity disorder (ADHD). *Clinical Psychology Review, 5*, 801–803. doi:10.1016/j.cpr.2007.10.008

Watemberg, N., Waiserberg, N., Zuk, L., & Lerman-Sagie, T. (2007). Developmental coordination disorder in children with attention-deficit-hyperactivity disorder and physical therapy intervention. *Developmental Medicine & Child Neurology, 49*, 920–925.

Yochman, A., Parush, S., & Ornoy, A. (2004). Responses of preschool children with and without ADHD to sensory events in daily life. *American Journal of Occupational Therapy, 58*, 294–302. doi:10.5014/ajot.58.3.294

Autism Spectrum Disorder

Sarah Stultz

Description and Diagnosis

Autism spectrum disorder (ASD) is an umbrella term to describe a group of complex impairments in social behaviors, communication skills, and restrictive repetitive patterns of behavior, interests, and activities (American Psychiatric Association [APA], 2000). ASDs are lifelong conditions and include three main diagnoses: autistic disorder, Asperger syndrome, and pervasive developmental disorder-not otherwise specified (PDD-NOS). Autistic disorder, or "classic autism," requires impairments in verbal and nonverbal communication, reciprocal social interaction, and the presence of repetitive or unusual behaviors.

Typically, children present with language delays, and some have comorbid intellectual disability. Individuals with Asperger syndrome have impairments in social and communication domains and show repetitive and focused behaviors, but they do not have a history of language delay or intellectual disability. PDD-NOS is used to describe other individuals with an ASD who display only some symptoms of ASDs. There is no medical test to diagnose an ASD, and diagnosis is based on educational and psychological testing and observations of communication and behavior.

Incidence and Prevalence

- 1 in every 110 children is diagnosed with an ASD.
- 1.5 million individuals are diagnosed in the United States, with tens of millions worldwide.
- Prevalence rate is increasing 10% to 17% annually.
- Boys are three to four times more likely to be diagnosed with an ASD than girls (Centers for Disease Control and Prevention [CDC], 2009).

Cause and Etiology

The cause of ASD is not completely understood (Autism Speaks, 2011). Theories about etiology include factors related to genetics, prenatal and perinatal events, and the environment. Genetic factors cannot be attributed to one particular genetic cause but are likely due to interactions among multiple genes or an interaction between genetic and environmental factors. Prenatal and perinatal events may include maternal history, abnormal presentation in labor, low birth weight, low Apgar score, or postterm birth.

Typical Course, Symptoms, and Related Conditions

Every individual with ASD has different symptoms, ranging from mild to severe, that include a range of communication difficulties, social symptoms, and repetitive behaviors.

Potential Symptoms

Communication	Social	Repetitive Behaviors
• Lack of or delay in language • Inability to form sentences or only speaks single words • Loss of early signs of communication • Precocious language or large vocabulary • Difficulty sustaining conversation • Difficulty with nonverbal language • Speaks with high-pitched or flat tone • Difficulty letting others know what they need • Difficulty understanding abstract or metaphorical language (humor, sarcasm)	• Little or no eye contact • Lack of interest in peer relationships, preference to be alone • Lack of spontaneous, make-believe, or appropriate play • Difficulty with friendships • Difficulty conforming to expected behavioral norms • Difficulty interpreting what others are thinking or feeling • Unusual parental attachment • Difficulty regulating emotions • Use of unconventional behaviors like biting • Difficulty with transitions • Use of monologues	• Repetitive use of language and/or motor mannerisms • Persistent fixation on parts of objects • Echolalia (repeating phrases over and over) • Repetitive motor behavior (like flapping arms or walking on toes)

Some of these symptoms may lead to disruptive behavior or physical aggression. If the child is aware of his or her social difficulties, there is a risk of anxiety or depression later in adolescence and adulthood (Whitehouse, Durkin, Jaquet, & Ziatas, 2009).

The symptoms of autism, particularly in behavioral domain, may decrease in severity in adulthood (Shattuck et al., 2007). Impairments in socialization remain particularly problematic in adulthood (Orsmond, Krauss, & Seltzer, 2004). Considerable research documents that most adults with an ASD experience problems with independent employment, living, and relationships (Billstedt, Gillberg, & Gillberg, 2007; Eaves & Ho 2008; Howlin, Goode, Hutton, & Rutter, 2004). Yet, given the heterogeneity in symptom severity and cognitive impairments, some adults are achieving independence in adulthood, success in postsecondary education and work, and in personal relationships.

Related Conditions

- Seizure disorders: As many as 39% of people with autism have seizure disorders, which commonly co-occur with cognitive impairments.
- Genetic disorders: These includes fragile X syndrome, Angelman's syndrome, tuberous sclerosis, or other chromosomal abnormalities. These conditions are often associated with intellectual disability.
- Gastrointestinal disorders: These includes gastritis, chronic constipation, colitis, celiac disease, and esophagitis. Discomfort from these disorders can cause changes in behavior.
- Sleep dysfunction: may be associated with co-occurring medical conditions and may impact performance
- Pica: eating disorder that involves eating things that aren't food
- Sensory integration (SI) dysfunction: a difficulty in processing and integrating sensory information (Asher et al., 2010; Audet, 2010; Seltzer et al, 2003)

Interdisciplinary Interventions

Applied Behavior Analysis

Applied behavior analysis (ABA) uses behavioral observation and positive reinforcement to promote behaviors and skills in context. ABA is customized for the client and can include discrete trail training, incidental teaching, pivotal response training, or fluency building to reinforce skill mastery.

Speech-Language Therapy

A speech therapist typically addresses the mechanics of speech and the social aspects of language to help clients communicate functionally, either verbally or nonverbally.

Physical Therapy

A physical therapist focuses on movement problems that cause functional limitations, such as poor muscle tone, balance, and coordination.

Complementary and Alternative Interventions

Some complementary and alternative interventions can include homeopathy; art, music, or dance therapy; yoga; gluten- and casein-free diets; or immunotherapy (Autism Speaks, 2011).

Occupational Therapy Evaluations

When evaluating individuals with ASD, it is important to understand clients' occupational performance in desired activities and occupations (Tomchek & Case-Smith, 2009). If clients have communication difficulties, evaluation information may be reported by parents or caregivers. The symptoms of autism may vary in different contexts; thus, evaluation in multiple settings is essential. Sample of assessments used during evaluation include the following:

Areas of Occupation

- Adaptive Behavior Assessment System-Second Edition: measures conceptual, social, and practical skills

- Pediatric Evaluation of Disability Inventory-Computer Adapted Testing (PEDI-CAT): measures self-care, mobility, social and cognitive domains, and management of life tasks
- Scales of Independent Behavior-Revised: assesses adaptive and maladaptive behavior
- School Function Assessment: evaluates functional task performance in schools
- Vineland Adaptive Behavior Scales-Second Edition: measures communication, daily living skills, socialization, motor skills, and adaptive behavior
- Canadian Occupational Performance Measure: measures self-perception of occupational performance
- Functional Independence Measure for Children (Wee-FIM II): measures performance in self-care, mobility, and cognition

Performance Skills

- Bruininks-Oseretsky Test of Motor Proficiency-Second Edition
- Peabody Developmental Motor Scales-Second Edition: measures gross and fine motor skills
- Sensory Integration and Praxis Tests: measures SI and praxis functions
- Sensory Processing Measure: measures sensory function in home, school, and community
- Beery-Buktenica Developmental Test of Visual-Motor Integration
- Bayley Scales of Infant Development: measures fine and gross motor skills, cognition, behavior, language, and social-emotional (Tomchek & Case-Smith, 2009; Watling, 2010)

Occupational Therapy Interventions

Occupational therapists focus on helping clients with an ASD maximize their ability to participate in home, school, work, and community activities by enhancing performance in all areas of occupation (Scott, 2011). Interventions may include occupation-based intervention, purposeful activities, and preparatory methods and involve collaboration with the client, family, caregivers, and teachers. Some occupational therapy interventions include SI or sensory-based interventions, relationship-based interactive interventions, developmental skill-based interventions, or social skills interventions (Case-Smith & Arbesman, 2008).

Sensory Integration or Sensory-Based Interventions

The goal of SI or sensory-based interventions is to improve the client's ability to process sensory information to increase function (Tomchek & Case-Smith, 2009). Based on the work of Dr. A. Jean Ayres, SI focuses on how sensory information is processed neurologically as a foundation for learning skills (Baranek, 2002). SI intervention can serve as a preparatory approach to help clients focus on participating in activities to enhance specific skills. One example of a sensory-based intervention is therapeutic listening, a program that involves listening to modulated music through headphones to help the client organize his or her nervous system to be more receptive to learning (Rimland & Edelson, 1994).

Relationship-Based Interactive Interventions

The goal of relationship-based interactive interventions is to establish a relationship with clients to promote social-emotional growth and behaviors important for learning (Tomchek & Case-Smith, 2009). This team approach includes the family, teachers, and therapy staff and engages clients in developmentally appropriate play activities, incorporating a challenge, and encouraging interaction.

Developmental Skill-Based Interventions

Developmental skill-based interventions use play-based activities to teach specific socialization, communication, and play skills for young children with an ASD. The therapist follows the child's lead in a play activity; then using direct instructions, challenges the child to try a new action and encourages practice of emerging skills. The goal is to motivate the child to initiate, develop self-efficacy, and generalize new skills (Tomchek & Case-Smith, 2009).

Social Skills Interventions

Social skills interventions are activity-based groups to teach social skills needed to interact with others and to conform to social conventions. Social skills groups provide an environment to facilitate interaction and learning and to practice social skills.

Social Stories

Social stories are written specifically for a certain client to guide social behavior before an event. To promote expected social behaviors, social stories describe a situation and desired behaviors for the upcoming situation (Reynhout & Carter, 2006).

Intervention, for people with an ASD across the life course, may also address the following:

- Regulation of emotional and behavioral responses
- Daily living skills (dressing, feeding, hygiene, sleep)
- Assistive technology for communication, school, or work functions
- Adjusting tasks and conditions to match clients' needs and abilities (adapting environment, computer software for communication)
- Job coaching and consulting with family, educators, employers, or team members
- Assisting with transitions between settings
- Teaching strategies to caregivers for stress and anxiety management, caring for individual with ASD, balancing life responsibilities
- Safe methods of community mobility (Asher et al., 2010; Scott, 2011)

Occupational therapists can provide intervention in many settings, including early intervention, child-care centers, schools, health centers, hospitals, private clinics, home health agencies, worksite, home, community-based programs, adult day care, or residential settings.

Occupational Therapy and the Evidence

Case-Smith and Arbesman's (2008) review of the intervention research evidence concluded the following:

- SI or sensory-based interventions enhance the child's ability to regulate behavior and create positive changes in social interaction and purposeful play. Following SI intervention, increased attention, and decreased sensitivity, maladaptive behaviors, hyperactivity, and self-stimulatory and stereotypic behaviors have been reported. However, according to Baranek (2002), the efficacy of these interventions needs further exploration.
- Relationship-based, interactive interventions have been shown to improve social interaction skills through modification of the environment and reinforcement of attempts to communicate. These interaction skills can promote joint attention, initiative, persistence, interest, cooperation, and positive affect.
- Developmental skill-based programs have been shown to be successful in promoting communication and learning through visual cueing and visual learning. Treatment and Education of Autistic and Related Communication Handicapped Children (TEACCH), a school-based program that guides students' behaviors by presenting information visually, has been effective in improving motor and cognitive performance, imitation, perception, gross motor skills, eye–hand coordination, and adaptive behaviors.
- Social skills training has been found effective when social-emotional skills are explained, modeled, and practiced. The use of social stories has also shown positive effects in increasing positive behaviors.
- Parent education about autism and behavior management has been shown to increase confidence and self-esteem in parents, subsequently improving the child's behavior.
- Intensive behavioral intervention, involving consistent instruction and consequences to behavior and modification of the environment to promote positive behavior, has been shown to be highly effective.

Caregiver Concerns

Caregivers are faced with many stresses, including difficulty obtaining an appropriate diagnosis, making intervention decisions, financial strain, grief, behavioral challenges, and strained marital relationships (Barker et al., 2010; Orsmond, Lin, & Seltzer, 2007). Research has shown that parents of children with an ASD experience more difficulty and frustration with caregiving and behavior management than parents of children with other disabilities. Mothers report higher levels of stress, depression, anxiety, and decreased marital satisfaction, especially when their children are young. As children get older, the emotional well-being of the mother may improve, which may be due to increased experience with parenting roles, changes in severity of symptoms and behavior problems, and changes in the child's residential status. However, mothers of grown children with an ASD continue to have higher stress and report spending more time caregiving and doing chores and less time participating in leisure activities (Barker et al., 2010). Because there is a higher risk of siblings of children with an ASD having a disability, some parents may be faced with caring for multiple children with disabilities. Mothers of multiple children with disabilities report more depressive symptoms, more anxiety, and decreased family cohesion and adaptability (Orsmond et al., 2007).

Resources

Websites

- Autism Speaks: http://www.austismspeaks.org
- Autism Society: http://www.autism-society.org
- Autism Today: http://www.autismtoday.com

Journals

- *Journal of Autism and Developmental Disorders*
- *Autism Research* (in association with International Society for Autism Research)

Books

- Maurice, C. (1994). *Let me hear your voice: A family's triumph over autism.* New York, NY: Random House.
- Lewis, C. (2008). *Rex: A mother, her autistic child, and the music that transformed their lives.* Nashville, TN: Thomas Nelson.
- Robinson, J. E. (2008). *Look me in the eye: My life with Asperger's.* New York, NY: Three Rivers Press.

References

American Psychiatric Association. (2000). *Diagnostic and statistical manual of mental disorders* (4th ed., text rev.). Washington, DC: Author.

Asher, A., Collins, A. L., Crabtree, L. A., Demchick, B. B., George, B. M., Harrington-Kane, E., . . . Watling, R. (2010). *What is occupational therapy's role in supporting persons with autism spectrum disorder?* Bethesda, MD: American Occupational Therapy Association.

Audet, L. R. (2010). Core features of autism spectrum disorders: Impairment in communication and socialization, and restrictive repetitive acts. In H. M. Kuhaneck & R. Watling (Eds.), *Autism: A comprehensive occupational therapy approach* (pp. 87–113). Bethesda, MD: American Occupational Therapy Association.

Autism Speaks. (2011). *Be informed.* Retrieved from http://www.autismspeaks.org/be_informed.php

Baranek, G. T. (2002). Efficacy of sensory and motor interventions for children with autism. *Journal of Autism and Developmental Disorders, 35*(5), 397–422.

Barker, E. T., Hartley, S. L., Seltzer, M. M., Floyd, F. J., Greenberg, J. S., & Orsmond, G. I. (2010). Trajectories of emotional well-being in mothers of adolescents and adults with autism. *Developmental Psychology.* doi:10.1037/a0021268

Billstedt, E., Gillberg, I. C., & Gillberg, C. (2007). Autism in adults: Symptom patterns and early childhood predictors. Use of the DISCO in a community sample followed from childhood. *Journal of Child Psychology and Psychiatry, 48,* 1102–1110.

Case-Smith, J., & Arbesman, M. (2008). Evidence-based review of interventions for autism used in or of relevance to occupational therapy. *American Journal of Occupational Therapy, 62,* 416–429.

Centers for Disease Control and Prevention. (2009). Prevalence of autism spectrum disorders—Autism and Developmental Disabilities Monitoring Network, United States, 2006. *Surveillance Summaries. Morbidity and Mortality Weekly Report,* 58 (No. SS-10). Retrieved from http://www.cdc.gov/mmwr/preview/mmwrhtml/ss5810a1.htm

Eaves, L. C., & Ho, H. H. (2008). Young adult outcome of autism spectrum disorders. *Journal of Autism and Developmental Disorders, 38,* 739–747.

Howlin, P., Goode, S., Hutton, J., & Rutter, M. (2004). Adult outcome for children with autism. *Journal of Child Psychology and Psychiatry, 45,* 212–229.

Orsmond, G. I., Krauss, M. W., & Seltzer, M. M. (2004). Peer relationships and social and recreational activities among adolescents and adults with autism. *Journal of Autism and Developmental Disorders, 34,* 245–256.

Orsmond, G. I., Lin, L. Y., & Seltzer, M. M. (2007). Mothers of adolescents and adults with autism: Parenting multiple children with disabilities. *Intellectual and Developmental Disabilities, 45,* 257–270.

Reynhout, G., & Carter, M. (2006). Social stories for children with disabilities. *Journal of Autism and Developmental Disorders, 36,* 445–469.

Rimland, B., & Edelson, S. M. (1994). The effects of auditory integration training on autism. *American Journal of Speech-Language Pathology, 3,* 16–24.

Seltzer, M. M., Krauss, M. W., Shattuck, P. T., Orsmond, G., Swe, A., & Lord, C. (2003). The symptoms of autism spectrum disorders in adolescence and adulthood. *Journal of Autism and Developmental Disorders, 33*(6), 565–581.

Scott, J. B. (2011). *Occupational therapy's role with autism.* Bethesda, MD: American Occupational Therapy Association.

Shattuck, P. T., Seltzer, M. M., Greenberg, J. S., Orsmond, G. I., Bolt, D., Kring, S., . . . Lord, C. (2007). Change in autism symptoms and maladaptive behaviors in adolescents and adults with an autism spectrum disorder. *Journal of Autism and Developmental Disorders, 37,* 1735–1747.

Tomchek, S. D., & Case-Smith, J. (2009). *Occupational therapy practice guidelines for children and adolescents with autism.* Bethesda, MD: American Occupational Therapy Association.

Watling, R. (2010). Occupational therapy evaluation for individuals with an autism spectrum disorder. In H. M. Kuhaneck & R. Watling (Eds.), *Autism: A comprehensive occupational therapy approach* (3rd ed., pp. 285–303). Bethesda, MD: American Occupational Therapy Association.

Whitehouse, A. J. O., Durkin, K., Jaquet, E., & Ziatas, K. (2009). Friendship, loneliness and depression in adolescents with Asperger's syndrome. *Journal of Adolescence, 32,* 309–322.

Burns

Anne LeBorgne

Description and Etiology

Burns involve tissue damage caused by heat, chemicals, electricity, sunlight, or radiation (National Institute of General Medical Science [NIGMS], 2008). Thermal burns, caused by contact with heat, flame, or scalding liquids, are the most common. Sixty-six percent of serious burns occur in the home, compared to 10% that occur in an employment setting. Children younger than the age of 4 years and adults older than age 65 years are most at risk for fire-related injuries and death. Serious burns can be complicated by postburn joint conformity, which can significantly impact function. Through reconstructive surgeries and subsequent rehabilitation in the months and years following a severe burn, individuals may return to optimal functioning (American Burn Association [ABA], 2010; Centers for Disease Control and Prevention [CDC], 2010; Sheridan, 2002).

Incidence and Prevalence

- There are 2.4 million burn injuries in the United States and Canada each year.
- Approximately 70% of people admitted to burn centers in the United States are male.
- About one million people annually sustain substantial or permanent disabilities from burn injuries.
- Between 2000 and 2009, the survival rate of people admitted to burn centers was 94.8% (ABA, 2010).

Symptoms and Related Conditions

Classifications

- First-degree, or superficial, burns: damage to the epidermis (outermost layer of skin) only. Signs of first-degree burns include pain, redness, and few, if any, blisters. First-degree burns usually heal within 3 to 6 days and do not result in scar formation.
- Second-degree, or partial-thickness, burns: The epidermis and dermis are damaged. Signs include blistering, wet or red appearance, and pain. If properly cared for, second-degree burns can heal in 7 to 20 days and will leave scarring.
- Third-degree, or full-thickness, burns: The most serious type of burn in which all layers of the skin are damaged; bones, tendons, nerves, and muscle tissues can be damaged as well. Skin is dry and may have small, thin-walled blisters; appearance varies from waxy white to cherry red to charred black. Pain may be limited due to destruction of dermal nerve endings. Healing is very slow and generally requires skin grafts. Extensive scarring is likely (ABA, 2010; NIGMS, 2008; Phillips, 2012).

Burn Size

Burns are typically described by the size of the affected total body surface area (TBSA). The "rule of nines" divides the body surface into percentages; for example, the front of one leg is 9% and the back of one arm is 4.5%. The rule of nines is a quick reference that health professionals use to describe how much of the body has been burned. The rule of nines is applicable for adults only; the percentage breakdown for children and infants is different due to the difference in body surface area. For children and infants, a modified rule of nines, the Lund-Browder chart, is used to describe the percentage of the burned body surface (Phillips, 2012; Sheridan, 2002).

Other Complications

Clients may experience pulmonary complications following a burn. These can be due to irritation of the airways caused by inhalation of toxic gases that are produced during combustion of many products. In addition, if the burns are on the client's abdomen and/or chest, inhalation and exhalation may be restricted. In the first 24 hours postburn, clients with severe burns may experience "burn shock." This is when the plasma levels within blood vessels decrease to dangerous levels as fluid shifts out of the vessels to swell in the burn area. Following a burn, the body's metabolic state drastically increases to accommodate the healing and infection-fighting process, resulting in the need for increased nutritional intake. Bacterial infection is a risk throughout the healing process. Finally, contractures may develop during the healing process due to a prolonged decrease in movement or to the tightening of the skin due to burn scars (Phillips, 2012).

Interdisciplinary Interventions

Surgical Interventions

Not all hospitals are equipped to provide care for significant burn injuries; in these cases, clients are treated at burn centers or hospitals with burn/trauma units.

- Escharotomy: a surgical incision through full-thickness eschar (necrotic tissue) on the arms, legs, or trunk to release tightness that can cut off circulation or prevent the lungs from being able to expand during breathing. Tightness occurs due to decreased elasticity of the eschar and increased internal pressure due to edema.
- Debridement: cleansing and removal of eschar from the wound to decrease potential for burn wound sepsis, facilitate healing, and prepare wound for grafting. Debridement may be surgical, chemical, mechanical, or autolytic. Because the process is painful, the client is premedicated with analgesics and sedative medication.
- Skin grafting: typically occurs in the acute phase and includes the removal of the necrotic tissue and the placement of healthy skin or a skin substitute over the wound. Grafting is usually performed for all full-thickness and large partial-thickness burns if regrowth of the burn site is not expected or has not occurred within 14 days. If the client has enough unburned skin, permanent autografts, in which skin is transplanted from unburned area of the patient to the burn site, are used. If the client does not have available donor sites, the burn can be temporarily closed using a synthetic dressing (e.g., Biobrane) or an allograft (donor skin that the body will naturally rejects in 10 to 14 days). In the meantime, other less severely burned areas of the body may heal enough to produce donor skin or cultured epithelium (new skin grown in a laboratory from a biopsy of unburned skin) can be produced (Phillips, 2012; Shakespeare, 2001; Sheridan, 2002).

Medications

Medications used for people who have experienced serious burns may include antimicrobial ointments to reduce the risk of infection and control bacteria growth, antibiotics to treat infections, and prescription pain medications. There may be additional medications depending on the other injuries, such as injuries to organs or to the respiratory system. The occupational therapist needs to ensure that the client is prepared for therapy and schedule therapy after pain medications have been administered (Sheridan, 2002). In addition to medications, clients may be administered intravenous fluids to prevent/treat burn shock. Nutritional support may be provided via nasogastric feeding to support the body's increased metabolic needs (Phillips, 2012).

Physical Therapy

The scope of physical and occupational therapy (OT) may overlap during the initial stages of burn recovery, particularly in relation to biomechanical interventions to maintain range of motion (ROM).

Scar Management

Hypertrophic scars are the primary type of scars that develop in deep dermal burns. These red, raised scars can be itchy, tender to the touch, and feel stiff. Massage, which includes stretching and slow, firm massage of the area, has been found to be effective in controlling scar formation. Massage techniques can be easily taught to clients and caregivers by the therapist (Sheridan, 2002). The use of compression garments, steroid injection, topical silicone, and surgery are other methods used, with the more conservative methods used first (Phillips, 2012).

Precautions

- Debridement can occur during therapy, which can cause pain or fear of pain as the body reacts to the removal of dead tissue.
- Postsurgical precautions (e.g., client may not be able to move certain joints or may be under heavy sedation)
- Abnormal burn patterns can indicate signs of abuse, such as localized burns with deep burn depth.
- Scar tissue development (Dalal, Saha, & Agarwal, 2010; Sheridan, 2002)

Complications

- Increased risk of tetanus
- Co-occurring injury to organs and/or the respiratory system
- Burned tissue at increased risk for infection
- Contractures due to decreased movement or scar development

Occupational Therapy Evaluations

The evaluation process focuses on what the client needs, wants, or is expected to do and analyzes what factors may impact desired occupational performance. The evaluation begins with occupation-focused assessments followed by specific evaluation of the potential impact of burns on occupational performance.

Occupation-Focused Assessments

- Activity Card Sort (ACS) (Baum & Edwards, 2008)
- Activity Measure for Post-Acute Care (AM-PAC) (Jette, Hayley, Coster, & Ni, 2007)
- Assessment of Motor and Process Skills (AMPS) (Fisher & Jones, 2010)
- Burn Specific Health Scale (Yoder, Nayback, & Gaylord, 2010)
- Canadian Occupational Performance Measure (COPM) (Law et al., 2005)
- Functional Independence Measure (FIM) (Uniform Data System for Medical Rehabilitation, 1997)
- WeeFIM (Serghiou et al., 2008)
- Functional Assessment Measure (FAM) (Wright, 2000)
- Kohlman Evaluation of Living Skills (KELS) (McGourty, 1999)
- Occupational Performance History Interview II (OPHI-II) (Kielhofner et al., 2004)
- Performance Assessment of Self-Care Skills (PASS) (Holm & Rogers, 2008)
- Role Checklist (Oakley, Kielhofner, Barris, & Reichler, 1986)
- Short Form-36 (SF-36) (Hays, Sherbourne, & Mazel, 1995)

Client Factor Assessments

- Burn Scar Index (Vancouver Scar Scale) (Sullivan, Smith, Kermode, McIver, & Courtemanche, 1990)
- Disabilities of the Arm, Shoulder, and Hand (DASH) Outcome Measure (Hudak, Amadio, Bombardier, & the Upper Extremity Collaborative Group, 1996)
- ROM
- Measures of pain (e.g., Visual Analog Scale [VAS])
- Measures of muscle strength
- Measures of edema

Occupational Therapy Interventions

Emergent

Within 24 to 48 hours after the burn, the occupational therapist helps to prevent early contracture formation by using antideformity splinting and positioning and maintaining joint movement. The therapist must be mindful of monitoring devices, including nasogastric tubes, central venous catheters, and endotracheal tubes when working with the client (Sheridan, 2002).

Acute

- Biomechanical
  - Splinting/positioning, exercises (active assistive range of motion [AAROM], active range of motion [AROM], and passive range of motion [PROM])
- Pain management
  - Monitor heart rate, blood pressure, and respiratory rate during treatment
- Discharge planning

Rehabilitation

- Biomechanical (ROM, strength/coordination training)
- Activities of daily living (ADL) and instrumental activities of daily living (IADL) training
- Psychosocial support
- Scar management (massage and pressure dressings)
- Patient and family education
- Plan for return to work, school, and community
- Leisure and social participation

Occupational Therapy and the Evidence

According to Whitehead and Sergiou's 2009 survey of therapeutic techniques for clients with burns, the number of burn centers that use positioning, AROM and PROM, and ambulation during interventions has significantly increased since 1994. In addition, therapy is being administered earlier during the acute stay and therefore results in earlier transition to outpatient rehabilitation services. Common outpatient rehabilitation focuses are on helping clients return to occupation. Hwang, Chen-Sea, and Chen (2009) recommend that OT services include return-to-work programs as they found that burn-related factors—that is, longer stay in hospital and burn injuries on both hands and trunk—increased the time required to return to work and may decrease the likelihood of return to work at all. Hill, O'Brien, and Yurt (2007) studied the effects of an OT cooking group for people who had sustained burns and found that not only did the group provide an opportunity for social participation and increase functional movement (e.g., using hands, standing for extended periods of time) but it also decreased burn-related anxiety in the kitchen and helped distract participants from their burns. Melchert-McKearnan, Deltz, Engel, and White (2000) concluded that, for children, purposeful activity and play were more effective than the use of rote activities postburn in rehabilitation.

Caregiver Concerns

Dorn, Yzermans, Spreeuwenberg, and van der Zee (2007) found that parents of children who have burns display significant increases in mental health issues, such as depression and anxiety, and cardiovascular problems years after their child experiences a burn. Parental adjustment to the burn injury was found to be a significant predictor of the child's psychological adjustment following a severe burn (Noronha & Faust, 2006). Caregivers may also take on rehabilitative responsibilities, including performing scar massage and stretching exercises (Sheridan, 2002).

Resources

Organizations

- American Burn Association
  ABA Central Office-Chicago
  625 N. Michigan Ave., Ste 2550
  Chicago, Illinois 60611
  Telephone: 312-642-9260
  Fax: 312-642-9130
  E-mail: info@ameriburn.org
  The organization provides information about burn awareness and prevention as well as advocates for those affected by burns.

- Phoenix Society for Burn Survivors
  1835 R W Berends Dr. SW
  Grand Rapids, MI 49519-4955
  Telephone: 1-800-888-2876 or (616) 458-2773
  Fax: (616) 458-2831
  E-mail: info@phoenix-society.org
  An organization devoted to supporting the needs of burns survivors and their families through connecting individuals in person and online.

Books

- Fisher, R. (2008). *After the fire: A true story of friendship and survival.* New York, NY: Little, Brown, & Company.
  An account of a fire at a college in New Jersey describing two friends' journey through recovery and rehabilitation including the involvement of occupational and physical therapists.

- Manning, G. (2002). *Love Greg and Lauren: A powerful true story of courage, hope, and survival.* New York, NY: Bantam Books.
  The story of one woman's rehabilitation and fight to recover from burns covering more than 80% of her body sustained in the September 11 attacks in New York City.

Websites

- Shriner's Hospital for Chidren
  http://www.shrinershospitalsforchildren.org/Education/BurnAwareness.aspx
- Children's Burn Trust
  http://www.cbtrust.org.uk/

Journals

- *Journal of Burn Care and Rehabilitation*
- *Journal of Burn Care & Research*

References

American Burn Association. (2010). *Burn incidence and treatment in the United States: 2011 fact sheet.* Retrieved from http://www.ameriburn.org/resources_factsheet.php

Baum, C. M., & Edwards, D. E. (2008). *Activity Card Sort* (2nd ed.). Bethesda, MD: AOTA Press.

Centers for Disease Control and Prevention. (2010). *Fire deaths and injuries: Fact sheet.* Retrieved from http://www.cdc.gov/HomeandRecreationalSafety/Fire-Prevention/fires-factsheet.html

Dalal, P. K., Saha, R., & Agarwal, M. (2010). Psychiatric aspects of burn. *Indian Journal of Plastic Surgery, 43,* 136–142. doi: 10.4103/0970-0358.70731

Dorn, T., Yzermans, J., Spreeuwenberg, P., & van der Zee, J. (2007). Physical and mental health problems in parents of adolescents with burns: A controlled, longitudinal study. *Journal of Psychosomatic Research, 63,* 381–389.

Fisher, A. G., & Jones, K. B. (2010). *Assessment of Motor and Process Skills. Vol. 1: Development, standardization, and administration manual* (7th ed.). Fort Collins, CO: Three Star Press.

Hays, R. D., Sherbourne, C. D., & Mazel, R. M. (1995). *User's manual for Medical Outcomes Study (MOS) core measures of health-related quality of life.* Santa Monica, CA: RAND.

Hill, K., O'Brien, K., & Yurt, R. (2007). Therapeutic efficacy of a therapeutic cooking group from the patients' perspective. *Journal of Burn Care & Research, 28,* 324–327.

Holm, M. B., & Rogers, J. C. (2008). The Performance Assessment of Self-Care Skills (PASS). In B. Hemphill-Pearson (Ed.), *Assessments in occupational therapy mental health* (2nd ed., pp. 101–110). Thorofare, NJ: Slack.

Hudak, P. L., Amadio, P. C., Bombardier, C., & the Upper Extremity Collaborative Group. (1996). Development of an upper extremity outcome measure: The DASH (disabilities of the arm, shoulder, and hand) [corrected]. *American Journal of Industrial Medicine, 29,* 602–608. Erratum in: *American Journal of Industrial Medicine, 30,* 372.

Hwang, Y., Chen-Sea, M., & Chen, C. (2009). Factors related to return to work and job modification after a hand burn. *Journal of Burn Care & Research, 30,* 661–667.

Jette, A., Hayley, S. M., Coster, W., & Ni, P. (2007). *Boston University Activity Measure for Post Acute Care: Instruction manual.* Retrieved from http://www.crecare.com/order/order.html

Kielhofner, G., Mallinson, T., Crawford, C., Nowak, M., Rigby, M., Henry, A., & Walens, D. (2004). *Occupational Performance History Interview II (OPHI-II).* Chicago, IL: MOHO Clearinghouse.

Law, M., Baptiste, S., Carswell, A., McColl, M., Polatajko, H., & Pollock, N. (2005). *Canadian Occupational Performance Measure* (4th ed.). Ottawa, Canada: CAOT Publications.

McGourty, L. K. (1999). *Kohlman Evaluation of Living Skills.* Bethesda, MD: AOTA Products.

Melchert-McKearnan, K., Deltz, J., Engel, J., & White, O. (2000). Children with burn injuries: Purposeful activity versus rote exercises. *American Journal of Occupational Therapy, 54,* 381–390.

National Institute of General Medical Science. (2008). *Burns fact sheet.* Retrieved from http://www.nigms.nih.gov/Education/Factsheet_Burns.htm

Noronha, D., & Faust, J. (2006). Identifying the variables impacting post-burn psychological adjustment: A meta-analysis. *Journal of Pediatric Psychology, 32,* 380–391.

Oakley, F., Kielhofner, G., Barris, R., & Reichler, R. (1986). The Role Checklist: Development and empirical assessment of reliability. *Occupational Therapy Journal of Research, 6,* 157–170.

Phillips, E. L. (2012). Burns. In B. J. Atchison & D. K. Dirette (Eds.), *Conditions in occupational therapy: Effect on occupational performance* (4th ed., pp. 199–208). Philadelphia, PA: Lippincott Williams & Wilkins.

Serghiou, M., Rose, M., Pidock, F., Esselman, P., Engrav, L., Kowalske, K., & Lezotte, D. (2008). The WeeFIM instrument: A paediatric measure of functional independence to predict longitudinal recovery of paediatric burn patients. *Developmental Neurorehabilitation, 11,* 39–50.

Shakespeare, P. (2001). Burn wound healing and skin substitutes. *Burns, 27,* 517–522.

Sheridan, R. (2002). Burns. *Critical Care Medicine, 30,* S500–S514.

Sullivan, T., Smith, J., Kermode, J., McIver, E., & Courtemanche, D. J. (1990). Rating the burn scar. *Journal of Burn Care and Rehabilitation, 3,* 256–260.

Uniform Data System for Medical Rehabilitation. (1997). *Guide for the uniform data set for medical rehabilitation* (Version 5.1). Buffalo, NY: State University of New York.

Whitehead, C., & Sergiou, M. (2009). A 12-year comparison of common therapeutic interventions in the burn unit. *Journal of Burn Care & Research, 30,* 281–287.

Wright, J. (2000). The Functional Assessment Measure. *The Center for Outcome Measurement in Brain Injury.* Retrieved from http://www.tbims.org/combi/FAM

Yoder, L., Nayback, A., & Gaylord, K. (2010). The evolution and utility of the burn specific health scale: A systematic review. *Burns, 36,* 1143–1156.

Cancer

Pamela Vaughn

Description and Diagnosis

According to the American Cancer Society (ACS; 2011a), "cancer is a group of diseases characterized by uncontrolled growth and spread of abnormal cells" (p. 1). If the growth is not controlled, cancer can be fatal. In the United States, cancer is the second leading cause of death, behind diseases of the heart, with more than 1,500 people dying every day and accounting for one in four deaths. There are over 100 forms of cancer that fall into one of four categories:

- Carcinomas: begin in the body's organs (including skin)
- Leukemias: begin in blood-forming tissues (e.g., bone marrow)
- Sarcomas: begin in connective tissue (e.g., bone, fat, muscle, or cartilage)
- Lymphomas: begin in the lymphatic system (National Cancer Institute [NCI], 2011)

The most common forms of cancer are breast, prostate, lung and bronchus, and colorectal cancers (Howlader et al., 2011; International Agency for Research on Cancer [IARC], 2010).

In most cases of cancer (the major exception being leukemia), the cancerous cells form a tumor. By performing regular and frequent self-exams or having a physician perform a physical screen, tumors can be identified, and a physician can from there determine whether the tumor is cancerous (malignant) and if it has spread (metastasized). To diagnose cancer, physicians may use imaging (e.g., computed tomography [CT] scans, X-rays, mammograms) and/or laboratory tests (e.g., blood tests, biopsies).

Incidence and Prevalence

- Between the years 2004 and 2008 in the United States, there was an average incidence of 464.4 cases per 100,000, or approximately 1.4 million new cases per year.
- As of January 2008, approximately 11.7 million Americans had a history of cancer (either were living with cancer or were in remission after a previous cancer diagnosis).

- In the United States, approximately one in two men and one in three women will develop or die from cancer.
- 78% of all cancers are diagnosed in persons aged 55 years or older.
- Breast cancer is the most common type of cancer diagnosed in women and prostate cancer is the most common in men, both accounting for ~30% of diagnoses in the respective gender.
- Lung and bronchus cancers are the second most common type of cancer among both genders in the United States (Howlader et al., 2011).
- Worldwide, cancer is the leading cause of death accounting for an estimated one in eight deaths.
- In 2008, an estimated 12.7 million people worldwide were diagnosed with cancer and 7.6 million people died from cancer; these numbers are expected to increase to an estimated 20.4 million and 13.2 million, respectively, in 2030.
- The 5-year relative survival rate for all cancers has increased—from 50% for those diagnosed between 1975 and 1977 to 68% for those diagnosed between 1999 and 2006.
- More than 60% of all cancer deaths occur in low- and middle-income countries (ACS, 2011a; IARC, 2010)

Cause and Etiology

Normally, when a "mutated" cell (a cell in which the DNA is damaged) is produced, the cell is either repaired or it dies. Cancer is the result of uncontrolled growth and spread of "mutated" cells. This abnormal growth can be caused by several internal and/or external factors. Internally, cancer can be caused by genetics (e.g., inherited cell mutations), immunological conditions, cell mutations produced via metabolism, and hormones. These factors cannot be controlled. External or environmental factors, however, are almost always modifiable; these include tobacco use, exposure to radiation (including sun exposure), poor nutrition and physical inactivity, certain infectious agents, certain medical treatments, and exposure to carcinogens (cancer-causing agents) via pollution, employment, and so forth. Seventy-five percent to 80% of cancer cases in the United States are caused by external factors, so prevention (e.g., via avoiding tobacco use and excessive sun exposure, preventing obesity) of many forms of cancer is possible (ACS, 2011a). Cancer is noncommunicable—you cannot "catch" it from another person.

Typical Course, Symptoms, and Related Conditions

Many forms of cancer are staged to describe the current status of the tumor and any metastases (regions to which the original cancerous site has spread). A common method of staging is the tumor, node, metastasis (TNM) system. Cancers of the nervous system and many lymphomas and leukemias do not use this system due to the nature in which they spread.

Tumor, Node, Metastasis System of Cancer Staging (NCI, 2010)	
T—extent of the primary tumor	• TX—primary tumor cannot be evaluated • T0—no evidence of primary tumor • Tis—carcinoma in situ (CIS; abnormal cells are present but have not spread to neighboring tissue; although not cancer, CIS may become cancer and is sometimes called preinvasive cancer) • T1, T2, T3, T4—size and/or extent of the primary tumor
N—extent of spread to lymph nodes	• NX—regional lymph nodes cannot be evaluated • N0—no regional lymph node involvement • N1, N2, N3—involvement of regional lymph nodes (number of lymph nodes and/or extent of spread)
M—presence of distant metastasis	• MX—distant metastasis cannot be evaluated • M0—no distant metastasis • M1—distant metastasis is present

The TNM system can allow the cancer itself to be staged; these more general stages vary between the different types of cancer:

Stage	Definition (NCI, 2010)
Stage 0	Cancer in situ (abnormal cells located only in layer in which they were originally detected)
Stage I, Stage II, and Stage III	Higher numbers indicate more extensive disease: larger tumor size and/or spread of the cancer beyond the organ/site in which it first developed to nearby lymph nodes and/or organs adjacent to the location of the primary tumor
Stage IV	The cancer has spread to another organ(s)

Generally, the earlier cancer is detected, the better chance of survival. Signs and symptoms vary between forms of cancer, between individuals, and depending on the stage of disease. Some forms of cancer do not have early symptoms, so regular screening is recommended.

General Symptoms of Cancer	Signs and Symptoms That May Indicate a Specific Form of Cancer
• Unexplained weight loss of 10 lb or more • Fever • Fatigue • Pain • Skin changes (color change, itching, excessive hair growth)	• Change in bowel habits or bladder function • Sores that do not heal • White patches inside the mouth or white spots on the tongue • Unusual bleeding or discharge • Thickening or lump in the breast or other parts of the body • Indigestion or trouble swallowing • Recent change in wart or mole or any new skin change • Nagging cough or hoarseness (ACS, 2010)

The treatment of cancer may cause exacerbation of cancer symptoms and/or additional symptoms, such as cognitive difficulties (e.g., confusion, memory problems, decreased executive functioning), decreased immunity, gastrointestinal problems (e.g., appetite changes, nausea or vomiting, diarrhea or constipation), edema/lymphedema, sleep disturbances, hormonal imbalances (leading to menopause, sexual problems, etc.), difficulty breathing, and nervous and musculoskeletal difficulties (e.g., pain, tremors, weakness, decreased range of motion [ROM], hearing loss) (ACS, 2011a; Brearley et al., 2011; Gilbertson-White, Aouizerat, Jahan, & Miaskowski, 2011). Symptoms of cancer most often result in a decrease in functional capacities and abilities, inhibiting an individual's occupational participation (Silver & Gilchrist, 2011). As a reaction to diagnosis, a result of decreased function or a side effect/result of treatment, cancer also affects individuals psychosocially (e.g., decreased coping, anxiety, and depression) (Shelton, Lipoma, & Oertli, 2008). Cancer can be fatal (the prognosis varies between individuals and types of cancer), but many treatment options have decreased mortality associated with a cancer diagnosis.

Interdisciplinary Interventions

Depending on the form and stage of cancer, the treatments used and members of the treatments team will vary. For example, an individual with lung cancer may have a respiratory therapist on his or her treatment team. Oncologists are the physicians that perform primary treatment to deal with the cancer itself, whereas other professionals work with the client to treat and/or alleviate symptoms (palliative care).

Primary Treatment Options (ACS, 2011b)	Examples of Palliative Care Treatments
• Surgery—to remove tumors or body parts affected by cancer • Chemotherapy—the use of medicine or drugs that destroy cancer cells • Radiation—the use of high-powered energy beams to damage or kill cancer cells • Targeted therapy—the use of drugs or other substances that directly block the growth and spread of cancerous cells • Biological therapy/immunotherapy—techniques to boost the immune system's response to cancer cells • Hyperthermia—the use of high temperatures to destroy cancer cells • Stem cell/bone marrow transplant—often used to replenish the body's supply of healthy cells after (or boost the supply before) chemotherapy or radiation treatment • Photodynamic therapy (PDT)—the use of drugs and light to destroy cancer cells • Hormone therapy—removal of hormones that fuel certain kinds of cancer (e.g., prostate and breast cancers)	• Pain medication • Respiratory therapy • Audiology • Physical therapy • Nutrition and dietary recommendations • Complementary and alternative medicines—for example, aromatherapy, art therapy, biofeedback, massage therapy, meditation, music therapy, tai chi, yoga • Social work

Occupational Therapy Evaluations

The evaluation process focuses on what the client needs, wants, or is expected to do and analyzes what factors may impact desired occupational performance. The evaluation begins with occupation-focused assessments followed by specific evaluation of the potential impact of cancer on occupational performance.

Occupation-Focused Assessments

- Functional Assessment of Cancer Therapy, General Scale (FACT-G) (Cella et al., 1993)
- Role Checklist (Oakley, Kielhofner, Barris, & Reichler, 1986)
- Occupational Performance History Interview II (OPHI—II) (Kielhofner et al., 2004)
- Assessment of Motor and Process Skills (AMPS) (Fisher & Jones, 2010)
- Occupational Self-Assessment, Version 2.2 (Baron, Kielhofner, Iyenger, Goldhammer, & Wolenski, 2006)
- Performance Assessment of Self-Care Skills (PASS) (Holm & Rogers, 2008)
- Canadian Occupational Performance Measure (COPM) (Law et al., 2005)
- Short Form-36 (SF-36) (Hays, Sherbourne, & Mazel, 1995)
- Activity Card Sort (ACS) (Baum & Edwards, 2008)

Client Factor Assessments

- M. D. Anderson Symptom Inventory (MDASI) (Cleeland et al., 2000)
- Brief Fatigue Inventory (Mendoza et al., 1999)
- Beck Depression Inventory-II (BDI-II) (Beck, Steer, & Brown, 1996)
- Allen Cognitive Level Screen-Fifth Version (ACLS-5) (Allen et al., 2007)
- ROM
- Measures of pain (e.g., Visual Analog Scale [VAS])
- Measures of edema
- Measures of muscle strength

Occupational Therapy Interventions

Interventions for clients with cancer vary depending on the individual's needs and desires, form and stage of cancer, symptoms, and treatment already received. Interventions may include the following:

- Retraining in activities of daily living (ADL)—environmental and/or task modifications, assistive technology; including suggestions to maintain satisfaction in sexual activity despite hormonal imbalances
- Environmental assessment to determine fall risk
- Cognitive retraining to address memory, concentration, and so forth, affected by treatment
- Development of the following coping strategies to address psychosocial and physical symptoms/effects:
  - Pain and/or edema management
  - Sleep regulation techniques
  - Energy conservation techniques to minimize fatigue when performing activities (particularly return to previous occupations); may include relaxation techniques, meaningful participation in exercise, time management skills to balance appointments, and other necessary activities (ADL, instrumental activities of daily living [IADL], employment, etc.) with leisure, play, social participation, and so forth
- Lifestyle modification—for example, identify new or alternate occupations that allow client to participate satisfactorily; may include employment
- Recommendations of support groups and resources within the community
- Consultation at end of life regarding strategies for maintaining productivity and finding closure in life, personal relationships, and so forth (Lemoignan, Chasen, & Bhargava, 2010; Shelton et al., 2008; Silver & Gilchrist, 2011)

Occupational Therapy and the Evidence

The most commonly used interventions for clients with cancer address the occupational domains of leisure and productive occupations (IADL, work, etc.) and involve teaching energy conservation techniques and goal setting (Lemoignan et al., 2010). Despite this knowledge, there is a paucity of evidence regarding the effectiveness of occupational therapy (OT) interventions for cancer. However, for clients with breast cancer, a specific OT-led exercise and relaxation intervention called the Breast Cancer Recovery Program was shown to safely decrease lymphedema while improving participant quality of life and mood when compared to controls (McClure, McClure, Day, & Brufsky, 2010).

Clients receiving OT services note that fatigue and the psychological stress associated with cancer impact their lives and ability to maintain life roles. They reported feeling satisfied with in-home OT interventions (Kealey & McIntyre, 2005). Despite difficulty obtaining referrals for OT, Lattanzi et al.'s (2010) study of women with breast cancer documents the participants' satisfaction with the individualized interventions and with the emotional support they received while in OT sessions.

Caregiver Concerns

According to van Ryn et al. (2011), caregivers of individuals with cancer who are currently undergoing treatment, who are in an advanced stage of cancer, and/or who have severe comorbidities report having to provide assistance to their family members significantly more than caregivers of clients with cancer who do not fit those characteristics. They predominantly assist with IADL and care-related tasks (e.g., medication administration, managing symptoms like vomiting). Only a small number of these caregivers reported receiving training to perform these tasks, and despite this, most said that they felt training was needed. Depending on the type of care provided and the details of each individual circumstance, caregivers have reported personal burden in many forms—for example, physical (pain, sleep problems, fatigue, etc.), social (financial difficulties, change in employment status, role strain, isolation, etc.), and emotional (anxiety, depression, fear, etc.) (Stenberg,

Ruland, & Miaskowski, 2010). In addition, caregivers report about the same amount of anxiety regarding death as their loved ones with cancer do (Sherman, Norman, & McSherry, 2010).

Resources

Organizations

- American Cancer Society
  1-800-227-2345
  http://www.cancer.org/
- National Comprehensive Cancer Network
  275 Commerce Dr., Suite 300
  Fort Washington, PA 19034
  Telephone: 215-690-0300
  http://www.nccn.org/

Books

- Hallerman, V. (2010). *How we survived prostate cancer: What we did and what we should have done.* New York, NY: Newmarket Press.
- Jarvis, D. (2008). *It's not about the hair: And other certainties of life and cancer.* Seattle, WA: Sasquatch Books.
- Siegfried, C. Z. (2010). *Cancer journey: A caregiver's view from the passenger seat.* Enumclaw, WA: Pleasant Word/WinePress.
- Silver, J. K. (Ed.). (2009). *What helped me get through: Cancer survivors share wisdom and hope.* Atlanta, GA: American Cancer Society.

Websites

- National Cancer Institute (at the National Institutes of Health)
  http://www.cancer.gov/
- Cancer.Net—patient information site from the American Society of Clinical Oncology
  http://www.cancer.net/
- Cancer Support Community—a support site for clients and caregivers
  http://cancersupportcommunity.org
- CancerCare—resource for clients to find professional and personal support and education regarding cancer
  http://www.cancercare.org/

References

Allen, C. K., Austin, S. L., David, S. K., Earhart, C. A., McCraith, D. B., & Riska-Williams, L. (2007). *Manual for the Allen cognitive level screen-5 (ACLS-5) and large Allen cognitive level screen-5 (LACLS-5).* Camarillo, CA: ACLS and LACLS Committee.

American Cancer Society. (2010). *Signs and symptoms of cancer.* Retrieved from http://www.cancer.org/Cancer/CancerBasics/signs-and-symptoms-of-cancer

American Cancer Society. (2011a). *Cancer facts and figures, 2011.* Retrieved from http://www.cancer.org/Research/CancerFactsFigures/CancerFactsFigures/index

American Cancer Society. (2011b). *Treatment types.* Retrieved from http://www.cancer.org/Treatment/TreatmentsandSideEffects/TreatmentTypes/index

Baron, K., Kielhofner, G., Iyenger, A., Goldhammer, V., & Wolenski, J. (2006). *Occupational Self-Assessment* (OSA; Version 2.2.). Chicago, IL: MOHO Clearinghouse.

Baum, C. M., & Edwards, D. E. (2008). *Activity Card Sort* (2nd ed.). Bethesda, MD: AOTA Press.

Beck, A. T., Steer, R. A., & Brown, G. K. (1996). *Beck Depression Inventory-Second edition manual.* San Antonio, TX: PsychCorp.

Brearley, S. G., Stamataki, Z., Addington-Hall, J., Foster, C., Hodges, L., Jarrett, N., . . . Amir, Z. (2011). The physical and practical problems experienced by cancer survivors: A rapid review and synthesis of the literature. *European Journal of Oncology Nursing, 15,* 204–212. doi:10.1016/j.ejon.2011.02.005

Cella, D. F., Tulsky, D. S., Gray, G., Sarafian, B., Linn, E., Bonomi, A., . . . Brannon, J. (1993). The Functional Assessment of Cancer Therapy scale: Development and validation of the general measure. *Journal of Clinical Oncology, 11,* 570–579.

Cleeland, C. S., Mendoza, T. R., Wang, X. S., Chou, C., Harle, M. T., Morrissey, M., & Engstrom, M. C. (2000). Assessing symptom distress in cancer patients. *Cancer, 89,* 1634–1646.

Fisher, A. G., & Jones, K. B. (2010). *Assessment of Motor and Process Skills. Vol. 1: Development, standardization, and administration manual* (7th ed.). Fort Collins, CO: Three Star Press.

Gilbertson-White, S., Aouizerat, B. E., Jahan, T., & Miaskowski, C. (2011). A review of the literature on multiple symptoms, their predictors, and associated outcomes in patients with advanced cancer. *Palliative & Supportive Care, 9,* 81–102. doi:10.1017/S147895151000057X

Hays, R. D., Sherbourne, C. D., & Mazel, R. M. (1995). *User's manual for Medical Outcomes Study (MOS) core measures of health-related quality of life.* Santa Monica, CA: RAND.

Holm, M. B., & Rogers, J. C. (2008). The Performance Assessment of Self-Care Skills (PASS). In B. Hemphill-Pearson (Ed.), *Assessments in occupational therapy mental health* (2nd ed., pp. 101–110). Thorofare, NJ: Slack.

Howlader, N., Noone, A. M., Krapcho, M., Neyman, N., Aminou, R., Waldron, W., . . . Edwards, B. K. (Eds). (2011). *SEER Cancer Statistics Review, 1975–2008.* Bethesda, MD: National Cancer Institute. Retrieved from http://seer.cancer.gov/csr/1975_2008/

International Agency for Research on Cancer. (2010). *GloboCan 2008.* Retrieved from http://globocan.iarc.fr/

Kealey, P., & McIntyre, I. (2005). An evaluation of the domiciliary occupational therapy service in palliative cancer care in a community trust: A patient and carers perspective. *European Journal of Cancer Care, 14,* 232–243. doi:10.1111/j.13652354.2005.00559.x

Kielhofner, G., Mallinson, T., Crawford, C., Nowak, M., Rigby, M., Henry, A., & Walens, D. (2004). *Occupational Performance History Interview II (OPHI-II).* Chicago, IL: MOHO Clearinghouse.

Lattanzi, J. B., Giuliano, S., Meehan, C., Sander, B., Wootten, R., & Zimmerman, A. (2010). Recommendations for physical and occupational therapy practice from the perspective of clients undergoing therapy for breast cancer-related impairments. *Journal of Allied Health, 39,* 257–264.

Law, M., Baptiste, S., Carswell, A., McColl, M., Polatajko, H., & Pollock, N. (2005). *Canadian Occupational Performance Measure* (4th ed.). Ottawa, Canada: CAOT Publications.

Lemoignan, J., Chasen, M., & Bhargava, R. (2010). A retrospective study of the role of an occupational therapist in the cancer nutrition rehabilitation program. *Supportive Care in Cancer, 18,* 1589–1596. doi:10.1007/s00520-009-0782-4

McClure, M. K., McClure, R. J., Day, R., & Brufsky, A. M. (2010). Randomized controlled trial of the breast cancer recovery program for women with breast cancer-related lymphedema. *American Journal of Occupational Therapy, 64,* 59–72.

Mendoza, T. R., Wang, X. S., Cleeland, C. S., Morrissey, M., Johnson, B. A., Wendt, J. K., & Huber, S. L. (1999). The rapid assessment of fatigue severity in cancer patients. *Cancer, 85,* 1186–1196.

National Cancer Institute. (2010). *Fact sheet: Cancer staging.* Retrieved from http://www.cancer.gov/cancertopics/factsheet/detection/staging

National Cancer Institute. (2011). *What is cancer?* Retrieved from http://www.cancer.gov/cancertopics/cancerlibrary/what-is-cancer

Oakley, F., Kielhofner, G., Barris, R., & Reichler, R. (1986). The Role Checklist: Development and empirical assessment of reliability. *Occupational Therapy Journal of Research, 6,* 157–170.

Shelton, M. L., Lipoma, J. B., & Oertli, E. S. (2008). Oncology. In M. V. Radomski & C. A. T. Latham (Eds.), *Occupational therapy for physical dysfunction* (6th ed., pp. 1358–1375). Philadelphia, PA: Lippincott Williams & Wilkins.

Sherman, D. W., Norman, R., & McSherry, C. B. (2010). A comparison of death anxiety and quality of life of patients with advanced cancer or AIDS and their family caregivers. *Journal of the Association of Nurses in AIDS Care, 21,* 99–112. doi:10.1016/j.jana.2009.07.007

Silver, J. K., & Gilchrist, L. S. (2011). Cancer rehabilitation with a focus on evidence-based outpatient physical and occupational therapy interventions. *American Journal of Physical Medicine & Rehabilitation, 90*(Supp. 1), S5–S15. doi:10.1097/PHM.0b013e31820be4ae

Stenberg, U., Ruland, C. M., & Miaskowski, C. (2010). Review of the literature on the effects of caring for a patient with cancer. *Psycho-Oncology, 19,* 1013–1025. doi:10.1002/pon.1670

van Ryn, M., Sanders, S., Kahn, K., van Houtven, C., Griffin, J., Martin, M., . . . Rowland, J. (2011). Objective burden, resources, and other stressors among informal cancer caregivers: A hidden quality issue? *Psycho-Oncology, 20,* 44–52. doi:10.1002/pon.1703

Cardiac Conditions

Pamela Vaughn

Description and Diagnosis

Cardiac conditions include any condition that originates in and/or affects the heart. These include, but are not limited to, the following:

- Coronary heart disease (CHD; also known as *coronary artery disease*): the most common type of heart disease (HD) in which there is a narrowing of the blood vessels that supply the heart due to the buildup of plaque, which can eventually lead to myocardial infarction (MI), angina (chest pain, discomfort, or tightness), or other complications.
- MI (also known as *heart attack*): damage or death to a portion of cardiac muscle as a result of insufficient oxygenated blood flow; during an MI, an individual may enter cardiac arrest.
- Heart failure (also known as *congestive heart failure* [CHF]; types are left-sided systolic heart failure, left-sided diastolic heart failure, and right-sided heart failure): a chronic and progressive condition in which the heart cannot sufficiently pump enough blood to meet the body's need for oxygenated blood; not to be confused with cardiac arrest.
- Congenital heart defects: defects that are present since birth due to abnormalities in the prenatal development of the structures or blood vessels of the heart; types of defects vary and may involve abnormal heart valves or holes in the wall of the heart.
- Arrhythmia: any change from the normal or expected electrical impulses that create the heartbeat; most are harmless but may result in cardiac arrest.
- Cardiac arrest: the sudden loss of heart function, resulting in death within minutes; cardiac arrest may be reversed and the person's life is saved if cardiopulmonary resuscitation (CPR) or an electrical shock using a defibrillator are administered immediately (American Heart Association [AHA], 2011a; Centers for Disease Control and Prevention [CDC], 2011).

Cardiac conditions are often diagnosed after an individual has experienced a cardiac event. However, if the condition is identified before this, the first stages of diagnosis are often made during physical exams conducted by a general practitioner that involve blood pressure, cholesterol, blood glucose tests, and an examination of family medical history. From there, a cardiologist may use one or more tests such as an electrocardiogram, ultrasound, chest X-ray, exercise stress test, angiogram, cardiac enzyme blood tests, or cardiac catheterization to further evaluate the condition of the client's heart to form a diagnosis and to develop a treatment plan (CDC, 2011). In the case of congenital heart defects, diagnosis is often made using similar techniques at birth or during infancy after the presentation of symptoms; sometimes, the diagnosis is made during pregnancy (AHA, 2011a).

Incidence and Prevalence

- Approximately 82.6 million—greater than one in three—U.S. adults have at least one cardiovascular disease (this includes cardiac conditions as well as stroke and hypertension); less than half of these (40.4 million) are among people aged 60 years or older.
- 16.3 million (7%) U.S. adults have CHD; men are slightly more affected than women.
- 5.7 million U.S. adults have heart failure (including CHF).
- 650,000 to 1.3 million U.S. adults are living with congenital heart defects.
- The estimated annual incidence of MI is 610,000 new attacks and 325,000 recurrent attacks; the average age at first MI is 64.5 years for men and 70.3 years for women.
- Among whites only, 11.9% have HD and 6.4% have CHD.
- Among blacks or African Americans, 11.2% have HD and 6.7% have CHD.
- Among Hispanics or Latinos, 8.5% have HD and 5.8% have CHD.
- Among Asians, 6.3% have HD and 3.9% have CHD.
- The average annual rates of first cardiovascular events rise from 3 per 1,000 men at 35 to 44 years of age to 74 per 1,000 men at 85 to 94 years of age; for women, comparable rates occur 10 years later in life. The gap narrows with advancing age.
- HD is the leading cause of death for both genders in the United States (Roger et al., 2011).

Cause, Etiology, and Risk Factors

- CHD is caused by atherosclerosis—a buildup of plaque (made of cholesterol) along the walls of the arteries that supply the heart, resulting in a narrowing of the vessels. The main risk factors for CHD are high cholesterol, hypertension, diabetes, cigarette smoking, overweight and obesity, poor diet, physical inactivity, and alcohol use. Genetics likely plays a role in the risk of an individual developing CHD, but it is as yet unclear whether this is simply because families tend to share common environments and lifestyle choices.
- MI is caused when a coronary artery's blood flow is stopped or impeded; this most often happens as a result of blood clots forming in the arteries after a portion of atherosclerotic plaque breaks, for example, in the case of CHD.
- CHF can be caused by several other compounding conditions, including hypertension, CHD, a history of MI, congenital heart defects, and diabetes.
- Congenital heart defects can develop as a result of genetics, environmental factors, and/or behaviors and lifestyle choices of the mother. There is an increased risk of birth defects if the mother uses drugs, smokes, or drinks alcohol during pregnancy.
- Arrhythmias can be caused by HD, MI, or any other condition in which the cells responsible for the electrical conduction of the heart are affected. They can also be a result of a congenital condition, a side effect of medication, or the use of addictive substances. Conversely, arrhythmias can *cause* MI, cardiac arrest, or stroke (AHA, 2011a; CDC, 2011; Eckert, 2007).

Typical Course, Symptoms, and Related Conditions

The course and symptoms for each cardiac condition will vary. However, the interrelatedness of these conditions should be noted—for example, CHD can cause MI and CHF; MI, CHF, and CHD can cause arrhythmias; arrhythmias can cause MI; and so forth. General signs and symptoms that an individual may be having a cardiac event include the following:

- Change in pattern of angina or shortness of breath
- Heart palpitations or "fluttering" feeling in chest
- Feeling lightheaded, dizzy, or confused; fainting or near-fainting spells
- Experiencing more fatigue than expected
- Unusual pain or discomfort in muscles or joints after exercise
- Sweating
- Blood pressure falls 20 mm Hg or more or heart rate is 20 beats per minute or more over resting heart rate (Eckert, 2007).

In addition, specific signs and symptoms for separate conditions include the following:

- CHD: MI is often the first sign (CDC, 2011).
- CHF: shortness of breath, persistent coughing or wheezing, edema, fatigue, lack of appetite, nausea, confusion, impaired thinking, and increased heart rate (AHA, 2011a)

- Congenital heart defects: blue skin, low blood pressure, difficulty breathing, feeding problems, and inability to gain weight. Minor heart defects often do not produce noticeable symptoms (AHA, 2011a).

It is crucial for the client as well as their family members and practitioners to particularly be aware of signs and symptoms of MI and cardiac arrest and to be able to obtain and/or provide immediate emergency care (call 911; if cardiac arrest occurs, have a trained individual begin CPR and/or provide electrical shock using a defibrillator) to increase the client's chance of survival. The major symptoms of MI are the following:

- Pain or discomfort in the jaw, neck, or back
- Feeling weak, light-headed, or faint
- Chest pain or discomfort
- Pain or discomfort in arms or shoulder
- Shortness of breath (CDC, 2011)

Signs of cardiac arrest, at which CPR and defibrillation should be administered by a trained individual, are sudden loss of responsiveness (e.g., no response when tapped on shoulder, no response when you ask if the person is okay) and no normal breathing (AHA, 2011a).

Being diagnosed with a cardiac condition takes an emotional and occupational toll on people. It is not uncommon for clients to experience symptoms of depression and anxiety, and the condition or their reaction to the condition may result in decreased cognitive functioning and occupational participation (Foster et al., 2011; Huntley, 2008).

Interdisciplinary Interventions

Surgery

The diagnosis of a cardiac condition, often only made during or after a medical emergency, may be followed closely by a surgical procedure to fix or alleviate the condition to prevent a (or another) cardiac emergency from occurring.

Surgeries for Cardiac Conditions (AHA, 2011c)

- Angioplasty (also known as percutaneous coronary intervention [PCI]): a deflated balloon is threaded into a coronary artery and then inflated (or a laser on the tip of the catheter vaporizes the plaque buildup) to widen a blocked area of the vessel and increase blood flow to the heart; often used in combination with stenting
- Stenting: insertion of a wire mesh tube to prop a coronary artery open
- Atherectomy: A catheter with a rotating shaver trims away plaque from artery walls.
- Coronary artery bypass graft (CABG, or "cabbage"; also known as *open-heart surgery*): grafting vessels from other parts of the body to the blocked coronary artery in order to reroute blood flow
- Minimally invasive bypass surgery: the use of video monitors and scopes inserted through small incisions ("ports") in the chest to perform bypasses
- Transmyocardial revascularization (TMR): the use of lasers to drill ~1 mm diameter holes directly into the walls of the heart to relieve severe angina when bypass is not an option
- Valve replacement: a replacement of an abnormal or diseased valve with an artificial valve
- Radiofrequency, or catheter, ablation: a procedure to correct arrhythmias by destroying a small amount of cardiac cells that are causing the abnormal heartbeat
- Insertion of left ventricular assist device (LVAD): assist the heart's pumping chamber
- Implantation of defibrillator or pacemaker: to maintain a normal heartbeat
- Cardiomyoplasty: Skeletal muscle is wrapped around the heart and stimulated for contraction with the use of a pacemaker-like device to assist the heart in pumping.
- Heart transplant: Organ donation can be used when a heart is irreversibly damaged.

Medication Therapy

There are many medications prescribed to either prevent a cardiac emergency or reduce the likelihood of experiencing another one. Because each medication treats a different symptom or performs a different function, clients are typically prescribed several. It should be noted that the medication adherence rate in the United States for various cardiovascular conditions is still not ideal (Brown & Bussell, 2011).

Classes of Medications for Cardiac Conditions (AHA, 2011b)

- Anticoagulants—decrease the clotting ability of blood
- Antiplatelet agents (e.g., aspirin)—prevent blood clots
- Angiotensin-converting enzyme (ACE) inhibitors—expand blood vessels to allow blood to flow more easily, decreasing the workload of the heart
- Angiotensin II receptor blockers—prevent vessel constriction and decrease blood pressure
- Beta-blockers—decrease heart rate and cardiac output to decrease blood pressure and angina
- Calcium channel blockers—decrease blood pressure and angina and treat some arrhythmias
- Diuretics—decrease blood pressure and reduce edema
- Vasodilators—expand vessels to decrease angina
- Digitalis preparations—increase the force of the heart's contractions to decrease symptoms and some arrhythmias
- Statins—decrease cholesterol levels

Cardiac Rehabilitation

After a person has a cardiac event (emergency, surgery, etc.), they are generally recommended for a cardiac rehab program. These programs use a combination of education and counseling to help people manage their condition by increasing physical fitness, reducing cardiac symptoms, and finding support. Techniques include individualized physical activity programs, smoking cessation counseling, dietary and nutrition counseling, and counseling for the psychological and emotional effects (e.g., stress, anxiety, depression) of the condition (AHA, 2011d; Huntley, 2008).

Occupational Therapy Evaluations

The evaluation process focuses on what the client needs, wants, or is expected to do and analyzes what factors may impact desired occupational performance. The evaluation begins with occupation-focused assessments followed by specific evaluation of the potential impact of cardiac conditions on occupational performance.

Occupation-Focused Assessments

- Role Checklist (Oakley, Kielhofner, Barris, & Reichler, 1986)
- Occupational Performance History Interview II (OPHI-II) (Kielhofner et al., 2004)
- Occupational Self-Assessment, Version 2.2 (Baron, Kielhofner, Iyenger, Goldhammer, & Wolenski, 2006)
- Performance Assessment of Self-Care Skills (PASS) (Holm & Rogers, 2008)
- Canadian Occupational Performance Measure (COPM) (Law et al., 2005)
- Short Form-36 (SF-36) (Hays, Sherbourne, & Mazel, 1995)
- Activity Card Sort (ACS) (Baum & Edwards, 2008)
- Reintegration to Normal Living (RNL) Scale (Wood-Dauphinee, Opzoomer, Williams, Marchand, & Spitzer, 1988)

Client Factor Assessments

- Beck Depression Inventory-II (BDI-II) (Beck, Steer, & Brown, 1996)
- Borg Rating of Perceived Exertion (RPE) scale (Borg, 1998)
- Measures of pain (e.g., Visual Analog Scale [VAS])
- Measures of muscle strength
- Monitoring of vital signs (i.e., heart rate, blood pressure)

Occupational Therapy Interventions

Occupational therapists are frequent members of cardiac rehab teams. Interventions provided depend on the condition, needs, and desires of the client. Precautions to prevent overexertion of the client should be taken, and the occupational therapist should monitor heart rate and blood pressure regularly and alert the appropriate members of the rehab team of any changes. Common interventions include the following:

- Teaching energy conservation techniques to minimize the stress placed on the heart
- Retraining in activities of daily living (ADL)—for example, grading activities to optimize participation without causing excessive strain, using assistive devices if necessary; includes suggestions to maintain satisfaction in sexual activity without overly exerting the heart
- Environmental adaptations
- Educating client and family members about the risk factors of cardiac conditions and measures to be taken to remain healthy and functional
- Lifestyle modification—for example, identify new or alternate occupations that allow client to participate satisfactorily without inducing cardiac stress
- Medication management
- Recommendations of support groups and resources within the community (Huntley, 2008)

Occupational Therapy and the Evidence

As the number of people living with cardiac conditions and surviving cardiac emergencies increases, there is a greater need for longer term rehabilitative and lifestyle occupational therapy (OT). Interdisciplinary cardiac rehab has been shown to consistently decrease cardiovascular-related causes of death and improve quality of life in clients of all ages and genders, increase likelihood of return to work, increase function in occupations such as ADL and instrumental activities of daily living (IADL), decrease length of stay in the hospital, and increase client independence after discharge (Vincent, Stephenson, Omli, & Vincent, 2008). Occupational performance declines in ADL and IADL are common, particularly in clients with CHF and CHD, and often result in the use of assistive devices and use of home and community help services (Foster et al., 2011; Norberg, Boman, & Löfgren, 2010). A review of OT for chronic conditions, including HD, showed that various interventions (e.g., in-home or group, occupation reteaching/adaptation or consulting) can improve function and quality of life for clients (Hand, Law, & McColl, 2011). Although most cardiac rehab programs take place in a hospital or other community setting, research has shown that in-home cardiac rehab is just as effective in increasing physical health and decreasing symptoms as center-based programs for older adults (Oerkild et al., 2011). Community-based group intervention sessions have been shown to provide clients with a mutual support system that assists in the transition to home- and community-dwelling after in-hospital acute cardiac rehab (Arndt, Murchie, Schembri, & Davidson, 2009). Despite the known occupational performance difficulties associated with congenital heart defects in children (Imms, 2004), there is a paucity of evidence regarding availability and use of OT services in schools or other settings (Majnemer et al., 2008).

Caregiver Concerns

Relatives of clients with cardiac conditions often experience stress, anxiety, and lowered quality of life as a result of their loved ones' conditions. There is also an increased risk of death following the diagnosis of a relative. These relatives may benefit from education regarding the best ways to support their family members and the importance of keeping themselves healthy and using their own support systems (Nissen, Madsen, & Zwisler, 2008).

Resources

Organizations

- American Heart Association
  7272 Greenville Ave.
  Dallas, TX 75231
  Website: http://www.heart.org

Books

- Jaworski, A. M., & Daigneault, B. (Eds.). (2009). *The heart of a father: Essays by men affected by congenital heart defects.* Temple, TX: Baby Hearts Press.
- Whitehead, J. (2008). *A heart too good to die: A shocking story of sudden cardiac arrest.* Bangor, ME: BookLocker.com.

Websites

- American College of Cardiology Foundation
  http://www.cardiosource.org/acc
- American Association of Cardiovascular and Pulmonary Rehabilitation
  http://www.aacvpr.org

References

American Heart Association. (2011a). *Conditions.* Retrieved from http://www.heart.org/HEARTORG/Conditions/Conditions_UCM_001087_SubHomePage.jsp

American Heart Association. (2011b). *Cardiac medications at-a-glance.* Retrieved from http://www.heart.org/HEARTORG/Conditions/HeartFailure/PreventionTreatmentofHeartFailure/Heart-Failure-Medications_UCM_306342_Article.jsp

American Heart Association. (2011c). *Cardiac procedures and surgeries.* Retrieved from http://www.heart.org/HEARTORG/Conditions/HeartAttack/PreventionTreatmentofHeartAttack/Cardiac-Procedures-and-Surgeries_UCM_303939_Article.jsp

American Heart Association. (2011d). *What is cardiac rehabilitation?* Retrieved from http://www.heart.org/HEARTORG/Conditions/More/CardiacRehab/What-is-Cardiac-Rehabilitation_UCM_307049_Article.jsp

Arndt, M., Murchie, F., Schembri, A. M., & Davidson, P. M. (2009). "Others had similar problems and you were not alone": Evaluation of an open-group mutual aid model in cardiac rehabilitation. *The Journal of Cardiovascular Nursing, 24,* 328–335. doi:10.1097/JCN.0b013e3181a1c236

Baron, K., Kielhofner, G., Iyenger, A., Goldhammer, V., & Wolenski, J. (2006). *Occupational Self-Assessment* (OSA; Version 2.2.). Chicago, IL: MOHO Clearinghouse.

Baum, C. M., & Edwards, D. E. (2008). *Activity Card Sort* (2nd ed.). Bethesda, MD: AOTA Press.

Beck, A. T., Steer, R. A., & Brown, G. K. (1996). *Beck Depression Inventory-Second edition manual.* San Antonio, TX: PsychCorp.

Borg, G. (1998). *Borg's Perceived Exertion and Pain Scale.* Champaign, IL: Human Kinetics.

Brown, M., & Bussell, J. (2011). Medication adherence: WHO cares? *Mayo Clinic Proceedings, 86,* 304–314. doi:10.4065/mcp.2010.0575

Centers for Disease Control and Prevention. (2011). *Division for heart disease and stroke prevention fact sheets.* Retrieved from http://www.cdc.gov/dhdsp/data_statistics/fact_sheets/hds_index.htm

Eckert, J. (2007). Cardiopulmonary disorders. In B. J. Atchison & D. K. Dirette (Eds.), *Conditions in occupational therapy: Effect on occupational performance* (3rd ed., pp. 195–218). Philadelphia, PA: Lippincott Williams & Wilkins.

Foster, E. R., Cunnane, K. B., Edwards, D. F., Morrison, M. T., Ewald, G. A., Geltman, E. M., & Zazulia, A. R. (2011). Executive dysfunction and depressive symptoms associated with reduced participation of people with severe congestive heart failure. *American Journal of Occupational Therapy, 65,* 306–313. doi:10.5014/ajot.2011.000588

Hand, C., Law, M., & McColl, M. A. (2011). Occupational therapy interventions for chronic diseases: A scoping review. *American Journal of Occupational Therapy, 65,* 428–436. doi:10.5014/ajot.2011.002071

Hays, R. D., Sherbourne, C. D., & Mazel, R. M. (1995). *User's manual for Medical Outcomes Study (MOS) core measures of health-related quality of life.* Santa Monica, CA: RAND.

Holm, M. B., & Rogers, J. C. (2008). The Performance Assessment of Self-Care Skills (PASS). In B. Hemphill-Pearson (Ed.), *Assessments in occupational therapy mental health* (2nd ed., pp. 101–110). Thorofare, NJ: Slack.

Huntley, N. (2008). Cardiac and pulmonary diseases. In M. V. Radomski & C. A. T. Latham (Eds.), *Occupational therapy for physical dysfunction* (6th ed., pp. 1295–1320). Philadelphia, PA: Lippincott Williams & Wilkins.

Imms, C. (2004). Occupational performance challenges for children with congenital heart disease: A literature review. *Canadian Journal of Occupational Therapy, 71,* 161–172.

Kielhofner, G., Mallinson, T., Crawford, C., Nowak, M., Rigby, M., Henry, A., & Walens, D. (2004). *Occupational Performance History Interview II (OPHI-II).* Chicago, IL: MOHO Clearinghouse.

Law, M., Baptiste, S., Carswell, A., McColl, M., Polatajko, H., & Pollock, N. (2005). *Canadian Occupational Performance Measure* (4th ed.). Ottawa, Canada: CAOT Publications.

Majnemer, A., Mazer, B., Lecker, E., Carter, A. L., Limperopoulos, C., Shevell, M., . . . Tchervenkov, C. (2008). Patterns of use of educational and rehabilitation services at school age for children with congenitally malformed hearts. *Cardiology in the Young, 18,* 288–296. doi:10.1017/S104795110800211

Nissen, N., Madsen, M., & Zwisler, A. (2008). Health service interventions targeting relatives of heart patients: A review of the literature. *Scandinavian Journal of Public Health, 36,* 818–826. doi:10.1177/1403494808092249

Norberg, E., Boman, K., & Löfgren, B. (2010). Impact of fatigue on everyday life among older people with chronic heart failure. *Australian Occupational Therapy Journal, 57,* 34–41. doi:10.1111/j.1440-1630.2009.00847.x

Oakley, F., Kielhofner, G., Barris, R., & Reichler, R. (1986). The Role Checklist: Development and empirical assessment of reliability. *Occupational Therapy Journal of Research, 6,* 157–170.

Oerkild, B., Frederiksen, M., Hansen, J., Simonsen, L., Skovgaard, L., & Prescott, E. (2011). Home-based cardiac rehabilitation is as effective as centre-based cardiac rehabilitation among elderly with coronary heart disease: Results from a randomised clinical trial. *Age & Ageing, 40,* 78–85. doi:10.1093/ageing/afq122

Roger, V. L., Go, A. S., Lloyd-Jones, D. M., Adams, R. J., Berry, J. D., Brown, T. M., . . . Wylie-Rosett, J. (2011). Heart disease and stroke statistics—2011 update: A report from the American Heart Association. *Circulation, 123,* e18–e209. doi:10.1161/CIR.0b013e3182009701

Vincent, H. K., Stephenson, M. L., Omli, M. R., & Vincent, K. R. (2008). Clinical outcomes following postacute comprehensive rehabilitative care in patients with cardiopulmonary disease. *Clinical Reviews in Physical and Rehabilitation Medicine, 20,* 127–158. doi:10.1615/CritRevPhysRehabilMed.v20.i2.30

Wood-Dauphinee, S. L., Opzoomer, M. A., Williams, J. I., Marchand, B., & Spitzer, W. O. (1988). Assessment of global function: The reintegration to normal living index. *Archives of Physical Medicine and Rehabilitation, 69,* 583–590.

Cerebral Palsy

Samantha Slocum

Description and Diagnosis

Cerebral palsy (CP) is a term that is used to describe motor disorders that are characterized by impaired voluntary movement and muscle control. CP can result from prenatal, perinatal, or postnatal brain injury occurring before the age of 5 years (Merck, 2006). There are four types of CP, characterized by the type of movement disturbance: spastic (muscles are stiff and weak; most common type), athetoid (slow, writhing, involuntary movement), ataxic (muscle weakness, poor coordination, and tremors), and mixed (combines spastic and athetoid) (Merck, 2006; United Cerebral Palsy Association [UCP], 2001a).

Incidence and Prevalence

Approximately 8,000 infants and 1,200 to 1,500 preschool-aged children are diagnosed with CP each year. An estimate of 764,000 children and adults in the United States demonstrate signs of CP (UCP, 2001a).

Cause and Risk Factors

There is no single cause of CP, and often more than one type of brain damage results in the condition. CP can be congenital and be caused by brain damage in utero or during the birthing process. Acquired CP occurs within the first few months or years of life and could be caused by brain infections, oxygen deprivation, brain injuries from motor vehicle accidents, falls, or child abuse (Merck, 2006; UCP, 2001a). Risk factors for CP include premature birth, low birth weight, inadequate nutrients in utero, blood type incompatibility between mother and infant, bacterial infections, oxygen deprivation, and severe jaundice (UCP, 2001a).

Typical Course, Symptoms, and Related Conditions

CP cannot be cured. Although the brain damage itself cannot get worse, the symptoms that occur as a result of the brain damage can change with maturity (Merck, 2006). Symptoms of CP can be managed through medical and therapeutic interventions, which help reduce the impact of symptoms and improve functional abilities in people with CP (Merck, 2006; UCP, 2001a).

Symptoms of CP can range from clumsiness to severe spasticity that causes deformities (i.e., contractures) and the need for mobility aids (Merck, 2006). Common difficulties associated with CP include cognitive delays, speech difficulty, seizure disorders, feeding problems, impaired vision and hearing, abnormal sensation and perception, difficulty with bowel control, breathing problems secondary to poor posture, and skin conditions as a result of pressure sores (UCP, 2001a).

Secondary conditions that are seen in adults with CP include musculoskeletal changes (increased spasticity and decreased strength, endurance, and flexibility), pain, fatigue, arthritis, fractures, and osteoporosis. People with CP typically live well into adulthood (Haak, Lenski, Hidecker, Li, & Paneth, 2009).

Precautions

- Seizure disorders
- Difficulty swallowing
- Impaired vision/hearing
- Abnormal sensation/perception
  (UCP, 2001a)

Interdisciplinary Interventions

Medical Interventions and Medication Therapy

- Anticonvulsant drugs: treat seizures (Merck, 2006; National Institute of Health [NIH], 2011)
- Baclofen pumps: relax muscles and control tremors and spasticity (Merck, 2006; NIH, 2011)
- Benzodiazepines: manage spasticity (Merck, 2006)
- Botulinum toxin (Botox): decrease muscle stiffness and allow for more controlled movement and increased function when used in conjunction with occupational therapy (OT) (Hoare et al., 2010; NIH, 2011)
- Selective dorsal rhizotomy surgery: reduce muscle tone (Goldstein, 2004; Merck, 2006)

Interdisciplinary Interventions

Children with CP may see physical and speech therapists on a regular basis (Merck, 2006).

Complementary Alternative Medicines

These are treatment approaches that have not been accepted by mainstream practice, and the evidence remains inconclusive[1]:

- Hyperbaric oxygen therapy (Collet et al., 2001; Hardy et al., 2002; Rosenbaum, Fehlings, & Iliffe, 2001)
- Therapeutic electrical stimulation (Dali et al., 2002; Sommerfelt, Markestad, Berg, & Saetesdal, 2001)
- Hippotherapy[1]
- Massage therapy
- Aquatherapy
- Chiropractic manipulation
- Conductive education (Carlson & Krahn, 2006; Hurvitz, Leonard, Ayyangar, & Nelson, 2003)

Occupational Therapy Evaluations

The basis of OT assessment for clients with CP is to determine the client's ability to participate in society and meaningful occupations. Evaluation of the need for assistive technology is important for clients across the life course because needs can change with age.

Pediatric Evaluations

Pediatric evaluations for CP may include the following:

Activities of Daily Living

- Pediatric Evaluation of Disability Inventory
- WeeFim: Functional Independence Measure for Children
- CHORES: Children Helping Out: Responsibility, Expectation, and Support
- AMPS: Assessment of Motor and Process Skills

School Specific

- School Function Assessment
- School Setting Interview
- School AMPS: School Assessment of Motor and Process Skills

Functional Mobility

- Gross Motor Function Classification System (GMFCS)

Play/Leisure

- Knox Preschool Play Scale
- Transdisciplinary Play-Based Assessment
- COSA: Children's Occupational Self Assessment
- Play History
- Children Assessment of Participation and Enjoyment (CAPE)
- Preferences for Activities of Children (PAC)

Adolescent/Adult Evaluations

Adolescent and adult evaluations for CP may include the following:

General Occupational Performance

- Canadian Occupational Performance Measure (COPM)
- Occupational Performance History Interview
- Occupational Circumstance Assessment Interview and Rating Scale
- Occupational Questionnaire

Activities of Daily Living

- Functional Independence Measure (FIM)

Work

- Work Environment Impact Scale

Leisure

- Adolescent Role Assessment
- Leisure Assessment Inventory

Additional client factors that may be assessed include cognition, tone, spasticity, sensation, fatigue, and range of motion (ROM) (Goldstein, 2004; Steultjens et al., 2004).

Occupational Therapy Interventions

When working with people who have CP, OT practitioners focus on adapting tasks and the environment to help enhance participation and quality of life. Occupational therapists aim to decrease disability, improve function, and maintain performance. OT practitioners may play a key role in helping people with CP to choose and access assistive devices and supports that will promote function. Practitioners can play an important role throughout the life course depending on the individual's needs and may be a part of early intervention, school, and rehabilitation services (Goldstein, 2004; Steultjens et al., 2004).

Interventions may include the following:

- Client and caregiver education on ROM to prevent contractures as well as finding ways to manage daily tasks and routines (Steultjens et al., 2004; UCP, 2001b)
- Fabrication of orthotics or splints (Goldstein, 2004; Steultjens et al., 2004)
- Provision of adaptive seating has been shown to enable engagement in meaningful occupations and may improve school performance (Rigby, Ryan, & Campbell, 2009).
- Constraint-induced therapy (Lam-Damji & Fehlings, 2006; Taub, Ramey, DeLuca, & Echols, 2004)

Occupational Therapy and the Evidence

Studies addressing the therapeutic approaches that are used by occupational therapists and other rehabilitation professionals have found that the motivation of the client, the degree of impairment, the therapist–client interaction and relationship, the intensity and duration of treatment, and the environment where therapy takes place can have more of an effect on the success of treatment than the particular intervention approach itself (Goldstein, 2004).

Interventions that focus only on physical capabilities and focus on changing the quality of movement, such as neurodevelopmental treatment, have been shown to provide only limited carryover (Butler & Darrah, 2001; Law et al., 1998; Law et al., 1997). Therefore, it is most appropriate to use a family-centered, functional approach that promotes functional performance, identifies and changes the primary constraints of the task, and encourages practice to improve performance in all areas of occupation. Providing treatment within the natural context has been shown to provide lasting effects in individuals with CP (Law et al., 1998; Law et al., 1997; Steultjens et al., 2004).

Caregiver Concerns

- Most people with CP will need at least some type of assistance from a caregiver throughout the life course. As parents age, they might become physically unable to care for their adult children and will need to find alternatives, such as group home placements.
- It is important for caregivers to allow their loved ones to maintain as much independence as possible. Allowing them opportunities to make choices and convey their preferences should be provided when feasible.
- It is important to make sure caregivers take care of themselves and seek assistance from others when needed (UCP, 2001b).

---

[1]Some research has produced beneficial results (Sterba, 2007).

Resources

Organizations

- United Cerebral Palsy Association
  1660 L Street, NW, Suite 700
  Washington, DC 20036
  Telephone: (800)-872-5827 or (202)-776-0406
  Fax: (202)-776-0414
  E-mail: info@ucp.org
  Website: http://www.ucp.org

- American Academy for Cerebral Palsy and Developmental Medicine
  555 East Wells, Suite 1100
  Milwaukee, WI 53202
  Telephone: (414)-918-3014
  Fax: (414)-276-2146
  E-mail: info@aacpdm.org
  Website: http://www.aacpdm.org

Books

- Brady, S. (2002). *Ten things I learned from Bill Porter*. Novato, CA: New World Library.
  Written by a close friend and assistant of Bill Porter, a man who worked as a door-to-door salesman despite the challenges presented to him by CP. The story shares the author's experiences with Bill Porter and the valuable lessons he learned from him.

- Brown, C. (1955). *My left foot*. New York, NY: Simon & Schuster.
  The author shares his story about growing up with CP and how he taught himself to use his foot to paint and write as a result of being unable to use his hands.

- Miller, F., & Bachrach, S. J. (2006). *Cerebral palsy: A complete guide for caregiving* (2nd ed.). Baltimore, MD: Johns Hopkins Press.
  This book, written by a team of experts, provides information about the diagnosis of CP, its course, treatment options, and implications. It provides parents information and advice on caregiving and advocacy.

- Sienkiewicz-Mercer, R., & Kaplan, S. (1996). *I raise my eyes to say yes*. Boston, MA: Houghton Mifflin.
  This is the true story of a woman who became paralyzed and unable to speak after contracting a disease in infancy. After she spent years in an institution, people around her finally realized that she was able to communicate via eye movements and facial expressions.

Journals

- *Developmental Medicine and Child Neurology*
- *Disability and Rehabilitation*

Websites

- 4MyChild (http://www.cerebralpalsy.org)—This is an easy-to-use Website that provides information about CP and provides resources for families. The site includes general information about the condition, discussion boards, and inspirational stories.

- American Academy for Cerebral Palsy and Developmental Medicine (http://www.aacpdm.org)—This Website provides information about news, events, and resources for professionals as well as parents of children with CP.

- United Cerebral Palsy Association (http://www.ucp.org)—This Website provides extensive information about various issues and services relevant to people with CP that is geared towards professionals as well as clients and their families.

References

Butler, C., & Darrah, J. (2001). Effects of neurodevelopmental treatment (NDT) for cerebral palsy: An AACPDM evidence report. *Developmental Medicine and Child Neurology, 43*, 778–790.

Carlson, M. J., & Krahn, G. (2006). Use of complementary and alternative medicine practitioners by people with physical disabilities: Estimates from a national US survey. *Disability and Rehabilitation, 28*, 505–513.

Collet, J. P., Vanasse, M., Marois, P., Amar, M., Goldberg, J., Lambert, J., . . . Majnemer, A. (2001). Hyperbaric oxygen for children with cerebral palsy: A randomized multicentre trial. *The Lancet, 357*, 582–586.

Dali, C., Haansen, F. J., Pedersen, S. A., Skov, L., Hilden, J., Bjornskov, I., . . . Lyskjaer, U. (2002). Threshold electrical stimulation (TES) in ambulant children with CP: A randomized double-blind placebo-controlled clinical trial. *Developmental Medicine and Child Neurology, 44*, 364–369.

Goldstein, M. (2004). The treatment of cerebral palsy: What we know, what we don't know. *Journal of Pediatrics, 145*(2, Suppl.), S42–S46. doi:10.1016/j.jpeds.2004.05.022

Hardy, P., Collet, J. P., Goldber, J., Ducruet, T., Vanasse, M., Lambert, J., . . . Lassonde, M. (2002). Neuropsychological effects of hyperbaric oxygen therapy in cerebral palsy. *Developmental Medicine and Child Neurology, 44*, 436–446.

Haak, P., Lenski, M., Hidecker, M. J. C., Li, M., & Paneth, N. (2009). Cerebral palsy and aging [Review]. *Developmental Medicine and Child Neurology, 51*(4, Suppl.), 16–23. doi:10.1111/j.1469-8749.2009.03428.x

Hoare, B. J., Wallen, M. A., Imms, C., Villanueva, E., Rawicki, H. B., & Carey, L., (2010). Botulinum toxin A as an adjunct to treatment in the management of the upper limb in children with spastic cerebral palsy (UPDATE) [Review]. *The Cochrane Database of Systematic Reviews*, (1), 1–160. doi:10.1002/14651858.CD003469.pub4

Hurvitz, E. A., Leonard, C., Ayyangar, R., & Nelson, V. S. (2003). Complementary and alternative medicine use in families of children with cerebral palsy. *Developmental Medicine and Child Neurology, 45*, 354–370.

Lam-Damji, S., & Fehlings, D. L. (2006). *An update on constraint therapy in children with hemiplegia*. Retrieved from http://www.canchild.ca/en/canchildresources/constrainttherapy.asp

Law, M., Darrah, J., Pollock, N., Gillian, K., Rosenbaum, P., Russell, D., . . . Watt, J. (1998). Family-centered functional therapy for children with cerebral palsy: An emerging practice model. *Physical and Occupational Therapy in Pediatrics, 18*, 83–102.

Law, M., Russell, D., Pollock, N., Rosenbaum, P., Walter, S., & King, G. (1997). A comparison of intensive neurodevelopmental therapy plus casting and a regular occupational therapy program for children with cerebral palsy. *Developmental Medicine and Child Neurology, 39*, 664–670.

Merck. (2006). *Cerebral palsy*. Retrieved from http://www.merckmanuals.com/home/sec23/ch284/ch284a.html

National Institute of Health. (2011). *Cerebral palsy*. Retrieved from http://www.nlm.nih.gov/medlineplus/ency/article/000716.htm

Rigby, P. J., Ryan, S. E., & Campbell, K. A. (2009). Effect of adaptive seating devices on the activity performance of children with cerebral palsy. *Archives of Physical Medicine and Rehabilitation, 90*, 1389–1395.

Rosenbaum, P., Fehlings, D., & Iliffe, C. (2001). *Hyperbaric oxygen therapy: Hot or not?* Retrieved from http://www.canchild.ca/en/canchildresources/hyperbaricoxygen.asp

Sommerfelt, K., Markestad, T., Berg, K., & Saetesdal, I. (2001). Therapeutic electrical stimulation in cerebral palsy: A randomized, controlled crossover trial. *Developmental Medicine and Child Neurology, 43*, 609–613.

Sterba, J. A. (2007). Does horseback riding therapy or therapist-directed hippotherapy rehabilitate children with cerebral palsy? [Review]. *Developmental Medicine and Child Neurology, 49*, 68–73.

Steultjens, E. M. J., Dekker, J., Bouter, L. M., van de Nes, J. C. M., Lambregts, B. L. M., & van den Ende, C. H. M. (2004). Occupational therapy for children with cerebral palsy: A systematic review. *Clinical Rehabilitation, 18*, 1–14. doi:10.1191/0269215504cr697oa

Taub, E., Ramey, S. L., DeLuca, S., & Echols, K. (2004). Efficacy of constraint-induced movement therapy for children with cerebral palsy with asymmetric motor impairment. *Pediatrics, 113*, 305–312.

United Cerebral Palsy Association. (2001a). *Cerebral palsy—Facts & figures*. Retrieved from http://ucp.org/ucp_generaldoc.cfm/1/9/37/37-37/447

United Cerebral Palsy Association. (2001b). *Caregiving basics*. Retrieved from http://www.ucp.org/ucp_channeldoc.cfm/1/11/54/54-54/2934

Cerebrovascular Accident

Larissa Sachs

Description

A *cerebrovascular accident* (CVA), also known as a stroke, results in anoxia and damage or death of brain tissue (Centers for Disease Control and Prevention [CDC], 2010). There are two forms of stroke. Ischemic strokes, which account for approximately 80% of all strokes, are caused by a blockage of a blood vessel supplying the brain. Hemorrhagic strokes result from the rupturing of an artery, causing blood to leak into the brain. Approximately 25% of people who have a stroke will have another stroke within 5 years (National Institute of Neurological Disorders and Stroke [NINDS], 2011).

Incidence and Prevalence

In 2008, an estimated 133,750 people died of stroke, making CVA the nation's fourth leading cause of death. Each year, about 795,000 people have a stroke in United States; about 610,000 are first attacks, and 185,000 are recurrent attacks. Incidence of stroke is higher among non-Caucasian groups (CDC, 2010).

Typical Course

Because some individuals regain full function and others regain very little, the course of recovery after stroke remains unpredictable (CDC, 2010). Although the location, size, and type of the brain lesion affect the prognosis for recovery, most people report decreased levels of activity, social interaction, and overall life satisfaction poststroke (Lai, Studenski, Duncan, & Perera, 2002). Research findings report a decline in functional status over time after an ischemic stroke (Dhamoon et al., 2009), but other evidence indicates that cortical reorganization and recovery of function remain possible for years after onset (Liepert, Bauder, Miltner, Taub, & Weiller, 2000).

Symptoms

Warning Signs of Stroke

- Sudden numbness or weakness of the face, arm, or leg, especially on one side of the body
- Sudden confusion or trouble speaking or understanding
- Sudden difficulty seeing in one or both eyes
- Sudden dizziness, trouble walking, or loss of balance or coordination
- Sudden severe headache with unknown cause (CDC, 2010; NINDS, 2011)

Effects of Stroke

- Hemiplegia/hemiparesis: decreased function on one side of the body
- Apraxia: motor planning problems
- Dysphagia: difficulty swallowing
- Dysarthria: oral motor difficulties characterized by poor articulation
- Aphasia: receptive and/or expressive language and communication deficits
- Cognitive deficits (e.g., impulsivity, decreased insight and judgment, memory loss)
- Visual-perceptual deficits (e.g., homonymous hemianopsia, unilateral neglect)
- Somatosensory deficits: impairment of sensation
- Psychosocial deficits (e.g., depression, denial, anger, emotional lability) (NINDS, 2011)

Precautions

- *Medical status/stability*: Assess daily before intervention during the acute stage of recovery and be attentive to the symptoms of progressing or recurrent stroke.
- *Cardiac and respiratory precautions*: Monitor for dizziness, breathing difficulties, chest pain, excessive fatigue, and altered heart rate or rhythm.
- *Fall prevention*: Provide supervision and assistance during all transitional movements.
- *Shoulder injury or pain*: Never move an individual by the affected upper extremity.
- *Skin integrity*: Monitor frequently, especially when client has decreased sensation, visual field deficits, and/or unilateral neglect.
- *Swallowing status*: Refer to a speech-language pathologist as needed to determine swallowing ability and follow safe techniques during feeding.
- *Poor safety awareness and impulsive behavior*: Provide appropriate level of supervision.
- *Contractures*: When appropriate, follow individualized preventative program of proper positioning, soft tissue and joint mobilization, and range of motion (ROM) exercises.
- *General safety concerns*: Educate the individual, family, and other health care providers regarding all precautions to maximize safety (Woodson, 2008).

Risk Factors and Prevention

Stroke risk factors include alcohol and tobacco use, physical inactivity, high blood pressure and cholesterol, heart disease, diabetes, sickle cell anemia, obesity, previous stroke, family history of stroke, and aging. Prevention practices include eating a healthy diet, maintaining a healthy weight, remaining physically active, avoiding tobacco use, limiting alcohol use, and managing or treating other medical conditions (CDC, 2010).

Interdisciplinary Interventions

Medications

- *Thrombolytic agents*: Treat an ongoing, acute ischemic stroke by dissolving the clot that is blocking the flow of blood to the brain; typically administered within 3 hours of stroke symptom onset, with effectiveness decreasing as times passes.
- *Antithrombotics (anticoagulants and antiplatelet agents)*: Prevent the formation of blood clots that create a blockage in a cerebral artery, decreasing the risk of a first or recurrent ischemic stroke when prescribed appropriately by a physician. Antiplatelet drugs, such as aspirin and clopidogrel, prevent clotting by reducing the activity of platelets in the blood. Anticoagulants, such as warfarin and heparin, decrease stroke risk by diminishing the blood's clotting property (NINDS, 2011).

Surgery

- *Carotid endarterectomy*: Plaque is removed from the walls of one of the carotid arteries, which are the primary suppliers of blood to the brain. This is an effective method of stroke prevention in individuals with constricted or narrowed blood vessels.
- *Angioplasty*: A less invasive procedure that involves inflating a small balloon to widen a clogged artery and inserting a small stent to prevent the artery from narrowing.
- *Extracranial/intracranial bypass*: A controversial procedure that reroutes a healthy artery in the scalp to an area of brain tissue deprived of blood by a blocked artery, restoring blood flow as a measure of prevention or treatment (NINDS, 2011).

Rehabilitation Therapies

- *Physical therapy*: Use of training, exercises, and physical manipulations to restore movement, balance, and coordination.
- *Speech-language pathology*: Address the relearning of language and speaking skills, communication, and swallowing.
- *Psychological/psychiatric therapy*: Use talk therapy and medications to address depression, anxiety, and other mental and emotional problems that result from stroke (NINDS, 2011).

Occupational Therapy Evaluations

Comprehensive Evaluations

- American Heart Association Stroke Outcome Classification (AHA. SOC): evaluates extent and severity of impairment and level of functional independence
- Functional Independence Measure (FIM): measures type and amount of assistance needed for safe and effective activity performance
- National Institutes of Health Stroke Scale (NIHSS): assesses level of impairment
- Chedoke-McMaster Stroke Assessment: assesses physical impairment and functional ability

Activities of Daily Living or Instrumental Activities of Daily Living/Leisure Evaluations

- Assessment of Motor and Process Skills (AMPS): observational assessment of activities of daily living (ADL) and instrumental activities of daily living (IADL) performance
- Barthel Index (BI): assesses self-care abilities and level of assistance needed
- Activity Card Sort (ACS): clients describe their instrumental, social, and leisure activities
- Frenchay Activities Index (FAI): measure of ADL and IADL participation

Upper Extremity Function Evaluations

- Fugl-Meyer Assessment of Motor Function (FMA)
- Functional Test for the Hemiplegic/Paretic Upper Extremity
- Modified Ashworth Scale (MAS): measure of muscle spasticity
- Goniometry: measures ROM
- Manual muscle testing, dynamometer, and pinch meter: assess strength
- Volumeter: measures edema

Balance Evaluations

- Berg Balance Scale (BBS)
- Postural Assessment Scale for Stroke Patients (PASS)
- Motor Assessment Scale (MAS)

Cognition/Perception Evaluations

- Behavioral Inattention Test (BIT)
- Rivermead Behavioral Memory Test (RBMT)
- Executive Function Performance Test (EFPT)
- Loewenstein Occupational Therapy Cognitive Assessment (LOTCA): assesses orientation, visual and spatial perception, visuomotor organization, and thinking operations
- Catherine Bergego Scale: behavioral assessment of unilateral neglect

Quality of Life Evaluations

- Canadian Occupational Performance Measure (COPM): self-report of performance and satisfaction with occupations
- Short-Form 36 Health Survey (SF-36): evaluates health-related quality of life
- Stroke Impact Scale (SIS): self-report health status measure
- Stroke-Specific Quality of Life Scale (SS-QOL): self-report questionnaire

Occupational Therapy Interventions

All of the following interventions may be used in conjunction with one another to facilitate participation in meaningful occupations.

- *Neuromuscular*: balance training, postural awareness, motor learning, constraint-induced movement therapy
- *Musculoskeletal*: strengthening, mobilization/manual therapy, stretching/passive ROM, edema control, aerobic exercise
- *Cognitive/perceptual/sensory*: cognitive therapy, perceptual training, visual training, sensory retraining, mental imagery
- *Physical agent modalities/orthotics/splinting*: pneumatic compression, compression stockings, electrical stimulation, biofeedback, robotic therapy
- *Skill acquisition/task-specific training*: in all areas of occupation
- *Adaptive/compensatory*: one-handed skills, energy conservation, environmental adaptation, adaptive equipment/assistive technology
- *Educational*: client, caregiver/family, and staff education and training
- *Psychosocial*: relaxation, stress management, coping skills (Hoffmann et al., 2008; Latham et al., 2006; Sabari & Lieberman, 2008)

Occupational Therapy and the Evidence

Research evidence supports the efficacy of various occupational therapy (OT) interventions in stroke rehabilitation. OT effectively improves role participation and performance in basic and IADL for individuals who have had a stroke (Trombly & Ma, 2002). Individuals poststroke demonstrated increased independence in ADL performance and maintenance of these abilities following OT intervention (Legg, Drummond, & Langhorne, 2006). Research findings indicate that provision of instruction and feedback, opportunities for practice of meaningful client-identified activities within natural contexts, and provision of necessary adaptations enhance occupational performance after stroke (Trombly & Ma, 2002). OT treatments focused on remediation of impairments, particularly those involving meaningful occupational tasks or functional goal-directed activity, have generally demonstrated beneficial outcomes (Ma & Trombly, 2002). Research findings also indicate that effective practices to improve upper limb motor recovery after stroke include a combination of mental and physical practice (Nilsen, Gillen, & Gordon, 2010) and the use of extrinsic feedback to enhance motor learning (Subramanian, Massie, Malcolm, & Levin, 2010). Current evidence supports the use of task-specific, task-oriented, and/or repetitive task practice. These interventions represent a shift away from facilitation models previously used in practice, such as neurodevelopmental treatment (NDT), proprioceptive neuromuscular facilitation (PNF), and Brunnstrom's or Rood's approaches.

Caregiver Concerns

Caregivers report that they experience various common challenges, which include lack of information and training, distress, uncertainty about the future, lack of support, social isolation, and lack of freedom. Although research more often focuses on caregiver burden, practitioners should also consider the satisfactions associated with the experience of caring, including pride and a sense of closeness (Greenwood, Mackenzie, Cloud, & Wilson, 2009). To successfully manage challenges, caregivers must be educated about taking care of their own physical, emotional, mental, spiritual, and interpersonal health. To support their own health and well-being, caregivers should be realistic about what they can and cannot do, think positively, take time for themselves, maintain a healthy lifestyle by practicing healthy eating and exercise habits, seek out support, and communicate with others (American Heart Association, 2011).

Resources

Organizations

- American Stroke Association
  7272 Greenville Avenue
  Dallas, TX 75231
  Telephone: 1-888-478-7653
  Website: http://www.strokeassociation.org/
  Offers comprehensive stroke information in a user-friendly format.

- National Stroke Association
  9707 E. Easter Lane, Suite B
  Centennial, CO 80112
  Telephone: 1-800-787-6537
  Website: http://www.stroke.org
  Educates and advocates for all people impacted by stroke.

- American Stroke Foundation
  5960 Dearborn Street, Suite 100
  Mission, KS 66202
  Telephone: 1-866-549-1776
  Website: http://www.americanstroke.org/
  Source of empowerment for individuals who have had a stroke and their families

Books

- Shapiro, A. B. (2009). *Healing into possibility*. Tiburon, CA: H. J. Kramer.
  This book recounts the recovery process of a businesswoman who had two major strokes. She shares the lessons she learned and how she found hope in the face of illness.

- Simon, S. (2002). *A stroke of genius: Messages of hope and healing from a thriving stroke survivor*. Delray Beach, FL: The Cedars Group.
  Written by a man who had a cerebral hemorrhage, this book shares personal anecdotes and offers advice on how to handle physical and psychosocial implications of stroke.

- Taylor, J. B. (2008). *My stroke of insight: A brain scientist's personal journey*. New York. NY: Viking.
  An account of a brain scientist's recovery from a debilitating stroke, this book offers a guide to understanding the experience of having a stroke and the rehabilitation process.

Journals

- *Archives of Physical Medicine and Rehabilitation*
- *Neurology*
- *Stroke*

Websites

- MedlinePlus
  http://www.nlm.nih.gov/medlineplus/stroke.html
  This Website provides comprehensive stroke-related information and links to helpful resources.

- National Institute of Neurological Disorders and Stroke
  http://www.ninds.nih.gov/
  This Website offers current stroke-related information, publications, research literature, and links.

References

American Heart Association. (2011). *Caregiver*. Retrieved from http://www.heart.org/HEARTORG/Caregiver/Caregiver_UCM_001103_SubHomePage.jsp

Centers for Disease Control and Prevention. (2010). *Stroke*. Retrieved from http://www.cdc.gov/stroke/

Dhamoon, M. S., Moon, Y. P., Paik, M. C., Boden-Albala, B., Rundek, T., Sacco, R. L., & Elkind, M. (2009). Long-term functional recovery after first ischemic stroke: The northern Manhattan study. *Stroke, 40*, 2805–2811. doi:10.1161/STROKEAHA.109.549576

Greenwood, N., Mackenzie, A., Cloud, G. C., & Wilson, N. (2009). Informal primary carers of stroke survivors living at home—Challenges, satisfactions and coping: A systematic review of qualitative studies. *Disability and Rehabilitation, 31*, 337–351.

Hoffmann, T., Bennett, S., McKenna, K., Green-Hill, J., McCluskey, A., & Tooth, L. (2008). Interventions for stroke rehabilitation: Analysis of the research contained in the OTseeker evidence database. *Topics in Stroke Rehabilitation, 15*, 341–350.

Lai, S.-M., Studenski, S., Duncan, P. W., & Perera, S. (2002). Persisting consequences of stroke measured by the Stoke Impact Scale. *Stroke, 33*, 1840–1844.

Latham, N. K., Jette, D. U., Coster, W., Richards, L., Smout, R. J., James, R. A., . . . Horn, S. D. (2006). Occupational therapy activities and intervention techniques for clients with stroke in six rehabilitation hospitals. *American Journal of Occupational Therapy, 60*, 369–378.

Legg, L., Drummond, A., & Langhorne, P. (2006). Occupational therapy for patients with problems in activities of daily living after stroke. *Cochrane Database of Systematic Reviews*, (4), CD003585. doi:10.1002/14651858.CD003585.pub2

Liepert, J., Bauder, H., Miltner, W., Taub, E., & Weiller, C. (2000). Treatment-induced cortical reorganization after stroke in humans. *Stroke, 31*, 1210–1216.

Ma, H.-I., & Trombly, C. A. (2002). Synthesis of the effects of occupational therapy for persons with stroke, part II: Remediation of impairments. *American Journal of Occupational Therapy, 56*, 260–274.

National Institute of Neurological Disorders and Stroke. (2011). *Stroke: Hope through research*. Retrieved from http://www.ninds.nih.gov/disorders/stroke/detail_stroke.htm#170781105

Nilsen, D. M., Gillen, G., & Gordon, A. M. (2010). Use of mental practice to improve upper-limb recovery after stroke: A systematic review. *American Journal of Occupational Therapy, 64*, 695–708. doi:10.5014/ajot.2010.09034

Sabari, J. S., & Lieberman, D. (2008). *Occupational therapy practice guidelines for adults with stroke*. Bethesda, MD: The American Occupational Therapy Association.

Subramanian, S. K., Massie, C. L., Malcolm, M. P., & Levin, M. F. (2010). Does provision of extrinsic feedback result in improved motor learning in the upper limb poststroke? A systematic review of the evidence. *Neurorehabilitation and Neural Repair, 24*, 113–124. doi:10.1177/1545968309349941

Trombly, C. A., & Ma, H.-I. (2002). A synthesis of the effects of occupational therapy for persons with stroke, part I: Restoration of roles, tasks, and activities. *American Journal of Occupational Therapy, 56*, 250–259.

Woodson, A. M. (2008). *Stroke*. In M. V. Radomski & C. A. Trombly Latham (Eds.), *Occupational therapy for physical dysfunction* (6th ed., pp. 1001–1041). Baltimore, MD: Lippincott Williams & Wilkins.

Chronic Fatigue Syndrome

Pamela Vaughn

Description and Diagnosis

Chronic fatigue syndrome (CFS), also known as chronic fatigue and immune dysfunction syndrome (CFIDS) and myalgic encephalomyelitis (ME), is characterized by extreme and persistent tiredness or weariness that is not alleviated by rest or sleep and is not caused by other medical conditions. Because there is currently no test for CFS, diagnosis entails the exclusion of other possible causes of symptoms and looks for the presence of four or more CFS symptoms over at least 6 months (Centers for Disease Control and Prevention [CDC], 2010).

Incidence and Prevalence

Prevalence reports vary from just under 1% to nearly 4% of the general adult population (Bhui et al., 2011; Fiest, Currie, Williams, & Wang, 2011; van't Leven, Zielhuis, van der Meer, Verbeek, & Bleijenberg, 2010). Although CFS tends to affect adults and older adults, some adolescents present with symptoms as well. One Dutch study reports a prevalence of adolescent CFS of 0.11% with an annual incidence of 12 per 100,000 (Nijhof et al., 2011). CFS occurs more frequently in women than in men (CDC, 2010).

Cause and Etiology

The cause of CFS is unknown. Although some studies (e.g., Lombardi et al., 2009) have reported links between the presence of certain viruses (i.e., xenotropic murine leukemia virus-related virus [XMRV], Epstein-Barr virus, and human herpesvirus 6 [HHV-6]) and a diagnosis of CFS, no definitive etiological connection has been established as of yet (e.g., Satterfield et al., 2011).

Typical Course, Symptoms, and Related Conditions

Symptoms of CFS significantly impair and reduce a client's level of activity and may include the following:

- Impaired memory or concentration
- Postexertional malaise (extreme, prolonged exhaustion and sickness following physical or mental activity)
- Unrefreshing sleep
- Muscle pain
- Multijoint pain without swelling or redness
- Headaches of a new type or severity
- Sore throat that is frequent or recurring
- Tender cervical or axillary lymph nodes (CDC, 2010)

There are many conditions that may have chronic fatigue as a symptom—for example, fibromyalgia, mononucleosis, hyperthyroidism, sleep apnea, AIDS, major depressive disorder, and so forth—but a diagnosis of CFS will only be made in the absence of such conditions. However, the emotional and psychological implications of CFS result in many clients being diagnosed with depression after the fact (Fiest et al., 2011).

Interdisciplinary Interventions

Medication Therapy

Medications to alleviate or treat the symptoms of CFS—for example, pain medication, sleep aids, and so forth—are frequently prescribed. Many clients may also take antidepressants (CDC, 2010).

Complementary and Alternative Medicine

Complementary and alternative medicine (CAM) techniques have been used to alleviate the symptoms of CFS as well as the associated emotional and psychological effects, for example, anxiety. One review of alternative medical interventions for CFS reported that many approaches (i.e., acupuncture, massage, and meditation) have resulted in decreased symptoms among clients (Porter, Jason, Boulton, Bothne, & Coleman, 2010).

Exercise Therapy

Gradual, guided physical activity is often used to maintain health and decrease severity of CFS symptoms over an extended period of time. It is important that exercise is carefully monitored to ensure that it does not increase fatigue. When compared to controls, individuals undergoing an exercise therapy intervention reported decreased fatigue after 12 weeks; when combined with other forms of intervention (e.g., education, medication), exercise therapy was found to be even more effective than any of the interventions alone (Edmonds, McGuire, & Price, 2010).

Occupational Therapy Evaluations

The evaluation process focuses on what the client needs, wants, or is expected to do and analyzes what factors may impact desired occupational performance. The evaluation begins with occupation-focused assessments followed by specific evaluation of the potential impact of CFS on occupational performance. For clients with CFS, it is particularly important to spread the evaluation period out so as not to exhaust the client in one sitting and also to gain insight regarding his or her capacity for endurance over an extended period of time.

Occupation-Focused Assessments

- National Institutes of Health (NIH) Activity Record (ACTRE) (Gerber & Furst, 1992)
- Role Checklist (Oakley, Kielhofner, Barris, & Reichler, 1986)
- Occupational Performance History Interview II (OPHI-II) (Kielhofner et al., 2004)
- Assessment of Motor and Process Skills (AMPS) (Fisher & Jones, 2010)
- Occupational Self-Assessment, Version 2.2 (Baron, Kielhofner, Iyenger, Goldhammer, & Wolenski, 2006)
- Performance Assessment of Self-Care Skills (PASS) (Holm & Rogers, 2008)
- Canadian Occupational Performance Measure (COPM) (Law et al., 2005)
- Short Form-36 (SF-36) (Hays, Sherbourne, & Mazel, 1995)
- Activity Card Sort (ACS) (Baum & Edwards, 2008)

Client Factor Assessments

- Chronic Fatigue Syndrome Screening Questionnaire (Jason et al., 1997)
- Functional Capacity Evaluations (FCEs) (see Barrows, 1995)
- Measures of endurance
- Range of motion (ROM)
- Measures of pain (e.g., Visual Analog Scale [VAS])
- Measures of muscle strength

Occupational Therapy Interventions

Cognitive Behavioral Therapy

Cognitive behavioral therapy (CBT) focuses on helping a client become aware of his or her thought processes to identify and change negative beliefs, behaviors, and emotions to become more functional by managing activity levels, stress, and symptoms. Professionals trained in and able to administer CBT may include psychologists and occupational therapists.

Energy Conservation

Because CFS can negatively affect all areas of occupation, developing energy conservation techniques can allow a client to maintain or improve participation. Techniques may focus on the individual (e.g., relaxation techniques) or on adapting the task and/or environment. This may involve the use of assistive and adaptive devices. Developing time management and pacing skills and prioritizing occupations can assist a client in reducing the occupational impact of CFS (Taylor & Kielhofner, 2003).

Consultation

In addition to working with clients to prevent occupational decline, occupational therapist can consult with clients and work with them to find alternative and potentially new occupations to help them fulfill their roles and increase participation. Referring clients to community support groups helps them access other resources pertaining to CFS. Occupational therapy (OT) consultation can also include an educational component for clients and their family members to learn more about CFS and its effects on occupation and about strategies for self-advocacy and assertiveness (Taylor & Kielhofner, 2003).

Occupational Therapy and the Evidence

Hughes (2009) reports the paucity of evidence-based research on the effects of OT for clients with CFS but notes that much research reports the occupational disruption that is caused by CFS. Highlighting this need for OT for clients with CFS, one qualitative study of women with CFS who participated in an art class as a means of occupational and social participation revealed the participants' desire for earlier access to OT (Reynolds, Vivat, & Prior, 2008).

An 8-week OT group focusing on developing empowerment and participatory action skills in clients with CFS was shown to significantly decrease CFS symptoms and increase quality of life compared to preintervention (Taylor, 2004). Increased occupational participation among clients with CFS has been associated with the coping strategy of maintaining activity as if they were feeling well; occupational participation negatively correlated with illness accommodation (rearranging life to deal with CFS symptoms) (Roche & Taylor, 2005). One case study that used energy conservation, time management, and education intervention techniques reports a drastic change in occupational functioning of one individual with CFS (Burley, Cox, & Findley, 2007).

CBT has been reported to decrease CFS symptoms postintervention when compared to usual care (i.e., medication) or other psychological interventions; reports of long-term benefits to CBT, however, are inconsistent (Price, Mitchell, Tidy, & Hunot, 2008).

Caregiver Concerns

Family members of individuals with CFS express frustration with trying to find a diagnosis that fits their loved one's condition and excitement when they learn that there is a name for it. They also often report feeling stigmatized against because their family member has a condition that is characterized by "being tired." Due to the potential loss of income, some families feel financial burden. Most report having to reassign family tasks to accommodate for the family member's inability to complete chores or roles without exacerbating symptoms (Donalek, 2009).

Resources

Organizations

- International Association for Chronic Fatigue Syndrome/Myalgic Encephalomyelitis (IACFS/ME)
  27 N. Wacker Drive Suite 416
  Chicago, IL 60606
  Telephone: 847-258-7248
  Fax: 847-579-0975
  E-mail: Admin@iacfsme.org
  Website: http://www.iacfsme.org

- The Chronic Fatigue and Immune Dysfunction Syndrome (CFIDS) Association of America
  PO Box 220398
  Charlotte, NC 28222-0398
  Telephone: 704-365-2343
  E-mail: cfids@cfids.org
  Website: http://www.cfids.org/

- National Chronic Fatigue Syndrome and Fibromyalgia Association (NCFSFA)
  PO Box 18426
  Kansas City, MO 64133
  Telephone: 816-737-1343
  Website: http://www.ncfsfa.org/

Books

- Barton, A. (2008). *Recovery from CFS: 50 personal stories*. Bloomington, IN: AuthorHouse.
- Skloot, F. (1996). *The night-side: Chronic fatigue syndrome & the illness experience*. Ashland, OR: Story Line Press.
- Wall, D. (2005). *Encounters with the invisible: Unseen illness, controversy, and chronic fatigue syndrome*. Dallas, TX: Southern Methodist University Press.

Websites

- Mayo Clinic: http://www.mayoclinic.com/health/chronic-fatigue-syndrome/DS00395
- PubMed: http://www.ncbinlm.nih.gov/pubmedhealth/PMH0002224/
- EndFatigue: http://www.endfatigue.com/

References

Baron, K., Kielhofner, G., Iyenger, A., Goldhammer, V., & Wolenski, J. (2006). *Occupational Self-Assessment* (OSA; Version 2.2.). Chicago, IL: MOHO Clearinghouse.

Barrows, D. (1995). Functional capacity evaluations of persons with chronic fatigue immune dysfunction syndrome. *American Journal of Occupational Therapy, 49*, 327–337.

Baum, C. M., & Edwards, D. E. (2008). *Activity Card Sort* (2nd ed.). Bethesda, MD: AOTA Press.

Bhui, K. S., Dinos, S., Ashby, D., Nazroo, J., Wessely, S., & White, P. D. (2011). Chronic fatigue syndrome in an ethnically diverse population: The influence of psychosocial adversity and physical inactivity. *BMC Medicine, 9*(26), 1–12.

Burley, L., Cox, D. L., & Findley, L. J. (2007). Severe chronic fatigue syndrome (CFS/ME): Recovery is possible. *British Journal of Occupational Therapy, 70*, 339–344.

Centers for Disease Control and Prevention. (2010). *Chronic fatigue syndrome: General information*. Retrieved from http://www.cdc.gov/cfs/general/

Donalek, J. G. (2009). When a parent is chronically ill: Chronic fatigue syndrome. *Nursing Research, 58*, 332–339. doi:10.1097/NNR.0b013e3181ac156f

Edmonds, M., McGuire, H., & Price, J. R. (2010). Exercise therapy for chronic fatigue syndrome. *Cochrane Database of Systematic Reviews*, (3), CD003200. doi:10.1002/14651858.CD003200.pub2

Fiest, K. M., Currie, S. R., Williams, J. V. A., & Wang, J. (2011). Chronic conditions and major depression in community-dwelling older adults. *Journal of Affective Disorders, 131*, 172–178. doi:10.1016/j.jad.2010.11.028

Fisher, A. G., & Jones, K. B. (2010). *Assessment of Motor and Process Skills. Vol. 1: Development, standardization, and administration manual* (7th ed.). Fort Collins, CO: Three Star Press.

Gerber, L., & Furst, G. (1992). Scoring methods and application of the Activity Record (ACTRE) for patients with musculoskeletal disorders. *Arthritis Care and Research, 5*, 151–156.

Hays, R. D., Sherbourne, C. D., & Mazel, R. M. (1995). *User's manual for Medical Outcomes Study (MOS) core measures of health-related quality of life*. Santa Monica, CA: RAND.

Holm, M. B., & Rogers, J. C. (2008). The Performance Assessment of Self-Care Skills (PASS). In B. Hemphill-Pearson (Ed.), *Assessments in occupational therapy mental health* (2nd ed., pp. 101–110). Thorofare, NJ: Slack.

Hughes, J. L. (2009). Chronic fatigue syndrome and occupational disruption in primary care: Is there a role for occupational therapy? *British Journal of Occupational Therapy, 72*, 2–10.

Jason, L. A., Ropacki, M. T., Santoro, N. B., Richman, J. A., Heatherly, W., Taylor, R., . . . Plioplys, S. (1997). A screening scale for chronic fatigue syndrome: Reliability and validity. *Journal of Chronic Fatigue Syndrome, 3*, 39–59.

Kielhofner, G., Mallinson, T., Crawford, C., Nowak, M., Rigby, M., Henry, A., & Walens, D. (2004). *Occupational Performance History Interview II (OPHI-II)*. Chicago, IL: MOHO Clearinghouse.

Law, M., Baptiste, S., Carswell, A., McColl, M., Polatajko, H., & Pollock, N. (2005). *Canadian Occupational Performance Measure* (4th ed.). Ottawa, Canada: CAOT Publications.

Lombardi, V. C., Ruscetti, F. W., Das Gupta, J., Pfost, M. A., Hagen, K. S., Peterson, D. L., . . . Mikovits, J. A. (2009). Detection of an infectious retrovirus, XMRV, in blood cells of patients with chronic fatigue syndrome. *Science, 326*, 585–589.

Nijhof, S. L., Maijer, K., Bleijenberg, G., Uiterwaal, C. S. P. M., Kimpen, J. L. L., & van de Putte, E. M. (2011). Adolescent chronic fatigue syndrome: Prevalence, incidence, and morbidity. *Pediatrics, 127*, e1169–e1175. doi:10.1542/peds.2010-1147

Oakley, F., Kielhofner, G., Barris, R., & Reichler, R. (1986). The Role Checklist: Development and empirical assessment of reliability. *Occupational Therapy Journal of Research, 6*, 157–170.

Porter, N. S., Jason, L. A., Boulton, A., Bothne, N., & Coleman, B. (2010). Alternative medical interventions used in the treatment and management of myalgic encephalomyelitis/chronic fatigue syndrome and fibromyalgia. *The Journal of Alternative and Complementary Medicine, 16*, 235–249. doi:10.1089/acm.2008.0376

Price, J. R., Mitchell, E., Tidy, E., & Hunot, V. (2008). Cognitive behaviour therapy for chronic fatigue syndrome in adults. *Cochrane Database of Systematic Reviews*, (3), CD001027. doi:10.1002/14651858.CD001027.pub2

Reynolds, F., Vivat, B., & Prior, S. (2008). Women's experiences of increasing subjective well-being in CFS/ME through leisure-based arts and crafts activities: A qualitative study. *Disability and Rehabilitation, 30*, 1279–1288. doi:10.1080/09638280701654518

Roche, R., & Taylor, R. R. (2005). Coping and occupational participation in chronic fatigue syndrome. *OTJR: Occupation, Participation, and Health, 25*, 75–83.

Satterfield, B. C., Garcia, R. A., Hongwei, J., Tang, S., Zheng, H., & Switzer, W. M. (2011). Serologic and PCR testing of persons with chronic fatigue syndrome in the United States shows no association with xenotropic or polytropic murine leukemia virus-related viruses. *Retrovirology, 8*(12), 1–7.
Taylor, R. R. (2004). Quality of life and symptom severity for individuals with chronic fatigue syndrome: Findings from a randomized clinical trial. *American Journal of Occupational Therapy, 58*, 35–43.
Taylor, R. R., & Kielhofner, G. W. (2003). An occupational therapy approach to persons with chronic fatigue syndrome: part two, assessment and intervention. *Occupational Therapy in Health Care, 17*, 63–87.
van't Leven, M., Zielhuis, G. A., van der Meer, J. W., Verbeek, A. L., & Bleijenberg, G. (2010). Fatigue and chronic fatigue syndrome-like complaints in the general population. *European Journal of Public Health, 20*, 251–257. doi:10.1093/eurpub/ckp113

Chronic Pain

Pamela Vaughn

Description and Diagnosis

Pain is "an unpleasant sensory and emotional experience associated with actual or potential tissue damage, or described in terms of such damage" (International Association for the Study of Pain [IASP] Task Force on Taxonomy, 1994/2011, p. 212). *Chronic pain*, differentiated from acute pain that is often due to a particular injury, is a persistent pain that lasts weeks to years and may or may not be related to a past injury or condition. It is often resistant to treatment, making it a condition that is very pervasive in clients' lives. Common types of chronic pain include low back pain, headaches and migraines, arthritis pain, and cancer pain. (National Institute of Neurological Disorders and Stroke [NINDS], 2001)

Incidence and Prevalence

The National Center for Health Statistics (2011) reported that in 2009, 16.1% of U.S. adults aged 18 years and older experienced severe headaches or migraines, 28.5% experienced low back pain, and 15.1% experienced neck pain in the past 3 months. One study (Tsang et al., 2008) reported prevalence rates of chronic pain conditions over the past 12 months among adults to be 37.3% in developed countries and 41.1% in developing countries. The prevalence of chronic pain tends to increase with age.

Cause and Risk Factors

Because pain is subjective and is a bodily response to several situations, it can be difficult for physicians to determine the exact cause of each instance of chronic pain. Patients are often asked to describe the location, type (e.g., stabbing, aching), and duration of the pain, which may then warrant further examination through neurological examination, magnetic resonance imaging (MRI), X-ray, electrocardiogram (EMG), and so forth (NINDS, 2001). Many cases of pain are symptoms of other chronic conditions (e.g., cancer pain and arthritis pain) or caused by injury or illness. Current research

> suggests that chronic non-cancer pain can develop as a result of persistent stimulation of or changes to nociceptors in receptors due to localized tissue damage from an acute injury or disease (e.g., osteoarthritis), or damage to the peripheral or central nervous system, or both (e.g., painful diabetic neuropathy, post stroke pain, spinal cord injury), which might not be readily detectable with currently available diagnostic technologies. (Cheng, 2010, as cited in Turk, Wilson, & Cahana, 2011, p. 2226)

A client's comfort and pain levels should be taken into account when planning an intervention so as to avoid exacerbating the pain.

Typical Course and Implications

Chronic pain, particularly low back pain, sometimes develops after the occurrence of an injury or as a result of a comorbid disease but persists past the expected recovery time (NINDS, 2001). As it is often resistant to treatment, clients experience barriers due to the pain in several areas of their lives, including activities of daily living (ADL) or instrumental activities of daily living (IADL), work, leisure, and social participation. These barriers can result in clients becoming frustrated, discouraged, and/or fearful to participate in activities that will exacerbate pain (Rochman & Kennedy-Spaien, 2007). Clients living with chronic pain have reported that it is "life changing" in that it affects numerous aspects of their lives, including "psychological state, occupational performance, relationships with others, and life satisfaction" (Fisher et al., 2007, p. 294).

Interdisciplinary Interventions

Medication Therapy and Other Medical Interventions

The use of medications, both prescription and over the counter, is one of the most common methods to control or alleviate pain (Turk et al., 2011). These include the following:

- Opioids
- Nonsteroidal anti-inflammatory drugs (NSAIDs) and acetaminophen-containing drugs
- Antidepressants
- Anticonvulsants
- Skeletal muscle relaxants
- Topical medications (including ones containing salicylate and capsaicin)

Other medical interventions that are commonly used include the following:

- Injection of anesthetics (e.g., epidural steroid injections)
- Surgery (e.g., lumbar fusion and disc replacement)
- Implantation of pain-relieving devices (medication or electrodes)

Physical Therapy

The overall goal of physical therapy for chronic pain is pain reduction. Techniques used to work towards this goal include muscle tension reduction and finding physical exercise activities that do not result in an increase in pain (NINDS, 2001).

Psychological Therapies

The focus of these intervention approaches is on the client's response to his or her pain (e.g., coping, adaptation, shift from hopelessness to self-management) and not necessarily on the reduction of the physical pain (Turk et al., 2011). Examples include the following:

- Operant conditioning
- Cognitive behavioral therapy (CBT)—for example, mindfulness
- Relaxation training

Complementary and Alternative Therapies

Although evidence supporting the use of complementary and alternative therapies for the control and alleviation of chronic pain is mixed, several techniques have been used, particularly when more traditional approaches fail to provide relief. Some common therapies include acupuncture, massage, biofeedback, and spinal manipulation (National Center for Complementary and Alternative Medicine, 2011).

Occupational Therapy Evaluations

Occupational therapy (OT) evaluations focus not only on individual daily functioning but also on the physical environment, social network, and quality of life for the client.

Participation and Activity

- Canadian Occupational Performance Measure (COPM) (Law et al., 2005): self-report of performance and satisfaction with occupations
- Health Status Questionnaire (SF-36): assesses patient's perceptions of health and physical limitations
- Activity Card Sort (ACS): helps clients describe instrumental and social activities

Client Factors

- Brief Pain Inventory (Cleeland & Ryan, 1994)
- Functional Capacity Evaluations
- Numerical Pain Rating Scale
- Wong-Baker FACES Pain Rating Scale (Wong & Baker, 1988)
- Face, Legs, Activity, Cry, Consolability (FLACC) Scale (Merkel, Voepel-Lewis, Shayevitz, & Malviya, 1997)

Occupational Therapy Interventions

The focus of OT interventions for clients with chronic pain is to increase participation and satisfaction with daily activities. Intervention may include various techniques, including the following:

- Increasing self-management of pain (e.g., teaching a client to use pain management tools independently and proactively)
- Task modification, for example, pacing or the use of adaptive devices to alter activities so that they can be completed without an increase in pain
- Environmental modification
- Assertiveness training and CBT to increase coping skills and self-efficacy
- Education regarding body mechanics and posture (Robinson, Kennedy, & Harmon, 2011a; Rochman & Kennedy-Spaien, 2007)

Occupational Therapy and the Evidence

Although a few intervention techniques commonly employed by occupational therapists for use with clients with chronic pain have shown to be effective—for example, CBT in increasing client self-management of pain (Turk, Swanson, & Tunks, 2008)—the vast majority of research in this area has not focused on occupation-based interventions (Robinson et al., 2011a, Robinson, Kennedy, & Harmon, 2011b). Occupational therapists are aware of the occupational needs of clients with chronic pain (Skjutar, Schult, Christensson, & Müllersdorf, 2010), but there appears to be a discrepancy between this knowledge and the clinical use of evidence-based interventions targeting these occupational needs. Therefore, Robinson et al. (2011a) call for an increase in the development and subsequent use of occupation-based interventions that are evidence based.

Evidence supporting the use of interdisciplinary teams and therapeutic approaches—including OT—has been reported frequently, but as the evidence does specify the efficacy of the individual approaches, it is difficult to conclude the effect that OT intervention has on alleviation of, adaptation to, and management of chronic pain (Oslund et al., 2009).

In research on the lived experience of clients with chronic pain conducted by Fisher et al. (2007), clients reported a reciprocal relationship between pain and occupation—that is, not only an increase in pain often decreased participation in occupations but also an increase in participation in new or different occupations often resulted in a decrease in and distraction from pain.

Caregiver Concerns

One major concern that caregivers have is that individuals with chronic pain will develop addiction to and/or overdose on certain prescription medications, namely, opioids (Morgan & Weaver, 2010). Suggestions to prevent this include enforcing stricter prescription criteria, educating users and caregivers about the dangers and signs of misuse, and choosing alternative therapeutic approaches to pain alleviation.

Resources

Organizations

- International Association for the Study of Pain (IASP)
  111 Queen Anne Ave N, Suite 501
  Seattle, WA 98109-4955
  Telephone: 206-283-0311
  E-mail: IASPdesk@iasp-pain.org
  http://www.iasp-pain.org
  IASP is the leading professional association for clinicians, researchers, and educators in the field of pain and aims to reduce the incidence of pain internationally through research and education.

- American Pain Society (APS)
  4700 W. Lake Ave.
  Glenview, IL 60025
  Telephone: 847-375-4715
  E-mail: info@ampainsoc.org
  http://www.ampainsoc.org/
  This is the United States' national chapter of IASP.

- The American Chronic Pain Association
  PO Box 850
  Rocklin, CA 95677
  Telephone: 1-800-533-3231
  E-mail: ACPA@pacbell.net
  http://www.theacpa.org
  A support and education resource for individuals with chronic pain and their caregivers.

Books

- Caudill, M. A. (2008). *Managing pain before it manages you* (3rd ed.). New York, NY: Guilford Press.

- Cochran, R. T., Jr. (2007). *Understanding chronic pain: A doctor talks to his patients.* Nashville, TN: Turner.

- Cochran, R. T., Jr. (2009). *Curing chronic pain: Stories of hope and healing.* Nashville, TN: Turner.

- Turk, D. C., & Winter, F. (2005). *The pain survival guide: How to reclaim your life.* Washington, DC: American Psychological Association.

Journals

- *PAIN* (the official journal of the IASP)
- *The Journal of Pain* (from APS)
- *Pain Physician*
- *Pain Practice*
- *Pain Research & Management*

Websites

- World Institute of Pain
  http://www.worldinstituteofpain.org

- American Pain Foundation
  http://www.painfoundation.org/

- National Pain Foundation
  http://www.nationalpainfoundation.org/

References

Cheng, H. T. (2010). Spinal cord mechanisms of chronic pain and clinical implications. *Current Pain and Headache Reports, 14,* 213–220. doi:10.1007/s11916-010-0111-0

Cleeland C. S., & Ryan, K. M. (1994). Pain assessment: Global use of the Brief Pain Inventory. *Annals of the Academy of Medicine, Singapore, 23,* 129–138.

Fisher, G. S., Emerson, L., Firpo, C., Ptak, J., Wonn, J., & Bartolacci, G. (2007). Chronic pain and occupation: An exploration of the lived experience. *American Journal of Occupational Therapy, 61,* 290–302.

International Association for the Study of Pain Task Force on Taxonomy (1994; updated 2011). Part III: Pain terms, a current list with definitions and notes on usage. In H. Merskey & N. Bogduk (Eds.), *Classification of chronic pain* (2nd ed., pp. 209–214). Seattle, WA: IASP Press.

Law, M., Baptiste, S., Carswell, A., McColl, M., Polatajko, H., & Pollock, N. (2005). *Canadian Occupational Performance Measure* (4th ed.). Ottawa, Canada: CAOT Publications.

Merkel, S. I., Voepel-Lewis, T., Shayevitz, J. R., & Malviya, S. (1997). The FLACC: A behavioral scale for scoring postoperative pain in young children. *Pediatric Nursing, 23*, 293–297.

Morgan, L. A., & Weaver, M. F. (2010). Preventing prescription opioid overdose. *Journal of Clinical Outcomes Management, 17*, 511–518.

National Center for Complementary and Alternative Medicines. (2011). *Chronic pain and CAM: At a glance* (NCCAM Publication No. D456). Retrieved from http://nccam.nih.gov/health/pain/chronic.htm#use

National Center for Health Statistics. (2011). *Health, United States, 2010: With special feature on death and dying* (Department of Health and Human Services Publication No. 2011-1232). Retrieved from http://www.cdc.gov/nchs/hus/diseases.htm#chronic

National Institute of Neurological Disorders and Stroke (2001). *Pain: Hope through research* (National Institutes of Health Publication No. 01-2406). Retrieved from http://www.ninds.nih.gov/disorders/chronic_pain/detail_chronic_pain.htm#175053084

Oslund, S., Robinson, R. C., Clark, T. C., Garofalo, J. P., Behnk, P., Walker, B., . . . Noe, C. E. (2009). Long-term effectiveness of a comprehensive pain management program: Strengthening the case for interdisciplinary care. *Baylor University Medical Center Proceedings, 22*, 211–214.

Robinson, K., Kennedy, N., & Harmon, D. (2011a). The issue is—Is occupational therapy adequately meeting the needs of people with chronic pain? *American Journal of Occupational Therapy, 65*, 106–113. doi:10.5014/ajot.2011.09160

Robinson, K., Kennedy, N., & Harmon, D. (2011b). Review of occupational therapy for people with chronic pain. *Australian Occupational Therapy Journal, 58*, 74–81. doi:10.1111/j.1440-1630.2010.00889.x

Rochman, D. L., & Kennedy-Spaien, E. (2007). Chronic pain management: Approaches and tools for occupational therapy. *OT Practice, 12*(13), 9–15.

Skjutar, A., Schult, M., Christensson, K., & Müllersdorf, M. (2010). Indicators of need for occupational therapy in patients with chronic pain: Occupational therapists' focus groups. *Occupational Therapy International, 17*, 93–103. doi:10.1002/oti.282

Tsang, A., Von Korff, M., Lee, S., Alonso, J., Karam, E., Angermeyer, M. C., . . . Watanabe, M. (2008). Common chronic pain conditions in developed and developing countries: Gender and age differences and comorbidity with depression-anxiety disorders. *The Journal of Pain, 9*, 883–891. doi:10.1016/j.jpain.2008.05.005

Turk, D. C., Swanson, K. S., & Tunks, E. R. (2008). Psychological approaches in the treatment of chronic pain patients—When pills, scalpels, and needles are not enough. *Canadian Journal of Psychiatry, 53*, 213–223.

Turk, D. C., Wilson, H. D., & Cahana, A. (2011). Treatment of chronic non-cancer pain. *The Lancet, 377*, 2226–2235. doi:10.1016/S0140-6736(11)60402-9

Wong, D., & Baker, C. (1988). *The Wong-Baker FACES Pain Rating Scale*. Retrieved from http://www.wongbakerfaces.org/

Developmental Coordination Disorder

Pamela Vaughn

Description and Diagnosis

Developmental coordination disorder (DCD), according to the *Diagnostic and Statistical Manual of Mental Disorders* (4th ed., text rev.; *DSM-IV-TR*; American Psychiatric Association [APA], 2000), is "a marked impairment in the development of motor coordination" (p. 56) and has the following diagnostic criteria:

- Performance in daily activities that require motor coordination is substantially below that expected given the person's chronological age and measured intelligence.
- Disturbance significantly interferes with academic achievement or activities of daily living (ADL).
- Disturbance is not due to a general medical condition (e.g., cerebral palsy, hemiplegia, or muscular dystrophy) and does not meet criteria for pervasive developmental disorder.
- If mental retardation is present, the motor difficulties are in excess of those usually associated with it (APA, 2000).

Although DCD is the term used to refer to this condition in most publications, other names that have been or are still used include *clumsy children, developmental dyspraxia, hand–eye coordination problems*, and *motor delay/impairment* (Cermak & Larkin, 2002; Magalhaes, Missiuna, & Wong, 2006).

Incidence and Prevalence

Reports of prevalence vary, but approximately 6% of otherwise typically developing school-aged children are estimated to have DCD (APA, 2000; Missiuna et al., 2011). Although recent studies have shown that incidence is about equal between boys and girls, other studies suggest a higher prevalence in boys (Chen, Tseng, Hu, & Cermak, 2009; Missiuna et al., 2011).

Cause and Etiology

The cause of DCD is unknown, although motor difficulties have been linked to central nervous system processing deficits (O'Brien, Williams, Bundy, Lyons, & Mittal, 2008), and a few functional magnetic resonance imaging (fMRI) studies have found differences in how information is processed in children with DCD (Kashiwagi, Iwaki, Narumi, Tamai, & Suzuki, 2009; Querne et al., 2008; Zwicker, Missiuna, & Boyd, 2009; Zwicker, Missiuna, Harris, & Boyd, 2011). Genetic predisposition has been cited as a potential causal factor as well (Lichtenstein, Carlstrom, Rastam, Gillberg, & Anckarsater, 2010). Prevalence is higher in individuals who were born extremely preterm or with extremely low birth weight (Roberts et al., 2011).

Typical Course, Symptoms, and Related Conditions

DCD, although commonly considered a childhood condition because it is often diagnosed at a young age, persists into adulthood (Kirby, Sugden, Beveridge, & Edwards, 2008). The presentation of symptoms and the degree that function and participation are limited, however, vary between adult individuals depending on intervention received, personality and activity preference, coping mechanisms, and adaptations used (Sugden & Chambers, 2007). Keeping the *DSM-IV-TR* diagnostic criteria of DCD in mind, symptoms of DCD may include the following:

- Marked delays in achieving motor milestones (i.e., crawling, sitting, walking)
- Difficulties learning new motor skills
- Dropping things; "clumsiness"
- Poor performance in sports/active leisure activities
- Difficulties in school tasks, for example, poor handwriting
- Difficulties with many ADL, such as feeding and dressing (APA, 2000; Missiuna et al., 2008)

DCD is often comorbid with diagnoses such as attention deficit/hyperactivity disorder (ADHD) and reading disabilities with approximately 50% overlap (Crawford & Dewey, 2008; Missiuna et al., 2011). Research has also shown that "children with DCD are likely to experience emotional, social and behavioural difficulties," which potentially "place them at risk of both current and long-term mental health problems" (Green, Baird, & Sugden, 2006, p. 748). Social participation of children with DCD is limited in home, community, and school settings, and it is thought that poor self-worth decreases their motivation to participate in activities (Chen & Cohn, 2003).

Interdisciplinary Interventions

Medication Therapy

A double-blind, placebo-controlled study reported the stimulant methylphenidate (MPH) to significantly decrease symptoms of ADHD and

DCD and increase health-related quality of life in children with both ADHD and DCD (Flapper & Schoemaker, 2008).

Physical Therapy

Physical therapists can help during the diagnostic process to differentiate DCD from other motor difficulties. Physical therapy intervention for DCD typically addresses low tone, gross motor, and physical endurance (Missiuna, Rivard, & Bartlett, 2006).

Other Disciplines

Some people with DCD seek the services of other professionals, for example, speech and language therapists, psychologists, and neurologists, depending on their individual needs and other diagnoses.

Occupational Therapy Evaluations

Assessments of Participation and Occupational Performance

- Children's Assessment of Participation and Enjoyment (CAPE) (King et al., 2004)
- School Function Assessment (SFA) (Coster, Deeney, Haltiwanger, & Haley, 1998)
- Children Activity Scale Parent & Teacher (ChAS–P/T) (Rosenblum, 2006)
- Canadian Occupational Performance Measure (COPM) (Law et al., 2005)
- Perceived Efficacy and Goal Setting System (PEGS) (Missiuna, Pollock, & Law, 2004)
- Child Occupational Self-Assessment (COSA) (Keller, Kafkes, Basu, Federico, & Kielhofner, 2005)
- Children Helping Out: Responsibilities, Expectations, and Supports (CHORES) (Dunn, 2004)
- Do-Eat (Goffer, Josman, & Rosenblum, 2009)

Assessments of Motor Skills

- Peabody Developmental Motor Scales (PDMS) (Folio & Fewell, 2000)
- Movement Assessment Battery for Children-Second Edition (Movement ABC-2) (Henderson, Sugden, & Barnett, 2007)
- The Developmental Coordination Disorder Questionnaire (DCDQ'07) (Wilson et al., 2009)
- Bruininks-Oseretsky Test of Motor Proficiency (BOT-2) (Bruininks & Bruininks, 2006)
- Sensory Integration and Praxis Tests (Ayres, 1989)

Occupational Therapy Interventions

Occupational therapists are the discipline that most frequently works with children with DCD, particularly within the school system. Occupational therapists contribute to the diagnostic process and provide intervention to facilitate skilled motor behavior.

Task-Oriented Approaches

Direct practice or teaching of motor tasks has been shown to improve the motor skills of children with DCD (Peens, Pienaar, & Nienaber, 2008). Neuromotor task training (NTT) is an example of this approach to intervention and has been shown to have positive results on motor performance (Niemeijer, Smits-Engelsman, & Schoemaker, 2007).

Cognitive and Performance-Based Approaches

These approaches, such as cognitive orientation to daily occupational performance (CO-OP), focus on the client identifying and using cognitive strategies through guided discovery to learn and perform tasks (Polatajko & Mandich, 2004).

Impairment-Oriented Approaches

Sensory integration (SI) has been used to address the underlying impaired sensory processing and sensory motor functions that are thought to be associated with DCD (Cermak & Larkin, 2002).

Consultation

Occupational therapists often provide consultation to help clients and their caregivers determine appropriate activities—particularly leisure and play activities—that will result in increased participation, success, and satisfaction of individuals with DCD (Missiuna et al., 2006).

Occupational Therapy and the Evidence

According to Bart, Jarus, Erez, and Rosenberg (2011), children with DCD not only exhibit poor motor performance and decreased participation but "also display decreased enjoyment in participation, and their parents are less satisfied with their children's participation" (p. 1322). Although there is no "cure" for DCD, there is an opportunity for improvement in occupational performance through occupational therapy interventions such as CO-OP (Banks, Rodger, & Polatajko, 2008). CO-OP has been shown to facilitate the use of strategies for task completion in children with DCD (Rodger & Liu, 2008). It has also been reported as an effective intervention strategy for improvement in occupational performance and satisfaction for both older and younger children (Taylor, Fayed, & Mandich, 2007). Overall, there is a call for practitioners to increase their awareness of DCD so that clients can be properly diagnosed and begin to receive services as early as possible (Missiuna et al., 2008).

If a child with DCD has sensory processing and praxis problems, use of an SI approach may be helpful in promoting motor skills. A systematic review of the research has indicated that SI may result in positive outcomes in sensory motor skills and motor planning (May-Benson & Koomar, 2010).

Caregiver Concerns

Caregivers of children with DCD have reported difficulties in getting their children diagnosed due to a lack of knowledge in the health care community of signs and symptoms of DCD, which results in delayed access to services (Maciver et al., 2011). Missiuna, Moll, King, King, and Law (2007) found that parents' concerns for their children with DCD tend to change as their children grow older—from worrying that they are not reaching motor milestones at very young ages to noticing differences in the way they play, to being concerned and even frustrated with their difficulties with self-care, academics, and physical activities, and to being concerned about their self-esteem and emotional health.

Resources

Organizations

- CanChild Centre for Child Disability Research—CanChild is a research and educational center located at McMaster University in Ontario, Canada that focuses on childhood disabilities including DCD.
  Institute for Applied Health Sciences, McMaster University,
  1400 Main Street West, Room 408
  Hamilton, Ontario
  Canada L8S 1C7
  Telephone: (905) 525-9140 ext. 27850
  E-mail: canchild@mcmaster.ca
  Website: http://dcd.canchild.ca/en/

- The Dyspraxia Foundation—The Dyspraxia Foundation is a resource in the United Kingdom for individuals with DCD as well as their caregivers and health professionals.
  8 West Alley
  Hitchin
  Herts, SG5 1EG
  United Kingdom
  Telephone: +44 01462 454 986 (help line)
  E-mail: dyspraxia@dyspraxiafoundation.org.uk
  Website: http://www.dyspraxiafoundation.org.uk/index.php

Books

- Ball, M. F. (2002). *Developmental coordination disorder: Hints and tips for the activities of daily living.* London, United Kingdom: Jessica Kingsley.
- Kirby, A. (2003). *The adolescent with developmental co-ordination disorder (DCD).* London, United Kingdom: Jessica Kingsley.
- Kurtz, L. A. (2003). *How to help a clumsy child: Strategies for young children with developmental motor concerns.* London, United Kingdom: Jessica Kingsley.
- Platt, G. (2011). *Beating dyspraxia with a hop, skip, and a jump: A simple exercise program for home and school.* London, United Kingdom: Jessica Kingsley.

References

American Psychiatric Association. (2000). *Diagnostic and statistical manual of mental disorders* (4th ed., text rev.). Washington, DC: Author.

Ayres, A. J. (1989). *Sensory Integration and Praxis Tests.* Los Angeles, CA: Western Psychological Services.

Banks, R., Rodger, S., & Polatajko, H. (2008). Mastering handwriting: How children with developmental coordination disorder succeed with CO-OP. *OTJR: Occupation, Participation & Health, 28,* 100–109.

Bart, O., Jarus, T., Erez, Y., & Rosenberg, L. (2011). How do young children with DCD participate and enjoy daily activities? *Research in Developmental Disabilities, 32,* 1317–1322. doi:10.1016/j.ridd.2011.01.039

Bruininks, R. H., & Bruininks, B. D. (2006). *Bruininks-Oseretsky Test of Motor Proficiency-second edition (BOT-2).* Bloomington, MN: Pearson.

Cermak, S. A., & Larkin, D. (Eds.). (2002). *Developmental coordination disorder.* Albany, NY: Delmar.

Chen, H., & Cohn, E. S. (2003). Social participation for children with developmental coordination disorder: Conceptual, evaluation, and intervention considerations. *Physical & Occupational Therapy in Pediatrics, 23*(4), 61–78.

Chen, Y., Tseng, M., Hu, F., & Cermak, S. A. (2009). Psychosocial adjustment and attention in children with developmental coordination disorder using different motor tests. *Research in Developmental Disabilities, 30,* 1367–1377. doi:10.1016/j.ridd.2009.06.004

Coster, W., Deeney, T., Haltiwanger, J., & Haley, S. (1998). *School Function Assessment.* San Antonio, TX, Psychological Corporation.

Crawford, S. G., & Dewey, D. (2008). Co-occurring disorders: A possible key to visual perceptual deficits in children with developmental coordination disorder? *Human Movement Science, 27,* 154–169. doi:10.1016/j.humov.2007.09.002

Dunn, L. (2004). Validation of the CHORES: A measure of school-aged children's participation in household tasks. *Scandinavian Journal of Occupational Therapy, 11,* 179–190. doi:10.1080/11038120410003673

Flapper, B., & Schoemaker, M. (2008). Effects of methylphenidate on quality of life in children with both developmental coordination disorder and ADHD. *Developmental Medicine & Child Neurology, 50,* 294–299. doi:10.1111/j.1469-8749.2008.02039.x

Folio, M. R., & Fewell, R. R. (2000). *Peabody Developmental Motor Scales* (2nd ed.). Austin, TX: Pro-Ed.

Goffer, A., Josman, N., & Rosenblum, S. (2009). *Do-Eat: Performance-based assessment tool for children.* Haifa, Israel: University of Haifa.

Green, D., Baird, G., & Sugden, D. (2006). A pilot study of psychopathology in developmental coordination disorder. *Child: Care, Health & Development, 32,* 741–750. doi:10.1111/j.1365-2214.2006.00684.x

Henderson, S. E., Sugden, D. A., & Barnett, A. L. (2007). *Movement Assessment Battery for Children-second edition (Movement ABC-2).* London, United Kingdom: Psychological Corporation.

Kashiwagi, M., Iwaki, S., Narumi, Y., Tamai, H., & Suzuki, S. (2009). Parietal dysfunction in developmental coordination disorder: A functional MRI study. *NeuroReport, 20,* 1319–1324. doi:10.1097/WNR.0b013e32832f4d87

Keller, J., Kafkes, A., Basu, S., Federico, J., & Kielhofner, G. (2005). *The Child Occupational Self Assessment* (Version 2.1). Chicago, IL: MOHO Clearinghouse.

King, G., Law, M., King, S., Hurley, P., Rosenbaum, P., Hanna, S., . . . Young, N. (2004). *Children's Assessment of Participation and Enjoyment (CAPE) and Preferences for Activities of Children (PAC).* San Antonio, TX: PsychCorp.

Kirby, A., Sugden, D., Beveridge, S., & Edwards, L. (2008). Developmental co-ordination disorder (DCD) in adolescents and adults in further and higher education. *Journal of Research in Special Educational Needs, 8,* 120–131. doi:10.1111/j.1471-3802.2008.00111.x

Law, M., Baptiste, S., Carswell, A., McColl, M., Polatajko, H., & Pollock, N. (2005). *Canadian Occupational Performance Measure* (4th ed.). Ottawa, Canada: CAOT Publications.

Lichtenstein, P., Carlstrom, E., Rastam, M., Gillberg, C., & Anckarsater, H. (2010). The genetics of autism spectrum disorders and related neuropsychiatric disorders in childhood. *American Journal of Psychiatry, 167,* 1357–1363. doi:10.1176/appi.ajp.2010.10020223

Maciver, D. D., Owen, C. C., Flannery, K. K., Forsyth, K. K., Howden, S. S., Shepherd, C. C., & Rush, R. R. (2011). Services for children with developmental co-ordination disorder: The experiences of parents. *Child: Care, Health and Development, 37,* 422–429. doi:10.1111/j.1365-2214.2010.01197.x

Magalhaes, L. C., Missiuna, C., & Wong, S. (2006). Terminology used in research reports of developmental coordination disorder. *Developmental Medicine & Child Neurology, 48,* 937–941. doi:10.1017/S0012162206002040

May-Benson, T. A., & Koomar, J. A. (2010). Systematic review of the research evidence examining the effectiveness of interventions using a sensory integrative approach for children. *American Journal of Occupational Therapy, 64,* 403–414. doi:10.5014/ajot.2010.09071

Missiuna, C., Cairney, J., Pollock, N., Russell, D., Macdonald, K., Cousins, M., . . . Schmidt, L. (2011). A staged approach for identifying children with developmental coordination disorder from the population. *Research in Developmental Disabilities, 32,* 549–559. doi:10.1016/j.ridd.2010.12.025

Missiuna, C., Gaines, R., Mclean, J., DeLaat, D., Egan, M., & Soucie, H. (2008). Description of children identified by physicians as having developmental coordination disorder. *Developmental Medicine & Child Neurology, 50,* 839–844. doi:10.1111/j.1469-8749.2008.03140.x

Missiuna, C., Moll, S., King, S., King, G., & Law, M. (2007). A trajectory of troubles: Parents' impressions of the impact of developmental coordination disorder. *Physical & Occupational Therapy in Pediatrics, 27*(1), 81–101.

Missiuna, C., Pollock, N., & Law, M. (2004). *Perceived efficacy and goal setting system* (PEGS). San Antonio, TX: Psychological Corporation

Missiuna, C., Rivard, L., & Bartlett, D. (2006). Exploring assessment tools and the target of intervention for children with developmental coordination disorder. *Physical & Occupational Therapy in Pediatrics, 26,* 71–89. doi:10.1080/J006v26n01_06

Niemeijer, A., Smits-Engelsman, B., & Schoemaker, M. (2007). Neuromotor task training for children with developmental coordination disorder: A controlled trial. *Developmental Medicine & Child Neurology, 49,* 406–411.

O'Brien, J., Williams, H. G., Bundy, A., Lyons, J., & Mittal, A. (2008). Mechanisms that underlie coordination in children with developmental coordination disorder. *Journal of Motor Behavior, 40,* 43–61.

Peens, A., Pienaar, A., & Nienaber, A. (2008). The effect of different intervention programmes on the self-concept and motor proficiency of 7- to 9-year-old children with DCD. *Child: Care, Health & Development, 34,* 316–328. doi:10.1111/j.1365-2214.2007.00803.x

Polatajko, H., & Mandich, A. (2004). *Enabling occupation in children: The cognitive orientation to daily occupational performance (CO-OP) approach.* Ottawa, Canada: CAOT Publications.

Querne, L., Berquin, P., Vernier-Hauvette, M., Fall, S., Deltour, L., Meyer, M., & de Marco, G. (2008). Dysfunction of the attentional brain network in children with developmental coordination disorder: A fMRI study. *Brain Research, 1244,* 89–102. doi:10.1016/j.brainres.2008.07.066

Roberts, G., Anderson, P. J., Davis, N., De Luca, C., Cheong, J., Doyle, L. W., & the Victorian Infant Collaborative Study Group. (2011). Developmental coordination disorder in geographic cohorts of 8-year-old children born extremely preterm or extremely low birthweight in the 1990s. *Developmental Medicine & Child Neurology, 53,* 55–60. doi:10.1111/j.1469-8749.2010.03779.x

Rodger, S., & Liu, S. (2008). Cognitive orientation to (daily) occupational performance: Changes in strategy and session time use over the course of intervention. *OTJR: Occupation, Participation & Health, 28,* 168–179.

Rosenblum, S. (2006). The development and standardization of the Children Activity Scales (ChAS-P/T) for the early identification of children with developmental coordination disorder. *Child: Care, Health, and Development, 32*, 619–632.

Sugden, D. A., & Chambers, M. E. (2007). Stability and change in children with developmental coordination disorder. *Child: Care, Health & Development, 33*, 520–528. doi:10.1111/j.1365-2214.2006.00707.x

Taylor, S., Fayed, N., & Mandich, A. (2007). CO-OP intervention for young children with developmental coordination disorder. *OTJR: Occupation, Participation & Health, 27*, 124–130.

Wilson, B. N., Crawford, S. G., Green, D., Roberts, G., Aylott, A., & Kaplan, B. J. (2009). Psychometric properties of the revised Developmental Coordination Disorder Questionnaire. *Physical and Occupational Therapy in Pediatrics, 29*(2), 182–202. doi:10.1080/01942630902784761

Zwicker, J. G., Missiuna, C., & Boyd, L. A. (2009). Neural correlates of developmental coordination disorder: A review of hypotheses. *Journal of Child Neurology, 24*, 1273–1281. doi:10.1177/0883073809333537

Zwicker, J. G., Missiuna, C., Harris, S. R., & Boyd, L. A. (2011). Brain activation associated with motor skill practice in children with developmental coordination disorder: An fMRI study. *International Journal of Developmental Neuroscience, 29*, 145–152. doi:10.1016/j.ijdevneu.2010.12.002

Developmental Delay

Alaina Krumbach

Description and Diagnosis

Developmental delay is an umbrella term used to describe a child that is maturing slowly in one or more areas of development: physical, cognitive, communication, social, and emotional. Common delays can be present in fine or gross motor skills, intellectual abilities or cognitive skills, speech and language, social skills, emotional control, or self-care skills (Boyse, 2010; National Dissemination Center for Children with Disabilities [NICHCY], 2009). Individuals with developmental disabilities typically experience symptoms of delay in early childhood but can be diagnosed until the age of 22 years. Individuals with an intellectual delay are diagnosed in early childhood and are later tested for an intellectual disability. Individuals with an intellectual disability are diagnosed before the age of 18 years (American Association of Intellectual and Developmental Disabilities [AAIDD], 2011).

Incidence and Prevalence

- Developmental or behavioral disability: 17% of children in the United States are diagnosed yearly.
- Intellectual disability: The most common developmental delay; approximately 1.5 million individuals between the ages of 6 and 64 years in the United States are diagnosed (Centers for Disease Control and Prevention [CDC], 2005).

Cause and Etiology

Developmental delay can be idiopathic or have a definite cause. Some possible causes of developmental delay can include the following:

- Chromosomal or genetic disorders: Down syndrome, fragile X syndrome, Prader-Willi syndrome, Williams syndrome, and phenylketonuria (PKU)
- Prenatal development: maternal alcohol use and infections (i.e., rubella)
- Perinatal: infections, premature birth, and anoxia
- Postnatal: malnutrition, lead or mercury poisoning, infections (i.e., whooping cough, measles, and meningitis), brain injury, anoxia, and epilepsy (AAIDD, 2011; Boyse, 2010; Children, Youth, and Women's Health Service [CYMHS], 2010; NICHCY, 2009)

Typical Course, Symptoms, and Related Conditions

Individuals with developmental delay can learn and develop with added supports and early intervention from health care professionals and caregivers. Individuals with developmental or intellectual delay typically have symptoms throughout the life course. Adaptations, modifications, and learned strategies can promote the individual's cognitive, social, physical, and communication skills (CYMHS, 2010). Possible symptoms or warning signs may be seen during the appropriate developmental milestone windows in different areas of development including:

- *Behavioral*: inability to focus or pay attention to tasks, frustrated at simple tasks, exhibits aggressive or violent behaviors, avoids making eye contact with others
- *Gross motor*: atypical muscle tone (hypertonia or hypotonia), experiences trouble maintaining proper posture, may be more clumsy than other children
- *Vision*: difficulty tracking, frequently rubs eyes, adjusts or strains head and neck to look at an object, eyes may be crossed or turned, difficulty finding or picking up small objects
- *Hearing*: atypical volume when talking, turns body toward sound to hear, difficulty following directions, may not startle at loud noise, may not develop sounds or words (Leslie et al., 2008)

Conditions related to developmental delay can include Down syndrome, fetal alcohol syndrome, autism, pervasive developmental disorder, cerebral palsy, and epilepsy (AAIDD, 2011; CYMHS, 2010). Other terms that are closely related to developmental delay include the following:

- *Global developmental delay*: used to describe limitations in all areas of development
- *Intellectual delay*: used for children, usually under the age of 5 years, to describe limitations in intellectual functioning and cognitive skills (reasoning, learning, problem solving) if it is uncertain that the delay is permanent
- *Intellectual disability*: term used for individuals with an intellectual delay that affects cognitive, social, and practical skills across the life course; IQ test results of 75 or less can indicate an intellectual disability classified as mild, moderate, severe, or profound (AAIDD, 2011)

Interdisciplinary Interventions

Special Education

Through special education, an individualized education plan (IEP) is developed to promote specific educational programming and resources for each student. Each IEP is designed specifically for the individual and includes detailed information about the student's needs and academic requirements (Boyse, 2010; NICHCY, 2009).

Audiology or Hearing Services

Interventions for children with developmental delay can include testing for hearing loss or hearing impairments. Audiologists may suggest a cochlear implant or introduce alternative forms of nonverbal communication (NICHCY, 2009).

Speech and Language Services

Interventions focus on improving verbal and introducing nonverbal communication. Nonverbal communication may include sign language, Mayer-Johnson symbols, or communication boards. Also, interventions may focus on muscular strength to help with dysphagia, a condition that results in difficulty with or inability to swallow (NICHCY, 2009).

Medical Services

Medical services include testing for chromosomal abnormalities, monitoring health, and prescribing antibiotics for infections in early childhood (NICHCY, 2009).

Nutrition Services

Intervention focuses on maternal and individual nutrition to help monitor symptoms. Specifically for individuals with PKU, a diet that is low in phenylalanine is prescribed during pregnancy and throughout the individual's life course to promote physical and mental health (NICHCY, 2009; Van Voorhees, 2009).

Physical Therapy

Physical therapists may work with individuals to improve gross motor skills including gait, range of motion, and strength (NICHCY, 2009).

Psychological Services

Counseling and training can be provided to the individual and family to educate caregivers and regulate emotional stress, aggressive behavior, and depressive symptoms (NICHCY, 2009).

Occupational Therapy Evaluations

Functional Screenings and Assessments

- Pediatric Evaluation of Disability Inventory (PEDI): assesses functional skills
- Functional Independence Measure for Children (WeeFIM)
- Screening Test for Evaluating Preschoolers (FirstSTEp): identifies risk for delays
- Hawaii Early Learning Profile (HELP): developmental skills and behaviors
- Bayley Scale of Infant Development-III (BSID-III): developmental functioning
- Miller Assessment for Preschoolers (MAP): assesses sensory, motor, and cognitive skills
- School Function Assessment (SFA): performance of student's tasks and activities

Motor Coordination

- Bruininks-Oseretsky Test of Motor Proficiency (BOT-2): gross and fine motor function
- Test of Infant Motor Performance (TIMP): posture and control functions
- Peabody Developmental Motor Scales-2 (PDMS): motor development
- Beery Test of Visual Motor Integration (Beery VMI): integration of vision and motor

Sensory and Sensory Motor Processing

- Sensory Integration and Praxis Test (SIPT): praxis, sensory processing, and integration
- Sensory Processing Measure (SPM): sensory processing abilities in the home or school
- Sensory Profile: the ability to process sensory information and the effects on function

Social Participation and Functioning

- Children's Assessment of Participation and Enjoyment (CAPE) and Performance for Activities of Children (PAC): participation and preferences in nonschool activities
- Canadian Occupational Performance Measure (COPM): activity and performance

Adolescent and Adult Activities of Daily Living and Instrumental Activities of Daily Living

- Functional Independence Measure (FIM): impact of disability of functional status
- Transition Planning Inventory (TPI): identifies comprehensive transitional needs
- Assessment of Motor and Process Skills (AMPS): personal and instrumental activities of daily living (ADL)
- Kohlman Evaluation of Living Skills (KELS): evaluates ability to live in the community
- Test of Grocery Shopping Skills (TOG-SS): ability to complete grocery shopping

Occupational Therapy Interventions

Early Intervention

Based on an individual family service plan (IFSP), therapy is provided for the family when the child is 3 years or younger in their natural environment. Interventions focus on the relationship of the infant and caregivers through play, identify strategies to implement during daily routines, suggest modifications for everyday activities, and introduce use of adaptive equipment (Frolek Clark, Jackson, & Polichino, 2011).

Specific Skills Training

Fine and gross motor interventions continue as the child matures and transitions from an IFSP onto an IEP. Interventions focus on increasing awareness and exploration of the environment; improving functional activities such as self-care, handwriting, and toileting; and education about safe and effective positioning (Frolek Clark et al., 2011).

Assistive Technology

Occupational therapists can work with the individual and family to determine special adaptive equipment and assistive technology to help with ADL (Boyse, 2010). Special considerations should be made for each individual and his or her caregiver to ensure that the equipment is the least restrictive device. Factors to consider include social implications of using equipment, the individual's ability to use and troubleshoot technological equipment, and the long-term influence on the individual's participation in the community (Hammel, 2003).

Sensory Integration

Sensory integration may help individuals with developmental delay who also have sensory modulation difficulties to help regulate emotions related to sensory stimuli in their environment (Roberts, King-Thomas, & Boccia, 2007; Shaaf & Miller, 2005).

Transition Planning

Transition planning begins when the individual is 14 years old and focuses on leaving the school environment and IEP for the community. The goal in transition planning is for the individual to be as independent as possible in the community (Kardos & White, 2006).

Supported Employment

Focusing on specific task training in a professional environment may increase individual self-efficacy, promote autonomy, and enhance productivity and participation within the community (Siporin & Lysack, 2004).

Occupational Therapy and the Evidence

Occupational therapists are part of an interdisciplinary team that includes caregivers, teachers, physical therapists, speech-language pathologists, nutritionists, and medical professionals (Frolek Clark et al., 2011). Occupational therapists may be included in the individual's IFSP for early intervention services because research has shown that early intervention therapy before the age of 3 years has the most significant improvement on an individual's development. Appropriately, recognizing a developmental delay early and identifying services has been shown to effectively enhance the lives of the individual and family throughout the life course (Edwards & Sarwark, 2005). As individuals age, it is important to include them in goal setting and intervention planning on their IEP because they can best express their needs and desires (Frolek Clark et al., 2011). Once individuals terminate the academic setting and IEP services, it is important to integrate them into the community through supportive employment opportunities to enhance their self-efficacy (Siporin & Lysack, 2004).

Interventions to increase fine and gross motor development early in an individual's life have shown to have lasting positive effects on physical, social, academic, and psychological skills (Riethmuller, Jones, & Okely, 2009). Using power mobility devices during early intervention therapy shows an increase later in life with skill transfer to powered wheelchairs (Deitz, Swinth, & White, 2002). Interventions to increase self-modulation and awareness of emotional regulation have significant positive effects on the individual's social and academic performances. Sensory integration may help individuals to regulate emotions and focus on tasks in the classroom and interactions with peers (Roberts et al., 2007; Schaaf & Miller, 2005). In combination with sensory integration techniques, sound therapy has positive effects on individual's emotional regulation (Hall & Case-Smith, 2007).

Caregiver Concerns

Often, being a caregiver to an individual with a developmental or intellectual delay is a lifelong role, and special considerations include seeking education for effective interventions and therapy, support from other families with developmental delay, and education on advocating for individuals and families with developmental delay (Hanson, 2003; O'Sullivan, 2007).

Resources

Organizations

- American Association of Intellectual and Developmental Disabilities
  501 3rd Street, NW Suite 200
  Washington, DC 20001
  Telephone: 1-202-387-1968
  Website: http://www.aaidd.org
  A national resource for publications and supports for individuals, caregivers, and researchers.

- National Down Syndrome Society
  666 Broadway
  New York, NY 10012
  Telephone: 1-800-221-4602
  Website: http://www.ndss.org
  A research and education on intellectual disabilities for individuals, caregivers, and professionals.

Books

- Fivozinsky LeComer, L. (2006). *A parent's guide to developmental delays: Recognizing and coping with missed milestones in speech, movement, learning, and other areas.* New York, NY: Penguin Group.
  A resource to help parents and educators spot "red flags" in development and learn to navigate treatment and education of a child with a developmental delay to lead a fulfilling life.

- Graf Groneberg, J. (2008). *Road map to Holland: How I found my way through my son's first two years with Down syndrome.* New York, NY: New American Library.
  A book written from a mother's perspective of raising a child with Down syndrome.

Journals

- *Journal of Intellectual Disability Research*
- *Research in Developmental Disabilities*

Websites

- How Kids Develop
  Website: http://www.howkidsdevelop.com/index.html
  A Website that offers parents an easy-to-read guide about developmental milestones and possible steps to take if a child seems to have a delay in achieving one or more developmental milestones.

- Parent to Parent USA (P2P USA)
  Website: http://www.p2pusa.org
  An online resource for parents of children with a developmental delay, to seek emotional and informational support.

References

American Association of Intellectual and Developmental Disabilities. (2011). *FAQs on intellectual disability.* Retrieved from http://www.aaidd.org

Boyse, K. (2010). *Developmental delay.* Retrieved from http://www.med.umich.edu/yourchild/topics/devdel.htm

Centers for Disease Control and Prevention. (2005). *Child development.* Retrieved from http://ghr.nlm.nih.gov/condition/down-syndrome

Children, Youth, and Women's Health Service. (2010). *Developmental delay.* Retrieved from http://www.cyh.com/HealthTopics/HealthTopicDetails.aspx?p=114&np=122&id=1633

Deitz, J., Swinth, Y., & White, O. (2002). Powered mobility and preschoolers with complex developmental delays. *American Journal of Occupational Therapy, 56,* 86–96.

Edwards, S. L., & Sarwark, J. F. (2005). Infant and child motor development. *Clinical Orthopaedics and Related Research, 434,* 33–39.

Frolek Clark, G., Jackson, L., & Polichino, J. (2011). Occupational therapy services in early childhood and school-based settings. *American Journal of Occupational Therapy, 65*(6, Suppl.), S46–S54. Retrieved from http://www.aota.org/Practitioners/PracticeAreas/Pediatrics.aspx

Hall, L., & Case-Smith, J. (2007). The effect of sound-based intervention on children with sensory processing disorders and visual-motor delays. *American Journal of Occupational Therapy, 61,* 209–215.

Hammel, J. (2003). Technology and the environment: Supportive resource or barrier for people with developmental disabilities? *The Nursing Clinics of North America, 38,* 331–349.

Hanson, M. J. (2003). Twenty-five years after early intervention: A follow up of children with Down syndrome, other developmental disabilities, and typically developing children. *American Journal of Occupational Therapy, 59,* 621–628.

Kardos, M. R., & White, B. P. (2006). Evaluation options for secondary transition planning. *American Journal of Occupational Therapy, 60,* 333–339.

Leslie, L., Bargallo, A., Gordon, J., Hayden-Wade, H., McDaniel, A., Hui Lui, Y., . . . Gist, K. (2008). *What is developmental delay and what services are available if I think my child might be delayed?* Retrieved from http://www.howkidsdevelop.com/index.html

National Dissemination Center for Children with Disabilities. (2009). *Developmental delay.* Retrieved from http://www.nichcy.org/Disabilities/Specific/Pages/DD.aspx

O'Sullivan, A. (2007). AOTA's statement on family caregivers. *American Journal of Occupational Therapy, 61,* 710. doi:10.5014/ajot.61.6.710

Riethmuller, A. M., Jones, R. A., & Okely, A. D. (2009). Efficacy of interventions to improve motor development in young children: A systematic review. *Pediatrics, 124,* 782–792. doi:10.1543/peds.2009-0333

Roberts, J. E., King-Thomas, L., & Boccia, M. L. (2007). Behavioral indexes of the efficacy of sensory integration therapy. *American Journal of Occupational Therapy, 61,* 555–562.

Schaaf, R. C., & Miller, L. J. (2005). Occupational therapy using a sensory integrative approach for children with developmental disabilities. *Mental Retardation and Developmental Disabilities Research Reviews, 11,* 143–148. doi:10.1002/mrdd.20067

Siporin, S., & Lysack, C. (2004). Quality of life and supported employment: A case study of three women with developmental disabilities. *American Journal of Occupational Therapy, 58,* 455–465. doi:10.5014/ajot.58.4.455

Van Voorhees, B. W. (2009). *Phenylketonuria.* Retrieved from http://www.ncbi.nlm.nih.gov/pubmedhealth/PMH0002150/

Eating Disorders

Theresa Griffin

Description

Severe changes in eating behavior and excessive concern about body shape or weight characterize eating disorders (Franco, 2011). As many as 24 million Americans and 70 million individuals worldwide have an eating disorder (The Renfrew Center Foundation, 2003). Women between the ages of 12 and 25 years make up 90% of Americans with eating disorders (Substance Abuse and Mental Health Services Administration [SAMHSA], 2010). According to a 10-year study, 86% of individuals with eating disorders reported onset by the age of 20 years, 10% at 10 years or younger, 33% between ages 11 and 15 years, and 43% between ages 16 and 20 years (National Association of Anorexia Nervosa and Associated Disorders [ANAD], 2011b). Additionally, 77% of those individuals reported a duration of 1 to 15 years (ANAD, 2011b). Eating disorders have the highest mortality rate of any mental illness (Sullivan, 1995). An estimated 480,000 individuals die each year due to eating disorders complications (The Renfrew Center Foundation, 2003).

Classifications

According to the American Psychiatric Association's (APA; 2000) *Diagnostic and Statistical Manual of Mental Health Disorders* (4th ed., text rev.; *DSM-IV-TR*), eating disorders can be classified into three categories: anorexia nervosa, bulimia nervosa, and eating disorders not otherwise specified (EDNOS).

Anorexia nervosa is characterized by severe dieting and/or purging, resulting in weight loss at least 15% below normal body weight (ANAD, 2011a). The disorder has two subtypes: a restrictive type and a binge eating or purging type. With the restrictive type, an individual will restrict food intake and possibly exercise excessively to maintain an unhealthy weight. With the binge eating or purging type, an individual simultaneously restricts food intake and engages in binge eating or purging behavior like self-induced vomiting or misuse of laxatives and diuretics (Franco, 2011). The average onset occurs between the ages of 17 and 19 years. Anorexia nervosa is the third most common chronic illness among adolescents (ANAD, 2011a). It has a higher mortality rate than any other cause of death among females aged 15 to 24 years (ANAD, 2011b).

Bulimia nervosa is characterized by recurrent binging and purging. Its two subtypes include a purging and nonpurging type. The purging type involves self-induced vomiting or misuse of laxatives, diuretics, or enemas to purge the body of calories consumed. The nonpurging type involves inappropriate compensatory behaviors like fasting and excessive exercise to prevent weight gain (Franco, 2011). As many as 7% of U.S. females have had bulimia nervosa at some point in their lives. At any given time, an estimated 5% of the U.S. population has undiagnosed bulimia nervosa (National Eating Disorders Association [NEDA], 2008).

The category EDNOS, the most common eating disorder diagnosis in clinical practice, encompasses all other eating disorders that exhibit symptoms of the other two categories but do not strictly fall into either category. This includes binge eating disorders. Current estimates suggest that binge eating disorders affect up to 4% of the U.S. population (NEDA, 2008).

Etiology

Although no defined cause has been established, it is believed that genetics can increase the risk of developing an eating disorder by 50% to 80% (The Alliance for Eating Disorder Awareness [The Alliance], 2011). Social factors, such as media; psychological factors, such as depression; and interpersonal factors, such as a history of abuse or traumatic life events, may all contribute to the development of an eating disorder (The Alliance, 2011).

Symptoms

Symptoms for anorexia nervosa include the following:

- Avoidance of food, eating foods in small amounts, weighing food, or counting calories
- Absent or irregular menstrual periods
- Hair loss
- Fatigue and fainting

Symptoms for bulimia nervosa include the following:

- Repeated episodes of binging and purging
- Broken blood vessels in the eyes
- Abuse of laxatives, diuretics, or diet pills
- Frequent dieting

Symptoms for EDNOS include the following:

- Periods of uncontrolled, impulsive, or continuous eating beyond the point of fullness
- Sporadic fasts or repetitive diets
- Anxiety, depression and loneliness, as well as feelings of shame after binge eating (ANAD, 2011a; NEDA, 2004; SAMHSA, 2010)

Course and Prognosis

The presentation of eating disorders varies substantially in every individual. Although the *DSM-IV-TR* allows for specific diagnosis of eating disorders, many individuals will demonstrate a mixture of symptoms from all of the categories. For instance, about 50% of individuals diagnosed with anorexia nervosa will develop bulimic symptoms, and about 40% of individuals diagnosed with bulimia nervosa will develop anorexic symptoms (PsychCentral, 2010). Without medical treatment, up to 20% of individuals with eating disorders die. With treatment, about 60% make full recoveries and 20% will make partial recoveries (Healthy Place, 2008).

Risk Factors

Factors increasing the risk of developing an eating disorder include the following:

- Gender: Being female increases one's risk.
- Age: Individuals in their teens and late 20s are at greater risk.
- Family history: Having a parent or a sibling with an eating disorder increases one's risk.
- Family influence: Individuals are more susceptible to developing an eating disorder if their parents or siblings are overly critical or if they get teased about their appearance.
- Emotional disorders: Individuals with depression, anxiety disorders, or obsessive-compulsive disorder are more likely to develop an eating disorder (Mayo Clinic, 2010).

Complications

Complications of eating disorders may include any of the following: stunted growth, heart disease, depression, suicidal thoughts or behaviors, bone loss, seizures, severe tooth decay, and kidney damage (Mayo Clinic, 2010; NEDA, 2005; The Renfrew Center Foundation, 2003).

Interdisciplinary Interventions

Treatment for eating disorders depends on the specific type that an individual has. Professionals from various disciplines may collaborate to address the medical, dental, and nutritional components of this disorder. Treatment typically includes psychotherapy, nutrition education, and medication (Mayo Clinic, 2010). Additionally, because depression, substance abuse, and anxiety disorders often co-occur with eating disorders, it is also important to seek medical treatment for these conditions if necessary (Healthy Place, 2008).

Psychotherapy

The emphasis of individual therapy is on replacing unhealthy thoughts, behaviors, and habits with healthy ones. One specific type of psychotherapy called *cognitive behavioral therapy* is often used because it addresses the disorder's behavioral components, as well as the irrational beliefs and illogical thought patterns related to body image, weight, and food (ANAD, 2011c).

Nutrition Education

Health care providers will help individuals establish an eating plan to achieve and maintain a healthy weight (ANAD, 2011c; SAMHSA, 2010). Emphasis is placed on a healthy diet and the development of normal eating habits.

Medication

Medications will not cure eating disorders, but they can help control binging and purging behaviors or manage preoccupation with weight loss. Additionally, antidepressants and antianxiety medications can help with any symptoms of depression or anxiety (Mayo Clinic, 2010).

Occupational Therapy Evaluations

Occupational Performance and Participation Level

- Canadian Occupational Performance Measure (COPM): self-report of performance and satisfaction with occupations
- Model of Human Occupational Screening Tool (MOHOST): overview of occupational functioning
- Occupational Self Assessment (OSA): self-report establishing priorities for change

Client Factors Level

- Depression, Anxiety, Stress Scale (DASS-42): self-report that measures the extent to which an individual has experienced these negative emotional states over the last week
- Domestic and Community Skills Assessment (DACSA): assesses an individual's performance on essential tasks for living in the community
- Eating Disorder Inventory: a self-report scale measuring symptoms of disordered eating

Occupational Therapy Intervention

Occupational Performance

- Menu planning and meal preparation
- Development of independent living skills and lifestyle redesign
- Learning and developing leisure interests
- Learning money and time management skills (Chipman, 2009)

Sensory

- Challenging distorted beliefs with accurate, multisensory information including touching, smelling, laughing, seeing, talking, and hearing (Chipman, 2009)
- Teaching sensory preferences (Chipman, 2009)

Psychosocial

- Body image improvement
- Stress management
- Reflective writing (Haerti, 2007)

Education and Advocacy

- Relapse prevention
- Communication and assertion training

Caregiver Concerns

Treasure et al. (2008) found that caregivers and family members are often confused by the meaning of an eating disorder because they may share the traits of anxiety, compulsivity, and abnormal eating behaviors that contribute to their loved one's eating disorder. Additionally, family members may become critical, hostile, or overprotective, and they may feel guilt and shame because of their loved one's eating disorder. Treasure et al. (2008) suggested that these reactions may cause family members to accommodate or enable symptoms of the disorder in their loved ones. Therefore, caregivers and family members may benefit from strategies to help them to cope with and assist with a family member's eating disorder. Johansson and Johansson (2009) highlighted the importance of offering support to caregivers by providing adequate information to them, and they found that strategies such as dinner arrangements and shared responsibility of food preparation helped caregivers handle the situation better. Balance among work, leisure, and rest is emphasized for both the caregiver and the individual with an eating disorder.

Occupational Therapy and the Evidence

Occupational therapy (OT) has a role in helping individuals cope with and recover from an eating disorder. Eating disorders can interfere with prior roles and occupations, as the new primary occupation becomes the unhealthy eating disorder and the rituals or behaviors needed to sustain it (Chipman, 2009). As further illustration, Singlehurst, Corr, Griffiths, and Beaulieu (2007) studied time use patterns of individuals with binge eating disorder in order to examine the disorder's impact on daily occupations. The results indicated that the time use patterns of individuals with binge eating disorder were similar to those of individuals without the disorder, with the exception of eating and socializing. The findings suggest that the disorder has an impact on self-care, leisure, and productivity occupations, all of which are areas wherein occupational therapists can address in therapy. It is important for occupational therapists to keep this in mind when trying to understand the meaning and purpose of occupational engagement of an individual with an eating disorder (Singlehurst et al., 2007).

Additionally, an occupational therapist can address low self-esteem, anxiety, and altered body image that may accompany an eating disorder. By looking specifically at OT's role in working with individuals with altered body images, Shearsmith-Farthing (2001) found that OT's perspective on activity, which indicates that activity can act as a facilitator of change in occupational performance, can adequately address concerns related to altered body image. However, it is recognized that education and training for occupational therapists are essential if OT is to expand to this area of practice.

Orchard (2003) discusses how conflicts can impinge a therapeutic relationship when a therapist and a client with an eating disorder have differing viewpoints. These differences can limit the client's engagement in the change process. It is suggested that motivational interviewing will enable the therapist and the client to work together towards reaching therapeutic goals (Orchard, 2003). Ultimately, occupational therapists can help a client with an eating disorder to explore new interests and to develop new behaviors while setting practical, healthy goals (Chipman, 2009).

Resources

Associations

- National Association of Anorexia Nervosa and Associated Disorders
  PO Box 7 Highland Park, IL 60035
  1-847-831-3438
  http://www.anad.org/
  A nonprofit organization dedicated to the prevention and alleviation of eating disorders.

- National Eating Disorders Association
  603 Stewart Street, Suite 803 Seattle, WA 98101
  1-800-931-2237
  http://www.nationaleatingdisorders.org
  An organization that promotes prevention and awareness of eating disorders.

Books

- Costin, C. (2007). *100 questions and answers about ED*. Sudbury, MA: Jones and Bartlett.
  A straightforward reference guide by a writer and therapist with more than 20 years of experience in treating eating disorders.

- de Rossi, P. (2010). *Unbearable lightness*. New York, NY: Atria.
  The memoir of an actress who writes candidly about having anorexia.

Journals

- *American Journal of Psychiatry*
- *Eating Disorders: The Journal of Treatment and Prevention*
- *International Journal of Eating Disorders*

Websites

- The Renfrew Center Foundation
  http://www.renfrew.org
  A nonprofit organization also connected to treatment facilities, which works on professional and consumer education, prevention, research, and access to treatment.

- The Elisa Project: Overcoming Eating Disorders Through Knowledge
  http://www.theelisaproject.org/
  An organization dedicated to the prevention and effective treatment of eating disorders through support, awareness, education, and advocacy.

References

The Alliance for Eating Disorder Awareness. (2011). *What causes eating disorders?* Retrieved from http://www.allianceforeatingdisorders.com/what-causes-eating-disorders

American Psychiatric Association. (2000). *Diagnostic and statistical manual of mental disorders* (4th ed., text rev.). Washington, DC: Author.

Chipman, J. (2009). *Occupational therapy for patients with eating disorders.* Retrieved from http://eatingdisorder.org/blog/2009/09/occupational-therapy-for-patients-with-eating-disorders/

Franco, K. (2011). *Eating disorders.* Retrieved from http://www.clevelandclinicmeded.com/medicalpubs/diseasemanagement/psychiatry-psychology/eating-disorders/#b0020

Haerti, K. (2007). Journaling as an assessment tool in mental health. In B. J. Hemphill-Pearson (Ed.), *Assessments in occupational therapy mental health: An integrative approach* (61–80). Thorofare, NJ: Slack.

Healthy Place. (2008). *For parents: Eating disorders are a serious mental health issue.* Retrieved from http://www.healthyplace.com/eating-disorders/main/for-parents-eating-disorders-are-a-serious-mental-health-issue/menu-id-58/

Johansson, A., & Johansson, U. (2009). Relatives' experiences of family members' eating difficulties. *Scandinavian Journal of Occupational Therapy, 16*(1), 25–32.

Mayo Clinic. (2010). *Eating disorders.* Retrieved from http://www.mayoclinic.com/print/eating-disorders/DS00294/DSECTION=all&METHOD=print

National Association of Anorexia Nervosa and Associated Disorders. (2011a). *Anorexia nervosa.* Retrieved from http://www.anad.org/get-information/about-eating-disorders/anorexia-nervosa/

National Association of Anorexia Nervosa and Associated Disorders. (2011b). *Eating disorders statistics.* Retrieved from http://www.anad.org/get-information/about-eating-disorders/eating-disorders-statistics/

National Association of Anorexia Nervosa and Associated Disorders. (2011c). *Therapeutic treatments.* Retrieved from http://www.anad.org/get-information/information-about-treatment/

National Eating Disorders Association. (2004). *What causes eating disorders?* Retrieved from http://www.nationaleatingdisorders.org/nedaDir/files/documents/handouts/WhatCaus.pdf

National Eating Disorders Association. (2005). *Health consequences of eating disorders.* Retrieved from http://www.nationaleatingdisorders.org/nedaDir/files/documents/handouts/HlthCons.pdf

National Eating Disorders Association. (2008). *Eating disorder information index.* Retrieved from http://www.nationaleatingdisorders.org/information-resources/index.php

Orchard, R. (2003). With you, not against you: Applying motivational interviewing to occupational therapy in anorexia nervosa. *British Journal of Occupational Therapy, 66*(7), 325–327.

PsychCentral. (2010). *Bulimia nervosa: Symptoms.* Retrieved from http://psychcentral.com/disorders/sx3.htm

The Renfrew Center Foundation. (2003). *Eating disorders 101 guide: A summary of issues, statistics and resources.* Retrieved from http://www.renfew.org

Shearsmith-Farthing, K. (2001). The management of altered body image: A role for occupational therapy. *British Journal of Occupational Therapy, 64*(8), 387–392.

Singlehurst, H., Corr, S., Griffiths, S., & Beaulieu, K. (2007). The impact of binge eating disorder on occupation: A pilot study. *British Journal of Occupational Therapy, 70*(11), 493–501.

Substance Abuse and Mental Health Services Administration. (2010). *Handout: Eating disorders.* Retrieved from http://www.ncsacw.samhsa.gov/files/TrainingPackage/MOD3/EatingDisorders.pdf

Sullivan, P. (1995). Mortality in anorexia nervosa. *American Journal of Psychiatry, 152,* 1073–1074.

Treasure, J., Sepulveda, A. R., MacDonald, P., Whitaker, W., Lopez, C., Zabala, M., . . . Todd, G. (2008). The assessment of the family of people with eating disorders. *European Eating Disorders Review, 16,* 247–255. doi:10.1002/erv.859

Hand and Wrist Conditions

Alissa Bonjuklian

Description

The American Occupational Therapy Association (AOTA) considers hand therapy a specialty practice area "concerned with treating orthopedic-based upper-extremity conditions to optimize the functional use of the hand and arm" (Amini, 2011b). Diagnostic conditions regularly treated by occupational therapists specializing in this area affect the integrity of all types of tissue present in the upper extremity. Fractures, particularly of the wrist, are commonly treated in the hand clinic. Nerve-related conditions include nerve entrapments, such as in carpal tunnel syndrome, and nerve lacerations and repair. Tendon- and ligament-related conditions include tendonitis, trigger finger, lateral and medial epicondylitis, De Quervain syndrome, and sprains. Care of postsurgical wounds as well as burns and accompanying complications represent common skin-related conditions treated by occupational therapists. Other soft tissue conditions, such as Dupuytren's disease, infections, and tumors, may present problems that require the expertise of an occupational therapist specializing in the treatment of the upper extremity (Cooper, 2007).

Prevalence

Epidemiological prevalence data related to general hand and wrist conditions typically pertains to the worker population. Hand injuries are consistently ranked as the second most common workplace injury; each year, 1,080,000 emergency room visits are generated by workers with hand injuries (Centers for Disease Control and Prevention, 2001). Injuries to the upper extremity account for over 23% of all workplace injuries, and carpal tunnel syndrome, in particular, accounts for an average of 28 days of lost work (U.S. Bureau of Labor Statistics, 2008). The prevalence rates of other hand or wrist conditions are as follows:

- Over one million adults, 50 years and older, were treated for fall-related forearm and/or wrist fractures in U.S. hospital emergency departments between 2001 and 2007 (Orces & Martinez, 2010). It has been estimated that fractures of the humerus, forearm, and wrist account for 27% of all fractures among older adults (Stevens, Corso, Finkelstein, & Miller, 2006).
- Dupuytren's disease is present in 2% to 42% of the international population. The wide range is due to its gross prevalence in Northern European countries and near absence in other regions (Kakar, Giuffre, Skeete, & Elhassan, 2010).
- Trigger finger, a common tendon disorder, is prevalent in roughly 2% of the general population (McAuliffe, 2010).
- Carpal tunnel syndrome, a common nerve disorder, is estimated to be present in 4 to 10 million American adults (Lawrence et al., 2008).
- Mild, moderate, or severe hand osteoarthritis is present in approximately 27% of American adults older than age 26 years. This number reaches 80% among older adults, although only a minority experience pain as a result (Lawrence et al., 2008).

Etiology and Risk Factors

Due to the diverse nature of hand and wrist conditions, the range of causes and risk factors is quite broad. These conditions may be caused by blatant trauma or more subtle origins. Hand and wrist conditions are sometimes idiopathic; clients may report symptoms beginning spontaneously, following mild local trauma or a minor change in routine, such as performing unaccustomed manual activity (McAuliffe, 2010). Other possible causes of and risk factors for hand and wrist conditions include the following:

- *Trauma*: Acute traumatic incidents such as falls or job-related accidents can directly result in crush injuries, nerve lacerations, or fractures or breaks in the bones of the upper extremity. Falling is indeed cited as the "strongest single risk factor for fractures in older adults" (Thompson, Evitt, & Whaley, 2010, p. 213). Experience of a past traumatic injury may serve as a risk factor for repeat or recurring incidents in two ways: the integrity of the local tissue may be jeopardized, rendering it more vulnerable to future damage, or, particularly in the case of fall-related fractures, the initial fall may serve as the "sentinel event" that precedes a "cascade of reduced mobility," which could lead to future falls and further injury (Thompson et al., 2010, p. 213).
- *Job-related factors*: Various aspects of occupational activity have been widely cited as both causes of and risk factors for upper extremity impairments in workers. Work factors, which have been linked with increased risk of upper extremity problems, include experience of physical strain during job performance (Aluoch & Wao, 2009), high perceived job-related stress, and monotonous or repetitive forceful work (Bongers, Kremer, & ter Laak, 2002).
- *Personal factors*: *Age* is a personal risk factor that may put an individual at greater risk for acquiring a particular hand or wrist condition. Older age has been associated with an increased risk of fall-related fractures (Thompson et al., 2010) and osteoarthritis (Lawrence et al., 2008), whereas middle age is considered a risk factor for tendon-related conditions such as carpal tunnel syndrome and tendonitis (Kakar et al., 2010; McAuliffe, 2010). *Preexisting conditions* may predispose individuals to other disorders; diabetes mellitus is considered a risk factor for both Dupuytren's disease (Kakar et al., 2010) and tendon disorders (McAuliffe, 2010), and low bone mineral density, such as in osteopenia or osteoporosis, is considered a risk factor for fractures (Thompson et al., 2010). An individual's *gender* may also alter his or her risk of developing an upper extremity condition: males were nine times more likely to exhibit signs and symptoms necessitating surgical intervention of Dupuytren's disease (Kakar et al., 2010), whereas females accounted for 80% of adults treated for fall-related forearm and/or wrist fractures from 2001 to 2007 (Orces & Martinez, 2010).
- *Lifestyle factors*: Certain lifestyle choices may alter the likelihood of developing hand or wrist conditions. Smoking and heavy alcohol consumption increase the likelihood of developing Dupuytren's disease (Kakar et al., 2010), and low dietary calcium intake is a risk factor for upper extremity fracture (Thompson et al., 2010).

Symptoms

Although clinical presentation of symptoms will vary by client and by specific diagnosis, common symptoms across many hand and wrist conditions include pain, swelling, tingling, numbness, weakness, and stiffness (Cooper, 2007). In addition to physical symptoms, disruption in the client's ability to manage daily occupations is a major complaint secondary to hand or wrist conditions.

Precautions

- *Skin integrity*—If a client's condition indicates provision of a splint or cast, it is important to regularly check the underlying skin for redness, irritation, or any irregularity.
- *Pain*—Pain experienced during therapy is a sign that injury is occurring. Irreversible damage can result when clients, caregivers, or therapists injure tissue by applying painful force during activities such as stretching (Cooper, 2007).
- *Modalities*—All physical agent modalities should be used with caution. For one example, cryotherapy should not be used for clients with nerve injury or repair, sensory impairment, peripheral vascular disease, Raynaud's phenomenon, lupus, leukemia, multiple myeloma, neuropathy, or cold intolerance (Cooper, 2007).

Interdisciplinary Interventions

Rehabilitation

Rehabilitation may be recommended for to maximize the client's level of functioning in the period of time following a surgery. Rehabilitation is provided by an occupational or physical therapist who specializes in the treatment of the upper extremity. The therapist may be a certified hand therapist (CHT). Responsibilities of therapists practicing in this specialty area include the following:

- Evaluation of relevant client factors, occupations, and environments
- Making recommendations about the client's prognosis and plan of care
- Preparing and implementing an evidence-based therapeutic intervention plan that is individually tailored for each client

Surgery

A hand or orthopedic surgeon may be consulted if a conservative approach to treatment is not effective. Common operative procedures include arthrodesis, arthroplasty, bone grafts, synovectomy, tenosynovectomy, tendon release, and tendon repair. The selection of the procedure is a function of the diagnosis's treatment protocol as well as client factors such as age and personal preference (Amadio, 2007).

Medications

Medications, administered orally or via injection or iontophoresis, may be prescribed to help alleviate problematic symptoms or to assist in the treatment of certain conditions. Commonly prescribed medications include the following:

- Pain relievers
- Anti-inflammatory agents, that is, nonsteroidal anti-inflammatory drugs (NSAIDs) or corticosteroids
- Disease-modifying antirheumatic drugs (DMARDs)
- Botulinum toxin A (Amadio, 2007)

Occupational Therapy Evaluations

Occupation-Based and Quality of Life

- Canadian Occupational Performance Measure (COPM): semistructured interview that elicits the client's self-assessment of performance and satisfaction in various areas of occupation over time
- Disabilities of the Arm, Shoulder, and Hand (DASH): a standardized questionnaire that rates disability and symptoms related to upper extremity musculoskeletal disorders
- Modified Hand Injury Severity Scale (MHISS): standardized scale to describe the pattern and severity of hand injury and to predict the amount of time needed to return to work
- Short Form-36 (SF-36): standardized scale that measures health related to quality of life

Biomechanical

- Range of motion, that is, goniometry
- Strength, grip, and pinch
- Sensory testing
- Edema
- Skin integrity
- Coordination testing

Occupational Therapy Intervention

Occupational therapy (OT) intervention for clients with upper extremity injuries or surgery focus on enabling clients to regain functional use of their affected body part so they may participate in necessary and desired occupations. Both biomechanical and occupation-based approaches should directly address clients' relevant functional goals. Adjunct therapies can be used to prepare clients for function-based activity, and task and environmental modifications to enhance occupational performance should supplement client factor interventions (Case-Smith, 2003; Jack & Estes, 2010; Skirven, Osterman, Fedorczyk, & Amadio, 2011).

- *Physical agent modalities.* Modalities such as heat or ice are typically applied as an adjunct to OT intervention. Applied heat via heat packs, paraffin baths, fluidotherapy, or whirlpool may decrease pain and stiffness and improve circulation. Cold modalities may reduce pain, inflammation, and metabolic activity of the area being iced. For clients with acute soft tissue injuries, a combination of ice and exercise may reduce poststrain and postsurgical pain (Amini, 2011a).
- *Scar management.* Scars, whether a direct result of the injury or corrective surgery, are common concern for clients with hand and wrist injuries. Scar management techniques include massage and silicone gel sheeting. Silicone gel sheeting reduces hypertrophic scarring and increases the elasticity of established scars. Scar massage can reduce pain and itching from scars associated with burns, decrease anxiety, and improve mood (Amini, 2011a).
- *Splinting.* Splints are typically fabricated for, or provided to, clients with hand injuries. Although the purpose of each splint is a function of the client's condition, common purposes are to provide support, immobilize specific joints, or block a specific motion. Splinting has been found to be a "beneficial preparatory technique" for reducing signs and symptoms of osteoarthritis and carpal tunnel syndrome (Amini, 2011a, p. 30).
- *Therapeutic exercise.* Therapeutic exercise typically includes range of motion, strengthening, endurance building, and motor control exercises. Depending on the client's needs, preferences, and ability, exercise may focus on only one body part or the whole body. For clients with rheumatoid arthritis, "appropriate exercise" may lead to long-term changes in strength and short-term changes in hand stiffness. For clients with osteoarthritis, aerobic exercise may improve functional status as determined by client reports of pain and ability to engage in desired activities. A 2-year full-body strengthening program including gripper exercise has been associated with improved static and dynamic grip strength among adults with osteoarthritis (Amini, 2011a).
- *Function-based activities.* Function-based activities are intervention activities that simulate activities of daily living (ADL) tasks as opposed to engaging clients in contrived therapeutic exercise (Amini, 2011a). In one randomized control trial, individuals with acute and chronic hand injuries who were given ADL simulations had statistically significant higher levels of improvement in areas assessed than did those who underwent traditional exercise-based treatment (Guzelkucuk, Duman, Taskaynatan, & Dincer, 2007).

Occupational Therapy and the Evidence

OT interventions have been found to generate positive functional outcomes in the area of hand and wrist rehabilitation. Case-Smith (2003) examined the effects of an OT intervention, which included splinting, therapeutic exercise, ADL, and physical agent modalities, for a group of 33 adults with various upper extremity conditions. Each client received an average of 13 hours of treatment. In addition, Case-Smith used the COPM to design intervention so that treatment remained consistent with the clients' goals and priorities. Comparison of preintervention and postintervention scores for three of the four outcome measures revealed statistically significant positive differences. Clinical interpretations of these data indicate improvement in the clients' self-ratings of performance and satisfaction in their chosen goal areas, improvement in ADL performance, decreased levels of perceived pain, and improvements in social participation and leisure activities. Of the 25 participants who were employed or were full-time students at baseline, 20 returned to their prior occupations. A recent systematic review of literature pertaining to OT interventions for conditions of the forearm, wrist, and hand supports general use of the intervention techniques used in the Case-Smith study (Amini, 2011a). Jack and Estes (2010) describe a case study to illustrate the positive outcomes generated when therapists apply a client-centered, occupation-based approach to all levels of OT services. In the case study, initial evaluation, goal setting, and intervention strictly adhered to a biomechanical approach. The client became discouraged and her motivation decreased due to only minimal objective gains on nonfunctional biomechanical measures. She expressed disappointment that the major functional gains she was experiencing were not reflected in the biomechanical goals. The focus of intervention then shifted to occupational adaptation, and the COPM was administered so the client could self-identify functional goals. Biomechanical intervention techniques were supplemented with collaborative problem solving and identification of compensatory techniques to address the functional goals. Upon reassessment, COPM scores demonstrated significantly improved self-ratings of performance and satisfaction in the identified functional goals. Combining biomechanical principles with a more function-oriented, client-centered approach improved the client's motivation and outlook and provided documentation that was more relevant to the functional gains experienced by the client.

Resources

Associations and Websites

- American Society of Hand Therapists: http://www.asht.org
- American Society for Surgery of the Hand: http://www.assh.org
- Hand Therapy Certification Commission: http://www.htcc.org
- National Institute for Occupational Safety and Health: http://www.cdc.gov/niosh/

Books

- Felstiner, M. (2007). *Out of joint: A private and public story of arthritis.* Lincoln, NE: University of Nebraska Press.
  A prize-winning history professor describes her experience with arthritis in a way that is as much poetry as powerful analysis.

References

Aluoch, M. A., & Wao, H. O. (2009). Risk factors for occupational osteoarthritis: A literature review. *American Association of Occupational Health Nurses, 57,* 283–290.

Amadio, P. C. (2007). Specialty update: What's new in hand surgery. *The Journal of Bone and Joint Surgery, 89A,* 460–465. doi:10.2106/JBJS.H.01697

Amini, D. (2011a). Occupational therapy interventions for work-related injuries and conditions of the forearm, wrist, and hand: A systematic review. *American Journal of Occupational Therapy, 65,* 29–36. doi:10.5014/ajot.2011.09186

Amini, D. (2011b). The unique role of occupational therapy in rehabilitation of the hand. Retrieved from http://www.aota.org/Practitioners/PracticeAreas/Rehab/Tools/Hand-Rehab.aspx?FT=.pdf

Bongers, P. M., Kremer, A. M., & ter Laak, J. (2002). Are psychosocial factors, risk factors for symptoms and signs of the shoulder, elbow, or hand/wrist?: A review of the epidemiological literature. *American Journal of Industrial Medicine, 41,* 315–342.

Case-Smith, J. (2003). Outcomes in hand rehabilitation using occupational therapy services. *American Journal of Occupational Therapy, 57,* 499–506.

Centers for Disease Control and Prevention. (2001). Nonfatal occupational injuries and illnesses treated in hospital emergency departments—United States, 1998. *Morbidity and Mortality Weekly Report, 50,* 313–317.

Cooper, C. (2007). Fundamentals of clinical reasoning: Hand therapy concepts and treatment techniques. In C. Cooper (Ed.), *Fundamentals of hand therapy: Clinical reasoning and treatment guidelines for common diagnoses of the upper extremity.* St. Louis, MO: Mosby Elsevier.

Guzelkucuk, U., Duman, I., Taskaynatan, M. A., & Dincer, K. (2007). Comparison of therapeutic activities with therapeutic exercises in the rehabilitation of young adult patients with hand injuries. *Journal of Hand Surgery,* 32, 1429–1435.

Jack, J., & Estes, R. I. (2010). Documenting progress: Hand therapy treatment shift from biomechanical to occupational adaptation. *American Journal of Occupational Therapy, 64,* 82–87.

Kakar, S., Giuffre, J., Skeete, K., & Elhassan, B. (2010). Dupuytren's disease. *Orthopaedics and Trauma,* 24, 197–206.

Lawrence, R. C., Felson, D. T., Helmick, C. G., Arnold, L. M., Choi, H., Deyo, R. A., . . . Wolfe, F. (2008). Estimates of the prevalence of arthritis and other rheumatic conditions in the United States. *Arthritis & Rheumatism, 58,* 26–35. doi:10.1002/art.23176

McAuliffe, J. (2010). Tendon disorders of the hand and wrist. *Journal of Hand Surgery, 35,* 846–853. doi:10.1016/j.jhsa.2010.03.001

Orces, A. O., & Martinez, F. J. (2010). Epidemiology of fall related forearm and wrist fractures among adults treated in US hospital emergency departments. *Injury Prevention, 17*(1), 33–36. doi:10.1136/ip.2010.026799

Skirven, T. M., Osterman, L., Fedorczyk, J., & Amadio, P. C. (2011). *Rehabilitation of the hand and upper extremity, 2-volume set* (6th ed.). Philadelphia, PA: Elsevier Mosby.

Stevens, J. A., Corso, P. S., Finkelstein, E. A., & Miller, T. R. (2006). The costs of fatal and non-fatal falls among older adults. *Injury Prevention, 12,* 290–295. doi:10.1136/ip.2005.011015

Thompson, M., Evitt, C. P., & Whaley, M. M. (2010). Screening for falls and osteoporosis: Prevention practice for the hand therapist. *Journal of Hand Therapy, 23,* 212–229. doi:10.1016/j.jht.2009.11.001

U.S. Bureau of Labor Statistics. (2008). *Nonfatal occupational injuries and illnesses requiring days away from work, 2007 (USDL 08–1716)* [News release]. Retrieved from www.bls.gov/news.release/archives/osh2_11202008.pdf

HIV/AIDS

Pamela Vaughn

Description and Diagnosis

Human immunodeficiency virus (HIV) affects the immune system by destroying white blood cells (specifically, T-cells expressing a specific protein known as CD4, also known as "CD4+ T cells"), which are central in fighting disease and infection. Acquired immunodeficiency syndrome (AIDS) is the final stage—stage 3—of HIV infection, at which point an individual has fewer than 200 remaining CD4+ T cells per μL of blood or has an AIDS-defining condition (Schneider et al., 2008). HIV is most commonly diagnosed using a blood test that detects the presence of HIV antibodies (created as a response to the presence of the virus); because it takes an average of 25 days for antibodies to develop, this type of test is not immediately accurate. Recently, blood tests that detect the presence of HIV antigens (the actual virus) have been used to provide more immediate diagnoses. A second blood test is used to confirm the diagnosis (Centers for Disease Control and Prevention [CDC], 2011a).

Incidence and Prevalence

- Each year, approximately 50,000 people in the United States become infected with HIV.
- Between 1999 and 2008, an average of 38,279 AIDS diagnoses were made per year.
- By the end of 2008, an estimated 1,178,350 U.S. adolescents and adults (aged 13 years and older) were living with HIV. Approximately 20% of these individuals are living undiagnosed.
- By the end of 2009, more than 33.3 million people worldwide were living with HIV.
- By the end of 2008, an estimated 479,161 U.S. adolescents and adults (aged 13 years and older) were living with AIDS.
- Between 1999 and 2008, 17,489 people in the United States with AIDS died per year.
- Men have higher HIV infection rates than women, with a ratio of about 3:1.
- Prevalence is highest among African Americans or Blacks (1.8%), followed by Hispanics and Latinos (0.6%) and non-Hispanic Whites (0.2%) (CDC, 2011b).

Cause and Etiology

The primary mode of HIV transmission is through unprotected sexual contact with someone who is infected with HIV. Transmission is highest among men who have sex with men. It can also be transmitted, in order of decreasing risk, via heterosexual anal sex, vaginal sex, and oral sex (both same sex and opposite sex). Correct and consistent use of latex condoms during sexual intercourse greatly decreases the chances of HIV transmission. Nonsexual modes of transmission include, but are not limited to, the following:

- Sharing needles/syringes used for injection of illicit drugs (the second most common mode after homosexual anal sex)
- Mother-to-child transmission during pregnancy, birth, or breastfeeding
- Accidental needle sticks (i.e., in medical settings)
- Unsafe or unsanitary blood transfusions or injections (less common in the United States)

HIV is *not* spread by air or water, insects, saliva, sweat, tears, casual contact, or anything that doesn't involve blood, semen, vaginal fluid, or breast milk (CDC, 2011a).

Typical Course, Symptoms, and Related Conditions

After infection with HIV occurs, a person typically begins to develop antibodies in 2 to 8 weeks; although in rare cases, this may take up to 6 months. Although tests for HIV may not detect the virus at this time, it is still active and very transmissible. Presentation of symptoms varies between individuals. Symptoms that may occur in early stages of HIV infection appear flulike and include fever, headache, tiredness, and enlarged lymph nodes (National Institute of Allergy and Infectious Diseases [NIAID], 2009a). As the virus continues to destroy the immune system, symptoms progress and often include the following:

- Rapid and extreme weight loss
- Recurring fever
- Extreme fatigue
- Prolonged swelling of lymph glands
- Extended bouts of diarrhea
- Sores in the mouth, anus, or genitals
- Pneumonia or other severe illnesses
- Coughing and shortness of breath
- Blotches on or under the skin or inside the mouth, nose, or eyelids
- Numbness or sensation loss, particularly in extremities
- Blurred and distorted vision
- Decrease in strength, range of motion (ROM)
- Memory loss, depression, and other neurological disorders (NIAID, 2009a)

Although there is no cure for HIV/AIDS, the virus can be controlled and the progression of symptoms slowed with the use of anti-HIV drugs. Infections and illnesses that would not be of major concern to healthy people are particularly dangerous and often fatal for people living with HIV/AIDS (PLWHA). Life expectancy for PLWHA in the United States has increased over the past few decades in large part due to advances in medication; following diagnosis, PLWHA in the United States have an estimated life expectancy of 20 to 25 years (Harrison, Song, & Zhang, 2010).

Considering the common modes of transmission of HIV, many PLWHA may have comorbid substance abuse addictions or participate in unsafe sexual activities that may lead to the acquisition of other sexually transmitted diseases. It is not unusual for clients to become stigmatized or marginalized due to these behaviors or as a result of their diagnosis of HIV/AIDS (Braveman & Suarez-Balcazar, 2009; Opacich, 2008).

Interdisciplinary Interventions

Medication Therapy

Individuals diagnosed with HIV will begin an antiretroviral (ARV) medication regimen in order to decrease levels of HIV to trace amounts and therefore decrease the severity and progression of symptoms. ARVs are taken to control HIV and protect the immune system as much as possible by preventing HIV from replicating itself within the body; there is no cure for HIV, and it is still transmissible even when controlled by medication (NIAID, 2009b). Typically, one person is prescribed two or three medications from different classes of ARVs to be taken in combination—what is considered highly active antiretroviral therapy (HAART).

Social Work or Counseling

Due to the impact that an HIV diagnosis can have on the emotional, psychological, and social well-being of an individual, PLWHA are frequently referred to counseling or social work to help them obtain medical care, transportation and housing, child care, financial and legal advice, and other services and resources as they learn to manage HIV.

Occupational Therapy Evaluations

The evaluation process focuses on what the client needs, wants, or is expected to do and analyzes what factors may impact desired occupational performance. The evaluation begins with occupation-focused assessments followed by specific evaluation of the potential impact of HIV/AIDS on occupational performance.

Occupation-Focused Assessments

- Pizzi Assessment of Productive Living for Adults with HIV Infection and AIDS (Pizzi, 1993)
- Role Checklist (Oakley, Kielhofner, Barris, & Reichler, 1986)
- Worker Role Interview (WRI) (Braveman et al., 2005)
- School Function Assessment (SFA) (Coster, Deeney, Haltiwanger, & Haley, 1998)
- Occupational Performance History Interview II (OPHI-II) (Kielhofner et al., 2004)
- Assessment of Motor and Process Skills (AMPS) (Fisher & Jones, 2010)
- Occupational Self-Assessment, Version 2.2 (Baron, Kielhofner, Iyenger, Goldhammer, & Wolenski, 2006)
- Performance Assessment of Self-Care Skills (PASS) (Holm & Rogers, 2008)
- Canadian Occupational Performance Measure (COPM) (Law et al., 2005)
- Short Form-36 (SF-36) (Hays, Sherbourne, & Mazel, 1995)
- Activity Card Sort (ACS) (Baum & Edwards, 2008)

Client Factor Assessments

- Whalen Symptom Index (Whalen, Antani, Carey, & Landefeld, 1994)
- The Revised Sign and Symptom Check-List for HIV (SSC-HIVrev) (Holzemer, Hudson, Kirksey, Hamilton, & Bakken, 2001)
- Pediatric Evaluation of Disability Inventory (PEDI) (Haley, Coster, Ludlow, Haltiwanger, & Andrellos, 1992)
- ROM
- Measures of pain (e.g., Visual Analog Scale [VAS])
- Measures of muscle strength

Occupational Therapy Interventions

Although interventions for PLWHA do not normally involve exposure to bodily fluids, occupational therapists should, as with any infectious disease, follow universal precautions to protect themselves from transmission of HIV. Interventions for PLWHA should always be client centered and have the goal of increasing their participation and satisfaction in occupations that are meaningful to and/or necessary for them. Because HIV/AIDS is a chronic disease, interventions tend to focus on lifestyle management to increase the potential for clients to participate fully. On the person level, common occupational therapy (OT) interventions include the following:

- Environmental and/or task adaptations, potentially including assistive or adaptive devices, to facilitate continued or return to independence in activities of daily living (ADL), instrumental activities of daily living (IADL), and so forth
- Training in energy conservation techniques and time management
- Pain management, including relaxation techniques
- Health preservation techniques, including medication management
- Recommendations for ambulatory devices
- Guidance through role changes, including time management and adjustments of daily living routines, coping strategies for role disruption, training for finding and using assistance, and so forth
- Strategies to compensate for difficulties related to physical symptoms (e.g., low vision, decreased strength, and coordination), particularly for children with HIV/AIDS, motor control, strength and balance exercises, and/or sensory integration techniques to address sensorimotor needs
- Education for the prevention of spreading HIV
- Recommendation of community resources (e.g., support groups, transportation, palliative care) to facilitate coping and occupational participation
- Helping clients learn how to be self-advocates (Kielhofner, Braveman, Fogg, & Levin, 2008; Opacich, 2008)

In addition, occupational therapists can provide intervention at an organization or population level by advocating for disability rights and social justice issues, such as equal access and equal opportunity, for PLWHA. This can help reduce the stigma that is often attributed to HIV/AIDS and ensure that PLWHA have access to resources necessary to participate occupationally (Braveman & Suarez-Balcazar, 2009).

Occupational Therapy and the Evidence

When compared to a control group receiving standard care, an OT intervention group for PLWHA that focused on needs related to productive participation (e.g., health management, independent living skills, role development, vocational skills, self-advocacy) resulted in significantly higher levels of postintervention productive participation—that is, employment, attending school or training, or volunteering (Kielhofner et al., 2008).

Caregiver Concerns

HIV-positive parents must choose whether or not they are going to disclose their diagnosis to their children; not wanting to worry or scare their children and wanting them to have a "carefree childhood" are among the top reasons why some parents choose to delay disclosure to their children. However, most parents do tell their children about their diagnosis because they feel their children have a right to know and want them to hear it directly from them; the vast majority of parents do not regret disclosing their diagnosis to their children (Ostrom Delaney, Serovich, & Lim, 2008).

There is a stigma associated with being a caregiver of PLWHA, and greater levels of perceived stigma are correlated with increased depressive symptoms. The greater number of people that these same caregivers disclosed their caregiver status to, however, the fewer the depressive symptoms they reported (Mitchell & Knowlton, 2009). Some caregivers report health difficulties as a result of caring for PLWHA, including tension, headaches, and low energy. Psychological concerns include feeling pressure as a result of caring for their loved ones and feeling down and/or lonely. Overall, there is a greater concern for the PLWHA that they are caring for than for their own well-being (Darling, Olmstead, & Tiggleman, 2010). Although anxiety concerning death is lesser for caregivers than for PLWHA, it still impacts the quality of life of caregivers (Sherman, Norman, McSherry, 2010). Support groups may be beneficial for caregivers.

In the case of serodiscordant couples (one has a diagnosis of HIV/AIDS and the other does not), a common concern is the potential of sexual transmission of HIV. In order to participate and enjoy sexual activities, these couples must make any and all precautions possible (i.e., correct use of condoms) to prevent the spread of HIV to the undiagnosed partner. For opposite-sex couples who wish to have children, fertility techniques—such as "sperm washing" to remove the HIV from the male's sperm prior to artificial insemination—and careful use of ARVs by an HIV-positive mother can decrease or eliminate the chance of a child being born with HIV (Gosselin & Sauer, 2011).

Resources

Organizations

- International AIDS Society—association for health professionals
  Ave. Louis Casaï 71
  PO Box 28
  CH-1216 Cointrin
  Geneva, Switzerland
  Telephone: +41-(0)22-7 100 800
  Fax: +41-(0)22-7 100 899
  E-mail: info@iasociety.org
  Website: http://www.iasociety.org
- Joint United Nations Programme on HIV/AIDS (UNAIDS)—international program to increase access to HIV prevention, treatment, care, and support
  20, Avenue Appia
  CH-1211 Geneva 27
  Switzerland
  Telephone: +41 22 791 36 66
  Fax: +41 22 791 4187
  Website: http://www.unaids.org

Books

- Brown, M., & Martin, C. (2008). *The naked truth: Young, beautiful, and (HIV) positive.* New York, NY: Amistad.
- Cameron, E. (2005). *Witness to AIDS.* New York, NY: I.B. Tauris.

Websites

- http://www.cdc.gov/hiv
- http://AIDS.gov
- http://www.aidsinfo.nih.gov/
- http://www.niaid.nih.gov/topics/hivaids
- http://www.avert.org/

References

Baron, K., Kielhofner, G., Iyenger, A., Goldhammer, V., & Wolenski, J. (2006). *Occupational Self-Assessment* (OSA; Version 2.2.). Chicago, IL: MOHO Clearinghouse.

Baum, C. M., & Edwards, D. E. (2008). *Activity Card Sort* (2nd ed.). Bethesda, MD: AOTA Press.

Braveman, B., Robson, M., Velozo, C., Kielhofner, G., Fisher, G. S., Forsyth, K., & Kerschbaum, J. (2005). *The Worker Role Interview (Version 10).* Chicago, IL: MOHO Clearinghouse.

Braveman, B., & Suarez-Balcazar, Y. (2009). Social justice and resource utilization in a community-based organization: A case illustration of the role of the occupational therapist. *American Journal of Occupational Therapy, 63,* 13–23.

Centers for Disease Control and Prevention. (2011a). *Basic information about HIV and AIDS.* Retrieved from http://www.cdc.gov/hiv/topics/basic/

Centers for Disease Control and Prevention. (2011b). HIV surveillance—United States, 1981–2008. *Morbidity and Mortality Weekly Report, 60,* 690–693.

Coster, W., Deeney, T., Haltiwanger, J., & Haley, S. (1998). *School Function Assessment.* San Antonio, TX: PsychCorp.

Darling, C. A., Olmstead, S. B., & Tiggleman, C. (2010). Persons with AIDS and their support persons: Stress and life satisfaction. *Stress and Health, 26,* 33–44. doi:10.1002/smi.1254

Fisher, A. G., & Jones, K. B. (2010). *Assessment of Motor and Process Skills. Vol. 1: Development, standardization, and administration manual* (7th ed.). Fort Collins, CO: Three Star Press.

Gosselin, J. T., & Sauer, M. V. (2011). Life after HIV: Examination of HIV serodiscordant couples' desire to conceive through assisted reproduction. *AIDS and Behavior, 15,* 469–478. doi:10.1007/s10461-010-9830-9

Haley, S. M., Coster, W. J., Ludlow, L. H., Haltiwanger, J. T., & Andrellos, P. J. (1992). *Pediatric Evaluation of Disability Inventory.* San Antonio, TX: PsycCorp.

Harrison, K. M., Song, R., & Zhang, X. (2010). Life expectancy after HIV diagnosis based on national HIV surveillance data from 25 states, United States. *Journal of Acquired Immune Deficiency Syndrome, 53,* 124–130.

Hays, R. D., Sherbourne, C. D., & Mazel, R. M. (1995). *User's manual for Medical Outcomes Study (MOS) core measures of health-related quality of life.* Santa Monica, CA: RAND.

Holm, M. B., & Rogers, J. C. (2008). The Performance Assessment of Self-Care Skills (PASS). In B. Hemphill-Pearson (Ed.), *Assessments in occupational therapy mental health* (2nd ed., pp. 101–110). Thorofare, NJ: Slack.

Holzemer, W. L., Hudson, A., Kirksey, K. M., Hamilton, M. J., & Bakken, S. (2001). The revised sign and symptom check-list for HIV (SSC-HIVrev). *Journal of the Association of Nurses in AIDS Care, 12,* 60–70. doi:10.1016/S1055-3290(06)60263-X

Kielhofner, G., Braveman, B., Fogg, L., & Levin, M. (2008). A controlled study of services to enhance productive participation among people with HIV/AIDS. *American Journal of Occupational Therapy, 61,* 36–45.

Kielhofner, G., Mallinson, T., Crawford, C., Nowak, M., Rigby, M., Henry, A., & Walens, D. (2004). *Occupational Performance History Interview II (OPHI-II).* Chicago, IL: MOHO Clearinghouse.

Law, M., Baptiste, S., Carswell, A., McColl, M., Polatajko, H., & Pollock, N. (2005). *Canadian Occupational Performance Measure* (4th ed.). Ottawa, Canada: CAOT Publications.

Mitchell, M. M., & Knowlton, A. (2009). Stigma, disclosure, and depressive symptoms among informal caregivers of people living with HIV/AIDS. *AIDS Patient Care & STDs, 23,* 611–617. doi:10.1089/apc.2008.0279

National Institute of Allergy and Infectious Diseases. (2009a). *HIV/AIDS: Symptoms.* Retrieved from http://www.niaid.nih.gov/topics/HIVAIDS/Understanding/Pages/symptoms.aspx

National Institute of Allergy and Infectious Diseases. (2009b). *HIV/AIDS: Treatment of HIV infection.* Retrieved from http://www.niaid.nih.gov/topics/HIVAIDS/Understanding/Pages/symptoms.aspx

Oakley, F., Kielhofner, G., Barris, R., & Reichler, R. (1986). The Role Checklist: Development and empirical assessment of reliability. *Occupational Therapy Journal of Research, 6,* 157–170.

Opacich, K. J. (2008). Human immunodeficiency virus. In M. V. Radomski & C. A. T. Latham (Eds.), *Occupational therapy for physical dysfunction* (6th ed., pp. 1345–1357). Philadelphia, PA: Lippincott Williams & Wilkins.

Ostrom Delaney, R. R., Serovich, J. M., & Lim, J. Y. (2008). Reasons for and against maternal HIV disclosure to children and perceived child reaction. *AIDS Care, 20,* 876–880. doi:10.1080/09540120701767158

Pizzi, M. (1993). HIV infection and AIDS. In H. L. Hopkins & H. D. Smith (Eds.), *Willard and Spackman's occupational therapy* (8th ed., pp. 716–729). Philadelphia, PA: Lippincott Williams & Wilkins.

Schneider, E., Whitmore, S., Glynn, M. K., Dominguez, K., Mitsch, A., McKenna, M. T., & Centers for Disease Control and Prevention. (2008). Revised surveillance case definitions for HIV infection among adults, adolescents, and children aged <18 months and for HIV infection and AIDS among children aged 18 months to <13 Years—United States, 2008. *Morbidity and Mortality Weekly Report, 57*(RR-10), 1–8. Retrieved from http://www.cdc.gov/mmwr/preview/mmwrhtml/rr5710a1.htm

Sherman, D. W., Norman, R., & McSherry, C. B. (2010). A comparison of death anxiety and quality of life of patients with advanced cancer or AIDS and their family caregivers. *Journal of the Association of Nurses in AIDS Care, 21,* 99–112. doi:10.1016/j.jana.2009.07.007

Whalen, C., Antani, M., Carey, J., & Landefeld, C. (1994). An index of symptoms for infection with human immunodeficiency virus: Reliability and validity. *Journal of Clinical Epidemiology, 47,* 537–546.

Homelessness

Pamela Vaughn

Description

According to the U.S. McKinney-Vento Homeless Assistance Act of 1987 (P.L. 100-77), a person who is *homeless* is defined as (1) an individual who lacks a fixed, regular, and adequate nighttime residence; and (2) an individual who has a primary nighttime residence—that is, (a) a supervised publicly or privately operated shelter designed to provide temporary living accommodations (including welfare hotels, congregate shelters, and transitional housing for the mentally ill); (b) an institution that provides a temporary residence for individuals intended to be institutionalized; or (c) a public or private place not designed for, or ordinarily used as, a regular sleeping accommodation for human beings.

Homelessness can be classified as either episodic (wherein an individual is homeless for one night or a few nights) or chronic (wherein an individual is unaccompanied [single adult], disabled, and homeless continuously for 1 year or more *or* for four or more episodes in the past 3 years) (McKinney-Vento Homeless Assistance Act, 1987). Information provided in this resource sheet generally refers to homelessness in the United States and uses the aforementioned definition of "homelessness" as a guide; homelessness may have similar characteristics in other developed countries. However, the definition and characteristics of homelessness vary by country and by culture.

Incidence and Prevalence

Determining exact numbers—or even close estimates—of people who are homeless in the United States is extremely difficult. This is in part due to the high turnover rate of the homeless population, but other factors that make it difficult are that some people who are homeless have living situations in which they are less likely to be counted (e.g., with a relative, in a hotel or motel) or are living in places where community officials would have a difficult time finding them (e.g., in a car, at a campground) (National Coalition for the Homeless, 2009). According to the most recent Annual Homeless Assessment Report to Congress made by the U.S. Department of Housing and Urban Development (HUD; 2011),

- On a single night in 2010, 649,917 people in the United States (407,966 individuals; 241,951 persons in families accounting for 79,446 families) were homeless.
  - 62% of these individuals were sheltered (in emergency shelters or transitional housing) and 38% were unsheltered (e.g., in streets, vehicles, abandoned buildings); families were more likely to be sheltered than individuals.
  - This is an increase of 1.1% from the single night in 2009.
  - Since 2007, however, this is a decrease of 3.3%.
  - 109,812 (16.9%) of these people met the criteria for chronic homelessness.
- On this single night count (one individual may fall into more than one category),
  - 26.2% of adults had a serious mental illness;
  - 34.7% of adults had substance abuse;
  - 3.9% of adults had HIV/AIDS;
  - 12.3% were survivors of domestic violence; and
  - 1.1% were unaccompanied youth.
- In 2010, over 1.59 million people in the United States spent at least one night in an emergency shelter or transitional housing.
  - Of these, 65% were individuals and 35% were persons in families.
  - Although this total number has remained relatively stable since 2007, it represents an increase of about 94,000 persons in families—a 20% increase—and a decrease in about 72,000 individuals—a 6% decrease—since 2007.
- Using the annual estimate to determine the characteristics of people who are homeless,
  - 78% are adults (62% of these are male);
  - 42% are white, non-Hispanic; 37% are black or African American; remaining 21% are members of other minority groups;
  - 21.8% are under the age of 18 years, 23.5% are aged 18 to 30 years, 37% are aged 31 to 50 years, 14.9% are aged 51 to 61 years, and 2.8% are 62 years and older; and
  - 36.8% of the adults have a disability.

Causes and Risk Factors

Homelessness can be caused by one or more personal, social, medical, or economic factors. People who are homeless make up a heterogeneous group—"they differ in demographics, subgroups, and their patterns of homelessness" (Helfrich, 2011, p. 611). The range of causes of and risk factors for homelessness include the following:

- Foreclosures and/or lack of affordable housing
- Poverty
- Domestic violence
- Unemployment
- Mental illness
- Substance addiction and abuse (Helfrich, 2011; Herzberg & Petrenchik, 2010; Schultz-Krohn, 2009)

Related Conditions

When people become homeless, drastic shifts in their physical environment are not all they experience. Their community and social environments have changed too, as have their affordances to participate in previous occupations. Because of the innumerable causes and effects of homelessness, it is necessary to look at each individual and/or family unit separately (Muñoz, Garcia, Lisak, & Reichenbach, 2006).

People may have medical and/or psychological conditions that either contributed to or came about as a result of becoming homeless. For example, individuals may develop depression, anxiety, or substance abuse after becoming homeless, but those same mental disorders can also be factors in individuals becoming homeless. Factors that may have contributed to an individual becoming homeless may have other implications (physical, mental, psychological, etc.) as well—for example, surviving domestic abuse or being a veteran.

As a result of living in shelters or transitional housing or of being unsheltered, many people are at an increased risk of contracting or developing medical conditions (e.g., general poor health and nutrition, lice, skin diseases, HIV/AIDS, physical injuries, tuberculosis, respiratory problems, high blood pressure, diabetes, cancer) and a lack of access to consistent and adequate health care may perpetuate these conditions (Herzberg & Petrenchik, 2010).

Due to stereotyping and stigma, individuals who are homeless frequently face barriers to receiving care and participating in necessary and/or meaningful occupations (Helfrich, 2011). In order to provide the best possible care, sensitivity to individual backgrounds and circumstances is essential.

Interdisciplinary Interventions

Interventions to Meet Basic Needs

When a person initially becomes homeless, he or she may be able to access local emergency assistance. Homeless shelters are more temporary than transitional housing; they provide a place to stay for 1 to 30 nights. Each shelter has different regulations and requirements (e.g., times that people must enter and exit, sobriety requirements, participation in events). Transitional housing programs provide temporary housing for up to 2 years. Some transitional housing programs have specific focuses (e.g., women and children survivors of domestic violence) and requirements for their inhabitants (e.g., participation in employment or education). Some shelters provide their clients with meals, facilities for bathing, and/or clothing donations.

Medical care or mental health counseling may be provided directly in these housing programs or through other community services. Organizations such as food pantries and soup kitchens can provide warm meals for people who may not have the resources to otherwise obtain them.

Medical Interventions

Medical needs of people who are homeless vary among individuals. Because there is an increased risk of developing medical conditions as a result of being homeless, medical services for this population may include the following:

- Prescription of medications
- Triage and wound care
- Immunizations
- HIV testing
- Screening for diseases such as tuberculosis
- Care of skin conditions
- Family planning and testing
- General health education

Mental Health Interventions

Mental health needs vary among individuals. Psychiatrists and psychologists may

- Perform mental health evaluations
- Provide psychotherapy and other interventions
- Psychiatrists and clinical nurse specialists may also provide prescriptions for medications

Social Work, Counseling, Advocates, Treatment Coordinators, or Case Managers

Assist people who are homeless by assessing their needs and finding appropriate resources, particularly financial entitlements when appropriate. They often act as liaisons among people who are homeless, other professionals, and shelters.

Other Interventions

Depending on the needs of the people or family who are homeless, other interventions may include substance cessation counseling, employment and education services, and legal representation.

Occupational Therapy Evaluations

The evaluation process focuses on what the person or family needs, wants, or is expected to do and analyzes what factors may impact desired occupational performance. The evaluation begins with occupation-focused assessments followed by specific evaluation of the potential impact of homelessness on occupational performance.

Occupation-Focused Assessments

- Role Checklist (Oakley, Kielhofner, Barris, & Reichler, 1986)
- Occupational Performance History Interview II (OPHI-II) (Kielhofner et al., 2004)
- Occupational Self-Assessment, Version 2.2 (Baron, Kielhofner, Iyenger, Goldhammer, & Wolenski, 2006)
- Canadian Occupational Performance Measure (COPM) (Law et al., 2005)
- Model of Human Occupation Screening Tool, Version 2.0 (MOHOST) (Parkinson, Forsyth, & Kielhofner, 2006)
- Activity Card Sort (ACS) (Baum & Edwards, 2008)
- Kohlman Evaluation of Living Skills (KELS) (McGourty, 1999)

Client Factor Assessments

- Allen Cognitive Level Screen (ACLS) (Allen et al., 2007)
- Beck Anxiety Inventory (BAI) (Beck, 1993)
- Beck Depression Inventory-II (BDI-II) (Beck, Steer, & Brown, 1996)
- Impact of Events Scale-Revised (IES-R) (Weiss & Marmar, 1996)

Occupational Therapy Interventions

Occupational therapy (OT) intervention for people who are homeless varies by individual. They may include direct OT services and/or consultations; examples may include the following (Helfrich, 2011; Herzberg & Petrenchik, 2010; Schultz-Krohn, 2009):

Direct Occupational Therapy Interventions

- Teach self-care skills (e.g., bathing, grooming, medication management).
- Teach food and nutrition management.
- Teach instrumental activities of daily living (IADL) skills (e.g., budgeting, shopping, home management, cleaning).
- Develop coping skills (e.g., stress management, anger management).
- For parents, develop strategies to maintain healthy parent–child relationships.
- For children, play intervention to promote positive socialization.
- Evaluate vocational skills and/or develop job-specific skills (including job-seeking skills and skills needed for the jobs themselves).
- Develop skills for self-advocacy.

Consultation

- Referral to other services
- Collaborate with shelter itself to assess the environment and identify potential barriers to occupational participation, develop programming, create effective documentation, and so forth.

Occupational Therapy and the Evidence

A systematic review of published OT interventions with people who are homeless reports that the most common OT needs of this population are in the areas of employment and education, money management, coping skills, and leisure skills. Although there are relatively few published intervention studies (due to many factors, including the fact that homelessness is a relatively new area of practice and that many people who are homeless are unable to participate in research studies for various reasons), OT interventions do show evidence of being effective (Thomas, Gray, & McGinty, 2011).

OT interventions focusing on life skills for people with mental illness, who are at risk for repeated homelessness, resulted in increased knowledge of many life skills, as tested by practical skills tests (e.g., money management, safe community participation); individuals with higher scores on the ACLS showed greater improvements in self-care skills after intervention (Helfrich, Chan, & Sabol, 2011). In another study focusing on individualized life skills interventions for persons with mental illness who are at risk for homelessness, participants were grouped according to their readiness to change based on the transtheoretical model. Placement of participants into either the "engaged" (higher readiness-to-change scores) or "preengaged" (lower readiness-to-change scores) study groups did not predict intervention outcome (which included some increases in scores on practical skills tests among both groups), indicating that individuals in various readiness-to-change classifications may benefit from OT intervention (Helfrich, Chan, Simpson, & Sabol, 2011). Interventions focused on professional development, specifically helping people who are homeless find and retain employment, resulted in more than 80% of the participants who completed the program becoming employed, and 40% choosing to pursue educational or vocational training in addition to their jobs (Muñoz, Dix, & Reichenbach, 2006).

Resources

Organizations

- National Coalition for the Homeless—a nonprofit organization for the advocacy of people who are homeless.
  2201 P St NW
  Washington, DC 20037
  Telephone: 202-462-4822
  info@nationalhomeless.org
  http://www.nationalhomeless.org

- United States Interagency Council on Homelessness—a government agency to coordinate policies and services regarding homelessness.
  Federal Center SW
  409 3rd Street SW, Suite 310
  Washington, DC 20024
  Telephone: 202-708-4663
  http://www.usich.gov

Books

- Liebow, E. (1995). *Tell them who I am: The lives of homeless women*. New York, NY: Penguin.
  The stories of several women living in homeless shelters in the Washington, DC, area, as told by an anthropologist and including social commentary.
- Hannah, R., & Soper, B. (2010). *A bum deal: An unlikely journey from hopeless to humanitarian*. Naperville, IL: Sourcebooks.
  The story of Rufus Hannah, an individual who was previously homeless and suffered from alcoholism, who is now an advocate for rights of homeless people.
- Skalitzky, K. M. (2007). *A recipe for hope: Stories of transformation by people struggling with homelessness*. Chicago, IL: ACTA.
  A collection of first-person accounts from men and women who are or were homeless in the Chicago area.

Websites

- U.S. Department of Housing and Urban Development (HUD)
  http://portal.hud.gov/hudportal/HUD?src=/topics/homelessness
  http://www.hudhre.info/index.cfm
- National Low Income Housing Coalition
  http://www.nlihc.org

References

Allen, C. K., Austin, S. L., David, S. K., Earhart, C. A., McCraith, D. B., & Riska-Williams, L. (2007). *Manual for the Allen cognitive level screen-5 (ACLS-5) and large Allen cognitive level screen-5 (LACLS-5)*. Camarillo, CA: ACLS and LACLS Committee.

Baron, K., Kielhofner, G., Iyenger, A., Goldhammer, V., & Wolenski, J. (2006). *Occupational Self-Assessment* (OSA; Version 2.2.). Chicago, IL: MOHO Clearinghouse.

Baum, C. M., & Edwards, D. E. (2008). *Activity Card Sort* (2nd ed.). Bethesda, MD: AOTA Press.

Beck, A. T. (1993). *Beck Anxiety Inventory (BAI) manual*. San Antonio, TX: PsycCorp.

Beck, A. T., Steer, R. A., & Brown, G. K. (1996). *Beck Depression Inventory-Second edition manual*. San Antonio, TX: PsychCorp.

Helfrich, C. (2011). Homeless and women's shelters. In C. Brown & V. C. Stoffel (Eds.), *Occupational therapy in mental health: A vision for participation* (pp. 610–624). Philadelphia, PA: F. A. Davis.

Helfrich, C. A., Chan, D. V., & Sabol, P. (2011). Cognitive predictors of life skill intervention outcomes for adults with mental illness at risk for homelessness. *American Journal of Occupational Therapy, 65*, 277–286. doi:10.5014/ajot.2011.001321

Helfrich, C. A., Chan, D. V., Simpson, E. K., & Sabol, P. (2011). Readiness-to-change cluster profiles among adults with mental illness who were homeless participating in a life skills intervention. *Community Mental Health Journal*. Advance online publication. doi:10.1007/s10597-011-9383-z

Herzberg, G., & Petrenchik, T. M. (2010). Health promotion for individuals and families who are homeless. In M. E. Scaffa, S. M. Reitz, & M. A. Pizzi (Eds.), *Occupational therapy in the promotion of health and wellness* (pp. 434–452). Philadelphia, PA: F. A. Davis.

Kielhofner, G., Mallinson, T., Crawford, C., Nowak, M., Rigby, M., Henry, A., & Walens, D. (2004). *Occupational Performance History Interview II (OPHI-II)*. Chicago, IL: MOHO Clearinghouse.

Law, M., Baptiste, S., Carswell, A., McColl, M., Polatajko, H., & Pollock, N. (2005). *Canadian Occupational Performance Measure* (4th ed.). Ottawa, Canada: CAOT Publications.

McGourty, L. K. (1999). *Kohlman Evaluation of Living Skills*. Bethesda, MD: AOTA Products.

McKinney-Vento Homeless Assistance Act of 1987, 101 Stat. 482, Pub. L. 100-77, 42 U.S.C. § 11301 (1987).

Muñoz, J. P., Dix, S., & Reichenbach, D. (2006). Building productive roles: Occupational therapy in a homeless shelter. *Occupational Therapy in Health Care, 20*(3–4), 167–187. doi:10.1080/J003v20n03_11

Muñoz, J. P., Garcia, T., Lisak, J., & Reichenbach, D. (2006). Assessing the occupational performance priorities of people who are homeless. *Occupational Therapy in Health Care, 20*(3–4), 135–148. doi:10.1080/J003v20n03_09

National Coalition for the Homeless. (2009). *How many people experience homelessness?* Retrieved from http://www.nationalhomeless.org/factsheets/index.html

Oakley, F., Kielhofner, G., Barris, R., & Reichler, R. (1986). The Role Checklist: Development and empirical assessment of reliability. *Occupational Therapy Journal of Research, 6*, 157–170.

Parkinson, S., Forsyth, K., & Kielhofner, G. (2006). *Model of Human Occupation Screening Tool (MOHOST), version 2.0*. Chicago, IL: Model of Human Occupation Clearinghouse.

Schultz-Krohn, W. (2009). There's no place like home: Occupational therapy services for people who are homeless. In E. B. Crepeau, E. S. Cohn, & B. A. B. Schell (Eds.), *Willard & Spackman's occupational therapy* (11th ed., pp. 610–624). Philadelphia, PA: Lippincott Williams & Wilkins.

Thomas, Y., Gray, M., & McGinty, S. (2011). A systematic review of occupational therapy interventions with homeless people. *Occupational Therapy in Health Care, 25*(1), 38–53. doi:10.3109/07380577.20 10.528554

U.S. Department of Housing and Urban Development. (2011). *The 2010 annual homeless assessment report to congress*. Retrieved from http://www.hudhre.info/documents/2010HomelessAssessmentReport.pdf

Weiss, D. S., & Marmar, C. R. (1996). The Impact of Event Scale—Revised. In J. Wilson & T. M. Keane (Eds.), *Assessing psychological trauma and PTSD* (pp. 399–411). New York, NY: Guilford Press.

Mood Disorders: Depression and Bipolar Disorder

Danielle Sotelo

Description

A *mood disorder* is the term used to refer to a group of psychiatric disorders characterized by a pervasive disturbance of mood that is not due to medication, substance abuse, or other psychiatric conditions. Two of the most common mood disorders are depression and bipolar disorder. *Depression* is a mood disorder that affects one's thoughts, moods, feelings, behavior, and physical health. The two most common forms of depression are major depression (which interferes with daily activities) and dysthymia (which lasts 2 years or longer with less severe symptoms). Less common forms of depression include seasonal affective disorder, psychotic depression, and postpartum depression (National Institute of Mental Health [NIMH], 2010a).

Bipolar disorder, also known as manic-depressive illness, is a brain disorder that causes unusual shifts in mood, energy, and activity levels—impeding the ability to function. Bipolar disorder is characterized by dramatic mood swings or episodes of mania and depression. Depending on the dominant mood, bipolar disorder is usually classified as bipolar I (symptoms of major depression, coupled with the occurrence of full-blown mania or mixed symptoms) or bipolar II (symptoms of major depression coupled with the reoccurrence of depressive episodes with hypomania) (NIMH, 2010b).

Incidence and Prevalence

Depression is the most common mental disorder and affects approximately 9.5% of adult Americans (20.9 million people) (American

Psychological Association [APA], 2011; NIMH, 2010a). Depression typically occurs between the ages of 15 and 30 years and is more likely to occur in women than men. Bipolar disorder affects approximately 5.7 million American adults, about 2.6% of the adult population. The median age of onset is 25 years. An equal number of men and women develop bipolar disorder (NIMH, 2010b).

Cause and Etiology

The exact cause of depression is unknown, but it likely results from a combination of genetic, biochemical, environmental, and psychological factors. Trauma or stressful situations may trigger a depressive episode (NIMH, 2010a). Research indicates that bipolar disorder is genetic in nature as it tends to run in families. Research also indicates that environmental and biochemical factors can influence the expression of the gene (NIMH, 2010b).

Course and Signs and Symptoms

The onset of depression typically occurs between the ages of 15 and 30 years but can appear at any point throughout the life course. Symptom-related criteria for depression include prolonged sadness, insomnia or hypersomnia, weight loss or gain, changes in appetite, feelings of guilt and worthlessness, fatigue or loss of energy, inability to concentrate, inability to take pleasure in former interests, social withdrawal, and suicidal ideation (NIMH, 2010a).

Bipolar disorder often occurs in a person's late teens or early adult years. At least half of all cases begin before age 25 years, but symptoms may appear at any point throughout the life course. Bipolar disorder lasts a lifetime, with alternating episodes of mania and depression recurring throughout the life course. Symptoms related to episodes of depression are similar to the depressive symptoms described previously. Symptom-related criteria for episodes of mania include increased physical and mental activity and energy, exaggerated optimism and self-confidence, decreased need for sleep, grandiose thoughts, impulsive behavior and poor judgment, and delusions or hallucinations (NIMH, 2010b).

Related Conditions

Depression often co-occurs with heart disease, stroke, diabetes, cancer, Parkinson's disease, and other serious illnesses that may precede depression, cause it, or are consequence of it. Substance abuse and anxiety disorders (such as posttraumatic stress disorder and obsessive-compulsive disorder) often coexist in people with depression and bipolar disorder. People with bipolar disorder are also at a higher risk for heart disease, diabetes, obesity, and other physical illnesses (NIMH, 2010a, 2010b).

Precautions

Individuals with mood disorders are at high risk for harming themselves, suicidal ideation, and substance abuse. The primary risk factor for suicide is a mood disorder combined with substance abuse. Substance abuse also increases the risk of developing depression (Ramsey, Engler, & Stein, 2005).

Interdisciplinary Interventions

Medications

Depression is often treated with selective serotonin reuptake inhibitors (SSRIs), tricyclic and tetracyclic antidepressants, monoamine oxidase inhibitors (MAOIs), and serotonin and norepinephrine reuptake inhibitors (SNRIs). Bipolar disorder is often treated with antidepressants, mood stabilizers, and antipsychotic medications such as lithium, Risperdal, and Seroquel (NIMH, 2010, 2010b).

Cognitive Behavioral Therapy

Cognitive behavioral therapy (CBT), focused directly on changing beliefs and psychoeducation, when combined with pharmacological treatment, may be beneficial in treating mood disorders (Beynon, Soares-Weiser, Woolacott, Duffy, & Geddes, 2008). CBT can help individuals with mood disorders learn how to obtain more satisfaction and rewards through their own actions. CBT helps clients change negative styles of thinking and behaviors often associated with depression or depressive symptoms (Beevers & Miller, 2005). Current evidence shows that computerized CBT for children, adults, and adolescents with depression is effective (Andrews, Cuijpers, Craske, McEvoy, & Titov, 2010; Richardson, Stallard, & Velleman, 2010).

Psychoeducation, as part of a multicomponent approach, can be effective in preventing relapse and hospitalization and increasing awareness of the illness and symptoms. Treatment includes teaching individuals with bipolar and depression (along with their family members or caregivers) about the illness and how it is treated as well as how to recognize symptoms and identify triggers (Hollon & Ponniah, 2010; Rouget & Aubry, 2007).

Electroconvulsive Therapy

Electroconvulsive therapy (ECT) is a psychiatric treatment in which electric currents sent through the brain induce seizures, often showing an immediate improvement in symptoms (Lisanby, 2007). It is used to treat people with severe depression or acute mania. The use of ECT is controversial, but some studies cite 80% improvement in symptoms for people with severe depression, although relapse usually occurs (Mental Health America [MHA], 2011).

Occupational Therapy Evaluations

Along with observations, interviews, and history taking, the following assessments can be used to evaluate the occupational performance of a person with a mood disorder:

Basic and Instrumental Activity of Daily Living Skills

- Kohlman Evaluation of Living Skills (KELS)
- Milwaukee Evaluation of Daily Living Skills (MEDLS)
- Routine Task Inventory-2 (RTI-2)
- Assessment of Living Skills and Resources (ALSAR)
- Cooking Assessment of Motor and Process Skills
- Test of Grocery Shopping Skills

Psychosocial Skills

- Role Activity Performance Scale (RAPS)
- Assessment of Occupational Functioning (AOF)
- Occupational Performance History Interview II (OPHI-II)

Cognition and Emotional

- Allen Cognitive Level Test-90 (ACLS-90)
- Loewenstein Occupational Therapy Cognitive Assessment (LOTCA)
- Mini-Mental State Exam (MMSE)
- Beck Depression Inventory

Self-Perception or Quality of Life

- Canadian Occupational Performance Measure (COPM)
- Occupational Questionnaire (OQ)
- Occupational Self-Assessment (OSA)
- Role Checklist

Occupational Therapy Interventions

Occupational therapists often assist with the remediation and maintenance of occupational performance of a client with a mood disorder. Both individual and group therapy is used in mental health settings and can focus on the following areas:

Activities of Daily Living or Instrumental Activities of Daily Living

- Establishment of routines or skills training for activities of daily living (ADL), including grooming, dressing, and hygiene
- Management of medication routines

- Management of finances
- Community mobility and safety, such as accessing public and knowing when to ask for help
- Establishment or reestablishment of normal routines
- Psychoeducation concerning symptoms and triggers

Social Participation and Leisure

- Assistance in the exploration of new leisure interests
- Encourage for self-exploration and self-expression
- Integration or reintegration into the community or social group

Work and Education

- Referral to work programs, such as supported employment programs
- Exploration of vocations based on skills, limitations, and interests
- Stress and time management skills
- Instruction on realistic goal setting

Occupational Therapy and the Evidence

Occupational therapists are among the many professionals who are qualified to use CBT during mental health interventions. The use of CBT is one of the most effective therapeutic modalities to treat depression, whether used alone or in combination with pharmacotherapy. CBT reduces negative thinking associated with depression, lessens symptoms, and decreases the chance of relapse (Beevers & Miller, 2005; Powell, Abreu, de Oliveira, & Sudak, 2008). CBT is a valuable tool for increasing self-control and increasing the amount of time between episodes for people with bipolar disorder. CBT, when combined with mood stabilizers, results in fewer bipolar episodes, fewer hospital admissions, better coping with manic symptoms, and higher functioning (Ball, Mitchell, & Corry, 2006; Lam et al., 2003). There is additional evidence that group psychoeducation combined with medication improves perceived quality of life in terms of physical functioning in individuals with bipolar disorder (De Andres et al., 2006; Huxley, Parikh, & Baldessarini, 2000).

Current evidence also suggests that participation in valued leisure activities, physical exercise, and meditation are valuable tools for immediately decreasing symptoms of depression (Arias, Steinberg, Banga, & Trestman, 2006; Tsang, Chan, & Cheung, 2008). Occupational therapists have the skill necessary to assist with supported employment. People with mood disorders often experience high rates of unemployment even though they desire to work. Supported employment is effective in helping people with mental illness obtain competitive employment (Crowther, Marshall, Bond, & Huxley, 2001). Occupational therapists have the skills to assist in job placement, job training, and supported employment for individuals with mood disorders.

Caregiver Concerns

Caring for people with mood disorders exacts a toll on their families and caregivers, often impacting their health and performance in work and leisure activities. Missed work hours and lower productivity caused by stress add a financial burden on the caregiver. As such, it is important for caregivers to make their mental and physical health a priority (National Alliance on Mental Illness [NAMI], 2011). They should also understand the signs and symptoms of mood disorders, the course of the disease, and the fact that the risk of suicide is always present.

Resources

Organizations and Websites

- American Psychiatric Association
  1000 Wilson Boulevard
  Suite 1825
  Arlington, VA 22209
  Telephone: 703-907-7300
  Website: http://www.psych.org

- Depression and Bipolar Support Alliance
  730 N. Franklin St.
  Suite 501
  Chicago, Illinois 60610
  Telephone: 800-826-3632
  Website: http://www.dbsalliance.org

- National Institute of Mental Health
  National Institutes of Health
  6001 Executive Blvd.
  Room 8184, MSC 9663
  Bethesda, MD 20892
  Telephone: 301-443-4513 or 866-615-6464
  Website: http://www.nimh.nih.gov

- National Foundation for Depressive Illness
  PO Box 2257
  New York, NY 10116
  Telephone: 800-248-4344
  Website: http://www.depression.org

Books

- Brampton, S. (2008). *Shoot the damn dog: A memoir of depression.* New York, NY: W. W. Norton.
  A memoir detailing the author's personal struggle with depression. It explores issues including stigma, hospitalizations, triggers, and suicide.

- Irwin, C. (1999). *Conquering the beast within: How I fought depression and won . . . and how you can, too.* New York, NY: Times Books.
  The author shares her personal experience of depression at age 14, including her experience with hospitalization, therapy, and medication.

- Jamison, K. R. (1995). *An unquiet mind: A memoir of moods and madness.* New York, NY: Vintage Books.
  A memoir that looks at bipolar disorder from the perspectives of both the client and the health care provider. The author details her personal experiences with this illness.

- Smith, H. (2010). *Welcome to the jungle: Everything you ever wanted to know about bipolar but were too freaked out to ask.* San Francisco, CA: Red Wheel/Weiser.
  This book targets young people diagnosed with bipolar disorder. It offers honest insight into living with bipolar and answers common questions.

References

American Psychological Association. (2011). *Depression and how psychotherapy and other treatments can help people recover.* Retrieved from http://www.apa.org/topics/depress/recover.aspx#

Andrews, G., Cuijpers, P., Craske, M. G., McEvoy, P., & Titov, N. (2010). Computer therapy for the anxiety and depressive disorders is effective, acceptable and practical health care: A meta-analysis. *PLoS ONE, 5,* 1–6.

Arias, A. J., Steinberg, K., Banga, A., & Trestman, R. L. (2006). Systematic review of the efficacy of meditation techniques as treatments for medical illness. *The Journal of Alternative and Complementary Medicine, 12,* 817–832.

Ball, J., Mitchel, P., & Corry, J. (2006). A randomized controlled trial of cognitive therapy for bipolar disorder: Focus on long-term change. *Journal of Clinical Psychiatry, 67,* 277–286.

Beevers, C., & Miller, I. (2005). Unlinking negative cognition and symptoms of depression: Evidence of a specific treatment effect for cognitive therapy. *Journal of Consulting and Clinical Psychology, 75,* 68–77.

Beynon, S., Soares-Weiser, K., Woolacott, N., Duffy, S., & Geddes, J. R. (2008). Psychosocial interventions for the prevention of relapse in bipolar disorder: Systematic review of controlled trials. *British Journal of Psychiatry, 192,* 5–11.

Crowther, R., Marshall, M., Bond, G., & Huxley, P. (2001). Vocational rehabilitation for people with severe mental illness. *Cochrane Database of Systematic Reviews,* (2).

De Andres, R., Aillon, N., Baridot, M., Bourgeois, P., Mertel, S., Nerfin, F., . . . Aubry, J. M. (2006). Impact of the life goals group therapy program for bipolar patients: An open study. *Journal of Affective Disorders, 93*, 253–257.

Hollon, S. D., & Ponniah, K. (2010). A review of empirically supported psychological therapies for mood disorders in adults. *Depression and Anxiety*, 27, 891–932.

Huxley, N., Parikh, S., & Baldessarini, R. (2000). Effectiveness of psychosocial treatments in bipolar disorder: State of the evidence. *Harvard Review of Psychiatry, 8*, 126–140.

Lam, D., Watkins, E., Hayward, P., Bright, J., Wright, K., Kerr, N., . . . Sham, P. (2003). A randomized controlled study of cognitive therapy for relapse prevention for bipolar affective disorder: Outcome of the first year. *Archives of General Psychiatry, 60*, 145–152.

Lisanby, S. H. (2007). Electroconvulsive therapy for depression. *The New England Journal of Medicine, 357*, 1939–1945.

Mental Health America. (2011). *Electroconvulsive therapy (ECT)*. Retrieved from http://www.nmha.org/go/information/get-info/treatment/electroconvulsive-therapy-ect

National Alliance on Mental Illness. (2011). *Impact and cost of mental illness: The case of bipolar disorder*. Retrieved from http://www.nami.org/Template.cfm?Section=bipolar_disorder&template=/ContentManagement/ContentDisplay.cfm&ContentID=42734

National Institute of Mental Health. (2010a). *Depression*. Retrieved from http://www.nimh.nih.gov/health/publications/depression/index.shtml

National Institute of Mental Health. (2010b). *Bipolar disorder*. Retrieved from http://www.nimh.nih.gov/health/publications/bipolar-disorder/index.shtml

Powell, V., Abreu, N., de Oliveira, I., & Sudak, D. (2008). Cognitive-behavioral therapy for depression. *Revista Brasileira de Psiquiatria, 30*, 73–80.

Ramsey, S., Engler, P., & Stein, M. (2005). Alcohol use among depressed patients: The need for assessment and intervention. *Professional Psychology: Research and Practice, 36*, 203–207.

Richardson, T., Stallard, P., & Velleman, S. (2010). Computerised cognitive behavioural therapy for the prevention and treatment of depression and anxiety in children and adolescents: A systematic review. *Clinical Child and Family Psychology Review, 13*, 275–290.

Rouget, B., & Aubry, J. (2007). Efficacy of psychoeducational approaches on bipolar disorders: A review of the literature. *Journal of Affective Disorders, 98*, 11–27.

Tsang, H. H., Chan, E. P., & Cheung, W. M. (2008). Effects of mindful and non-mindful exercises on people with depression: A systematic review. *British Journal of Clinical Psychology, 47*, 303–322.

Multiple Sclerosis

Sarah Stultz

Multiple sclerosis (MS) is a chronic, progressive neurological condition characterized by patches of demyelination of nerves in areas of the brain and the spinal cord, which results in distorted or interrupted transmission of nerve impulses to and from the brain (Beers & Berkow, 1999). MS is considered to be an autoimmune disease in which the body's own defense system attacks the myelin sheath that surrounds and protects the nerve fibers of the central nervous system (CNS). The sites where myelin is lost appear as hardened sclerotic (scarred) areas in the CNS and cause various physical and neurological symptoms (Reed, 2001).

Prevalence/Incidence

Approximately 400,000 Americans and 2.5 million people worldwide have MS, and approximately 200 more people are diagnosed each week. Most people with MS are diagnosed between the ages of 20 and 50 years, and it is two to three times more common in women than in men. The cause of MS is not completely understood, but it is likely that genetics and the environment play a role. Although MS occurs predominantly in adults, there are an estimated 8,000 to 10,000 children (defines as younger than 18 years of age) diagnosed with MS, and another 10,000 to 15,000 who have experienced at least one symptom of the disease (National Multiple Sclerosis Society [NMSS], n.d.). Due to the unique nature of pediatric MS, the NMSS has established six Pediatric MS Centers of Excellence across the country to study and treat this population.

Course

MS is characterized by four different disease courses, each of which can be mild, moderate, or severe (NMSS, n.d.).

Relapsing-Remitting

Clearly defined and unpredictable relapses or exacerbations and episodes of acute worsening of neurological function. During these episodes, which can last days or months, present symptoms may worsen and new ones may appear. There are also partial or complete recovery periods (remissions) during which the person is free of disease progression. This is the most common form of MS at time of initial diagnosis (~85%).

Primary-Progressive

A slow but nearly continuous worsening of the disease from the onset, with no distinct relapses or remissions. However, there are variations in rates of progression over time, occasional plateaus, and temporary minor improvements. This course is relatively rare (~10%).

Secondary-Progressive

An initial period of relapsing-remitting disease followed by a steadily worsening, unpredictable disease course. About 50% of people with relapsing-remitting MS developed this form of the disease within 10 years of their initial diagnosis.

Progressive-Relapsing

A steadily worsening disease from the onset but also has clear acute relapses, with or without recovery. In contrast to relapsing-remitting MS, the periods between relapses are characterized by continuous disease progression. This course is relatively rare (~5%).

Prognosis

MS is not a fatal diagnosis, and a normal life course can usually be expected. Most people die from the similar causes as the rest of the population (Simon, 2009). In rare cases, some people with a more severe disability may die of infectious complications (NMSS, n.d). Because of the symptoms of the condition, which are unpredictable and vary widely from one individual to another, there is a negative effect on quality of life (QOL). Most individuals do not become severely disabled, and about two-thirds of people remain ambulatory 20 years after being diagnosed (Simon, 2009).

Symptoms

- Fatigue and weakness
- Vision problems, including vision loss, optic neuritis, blurred vision, double vision, or involuntary rapid eye movement
- Balance and coordination problems: loss of balance, tremors, ataxia, vertigo, or clumsiness
- Spasticity
- Pain and altered sensations, including tingling, numbness, burning, or sensitivity to heat
- Bladder and bowel problems
- Problems with sexual functioning: impotence, decreased arousal, and loss of sensation
- Cognitive problem: mainly executive function such as loss of short-term memory, concentration, judgment, or problem solving
- Emotional changes: depression, mood swings, irritability, or pseudobulbar affect (uncontrollable laughing and crying)

- Slowed or slurred speech or dysphagia
- Other symptoms can include headaches, seizures, hearing problems, respiration problems, and itching

Interdisciplinary Intervention

Intervention focuses on modifying the disease course, treating exacerbations, managing symptoms, and improving function and safety.

Medications

- There are nine U.S. Food and Drug Administration (FDA)–approved disease-modifying treatments for use with relapsing MS and one specifically for secondary-progressive MS. Eight of these medications are administered by injection, and one (Gilenya) is an oral medication. These medications have shown effectiveness in modifying the natural course of MS by altering the rate and/or extent of disease progression and reducing the frequency and severity of relapses. Medication management with these "disease modifiers" is recommended as early as possible for individuals with a relapsing course (NMSS, n.d.).
- Corticosteroids shorten acute attacks, reduce inflammation, and ease symptoms (for exacerbations). More potent medications are being developed that are effective in slowing down MS that is rapidly worsening or becoming progressive (Beers & Berkow, 1999).
- Various medications are available to help manage specific symptoms.
- Complementary and alternative medicines (CAMs) may include exercise, diet, food, supplements, stress management, and lifestyle changes. Because CAMs have not been thoroughly tested by the FDA, the safety of these methods remains inconclusive (NMSS, n.d.).

Rehabilitation

Physical Therapy

Physical therapy focuses primarily on mobility and the use of mobility aids, muscle strength and tone, and physical fitness. Personalized exercise programs may help people recover muscle control and strength after an exacerbation. There is significant evidence associating aerobic exercise with improved QOL, mobility, endurance, and reduction in fatigue (Mostert & Kesselring, 2002).

Speech Therapy

In progressive forms of MS, problems with speech or swallowing due to muscle weakness or a lack of coordination may need to be addressed.

Psychosocial Support or Counseling

Individual or group therapy can help individuals with MS and their families to deal with depression, anxiety, and the unpredictability of the disease process. Evidence suggests that a personalized psychosocial rehabilitation program encourages active participation, increased autonomy, and improved QOL (Ferriani et al., 2002).

Occupational Therapy Evaluations

The evaluation process focuses on what the client needs, wants, or is expected to do and analyzes what factors may impact desired occupational performance. The evaluation begins with occupation-focused assessments followed by specific evaluation of the potential impact of MS on occupational performance.

Occupation-Focused Assessments

- Functional Independence Measure (FIM): measures functional status and assistance needs (used primarily in rehabilitation hospitals)
- MS Impact Scale (MSIS-29): measures physical and psychological impact of MS
- Barthel Index (BI): assesses activities of daily living (ADL) function
- Fatigue Impact Scale and the Modified Fatigue Impact Scale (MFIS): measures impact of fatigue on daily life
- Canadian Occupational Performance Measure (COPM): self-report of performance and satisfaction with occupations
- Health Status Questionnaire (SF-36): patient's perception of health and physical limitations
- Multiple Sclerosis Quality of Life Inventory (MSQLI): multidimensional QOL measure
- Occupational Performance History Interview (OPHI): life history and impact of disability
- Occupational Self Assessment (OSA): explores a client's performance, habits, roles, volition, and interests

Client Factors Assessments

- Berg Balance Scale: measures balance among older people
- The Dallas Pain Questionnaire: assesses how pain affects daily function
- Minimal Assessment of Cognitive Function in MS (MACFIMS): assesses cognitive domains affected by MS
- Behavioral Rating Inventory or Executive Function for Adults (BRIEF-A): client and caregiver self-report of executive function
- Range of Motion (ROM), Manual Muscle Test (MMT) and Grasp Dynamometry
- Tinetti Assessment Tool: used to measure gait and balance

Occupational Therapy Interventions

The role of the occupational therapist is to provide assessment and intervention to improve functional performance in ADL and instrumental activities of daily living (IADL), manage fatigue and cognitive symptoms, and support the client to effectively participate in desired roles (Finlayson, Shevil, & Cho, 2009).

Interventions

- ADL and cognitive retraining
- Energy conservation
- Assistive technology
- Environmental, employment, and home modifications
- Pain and stress management
- ROM/endurance/strengthening for desired activities
- Safety awareness
- Splinting

Educating Clients and Care Providers About

- Disease process
- Energy conservation strategies
- Cognitive strategies
- Grading activities
- Use of mobility aids and assistive technology
- Safety awareness
- Work or home modification

Occupational Therapy Evidence

Meta-analysis suggests that occupational therapy (OT) is effective in treating the deficits associated with MS, particularly for outcomes in the capacity and ability, and task and activity levels of performance. Studies that examined a specific intervention method, such as exercise, fatigue management, and cooling and transcutaneous electrical nerve stimulator application for pain, were effective for capacities and ability outcomes (Baker & Tickle-Degnen, 2001).

In a study designed to understand how people with MS experience engagement in occupations, participants reported decreased engagement in meaningful occupations, which led to a belief they were different people and now live their lives differently than they did before (Lexell, Lund, & Iwarsson, 2009). One reason for this life shift is fatigue, a symptom reported in 75% to 90% of individuals with MS and described as the most disabling symptom interfering with performance in daily occupations (Matuska, Mathiowetz, & Finlayson, 2007).

Although courses to teach energy conservation have been effective for individuals with mild-to-severe MS, some studies suggest that participants do not use the strategies (Holberg & Finlayson, 2007). The progressive nature and variability of the disease, effect of fatigue on everyday life, amount of social supports, struggles with sense of self, lack of resources, and physical and social environments may all influence strategy use. Strategies involving rest were the most effective, and peer interaction was beneficial (Holberg & Finlayson, 2007; Matuska et al., 2007; Vanage, Gilbertson, & Mathiowetz, 2003). Research has also demonstrated that OT can be beneficial in the areas of balance and mobility, self-care, transfers, and homemaking tasks. Specifically, inpatient OT can help increase independence in ADL, particularly tub and toilet transfers, toileting, bathing, and dressing (Maitra et al., 2010). Although individual studies document positive outcomes related to OT interventions, a meta-analysis suggests more inconclusive findings. Due to the constantly changing nature of the disease, it is challenging to conduct randomized controlled trials with this population (Steultjens et al., 2004). However, Finlayson and colleagues (2009) found that OT services to discuss cognitive symptoms were useful for mental health and well-being among people aging with MS. More definitive intervention effectiveness research is indicated.

Caregiver Concerns

MS affects people in their most productive years: young adults readying themselves to leave home in pursuit of academic, vocational, or social goals; men and women starting their careers and families of their own; and those in middle age who are enjoying their productive years and planning for retirement. Because individuals with MS report that their ability to engage in occupations is dependent on other people, caregiver support is critical to enable people with MS to continue living in the community (Finlayson et al., 2009; Khan, Pallant, & Brand, 2007). Occupational therapists may educate the client's family about the disease process, including the client's and caregiver's perceptions of cognitive symptoms. Caregivers of those with cognitive symptoms reported spending more time caregiving, and discrepant perceptions could increase caregiver distress (Finlayson et al., 2009). Interventions for caregivers that focused on reducing caregiver strain are important for the well-being of the care recipient, thus a combined patient–caregiver intervention approach is recommended.

Resources

Associations

- National Multiple Sclerosis Society
  733 Third Avenue
  New York, NY 10017
  Telephone: 800-344-4867
  Website: http://www.nmss.org
- Multiple Sclerosis Association of America
  706 Haddonfield Road
  Cherry Hill, NJ 08002
  Telephone: 856-488-4500
  Website: http://www.msassociation.org
- Multiple Sclerosis Foundation
  6520 North Andrews Avenue
  Fort Lauderdale, Florida 33309-2130
  Telephone: 888-MSFOCUS
  http://www.msfocus.org
- Consortium of Multiple Sclerosis Centers
  359 Main Street, Suite A
  Hackensack, NJ 07601
  Telephone: 201-487-1050
  http://www.mscare.org/
- Through the Looking Glass
  3075 Adeline Street, Suite 120
  Berkeley, CA 94703
  Telephone: (510) 848-1112
  Website: http://www.lookingglass.org

First-Person Accounts

- Davis, A. (2004). *My story: A photographic essay on life with multiple sclerosis.* New York, NY: Demos Medical.
- Williams, M. (2004). *Climbing higher.* New York, NY: NAL Trade.
- Mackie, C. (1999). *Me and my shadow.* London, United Kingdom: Aurum Press.
- Garr, T. (2005). *Speedbumps: Flooring it through Hollywood.* New York, NY: Hudson Street Press.

Websites

- Multiple Sclerosis International Federation: http://www.msif.org
- MS Neighborhood: http://www.msneighborhood.com
- MS Active Source: http://www.msactivesource.com

References

Baker, N., & Tickle-Degnen, L. (2001). The effectiveness of physical, psychological, and functional interventions in treating clients with multiple sclerosis: A meta-analysis. *The American Journal of Occupational Therapy, 55,* 324–331.

Beers, M., & Berkow, R. (1999). *The Merck manual of diagnosis and therapy* (17th ed.). Whitehouse Station, NJ: Merck Research Laboratories.

Ferriani, E., Ravaioli, C., Trombetti, M., Balugani, R., Battaglia, S., & Stecchi, S. (2002). Psychological rehabilitation: An integrated approach to provide the best quality of life in multiple sclerosis patients. *Multiple Sclerosis, 8,* S129–S129.

Finlayson, M., Shevil, E., & Cho, C. C. (2009). Perceptions of cognitive symptoms among people aging with multiple sclerosis and their caregivers. *American Journal of Occupational Therapy, 63,* 151–159.

Holberg, C., & Finlayson, M. (2007). Factors influencing the use of energy conservation strategies by persons with multiple sclerosis. *American Journal of Occupational Therapy, 61,* 96–107.

Khan, F., Pallant, J., & Brand, C. (2007). Caregiver strain and factors associated with caregiver self-efficacy and quality of life in a community cohort with multiple sclerosis. *Disability and Rehabilitation, 29*(16), 1241–1250. doi:10.1080/01443610600964141

Lexell, E. M., Lund, M. L., & Iwarsson, S. (2009). Constantly changing lives: Experiences of people with multiple sclerosis. *American Journal of Occupational Therapy, 63,* 772–781.

Maitra, K., Hall, C., Kalish, T., Anderson, M., Dugan, E., Rehak, J., . . . Zeitlin, D. (2010). Research scholars initiative—Five-year retrospective study of inpatient occupational therapy outcomes for patients with multiple sclerosis. *American Journal of Occupational Therapy, 64,* 689–694. doi:10.5014/ajot.2010.090204

Matuska, K., Mathiowetz, V., & Finlayson, M. (2007). Use and perceived effectiveness of energy conservation strategies for managing multiple sclerosis fatigue. *American Journal of Occupational Therapy, 61,* 62–69.

Mostert, S., & Kesselring, J. (2002). Effects of a short-term exercise training program on aerobic fitness, fatigue, health perception and activity level of subjects with multiple sclerosis. *Multiple Sclerosis, 8,* 161–168.

National Multiple Sclerosis Society. (n.d.). *National Multiple Sclerosis Society.* Retrieved from http://www.nationalmssociety.org/index.aspx

Reed, K. (2001). *Quick reference to occupational therapy* (2nd ed). Gaithersburg, MD: Aspen.

Simon, H. (2009). *Multiple sclerosis-prognosis.* Retrieved from http://www.umm.edu/patiented/articles/what_causes_multiple_sclerosis_000017_4.htm

Steultjens, E. M. J., Dekker, J., Bouter, L. M., Cardol, M., Van de Nes, J. C. M., & Van den Ende, C. H. M. (2004). Occupational therapy for multiple sclerosis (Cochrane review). *The Cochrane Library,* (1).

Vanage, S. M., Gilbertson, K. K., & Mathiowetz, V. (2003). Effects of an energy conservation course on fatigue impact for persons with progressive multiple sclerosis. *American Journal of Occupational Therapy, 57,* 315–323.

Obesity, Diabetes, and Hypertension

Danielle Sotelo

Description

Overweight (body mass index [BMI] of 25 to 29.9) and *obesity* (BMI of 30 or higher) are terms used to describe the ranges of weight that are considered to be unhealthy for a certain height. These ranges are also associated with increased risk for certain diseases and health problems, such as diabetes and hypertension (Centers for Disease Control and Prevention [CDC], 2010b).

Diabetes mellitus (or "diabetes") is a condition that causes blood sugar to rise to dangerous levels (fasting blood glucose of 126 mg/dL or more). Type 1 diabetes, previously known as *juvenile diabetes*, is diagnosed in children and young adults and occurs when the body does not produce insulin—a hormone needed to convert sugar, starches, and other foods into energy. Type 2 diabetes, which is closely associated with obesity and physical inactivity, occurs when the pancreas does not make enough insulin or when the body develops insulin resistance (occurs when the body cannot use insulin efficiently) (American Diabetes Association [ADA], 2011a; American Heart Association [AHA], 2011a).

Hypertension, or high blood pressure, is a common condition in which the force of blood against the artery walls is elevated (140/90 mm Hg or higher), causing damage to the artery walls over time. There are two types: primary and secondary hypertension (AHA, 2011b).

Incidence and Prevalence

In 2008, 1.5 billion adults aged 20 years or older were classified as overweight. Of these, nearly 200 million men and 300 million women were obese (World Health Organization [WHO], 2011). In the United States, 68% of adults and 17% of children are overweight (CDC, 2010a).

The 15.8 million children and adults in the United States (8.3% of the population) have diabetes, with 7 million of those people undiagnosed. Additional 79 million people are prediabetic. The majority of this population is 65 years or older (26.9%). Hispanic and African Americans are more likely to be diagnosed with diabetes (ADA, 2011b).

About 74.5 million people in the United States aged 20 years and older have high blood pressure (one in three adults). It is more common in people who are middle aged or older, overweight or obese, physically inactive, or have diabetes (AHA, 2011b).

Cause and Etiology

The cause of obesity is complex, but it is believed to result from various factors including genes, metabolism, behavior, environment, culture, and socioeconomic status. Behavior and environment play a large role in obesity and are the greatest areas for focus and treatment (CDC, 2010b). There are several factors that increase a person's risk for developing type 2 diabetes, including family history, ethnic background, age, overweight or obesity, physical inactivity, hypertension, smoking, and excessive alcohol consumption (AHA, 2011a). Risk factors for developing high blood pressure include family history, advanced age, gender-related risk patterns (more men than women until 45 years; more women than men after 64 years), lack of physical activity, poor diet (especially too much salt), overweight and obesity, and excessive alcohol consumption. Possible contributing factors include stress, smoking and second-hand smoke, and sleep apnea (AHA, 2011b).

Course and Signs and Symptoms

Insulin resistance and prediabetes are precursors to full-blown diabetes. In response to insulin resistance, the pancreas releases excessive amounts of insulin to keep blood sugar levels normal. Over time, the cells in the pancreas become defective and are unable to regulate blood sugar levels, causing prediabetes and, eventually, full-blown diabetes (AHA, 2011a). The symptoms of type 2 diabetes are as follows:

- Frequent urination
- Unusual thirst
- Extreme hunger
- Unusual weight loss
- Extreme fatigue and irritability
- Frequent infections
- Blurred vision
- Cuts/bruises that are slow to heal
- Peripheral neuropathy: tingling, numbness, or sensation loss in the hands or feet
- Recurring skin, gum, or bladder infections (ADA, 2011a)

Most people do not realize they have hypertension because they have little or no symptoms. People with advanced cases of hypertension may have the following symptoms:

- Severe headache
- Confusion
- Nausea
- Visual disturbances
- Seizure (AHA, 2011b)

Related Conditions

Obesity, diabetes, and hypertension can lead to serious health risks, such as heart disease, stroke, musculoskeletal disorders (osteoarthritis), and certain types of cancer (endometrial, breast, and colon) (WHO, 2011). Adult obesity is associated with psychosocial and societal problems, such as reduced quality of life, stigmatization, social isolation, and discrimination (CDC, 2010a, 2010b). Individuals who are obese may face limitations in performing daily activities, especially if they have medical complications such as diabetes or heart disease (American Occupational Therapy Association [AOTA], 2010). Over time, diabetes may damage and cause blindness, glaucoma, cataracts, kidney disease, neuropathy, and amputation, whereas chronic hypertension causes the walls of the arteries to stretch, resulting in vascular weakness and scarring (ADA, 2011a; AHA, 2010a). It also increases the risk of blood clots, plaque buildup, tissue or organ damage, and increases the workload on the circulatory system. Chronic hypertension can cause changes in the blood vessels in the retina, thickening of the heart muscle, kidney failure, and brain damage (AHA, 2011b).

Precautions

People who are obese are at a higher risk for developing depression (ADA, 2011b). People who are obese or overweight must pay special attention to their nutrition and lifestyle choices because they are more likely to develop heart disease and related conditions like diabetes or hypertension (AHA, 2011a). In addition, people with diabetes must take special care to keep their feet clean, dry, and free of cuts or wounds (ADA, 2011a). Other precautions include special attention to one's diet, participation in physical activity, and adherence to their medication schedule. People with hypertension should pay special attention to monitoring their blood pressure because they are at increased risk for stroke (AHA, 2011b).

Interdisciplinary Interventions

Many health care settings use a multidisciplinary team approach to provide intervention for people with chronic conditions such as overweight, obesity, diabetes, and hypertension. Team members may include physicians (bariatric, cardiologists, endocrinologists), nurses, dieticians, social workers, case managers, pharmacists, physical therapists, and occupational therapists (AOTA, 2010). The treatment of obesity usually focuses on shaping people's behavior choices so that they make healthier lifestyle choices (WHO, 2011). Common medications used to reduce weight include appetite suppressants, lipase inhibitors, and medications for depression. Surgical interventions include gastric bypass surgery and the LAP-BAND System (CDC, 2010b). Diabetes is treated by close monitoring of blood glucose levels, healthy lifestyle choices, and medications such as insulin, sulfonylureas, meglitinides, and biguanides (ADA, 2011a). Control and treatment for hypertension includes adopting a healthy lifestyle (nutrition and exercise) and taking medication such as diuretics, angiotensin-converting enzyme (ACE) inhibitors, beta-blockers, or angiotensin II receptor blockers (AHA, 2011b).

Occupational Therapy Evaluations

Along with observations, interviews, and history taking, the following assessments can be used to evaluate the ability of a person with a chronic illness to perform relevant occupations:

Participation and Activity

- Canadian Occupational Performance Measure (COPM) (Law et al., 2005): self-report of performance and satisfaction with occupations
- Health Status Questionnaire (SF-36): assesses patient's perceptions of health and physical limitations
- Activity Card Sort (ACS): helps clients describe instrumental and social activities
- Assessment of Occupational Functioning-Collaborative Version (AOF-CV): identifies factors likely to influence functional ability by looking at personal causation, values, roles, habits, and skills
- Occupational Performance History Interview II (OPHI II): gathers information about client's occupational adaptation over time by looking at critical life events, daily routines, and occupational roles
- Occupational Questionnaire (OQ): assesses time use patterns
- Occupational Profile of Sleep (Pierce & Summers, 2011)
- Stress diary

Basic and Instrumental Activity of Daily Living Skills

- Kohlman Evaluation of Living Skills (KELS): assesses the ability to live safely and independently in the community by looking at self-care, safety, work, and leisure
- Assessment of Motor and Process Skills (AMPS): assesses motor and process skill in context of performing familiar functional tasks

Client Factors

- Beck Depression Inventory-II (BDI-II): assesses the intensity of depression

Occupational Therapy Interventions

Occupational therapy (OT) practitioners can provide services to enhance the functional capabilities and self-management of individuals who have chronic conditions. Intervention can focus on the following:

- Activities of daily living (ADL), such as bathing, dressing, and toileting, especially for activities that require reach and flexibility
- Instrumental activities of daily living (IADL), such as cleaning, meal preparation, and child care
- The use of proper and safe, durable medical equipment
- Therapeutic exercises to increase strength for improved stamina and fitness
- Grading of functional tasks to gradually improve physical endurance
- Functional mobility, such as transfers out of bed and during bathing
- Safety in the home and community, especially in car transfers and moving in small spaces
- Home modifications to improve access to environment
- Task modifications to safely increase energy expenditure to enhance weight loss/management
- Establishment of healthy routines for food shopping and meal preparation
- Energy conservation
- Wellness groups for individuals and their families to support health promotion through lifestyle change (AOTA, 2010)

OT interventions specifically for clients with diabetes include the following:

- Patient and family education about monitoring of blood glucose levels, blood pressure, weight, and skin/foot health (including self-inspections)
- Techniques for medication management
- Protective or compensatory techniques for sensory loss in activities involving exposure to heat, cold, sharp, and so forth
- Interventions for secondary complications such as vision impairments, sensation loss, and amputations
- Education for techniques to structure time and prevent depression (Sokol-McKay, 2011)

Occupational Therapy and the Evidence

Occupational therapists support health promotion, disease prevention, and occupational performance in people who have chronic conditions, such as overweight and obesity, diabetes, and hypertension. Occupational therapists create individualized, client-centered interventions to address performance skills to enable people to engage in meaningful activities and occupations and identify barriers that may interfere with performance (Cozzolino, Henshaw, Kleumper, & Hermann, 2010; Sokol-McKay, 2011). They can assist and support lifestyle changes for individuals with obesity through interventions that focus on health promotion, prevention, remediation, adaptation, and maintenance (Clark, Reingold, & Salles-Jordan, 2007). The focus on living healthy lifestyles and managing weight can also be applied to the management of other chronic conditions such as diabetes and hypertension.

Specifically, occupational therapists help individuals with these conditions modify their lifestyle, control their weight, and engage in meaningful activities (Clark et al., 2007). Intervention approaches address health-related concerns, such as lifestyle change, weight control, and medication management. Client education, coupled with individualized and collaborative intervention planning, may promote effective health promoting routines and habit (Clark et al., 2007; Cohn et al, in press). Intervention also considers environmental adaptations or modifications that make engagement of meaningful activities of everyday life possible (Bondoc & Siebert, 2011; Forhan, Law, Vrkljan, & Taylor, 2010).

Caregiver Concerns

Caring for a family member with diabetes can be challenging. Special care must be paid to blood sugar monitoring, administration of medication, the nutritional content of food, and skin and foot care (Caswell, 2009). Caregivers of people with hypertension should be well informed of their loved one's physical, mental, and medical needs (Pulmonary Hypertension Association [PHA], 2011).

Resources

Organizations and Websites

- American Diabetes Association
  1701 North Beauregard Street
  Alexandria, VA 22311
  Website: http://www.diabetes.org

- American Heart Association
  7272 Greenville Ave.
  Dallas, TX 75231
  Website: http://www.heart.org

- The Obesity Society
  8757 Georgia Avenue, Suite 1320
  Silver Spring, MD 20910
  Website: http://www.obesity.org

- Pulmonary Hypertension Association
  801 Roeder Road, Ste. 1000
  Silver Spring, MD
  Website: http://www.phassociation.org

Journals

- *International Journal of Obesity*
- *International Journal of Pediatric Obesity*
- *Obesity*
- *Diabetes*
- *Diabetes Care*
- *Hypertension*

Books

- Becker, G. (2006). *The first year: Type 2 diabetes: An essential guide for the newly diagnosed.* Cambridge, MA: Da Capo Press.
  A clear, concise, step-by-step guide for living through your first year with diabetes.

- Lipsky, M., Mendelson, M., Havas, S., & Miller, M. (2008). *American Medical Association guide to preventing and treating heart disease: Essential information you and your family need to know about having a healthy heart.* Hoboken, NJ: Wiley.
  A comprehensive guide for learning about your heart and the importance of a healthy lifestyle, as well as critical warning signs.

- Chilnick, L. D. (2008). *The first year: Heart disease: An essential guide for the newly diagnosed.* Cambridge, MA: Da Capo Press.
  This book contains information about risk factors, circulatory system anatomy, and medications as well as a living section that addresses healthy lifestyle habits.

- Hurley, D. (2010). *Diabetes rising: How a rare disease became a modern pandemic, and what to do about it.* New York, NY: Kaplan.
  The author examines why both types of diabetes are rising, and what can be done to reverse the trend.

References

American Diabetes Association. (2011a). *Diabetes basics.* Retrieved from http://www.diabetes.org/diabetes-basics/

American Diabetes Association. (2011b). *Diabetes statistics.* Retrieved from http://www.diabetes.org/diabetes-basics/diabetes-statistics/

American Heart Association. (2011a). *Diabetes.* Retrieved from http://www.heart.org/HEARTORG/Conditions/Diabetes/Diabetes_UCM_001091_SubHomePage.jsp

American Heart Association. (2011b). *High blood pressure.* Retrieved from http://www.heart.org/HEARTORG/Conditions/HighBloodPressure/High-Blood-Pressure_UCM_002020_SubHomePage.jsp

American Occupational Therapy Association. (2010). *AOTA's Societal Statement on Obesity.* Retrieved from http://www.aota.org

Bondoc, S., & Siebert, C. (2011). *The role of occupational therapy in chronic disease management. AOTA fact sheet.* Retrieved from http://www.aota.org/Practitioners/PracticeAreas/Aging/Tools/Chronic-Disease-Management.aspx

Caswell, J. (2009). Caregivers and diabetes. *Stroke Connection.* Retrieved from http://www.nxtbook.com/nxtbooks/aha/strokeconnection_20091112/index.php#/10

Centers for Disease Control and Prevention. (2010a). *Morbidity and mortality weekly report: Vital signs: State-specific obesity prevalence among adults—United States, 2009.* Retrieved from http://www.cdc.gov/mmwr/preview/mmwrhtml/mm59e0803a1.htm

Centers for Disease Control and Prevention. (2010b). *Overweight and obesity.* Retrieved from http://www.cdc.gov/obesity/index.html

Clark, F., Reingold, F., & Salles-Jordan, K. (2007). Obesity and occupational therapy position paper. *American Journal of Occupational Therapy*, 61, 701–703.

Cohn, E., Cortés, D., Fix, G., Mueller, N., Soloman, J., & Bokhour, B. (in press). Habits and routines in the daily management of hypertension. *Journal of Health Psychology.*

Cozzolino, M., Henshaw, E., Kleumper, S., & Hermann, V. (2010). *Occupational therapy's role in bariatric care.* Retrieved from http://www.aota.org/Practitioners/PracticeAreas/Wellness/Tools/Bariatric.aspx

Forhan, M., Law, M., Vrkljan, B., & Taylor, V. (2010). The experience of participation in everyday occupations for adults with obesity. *Canadian Journal of Occupational Therapy, 77,* 210–218.

Law, M., Baptiste, S., Carswell, A., McColl, M., Polatajko, H., & Pollock, N. (2005). *Canadian Occupational Performance Measure* (4th ed.). Ottawa, Canada: CAOT Publications.

Pierce, D., & Summers, K. (2011). Rest and Sleep. In C. Brown & V. C. Stoffel (Eds.), Occupational Therapy in Mental Health (pp. 736–754). Philadelphia: F. A. Davis Company.

Pulmonary Hypertension Association (2011). *Caregivers.* Retrieved from http://www.phassociation.org/page.aspx?pid=870

Sokol-McKay, D. (2011). *Occupational therapy's role in diabetes self-management.* Retrieved from http://www.aota.org/Practitioners/PracticeAreas/Wellness/Tools/Diabetes.aspx?FT=.pdf

World Health Organization. (2011). *Obesity.* Retrieved from http://www.who.int/topics/obesity/en

Orthopedic Conditions

Pamela Vaughn

Description and Diagnosis

Orthopedic conditions pertain to the musculoskeletal system and include any injury, disease, or deformity of bones, joints, and their related structures (muscles, tendons, ligaments, nerves). Conditions that occupational therapists commonly encounter are fractures—particularly of the upper extremity and hip—and joint replacements (Javaherian, 2007). Orthopedic surgeons and physicians refer clients to occupational therapy (OT) after surgery or initial stabilization or diagnosis of the condition.

Incidence and Prevalence

- The number of annual fractures among children has increased over the past several decades and has a current prevalence of over 2% of children per year; the forearm and wrist are the most common fracture locations in children (Hedström, Svensson, Bergström, & Michno, 2010).
- Hip fractures among older adults have declined in recent years but still occur in approximately 1.5% to 3% of U.S. older adult population; the incidence increases with age (Stevens & Rudd, 2010).
- In the United States, total knee replacement (TKR) and total hip replacement (THR) surgeries have increased over the past two decades, with 25.9 TKRs and 11.7 THRs among adults aged 45 to 64 years per 10,000 population in the year 2006 to 2007; the figures increase to 82.1 and 33.3 per 10,000, respectively, among adults aged 65 years and older (National Center for Health Statistics, 2011).

Cause and Etiology

Falls are the leading cause of nonfatal injuries in the United States (Office of Statistics and Programming, National Center for Injury Prevention and Control, Centers for Disease Control and Prevention, 2009) and are the most common mechanism of fractures in children and adolescents (Hedström et al., 2010). Other common traumatic events that cause orthopedic conditions are motor vehicle accidents, sports injuries, and work-related accidents; cumulative trauma (e.g., stress fractures) can also result in these conditions. There may be circumstances in which clients, particularly children, sustained orthopedic injuries as a result of abuse; it is necessary to follow protocol for mandatory reporting if this is suspected (Javaherian, 2007).

Orthopedic conditions can be secondary to diseases, such as osteoarthritis and osteoporosis, or due to congenital anomalies as well (Javaherian, 2007; Maher & Bear-Lehman, 2008).

Typical Course, Symptoms, and Related Conditions

Because orthopedic conditions involve the musculoskeletal system, they tend to affect occupations that involve the use of that body part.

Fractures

Some fractures—including most hip fractures—require initial surgical repair to set the bone. Physical healing time depends on the location and extent of the injury and can last weeks to months (Maher & Bear-Lehman, 2008). Symptoms of a fracture typically include pain at the site of injury, swelling, bruising, deformity, and an inability to bear weight or experience pressure on the bone/joint (Javaherian, 2007). Individuals with osteoporosis are particularly at risk for fractures (Oyen et al., 2011).

Joint Replacements

A severe fracture or significant and lasting decrease in functionality—potentially caused by osteoarthritis—of a joint often indicate the need for joint replacement surgery (Javaherian, 2007). The prosthetic joint, made of metal and plastic and designed to perform like a healthy joint, can last for more than 10 years (American Academy of Orthopaedic Surgeons, 2007).

Interdisciplinary Interventions

Medication Therapy

Postoperative procedures, that is, pain management medications, antibiotics, and anticoagulants, are standardly used following joint replacement procedures.

Physical Therapy

General strengthening and range of motion (ROM) exercises to rehabilitate the affected and adjoining body structures are the focus of physical therapy interventions. The physical therapist will also train the client to properly use any ambulatory devices (crutches, walker, and/or cane) required for lower extremity conditions.

Occupational Therapy Evaluations

The evaluation process focuses on what the client needs, wants, or is expected to do and analyzes what factors make impact desired occupational performance. The evaluation begins with occupation-focused assessments followed by specific evaluation of the orthopedic condition on occupational performance.

Occupation-Based Assessments

- Role Checklist (Oakley, Kielhofner, Barris, & Reichler, 1986): assesses clients' participation in and value placed on occupational roles
- Occupational Performance History Interview II (OPHI-II) (Kielhofner et al., 2004): a semistructured interview used to gather occupational performance and participation over time
- Assessment of Motor and Process Skills (AMPS) (Fisher & Jones, 2010): assessment of skills in the context of performing functional tasks
- Activity Measure for Post-Acute Care (AM-PAC) (Jette, Hayley, Coster, & Ni, 2007): used in rehabilitation settings to assess mobility, daily activities, and cognition
- Performance Assessment of Self-Care Skills (PASS) (Holm & Rogers, 2008): an observational tool to assess client's functional mobility, personal care, and home management
- Canadian Occupational Performance Measure (COPM) (Law et al., 2005): a semistructured interview that elicits the client's self-assessment of performance and satisfaction in various areas of occupation over time
- Short Form-36 (SF-36) (Hays, Sherbourne, & Mazel, 1995): a standardized scale that measures health-related quality of life

Assessments of Client Factors

- Disability of Arm, Shoulder, and Hand (DASH) (Hudak, Amadio, Bombardier, & the Upper Extremity Collaborative Group, 1996): a standardized questionnaire that rates disability and symptoms related to upper extremity musculoskeletal disorders
- ROM
- Measures of pain (e.g., Visual Analog Scale [VAS])
- Manual muscle testing
- Measures of grasp and pinch strength
- Measures of edema

Occupational Therapy Interventions

The primary goal of OT intervention in orthopedics is to restore clients to occupational functioning. This takes different forms depending on the condition and stage of recovery. Proper precautions, for example, movement and weight-bearing restrictions after surgery, should be considered at all times and communicated regularly to clients (Maher & Bear-Lehman, 2008).

Acute Stage of Recovery

Following surgery or medical stabilization, occupational therapists help educate clients on safe and proper methods to keep their injury/surgery site clean and protected in order to facilitate healing. When medically cleared, occupational therapists evaluate client factors and therapeutic goals (e.g., current ROM and strength, desire to return to previous roles and occupations) and begin to help remediate the muscles and joints surrounding the site via controlled movement and strengthening exercises. Splints, braces, and slings may be used to provide the client with additional support and/or comfort throughout the healing and early rehabilitative process (Javaherian, 2007).

Activities of Daily Living Retraining

Occupational therapists develop and teach clients compensatory strategies for dressing, feeding, bathing, toileting, functional mobility, personal care, and participating in sexual activities. These compensatory strategies may include the use of adaptive devices (e.g., long-handled equipment, pump bottles), task modification, or environmental modification. Depending on the condition, these strategies will either be temporarily or permanently implemented (Maher & Bear-Lehmen, 2008).

Environmental Assessment and Fall Prevention

Just prior to or immediately following discharge after surgery, occupational therapists may visit the home or workplace of the client in order to perform an environmental assessment and, if necessary, recommend modifications to increase mobility and participation following injury. In the case of lower extremity conditions, suggestions for community mobility can be made (Maher & Bear-Lehman, 2008). Fall prevention education may be beneficial, particularly for older adults, in preventing exacerbation or a repeat of the current condition.

Occupational Therapy and the Evidence

OT in acute care settings for older adult clients with hip fractures has been shown to be effective in increasing recovery of ambulatory ability, improving functional recovery, decreasing length of stay in hospital, increasing lower extremity strength, and increasing fall-related self-efficacy (Chudyk, Jutai, Petrella, & Speechley, 2009). The use of the COPM was reported as an effective outcome measures with this population as well, although it should be noted that most clients do not return to the same level of function that they were at prior to injury (Edwards, Baptiste, Stratford, & Law, 2007).

Early mobilization following orthopedic injuries of upper extremity joints via ROM exercises has been shown to be somewhat effective in decreasing pain and swelling and facilitating quicker return to previous occupations (Amini, 2011; von der Heyde, 2011).

Caregiver Concerns

Nahm, Resnick, Orwig, Magaziner, and DeGrezia (2010) reported that caregivers of individuals with hip fractures reported the following:

- Concern about their loved ones now being in a state of frailty
- Feeling tired and overwhelmed by the demands placed on them as caregivers
- Frustration with the health care system—lack of communication from health care providers and rough transitions between stages of recovery (e.g., acute care to rehabilitation facility)
- Wanting more information and resources

Resources

Organizations

- American Association of Orthopaedic Surgeons: a research and advocacy organization for patients and health care practitioners in the field of orthopedics.
  6300 North River Road
  Rosemont, IL 60018
  Telephone: (847) 823-7186
  Fax: (847) 823-8125
  E-mail: orthoinfo@aaos.org
  Website: http://www.aaos.org

Books

- Cobb, V. (2008). *Your body battles a broken bone*. Minneapolis, MN: Millbrook Press.
  A children's book about broken bones and the healing process.
- McQuaig, J. (2010). *How strong is your titanium? The real life misadventures of a knee and hip replacement survivor*. Bloomington, IL: AuthorHouse.

Websites

- http://orthoinfo.aaos.org/

References

American Academy of Orthopaedic Surgeons. (2007). *Total joint replacements*. Retrieved from http://orthoinfo.aaos.org/topic.cfm?topic=A00233

Amini, D. (2011). Occupational therapy interventions for work-related injuries and conditions of the forearm, wrist, and hand: A systematic review. *American Journal of Occupational Therapy, 65*, 29–36. doi:10.5014/ajot.2011.09186

Chudyk, A. M., Jutai, J. W., Petrella, R. J., & Speechley, M. (2009). Systematic review of hip fracture rehabilitation practices in the elderly. *Archives of Physical Medicine and Rehabilitation, 90*, 246–262. doi:10.1016/j.apmr.2008.06.036

Edwards, M., Baptiste, S., Stratford, P. W., & Law, M. (2007). Recovery after hip fracture: What can we learn from the Canadian Occupational Performance Measure? *American Journal of Occupational Therapy, 61*, 335–344.

Fisher, A. G., & Jones, K. B. (2010). *Assessment of Motor and Process Skills. Vol. 1: Development, standardization, and administration manual* (7th ed.). Fort Collins, CO: Three Star Press.

Hays, R. D., Sherbourne, C. D., & Mazel, R. M. (1995). *User's manual for Medical Outcomes Study (MOS) core measures of health-related quality of life*. Santa Monica, CA: RAND.

Hedström, E. M., Svensson, O., Bergström, U., & Michno, P. (2010). Epidemiology of fractures in children and adolescents: Increased incidence over the past decade: A population-based study from northern Sweden. *Acta Orthopaedica, 81*, 148–153. doi:10.3109/17453671003628780

Holm, M. B., & Rogers, J. C. (2008). The Performance Assessment of Self-Care Skills (PASS). In B. Hemphill-Pearson (Ed.), *Assessments in occupational therapy mental health* (2nd ed., pp. 101–110). Thorofare, NJ: Slack.

Hudak, P. L., Amadio, P. C., Bombardier, C., & the Upper Extremity Collaborative Group. (1996). Development of an upper extremity outcome measure: The DASH (disabilities of the arm, shoulder, and hand) [corrected]. *American Journal of Industrial Medicine, 29*, 602–608. Erratum in: *American Journal of Industrial Medicine, 30*, 372.

Javaherian, H. G. (2007). Orthopaedics. In B. J. Atchison & D. K. Dirette (Eds.), *Conditions in occupational therapy: Effect on occupational performance* (3rd ed., pp. 341–355). Philadelphia, PA: Lippincott Williams & Wilkins.

Jette, A., Hayley, S. M., Coster, W., & Ni, P. (2007). *Boston University Activity Measure for Post Acute Care: Instruction manual*. Retrieved from http://www.crecare.com/order/order.html

Kielhofner, G., Mallinson, T., Crawford, C., Nowak, M., Rigby, M., Henry, A., & Walens, D. (2004). *Occupational Performance History Interview II (OPHI-II)*. Chicago, IL: MOHO Clearinghouse.

Law, M., Baptiste, S., Carswell, A., McColl, M., Polatajko, H., & Pollock, N. (2005). *Canadian Occupational Performance Measure* (4th ed.). Ottawa, Canada: CAOT Publications.

Maher, C., & Bear-Lehman, J. (2008). Orthopaedic conditions. In M. V. Radomski & C. A. T. Latham (Eds.), *Occupational therapy for physical dysfunction* (6th ed., pp. 1107–1130). Philadelphia, PA: Lippincott Williams & Wilkins.

Nahm, E., Resnick, B., Orwig, D., Magaziner, J., & DeGrezia, M. (2010). Exploration of informal caregiving following hip fracture. *Geriatric Nursing, 31*, 254–262. doi:10.1016/j.gerinurse.2010.01.003

National Center for Health Statistics. (2011). *Health, United Stated, 2010: With special feature on death and dying* (Department of Health and Human Services Publication No. 2011-1232). Retrieved from http://www.cdc.gov/nchs/hus/diseases.htm#chronic

Oakley, F., Kielhofner, G., Barris, R., & Reichler, R. (1986). The Role Checklist: Development and empirical assessment of reliability. *Occupational Therapy Journal of Research, 6*, 157–170.

Office of Statistics and Programming, National Center for Injury Prevention and Control, Centers for Disease Control and Prevention. (2009). *10 leading causes of nonfatal injury, United States*. Retrieved from http://www.cdc.gov/injury/wisqars/nonfatal.html

Oyen, J., Brudvik, C., Gjesdal, C., Tell, G., Lie, S., & Hove, L. (2011). Osteoporosis as a risk factor for distal radial fractures: A case-control study. *Journal of Bone & Joint Surgery, American Volume, 93*, 348–356. doi:10.2106/JBJS.J.00303

Stevens, J. A., & Rudd, R. A. (2010). Declining hip fracture rates in the United States. *Age and Ageing, 39*, 500–503. doi:10.1093/ageing/afq044

von der Heyde, R. L. (2011). Occupational therapy interventions for shoulder conditions: A systematic review. *American Journal of Occupational Therapy*, 65, 16–23. doi:10.5014/ajot.2011.09184

Parkinson's Disease

Theresa Griffin

Description

Parkinson's disease (PD) is a chronic, idiopathic, progressive neurodegenerative disorder of the central nervous system characterized by damage to dopamine-producing brain cells. The four primary symptoms include tremors at rest; bradykinesia; stiffness or rigidity of arms, legs, or trunk; and postural instability (National Parkinson Foundation, 2011). The average age of onset of PD is 60 years; however, estimates indicate the incidence has increased by 10% for those younger than the age of 40 years. Currently, 1.5 million Americans are living with PD, and there are 50,000 to 60,000 new cases of PD diagnosed each year (National Institute of Neurological Disorders and Stroke [NINDS], 2011).

Hoehn and Yahr Stages of Parkinson's Disease

Doctors categorize the severity of the disease based on the Hoehn and Yahr staging system, with stage 1 representing the earliest form and stage 5 representing the end stage.

- Stage 1: There are mild movement-related symptoms on one side of the body, but the individual is able to function without disability.

- Stage 2: Both sides of the body are affected by movement-related symptoms, but balance remains intact. Typically, there will be symptom improvement in response to medication.
- Stage 3: There is mild imbalance during walking or standing. The individual has moderately severe generalized dysfunction but typically remains physically independent.
- Stage 4: The motor symptoms are advanced and severe. There is a disabling instability while walking or standing, and the individual is no longer able to live alone. Changes in speech and swallowing are also apparent.
- Stage 5: The disease is severe and fully developed. The individual is unable to stand or walk and requires constant care (Hoehn & Yahr, 1967).

Interdisciplinary Interventions

Medications

There are three categories of medications for PD. The first category aims to increase the dopamine levels in the brain. For example, levodopa converts into dopamine in the brain; however, its benefits may become less stable as PD progresses (National Library of Medicine, 2011). The second category influences neurotransmitters to ease symptoms of PD. For example, an anticholinergic drug inhibits the uptake of acetylcholine, which helps to reduce tremors. Medication side effects from the first two categories can include orthostatic hypotension, cardiac arrhythmias, and dystonic movements. The third category of medication controls nonmotor symptoms such as depression (NINDS, 2011).

Surgery

Surgery is used for individuals with PD that has progressed to the point wherein medications are not effective. A pallidotomy destroys the globus pallidus in the brain, which reduces symptoms of tremor, bradykinesia, and rigidity and improves gait and balance. A thalamotomy involves the removal of part of the thalamus, which may reduce tremors. Deep brain stimulation, which is often used because it does not involve the removal of brain tissue, stops the symptoms of PD by exciting an electrode implanted in the brain (NINDS, 2011).

Therapies

Physical therapy focuses on improving activities of daily living (ADL), stride length, and walking speed (Ellis et al., 2005). Speech therapy focuses on improving voice and speech function (de Swart, Willemse, Maassen, & Horstink, 2003).

Occupational Therapy Evaluations

PD specific and some general occupational therapy (OT) assessments may be appropriate for evaluating reduced control of muscular movements, strength, endurance, speech, and psychosocial functions.

Participation and Activity Level

- Canadian Occupational Performance Measure (COPM): self-report of performance and satisfaction with occupations
- Parkinson's Disease Quality of Life Questionnaire-39 Item Version (PDQ-39): self-report that includes the following:
  - Assessment of problems with health and well-being during the last month
  - Eight subscales including mobility, ADL, emotional well-being, stigma, social support, cognition, communication, and bodily discomfort
- Unified Parkinson's Disease Rating Scale (UPDRS): a rating tool that follows the longitudinal course of PD and offers insight about disease progression
  - Categories include evaluation of mentation, behavior, and mood; self-evaluation of ADL; and clinician-scored motor evaluation
- Functional Independence Measure (FIM): assesses functional performance in self-care, transfers, locomotion, communication, and social cognition

Client Factor Level

- Hoehn and Yahr staging of PD
- Unified Parkinson's Disease Rating Scale Balance Test
- Range of motion (ROM) testing
- Manual muscle testing
- Rigidity testing
- Mini-Mental State Examination (MMSE): assesses cognition
- Geriatric Depression Scale (GDS): basic screening measure for depression in older adults
- Fatigue Severity Scale (FSS): self-report questionnaire evaluating the impact of fatigue

Occupational Therapy Intervention

OT intervention helps individuals with PD function optimally in daily life and enables individuals to participate in meaningful occupations (American Occupational Therapy Association, 2007).

Activities of Daily Living or Instrumental Activities of Daily Living

- Teach use of adaptive techniques and tools to reduce the effect of tremors (Lyons, 2003).
- Provide strategies to assist with medication routines.

Sensorimotor

- Facilitate joint movement, maintain ROM, and prevent contractures by stretching.
- Improve motor planning and increase speed by adding cues such as music with beats (Marchese, Diverio, Zucchi, Lentino, & Abbruzzese, 2000).

Psychosocial

- Group intervention can increase client functioning and perceptions of capabilities and self-esteem (Kimchi, Tamir, & Pessach, 2010).
- Educate in self-management skills, such as knowing how to respond to changing symptom displays, when to seek medical help, and how to improve self-efficacy (Lyons, 2003; Tickle-Degnen, Ellis, Saint-Hilaire, Thomas, & Wagenaar, 2010).
- Promote engagement in productive activities and leisure with suitable challenges (Sunvisson & Ekman, 2001).
- Encourage discussion of roles within the family and living unit.
- Educate the family about difficulties affecting social interaction, such as facial masking and oral rigidity (Lyons & Tickle-Degnen, 2003).

Environment

- Suggest home modifications for increased safety.
- Encourage client and family to participate in support groups.
- Help client and family explore the community for resources.

Caregiver Concerns

Caregivers may experience financial strains, fear of losing employment, depression, and social isolation. Additionally, when neuropsychiatric conditions such as dementia and depression co-occur with PD, there is an increase in caregiver burden (Stella, Banzato, Barasnevicius Quagliato, Aparecida Viana, & Christofoletti, 2009). Caregivers may need support to effectively manage this new role (Bhatia & Gupta, 2003). Frequent breaks and social support can decrease the effects of caregiver burden and improve caregiver quality of life (Goldsworthy & Knowles, 2008).

Occupational Therapy and the Evidence

Because disability can advance in this progressive disease even with optimal pharmacological treatment, OT has a role in rehabilitation anywhere along the continuum of care. Recognizing this, it is important to consider what therapeutic techniques and OT interventions may be effective in supporting individuals living with PD. Evidence supports the use of external cueing during functional tasks, such as sit to stand (Mak & Hui-Chan, 2004), reaching (Ma, Trombly, Tickle-Degnen, & Wagenaar, 2004), and walking (Rochester et al., 2004), indicating that this may be an effective technique to use in order to help individuals reach their therapeutic goals. Meek et al. (2010) determined that a large portion of OT interventions developed to optimize independence involved goals related to equipment provision and environmental adaptations; mobility, transfer, and ADL training; and review, discussion, and teaching of new techniques. Additionally, these goals correspond with the OT outcomes of functional independence and mobility that Clarke et al. (2009) found to be the most relevant for optimizing independence in individuals with PD.

Multidisciplinary interventions are used with individuals throughout the progression of PD to address various motor and nonmotor outcomes; yet, research does not substantiate an impact on motor outcomes. Johnston and Chu's (2010) review of available literature indicates that motor outcomes will continue to decline over time despite the use of multidisciplinary intervention. However, Tickle-Degnen et al. (2010) found that an interdisciplinary self-management rehabilitation program may improve health-related quality of life. Additionally, they hypothesized that the self-management strategies and skills could continue to help individuals manage changes in their lives as the PD progressed. Therefore, motor problems may remain constant or continue to decline with intervention, but despite motor challenges, an individual's health and well-being can improve over time. These findings suggest that a self-management program should be considered in early to middle stages of PD to improve and sustain health-related quality of life. Ultimately, Tickle-Degnen et al. (2010) recognized that a theory- and evidence-based self-management program that takes a client-centered, goal-directed approach leads to successful rehabilitation outcomes. It is important to keep in mind that PD can affect facial, gestural, and vocal expression of motivation. Therefore, to be client-centered, OT practitioners should vary their emotional tone when questioning clients with PD and assessing motivation (Takahashi, Tickle-Degnen, Coster, & Latham, 2010).

Resources

Associations

- American Parkinson Disease Association, Inc.
  135 Parkinson Ave
  Staten Island, NY 10305
  Telephone: 800-223-2732
  Website: http://www.apdaparkinson.org
  An association dedicated to funding PD research. They offer medical information, as well as public or professional education and support services.

- Michael J. Fox Foundation for Parkinson's Research
  Church Street Station
  PO Box 780
  New York, NY 10163
  Telephone: 800-708-7644
  Website: http://www.michaeljfox.org/
  A foundation dedicated to finding a cure for PD by funding current research. This foundation is also interested in the development of improved therapies.

- National Parkinson Foundation
  1501 N.W. 9th Avenue
  Bob Hope Road
  Miami, Florida 33136-1494
  Telephone: 800-327-4545
  Website: http://www.parkinson.org
  A nationwide network of chapters and support groups that offer patient services, clinical studies and research, and public and professional education.

Books

- Fox, M. J. (2002). *Lucky man.* New York, NY: Hyperion.
  An autobiography chronicling Fox's life; he shares his first symptoms of PD and what life is like living with PD.

- Havemann, J. (2002). *A life shaken: My encounter with Parkinson's disease.* Baltimore, MD: Johns Hopkins University Press.
  A true story with scientific and medical information interwoven with the personal story of a man with PD.

- Newsom, H. (2002). *Hope: Four keys to a better quality of life for Parkinson's people.* Mercer Island, WA: The Northwest Parkinson's Foundation.
  Personal guidelines and tips on how to live with PD by a man who has PD.

Journals

- *Archives of Neurology*
- *Journal of Gerontology*
- *Journal of Neurology, Neurosurgery, and Psychiatry*
- *Movement Disorders*
- *Neurology*
- *Parkinsonism and Rehabilitation*

Websites

- Parkinson's Disease Foundation (PDF)
  http://www.pdf.org
  This is a national foundation that focuses on research, education, and advocacy for PD. One of the primary goals of the foundation's Website is to disseminate accurate, accessible information about PD to individuals with the disease and their families.

- Parkinson's Resource Organization
  http://www.parkinsonsresource.org
  This organization helps families affected by PD by offering emotional and educational support programs, providing information and referral services, promoting public awareness, and publishing a monthly newsletter about family issues.

References

American Occupational Therapy Association. (2007). *Living with Parkinson's disease.* Retrieved from http://www.aota.org/Consumers/consumers/Health-and-Wellness/Parkinsons/35188.aspx

Bhatia, S., & Gupta, A. (2003). Impairments in activities of daily living in Parkinson's disease: Implications for management. *NeuroRehabilitation, 18,* 209–214.

Clarke, C., Furmston, A., Morgan, E., Patel, S., Sackley, C., Walker, M., . . . Wheatley, K. (2009). Pilot randomised controlled trial of occupational therapy to optimise independence in Parkinson's disease: The PD OT trial. *Journal of Neurology, Neurosurgery & Psychiatry, 80*(9), 976–978.

de Swart, B. J. M., Willemse, S. C., Maassen, B. A. M., & Horstink, M. W. I. M. (2003). Improvement of voicing in patients with Parkinson's disease by speech therapy. *Neurology, 60,* 498–500.

Ellis, T., de Goede, C. J., Feldman, R. G., Wolters, E. C., Kwakkel, G., & Wagenaar, R. C. (2005). Efficacy of a physical therapy program in patients with Parkinson's disease: A randomized controlled trial. *Archives of Physical Medicine and Rehabilitation, 86,* 626–632.

Goldsworthy, B., & Knowles, S. (2008). Caregiving for Parkinson's disease patients: An exploration of a stress-appraisal model for quality of life and burden. *The Journals of Gerontology Series B Psychological Sciences and Social Sciences, 63,* P372–P376.

Hoehn, M. M., & Yahr, M. D. (1967). Parkinsonism: Onset, progression and mortality. *Neurology, 17,* 427–442.

Johnston, M., & Chu, E. (2010). Does attendance at a multidisciplinary outpatient rehabilitation program for people with Parkinson's disease produce quantitative short term or long term improvements? A systematic review. *NeuroRehabilitation, 26*(4), 375–383. doi:10.3233/NRE-2010-0575

Kimchi, O., Tamir, R., & Pessach, L. (2010). "Think big" and "feel big" with Parkinson's disease. *Israel Journal of Occupational Therapy, 19*(3–4), E79–E80.

Lyons, K. D. (2003). Self-management of Parkinson's disease: Guidelines for program development and evaluation. *Physical & Occupational Therapy in Geriatrics, 21*, 17–31.

Lyons, K. D., & Tickle-Degnen, L. (2003). Dramaturgical challenge of Parkinson's disease. *Occupational Therapy Journal of Research, 23*, 27–34.

Ma, H., Trombly, C., Tickle-Degnen, L., & Wagenaar, R. (2004). Effect of one single auditory cue on movement kinematics in patients with Parkinson's disease. *American Journal of Physical Medicine & Rehabilitation, 83*, 530–536.

Mak, M., & Hui-Chan C. (2004). Audiovisual cues can enhance sit-to-stand in patients with Parkinson's disease. *Movement Disorders, 19*, 1012–1019.

Marchese, R., Diverio, M., Zucchi, F., Lentino, C., & Abbruzzese, G. (2000). The role of sensory cues in the rehabilitation of Parkinson patients: A comparison of two physical therapy protocols. *Movement Disorders, 15*, 879–883.

Meek, C., Morgan, E., Walker, M., Furmston, A., Aragon, A., Birleson, A., . . . Sackley, C. (2010). Occupational therapy to optimize independence in Parkinson's disease: The designing and recording of a randomized controlled trial intervention. *British Journal of Occupational Therapy, 73*, 178–185.

National Institute of Neurological Disorders and Stroke. (2011). *Parkinson's disease: Hope through research.* Retrieved from http://www.ninds.nih.gov/disorders/parkinsons_disease/detail_parkinsons_disease.htm#171663159

National Library of Medicine. (2011). *Levodopa and carbidopa.* Retrieved from http://www.nlm.nih.gov/medlineplus/druginfo/meds/a601068.html#why

National Parkinson Foundation. (2011). *What is Parkinson's disease?* Retrieved from http://www.parkinson.org/Parkinson-s-Disease/PD-101/What-is-Parkinson-s-disease

Rochester, L., Hetherington, V., Jones, D., Nieuwboer, A., Willems, A., Kwakkel, G., & Van Wegen, E. (2004). Attending to the task: Interference effects of functional tasks on walking in Parkinson's disease and the roles of cognition, depression, fatigue, and balance. *Archives of Physical Medicine & Rehabilitation, 85*, 1578–1585.

Stella, F., Banzato, C., Barasnevicius Quagliato, E., Aparecida Viana, M., & Christofoletti, G. (2009). Psychopathological features in patients with Parkinson's disease and related caregivers' burden. *International Journal of Geriatric Psychiatry, 24*(10), 1158–1165.

Sunvisson, H., & Ekman, S. (2001). Environmental influences on the experiences of people with Parkinson's disease. *Nursing Inquiry, 8*, 41–50.

Takahashi, K., Tickle-Degnen, L., Coster, W., & Latham, N. (2010). Expressive behavior in Parkinson's disease as a function of interview context. *American Journal of Occupational Therapy, 64*, 484–495.

Tickle-Degnen, L., Ellis, T., Saint-Hilaire, M., Thomas, C., & Wagenaar, R. (2010). Self-management rehabilitation and health-related quality of life in Parkinson's disease: A randomized controlled trial. *Movement Disorders, 25*, 194–204. doi:10.1002/mds.22940

Peripheral Nerve Injury

Pamela Vaughn

Description and Diagnosis

Peripheral nerve injury (PNI) is any injury that affects the nerves outside of the brain and spinal cord, including nerve roots, ganglia, plexi, autonomic nerves, and sensory and motor nerves. A *mononeuropathy* is when one nerve is affected; *polyneuropathies* involve multiple nerves. Examples of PNIs include carpal tunnel and brachial plexus injuries (e.g., Erb's palsy). PNIs are diagnosed via neurological examinations that may also include the use of magnetic resonance imaging (MRI), electromyography (EMG), computed tomography (CT) scans, or nerve conduction velocity (NCV) tests to determine location, cause, extent, and type of injury (National Institute of Neurological Disorders and Stroke [NINDS], 2004).

Incidence and Prevalence

Approximately 60,000 Americans experience upper extremity PNIs per year (Lad, Nathan, Schubert, & Boakye, 2010). Injuries to upper extremity nerves (i.e., ulnar, brachial plexus, median, and radial) account for 70% to 80% of PNIs, followed by lower extremity nerve (~20%) and facial nerve injury (Ciaramitaro et al., 2010; Kouyoumdjian, 2006; Lad et al., 2010; Scholz et al., 2009). The 1.68% of individuals who experience a limb trauma develop PNIs within 90 days (Taylor, Braza, Rice, & Dillingham, 2008). Males account for the around 70% of clients with PNI (Ciaramitaro et al., 2010; Kouyoumdjian, 2006; Lad et al., 2010), and incidence is highest among emerging young and middle adults (Ciaramitaro et al., 2010; Kouyoumdjian, 2006; Lad et al., 2010; Taylor et al., 2008).

Cause and Etiology

Seddon (1943) divided nerve injuries into three classifications (as outlined in Campbell, 2008, p. 1952):

- Neurapraxia—"the nerve is intact but cannot transmit impulses"
- Axonotmesis—"the axon is damaged or destroyed, but most of the connective tissue framework is maintained"
- Neurotmesis—"the nerve trunk is disrupted and not in anatomical continuity. Most of the connective tissue framework is lost or badly distorted"

Among the many causes of PNI are traumas (automobile and motorcycle accidents, penetrations [e.g., deep cuts], falls, dislocations, burns, etc.), repetitive stress (e.g., at work or in sports), and anesthetization; automobile accidents account for the largest percentage of PNIs (Ciaramitaro et al., 2010; Kouyoumdjian, 2006). Common mechanisms of injury include stretch, compression, section, and ischemia (Campbell, 2008).

Typical Course, Symptoms, and Related Conditions

The nature, severity, and time until onset of symptoms depends on the nature of the injury, but symptoms (often anatomically distal to the site of injury) may include one or more of the following:

- Numbness
- Tingling
- Burning sensation
- Muscle weakness
- Sensitivity to touch
- Pain (NINDS, 2004)

The more severe the injury, the longer it will take for maximal outcomes due to intervention to be reached (Scholz et al., 2009). As long as the nerve cell has not died, regeneration, repair, and symptom alleviation to some extent is possible, although full recovery may not occur (Martinez de Albornoz, Delgado, Forriol, & Maffulli, 2011; NINDS, 2004). Due to the occupational limitations that many individuals with PNI experience, high levels of disability after injury are reported (Novak, Anastakis, Beaton, Mackinnon, & Katz, 2011).

Although not considered to be injuries, neuropathies caused by illnesses (e.g., diabetes), infections (e.g., shingles), and so forth may present with the same or similar symptoms as PNI.

Interdisciplinary Interventions

Medication Therapy and Other Medical Interventions

Scholz et al. (2009) report that surgeons are able to surgically, directly repair just under 80% of PNIs and perform other surgical techniques (e.g., nerve graft, nerve transplants) in ~18% of patients but are unable to surgically repair injuries in ~2.5%. For clients who experience pain due to their PNI, medications such as over-the-counter analgesics or injections of local anesthetics can be used (NINDS, 2004).

Physical Therapy

Although evidence is mixed regarding efficacy, physical therapy after PNI focuses on strengthening muscles and maintaining range of motion (ROM) of joints affected by the injured nerve as well as on facilitating nerve regeneration with techniques such as phototherapy and electrical stimulation (Deumens et al., 2010).

Occupational Therapy Evaluations

The evaluation process focuses on what the client needs, wants, or is expected to do and analyzes what factors may impact desired occupational performance. The evaluation begins with occupation-focused assessments followed by specific evaluation of the potential impact of PNI on occupational performance.

Occupation-Focused Assessments

- Role Checklist (Oakley, Kielhofner, Barris, & Reichler, 1986): assesses client's participation in and value placed on occupational roles
- Occupational Performance History Interview II (OPHI-II) (Kielhofner et al., 2004): a semistructured interview used to gather occupational performance and participation over time
- Assessment of Motor and Process Skills (AMPS) (Fisher & Jones, 2010): assessment of skills in the context of performing functional tasks
- Activity Measure for Post-Acute Care (AM-PAC) (Jette, Hayley, Coster, & Ni, 2007): used in rehabilitation settings to assess mobility, daily activities, and cognition
- Performance Assessment of Self-Care Skills (PASS) (Holm & Rogers, 2008): an observational tool to assess client's functional mobility, personal care, and home management
- Canadian Occupational Performance Measure (COPM) (Law et al., 2005): a semistructured interview that elicits the client's self-assessment of performance and satisfaction in various areas of occupation over time
- Short Form-36 (SF-36) (Hays, Sherbourne, & Mazel, 1995): a standardized scale that measures health-related quality of life
- Activity Card Sort (ACS) (Baum & Edwards, 2008): a tool to help clients describe instrumental activities of daily living (IADL), leisure, and social activities.

Client Factor Assessments

- Disabilities of the Arm, Shoulder, and Hand (DASH) Outcome Measure (Hudak, Amadio, Bombardier, & the Upper Extremity Collaborative Group, 1996): a standardized questionnaire that rates disability and symptoms related to upper extremity musculoskeletal disorders
- Various sensory tests (e.g., two-point discrimination tests, Moberg Pickup Test [Ng, Ho, & Chow, 1999])
- ROM
- Measures of pain (e.g., Visual Analog Scale [VAS])
- Measures of muscle strength, grasp, and pinch strength

Occupational Therapy Interventions

Sensory Reeducation

Sensory reeducation is a commonly used technique, particularly in hand therapy, in which therapists assist clients to "relearn" tactile sensations that, as a result of the injury, were no longer recognized by the clients—Dellon's (1988) clinical example was of patients with upper extremity PNI who could not correctly identify coins using only touch sensation in their hands. The neurological mechanism that facilitates this relearning is the retraining of the cortical map that correlates with touch sensation in the affected part of the body (Oud, Beelen, Eijffinger, & Nollet, 2007).

Hand Therapy

When PNI occurs in the distal upper extremity, occupational therapists trained in hand therapy use splinting to maintain correct anatomical positioning during the initial stages of recovery. Later, therapists can use occupation-based strategies (e.g., handwriting, holding and using kitchen utensils to cook a meal) to strengthen muscles and tendons of the hand for functional use (Guzelkucuk, Duman, Taskaynatan, & Dincer, 2007).

Prevention

Occupational therapists can educate clients in preventive measures—such as proper ergonomics, work station adjustments, and body mechanics—to reduce the likelihood of incurring PNI due to misuse or repetitive stress (Shiri et al., 2011).

Consultation

Because individuals with PNI report a temporary decrease in participation in employment, activities of daily living (ADL), and IADL as well as a prolonged decrease in participation in leisure activities (Novak et al., 2011), occupational therapists can assist clients in the process of finding new and alternative occupations to increase and enhance their participation after injury (Meiners, Coert, Robinson, & Meek, 2005).

Occupational Therapy and the Evidence

Although limited, the evidence regarding sensory reeducation after PNI shows that this technique results in improved functional sensation in the upper limb (Oud et al., 2007). Amini (2011) reports that many intervention approaches commonly used in occupational therapy for clients with upper extremity injuries and conditions, including PNI, show positive outcomes—for example, decreased pain, increased function—including the use of sensory reeducation, and that occupation-based interventions resulted in improvements in affected areas of occupation.

Resources

Organizations

- Foundation for Peripheral Neuropathy (FPN)
  485 Half Day Road
  Suite 200
  Buffalo Grove, IL 60089
  Telephone: 877-883-9942
  E-mail: info@tffpn.org
  http://www.foundationforpn.org/
  FPN is an educational resource for clients and professionals and raises funds to further research of neuropathy.

Books

- Berman, S. I. (2007). *Coping with peripheral neuropathy: How to handle stress, disability, anxiety, fatigue, depression, pain, and relationships.* New York, NY: iUniverse.
- Cushing, M., & Latov, N. (2009). *You can cope with peripheral neuropathy: 365 tips for living a full life.* New York, NY: Demos Medical.

Websites

- http://www.neuropathy.org

References

Amini, D. (2011). Occupational therapy interventions for work-related injuries and conditions of the forearm, wrist, and hand: A systematic review. *American Journal of Occupational Therapy, 65,* 29–36. doi:10.5014/ajot.2011.09186

Baum, C. M., & Edwards, D. E. (2008). *Activity Card Sort* (2nd ed.). Bethesda, MD: AOTA Press.

Campbell, W. W. (2008). Evaluation and management of peripheral nerve injury. *Clinical Neurophysiology, 119,* 1951–1965. doi:10.1016/j.clinph.2008.03.018

Ciaramitaro, P., Mondelli, M., Logullo, F., Grimaldi, S., Battiston, B., Sard, A., . . . Cocito, D. (2010). Traumatic peripheral nerve injuries: Epidemiological findings, neuropathic pain and quality of life in 158 patients. *Journal of the Peripheral Nervous System, 15,* 120–127.

Dellon, A. L. (1988). *Evaluation of sensibility and re-education of sensation in the hand*. Baltimore, MD: Lucas.

Deumens, R., Bozkurt, A., Meek, M. F., Marcus, M. A. E., Joosten, E. A. J., Weis, J., & Brook, G. A. (2010). Repairing injured peripheral nerves: Bridging the gap. *Progress in Neurobiology, 92*, 245–276. doi:10.1016/j.pneurobio.2010.10.002

Fisher, A. G., & Jones, K. B. (2010). *Assessment of Motor and Process Skills. Vol. 1: Development, standardization, and administration manual* (7th ed.). Fort Collins, CO: Three Star Press.

Guzelkucuk, U., Duman, I., Taskaynatan, M. A., & Dincer, K. (2007). Comparison of therapeutic activities with therapeutic exercises in the rehabilitation of young adult patients with hand injuries. *Journal of Hand Surgery, 32*, 1429–1435.

Hays, R. D., Sherbourne, C. D., & Mazel, R. M. (1995). *User's manual for Medical Outcomes Study (MOS) core measures of health-related quality of life*. Santa Monica, CA: RAND.

Holm, M. B., & Rogers, J. C. (2008). The Performance Assessment of Self-Care Skills (PASS). In B. Hemphill-Pearson (Ed.), *Assessments in occupational therapy mental health* (2nd ed., pp. 101–110). Thorofare, NJ: Slack.

Hudak, P. L., Amadio, P. C., Bombardier, C., & the Upper Extremity Collaborative Group (1996). Development of an upper extremity outcome measure: The DASH (disabilities of the arm, shoulder, and hand) [corrected]. *American Journal of Industrial Medicine, 29*, 602–608. Erratum in: *American Journal of Industrial Medicine, 30*, 372.

Jette, A., Hayley, S. M., Coster, W., & Ni, P. (2007). *Boston University Activity Measure for Post Acute Care: Instruction manual*. Retrieved from http://www.crecare.com/order/order.html

Kielhofner, G., Mallinson, T., Crawford, C., Nowak, M., Rigby, M., Henry, A., & Walens, D. (2004). *Occupational Performance History Interview II (OPHI-II)*. Chicago, IL: MOHO Clearinghouse.

Kouyoumdjian, J. A. (2006). Peripheral nerve injuries: A retrospective survey of 456 cases. *Muscle & Nerve, 34*, 785–788. doi:10.1002/mus.20624

Lad, S. P., Nathan, J. K., Schubert, R. D., & Boakye, M. (2010). Trends in median, ulnar, radial, and brachioplexus nerve injuries in the United States. *Neurosurgery, 66*, 953–960. doi: 10.1227/01.NEU.0000368545.83463.91

Law, M., Baptiste, S., Carswell, A., McColl, M., Polatajko, H., & Pollock, N. (2005). *Canadian Occupational Performance Measure* (4th ed.). Ottawa, Canada: CAOT Publications.

Martinez de Albornoz, P., Delgado, P. J., Forriol, F., & Maffulli, N. (2011). Non-surgical therapies for peripheral nerve injury. *British Medical Bulletin*. Advance online publication. doi:10.1093/bmb/ldr005

Meiners, P. M., Coert, J. H., Robinson, P. H., & Meek, M. F. (2005). Impairment and employment issues after nerve repair in the hand and forearm. *Disability and Rehabilitation, 27*, 617–623.

National Institute of Neurological Disorders and Stroke. (2004). *Peripheral neuropathy fact sheet* (National Institutes of Health Publication No. 04-4853). Retrieved from http://www.ninds.nih.gov/disorders/peripheralneuropathy/detail_peripheralneuropathy.htm

Ng, C. L., Ho, D. D., & Chow, S. P. (1999). The Moberg pickup test: Results of testing with a standard protocol. *Journal of Hand Therapy, 12*, 309–312.

Novak, C. B., Anastakis, D. J., Beaton, D. E., Mackinnon, S. E., & Katz, J. (2011). Biomedical and psychosocial factors associated with disability after peripheral nerve injury. *The Journal of Bone and Joint Surgery, 93*, 929–936. doi:10.2106/JBJS.J.00110

Oakley, F., Kielhofner, G., Barris, R., & Reichler, R. (1986). The Role Checklist: Development and empirical assessment of reliability. *Occupational Therapy Journal of Research, 6*, 157–170.

Oud, T., Beelen, A., Eijffinger, E., & Nollet, F. (2007). Sensory re-education after nerve injury of the upper limb: A systematic review. *Clinical Rehabilitation, 21*, 483–494.

Scholz, T., Krichevsky, A., Sumarto, A., Jaffurs, D., Wirth, G. A., Paydar, K., & Evans, G. R. D. (2009). Peripheral nerve injuries: An international survey of current treatments and future perspectives. *Journal of Reconstructive Microsurgery, 25*, 339–344. doi:10.1055/s-0029-1215529

Seddon, H. (1943). Three types of nerve injury. *Brain, 66*, 237–288.

Shiri, R., Martimo, K. P., Miranda, H., Ketola, R., Kaila-Kangas, L., Liira, H., . . . Viikari-Juntura, E. (2011). The effect of workplace intervention on pain and sickness absence caused by upper-extremity musculoskeletal disorders. *Scandinavian Journal of Work Environment & Health, 37*, 120–128. doi:10.5271/sjweh.3141

Taylor, C., Braza, D., Rice, J., & Dillingham, T. (2008). The incidence of peripheral nerve injury in extremity trauma. *American Journal of Physical Medicine & Rehabilitation, 87*, 381–385.

Prematurity

Samantha Slocum

Description and Diagnosis

Infants who are born prior to 37 weeks of gestation are considered premature and often referred to as preterm infants or "preemies" (Lee, 2010). Babies who are born preterm are at risk for a wide range of serious health problems and medical complications as a result of low birth weights and underdeveloped organs (March of Dimes, 2010). Premature infants typically receive care in the neonatal intensive care unit (NICU) until they are strong and stable enough to go home (Lee, 2010; March of Dimes, 2010; Torpy, 2003).

Incidence and Prevalence

Approximately 12% of infants (500,000) born in the United States each year are preterm (March of Dimes, 2010). Certain risk factors may increase the likelihood of delivering prematurely including previous preterm births, birth defects of the infant, and maternal uterine or cervical abnormalities (Lee, 2010; March of Dimes, 2010; Nemours Foundation, 2011). Premature births are more likely to occur in women who are African American, younger than 17 years or older than 35 years, and of low socioeconomic status (Lee, 2010; March of Dimes, 2010).

Cause and Etiology

The cause of premature birth is often unknown, and various factors could lead to prematurity. Early labor may be induced intentionally as a result of pregnancy complications or health problems; however, most premature births result from spontaneous preterm labor (March of Dimes, 2010). Multiple pregnancies (twins, triplets, etc.) are a major cause of prematurity, accounting for approximately 15% of all preemies. Other health conditions and pregnancy-related issues that may increase the likelihood of preterm labor include diabetes, heart disease, infections (especially of amniotic membranes or urinary tract), use of drugs or alcohol, lack of prenatal care, poor nutrition before and during pregnancy, stress, preeclampsia, placenta previa, obesity, working for long hours, and being underweight (Lee, 2010; March of Dimes, 2010; Nemours Foundation, 2011).

Typical Course, Symptoms, and Related Conditions

As a result of medical advancements, the survival rate of preterm infants has increased significantly; of babies born at 28 weeks or later, 90% survive. Some premature infants develop typically and have no long-term health complications caused by their prematurity. However, most preemies will likely present with transient developmental differences because they will be exposed to unique extrauterine experiences at gestational ages in which full-term infants would experience in utero. These differences vary but may include thin and wrinkled skin with a transparent appearance, soft body hair known as lanugo—covering the face and body, difficulty breathing due to underdeveloped lungs, less activity and lower muscle tone than full-term infants, feeding difficulties, and decreased body fat (Lee, 2010; March of Dimes, 2010). Once premature infants reach the age of 2 years, they are expected to reach the typical growth patterns and developmental milestones of full-term infants.

Related conditions that a premature infant may experience include the following:

- Difficulty maintaining body temperature (Lee, 2010; Torpy, 2003)
- Bradycardia: low heart rate (Torpy, 2003)
- Respiratory distress syndrome (RDS): difficulty breathing caused by the absence of pulmonary surfactant, a detergent-like protein that prevents the collapse of air sacs
- Apnea: interruption or cessation of breathing
- Intraventricular hemorrhage (IVH): bleeding in the brain
- Patent ductus arteriosus (PDA): heart condition resulting from an arterial duct not closing properly after birth
- Necrotizing enterocolitis (NEC): intestinal problem that may lead to feeding problems and abdominal swelling
- Retinopathy of prematurity (ROP): damage to retinas that may lead to visual impairment
- Jaundice
- Anemia
- Infections (Lee, 2010; March of Dimes, 2010)

Long-term complications of prematurity may include delayed growth and development, mental or physical disabilities or delays (e.g., mental retardation, cerebral palsy, learning disabilities, behavior problems), chronic lung disease, continuing health/medical complications, and hearing or visual impairments (Lee, 2010; March of Dimes, 2010; Torpy, 2003).

Precautions

It is important to closely monitor a preemie's vital signs and be aware of possible abnormalities; some irregularities may affect respiratory, cardiovascular, visual, and auditory functioning. Feeding problems, as a result of swallowing and sucking difficulties due to immaturity, and hypoglycemia are also common in premature infants (Lee, 2010).

Interdisciplinary Interventions

Medical Interventions

- Body temperature: Incubators and warming pads may be used to keep temperature within a normal range, which is crucial to development (Lee, 2010; Nemours Foundation, 2011).
- Nutrition and growth: Most preemies cannot feed directly from breast or bottle until after 32 weeks, so feeding tubes may be placed through the nose or mouth to the stomach. In very preterm or sick infants, nutrition may also be provided intravenously (Lee, 2010; Nemours Foundation, 2011).
- Breathing and lungs: Mechanical ventilation, continuous positive airway pressure (CPAP), or oxygen delivered through nasal prongs or an oxygen hood may be used (Lee, 2010).
- Continuous monitoring of vital signs (Lee, 2010)
- Synthetic surfactant may be given to premature infants experiencing breathing difficulties and has been shown to be effective to prevent respiratory distress syndrome (RDS) as well as in reducing pneumothorax and death in preemies (Soll, 2009).
- Sucrose (sugar) given to babies, often on pacifiers, during painful procedures, such as needles or heel pricks, has been shown to be effective in decreasing pain, crying time, and behaviors such as grimacing (Stevens, Yamada, & Ohlsson, 2010). Local analgesics may also be used for pain prevention.

Interdisciplinary Interventions

Care in the NICU is family centered and focuses on caregivers as well as the premature infant. Most of the care and treatment provided in the NICU is interdisciplinary and, therefore, role crossover is very common. A preemie's interdisciplinary care team may include physical therapy (to address mobility needs and assist with improving lung function), speech therapy (to address feeding and swallowing needs), respiratory therapy (to provide equipment and monitoring devices to help with breathing), and nursing (to provide constant care and monitoring). Skin-to-skin care, also known as *kangaroo care*, has been found to be very successful in keeping infants warm and content, decreasing stress, and promoting development among other benefits (Vergara & Bigsby, 2004; Zieve, 2009).

Occupational Therapy Evaluations

- Neurobehavioral Assessment of the Preterm Infant (NAPI): assesses neurobehavioral maturity for stable preemies functioning in range of 32 to 42 weeks (Stanford School of Medicine, 2011)
- Naturalistic Observations of Newborn Behaviors (NONB): for infants who are too fragile for handling (Vergara & Bigsby, 2004)
- Assessment of Preterm Infant Behavior (APIB): for stable preterm infants (<30 to 32 weeks) (Als, Butler, Kosta, & McAnulty, 2005)
- NICU Network Neurobehavioral Scale (NNNS): assesses neurological and behavioral function of stable preterm infants (Lester & Tronick, 2004)
- Neurologic Assessment of the Preterm and Full-Term Newborn Infant (NAPFI): assesses function of the nervous system in infants who can tolerate handling (Dubowitz, Dubowitz, & Mercuri, 1999)

Occupational Therapy Interventions

Occupational therapists in the NICU focus on promoting and enabling preemies to engage in the expected neonatal and infant occupations. Because the safety and comfort of the preemie should be taken into consideration first and foremost, interventions may be implemented by the member of the transdisciplinary team who is available at the most appropriate time (March of Dimes, 2010; Vergara & Bigsby, 2004).

Several of the following interventions fall into the category of developmental care, targeted to minimize the impact of stressors in the NICU environment on the preemie: environmental modulation, positioning, cue-based care, and so forth. Programs such as the Newborn Individualized Developmental Care and Assessment Program (NIDCAP) are designed to use a combination of developmental care strategies, individualized to the needs of each preemie (Symington & Pinelli, 2009).

- *Family and caregiver support and education*: Occupational therapists may teach parents appropriate handling and holding techniques, ways to position and interact with their baby as well as read and understand the preemie's cues and reactions to the environment to reduce stress (Vergara & Bigsby, 2004; Zieve, 2009).
- *Monitoring sensory environment*: Establishing a NICU environment that resembles the intrauterine environment as closely as possible and protects the infant from the aversive sensory stimulation of the NICU is most appropriate to promote neurobehavioral, motor, and sensory development of preemies and minimize stress. Eliminating excessive stimulation when possible, minimizing handling, clustering care activities, and providing longer rest periods are important to decrease stress for the infant. Aspects of the environment that should be considered are lighting, sound, temperature, humidity, and movement. Modifications of the environment and sensory stimulation should be constantly assessed and modified to provide individualized, developmentally supportive care that compliments the infant's age, medical status and stability, and state of readiness (Symington & Pinelli, 2009; Vergara & Bigsby, 2004).
- *Therapeutic positioning*: Crucial for infants to foster growth and development, reduce the risk of acquired positional deformities, and allow for neurobehavioral organization. Positioning should be comfortable and secure with extremities flexed and toward the midline to promote hand-to-mouth activity. This position will also help the infant feel calm, peaceful, and organized. Use of soft-rolled blankets create a secure "nest" that closely resembles the intrauterine environment. Positioning should be individualized and based on infant cues (Hellman, 2009).
- *Promote infant suck reflex*: For nipple feeding and oral-motor skills. The occupational therapist can provide alternative feeding strategies,

equipment, methods, techniques, feeding position, or changing the type or flow rate of liquid (Lee, 2010; Vergara & Bigsby, 2004).

- *Early intervention*: Long-term risks or disabilities as a result of prematurity may indicate the need for early intervention services once the premature infant has been discharged home (Vergara & Bigsby, 2004).

Occupational Therapy and the Evidence

Individualized developmentally supportive care has been shown to be effective in improving various outcomes for premature infants in the NICU. Modification of external stimuli, specifically when congruent with the intrauterine environment at the gestational age of the preemie, may improve short-term growth outcomes, decreased lengths of stay, and enhanced neurodevelopmental outcomes such as organization and self-regulation. Some research has shown that preemies receiving NIDCAP required less respiratory support (McAnulty et al., 2009; Symington & Pinelli, 2009). McAnulty et al. (2009) also found that NIDCAP resulted in decreased morbidity, as well as improved posture, motility, quality of life, and response rate in preemies. There is also some evidence that shows NIDCAP interventions provide long-term effects. Children who received NIDCAP as preemies showed better medical outcomes, behavioral functioning (organization and self-regulation), and motor responses at 8 years of age (McAnulty et al., 2010). Overall, individualized developmental care for preemies in the NICU has been shown to provide beneficial short- and long-term outcomes for premature infants (McAnulty et al., 2009; Symmington & Pinelli, 2009).

Caregiver Concerns

Premature infants will likely spend a significant amount of time in the NICU, and this experience can be physically and emotionally stressful for caregivers. It is important for caregivers to become familiar with the specific needs of their infant and be aware of the subtle cues, signs, and symptoms their preemie gives. It is also helpful for caregivers to learn as much as they can about their baby's condition, medications, and care schedule. Involvement in his or her care in the NICU will promote increased knowledge and preparedness for when the preemie is discharged. Caregivers need to understand that their preemie may be difficult to console. The needs and delays of a preterm infant may continue to change and develop as they age. Keeping in touch with other families from the NICU or joining support groups may also be beneficial (March of Dimes, 2010; Vergara & Bigsby, 2004).

Resources

Organizations

- March of Dimes (National Office)
  1275 Mamaroneck Avenue
  White Plains, NY 10605
  Telephone: (914)-997-4488
  Website: http://www.marchofdimes.com
  Local chapter contact information may be obtained from the Website.

- The American Academy of Pediatrics
  141 Northwest Point Boulevard
  Elk Grove Village, IL 60007
  Telephone: (847)-434-4000
  Fax: (847)-434-4000
  Website: http://www.aap.org

Books

- Davis, D. L., & Stein, M. T. (2004). *Parenting your premature baby and child: The emotional journey*. Golden, CO: Fulcrum.
  This book provides information and suggestions on all aspects of raising a premature infant from birth to long-term parenting. It focuses on experiences, feelings, and relationships.

- Davis, H., & Davis, P. (2011). *The story of Katie Rose: A preemie's journey*. Berkeley, CA: Never Surrender Productions.
  This book is a first-hand account of one preemie's journey, targeted for siblings of preterm infants. The book details the complexities of preterm birth, life in the NICU, and bringing home a preemie in clear and simple language for children to understand.

- Vergara, E. R., & Bigsby, R. (2004). *Developmental and therapeutic interventions in the NICU*. Baltimore, MD: Brookes.
  This book is a great resource for practitioners. It uses easy-to-understand terminology and provides various information and techniques to use when working with preterm infants in the NICU.

Journals

- *Pediatrics*
- *Physical and Occupational Therapy in Pediatrics*
- *Infants and Young Children*

Websites

- March of Dimes (http://www.marchofdimes.org)—This Website provides news, events, and resources to support caregivers of preterm infants as well as professionals. It provides an online community for families of preemies to connect and support each other. This Website has a wide range of information on prematurity facts and what to expect when caring for a preterm infant.

- Premature Baby, Premature Child (http://www.prematurity.org)—This Website provides resources for parents and caregivers of preterm infants and children. It offers information on raising preemies as well as connections with other families of premature children and resources such as books, research, and personal stories.

Occupational Therapy Resources

- AOTA's NICU Knowledge and Skills Paper: A thorough outline of the advanced skills and knowledge necessary to provide quality care to preemies and their families in the NICU. Available from the AOTA Website.

References

Als, H., Butler, S., Kosta, S., & McAnulty, G. (2005). The Assessment of Preterm Infants' Behavior (APIB): Furthering the understanding and measurement of neurodevelopmental competence in preterm and full-term infants. *Mental Retardation and Developmental Disabilities Research Reviews, 11*, 94–102. doi:10.1002/mrdd.20053

Dubowitz, L. M., Dubowitz, V., & Mercuri, E. (1999). The neurological assessment of the pre-term & full-term newborn infant. *Clinics in Developmental Medicine, 148*, 1–172.

Hellman, J. (2009). *Premature babies: Overview of treatment*. Retrieved from http://www.aboutkidshealth.ca/En/ResourceCentres/PrematureBabies/OverviewofTreatment/Pages/default.aspx

Lee, K. (2010). *Premature infant*. Retrieved from http://www.nlm.nih.gov/medlineplus/ency/article/001562.htm

Lester, B. M., & Tronick, E. (2004). The neonatal intensive care unit network neurobehavioral scale procedures. *Pediatrics, 113*, 641–667.

March of Dimes. (2010). *Your premature baby*. Retrieved from http://www.marchofdimes.com/baby/premature_indepth.html

McAnulty, G. B., Duffy F. H., Butler, S. C., Bernstein, J. H., Zurakowski, D. & Als, H. (2010). Effects of the newborn individualized developmental care and assessment program (NIDCAP) at age 8 years: Preliminary data. *Clinical Pediatrics, 49*, 258–270. doi:10.1177/0009922809335668

McAnulty, G. B., Duffy, F. H., Butler, S., Parad, R., Ringer, S., Zurakowski, D., & Als, H. (2010). Individualized developmental care for a large sample of very preterm infants: health, neurobehavior and neurophysiology. *Acta Paediatrica, 98*, 1920–1926. doi:10.1111/j.1651-2227.2009.01492.x

Nemours Foundation. (2011). *Primer on preemies*. Retrieved from http://kidshealth.org/parent/growth/growing/preemies.html#

Soll, R. (2009). Synthetic surfactant for respiratory distress syndrome in preterm infants [Review]. *The Cochrane Database of Systematic Reviews*, (1), 1–27. doi:10.1002/14651858.CD001149

Stanford School of Medicine. (2011). *Neurobehavioral Assessment of the Preterm Infant (NAPI)*. Retrieved from http://med.stanford.edu/NAPI/

Stevens, B., Yamada, J., & Ohlsson, A. (2010). Sucrose for analgesia in newborn infants undergoing painful procedures (review). *The Cochrane Database of Systematic Reviews*, (1), 1–112. doi:10.1002/14651858.CD001069.pub3

Symington, A. J., & Pinelli, J. (2009). Developmental care for promoting development and preventing morbidity in preterm infants [Review]. *The Cochrane Database of Systematic Reviews*, (1), 1–72. doi:10.1002/14651858.CD001814.pub2

Torpy, J. M. (2003). Care of premature infants. *The Journal of the American Medical Association, 289*, 796.

Vergara, E. R., & Bigsby, R. (2004). *Developmental and therapeutic interventions in the NICU*. Baltimore, MD: Brookes.

Zieve, D. (2009). *NICU consultants and support staff* (National Institutes of Health). Retrieved from http://www.nlm.nih.gov/medlineplus/ency/article/007249.htm

Pulmonary Conditions

Pamela Vaughn

Description and Diagnosis

Any condition or disease that affects or is located in the lungs is considered a pulmonary condition. Examples include chronic obstructive pulmonary disease (COPD), which includes both emphysema and chronic bronchitis, asthma, cystic fibrosis, pneumonia, and tuberculosis. Of these conditions, occupational therapists are most likely to encounter clients with COPD.

- COPD: a condition in which airflow blockages that create breathing-related problems; includes emphysema and/or chronic bronchitis
- Emphysema: a type of COPD characterized by permanent damage to the alveoli (air sacs that are responsible for the carbon dioxide–oxygen exchange) in the lungs, resulting in shortness of breath and difficulty exhaling
- Chronic bronchitis: a type of COPD characterized by the inflammation (and eventual scarring) of the lining of the bronchial tubes, producing thick mucus and restricting airflow. Chronic bronchitis is diagnosed when a person has a mucus-producing cough most days of the month, 3 months of a year for two successive years without other underlying disease to explain the cough (American Lung Association [ALA], 2011; Centers for Disease Control and Prevention [CDC], 2011; National Heart Lung and Blood Institute [NHLBI], 2010).

When an individual presents with symptoms, a physician will perform tests to determine whether the symptoms are caused by COPD or other conditions (e.g., heart failure or asthma). Tests may include lung function tests (e.g., spirometry to measure the volume and velocity of exhaled air), computed tomography (CT) scans, chest X-rays, and arterial blood gas level tests (NHLBI, 2010).

Prevalence

- In 2009, more than 2% of U.S. adults aged 18 years and older (n = 4.9 million) were living with a diagnosis of emphysema.
- In 2009, more than 4% of U.S. adults aged 18 years and older (n = 9.9 million) were living with a diagnosis of chronic bronchitis (Pleis, Ward, & Lucas, 2010).
- Chronic lower respiratory diseases are the fourth leading cause of death in the United States. The death rate of people with these diseases has remained stable over the past decade at just more than 5% of all deaths annually; with a growing population, this indicates that the number of deaths due to COPD is increasing annually (National Center for Health Statistics, 2011).

Cause and Etiology

Almost all cases of COPD are due to long-term exposure to and inhalation of lung irritants. The most common COPD-causing irritant in the United States is cigarette smoke, although other forms of tobacco smoke (e.g., cigar, pipe) can cause the disease as well. The risk of developing COPD is greater with first-hand inhalation than second-hand exposure, but both modes are common. Examples of other substances that can cause COPD with long-term inhalation are air pollution, dust, and chemical fumes. Individuals who have the genetic condition alpha-1 antitrypsin (AAT) deficiency—a condition in which the body produces low levels of a lung-protective protein—have an increased risk of developing COPD, especially if they smoke (NHLBI, 2010).

Typical Course, Symptoms, and Related Conditions

There are four stages of COPD (I to IV, corresponding with mild, moderate, severe, and very severe COPD) according to the extent to which airflow is limited based on spirometry. The symptoms at each stage vary between individuals. In the mild stage, clients may not even be aware that their lung functioning is atypical. Most often, the symptoms develop slowly and may not initially interfere with daily activity. Some individuals may attribute symptoms to having a cold, ageing, or being physically out of shape (Eckert, 2007).

Symptoms of Chronic Obstructive Pulmonary Disease (NHLBI, 2010)

Initial	• Persistent cough or a cough that produces large amounts of mucus • Shortness of breath ("dyspnea"), particularly during and after physical activity • Wheezing • Chest tightness
With disease progression	• Edema in the ankles, feet, or legs • Weight loss and muscle atrophy • Decreased endurance, fatigue • Bluish-colored lips and/or fingernails • Severe and constant dyspnea that inhibits even talking • Rapid heartbeat • Decreased alertness

As a result of COPD, many individuals contract colds, the flu, or other illnesses frequently. In addition, clients will experience decreases in occupational performance and participation—because of lack of energy, inability to increase respiratory rate to keep up with activities, and so forth—often leading to decreased quality of life and self-efficacy. Even eating becomes exhausting (Huntley, 2008). Many clients develop a comorbid diagnosis of depression. Other common comorbid conditions include hypertension, high cholesterol, and osteoporosis (Barr et al., 2009).

Interdisciplinary Interventions

Pulmonary rehabilitation is a comprehensive and multidisciplinary individualized therapeutic and educational program that educates clients about their pulmonary condition and teaches both physical and psychosocial strategies and techniques to live functionally with the condition. Smoking cessation programs are often one aspect of pulmonary rehab. Occupational therapists play an integral role on the multidisciplinary team. Other team members may include respiratory therapists, thoracic surgeons, physicians, nurses, physical therapists, psychologists, social workers, nutritionists, and so forth (Ries et al., 2007).

Medication Therapy

Inhalers containing bronchodilators and/or anti-inflammatory drugs are commonly prescribed for COPD. These are used either on a maintenance level to control symptoms or on an as-needed basis when symptoms are acutely exacerbated. To combat the potential contraction of illnesses, antibiotics may be prescribed as well (Eckert, 2007; Garvey, 2011).

Oxygen Therapy

When lung function declines to the point that an individual is no longer able to consistently inhale sufficient oxygen to meet the body's needs and meet the demands of activities, oxygen supplementation may be used. A physician or respiratory therapist will work with a client to determine the best form of supplemental oxygen to meet his or her lifestyle needs. Forms include compressed oxygen containers, liquid oxygen containers, and oxygen concentrators. These come in various sizes and can be stationary or portable (Garvey, 2011).

Surgery

Some clients may be candidates for lung surgery. Types of surgery used include lung transplants, lung volume reduction (removes damaged portions to increase ventilation ability), and removal of damaged or diseased alveoli (Garvey, 2011).

Occupational Therapy Evaluations

The evaluation process focuses on what the client needs, wants, or is expected to do and analyzes what factors may impact desired occupational performance. The evaluation begins with occupation-focused assessments followed by specific evaluation of the potential impact of pulmonary conditions on occupational performance.

Occupation-Focused Assessments

- Role Checklist (Oakley, Kielhofner, Barris, & Reichler, 1986)
- Occupational Performance History Interview II (OPHI-II) (Kielhofner et al., 2004)
- Occupational Self-Assessment (OSA) Version 2.2 (Baron, Kielhofner, Iyenger, Goldhammer, & Wolenski, 2006)
- Performance Assessment of Self-Care Skills (PASS) (Holm & Rogers, 2008)
- Canadian Occupational Performance Measure (COPM) (Law et al., 2005)
- Short Form-36 (SF-36) (Hays, Sherbourne, & Mazel, 1995)
- Activity Card Sort (ACS) (Baum & Edwards, 2008)

Client Factor Assessments

- Chronic Respiratory Disease Questionnaire Self-Administered Standardized (CRQ-SAS) (Schünemann et al., 2003)
- Beck Depression Inventory-II (BDI-II) (Beck, Steer, & Brown, 1996)
- Borg Rating of Perceived Exertion (RPE) scale (Borg, 1998)
- Range of motion (ROM)
- Measures of pain (e.g., Visual Analog Scale [VAS])
- Measures of muscle strength
- Monitoring of vital signs (particularly respiratory rate and blood oxygen saturation)

Occupational Therapy Interventions

Separately or as part of a pulmonary rehab team, occupational therapists provide interventions to assist clients in maintaining or increasing their occupational performance and participation while living with pulmonary conditions. Depending on the clients' needs and desires, intervention may include the following:

- Teaching energy conservation techniques: to minimize respiratory exertion; may include environmental adaptations, breathing techniques, and so forth
- Retraining in activities of daily living (ADL): for example, grading activities to optimize participation without causing excessive strain; using assistive devices, if necessary
- Upper extremity strength and ROM training: Some medications for pulmonary conditions weaken muscles. Because clients with these conditions often use their shoulder girdle muscles to assist in inhalation, maintaining strength in these muscles is necessary.
- Educating client and family members about the risk factors of respiratory conditions and measures to be taken to remain healthy and functional (i.e., smoking cessation)
- Lifestyle modification: for example, identify new or alternate occupations that allow client to participate satisfactorily without exacerbating the pulmonary condition
- Environmental assessment, particularly if supplemental oxygen is prescribed
- Medication management
- Recommendations of support groups and resources within the community (Eckert, 2007; Huntley, 2008)

Occupational Therapy and the Evidence

In a qualitative study on the lived experience of clients with COPD, participants revealed that they needed to change their occupations (i.e., ADL, instrumental activities of daily living [IADL], and leisure) to accommodate for their symptoms and that they often viewed this change as a loss. However, many techniques learned and suggestions garnered in therapy helped them maintain or return to occupational satisfaction (Kerr & Ballinger, 2010).

Occupational therapy (OT) interventions (or multidisciplinary pulmonary rehab including OT) has been shown to increase physical function, quality of life, and independence and efficiency in ADL and IADL and to decrease dyspnea in clients with COPD (Chan, 2004; Puhan et al., 2009; Vincent, Stephenson, Omli, & Vincent, 2008). OT for COPD also can result in improvements in social functioning, overall physical health, and psychological health (Hand, Law, & McColl, 2011). Pulmonary rehab provides clients with a positive support system and relevant social outlet (Halding, Wahl, & Heggdal, 2010).

Caregiver Concerns

As COPD increases in severity, client reliance on friends and family members increases as well. This often results in caregivers experiencing decreased quality of life and/or depression, feeling burdened with the task of assisting their loved ones to complete occupations, and becoming one of the client's only emotional and social outlets. Caregivers need to be supported and educated regarding the best ways to help their loved ones while still keeping themselves physically and emotionally healthy (Caress, Luker, Chalmers, & Salmon, 2009).

Resources

Organizations

- American Association of Cardiovascular and Pulmonary Rehabilitation
  401 North Michigan Avenue, Suite 2200
  Chicago, IL 60611
  Telephone: 312-321-5146
  E-mail: aacvpr@aacvpr.org
  Website: http://www.aacvpr.org

- American Lung Association
  1301 Pennsylvania Ave. NW, Suite 800
  Washington, DC 20004
  Telephone: 202-785-3355
  E-mail: info@lungusa.org
  Website: http://www.lungusa.org

- American Thoracic Society
  25 Broadway, 18th Floor
  New York, NY 10004
  Telephone: 212-315-8600
  E-mail: atsinfo@thoracic.org
  Website: http://www.thoracic.org

- COPD Foundation
20 F Street NW, Suite 200-A
Washington, DC 20001
Telephone: 866-731-COPD (2673) (general office); 866-316-COPD (COPD information line)
E-mail: info@copdfoundation.org
Website: http://www.copdfoundation.org

Books

- Martin, R. D. (2010). *The complete guide to understanding and living with COPD: From a COPDer's perspective*. Rye Brook, NY: EveryBreath, LLC.
- Vogel, L. G. (2004). *Huffin' n' puffin': Living with COPD*. West Conshohocken, PA: Infinity.

Websites

- Global Initiative for Chronic Obstructive Lung Disease (GOLD)
http://www.goldcopd.org/
- National Heart Lung and Blood Institute (NHLBI; part of National Institutes of Health [NIH])
http://www.nhlbi.nih.gov/

References

American Lung Association. (2011). *Chronic obstructive pulmonary disease (COPD) fact sheet*. Retrieved from http://www.lungusa.org/lung-disease/copd/resources/facts-figures/COPD-Fact-Sheet.html

Baron, K., Kielhofner, G., Iyenger, A., Goldhammer, V., & Wolenski, J. (2006). *Occupational Self-Assessment* (OSA; Version 2.2.). Chicago, IL: MOHO Clearinghouse.

Barr, R. G., Celli, B. R., Mannino, D. M., Petty, T., Rennard, S. I., Sciurba, F. C., . . . Turino, G. M. (2009). Comorbidities, patient knowledge, and disease management in a national sample of patients with COPD. *The American Journal of Medicine, 122*, 348–355. doi:10.1016/j.amjmed.2008.09.042

Baum, C. M., & Edwards, D. E. (2008). *Activity Card Sort* (2nd ed.). Bethesda, MD: AOTA Press.

Beck, A. T., Steer, R. A., & Brown, G. K. (1996). *Beck Depression Inventory-Second edition manual*. San Antonio, TX: PsychCorp.

Borg, G. (1998). *Borg's Perceived Exertion and Pain Scale*. Champaign, IL: Human Kinetics.

Caress, A., Luker, K., Chalmers, K., & Salmon, M. (2009). A review of the information and support needs of family carers of patients with chronic obstructive pulmonary disease. *Journal of Clinical Nursing, 18*, 479–491. doi:10.1111/j.1365-2702.2008.02556.x

Centers for Disease Control and Prevention. (2011). *Chronic obstructive pulmonary disease*. Retrieved from http://www.cdc.gov/copd/

Chan, S. C. C. (2004). Chronic obstructive pulmonary disease and engagement in occupation. *American Journal of Occupational Therapy, 58*, 408–415.

Eckert, J. (2007). Cardiopulmonary disorders. In B. J. Atchison & D. K. Dirette (Eds.), *Conditions in occupational therapy: Effect on occupational performance* (3rd ed., pp. 195–218). Philadelphia, PA: Lippincott Williams & Wilkins.

Garvey, C. (2011). Best practices in chronic obstructive pulmonary disease. *The Nurse Practitioner, 36*, 16–22. doi:10.1097/01.NPR.0000396473.61188.11

Halding, A., Wahl, A., & Heggdal, K. (2010). 'Belonging'. 'Patients' experiences of social relationships during pulmonary rehabilitation. *Disability & Rehabilitation, 32*, 1272–1280. doi:10.3109/09638280903464471

Hand, C., Law, M., & McColl, M. A. (2011). Occupational therapy interventions for chronic diseases: A scoping review. *American Journal of Occupational Therapy, 65*, 428–436. doi:10.5014/ajot.2011.002071

Hays, R. D., Sherbourne, C. D., & Mazel, R. M. (1995). *User's manual for Medical Outcomes Study (MOS) core measures of health-related quality of life*. Santa Monica, CA: RAND.

Holm, M. B., & Rogers, J. C. (2008). The Performance Assessment of Self-Care Skills (PASS). In B. Hemphill-Pearson (Ed.), *Assessments in occupational therapy mental health* (2nd ed., pp. 101–110). Thorofare, NJ: Slack.

Huntley, N. (2008). Cardiac and pulmonary diseases. In M. V. Radomski & C. A. T. Latham (Eds.), *Occupational therapy for physical dysfunction* (6th ed., pp. 1295–1320). Philadelphia, PA: Lippincott Williams & Wilkins.

Kerr, A., & Ballinger, C. (2010). Living with chronic lung disease: An occupational perspective. *Journal of Occupational Science, 17*, 34–39.

Kielhofner, G., Mallinson, T., Crawford, C., Nowak, M., Rigby, M., Henry, A., & Walens, D. (2004). *Occupational Performance History Interview II (OPHI-II)*. Chicago, IL: MOHO Clearinghouse.

Law, M., Baptiste, S., Carswell, A., McColl, M., Polatajko, H., & Pollock, N. (2005). *Canadian Occupational Performance Measure* (4th ed.). Ottawa, Canada: CAOT Publications.

National Center for Health Statistics. (2011). *Health, United Stated, 2010: With special feature on death and dying*. (Department of Health and Human Services Publication No. 2011-1232). Retrieved from http://www.cdc.gov/nchs/hus/diseases.htm#chronic

National Heart Lung and Blood Institute. (2010). *COPD*. Retrieved from http://www.nhlbi.nih.gov/health/dci/Diseases/Copd/Copd_WhatIs.html

Oakley, F., Kielhofner, G., Barris, R., & Reichler, R. (1986). The Role Checklist: Development and empirical assessment of reliability. *Occupational Therapy Journal of Research, 6*, 157–170.

Pleis J. R., Ward B. W., & Lucas J. W. (2010). Summary health statistics for U.S. adults: National Health Interview Survey, 2009. National Center for Health Statistics. *Vital and Health Statistics, 10*(249), 1–217.

Puhan, M. A., Gimeno-Santos, E., Scharplatz, M., Troosters, T., Walters, E. H., & Steurer J. (2009). Pulmonary rehabilitation following exacerbations of chronic obstructive pulmonary disease. *Cochrane Database of Systematic Reviews*, (1). doi:10.1002/14651858.CD005305.pub2

Ries, A. L., Bauldoff, G. S., Carlin, B. W., Casaburi, R., Emery, C. F., Mahler, D. A., . . . Herrerias, C. (2007). Pulmonary rehabilitation: Joint ACCP/AACVPR evidence-based clinical practice guidelines. *CHEST, 131*, 4S–42S. doi:10.1378/chest.06-2418

Schünemann, H. J., Griffith, L., Jaeschke, R., Goldstein, R., Stubbing, D., Austin, P., & Guyatt, G. H. (2003). A comparison of the original Chronic Respiratory Questionnaire with a standardized version. *CHEST, 124*, 1421–1429.

Vincent, H. K., Stephenson, M. L., Omli, M. R., & Vincent, K. R. (2008). Clinical outcomes following postacute comprehensive rehabilitative care in patients with cardiopulmonary disease. *Clinical Reviews in Physical and Rehabilitation Medicine, 20*, 127–158. doi:10.1615/CritRevPhysRehabilMed.v20.i2.30

Schizophrenia and Schizoaffective Disorder

Alissa Bonjuklian

Description

Schizophrenia is a mental illness that typically occurs in late adolescence or adulthood and may affect an individual's perceptions and behaviors in all facets of life. Disturbed thought patterns or psychotic symptoms leading to severe difficulties in social or occupational functioning must be present for a minimum of 6 months for diagnosis.

Schizoaffective disorder is a mental illness in which schizophrenia-like symptoms are present for at least 2 weeks and are accompanied by abnormal mood patterns, such as mood swings or prolonged depression or mania (American Psychiatric Association [APA], 2000).

Prevalence

- The lifetime prevalence rate of schizophrenia is 0.87%.
- The lifetime prevalence rate of schizoaffective disorder is 0.32% (Perala et al., 2007).

Etiology and Risk Factors

The cause of schizophrenia is a debated topic; yet, it is generally attributable to various genetic, biological, and environmental risk factors during brain development. However, the specific genes responsible for schizophrenia have not yet been identified. Later environmental stressors, such as urbanicity, cannabis use, or exposure to trauma, coupled with early risk factors, are more associated with the development of positive psychotic symptoms, such as hallucinations and delusions (Dominguez, Saka, Lieb, Wittchen, & van Os, 2010).

Symptoms

Characteristic symptoms of schizophrenia include delusions, hallucinations, disorganized speech (e.g., frequent derailment or incoherence), grossly disorganized or catatonic behavior, and negative symptoms, for example, affective flattening, alogia, or avolition. Characteristic symptoms of schizoaffective disorder include the symptoms of schizophrenia, with the addition of any of the following:

- Major depressive episode, which may include depressed mood for most of the day, diminished interest or pleasure in activities, weight loss or gain, change in sleep pattern, or feelings of worthlessness or guilt
- Manic episode, which may include inflated self-esteem or grandiosity, decreased need for sleep, increased talkativeness, increased distractibility, or excessive involvement in pleasurable activities with high potential for painful consequences
- Mixed episode, which is characterized by criteria met for both a major depressive and manic episode nearly every day for at least 1 week (APA, 2000)

Precautions

- Suicide
- Cigarette smoking
- Cannabis use
- Weight gain

Interdisciplinary Interventions

The treatment of schizophrenia requires various approaches. Psychiatrists, psychologists, nurses, case managers, social workers, occupational therapists, and other health care professionals make unique contributions to the recovery process based on their training and expertise. Combining pharmacological and psychosocial intervention yields the most effective outcomes in improving clients' overall functioning and quality of life (Dixon, Perkins, & Calmes, 2009).

Medication

Antipsychotic medications are prescribed by psychiatrists to manage symptoms and help clients establish a stable base to benefit from other interventions. The first generation of drugs, conventional neuroleptic agents, were introduced in the 1950s; these drugs are referred to as "typical" antipsychotics. A second generation of antipsychotic tranquilizing medications were developed in the 1990s; these drugs are referred to as "atypical." Both generations of drugs act as antagonists of dopamine in the frontal context and limbic system, impacting behavior and affect. The atypical drugs are less likely to cause problematic extrapyramidal motor control side effects. The advantages and disadvantages of the two categories are debated, and although atypical are preferred, typical agents may be more appropriate for some clients. "Medication selection is informed by current symptoms, co-occurring conditions, the client's medication history, concurrent treatments, and preferences" (Dixon, Perkins, et al., 2009, p. 2).

Commonly prescribed first generation drugs include the following:

- Chlorpromazine
- Molindone
- Perphenazine
- Haloperidol

Commonly prescribed second generation drugs include the following:

- Amisulpride
- Aripiprazole
- Clozapine
- Olanzapine
- Quetiapine
- Risperidone
- Ziprasidone

Side effects are common among both generations of medications, which may include the following:

- Metabolic changes (weight gain)
- Extrapyramidal symptoms (tardive dyskinesia, akinesia, or other movement disorders)
- Sedation or drowsiness
- Cardiac effects (hypertension or hypotension)
- Anticholinergic symptoms (blurred vision, dry mouth, constipation, urinary retention) (Dixon, Perkins, et al., 2009)

Because schizoaffective disorder is characterized by abnormal mood patterns in addition to psychotic symptoms, these individuals are often prescribed a supplementary mood stabilizer. A newer atypical antipsychotic, paliperidone, has been found to be particularly helpful in managing both the psychosis- and mood-related symptoms of schizoaffective disorder (Canuso, Turkoz, Fu, & Bossie, 2010).

Occupational Therapy Evaluation

Activities of Daily Living or Instrumental Activities of Daily Living

- Independent Living Scales (ILS)
- Independent Living Skills Survey (ILSS)
- Kohlman Evaluation of Living Skills (KELS)
- Medication Management Ability Assessment (MMAA)
- Milwaukee Evaluation of Daily Living Skills (MEDLS)
- Test of Grocery Shopping Skills (TOG-SS)
- UCSD Performance-Based Skills Assessment (UPSA)

Client, Caregiver, and Staff Perceptions of Impact on Occupational Performance

- Canadian Occupational Performance Measure (COPM)
- Client Assessment of Strengths, Interests, and Goals/Staff Observations and Client Information (CASIG/SOCI)
- Illness Perception Questionnaire for Schizophrenia—Relatives Version (IPQS—Relatives)
- Profile of Occupational Engagement for Schizophrenia (POES)

Cognition

- Allen's Cognitive Levels (ACL)
- Assessment of Motor and Process Skills (AMPS)
- Cognitive Assessment Interview (CAI)
- Schizophrenia Cognition Rating Scale (SCoRS)

Occupational Therapy Intervention

Occupational therapists may use the following interventions to enable clients with schizophrenia or schizoaffective disorder to participate in meaningful occupations.

Assertive Community Treatment

Assertive community treatment (ACT) is a multidisciplinary team-based approach for clients living in the community to improve their psychiatric and social functioning and quality of life. Key elements of ACT include a medicine prescriber, a shared caseload among team members, direct service provision by team members, a high frequency of client contact, low client-to-staff ratios, and outreach to individuals in the community. ACT has been found to reduce hospitalization rates and homelessness; improve outcomes in the areas of accommodation, employment, and client satisfaction; and increase the likelihood of clients staying in contact with mental health services (Dixon, Dickerson, et al., 2009; Dixon, Perkins, et al., 2009; Jung & Newton, 2009).

Peer Support

Peer support involves consumers in the planning, provision, and evaluation of mental health services (Dixon, Dickerson, et al., 2009). Consumers may run their own independent agencies, serve as members of regular clinical teams, or be providers of peer-to-peer services, which may include Internet support groups, clubhouses, and peer partnerships (Dixon, Dickerson, et al., 2009; Dixon, Perkins, et al., 2009). Although research examining the effects of peer support is limited, it is hypothesized that empowering consumers facilitates the sharing of lived experiences, helps consumers serve as role models for one another, and helps remove "inappropriate hiring barriers" faced by individuals with mental illness (Dixon, Dickerson, et al., 2009, p. 61).

Cognitive Behavioral Therapy

Cognitive behavioral therapy (CBT) aims to change behavior through the collaborative identification of target problems or symptoms, such as negative thought patterns, and developing rational or adaptive coping responses. Sessions may be conducted in an individual or group format and typically last for approximately 4 to 9 months (Dixon, Dickerson, et al., 2009; Jung & Newton, 2009). Although there is a limited evidence that CBT is effective for individuals experiencing acute psychotic symptoms at the time of intervention (Dixon, Perkins, et al., 2009), recent evidence supports the role of CBT in improving clients' short-term mental state (Jung & Newton, 2009), reducing positive and negative symptoms, and improving social functioning (Dixon, Dickerson, et al., 2009).

Family-Based Services

Family-based services involve engaging and collaborating with clients and their family members during an acute episode and may include illness education, emotional support, and training in how to cope with illness symptoms and how to access providers during crises (Dixon, Dickerson, et al., 2009; Dixon, Perkins, et al., 2009). Outcomes of family-based services include decreased rates of relapse and hospitalization, increased treatment adherence, and improved social and vocational outcomes for clients. For families, outcomes include decreased family burden and levels of perceived stress, increased knowledge about schizophrenia, and improved family relationships and perceptions of professional support (Dixon, Dickerson, et al., 2009; Dixon, Perkins, et al., 2009; Jung & Newton, 2009).

Social Skills Training

Social skills training uses behavioral demonstrations, role-play activities, feedback, prompting, coaching, modeling, shaping, and out-of-session assignments to help participants develop the skills necessary for communication, social adaptation, and interpersonal relationships. Interventions focus on the specific needs of the participants and are supplemented with strategies to apply learned skills in the context of everyday life (Dixon, Dickerson, et al., 2009). Social skills training improved participants' knowledge about social interaction and participation, social skills performance within the clinic, as well as broader functional outcomes regarding communication in the workplace and with health care professionals (Dixon, Perkins, et al., 2009).

Supported Employment

Supported employment helps individuals obtain and retain competitive employment by individually tailoring job development and engaging the client in a rapid job search and placement, rather than an extended period of preemployment preparation. Other key components include an emphasis on client preference, availability of ongoing supports, and integration of vocational and mental health services. Supported employment programs are consistently supported by research in yielding positive vocational outcomes for individuals with schizophrenia, such as an increase in hours worked, wages earned, and likelihood of obtaining competitive employment (Dixon, Dickerson, et al., 2009).

Healthy Living

Evidence consistently indicates that individuals with mental illness commonly practice unhealthy habits, such as smoking and poor nutritional and exercise routines, which lead to medical problems such as obesity and cardiovascular disease. Healthy living interventions typically focus on smoking cessation and weight and nutrition management (Bradshaw, Lovell, & Harris, 2005). Interventions typically consist of individual or group education sessions, although smoking cessation interventions may include the prescription of bupropion. Although the body of literature surrounding healthy living interventions is small, Bradshaw et al. (2005) found that smoking cessation interventions, which provided nicotine replacement, and group therapy reduced smoking.

Occupational Therapy and the Evidence

Numerous studies demonstrate that occupational therapy (OT) interventions have resulted in positive functional outcomes for individuals with schizophrenia and schizoaffective disorder. In a systematic review of the literature, Arbesman and Logsdon (2011) found that OT intervention is particularly helpful in preparing this population for vocational pursuits. Supported employment programs, particularly those with high fidelity to an individual placement and support model, have demonstrated outcomes such as increases in earnings, hours worked, and rate of employment. These outcomes are stronger when combined with cognitive or social skills training. The evidence supporting the effectiveness of supported education programs is also strong. A biweekly, 12-session OT intervention based on supported education principles helped participants improve their professional behaviors and social skills. This intervention consisted of classroom–laboratory group modules and individual mentoring on time management, public speaking, computer use, and other topics that support vocational efforts (Gutman, Kerner, Zombek, Dulek, & Ramsey, 2009). In a systematic review of available evidence, Gibson, D'Amico, Jaffe, and Arbesman (2011) reported several effective OT interventions that support recovery in the areas of community integration and normative life roles for people with serious mental illness. Moderate-to-strong evidence was reported for interventions addressing social participation, such as social skills training and assertiveness training. Moderate evidence for the effectiveness of life skills and instrumental activities of daily living (IADL) training was found, although Arbesman and Logsdon (2011) note more positive outcomes when life skills interventions are highly structured, manual driven, and combined with social skills training. In a longitudinal study investigating the effectiveness of a manualized life skills intervention based on skills training for individuals with mental illness who have been homeless, Helfrich, Chan, and Sabol (2011) reported increases in and maintenance of life skills knowledge over time.

Resources

Associations and Websites

- National Alliance on Mental Illness (NAMI)
  http://www.nami.org/
- National Alliance for Research on Schizophrenia and Depression (NARSAD)
- http://www.narsad.org/
- National Institute of Mental Health (NIMH)
- http://www.nimh.nih.gov/
- Schizophrenia International Research Society (SIRS)
- http://www.schizophreniaresearchsociety
- Schizophrenia and Related Disorders Alliance of America (SARDAA)
  http://www.sardaa.org/

Books

- Earley, P. (2006). *Crazy: A father's search through America's mental health madness*. New York, NY: Penguin.
  A journalist of more than 30 years, Pete Earley writes of his experiences with his son, who was diagnosed with schizophrenia, and of the mental health care system and its ties to the criminal justice system.
- Torrey, E. F. (2006). *Surviving schizophrenia: A manual for families, patients, and providers*. New York, NY: Harper Paperbacks.
  A useful reference book written in clear language, this book describes the nature, causes, symptoms, treatment, and course of schizophrenia and also explores living with it from both the client and the family's point of view.

Journals

- *American Journal of Psychiatry*
- *Journal of Abnormal Psychology*
- *Journal of Mental Health*
- *Schizophrenia Bulletin*
- *Schizophrenia Research*

References

American Psychiatric Association. (2000). *Diagnostic and statistical manual of mental disorders* (4th ed., text rev.). Washington, DC: Author.

Arbesman, M., & Logsdon, D. W. (2011). Occupational therapy interventions for employment and education for adults with serious mental illness: A systematic review. *American Journal of Occupational Therapy, 65*, 238–246. doi:10.5014/ajot.2011.001289

Bradshaw, T., Lovell, K., & Harris, N. (2005). Healthy living interventions and schizophrenia: A systematic review. *Journal of Advanced Nursing, 49*, 634–654. doi:10.1111/j.1365-2648.2004.03338.x

Canuso, C. M., Turkoz, I., Fu, D. J., & Bossie, C. A. (2010). Role of paliperidone extended-release in treatment of schizoaffective disorder. *Neuropsychiatric Disease and Treatment, 6*, 667–679. doi:10.2147/NDT.S12612

Dixon, L. B., Dickerson, F., Bellack, A. S., Bennett, M., Dickinson, D., Goldberg, R. W., . . . Kreyenbuhl, J. (2009). The 2009 schizophrenia PORT psychosocial treatment recommendations and summary statements. *Schizophrenia Bulletin, 36*, 48–70. doi:10.1093/schbul/sbp115

Dixon, L., Perkins, D., & Calmes, C. (2009). *Guideline watch (September 2009): Practice guideline for the treatment of patients with schizophrenia*. Retrieved from http://www.psychiatryonline.com/pracGuide/PracticePDFs/Schizophrenia_Guideline%20Watch.pdf

Dominguez, M. D., Saka, M. C., Lieb, R., Wittchen, H. U., & van Os, J. (2010). Early expression of negative/disorganized symptoms predicting psychotic experiences and subsequent clinical psychosis: A 10-year study. *American Journal of Psychiatry, 167*, 1075–1082. doi:10.1176/appi.ajp.2010.09060883

Gibson, W. R., D'Amico, M., Jaffe, L., & Arbesman, M. (2011). Occupational therapy interventions for recovery in the areas of community integration and normative life roles for adults with serious mental illness: A systematic review. *American Journal of Occupational Therapy, 65*, 247–256. doi:10.5014/ajot.2011.001297

Gutman, S. A., Kerner, R., Zombek, I., Dulek, J., & Ramsey, C. A. (2009). Supported education for adults with psychiatric disabilities: Effectiveness of an occupational therapy program. *American Journal of Occupational Therapy, 63*, 245–254.

Helfrich, C. A., Chan, D. V., & Sabol, P. (2011). Cognitive predictors of life skill intervention outcomes for adults with mental illness at risk for homelessness. *American Journal of Occupational Therapy, 65*, 277–286. doi:10.5014/ajot.2011.001321

Jung, X. T., & Newton, R. (2009). Cochrane Reviews of non-medication-based psychotherapeutic and other interventions for schizophrenia, psychosis, and bipolar disorder: A systematic literature review. *International Journal of Mental Health Nursing, 18*, 239–249. doi:10.1111/j.1447-0349.2009.00613.x

Perala, J., Suvisaari, J., Saarni, S. I., Kuoppasalmi, K., Isometsa, E. Pirkola, S., . . . Lonnqvist, J. (2007). Lifetime prevalence of psychotic and bipolar I disorders in a general population. *Archives of General Psychiatry, 64*, 19–28.

Sensory Processing Disorder

Pamela Vaughn

Description and Diagnosis

Sensory processing disorder (SPD) is a condition in which a person has difficulty organizing and integrating sensory information for use. As a result, individuals with SPD experience challenges in acting on and adapting to sensory information, making it difficult to participate in and enjoy many everyday tasks (Miller, Nielsen, Schoen, & Brett-Green, 2009). SPD can affect one or multiple sensory systems—vision, auditory, gustatory (taste), olfactory (smell), tactile (touch), proprioceptive (joint position sense), and vestibular (balance and movement). Three proposed subtypes of SPD are the following:

- Sensory modulation disorder (SMD), including sensory underresponsivity, sensory overresponsivity, and sensory seeking responses
- Sensory discrimination disorder (SDD)
- Sensory-based motor disorder (SBMD), including postural disorders and dyspraxia (Miller, Anzalone, Lane, Cermak, & Osten, 2007)

SPD, first described by A. Jean Ayres (1972) as "sensory integration dysfunction," is not considered a stand-alone diagnosis according to the latest editions of medical diagnostic manuals, such as the American Psychiatric Association's *Diagnostic and Statistical Manual*. Some occupational therapists are among those advocating for SPD to be included as a separate and valid disorder in future editions; others hold the perspective that sensory processing is a client factor—a neurological function—that can affect all human performance but is not a specific diagnostic condition. SPD may occur alone but is sometimes comorbid with or contributing to other conditions, such as autism spectrum disorders, attention deficit disorder, learning disabilities, and anxiety and panic disorders (American Occupational Therapy Association [AOTA], 2011; Gouze, Hopkins, LeBailly, & Lavigne, 2009).

Incidence and Prevalence

The conservative estimated prevalence of SPD among kindergarteners in 2000 was 5.3% or 1 out of 20 (Ahn, Miller, Milberger, & McIntosh, 2004). Sensory overresponsivity of school-aged children has been estimated to be 16.5% or 1 out of 6 children (Ben-Sasson, Carter, & Briggs-Gowan, 2009). The incidence of sensory processing challenges is higher in males and in individuals with other disorders, including autism spectrum disorders and attention deficit/hyperactivity disorder (Cheung & Siu, 2009; Gouze et al., 2009; Rogers & Ozonoff, 2005).

Cause and Etiology

The cause of SPD is still undetermined, although various studies have cited genetics, environmental factors, and prenatal factors such as stress or alcohol exposure as potential influencing factors (Goldsmith, Van Hulle, Arneson, Schreiber, & Gernsbacher, 2006; Schneider et al., 2008). As Ayres (1972) and many others have proposed that SPD is caused by atypical brain processing and/or an immature brain, recent research has focused on determining whether SPD presents neurologically. In one study, electroencephalographic (EEG) measurements were taken while typically developing children, and children with an occupational therapy (OT) diagnosis of SPD were presented with auditory stimuli (Davies & Gavin, 2007). Results revealed a difference between the two groups—based on interpretation of EEG measurements, children with SPD were found to be "deficient in their ability to suppress (i.e., filter out) repeated or irrelevant sensory input and failed to selectively regulate the sensitivity of cortical responses to additional incoming sensory stimuli" when compared to their age-matched typically developing peers (Davies & Gavin, 2007, p. 186).

Typical Course, Symptoms, and Related Conditions

Although SPD is considered to be a lifelong condition that can affect people of all ages due to the impact it has on everyday functioning, SPD is usually identified in childhood (AOTA, 2011). Sensory sensitivity in infants and change in early sensitivities were found to be associated with the presence of sensory overresponsivity (one of the classifications under subtype SMD) in the same children at school age (Ben-Sasson, Carter, & Briggs-Gowan, 2010). Adults who go undiagnosed or who do not learn coping mechanisms at a younger age may experience mental health symptoms, such as depression and anxiety as well as decreased quality of life and participation (Kinnealey, Koenig, & Smith, 2011). Symptoms vary depending on the individual but only constitute SPD if they interfere or inhibit function and participation in occupations (Koenig & Rudney, 2010). Examples of symptoms may include, but are not limited to, the following:

- Frequent distraction from tasks; restlessness
- Poor motor skills and praxis; poor posture
- Distress or aversion to sensory stimuli present in daily activities
- Irritation, pain, or unpleasant feelings when experiencing a sensation
- Lack of expected response to sensory stimuli (e.g., does not pull finger back when pricked with a pin)
- Seeks opportunities for excessive or extreme sensory stimulation
- Difficulty discriminating between sensory stimuli
- Inability to self-regulate emotions, behaviors, and so forth (AOTA, 2009, 2011)

Interdisciplinary Interventions

Physical Therapy and Speech-Language Therapy

Although occupational therapists most frequently provide intervention for SPD, physical therapists and speech-language pathologists may also be included on an intervention team depending on the needs of the client.

Occupational Therapy Evaluations

The evaluation process focuses on what the client needs, wants, or is expected to do and analyzes what factors may impact desired occupational performance. The evaluation begins with occupation-based assessments followed by specific evaluation of the potential impact of sensory processing on occupational performance.

Evaluations of Sensory Processing

- Sensory Integration and Praxis Tests (SIPT) (Ayres, 1989)
- Sensory Profiles: Infant/Toddler Sensory Profile (Dunn, 2002), Sensory Profile (Dunn, 1999), Adolescent/Adult Sensory Profile (Brown & Dunn, 2002)
- Sensory Processing Measure (Miller-Kuhaneck, Henry, Glennon, Parham, & Ecker, 2007)
- Direct and clinical observation
- Parent/caregiver/teacher interviews

Occupational Therapy Interventions

Ayres Sensory Integration

Ayres Sensory Integration (ASI), based on theory and research originally done by Ayres (1972), is the most intensive form of OT using sensory integration (SI) theories. The goal of ASI is for clients to create adaptive responses to sensory stimuli in their environment so they can more fully participate in desired occupations. Using specialized suspended equipment and providing opportunities for exploration of various sensory stimuli, the therapist adjusts therapeutic activities, customized for the client, to improve the efficiency of the client's nervous system to interpret and use sensory information. Some major elements of ASI intervention are the following:

- It occurs within an environment that is rich in tactile, proprioceptive, and vestibular opportunities and that creates both physical and emotional safety for the child.
- Therapist presents or modifies activities so child can experience success in response to a challenge.
- All therapeutic activities are child directed and therapist supported.
- Therapeutic activities will challenge the child to develop ideas about what to do; the therapist encourages the child to plan out these ideas and then successfully carry out the plans.
- Therapeutic activities are conducive to attaining or sustaining client's optimum level of arousal by modifying the environment (Parham et al., 2007).

Best practice guidelines recommend that practitioners obtain additional training in ASI before administering this intervention.

Sensory-Based and Sensorimotor Approaches

Sensory-based and sensorimotor approaches also focus on remediating impaired sensory processing in order to increase occupational performance and participation in desired activities.

Examples of Sensory-Based Approaches	Evidence
Weighted vests—Wearing weighted vests provides calming deep pressure to meet tactile and proprioceptive needs.	Students were able to focus on tasks for increased periods of time after wearing weighted vests (VandenBerg, 2001).
Sensory diets—A carefully designed, customized activity plan that provides sensory input a client can use throughout the day to meet sensory needs.	Uses sensory diet framework to improve quality of life for adults with neurological conditions (Fenech & Baker, 2008).
Therapeutic listening—The use of music and auditory stimuli, modified to include different frequencies, to "train" the auditory system to more effectively modulate sounds.	Children showed improvements in behaviors related to sensory processing after undergoing an 8-week therapeutic listening program (Hall & Case-Smith, 2007).
Hippotherapy—Therapeutic horse riding to increase posture, balance, and muscle tone and to increase participation and socialization.	Children attended a camp that featured therapeutic riding; parents reported positive changes in children's behaviors related to sensory processing after attending camp (Candler, 2003).

Sensory intervention approaches have also been used in mental health settings; for example, with individuals with schizophrenia or posttraumatic stress disorder, with the rationale that when an individual's sensory processing (viewed as a neurological function) is impaired, "such activities may provide calming and/or alerting sensory experiences . . . and become meaningful ways to help [a] person self-organize, remain safe and in control" (Champagne, 2005, p. 2).

Performance-Oriented Approaches

These approaches focus on directly improving performance and participation and include the following:

- Direct skills teaching (e.g., teaching a client to ride a bike)
- Cognitive-based approaches (e.g., Cognitive Orientation to daily Occupational Performance [CO-OP], a program to help client identify and use cognitive strategies in order to learn and perform tasks) (Polatajko & Cantin, 2010)

Compensatory Lifestyle Approaches

Compensatory approaches help clients develop specific skills or coping skills that use environmental and task adaptations to regulate their sensory needs. Sensory diets and the Alert Program: "How Does Your Engine

Run?" help children increase self-regulatory skills by teaching them to recognize their internal arousal states and use strategies (e.g., activities, environment changes) to meet their sensory needs (Shellenberger & Williams, 2007).

Consultation

Occupational therapists can also provide an indirect form of intervention to help family members, teachers, or others understand the nature of sensory processing and how it influences occupational performance.

Occupational Therapy and the Evidence

A systematic review of the effectiveness of SI interventions based on 27 studies concluded that "there is a trend for positive results from the SI approach, especially in contrast to no treatment" and that "occupational therapists can use this information to begin to support the use of the SI approach within their professional domain of practice with a variety of outcomes, particularly sensory and motor outcomes and individually identified client-centered goals" (May-Benson & Koomar, 2010, p. 411). Although this research is promising, low sample sizes and lack of fidelity to the theoretical postulates of SI intervention principles highlight the need for further research (May-Benson & Koomar, 2010). Polatajko and Cantin (2010) reviewed studies using non-SI approaches to intervention and found performance-oriented approaches to show positive outcomes as measured by increases in motor skills and coordination.

Caregiver Concerns

Many parents of children with SPD report concerns about their children's social participation. Parents are seeking help in order to understand their children's behavior, to support their children's growth, and to advocate for their children. Gaining an appreciation for sensory processing and how it may impact occupational performance helps parents develop realistic expectations for their children (Cohn, 2001).

Resources

Organizations

- The Spiral Foundation at OTA-Watertown: a nonprofit organization to further the understanding of SPD through research and community education.
  124 Watertown Street
  Watertown, MA 02472
  (617) 923-4410
  http://www.thespiralfoundation.org/index.html

- Sensory Processing Disorder Foundation: conducts research about, provides education to professionals and caregivers regarding, and advocates for the recognition of SPD.
  5420 S. Quebec Street, Suite 135
  Greenwood Village, CO 80111
  (303) 794-1182
  http://www.spdfoundation.net

- Pediatric Therapy Network: a therapy and research center with resources for professionals and parents of children with special needs.
  1815 W 213th St. Suite 100
  Torrance, CA 90501
  Telephone: 310.328.0276
  http://www.pediatrictherapynetwork.org/

Books

- Dunn, W. (2008). *Living sensationally: Understanding your senses.* Philadelphia, PA: Jessica Kingsley.

- Heller, S. (2003). *Too loud, too bright, too fast, too tight: What to do if you are sensory defensive in an overstimulating world.* New York, NY: Harper Collins.

- Kranowitz, C. (2006). *The out-of-sync child: Recognizing and coping with sensory processing disorder.* New York, NY: Perigee.

- Laird, C. T. (2009). *Not just spirited: A mom's sensational journey with sensory processing disorder (SPD).* Ann Arbor, MI: Loving Healing Press.

- Miller, L. J. (2006). *Sensational kids: Hope and help for children with sensory processing disorder.* New York, NY: Perigee.

- Renna, D. M. (2007). *Meghan's world: The story of one girl's triumph over sensory processing disorder.* Speonk, NY: Indigo Impressions.

Websites

- Sensory Integration Global Network (SIGN)
  http://www.siglobalnetwork.org

References

Ahn, R., Miller, L., Milberger, S., & McIntosh, D. (2004). Prevalence of parents' perceptions of sensory processing disorders among kindergarten children. *American Journal of Occupational Therapy, 58,* 287–302.

American Occupational Therapy Association. (2009). Providing occupational therapy using sensory integration theory and methods in school-based practice. *American Journal of Occupational Therapy, 63,* 823–842. doi:10.5014/ajot.63.6.823

American Occupational Therapy Association. (2011). *Occupational therapy using a sensory-integration approach with adult populations: Fact sheet.* Retrieved from http://www.aota.org/Consumers/Professionals/WhatIsOT/HW.aspx

Ayres, A. J. (1972). *Sensory integration and learning disorders.* Los Angeles, CA: Western Psychological Services.

Ayres, A. J. (1989). *Sensory Integration and Praxis Tests.* Los Angeles, CA: Western Psychological Services.

Ben-Sasson, A., Carter, A. S., & Briggs-Gowan, M. J. (2009). Sensory over-responsivity in elementary school: Prevalence and social-emotional correlates. *Journal of Abnormal Child Psychology, 37,* 705–716. doi:10.1007/s10802-008-9295-8

Ben-Sasson, A., Carter, A. S., & Briggs-Gowan, M. J. (2010). The development of sensory over-responsivity from infancy to elementary school. *Journal of Abnormal Child Psychology, 38,* 1193–1202. doi:10.1007/s10802-010-9435-9

Brown, C., & Dunn, W. (2002). *The adolescent/adult sensory profile.* San Antonio, TX: Psychological Corporation.

Candler, C. (2003). Sensory integration and therapeutic riding at summer camp: Occupational performance outcomes. *Physical and Occupational Therapy in Pediatrics, 23*(3), 51–64. doi:10.1300/J006v23n03_04

Champagne, T. (2005, March). Expanding the role of sensory approaches in acute psychiatric settings. *Mental Health Special Interest Section Quarterly, 28,* 1–4.

Cheung, P. P. P., & Siu, A. M. H. (2009). A comparison of patterns of sensory processing in children with and without developmental disabilities. *Research in Developmental Disabilities, 30,* 1468–1480. doi:10.1016/j.ridd.2009.07.009

Cohn, E. S. (2001). Parent perspectives of occupational therapy using a sensory integration approach. *American Journal of Occupational Therapy, 55,* 285–294.

Davies, P. L., & Gavin, W. J. (2007). Validating the diagnosis of sensory processing disorder using EEG technology. *American Journal of Occupational Therapy, 61,* 176–189.

Dunn, W. (1999). *The sensory profile.* San Antonio, TX: Psychological Corporation.

Dunn, W. (2002). *The infant/toddler sensory profile.* San Antonio, TX: Psychological Corporation.

Fenech, A., & Baker, M. (2008). Casual leisure and the sensory diet: A concept for improving quality of life in neuropalliative conditions. *NeuroRehabilitation, 23,* 369–376.

Goldsmith, H. H., Van Hulle, C. A., Arneson, C. L., Schreiber, J. E., & Gernsbacher, M. A. (2006). A population-based twin study of parentally reported tactile and auditory defensiveness in young children. *Journal of Abnormal Child Psychology, 34,* 393–407. doi:10.1007/s10802-006-9024-0

Gouze, K. R., Hopkins, J., LeBailly, S. A., & Lavigne, J. V. (2009). Re-examining the epidemiology of sensory regulation dysfunction and comorbid psychopathology. *Journal of Abnormal Child Psychology, 37,* 1077–1087. doi:10.1007/s10802-009-9333-1

Hall, L., & Case-Smith, J. (2007). The effect of sound-based intervention on children with sensory processing disorders and visual-motor delays. *American Journal of Occupational Therapy, 61*, 209–215. doi:10.5014/ajot.61.2.209

Kinnealey, M., Koenig, K. P., & Smith, S. (2011). Relationships between sensory modulation and social supports and health-related quality of life. *American Journal of Occupational Therapy, 65*, 320–327. doi:10.5014/ajot.2011.001370

Koenig, K. P., & Rudney, S. G. (2010). Performance challenges for children and adolescents with difficulty processing and integrating sensory information: A systematic review. *American Journal of Occupational Therapy, 64*, 430–442. doi:10.5014/ajot.2010.09073

May-Benson, T. A., & Koomar, J. A. (2010). Systematic review of the research evidence examining the effectiveness of interventions using a sensory integrative approach for children. *American Journal of Occupational Therapy, 64*, 403–414. doi:10.5014/ajot.2010.09071

Miller, L. J., Anzalone, M. E., Lane, S. J., Cermak, S. A., & Osten, E. T. (2007). Concept evolution in sensory integration: A proposed nosology for diagnosis. *American Journal of Occupational Therapy, 61*, 135–140. doi:10.5014/ajot.61.2.135

Miller, L. J., Nielsen, D. M., Schoen, S. A., & Brett-Green, B. A. (2009). Perspectives on sensory processing disorder: A call for translational research. *Frontiers in Integrative Neuroscience, 3*(22), 1–12. doi:10.3389/neuro.07.022.2009

Miller-Kuhaneck, H., Henry, D., Glennon, T., Parham, D., & Ecker, C. (2007). *Sensory processing measure: Home form, main classroom form, and school environments form.* Los Angeles, CA: Western Psychological Services.

Parham, L. D., Cohn, E. S., Spitzer, S., Koomar, J. A., Miller, L. J., Burke, J. P., . . . Summers, C. A. (2007). Fidelity in sensory integration intervention research. *American Journal of Occupational Therapy, 61*, 216–227. doi:10.5014/ajot.61.2.216

Polatajko, H. J., & Cantin, N. (2010). Exploring the effectiveness of occupational therapy interventions, other than the sensory integration approach, with children and adolescents experiencing difficulty processing and integrating sensory information. *American Journal of Occupational Therapy, 64*, 415–429. doi:10.5014/ajot.2010.09072

Rogers, S. J., & Ozonoff, S. (2005). Annotation: What do we know about sensory dysfunction in autism? A critical review of the empirical evidence. *Journal of Child Psychology and Psychiatry, 46*, 1255–1268. doi:10.1111/j.1469-7610.2005.01431.x

Schneider, M. L., Moore, C. F., Gajewski, L. L., Larson, J. A., Roberts, A. D., Converse, A. K., & DeJesus, O. T. (2008). Sensory processing disorder in a primate model: Evidence from a longitudinal study of prenatal alcohol and prenatal stress effects. *Child Development, 79*, 100–113. doi:10.1111/j.1467-8624.2007.01113.x

Shellenberger, S., & Williams, M. S. (2007). How does your engine run? Albuquerque, NM: Therapy Works.

VandenBerg, N. L. (2001). The use of a weighted vest to increase on-task behavior in children with attention difficulties. *American Journal of Occupational Therapy, 55*, 621–628.

Spinal Cord Injury

Larissa Sachs

Description and Classification

Spinal cord injury (SCI) involves damage to the axons of spinal nerve cells due to compression, bruising, tearing, or severing of spinal cord tissue. The damage results in impairment or loss of sensory and motor function corresponding with the level at which the injury occurs. SCIs are classified as either complete or incomplete, and the resulting paralysis is categorized as either tetraplegia or paraplegia. A complete injury indicates a lack of all sensory and motor function below the level of injury, and an incomplete injury indicates some remaining sensory or motor function below the affected area. Tetraplegia involves an impairment of function in the upper and lower extremities, trunk, and pelvic organs; depending on the level of injury, paraplegia involves functional impairment of the trunk, legs, and pelvic organs but spares the upper extremities (Mayo Clinic, 2009; National Institute of Neurological Disorders and Stroke [NINDS], 2011).

Etiology

An SCI may be either traumatic or nontraumatic. SCIs in the United States are most often caused by trauma. Motor vehicle crashes are the leading cause, accounting for over 40% of SCIs. Falls, the most common cause after age 65 years, account for 27.3% of SCIs. Acts of violence, often involving gunshot and knife wounds, account for 15% of SCIs, and recreational sporting activities cause 7.9% of SCIs. Alcohol use is a contributing factor in about one-quarter of all cases. Common causes of nontraumatic SCI include arthritis, cancer, inflammation or infections of the spinal cord, and disk degeneration of the spine (Mayo Clinic, 2009; National Spinal Cord Injury Statistical Center [NSCISC], 2010).

Incidence and Prevalence

There are approximately 262,000 people living with an SCI in the United States, and about 12,000 new cases occur each year. Males account for 80.8% of all SCIs. SCI predominantly affects young adults, and, among those affected, 66% are Caucasian and 27% are African American (NSCISC, 2010).

Typical Course

The median length of stay in an acute care unit immediately after injury is 12 days followed by a median stay of 38 days on a rehabilitation unit. The length of overall hospitalization in both acute care and rehabilitation units depends on the severity of the SCI and any related injuries. Individuals with higher level or complete injuries often require longer and more intensive treatment than do individuals with lower level or incomplete injuries (NSCISC, 2010). Furthermore, individuals with an incomplete injury have a better prognosis than those with a complete injury (Kirshblum, Millis, McKinley, & Tulsky, 2004). Mortality rates significantly decrease after the first year postinjury, but life expectancies of individuals with SCI remain less than those of individuals without SCI (NSCISC, 2010). Although neural recovery commonly occurs after SCI, most motor and sensory return takes place within the first 6 months postinjury, and the recovery rate decreases with time (Kirshblum et al., 2004). Individuals with SCI will continue to live with functional limitations based on their level and type of injury. They may also continue to experience chronic pain, bladder and bowel dysfunction, and other secondary medical complications, all of which must be handled daily to promote successful recovery. Advancements in interventions, rehabilitation, and technology continue to promote improvements in the functional capabilities of people with SCIs (NINDS, 2011).

Symptoms and Complications

Major Signs

- Paralysis: loss of motor function
- Paresis: impairment of motor function
- Sensory deficits: impairment or loss of sensory function
- Spasticity: increase in excitability of the stretch reflex
- Respiratory dysfunction: compromised breathing resulting from paralysis of diaphragm and respiratory muscles (most common for individuals with high level injuries)
- Orthostatic hypotension: sudden drop in blood pressure upon assuming an upright position
- Bladder and bowel dysfunction
- Pain
- Reproductive and sexual dysfunction (Mayo Clinic, 2009; NINDS, 2011)

Complications

- Autonomic dysreflexia: sudden dangerous rise in blood pressure in response to a noxious stimulus below the level of injury
- Heterotopic ossification: abnormal bone growth at joints
- Deep vein thrombosis: formation of a blood clot
- Skin breakdown and pressure sores
- Pain
- Urinary tract infection
- Pneumonia
- Cardiovascular disease (Atkins, 2008; NINDS, 2011)

Precautions

- Monitor the client's skin for redness or pressure ulcers; individuals with SCI must perform pressure relief regularly to reduce the risk of skin breakdown.
- Monitor blood pressure, check for dizziness, and encourage the client to move slowly when shifting positions to prevent orthostatic hypotension.
- Observe body temperature; people with SCI often have problems with temperature regulation.
- Watch for signs of autonomic dysreflexia, including headache, hypertension, sweating, congestion, blurred vision, difficulty breathing, and chest tightness; if signs are present, immediately move the client into an upright position and remove any constricting materials or obvious noxious stimuli.
- Monitor the respiration of clients with high-level injuries, especially those on a ventilator.
- Assess the client for pain, spasticity, hypertonia, decreased range of motion, and subluxation to prevent further injury during treatment (Atkins, 2008).

Interdisciplinary Interventions

- *Immobilization*: The spine and neck are immobilized immediately following injury to prevent further damage.
- *Medication*: Corticosteroids, such as methylprednisolone, reduce inflammation near the site of injury and decrease damage to nerve cells; if administered within 8 hours of injury onset, individuals may experience mild improvement in recovery. Medications are also used to address SCI symptoms, helping with pain management, control of muscle spasticity, and improvement in bladder and bowel control.
- *Surgery*: It is often needed to decrease compression of the spine by removing bone fragments, foreign objects, herniated disks, or fractured vertebrae.
- *Rehabilitation*: In addition to receiving continuing medical care during the postacute phase of recovery, the rehabilitation team for individuals with SCI often includes physical therapists, occupational therapists, social workers, recreational therapists, rehabilitation psychologists, rehabilitation nurses, and dietitians. The focus of rehabilitation is on maintaining health, restoring strength and function, redeveloping fine motor skills, using equipment and technology, addressing psychosocial concerns, providing client and caregiver education, and developing compensatory strategies to promote as much client independence as possible (Mayo Clinic, 2009; NINDS, 2011).

Occupational Therapy Evaluations

Motor and Sensory Function Evaluations

- American Spinal Injury Association (ASIA) Impairment Scale
- Manual muscle testing
- Range of motion testing using a goniometer
- Pinch and grip strength using a dynamometer

Activities of Daily Living and Instrumental Activities of Daily Living Evaluations

- Functional Independence Measure (FIM): measures type and amount of assistance needed for safe and effective activity performance
- Self-Reported Functional Measure (SRFM): measure of activities of daily living (ADL) and instrumental activities of daily living (IADL) performance
- Barthel Index (BI): assesses self-care abilities and level of assistance needed
- Klein-Bell ADL Scale: measure of ADL independence
- Frenchay Activities Index (FAI): measure of ADL and IADL participation
- Quadriplegia Index of Function (QIF): assessment of performance in functional activities in interview format
- Tetraplegia Hand Activity Questionnaire (THAQ): measure of arm and hand function in ADL and IADL
- Spinal Cord Independence Measure (SCIM): evaluates ADL performance

Quality of Life Evaluations

- Canadian Occupational Performance Measure (COPM): self-report of performance and satisfaction with occupations
- Quality of Life Profile for Adults with Physical Disabilities (QOLP-PD): measures quality of life in the domains of being, belonging, and becoming
- Short-Form Health Survey (SF-36): evaluates health-related quality of life

Occupational Therapy Interventions

Occupational therapists use a combination of intervention approaches to facilitate participation in meaningful occupations and desired contexts.

- *Biomechanical*: improve strength, range of motion, endurance, balance, and mobility
- *Skill acquisition*: promote skills necessary for participation in ADL, IADL, work, education, leisure, and social participation
- *Adaptive/Compensatory*: energy conservation, environmental adaptation, and adaptive equipment/assistive technology to support participation in occupations
- *Educational*: client, caregiver, family, and staff education and training
- *Psychosocial*: enhance self-efficacy, self-esteem, and self-management skills (Atkins, 2008)

Caregiver Concerns

Between 40% and 45% of individuals with SCI require assistance with daily activities, and family members often face numerous challenges as the primary caregivers for their loved ones. Caregivers commonly experience stress resulting from concerns about finances, work, home accessibility, providing appropriate care, and lifestyle adjustments. To enhance quality of life and promote healthy relationships, caregivers must take time to manage their own health. Important approaches for maintaining caregiver well-being include adopting a healthy lifestyle, practicing stress management techniques, finding time to relax, seeking the help of others, and learning to solve problems effectively (Lindsey, 2008).

Occupational Therapy and the Evidence

Research evidence supports the efficacy and importance of various occupational therapy interventions throughout the rehabilitation process to facilitate the occupational and social participation of individuals with SCI (Guidetti, Asaba, & Tham, 2009; Pillastrini et al., 2008; Ward, Mitchell, & Price, 2007). Occupational therapists use various approaches to support overall occupational participation (Ward et al., 2007), to promote independence in self-care activities (Guidetti et al., 2009), and to improve independence in performance of functional tasks, such as transfers and wheelchair use (Pillastrini et al., 2008). Effective approaches include the use of occupation-based, client-centered practices (Ward et al., 2007) and the development of a positive therapeutic relationship (Guidetti et al., 2009).

Research evidence also documents the effectiveness of more specific interventions for clients with SCI. Functional electrical stimulation, used to restore useful movements, has been found to promote positive health and fitness outcomes among individuals with SCI (Hamzaid & Davis, 2009). Effective strategies to improve arm and hand functioning in individuals with SCI include motor training (Spooren, Janssen-Potten, Kerckhofs, & Seelen, 2009) and activity-based interventions, which combine intense and repetitive input to the central nervous system (Backus, 2008). Harvey, Lin, Glinsky, and De Wolf (2009) suggest that fitness training, strength training, and gait training demonstrate the greatest effectiveness among physical interventions for individuals with SCI. Furthermore, cognitive behavior therapy approaches following SCI have a significant positive impact on clients' short-term psychological outcomes, including assertiveness, coping, self-efficacy, depression, and quality of life (Dorstyn, Mathias, & Denson, 2011).

Resources

Associations

- National Spinal Cord Injury Association
  1 Church Street #600
  Rockville, MD 20850
  Helpline: (800) 962-9629
  Fax: (866) 387-2196
  Website: http://www.spinalcord.org/
- United Spinal Association
  75-20 Astoria Boulevard, Suite 120
  Jackson Heights, NY 11370
  Telephone: (800) 404-2898
  Fax: (718) 803-0414
  Website: http://www.unitedspinal.org
- Christopher Reeve Spinal Cord Injury and Paralysis Foundation
  636 Morris Turnpike, Suite 3A
  Short Hills, NJ 07078
  Telephone: (800) 225-0292
  Website: http://www.christopherreeve.org

Books

- Ahrens, G. S. (2009). *Shattered, shaken and stirred.* Los Altos, CA: Positano Press.
  This book chronicles the effects of a car accident on an entire family, discussing the wife's process of recovery from an SCI and the struggles they encounter while trying to put their lives back together.
- Ellison, J., & Ellison, B. (2004). *The Brooke Ellison story: One mother, one daughter, one journey.* New York, NY: Hyperion Books.
  This is the story of Brooke Ellison's life, from the automobile accident that left her paralyzed as a young girl to her graduation from Harvard University. Brooke and her mother cowrote this book, detailing their individual experiences with the situation and their journey together.
- Reeve, C. (1999). *Still me.* New York, NY: Ballantine Books.
  Christopher Reeve's autobiography chronicles his life with tetraplegia after a horseback riding accident, offers insights into his recovery, and details his journey to reclaim his life.
- Reeve, C. (2005). *Nothing is impossible: Reflections on a new life.* New York, NY: Ballantine Books.
  In this sequel, Christopher Reeve shares aspects of how to successfully live with an SCI and deal with major life issues. Snippets from speeches, personal anecdotes, and remarks from talk shows are interspersed throughout Reeve's book.

Journals

- *Spinal Cord*
- *American Journal of Physical Medicine & Rehabilitation*
- *Journal of Rehabilitation Research & Development*
- *Journal of Neurotrauma*

Websites

- Spinal Cord Injury Information Network
  http://www.spinalcord.uab.edu
  This Website provides educational and research information about various issues along the spectrum of SCI care and contains helpful links to other organizations, publications, and resources.
- Foundation for Spinal Cord Injury Prevention, Care, and Cure
  http://www.fscip.org/index.html
  Promoting SCI public awareness, education, and research, this is a helpful resource for individuals living with SCI and their family members to locate information and support.
- National Institute of Neurological Disorders and Stroke
  http://www.ninds.nih.gov/disorders/sci/sci.htm
  This Website is a useful resource for locating current SCI-related information, publications, organizations, news, and research.
- MedlinePlus
  http://www.nlm.nih.gov/medlineplus/spinalcordinjuries.html
  This Website provides comprehensive SCI information and links to several other helpful resources, including organizations, journal articles, tutorials, and client handouts.

References

Atkins, M. S. (2008). Spinal cord injury. In M. V. Radomski & C. A. Trombly Latham (Eds.), *Occupational therapy for physical dysfunction* (6th ed., pp. 1171–1213). Baltimore, MD: Lippincott Williams & Wilkins.

Backus, D. (2008). Activity-based interventions for the upper extremity in spinal cord injury. *Topics in Spinal Cord Injury Rehabilitation, 13,* 1–9. doi:10.1310/sci1304-1

Dorstyn, D., Mathias, J., & Denson, L. (2011). Efficacy of cognitive behavior therapy for the management of psychological outcomes following spinal cord injury: A meta-analysis. *Journal of Health Psychology, 16,* 374–391. doi:10.1177/1359105310379063

Guidetti, S., Asaba, E., & Tham, K. (2009). Meaning of context in recapturing self-care after stroke or spinal cord injury. *American Journal of Occupational Therapy, 63,* 323–332.

Hamzaid, N. A., & Davis, G. M. (2009). Health and fitness benefits of functional electrical stimulation-evoked leg exercise for spinal cord-injured individuals: A position review. *Topics in Spinal Cord Injury Rehabilitation, 14,* 88–121. doi:10.1310/sci1404-88

Harvey, L. A., Lin, C.-W. C., Glinsky, J. V., & De Wolf, A. (2009). The effectiveness of physical interventions for people with spinal cord injuries: A systematic review. *Spinal Cord, 47,* 184–195. doi:10.1038/sc.2008.100

Kirshblum, S., Millis, S., McKinley, W., & Tulsky, D. (2004). Late neurologic recovery after traumatic spinal cord injury. *Archives of Physical Medicine and Rehabilitation, 79,* 20–23.

Lindsey, L. (2008). *Caring for caregivers—SCI infosheet #17.* Retrieved from http://www.spinalcord.uab.edu/show.asp?durki=22479

Mayo Clinic. (2009). *Spinal cord injury.* Retrieved from http://www.mayoclinic.com/health/spinal-cord-injury/DS00460

National Institute of Neurological Disorders and Stroke. (2011). *Spinal cord injury: Hope through research.* Retrieved from http://www.ninds.nih.gov/disorders/sci/detail_sci.htm

National Spinal Cord Injury Statistical Center. (2010). *Spinal cord injury facts and figures at a glance.* Retrieved from https://www.nscisc.uab.edu/

Pillastrini, P., Mugnai, R., Bonfiglioli, R., Curti, S., Mattioli, S., Maioli, M. G., . . . Violante, F. S. (2008). Evaluation of an occupational therapy program for patients with spinal cord injury. *Spinal Cord, 46,* 78–81. doi:10.1038/sj.sc.3102072

Spooren, A. I. F., Janssen-Potten, Y. J. M., Kerckhofs, E., & Seelen, H. A. M. (2009). Outcome of motor training programmes on arm and hand functioning in patients with cervical spinal cord injury according to different levels of the ICF: A systematic review. *Journal of Rehabilitation Medicine, 41,* 497–505. doi:10.2340/16501977-0387

Ward, K., Mitchell, J., & Price, P. (2007). Occupation-based practice and its relationship to social and occupational participation in adults with spinal cord injury. *Occupational Therapy Journal of Research: Occupation, Participation and Health, 27*, 149–156.

Substance Use Disorders

Christine M. Carifio

Description and Diagnosis

Substance use disorders are the harmful and hazardous use of psychoactive substances, which includes alcohol, illicit drugs, and psychotherapeutics (National Institute on Drug Abuse [NIDA], 2010). Illicit drugs include marijuana, cocaine, heroin, hallucinogens, and inhalants. Psychotherapeutic use refers to the nonmedical use of pain relievers, tranquilizers, stimulants, and sedatives (Substance Abuse and Mental Health Services Administration [SAMHSA], 2007). Substance use disorders according to the *Diagnostic and Statistical Manual of Mental Disorders* (4th ed., text rev.; *DSM-IV-TR*; American Psychiatric Association [APA], 2000) can either be classified as abuse or dependence. Substance dependence is the more serious condition. Its key characteristics include the individual having the strong desire to continue using the substance regardless of negative consequences, difficulty in controlling use, increased tolerance, prioritizing the substance, and experiencing a physical withdrawal from the substance. Substance abuse, in contrast, does not reach the point of increased tolerance or withdrawal symptoms; yet, the individual does experience negative consequences and continues to use (APA, 2000).

Incidence and Prevalence

The following are statistics according to the 2006 National Survey on Drug Use and Health (NSDUH) about substance use disorders:

- The 52% of Americans (125 million people) aged 12 years and older are current regular drinkers (at least 12 drinks in the past year).
- The 23.7% of Americans aged 12 years and older participated in binge drinking, which is defined as having five or more drinks on the same occasion on at least 1 day in the past 30 days.
- The harmful use of alcohol leads to 2.5 million deaths each year.
- The 20.4 million Americans (8.7% of the population) aged 12 years and older are current illicit drug users (SAMHSA, 2007).
- The 16.7 million people have used marijuana, 7 million people have used psychotherapeutics, 1.6 million people have used cocaine, 1.3 million people have used hallucinogens, and 502,000 people have used methamphetamines in the past month (SAMHSA, 2007).

Cause and Prognosis

Substance use disorders are chronic, addictive disorders that may develop over a period of years and can begin at any age. The exact cause is not known; however, genetics, the preferred drug, temperament, sociocultural influences, emotional distress, anxiety, depression, and environmental factors can all contribute. Oftentimes, substance use will co-occur with other mental health conditions (APA, 2000; SAMHSA, 2007). There is no cure, and the individual with a substance use disorder may go through intermittent periods of sobriety, remission, and relapse. Relapse rates range widely from 50% to 90%. Relapse depends on many variables including, but not limited to, substance abused, severity of addiction, length of treatment, gender, readiness for change, environmental and societal factors, and many other elements (SAMHSA, 2007). Substance dependence and abuse may lead to a fatal drug overdose (United States National Library of Medicine, 2010).

Stages of Substance Use

Substance use can be divided into four categories:

- Experimental use is typically done recreationally with peers.
- Regular use is when the user may increasingly prioritize the substance over other things, isolate self from family or friends not involved with the substance, or show increased tolerance to the substance.
- Daily preoccupation occurs when the user loses all motivation for other things besides the substance. The user may experience behavior or relationship changes and may start using more dangerous substances.
- Dependence is when the user cannot face his or her daily life without drugs and loses control over use (United States National Library of Medicine, 2010).

Symptoms of Substance Abuse

Substance use disorders influence the individual in a myriad of ways depending on the substance and severity of use. Symptoms include, but are not limited, to changes in the following:

- Cognition: includes confusion, distorted perception, or decreased emotional regulation
- Personality: violent or hostile when confronted about substance use
- Behavior: continuation of drugs despite negative consequences, lack of control
- Performance patterns: missing work, school, changes in eating or sleeping habits, unkempt in self-care, lack of enjoyment in activities (American Occupational Therapy Association [AOTA], 2008; National Institute of Drug Abuse, 2010).

Symptoms of Withdrawal

Withdrawal symptoms exhibit the overreactivity of the autonomic nervous system and may include headache, nausea, anxiety, agitation, insomnia, rapid heart rate, fever, convulsions, and hallucinations (National Institute of Health, 2010).

Effects of Substance Abuse on the Body

Heavy substance abuse can negatively affect almost every body structure and system and is linked to serious medical conditions such as heart disease, cancer, HIV/AIDS, and mental illness. Substance abuse can lead to the following complications:

- Internal organ damage, especially the liver and pancreas; cancers of the mouth, lungs, stomach, breast, liver, and pancreas
- Lung and heart disease including cardiac damage, elevated heart rates, heart attack, and stroke
- Decreased immune system
- Cognitive functioning impairments including mental health issues, hallucinations, memory loss, paranoia, and aggression
- Psychosocial functioning impairments including anxiety and depression
- Respiratory depression including difficulty breathing
- Sexually transmitted diseases
- Bacterial endocarditis, blood clots, pulmonary emboli, and many other issues (United States National Library of Medicine, 2010)

Treatment

Treatment for individuals with substance use disorders can occur in various settings such as hospitals, emergency rooms, drug or alcohol rehabilitation centers, mental health facilities, private medical or psychological offices, prisons, and self-help groups (SAMHSA, 2007). The most effective treatment for a substance-related disorder is a dual approach of both pharmaceutical and psychosocial interventions. Medications can reduce the positive effects of the illicit drug and decrease cravings, whereas the psychosocial cognition component of treatment addresses readiness to change, mental illness, and addiction (Carey, Carey, Maisto, & Purnine, 2002; Gutman, 2006). Interdisciplinary care is common and includes a team of doctors, psychologists, social workers, occupational therapists and other appropriate allied health professionals for the individual (Gutman, 2006). After care, outpatient facilities and support groups are key factors in preventing relapse (United States National Library of Medicine, 2010).

Occupational Therapy Evaluations

The type and method of evaluation used in practice will be determined by the client's treatment preferences, the presence of cognitive impairments, and comorbid conditions (Stoffel & Moyers, 2004).

- Alcohol Use Disorders Identification Test: a screening that identifies people whom are alcohol dependent and at risk for alcohol abuse (Babor, Higgins-Biddle, Saunders, & Monteiro, 2010)
- Addiction Severity Index (ASI): a semistructured interview about client's life
- Beck Depression Inventory II (BDI-II): a self-report measure of depression
- CAGE-AID Screening Test: a screening to determine further alcohol testing
- Coping Behaviors Inventory (CBI): assesses behaviors and thoughts of clients
- Canadian Occupational Performance Measure (COPM): a self-report of performance and satisfaction with occupations
- Occupational Questionnaire: evaluates how substance use affects a client's weekly schedule and routine
- Role Checklist: assesses occupational roles
- Routine Task Inventory 2 (RTI-2): assesses function through everyday tasks with self-report or observation
- University of Rhode Island Change Assessment Scale (URICA): evaluates motivation for change

Occupational Therapy Interventions

Occupational therapy (OT) must recognize and respect the individual's stage of recovery and should be sensitive to a client's particular needs (SAMHSA, 2007). OT intervention goals with clients that have substance use disorders may include improving health habits and routines; self-care; developing skills in self-regulation and impulse control; experiencing group participation; learning communication strategies; preparing for a vocational role; and education about job, leisure, life management, coping, social skills, life roles, identity, and community resources (Stoffel & Moyers, 2004).

Types of Occupational Therapy Interventions

- Brief intervention: One or several sessions may provide the client with screening; education about the risks of substance abuse and coping strategies; group therapy sessions; goal setting; referrals; encouragement to change; and participation in meaningful, healthy activities (Stoffel & Moyers, 2004).
- Cognitive behavioral therapy (CBT): It emphasizes the development of coping behaviors and self-efficacy to change what a person thinks and does regarding substance abuse. This approach connects to relapse prevention (Stoffel & Moyers, 2004).
- Motivational techniques: They facilitate the client's motivation for change (Stoffel & Moyers, 2004).
- Twelve-step facilitation: Social and spiritual support groups encourage maintenance of abstinence. Occupational therapists may assist an individual with finding support groups in his or her area and incorporating them into his or her schedule (Stoffel & Moyers, 2004).
- Harm reduction model: It is a controversial approach; clients learn practical strategies that help reduce the negative results of substance use. Although individuals do not completely abstain from substances, the goal is to increase an individual's readiness to change behaviors (Harm Reduction Coalition, n.d.).

Occupational Therapy and the Evidence

Substance dependence and abuse may impact an individual's performance in almost all areas of occupation. Through working with OT, clients may identify how their substance use is affecting performance patterns, daily routines, and life roles. Occupational therapists should emphasize helping the individual engage, without the use of substances, in meaningful and healthy occupations within various contexts. Individuals may also learn coping, self-regulation, and other educational strategies. Interventions that are modified to include an occupational perspective, such as brief interventions, CBT, motivational strategies, and 12-step programs are effective treatments that occupational therapists may use. In addition, peer-supported community programs run by occupational therapists, with opportunities for socialization, mutual support, and self-determination, may provide a significant reduction in relapse. Although positive change in occupational performance may occur in supportive environments, sustaining a healthy lifestyle may be challenged when clients confront obstacles, therefore emphasizing OT's important role in empowering clients to engage in healthy occupations and use strategies to maintain healthy living behaviors (AOTA, 2008; Boisvert, Martin, Grosek, & Clarie, 2008; Huhman, 2008; Stoffel & Moyers, 2004).

Caregiver Concerns

Family members and friends play a pivotal role in the treatment and recovery of individuals who abuse substances. Families are the key in an alcohol or drug intervention. A professional interventionist may guide family members to speak openly and honestly about the individual and how his or her substance abuse influences everyone around them. The goal is for the individual to enter a rehabilitation program to receive treatment. Family and friends can also help an individual with substance abuse by attending family and group counseling where concerns can be discussed and where family members can receive advice and support for living with and promoting a healthy lifestyle for a person with substance use challenges. Finally, rehabilitation after care, such as 12-step programs and follow-up counseling are important resources that families and other loved ones can use for support (Croft, 2009, NIDA, 2010).

Resources

Associations

All of the following are spiritual support group organizations with a 12-step focus for individuals experiencing substance abuse and their family and friends.

- Al-Anon/Alateen
  Al-Anon World Service Office
  1600 Corporate Landing Parkway
  Virginia Beach, VA 23454-5617
  Telephone: 1-800-4AL-ANON
  Website: http://www.al-anon.alateen.org/

- Narcotic Anonymous
  NA World Services, Inc.
  PO Box 9999
  Van Nuys, CA 91409-9099
  Telephone: 1-818-773-9999
  Website: http://www.na.org

Books

- Franklin, K., & King, L. (2009). *Addicted like me: A mother–daughter story of substance abuse and recovery.* New York, NY: Seal Press.
  This book details how addiction can affect an entire family through the generations.

- McCully, C. B. (2004). *Goodbye, Mr. Wonderful: Alcoholism, addiction, and early recovery.* New York, NY: Jessica Kingsley.
  This book is about a young man's struggle with the physical and mental addictions of alcoholism.

Journals

- *Addiction*
- *Drug & Alcohol Dependence*
- *Journal of Substance Abuse Treatment*

Websites

- Drugfree America
  http://www.drugfree.org/about
  This Website offers science-based resources and creates public awareness campaigns to help parents prevent, intervene, and find treatment for children.

- SAMHSA: Substance Abuse and Mental Health Services Administration
  http://www.samhsa.gov
  A resource for those with substance abuse and mental health concerns.

References

American Occupational Therapy Association. (2008). Occupational therapy practice framework: Domain and process, second edition. *American Journal of Occupational Therapy, 62*, 625–683.

American Psychiatric Association. (2000). *Diagnostic and Statistical Manual of Mental Disorders* (4th ed., text rev.). Washington, DC: Author.

Babor, T., Higgins-Bindle, J. C., Saunders, J., & Monteiro, M. (2001). The Alcohol Use Disorders Identification Test. *World Health Organization, 2*, 1–41

Boisvert, R. A., Martin, L. M., Grosek, M., & Clarie, A. J. (2008). Effectiveness of a peer-support community in addiction recovery: Participation as intervention. *Occupational Therapy International, 15*(4), 205–220.

Carey, K. B., Carey, M. P., Maisto, S. A., & Purnine, D. M. (2002). The feasibility of enhancing psychiatric outpatients' readiness to change their substance abuse. *Psychiatric Services, 53*, 602–608.

Croft, H. (2009). *Effects of substance abuse on family members*. Retrieved from http://www.healthyplace.com/about-hptv/croft-blog/effects-of-substance-abuse-on-family-members/menu-id-1824/

Gutman, S. A. (2006). Why addiction has a chronic, relapsing course. The neurobiology of addiction: Implications for occupational therapy practice. *Occupational Therapy in Mental Health, 22*(2), 1–29.

Harm Reduction Coalition. (n.d.). *Principles of harm reduction*. Retrieved from http://harmreduction.org/article.Php?list=type&type=62

Huhman, H. (2008). *Study: Occupational therapy reduces substance abuse, homelessness relapses*. Retrieved from http://www.aota.org/Archive/PrArchive/2008Releases/SubstanceAbuse.aspx

National Institute on Drug Abuse. (2010). *Substance use* (NIH Publication). Retrieved from http://www.nida.nih.gov/DrugPages/DrugsofAbuse.html

Stoffel, V. C., & Moyers, P. A. (2004). An evidence-based and occupational perspective of interventions for persons with substance-use disorders. *American Journal of Occupational Therapy, 58*(5), 570–586.

Substance Abuse and Mental Health Services Administration. (2007). *Results from the 2006 National Survey on Drug Use and Health: National findings* (Office of Applied Studies, NSDUH Series H-32, DHHS Publication No. SMA 07-4293). Rockville, MD: Author.

United States National Library of Medicine. (2010). *Drug dependence*. Retrieved from http://www.nlm.nih.gov/medlineplus/ency/article/001522.htm

Traumatic Brain Injury

Anne LeBorgne

Description

A *traumatic brain injury* (TBI) is an alteration in brain function, or other evidence of brain pathology, caused by an external force. A TBI may produce a diminished or altered state of consciousness that results in impairment of cognitive abilities or physical functioning as well as disturbances of behavioral, sensory, and emotional function. These impairments may be either temporary or permanent and may cause partial or total functional disability or psychosocial maladjustment (American Occupational Therapy Association [AOTA], 2011; Brain Injury Association of America [BIAA], 2011).

Types of Traumatic Brain Injury

- Penetrating or missile (open) injuries: result from penetration of the skull. The injury usually results in various types of skull fracture. Firearms are the single largest cause of death from TBI.
- Nonpenetrating, closed head injuries: result from rapid acceleration or deceleration of the brain within the skull, causing damage at the point of impact (coup injuries) or at the opposite pole (contracoup injuries). Closed head injuries include diffuse axonal injury, concussion, contusion, second impact syndrome, or recurrent TBI locked in syndrome. Overall closed head injuries involve large amounts of swelling and an increase in intracranial pressure; brain tissue can also be compressed, which causes further injury (BIAA, 2011).

Incidence and Prevalence

- Each year, an estimated 1.4 million Americans sustain a TBI.
- More than 5 million Americans currently live with a TBI, resulting in a permanent need for help in performing daily living activities.
- The 75% of TBIs that occur each year are mild brain injuries, such as concussions.
- Most TBIs are seen primarily in males between the ages of 18 and 25 years (BIAA, 2011; Centers for Disease Control and Prevention [CDC], 2010; National Institute of Neurological Disorders and Stroke [NINDS], 2011).
- Due to the fact that most TBIs occur during young adulthood, there is a major impact on role development, specifically in the realm of education, social, employment, marital relationships, and adult independence (Golisz, 2009).

Primary Causes

The primary causes leading to TBI are falls, motor vehicle traffic crashes, struck by or against events (colliding with a moving or stationary object), and assaults (CDC, 2010).

Typical Prognosis

No two brain injuries are exactly the same; the course of a TBI is complex and can vary greatly between individuals. Early prediction of outcome and prognosis is difficult because of the complex interaction of various factors, including the cause, location, and severity of injury; age; length of posttraumatic amnesia; increased intracranial pressure; and/or alteration of consciousness. Accurate prognosis requires repeated observations over weeks or months to predict the level of recovery and the amount of rehabilitation needed (BIAA, 2011).

Possible Symptoms/Deficits

Depending on the location and severity of the injury, deficits may be present in the areas of cognition, behavioral/emotional, physical, and/or sensory functioning. Symptoms and deficits range widely and can include aphasia, dysarthria, blurred vision, seizures, numbness in extremities, decreased balance/coordination, as well as changes in visual and auditory functions (AOTA, 2011; NINDS, 2011).

Ranchos Los Amigos Levels of Cognitive Functioning Scale

The Rancho Los Amigos Scale, a nonstandardized method of organizing and describing clinical observations of cognitive performance in individuals with TBI, allows for assessment of recovery and communication with families.

- Level I: no response, total assistance
- Level II: generalized response, total assistance
- Level III: localized response, total assistance
- Level IV: confused, agitated, maximal assistance
- Level V: confused, inappropriate, maximal assistance
- Level VI: confused, appropriate, moderate assistance
- Level VII: automatic, appropriate, minimal assistance for daily living skills
- Level VIII: purposeful, appropriate, with standby assistance
- Level IX: purposeful, appropriate, with standby assistance on request
- Level X: purposeful, appropriate, modified independence (Hagan, 1998)

Occupational Therapy Evaluations

- Rancho Los Amigos Levels of Cognitive Functioning Scale

Acute Stages of Recovery

- Glasgow Coma Scale (GCS): not administered by occupational therapists but important for quantifying level of consciousness and predicting recovery with early treatment and prognostic indicators
- Western Neuro Sensory Stimulation Profile (WNSSP): objective assessment of arousal and attention, expressive communication, and response to stimulation.
- Coma Recovery Scale-Revised (CRS-R): monitors level of responsiveness

Inpatient Rehabilitation

- Functional Independence Measure (FIM): performance-based measure of disability measuring basic activities of daily living (BADL)
- Functional Assessment Measure (FAM): an addition to the FIM, evaluating cognitive, behavioral, communication, and community functioning measures
- Assessment of Motor and Process Skills (AMPS): observational measure of performance of functional tasks, assesses quality of person's activities of daily living (ADL) performance; requires certification
- Loewenstein Occupational Therapy Cognitive Assessment (LOTCA): standardized assessment of cognitive-perceptual abilities and disabilities, assists in developing intervention goals
- Kohlman Evaluation of Living Skills (KELS): assesses basic living skills by interview and task performance
- Family Needs Questionnaire (FNQ): explores the needs of family members during acute rehabilitation including their perception of needs and extent to which needs are met
- Kitchen Task Assessment (KTA): a functional measure of the levels of cognitive support required by a person with dementia to successfully cook.
- Rivermead Behavioral Memory Test-Extended Version (RBMT-E): assesses visual and verbal memory in order to predict everyday memory tasks that will be difficult

Postacute Rehabilitation

- Canadian Occupational Performance Measure (COPM): self-report of performance and satisfaction with occupations
- Safety Assessment of Function and the Environment for Rehabilitation (SAFER): assesses cognitive abilities to function in the environment and perform tasks
- Community Integration Questionnaire (CIQ): assesses home and social integration, productivity in employment, volunteer, work, or school
- Brain Injury Community Reintegration Outcome (BICRO-39): measures personal care, mobility self-organization, partner/child and parent/sibling contact, socializing, productive employment, and psychological well-being

Occupational Therapy Intervention

Acute Stages of Recovery

- Biomechanical approaches including positioning; active range of motion (AROM), active assistive range of motion (AAROM), and passive range of motion (PROM) exercises; splinting; and casting
- Sensory stimulation
- Patient and family education and support

Inpatient Rehabilitation

- Optimize gross and fine motor functioning and abilities through meaningful tasks and activities.
- Optimize visual-perceptual functioning and abilities through environmental adaptations, compensatory techniques, and assistive devices such as low-vision aids.
- Maximize cognitive functioning and abilities with compensatory or remedial strategies that optimize the areas of orientation, attention, and memory.
- Increase independence in ADL and instrumental activities of daily living (IADL).

Postacute Rehabilitation

- Community reintegration including the development of effective routines and schedules, relearning social skills, and memory compensation techniques
- Environmental modifications such as using lighting to improve attention and vision or labeling drawers to help with cognitive challenges and the use of adaptive equipment
- Restore competence in ADL and IADL through training and adaptation
- Participation in previous or new leisure and/or work activities, as well as social skills training
- Patient and family education and support including consulting with employers or educational systems (AOTA, 2011)

Occupational Therapy and the Evidence

Occupational therapy (OT) plays an integral role as a part of an interdisciplinary rehabilitation team for individuals with TBI in multiple settings, including inpatient, outpatient, and community settings. Evidence has shown OT to be effective in improving occupational performance through participation in functional tasks and activities for individuals with TBI. Trombly, Radomski, Trexel, and Burnett-Smith (2002) concluded that participation in goal-specific outpatient OT that focuses on teaching compensatory strategies is strongly associated with the achievement of self-identified goals and the reduction of disability in adults with mild-to-moderate brain injury. Dirette (2002) found that clients with brain injury slowly developed awareness of their deficits when they were in situations that enabled them to compare current performance to performance prior to brain injury. Giles (2010) determined that the use of neurofunctional techniques such as task analysis, cue experimentation, and errorless learning programs for skill acquisition can be effective in the development of independent living skills for clients who have had a TBI when implemented in addition to standard care. These techniques are especially relevant for clients whose short-term goals relate to independent living rather than return to work or school. A goal-setting process that consists of a collaboration between the client, therapist, and significant others can enhance goal-directed rehabilitation in a community setting (Doig, Fleming, Cornwell, & Kuipers, 2009).

Caregiver Concerns

Families and caregivers require education and support for the many behavioral, emotional, and personality changes that can occur in an individual following a TBI. A study by Verhaeghe, Defloor, and Grypdonk (2005) concluded that the better the family members can cope with the situation following a TBI, the better the patient's recovery. This has clinical implications as therapists work with the entire family not only the individual with the TBI. Caregivers may have numerous concerns during the recovery of a loved one following TBI, possibilities include management of agitation and low frustration tolerance; personality and behavioral changes following injury; difficulty with communicating; concerns about reintegration and adaptation; lack of awareness of deficits/denial; deficits in higher level executive cognitive functions, including orientation, attention, and memory; disinhibition of inappropriate behavior; depression; long-term need for assistance/care; a change in family and societal roles; or safety concerns/awareness (BIAA, 2011).

Resources

Associations

- Brain Injury Association of America
  105 North Alfred Street
  Alexandria, VA 22314
  Telephone: 800-444-6443
  Family Helpline: 703-236-6000
  Fax: 703-236-6001
  Website: http://www.biusa.org

- Family Caregiver Alliance
  690 Market Street
  Suite 600
  San Francisco, CA 94104
  Telephone: 415-434-3388 or 800-445-8106
  Website: http://www.caregiver.org

Books

- Woodruff, L., & Woodruff, B. (2007). *In an instant: A family's journey in love and healing.* New York, NY: Random House.
  Woodruff and her husband describe his accident as a news anchor after he hit an explosive device in Iraq and sustained a TBI. The book is focused on Bob's rehabilitation and the family's experience of TBI from both private and public perspectives.

- Crimmins, C. (2001). *Where is the mango princess?* New York, NY: Random House.
  Crimmins tells her personal story of the victories and losses that she endured as the caregiver of an individual recovering from a severe brain injury. She describes issues ranging from the frustrations of dealing with doctors and insurance plans to the pain of caregiver issues.

- Meili, T. (2003). *I am the Central Park jogger: A story of hope and possibility.* Waterville, ME: Thorndike Press.
  Meili tells her personal experience of recovery from a violence-related TBI following an attack in Central Park. She focuses her book on the rehabilitation process, how brain injury affected her personal and professional life, and her outlook on living with a brain injury.

Journals

- *Brain*
- *Journal of Head Trauma Rehabilitation*

Websites

- Brain Injury Association of America
  http://www.biusa.org
  This is a thorough and accessible Website that provides information and resources relating to TBI for families, professionals, and individuals with brain injuries including a guide for patients or caregivers to guide long-term therapy and care.

- Traumatic Brain Injury Resource Guide
  http://www.neuroskills.com
  This Website provides a review of information, services, and products relating to TBI, brain injury recovery, and postacute rehabilitation.

References

American Occupational Therapy Association. (2011). *Fact sheet: Occupational therapy and community reintegration of persons with brain injury.* Retrieved from http://www.aota.org/Practitioners/PracticeAreas/Rehab/Tools/Reintegration.aspx?FT.pdf

Brain Injury Association of America. (2011). *About brain injury.* Retrieved from http://www.biausa.org/Default.aspx?PageID=3597010&A=SearchResult&SearchID=1981228&ObjectID=3597010&ObjectType=1

Centers for Disease Control and Prevention. (2010). *Traumatic brain injury.* Retrieved from http://www.cdc.gov/TraumaticBrainInjury/index.html

Dirette, D. (2002). The development of awareness and the use of compensatory strategies for cognitive deficits. *Brain Injury, 16,* 861–871.

Doig, E., Fleming, J., Cornwell, P. L., & Kuipers, P. (2009). Qualitative exploration of a client-centered, goal-directed approach to community-based occupational therapy for adults with traumatic brain injury. *American Journal of Occupational Therapy, 63,* 559–568.

Giles, G. M. (2010). Cognitive versus functional approaches to rehabilitation after traumatic brain injury: Commentary on a randomized controlled trial. *American Journal of Occupational Therapy, 64,* 182–185.

Golisz, K. (2009). *Occupational therapy practice guidelines for adults with traumatic brain injury.* Bethesda, MD: AOTA Press.

National Institute of Neurological Disorders and Stroke. (2011). *Traumatic brain injury: Hope through research.* Retrieved from http://www.ninds.nih.gov/disorders/tbi/detail_tbi.htm

Trombly, C. A., Radomski, M. V., Trexel, C., & Burnett-Smith, S. E. (2002). Occupational therapy and achievement of self-identified goals by adults with acquired brain injury: Phase II. *American Journal of Occupational Therapy, 56,* 489–498.

Verhaeghe, S., Defloor, T., & Grypdonck, M. (2005). Stress and coping among families of patients with traumatic brain injury: A review of the literature. *Clinical Nursing, 14,* 1004–1012.

References for Assessments

Hagan, C. (1998). *The Ranchos Levels of Cognitive Functioning: The revised levels* (3rd ed.). Retrieved from http://www.rancho.org/research/cognitive_levels.pdf

Jang, Y., Chern, J., & Lin, K. (2009). Validity of the Loewenstein Occupational Therapy Cognitive Assessment in people with intellectual disabilities. *American Journal of Occupational Therapy, 63,* 414–422.

Kim, H., & Colantonio, A. (2010). Effectiveness of rehabilitation in enhancing community integration after acute traumatic brain injury: A systematic review. *American Journal of Occupational Therapy, 64,* 709–719.

Klyczek, J. P., Bauer-Yox, N., & Fiedler, R. C. (1997). The Interest Checklist: A factor analysis. *American Journal of Occupational Therapy, 51,* 815–823.

Linden, A., Boschian, K., Eker, C., Schalen, W., & Nordstrom, C. H. (2005). Assessment of Motor and Process Skills reflects brain injured patients' ability to resume independent living better than neuropsychological tests. *Acta Neurologica Scandinavica, 111,* 364–369.

McNett, M. (2007). A review of the predictive ability of the Glasgow Coma Scales in head-injured patients. *Journal of Neuroscience Nursing, 39,* 68–75.

Oliver, R., Blathwayt, J., Brackley, C., & Tamaki, T. (1993). Development of the Safety Assessment of Function and the Environment for Rehabilitation (SAFER) tool. *Canadian Journal of Occupational Therapy, 60,* 78–82.

Patrick, P., Wamstad, J. B., Mabry, J. L., Smith-Janik, S., Gurka, M., Buck, M. L., & Blackman J. A. (2009). Assessing the relationship between the WNSSP and therapeutic participation in adolescents in low response states following severe traumatic brain injury. *Brain Injury, 23,* 528–534.

Phipps, S., & Richardson, P. (2007). Occupational therapy outcomes for clients with traumatic brain injury and stroke using the Canadian Occupational Performance Measure. *American Journal of Occupational Therapy, 61,* 328–334.

van Baalen, B., Odding, E., van Hoensel, M. P., van Kessel, M. A., Roebroeck, M. E., & Stam, H. J. (2006). Reliability and sensitivity to change of measurement instruments used in a traumatic brain injury population. *Clinical Rehabilitation, 20,* 686–700.

Visual Impairments

Emily Meibeyer

Description and Diagnosis

Low vision is characterized as a visual impairment that cannot be corrected by medical or surgical intervention and is severe enough to interfere with daily functioning but allows some usable vision. Low vision includes having decreased acuity and/or a decreased visual field. *Legal blindness* is defined as having best corrected vision of at least 20/200 or a visual field of 20 degrees or less. *Blindness* is a visual impairment in which the person has no object or light perception and cannot use vision to complete daily occupations (Warren, 2008). Low vision can result from various ophthalmologic and neurologic disorders; the most common causes of low vision in the United States include the following:

- *Age-related macular degeneration* (AMD): a disease associated with aging that affects the macula and gradually destroys sharp, central vision, and ability to see fine detail (American Optometric Association [AOA], 2011d).
- *Glaucoma*: a group of diseases that causes damage to the eye's optic nerve when there is an increase of fluid pressure inside the eye; causes gradual failing of peripheral vision (AOA, 2011c).
- *Diabetic retinopathy*: a disease associated with both type 1 and 2 diabetes caused by damage to the blood vessels in the retina, resulting in blurred vision or spotty areas of vision loss called *scotomas* (AOA, 2011b).
- *Cataracts*: clouding of the lens in the eye, causing blurred vision; generally related to aging; dulls color and blurs visual details throughout the visual field (AOA, 2011a).

Incidence and Prevalence

Over 2.4 million people older than 40 years old in the United States have low vision, and approximately 937,000 people older than 40 years are blind (Congdon et al., 2004). AMD is the leading cause of vision loss in Americans 60 years of age and older; the number of Americans with AMD is estimated at 1.8 million. Two million Americans presently have glaucoma, and approximately 40% of the 10.2 million Americans with diabetes have diabetic retinopathy (National Eye Institute [NEI], 2008).

Cause and Etiology

Aging is the single best predictor of low vision and blindness. Other risk factors associated with glaucoma include race, family history of glaucoma, medical conditions (e.g., diabetes, hypertension, and heart disease), physical injuries to the eye, and corticosteroid use (AOA, 2011c). Severe hyperopia (farsightedness), smoking, nutrition, light eye color, and family history are risk factors of AMD (NEI, 2010). Caucasians are at higher risk for AMD than other races; however, glaucoma is the leading cause of low vision for African Americans and Hispanic Americans. Sunlight exposure, smoking, alcohol intake, and poor nutrition are additional risk factors for cataracts (AOA, 2011a). For diabetic retinopathy, diabetes is the most prevalent risk factors, especially related to severity of diabetic disease, age of onset, and poorly controlled blood sugar; other risk factors involve obesity and high blood pressure.

Typical Course and Symptoms

- *AMD*: gradual loss of ability to see objects clearly, objects appear distorted in shape, straight lines look wavy or crooked, loss of clear color vision, dark or empty area appears in the center of vision, difficulty with reading (AOA, 2011d)
- *Glaucoma*: peripheral vision is lost first; central vision is lost, and total blindness can result if left untreated; difficulty with mobility (AOA, 2011c)
- *Diabetic retinopathy*: seeing spots or floaters in your field of vision, blurred vision, having a dark or empty spot in the center of vision, difficulty seeing well at night (AOA, 2011b)
- *Cataracts*: blurred or hazy vision, reduced intensity of colors, increased sensitivity to glare from lights, increased difficulty seeing at night, change in the eye's refractive error (AOA, 2011a)

Precautions

There are many safety precautions for individuals with vision loss, including:

- Falls and safety with mobility
- Safety with using kitchen appliances (e.g., stove)
- Medication management
- Driving: Adults with low vision need to be evaluated before they should be permitted to continue driving.

Interdisciplinary Interventions

Medical/Surgical Interventions

Ophthalmologists and optometrists are the medical professionals most involved in the treatment of visual impairments. Medical treatments for AMD include laser surgery, macular translocation surgery, and injections that reduce inflammation and stop blood vessel growth (NEI, 2010). However, no cure exists for AMD. Glaucoma can be treated with eye drops to slow progression of disease, if diagnosed early, before significant damage is done to the optic nerve. Laser surgery and other surgical techniques are also used to treat glaucoma. Diabetic retinopathy can be treated with laser photocoagulation or intraocular surgery to destroy the leaking blood vessels in the retina, but minimal gains are typically seen. Surgical treatment of cataracts consists of removing the existing lens and replacing it with a synthetic intraocular lens; this is generally successful in restoring vision (AOA, 2011a; NEI, 2010). It is important that clients with low vision are provided with best correct vision through refraction by optometrists or ophthalmologists before receiving services from occupational therapy (OT).

Occupational Therapy Evaluations

For clients with low vision, occupational therapists should collaborate with clients to identify the activities and occupations that provide meaning and purpose to the client's life. The occupational therapists should also complete a visual assessment in coordination with optometry/ophthalmology. Evaluation of the client's living context and environment, as well as his or her occupational performance in activities of daily living (ADL) and/or instrumental activities of daily living (IADL), are also necessary to assess the client's abilities and limitations, as well as barriers and supports in his or her environment.

Visual Skills Assessments

- Amsler grid testing: assesses central vision and visual fields; determine areas of scotoma or distortion
- Pursuits/tracking: assesses ability to track a moving object with a stationary head
- Saccades: assesses ability for sequenced, rapid eye movements
- Convergence: assesses ability of eyes to work together by following a target
- Ocular alignment: measures alignment of the reflection in corneas with pen light
- Confrontation field testing: assessment of peripheral visual field function
- Mars Letter Contrast Sensitivity Test: assessment of contrast sensitivity (Scheiman, Scheiman, & Whittaker, 2007)

Occupation-Based Assessments

- Canadian Occupational Performance Measure (COPM): self-report of performance and satisfaction with occupations
- Environmental assessment: assess supports and barriers in home environment, including lighting (using a light meter), contrast, and organization (Gilbert & Sikes Baker, 2011)
- Geriatric Depression Scale (GDS): self-report scale assessing risk for depression

- Impact of Visual Impairment Questionnaire (IVI): measures impact of visual impairment on ADL, IADL, and leisure (Weih, Hassell, & Keeffe, 2002)
- National Eye Institute Visual Function Questionnaire: self-report measuring impact of visual impairment on daily functioning related to ADL, leisure, and psychosocial issues (Mangione et al., 1998)
- Pepper Visual Skills for Reading Test: assessment of reading speed and performance (Scheiman et al., 2007)
- Self-Report Assessment of Functional Visual Performance: a self-report questionnaire with an observational component for ADL/IADL (Gilbert & Sikes Baker, 2011)

Occupational Therapy Interventions

OT in low-vision rehabilitation focuses on training the client to optimize use of his or her remaining vision for daily occupational engagement and safety. Interventions may include environmental adaptations, use of compensatory strategies, and client and family education. Specific OT interventions for low vision include the following:

- *Visual strategies*: eccentric viewing (moving the scotoma out of line of vision by turning head to side); scanning techniques for decreased visual field
- *Contrast enhancement*: increase visibility of objects by providing high contrast between foreground and background; useful for stairs, for eating (white plates on dark-colored placemats), and in the bathroom
- *Lighting*: increase general light to at least 300 lux; increase task lighting at least 750 to 1,000 lux for reading; minimize glare (Figueiro, 2001)
- *Magnification*: use of large print; teaching use of optical devices, such as magnifiers (e.g., stand, hand held) and telescopes
- *Sensory substitutions*: use of tactile markings on pill bottles, oven dials, faucets, and so forth; check writing or signature guides; use of auditory strategies (i.e., talking clocks, talking glucose meters); liquid level indicators
- *Falls prevention*: elimination of clutter; installation of handrails and grab bars; removal of environmental hazards
- *ADL/IADL retraining/adaptation*: teaching the use of strategies for problem areas, such as matching clothing, identifying spoiled foods, dialing emergency numbers, using knives to cut foods, and so forth
- *Caregiver training*: sighted guide training (technique of guiding someone with visual impairments safely); education and training on how to facilitate independence and participation (Bartmann, Bettenhausen, Sikes-Baker, Kern, & Storm-Weiss, 2008; Gilbert & Sikes Baker, 2011; Riddering, 2008)

Occupational Therapy and the Evidence

Adults with visual impairments are at risk for social isolation and depression due to dissatisfaction with performance in valued occupations, restricted participation in daily activities, and decreased social interactions (Alma et al., 2011; Rovner, Casten, Hegel, Hauck, & Tasman, 2007). OTs can address isolation by identifying those at risk for depression, by enabling engagement in meaningful activities, and by encouraging positive adaptation to vision loss through teaching cognitive and adaptive strategies (Girdler, Packer, & Boldy, 2008; Rovner et al., 2007). Self-management programs that include cognitive behavioral techniques, problem solving, health education, and/or an emphasis on self-efficacy may be effective for reducing depression in older adults with AMD (Brody et al., 2006; Girdler, Boldy, Dhaliwal, Crowley, & Packer, 2010).

Eccentric viewing training was found to be useful in improving ADL performance with older adults with AMD (Vukicevic & Fitzmaurice, 2009). Improved overall and task lighting was cited as effective in increasing participation in kitchen tasks (e.g., pouring a drink), leisure, and social participation (Brunnstrom, Sorensen, Alsterstad, & Sjostrand, 2004).

Caregiver Concerns

A person adjusting to low vision or vision loss often faces threat to his or her independence and loss of life roles and responsibilities (Girdler et al., 2008). Families often experience difficulty adjusting and adapting to their loved one's change in roles and abilities (Bambara et al., 2009). Additionally, the loss of vision has been shown to profoundly affect the individual's spouse, increasing his or her risk for depression, and minimizing physical and emotional well-being and marital quality (Strawbridge, Wallhagen, & Shema, 2007). Occupational therapists can provide education, training, and resources to caregivers and families of individuals with visual impairments to support them and to enable productive adjustment to the shift in family functioning and roles.

Resources

Organizations

- American Foundation for the Blind
  2 Penn Plaza, Suite 1102
  New York, NY 10121
  Telephone: 888-545-8331

- American Optometric Association
  243 N. Lindbergh Blvd.
  St. Louis, MO 63141
  Telephone: 800-365-2219

Books

- Alexander, S. H. (1994). *Taking hold: My journey into blindness.* New York, NY: Macmillian.
  Alexander, a third-grade teacher and author, details her adjustment to blindness and what it is like to live in a sighted world.

- Neer, F. L. (1998). *Perceiving the elephant: Living creatively with loss of vision.* Berkeley, CA: Creative Arts Book.
  This collection of essays, letters, and vignettes provides inspiration on how to cope with vision loss and how to live creatively with it.

Journals

- *Archives of Ophthalmology*
- *Journal of Visual Impairment and Blindness*
- *Journal of the American Optometric Association*
- *Ophthalmic and Physiological Optics*

Websites

- American Foundation for the Blind (AFB)
  http://www.afb.org/
  AFB is a nonprofit organization that works to deliver services and access to technology to persons living with vision loss, as well as makes relevant eye health resources available to health professionals and families.

- National Eye Institute (NEI)
  http://www.nei.nih.gov/
  NEI, as part of the federally funded National Institutes of Health, seeks to disseminate eye health information, support research, and provide programs and training related to vision loss and blindness.

- Prevent Blindness America (PBA)
  http://www.preventblindness.org/
  PBA, the nation's leading eye health and safety organization, provides education, advocacy, vision screenings, training, and research with the goal of preventing blindness and preserving sight.

References

Alma, M. A., Van Der Mei, S. F., Melis-Dankers, B. J. M., Van Tilburg, T. G., Groothoff, J. W., & Suurmeijer, T. P. B. M. (2011). Participation of the elderly after vision loss. *Disability and Rehabilitation, 33*, 63–72.

American Optometric Association. (2011a). *Cataract.* Retrieved from http://www.aoa.org/glaucomafxml

American Optometric Association. (2011b). *Diabetic retinopathy.* Retrieved from http://www.aoa.org/glaucoma.xml

American Optometric Association. (2011c). *Glaucoma.* Retrieved from http://www.aoa.org/glaucoma.xml

American Optometric Association. (2011d). *Macular degeneration.* Retrieved from http://www.aoa.org/glaucoma.xml

Bambara, J. K., Wadley, V., Owsley, C., Martin, R. C., Porter, C., & Dreer, L. E. (2009). Family functioning and low vision: A systematic review. *Journal of Visual Impairment & Blindness, 103,* 137–149.

Bartmann, L., Bettenhausen, D., Sikes-Baker, S., Kern, T., & Storm-Weiss, D. (2008). Evaluation and intervention for basic and instrumental activities of daily living. In M. Warren (Ed.), *Low vision: Occupational therapy evaluation and intervention with older adults* (pp. 163–204). Bethesda, MD: AOTA Press.

Brody, B. L., Roch-Levecq, A. C., Kaplan, R. M., Moutier, C. Y. & Brown, S. I. (2006). Age related macular degeneration: Self-management and reduction of depressive symptoms in a randomized, controlled study. *Journal of the American Geriatrics Society, 54,* 1557–1562.

Brunnstrom, G., Sorensen, S., Alsterstad, K., & Sjostrand, J. (2004). Quality of light and quality of life-the effect of lighting adaptation among people with low vision. *Ophthalmic and Physiological Optics, 24,* 274–280.

Congdon, N., O'Colmain, B., Klaver, C. C., Klein, R., Munoz, B., Friedman, D. S., . . . Mitchell, P. (2004). Causes and prevalence of visual impairment among adults in the United States. *Archives of Ophthalmology, 122,* 477–485.

Figueiro, M. G. (2001). *Lighting the way: A key to independence.* Retrieved from http://www.lrc.rpi.edu/programs/lightHealth/AARP/pdf/AARPbook3.pdf

Gilbert, M. P., & Sikes Baker, S. (2011). Evaluation and intervention for basic and instrumental activities of daily living. In M. Warren & E. A. Barstow (Eds.), *Occupational therapy interventions for adults with low vision* (pp. 227–267). Bethesda, MD: AOTA Press.

Girdler, S. J., Boldy, D. P., Dhaliwal, S. S., Crowley, M., & Packer, T. L. (2010). Vision self-management for older adults: A randomized controlled trial. *British Journal of Ophthalmology, 94,* 223–228.

Girdler, S., Packer, T. L., & Boldy, D. (2008). The impact of age-related vision loss. *OTJR: Occupation, Participation and Health, 28,* 110–120.

Mangione, C., Lee, P., Pitts, J., Gutierrez, P., Berry, S., & Hays, R. (1998). Psychometric properties of the National Eye Institute Visual Functioning Questionnaire (NEI-VFQ). *Archives of Ophthalmology, 116,* 1496–1504.

National Eye Institute. (2008). *Statistics and data: Prevalence of blindness data.* Retrieved from http://www.nei.nih.gov/eyedata/pbd.asp

National Eye Institute. (2010). *Facts about age-related macular degeneration.* Retrieved from http://www.nei.nih.gov/health/maculardegen/armd_facts.asp

Riddering, A. (2008). Evaluation and intervention for deficits in home and community mobility. In M. Warren (Ed.), *Low vision: Occupational therapy evaluation and intervention with older adults* (pp. 131–162). Bethesda, MD: AOTA Press.

Rovner, B. W., Casten, R. J., Hegel, M. T., Hauck, W. W., & Tasman, W. S. (2007). Dissatisfaction with performance of valued activities predicts depression in age-related macular degeneration. *International Journal of Geriatric Psychiatry, 22,* 789–793.

Scheiman, M., Scheiman, M., & Whittaker, S. G. (Eds.). (2007). Occupational therapy low vision rehabilitation evaluation. In *Low vision rehabilitation: A practical guide for occupational therapists* (pp. 103–131). Thorofare, NJ: Slack.

Strawbridge, W., Wallhagen, M., & Shema, S. (2007). Impact of spouse vision impairment on partner health and well-being: A longitudinal analysis of couples. *Journals of Gerontology, Series B: Psychological Sciences and Social Sciences, 62,* S315–S322.

Vukicevic, M., & Fitzmaurice, K. (2009). Eccentric viewing training in the home environment: Can it improve the performance of activities of daily living? *Journal of Visual Impairment and Blindness, 103,* 277–290.

Warren, M. (Ed.). (2008). An overview of low vision rehabilitation and the role of occupational therapy. In *Low vision: Occupational therapy evaluation and intervention with older adults* (pp. 1–23). Bethesda, MD: AOTA Press.

Weih, L. M., Hassell, J. B., & Keeffe, J. (2002). Assessment of the impact of vision impairment. *Investigative Ophthalmology & Visual Science, 43,* 927–935.

APPENDIX II

Table of Assessments: Listed Alphabetically by Title

Cheryl Lynne Trautmann Boop

Assessment Title and Author(s)	Publisher and/or Contact Information	Ages	Stated Purpose	Areas Assessed
ABILHAND Questionnaire/ ABILHAND-Kids Questionnaire *Penta, M., Thonnard, J. L., and Tesio, L.*	http://www.rehab-scales.org/ abilhand.html	Adults/children ages 6–15 years	Measure ability to perform ADL that require the use of upper extremities, including any strategies	ADL
Academic Performance Rating Scale *DuPaul, G. J., Rapport, M. D., and Perriello, L. M.*	DuPaul, G. J., Rapport, M. D., & Perriello, L. M. (1991). Teacher Ratings of Academic Skills: The Development of the Academic Performance Rating Scale. *School Psychology Review*, *20*, 284–300.	School age	Measure academic performance on three factors	Academic success, impulse control, academic productivity
Action Research Arm Test *Lyle, R.*	Lyle, R. (1981). A performance test for assessment of upper limb function in physical rehabilitation treatment and research. *International Journal of Rehabilitation Research*, *4*, 483–492.		Assess "specific changes in limb function among individuals who sustained cortical damage resulting in hemiplegia"	Upper extremity functioning
Activity Card Sort (ACS) *Baum, C. M., and Edwards, D.*	Baum, C. M., & Edwards, D. (2008). *Activity Card Sort* (2nd ed.). Bethesda, MD: AOTA Press.	Adults	Used as an interview-based tool to measure participation in leisure, social, and instrumental activities	Social, leisure, ADL
Activity Index & Meaningfulness of Activity Scale *Gregory, M. D.* *Nystrom, E. P.*	Gregory, M. D. (1983). Occupational behavior and life satisfaction among retirees. *American Journal of Occupational Therapy*, *37*, 548–553. Nystrom, E. P. (1974). Activity patterns and leisure concepts among the elderly. *American Journal of Occupational Therapy*, *28*, 337–345.	Older adults	Examine the meaning and significance of activity and activity patterns among the elderly	Activity/leisure

Assessment Title and Author(s)	Publisher and/or Contact Information	Ages	Stated Purpose	Areas Assessed
Activity Measures for Post-Acute Care (AM-PAC) *Jette, A., Haley, S. M., Coster, W. J., and Ni, P.*	Jette, A., Haley, S. M., Coster, W. J., & Ni, P. (2008). *Instruction Manual. Activity Measures for Post-Acute Care (AM-PAC): Basic mobility, daily activity, applied cognitive functional domains.* Boston, MA: Boston University Health and Disability Research Institute. Jette, A., Haley, S. M., Coster, W. J., & Ni, P. (2007). *Instruction Manual. AM-PAC computerized adaptive testing (AM-PAC CAT™) personal computer version: Basic mobility, daily activity, applied cognitive functional domains.* Boston, MA: Boston University Health and Disability Research Institute. http://www.crecare.com/am-pac/ampac.html For information, e-mail: information@crecare.com or call 617-780-8815		Designed as an outcomes measuring instrument to measure function in three domains; can be used for quality improvement, outcomes monitoring, and research activities	Basic mobility, ADL, applied cognitive functioning
Adaptive Behavior Assessment System-Second Edition (ABAS-II) *Harrison, P., and Oakland, T.*	Pearson Assessments Attention: Inbound Sales and Customer Support 19500 Bulverde Road San Antonio, TX 78259-3701 ClinicalCustomerSupport@Pearson.com 800-627-7271	Infant/child school adult	Assess adaptive skills functioning in three areas of adaptive behavior (conceptual, social, and practical)	Behavior
Addiction Severity Index (ASI) *Fureman, I., and McLellan, A. T.*	Fureman, I., & McLellan, A. T. (1999). *Addiction Severity Index Checker's Manual: A guide to checking data collected with the addiction severity index.* Philadelphia, PA: University of Pennsylvania/Philadelphia VAMC Center for Studies of Addiction.	Adults	Assist in substance abuse treatment and intervention	Substance abuse
ADHD Behavior Checklist for Adults *Barkley, R. A., and Murphy, K. R.*	Barkley, R. A., & Murphy, K. R. (1998). *Attention deficit hyperactivity disorder: A clinical workbook* (2nd ed.). New York, NY: Guilford.	Adults	Used as a self-report symptom checklist to help diagnose ADHD in adults	Attention
Adolescent Behavior Checklist *Demb, H. B., Brier, N., Huron, R., and Tomor, E.*	Demb, H. B., Brier, N., Huron, R., & Tomor, E. (1994). The adolescent behavior checklist: Normative data and sensitivity and specificity of a screening tool for diagnosable psychiatric disorders in adolescents with mental retardation and other developmental disabilities. *Research in Developmental Disabilities, 15,* 151–165.	12–21 years "with mild mental retardation or borderline intelligence"	To identify adolescents at risk for having a diagnosable psychiatric disturbance	Behavior
Adolescent Role Assessment (ARA) *Black, M. M.*	Black, M. M. (1976). Adolescent Role Assessment. *American Journal of Occupational Therapy, 30,* 73–79.	Adolescents	Gather information on the adolescent's occupational role involvement over time and across domains	Childhood play, socialization with family, socialization with peers, school functioning, occupational choice, anticipated adult work

(*continued*)

Assessment Title and Author(s)	Publisher and/or Contact Information	Ages	Stated Purpose	Areas Assessed
Adolescent/Adult Sensory Profile *Brown, C., and Dunn, W.*	Pearson Assessments Attention: Inbound Sales and Customer Support 19500 Bulverde Road San Antonio, TX 78259-3701 ClinicalCustomerSupport@Pearson.com 800-627-7271	11 years and older	To determine how well a person processes sensory information in everyday situations and to profile the sensory system's effect on functional performance	Sensory processing, modulation, and behavioral and emotional responses
Adult Playfulness Scale *Glynn, M. A., and Webster, J.*	Glynn, M. A., & Webster, J. (1992). The Adult Playfulness Scale: An initial assessment. *Psychological Reports*, *71*, 83–103.	Adults	Measure adult play behavior in the workplace	Play/leisure
Alcohol Use Disorders Identification Test (AUDIT)-Second Edition *Babor, T. F., Higgins-Biddle, J. C., Saunders, J. B., and Monteiro, M.*	Babor, T. F., Higgins-Biddle, J. C., Saunders, J. B., & Monteiro, M. (2001). *AUDIT: The Alcohol Use Disorders Identification Test. Guidelines for use in primary care.* Geneva, Switzerland: World Health Organization.	Adults	Identify those who are at risk for alcohol dependency and at risk for alcohol abuse	Alcohol use
Allen Cognitive Level Screen-5 (ACLS-5) (also see Large Allen Cognitive Level Screen-5) *Allen, C. K., et al.*	Allen, C. K., Austin, S. L., David, S. K., Earhart, C. A., McCraith, D. B., & Riska-Williams, L. (2007). *Manual for the Allen cognitive level screen-5 (ACLS-5) and large Allen cognitive level screen-5 (LACLS-5).* Camarillo, CA: ACLS and LACLS Committee. ACLS and LACLS Committee PO Box 3144 Camarillo, CA 93011 http://www.allencognitivelevelscreen.org/products.htm	All ages	To provide a quick measure of learning potential, global cognitive processing capacities, and performance abilities	Problem solving, following directions
Allen Diagnostic Module-Second Edition (ADM-2): Manual and Assessment Tasks *Earhart, C. A.*	Earhart, C. A. (2006). *Allen Diagnostic Module* (2nd ed.). Colchester, CT: S&S Worldwide.	All ages	To assess cognitive disability and suggest treatment approach	Problem solving, following direction
ALS Functional Rating Scale-Revised (ALSFRS-R) *Cedarbaum, J., et al.*	Cedarbaum, J., Stambler, N., Malta, E., Fuller, C., Hilt, D., Thurmond, B., Nakanishi, A., & BDNF ALS Study Group (Phase III). (1999). The ALSFRS-R: A revised ALS functional rating scale that incorporates assessments of respiratory function. *Journal of the Neurological Sciences*, *169*, 13–21.	Adults	Evaluate the functional status of individuals diagnosed with ALS	ADL, IADL
American Heart Association Stroke Outcome Classification (AHA:SOC) *Kelly-Hayes, M., et al.*	Kelly-Hayes, M., Robertson, J. T., Broderick, J. P., Duncan, P. W., Hersehy, L. A., Roth, E. J., . . . Trombly, C. A. (1998). The American Heart Association Stroke Outcome Classification. *Stroke*, *29*, 1274–1280.	Adults	Classify the severity and extent of neurological impairments following survival of a stroke, identify the level of independence in BADL and IADL	Motor impairments, sensory deficits, vision issues, language, cognition, affect, BADL, IADL
American Spinal Injury Association (ASIA) Impairment Scale *American Spinal Injury Association*	http://www.asia-spinalinjury.org/publications/59544_sc_Exam_Sheet_r4.pdf	All ages	Classify neurological impairments in individuals with spinal injuries	Motor impairments, sensory impairments

Assessment Title and Author(s)	Publisher and/or Contact Information	Ages	Stated Purpose	Areas Assessed
Arm Motor Ability Test (AMAT) *Kopp, B., et al.*	Kopp, B., Kunkel, A., Flor, H., Platz, T., Rose, U., Mauritz, K. H., . . . Taub, E. (1997). The Arm Motor Ability Test: Reliability, validity, and sensitivity to change of an instrument for assessing disabilities in activities of daily living. *Archives of Physical Medicine and Rehabilitation, 78*, 615–620.	Adults	Measure upper extremity movement using daily activity tasks	ADL, IADL
Árnadóttir OT-ADL Neurobehavioral Evaluation (A-ONE) also known as ADL-Focused Occupation-Based Neurobehavioral Evaluation *Árnadóttir, G.*	Árnadóttir, G. (1990). *The brain and behavior: Assessing cortical dysfunction through activities of daily living*. St. Louis, MO: Mosby.	Adults	To provide a structured guideline for clinical observation of ADL performance and underlying neurobehavioral components	ADL, neurobehavioral components
Arthritis Hand Function Test *Backman, C., Mackie, H., and Harris, J.*	Backman, C., Mackie, H., & Harris, J. (1991). Arthritis Hand Function Test: Development of a standardized assessment tool. *The Occupational Therapy Journal of Research, 11*, 245–256. The School of Rehabilitation Sciences University of British Columbia T325-2211 Wesbrook Mall Vancouver, BC Canada V6T 2B5	Adults	Assess pure and applied strength and dexterity of both hands in adults with rheumatoid arthritis and osteoarthritis	Hand strength and dexterity, ADL
Arthritis Impact Measurement Scale (AIMS) Arthritis Impact Measurement Scale, Expanded (AIMS2)—also a children's version and a geriatric version *Meenan, R. F.*	Meenan, R. F., Gertman, P. M., & Mason, J. H. (1980). Measuring health status in arthritis: The Arthritis Impact Measurement Scales. *Arthritis Rheumatism, 23*, 146–152. Robert F. Meenan, Dean, Boston University School of Public Health, 715 Albany St., T-C-306, Boston, MA 02118. E-mail: rmwwnan@bu.edu	All ages	Measure physical, social, and emotional well-being as an outcome measure in people diagnosed with arthritis	Physical activity, dexterity, household activities, social activities, ADL, pain, depression, anxiety
Ashworth Scale *Ashworth, B.*	Ashworth, B. (1964). Preliminary trial of carisprodal in multiple sclerosis. *Practitioner, 192*, 540–542.	Adults	Measure the resistance to stretch of a limb that is passively ranged	Spasticity
Assessment of Communication and Interaction Skills (ACIS) *Forsyth, K., Salamy, M., Simon, S., and Kielhofner, G.*	http://www.uic.edu/depts/moho/assess/acis.html	Adults	Assess the communication/interaction skills of adults who have physical or mental illness	Communication, social interaction skills
Assessment of Life Habits (LIFE-H) *Fougeyrollas, P., and Noreau, L.*	Fougeyrollas, P., & Noreau, L. (2003). *Assessment of Life Habits (LIFE-H, 3.0): General long form*. Quebec, Canada: INDCP.	Adults	Assess the level of performance in life habits in various contexts	Nutrition, fitness, personal care, communication, housing, mobility, responsibility, interpersonal relationships, community, education, employment, recreation

(continued)

Assessment Title and Author(s)	Publisher and/or Contact Information	Ages	Stated Purpose	Areas Assessed
Assessment of Life Habits in Children (LIFE-H Child) *Noreau, L., Fougeyrollas, P. and Lepage, C.*	Noreau, L., Fougeyrollas, P., & Lepage, C. (2003). *Assessment of Life Habits (LIFE-H for children 5–13, 1.0): Adapted for children 5 to 13 years, short form*. Quebec, Canada: INDCP. Noreau, L., Fougeyrollas, P., & Lepage, C. (2004). *Assessment of Life Habits (LIFE-H for children 5–13, 1.0): Adapted for children 5 to 13 years, long form*. Quebec, Canada: INDCP. Fougeyrollas, P., Noreau, L., & Lepage, C. (2007). *Assessment of Life Habits (LIFE-H for children 0–4, 1.0): Adapted for children birth to 4 years*. Quebec, Canada: INDCP.	5–13 years Birth to 4 years	Assess the level of performance of life habits in various contexts	Daily activities
Assessment of Living Skills and Resources (ALSAR)-Revised Format *Williams, J. H., et al.*	Madison Geriatric Research, Education, and Clinical Center VA Medical Center 2500 Overlook Terrace Madison, WI 53705	Adults	Used as an interview-based assessment of personal independence	IADL
Assessment of Living Skills and Resources-Revised 2 (ALSAR-R2) *Clemson, L., Bundy, A., Unsworth, C., and Fiatarone Singh, M.*	http://sydney.edu.au/health_sciences/ageing_work_health/docs/Clemson_ALSAR.pdf	Adults	Used as an interview-based assessment of personal independence	IADL
Assessment of Ludic Behaviors (ALB) *Ferland, F.*	Ferland, F. (1997). *Play, children with physical disabilities and occupational therapy: The Ludic model*. Ottawa, ON: University of Ottawa Press	Children	Assess play behaviors of children with disabilities	Play/leisure
Assessment of Motor and Process Skills (AMPS) *Fisher, A. G., and Bray Jones, K.*	Fisher, A. G., & Bray Jones, K. (2012). *Assessment of Motor and Process Skills: Development, standardization, and administration manual* (Vol. 1, 7th ed., Rev. ed.). Fort Collins, CO: Three Star Press. Fisher, A. G., & Bray Jones, K. (2012). *Assessment of Motor and Process Skills: User manual* (Vol. 2, 7th ed., Rev. ed.). Fort Collins, CO: Three Star Press. http://www.ampsintl.com/	3 years and older	Provide an objective assessment of motor and process skills in the context of performing several familiar functional tasks of the subject's choice	Motor and process skills, such as the ability to initiate, inquire, notice and respond, pace, sequence, organize, and terminate
Assessment of Occupational Functioning-Collaborative Version (AOF-CV) *Watts, J. H.*	http://www.sahp.vcu.edu/occu/ot/aofinstrument2.pdf Janet H. Watts, PhD, OTR/L Virginia Commonwealth University/Department of OT VCU Box 980008 Richmond, VA 23298-0008 jhwatts@hsc.vcu.edu	Adults	Used to inform intervention by indicating the factors likely to influence a person's ability to function	Personal causation, values, roles, habits, skills
Assessment of Occupational Functioning (AOF)-Second Revision *Watts, J. H., Brollier, C., Bauer, D., and Schmidt, W.*	Watts, J. H., Brollier, C., Bauer, D., & Schmidt, W. (1989). The Assessment of Occupational Functioning: The second revision. In J. H. Watts & C. Brollier (Eds.), *Instrument development in occupational therapy* (pp. 61–88). New York, NY: Haworth.	Adults	Screen overall occupational function of residents in long-term care settings	Volition, habituation, performance, values, personal causation, interests, roles, habits, skills, school and job history

Assessment Title and Author(s)	Publisher and/or Contact Information	Ages	Stated Purpose	Areas Assessed
Assessment of Preschool Children's Participation *Law, M., King, G., Petrenchik, T., and Kertoy, M.*	Law, M., King, G., Petrenchik, T., Kertoy, M., & Anaby, D. (2012). The Assessment of Preschool Children's Participation: Internal consistency and validity. *Physical & Occupational Therapy in Pediatrics, 32,* 272–287.	2–6 years	Measure participation in activities	Play skills, skill development, active physical recreation, social activities
Assessment of Preterm Infant Behavior (APIB) *Als, H., Butler, S., Kosta, S., and McAnulty, G.*	Als, H., Butler, S., Kosta, S., & McAnulty, G. (2005). The Assessment of Preterm Infants' Behavior (APIB): Furthering the understanding and measurement of neurodevelopmental competence in preterm and full-term infants. *Mental Retardation and Developmental Disabilities Research Reviews, 11,* 94–102.	Preterm, at-risk, and full-term infants from birth to 1 month after expected due date	Assess "mutually interacting behavioral subsystems in simultaneous interaction with the environment"	Autonomic, motor, state of organization, attention, self-regulation
Asset-Based Context Matrix (ABCM) *Wilson, L. L., and Mott, D. W.*	Wilson, L. L., Mott, D. W., & Batman, D. (2004). The Asset-Based Context Matrix: A tool for assessing children's learning opportunities and participation in natural environments. *Topics in Early Childhood Special Education, 24,* 110–120. Linda L. Wilson, Family, Infant and Preschool Program J. Iverson Riddle Developmental Center 300 Enola Rd., Morganton, NC 28655 E-mail: Linda.L.Wilson@ncmail.net	Infants and young children	Assess a child's participation in family life, community, and early childhood program participation	Activity settings, interests, assets, functional and meaningful activities, opportunity, participation, possibilities
Barthel Index *Mahoney, F. I., and Barthel, D. W.*	Mahoney, F. I., & Barthel, D. W. (1965). Functional evaluation: The Barthel index. *Maryland State Medical Journal, 14,* 56–61.	Adults	Reflect the functional status of hospital patients in ADL and to assess change	ADL
Bay Area Functional Performance Evaluation (BaFPE)-Second Edition *Williams, S. L., and Bloomer, J.*	Williams, S. L., & Bloomer, J. (1987). *Bay area functional performance evaluation* (2nd ed.). Palo Alto, CA: Consulting Psychologists Press.	Late adolescence to adult	To assess cognitive, affective, and performance skills in daily living tasks and social interaction skills; evaluate the effectiveness of OT interventions	Social interaction/behavior; ADL skills, cognitive, affective, and performance skills
Bayley Scales of Infant Development-Third Edition (BSID-III) *Bayley, N.*	Pearson Assessments Attention: Inbound Sales and Customer Support 19500 Bulverde Road San Antonio, TX 78259-3701 ClinicalCustomerSupport@Pearson.com 800-627-7271	Birth to 42 months	To assess the current developmental functioning of infants and children	Mental, cognitive, motor, and adaptive behaviors
Beck Anxiety Inventory (BAI) *Beck, A. T.*	Pearson Assessments Attention: Inbound Sales and Customer Support 19500 Bulverde Road San Antonio, TX 78259-3701 ClinicalCustomerSupport@Pearson.com 800-627-7271	17–80 years	To screen for anxiety	Anxiety

(*continued*)

Assessment Title and Author(s)	Publisher and/or Contact Information	Ages	Stated Purpose	Areas Assessed
Beck Depression Inventory-II (BDI-II) *Beck, A. T., Steer, R. A., and Brown, G. K.*	Pearson Assessments Attention: Inbound Sales and Customer Support 19500 Bulverde Road San Antonio, TX 78259-3701 ClinicalCustomerSupport@Pearson.com 800-627-7271	13–80 years	To assess the intensity of depression	Depression
Beery-Buktenica Developmental Test of Visual-Motor Integration-Sixth Edition (BEERY VMI) *Beery, K. E., Buktenica, N. A., and Beery, N. A.*	Pearson Assessments Attention: Inbound Sales and Customer Support 19500 Bulverde Road San Antonio, TX 78259-3701 ClinicalCustomerSupport@Pearson.com 800-627-7271	2–100 years	Screen for visual-motor deficits	Visual-motor integration skills, visual perceptual skills, motor coordination skills
Behavior Assessment System for Children-Second Edition (BASC-2) *Reynolds, C. R., and Kamphaus, R.*	Reynolds, C. R., & Kamphaus, R. (2004). *BASC-2: Behavior assessment system for children, second edition manual.* Circle Pines, MN: American Guidance Service.	2–21 years and 11 months	Assess behaviors and emotions of children and teens	Behavior in school and home environments
Behavior Rating Inventory of Executive Function-Adult Version (BRIEF-A) *Roth, R., Isquith, P., and Gioia, G.*	Psychological Assessment Resources, Inc. 16204 N. Florida Avenue Lutz, FL 33549 800-331-8378	Adults and older adults	To assess adult executive functioning/self-regulation in individuals ages 18–90 years	Executive functioning
Behavioral Inattention Test (BIT) *Wilson, B., Cockburn, J., and Halligan, P.*	Pearson Assessments Attention: Inbound Sales and Customer Support 19500 Bulverde Road San Antonio, TX 78259-3701 ClinicalCustomerSupport@Pearson.com 800-627-7271	Adults	To identify unilateral visual neglect and how it affects daily life	Nine subtests reflecting daily life activities, Six conventional pencil-and-paper tasks
Bennett Hand-Tool Dexterity Test *Bennett, G. K.*	Access Health Unit 1 Rear 194-196 Whitehorse Rd BLACKBURN VIC 3130 Australia http://www.accesshealth.com.au/	Adults	To provide a measure of proficiency in using ordinary mechanics tools.	Manipulative skills independent of intellectual skills
Borg Scale of Rating of Perceived Exertion (RPE) *Borg, G.*	Borg, G. (1998). *Borg's Perceived Exertion and Pain Scale.* Champaign, IL: Human Kinetics.	Adults	Used as self-assessment of exertion during activities	Perceived exertion
Box and Block Test *Mathiowetz, V., Volland, G., Kashman, N., and Weber, K.* *Mathoiwetz, V., Federman, S., and Wiemer, D.*	Mathiowetz, V., Volland, G., Kashman, N., & Weber, K. (1985). Adult norms for the Box and Block Test of Manual Dexterity. *American Journal of Occupational Therapy, 39*, 386–391. Mathoiwetz, V., Federman, S., & Wiemer, D. (1985). Box and Block Test of Manual Dexterity: Norms for 6–19 year olds. *Canadian Journal of Occupational Therapy, 52*, 241–245.	7 years and older	To provide a baseline for upper extremity manual dexterity and gross motor coordination	Manual dexterity

Assessment Title and Author(s)	Publisher and/or Contact Information	Ages	Stated Purpose	Areas Assessed
Brain Injury Community Reintegration Outcome (BICRO-39) *Beckers, K., Greenwood, R. J., and Powell, J. H.*	Beckers, K., Greenwood, R. J., & Powell, J. H. (1998). Measuring progress and outcome in community rehabilitation after brain injury with a new assessment instrument—the BICRO-39 Scales. *Archives of Physical Medicine and Rehabilitation, 79*, 1213–1215.	Adults	Assess problems experienced in the community by people with brain injuries	Personal and social functioning
Brief Fatigue Inventory *Mendoza, T., et al.*	Mendoza, T., Wang, X. S., Cleeland, C. S., Morrissey, M., Johnson, B. A., Wendt, J. K., & Huber, S. L. (1999). The rapid assessment of fatigue severity in cancer patients: Use of the Brief Fatigue Inventory. *Cancer, 85*, 1186–1196. For permission to use the assessment, contact The Department of Symptom Research Attn: Assessment Tools The University of Texas MD Anderson Cancer Center 1515 Holcombe Boulevard, Unit 1450 Houston, Texas 77030 713-745-3805	Adults	Assess the severity of fatigue and its effect on daily function	Fatigue
Brief Pain Inventory *Cleeland, C. S.*	Cleeland, C. S. (1991). Research in cancer pain: What we know and what we need to know. *Cancer, 67*, 823–827. For permission to use the assessment, contact The Department of Symptom Research Attn: Assessment Tools The University of Texas MD Anderson Cancer Center 1515 Holcombe Boulevard, Unit 1450 Houston, Texas 77030 713-745-3805	Adults	Assess how much pain interferes with occupational performance and mood	Pain and its relationship to occupational performance
Bruininks-Oseretsky Test of Motor Proficiency-Second Edition (BOT-2) *Bruininks, R. H., and Bruininks, B. D.*	Pearson Assessments Attention: Inbound Sales and Customer Support 19500 Bulverde Road San Antonio, TX 78259-3701 ClinicalCustomerSupport@Pearson.com 800-627-7271	4–21 years	To assess the gross and fine motor functioning of school-age clients	Fine motor control, manual dexterity, body coordination, strength and agility
BTE Work Simulator *BTE Technologies, Inc.*	BTE Technologies, Inc. 7455-L New Ridge Road Hanover, MD 21076-3105 800-331-8845	Adults	Used in work capacity evaluations to determine whether clients have the capabilities to return to work	Physical strength and endurance using a variety of attachments simulating tools
Canadian Occupational Performance Measure (COPM)-Fourth Edition *Law, M., et al.*	Canadian Association of Occupational Therapists CTTC Bldg. 3400-1125 Colonel By Drive Ottawa, ON K1S 5R1 613-523-2268 http://www.caot.ca/copm	7 years and older	Measure client's perception of his or her occupational performance over time	Self-care, productivity, leisure

(*continued*)

Assessment Title and Author(s)	Publisher and/or Contact Information	Ages	Stated Purpose	Areas Assessed
Catherine Bergego Scale (CBS) *Azouvi, P.*	Azouvi, P. (1996). Functional consequences and awareness of unilateral neglect: Study of an evaluation scale. *Neuropsychological Rehabilitation*, *6*, 133–150.	Adults	Assess the presence and severity of unilateral neglect in daily activities	ADL, unilateral neglect
Chedoke Arm and Hand Activity Inventory (CAHAI), Version 2 *Barreca, S.*	Barreca, S., Gowland, C., Stratford, P., Huijbregts, M., Griffiths, J., Torresin, W., . . . Masters, L. (2004). Development of the Chedoke Arm and Hand Activity Inventory: Theoretical constructs, item generation, and selection. *Topics in Stroke Rehabilitation*, *11*, 31–42. http://www.cahai.ca/	Adults	Assess functional use of a hemiplegic upper extremity	ADL, IADL
Chedoke-McMaster Stroke Assessment *Miller, P., et al.*	Miller, P., Huijbregts, M., Gowland, C., Berreca, S., Torresin, W., Moreland, J., . . . Barclay-Goddard, R. (2008). *Chedoke-McMaster Stroke Assessment—development, validation, and administration manual.* Ontario, Canada: McMaster University and Hamilton Health Sciences. School of Rehabilitation Sciences, McMaster University, Building T-16, 1280 Main Street West, Hamilton, ON http://www.chedokeassessment.ca/	Adults	Assess physical impairment and disability in people who have had strokes or other neurological impairment	Physical impairment, ADL
Child and Adolescent Scale of Environment (CASE) *Bedell, G.*	Bedell, G. (2009). Further validation of the Child and Adolescent Scale of Participation (CASP). *Developmental Neurorehabilitation*, *12*, 342–351.	3–22 years	Assess environmental issues that could affect participation at home, school, and in the community	Physical environment, social environment, attitudinal environment
Child and Adolescent Scale of Participation (CASP) *Bedell, G.*	Bedell, G. (2009). Further validation of the Child and Adolescent Scale of Participation (CASP). *Developmental Neurorehabilitation*, *12*(5), 342–351.	3–22 years	Measure participation in children and adolescents with brain injuries and other types of disabilities	Participation in home, school, and community activities
Child and Adolescent Social Perception (CASP) Measure *Magill-Evans, J., Koning, C., Cameron-Sadava, A., and Manyk, K.*	Magill-Evans, J., Koning, C., Cameron-Sadava, A., & Manyk, K. (1995). The Child and Adolescent Social Perception Measure. *Journal of Nonverbal Behavior*, *19*, 151–169.	6–15 years	To measure a child's sensitivity to nonverbal aspects of communication	Ability to interpret nonverbal aspects of communication
Child Behavior Checklist- Preschool School Age Multicultural *Achenbach, T. M.*	ASEBA Research Center for Children, Youth, and Families 1 South Prospect Street Burlington, VT 05401-3456 802-656-5130 www.ASEBA.org	Preschool: 1.5–5 years School age: 6–18 years Multicultural: 1.5–5 years	To record a child's competencies and problems as reported by parent or caregiver, teacher, and self	Internalizing and externalizing psychological symptoms for children and adolescents
Child Behaviors Inventory of Playfulness (CBI) *Rogers, C. S., et al.*	Rogers, C. S., Impara, J. C., Frary, R. B., Harris, T., Meeks, A., Semanic-Lauth, S., & Reynolds, M. R. (1998). Measuring playfulness: Development of the Child Behaviors Inventory of Playfulness. In M. C. Duncan, G. Chick, & A. Aycock (Eds.), *Play & culture studies: Diversions and divergences in fields of play* (Vol. 1). Greenwich, CT: Ablex.	Children	Examine playful behaviors of children	Play/leisure

Assessment Title and Author(s)	Publisher and/or Contact Information	Ages	Stated Purpose	Areas Assessed
Child Occupational Self Assessment (COSA) *Keller, J., Kafkes, A., Basu, S., Federico, J., and Kielhofner, G.*	http://www.uic.edu/depts/moho/assess/cosa.html	Children and youth	To understand how a child/youth perceives his or her own sense of occupational competence in everyday activities as well as the importance of those activities in his or her life	ADL
Children Activity Scales-Parent and Teacher (ChAS-P/T) *Rosenblum, S.*	Rosenblum, S. (2006). The development and standardization of the Children Activity Scales (ChAS-P/T) for the early identification of children with developmental coordination disorders. *Child Care Health and Development, 32*, 619–632.	4–8 years	To identify children with developmental coordination disorder	Gross and fine motor skills; organization in space and time during ADL, mobility, ball skills, play, and school activities
Children's Assessment of Participation and Enjoyment (CAPE) and Preferences for Activities of Children (PAC) *King, G., et al.*	Pearson Assessments Attention: Inbound Sales and Customer Support 19500 Bulverde Road San Antonio, TX 78259-3701 ClinicalCustomerSupport@Pearson.com 800-627-7271	6–21 years	Gather information on child's participation and engagement in everyday activities outside of mandated school activities	Social participation in nonschool activities
Children Helping Out: Responsibilities, Expectations, and Supports (CHORES) *Dunn, L.*	Dunn, L. (2004). Validation of the CHORES: A measure of school-aged children's participation in household tasks. *Scandinavian Journal of Occupational Therapy, 11*, 179–190.	School-age children and adolescents	To assess a child's participation in household tasks and changes in the amount of assistance needed to participate	ADL, IADL
Children's Kitchen Task Assessment (CKTA) *Rocke, K., Hays, P., Edwards, D., and Berg, C.*	Rocke, K., Hays, P., Edwards, D., & Berg, C. (2008). Development of a performance assessment of executive function: The Children's Kitchen Task Assessment. *American Journal of Occupational Therapy, 62*, 528–537.	Children	Assess executive function skills using kitchen activities	Executive function
Children's Participation Questionnaire (CPQ) *Rosenberg, L., Jarus, T., and Bart, O.*	Rosenberg, L., Jarus, T., & Bart, O. (2010). Development and initial validation of the Children's Participation Questionnaire (CPQ). *Disability and Rehabilitation, 32*, 1633–1644.	4–6 years	Measure participation of preschool children	ADL
Chronic Fatigue Syndrome Screening Questionnaire *Jason, L. A., Ropacki, M. T., and Santoro, N. B.*	Jason, L. A., Ropacki, M. T., & Santoro, N. B. (1997). A screening scale for chronic fatigue syndrome: Reliability and validity. *Journal of Chronic Fatigue Syndrome, 3*, 39–59.	Adults	Assess fatigue and its impact on daily activities	Fatigue
Chronic Respiratory Disease Questionnaire Self-Administered Standardized (CRQ-SAS) *Schünemann, H. J., Puhan, M., Goldstein, R., Jaeschke, R., and Guyatt, G. H.*	Schünemann, H. J., Puhan, M., Goldstein, R., Jaeschke, R., & Guyatt, G. H. (2005). Measurement properties and interpretability of the Chronic Respiratory Disease Questionnaire (CRQ). *COPD, 2*, 81–89.	Adults	Assess the effects of chronic respiratory disease on daily activities and function	Dyspnea, fatigue, emotional function, mastery

(*continued*)

Assessment Title and Author(s)	Publisher and/or Contact Information	Ages	Stated Purpose	Areas Assessed
Client Assessment of Strengths, Interests, and Goals (CASIG)-Self-Report (SR) and Informant (I) *Wallace, C. J., Lecomte, T., Wilde, J., and Liberman, R. P.*	Psychiatric Rehabilitation Consultants 9259 Louise Avenue Northridge, CA 91325-2426 Psych_rehab@yahoo.com 818-671-5792	Adults	Used for treatment planning and outcomes assessment of individuals with mental illness	Community functioning, social and independent living skills, medication compliance and side effects, quality of life, quality of treatment, symptoms, performance of unacceptable community behaviors
Clinical Dementia Rating Scale *Morris, J. C.*	Morris, J. C. (1993). The Clinical Dementia Rating (CDR): Current version and scoring rules. *Neurology, 43*, 2412–2414.	Older adults	Assist in staging dementia	Memory, orientation, judgment and problem solving, community affairs, home and hobbies, personal care
Clinical Observation of Motor and Postural Skills (COMPS)-Second Edition *Wilson, B., Kaplan, B., Pollack, N., and Law, M.*	Wilson, B., Kaplan, B., Pollack, N., & Law, M. (2000). *Clinical observation of motor and postural skills—administration and scoring manual* (2nd ed.). Framingham, MA: Therapro.	6–12.5 years	Assess motor coordination in children	Motor skills, postural skills
Cognitive Assessment Interview (CAI) *Ventura, J., et al.*	Ventura, J., Reise, S. P., Keefe, R. S., Baade, L. E., Gold, J. M., Green, M. F., . . . Bilder R. M. (2010). The Cognitive Assessment Interview (CAI): Development and validation of an empirically derived, brief interview-based measure of cognition. *Schizophrenia Research, 121*, 24–31.	Adults	Rate cognitive functioning	Cognition
Cognitive Assessment of Minnesota (CAM) *Rustad, R. A., et al.*	Pearson Assessments Attention: Inbound Sales and Customer Support 19500 Bulverde Road San Antonio, TX 78259-3701 ClinicalCustomerSupport@Pearson.com 800-627-7271	Adults	Screen a wide range of cognitive skills in order to identify general problem areas	Attention, memory, visual neglect, math, ability to follow directions, judgment
Cognitive Performance Test (CPT) *Burns, T.*	North Coast Medical, Inc. 8100 Camino Arroyo Gilroy, CA 95020 U.S.A. 800-821-9319	Adults	Assess how cognitive processing deficits affect performance of common activities	Cognitive processing
Coma Recovery Scale-Revised (CRS-R) *Giacino, J., and Kalmar, K.*	Giacino, J., & Kalmar, K. (2004). *CRS-R: Coma Recovery Scale-Revised: Administration and Scoring Guidelines.* Edison, NJ: Center for Head Injuries.	All ages	To assist with differential diagnosis, assessment of prognosis, and treatment planning	Auditory, visual, motor, oral motor, communication, arousal
Community Integration Questionnaire *Willer, B., Rosenthal, M., Kreutzer, J., Gordon, W., and Rempel, R.*	Centre for Research on Community Integration at the Ontario Brain Injury Association 3550 Schmon Parkway Thorold, Ontario L2V 4Y6, Canada	Adults	Help clients examine the extent of their community participation	Household activities, shopping, errands, leisure activities, visiting friends, social events, productive activities
Complete Minnesota Manual Dexterity Test *Lafayette Instrument Company*	Lafayette Instrument Company, USA PO Box 5729 Lafayette, IN 47903 USA U.S. Toll Free: 800-428-7545 sales@lafayetteinstrument.com	Adults	Used as a vocational evaluation, preemployment screening, and tests unilateral and bilateral movements	Simple hand-eye coordination and gross motor skills

Assessment Title and Author(s)	Publisher and/or Contact Information	Ages	Stated Purpose	Areas Assessed
Comprehensive Occupational Therapy Evaluation (COTE) *Brayman, S., Kirby, T., Misenheimer, A., and Short, M.*	Brayman, S., Kirby, T., Misenheimer, A., & Short, M. (1976). Comprehensive Occupational Therapy Evaluation Scale. *American Journal of Occupational Therapy, 30,* 95–100.	Adults	Can be used as an initial evaluation and as a measure of progress	ADL, IADL, work, play, leisure, social participation
Comprehensive Trail-Making Test (CTMT) *Reynolds, C. R.*	PRO-ED, Inc. 8700 Shoal Creek Blvd. Austin, TX 78757 800-897-3202	11–74 years	To evaluate and diagnose brain injury and other forms of central nervous system compromise	Visual search and sequencing, attention, concentration, resistance to distraction, and cognitive flexibility (or set shifting)
Coping Behaviors Inventory (CBI) *Litman, G. K., Stapleton, J., Oppenheim, A. N., and Peleg, M.*	Litman, G. K., Stapleton, J., Oppenheim, A. N., & Peleg, M. (1983). An instrument for measuring coping behaviours in hospitalized alcoholics: Implications for relapse prevention treatment. *British Journal of Addiction, 78,* 269–276.	Adolescent to older adult	Assess the thoughts and behaviors of alcoholics	Alcohol use
Coping Inventory *Zeitlin, S.*	Scholastic Testing Service 480 Meyer Road Bensonville, IL 60106-1617 800-642-6787	Observation form for 3–16 years Self-rated form for 15 years to adult	To assess adaptive and maladaptive coping habits, skills, and behaviors	Coping with self, coping with environment, use of personal resources, initiation of activity
Craig Handicap Assessment and Report Technique (CHART) *Whiteneck, G., Charlifue, S., Gerhart, K., Overholser, J., and Richardson, G.*	Craig Hospital Research Department 3425 S. Clarkson Street Englewood, Colorado 80113 (303) 789-8202 Dave Mellick, MA	Adult	Assess behaviors related to participation	Orientation, physical independence, mobility, occupation, social integration, economic self-sufficiency
Crawford Small Parts Dexterity Test (CSPDT) *Crawford, J.*	This test is no longer available through Pearson Assessments. They have indicated that it has been discontinued.	Adult	Assess dexterity and fine motor skills in handling small tools and parts Determine whether your applicant has the skills vital in positions requiring agility and strong dexterity	Eye–hand coordination, fine motor skills
Dallas Pain Questionnaire *Lawlis, G. F., Cuencas, R., Selby, D., and McCoy, C. E.*	Lawlis, G. F., Cuencas, R., Selby, D., & McCoy, C. E. (1989). The development of the Dallas Pain Questionnaire: An assessment of the impact of spinal pain on behavior. *Spine, 14,* 511–516.	Adult	Assess the amount of chronic spinal pain that affects daily life	Daily and work-leisure activities, anxiety-depression, social interest
DeGangi-Berk Test of Sensory Integration (TSI) *DeGangi, G. A., and Berk, R. A.*	Western Psychological Services 625 Alaska Avenue Torrance, CA 90503-5124 800-648-8857	3–5 years	Identify sensory integrative dysfunction in young children	Sensory integration, postural control, bilateral motor integration, and reflex integration
Depression, Anxiety, Stress Scale (DASS-42) *Psychology Foundation of Australia*	Psychology Foundation of Australia http://www2.psy.unsw.edu.au/groups/dass/	12 years and older	To assess the severity of the core symptoms of depression, anxiety, and stress	Depression, anxiety, stress

(*continued*)

Assessment Title and Author(s)	Publisher and/or Contact Information	Ages	Stated Purpose	Areas Assessed
Developmental Coordination Disorder Questionnaire 2007 (DCDQ 2007) *Wilson, B. N., Kaplan, B. J., Crawford, S. G., and Roberts, G.*	Wilson, B. N., Kaplan, B. J., Crawford, S. G., & Roberts, G. (2007). *The Developmental Coordination Disorder Questionnaire 2007© (DCDQ'07)*. Calgary, AB: Author. Alberta Children's Hospital Decision Support Research Team 2888 Shaganappi Trail NW Calgary, Alberta, Canada T3B 6A8 http://www.dcdq.ca	5–15 years	Uses parental reports to identify developmental coordination disorder	Motor coordination skills
Developmental Test of Visual Perception-Second Edition *Hammill, D. D., Pearson, N. A., and Voress, J. K.*	Pearson Assessments Attention: Inbound Sales and Customer Support 19500 Bulverde Road San Antonio, TX 78259-3701 ClinicalCustomerSupport@ Pearson.com 800-627-7271	4–9 years	Test visual perception and visual-motor integration skills of children	Eye–hand coordination, copying, spatial relations, position in space, figure-ground, visual closure, visual-motor speed, and form constancy
Developmental Test of Visual Perception-Adolescent and Adult *Reynolds, C. R., Pearson, N. A., and Voress, J. K.*	PRO-ED, Inc. 8700 Shoal Creek Boulevard Austin, Texas 78757-6897 800-897-3202	11–74 years	Measure different but interrelated visual-perceptual and visual-motor abilities	Copying, figure–ground, visual-motor speed, visual-motor search, visual closure, and form constancy
Difficulties in Emotion Regulation Scale *Gratz, K.L., and Roemer, L.*	Gratz, K. L., & Roemer, L. (2004). Multidimensional assessment of emotion regulation and dysregulation: Development, factor structure, and initial validation of the difficulties in emotion regulation scale. *Journal of Psychopathology & Behavioral Assessment, 26*, 41–54.	18–60 years	Assess multiple aspects of emotion dysregulation	Emotion regulation
Disabilities of the Arm, Shoulder, and Hand (DASH) Outcome Measure *Hudak, P., Amadio, P. C., Bombardier, C., and the Upper Extremity Collaborative Group*	Hudak, P., Amadio, P. C., Bombardier, C., & the Upper Extremity Collaborative Group. (1996). The development of an upper extremity outcome measure: The DASH (Disabilities of the Arm, Shoulder, and Hand). *American Journal of Industrial Medicine, 29*, 602–608. Copyright owned by the Institute for Work & Health (IWH) DASH Outcome Measure Institute of Work & Health 481 University Avenue, Suite 800 Toronto, Ontario Canada M5G 2E9 http://www.dash.iwh.on.ca/home	Adults	To measure physical function and symptoms in people with various upper extremity musculoskeletal disorders	ADL, IADL, pain
Disability Assessment for Dementia (DAD) *Gelinas, I., Gauthier, L., and McIntyre, M.*	Gelinas, I., Gauthier, L., & McIntyre, M. (1999). Development of a functional measure for persons with Alzheimer's disease: The Disability Assessment for Dementia. *American Journal of Occupational Therapy, 53*, 471–481. http://www.dementia-assessment .com.au/function/DAD_manual.pdf	Adults	Assess BADL and IADL of people diagnosed with Alzheimer's disease	ADL, IADL

Assessment Title and Author(s)	Publisher and/or Contact Information	Ages	Stated Purpose	Areas Assessed
Do-Eat *Josman, N., Goffer, A., and Rosenblum, S.*	Josman, N., Goffer, A., & Rosenblum, S. (2010). Development and standardization of a "Do-Eat" activity of daily living performance test for children. *American Journal of Occupational Therapy, 64*, 47–58.	Children	To identify children at risk for developmental coordination disorder	ADL
Domestic and Community Skills Assessment (DACSA) *Collister, L., Wood, S., and Alexander, K.*	Collister, L., Wood, S., & Alexander, K. (1987). *The Domestic and Community Skills Assessment (DACSA)*. Macleod, Victoria: Mond Park Hospital.	Adults	To assess performance of essential tasks for living in the community	Behavioral rating scale, qualitative aspects of performance
Dyadic Adjustment Scales (DAS) *WALMYR Publishing Company*	WALMYR Publishing Company PO Box 12217 Tallahassee, FL 32317-2217 walmyr@walmyr.com	Adults	Assess both partners perceptions of relationship adjustment	Relationship satisfaction
Early Coping Inventory *Zeitlin, S., Williamson, G. G., and Szczepanski, M.*	Scholastic Testing Service, Inc. www.ststesting.com 1-800-642-6787	4–36 months	Assess the coping-related behavior of children whose chronological or developmental age is between 4 and 36 months	Sensorimotor organization, reactive behavior, and self-initiated behavior
Eating Disorder Inventory-3 (EDI-3) *Garner, D. M.*	Psychological Assessment Resources, Inc. (PAR) 16204 N. Florida Avenue Lutz, FL 33549 800-331-8378	13–53 years	To provide a standardized clinical assessment of symptomatology associated with eating disorders	Eating habits
Engagement in Meaningful Activity Scale (EMAS) *Goldberg, B., Brintnell, E. S., and Goldberg, J.*	Goldberg, B., Brintnell, E. S., & Goldberg, J. (2002). The relationship between engagement in meaningful activities and quality of life in persons disabled by mental illness. *Occupational Therapy in Mental Health, 18*, 17–44.	Adults	Assess the meaningfulness of activities of everyday life	Meaningfulness of activities
Environmental Restriction Questionnaire (ERQ) *Rosenberg, L., Ratzon, N. Z., Jarus, T., and Bart, O.*	Rosenberg, L., Ratzon, N. Z., Jarus, T., & Bart, O. (2010). Developmental and initial validation of the Environmental Restriction Questionnaire (ERQ). *Research in Developmental Disabilities, 31*, 1323–1331.	4–6 years	Measure perceived environmental restrictions to participation in young children	Environmental restrictions
Epworth Sleepiness Scale *Johns, M. W.*	Johns, M. W. (1991). A new method for measuring daytime sleepiness: The Epworth Sleepiness Scale. *Sleep, 14*, 540–545. http://epworthsleepinessscale.com/	Adults	Measure daytime sleepiness	Sleepiness
Erhardt Developmental Prehension Assessment (EDPA) *Erhardt, R. P.*	Erhardt Developmental Products 2379 Snowshoe Court E Maplewood, MN 55119 http://www.erhardtproducts.com/index.html	Children	To measure components and skills of hand function development in children with disabilities	Arm and hand development
Evaluation of Social Interaction (ESI)-Second Edition *Fisher, A. G., and Griswold, L. A.*	Fisher, A. G., & Griswold, L. A. (2010). *Evaluation of social interaction* (2nd ed.). Fort Collins, CO: Three Star Press. http://www.ampsintl.com/ESI/	2 years to adult	To evaluate the quality of social interaction during natural social exchanges with typical social partners	Social interaction

(*continued*)

Assessment Title and Author(s)	Publisher and/or Contact Information	Ages	Stated Purpose	Areas Assessed
Executive Function Performance Test (EFPT) *Baum, C., Edwards, D., Morrison, T., and Hahn, M.*	Baum, C., Edwards, D., Morrison, T., & Hahn, M. (2003). *Executive Function Performance Test*. St. Louis, MO: Washington University School of Medicine. Baum, C., Connor, L. T., Morrison, T., Hahn, M., Dromerick, A. W., & Edwards, D. F. (2008). Reliability, validity, and clinical utility of the Executive Function Performance Test: A measure of executive function in a sample of people with stroke. *American Journal of Occupational Therapy*, *62*, 446–455.	Adults	To assess executive functions via ADL performance	ADL, IADL
FICA Spiritual History Tool© *Puchalski, C. M.*	The George Washington Institute for Spirituality & Health 2300 K Street NW, Warwick Building Suite 313 Washington, DC 20037 http://www.gwumc.edu/gwish/clinical/fica.cfm		To help physicians and other health care professionals address spiritual issues with their clients	Spirituality
Family Environment Scale *Moos, B. S., and Moos, R. H.*	Mind Garden, Inc. 855 Oak Grove Ave., Suite 215 Menlo Park, CA 94025 USA Telephone: (650) 322-6300	Children and adults	Give counselors and researchers a way of examining each family member's perceptions of the family	Family dynamics and interactions
Family Needs Questionnaire (FNQ) *Kreutzer, J., and Marwitz, J.*	Kreutzer, J., & Marwitz, J. (1989). *The Family Needs Questionnaire*. Richmond, VA: The National Resource Center for Traumatic Brain Injury.	Adults	To provide information regarding the family's needs following traumatic brain injury	Health information, emotional support, instrumental support, professional support, community support network, involvement with care
Family Needs Scale *Dunst, C. J., Cooper, C. S., Weeldreyer, J. C., Synder, K. D., and Chase, J. H.*	Brookline Books 617-558-8010, 800-666-BOOK www.brooklinebooks.com/	Adults	Measure a family's needs	Financial, food and shelter, vocation, child care, transportation, communication, and so forth
Family Routines Inventory *Jensen, E. W., James, S. A., Boyce, W. T., and Hartnett, S. A.*	Jensen, E. W., James, S. A., Boyce, W. T., & Hartnett, S. A. (1983). The Family Routines Inventory: Development and validation. *Social Science and Medicine*, *17*, 201–211.	All ages	Measure family routines	Positive family routines
Fatigue Impact Scale (FIS©) (also see the Modified Fatigue Impact Scale [MFIS]) *Fisk, J.*	Fatigue Impact Scale (FIS©), Dr. John Fisk, 1994. MAPI Research Trust 27 rue de la Villette F–69003 Lyon PROinformation@mapi-trust.org	Adult	To assess the problems in clients' quality of life that they attribute to their symptoms of fatigue	Quality of life
FirstSTEP Developmental Screening Test *Miller, L. J.*	Pearson Assessments Attention: Inbound Sales and Customer Support 19500 Bulverde Road San Antonio, TX 78259-3701 ClinicalCustomerSupport@Pearson.com 800-627-7271	2 years and 9 months to 6 years and 2 months	Identify preschoolers at risk for developmental delays	Cognition, communication, motor skills

Assessment Title and Author(s)	Publisher and/or Contact Information	Ages	Stated Purpose	Areas Assessed
Face, Legs, Activity, Cry, Consolability (FLACC) Scale *Merkel, S., Voepel-Lewis, T., Shayevitz, J. R., and Malviya, S.*	Merkel, S., Voepel-Lewis, T., Shayevitz, J. R., & Malviya, S. (1997). The FLACC: A behavioral scale for scoring postoperative pain in young children. *Pediatric Nurse, 23*, 293–297.	2 months to 7 years	Assess pain in children and in people who are nonverbal	Pain
Frenchay Activities Index *Holbrook, M., and Skilbeck, C. E.*	Holbrook, M., & Skilbeck, C. E. (1983). An activities index for use with stroke patients. *Age and Ageing, 12*, 166–170.	Adults	To assess functional status poststroke	ADL, IADL
Frenchay Arm Test *De Souza, L. H., Langton Hewer, R., and Miller, S.*	De Souza, L. H., Langton Hewer, R., & Miller, S. (1980). Assessment of recovery of arm control in hemiplegic stroke patients: Arm Function Test. *International Rehabilitation Medicine, 2*, 3–9.	Adults	Assess the functional use of an upper extremity affected by hemiplegia	Five tasks using the more affected upper extremity
Fugl-Meyer Evaluation of Physical Performance *Fugl-Meyer, A. R., Jaasko, L., Leyman, I., Olsson, S., and Steglind, S.*	Fugl-Meyer, A. R., Jaasko, L., Leyman, I., Olsson, S., & Steglind, S. (1975). The post-stroke hemiplegic patient. I. A method for evaluation of physical performance. *Scandinavian Journal of Rehabilitation Medicine, 7*, 13–31. Fugl-Meyer, A. R., Jaasko, L., Leyman, I., Olsson, S., & Steglind, S. (1975). Post-stroke hemiplegic patient: Assessment of physical properties. *Scandinavian Journal of Rehabilitation Medicine, 7*, 83–93.	Adults	To quantify motor recovery stages based on the Brunnstrom and Twitchell scales	Motor recovery, balance, sensation, range of motion, pain
Fugl-Meyer Sensorimotor Assessment *Fugl-Meyer, A. R.*	Fugl-Meyer, A. R., Jaasko, L., Leyman, I., Olsson, S., & Steglind, S. (1975). The post-stroke hemiplegic patient: A method for evaluation of physical performance. *Scandinavian Journal of Rehabilitation Medicine, 7*, 13–31.		Assess body function impairment following stroke	Motor, sensory, balance, range of motion, joint pain
Functional Assessment Measure (FAM) *Rehabilitation Research Center for TBI & SCI at Santa Clara Valley Medical Center*	Wright, J. (2000). The Functional Assessment Measure. *The Center for Outcome Measurement in Brain Injury*. Retrieved from http://www.tbims.org/combi/FAM http://www.birf.info/home/bi-tools/tests/fam.html	Adults	Served as an adjunct to the FIM—the areas addressed in the FAM are to be added to the scores from the FIM. The FAM does not stand alone.	Cognition, behavior, communication, community functioning
Functional Assessment of Cancer Therapy, General Scale (FACT-G) *Cella, D. F.*	Cella, D. F., Tulsky, D. S., Gray, G., Sarafian, B., Linn, E., Bonomi, A., . . . Brannon, J. (1993). The Functional Assessment of Cancer Therapy Scale: Development and validation of the general measure. *Journal of Clinical Oncology, 11*, 570–579.	Adults	Assess quality of life for people undergoing treatment for cancer	Quality of life
Functional Emotional Assessment Scale *Greenspan, S., DeGangi, G., and Wieder, S.*	Interdisciplinary Council on Developmental and Learning Disorders http://www.icdl.com	7 months to 4 years	Assess a child's emotional and social functioning	Social and emotional development

(*continued*)

Assessment Title and Author(s)	Publisher and/or Contact Information	Ages	Stated Purpose	Areas Assessed
Functional Independence Measure (FIM) *The Center for Functional Assessment Research at State University of New York (SUNY), Buffalo*	Uniform Data System for Medical Rehabilitation 270 Northpointe Parkway Suite 300 Amherst, NY 14228 (716) 817-7800	Adults with various physical impairments	Measure functional status, reflects the impact of disability on the individual and on human and economic resources in the community	18 activities (13 with a motor emphasis related to self-care and 5 with a cognitive emphasis involving communication)
Functional Reach Test *Duncan, P. W., Weiner, D. K., Chandler, J., and Studenski, S.*	Pamela W. Duncan Graduate Program in Physical Therapy PO Box 3965, Duke University Medical Center Durham, NC 27710 http://www.ohcponline.com/tools/functionalreach.html	Adults	To assess balance impairment, detect chance in balance performance over time, and to aid in designing modified environments for impaired persons	Balance and maximum forward reach
Functional Test for the Hemiplegic/Paretic Upper Extremity *Wilson, D. J., Baker, L. L., and Craddock, J. A.*	Wilson, D. J., Baker, L. L., & Craddock, J. A. (1984). Functional test for the hemiparetic upper extremity. *American Journal of Occupational Therapy*, *38*, 159–164. Wilson, D. J., Baker, L. L., & Craddock, J. A. (1984). *Protocol-Functional Test for the Hemiplegic/Paretic Upper Extremity*. Downey, CA: Rancho Los Amigos Occupational Therapy Department and Rehabilitation Engineering Center.	Adults	To evaluate motor capability for function	Motor coordination, ADL
Geriatric Depression Scale *Yesavage, J. A., et al.*	Yesavage, J. A., Brink, T. L., Rose, T. L., Lum, O., Huang, V., Adey, M. B., & Leirer, V. O. (1983). Development and validation of a Geriatric Depression Screening Scale: A preliminary report. *Journal of Psychiatric Research*, *17*, 37–49.	Older adults	Measure depression in older adults	Depression
Glascow Coma Scale *Teasdale, G., and Jennett, B.*	Teasdale, G., & Jennett, B. (1994). Assessment of coma and impaired consciousness: Practical scale. *Lancet*, *2*, 81–84.	Adult	To monitor levels of consciousness in people with traumatic brain injury	Motor, verbal, and eye-opening responses
Grooved Pegboard Test *Trites, R.*	Lafayette Instrument Co. 3700 Sagamore Parkway North PO Box 5729 Lafayette, IN 47903-5729 Phone No.: 765-423-1505 Fax No.: 765-423-4111 Toll Free: 800-428-7545	5 years to adult	To test manipulative dexterity; this test requires more complex visual-motor coordination than other pegboard tests	Eye–hand coordination, fine motor dexterity
Gross Motor Function Classification System-Expanded and Revised (GMFCS-E & R) *Palisano, R., Rosenbaum, P., Bartlett, D., and Livingston, M.*	Palisano, R., Rosenbaum, P., Bartlett, D., & Livingston, M. (2007). *GFMCS-E & R*. Hamilton, Canada: CanChild Centre for Childhood Disability Research, McMaster University. Palisano, R., Rosenbaum, P., Walter, S., Russell, D., Wood, E., & Galuppi, B. (1997). Development and reliability of a system to classify gross motor function in children with cerebral palsy. *Developmental Medicine and Child Neurology*, *39*, 214–223.	2–18 years	To provide a standardized system to classify the self-initiated movement of children with cerebral palsy	Gross motor function

Assessment Title and Author(s)	Publisher and/or Contact Information	Ages	Stated Purpose	Areas Assessed
Gross Motor Function Measure (GMFM-66 and GMFM-88) *Russell, D., Rosenbaum, P., Avery, L., and Lane, M.*	Russell, D., Rosenbaum, P., Avery, L., & Lane, M. (2002). *Gross Motor Function Measure (GMFM-66 and GMFM-88) User's Manual.* London, United Kingdom: Mac Keith Press. Blackwell Publishing AIDC PO Box 20 Williston, VT 05495-9957 800-216-2522 www.blackwellpublishing.com	5 months to 16 years	Evaluate change in motor function for children with cerebral palsy (has also been used for children with Down syndrome)	Lying and rolling, sitting, crawling and kneeling, standing, walking, running, and jumping
Handwriting File *Alston, J., and Taylor, J.*	Alston, J., & Taylor, J. (1988). *The handwriting file* (2nd ed.). Wisbech, United Kingdom: LDA.	School age	Used as a standardized handwriting assessment	Handwriting
Hawaii Early Learning Profile (HELP) *Furuno, S., et al.*	VORT Corporation PO Box 60132-W Palo Alto, CA 94306 650-322-8282	Birth to 3 years	To assess developmental skills and behaviors	Cognitive, language, gross motor, fine motor, social, and self-help skills
Home Observation for Measurement of the Environment *Caldwell, B. M., and Bradley, R. H.*	University of Arkansas http://ualr.edu/case/index.php/home/home-inventory/ (501) 565-7627	Birth to 3 years	Measure the quality and extent of stimulation available to a child in the home environment	Quality and quantity of stimulation and support available to a child in the home environment
Home Situations Questionnaire (HSQ) *Barkley, R. A.*	Barkley, R. A., & Murphy, K. R. (1998). *Attention deficit hyperactivity disorder: A clinical workbook* (2nd ed.). New York, NY: Guilford.	School age	Identify how symptoms of ADD/ADHD disrupt the home environment and the child's ability to participate in ADL	ADL
Illness Perception Questionnaire for Schizophrenia (IPQS) *Lobban, F., Barrowclough, C., and Jones, S.*	Lobban, F., Barrowclough, C., & Jones, S. (2005). Assessing cognitive representations of mental health problems. I. The illness perception questionnaire for schizophrenia. *British Journal of Clinical Psychology*, *44*, 147–162.	Adults	To assess how an individual diagnosed with schizophrenia perceives himself or herself and the impact of his or her perceptions on his or her health and performance	Self-perception
Illness Perception Questionnaire for Schizophrenia-Relatives' Version (IPQS-Relatives) *Lobban, F., Barrowclough, C., and Jones, S.*	Lobban, F., Barrowclough, C., & Jones, S. (2005). Assessing cognitive representations of mental health problems. II. The illness perception questionnaire for schizophrenia: Relatives' version. *British Journal of Clinical Psychology*, *44*, 163–179.	Adults	To assess the perceptions of relatives of individuals diagnosed with schizophrenia to understand how they impact the individual's health and performance	Illness perception
Impact of Events Scale-Revised (IES-R) *Weiss, D. S., and Marmar, C. R.*	Weiss, D. S., & Marmar, C. R. (1996). The Impact of Event Scale—revised. In J. Wilson & T. M. Keane (Eds.), *Assessing psychological trauma and PTSD* (pp. 399–411). New York, NY: Guilford.		Measure subjective stress brought on by traumatic events	Stress
Impact of Vision Impairment (IVI) Questionnaire *Weih, L. M., Hassell, J. B., and Keeffe, J. E.*	Weih, L. M., Hassell, J. B., & Keeffe, J. E. (2002). Assessment of the Impact of Vision Impairment. *Investigative Ophthalmology and Visual Science*, *43*, 927–935.	Adults	Measure the impact of vision impairment on restriction of participation in ADL	ADL

(*continued*)

Assessment Title and Author(s)	Publisher and/or Contact Information	Ages	Stated Purpose	Areas Assessed
Independent Living Scales (ILS) *Loeb, P. A.*	Pearson Assessments Attention: Inbound Sales and Customer Support 19500 Bulverde Road San Antonio, TX 78259-3701 ClinicalCustomerSupport@Pearson.com 800-627-7271	Adults aged 65 years and older	Determine to what degree adults are capable of caring for themselves and their property	Memory and orientation, managing money, managing home and transportation, health and safety, and social adjustment
Independent Living Skills Survey (ILSS) *Wallace, C. J., Liberman, R. P., Tauber, R., and Wallace, J.*	Psychiatric Rehabilitation Consultants 9259 Louise Avenue Northridge, CA 91325-2426 Psych_rehab@yahoo.com 818-671-5792	Adults	Assess social and independent living skills	Personal hygiene, appearance and care of clothing, care of personal possessions and living space, food preparation, care of one's own health and safety, money management, transportation, leisure and recreational activities, job seeking, job maintenance
Infant Neurological International Battery (INFANIB) *Ellison, P. H.*	Pearson Assessments Attention: Inbound Sales and Customer Support 19500 Bulverde Road San Antonio, TX 78259-3701 ClinicalCustomerSupport@Pearson.com 800-627-7271	4- to 18-month-old infants	Used as a reliable method for the neuromotor assessment of infants	Tone and posture in infants
Infant/Toddler Symptom Checklist *DeGangi, G., Poisson, S., Sickel, R., and Wiener, A.*	Pearson Assessments Attention: Inbound Sales and Customer Support 19500 Bulverde Road San Antonio, TX 78259-3701 ClinicalCustomerSupport@Pearson.com 800-627-7271	7- to 30-month-old infants	Screen infants and toddlers for sensory and regulatory disorders	Self-regulation, attention, sleep, eating or feeding, dressing, bathing, touch, movement, listening and language, looking and sight, and attachment and emotional functioning
Instrumental Activities of Daily Living (IADL) Scale *Lawton, M. P., and Brody, E. M.*	Lawton, M. P., & Brody, E. M. (1969). Assessment of older people: Self-maintaining and instrumental activities of daily living. *Gerontologist*, *9*, 179–186.	Older adults	Assess independence in IADL	IADL
Interest Checklist/NPI Interest Checklist *Matsutsuyu, J.* Revised by *Rogers, J., Weinstein J., and Figone, J.*	Matsutsuyu J. S. (1969). The interest check list. *American Journal of Occupational Therapy*, *23*, 323–328. Rogers, J. C., Weinstein, J. M., & Figone, J. J. (1978). The Interest Checklist: An empirical assessment. *American Journal of Occupational Therapy*, *32*, 628–630.	Adolescents to adults	Gather data about a person's interest patterns and characteristics	ADL, manual skills, cultural and educational activities, physical sports, social and recreational activities

Assessment Title and Author(s)	Publisher and/or Contact Information	Ages	Stated Purpose	Areas Assessed
Jebsen-Taylor Hand Function Test *Jebsen, R. H., Taylor, N., Trieschmann, R. B., Trotter, M. J., and Howard, L. A.*	Jebsen, R. H., Taylor, N., Trieschmann, R. B., Trotter, M. J., & Howard, L. A. (1969). An objective and standardized test of hand function. *Archives of Physical Medicine & Rehabilitation*, *50*, 311–319. Bovend Eerdt, T. J. H., Dawes, H., Johansen-Berg, H., & Wade, D. T. (2004). Evaluation of the Modified Jebsen Test of Hand Function and the University of Maryland Arm Questionnaire for Stroke. *Clinical Rehabilitation*, *18*, 195–202.	5 years and older	To assess effective use of the hands in everyday activity by performing tasks representative of functional manual activities	Writing, card turning, picking up small objects, simulated feeding, stacking checkers, picking up light and heavy objects
Katz Index of Independence in Activities of Daily Living *Katz, S., Down, T. D., Cash, H. R., and Grotz, R. C.*	Katz, S., Down, T. D., Cash, H. R., & Grotz, R. C. (1970). Progress in the development of the index of ADL. *The Gerontologist*, *10*(1), 20–30.	Older adults	Assess functional status of older adults	ADL
Kitchen Task Assessment (KTA) *Baum, C., and Edwards, D. F.*	Baum, C., & Edwards, D. F. (1993). Cognitive performance in senile dementia of the Alzheimer's type: The Kitchen Task Assessment. *American Journal of Occupational Therapy*, *47*, 431–436.	Adults	Measure the level of cognitive support required by a person diagnosed with dementia	ADL
Klein-Bell Activities of Daily Living Scale *Klein, R. M., and Bell, B.*	Klein, R. M., & Bell, B. J. (1979). *Klein-Bell Activity of Daily Living Scale: Manual*. Seattle, WA: Division of Occupational Therapy, University of Washington. Marie Gary HSCER Distribution HSBT 281 SB 56 University of Washington Seattle, Washington 98195	Children and adults	Measure ADL independence to determine current status, change in status, and subactivities to focus on in rehabilitation	Dressing, mobility, elimination, bathing and hygiene, eating, and emergency communication
Kohlman Evaluation of Living Skills (KELS) *McGourty, L. K. (1979, 1999)*	AOTA Products PO Box 0151 Annapolis Junction, MD 20701-0151 877-404-AOTA http://www.aota.org	Adults with cognitive impairments	Evaluate the ability to live independently and safely in the community	Self-care, safety and health, money management, transportation and telephone, work and leisure; tends to emphasize the knowledge component of activities
Large Allen Cognitive Level (ACLS-5) Screen *Allen, C. K., et al.*	Allen, C. K., Austin, S. L., David, S. K., Earhart, C. A., McCraith, D. B., & Riska-Williams, L. (2007). *Manual for the Allen cognitive level screen-5 (ACLS-5) and large Allen cognitive level screen-5 (LACLS-5)*. Camarillo, CA: ACLS and LACLS Committee. ACLS and LACLS Committee PO Box 3144 Camarillo, CA 93011 http://www.allencognitivelevelscreen.org/products.htm	All ages	To provide a quick measure of learning potential, global cognitive processing capacities, and performance abilities	Problem solving, following directions

(*continued*)

Assessment Title and Author(s)	Publisher and/or Contact Information	Ages	Stated Purpose	Areas Assessed
Leisure Assessment Inventory (LAI) *Hawkins, B. A., Ardovino, P., Brattain Rogers, N., Foose, A., and Ohlsen, N.*	Idyll Arbor 39129 264th Ave SE Enumclaw, WA 98022 Voice: 360-825-7797 Fax: 360-825-5670 sales@idyllarbor.com	Adults	Measure the leisure behavior of adults through its four components: (1) the leisure activity participation index (LAP), (2) the leisure preference index (L-PREF), (3) the leisure interest index (L-INT), and (4) the leisure constraints index (L-CON)	Leisure skills, social skills
Leisure Boredom Scale (LBS) *Iso-Ahola, S. E., and Weissinger, E.*	Iso-Ahola, S. E., & Weissinger, E. (1990). Perceptions of boredom in leisure: Conceptualization, reliability and validity of the leisure boredom scale. *Journal of Leisure Research*, *22*, 17–25.	All ages	Measure constraints on achieving enjoyment from leisure activities	Play/leisure
Leisure Competence Measure *Kloseck, M., and Crilly, R.*	Kloseck, M., & Crilly, R. (1997). *Leisure Competence Measure (LCM): Professional Manual and User Guide*. London, United Kingdom: Leisure Competence Measure Data System. Kloseck, M., Crilly, R., Ellis, G. D., & Lammers, E. (1996). Leisure Competence Measure: Development and reliability testing of a scale to measure functional outcomes in therapeutic recreation. *Therapeutic Recreation Journal*, *30*, 13–26.	All ages	Measure outcomes in leisure/play activities	Leisure awareness, leisure attitude, leisure skills, cultural/social behaviors, interpersonal skills, community integration skills, social contact, and community participation
Leisure Diagnostic Battery *Witt, P., Widmer, M., and Ellis, G.*	Venture Publishing, Inc. 1999 Cato Avenue State College, PA 16801 814-234-4561	Adolescents and adults	Assess an individual's "leisure functioning"	Perceived Leisure Competency Scale, Perceived Leisure Control Scale, Leisure Needs Scale, Depth of Involvement in Leisure Scale, Playfulness Scale, Perceived Freedom in Leisure-Total Score, Barriers to Leisure Involvement Scale, Knowledge of Leisure Opportunities Test, and Leisure Preference Inventory
Leisure Satisfaction Scale *Beard, J. G., and Ragheb, M. G.*	Beard, J. G., & Ragheb, M. G. (1980). The leisure satisfaction measure. *Journal of Leisure Research*, *12*, 20–33.	All ages	Measure a client's level of satisfaction in leisure activities	Play/leisure
Life Balance Inventory *Matuska, K.*	Matuska, K. (2012). Description and development of the Life Balance Inventory. *OTJR: Occupation, Participation, and Health*, *32*, 220–228.	Adults	To assess balances and imbalances in a person's life	Perceived balance in health, relationships, challenge, and identity
Locke-Wallace Marital Adjustment Scale (MAT) *Locke, H. J., and Wallace, K. M. (1959)*	Corcoran, K., & Fischer, J. (2000). *Measures for clinical practice: A sourcebook* (Vol. 1, 3rd ed., pp. 133–135.). New York, NY: Free Press.	Adults	To measure marital adjustment	Relationship

Assessment Title and Author(s)	Publisher and/or Contact Information	Ages	Stated Purpose	Areas Assessed
Lowenstein Occupational Therapy Cognitive Assessment (LOTCA)-Second Edition (dynamic version is available) *Itzkovich, M., Elazar, B., Averbuch, S., and Katz, N.*	Maddak, Inc. 661 Route 23 South Wayne, NJ 07470 800-443-4926 http://www.maddak.com	6 years and older	To identify abilities and limitations in areas of cognitive processing	Orientation, perception, visuomotor organization, thinking operations
Lowenstein Occupational Therapy Cognitive Assessment-Geriatric (LOTCA-G) *Elazar, B., Itzkovich, M., and Katz, N.*	Maddak, Inc. 661 Route 23 South Wayne, NJ 07470 800-443-4926 http://www.maddak.com	Older adults	To identify abilities and limitations in areas of cognitive processing	Orientation, perception, visuomotor organization, thinking operations
Manual Ability Measure (MAM) *Chen, C., and Bode, R. K.*	Chen, C., & Bode, R. K. (2010). Psychometric validation of the Manual Ability Measure (MAM-36) in patients with neurological and musculoskeletal disorders. *Archives of Physical Medicine and Rehabilitation, 91,* 414–420.	Adults	Assess functional ability to perform meaningful occupation-based activities	ADL, IADL
Matson Evaluation of Social Skills in Individuals with Severe Retardation (MESSIER) *Matson, J. L., and LeBlanc, L. A.*	Matson, J. L. (1995). *Matson Evaluation of social skills for individuals with severe retardation.* Baton Rouge, LA: Scientific.	All ages	To measure social skills of people with severe developmental delays	Social skills
Mayer-Salovey-Caruso Emotional Intelligence Test *Mayer, J. D., Caruso, D. R., and Salovey, P.*	Multi-Health Systems Inc. P.O. Box 950 North Tonawanda, NY 14120-0950 1-800-456-3003	17 years and older	To measure emotional intelligence through a series of objective and impersonal questions	Emotion regulation
McGill Pain Questionnaire *Melzack, R.*	Melzack, R. (Ed.). (1983). The McGill Pain Questionnaire. In *Pain measurement and assessment* (pp. 41–48). New York, NY: Raven Press.	Adults	Self-assessment of pain	Pain
M. D. Anderson Symptom Inventory (MDASI) *Cleeland, C. S., et al.*	Cleeland, C. S., Mendoza, T. R., Wang, X. S., Chou, C., Harle, M., Morrissey, M., & Engstrom, M. C. (2000). Assessing Symptom Distress in Cancer: The M. D. Anderson Symptom Inventory. *Cancer, 89,* 1634–1646. http://www.mdanderson.org	Adults	Assess the severity of multiple symptoms and the impact of symptoms on daily functioning	Symptoms
Meaningful Activity Participation Assessment (MAPA) *Eakman, A., Carlson, M., and Clark, F.*	Eakman, A., Carlson, M., & Clark, F. (2010). The Meaningful Activity Participation Assessment: A measure of engagement in personally valued activities. *International Journal of Aging and Human Development, 70,* 299–317.	Older adults	Assess the meaningfulness of activity	IADL
Medication Management Ability Assessment (MMAA) *Patterson, T. L., Lacro, J., McKibben, C. L., Moscona, S., Hughes, T., and Jeste, D. V.*	Patterson, T. L., Lacro, J., McKibben, C. L., Moscona, S., Hughes, T., & Jeste, D. V. (2002). Medication Management Ability Assessment: Results from a performance-based measure in older outpatients with schizophrenia. *Journal of Clinical Psychopharmacology, 22,* 11–19.	Older adults	Assess the ability of adults with schizophrenia to manage their medications	Medication management

(*continued*)

Assessment Title and Author(s)	Publisher and/or Contact Information	Ages	Stated Purpose	Areas Assessed
Melville-Nelson Self-Care Assessment (SCA) *Nelson, D. L., and Melville, L. L.*	Nelson, D. L., Melville, L. L., Wilkerson, J. D., Magness, R. A., Grech, J. L., & Rosenberg, J. A. (2002). Interrater reliability, concurrent validity, responsiveness, and predictive validity of the Melville-Nelson Self-Care Assessment. *American Journal of Occupational Therapy*, *56*, 51–59. http://www.utoledo.edu/eduhshs/depts/rehab_sciences/ot/melville.html	Adults in subacute rehab and nursing homes	To objectively assess self-care skills	Bed mobility, transfers, dressing, eating, toileting, personal hygiene, and bathing
Miller Assessment for Preschoolers (MAP) *Miller, L. J.*	Pearson Assessments Attention: Inbound Sales and Customer Support 19500 Bulverde Road San Antonio, TX 78259-3701 ClinicalCustomerSupport@Pearson.com 800-627-7271	2–6 years	To identify children who exhibit moderate "preacademic problems"	Sensory, motor, and cognitive skills through verbal and nonverbal tasks
Miller Function & Participation Scales *Miller, L. J.*	Pearson Assessments Attention: Inbound Sales and Customer Support 19500 Bulverde Road San Antonio, TX 78259-3701 ClinicalCustomerSupport@Pearson.com 800-627-7271	2 years and 6 months to 7 years and 11 months	Assess development in fine, gross, and visual-motor skills	Fine motor, gross motor, visual motor, play
Milwaukee Evaluation of Daily Living Skills (MEDLS) *Leonardelli, C.*	Leonardelli, C. (1988). *The Milwaukee evaluation of daily living skills: Evaluation in long-term psychiatric care.* Thorofare, NJ: Slack. Slack, Inc. 6900 Grove Road Thorofare, NJ 08086 800-257-8290	Adults with chronic mental health problems	Establish baseline behaviors to develop treatment objectives related to daily living skills	Communication, personal care, clothing care, home and community safety, money management, personal health care, medication management, telephone use, transportation usage, time awareness; subtests can be used individually or in combination
Mini-Mental State Exam (MMSE) *Folstein, M. F., Folstein, S. E., and McHugh, P. R.*	Folstein, M. F., Folstein, S. E., & McHugh, P. R. (1975). "Mini-mental state": A practical method for grading the cognitive-state of patients for the clinician. *Journal of Psychiatric Research*, *12*, 89–198.	Adolescents and adults	To quantitatively measure cognitive performance	Orientation, memory, attention, calculation, recall, language
Minimum Data Set—Section G. Physical Functioning and Structural Problems Scale, Version 2.0 *Health Care Financing Administration*	U.S. Government Printing Office Washington, DC http://www.cms.hhs.gov/NursingHomeQualityInits/downloads/MDS20MDSAllForms.pdf	Residents in long-term care Clients in home care	To describe baseline ADL and track changes in ADL	Bed mobility, transfer, walk in room, walk in corridor, locomotion on unit, locomotion off unit, dressing, eating, toilet use, personal hygiene and bathing
Minnesota Rate of Manipulation Tests (MRMT) *American Guidance Services*	American Guidance Services. (1969). *Minnesota Rate of Manipulation Tests.* Circle Pines, MN: Author.	13 years and older	To measure manual dexterity (speed of gross arm and hand movements during rapid eye–hand coordination tasks)	Placing test, turning test, displacing test, one-hand turning and placing, two-handed turning and placing

Assessment Title and Author(s)	Publisher and/or Contact Information	Ages	Stated Purpose	Areas Assessed
Model of Human Occupation Screening Tool (MOHOST), Version 2.0 *Parkinson, S., Forsyth, K., and Kielhofner, G.*	http://www.uic.edu/depts/moho/assess/mohost.html	Adults	To assess an individual's capacity for occupational functioning	Volition, habituation, motor skills, and environment
Modified Ashworth Scale (MAS) *Bohannon, R., and Smith, M.*	Bohannon, R., & Smith, M. (1987). Interrater reliability of a Modified Ashworth Scale of muscle spasticity. *Physical Therapy, 67*, 206.	Adults	Assess muscle tone	Muscle spasticity
Modified Fatigue Impact Scale (MFIS) *Ritvo, P. G., Fischer, J. S., Miller, D. M., Andrews, H., Paty, D. W., and LaRocca, N. G.*	Ritvo, P. G., Fischer, J. S., Miller, D. M., Andrews, H., Paty, D. W., & LaRocca, N. G. (1997). *MSQLI: Multiple Sclerosis Quality of Life Inventory: A user's manual*. New York, NY: National Multiple Sclerosis Society.	Adults	Assess the effects of fatigue on physical, cognitive, and psychosocial functioning	Fatigue
Modified Hand Injury Scoring System (MHISS) *Urso-Baiarda, F., Lyons, R. A., Laing, J. H., Brophy, S., Wareham, K., and Camp, D.*	Urso-Baiarda, F., Lyons, R. A., Laing, J. H., Brophy, S., Wareham, K., & Camp, D. (2008). A prospective evaluation of the Modified Hand Injury Severity Score in predicting return to work. *International Journal of Surgery, 6*, 45–50.	Adults	Quantify hand, wrist, and forearm injuries; can be used to predict return to work abilities	Injury severity
Motor Activity Log *Uswatte, G., Taub, E., Morris, D., Light, K., and Thompson, P. A.*	Uswatte, G., Taub, E., Morris, D., Light, K., & Thompson, P. A. (2006). The Motor Activity Log-28: Assessing daily use of the hemiparetic arm after stroke. *Neurology, 67*, 1189–1194.	Adults	Provide information about actual use of the limb in everyday life situations	ADL, IADL
Motor Assessment Scale (MAS) *Carr, J., and Shepherd, R.*	Carr, J. H., Shepherd, R. B., Nordholm, L., & Lynne, D. (1985). Investigation of a new motor assessment scale for stroke patients. *Physical Therapy, 65*, 175–180.	Adults	Assess everyday motor function in people affected by strokes	ADL
Motor-Free Visual Perception Test-Third Edition (MVPT-3) *Colarusso, R. P., and Hammill, D. D.*	Academic Therapy Publications 20 Commercial Blvd. Novato, CA 94949 800-422-7249	4–11 years	To test visual perception without motor involvement	Spatial relationships, visual discrimination, visual figure-ground, visual closure, and visual memory
Movement Assessment Battery for Children-Second Edition (Movement ABC-2) *Henderson, S. E., Sugden, D. A., and Barnett, A.*	Pearson Assessments Attention: Inbound Sales and Customer Support 19500 Bulverde Road San Antonio, TX 78259-3701 ClinicalCustomerSupport@Pearson.com 800-627-7271	3–16 years and 11 months	To assess children's motor skills in children with motor impairments	Static balance, dynamic balance, manual dexterity, speed of movement, eye–hand coordination, problem-solving skills
Mullen Scales of Early Learning *Mullen, E. M.*	Pearson Assessments Attention: Inbound Sales and Customer Support 19500 Bulverde Road San Antonio, TX 78259-3701 ClinicalCustomerSupport@Pearson.com 800-627-7271	Birth to 68 months	Assess the cognitive, motor, and language functioning of young children	Gross motor, expressive language, visual reception, receptive language, and fine motor

(*continued*)

Assessment Title and Author(s)	Publisher and/or Contact Information	Ages	Stated Purpose	Areas Assessed
Multidimensional Fatigue Inventory *Smets, E. M., Garssen, B., Bonke, B., and DeHaes, J. C.*	Smets, E. M., Garssen, B., Bonke, B., & DeHaes, J. C. (1995). The Multidimensional Fatigue Inventory (MFI) psychometric qualities of an instrument to assess fatigue. *Journal of Psychomatic Research*, *39*, 315–325.	Adults	Measure various types of fatigue	General fatigue, physical fatigue, mental fatigue, reduced motivation, reduced activity
Multi-directional Reach Test (MDRT) *Newton, R.*	Newton, R. A. (1997). Validity of the multi-directional reach test: A practical measure of limits of stability in older adults. *Journal of Gerontology Series: Biological Sciences, Medical Sciences*, *56A*, 248–252.	Adults	Measure stability of the body during reaching activities	Stability in a variety of directional movement
Multiple Sclerosis Impact Scale (MSIS-29) *Hobart, J., Lamping, D., Fitzpatrick, R., Riazi, A., and Thompson, A.*	Hobart, J., Lamping, D., Fitzpatrick, R., Riazi, A., & Thompson, A. (2001). The Multiple Sclerosis Impact Scale (MSIS-29): A new patient-based outcome measure. *Brain*, *124*, 962–973.	Adults	To measure the physical and the psychological impact of multiple sclerosis from the patient's perspective	Disability/physical functioning, quality of life
Multiple Sclerosis Quality of Life Inventory (MSQLI) *National Multiple Sclerosis Society Consortium of Multiple Sclerosis Centers*	Director of Health Care Delivery and Policy Research National Multiple Sclerosis Society Nicholas LaRocca, PhD 733 Third Avenue 3rd floor New York, NY 10017 212-476-0414 nicholas.larocca@nmss.org http://www.nationalmssociety.org/docs/HOM/MSQLI_Manual_and_Forms.pdf	Adults	Measure quality of life in adults with multiple sclerosis	Quality of life
National Eye Institute-Visual Function Questionnaire (NEI-VFQ-25) *Mangione, C. M., Lee, P. P., Gutierrez, P. R., Spritzer, K., Berry S., and Hays, R. D.*	Mangione, C. M., Lee, P. P., Gutierrez, P. R., Spritzer, K., Berry S., & Hays, R. D. (2001). Development of the 25-item National Eye Institute Visual Function Questionnaire. *Archives of Ophthalmology*, *119*, 1050–1058.	Adults	Assess the impact of visual impairment on daily functioning	ADL, leisure, psychosocial
National Institutes of Health Activity Record (ACTRE) *Furst, G.*	National Institutes of Health Building 10, Room 6s235 10 Center Drive MSC 1604 Bethesda, MD 20892-1604 hodsdonb@cc.nih.gov	Adolescents to adults	To identify changes in role activities	ADL
National Institutes of Health Pain Scales *National Institutes of Health*	http://painconsortium.nih.gov/pain_scales/index.html	Adults and children (>3 years old)	Quantify pain	Pain intensity
National Institutes of Health Stroke Scale (NIHSS) *National Institutes of Health*	http://www.nihstrokescale.org/ http://www.ninds.nih.gov/doctors/NIH_Stroke_Scale.pdf	Adults	Provide a quantitative measure of stroke-related neurological deficits	Consciousness, language, neglect, visual field loss, extraocular movement, motor strength, ataxia, dysarthria, sensory loss
Naturalistic Observations of Newborn Behavior (NONB) *Als, H.*	Als, H. (1984). *Manual for the naturalistic observations of newborn behavior: Preterm and fullterm infants*. Boston, MA: The Children's Hospital.	Preterm to full-term infants	Assess infant behaviors through formal observation; can be used with infants, who are too fragile to handle	Behaviors, including approach and withdrawal

Assessment Title and Author(s)	Publisher and/or Contact Information	Ages	Stated Purpose	Areas Assessed
Neurobehavioral Assessment of the Preterm Infant (NAPI) *Korner, A. F., Brown, J. V., Thom, V. A., and Constantinou, J. C.*	Korner, A. F., Brown, J. V., Thom, V. A., & Constantinou, J. C. (2000). *Neurobehavioral Assessment of the Preterm Infant Revised* (2nd ed.). Van Nuys, CA: Child Development Media. http://med.stanford.edu/NAPI/	32-week postconceptional age to term	Monitor developmental progress in preterm infants to identify persistent lags in development; can be used at outcomes measurement for intervention	Developmental milestones
Neurobehavioral Functioning Inventory *Kreutzer, J. S., Seel, R. T., and Marwitz, J. H.*	Pearson Assessments Attention: Inbound Sales and Customer Support 19500 Bulverde Road San Antonio, TX 78259-3701 ClinicalCustomerSupport@Pearson.com 800-627-7271	17–80 years	To develop treatment plans and measure change for people with neurological deficits	Depression, somatic, memory/attention, communication, aggression, motor
Neurological Assessment of the Preterm and Full-Term Newborn Infant (NAPFI) *Dubowitz, L. M. S., Dubowitz, V., and Mercuri, E.*	Dubowitz, L. M. S., Dubowitz, V., & Mercuri, E. (2000). *Neurological Assessment of the Preterm and Full-Term Infant*. London, United Kingdom: Mac Keith Press.	Preterm to full-term infants	Used as a clinical neurological assessment	Neurological systems
NICU Network Neurobehavioral Scale (NNNS) *Lester, B. M., and Tronick, E. Z.*	Lester, B. M., & Tronick, E. Z. (2004). *NICU Network Neurobehavioral Scale (NNNS)*. Baltimore, MD: Brookes.	Preterm and full-term infants	Assess neurobehavioral functioning	Neurological items, behavioral state, stress/abstinence items
Nine Hole Peg Test	Mathiowetz, V., Weber, K., Kashman, N., & Volland, G. (1985). Adult norms for the Nine Hole Peg Test of finger dexterity. *Occupational Therapy Journal of Research*, *5*, 24–38.	Adults	Assess finger dexterity	Fine motor dexterity
Nottingham Extended Activities of Daily Living Scale (NEADL Scale) *Nouri, F. M., and Lincoln, N. B.*	Nouri, F. M., & Lincoln, N. B. (1987). An extended activities of daily living scale for stroke patients. *Clinical Rehabilitation*, *1*(4), 301–305. http://www.nottingham.ac.uk/iwho/research/publishedassessments.aspx	Older adults	Assess activities which may be important to individuals with strokes who are discharged to home	IADL
Occupational Circumstances Assessment-Interview Rating Scale (OCAIRS), Version 4.0 *Forsyth, K., et al.*	http://www.uic.edu/depts/moho/assess/ocairs.html	Adolescents to adults	Gather data on a client's occupational adaptation	Personal causation, values and goals, interests, roles, habits, skills, previous experiences, physical and social environments, overall occupation participation and adaptation
Occupational Performance History Interview-Second Version (OPHI-II) *Kielhofner, G., et al.*	http://www.uic.edu/depts/moho/assess/ophi%202.1.html	Adolescents to adults	Gather data on a client's occupational adaptation over time	Activity/occupational choices, critical life events, daily routines, occupational roles, occupational behavior settings
Occupational Profile of Sleep *Pierce, D., and Summers, K.*	Pierce, D., & Summers, K. (2011). Rest and sleep. In C. Brown & V. C. Stoffel (Eds.), *Occupational therapy in mental health: A vision for participation* (pp. 736–754). Philadelphia, PA: F. A. Davis.	Adults	Develop sleep profile	Sleep

(continued)

Assessment Title and Author(s)	Publisher and/or Contact Information	Ages	Stated Purpose	Areas Assessed
Occupational Questionnaire (OQ) *Smith, N. R., Kielhofner, G., and Watts, J. H.*	http://www.uic.edu/depts/moho/mohorelatedrsrcs.html	Adolescents and Adults	Gather data on time use patterns and feelings about time use	Time use
Occupational Self-Assessment (OSA), Version 2.2 *Baron, K., Kielhofner, G., Iyenger, A., Goldhammer, V., and Wolenski, J.*	http://www.uic.edu/depts/moho/assess/osa.html	14 years and older	Used as a self-report of client's perception of his or her occupational competence on his or her occupational adaptation	Volition, habituation, performance, values, personal causation, interests, roles, habits, skills
Occupational Therapy Psychosocial Assessment of Learning (OT PAL), Version 2.0 *Townsend, S., et al.*	http://www.uic.edu/depts/moho/assess/otpal.html	6–12 years	Gather information about the student and how they interact with their physical and social environments	Volition, habitation, environmental fit
O'Connor Finger Dexterity Test *O'Connor, J.*	Lafayette Instrument Company, USA PO Box 5729 Lafayette, IN 47903 USA U.S. Toll Free: 800-428-7545 sales@lafayetteinstrument.com	Adults	Used successfully as a predictor for rapid manipulation of small objects work, filling vials, and small lathe work	Manipulative skills, dexterity, eye–hand coordination
Outcome and Assessment Information Set, B-1, M0640-M0800 (OASIS) *Centers for Medicare & Medicaid Services*	http://www.cms.gov/Medicare/Quality-Initiatives-Patient-Assessment-Instruments/OASIS/index.html	Adults	Measure the ability to perform ADL and IADL in people in home care	Dressing, toileting, transferring, ambulation/locomotion, feeding/eating, grooming Meal preparation, transportation, laundry, housekeeping, telephone use, medication management
Parenting Stress Index *Abidin, R. A.*	PAR, Inc. 16204 North Florida Avenue Lutz, FL 33549 1-800-331-8378	18–60 years	Identify characteristics that fail to promote normal functioning in children, children with behavioral and emotional problems, and parents who are at risk for dysfunctional parenting	Parental distress, parent–child dysfunctional interaction, and difficult child
Parkinson's Disease Quality of Life Questionnaire (PDQ-39) *University of Oxford Health Services Research Unit*	Jenkinson, C., Fitzpatrick, R., & Peto, V. (1998). *The Parkinson's Disease Questionnaire: User Manual for the PDQ-39, PDQ-8, and the PDQ Summary Index.* Oxford, United Kingdom: Health Services Research Unit. http://www.publichealth.ox.ac.uk/units/hsru/PDQ/Intro%20pdq	Adults with Parkinson's disease	To measure health-related quality of life in patients diagnosed with Parkinson's disease	ADL, emotions, stigma, social support, cognition, communication, bodily discomfort
Participation and Environment Measure for Children and Youth (PEM-CY) *Coster, W., Law, M., and Bedell, G.*	Coster, W., Law, M., Bedell, G., Khetani, M. A., Cousins, M., & Teplicky, R. (2012). Development of the Participation and Environment Measure for Children and Youth: Conceptual basis. *Disability and Rehabilitation*, *34*, 238–246. http://www.canchild.ca/en/ourresearch/pep.asp	5–17 years	Assess participation and environment	Activities in the home, school, and community

Assessment Title and Author(s)	Publisher and/or Contact Information	Ages	Stated Purpose	Areas Assessed
Participation Objective, Participation Subjective (POPS) *Brown, M., Dijkers, M. P. J. M., Gordon, W. A., Ashman, T., Charatz, H., and Cheng, Z.*	Brown, M., Dijkers, M. P. J. M., Gordon, W. A., Ashman, T., Charatz, H., & Cheng, Z. (2004). Participation Objective, Participation Subjective: A measure of participation combining insider and outsider perspectives. *Journal of Head Trauma Rehabilitation, 19*, 459–481.	Adults	Use two perspectives (the person with a disability and a normative "outsider") to measure participation in ADL and IADL	ADL, IADL, community integration
Peabody Developmental Motor Scales-Second Edition (PDMS-2) *Folio, M. R., and Fewell, R. R.*	Academic Therapy Publications 20 Commercial Blvd. Novato, CA 94949-6191 800-422-7249 Fax: 415-883-3720 http://www.academictherapy.com	Birth to 7 years	To quantitatively assess motor development of children	Gross and fine motor skills
Pediatric Evaluation of Disability Inventory (PEDI) *Haley, S. M., Coster, W. J., Ludlow, L. H., Haltiwanger, J. T., and Andrellos, P. J.*	http://crecare.com/home.html	6 months to 7.5 years	To assess functional skills of young children, monitor progress, or evaluate the outcome of a therapeutic program	Self-care, mobility, social function
Pediatric Evaluation of Disability Inventory (PEDI)-CAT	http://crecare.com/home.html	6 months to 14 years	Assess key functional capabilities and performance; can be used on older children whose functional abilities are less than that of a 7-year-old	Self-care, mobility, social function
Pediatric Interest Profiles (PIPs): Kid's Play Profile Preteen Play Profile Adolescent Leisure Interest Profile *Henry, A. D.*	http://www.uic.edu/depts/moho/images/assessments/PIPs%20Manual.pdf	Kid's play: 6–9 years Preteen play: 9–12 years Adolescent leisure interest: 12–21 years	To select specific play/leisure activities with which to engage a child by assessing the child's interest and participation in play and leisure activities	Interest and participation in play and leisure activities
Pediatric Volitional Questionnaire (PVQ), Version 2.1 *Basu, S., Kafkes, A., Schatz, R., Kiraly, A., and Kielhofner, G.*	http://www.uic.edu/depts/moho/assess/pvq.html	2–7 years	Evaluate a young child's volition	Motivation, values, interests, environmental impact
Pepper Visual Skills for Reading Test (VSRT) *Baldasare, J., and Watson, G. R.*	Baldasare, J., & Watson, G. R. (1986). The development and evaluation of a reading test for low vision individuals with macular loss. *Journal of Visual Impairment and Blindness, 80*, 785–789.	Adults	Assess reading speed and performance based on vision	Visual motor, acuity
Perceive, Recall, Plan, and Perform (PRPP) System of Task Analysis *Aubin, G., Chapparo, C., Gelinas, I., Stip, E., and Rainville, C.*	Aubin, G., Chapparo, C., Gelinas, I., Stip, E., & Rainville, C. (2009). Use of the Perceive, Recall, Plan, and Perform System of Task Analysis for persons with schizophrenia: A preliminary study. *Australian Occupational Therapy Journal, 56*, 189–199.	Adults	To assess work behaviors and function in daily activities	ADL, IADL
Perceived Efficacy and Goal Setting System (PEGS) *Missiuna, C., Pollock, N., and Law, M.*	Pearson Assessments Attention: Inbound Sales and Customer Support 19500 Bulverde Road San Antonio, TX 78259-3701 ClinicalCustomerSupport@Pearson.com 800-627-7271	5–10 years	To assess a child's daily activities in the home, school, and community environments	ADL, IADL

(*continued*)

Assessment Title and Author(s)	Publisher and/or Contact Information	Ages	Stated Purpose	Areas Assessed
Performance Assessment of Self-Care Skills (PASS), Version 3.1 *Holm, M. B., and Rogers, J. C.*	University of Pittsburgh School of Health and Rehabilitation Sciences Pittsburgh, PA 15260	Adults with various impairments	Evaluate independent living skills in client's home and in the clinic and to assess change	Functional mobility, personal care, home management
Playform *Sturgess, J., and Ziviani, J.*	Sturgess, J., & Ziviani, J. (1995). Development of self-report play questionnaire for children aged 5 to 7 years: A preliminary report. *Australian Occupational Therapy Journal, 42*, 107–117.	5–7 years	Assess self-reported play skills	Play
Play History *Takata, N.*	Behnke, C., & Fetkovich, M. (1984). Examining the reliability and validity of the Play History. *American Journal of Occupational Therapy, 38*, 94–100.	Children and adolescents	To identify a child's play experiences and play opportunities	Previous play experiences, actual play and opportunity for play
Positive and Negative Affect Schedule *Watson, D., and Clark, L. A.*	Watson, D., & Clark, L. A. (1994). *Manual for the positive and negative affect schedule—expanded form.* Retrieved from University of Iowa website: http://www.psychology.uiowa.edu/faculty/clark/panas-x.pdf	Adults	Assesses specific emotional states	Emotion regulation
Postural Assessment Scale for Stroke Patients (PASS) *Benaim, C., Perennou, D. A., Villy, J., Rousseaux, M., and Pelissier, J. Y.*	Benaim, C., Perennou, D. A., Villy, J., Rousseaux, M., & Pelissier, J. Y. (1999). Validation of a standardized assessment of postural control for stroke patients: The Postural Assessment Scale for Stroke Patients (PASS). *Stroke, 30*, 1862–1868.	Adults	To assess postural abilities specifically for people with hemiplegia	Postural abilities in a variety of positions
Preferences for Activities of Children (PAC)	See information for Children's Assessment of Participation and Enjoyment (CAPE).			
Preschool Activity Card Sort (PACS) *Berg, C., and LaVesser, P.*	Berg, C., & LaVesser, P. (2006). The Preschool Activity Card Sort. *Occupational Therapy Journal of Research, 26*, 143–151.	3–6 years	Use pictures to help assess participation in activities	ADL, community, mobility, leisure, social interaction, domestic chores, education
Profile of Mood States, edition 2 *Heuchert, J. P., and McNair, D. M.*	Multi-Health Systems Inc. P.O. Box 950 North Tonawanda, NY 14120-0950 1-800-456-3003	13 years and older	Assess mood states via self-report	Emotional regulation
Profile of Occupational Engagement in People with Schizophrenia (POES) *Bejerholm, U., Hansson, L., and Eklund, M.*	Bejerholm, U., Hansson, L., & Eklund, M. (2006). Profiles of Occupational Engagement in people with Schizophrenia, POES: Development of a new instrument based on time-use diaries. *British Journal of Occupational Therapy, 69*, 1–11.	Adults	Identify how persons engage in occupation throughout a typical day	Daily rhythm of activity and rest, variety and range of occupations, place, social environment, social interplay, interpretation, extent of meaningful occupations, routines, initiation of performance
Purdue Pegboard *Tiffin, J.*	Lafayette Instrument Company 3700 Sagamore Parkway North PO Box 5729 Lafayette, IN 47903 800-428-7545	5 years and older	To measure dexterity of fingertip activity and finger/hand/arm activity	Finger dexterity, fine motor coordination, and speed

Assessment Title and Author(s)	Publisher and/or Contact Information	Ages	Stated Purpose	Areas Assessed
Quadriplegia Index of Function (QIF) *Gresham, G. E., Labi, M. L., Dittmar, S. S., Hicks, J. T., Joyce, S. Z., and Stehlik, M. A.*	Gresham, G. E., Labi, M. L., Dittmar, S. S., Hicks, J. T., Joyce, S. Z., & Stehlik, M. A. (1986). The Quadriplegia Index of Function (QIF): Sensitivity and reliability demonstrated in a study of thirty quadriplegic patients. *Paraplegia, 24*(1), 38–44.	18 years and older	Document small but significant gains in function of people with spinal cord injuries	ADL
Quality of Life Inventory (QOLI) *Frisch, M. B.*	Pearson Assessments Attention: Inbound Sales and Customer Support 19500 Bulverde Road San Antonio, TX 78259-3701 ClinicalCustomerSupport@Pearson.com 800-627-7271	17 years and older	Assess positive health, well-being, and quality of life	Quality of life in 16 areas
Quality of Life Profile for Adults with Physical Disabilities (QOLP-PD) *Renwick, R., Nourhaghighi, N., Manns, P. J., and Rudman, D. L.*	Renwick, R., Nourhaghighi, N., Manns, P. J., & Rudman, D. L. (2003). Quality of life for people with physical disabilities: A new instrument. *International Journal of Rehabilitation Research, 26*(4), 279–287.	Adults	Measure quality of life for people with physical disabilities	Quality of life in being, belonging, and becoming
Quick Neurological Screening Test-Third Edition (QNST-3) *Mutti, M., Martin, N. A., Sterling, H. M., and Spalding, N. V.*	Academic Therapy Publications 20 Commercial Blvd. Novato, CA 94949-6191 800-422-7249 Fax: 415-883-3720 http://www.academictherapy.com	4–80 years	Identify neurological soft signs and associated motor impairments, learning difficulties, and problems in daily functioning	Large and small muscle control, motor planning, sequencing, sense of rate and rhythm, spatial organization, visual and auditory perceptual skills, balance, cerebellar-vestibular function, disorders of attention
Rancho Los Amigos Levels of Cognitive Functioning Scale-Revised *Hagen, C.*	Hagen, C. (1998). *The Rancho Levels of Cognitive Functioning: The revised levels* (3rd ed.). Downey, CA: Rancho Los Amigos Medical Center.	All ages	Assess levels of consciousness and cognitive functioning	Cognitive functioning
Reintegration to Normal Living (RNL) Index *Wood-Dauphinee, S., Opzoomer, M. A., Williams, J. I., Marchand, J., and Spitzer, W. O.*	Wood-Dauphinee, S., Opzoomer, M. A., Williams, J. I., Marchand, B., & Spitzer, W. O. (1988). Assessment of global function: The Reintegration to Normal Living Index. *Archives of Physical Medicine and Rehabilitation, 69*, 583–590.	Adults	To assess how well individuals return to normal living patterns following incapacitating diseases or injury	ADL
Residential Environmental Impact Scale (REIS) *Fisher, G., Arriaga, P., Less, C., Lee, J., and Ashpole, E.*	http://www.uic.edu/depts/moho/REISinformation.html	Adults living in community residential facilities	Assess how well the home environment is meeting the needs of the residents as a whole	Accessibility, cognitive and physical supports, physical environment, natural environment, furniture, sensory environment, home-like qualities, presence of objects, personal preferences
Revised Children's Manifest Anxiety Scale-Second Edition (RCMAS-2) *Reynolds, C. R., and Richmond, B. O.*	Western Psychological Services 625 Alaska Ave. Torrance, CA 90503-5124 424-201-8800	6–19 years	Measure the level and nature of anxiety as experienced by children	Anxiety

(*continued*)

Assessment Title and Author(s)	Publisher and/or Contact Information	Ages	Stated Purpose	Areas Assessed
Revised Knox Preschool Play Scale (RKPPS) *Knox, S.*	Knox, S. (1997). Development and current use of the Knox Preschool Play Scale. In L. Parham & L. Fazio (Eds.), *Play in occupational therapy for children* (pp. 35–51). St. Louis, MO: Mosby.	Birth to 6 years	Used as an observational assessment of play skills	Space management, material management, pretense or symbolic play, participation in play
Rivermead Behavioral Memory Test-Extended Version (RBMT-E) *Wilson, B., Clare, L., Baddeley, A., Watson, P., and Tate, R.*	Pearson Assessments Attention: Inbound Sales and Customer Support 19500 Bulverde Road San Antonio, TX 78259-3701 ClinicalCustomerSupport@Pearson.com 800-627-7271	16–65 years	To detect and identify memory impairments that occur in every activity, with a broader cultural sensitivity	Memory
Rivermead Behavioral Memory Test for Children (RBMT-C) *Wilson, B., Ivani-Chalian, R., and Aldrich, F.*	Pearson Assessments Attention: Inbound Sales and Customer Support 19500 Bulverde Road San Antonio, TX 78259-3701 ClinicalCustomerSupport@Pearson.com 800-627-7271	Children, 5–11 years	To detect and identify memory impairments that occur in every activity	Verbal recall, remember to do a task later in the test, remember and identify pictures, remember and retell a story, retrace a route around the room, memory
Rivermead Behavioral Memory Test-Third Edition (RBMT-3) *Wilson, B., et al.*	Pearson Assessments Attention: Inbound Sales and Customer Support 19500 Bulverde Road San Antonio, TX 78259-3701 ClinicalCustomerSupport@Pearson.com 800-627-7271	16–96 years	Detect and identify memory impairments	Memory
Rivermead Motor Assessment (RMA) *Institute of Work, Health, & Organisations*	Institute of Work, Health, & Organisations International House Jubilee Campus, Wollaton Road Nottingham, NG8 1BB http://www.nottingham.ac.uk/iwho/research/publishedassessments.aspx	Adults	Evaluate function after stroke	Gross motor, fine motor
Role Activity Performance Scale (RAPS) *Good-Ellis, M. A.*	Good-Ellis, M. A. (1999). The Role Activity Performance Scale. In B. J. Hemphill-Pearson (Ed.), *Assessments in occupational therapy mental health: An integrative approach* (pp. 205–230). Thorofare, NJ: Slack.	Adults	Assess role activity performance history over time (up to 18 months)	ADL, IADL
Role Change Assessment *Jackoway, I. S., Rogers, J. C., and Snow, T. L.*	Jackoway, I. S., Rogers, J. C., & Snow T. L. (1987). The Role Change Assessment: An interview tool for evaluating older adults. *Occupational Therapy in Mental Health*, *7*, 17–37.	Older adults	Evaluate the role performance of older adults	Family and social, vocational, self-care, organizational, leisure, health care
Role Checklist (RC) *Oakley, F.*	http://www.uic.edu/depts/moho/mohorelatedrsrcs.html E-mail Fran Oakley to request the Role Checklist at foakley@nih.gov. Please include the following information in your e-mail request: first and last name; type of facility in which you work; type of clients served; and city, state, and country of residence.	Adults	To assess productive roles in adult life	Roles significant to the client, motivation to engage in tasks necessary to those roles, perceptions of role shifting

Assessment Title and Author(s)	Publisher and/or Contact Information	Ages	Stated Purpose	Areas Assessed
Routine Task Inventory-2 (RTI-2) *Allen, C. K., Kehrberg, K., and Burns, T.*	Allen, C. K., Kehrberg, K., & Burns, T. (1992). Evaluation instruments. In C. K. Allen, C. A. Earhart, & T. Blue (Eds.), *Occupational therapy treatment goals for the physically and cognitively disabled* (pp. 30–84). Bethesda, MD: American Occupational Therapy Association.	Adults	To assess functional behavior during typical tasks using self-report or observation	Self-awareness (e.g., grooming, dressing, bathing), situational awareness (e.g., housekeeping, spending money, shopping), occupational role (e.g., planning/doing major role activities, pacing and timing actions), social role (e.g., communicating, meaning, following directions)
Routines-Based Interview (RBI) *McWilliam, R., Casey, A., and Sims, J.*	McWilliam, R., Casey, A., & Sims, J. (2009). The Routines-Based Interview: A method for gathering information and assessing needs. *Infants and Young Children, 22,* 224–233. Siskin Children's Institute http://www.siskin.org/www/docs/112.190/	Children	To gather information for improved IFSP and IEP goals	Daily routine, family concerns and needs, social engagement
Safety Assessment of Function and the Environment for Rehabilitation (SAFER) *Oliver, R., Blathwayt, J., Brackley, C., and Tamaki, T.*	Oliver, R., Blathwayt, J., Brackley, C., & Tamaki, T. (1993). Development of the Safety Assessment of Function and the Environment for Rehabilitation (SAFER) tool. *Canadian Journal of Occupational Therapy 60*, 78–82.	Older adults	To evaluate home safety for elders	Risks in various rooms of the home as well as general risks such as fire hazards; examines safety issues in how the individual performs various self-care and household tasks; examines the potential for wandering and the use of memory aids; and identifies how help could be summoned
Satisfaction with Life Scale (SWLS) *Diener, E., Emmons, R. A., Larsen, R. J., and Griffin, S.*	Diener, E., Emmons, R. A., Larsen, R. J., & Griffin, S. (1985). The Satisfaction with Life Scale. *Journal of Personality Assessment, 49*, 71–75.	Adults	To assess global life satisfaction	Quality of life
Scales of Independent Behavior-Revised (SIB-R) *Bruininks, R. H., Woodcock, R. W., Weatherman, R. F., and Hill, B. K.*	Riverside Publishing Company 3800 Golf Road, Suite 200 Rolling Meadows, IL 60008 800-323-9540	All ages	Provide a comprehensive assessment of adaptive behavior and identifies areas of problem behaviors	Adaptive behavior
Scale of Older Adults' Routine (SOAR) *Zisberg, A., Young, H. M., and Schepp, K.*	Zisberg, A., Young, H. M., & Schepp, K. (2009). Development and psychometric testing of the Scale of Older Adults' Routine. *Journal of Advanced Nursing, 65*, 672–683.	Older adults	Assess routine stability across time	BADL, IADL, social activities, leisure activities, rest activities
Schizophrenia Cognition Rating Scale (SCoRS) *Keefe, R. S. E., Poe, M., Walker, T. M., Kang, J. W., and Harvey, P. D.*	Keefe, R. S. E., Poe, M., Walker, T. M., Kang, J. W., & Harvey, P. D. (2006). The Schizophrenia Cognition Rating Scale: An interview-based assessment and its relationship to cognition, real-world functioning, and functional capacity. *The American Journal of Psychiatry, 163*, 426–432.	Adults	Assess how cognitive deficits affect daily functioning	Attention, memory, reasoning and problem solving, working memory, language production, motor skills

(*continued*)

Assessment Title and Author(s)	Publisher and/or Contact Information	Ages	Stated Purpose	Areas Assessed
School Function Assessment (SFA) *Coster, W., Deeney, T., Haltiwanger, J., and Haley, S.*	Pearson Assessments Attention: Inbound Sales and Customer Support 19500 Bulverde Road San Antonio, TX 78259-3701 ClinicalCustomerSupport@Pearson.com 800-627-7271	Kindergarten to sixth grade	To evaluate and monitor a student's performance of functional tasks and activities that support his or her participation in elementary school	Participation in elementary school setting, task supports, activity performance
School Observation-Environment *Hanft, B., and Place, P.*	Pearson Assessments Attention: Inbound Sales and Customer Support 19500 Bulverde Road San Antonio, TX 78259-3701 ClinicalCustomerSupport@Pearson.com 800-627-7271	Environmental assessment	Identify environmental factors that facilitate or interfere with learning	Student's environment: classrooms, gym, cafeteria, bathrooms, playground, and hallways
School Setting Interview (SSI), Version 3.0 *Hemmingsson, H., Egilson, S., Hoffman, O. R., and Kielhofner, G.*	http://www.uic.edu/depts/moho/assess/ssi.html	9 years to high school	Allow children and adolescents with disabilities to describe the impact of the environment on their functioning in multiple school settings	Impact of school environment on functional performance of children and adolescents with disability
School Situations Questionnaire (SSQ) *Barkley, R.*	Barkley, R. A., & Murphy, K. R. (1998). *Attention deficit hyperactivity disorder: A clinical workbook* (2nd ed.). New York, NY: Guilford.	School age	Identify how symptoms of ADD/ADHD disrupt the school environment and the child's ability to participate in ADL	ADL
School Version of the Assessment of Motor and Process Skills (School AMPS) *Fisher, A. G., Bryze, K., Hume, V., and Griswold, L. A.*	Fisher, A. G., Bryze, K., Hume, V., & Griswold, L. A. (2005). *School AMPS: School version of the Assessment of Motor and Process Skills* (2nd ed.). Fort Collins, CO: Three Star Press.	3–12 years	Assess a student's schoolwork performance	Motor skills, process skills
Self-Directed Search *Holland, J. L.*	Psychological Assessment Resources, Inc. 16204 N. Florida Avenue Lutz, FL 33549 813-968-3003 http://www.self-directed-search.com/	14 years and older	Assess career interests	Aspirations, activities, competencies, occupations
Self-Discovery Tapestry *Meltzer, P.*	Meltzer, P. (2003). *Self-Discovery Tapestry: A Colorful, Interactive, Life-Review Instrument.* Baltimore, MD: Health Professions Press.	Adults	Used as a self-assessment of interests; recognize adaptations	Interests, self-awareness
Self-Perception Profile for Adolescents *Harter, S.*	Harter, S. (1988). *Manual for the Adolescent Self-Perception Profile.* Denver, CO: Author.	Adolescents	To measure self-esteem and perceived competence in adolescents	Scholastic competence, social acceptance, athletic competence, physical appearance, behavioral conduct, self-worth
Self-Perception Profile for Children *Harter, S.*	Harter, S. (1985). *The Self-Perception Profile for Children: Revision of the Perceived Competence Scale for Children.* Denver, CO: University of Denver.	Children 8 years and older	To measure self-esteem and perceived competence in children	Scholastic competence, social acceptance, athletic competence, physical appearance, behavioral conduct, self-worth

Assessment Title and Author(s)	Publisher and/or Contact Information	Ages	Stated Purpose	Areas Assessed
Self-Report Assessment of Functional Visual Performance *Warren, M., Velozo, C. A., and Hicks, E.*	Warren, M., Velozo, C. A., & Hicks, E. (2008, April). *Self-Report Evaluation to Identify and Predict Occupational Performance in Aadults with Low Vision*. Paper presented at the American Occupational Therapy Annual Conference, Long Beach, CA.	Adults	Used as a self-report with an observational component regarding functional vision	ADL, IADL
Self-Reported Functional Measure (SRFM) *Hoenig, H.*	Hoenig, H., McIntyre, L., Sloane, R., Branch, L. G, Truncali, A., & Horner, R. D. (1998). The reliability of a Self-reported measure of disease, impairment, and function in persons with spinal cord dysfunction. *Archives in Physical Medicine and Rehabilitation, 79*, 378–387.		Used as a self-assessment of function; can be used to measure efficacy of treatment, readiness for community reentry	BADL, IADL, amount of support required
Semmes-Weinstein Monofilament Test *Weinstein, S.*	Weinstein, S. (1993). Fifty years of somatosensory research: From the Semmes-Weinstein monofilaments to the Weinstein enhanced sensory test. *Journal of Hand Therapy*, 6, 11–22.	All	Identify skin pressure thresholds useful in determining degree of normal and protective sensation	Skin sensation
Sensory Integration and Praxis Tests (SIPT) *Ayres, A. J.*	Western Psychological Services 625 Alaska Ave Torrance, CA 90503-5124 800-648-8857	4–8 years and 11 months	To assess praxis and sensory processing and integration of vestibular, proprioceptive, tactile, kinesthetic, and visual systems	Sensory processing, visual-spatial perception, coordination, motor planning
Sensory Integration Observation Guide *Schaaf, R., Burke, J., and Anzalone, M.*	Sensory Processing Disorder Foundation http://www.sinetwork.org/	0–2 months	Measure parent's report regarding infant sensory responsiveness	Tactile-kinesthetic, vestibular-proprioceptive, adaptive motor, regulatory
Sensory Organization Test (SOT) *Nashner, L. M.*	NeuroCom 9570 SE Lawnfield Road Clackamas, OR 97015 800-767-6744	Adult	To objectively identify abnormalities in a patient's use of somatosensory, visual and vestibular systems that contribute to postural control	Postural stability in various sensory conditions/environments
Sensory Processing Measure (SPM) Home Form *Parham, L. D., and Ecker, C.*	Western Psychological Services 625 Alaska Ave. Torrance, CA 90503-5124 800-648-8857	5–12 years	To provide a complete picture of a child's sensory processing difficulties in the home	Visual, auditory, tactile, proprioceptive, vestibular
Sensory Processing Measure (SPM) School Form *Miller-Kuhaneck, H., Henry, D., and Glennon, T.*	Western Psychological Services 625 Alaska Ave Torrance, CA 90503-5124 800-648-8857	5–12 years	To provide a complete picture of a child's sensory processing difficulties at school	Visual, auditory, tactile, proprioceptive, vestibular
Sensory Profile Adolescent/Adult Sensory Profile Infant/Toddler Sensory Profile *Dunn, W.*	Pearson Assessments Attention: Inbound Sales and Customer Support 19500 Bulverde Road San Antonio, TX 78259-3701 ClinicalCustomerSupport@Pearson.com 800-627-7271	Sensory profile: 3–10 years Adolescent/adult: 10 years and older Infant/Toddler: 0–36 months	To determine how well a subject processes sensory information in everyday situations and to profile the sensory system's effect on functional performance	Sensory processing, modulation, and behavioral and emotional responses

(continued)

Assessment Title and Author(s)	Publisher and/or Contact Information	Ages	Stated Purpose	Areas Assessed
Short Child Occupational Profile (SCOPE), Version 2.2 *Bowyer, P., et al.*	http://www.uic.edu/depts/moho/assess/scope.html	Birth to 21 years	Assess a child's ability to participate	Volition, habituation, skills, environment
Short Form-36 *Ware, J. E.*	http://www.qualitymetric.com/WhatWeDo/GenericHealthSurveys/tabid/184/Default.aspx?gclid=CNHFq4fPuK8CFSzptgodyiN5iw	14 years and older	To assess general health	Physical activities, social activities, role activities, bodily pain, mental health, emotional health, vitality, general health
Sign and Symptom Checklist for HIV, Revised (SSC-HIVrev) *Holzemer, W. L., Hudson, A., Kirksey, K. M., Hamilton, M. J., and Bakken, S.*	Holzemer, W. L., Hudson, A., Kirksey, K. M., Hamilton, M. J., & Bakken, S. (2001). The Revised Sign and Symptom Checklist for HIV (SSC-HIVrev). *Journal of the Association of Nurses in AIDS Care, 12*, 60–70.	Adults	To identify signs and symptoms related to HIV	Physical signs and symptoms of HIV
Simulator Sickness Questionnaire (SSQ) *Kennedy, R. S., Lane, N. E., Berbaum, K. S., and Lilienthal, M. G.*	Kennedy, R. S., Lane, N. E., Berbaum, K. S., & Lilienthal, M. G. (1993). Simulator Sickness Questionnaire: An enhanced method for quantifying simulator sickness. *The International Journal of Aviation Psychology, 3*, 203–220.	Adults	Assess simulator sickness; can be used during driving simulation	Symptoms of motion sickness in oculomotor, disorientation, and nausea domains
Social Rhythm Metric (SRM-5) *Monk, T. H., Frank, E., Potts, J. M., and Kupfer, D. J.*	Monk, T. H., Frank, E., Potts, J. M., & Kupfer, D. J. (2002). A simple way to measure daily lifestyle regularity. *Journal of Sleep Research, 11*, 183–190.	19–92 years	To quantify lifestyle regularity	Record timing of morning and afternoon/evening events
Social Skills Rating System (SSRS) *Gresham, F. M., and Elliot, S. N.*	Pearson Assessments Attention: Inbound Sales and Customer Support 19500 Bulverde Road San Antonio, TX 78259-3701 ClinicalCustomerSupport@Pearson.com 800-627-7271	3–18 years	Rate social behaviors believed to affect areas such as teacher–student relationships, peer acceptance, and academic performance	Social skills (cooperation, assertion, responsibility, empathy, and self-control), problem behaviors, and academic competence (teacher ratings of reading, math performance, general cognitive functioning, motivation, and parental support)
Spinal Cord Independence Measure (SCIM) *Catz, A., Itzkovich, M., Agranov, E., Ring, H., and Tamir, A.*	Catz, A., Itzkovich, M., Agranov, E., Ring, H., & Tamir, A. (1997). SCIM—Spinal Cord Independence Measure: A new disability scale for patients with spinal cord lesions. *Spinal Cord, 35*(12), 850–856.	Adults	Measure independence in ADL; can be used for goal determination and outcomes assessment	ADL
Stroke Impact Scale (SIS), Version 3.0 *Duncan, P. W.*	Ms. Elaine Spildbusch University of Kansas Medical Center Research Institute, Inc. 3901 Rainbow Blvd, Kansas City, Kansas 66160-7702 espielbu@kumc.edu	Adults	Measure stroke recovery in eight domains: strength, hand function, mobility, ADL, emotion, memory, communication, and social participation	Strength, hand function, mobility, ADL, emotion, memory, communication, social participation
Stroke Specific Quality of Life (SS-QOL) Scale *Williams, L. S., Weinberger, M., Harris, L. E., Clark, D. O., and Biller, J.*	Williams, L. S., Weinberger, M., Harris, L. E., Clark, D. O., & Biller, J. (1999). Development of a Stroke-Specific Quality of Life Scale. *Stroke, 30*(7), 1362–1369. http://www.strokecenter.org/trials/scales/ssqol.html	Adults	To measure quality of life of individuals poststroke	Mobility, energy, upper extremity function, work/productivity, mood, self-care, social roles, family roles, vision, language, thinking, personality

Assessment Title and Author(s)	Publisher and/or Contact Information	Ages	Stated Purpose	Areas Assessed
Swallowing Ability and Function Evaluation (SAFE) *Kipping, P., Ross-Swain, D., and Yee, P.*	PRO-ED, Inc. 8700 Shoal Creek Blvd. Austin, TX 78757 800-897-3202	Adolescents to adults	Evaluate swallowing	Swallowing
Tardieu Scale and Modified Tardieu Scale *Tardieu, G.*	Haugh, A. B., Pandyan, A. D., & Johnson, G. R. (2006). A systematic review of the Tardieu Scale for the measurement of spasticity. *Disability and Rehabilitation, 28*, 899–907.	Children and adults	Quantify spasticity level	Spasticity
Tennessee Self-Concept Scale-Second Edition (TSCS-2) *Fitts, W. H., and Warren, W. L.*	Western Psychological Services 625 Alaska Ave Torrance, CA 90503-5124 800-648-8857	7–90 years	Measure self-concept across the life span	Motor skills, values, social skills, academics
Test d'Evaluation des Membres supérieurs des Personnes Agées (TEMPA) *Desrosiers, J., Hébert, J., Dutil, E., and Bravo, G.*	Desrosiers, J., Hébert, J., Dutil, É., Bravo, G., & Mercier, L. (1994). Validity of a measurement instrument for upper extremity performance: The TEMPA. *Occupational Therapy Journal of Research 14*, 267–281.	Adults	Measure upper extremity performance using ADL	Upper extremity performance
Test of Environmental Supportiveness (TOES) *Bundy, A.*	Bundy, A. C., Waugh, K., & Brentnall, J. (2009). Developing assessments that account for the role of the environment: An example using the Test of Playfulness and Test of Environmental Supportiveness. *Occupational Therapy Journal of Research, 29*, 135–143.	Children	Assess the extent to which the environment supports an individual's play	Caregiver's actions, rules, and boundaries; peer, younger, and older playmates' use of cues and domination of interaction; natural and fabricated objects; amount and configuration of space; sensory environment; safety and accessibility of space
Test of Grocery Shopping Skills (TOGSS) *Brown, C., Rempfer, M., and Hamera, E.*	Brown, C., Rempfer, M., & Hamera, E. (2009). *The Test of Grocery Shopping Skills*. Bethesda, MD: AOTA Press.	Adults	Measure a consumer's ability to complete a grocery shopping task	IADL
Test of Ideational Praxis *May-Benson, T. A.*	TMB Educational Enterprises http://www.tmbeducational enterprises.com/	5–8 years	Measure ideational abilities in children	Demonstration of various actions with and on specified objects that indicate recognition of the specific affordances offered by the individual objects
Test of Infant Motor Performance (TIMP) *Campbell, S. K., Girolami, G., Kolobe, T., Osten, E., and Lenke, M.*	Infant Motor Performance Scales, LLC 1301 W. Madison St. #526 Chicago, IL 60607-1953 http://thetimp.com	34 weeks postconceptional to 4 months postterm	Assess postural and selective control of movement	Postural control, motor control
Test of Playfulness (ToP) *Bundy, A.*	Bundy, A. C. (2000). *The Test of Playfulness (revised version 3.5) manual*. Fort Collins, CO: Colorado State University.	15 months to 10 years	Assess a child's play behavior based on playfulness rather than on motor, cognitive, or language skills	Playfulness
Test of Sensory Functions in Infants *DeGangi, G., and Greenspan, S. I.*	Western Psychological Services 625 Alaska Avenue Torrance, CA 90503-5124 800-648-8857	4–18 months	Determine whether and to what extent an infant has sensory processing deficits	Reactivity to tactile deep pressure, visual tactile integration, adaptive motor function, ocular-motor control, reactivity to vestibular stimulation

(*continued*)

Assessment Title and Author(s)	Publisher and/or Contact Information	Ages	Stated Purpose	Areas Assessed
Test of Visual-Motor Skills-Third Edition (TVMS-3) *Martin, N.*	Academic Therapy Publications 20 Commercial Blvd. Novato, CA 94949-6191 800-422-7249 Fax: 415-883-3720 http://www.academictherapy.com	3–90 years	To assess how a person visually perceives nonlanguage forms and translates what is perceived through hand function	Visual-motor skills
Test of Visual-Perceptual Skills-Third Edition (TVPS-3) *Martin, N.*	Academic Therapy Publications 20 Commercial Blvd. Novato, CA 94949-6191 800-422-7249 Fax: 415-883-3720 http://www.academictherapy.com	4–18 years and 11 months	To determine visual-perceptual strengths and weaknesses without the use of motor responses	Visual discrimination, visual memory, visual-spatial relations, visual form constancy, visual sequential memory, visual figure–ground; visual closure
Tetraplegia Hand Activity Questionnaire (THAQ) *Land, N. E., Odding, E., Duivenvoorden, H. J., Bergen, M. P., and Stam, H. J.*	Land, N. E., Odding, E., Duivenvoorden, H. J., Bergen, M. P., & Stam, H. J. (2004). Tetraplegia Hand Activity Questionnaire (THAQ): The development, assessment of arm–hand function-related activities in tetraplegic patients with a spinal cord injury. *Spinal Cord*, 42, 294–301.	Adults	Measure arm and hand function in individuals with tetraplegia	ADL
The Experience of Leisure Scale (TELS) *Bundy, A., Gliner, J., and Meakins, C. R. H.*	Bundy, A., Gliner, J., & Meakins, C. R. H. (2005). Validity and reliability of The Experience of Leisure Scale (TELS). In F. McMahon, D. E. Lytle, & B. Sutton-Smith (Eds.), *Play: An interdisciplinary synthesis—play & culture studies* (Vol. 6, pp. 255–278). Lanham, MD: University Press of America.	Adolescents and adults	Examine play and leisure experiences of adults and adolescents	Play/leisure
Timed Up and Go Test *Posiadlo, D., and Richardson, S.*	Podsiadlo, D., & Richardson, S. (1991). The timed "up & go": A test of basic functional mobility for frail elderly persons. *Journal of the American Geriatrics Society, 39*, 142–148.	Older adults	Predict fall risk in elderly patients	Fall risk
Tinetti Assessment Tool *Tinetti, M.*	Tinetti, M. E. (1986). Performance-oriented assessment of mobility problems in elderly patients. *Journal of the American Geriatrics Society, 34*, 119–126.	Adult	To measure fall risk in adult and geriatric populations	Gait, balance
Toglia Category Assessment (TCA) *Toglia, J. P.*	Maddak, Inc. 661 Route 23 South Wayne, NJ 07470 800-443-4926 http://www.maddak.com	All ages	To assess category flexibility	Categorization, strategies, problem solving
Transdisciplinary Play-Based Assessment-Second Edition (TPBA-2) and Transdisciplinary Play-Based Intervention-Second Edition (TPBI-2) *Linder, T. W.*	Customer Service Department Brookes Publishing Co. PO Box 10624 Baltimore, MD 21285-0624 800-638-3775	0–6 years	Use play to assess a child's development	Cognition, communication, language, movement skills, social and emotional development

Assessment Title and Author(s)	Publisher and/or Contact Information	Ages	Stated Purpose	Areas Assessed
Transition Planning Inventory (TPI)-Updated Version *Clark, G. M., and Patton, J. R.*	PRO-ED, Inc. 8700 Shoal Creek Blvd. Austin, TX 78757 800-897-3202	14–22 years	To identify and plan for the comprehensive transitional needs of students; designed to provide school personnel with a systematic way to address mandates of the Individuals with Disabilities Education Act (IDEA)	School skills, interests, environmental requirements
Trunk Control Test *Collin, C., and Wade, D.*	Collin, C., & Wade, D. (1990). Assessing motor impairment after stroke: A pilot reliability study. *Journal of Neurology, Neurosurgery, and Psychiatry, 5,* 576–579.	Adults	Assess bed mobility, correlate with eventual walking ability	Bed mobility
UCSD Performance-Based Skills Assessment (UPSA) *Patterson, T. L., Goldman, S., McKibbin, C. L., Hughs, T., and Jeste, D. V.*	Patterson, T. L., Goldman, S., McKibbin, C. L., Hughs, T., & Jeste, D. V. (2001). UCSD Performance-Based Skills Assessment: Development of a new measure of everyday functioning for severely mentally ill adults. *Schizophrenia Bulletin, 27,* 235–245.	Adults	Assess ability to independently function in a community	Household chores, communication, finance, transportation, planning recreational activities
Unified Parkinson's Disease Rating Scale (UPDRS) *Fahn, S., Elton, R., and the Members of the UPDRS Development Committee*	http://www.mdvu.org/library/ratingscales/pd/ Fahn, S., Marsden, C. D., Calne, D. B., & Goldstein, M. (Eds.). (1987). *Recent developments in Parkinson's disease* (Vol. 2., pp. 153–163, 293–304). Florham Park, NJ: Macmillan Health Care Information.	Adults	Follow the longitudinal course of Parkinson's disease	Mentation, behavior, and mood; ADL; motor skills
University of Rhode Island Change Assessment (URICA) Scale *Levesque, D. A., Gelles, R. J., and Velicer, W. F.*	Levesque, D. A., Gelles, R. J., & Velicer, W. F. (2000). Development and validation of a stages of change measure for men in batterer treatment. *Cognitive Therapy and Research, 24,* 175–199.	Adults	Evaluate motivation for change	Motivation
Useful Field of View (UFOV) *Ball, K., and Roenker, D.*	Visual Awareness Research Group, Inc. 2580 Tarpon Cove Suite 922 Punta Gorda, FL 33950 859-523-8007	Older adults	Assess visual attention	Visual processing capabilities, visual attention
Vineland Adaptive Behavior Scales-Second Edition (VABS-II) *Sparrow, S. S., Cicchetti, D. V., and Balla, D. A.*	Sparrow, S., Cicchetti, D., & Balla, D. (2005). *Vineland Adaptive Behavior Scales* (2nd ed.). Minneapolis, MN: Pearson Assessments. Pearson Assessments Attention: Inbound Sales and Customer Support 19500 Bulverde Road San Antonio, TX 78259-3701 ClinicalCustomerSupport@Pearson.com 800-627-7271	Birth to 90 years	To assess personal and social sufficiency of individuals from birth to adulthood	Communication, ADL, socialization, motor skills, adaptive behavior, maladaptive behavior

(*continued*)

Assessment Title and Author(s)	Publisher and/or Contact Information	Ages	Stated Purpose	Areas Assessed
Volitional Questionnaire (VQ), Version 4.1 *de la Heras, C. G., Geist, R., Kielhofner, G., and Li, Y.*	http://www.uic.edu/depts/moho/assess/vq.html	Adults	Measure how a person reacts to and acts within his or her environment	Motives, environment
WeeFIM (Guide for the Uniform Data Set for Medical Rehabilitation for Children), Version 6.0 *The Center for Functional Assessment Research*	Uniform Data System for Medical Rehabilitation. (2005). *The WeeFIM II System Clinical Guide* (Version 6.0). Buffalo, NY: Author. Information Resource Center Uniform Data System for Medical Rehabilitation 270 Northpointe Parkway, Suite 300 Amherst, NY 14228 716-817-7800 info@udsmr.org	Children from 6 months to 7 years	Measure disability severity related to physical impairment, across health, development, educational, and community settings	18 activities (13 with a motor emphasis related to self-care and 5 with a cognitive emphasis involving communication)
Western Neuro Sensory Stimulation Profile (WNSSP) *Ansell, B. J., and Keenan, J. E.*	Ansell, B. J., & Keenan, J. E. (1989). The Western Neuro Sensory Stimulation Profile: A tool for assessing slow-to-recover head-injured patients. *Archives of Physical Medical Rehabilitation, 70*(2), 104–108.	Adults	To assess cognitive function in severely impaired head-injured adults (Rancho levels II-V) and to monitor and predict change in slow-to-recover patients	Arousal/attention; expressive communication; response to auditory, visual, tactile, and olfactory stimulation
Whalen HIV Symptom Index *Whalen, C. C., Antani, M., Carey, J., and Landefeld, C. S.*	Whalen, C. C., Antani, M., Carey, J., & Landefeld, C. S. (1994). An index of symptoms for infection with human immunodeficiency virus: Reliability and validity. *Journal of Clinical Epidemiology, 47*(5), 537–546.	Adults	Measure symptoms in individuals affected with HIV	Symptoms
Wolf Motor Function Test (modified) *Wolf, S.*	Wolf, S., Lecraw, D. E., Barton, L. A., & Jann, B. B. (1989). Forced use of hemiplegic upper extremities to reverse the effect of learned nonuse among chronic stroke and head-injured patients. *Exploring Neurology, 104*, 125–132. Taub, E., Morris, D.M., & Crago, J. (2011). *Wolf Motor Function Test (WMFT) Manual: UAB CI Therapy Research Group*. Retrieved from http://www.uab.edu/citherapy/images/pdf_files/CIT_Training_WMFT_Manual.pdf	Adults	Assess the motor ability of patients with moderate-to-severe upper extremity motor deficits	Positional movement, object manipulation
Wong-Baker FACES Pain Rating Scale *Wong, D., and Baker C.*	http://www.wongbakerfaces.org/	Children to adults	Allow nonverbal assessment of pain on a scale	Pain
Work Environmental Impact Scale (WEIS), Version 2.0 *Moore-Corner, R. A., Kielfhofner, G., and Olson, L.*	http://www.uic.edu/depts/moho/assess/weis.html	Adults	Identify environmental characteristics that facilitate successful employment experiences	Social and physical environment, supports, temporal demands, objects used, daily job functions
Worker Role Interview (WRI), Version 10.0 *Braveman, B., et al.*	http://www.uic.edu/depts/moho/assess/wri.html	Adults	Gather data on psychosocial and environmental factors related to work	Personal causation, values, interests, roles and habits related to work, influence of the environment

ADD, attention deficit disorder; ADHD, attention deficit/hyperactivity disorder; ADL, activities of daily living; ALS, amyotrophic lateral sclerosis; BADL, basic activities of daily living; CAT, computer-assisted test; FICA, faith and belief, importance, community, and address in care; IADL, instrumental activities of daily living; IEP, Individualized Education Program; IFSP, Individual Family Service Plan; NICU, neonatal intensive care unit; OT, occupational therapy.

Glossary

The following definitions are drawn from the chapters in this book and are intended as a resource for understanding. Chapter numbers appear in parentheses at the end of each definition so that readers can refer to the cited chapters for concepts and definitions listed here. The Glossary also includes definitions from the American Occupational Therapy Association (AOTA) "Occupational Therapy Practice Framework, 2nd Edition." These definitions are indicated by the abbreviations OTPF-II. Likewise, there are definitions from the World Health Organization (indicated by WHO) and the WHO International Classification of Functioning, Disability, and Health (indicated by the abbreviation ICF). Readers should cite the appropriate authors or original citations when referring to these constructs.

Accessible design Also referred to as barrier-free design, adds accessibility to otherwise inaccessible buildings, products, and services to enable persons with disabilities to function independently (29).

Accountable care organization An organization of health care providers that agrees to be accountable for the quality, cost, and overall care of Medicare beneficiaries who are enrolled in the traditional fee-for-service program who are assigned to it (71).

Acquisitional occupation Using occupations to promote the person to develop or reacquire skills (58).

Actigraphy The use of recordings of body motion to display activity patterns across many consecutive days and nights (51).

Active assistive range of motion (AROM) Arc of motion through which the joint passes when moved by muscles acting on the joint in conjunction with external assistance (54).

Active range of motion (AROM) Arc of motion through which the joint passes when moved by muscles acting on the joint in conjunction with external resistance (54).

Activities of daily living (ADL) Activities that are oriented toward taking care of one's own body such as bathing/showering, bowel and bladder management, dressing, feeding, functional mobility, personal device care, personal hygiene and grooming, sexual activity, and toilet hygiene (47).

Activity The execution of a task or series of actions (ICF, 21, 46).

Activity analysis An analytical analysis intended for purposes of determining the typically required demands of a task within a given culture; addresses the required body functions, personal factors, and environmental characteristics needed to successfully perform the task. It is used in occupational therapy to design therapeutic activities and identify ways to modify activities for improved performance (21, 22).

Activity choices Activities that are engaged in during play and leisure (50).

Activity interests/preferences Affective responses to play and leisure activities, perceptions and awareness of self and environments in relation to play and leisure activities, and motivation to participate in specific play and leisure activities (50).

Activity limitations Difficulties an individual may have in executing activities (ICF, 46).

Acute care Short-term medical treatment, usually in a hospital, for individuals having an acute illness of injury, recovering from surgery, or requiring medical stabilization due to safety concerns (59).

Adaptation A change in response approach generated when encountering a challenge. It also refers to therapeutic intervention in which task demands are changed to be consistent with the individual's ability level; may involve modification by reducing demands, use of assistive devices, or changes in the physical or social environment (26, 40).

Adaptation gestalt Relative balance of sensorimotor, cognitive, and psychosocial functioning that the individual creates internally in order to carry out an adaptive response (40).

Adaptation rate The rate at which afferent sensory receptors discharge into their afferent axons (56).

Adaptive capacity Apparent capability of the individual to perceive the need for change and draw from a repertoire of adaptive responses that will enable him or her to experience mastery over the environment (40).

Adaptive response (adaptiveness) A successful environmental interaction in which the individual meets the demands of the task demand; requires adequate sensory integration (40, 56).

Adenotonsillar hypertrophy Adenoid and tonsillar enlargement that may cause airway obstruction (51).

Administration The process of guiding an organization through the authoritative control of others completed by the governing body of the organization (69).

Administrative controls Changes in the nature of work such as scheduling, worker rotation, or the assignment of work tasks (49).

Administrative supervision Aspect of supervision directed toward managing the day-to-day work performance and process; includes tasks such as scheduling, monitoring performance, and delegating (72).

Advocacy (advocating, advocating mode) The act or process of supporting a cause or proposal such as public policy or resource allocation within political, economic, and social systems and institutions to directly affect people's lives. In occupational therapy, it often refers to actions to advance a profession and to assure that the client rights and resources are secured (29, 33, 68).

Affect Description of general observable emotional expression (33).

Affordances Qualities or properties of objects or the environment that elicit action possibilities (56).

Ageism Stereotypic and often negative bias against older adults; a form of discrimination based on age (17).

Aging in place Designing dwelling units such that residents, if they so choose, can occupy their home from childhood to old age unless illness or impairment come into play (18).

Agnosia Inability to recognize incoming sensory information in spite of intact sensory capacities (55).

Allopathic medicine See *Biomedical model.*

Alternative plausible explanations Scientific explanations for the findings beyond the conclusions drawn from the study and its researchers (31).

Americans with Disabilities Act Federal law preventing discrimination against persons with disabilities (2).

Apnea A cessation of breathing (51).

Apnea/hypopnea index (AHI) An index of obstructive sleep apnea severity (51).

Apraxia Inability to perform motor activities, although sensory motor function is intact and the individual understands the requirements of the task (55).

Areas of occupation Various kinds of life activities in which people engage, including the following categories: ADL, IADL, rest and sleep, education, work, play, leisure, and social participation (46).

Arena Describes the places in which activities occur, such as a library, school, or hospital (21).

Arousal Level of alertness and responsiveness to stimuli (56).

Arts and Crafts Movement A movement originating in England that championed design and manual craftsmanship as a form of cultural resistance to the mechanization and impersonal production of industrialism (2, 41).

Assessment Specific method, instrument, tool, or strategy that is used as part of the evaluation process (24, 47, 48).

Assets Resources and attributes that might be used to achieve desired intervention outcomes (27).

Assistive technology(ies) Devices, adaptive equipment, or products that are designed to enable persons with disabilities to engage in daily occupations within their home, school, workplace, and communities (29).

Assumptions Thoughts, ideas, beliefs, values, and habits that are taken for granted as true or correct; often form the foundation for a viewpoint or action; may include ideas that cannot be demonstrated to be true or false (3, 37).

Ataxia An inability to coordinate voluntary muscular movements that is symptomatic of some central nervous system disorders and injuries and not due to muscle weakness (47).

At-homeness The taken-for-granted situation of feeling completely comfortable and intimately familiar with the world in which one lives his or her everyday life (18).

Atonia Muscle paralysis (51).

Atopic dermatitis An inflammatory, chronically relapsing, noncontagious, and pruritic skin disorder (51).

Attention The cognitive ability to focus on a task, issue, or object (55).

Attrition In the context of research, it refers to loss of participants from a sample during the course of data collection (31).

Axiology The theory of values (3).

Background question A type of question used to obtain general knowledge about a disorder or condition (31).

Beliefs Cognitive content, such as ultimate principles, that are accepted as true (3, 20).

Benign prostatic hypertrophy Benign enlargement of the prostate (51).

Bias In quantitative research designs, it refers to systematic (as compared to a random) distortion of the results (31).

Biofeedback The process of becoming aware of various physiological functions using instruments that provide information on the activity of those same systems, with a goal of being able to manipulate them at will (51).

Biological needs Requirements for survival, such as air, water, food, and shelter (6).

Biomechanical approach Therapeutic intervention focused on improving body movement and strength; typically identified with remediation or improvements in strength, range of motion, or endurance (49, 54).

Biomechanics (biomechanical) The study of mechanical laws and their application to living organisms, especially the human body and its locomotor system (49).

Biomedical model Model based on scientific knowledge that attributes health and illness to physiological, biological, and scientifically explainable changes in one's body (16).

Bipolar disorder A mental illness characterized by severe mood swings, episodes of depression, and at least one episode of mania (62).

Blinding Research term use for when a subject and/or researcher is not aware of the status of the subject in the study (31).

Body functions Physiological processes of the body (ICF, 19).

Body routines Sets of coordinated, habitual bodily actions sustaining a specific task or aim, for example, driving, cooking, or lawn mowing; see also *Body-subject* and *Time-space routines* (18).

Body structures Anatomical parts of the body such as bones and organs (ICF, 19).

Body-subject The pre-reflective but intelligent awareness of the body manifested through habitual action and typically in sync with the environment in which the action unfolds; plays a major role in the habitual, routine aspects of the lifeworld; see also *Body routines* and *Time-space routines* (18).

Boundary crossing Ways in which people who come from different lived worlds and have different life experiences find commonalities and areas of mutual interest, bridge differences, negotiate multiple and diverse perspectives, develop understandings, and respect multiple and, at times, divergent perspectives (14).

Brain-computer interface (BCI) A developing digital and electronic technology that allows objects and images to be manipulated via sensory devices registering brain waves or eye and facial movements (18).

Broad theory Overarching model that helps to explain a large set of findings or observations (37).

Bruxism Grinding of the teeth (during sleep); typically includes the clenching of the jaw (51).

Capacities Refers to a person's potential for occupation and includes aspects of human anatomy (e.g., bipedal locomotion, opposable thumbs, binocular vision), cognitive functions (e.g., consciousness, attention), and the abilities developed through maturational processes (e.g., strength, coordination, language, problem solving). Capacities are age and gender specific, may not yet be developed, and are shaped by a person's genetic heritage, aptitudes, traits, context, and occupational history (6).

Case-control studies A retrospective study in which subjects with the outcome of interest (cases) are selected and matched to subjects without the outcome of interest (controls). The presence of risk factors or predictors is determined through self-report or chart review, and the relationship between these retrospective predictors and the outcome of interest is determined (31).

Case management A collaborative process that assesses, plans, implements, coordinates, monitors, and evaluates options and services to meet an individual's health needs through communication and available resources to promote quality cost-effective outcomes (49).

Case series A study that tracks several patients over the course of a disease. The results are not aggregated and detailed information on the diagnosis, treatment, and outcomes is provided for each individual patient (a case study tracks a single patient in a like manner) (31).

Cataplexy An abnormal sudden paralysis of some or all skeletal muscles brought on by strong emotions such as accompany laughter and anger (51).

Centers for independent living A nonresidential, private, nonprofit agency, providing an array of independent living services that are consumer controlled, community based, cross disability, designed and operated within a local community by individuals with disabilities. Core services include information and referral, independent living skills training, individual and systems advocacy, and peer counseling (59).

Chaining A stepwise process for teaching a multistep task (45).

Change talk Statements made by the client revealing consideration of, motivation for, or commitment to change (45).

Circadian biological clock See *Suprachiasmic nucleus (SCN).*

Class Ranking of people into a hierarchy within a culture, arising from interdependent economic relationships such as "middle class," "upper class," or "lower class" (17).

Classical test theory (CTT) Also called classical reliability theory; centers around the notion that each observation or test score has a single true score and yields a single reliability coefficient and that the observed or test score has two components: the true score and the measurement error score (25).

Classroom model A supported education model where students attend closed classes on campus (62).

Client-centered care (client-centered practice) An approach to service that incorporates respect for and partnership with clients as active participants in the therapy process. This approach emphasizes clients' knowledge and experience, strengths, capacity for choice, and overall autonomy (16, 33, 54).

Client characteristics Features of a client's interpersonal behavior that are important to observe and understand during therapy (33).

Clinical reasoning Process used by practitioners to plan, direct, perform, and reflect on client care. See *Professional reasoning* for a term that is considered to be broader (30).

Clinical supervision Supervision that is aimed at providing support, training, and evaluation of a supervisee's professional performance and development (72).

Code of ethics A set of conventional principles and expectations based on values and the standards of conduct to which practitioners of a profession are expected to conform; a public statement of principles used to promote and maintain high standards of conduct within the profession (68).

Cognition Mental processes including attention, memory, motivation, emotional control, motor control, sensory processing, and thinking; ability to think and reason to solve problems (55).

Cognitive behavioral therapy (CBT) A psychotherapeutic approach that combines cognitive and behavioral therapy techniques, aiming to solve problems concerning dysfunctional emotions, behaviors, and cognitions through a goal-oriented, systematic procedure (59).

Cohort studies A study in which subjects who represent a particular population are measured on suspected risk factors/predictors of outcome(s) of interest and are followed over time to determine (a) the incidence/natural history of the outcome and (b) the relationship between the predictors and the outcome(s) (31).

Collaboration A spirit of egalitarianism and mutual participation and exchange within the therapeutic relationship. It includes providing choice, involving clients in decision making, and encouraging clients to actively contribute and to set their own goals for therapy (33).

Collaborative supervision (in fieldwork) Involves one or more supervisors working with multiple students with all participants viewed as more equal partners in the learning process (66).

Collectivist societies Those that put more value on the family structure than the individual. Interdependence is valued, and decisions are made by the group or family who consider what is good for the entire group before focusing on the individual (16).

Communication style Interpersonal characteristic that describes a person's ability and approach to communication. In therapy, it can refer to therapist or client's style (33).

Community(ies) Collective(s) of people who share common values and demonstrate mutual concern for the development and well-being of the group; may share interests, interactions, and sense of identity (27, 29).

Community agencies Provide services for all ages of individuals, often funded by local communities or states or private payment. For children, services may include early intervention, school based, and/or private practice. For adults, services are often supplemental for individuals who are living at home with the need for socialization and supervision, medical services, and/or dementia supports. Such services may be available in freestanding agencies but may be associated with other community programs or health agencies such as senior centers, assisted living facilities, mental health centers, rehabilitation centers, nursing homes, or hospitals (59).

Community development Community consultation, deliberation, and action to promote individual, family, and community-wide responsibility for self-sustaining development, health, and well-being (29).

Community level Social networks, norms, trends, and standards that facilitate or constrain desired occupational performance and/or participation and impact health (27).

Community participation Participation refers to active participation of individuals who both benefit and contribute to the community through their actions, ideas, knowledge, or skills. And so, community participation is about relating to others, to be in some sort of relationship with them (29).

Compassion fatigue Painful emotional reaction that occurs when the helper (volunteer or professional) becomes preoccupied with the suffering and distress being experienced by the recipients of care, resulting in deep physical, emotional, and spiritual exhaustion; sometimes referred to as secondary traumatic stress reaction (65).

Compelling occupations Occupational pursuits that evoke a deep, intense sense of engagement and meaningfulness (7).

Competence An individual's capacity to perform his or her responsibilities; commonly used in reference to demonstrated performance on a job or in professional practice (67, 73).

Complementarity Supplying mutual needs and/or offsetting mutual lacks, bringing together, or completing as a whole (14).

Concealed random allocation In randomized control trials (RCTs), it refers to the a priori development of a randomization sequence so as to prevent investigators and subjects from knowing beforehand to which group a subject will be assigned (31).

Conditioning Designing situations that increase or decrease the likelihood of a behavior being performed (45).

Confidence interval Based on sample scores or outcomes, it is the likely range within which the population scores or outcomes would occur (31).

Conservatorship A legal relationship, like guardianship, but is limited to managing the protected individual's financial affairs and property (47).

Constraint-induced movement therapy (CI or CI therapy) A form of rehabilitation therapy that improves limb function after central nervous system damage and is aimed at increasing the use of the affected upper limb (54).

Construct validity Establishes whether the assessment measures a construct and the theoretical components underlying the construct. A construct is an abstract idea that cannot be observed directly (25).

Consultation A collaborative process completed with clients, families, other professionals, organizations, or communities to identify and solve problems with participation in occupations (73).

Consumer-directed health plan A type of health care financing designed to reduce health spending by providing a financial incentive for consumers to choose the best health care value. One example of a consumer-directed health plan is the health savings account (HSA), linked with a high-deductible health plan (71).

Content validity The extent to which an empirical measurement reflects a specific domain of content (25).

Context A variety of interrelated conditions (cultural, physical, social, spiritual, temporal, and virtual) within and surrounding individuals and which influence performance; includes the external physical, social, economic, political, and cultural environments in which people function; sometimes referred to a contextual or environmental features or influences (21, 29, 50, 55).

Context-focused therapy Occupational therapy in which the environment and environmentally situated occupations are modified as the mode of intervention (7).

Contextual interference A learning phenomenon where interference during practice is beneficial to skill learning (54).

Contextualism A view in which the person and situation are seen as integrated and cannot be understood separately (5).

Continuous positive airway pressure (CPAP) A treatment for obstructive sleep apnea in which a continuous stream of air under pressure is delivered through a mask worn over the nose, or nose and mouth, to keep the sleeper's airway open (51).

Continuous reinforcement Reinforcement for every instance of the behavior (45).

Continuum of care Term used to summarize the range of health care, educational, residential, employment, and social settings, which may be necessary to meet a client's needs over time (59).

Contraindications A therapeutic procedure that should be avoided because it could potentially harm a client because of the client's condition or medications (36).

Control group (control arm) Group in experimental research that receives the placebo or other comparison treatment against which the intervention is being tested (31).

Convergence Coming together, joining; applied to neural processes, convergence occurs when input from multiple sources synapse together in one region (56).

Co-occupation An occupation that implicitly involves two or more individuals (21).

Coping Conscious, volitional efforts to regulate emotion, cognition, behavior, physiology, and the environment in response to stressful events or circumstances (57).

Core values (organizational) Values that provide purpose and guide an organization's decisions and future direction (68).

Covariate A variable that is possibly predictive of the outcome (31).

Credentials Abbreviations after a person's name that designate that person's educational level and/or professional designation (36).

Criterion-referenced tests Assessments that measure activity mastery and often incorporate activity analyses. The degree of structure that is imposed on testing is usually more flexible than those for norm-referenced testing, allowing therapists to tailor tests appropriately (47).

Criterion validity Implies that the outcome of one assessment can be used as a substitute test for the established gold standard criterion test. Criterion validity can be tested as concurrent validity or predictive validity (25).

Cross-sectional studies A study in which subjects who represent a particular population are measured simultaneously for suspected risk factors/predictors and outcome(s) of interest to determine the prevalence of the outcome and the relationship between the predictors and the outcome(s) (31).

Cryotherapy The use of therapeutic low temperatures such as ice packs to relieve symptoms (54).

Cultural competence The ability to effectively interact with those who differ from oneself (16).

Cultural congruence The degree to which health professionals think and act in ways that "fit" with a person or group's beliefs and cultural style (16).

Cultural emergent A model that suggests that the symbolic aspects of culture and cultural identity emerge in interaction and are displayed primarily through talk and through action (16).

Culturally responsive care An approach that communicates a state of being open to the process of building mutuality with a client and to accepting that the cultural-specific knowledge one has about a group may or may not apply to the client they were currently treating (16).

Culture The sum total of a way of living, including values, beliefs, standards, linguistic expression, patterns of thinking, behavioral norms, and styles of communication that influence the behavior(s) of a group of people [and] is transmitted from generation to generation (16).

Day programs A subset of an outpatient rehabilitation facility in which a patient spends a major part of the day in an outpatient rehabilitation facility (59).

Deinstitutionalization The process of releasing institutionalized individuals from an institution such as a state hospital (2).

Delayed sleep phase syndrome A daily sleep/wake rhythm in which the onset of sleep and the time of awakening are later than desired (51).

Descriptive research A type of research whose purpose is to provide information about a population, for example, the prevalence of a disorder or specific characteristics of a disorder (31).

Diagnosis The process of assessing the presence and degree of disorders and their effect on a client's current status (31).

Diagnostic-related group (DRG) Classification system for Medicare Part A payments based on groups of diagnoses and procedures (71).

Differential reinforcement A technique that teaches individuals to discriminate between desired and undesired behavior and can be used to increase or decrease behavior (45).

Disaster A dangerous accidental or uncontrollable situation or event that causes significant environmental destruction, loss of life, and disruption of social structure and normal daily life routines (65).

Discontinuation (discharge) summary Documentation written at the termination of services to summarize the course of a client's intervention (36).

Discrimination Denial of equal treatment to people because of their membership in some group that occurs at many levels including individual, institutional or organizational, or structural (16).

Distributive occupations Elements that produce occupation distributed among multiple individuals working within a particular system (42).

Divergence Moving apart or separating; applied to neural processes, divergence occurs when fibers from one source split, connecting to many other regions (56).

Diversity Having distinct forms and qualities (16).

Domotics The science of using digital applications to integrate home services with technology in order to improve residents' comfort, communication, safety, and health; see also *Smart house* (18).

Dual diagnosis A comorbid condition of a person who has been diagnosed with substance abuse and a concurrent mental health issue, such as a mood disorder, anxiety, or other mental illness (59).

Dyspraxia A developmental condition in which the ability to plan unfamiliar motor tasks is impaired (56).

Early intervention (early intervening) services Multidisciplinary academic and support services provided to children who have developmental delays or special needs, generally from birth until the child turns three, or five, dependent upon individual state laws/regulations. State law also determines context for service delivery, provided either in a child's home or in an early intervention program facility (48, 59).

Effect size The strength of an association between variables or the strength of the difference between the outcomes of different conditions (31).

Effectiveness The effect of an intervention in the real world (e.g., clinical settings) under nonideal conditions (31).

Effectiveness evidence Evidence obtained from effectiveness studies (31).

Efficacy The effect of an intervention under ideal conditions (31).

Efficacy expectations A person's belief about how successful or unsuccessful he or she will be at performing a skill or occupation (45).

Effortful control A volitional ability to shift attention, inhibit the tendency to enact a dominant response, and/or activate an alternative response as needed (57).

Eleanor Clarke Slagle Lectureship An AOTA academic honor established as a memorial to Eleanor Clarke Slagle, a pioneer in the profession of occupational therapy (2).

Electroencephalogram (EEG) A recording of brain waves obtained by attaching flat metal discs (electrodes) to the scalp (51).

Electromyogram Technology that measures motor activity through electrodes placed on the skin over muscles (51).

Electronic aid to independent living (EADL) Provides the user with control over appliances and other electronic devices within the environment; a wide variety of switches interface with EADLs to allow individuals with a variety of skills and impairments to use them (47).

Electronic health record Computerized medical record created in an organization that delivers care (36).

Electrooculogram Technology that measures eye movements through electrodes placed on the skin around the eyes (51).

Embodied action A view of action in which thoughts, sociality, and emotions are considered part of the lived body as opposed to the dualistic view of the mind as planning actions and the body carrying out actions (5).

Emergency A situation that poses an immediate risk to health, life, property, or environment (59).

Emergent performance The process whereby a person puts together actions to engage in a way that is functional drawing on intrinsic capacities and an understanding of the dynamics of the situation as performance unfolds (5).

Emmanuelism A community-based health care approach started in the early 19th century that incorporated the use of volunteer providers, education, and arts and crafts as part of its regimen for treating chronic illnesses, including tuberculosis and alcoholism (2).

Emotion An evaluative mental state that occurs in the present moment and consists of neurobiological arousal, perceptual-cognitive processes, subjective experience, and affective expression (57).

Emotion dysregulation Actions or behaviors related to emotional experience that interfere with goal-directed pursuits, interpersonal relationships, or healthy adaptation (57).

Emotional regulation skills Actions or behaviors a client uses to identify, manage, and express feelings while engaging in activities or interacting with others (57).

Empathy Awareness of and insight into the feelings, emotions, and behavior of another person and their meaning and significance; not the same as sympathy, which is usually nonobjective and noncritical (32, 33).

Engineering controls Equipment and workplace designs or changes that reduce the human efforts needed (49).

Entry-level competence Denotes successful completion of academic program requirements, classroom, and fieldwork, resulting in eligibility to apply for professional credentials required for employment (66).

Environment(s) Particular physical, social, cultural, economic, and political features within a person's everyday life that affects the motivation, organization, and performance (29, 38, 39).

Environmental embodiment The various ways, both sensorially and movement wise, that the lived body engages and coordinates with the world at hand, especially its environmental aspects (18).

Environmental modifications Internal and external physical adaptations to environments that are necessary to maximize independence and to ensure health and safety (26).

Epidemiology (epidemiological) The study of the distribution and determinants of disease, injury, or dysfunction in human populations (49).

Epistemology The theory of knowledge (3).

Epworth Sleepiness Scale A self-report scale intended to measure daytime sleepiness (51).

Ergonomics The scientific discipline concerned with the understanding of interactions among humans and other elements of a system, and the profession that applies theory, principles, data, and methods to design in order to optimize human well-being and overall system performance (49).

Essential tasks The basic job duties that all employees must be able to perform with or without reasonable accommodation (49).

Ethnicity A social grouping of people who share cultural or national similarities. The most common characteristics of an ethnic group include kinship, family rituals, food preferences, special clothing, and particular celebrations (16).

Ethnocentrism Tendency of people to put their own group (*ethnos*) at the center; to see things through the narrow lens of their own culture and use the standards of that culture to judge others (16).

Evaluation Process of gathering and interpreting qualitative and/or quantitative data to understand client needs and desires, describe function, predict future function, plan intervention, or measure outcome of OT intervention (23, 24, 36, 47, 48). The process of obtaining and interpreting data necessary for intervention. This includes planning for and documenting the evaluation process and results (OTPF-II).

Evidence-based practice Professional practices that integrates the results of scientific research into the clinical decision-making process (31, 35).

Existentialism A philosophy (often associated with Kierkgaard) that focuses on the essence of a human that is realized through self-determination (3).

Experimental research Compares two or more conditions in order to determine cause and effect relationships (31).

Exploratory research Research that examines a specific phenomenon and its relationship to other factors (31).

External validity Refers to whether generalizations be made to the general population (25).

Extinction (in behavioral theory) The process of reducing the frequency of a behavior by withholding reinforcement (45).

Extinction burst In behavioral theory, term is used for the phenomenon in which the behavior being extinguished gets worse before it gets better (45).

Face validity Indicates that a measure's items are viewed as plausible (25).

Facilitation A neural process that promotes the conduction of impulses or a response to them. Facilitation is the opposite of inhibition (56).

Fading Systematic reduction of support (scaffold) to clients so that task demands increase; used when clients improve their skills (45).

Family-centered care Service provision that tends to the concerns of family members (14).

Family routines Observable and repetitive patterns involving two or more family members and occur with predictable regularity in family life (15).

Feed forward Neural information sent from the motor cortex to the cerebellum in parallel with the motor command sent to the alpha motor neurons; a "preview" of the intended motor action. It permits the cerebellum to exert its role as comparator of expected movement with actual movement (56).

Feedback Information arising from the response itself (i.e., production feedback) or from changes that occur in the environment as a result of the response (outcome feedback) (56).

Fee-for-service Retrospective reimbursement for medical services based on "reasonable and necessary" criteria (71).

Fiber diameter Neuronal diameter; fiber diameter plays a role in determining how fast a neural signal is transmitted; bigger fibers transmit information more quickly because there is less resistance to the flow of ions (56).

Fieldwork (practice placements) Structured learning experiences that are formally administered by academic programs in partnership with facilities that offer supervised training experiences (66).

Fieldwork educator Person responsible for providing student supervision; interchangeable terms include clinical educator, fieldwork supervisor, student supervisor, or practice educator (66).

Folk healer A person who is recognized within the culture who uses traditional magico-religious practices and rituals to help heal the sick (16).

Folk practices Traditional home remedies used by certain family, ethnic, and cultural groups to counteract illness and support wellness (16).

Foreground questions A type of question used to obtain current knowledge related to best practice treatment of a disorder/condition (31).

Form (of an occupation) The observable features of an occupation such as the sequence of actions in doing an occupation (7).

Fraud (in relation to therapy billing) The act of intentionally being deceptive in relation to the provision of services; can include fabricating documentation for services that were not really rendered, billing for more services than were provided in a visit, or accepting bribes or kickbacks for referrals (36).

Free appropriate public education (FAPE) Special education and related services provided at public expense that meets the standards of the state education agency (SEA) (48, 71).

Freestanding model A supported education model that provides support at the organization which sponsors program (62).

Function (of an occupation) Is what an occupation achieves, such as volunteering for a local service might achieve integration into the community (7).

Functional assessment Observation of behavior in a natural context or one that closely simulates the natural context in order to understand how environmental factors affect performance or specific behaviors (45).

Functional capacity evaluation An individual's functional abilities and/or limitations in the context of safe, productive work tasks (49).

Functional group A group designed to promote adaptation and health through group action and engagement in occupation (34).

Functional supervision Supervision over a specific aspect of work or job function (72).

Functionally illiterate Reading below the fifth-grade level (28).

Generalizability (in research) The applicability of a study result to the population (31).

Generalizability theory A measurement theory that recognizes multiple different sources of error and attempts to quantify the sources from those various errors (25).

Generalize The ability to apply what has been learned in therapy to a variety of new situations and environments (55).

Grading Systematically increasing the demands of an activity or occupation to stimulate improved function or reducing the demands to respond to client difficulties in performance (26).

Group An aggregate of people who share a common purpose that can only be achieved through collaboration (34).

Group-centered action Member actions that are interdependent (34).

Group cohesiveness The degree of understanding, acceptance, and feelings of closeness group members have toward each other and the value they place on the group (34).

Group goal A future state toward which a majority of group members' efforts are directed (34).

Group home Small, residential facilities located within a community, designed to serve children or adults with chronic disabilities. These homes usually have six or fewer occupants and are staffed 24 hours a day by trained caregivers (59).

Group norms The value system of the group; what members believe are appropriate ways of thinking, feeling, and behaving (34).

Group process The interrelationships and interactions among members, leaders, and within the group as a whole (34).

Group protocol (in therapy) An intervention plan for a specific client population (34).

Guardianship A legal association in which a protected individual's personal affairs are managed by one or more people or an agency. Conservatorship is a legal relationship, like guardianship, but is limited to managing the protected individual's financial affairs and property (47).

Habits Acquired tendencies to respond and perform in certain consistent ways in familiar environments or situation; specific, automatic behaviors performed repeatedly, relatively automatically, and with little variation (15, 39).

Habituation Internalized readiness to exhibit consistent patterns of behavior guided by habits and roles and fitted to the characteristics of routine temporal, physical, and social environment. It also refers to a decrease in neural response as a result of continued presentation of a stimulus and to the personal responses in which there is a decreased behavioral response to a repeated stimulus (39, 56).

Health The complete state of physical, mental, and social well-being and not just the absence of disease or infirmity (WHO, 44).

Health disparity Gaps in the quality of health and health care across racial and ethnic groups; population-specific differences in the presence of disease, health outcomes, or access to health care (17).

Health literacy The degree to which individuals have the capacity to obtain, process, and understand basic health information and services needed to make appropriate health decisions (28).

Health promotion The movement toward optimal health and high-level wellness; the use of discipline-specific techniques to assist people in achieving their health-related goals (44, 49).

Health savings account Savings account used for medical bills that is not subject to income tax (synonym: *Health reimbursement accounts*) (71).

High-deductible health plan A health insurance plan with lower premiums and higher deductibles than a traditional health plan. Being covered by an HDHP is also a requirement for having a health savings account (71).

High-touch societies Those whose members may seek out touch as a means of communication and are comfortable with casual touch (16).

Historically controlled study The control group of the experimental trial is a group of patients observed sometime in the past or for whom data are available only through records (31).

Home health care Provision of predominantly medically related services to patients in a home setting rather than in a medical facility (59).

Homeostatic sleep drive The drive to sleep that accumulates during prolonged wakefulness and lessens during sleep. Sleep homeostasis is one of the primary modulators of sleep in humans (51).

Hospice Palliative care designed to provide medical, emotional, social, and spiritual support to individuals in the final phase of a terminal illness, focusing on comfort and quality of life, rather than curative interventions. Aggressive methods of pain control may be used. It is generally provided as home care but can be delivered in freestanding facilities, nursing homes, or within hospitals (59).

Humanism A philosophy of human nature, human interests, welfare, and dignity that upholds humans as having inherent worth and potential (3).

Hyperalgesia An increased sensitivity to pain (51).

Hypertension High blood pressure (51).

Hypnagogic hallucinations Vivid, sometimes frightening images in transition to sleep (51).

Hypnogram A graph that summarizes the pattern of sleep stages across a night, for instance, as recorded in the sleep laboratory (51).

Impairment A problem with part of a person's anatomy or his or her physiological or psychological functioning due to a significant deviation from normal or loss (ICF, 6).

Inception cohort study A cohort study in which all subjects are in the early stages of their disorder when they enter the study (31).

Incompetence Acting without appropriate knowledge, skill, or ability (36).

Indemnity plans Insurance plans that pay for costs associated with a medical condition or injury; associated with fee-for-service method of payment (71).

Indirect assessment Includes interviews, questionnaires, role-playing, consulting with other professionals, and client self-monitoring (45).

Individual controls The physical, cognitive, and social skills and performance of the workers. Safe, efficient job design is dependent upon coordination of all aspects of the system (49).

Individualistic societies Societies that value self-expression, personal choice, autonomy, individual responsibility, and independence (16).

Individualized Education Programs (IEPs) Written plan for the delivery of educationally related services to children ages 3 to 21 years with disabilities, as mandated by IDEA (36).

Individualized Family Service Plans (IFSPs) Written plan for the delivery of services to children with disabilities ages birth through 2 years; prepares children with disabilities to enter the educational system at age 3 years (36).

Individuals with Disabilities Education Act (IDEA) Federal law that mandates that educational services must be provided to a child with a disability from birth to age 21 years (2, 71).

Inevitable interpersonal events Naturally occurring communications, reactions, processes, tasks, or general circumstances of therapy that carry an emotional valence (33).

Inferential statistics Statistics that are used to infer the degree to which a study result from a sample can confidentially be applied to the population (31).

Information and communication technologies (ICT) An umbrella term referring to broadband, wireless, and mobile computing as they combine with the Internet and with social media such as blogging, social networking, gaming, and e-mail (18).

Inhibition A neural process that reduces the likelihood that the postsynaptic neuron will reach threshold (signal level) required for an action potential to occur (56).

Inner drive Motivation and self-direction that come from within a child to develop sensory integration (56).

Inpatient rehabilitation Intensive interdisciplinary services (at least 3 hours a day, 5 to 7 days a week of at least two different types of therapy) performed on a discrete, licensed unit either within a hospital or in a freestanding hospital. Specific admission criteria must be met in order for individuals to be eligible for inpatient rehabilitation (59).

Insomnia Trouble falling asleep, staying asleep, or waking up too early (51).

Institutional review board (IRB) A panel of diverse individuals, including organization staff and at least one community member, who are responsible for reviewing all research proposals and grants to ensure that adequate protections for research participants are in place (32).

Instructing mode One of the six therapist interpersonal modes defined by a therapist's efforts to carefully structure therapy activities and to be explicit with clients about the plan, sequence, and events of therapy (33).

Instrumental activities of daily living (IADL) Activities to support daily life within the home and community that often require more complex interactions than self-care used in ADL. IADL include 12 activity categories: care of others, care of pets, child rearing, communication management, community mobility, financial management, health management and maintenance, home establishment and management, meal preparation and clean up, religious observance, safety and emergency maintenance, and shopping (47).

Intensive outpatient programs (IOPs) A step down from partial hospitalization programs. Persons at this level may be functioning adequately in one or more of their occupational roles but need more support or therapy than traditional outpatient treatment (62).

Intentional use of self The therapist's ability to deliberately anticipate, formulate, reason, and reflect about the use of modes and other interpersonal skills in light of the client's unique interpersonal characteristics and the inevitable interpersonal events that emerge during the therapy process (33).

Interdisciplinary team Individuals representing different professional disciplines that work together to identify goals and plan intervention collaboratively (35).

Interests What one finds enjoyable and satisfying (39).

Intermittent reinforcement Reinforcement only after certain demonstrations of the behavior (45).

Internal validity Refers to whether or not the assessment measure what it is supposed to measure, that is, a specific trait, behavior, construct, or performance (25).

International Code of Sleep Disorders (ICSD-2) Published by the American Academy of Sleep Medicine. This system classifies sleep disorders into eight major categories (51).

Interpersonal event A naturally occurring communication, reaction, process, task, or general circumstance that occurs during therapy and that has the potential to fortify or weaken the therapeutic relationship, depending on how it is handled (33).

Interpersonal level Relationships among family, friends, peers, and groups that provide support, identity, and role definition and facilitate or constrain occupational performance and/or participation and impact health (27).

Interpersonal reasoning A stepwise process by which a therapist decides what to say, do, or otherwise express in reaction to a client's interpersonal characteristics and behavior (33).

Interpersonal style Defined by the therapist's primary mode or set of modes used during therapy (33).

Interrater reliability With a statistical approach, it is used to detect differences in scoring between two or more raters who measure the same clients on the same attributes (25).

Intervention Process and skilled actions taken by occupational therapy practitioners in collaboration with the client to facilitate engagement in occupations related to health and participation. The intervention process includes the plan, implementation, and review (OTPF-II, 23).

Intrapersonal level Characteristics of individuals within the organization or population that influence behavior and impact occupational performance, participation, and health (27).

Intrarater reliability A statistical approach used to detect differences in scoring obtained by the same rater when measuring the same client on the same attributes (25).

Job accommodations Accommodations may involve the office, industrial, service, and medical industries and can extend to personal needs (29).

Job analysis Includes a formal methodology that details the interaction between the worker and the equipment of a system (49).

Job description A statement that defines the essential functions of the job and how the job relates to other jobs and to the workplace (49).

Just-right challenge A task that is manageably demanding, neither too difficult nor too easy; promotes central nervous system integration (56).

Leadership The process of creating structural change where the values, vision, and ethics of individuals are integrated into the culture of a community as a means of achieving sustainable change (69).

Learned nonuse A learning phenomenon whereby movement is suppressed initially due to adverse reactions and failure of any activity attempted with the affected limb, which then results in the suppression of behavior (54).

Least restrictive environment (LRE) Environment that provides maximum interaction with nondisabled peers and is consistent with the needs of the child/student (48).

Level I fieldwork Experiences designed to enrich didactic course work through directed observation and participation in selected aspects of the occupational therapy process (66).

Level II fieldwork An in-depth experience in delivering occupational therapy services to clients, focusing on the application of purposeful and meaningful occupation, as integral to the academic program's curriculum design (66).

Liability A legal term pertaining to personal responsibility (73).

Life balance A satisfying pattern of daily activity that is healthful, meaningful, and sustainable to an individual within the context of his or her current life circumstances (15).

Life coaches Professionals who facilitate positive life changes in their clients using a conversation and question-based process to help clients become more self-aware, assess their values and strengths that lead to self-directed change (15).

Life course A term (and a field of study) used to describe the patterns of people's lives in context. It considers the determinants and consequences of social relationships, historic events, and government policy for how people live their lives (5).

Life imbalance A state in which one's activity configurations limit or compromise participation in valued relationships; are incongruent for establishing or maintaining physiological health and a satisfactory identity; or are mundane, uninteresting, or unchallenging (15).

Life span development A broad phrase from developmental psychology and developmental science that connotes systematic changes within a person from conception to the end of life as they are reflected by changes in behavior. Although change occurs through interacting with the social and physical world, the focus is on the changing functions of the person (5).

Lifeworld The tacit, taken-for-granted context, tenor, and pace of daily life to which normally people give no reflective attention; a major focus of phenomenological investigation (18).

Lived body A phenomenological concept referring to the ways in which our existence as bodily beings contributes to the constitution of human experience and to the human lifeworld; the phenomenologist argues that the lived body is the primary means of being in, experiencing, and encountering the world; see also *Body-subject* (18).

Local independence An indication of whether the items of an assessment independently contribute to the measurement of a particular trait. That is, some items are redundant or not adding anything new to the measuring of a particular trait (25).

Long-term acute care (LTAC) Specialized acute care for medically complex patients who are critically ill with multisystem complications or failures and require long-term hospitalizations, performed on a discrete, licensed unit either within a hospital or in a freestanding hospital (59).

Long-term care (LTC) A combination of medical, nursing, custodial, social, and community services designed to help people who have disabilities or chronic care needs, including dementia, who cannot care for themselves for long periods of time. Services may be provided in the person's home, in the community, in assisted living facilities, or in nursing homes (59).

Low-touch societies Those that tend to avoid touch, especially in public, except in prescribed situations such as the handshake during a greeting. For many, a casual touch between members of the opposite sex may be interpreted as a sexual overture and should be avoided (16).

Lures Use of play, leisure, or other incentives as motivation to participate in therapeutic activities or as rewards for participation in them (50).

Macro level The broadest factors from the external environment that affect policy, funding, services, and sociopolitical influences on the consultation process (73).

Major depressive disorder A mental illness characterized by depressed mood, reduced interest in activities that used to be enjoyed, sleep disturbances, loss of energy, difficulty concentrating, holding a conversation, paying attention, making decisions that used to be made fairly easily, and suicidal thoughts or intentions (62).

Malpractice Misconduct on the part of a professional that results in harm to a client (36).

Managed care Comprehensive health care system that provides a variety of health services and facilities with a focus on controlling costs (71).

Management The process of guiding a work unit by planning for future work obligations, organizing employees into functional units, directing employees in the process of completing daily work tasks, and controlling work processes and systems to assure adequate quality of work output (69).

Marginal functions Tasks that are not essential to the specific job or tasks that could, if necessary, be completed by another worker (49).

Meaning (of an occupation) The significance of an occupation and what is expressed through doing; includes personal, societal, cultural, and historical expressions (7).

Measurement Process of assigning numbers to represent quantities of a trait, attribute, or characteristic or to classify objects (25).

Mechanism-based reasoning Obtaining evidence by extrapolating the results of basic science and applying them to clinical situations (31).

Mechanisms of action An understanding of how specific intervention strategies lead to particular outcomes including how change proceeds and the particular conditions under which an intervention achieves the desired results (37).

Medicaid A governmental insurance program in the United States for older adults, children and parents of dependent children, pregnant women, and people with disabilities who meet the eligibility requirements (71).

Medicare A U.S. national social insurance program that guarantees access to health insurance for Americans ages 65 years and older and younger people with disabilities as well as people with end-stage renal disease (71).

Medigap policy Private health insurance designed to supplement original Medicare; helps pay some of the health care costs ("gaps") that original Medicare does not cover (e.g., copayments, coinsurance, and deductibles) (71).

Melatonin A hormone secreted by the pineal gland in the brain. It helps regulate other hormones and maintains the body's circadian rhythm (51).

Memory Ability to register, retain, and recall past experience, knowledge, and sensation (55).

Mental status examinations Formal procedure to examine and diagnose mental functioning, including a general description of a person, notation of emotional expression, identification of perceptual disturbances, and exploration of thought processes and thought content (55).

Metacognitive Form of cognitive process in which one thinks about one's own thinking (30).

Methods (methodology) A general approach to practice; the design and approach used to collect data in research (3, 31).

Mezzo level The factors of the environment external to the client receiving consultation services including cultural, physical, temporal, and virtual elements (73).

Micro level The person, interpersonal factors, cultural, and personal contexts of the individual receiving occupational therapy services (73).

Minimal clinically important difference (MCID) The smallest change in an outcome that indicates a clinically important change in a client's condition (31).

Mission The core purpose of an organization, often includes why an organization exists, who the organization serves, and how an organization goes about achieving its purpose (68).

Mission statement A written summary of the core purpose of an organization, often includes why an organization exists, who the organization serves, and how an organization goes about achieving its purpose (69).

Mobile support model A supported education model that meets students with psychiatric disabilities in the community to provide individualized educational support (62).

Mode An aspect of the therapist's therapeutic personality that defines a specific approach to relating with a client (33).

Mode shift A conscious change in one's way of relating to a client when a therapist changes the communication approach from one approach to another (33).

Mood disorder A category of disorders that includes those where the primary symptom is inappropriate, exaggerated, or limited range of feelings or moods; includes depression and bipolar disorders (59).

Moral distress A problem that occurs when practitioners know the right thing to do but cannot achieve it because of external barriers or uncertainty about the outcome (32).

Moral reasoning The process of reflecting on ethical issues; includes reasoning about norms and values, ideas of right and wrong, and how practitioners make decisions in professional work (32).

Moral treatment Term given for a movement characterized by the provision of humane conditions of care for persons with mental illness, influenced by the ideas emanating from the age of enlightenment (2).

Motor control Ability to direct the movement (static or dynamic) of the body through conscious or unconscious motor and sensory processes (54).

Motor learning Set of processes associated with practice or experience leading to permanent changes in the capability for skilled acts (54).

Motor planning Ability to carry out a skilled, nonhabitual motor activity; process that bridges ideation and motor execution to enable an adaptive response (55).

Motor skills Occupational performance skills observed as the person interacts with and moves task objects and moves oneself around the task environment (22).

Multiculturalism An ideal in which diverse groups in a society coexist amicably, retaining their individual cultural identities (16).

Multidisciplinary team A group of individuals from different professional disciplines that serves the client; each are responsible for identifying and carrying out one's own discipline-related assessment, intervention plan and implementation, and communicating with each other (35).

Multimodal An interpersonal style that describes therapists who have an ability to use all six of the modes flexibly and comfortably and an ability to match those modes to the client and the situation (33).

Muscle tone The continuous and passive partial contraction of the muscles or the muscle's resistance to passive stretch during resting state (56).

Narcolepsy A rare sleep disorder marked by excessive sleepiness or sudden sleep attacks (51).

National Board for Certification in Occupational Therapy (NBCOT) The credentialing body for occupational therapists and occupational therapy assistants practicing in the United States; organization which develops and administers the initial certification examinations for occupational therapists and occupational therapy assistants (32, 67, 68).

National Society for the Promotion of Occupational Therapy The name given to the professional society founded in 1917 that organized workers in the curative occupations, leading to what is now known as the American Occupational Therapy Association (2).

Need for control An interpersonal characteristic describing the role taken within a relationship; ranges from active versus passive (33).

Negative predictive value A statistic indicating the likelihood that people with a negative test result would not have a condition (25).

Negligence Failing to do something that ought to be done to prevent harm to a client (36).

Neurasthenia The name given to a nervous condition characterized by fatigue and listlessness that was widely diagnosed during the period from 1880 to 1910. Originally, neurasthenia was treated using "the rest cure," but the rise of the curative occupation movement and its success with these patients helped create legitimacy for this approach to therapy, helping lead to the founding of occupational therapy (2).

Neurologic threshold The smallest change in membrane potential required for the production of an action potential (56).

Neuroplasticity Brain's ability to reorganize itself by forming new neural connections; may be either developmental (occurring throughout life) or reactive (in response to insult or injury). Neuroplasticity entails the activity-dependent shaping of connections at synapses where information is transferred from one nerve cell to another. It is influenced profoundly by sensory input, behavioral output, and practice (56).

New poor Unexpected poverty with inability to meet most basic needs; major factors contributing to growing numbers of new poor are job layoffs, family breakdown, and sudden illness (17).

Night terrors Episodes of fear, flailing, and screaming while asleep; also known as sleep terrors, night terrors often are paired with sleepwalking (51).

Nocturia The need to get up in the night to urinate, thus interrupting sleep (51).

Noncompete clause A statement limiting a person, or company, from competing in a stated business after termination, or resignation, for a specific time, in a particular geographic area, or other specified way (73).

Nonconsecutive cohort study A cohort study in which the sample includes only some of the eligible patients identified during the study recruitment period (31).

Nonrapid eye movement sleep (NREM) The stages of sleep that do not include rapid eye movement patterns. According to current guidelines for sleep stage classification, NREM consists of three different stages: N1, N2, and N3 (51).

Nonstandardized assessments Assessments that do not follow a standard approach or protocol. For instance, they may not involve a consistent set of questions, directions, or conditions for administration, testing, or scoring (25).

Nonverbal cues Communications that do not involve the use of formal language. Some examples of these are facial expressions, movement patterns, body posture, and eye contact (33).

Norm-referenced test A type of test, assessment, or evaluation that yields an estimate of the position of the tested individual in a predefined population, with respect to the trait being measured. This estimate is derived from the analysis of test scores and possibly other relevant data from a sample drawn from the population (47).

Normative expectations Activities or occupations viewed as standard behavior expected of other people in the same circumstances; may be encouraged by members of the community (5).

Objective Not influenced by personal feelings, interpretations, or prejudice; based on facts; unbiased (19).

Observational study Another term for either an associative or descriptive research; called observational studies because the subjects do not receive an experimental intervention but are simply observed (31).

Obstructive sleep apnea (OSA) Apnea caused by partial or complete blockage of airway passages during sleep (51).

Occupation The things that people do that occupy their time and attention; meaningful, purposeful activity; the personal activities that individuals choose or need to engage in and the ways in which each individual actually experiences them (6, 21, 49).

Occupation as end Occupations that constitute the end product of therapy, that is, the occupations to be learned or relearned (26).

Occupation as means Occupations that act as the therapeutic change agent to remediate impaired abilities or capacities (26).

Occupational activities Tasks that are directly related to the individual's preferred occupational role. Such tasks must have personal meaning and occupational relevance; the individual must be the primary actor in the activity (40).

Occupational adaptation Normative internal process that is activated by the individual when approaching and adapting to challenges in life; constructing a positive occupational identity and achieving occupational competence over time in the context of one's environment (39, 40).

Occupational analysis Analysis of an occupation that is relevant to an individual within the actual context of performance. Occupational analysis refers to systematically analyzing what and how a person or groups of people actually do an activity (21, 22, 36).

Occupational apartheid Separation between those who have meaningful, useful occupations and those who are deprived of, isolated from, or otherwise constrained in their daily life occupations (17).

Occupational choice Determination of meaningful activities based on one's values; interests and beliefs; social situation; gender and gender identity; age; and physical, cognitive, and emotional abilities (16).

Occupational competence The degree to which one is able to sustain a pattern of occupational participation that reflects one's occupational identity (39).

Occupational deprivation Lack of access to engagement in an array of self-selected occupations that have meaning to the individual, family, or community (44).

Occupational engagement One's doing, thinking, and feeling under certain environmental conditions in the midst of or as a planned consequence of therapy (39).

Occupational environment One of the three primary elements in the theory of occupational adaptation. In contrast with other environments, the occupational environment calls for an occupational response from the individual in the context of work, play/leisure, or self-maintenance. The contexts are shaped by unique physical, social, and cultural influences (40).

Occupational identity Composite sense of who one is and wishes to become as an occupational being generated from one's history of occupational participation (39).

Occupational orchestration The capacity of individuals to enact their occupations on a daily basis to meet their own needs and the expectations of the many environments in which they are required to function. This may include attention to habits and routines and the interface of these with the needs and expectations of others (21).

Occupational participation Engagement in work, play, or activities of daily living that are part of one's sociocultural context and that are desired and/or necessary to one's well-being (39).

Occupational patterns Habits, routines, roles, and rituals used in the process of engaging in occupations or activities (OTPF-II, 15).

Occupational performance Doing a task related to participation in a major life area; the accomplishment of the selected occupation resulting from the dynamic transaction among the client, the context and environment, and the activity (16, 38, 39).

Occupational profile A summary of information that describes the client's occupational history and experiences, patterns of daily living, interests, values, and needs (OTPF-II, 26).

Occupational readiness A term that characterizes interventions that are designed to affect the individual's sensorimotor, cognitive, and/or psychosocial deficits (40).

Occupational rights Ethical, moral, and civic issues such as equity and fairness for both individuals and collectives specific to engagement in diverse and meaningful occupation (41).

Occupational role The personally experienced situation of the individual (21).

Occupational science The study of the things people do; interdisciplinary academic discipline in the social and behavioral sciences dedicated to the study of the form, the function, and the meaning of human occupations (OTPF-II, 7).

Occupational skill acquisition Increased proficiency in performance and skill related to a meaningful occupation (26).

Onsite model A supported education model that provides individualized support sponsored by an educational institution (62).

Ontology An element of philosophy that is concerned with the nature of reality (3).

Operant conditioning Skinner's basic principle that a response followed by some reinforcement is likely to be strengthened (45).

Organizational level (of ecologically based interventions) Rules, regulations, policies, procedures, programs, and resources within agencies and organizations that impact occupational performance and/or participation and impact health (27).

Orientation Awareness of self in relation to time, place, and identification of others (55).

Orientation toward relating Personal characteristic that describes a client's need for interpersonal closeness versus professional distance within the therapeutic relationship (33).

Orthosis (splint) An orthopedic appliance or apparatus used to support, align, prevent, or correct deformities or to improve function of movable parts of the body (54).

Outcome(s) Measurable result(s) or consequence(s) of an intervention or other factors (23, 31).

Outpatient rehabilitation Rehabilitation performed in an outpatient facility that is either attached to an acute care hospital, rehabilitation hospital, or freestanding facility (59).

Oxygen saturation A measure of how much oxygen the blood is carrying (51).

p value The probability that a study effect, or a larger effect, would be found if in actuality there were no true effect or the effect was due to chance (31).

Palliative (palliation) Providing clients with relief from the symptoms, pain, and stress of a serious illness regardless of the diagnosis with a goal of improving quality of life for both the clients and their family (26).

Paradigm A set of broad assumptions and perspectives that unifies a field and defines its purpose and nature. These assumptions and perspectives are believed to underlie a discipline's science and practice at a given time (1, 2).

Parasomnias Non-sleep behaviors that intrude during sleep, such as sleepwalking and sleep eating (51).

Parasympathetic Relating to the division of the autonomic nervous system that acts in opposition to the sympathetic system by slowing the heartbeat, constricting the bronchi of the lungs, stimulating the smooth muscles of the digestive tract, etc. (56).

Partial hospitalization programs (PHPs) Programs that are intended to divert the person from hospitalization or serve as an intermediary step toward community living after an acute inpatient course of treatment. Also, an outpatient program specifically designed for the diagnosis or active treatment of a serious mental disorder when there is a reasonable expectation for improvement or when it is necessary to maintain an individual's functional level and prevent relapse or full hospitalization (59, 62).

Participation Involvement in life situations (e.g., self-care tasks, domestic life, education, employment, social, and civic life). Participation encompasses passive participation (e.g., observing others or listening). Occupational therapists generally include additional elements such as the meaning of participation and people's subjective experience of participating (ICF, 6, 46, 52).

Passive range of motion (PROM) Arc of motion through which the joint passes when moved by an outside force (54).

Peer-operated services Part of the continuum of services available in the community for people with psychiatric disabilities and are based on a belief that people who have faced, endured, or overcome adversity can offer useful support, hope, and encouragement to others in similar situations (62).

Peer review When work is reviewed by experts in the field who provide feedback and contribute to the decision of whether or not the work meets specified criteria for dissemination (35).

Perception(s) The identification, organization, and interpretation of sensation, leading to a mental representation (56).

Performance analysis The evaluation of the quality or effectiveness of the motor, process, and/or social interaction skills based on the observation of a person as he or she is engaged in the performance of a desired or needed daily life task and with the goal of evaluating the person's quality of occupational performance (22).

Performance capacity Ability to do things provided by the status of underlying objective, physical and mental components, and corresponding subjective experience (39).

Performance skills The smallest observable units of occupational performance; goal-directed actions a person carries out one by one when engaged in naturalistic and relevant daily life task performances (22).

Periodic limb movement disorder (PLMD) A sleep disorder characterized by leg movements or jerks that typically occur every 20 to 40 seconds during sleep, causing sleep to be disrupted and leaving the person with excessive daytime sleepiness (51).

Perseveration Unnecessary and prolonged repetition of a word, phase, or movement (55).

Personal causation Sense of capacity and effectiveness (39).

Personal factors Aspects of the human condition such as body structures and body functions (19).

Personal meaning Satisfaction of conscious or unconscious needs and/or attribution of benefits derived from activities (50).

Phenomenology (phenomenological) A philosophical tradition that focuses on describing and interpreting human experience. It is also used to indicate experience of occupation (7, 18).

Philosophy An academic discipline that studies the essence and limits of human beings, reality, knowledge, and action among other fundamental principles pertaining to existence (3).

Physical agent modalities (PAM) Treatment that uses energy in the form of heat, light, sound, cold, electricity, or mechanical devices (54).

Physical environment The natural and built nonhuman environment and objects in them; particular physical features (i.e., spaces and objects) of the specific context in which one does something, which impacts upon what one does, and how it is done (OTPF-II, 39).

Physiological Pertaining to the functioning of an organ as governed by the interactions between its physical and chemical conditions (49).

Place Any environmental locus that gathers individual or group meanings, intentions, and actions spatially; a fusion of human and natural order and any significance spatial center of a person or group's lived experience; see also *Lifeworld* (18).

Plan of care A written document that describes the client's occupational therapy goals and how those goals will be achieved; can also be called a care plan, intervention plan, or treatment plan (36).

Play and leisure activity Activity interests/preferences and activity choices related to play and leisure performance (50).

Play and leisure experience Subjective experience, personal meaning, and satisfaction with experience related to play and leisure performance (50).

Policies Written statements of direction and responsibility (36).

Political Action Committee A committee in the United States that provides fiscal support to political candidates. In the United States, the Occupational Therapy Political Action Committee (OTPAC) supports candidate with positions important to occupational therapy and its clients (69).

Polysomnography (PSG) The recording of a person's sleep using several physiologic signals such as the brain waves (electroencephalography), eye movements (electrooculography), muscle activity (electromyography), as well as breathing, the amount of oxygen in the bloodstream, heart rate, etc.; used to evaluate patients in a sleep laboratory for potential sleep disorders (51).

Populations Groups of people within a community who share common characteristics, for example, homeless persons, veterans, refugees, and people with chronic mental and/or physical disabilities (27).

Positive predictive value Indicates the likelihood that a person with a positive test result would actually have the condition for which the test is used (25).

Posttraumatic growth Occurs when survivors find something positive in a tragedy and try to make sense of it. Personal growth may manifest as increased emotional closeness to loved ones, faith in the ability to reconstruct life, spirituality, meaning or purpose in life, and/or recognition of inner strength (65).

Postural control Controlling or regulating the body's position in space to maintain stability and orientation (54).

Postural disorder Deficits characterized by difficulty with proximal stability, low extensor muscle tone, poor prone extension, poor neck flexion against gravity, and, often, poor equilibrium (56).

Pragmatism A philosophic perspective that focuses in experience, science, and logic as the basis for knowledge; associated with the progressive movement (3).

Praxis The ability to conceptualize, plan, and execute skilled tasks. It is goal-directed motor action, supported through the processing of sensation (56).

Precautions Actions to prevent harm to an individual (36).

Predictor variables Variables expected to have an effect on an outcome (31).

Predisposition to giving feedback An interpersonal characteristic that describes a person's ability to provide another with appropriate negative or positive comments about his or her reactions and experiences (33).

Preference for touch An interpersonal characteristic that describes a person's observed or expressed comfort or discomfort with or expressed reaction to any type of physical touch, whether it be a necessary part of treatment or an expression of caring (33).

Prejudice Preconceived ideas and attitudes—usually negative about a particular group of people, often without full examination of the facts (16).

Preparatory interventions Methods and techniques that prepare the client for occupational performance (OTPF-II, 26).

Press The demands of the environment (38).

Preventative strategies Actions people take to avoid negative health consequences (7).

Prevention Measures not only taken to prevent disease but also to arrest its progress and reduce its consequences once established. This also refers to injury prevention and prevention of secondary impairments (26, 64).

Problem solving mode An interpersonal mode defined by a therapist's efforts to facilitate pragmatic thinking and solve dilemmas by outlining choices, posing strategic questions, and providing opportunities for comparative or analytical thinking (33).

Procedures Written statements that describe how policies should be implemented (36).

Process skills Occupational performance skills observed as a person (a) selects, interacts with, and uses task tools and materials; (b) carries out individual actions and steps; and (c) modifies performance when problems are encountered (22).

Professional development Continuous process of acquiring new knowledge and skills that relate to one's profession (68).

Professional identity formation A socialization process that involves both the acquisition of specific knowledge and skills required for professional practice as well as the internalization of attitudes, dispositions, and self-identity that connect the individual to the larger profession (68).

Professional organizations Nonprofit organizations seeking to further a profession, the interests of individuals engaged in that profession, and the public interest by building a strong community of students and practitioners that collectively contribute power in numbers (68).

Professional practice supervision Supervision of others in the same profession undertaken with an understanding of the profession's values, standards, and ethics aimed at providing support, training, and evaluation of the supervisee's professional performance (73).

Professional reasoning Process used by practitioners to plan, direct, perform, and reflect on client care; includes processes by supervisors, fieldwork educators, and occupational therapy managers as they conceptualize occupational therapy practice (30).

Professionalism The embodiment and demonstration of characteristics that exemplify a profession and its members (35).

Prognosis An estimate of the probable course and outcome of a disorder/condition (31).

Programs Systematic efforts to achieve preplanned objectives such as changes in knowledge, attitudes, skills, and behaviors to maintain or improve function and/or health (27).

Progress notes Any note written about a client that explains what the client did in occupational therapy (36).

Progressive era A period during the early 20th century in the United States characterized by bold ideas, ambitious projects, life-changing inventions, and reforms that created general social optimism and confidence in the future (2).

Project-focused fieldwork A field-based learning experience in which the learner manages a project, such as developing new programs or resources, or evaluating an existing program, involving skill acquisition of conducting a needs assessment/

analysis, proposal preparation, and development of reporting structures and time lines (66).

Propositions Formal statements about causes and effects or the nature of relationships among features of the world (37).

Prospective payment system (PPS) A method of reimbursement commonly associated in the United States with Medicare. Payment is made based on a predetermined, fixed amount; derived from the classification system of that service (e.g., diagnosis-related groups for inpatient hospital services) (71).

Proxemics The measureable distance between people as they interact (16).

Psychiatric overlay The circumstance where a client being treated for a primary illness or impairment might also have a coexisting psychiatric diagnosis or other psychosocial issue (33).

Psychosis A thought disorder in which reality testing is grossly impaired. Symptoms can include seeing, hearing, smelling, or tasting things that are not there; paranoia; and delusional thoughts (62).

Psychosocial Referring to the mind's ability to, consciously or unconsciously, adjust and relate the body to its social environment (49).

Public policy level Local, state, and federal policies, laws, and programs that regulate, support, or constrain desired occupational performance and/or participation and impact health (27).

Punishment A negative response to an undesired behavior (45).

Purposeful action Activities that have meaning for individuals and/or groups as a whole (34).

Purposeful activities Specifically selected activities that allow the client to develop skills that enhance occupational engagement (21).

Qualitative studies A research paradigm based on the assumption that there are multiple constructed realities and that the purpose of research is to describe and analyze these realities to facilitate the understanding of the phenomena (31).

Quality of life A measure of well-being and encompasses individuals' perceptions of their position in life in the context of culture and value systems in which they live and in relation to their goals, expectations, standards, and concerns (52).

Quasi-experimental studies An intervention study in which subjects are nonrandomly assigned to the experimental treatment group or the control group (31).

Race A social construction that separates people into groups based on physical characteristics, especially skin color (16).

Racism The assessment of individual worth on the basis of real or imputed group characteristics, most notably skin color (16).

Randomized clinical trials (RCTs) An intervention study in which subjects are randomly assigned to the experimental treatment group or the control group (31).

Range of motion (ROM) Arc of motion through which a joint moves (54).

Rapid eye movement sleep (REM) The stage of sleep characterized by a period of intense brain activity often associated with dreams; named for the rapid eye movements that occur during this time. It is also called paradoxical or dreaming sleep (51).

Reading level Grade level at which one reads; academic level and reading level are often not equivalent (28).

Reasonable and necessary Terms used by payers to determine if services should be covered; based on payer criteria about the likelihood of client change and importance of that change (71).

Receptive fields Region of space in which the presence of a stimulus will alter neural firing (56).

Reconstruction aides Volunteer workers recruited to help care for wounded soldiers in World War I using physical agents and curative occupations. The traditions of this approach to treatment led to the development of physical therapy, occupational therapy, and, eventually, rehabilitation medicine (2).

Recovery (in mental health) A process of change through which individuals with mental disorders and substance abuse disorders improve their health and wellness, live a self-directed life, and strive to reach their full potential (62).

Reductionism A simplification and narrowing of phenomena in which the whole is understood in terms of its parts. In occupational therapy, reductionism refers to focusing intervention on the parts of the person (physical, emotional, or cognitive) or parts of the occupation rather than the whole person and related context (1, 3).

Reevaluation A systematic evaluation conducted to determine change from initial evaluation; typically performed to determine need for changes in course of intervention (23).

Reference standard An existing diagnostic test that can most accurately identify the disease. The results of the assessment being studied are compared to the results of the reference standard (31).

Reflection A form of self-assessment that can be used to improve practice. Developing reflective capacity is a critical element in professional development and competence (32).

Rehabilitation approach A therapeutic approach aimed at making people as independent as possible in spite of any residual impairment (54).

Reinforcement Something that causes a behavior to be strengthened and performed again (45).

Reinforcement schedule A schedule that indicates which instances of behavior, if any, will be reinforced (45).

Related services (in schools) In a school setting, services that help a child with a disability to benefit from special education, such as those provided by occupational or physical therapy practitioners, school nurse, psychologist, or social worker or special transportation services (36, 48).

Relative mastery A person's phenomenological evaluation of the quality of his or her occupational response. This evaluation has four aspects: efficiency (use of time, energy, resources), effectiveness (the extent to which the desired goal was achieved), satisfaction to self, and satisfaction to society (40).

Relevance The degree to which a research study answers the clinical question and how well its methods fit within the constraints and resources of the practitioner's context of practice (31).

Reliability Consistency and repeatability of the outcome of administration of a test across time, parallel forms of the test, and raters. It also refers to the consistency of the internal structure of the test (25, 31).

REM sleep behavior disorder (RBD) A sleep disorder in which one appears to physically act out vivid, often unpleasant dreams with abnormal vocal sounds and movements during REM sleep (51).

Remediation An intervention approach designed to change client variables to establish a skill or ability that has not yet developed or to restore a skill or ability that has been impaired (26).

Requisite managerial authority The level of control and discretion that a manager must have to be fairly held responsible for the outcomes of work groups (69).

Response The reaction to the stimulus (45).

Response to change and challenge The ability to adapt to things that are new or challenging (33).

Response to human diversity A reaction to another based on how much the other is the same or different. These differences may occur in terms of observable sociodemographic characteristics (e.g., race, ethnicity, gender, age) or other interpretations of outward appearance or perceived worldview (33).

Rest Period of relaxing or ceasing to engage in strenuous or stressful activity (51).

Restless leg syndrome (RLS) A disorder in which there is an urge to move the legs to stop unpleasant sensations (51).

Restorative occupation Using occupations to facilitate restoring person factors and/or body functions (58).

Retrospective payment Payment made based on what was billed; contrasted with prospective payment in which payment is set in advance of intervention (71).

Role(s) A set of socially agreed-upon behavioral expectations, rights, and responsibilities for a specific position or status in a group or in society. These may be further conceptualized and defined by individuals enacting the role(s) (21, 34, 39).

Role-emerging supervision A form of fieldwork in which placement occurs where there is no occupational therapist on-site; generally provides opportunities for students to be more autonomous and independent, promoting increased professional growth (66).

Routines A type of higher order habits that involves sequencing and combining processes, procedures, steps, or occupations and provide a structure for daily life (15).

Same-site model of fieldwork Entails students completing a Level I and Level II fieldwork experience at the same training site (66).

Satisfaction with experience Overall feelings and perceptions related to experiences (50).

Schizophrenia One of several brain diseases whose symptoms may include loss of personality (flat affect), agitation, catatonia, confusion, psychosis, unusual behavior, and withdrawal. The illness usually begins in early adulthood (62).

Screening Obtaining and reviewing data that are relevant to a potential client to determine the need for further evaluation and intervention (24, 36).

Secondary insomnia When insomnia is a result of another medical condition, a side effect of a drug, or another similar cause, it is called secondary insomnia (51).

Self-efficacy Confidence in one's ability to take action (44).

Self-initiated action Individual takes initiative verbally or nonverbally (34).

Self-regulation The individual's ability to alter behavior to match environmental demand; in relationship to sensory integration and processing, this involves intake, integration, and processing of sensation and using it as a foundation for appropriate environmental interaction (56).

Sensitivity The predictor test's ability to obtain a positive test when the condition really exists (a true positive) (25).

Sensitization Progressive increases in response to a stimulus with repeated exposure (56).

Sensory modulation The ability to regulate and organize reactions to sensory input in a graded and adaptive manner; the balancing of excitatory and inhibitory inputs and adapting to environmental changes (56).

Sensory registration Detection of sensory information by the central nervous system (56).

Sensory-related affordances The sensory possibilities or qualities of things in the environment and of the environment itself (56).

Serious mental illness (psychiatric disability) (SMI) A diagnosable mental disorder found in persons aged 18 years and older that is so long lasting and severe that it seriously interferes with a person's ability to take part in major life activities (62).

Service competency The specific knowledge, skills, and attitudes to perform at an expected level that matches the requirements of the area of practice or service (73).

Service coordinators In educational settings, the person responsible for managing a student's IFSP or IEP (36).

Service learning Learning experiences, based on a community-identified need, that tend to be aligned with academic course objectives. Learning activities can involve more than one visit and may evolve during a semester or at multiple points across a curriculum in a programmatic approach (66).

Setting Describes those aspects of the context or arena to which the person attends (21).

Shaping A strategy to develop closer and closer approximations of behavior (45, 54).

Sheltered workshops Noncompetitive employment settings intended to provide many of the positive benefits of a work atmosphere for individuals with disabilities (49).

Shift work A general term to describe a job that requires an individual to work other than the standard working hours of midmorning to late afternoon, Monday through Friday. For instance, shift work may involve working from midnight until 7:00 a.m. (51).

Single subject (*n* of 1) studies An intervention study in which a single subject is the total population of the study (31).

Situated activities This concept calls for the study of activities in the real life contexts and examination of the practices of social institutions where activities occur naturally. To understand situated activities, the practitioner pays special attention to the innovative solutions that unfold as the activities are carried out in that particular context (5).

Skilled nursing facility (SNF) A hospital unit, nursing home, or distinct part of a nursing home that provides skilled nursing care, medical treatments, and rehabilitation services (59).

Skills (skilled) Observable, goal-directed actions that a person uses while performing (39, 71).

Sleep debt An individual's accumulated sleep loss from insufficient sleep, regardless of cause (51).

Sleep diary Self-report system for tracking sleep time and restorative experience (51).

Sleep disordered breathing (SDB) Describes a group of disorders characterized by abnormalities of respiratory pattern (pauses in breathing) or the quantity of ventilation during sleep (51).

Sleep hygiene Habits, environmental factors, and practices that may influence the length and quality of one's sleep (51).

Sleep inertia Period after awakening before full alertness (51).

Sleep latency Period awake in bed before falling asleep (51).

Sleep-wake homeostasis Regulated balance between sleep and waking (51).

Slow wave sleep (SWS) Often referred to as deep sleep, consists of stages 3 and 4 of NREM sleep (51).

Smart house (smart house technology) Dwelling design using computer technologies to incorporate robotics, networked appliances, and other digital devices connecting residents with their home and wider community; the house is "smart" in the sense that it can respond, through digital directives, to the residents' everyday needs in terms of lighting, thermal comfort, security, and so forth; see also *Domotics* (18, 29).

SOAP note A type of progress note written in a standard format of subjective, objective, assessment, and plan so that specific information is easy to find (36).

Social environment Particular social features (i.e., social groups and occupational tasks) of the specific context in which one does something that impacts upon what one does and how it is done (39).

Social health Having a standard of living adequate for health and well-being, with equal rights to work, to free choice of employment; to rest, leisure, and holidays; to participate in the cultural life of a community; to the arts and scientific advancement; to take part in national governments; and to education directed to the full development of the human personality (41).

Social inequality Unequal rewards and opportunities that accrue to different individuals and groups, particularly rewards and opportunities that are judged to be unfair, unjust, avoidable, and unnecessary; often linked to unequal distribution of economic assets and power within a society (17).

Social interaction skills Occupational performance skills observed during the ongoing stream of a social exchange (22).

Social justice Ethical distribution and sharing of resources, rights, and responsibilities between people recognizing their equal worth as citizens (OTPF-II, 41).

Social media Internet-based tools that enable one to communicate quickly and to a very wide audience (35).

Social mobility The degree to which, in a given society, an individual's social status can change throughout the life course or the degree to which that individual's offspring and subsequent generations move up and down the class system (17).

Social participation Involvement in a subset of activities that involve social interactions with others and that support social interdependence; organized patterns of behavior that are characteristic and expected of an individual or a given position within a social system and encompasses the individual's engagement with family, peers and friends, and community members (52).

Social supports Support systems that provide assistance and encouragement to individuals with physical or emotional disabilities in order that they may better cope. Informal social support is usually provided by friends, relatives, or peers, whereas formal assistance is provided by churches, groups, etc. (29).

Socioeconomic status (SES) Status- or prestige-based measure of place in the social hierarchy; measurement of SES includes occupational attainment, education, and income (17).

Somatodyspraxia A relatively severe form of sensory integrative–based dyspraxia characterized by difficulty with both easy (feedback dependent) and more difficult (feed forward dependent) motor tasks; thought to be based on poor processing of tactile and likely vestibular and proprioceptive sensations (56).

Spatial neglect A condition in which, after damage to one hemisphere of the brain (usually right) is sustained, a deficit in attention to and awareness of the opposite side (usually left) of space is observed (55).

Spatial summation Involves activating several receptors and summing the excitation from each to produce a response (56).

Special education Educational services that are designed to help a child with a disability learn in a way that is consistent with that child's unique needs (36).

Specificity The predictor test's ability to obtain a negative result when the condition is really absent (a true negative) (25).

Spirituality The personal quest for understanding answers to ultimate questions about life, about meaning, and about relationship with the sacred or transcendent, which may (or may not) lead to or arise from the development of religious rituals and the formation of community (20).

Spontaneous action Action occurs in the here and now (34).

Stage theory Assumes that there are discontinuous, qualitative shifts that reflect a transition from one stage into the next stage in a predictable manner. The focus is on different organizational or structural change over age-related phases such as infancy, early adulthood, and late adulthood. Classic theorists include Erikson, Kohlberg, and Piaget that provide descriptions of distinctly different psychosocial issues, moral reasoning, and cognition (5).

Standard setting A professional association's role and methodology for defining levels of achievement (68).

Standardized assessments Measurement instrument that has been developed in a rigorous, scientific manner for a defined construct and population with a prescribed process of administration and scoring and with demonstrated psychometric properties (25, 47).

State professional associations Nonprofit organizations in the United States that seek to further a profession, the interests of individuals engaged in that profession, and the public interest by building a strong community of students and practitioners that collectively contribute power in numbers (68).

Stereotyping Preconceived ideas and attitudes, usually negative, about a particular group of people, often without full examination of the facts (16).

Stimulus Something that prompts a behavior (45).

Stimulus discrimination learning A procedure by which an individual can learn to emit a behavior under certain conditions instead of others (45).

Stimulus generalization Occurs when a behavior becomes more probable in the presence of one stimulus as a result of being reinforced in the presence of another similar stimulus (45).

Strategic planning The process of ensuring that an organization's current purpose, aspirations, goals, activities, and strategies connect to plans and support its mission (68).

Strengthening A variety of techniques aimed at increasing the amount of force a muscle can produce (54).

Structuralism Philosophical inquiry focused on understanding the elements that comprise a phenomenon or system (3).

Subjective experience (subjectively experienced) State of mind with which activities are approached and the affective experience of engaging in them (19, 50).

Substrates of occupation The human capacities required for engagement in an occupation (7).

Successful aging Moving through late life in a way that enables participation in valued activities and sustains life satisfaction (64).

Sundowning Increased confusion or disorientation that occurs at the end of the day; typically seen in people with Alzheimer's disease or other dementias (55).

Supervision The process of guiding individuals or an organization through the authoritative control of others authorized by the governing body of the organization (69, 72).

Supported employment Competitive work in an integrated work environment consistent with the strengths, resources, priorities, concerns, abilities, capabilities, interests, and informed choice of the individuals (49).

Suprachiasmic nucleus (SCN) Also referred to as circadian clock, circadian pacemaker, or internal biological clock. The internal circadian pacemaker is a small group of nerve cells located in the hypothalamus that controls the circadian cycles and influences many physiological and behavioral rhythms occurring over a 24-hour period, including the sleep/wake cycle (51).

Sympathetic nervous system Part of the autonomic nervous system. The sympathetic nervous system activates what is often termed the fight-or-flight response. Like other parts of the nervous system, the sympathetic nervous system operates through a series of interconnected neurons (56).

Synaptic activity Transfer of information from one cell to another at a synapse; facilitated if the firing of the presynaptic cell increases the likelihood that the postsynaptic cell with reach threshold and fire an action potential (excitatory synapse) or inhibited if the firing of the presynaptic cell reduces the likelihood of the postsynaptic cell firing (inhibitory synapse) (56).

Synaptic function Entails the transfer of information from one cell (presynaptic neuron) to another (postsynaptic neuron) at the synaptic cleft; commonly referred to as synaptic transmission (56).

Systematic review A literature review pertinent to a specific question that aims at identifying, appraising, and synthesizing all the research evidence relevant to that question (31).

Systems approach Views the properties of the "whole," or system, as arising from interactions and relationships among the parts (49).

Tacit Implicit or based on information or experiences that we cannot easily put into language (37).

Tactile defensiveness A sensory integrative dysfunction in which the tactile sensations cause excessive emotional reactions, hyperactivity, or other behavioral problems (56).

Task analysis An analytical analysis intended for purposes of identifying what environmental, task-related, person-related (i.e., person factors and body functions), and/or societal and cultural factors may have been the reason for a person's diminished quality of occupational performance; most often based on professional reasoning and speculation following the occupational therapist's observation of the person's task performance (22).

Task-oriented training Includes a wide range of interventions such as treadmill training, walking training on the ground, bicycling programs, endurance training and circuit training, sit-to-stand exercises, and reaching tasks for improving balance. In addition, use is made of arm training using functional tasks such as grasping objects, CI therapy, and mental imagery. Such training is task and patient focused and not therapist focused (54).

Taxonomies Broad classifications; a way to group things together (4).

Teamwork When more than one health care provider collaborates on the care of the client (35).

Temporal Denoting time (7).

Temporal summation Occurs when a stimulus of limited strength is repeated in quick succession, such that the strength of the second stimulus is "added to" the strength of the first stimulus, and so forth, until threshold is reached and the signal is sent forward (56).

Therapeutic mode A specific way of relating to a client (33).

Therapeutic relationship Client–therapist interactions (33).

Therapeutic use of self Planned use of practitioner's personality, insights, perceptions, and judgments as part of the therapeutic process (26, 33).

Third-party payer Private company or government agency that provides payment for medical expenses (47).

Time-space routines Sets of more or less habitual bodily actions extending through a considerable portion of time, for example, a getting-up routine, a going-to-the-gym routine, or a going-to-church-and-lunch routine; see also *Body-subject* and *Body routines* (18).

Tort law limits The parameters a court can award for a wrongful act or injury. These usually fluctuate based on state law and severity of the type of injury or act (73).

Transactional perspective of occupations Offered as an alternative to individualism that presumes the person is separate from life situations; a transactional way of thinking sees interrelated elements where occupations forms relationships between the person and life situations. This idea is compatible with contextualism (5).

Transdisciplinary team Individuals representing different professional disciplines whose role-related functions become interchangeable (35).

Transduction With respect to neural activity, the process of changing stimulus energy into a coded action potential that can be propagated and interpreted by the central nervous system (56).

Transition planning The education and rehabilitation team prepare the student to leave the school setting and enter into employment and community living (49).

Transitional portfolio A dynamic, flexible, and reflective tool for one to self-direct and document professional development through thoughtful engagement with artifacts created and accumulated during one's career in relationship to professional goals and desired roles (67).

Translational science Theory-driven research focused on developing practical applications that resolve peoples' real-world needs (7).

Trauma-informed care Assessment and intervention services that include attention to the impact of trauma on client lives, designed to minimize trauma and avoid retraumatization (65).

Treatment group (intervention group) In experimental research, it is the group that receives the treatment or intervention being tested (31).

Unidimensionality The determination of whether an assessment measures a single trait (25).

Universal design (UD) Also called "inclusive design" and "life-span design"; design of environments and products to be usable by all people to the greatest extent possible without the need for special arrangements or adaptations; intended to simplify life for everyone by making products, communications, and the built environment more usable by as many people as possible at little or no extra cost (18, 29).

Universal housing Dwellings, housing, and neighborhoods that address the needs of all users, whatever their age or ability (18).

Validation study A second study, using either a subset of data or collecting new data, which is used to confirm the results of a previous study. This term is most often used with prognostic studies (31).

Validity The degree to which a measurement tool measures what it is supposed to measure (accuracy) (31).

Values That which is perceived to be inherently desirable and good; concerned with ideals; it is also the principles, standards, or qualities considered worthwhile by the client who holds them (OTPF-II, 3, 20, 39).

Vestibular-based bilateral integration and sequencing disorder A sensory integrative dysfunction characterized by shortened duration nystagmus, poor integration of the two sides of the body and brain, and difficulty in learning to read or compute (56).

Vision (vision statement) in management An aspirational statement about what a department or organization would like to become as it seeks to fulfill its mission (68, 69).

Visual perceptual Cognitive process of obtaining and interpreting visual information from the environment (55).

Vocational rehabilitation A multiprofessional evidence-based approach that is provided in different settings, services, and activities to working age individuals with health-related impairments, limitations, or restrictions with work functioning and whose primary aim is to optimize work participation (49).

Volition Pattern of thoughts and feelings about oneself as an actor in one's world that occurs as one anticipates, chooses, experiences, and interprets what one does (39).

Wake after sleep onset (WASO) The time spent awake from sleep onset to final awakening (51).

Well-being Implies that basic survival needs are met and encompasses ideas such as health, happiness, and prosperity (6).

Wellness The individual's perception of and responsibility for psychological and physical well-being as these contribute to overall satisfaction with one's life situation. It is also the outcome of health promotion (44, 49, 64).

Work Exertion or effort directed to produce or accomplish something (49).

Work conditioning Intervention that emphasizes physical conditioning and addresses issues of strength, endurance, flexibility, motor control, and cardiopulmonary function (49).

Work hardening A highly structured, goal-oriented, individualized treatment program designed to maximize the individual's ability to return to work (49).

Work integration programs A program designed to coordinate the clinical features of the injured worker into the organizational and ergonomic aspects of the system (49).

Workers' compensation State programs that pay for care of workers who have injuries or illnesses due to work-related causes (71).

Working poor People who maintain full-time jobs but remain in relative poverty according to government-established poverty standards; may have negative net worth and lack the ability to escape their situations (17).

Index

Page numbers followed by *f* denote figures, those followed by *t* denote tables, and those followed by *b* denote boxes.

B

C

N

O

Q